SECOND EDITION

Volume 2

HEART DISEASE

A Textbook of Cardiovascular Medicine

Edited by

EUGENE BRAUNWALD, M.D.

Hersey Professor of the Theory and Practice of Physic;
Herman Ludwig Blumgart Professor of Medicine, Harvard Medical School;
Chairman, Department of Medicine,
Brigham and Women's and Beth Israel Hospitals, Boston

W. B. SAUNDERS COMPANY

PHILADELPHIA · LONDON · TORONTO · MEXICO CITY · RIO DE JANEIRO · SYDNEY · TOKYO

W. B. Saunders Company: West Washington Square
Philadelphia, PA 19105

1 St. Anne's Road
Eastbourne, East Sussex BN21 3UN, England

1 Goldthorne Avenue
Toronto, Ontario M8Z 5T9, Canada

Apartado 26370 — Cedro 512
Mexico 4, D.F., Mexico

Rua Coronel Cabrita, 8
Sao Cristovao Caixa Postal 21176
Rio de Janeiro, Brazil

9 Waltham Street
Artarmon, N.S.W. 2064, Australia

Ichibancho, Central Bldg., 22-1 Ichibancho
Chiyoda-Ku, Tokyo 102, Japan

Library of Congress Cataloging in Publication Data
    Main entry under title:

Heart disease.

    Includes bibliographical references and index.
    1. Heart—Diseases. I. Braunwald, Eugene.
[DNLM: 1. Heart diseases—Complications. WG 200
H4364]
RC681.H362   1984   616.1'2   83-2850
ISBN 0-7216-1938-X (single v.)
ISBN 0-7216-1939-8 (v. 1)
ISBN 0-7216-1940-1 (v. 2)
ISBN 0-7216-1941-X (set)

ISBN: SINGLE VOLUME   0-7216-1938-X

ISBN: VOLUME 1   0-7216-1939-8

ISBN: VOLUME 2   0-7216-1940-1

ISBN: SET   0-7216-1941-X

HEART DISEASE

Last digit is the print number: 9   8   7   6   5   4   3   2

Dedicated to the memory of my father,

WILLIAM BRAUNWALD

CONTRIBUTORS

JOSEPH S. ALPERT, M.D.

Professor of Medicine, University of Massachusetts Medical School. Director, Division of Cardiovascular Medicine, University of Massachusetts Medical Center, Worcester, Massachusetts.

Pulmonary Hypertension; Congenital Heart Disease in the Adult; Acute Myocardial Infarction: Pathological, Pathophysiological, and Clinical Manifestations

MURRAY G. BARON, M.D.

Professor of Radiology, Emory University School of Medicine. Associate Chairman of Radiology, Emory University Hospital, Atlanta, Georgia.

Radiological and Angiographic Examination of the Heart

WILLIAM H. BARRY, M.D.

Associate Professor of Medicine, Harvard Medical School. Director, Cardiac Catheterization Laboratory, Brigham and Women's Hospital, Boston, Massachusetts.

Cardiac Catheterization

EUGENE H. BLACKSTONE, M.D.

Cardiovascular Surgical Research Professor, The University of Alabama School of Medicine, University of Alabama, Birmingham, Alabama.

General Principles of Cardiac Surgery

KENNETH M. BOROW, M.D.

Associate Professor of Medicine, Cardiology, University of Chicago. Director, Cardiac Noninvasive Imaging Laboratory, University of Chicago Hospitals and Clinics, Chicago, Illinois.

Congenital Heart Disease in the Adult

EUGENE BRAUNWALD, M.D.

Hersey Professor of the Theory and Practice of Physic, and Herrman Ludwig Blumgart Professor of Medicine, Harvard Medical School. Chairman, Department of Medicine, Brigham and Women's and Beth Israel Hospitals, Boston, Massachusetts.

The History; The Physical Examination; Contraction of the Normal Heart; Pathophysiology of Heart Failure; Assessment of Cardiac Function; Clinical Manifestations of Heart Failure; The Management of Heart Failure; Pulmonary Edema: Cardiogenic and Noncardiogenic; Pulmonary Hypertension; Congenital Heart Disease in the Adult; Valvular Heart Disease; Coronary Blood Flow and Myocardial Ischemia; Acute Myocardial Infarction: Pathological, Pathophysiological, and Clinical Manifestations; The Management of Acute Myocardial Infarction; Chronic Ischemic Heart Disease; The Cardiomyopathies and Myocarditides; Primary Tumors of the Heart; Pericardial Disease; Traumatic Heart Disease; Cor Pulmonale and Pulmonary Thromboembolism; Hematologic-Oncologic Disorders and Heart Disease; Endocrine and Nutritional Disorders and Heart Disease; Renal Disorders and Heart Disease; General Anesthesia and Noncardiac Surgery in Patients with Heart Disease

MICHAEL S. BROWN, M.D., D.Sc. (Hon.)

Professor, Department of Molecular Genetics, and Director, Center for Genetic Diseases, University of Texas Health Science Center at Dallas. Senior Attending Physician, Parkland Memorial Hospital, Dallas, Texas.

Genetics and Cardiovascular Disease

PETER F. COHN, M.D.

Professor of Medicine and Chief of Cardiology Division, State University of New York Health Sciences Center, Stony Brook, New York.

Chronic Ischemic Heart Disease; Traumatic Heart Disease

WILSON S. COLUCCI, M.D.

Assistant Professor of Medicine, Harvard Medical School. Associate Physician, Brigham and Women's Hospital, Boston, Massachusetts.

Primary Tumors of the Heart

ERNEST CRAIGE, M.D.

Henry A. Foscue Distinguished Professor of Cardiology, University of North Carolina School of Medicine. Director, Cardiac Graphics Laboratory, North Carolina Memorial Hospital, Chapel Hill, North Carolina.

Heart Sounds; Echophonocardiography and Other Noninvasive Techniques to Elucidate Heart Murmurs

ROMAN W. DE SANCTIS, M.D.

Professor of Medicine, Harvard Medical School. Physician and Director of Clinical Cardiology, Massachusetts General Hospital, Boston, Massachusetts.

Diseases of the Aorta

EDWIN G. DUFFIN, Ph.D.

Clinical Research Manager, Pacing Division, Medtronic, Inc., Minneapolis, Minnesota.

Cardiac Pacemakers

HARVEY FEIGENBAUM, M.D.

Distinguished Professor of Medicine, Indiana University School of Medicine. Senior Research Associate, Krannert Institute of Cardiology, Indianapolis, Indiana.

Echocardiography

MANNING FEINLEIB, M.D., Dr. P.H.

Clinical Professor, Georgetown University of Medicine, Washington, D.C. Visiting Lecturer on Epidemiology, Harvard School of Public Health, Boston, Massachusetts. Associate, Johns Hopkins University, Baltimore, Maryland. Director, National Center for Health Statistics, Hyattsville, Maryland.

Risk Factors for Coronary Artery Disease and Their Management

CHARLES FISCH, M.D.

Distinguished Professor of Medicine, Indiana University School of Medicine. Director, Krannert Institute of Cardiology and Division of Cardiology, Indiana University School of Medicine, Indianapolis, Indiana.

Electrocardiography and Vectorcardiography

WILLIAM F. FRIEDMAN, M.D.

J. H. Nicholson Professor of Pediatric Cardiology, University of California, Los Angeles, School of Medicine. Professor and Chairman, Department of Pediatrics, U.C.L.A. Center for Health Sciences, Los Angeles, California.

Congenital Heart Disease in Infancy and Childhood; Acquired Heart Disease in Infancy and Childhood

GOFFREDO G. GENSINI, M.D.

Clinical Professor of Medicine, State University of New York Upstate Medical Center College of Medicine. Director, Monseigneur Toomey Cardiovascular Laboratory and Research Department, Saint Joseph Hospital Health Center, Syracuse, New York.

Coronary Arteriography

JOSEPH L. GOLDSTEIN, M.D., D.Sc. (Hon.)

Paul J. Thomas Professor and Chairman, Department of Molecular Genetics, University of Texas Health Science Center at Dallas. Senior Attending Physician, Parkland Memorial Hospital, Dallas, Texas.

Genetics and Cardiovascular Disease

MICHAEL N. GOTTLIEB, M.D.

Assistant Clinical Professor of Medicine, Harvard Medical School. Associate Physician, Brigham and Women's Hospital, Boston, Massachusetts.

Renal Disorders and Heart Disease

WILLIAM GROSSMAN, M.D.

Professor of Medicine, Harvard Medical School. Chief, Cardiovascular Division, Beth Israel Hospital, Boston, Massachusetts.

Cardiac Catheterization; High–Cardiac Output States; Pulmonary Hypertension

THOMAS P. HACKETT, M.D.

Eben S. Draper Professor of Psychiatry, Harvard Medical School. Chief of Psychiatry, Massachusetts General Hospital, Boston, Massachusetts.

Emotion, Psychiatric Disorders, and the Heart

ROBERT I. HANDIN, M.D.

Associate Professor of Medicine, Harvard Medical School. Director, Hematology Division, Brigham and Women's Hospital, Boston, Massachusetts.

Hematologic-Oncologic Disorders and Heart Disease

B. LEONARD HOLMAN, M.D.

Professor of Radiology, Harvard Medical School. Director, Clinical Nuclear Medicine Services, Brigham and Women's Hospital, Boston, Massachusetts.

Nuclear Cardiology

ROLAND H. INGRAM, Jr., M.D.

Parker B. Francis Professor of Medicine, Harvard Medical School. Director, Respiratory Divisions, Brigham and Women's and Beth Israel Hospitals, Boston, Massachusetts.

Pulmonary Edema: Cardiogenic and Noncardiogenic; Relationship Between Diseases of the Heart and Lungs

NORMAN M. KAPLAN, M.D.

Professor of Internal Medicine, University of Texas Southwestern Medical School. Chief, Hypertension Section, Parkland Memorial Hospital, Dallas, Texas.

Systemic Hypertension: Mechanisms and Diagnosis; Systemic Hypertension: Therapy

JAMES K. KIRKLIN, M.D.

Assistant Professor of Surgery, University of Alabama School of Medicine. Staff Physician, Department of Surgery, University of Alabama Medical Center, Birmingham, Alabama.

General Principles of Cardiac Surgery

JOHN W. KIRKLIN, M.D.

Professor of Surgery, University of Alabama School of Medicine. Director, Division of Cardiothoracic Surgery, Department of Surgery, and Director, Alabama Congenital Heart Disease Diagnosis and Treatment Center, University of Alabama Medical Center, Birmingham, Alabama.

General Principles of Cardiac Surgery

ROBERT I. LEVY, M.D.

Vice President for Health Sciences, Columbia University College of Physicians and Surgeons, New York, New York.

Risk Factors for Coronary Artery Disease and Their Management

BEVERLY H. LORELL, M.D.

Assistant Professor of Medicine, Harvard Medical School. Co-Director, Hemodynamic Research Laboratory, and Attending Cardiologist, Beth Israel Hospital, Boston, Massachusetts.

Pericardial Disease

BERNARD LOWN, M.D.

Professor of Cardiology, Harvard School of Public Health. Senior Physician, Brigham and Women's Hospital, Boston, Massachusetts.

Cardiovascular Collapse and Sudden Cardiac Death

E. REGIS McFADDEN, Jr., M.D.

Associate Professor of Medicine, Harvard Medical School. Director of Research, Shipley Institute of Medicine, Brigham and Women's Hospital, Boston, Massachusetts.

Cor Pulmonale and Pulmonary Thromboembolism; Relationship Between Diseases of the Heart and Lungs

ALBERT OBERMAN, M.D., M.P.H.

Professor and Chairman, Department of Preventive Medicine, The University of Alabama School of Medicine. Active Medical Staff, University of Alabama Hospitals, Birmingham, Alabama.

Rehabilitation of Patients with Coronary Artery Disease

JOSEPH K. PERLOFF, M.D.

Professor of Medicine and Pediatrics, University of California, Los Angeles, School of Medicine. Attending Physician, U.C.L.A. Center for Health Sciences, Los Angeles, California.

Neurological Disorders and Heart Disease; Pregnancy and Cardiovascular Disease

GERALD M. POHOST, M.D.

Associate Professor of Medicine, Harvard Medical School. Director of Nuclear Cardiology, Cardiac Unit, Massachusetts General Hospital, Boston, Massachusetts.

Nuclear Magnetic Resonance Imaging of the Heart

ADAM V. RATNER, B.A.

Special Fellow in Cardiac NMR, Massachusetts General Hospital, Boston, Massachusetts. Fellow, Stanley J. Sarnoff Society of Fellows for Cardiovascular Research, Medical Student, University of Texas Southwestern Medical School, Dallas, Texas.

Nuclear Magnetic Resonance Imaging of the Heart

ROBERT ROBERTS, M.D.

Professor of Medicine, Baylor College of Medicine. Chief of Cardiology, The Methodist Hospital, Houston, Texas.

Hypotension and Syncope

JERROLD F. ROSENBAUM, M.D.

Assistant Professor of Psychiatry, Harvard Medical School. Chief, Clinical Psychopharmacology Unit, Massachusetts General Hospital, Boston, Massachusetts.

Emotion, Psychiatric Disorders, and the Heart

DAVID S. ROSENTHAL, M.D.

Associate Professor of Medicine, Harvard Medical School. Clinical Director, Hematology Division, Brigham and Women's Hospital, Boston, Massachusetts.

Hematologic-Oncologic Disorders and Heart Disease

JOHN ROSS, Jr., M.D.

Professor of Medicine, University of California, San Diego, School of Medicine. Cardiologist, University of California Medical Center, San Diego, California.

Contraction of the Normal Heart

L. THOMAS SHEFFIELD, M.D.

Professor, Department of Medicine, The University of Alabama School of Medicine. Director, ECG Laboratory and Allison Laboratory of Exercise Electrophysiology, University Hospital. Attending Cardiologist, University Hospital and Veterans Administration Hospital, Birmingham, Alabama.

Exercise Stress Testing

EVE E. SLATER, M.D.

Assistant Professor of Medicine, Harvard Medical School. Chief, Hypertension Unit, Massachusetts General Hospital, Boston, Massachusetts.

Diseases of the Aorta

THOMAS W. SMITH, M.D.

Professor of Medicine, Harvard Medical School. Chief, Cardiovascular Division, Brigham and Women's Hospital, Boston, Massachusetts.

The Management of Heart Failure

BURTON E. SOBEL, M.D.

Professor of Medicine and Director of Cardiovascular Division, Washington University School of Medicine. Cardiologist-in-Chief, Barnes Hospital, St. Louis, Missouri.

Cardiac and Noncardiac Forms of Acute Circulatory Failure (Shock); Hypotension and Syncope; Coronary Blood Flow and Myocardial Ischemia; The Management of Acute Myocardial Infarction

EDMUND H. SONNENBLICK, M.D.

Professor of Medicine, The Albert Einstein College of Medicine. Chief, Division of Cardiology, Hospital of the Albert Einstein College of Medicine and The Bronx Municipal Hospital Center, Bronx, New York.

Contraction of the Normal Heart

GENE H. STOLLERMAN, M.D.

Professor of Medicine, Boston University School of Medicine. Attending Physician, University Hospital, Boston, Massachusetts.

Rheumatic and Heritable Connective Tissue Diseases of the Cardiovascular System

LOUIS WEINSTEIN, M.D., Ph.D.

Lecturer in Medicine, Harvard Medical School. Physician and Director of the Clinical Services of the Division of Infectious Disease, Department of Medicine, Brigham and Women's Hospital, Boston, Massachusetts.

Infective Endocarditis

GORDON H. WILLIAMS, M.D.

Professor of Medicine, Harvard Medical School. Chief, Endocrinology-Hypertension Service, Brigham and Women's Hospital, Boston, Massachusetts.

Endocrine and Nutritional Disorders and Heart Disease

ROBERT W. WISSLER, Ph.D., M.D.

Donald N. Pritzker Distinguished Service Professor of Pathology, The Pritzker School of Medicine of the University of Chicago. Physician, University of Chicago Medical Center, Chicago, Illinois.

Principles of the Pathogenesis of Atherosclerosis

MARSHALL A. WOLF, M.D.

Associate Professor of Medicine, Harvard Medical School, Associate Physician-in-Chief, Brigham and Women's Hospital, Boston, Massachusetts.

General Anesthesia and Noncardiac Surgery in Patients with Heart Disease

JOSHUA WYNNE, M.D.

Assistant Professor of Medicine, Harvard Medical School. Director, Noninvasive Cardiac Laboratory, and Associate Physician, Brigham and Women's Hospital, Boston, Massachusetts.

The Cardiomyopathies and Myocarditides

DOUGLAS P. ZIPES, M.D.

Professor of Medicine, Indiana University School of Medicine. Senior Research Associate, Krannert Institute of Cardiology. Attending Physician, University Hospital, Veterans Administration Medical Center, and Wishard Memorial Hospital, Indianapolis, Indiana.

Genesis of Cardiac Arrhythmias: Electrophysiological Considerations; Management of Cardiac Arrhythmias; Specific Arrhythmias: Diagnosis and Treatment; Cardiac Pacemakers

CONTENTS

PART II
ABNORMALITIES OF CIRCULATORY FUNCTION

PART
III

DISEASES OF THE HEART, PERICARDIUM, AORTA, AND PULMONARY VASCULAR BED

29 CONGENITAL HEART DISEASE IN INFANCY AND CHILDHOOD

by William F. Friedman, M.D.

INTRODUCTION

DEFINITION. Congenital cardiovascular disease is defined as an abnormality at birth in cardiocirculatory structure or function.

Congenital cardiovascular malformations result generally from altered embryonic development of a normal structure or failure of such a structure to progress beyond an early stage of embryonic or fetal development. The aberrant patterns of flow created by an anatomical defect may, in turn, significantly influence the structural and functional devel-

opment of the rest of the circulation. For instance, the presence in utero of mitral atresia may not permit normal development of the left ventricle, aortic valve, and ascending aorta. Similarly, speculation exists that constriction of the fetal ductus arteriosus may result directly in right ventricular dilatation and tricuspid regurgitation in the fetus and newborn, contribute importantly to the development of pulmonary arterial aneurysms in the presence of ventricular septal defect and absent pulmonic valve, or, further, result in an alteration in the number and caliber of fetal and newborn pulmonary vascular resistance vessels. In this

941

same regard, postnatal events may markedly influence the clinical presentation of a specific "isolated" malformation. The infant with Ebstein's malformation of the tricuspid valve may improve dramatically as the magnitude of tricuspid regurgitation diminishes with normal fall in pulmonary vascular resistance after birth; the infant with hypoplastic left heart syndrome or interrupted aortic arch may not exhibit circulatory collapse, and the baby with pulmonic atresia or severe stenosis may not become cyanotic until normal spontaneous closure occurs of a patent ductus arteriosus. Ductal constriction many days after birth may also be a central factor in some infants in the development of coarctation of the aorta. Still later in life the patient with a ventricular septal defect may experience spontaneous closure of the abnormal communication, or develop right ventricular outflow tract obstruction and/or aortic regurgitation, or pulmonary vascular obstructive disease. These selected examples serve to emphasize that anatomical and physiological changes in the heart and circulation may continue indefinitely from prenatal life in association with any specific congenital cardiocirculatory lesion.

It should be recognized further that certain congenital defects are not apparent on gross inspection of the heart or circulation. Examples include the electrophysiological pathways for ventricular preexcitation or interruptions in the cardiac conduction system giving rise to paroxysmal supraventricular tachycardia or congenital complete heart block, respectively. Similarly, abnormalities in the development of myocardial autonomic innervation or in the ultrastructure of myocardial cells may ultimately prove to contribute to asymmetrical septal hypertrophy and left ventricular outflow tract obstruction. These examples make clear that occasional difficulties arise in distinguishing between congenital anomalies that are readily apparent at or shortly after birth and lesions that may have as their basis a subtle or undetectable abnormality that is present at birth.

INCIDENCE. The true incidence of congenital cardiovascular malformations is difficult to determine accurately, partly because of the difficulties in definition discussed above. It has been estimated that approximately 0.8 per cent of live births are complicated by a cardiovascular malformation.[1] This figure does not take into account what may be the two most common cardiac anomalies: the congenital, nonstenotic bicuspid aortic valve[2] and the leaflet abnormality associated with mitral valve prolapse.[3] Moreover, the widely quoted 0.8 per cent incidence figure fails to include small preterm infants, almost all of whom have persistent patent ductus arteriosus, or the prevalence of cardiovascular abnormalities in stillborn infants. Thus, it is clear that past statistical analyses have seriously underestimated the incidence of congenital heart disease.

Precise data concerning frequency of individual congenital lesions are also lacking, and the results of many analyses differ, depending upon the source (living or dead) and the selection of the study population.[4] Table 29–1 is a compilation from both clinical and pathological studies that approximates the frequency of occurrence of specific cardiovascular malformations.[5,6]

Taken in toto, children with congenital heart disease are predominantly male. Moreover, specific defects may show

TABLE 29–1   FREQUENCY OF OCCURRENCE OF CARDIAC MALFORMATIONS AT BIRTH

DISEASE	PERCENTAGE
Ventricular septal defect	30.5
Atrial septal defect	9.8
Patent ductus arteriosus	9.7
Pulmonic stenosis	6.9
Coarctation of the aorta	6.8
Aortic stenosis	6.1
Tetralogy of Fallot	5.8
Complete transposition of the great arteries	4.2
Persistent truncus arteriosus	2.2
Tricuspid atresia	1.3
All others	16.5

Data based on 2310 cases.

a definite sex preponderance; patent ductus arteriosus and atrial septal defect are more common in females, whereas valvular aortic stenosis, coarctation of the aorta, tetralogy of Fallot, and transposition of the great arteries are more common in males.

Extracardiac anomalies occur in approximately 25 per cent of infants with significant cardiac disease,[7] and their presence may significantly increase mortality. Often the extracardiac anomalies are multiple, in part involving the musculoskeletal system; one third of infants with both cardiac and extracardiac anomalies have some established syndrome.

ETIOLOGY.   Malformations appear to result from an interaction between multifactorial genetic and environmental systems too complex to allow a single specification of etiology.[8] In most instances, a causal factor cannot be identified. Maternal rubella, ingestion of thalidomide early during gestation, and chronic maternal alcohol abuse are environmental insults known to interfere with normal cardiogenesis in man.[9–12] *Rubella syndrome* consists of cataracts, deafness, microcephaly, and, either singly or in combination, patent ductus arteriosus, pulmonic valvular and/or arterial stenosis, and atrial septal defect. *Thalidomide* is associated with major limb deformities and occasionally with cardiac malformations without predilection for a specific lesion. The *fetal alcohol syndrome* consists of microcephaly, micrognathia, microphthalmia, prenatal growth retardation, developmental delay, and cardiac defects. The latter—often defects of the ventricular septum—occur in approximately 45 per cent of affected infants. *Maternal lupus erythematosus* during pregnancy has recently been linked to congenital complete heart block (p. 1014). Animal experiments have incriminated hypoxia, deficiency or excess of several vitamins, intake of several categories of drugs, and ionizing irradiation as teratogens capable of causing cardiac malformations.[10] The precise relationship of these animal teratogens to human malformations is not clear.

The genetic aspects of congenital heart disease are discussed extensively in Chapter 47. A single gene mutation may be causative in the familial forms of atrial septal defect with prolonged AV conduction, mitral valve prolapse, ventricular septal defect, congenital heart block, situs inversus, pulmonary hypertension, the combination of supravalvular aortic stenosis and peripheral pulmonary arterial stenosis, and the syndromes of Noonan, LEOPARD, Holt-Oram, Ellis–van Creveld, and Kartagener. Table 29–

TABLE 29–2 SYNDROMES WITH ASSOCIATED CARDIOVASCULAR INVOLVEMENT

SYNDROME	MAJOR CARDIOVASCULAR MANIFESTATIONS	MAJOR NONCARDIAC ABNORMALITIES
Heritable and Possibly Heritable		
Ellis–van Creveld	Single atrium or atrial septal defect	Chondrodystrophic dwarfism, nail dysplasia, polydactyly
TAR (thrombocytopenia-absent radius)	Atrial septal defect, tetralogy of Fallot	Radial aplasia or hypoplasia, thrombocytopenia
Holt-Oram	Atrial septal defect (other defects common)	Skeletal upper limb defect, hypoplasia of clavicles
Kartagener	Dextrocardia	Situs inversus, sinusitis, bronchiectasis
Laurence-Moon-Biedl-Bardet	Variable defects	Retinal pigmentation, obesity, polydactyly
Noonan	Pulmonic valve dysplasia	Webbed neck, pectus excavatum, cryptorchidism
Tuberous sclerosis	Rhabdomyoma, cardiomyopathy	Phakomatosis, bone lesions, hamartomatous skin lesions
Multiple lentigenes (LEOPARD)	Pulmonic stenosis	Basal cell nevi, broad facies, rib anomalies
Rubinstein-Taybi	Patent ductus arteriosus (others)	Broad thumbs and toes, hypoplastic maxilla, slanted palpebral fissures
Familial deafness	Arrhythmias, sudden death	Sensorineural deafness
Friedreich's ataxia	Cardiomyopathy and conduction defects	Ataxia, speech defect, degeneration of spinal cord dorsal columns
Muscular dystrophy	Cardiomyopathy	Pseudohypertrophy of calf muscles, weakness of trunk and proximal limb muscles
Weber-Osler-Rendu	Arteriovenous fistulas (lung, liver, mucous membranes)	Multiple telangiectasias
Cystic fibrosis	Cor pulmonale	Pancreatic insufficiency, malabsorption, chronic lung disease
Sickle cell anemia	Cardiomyopathy, mitral regurgitation	Hemoglobin SS
Conradi-Hünermann	Ventricular septal defect, patent ductus arteriosus	Asymmetrical limb shortness, early punctate mineralization, large skin pores
Cockayne	Accelerated atherosclerosis	Cachectic dwarfism, retinal pigment abnormalities, photosensitivity dermatitis
Progeria	Accelerated atherosclerosis	Premature aging, alopecia, atrophy of subcutaneous fat, skeletal hypoplasia
Apert	Ventricular septal defect	Craniosynostosis, midfacial hypoplasia, syndactyly
Incontinentia pigmenti	Patent ductus arteriosus	Irregular pigmented skin lesions, patchy alopecia, hypodontia
Connective Tissue Disorders		
Cutis laxa	Peripheral pulmonic stenosis	Generalized disruption of elastic fibers, diminished skin resilience, hernias
Ehlers-Danlos	Arterial dilatation and rupture, mitral regurgitation	Hyperextensible joints, hyperelastic and friable skin
Marfan	Aortic dilatation, aortic and mitral incompetence	Gracile habitus, arachnodactyly with hyperextensibility, lens subluxation
Osteogenesis imperfecta	Aortic incompetence	Fragile bones, blue sclerae
Pseudoxanthoma elasticum	Peripheral and coronary arterial disease	Degeneration of elastic fibers in skin, retinal angioid streaks
Inborn Errors of Metabolism		
Pompe's disease	Glycogen storage disease of heart	Acid maltase deficiency, muscular weakness
Homocystinuria	Aortic and pulmonary artery dilatation, intravascular thrombosis	Cystathionine synthetase deficiency, lens subluxation, osteoporosis
Mucopolysaccharidoses: Hurler; Hunter	Multivalvular and coronary and great artery disease, cardiomyopathy	Hurler: Deficiency of α-L-iduronidase, corneal clouding, coarse features, growth and mental retardation Hunter: Deficiency of L-idurano-sulfate sulfatase, coarse facies, clear cornea, growth and mental retardation
Morquio; Scheie; Maroteaux-Lamy	Aortic incompetence	Morquio: Deficiency of N-acetylhexosamine sulfate sulfatase, cloudy cornea, normal intelligence, severe bone changes involving vertebrae and epiphyses Scheie: Deficiency of α-L-iduronidase, cloudy cornea, normal intelligence, peculiar facies Maroteaux-Lamy: Deficiency of arylsulfatase B, cloudy cornea, osseous changes, normal intelligence
Chromosomal Abnormalities		
Trisomy 21 (Down's syndrome)	Endocardial cushion defect, atrial or ventricular septal defect, tetralogy of Fallot	Hypotonia, hyperextensible joints, mongoloid facies, mental retardation
Trisomy 13 (D)	Ventricular septal defect, double-outlet right ventricle	Single midline intracerebral ventricle with midfacial defects, polydactyly, nail changes, mental retardation
Trisomy 18 (E)	Ventricular septal defect, patent ductus arteriosus, pulmonic stenosis	Clenched hand, short sternum, low arch dermal ridge pattern on fingertips, mental retardation
Cri du chat (short-arm deletion-5)	Ventricular septal defect	Cat cry, microcephaly, antimongoloid slant of palpebral fissures, mental retardation
XO (Turner)	Coarctation of aorta	Short female, broad chest, lymphedema, webbed neck
XXXY and XXXXX	Patent ductus arteriosus	XXXY: Hypogenitalism, mental retardation, radial-ulnar synostosis XXXXX: Small hands, incurving of fifth fingers, mental retardation

Modified from Friedman, W. F.: Congenital heart disease. *In* Isselbacher, K. J., Adams, R. D., Braunwald, E., Petersdorf, R. G., and Wilson, J. D. (eds.): Harrison's Principles of Internal Medicine. 10th ed. New York, McGraw-Hill Book Co., 1983, p. 1383.

TABLE 29–3   RECURRENCE RISK IN SIBLINGS OF PROBANDS WITH CONGENITAL HEART LESIONS

DEFECT	AFFECTED SIBLINGS (%)
Ventricular septal defect	4.4
Patent ductus arteriosus	3.4
Tetralogy of Fallot	2.7
Atrial septal defect	3.2
Pulmonic stenosis	2.9
Aortic stenosis	2.2
Atrioventricular canal	2.6
Transposition of great arteries	1.9
Coarctation of aorta	1.8

Modified from Nora, J. J., et al.: Etiologic aspects of cardiovascular disease and pre-disposition detectable in the infant and child. *In* Friedman, W. F., et al. (eds.): Neonatal Heart Disease. New York, Grune and Stratton, 1973, p. 279.

2 provides a partial list of syndromes in which cardiovascular anomalies may be manifestations of the pleiotropic effects of single genes or examples of gross chromosomal defects. Less than 5 to 10 per cent of all cardiac malformations can be accounted for by chromosomal aberrations or genetic mutations or transmission.

The finding that, with some exceptions, only one of a pair of monozygotic twins is affected by congenital heart disease indicates that the vast majority of cardiovascular malformations are not inherited in a simple manner.[13] Family studies indicate a two- to five-fold increase in the incidence of congenital heart disease in siblings of affected patients or in the offspring of an affected parent. Malformations are often concordant or partially concordant within families.[13a] Table 29–3 provides the recurrence risks observed in 3400 siblings of probands with various congenital heart lesions. Because the incidence of congenital heart disease in the offspring or siblings of an index patient is only 2 to 5 per cent, it is rarely wise to discourage the parents of one affected child from having additional children if either parent is free of a cardiovascular anomaly.[14] Moreover, the low recurrence rate and the increasing possibilities for effective treatment for nearly all cardiac lesions usually justify a positive approach to family counseling. When two or more members of the family are affected, the recurrence risk may be quite high, and a pedigree should be obtained before further counseling. If a dominant or recessive mendelian pattern is established, the mendelian laws apply, and the risk of recurrence in each pregnancy is equal.

Prevention. The feasibility of preventive programs will depend upon what is learned in the future about the cause of the 90 per cent or more of cardiovascular anomalies for which no cause is currently known. Strict testing in animals of new drugs that may be teratogenic when taken during pregnancy may be expected to reduce the chances of another thalidomide tragedy. In this regard, the dictum cannot be emphasized too strongly that no medication should be taken during pregnancy without prior consultation with a physician. Physicians dealing with pregnant women should be aware of known teratogens as well as of drugs that may have a functional rather than a structural damaging influence on the fetal and newborn heart and circulation and should recognize that drugs abound for which there is inadequate information concerning their teratogenic potential. Similarly, appropriate use of radiological equipment and techniques for reducing gonadal and fetal radiation exposure should always be employed to reduce the potential hazards of this likely cause of birth defects.

Detection of abnormal chromosomes in fetal cells obtained from amniotic fluid (Chap. 47) may occasionally predict cardiac malformation as one component of the multiple system involvement that may exist in Down's, Turner's, or trisomy 13–15 (D1) and 16–18 (E) syndrome. Similarly, identification in such cells of the enzyme disorders observed in the mucopolysaccharidoses, homocystinuria, or type II glycogen storage disease may allow one to predict the ultimate presence of cardiac disease. Lastly, immunization of children with rubella vaccine may be anticipated to minimize the effects of maternal rubella and its cardiac consequences.

Embryology

Correlation of anatomical features of malformed hearts and embryonic cardiac morphology allows a developmental analysis of various anomalies. Detailed accounts of the normal development of the cardiovascular system are provided elsewhere.[15-17] In brief, during the first month of gestation the primitive, straight cardiac tube is formed, comprising the sinuatrium, the primitive ventricle, the bulbus cordis, and the truncus arteriosus in series (Fig. 29–1). In the second month of gestation this tube doubles over on itself to form two parallel pumping systems, each with two chambers and a great artery. The two atria develop from the sinuatrium; the atrioventricular canal is divided by the endocardial cushions into tricuspid and mitral orifices; and the right and left ventricles develop from the primitive ventricle and bulbus cordis. Differential growth of myocardial cells causes the straight cardiac tube to bear to the right, and the bulboventricular portion of the tube doubles over on itself, bringing the ventricles side by side (Fig. 29–2). Migration of the atrioventricular canal to the right and of the ventricular septum of the left serves to align each ventricle with its appropriate atrioventricular valve. At the distal end of the cardiac tube the bulbus cordis divides into a subaortic muscular conus and a subpulmonic muscular conus; the subpulmonic conus elongates, and the subaortic conus reabsorbs, allowing the aorta to move posteriorly and connect with the left ventricle.

A host of anomalies may result from defects in this basic developmental pattern. Thus, double-inlet left ventricle (p. 1012) is observed

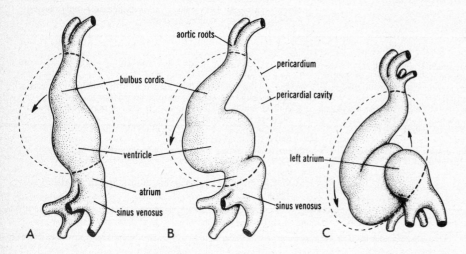

FIGURE 29–1   Formation of the cardiac loop as seen from the left side at 32 days *(A)*, 34 days *(B)*, and 38 days *(C)*. Dashed line indicates parietal pericardium. The atrium gradually assumes an intrapericardial position. (From Langman, J., and van Mierop, L. H. S.: Development of the cardiovascular system. *In* Moss, A. J., and Adams, F. H. (eds.): Heart Disease in Infants, Children and Adolescents. Baltimore, Williams and Wilkins, 1968.)

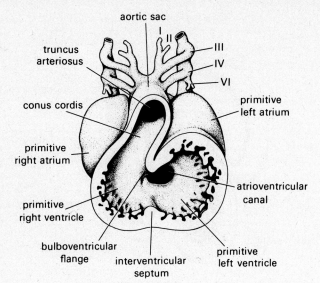

FIGURE 29–2 Frontal section through the heart of 5-mm embryo showing the side-by-side primitive ventricles and the single opening of the atrium into the ventricles. (From Langman, J., and van Meirop, L. H. S.: Development of the cardiovascular system. *In* Moss, A. J., and Adams, F. H. (eds.): Heart Disease in Infants, Children and Adolescents. Baltimore, Williams and Wilkins, 1968.)

if the tricuspid orifice does not align over the right ventricle. The various types of persistent truncus arteriosus (p. 969) result from failure of the truncus to divide into main pulmonary artery and aorta. Double-outlet anomalies of the right ventricle (p. 1005) are produced by failure of either the subpulmonic or subaortic conus to resorb, whereas resorption of the subpulmonic instead of the subaortic conus may be central to transposition of the great arteries (p. 997).

The primitive sinuatrium is separated into right and left atria by the downgrowth from its roof of the septum primum toward the atrioventricular canal, thereby creating an inferior intraatrial ostium primum opening (Fig. 29–3). Multiple perforations form in the anterosuperior portion of the septum primum as the septum secundum begins to develop to the right of the former. The coalescence of these perforations forms the ostium secundum. The septum secundum completely separates the atrial chambers except for a central opening—the fossa ovalis—which is covered by tissue of the septum primum forming the valve of the foramen ovale. Fusion of the endocardial cushions anteriorly and posteriorly divides the atrioventricular canal into tricuspid and mitral inlets (Fig. 29–4). The inferior portion of the atrial sep-

tum, the superior portion of the ventricular septum, and portions of the septal leaflets of both the tricuspid and mitral valves are formed from the endocardial cushions. The integrity of the atrial septum depends on growth of the septum primum and septum secundum and proper fusion of the endocardial cushions. Atrial septal defects (p. 958) and varying degrees of endocardial cushion defect (p. 961) are the result of developmental deficiencies of this process.

Partitioning of the ventricles occurs as cephalad growth of the main ventricular septum results in its fusion with the endocardial cushions and the infundibular or conus septum. Defects in the ventricular septum may occur owing to a deficiency of septal substance; malalignment of septal components in different planes, preventing their fusion; or an overly long conus, keeping the septal components apart. Isolated defects (p. 963) probably result from the former mechanism, while the latter two appear to generate the ventricular defects seen in tetralogy of Fallot (p. 990) and transposition complexes (p. 967).

The lungs arise from the primitive foregut and are drained early in embryogenesis by channels from the splanchnic plexus to the cardinal and umbilicovitelline veins. An outpouching from the posterior left atrium forms the common pulmonary vein, which communicates with the splanchnic plexus, establishing pulmonary venous drainage to the left atrium. The umbilicovitelline and anterior cardinal vein communications atrophy as the common pulmonary vein is incorporated into the left atrium. Anomalous pulmonary venous connections (p. 1008) to the umbilicovitelline (portal) venous system or to the cardinal system (superior vena cava) result from failure of the common pulmonary vein to develop or establish communications to the splanchnic plexus. Cor triatriatum (p. 984) results from a narrowing of the common pulmonary vein–left atrial junction.

The truncus arteriosus is connected to the dorsal aorta in the embryo by six pairs of aortic arches. Partition of the truncus arteriosus into two great arteries is a result of the fusion of tissue arising from the back wall of the vessel and the truncus septum. Rotation of the truncus coils the aorticopulmonary septum and creates the normal spiral relationship between aorta and pulmonary artery. Semilunar valves and their related sinuses are created by absorption and hollowing out of tissue at the distal side of the truncus ridges. Aorticopulmonary septal defect (p. 969) and persistent truncus arteriosus (p. 969) represent varying degrees of partitioning failure.

Although the six aortic arches appear sequentially, portions of the arch system and dorsal aorta disappear at different times during embryogenesis (Fig. 29–5). The first, second, and fifth sets of paired arches regress completely. The proximal portions of the sixth arches become the right and left pulmonary arteries and the distal left sixth arch becomes the ductus arteriosus. The third aortic arch forms the connection between internal and external carotid arteries, while the left fourth arch becomes the arterial segment between left carotid and subclavian arteries; the proximal portion of the right subclavian

FIGURE 29–3 Diagrammatic representation of the atrial septa at 30 days *(A)*, at 33 days *(B)*, at 33 days (seen from the right side) *(C)*, at 37 days *(D)*, and in the newborn *(E)*; the newborn atrial septum viewed from the right *(F)*. (From Langman, J., and van Meirop, L. H. S.: Development of the cardiovascular system. *In* Moss, A. J., and Adams, F. H. (eds.): Heart Disease in Infants, Children and Adolescents. Baltimore, Williams and Wilkins, 1968.)

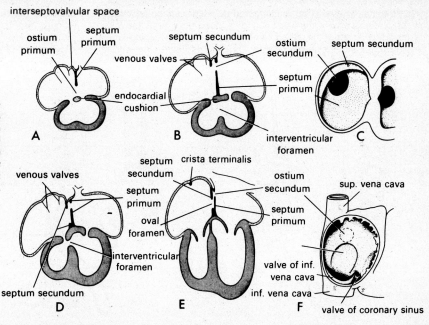

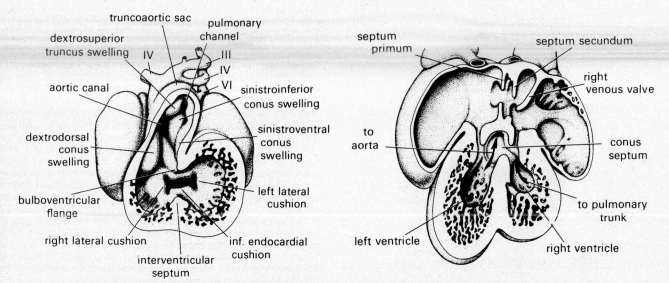

FIGURE 29–4   Frontal section through the heart of a 9-mm embryo (*left panel*) and 15-mm embryo (*right panel*). At 9 mm, development is noted of the cushions in the atrioventricular canal, and the truncus and conus swellings are visible. At 15 mm, the conus septum is completed; note the septation in the atrial region. (From Langman, J., and Van Mierop, L. H. S.: Development of the cardiovascular system. *In* Moss, A. J., and Adams, F. H. (eds.): Heart Disease in Infants, Children and Adolescents. Baltimore, Williams and Wilkins, 1968.)

artery forms from the right fourth arch. An abnormality in regression of the arch system in a number of sites can produce a wide variety of arch anomalies, whereas a failure of regression results generally in a double aortic arch malformation (p. 1013).

Fetal and Transitional Circulations

Although the illness created by the presence of a cardiac malformation is almost always recognized only after an affected baby is born, important effects on the circulation have existed from early in pregnancy until the time of delivery.[18] Thus, knowledge of the changes in cardiocirculatory structure, function, and metabolism that accompany development is central to a systematic comprehension of congenital heart disease.

Dynamic alterations occur in the circulation during the transition from fetal to neonatal life when the lungs, rather than the placenta, take over the function of gas exchange.[19] The single fetal circulation consists of parallel pulmonary and systemic pathways (Fig. 29–6) in contrast to the two-circuit system in the newborn and adult in whom the pulmonary vasculature exists in series with the systemic circulation. Prenatal survival is not endangered by major cardiac anomalies as long as one side of the heart can drive blood from the great veins to the aorta; in the fetus, blood can bypass the nonfunctioning lungs both proximal and distal to the heart. Oxygenated blood returns from

the placenta through the umbilical vein and enters the portal venous system. A variable amount of this stream bypasses the hepatic microcirculation and enters the inferior vena cava via the ductus venosus. Inferior vena caval blood is composed of flow from the ductus venosus, hepatic vein, and lower body venous drainage, which is summarily deflected to a significant extent across the foramen ovale into the left atrium. Almost all superior vena caval blood passes directly through the tricuspid valve entering the right ventricle. Most of the blood that reaches the right ventricle bypasses the high-resistance, unexpanded lungs and passes through the ductus arteriosus into the descending aorta. The output of the right and left ventricles contributes to the total fetal cardiac output in an approximate ratio of 2/3 to 1/3. The major portion of blood ejected from the left ventricle supplies the brain and upper body, with lesser flow to the coronary arteries; the balance passes across the aortic isthmus to the descending aorta where it joins with the large stream from the ductus arteriosus before flowing to the lower body and placenta.

In fetal life pulmonary arteries and arterioles are surrounded by a fluid medium, have relatively thick walls and small lumina, and resemble comparable arteries in the systemic circulation. The low pulmonary blood flow in the fetus (7 to 10 per cent of the total cardiac output) is the result of high pulmonary vascular resistance. Fetal pulmonary vessels are highly reactive to changes in oxygen tension or in the pH of blood perfusing them as well as to a number of other physiological and pharmacological influences.

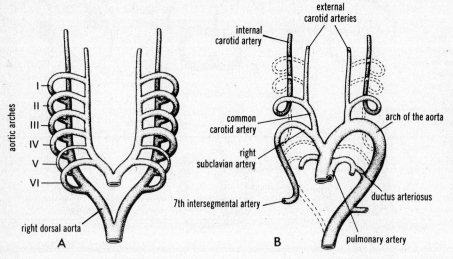

FIGURE 29–5   *A,* Aortic arches and dorsal aortas before transformation into the definitive vascular pattern. *B,* Aortic arches and dorsal aortas after transformation. The obliterated components are indicated by broken lines. (From Langman, J., and van Mierop, L. H. S.: Development of the cardiovascular system. *In* Moss, A. J., and Adams, F. H. (eds.): Heart Disease in Infants, Children and Adolescents. Baltimore, Williams and Wilkins, 1968.)

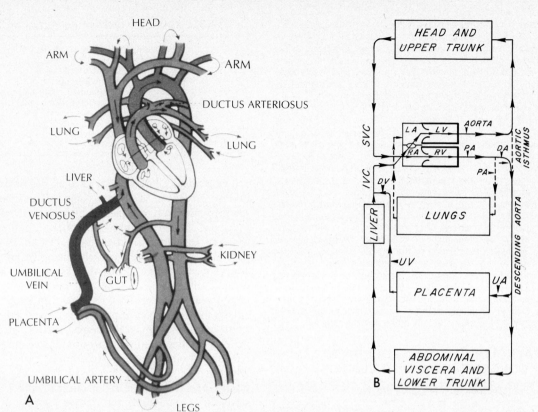

FIGURE 29–6 *A*, The fetal circulation. Shading shows the relative oxygenation of the blood, and arrows indicate its direction of flow. *B*, Prenatally, a fraction of umbilical venous (UV) blood enters the ductus venosus (DV) and bypasses the liver. This relatively well-oxygenated blood flows across the foramen ovale to the left heart, preferentially perfusing the coronary arteries, head, and upper trunk. Superior vena caval (SVC) blood is ejected by the right heart into the pulmonary artery (PA) and ductus arteriosus (DA). This stream circulates to the placenta as well as to the abdominal viscera and lower trunk. Dashed lines indicate diminished blood flow to and from the lungs and across the aortic isthmus. IVC = inferior vena cava, RA = right atrium, LA = left atrium, RV = right ventricle, LV = left ventricle, PA = pulmonary artery. (From Kaplan, S.: Congenital heart disease. *In* Vaughan, V. C., and McKay, R. J. (eds.): Nelson Textbook of Pediatrics. 10th ed. Philadelphia, W. B. Saunders Co., 1975.)

Although fetal somatic growth may be unimpaired, the hemodynamic effects in utero of many cardiac malformations may alter the development and structure of the fetal heart and circulation.[18] Thus, total anomalous pulmonary venous connection in utero may result in underdevelopment of the left atrium and left ventricle (p. 983), and premature closure of the foramen ovale may result in hypoplasia of the left ventricle (p. 983). Moreover, postnatally the caliber of the aortic isthmus may be reduced (p. 973) in the presence of lesions in utero that create left ventricular hypertrophy and impede filling because of reduced compliance of that chamber or that interfere with left ventricular filling directly (e.g., mitral stenosis) or indirectly by diverting a proportion of left ventricular output away from the ascending aorta while increasing right ventricular output and ductus arteriosus flow (e.g., endocardial cushion defect with left ventricular–right atrial shunt or aortic or subaortic stenosis with ventricular septal defect). Similarly, obstruction in utero to right ventricular outflow is associated with an increase in proximal aortic flow and diameter and almost never with aortic coarctation (p. 973). In these and other examples it is important to recognize that malformations compatible with fetal survival may nonetheless result in abnormal development of the circulation in utero and also affect circulatory adjustments after birth.

Compared to the adult heart, the fetal and newborn heart is unique with respect to its ultrastructural appearance,[20] its mechanical and biochemical properties,[21–23] and its autonomic innervation.[22–25] During late fetal and early neonatal development there is maturation of the biochemical composition of the heart's energy-utilizing myofibrillar proteins and of ATP and creatine phosphate energy-producing proteins.[23] Moreover, fetal and neonatal myocardial cells are small in diameter and reduced in density, so that the young heart contains relatively more noncontractile mass (primarily mitochondria, nuclei, and surface membranes) than later in postnatal life. As a result, force

generation and the extent and velocity of shortening are decreased, and stiffness and water content of ventricular myocardium are increased in the fetal and early newborn periods. The diminished function of the young heart is reflected in its limited ability to increase cardiac output in the presence of either a volume load or a lesion that increases resistance to emptying.[26] Although functional integrity exists of efferent and afferent cardiac autonomic pathways early in life, fetal and newborn myocardium lacks the complete development of sympathetic but not cholinergic innervation. Thus, adaptation to cardiocirculatory stress in fetal or early newborn life may be less effective than in the adult.

Normally, the fundamental change that occurs at birth is a division of the single parallel fetal circulation into separate, independent circulations. Inflation of the lungs at the first inspiration produces a marked reduction in pulmonary vascular resistance owing partly to the sudden suspension in air of fetal pulmonary vessels previously supported by fluid media. The reduced extravascular pressure assists new vessels to open and already patent vessels to enlarge. The rapid decrease in pulmonary vascular resistance is related more importantly to vasodilatation due to the increase in oxygen tension to which pulmonary vessels are exposed than to physical expansion of alveoli with gas. Pulmonary arterial pressure falls, and pulmonary blood flow increases greatly. Systemic vascular resistance rises when clamping of the umbilical cord removes the low-resistance placental circulation. Increased pulmonary blood flow increases the return of blood to the left atrium and raises left atrial pressure, which in turn closes the foramen ovale. The shift in oxygen dependence from the placenta to the lungs produces a sudden increase in arterial blood oxygen tension, which, in concert with alterations in the local prostaglandin milieu, initiates constriction of the ductus arteriosus.[27] Pulmonary pressure falls further as the ductus constricts. In mature infants the ductus arteriosus is closed functionally within 10 to 15 hours, with total anatomical closure following within a few weeks by a process of thrombosis, intimal proliferation, and fibrosis. A high incidence exists in preterm infants of persistent patency of the ductus arteriosus, probably because of an immaturity of those mechanisms responsible for constriction (p. 967). Surviving preterm infants spontaneously close the ductus arteriosus within 4 to 6 months of birth.

The ductus venosus, ductus arteriosus, and foramen ovale remain potential channels for blood flow after birth. Thus, persistent patency of the ductus venosus may mask the most marked signs of pulmonary venous obstruction in infants with total anomalous pulmonary venous connection below the diaphragm (p. 1008). Similarly, lesions producing right or left atrial volume or pressure overload may stretch the foramen ovale and render incompetent the flap valve mechanism for its closure (p. 958). Anomalies that depend on patency of the ductus arteriosus for preserving pulmonary or systemic blood flow remain latent until the ductus arteriosus constricts. A common example is the sudden intensification of cyanosis observed in the infant with tetralogy of Fallot when the magnitude of pulmonary hypoperfusion is unmasked by spontaneous closure of the ductus arteriosus. Moreover, there is increasing evidence that ductal constriction is a key factor in the postnatal development of coarctation of the aorta (p. 973). Lastly, it should be recognized that because the ductus arteriosus is potentially patent after birth and the pulmonary resistance vessels are hyperreactive, hypoxic pulmonary vasoconstriction of diverse etiologies may result in a right-to-left shunt through the ductus.

PATHOLOGICAL CONSEQUENCES OF CONGENITAL CARDIAC LESIONS

Congestive Heart Failure

Although the basic mechanisms of cardiac failure, as outlined in Chapter 13, are the same for all ages, the pediatric cardiologist should recognize clearly that the common causes, time of onset, and often the approach to treatment vary with age.[28–30,30a] Infants under one year of age with cardiac malformations account for 80 to 90 per cent of pediatric patients who develop congestive failure. Moreover, cardiac decompensation in the infant is a medical emergency necessitating immediate treatment if the patient is to be saved.

In the preterm infant, especially under 1500 grams birthweight, persistent patency of the ductus arteriosus is the most common cause of cardiac decompensation, and other forms of structural heart disease are rare. In the full-term newborn the earliest important causes of heart failure are the hypoplastic left heart and coarctation of the aorta syndromes, paroxysmal atrial tachycardia, cerebral or hepatic arteriovenous fistula, and myocarditis. Among the lesions commonly producing heart failure beyond age 1 to 2 weeks, when diminished pulmonary vascular resistance allows substantial left-to-right shunting, are ventricular septal and endocardial cushion defects, transposition of the great arteries, truncus arteriosus, and total anomalous pulmonary venous connection, often with pulmonary venous obstruction. Although heart failure is most usually the result of a structural defect or of myocardial disease, it should be recognized that the newborn myocardium may be depressed severely by such abnormalities as hypoxemia and acidemia, anemia, septicemia, marked hypoglycemia, hypocalcemia, and polycythemia. In the older child, heart failure is often due to acquired disease (Chap. 31) or is a complication of open-heart surgical procedures. In the acquired category are rheumatic and endomyocardial diseases, infective endocarditis, hematological and nutritional disorders, and severe cardiac arrhythmias.

TABLE 29–4   FEATURES OF HEART FAILURE IN INFANTS

Poor feeding and failure to thrive
Respiratory distress—mainly tachypnea
Rapid heart rate (160 to 180 beats/min)
Pulmonary rales or wheezing
Cardiomegaly and pulmonary edema on x-ray
Hepatomegaly (peripheral edema unusual)
Gallop sounds
Color—ashen pale or faintly cyanotic
Excessive perspiration
Diminished urine output

The clinical expression of cardiac decompensation in the infant consists of distinctive signs of pulmonary and systemic venous congestion and altered cardiocirculatory performance that resemble, but often are not identical to, those of the older child or adult (Table 29–4).[31] These reflect the interplay between the hemodynamic burden and adaptive responses. Common symptoms and signs are feeding difficulties and failure to gain weight and grow, tachypnea, tachycardia, pulmonary rales and rhonchi, liver enlargement, and cardiomegaly. Less frequent manifestations include peripheral edema, ascites, pulsus alternans, gallop rhythm, and inappropriate sweating. Pleural and pericardial effusions are exceedingly rare. The distinction between left and right heart failure is less obvious in the infant than it is in the older child or adult, since most lesions that create a left ventricular pressure or volume overload also result in left-to-right shunting of blood through the foramen ovale and/or patent ductus arteriosus as well as pulmonary hypertension due to elevated pulmonary venous pressures. Conversely, augmented filling or elevated pressure of the right ventricle in the infant reduces left ventricular compliance disproportionately when compared to the older child or adult and gives rise to signs of both systemic and pulmonary venous congestion.[22]

Fatigue and dyspnea on exertion express themselves as a feeding problem in the infant. Characteristically, the respiratory rate in heart failure is rapid (50 to 100 breaths/min). In the presence of left ventricular failure, interstitial pulmonary edema reduces pulmonary compliance and results in tachypnea and retractions. Excessive pulmonary blood flow via significant left-to-right shunts may further decrease lung compliance. Moreover, upper airway obstruction may be produced by selective enlargement of cardiovascular structures. In patients with large left-to-right shunts and left atrial and main pulmonary artery enlargement, the left main stem bronchus may be compressed, resulting in emphysematous expansion of the left upper or lower lobe or left lower lobe collapse.[32] Respiratory distress with grunting, flaring of the alae nasi, and intercostal retractions is observed when failure is severe and especially when pulmonary infection precipitates cardiac decompensation, which is often the case. Under these circumstances pulmonary rales may be due to the infection or failure or both. A resting heart rate with little variability is characteristic of heart failure. Hepatomegaly is seen regularly in infants in failure, although liver tenderness is uncommon. Cardiomegaly may be assessed roentgenographically, but it must be recognized that in the normal newborn infant the cardiac diameter may be as much as 60 per cent of the thoracic diameter, and the large thymus gland in infants interferes occasionally with evaluation of heart size.

Echocardiography provides a good estimate of cardiac chamber dimensions, and values may be compared to data derived from normal infants.[33-36]

Cardiac decompensation may progress with extreme rapidity in the first hours and days of life, producing a clinical picture of advanced cardiogenic shock and a profoundly obtunded infant. The presence of marked hepatomegaly and gross cardiomegaly usually allows distinction from noncardiac causes of diminished systemic perfusion.

Cyanosis
(See also page 7)

Cyanosis is produced by an increased amount of reduced hemoglobin in cutaneous vessels in excess of 3 gm/dl. Peripheral cyanosis usually reflects an abnormally great extraction of oxygen from normally saturated arterial blood, commonly the result of peripheral cutaneous vasoconstriction. Central cyanosis is a result of arterial blood oxygen unsaturation, most often in patients with congenital heart disease caused by shunting of systemic venous blood into the arterial circuit. Infants especially may appear cyanotic when in heart failure because of both peripheral and central factors; the latter may include severe impairment of pulmonary function that commonly exists with alveolar hypoventilation, ventilation-perfusion inequality, or impaired oxygen diffusion. In patients with central cyanosis due to arterial oxygen unsaturation, the degree of cutaneous discoloration depends upon the absolute amount of reduced hemoglobin, the magnitude of the right-to-left shunt relative to systemic flow, and the oxyhemoglobin saturation of venous blood. The last of these depends in turn upon the tissue extraction of oxygen. Commonly, cyanosis appears or intensifies with physical activity or exercise as the saturation of systemic venous blood declines concurrent with an increase in right-to-left shunting across a defect as peripheral vascular resistance decreases. Oxygen transfer to the tissues is affected by shifts in the oxygen-hemoglobin dissociation relationship, which may be altered by blood pH and levels of red blood cell 2,3 diphosphoglycerate concentration.[37]

CLUBBING AND POLYCYTHEMIA. Prominent accompaniments of arterial hypoxemia are polycythemia and clubbing of the digits. The latter is associated with an increased number of capillaries with increased blood flow through extensive arteriovenous aneurysms and an increase of connective tissue in the terminal phalanges of the fingers and toes. Polycythemia is a physiological response to chronic hypoxemia that stimulates erythrocytosis. The extremely high hematocrits observed in patients with arterial oxygen unsaturation cause a progressive increase in blood viscosity, especially beyond packed red blood cell volumes of 60 per cent. Both the hematocrit and the circulating whole blood volume are increased in polycythemia accompanying cyanotic congenital heart disease; the hypervolemia is the result of an increase in red cell volume. The augmented red blood cell volume provoked by hypoxemia provides an increased oxygen-carrying capacity and enhanced oxygen supply to the tissues. The compensatory polycythemia is often of such severity that it becomes a liability and produces adverse physiological effects such as thrombotic lesions in diverse organs and a hemorrhagic diathesis.[38] In this regard, oral steroid contraceptives are contraindicated in the adolescent cyanotic female because of the enhanced risk of cerebral thrombosis. Red cell volume reduction and replacement with plasma or albumin (erythrophoresis) lowers blood viscosity and increases systemic blood flow and systemic oxygen transport and thus may be helpful in the management of patients with severe hypoxic polycythemia (hematocrit $\geq$ 65 per cent). A final hematocrit of 55 to 63 per cent should be achieved; the higher level is necessary in patients with low initial oxygen saturation in order to avoid a severe reduction in arterial oxygen content. Acute phlebotomy without fluid replacement is contraindicated.

CEREBRAL AND PULMONARY COMPLICATIONS. Cerebral vascular accidents and brain abscesses occur particularly in cyanotic patients with substantial arterial desaturation.[39-41] *Cerebral thrombosis* is most common under age 2 years in severely cyanotic children, even in the presence of relatively low hematocrits, and occurs especially in a clinical setting in which oxygen requirements are raised by fever or, if blood viscosity is increased, by dehydration.

Brain abscesses are an important complication of cyanotic heart disease.[40,41] They are rare under 18 months of age and commonly are of insidious onset marked by headache, low-grade fever, vomiting, and a change in personality. Seizures or paralysis less frequently heralds the onset of a brain abscess. Abscess must be suspected in any cyanotic child with focal neurological signs. Morbidity and mortality are related inversely to oxygen saturation levels. Brain abscess is thought to occur in approximately 2 per cent of the population with cyanotic congenital heart disease; a mortality rate of 30 to 40 per cent is often related to delay in diagnosis and treatment.

Paradoxical embolus is a rare complication of cyanotic heart disease, usually observed only at necropsy.[42] Emboli arising in systemic veins may pass directly to the systemic circulation, since right-to-left intracardiac shunts allow venous blood to bypass the normal filtering action of the lungs.

Retinopathy consisting of dilated tortuous vessels progressing to papilledema and retinal edema is occasionally observed in cyanotic patients and appears to be related to decreased arterial oxygen saturation and/or to erythrocytosis but not to hypercapnea.

Hemoptysis is an uncommon but major complication in cyanotic patients with congenital heart disease and occurs most often in the presence of pulmonary vascular obstructive disease or in patients with an extensive bronchial collateral circulation or pulmonary venous congestion.[43] Massive hemoptysis almost always represents rupture of a dilated bronchial artery.

SQUATTING. After exertion, patients with cyanotic heart disease, especially tetralogy of Fallot, typically assume a squatting posture in order to obtain relief from breathlessness.[44] Squatting appears to improve arterial oxygen saturation by increasing systemic vascular resistance, thereby diminishing the right-to-left shunt, and also by the pooling of markedly desaturated blood in the lower extremities. In addition, systemic venous return and therefore pulmonary blood flow may increase.

HYPOXIC SPELLS. Hypercyanotic or hypoxemic

spells commonly complicate the clinical course in younger children with certain types of cyanotic heart disease, especially tetralogy of Fallot (p. 990).[44,45] The spells are characterized by anxiety, hyperpnea, and a sudden marked increase in cyanosis; they are the result of an abrupt reduction in pulmonary blood flow. Unless terminated, the hypercyanotic episodes may lead to convulsions and may even be fatal. The sudden reduction in pulmonary blood flow may be precipitated by fluctuations in arterial pCO_2 and pH, a sudden fall in systemic or increase in pulmonary vascular resistance, or an acute increase in the severity of right ventricular outflow tract obstruction either by augmented contraction of the hypertrophied muscle in the right ventricular outflow tract or by a decrease in right ventricular cavity volume due to tachycardia. *Treatment* consists of oxygen administration, placing the child in the knee-chest position, and administration of morphine sulfate. Additional medications that may prove of value include the intravenous administration of sodium bicarbonate to correct the accompanying acidemia, alpha-adrenergic receptor stimulants such as neosynephrine or methoxamine to raise peripheral resistance and diminish right-to-left shunting, and beta-adrenergic blocking agents that reduce cardiac sympathetic tone and depress cardiac contractility directly and that increase ventricular volume by reducing heart rate.

Acid-base Imbalance

Disturbances in blood gas and acid-base equilibrium are noted particularly in infants with either congestive heart failure or cyanosis.[46] Large-volume left-to-right shunts, especially with pulmonary edema, may be associated with moderate respiratory acidemia and a lowering of arterial oxygen tensions, reflecting an increase in the alveolar-arterial oxygen tension gradient and ventilation-perfusion imbalance. Interference with carbon dioxide transport implies moderate to severe failure in these infants. Lesions associated with a reduced systemic cardiac output, such as severe coarctation of the aorta or critical aortic stenosis in infancy, present often with cardiac failure complicated by a severe metabolic acidemia and relatively high values of arterial oxygen tension. The latter finding, even in the presence of right-to-left shunting across a patent ductus arteriosus, is a result of diminished systemic perfusion and an elevated pulmonary-to-systemic blood flow ratio. Respiratory acidemia and depressed levels of oxygen tension are observed in infants with obstruction to pulmonary venous return and right-to-left atrial shunting. Infants with severe hypoxemia due to lesions such as transposition of the great arteries or pulmonic atresia often show metabolic acidemia and marked reductions in carbon dioxide tension secondary to hyperventilation resulting from hypoxic stimulation of peripheral chemoreceptors.

Impaired Growth

Impaired growth and physical development and delayed onset of adolescence are common features of many cyanotic and, to a lesser extent, acyanotic forms of congenital heart disease.[47] Mental development is rarely affected. In general, the severity of growth disturbance depends upon the anatomical lesion and its functional effect. Most chil-

dren with mild defects grow normally. Weight gain is commonly slower than linear growth in acyanotic patients with large left-to-right shunts, whereas in cyanotic congenital heart disease height and weight usually parallel each other. Boys appear to be more retarded in growth than girls, especially in the second decade. Skeletal maturity (i.e., bone age) is delayed in cyanotic children in relation to the severity of hypoxemia. In some children, prenatal factors such as intrauterine infection and chromosomal or other hereditary and nonhereditary syndromes are responsible for growth retardation. In other patients, extracardiac malformations may contribute to poor weight gain and linear growth. Additional explanations for the mechanisms of growth interference have implicated malnutrition as a result of anorexia and inadequate nutrients and caloric intake, hypermetabolic state, acidemia and cation imbalance, tissue hypoxia, diminished peripheral blood flow, chronic cardiac decompensation, malabsorption or protein loss, recurrent respiratory infections, and endocrine or genetic factors. In some instances, the underdevelopment is influenced little by operative correction of the underlying cardiac anomaly. Among factors that may be responsible for persistent growth retardation postoperatively are age at operation, hemodynamically significant residual lesions, and sequelae or complications of operation. As a general rule, it is unwise preoperatively to guarantee to the parents of a child with heart disease that surgery will result in accelerated growth and development.

Pulmonary Hypertension
(See also Chapter 25)

Pulmonary hypertension is a common accompaniment of many congenital cardiac lesions, and the status of the pulmonary vascular bed is often the principal determinant of the clinical manifestations, course, and whether surgical treatment is feasible.[48] Increases in pulmonary arterial pressure result from elevations of pulmonary blood flow and/or resistance, the latter due sometimes to an increase in vascular tone, but usually the result of obstructive, obliterative structural changes within the pulmonary vascular bed.[49]

Normally, pulmonary vascular resistance falls rapidly immediately after birth owing to onset of ventilation and subsequent release of hypoxic pulmonary vasoconstriction. Subsequently the medial smooth muscle of pulmonary arterial resistance vessels thins gradually.[50] This latter process is delayed often by several months in infants with large aorticopulmonary or ventricular communications, at which time levels of pulmonary vascular resistance are still somewhat elevated. In patients with high pulmonary arterial pressure from birth, failure of normal growth of the pulmonary circulation may occur, and anatomical changes in the pulmonary vessels in the form of proliferation of intimal cells and intimal and medial thickening often progress, so that in the older child or adult vascular resistance may ultimately become fixed by obliterative changes in the pulmonary vascular bed. The causes of pulmonary vascular obstructive disease remain unknown, although increased pulmonary blood flow, increased pulmonary arterial blood pressure, elevated pulmonary venous pressure, polycythemia, systemic hypoxia, acidemia, and the nature of the bronchial circulation have all been implicated. There are many patients with pulmonary vascular obstruction whose cardiac anomaly places them at particular risk quite early in life, precluding survival to adulthood. Patients at particularly high risk for the development of significant pulmonary vascular obstruction are those with certain forms of cyanotic congenital heart disease, such as complete transposition of the great arteries with or without ventricular septal defect or patent ductus arteriosus, single ventricle without pulmonary stenosis, double outlet right ventricle, and truncus arteriosus. Other conditions in which pulmonary vascular obstruction appears to progress rapidly include large ventricular septal defect, as well as the less common conditions of unilateral pulmonary artery absence, congenital left-to-right shunts in an environment of high altitude or in association with the Down's syndrome of trisomy 21, and complete atrioventricular canal defects, even unassociated with a chromosomal anomaly.

Intimal damage appears to be related to shear stresses, since endothelial cell damage occurs at high-flow shear rates. A reduction in pulmonary arteriolar lumen size due to either thickened medial muscle or vasoconstriction increases the velocity of flow. Shear stress also increases as blood viscosity rises; therefore, infants with hypoxemia and high hematocrits as well as increased pulmonary blood flow are at increased risk of developing pulmonary vascular disease. In patients with left-to-right shunts, pulmonary arterial hypertension, if not present in infancy or childhood, may never occur or may not develop until the third or fourth decade or later. Once developed, intimal proliferative changes with hyalinization and fibrosis are not reversible by repair of the underlying cardiac defect. In severe pulmonary vascular obstructive disease, arteriovenous malformations may develop and predispose to massive hemoptysis.

Most vexing is the variability among patients with the same or similar cardiac lesions in both the time of appearance and rate of progression of their pulmonary vascular obstructive process. While genetic influences may be operative (an example is the apparent acceleration of pulmonary vascular disease in patients with congenital heart disease and trisomy 21), evidence is now accumulating for important pre- and postnatal modifiers of the pulmonary vascular bed that appear, at least in part, to be lesion-dependent. Thus, a quantitative variability exists in the pulmonary vascular bed related to the *number*, not just the size and wall structure, of arterial vessels within the pulmonary circulation.[51] Modeling of the blood vessels occurs proximal to and within terminal bronchioles (pre- and intra-acinar vessels, respectively) continuously from before birth. The intra-acinar vessels, in particular, increase in size and number from late fetal life throughout childhood with minimal muscularization of their walls. The ensuing increase in the cross-sectional area of the pulmonary arterial circulation allows the cardiac output to rise substantially without an increase in pulmonary arterial pressure. If, however, the presence of a cardiac lesion interferes with the normal growth and multiplication of these most peripheral arteries, the resulting elevation of pulmonary vascular resistance may first be related to failure of the intra-acinar pulmonary circulation to develop fully, and then secondarily to the morphological changes of obliterative vascular disease—medial thickening, intimal proliferation,

hyalinization and fibrosis, and angiomatoid and plexiform lesions, and, ultimately, arterial necrosis.[49]

Since pulmonary vascular obstructive disease may be the factor limiting a decision concerning the advisability of operation, it is important to quantify and compare pulmonary-to-systemic flow and resistance in patients with severe pulmonary hypertension. Moreover, the reactivity of the pulmonary vascular bed should be evaluated. A marked reduction in pulmonary vascular resistance with infusion of tolazoline or the inhalation of oxygen suggests that the resistance is not fixed and may fall after successful operation. Some defects between the left and right sides of the heart should be closed in order to eliminate a sizable left-to-right shunt, which may in turn result in a significant drop in pulmonary arterial pressure. Conversely, little or no benefit and high mortality rates may be expected from closure of defects associated with bidirectional or predominantly right-to-left shunts in patients with high resistance and obstructive pulmonary hypertension.

The clinical manifestations of pulmonary hypertension associated with a large left-to-right shunt reflect the specific malformation responsible. When pulmonary vascular resistance is elevated and a significant right-to-left shunt exists, the patient is cyanotic, and polycythemia and clubbing are noted. A dominant *a* wave in the jugular venous pulse may be seen reflecting vigorous right atrial contraction due to diminished compliance of the right ventricle. In some instances there are large systolic *c-v* waves, which suggest tricuspid regurgitation. A prominent right ventricular parasternal lift and palpable systolic expansion of the pulmonary artery are present. A soft pulmonary systolic ejection murmur preceded by an ejection sound and followed by a markedly accentuated pulmonic component of the second heart sound are often audible on auscultation; an early diastolic decrescendo blowing murmur of pulmonary regurgitation may be heard. If right ventricular failure and dilatation supervene, the systolic murmur of tricuspid regurgitation may be audible at the lower left, sternal border. Right ventricular enlargement may be evident on the chest roentgenogram and electrocardiogram. The former examination also reveals a conspicuously enlarged pulmonary artery, prominent hilar pulmonary vascular markings, and attenuated peripheral vessels. The site of the underlying defect may be localized by means of cardiac catheterization and angiocardiography. Pressures in the right side of the heart are essentially identical to systemic pressures in cyanotic patients if the shunt is at the ventricular or aorticopulmonary levels, but they are usually lower than systemic pressures in patients with an intraatrial shunt. No specific treatment has proved beneficial for obstructive pulmonary vascular disease.

Infective Endocarditis
(See also Chapter 33)

Infective endocarditis is uncommon under age 2 years and thereafter most often affects children with tetralogy of Fallot (especially after systemic-pulmonary anastomosis), ventricular septal defect, aortic stenosis, and patent ductus arteriosus. Postsurgical patients with prosthetic heterograft or homograft valves or conduits are at particular risk. A causative organism can be isolated in approximately 90 per cent of children, usually either alpha-streptococci (usually

Strep. viridans) or *Staphylococcus aureus*.[52] Fungal endocarditis is quite rare in the pediatric age group. Mortality appears to be highest when coagulase-positive staphylococcus is the offending organism and when the endocarditis involves the left, rather than the right, side of the heart. Most recent data suggest 75 to 80 per cent overall survival.[52,53] Factors predisposing to endocarditis may be identified in approximately one third of cases; these include cardiovascular surgery with infection during the perioperative period; respiratory tract infections; and ear, nose, throat, and dental procedures. Less often, contamination during a surgical procedure or cardiac catheterization or an infection involving the skin, genitourinary tract, or other organ system has been the cause.

Although routine antimicrobial prophylaxis is recommended for all children with congenital heart disease and for the majority of patients after operative repair of the lesion, it should be recognized that many different microbes are responsible for the disease and that an effective preventive approach may center ultimately on active immunization rather than antibiotics. Currently, antibiotic prophy-laxis is recommended for all dental procedures except minor readjustments of braces, oral trauma, and other procedures such as tonsillectomy, gastrointestinal surgery, and genitourinary surgery, or diagnostic procedures such as proctosigmoidoscopy and cystoscopy (Table 29–5).[54] The risk of endocarditis is undoubtedly related both to the magnitude of bacteremia and to the type of underlying heart disease. Since infection on a prosthetic heart valve or conduit may be devastating, combinations of antibiotics given parenterally are advisable in these patients.

Chest Pain
(See also pages 5 and 1335)

Angina pectoris is an uncommon symptom of cardiac disease in infants and children, occurring in association with anomalous pulmonary origin of a coronary artery or occasionally in association with severe aortic stenosis, pulmonic stenosis, or pulmonary hypertension due to pulmonary vascular obstruction. Cardiac pain in the infant with anomalous coronary artery (p. 971) most usually takes the

TABLE 29–5 PROPHYLACTIC ANTIBIOTICS FOR PROTECTION FROM BACTERIAL ENDOCARDITIS

For Dental Procedures and also for Tonsillectomy, Adenoidectomy, and Bronchoscopy

I. For most patients: PENICILLIN	**a) Intramuscular plus Oral** **Adults:** 600,000 units or procaine penicillin G mixed with 1,000,000 units or aqueous crystalline penicillin G intramuscularly 30–60 minutes prior to procedure, followed by 500 mg penicillin V orally every 6 hours for 8 doses. **Children:** 30,000 units aqueous penicillin G/kg mixed with 600,000 units of procaine penicillin intramuscularly (not to exceed adult dose). For children less than 60 lbs the dose of penicillin V is 250 mg every 6 hours for 8 doses. **b) Oral only** **Adults:** 2.0 gm of penicillin V 30–60 minutes prior to procedure and then 500 mg every 6 hours for 8 doses. **Children less than 60 lbs:** 1.0 gm of penicillin V orally 30 minutes to one hour prior to procedure and then 250 mg orally every 6 hours for 8 doses.	continuous rheumatic fever prophylaxis): ERYTHROMYCIN	**Children:** 20 mg/kg orally one and one-half to two hours prior to procedure and then 10 mg/kg (not to exceed adult dosage) every 6 hours for 8 doses (or Regimen IV).
		III. For those patients at higher risk of infective endocarditis (especially those with prosthetic heart valves) who are not allergic to penicillin: PENICILLIN plus STREPTOMYCIN	**Adults:** IM penicillin as outlined above in I.a, **plus** streptomycin 1.0 gm IM, both given 30–60 minutes before procedure; then penicillin V 500 mg orally every 6 hours for 8 doses. **Children:** Timing of doses is same as for adults. Aqueous penicillin dose is 30,000 units/kg mixed with 600,000 units procaine penicillin. Streptomycin dose is 20 mg/kg (not to exceed adult dosage). For children less than 60 lbs, the dose of penicillin V is 250 mg every 6 hours for 8 doses.
II. For those allergic to penicillin (may also be selected for those receiving oral penicillin as	**Adults:** 1.0 gm orally one and one-half to two hours prior to procedure and then 500 mg every 6 hours for 8 doses (or Regimen IV).	IV. For higher risk patients (especially those with prosthetic heart valves) who are allergic to penicillin: VANCOMYCIN intravenously and ERYTHROMYCIN orally	**Adults:** Vancomycin 1 gm IV over 30–60 minutes, begun 30–60 minutes before procedure; then erythromycin 500 mg orally every 6 hours for 8 doses. **Children:** Timing of doses is same as for adults. Dose of vancomycin is 20 mg/kg. Dose of erythromycin is 10 mg/kg every 6 hours for 8 doses (not to exceed adult dose).

For Gastrointestinal and Genitourinary Tract Surgery and Instrumentation and also for Any Surgery of Infected Tissues

I. For most patients: PENICILLIN or AMPICILLIN plus STREPTOMYCIN or GENTAMICIN	**Adults:** 2 million units of aqueous penicillin G IM or IV **or** 1.0 gm ampicillin IM or IV **plus** gentamicin 1.5 mg/kg (not to exceed 80 mg) IM or IV **or** streptomycin 1.0 gm IM. This should be given 30–60 minutes before procedure. Repeat every 8 hours for 2 additional doses if gentamicin is used, or every 12 hours for 2 additional doses if streptomycin is used. **Children:** Same timing of medications as adult schedule. Dosages are aqueous penicillin G 30,000 units/kg **or** ampicillin 50 mg/kg; gentamicin 2.0 mg/kg (not to exceed adult dosage).	II. For patients allergic to penicillin: VANCOMYCIN plus STREPTOMYCIN	**Adults:** 1.0 gm vancomycin IV given over 30–60 minutes **plus** 1.0 gm streptomycin IM, each given 30–60 minutes before procedure. Doses may be repeated in 12 hours. **Children:** Timing as above. Doses are vancomycin 20 mg/kg and streptomycin 20 mg/kg (not to exceed adult dosage).

NOTE: In patients with significantly compromised renal function, antibiotic dosages may need to be modified. Intramuscular injections may be contraindicated in patients receiving anticoagulants.

Adapted from The Report of the Committee on Rheumatic Fever and Bacterial Endocarditis, American Heart Association, 1977.[54]

form of irritability and crying during feeding or straining at bowel movement. In children with severe left or right ventricular outflow tract obstruction chest pain commonly follows effort and is identical to angina observed in adults. Cardiac pain associated with *pulmonary vascular obstruction* may be anginal in nature but often is evanescent and pleuritic in type. Atypical forms of chest pain associated with the syndrome of *mitral valve prolapse* are much less usual in children than adults. A sensation of chest discomfort or cardiac awareness is frequently interpreted as pain by the parents of children with cardiac arrhythmias. Careful questioning serves to identify palpitations rather than pain as the symptom and often elicits an additional history of anxiety, pallor, and sweating. Pain due to *pericarditis* is commonly of acute onset, is associated with fever, and can be identified by specific physical, roentgenographic, and echocardiographic findings.

Most commonly, chest pain in children is *musculoskeletal* in origin and may be reproduced upon upper extremity movement or by palpation; often, chest wall pain is the result of *costochondritis*. Lastly, children, like adults, may suffer chest pain of nonspecific pattern owing to *anxiety* in the presence or absence of hyperventilation; often a history is elicited of a family member or friend who had died recently or suffered myocardial infarction.

Syncope
(See also Chapter 28)

Syncope is an unusual feature of heart disease in children; its presence suggests specific diagnoses, the most common being an arrhythmia. The symptom is observed in children with complete atrioventricular block that is less often of congenital origin than a sequela of cardiac operation. Syncope due to abrupt episodes of either bradycardia or tachycardia occurs in association with the sick sinus syndrome. The latter is most commonly produced in children after surgical procedures involving the region of the sinoatrial node, e.g., atrial septal defect closure or Mustard's procedure for transposition of the great arteries (p. 1001). Syncope is an occasional but ominous symptom if associated with severe aortic stenosis, pulmonary vascular obstruction, or a left atrial myxoma that transiently occludes left ventricular inflow.

Sudden Death
(See also Chapter 23)

In contrast to adults, children seldom die suddenly and unexpectedly from cardiovascular disease. Arrhythmias, hypoxemia, and coronary insufficiency secondary to left ventricular outflow tract obstruction are the most frequent causes of death.[55] Sudden death is most often reported in patients with aortic stenosis or hypertrophic obstructive cardiomyopathy, the Eisenmenger syndrome of pulmonary vascular obstruction, myocarditis, congenital complete heart block, primary endocardial fibroelastosis, anomalies of the coronary arteries, and cyanotic congenital heart disease with pulmonic stenosis or atresia. A relationship exists between strenuous exercise and sudden demise in patients with aortic stenosis or obstructive cardiomyopathy, thus providing justification for restricting patients with these lesions from gymnastic activities and strenuous competitive sports.

APPROACH TO THE HIGH-RISK INFANT

Approximately one-third of all infants born with congenital heart disease will die in the first months of life without prompt recognition, accurate diagnosis, or treatment of their life-threatening anomaly. Heart failure and cyanosis are the two cardinal signs of the high-risk infant with heart disease, and this section will provide an approach for the management of each.

Heart Failure
(See also Chapter 16)

Care of the infant with heart failure must include careful consideration of the underlying structural or functional disturbance. The general aims of treatment are to achieve an increase in cardiac performance, augment peripheral perfusion, and decrease pulmonary and systemic venous congestion. It must be emphasized, however, that under many conditions medical management cannot control the effects of the abnormal loads imposed by a host of congenital cardiac lesions. Under these circumstances cardiac catheterization and operative intervention may be urgently required.[56] Thus, initial therapy is aimed at stabilizing the infant for diagnostic hemodynamic and angiocardiographic study as soon as possible. In almost all situations the decision to intervene surgically or to continue medical management requires a definitive anatomical diagnosis.

Table 29–6 lists supportive and pharmacological measures in the treatment of the newborn with heart failure. Digitalis glycosides and certain diuretic agents provide the most important elements of medical therapy, but it is important to recognize that the dosage regimen of drugs administered to young patients must be adjusted to take into account the age and size of the patient and the maturity-dependent pharmacological properties of cardioactive drugs.[57,58] Since this is especially true in early infancy, Table 29–7 provides the dosages of digoxin and diuretics commonly employed. Digoxin is the glycoside used exclusively to treat pediatric patients in most cardiac centers, since it is readily absorbed, is available in convenient dosage form, and is excreted rapidly from the body. Premature infants are more sensitive to digitalis than are full-term newborns who, in turn, are more sensitive than older infants. Infants absorb and excrete digoxin as well as adults

---

TABLE 29–6 TREATMENT OF CONGESTIVE HEART FAILURE

I. Rest (occasional sedation)
    Semi-Fowler position
    Temperature and humidity control
    Oxygen
II. Diet—Decrease NaCl load, recognize danger of aspiration
III. Medications
    Correct hypoglycemia, anemia, or acidemia, if present
    Treat infection, if contributing factor
    Diuretics
    Digitalis
    Occasional need for catecholamine infusion, mechanical ventilation, peritoneal dialysis, afterload reduction, prostaglandin infusion or blocker
IV. Surgery

TABLE 29–7   DIURETIC AND DIGITALIS DOSAGES FOR INFANTS

PREPARATION	DOSAGE AND ROUTE OF ADMINISTRATION
Furosemide	IV, 1 mg/kg/dose; oral, 2 to 3 mg/kg/day
Ethacrynic acid	IV, 1 mg/kg/dose; oral, 2 to 3 mg/kg/day
Hydrochlorothiazide	Oral, 2 to 5 mg/kg/day
Spironolactone	Oral, 1 to 2 mg/kg/day
Triamterene	Oral, 2 to 4 mg/kg/day
Digoxin	
Elixir	0.05 mg/ml

Parenteral	0.10 mg/ml Loading dose
	Premature infants: 0.03 mg/kg IV or IM
	Term infants:
	   Oral: Up to 2 weeks, 0.03 mg/kg
	       2 weeks to 6 months, 0.06 mg/kg
	       6 months to 2 years, 0.045 mg/kg
	       Beyond 2 years, 0.03 mg/kg
	Parenteral: 75% of oral dose
	Maintenance dosage: $^1/_3$ to $^1/_4$ loading dose,
	   given in 2 divided doses every 24 hours

do, and the relative distribution of the glycoside to different body tissues is also similar. The prevailing dose schedules for digoxin produce higher serum concentrations in infants than would be considered optimum for adults.[18,58] The basis for the higher digitalis requirement in infancy is unclear, although it may relate to an age-dependent alteration in the sensitivity of the myocardium per se to the glycosides. In this regard, infants tolerate higher serum digoxin concentrations than adults without developing signs of toxicity. In the adult, the usual therapeutic concentrations of digoxin are less than 2 ng/ml blood, and toxicity commonly occurs above that level. In contrast, in infants, therapeutic levels of digoxin range from 1 to 5 ng/ml (mean = 3.5), while toxicity is associated with concentrations in excess of 3 ng/ml. Older children have therapeutic and toxic levels similar to those of adults.

A restricted fluid intake (65 ml/kg/day) and a low-sodium diet (1 to 2 mEq/kg/day) should accompany diuretic therapy in the most seriously ill infants with heart failure. Furosemide is the agent of choice when the rapid elimination of excess salt and water is needed. Hydrochlorothiazide, occasionally in conjunction with spironolactone or triamterene to reduce potassium loss and sodium retention, is convenient for long-term therapy.

Other pharmacological approaches may prove to be of significant benefit in selected instances in which digitalis and diuretics are relatively ineffective. In situations in which cardiac decompensation is not the result of an obstructive lesion, catecholamines may be employed temporarily to alleviate cardiac failure while awaiting more definitive operative treatment.[18] Isoproterenol (0.05 to 0.50 μg/kg/min), norepinephrine (0.25 to 1 μg/kg/min), and dopamine (5 to 15 μg/kg/min) have all been employed by titrating their infusion until a beneficial effect is reached or until ventricular ectopic beats occur. In infants with the coarctation of the aorta syndrome, in whom ductal constriction unmasks the aortic branch point producing aortic narrowing (p. 973), heart failure may be reversed dramatically by the intravenous infusion of prostaglandin E_1 (0.03–0.1 mg/kg/min), which results in dilatation of the ductus arteriosus and relief of the obstruction.[59,60] Conversely, in preterm infants in whom patent ductus arteriosus is responsible for profound cardiopulmonary deterioration, constriction for the ductus arteriosus may be accomplished by inhibition of prostaglandin synthesis with the nonsteroidal anti-inflammatory agent indomethacin (0.2 mg/kg IV).[27,61] Vasodilator therapy is also employed in infants or children with heart disease in whom afterload reduction may be expected to improve cardiac performance.[62,63] We usually employ sodium nitroprusside for acute intravenous use, administered as a continuous infusion in a dose ranging from 1 to 8 μg/kg/min. Hydralazine may also be effective acutely by intravenous administration (0.05–0.2 mg/kg/day q4–6h) or chronically by the oral route (0.7–7.0 mg/kg/day divided q6–12h). In this regard, it may be anticipated that a pharmacological reduction in systemic vascular resistance will diminish the pulmonary-to-systemic flow ratio in patients in whom the magnitude of left-to-right shunting depends on the relationship between pulmonary and systemic vascular resistance (e.g., ventricular septal defect). The additional supportive measures listed in Table 29–5 are designed to increase tissue oxygen supply, decrease tissue oxygen consumption, and correct metabolic abnormalities.

Cyanosis

Cyanosis in the infant often presents as a diagnostic emergency, necessitating prompt detection of the underlying cause. The schema in Figure 29–7 outlines a general approach to diagnosis. The cardiologist must distinguish between three types of cyanosis—peripheral, differential, and central—while recognizing that cyanosis may accompany diseases of the central nervous, hematological, respiratory, and cardiac systems.

PERIPHERAL CYANOSIS. Peripheral cyanosis (normal arterial oxygen saturation and widened arteriovenous oxygen differences) usually indicates stasis of blood flow in the periphery. The level of reduced hemoglobin in the capillaries of the skin usually exceeds 3 gm/100 ml. The most prominent causes of peripheral cyanosis in the newborn are autonomically controlled alterations in the cutaneous distribution of capillary blood flow (acrocyanosis) and septicemia associated with evidence of a low cardiac output, i.e., hypotension, weak pulse, and cold extremities. In many instances peripheral cyanosis is clearly the result of a cold environment or high hemoglobin content. When caused by the former, vasodilatation produced by immersing the extremity in warm water for several minutes will reverse the cyanosis.

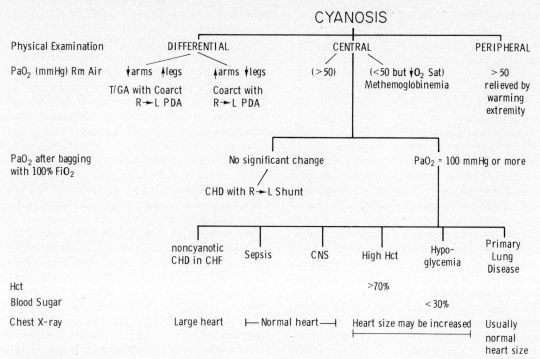

FIGURE 29–7 Flow chart for the evaluation of cyanotic infants. Tests to be done are listed at the left. The response to each of these tests leads along the line to the proper diagnostic category. CHD = congenital heart disease, CHF = congestive heart failure, CNS = central nervous system, Hct = hematocrit, PDA = patent ductus arteriosus. T/GA = transpoitim great arteries (From Kirkpatrick, S. E., et al.: Differential diagnosis of congenital heart disease in the newborn—University of California, San Diego, School of Medicine, and University Hospital, San Diego (Specialty Conference). West. J. Med. *128*:127, 1978.)

CENTRAL CYANOSIS. Oxygen unsaturation in central cyanosis may result from inadequately oxygenated pulmonary venous blood, in which case inhalation of 100 per cent oxygen may diminish or clear the discoloration (see below). Conversely, in instances in which cyanosis is due to an intra- or extracardiac right-to-left shunt, pulmonary venous blood is fully saturated, and inhalation of 100 per cent oxygen generally will not improve the infant's color. It is necessary to qualify the latter statement because oxygen may act directly in infants with elevated pulmonary vascular resistance to dilate the pulmonary blood vessels and thus reduce the magnitude of the venoarterial shunt. Central cyanosis may also be due to the replacement of normal by abnormal hemoglobin, as in methemoglobinemia.

Several factors influence the oxygen saturation produced at any given arterial pO$_2$. These include temperature, pH, ratio of fetal-to-adult hemoglobin, and erythrocyte concentration of 2,3-diphosphoglycerate. For example, fetal hemoglobin has a higher affinity for oxygen than does adult hemoglobin and therefore would be more highly saturated at any given pO$_2$. Thus, determination of the systemic arterial oxygen tension may provide a more accurate picture of the underlying pathophysiology than simply measuring the oxygen saturation.

DIFFERENTIAL CYANOSIS. Differential cyanosis virtually always indicates the presence of congenital heart disease, often with patency of the ductus arteriosus and coarctation of the aorta as components of the abnormal anatomical complex. If the upper part of the body is pink and the lower part of the body blue, coarctation of the aorta or interruption of the aortic arch is probable, with oxygenated blood supplying the upper body and desatu-

rated blood supplying the lower body via right-to-left flow through the ductus arteriosus. The latter occurs also in patients with patent ductus arteriosus and markedly elevated pulmonary vascular resistance. A patient with transposition of the great arteries and coarctation of the aorta with retrograde flow through a patent ductus arteriosus demonstrates the reverse situation, i.e., the lower part of the body is pink and the upper part blue. Simultaneous determinations of oxygen saturation in the temporal or right brachial artery and the femoral artery are helpful in confirming the presence of differential cyanosis.

Central Nervous System and Hematological Causes

Irregular, shallow breathing secondary to central nervous system depression results in reduced alveolar ventilation and an abnormally low alveolar oxygen tension. Alveolar arterial pCO$_2$ becomes elevated, and arterial pO$_2$ is reduced. Sedatives and hypnotics administered to the mother during labor cause central nervous system depression in the newborn and intracranial hemorrhage secondary to birth trauma, accounting for most cases.

Methemoglobinemia, either congenital or acquired, is a rare cause of cyanosis in the newborn, with recognizable cyanosis occurring in affected babies when 15 per cent or more of the total hemoglobin is replaced by methemoglobin. Venous blood exposed to room air normally becomes pink but remains dark in infants with methemoglobinemia. Arterial blood with a normal partial pressure of oxygen but a low oxygen saturation should suggest the diagnosis, which may be established conclusively by spectrophotometry.

Pulmonary vs. Cardiac Causes

The distinction between respiratory signs and symptoms arising from cyanotic cardiac disease and those associated with a primary pulmonary disorder is an important challenge to the cardiologist.[31] Upper airway obstruction precipitates cyanosis by producing alveolar hypoventilation due to reduced pulmonary ventilation. Mechanical obstruction may occur from the nares to the carina, and the important diagnostic possibilities among congenital abnormalities are choanal atresia, vascular ring, laryngeal web, and tracheomalacia. Acquired causes include vocal cord paresis, obstetrical injury to the cricothyroid cartilage, and foreign body. Structural abnormalities in the lungs due to intrapulmonary disease are more frequently a basis for cyanosis among newborns than is upper airway obstruction. Hyaline membrane disease, atelectasis, or pneumonitis causing inflammation, collapse, and fluid accumulation in the alveoli results in incompletely oxygenated blood reaching the systemic circulation.

Successfully distinguishing between these various causes of cyanosis depends upon interpretation of the respiratory pattern, the cardiac physical examination, evaluation of arterial blood gases, and interpretation of the electrocardiogram, chest x-ray, and echocardiogram.

RESPIRATORY PATTERNS. The key to differential diagnosis at the bedside is commonly the proper evaluation of the pattern of respiration. Normally, term infants exhibit a progressive reduction in respiratory rate during the first day of life from 60 to 70/minute to 35 to 55/minute. Moreover, mild intercostal retractions and minimal expiratory grunting disappear within several hours of birth. An increased depth of respiration in the presence of cyanosis, but without other signs of respiratory distress, is often associated with congenital cardiac disease in which inadequate pulmonary blood flow is the most important functional component.

The most important variations from normal respiratory patterns are apnea and bradypnea, and tachypnea. Intermittent apneic episodes are common in premature infants with central nervous system immaturity or disease. In addition, higher centers may be depressed as a result of severe hypoxemia, acidemia, or the administration of pharmacological agents to mother or baby. The association of apneic episodes, lethargy, hypotonicity, and a reduction in spontaneous movements most often point to intracranial disease as an underlying cause.

Diverse conditions result in tachypnea in the newborn period. Tachypnea in the presence of intrinsic pulmonary disease with upper or lower airway obstruction is usually accompanied by flaring of the alae nasi, chest wall retractions, and grunting. In contrast, tachypnea associated with intense cyanosis in the absence of obvious respiratory distress suggests the presence of cyanotic congenital heart disease. In general, highest respiratory rates (80 to 110/min) are seen in association with primary lung, and not heart, disease. Frequently, an initial chest x-ray is diagnostic, especially if the problem is aspiration, mucous plug, adenomatoid malformation, lobar emphysema, diaphragmatic hernia, pneumothorax, lung agenesis, pulmonary hemorrhage, or an abnormal thoracic cage configuration. Choanal atresia may be excluded by passing a feeding tube through the nares, and the more common types of esopha-

geal atresia and tracheoesophageal fistula may be excluded by passing the tube farther into the stomach.

CARDIAC EXAMINATION. Specific findings upon cardiovascular examination may direct attention to a cardiac etiology for cyanosis.[64] Peripheral perfusion is poor in the presence of severe primary myocardial disease or the hypoplastic left heart syndrome. In contrast, peripheral pulses are bounding and the dorsalis pedis and palmar pulses are easily palpable in infants with patent ductus arteriosus, truncus arteriosus, or aorticopulmonary window. A marked discrepancy between upper and lower extremity blood pressures help identify the infant with coarctation of the aorta. Inspection and palpation of the precordium allows an overall estimate of cardiac activity. A suprasternal notch and precordial thrill may occasionally be felt in the infant with patent ductus arteriosus, critical aortic stenosis, or coarctation of the aorta. Characterization of the second heart sound may be of help, since it is often single in infants with a hypoplastic left heart complex, pulmonary atresia with or without an intact ventricular septum, and truncus arteriosus. Wide splitting of the second heart sound may occur in infants with total anomalous pulmonary venous return. Ejection sounds are often detectable in infants with persistent truncus arteriosus and occasionally with critical aortic or pulmonic stenosis. The presence of a third heart sound is normal, but a gallop rhythm may provide a clue to myocardial failure. Wide splitting of the first and second heart sounds and prominent third and fourth heart sounds may produce the characteristically rhythmic auscultatory cadence of Ebstein's anomaly of the tricuspid valve (p. 996). The presence of a cardiac murmur may point clearly to underlying cardiac disease, but the absence of a murmur does not exclude the presence of a cardiac malformation. Moreover, cardiac murmurs of specific anomalies are often atypical in the newborn period. However, certain cardiac murmurs such as the decrescendo holosystolic murmur of tricuspid regurgitation in Ebstein's anomaly or transient tricuspid regurgitation of infancy may point clearly to a proper diagnosis. Auscultation of the head and abdomen may detect the murmur of an arteriovenous malformation at those sites in infants who present with findings of severe heart failure.

BLOOD GAS AND pH PATTERNS. Arterial blood gases may be a reliable method of evaluating cyanosis, suggesting the type of altered physiology, and assessing responses to therapeutic maneuvers.[28,46] Blood gases should be obtained in room air and in 100 per cent oxygen. Stick capillary samples from the patient's warmed heel may be employed, although determinations obtained by arterial puncture are preferable for evaluation of oxygenation, since they are less susceptible to alterations in regional blood flow in the critically ill infant. Sampling of right radial or temporal arterial blood is preferable, since these sites are proximal to flow through a ductus arteriosus and do not reflect right-to-left ductal shunting, as would a sample from the descending aorta obtained via an umbilical artery catheter. A trial of continuous positive airway pressure may improve oxygenation in infants with either hyaline membrane disease or pulmonary edema. Arterial blood gas patterns in various pathophysiological conditions are listed in Table 29–8. Pattern 1 is typically observed in infants with ventilation-perfusion abnormalities on the basis of primary respiratory disease often associated

TABLE 29–8 ARTERIAL BLOOD GASES IN VARIOUS DISORDERS

Pattern	pH	pO$_2$	pCO$_2$	Response to O$_2$	Venous pH	Suggested Condition
1	↓	↓↓	↑	↑↑	↓	Hyaline membrane or other pulmonary parenchymal disease
2	↓	↓	↑↑↑	↑	↓	Hypoventilation
3	—	↓	—	↑	—	Venous admixture
4	↓	↓↓	—	—	↓	Decreased or ineffective pulmonary blood flow
5	↓↓↓	↓	—↑	—↑	↓↓↓↓	Systemic hypoperfusion

with elevated pulmonary vascular resistance and venoarterial shunting across a patent foramen ovale or patent ductus arteriosus. Pulmonary hypoventilation with CO_2 retention produces pattern 2. In the presence of a lesion causing obligatory venous admixture, such as total anomalous pulmonary venous connection (pattern 3), the response to oxygen may reflect an increase in pulmonary venous return secondary to a fall in pulmonary vascular resistance. Pattern 4 is seen typically in infants with a cardiac malformation that results in reduced pulmonary blood flow. Oxygen administration in these infants does not alter the arterial pO_2. The alterations of pattern 5 are observed when systemic hypoperfusion is the principal hemodynamic problem. In these babies the arteriovenous oxygen difference is high, and the acidemia may be progressive and unrelenting.

ELECTROCARDIOGRAM. The electrocardiogram is less helpful in suggesting a diagnosis of heart disease in the premature and newborn infant than in the older child. Right ventricular hypertrophy is a normal finding in the neonate, and the range of normal voltages is wide. However, specific observations may offer major clues to the presence of a cardiovascular anomaly. A counterclockwise, superiorly oriented frontal QRS loop with absent or reduced right ventricular forces suggests the diagnosis of tricuspid atresia (p. 994). In contrast, when the QRS axis is normal but left ventricular forces predominate, the diagnosis of pulmonic atresia must be considered (p. 988). The counterclockwise, superior QRS orientation is also observed in infants with an endocardial cushion defect (p. 961) and in some with double-outlet right ventricle (p. 1005); right ventricular forces in these babies are increased. The initial septal vector should be assessed from the electrocardiogram. Often Q waves are not clearly seen in the lateral precordial leads in the first 72 hours of life. A leftward, posteriorly directed septal vector giving rise to Q waves in the right precordial leads is abnormal and suggests the presence of marked right ventricular hypertrophy, single ventricle (p. 1012), or inversion of the ventricles (p. 1003). T-wave alterations may be seen in a normal neonatal electrocardiogram and may be of no specific consequence. However, by 72 hours of age the T waves should be inverted in V$_3$ and V$_1$ and upright in the lateral precordium; persistently upright T waves in the right precordial leads are a sign of right ventricular hypertrophy. Depressed or flattened T waves in the lateral precordium may suggest subendocardial ischemia and a left heart outflow tract obstructive lesion, electrolyte disturbance, acidosis, or hypoxemia. An electrocardiographic pattern of myocardial infarction suggests a diagnosis of anomalous pulmonary origin of the coronary artery (p. 971). Lastly, rhythm disturbances such as complete heart block or supraventricular tachycardia can be detected readily by electrocardiography.

RADIOGRAPHIC EXAMINATION (see also pages 166 to 171). The chest x-ray is often the single most useful examination in differentiating between respiratory and cardiac causes of cyanosis in the newborn period. Determination of a normal cardiac and abdominal situs aids in ruling out several kinds of complex cyanotic cardiac malformations associated with asplenia or polysplenia with abdominal heterotaxy and dextrocardia (p. 1011). The distinct appearance of pulmonary parenchymal disease such as the classic reticulogranular pattern of hyaline membrane disease may allow a specific radiological diagnosis. In those premature infants with a large ductus arteriosus the x-ray appearance often evolves from the typical findings of hyaline membrane disease to increased pulmonary vascular markings and finally to perihilar and generalized pulmonary edema. Most importantly, the pediatric cardiologist depends heavily on the evaluation of pulmonary vascular markings to categorize congenital cardiac malformations in the newborn infant according to function. In the presence of cyanosis, diminished pulmonary vascular markings call attention to the group of anomalies that includes tetralogy of Fallot, pulmonic stenosis with intact ventricular septum, pulmonic atresia, tricuspid atresia, and Ebstein's malformation of the tricuspid valve. Reduced pulmonary blood flow is responsible for the systemic arterial desaturation in these babies. Increased pulmonary vascular markings in the cyanotic infant are associated with lesions in which an obligatory admixture of systemic venous and pulmonary venous blood occurs. The more common anomalies in this category include transposition of the great arteries, hypoplastic left heart syndrome, truncus arteriosus, and total anomalous pulmonary venous drainage.

As mentioned earlier, overall heart size in the normal newborn infant is greater than in the older child, and cardiothoracic ratios up to 0.60 are within normal limits. Occasionally, the thymus shadow obscures the cardiac silhouette and prohibits accurate estimation of heart size. An enlarged heart on x-ray examination suggests a cardiac disorder. However, in the presence of severe respiratory difficulties with an increase in carbon dioxide tension and a decrease in both pH and arterial oxygen tension, cardiomegaly may be only moderate. A right aortic arch suggests the presence of either tetralogy of Fallot or persistent truncus arteriosus. An ovoid heart with a narrow base associated with increased pulmonary vascular marking is typical of transposition of the great arteries. A boot-shaped heart with concavity of the pulmonary outflow tract suggests tetralogy of Fallot, pulmonic atresia, or tricuspid atresia.

ECHOCARDIOGRAPHY (see also pages 117 to

125). Echocardiography is of immense value in distinguishing heart disease from lung disease in the newborn.[33-36,65] Ultrasound techniques are now sufficiently accurate to allow visualization of cardiac anatomy and function even before birth.[66] Single-crystal techniques must employ high-frequency piezoelectrical crystals with low cross-sectional area to increase the definition of cardiac structures in the small newborn. Most importantly, especially in infants with complicated cardiac malformations, cross-sectional echocardiographic techniques provide a real-time, two-dimensional format that allows a substantially enhanced appreciation of spatial intra- and extracardiac structural interrelationships.[67] The latter is provided whether the cross-sectional images result from the mechanical motion of a single transducer to provide a real-time sector scan or from systems employing phased-array principles to steer the ultrasound beam rapidly through the structures under investigation. In addition, saline contrast echocardiography (in which normal saline is injected into the peripheral or central venous system of the infant) may be of value in identifying the site of intercirculatory shunting in the sick newborn in whom the differentiation of cardiac from noncardiac causes of cyanosis is urgent.[65] Echocardiographic diagnoses that can often be made with certainty include hypoplastic left heart syndrome, aortic valve stenosis, membraneous subvalvar aortic stenosis, hypertrophic cardiomyopathy, cor triatriatum, tricuspid atresia, Ebstein's anomaly of the tricuspid valve, endocardial cushion defect, single ventricle, double-outlet right ventricle, transposition of the great arteries, and patent ductus arteriosus. The echocardiogram provides suggestive evidence for tetralogy of Fallot, truncus arteriosus, total anomalous pulmonary venous connection, valvar pulmonic stenosis, and pulmonary atresia with an intact ventricular septum.

CARDIAC CATHETERIZATION (see also Chap. 9). If a cardiac anomaly is identified by noninvasive studies or if a clear-cut differentiation cannot be made between cardiac and pulmonary disease, heart catheterization and angiocardiography are required to define the underlying state precisely. Hemodynamic study of the newborn infant carries a small but distinct risk.[68] As a general rule, cardiac catheterization is not performed unless the information sought is central to the management of the infant. Infants with serious heart disease usually require therapeutic intervention, and thus catheterization should be performed only when surgical support is readily available. Cardiac catheterization is indicated in almost all newborns who experience congestive heart failure in the first days after birth if the cause is an anatomical abnormality rather than an arrhythmia or a metabolic disturbance. Preferably, medical measures will have been instituted to stabilize the clinical state before a hemodynamic study is performed.

It is generally agreed that newborns with cyanotic congenital heart disease require immediate cardiac catheterization, since there is considerable risk of rapid deterioration.[56] Under these circumstances hemodynamic and angiographic study may not only provide the anatomical diagnosis required prior to emergency operation but may also allow the opportunity for therapeutic maneuvers such as balloon atrial septostomy to facilitate intercirculatory mixing in patients with complete transposition of the great arteries or to augment interatrial shunting in patients with a restrictive patent foramen ovale and either tricuspid, pulmonic, or mitral atresia, or total anomalous pulmonary venous connection. In addition, the selective infusion of low doses of prostaglandin E_1 (0.05–0.1 μg/kg/min) intravenously has been employed at cardiac catheterization for the emergency palliation of ductus-dependent cardiac lesions such as pulmonic atresia or interruption of the aortic arch.[59] Since a patent ductus arteriosus maintains pulmonary and systemic blood flow, respectively, in these infants, dilatation of the ductus with vasodilatory prostaglandins may retard their clinical deterioration. Thus, prostaglandin E_1 infusion has been shown to be an effective short-term measure to correct hypoxemia and acidemia and to improve the pre- and intraoperative status of infants requiring surgical relief of the congenital cardiac lesion that is causing pulmonary or systemic hypoperfusion.

SPECIFIC CARDIAC DEFECTS

Many classifications of congenital cardiovascular lesions have been proposed based upon hemodynamic, anatomical, and radiographic factors. Although there is overlapping between groups, the following arrangement of cardiac anomalies is used in this chapter: (1) communications between the systemic and pulmonary circulations without cyanosis (left-to-right shunts), (2) obstructing valvular and vascular lesions with or without associated right-to-left shunt, (3) abnormalities in the origins of the great arteries and veins (the transposition complexes), (4) malpositions of the heart and cardiac apex, and (5) miscellaneous anomalies.

COMMUNICATIONS BETWEEN THE SYSTEMIC AND PULMONARY CIRCULATIONS WITHOUT CYANOSIS (LEFT-TO-RIGHT SHUNTS)

Atrial Septal Defect

MORPHOLOGY. Atrial septal defect is one of the most commonly recognized congenital cardiac anomalies in adults but is very rarely diagnosed and even less commonly results in disability in infants.[69-71] The anatomical sites of interatrial defects are depicted in Figure 29–8. Defects of the sinus venosus type are high in the atrial septum near the entry of the superior vena cava and are frequently associated with, and may be a consequence of, anomalous connection of pulmonary veins from the right lung to the junction of the superior vena cava and right atrium.[72] Most often the atrial septal defect involves the fossa ovalis, is midseptal in location, and is of the ostium secundum type. This type of defect is a true deficiency of the atrial septum and should not be confused with a patent foramen ovale.[73] Embryologically the left side of the atrial septum is derived from the septum primum, which possesses an opening—the interatrial ostium secundum (see Fig. 29–3). The ostium secundum lies forward of the superior to the position of the foramen ovale. The latter is formed by the septum secundum and occupies the right side of the atrial septum. Tissue of the septum primum lying to the left of the foramen ovale serves as a flap valve

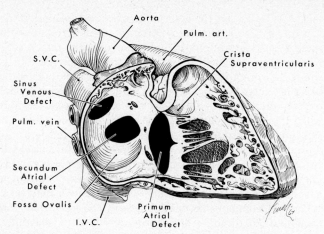

FIGURE 29–8 Composite locations of atrial defects. S.V.C. = superior vena cava; I.V.C. = inferior vena cava.

that usually becomes fused postnatally with the side of the foramen ovale yielding an anatomically closed or sealed foramen. "Probe patency" or an incomplete seal of the foramen ovale occurs in approximately 25 per cent of adults. A widely patent foramen ovale may be considered an acquired form of atrial septal defect that occurs especially when a disproportion exists between the size of the foramen ovale and the effective length of its valve. Enlargement of the foramen ovale per se is commonly associated with obstructive lesions of the right side of the heart, whereas a short valve relative to the size of the foramen is often seen in large-volume left-to-right shunts in which left atrial dilatation is prominent.

Ostium primum atrial septal anomalies are a form of endocardial cushion defect and will be dealt with in the following section. Lutembacher's syndrome is a designation applied to the rare combination of atrial septal defect and mitral stenosis, which is almost invariably the result of acquired rheumatic valvulitis. Recently it has been recognized that 10 to 20 per cent of patients with ostium secundum atrial septal defect also have prolapse of the mitral valve as an associated anomaly.[74]

HEMODYNAMICS. The magnitude of the left-to-right shunt through an atrial septal defect depends on the size of the defect and the relative compliance of the ventricles, and the relative resistance in the pulmonary and in the systemic circulation.[75] In patients with a small atrial septal defect or patent foramen ovale, the left atrial pressure may exceed the right by several mm Hg, whereas the mean pressure in both atria is nearly identical when the defect is large. Left-to-right shunting occurs predominantly in late ventricular systole and early diastole with some augmentation during atrial contraction. The shunt results in diastolic overloading of the right ventricle and increased pulmonary blood flow. During the first few days and weeks of life pulmonary resistance falls and systemic resistance rises, facilitating right ventricular emptying and impeding left ventricular emptying; the left-to-right shunt rises. Early in infancy left-to-right flow through even a large interatrial communication is commonly limited by both the reduced chamber compliance of thickened neonatal right ventricle and the elevated pulmonary and reduced systemic vascular resistance of the neonate. The pulmonary vascular resistance is commonly normal or low in the older infant or child with atrial septal defect, and the volume load is usually well tolerated, even though pulmonary blood flow may be two to five times greater than systemic. A transient and small right-to-left shunt occurring with the onset of left ventricular contraction and especially during respiratory periods of decreasing intrathoracic pressure is common in patients with ostium secundum defect, even in the absence of pulmonary hypertension.

CLINICAL FINDINGS. Patients with atrial septal defect are usually asymptomatic in early life, although occasional reports exist of congestive heart failure and recurrent pneumonia in infancy.[69,70] Children with atrial septal defect may experience easy fatigability and exertional dyspnea. They tend to be somewhat underdeveloped physically and prone to respiratory infection. In contrast to their common appearance in adults with atrial septal defect, atrial arrhythmias, pulmonary arterial hypertension, development of pulmonary vascular obstruction, and heart failure are exceedingly uncommon in the pediatric age range. In the latter group, diagnosis is entertained often after detection of a heart murmur on routine physical examination prompts a more extensive cardiac evaluation.

Common findings on *physical examination* include a prominent right ventricular cardiac impulse and palpable pulmonary artery pulsation. The first heart sound is normal or split, with accentuation of the tricuspid valve closure sound. Increased flow across the pulmonic valve is responsible for a midsystolic pulmonary ejection murmur. After the normal, postnatal drop in pulmonary vascular resistance, the second heart sound is split widely and is relatively fixed in relation to respiration in patients with normal pulmonary pressures and low pulmonary vascular impedance because of a delay in pulmonic valve closure. With pulmonary hypertension the splitting interval is a function of the electromechanical intervals of each ventricle; wide splitting occurs with shortening of the left and/or lengthening of the right ventricular electromechanical interval.[76] If the shunt is large; increased blood flow across the tricuspid valve is responsible for a mid-diastolic rumbling murmur at the lower left sternal border. In patients with associated prolapse of the mitral valve an apical holosystolic or late systolic murmur radiating to the axilla is often heard, but a midsystolic click may be difficult to discern. Moreover, left ventricular precordial overactivity is usually absent because mitral regurgitation is mild in most patients.

In the teenage patient, the physical findings may be altered when an increase in pulmonary vascular resistance results in diminution of the left-to-right shunt. Both the pulmonary and tricuspid murmurs decrease in intensity, whereas the pulmonic component of the second heart sound becomes accentuated and the two components of the second heart sound may fuse; a diastolic murmur of pulmonic incompetence appears. Cyanosis and clubbing accompany development of a right-to-left shunt.

The *electrocardiogram* in patients with an ostium secundum defect usually shows right-axis deviation, right ventricular hypertrophy, and rSR' or rsR' pattern in the right precordial leads with a normal QRS duration (Fig. 29–9). It is not clear whether the delay in right ventricular activation is a manifestation of right ventricular volume overload or a true conduction delay in the right bundle branch and

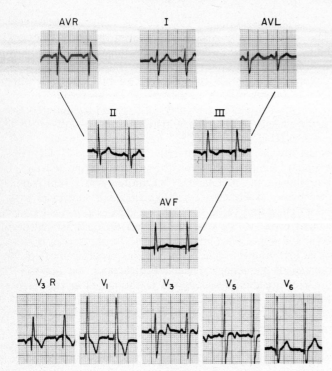

FIGURE 29–9 Typical electrocardiographic tracing in secundum atrial septal defect showing right axis deviation, rSR' in the right precordial leads and right ventricular hypertrophy. Contrast this with Figure 29–11. (Courtesy of Delores A. Danilowicz, M.D.)

peripheral Purkinje system.[77] Left-axis deviation of the P wave in the frontal plane (manifested by a negative P wave in lead III) suggests the presence of a sinus venosus rather than an ostium secundum type of atrial septal defect. Left-axis deviation and superior orientation and counterclockwise rotation of the QRS loop in the frontal plane suggests the presence of either an ostium primum defect or a secundum atrial septal defect in association with mitral valve prolapse. Prolongation of the P-R interval may be seen with all types of atrial septal defects; the prolonged internodal conduction time may be related to both the increased size of the atrium and the increased distance for internodal conduction produced by the defect itself.[77] *Chest roentgenograms* reveal enlargement of the right atrium and ventricle, dilatation of the pulmonary artery and its branches, and increased pulmonary vascular markings (Fig. 29–10). Dilatation of the proximal portion of the superior vena cava is noted occasionally in patients with a sinus venosus defect. Left atrial dilatation is extremely rare but may be observed when significant mitral regurgitation exists. Echocardiographic features include pulmonary arterial and right ventricular dilatation and anterior systolic (paradoxical) or "flat" interventricular septal motion if significant right ventricular volume overload is present.[34] The defect may be visualized directly by two-dimensional echo imaging, particularly from a subcostal view of the interatrial septum[34] (see Fig. 5–57, p, 121). Mitral valve prolapse may also be identified by echocardiographic examination.

Diagnosis may be readily confirmed at *cardiac catheterization* by passage of the catheter across the atrial defect. The site at which the catheter crosses, if high in the cardiac silhouette, may suggest a sinus venosus defect; if

midseptal, a patent foramen ovale or ostium secundum defect; or, if low, a primum defect.[78] Serial determinations of the oxygen saturation or indicator dilution curve techniques may be used to estimate the magnitude of the shunt. In young patients, pressures on the right side of the heart are often normal, despite a large shunt. When a high oxygen saturation is found in the superior vena cava or when the catheter enters pulmonary veins directly from the right atrium, a sinus venosus defect is likely, and indicator dilution curves and selective angiography will aid in identifying the number and location of the anomalous veins. Partial anomalous pulmonary venous connection, although generally associated with sinus venosus defect, may occasionally accompany secundum defects. Selective left ventricular angiography will identify prolapse of the mitral valve and allow assessment of the magnitude of mitral regurgitation that may be present in such patients.

In contrast to adults, children with sinus venosus or secundum types of atrial septal defect rarely require treatment for heart failure or antiarrhythmic medications for atrial fibrillation or supraventricular tachycardia. Respiratory tract infections should be treated promptly. Although the risk of infective endocarditis is low, antibiotics should be administered prophylactically prior to dental procedures.

MANAGEMENT. *Operative repair*, ideally in patients 3 to 6 years of age, should be advised for all patients with uncomplicated atrial septal defects in whom there is evidence of significant left-to-right shunting, i.e., with pulmonary to systemic flow ratios exceeding approximately 1.5:1.0.[79] The defect is closed by suture or with a patch of prosthetic material with the patient on cardiopulmonary

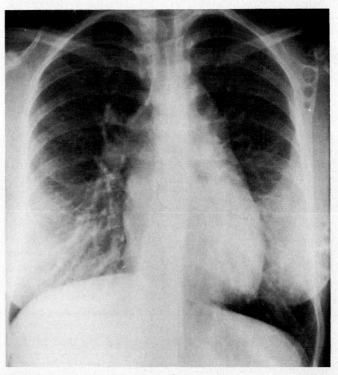

FIGURE 29–10 Anteroposterior chest roentgenogram in a patient with atrial septal defect. The right ventricular outflow tract and main pulmonary artery are enlarged and the pulmonary vascular markings are increased without enlargement of the left atrium.

bypass. Earlier surgical repair is definitive treatment for the small number of infants and young children with significant symptoms or congestive failure. The surgical mortality rate is less than 1 per cent, and results are generally excellent. While the mitral valve may be examined directly at operation, it is rarely necessary in childhood to attempt plication or replacement of a ballooning or prolapsing mitral valve. Operation should not be carried out in patients with small defects and trivial left-to-right shunts (pulmonary-to-systemic flow ratio $\leq$ 1.5:1.0) or in those with severe pulmonary vascular disease (pulmonary-to-systemic resistance ratio $\geq$ 0.7:1.0) without a significant left-to-right shunt. Subtle evidence of left ventricular dysfunction may be observed preoperatively at cardiac catheterization in children with isolated large atrial septal defects but without overt left or right ventricular failure.[80] Thus, decreased left ventricular stroke volume and cardiac output have been observed in children with both low and normal left ventricular end-diastolic volumes. In this regard, in essentially normal routine catheterization studies patients with operatively closed atrial septal defects have been shown to have a residual reduced cardiac output response to intense upright exercise in the absence of residual shunts, arrhythmias, or pulmonary arterial hypertension.[81,82] These findings are observed in patients who undergo operation as preadolescents or older, and one must wonder if normal myocardial function is preserved in children for whom the defects were closed at a substantially younger age.

Endocardial Cushion Defects

Endocardial cushion defects comprise a range of malformations that involve—singly or in combination—the atrial septum, the ventricular septum, and one or both atrioventricular valves[82,83] (see Fig. 29–3). They range in severity from a small ostium primum atrial septal defect to a complete atrioventricular canal. The anomalies result from failure of the common channel between the atria and ventricles to partition during development of the embryonic heart. Often endocardial cushion defects are encountered in association with other congenital abnormalities such as asplenia or polysplenia syndromes, trisomy 21 (Down's syndrome), and Ellis–van Creveld syndrome of ectodermal dysplasia and polydactyly.

OSTIUM PRIMUM DEFECT (PARTIAL ATRIOVENTRICULAR CANAL). Ostium primum atrial septal defects lie immediately adjacent to the atrioventricular valves, either of which may be deformed and incompetent. Most often, only the anterior or septal leaflet of the mitral valve is displaced and is commonly cleft; the tricuspid valve is usually not involved. The ostium primum defect occurs as a result of incomplete fusion between the septum primum and the endocardial cushions. A cleft is usually present in the mitral valve because of a lack of fusion of the endocardial cushions themselves. The interatrial defect is often large, and the size of the left-to-right interatrial shunt in these patients is controlled by the same factors that exist in patients with ostium secundum atrial septal defect. Moreover, the clinical features are quite similar and consist principally of right ventricular precordial hyperactivity, a wide and persistently split second heart sound, a right ventricular outflow tract systolic ejection murmur,

and a mid-diastolic tricuspid flow rumble. The murmurs of atrioventricular valve regurgitation may be audible if either valve is cleft significantly; usually, however, significant AV valve regurgitation is absent. In the occasional patient, mitral regurgitation is substantial and creates prominent signs of left ventricular overload.

Chest roentgenography usually reveals right atrial and ventricular cardiomegaly, prominence of the right ventricular outflow tract, and increased pulmonary vascular markings. The *electrocardiogram* is characteristic and shows a right ventricular conduction defect accompanied by left-axis deviation and by superior orientation and counterclockwise rotation of the QRS loop in the frontal plane (Fig. 29–11).[84] Hemodynamic factors do not appear to be important in producing the characteristic electrocardiogram. Rather, the superior QRS vector in patients with a shortened H-V interval appears to be related to early activation of the posterobasal left ventricular wall; in other

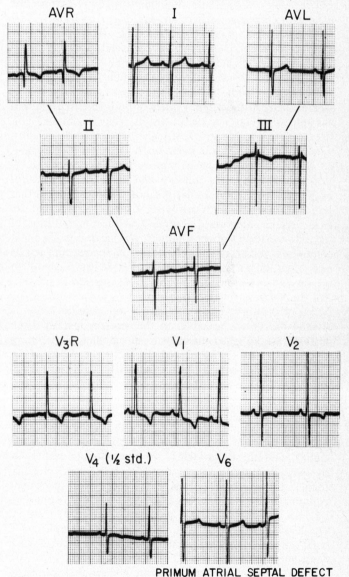

PRIMUM ATRIAL SEPTAL DEFECT

FIGURE 29–11 Primum atrial septal defect. The QRS loop in the frontal plane is counterclockwise, and the axis is leftward and superiorly oriented. In addition, the patient has biventricular hypertrophy, predominantly right. Contrast this with Figure 29–9. (Courtesy of Delores A. Danilowicz, M.D.)

patients with a normal conduction time between the bundle of His and the ventricles, the counterclockwise superior inscription of the frontal plane vector appears to be related to late activation of the anterolateral left ventricular wall.[85,86] A prolonged P-R interval is observed in many patients with an ostium primum atrial septal defect; prolonged internodal conduction may be related to displacement of the AV node in a posteroinferior direction in some patients or to the enlarged right atrium, or both.[87]

Echocardiographic features include enlargement of both the right ventricle and the pulmonary artery, systolic anterior ventricular septal motion, prolonged mitral-septal apposition in diastole, and various abnormalities in mitral valve motion.[88-90] Using the subxiphoid or apical views, the two-dimensional echocardiogram detects the absence of interatrial septal tissue in the region of the crest of the interventricular septum; the anterior leaflet of the mitral valve may also be examined and a cleft identified. The *angiographic features* resemble those in the complete form or atrioventricular canal defect and are discussed below.

COMPLETE ATRIOVENTRICULAR CANAL DEFECT. The complete form of persistent common atrioventricular (AV) canal includes, an addition to the ostium primum atrial septal defect, a ventricular septal defect in the posterior basal portion of the ventricular septum as well as clefts in the septal leaflets of both the tricuspid and the mitral valves. The defect results from a complete failure to fuse of the atrioventricular endocardial cushions. The extent to which the common AV canal was partitioned during development determines the severity of the lesion anatomically. The anterior and posterior segments of each septal AV valve leaflet are not separated, but rather join each other through the defect. Complete AV canal defects may be categorized according to the configuration of the anterior leaflet of the common AV valve.[91] In the most common, Type A, the anterior leaflet is divided into mitral and triscupid portions that are both attached medially to the muscular septum, the membranous septum is present, and the ventricular communication does not extend to the region of the aortic cusps. In Type B, the anterior leaflet is divided but is not attached to the septum; instead, both portions are attached medially to an anomalous papillary muscle adjacent to the septum in the right ventricle. In Type C the anterior leaflet is undivided and unattached and floats freely above the muscular septum. Types B and C have in common a deficiency of the membranous ventricular septum, and the interventricular communication therefore extends to the proximity of the aortic cusps. The posterior common leaflet is usually rudimentary and shows similar anatomical variability to the anterior leaflet. A high incidence exists (approximately 35 per cent) of additional cardiovascular lesions in patients with persistent common AV canal. Principal among these are ostium secundum atrial septal defect, pulmonic stenosis, and persistent left superior vena cava. Moreover, the complete AV canal anomaly is seen commonly in patients with Down's syndrome.

Patients with persistent common AV canal defects present clinically under age one year with a history of frequent respiratory infections and poor weight gain. Heart failure in infancy is extremely common. The *physical findings* are similar to those observed in patients with ostium primum atrial septal defect but may include as well the holosystolic, lower left sternal border murmur of an interventricular communication and/or the decrescendo, holosystolic apical murmur of mitral regurgitation. The *electrocardiographic features* of complete AV canal defects resemble those in the partial ostium primum variety of endocardial cushion anomalies. *Radiographically,* the usual findings are generalized cardiomegaly and engorged pulmonary vessels. Single-crystal *echocardiographic findings* do not often allow a distinction between an ostium primum atrial septal defect and the more complete forms of AV canal malformations to be made with confidence. In contrast, cross-sectional echocardiographic techniques may be especially useful in making this distinction, since the apical and subcostal views permit visualization of the interatrial and interventricular septa and allow differentiation of leaflet morphology, clefting, and the types of ventricular insertion of the chorda tendineae. Thus the type and extent of the defect and the atrioventricular valve morphology may be characterized.[88,89] On *hemodynamic study,* patients with persistent common AV canal invariably have elevated pulmonary arterial pressures; beyond age two years a significant number of these patients have progressively severe pulmonary vascular obstructive disease.

Diagnosis is established reliably by selective left ventricular *angiocardiography* using rapid injection of relatively large quantities of contrast material.[90] The anterior-inferior portion of the anterior mitral leaflet is abnormally anchored in all forms of endocardial cushion defect. The absence of the atrioventricular septum results in an abnormal line of attachment of the anterior mitral leaflet, which is displaced inferiorly and anteriorly. This displacement results in a shift of the orifice of the valve toward the right side of the left ventricle and a rotation toward the sagittal plane. The change in position of the mitral orifice and the associated elongation of the left ventricular outflow tract produces a pathognomonic "gooseneck" deformity seen angiographically in diastole (Fig. 29–12). Additional findings include visualization of the cleft in the mitral valve, mitral incompetence, and a jet of contrast material from left ventricle directly to right atrium or via mitral regurgitation and left-to-right atrial shunting. Conventional anteroposterior and lateral left ventricular angiographic views may not always differentiate between the partial and complete types of AV canal defects because all have the characteristic "gooseneck" left ventricular outflow tract deformity and because mitral regurgitation into the right atrium may obscure the presence or absence of a defect in the ventricular septum. Axial cineangiography, however, permits a more accurate distinction between types of endocardial defects, since the hepato-clavicular view helps greatly in separating a left ventricular–right atrial communication and shunt from left ventricular–left atrial regurgitation with subsequent left-to-right atrial shunt. In addition, the long axial oblique view portrays the atrioventricular portion of the ventricular septum.[92]

Management of infants with the complete form of endocardial cushion defect consists initially of controlling cardiac decompensation. If an adequate response to medical therapy occurs early in life, a second hemodynamic study is indicated at approximately age 6 to 9 months to determine

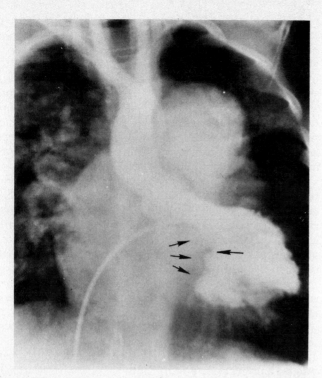

FIGURE 29–12 Left ventriculogram in systole in a patient with an endocardial cushion defect. The concavity of the right border of the left ventricle (left arrows) is caused by the abnormal position of the mitral orifice.

the level of pulmonary vascular resistance, since infants with the complete form of the AV canal defect are at high risk of obstructive pulmonary vascular disease.[93] The level of major shunting should be determined during the initial hemodynamic and angiographic study, since, if it is mainly at the ventricular level, pulmonary artery banding may be advised for intractable heart failure and failure to thrive. Often, however, there is a significant left ventricular–right atrial shunt either directly or indirectly via mitral regurgitation and left-to-right interatrial shunting, which will be unaffected by pulmonary artery banding and requires complete surgical correction. In many centers primary repair in patients who have either intractable heart failure or severe pulmonary hypertension is the preferred approach at any age.[94–97,97a] Mild to moderate mitral regurgitation often persists after surgical repair despite efforts to align the anterior and posterior halves of the anterior mitral leaflet accurately. Rarely, if leaflet tissue is remarkably deficient or deformed, mitral valve replacement may be required. Recent advances in the surgical approach to complex forms of AV canal defects have greatly improved the outlook for patients born with this malformation.

Ventricular Septal Defect (VSD)

Among the most prevalent of cardiac malformations, defects of the ventricular septum occur commonly, both as isolated anomalies and in combination with other anomalies. The ventricular septum consists of a fibrous component, the membranous septum, and a muscular portion; the latter has three components—the inlet, trabecular, and outlet parts (see Fig. 29–4). Defects result when a deficiency of growth or a failure of alignment or fusion exists of component parts. Most often there is a single opening in

the membranous portion of the septum, although, as Figure 29–13 shows, a defect may occur anywhere in the interventricular septum. Defects vary in size from barely visible openings to almost complete absence of the interventricular septum. In the extremely common type of membranous ventricular septal defect that lies below the crista supraventricularis, the bundle of His is contiguous with the posterior-inferior aspect of the defect, while the proximal right bundle branch is close to the inferior edge. Supracristal (subpulmonic) VSD's lie beneath the pulmonic valve and are remote from the conduction system. Supracristal defects may occur as isolated lesions but more often are combined with other malformations related to defects in truncal development, such as persistent truncus arteriosus, transposed aorta with overriding pulmonary artery (Taussig-Bing variety of double-outlet right ventricle), and complete transposition of the great arteries. Muscular defects, when single, are usually located in the posterior portion of the ventricular septum; they are often multiple, however, and have no predilection for a particular site.[98]

In general, the functional disturbance caused by a ventricular septal defect depends primarily on its size and the status of the pulmonary vascular bed rather than on the location of the defect. A small VSD with high resistance to flow permits only a small left-to-right shunt. A large interventricular communication allows a large left-to-right shunt only if there is no pulmonic stenosis or high pulmonary vascular resistance, since these factors also determine shunt flow. Resistance to left ventricular emptying also affects shunt flow because it is an important factor in determining left ventricular pressure. Large defects allow both ventricles to function hemodynamically as a single pumping chamber with two outlets, equalizing the pressure in

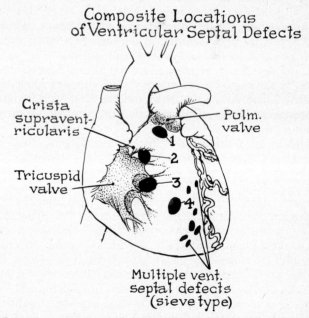

FIGURE 29–13 Anatomical classification of defects of the interventricular septum. Type 1 defects are superoanterior to the crista supraventricularis; Type 2 defects are posteroinferior to the crista supraventricularis; Type 3 defects are located under the septal leaflet of the tricuspid valve; Type 4 defects are multiple and involve the muscular septum. (From Friedman, W. F., et al.: Multiple muscular ventricular septal defects. Circulation *32*:35, 1965, by permission of the American Heart Association, Inc.)

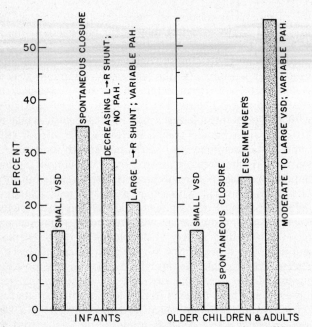

FIGURE 29–14 Natural history of ventricular septal defect. Approximate percentages are depicted for the various events that may occur in infants *(left)* and older children and adults *(right)* with VSD. PAH = pulmonary arterial hypertension, L-R = left to right. (From Friedman, W. F., and Pitlick, P. T.: Ventricular septal defect in infancy — University of California, San Diego (Specialty Conference). West. J. Med. *120*:295, 1974.)

the systemic and pulmonary circulations. In such patients the magnitude of the left-to-right shunt varies inversely with pulmonary vascular resistance.

A wide spectrum exists in the natural history of VSD, ranging from spontaneous closure to congestive cardiac failure and death in early infancy (Fig. 29–14). Within this spectrum are possible development of pulmonary vascular obstruction, right ventricular outflow tract obstruction, aortic regurgitation, and infective endocarditis.[98–107]

INFANCY. It is unusual for a VSD to cause difficulties in the immediate postnatal period, although congestive heart failure during the first 6 months of life is a frequent occurrence. Early diagnosis is helpful in order to ensure more careful observation of the affected infant.[107] The examining physician usually suspects the diagnosis because of a harsh systolic murmur at the lower left sternal border. The electrocardiogram and chest roentgenogram are within normal limits in the immediate neonatal period because appreciable left-to-right shunting occurs only after the pulmonary vascular resistance decreases as the pulmonary vessels lose their fetal characteristics. It is desirable to follow these infants continually. A VSD that either decreases in size or closes completely during the first year of life presents no problems to the practicing physician. Spontaneous closure occurs by age 3 years in approximately 40 per cent of patients born with VSD; occasional patients, however, do not experience spontaneous closure until age 8 to 10 years.[103] Closure is more common in patients born with a small VSD; nonetheless, approximately 7 per cent of infants with a large defect and congestive heart failure early in life may also experience spontaneous closure. Partial rather than complete closure is common in patients with both large and small VSD's.[98] Anatomically, reduction of the VSD is often based on adherence of the tricus-

pid valve to the VSD, hypertrophy of septal muscle, or ingrowth of fibrous tissue; rarely, VSD closure is the result of prolapse of an aortic cusp[108] or infective endocarditis.[109] Some defects close when an aneurysm forms in the ventricular septum. On auscultation a click may be heard in early systole as the aneurysm tenses toward the right; the septal aneurysm may be detected by echocardiography as an anterior systolic bulge in the right ventricular outflow tract. A persistent minute VSD is not life-threatening unless bacterial endocarditis develops. With proper precautions the incidence of this complication is less than 1 per cent.

If a moderate or large defect maintains its size after birth, the net left-to-right shunt increases during the first month of life as pulmonary vascular resistance falls. *Physical examination* during this time usually reveals a thrill along the lower left sternal border, and the holosystolic murmur of flow across the interventricular defect is accompanied by a low-pitched diastolic rumble at the apex, reflecting increased flow across the mitral valve. *Chest roentgenograms* reveal increased pulmonary vascular markings; evidence of left or biventricular hypertrophy may be observed on the electrocardiogram. Infants with a large left-to-right shunt tend to do poorly, with recurrent upper and lower respiratory tract infections, failure to gain weight, and congestive heart failure. Congestive heart failure may be severe and intractable despite intensive medical management.[105,106] For these infants we currently recommend primary intracardiac repair of the VSD rather than surgical banding of the pulmonary artery[107,110] in order to reduce pulmonary blood flow and alleviate heart failure. Primary VSD closure may be performed in infancy employing cardiopulmonary bypass, profound hypothermia and cardiocirculatory arrest, or a combination of the two techniques. Mortality is less than 10 per cent if the defect is single but approaches 25 per cent if multiple defects are present.[111–114]

Fortunately, medical treatment often is successful in controlling congestive heart failure. Nevertheless, these infants should be referred for cardiac catheterization to evaluate pulmonary vascular resistance and to detect associated defects that may require operation, such as patent ductus arteriosus and coarctation of the aorta.

It is of utmost importance to identify patients who may develop irreversible pulmonary vascular obstructive disease (the Eisenmenger reaction).[115–117] Retrospective analyses of children who develop this complication indicate that infants with systemic or near systemic pressures in the pulmonary artery at the time of initial hemodynamic study are most at risk. Recatheterization before age 18 months and a second determination of pulmonary vascular resistance should be performed in these patients in order to decide whether surgical intervention is necessary to prevent development of fixed obliterative changes in the pulmonary vessels. It is likely that multiple factors are involved in the development of pulmonary vascular disease (p. 832 and 950). The anatomically large VSD allows some or all of the systemic pressure to be transmitted to the pulmonary arteries, thereby retarding regression of their muscular media. Medial hypertrophy in the first months of life is responsible for higher pulmonary vascular resistance than would be anticipated for the amount of pulmonary blood flow. The shearing forces created by the high velocity of flow through narrowed pulmonary arterioles cause endothelial damage that is progressive. While an evalation in left atrial pressure may contribute to the rise in pulmonary vascular resistance, it is not an essential factor, since pulmonary venous pressures can be low in patients who later develop pulmonary vascular disease. Nonetheless, pulmonary venous hypertension may also contribute to pulmonary arterial vasoconstriction and thus to increased shear forces. In this same regard, pulmonary vasoconstriction enhancing the risk of pulmonary vascular obstruction may also be caused by hypoxia due to either high altitude or lung disease. At high altitude, large VSD's have higher pulmonary vascular resistances and smaller shunts than at low altitude.

CHILDHOOD. Beyond the first year of life a variable clinical picture emerges in children with VSD.[98-107] If a small defect is present, the child is usually asymptomatic, the electrocardiogram is generally normal, and the chest roentgenogram shows normal or only a mild increase in pulmonary vascular markings. Effort intolerance and fatigue are associated with moderate left-to-right shunts. These children exhibit cardiomegaly with a forceful left ventricular impulse and a prominent systolic thrill along the lower left sternal border. The second heart sound is normally split, with moderate accentuation of the pulmonic component; a third heart sound and rumbling diastolic murmur that reflects increased flow across the mitral valve are audible at the cardiac apex. The characteristic murmur resulting from flow across the defect is harsh and holosystolic, is best heard along the third and fourth interspaces to the left of the sternum, and is widely transmitted over the precordium. A basal midsystolic ejection murmur due to increased flow across the pulmonic valve may also be heard. The electrocardiogram reveals left or combined ventricular hypertrophy, and the chest roentgenogram shows cardiomegaly, left atrial enlargement, and vascular engorgement.

RIGHT VENTRICULAR OUTFLOW TRACT OBSTRUCTION. With time, the clinical picture changes in 8 to 15 per cent of patients with VSD and a moderate to large left-to-right shunt early in life. It begins to resemble more closely the tetralogy of Fallot (p. 990), i.e., subvalvular right ventricular outflow tract obstruction due to progressive hypertrophy of the crista supraventricularis develops. Depending on the severity of the latter process, it may result ultimately in reduced blood flow and a right-to-left shunt across the VSD. As right ventricular outflow tract obstruction develops, the holosystolic VSD murmur is replaced by the crescendo-decrescendo ejection systolic murmur of pulmonic stenosis, and the pulmonary closure sound becomes softer. Right ventricular hypertrophy is evident on the electrocardiogram, while the chest x-ray shows a reduction in pulmonary vascular markings and a smaller heart size with a right ventricular configuration. Infundibular hypertrophy may progress quite rapidly within the first year of life, but the typical evolution to a clinical picture of cyanotic tetralogy of Fallot often takes 1 to 4 years. In those infants who develop right ventricular outflow obstruction the incidence of spontaneous closure or reduction in size of a ventricular septal defect is low.

AORTIC REGURGITATION (AR). This is a well-described complication of VSD that occurs in approximately 5 per cent of patients.[118-123] It is usually noted after age 5 years when a physician detects the early diastolic blowing murmur and wide pulse pressure of aortic regurgitation while following a patient with a VSD. In such patients, AR may become the predominant hemodynamic abnormality. It is of interest that VSD with AR is rare in Europe and America, with an incidence of approximately 4 per cent of all cases of isolated VSD, whereas in Japan the incidence is substantially higher (approximately 10 per cent). In the Japanese, in particular, AR is the result of herniation of an aortic leaflet (usually the right coronary) through a subpulmonic supracristal VSD. In these patients, closure of the VSD may be all that is required to relieve aortic regurgitation. In many patients, however, especially in the western world, the VSD is below the crista supraventricularis. While aortic leaflet herniation, especially of the right or noncoronary cusp, may occur in some of these patients, quite often AR results from a primary abnormality of the valve, usually one defective commissure. In the latter situation, plication of the elongated leaflet may lessen, but not abolish, the aortic regurgitation; in some patients prosthetic aortic valve replacement may be necessary to provide hemodynamic relief. In most patients with VSD and AR, the VSD is small to moderate in size, and mild right ventricular outflow tract obstruction exists. The latter is caused either by subpulmonic infundibular stenosis or projection of the herniated aortic cusp into the right ventricular outflow tract. The distinction between types of VSD with AR can usually be made by selective left ventricular angiocardiography to define the site of the interventricular communication in combination with retrograde aortography to assess the anatomy and competence of the aortic valve (Fig. 29–15).

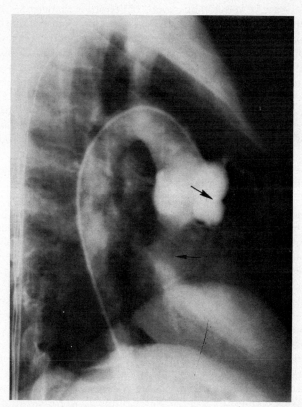

FIGURE 29–15 Retrograde aortogram showing herniation of the right coronary cusp through a supracristal ventricular septal defect (upper arrow) and the jet of aortic regurgitation (lower arrow). (Courtesy of Robert White, M.D.)

Currently, optimal management of the patient with VSD and AR is controversial. In patients with a large, hemodynamically significant left-to-right shunt, repair of the VSD is indicated, but AR is repaired only if at least moderate aortic regurgitation exists. If a supracristal VSD without AR is identified at cardiac catheterization in early childhood, a sensible argument for prophylactic closure of the VSD can be put forth to prevent the potential complication of aortic valve incompetence. In the presence of moderate or severe AR, valvuloplasty is preferred to valve replacement, in recognition of the fact that the severity of aortic regurgitation may increase in subsequent years and that reoperation with valve replacement may be necessary. Operation should probably be deferred in asymptomatic patients with a subcristal VSD and an insignificant left-to-right shunt in whom AR is not severe. If the defect is supracristal in the same clinical setting, its closure may not alleviate the mild degree of aortic incompetence but may retard its progression.

It is rarely necessary to restrict the activities of a child with an isolated VSD in any way. Subacute bacterial endocarditis is always a threat, and antibiotic prophylaxis for dental procedures and minor surgery is indicated.[124] Respiratory infections require prompt evaluation and treatment. These children should be seen at least once or twice yearly to detect changes in the clinical picture that suggest the development of pulmonary vascular obliterative changes.

PULMONARY VASCULAR OBSTRUCTION. If a child who previously had a loud murmur and thrill associated with poor growth suddenly has a growth spurt, fewer respiratory infections, and a diminution of the intensity of the cardiac murmur and disappearance of the thrill, he or she may be developing severe obliterative changes in the pulmonary vascular bed. An increase in intensity of the pulmonic component of the second heart sound, a reduction in heart size on chest roentgenograms, and more pronounced right ventricular hypertrophy on the electrocardiogram are also noted. These changes occur because the increased pulmonary vascular resistance causes a decrease in the left-to-right shunt. If these changes are suspected, cardiac catheterization should be repeated; if they are confirmed, prompt surgical repair is indicated before an inoperable predominant right-to-left shunt ensues. If operation is performed under age 2 years, pulmonary vascular resistance may be expected to fall to normal levels.[117] In older patients the degree to which pulmonary vascular resistance is elevated before operation is a critical factor determining prognosis. If the pulmonary vascular resistance is one third or less of the systemic value, progressive pulmonary vascular disease after operation is unusual. However, if a moderate-to-severe increase in pulmonary vascular resistance exists preoperatively, either no change or progression of pulmonary vascular disease is common postoperatively. Moreover, the presence of increased pulmonary vascular resistance results in a higher immediate postoperative mortality rate for closure of VSD. These observations make it clear that a large VSD should be approached surgically very early in life when pulmonary vascular disease is still reversible or has not yet developed.

Miscellaneous Ventricular Defects. Unusual forms of VSD include multiple muscular defects and left ventricular–right atrial communications. Defects in the muscular ventricular septum frequently are multiple small fenestra-tions that produce a large net left-to-right shunt.[98] Their recognition is a necessary preliminary to successful operation, since incomplete repair may result in post-operative cardiac failure and death. A shunt from the left ventricle to right atrium may occur with a VSD in the most superior portion of the ventricular septum, since the tricuspid valve is lower than the mitral valve. The clinical, electrocardiographic, and radiological findings in these patients do not differ appreciably from those of a simple VSD, although right atrial enlargement may provide a clue to correct diagnosis of left ventricular–right atrial communication. The pathophysiology of single or common ventricle (p. 1012) resembles that of a large VSD, although these defects are dissimilar embryologically. The single chamber frequently is the morphological left ventricle; transposition of the great arteries is quite common. There may be no detectable cyanosis if selective streaming and increased pulmonary blood flow rather than complete mixing occurs. Pulmonary hypertension invariably is present unless pulmonic stenosis exists. It is imperative to differentiate a single ventricle from a large VSD by echocardiography[125] and angiography[126] because corrective operation of the former malformation has had only limited success.

MANAGEMENT. Whenever clinical findings suggest a moderate shunt but no pulmonary hypertension, elective hemodynamic evaluation should be advised between ages 3 and 6 years. Of prime importance in the hemodynamic evaluation is a determination of pressure and blood flow in the pulmonary artery.[107,127] We do not recommend surgical treatment for children who have normal pulmonary arterial pressures with small shunts (pulmonary-systemic flow ratios of less than 1.5 to 2.0:1). In such patients the remaining risk of infective endocarditis[124] does not exceed the risk of operation. Moreover, although the inherent risk of operation is small, the possibility of postoperative heart block, infection, or other complications of operation and cardiopulmonary bypass dictates a conservative approach when the cardiac defect may be well tolerated for life.

With larger shunts, elective operation may be advised before the child enters school, thus minimizing any subsequent distinction of these patients from their normal classmates.[127a] A total assessment of the psychosocial dynamics of the family and child is obviously helpful in determining the proper age for elective operation in each patient.

Complete heart block is the most significant surgically induced conduction system abnormality, occurring immediately following surgery in less than 1 per cent of patients. Late-onset complete heart block is occasionally a problem, especially in the 10 to 25 per cent of patients whose postoperative electrocardiographic findings show complete right bundle branch block with left anterior hemiblock.[128] When the latter electrocardiographic pattern is observed in patients with transient complete heart block in the early postoperative period, electrophysiological studies should be conducted at postoperative cardiac catheterization. It would appear that patients presenting postoperatively with right bundle branch block and left anterior hemiblock fall into two different populations, defined by either peripheral damage to the conduction system or damage to the bundle of His or its proximal branches.[129] The former has not been associated with transient postoperative complete heart block, and these patients have been found to have a generally benign course. Trifascicular damage may be demonstrated in the latter population by a prolonged H-V interval, which implies a higher risk of complete heart block later in life. Although the prophylactic use of permanent pacemakers in asymptomatic patients with evidence of trifascicular damage is not currently recommended, this group certainly requires careful follow-up and continued study.

Intense treadmill exercise studies in patients who preoperatively had normal or only moderately elevated pulmonary vascular resistance and essentially normal postoperative cardiac catheterization data may uncover late abnormalities in circulatory function.[130] Despite normal cardiac output at rest, an impaired cardiac output response to exercise is noted in some. Moreover, despite a normal pulmonary arterial pressure at rest, markedly abnormal increases in pulmonary arterial pressure may be noted during exercise. These findings may be related to abnormal left ventricular function after closure of the VSD and/or to persistent pathological changes in the pulmonary arterioles or to abnormal pulmonary vascular reactivity.[131,132] A direct relation exists between age at operation and the magnitude of the pulmonary arterial pressure response to intense exercise, suggesting that early operation may prevent permanent impairment of the functional capacity of the myocardium and pulmonary vascular bed.

Occasionally a child may come to medical attention who has already developed pulmonary vascular obstruction and a net right-to-left shunt across the VSD. Symptoms may consist of exertional dyspnea, chest pain, syncope, and hemoptysis; the right-to-left shunt leads to cyanosis, clubbing, and polycythemia. At present there is little to offer this group of patients other than continuing support to the patient and family.

Patent Ductus Arteriosus

The ductus arteriosus exists normally in the fetus as a widely patent vessel connecting the pulmonary trunk and the descending aorta just distal to the left subclavian artery (Fig. 29–5). In the fetus most of the output of the right ventricle bypasses the unexpanded lungs via the ductus arteriosus and enters the descending aorta where it travels to the placenta, the fetal organ of oxygenation. Until recently it was assumed that during fetal life the ductus arteriosus was a passively open channel that constricted postnatally by means of undefined molecular mechanisms in response to the abrupt rise in arterial pO_2 accompanying the first breath of life.[133] Evidence now exists that even in utero the size of the ductus arteriosus lumen may be influenced by vasoactive substances, particularly prostaglandins.[61,134,135] Thus, inhibition of prostaglandin synthesis causes profound constriction of the ductus arteriosus in the mammalian fetus that may be reversed by administration of vasodilatory E-type prostaglandins. Initial contraction and functional closure of the ductus arteriosus immediately after birth may be related to both the sudden increase in arterial oxygen saturation that accompanies ventilation and the synthesis, release, or inhibition of vasoactive substances. Intimal proliferation and fibrosis proceed more gradually, so that anatomical closure may take as long as several weeks for completion.

The ductus arteriosus is a unique structure after birth, since its patency may, on the one hand, result in cardiac decompensation but may, on the other hand, provide the only life-sustaining conduit to preserve systemic or pulmonary arterial blood flow in the presence of certain cardiac malformations.[59] Appreciable left-to-right shunting across the patent ductus arteriosus frequently complicates the clinical course of infants born prematurely.[27,136] The ductal shunt has been implicated specifically in the deterioration of pulmonary function in infants with the respiratory distress syndrome in whom severe congestive heart failure is often unresponsive to digitalis and diuretics.

A distinction should be made between patency of the ductus arteriosus in the *preterm* infant, who lacks the normal mechanisms for postnatal ductal closure because of immaturity, and the full-term newborn, in whom patency of the ductus is a true congenital malformation, related most likely to a primary anatomical defect of the elastic tissue within the wall of the ductus.[137] In the former circumstance, delayed spontaneous closure of the ductus may be anticipated if the infant does not succumb to the cardiopulmonary difficulties caused by the ductus itself or to some lethal complication of prematurity, such as hyaline membrane disease, intraventricular hemorrhage, or necrotizing enterocolitis. In similar fashion, some full-term newborns have persistent patency of the ductus arteriosus for weeks or months because their relative hypoxemia contributes to vasodilatation of the channel. In the latter category are infants born at high altitude; those born with congenital malformations causing hypoxemia, such as pulmonic atresia with and without ventricular septal defect; or malformations in which ductal flow supplies the systemic circulation, such as hypoplastic left heart syndrome, interruption of the aortic arch, or some examples of coarctation of the aorta syndrome. In the clinical settings in which the ductus preserves pulmonary blood flow, the essentially inevitable spontaneous closure of the vessel is associated with profound clinical deterioration. The latter may be reversed medically by infusion of vasodilatory prostaglandins intravenously or via an aortic catheter at the level of the ductus. By dilating the constricted ductus arteriosus, this results in a temporary increase in arterial blood oxygen tension and oxygen saturation and correction of acidemia.[59,138] These infants can then undergo operation, usually a systemic-pulmonary anastomosis, under more optimal circumstances. Pharmacological dilation of the ductus arteriosus may also be effective in the preoperative restoration of systemic blood flow and the alleviation of heart failure, especially in infants with aortic coarctation, and in infants with complete transposition of the great arteries in whom intercirculatory mixing is augmented.[59]

PREMATURE INFANTS. In most, if not all, preterm infants under 1500 grams birthweight, persistence of a patent ductus arteriosus is prolonged, and in approximately one third of these infants a large aorticopulmonary shunt is responsible for significant cardiopulmonary deterioration.[139–143] Radiographic and echocardiographic signs of significant left-to-right shunting usually precede the appearance of physical findings suggesting ductal patency.[144] A significant increase in the cardiothoracic ratio is seen on sequential radiographs as well as increased pulmonary arterial markings progressing to perihilar and generalized

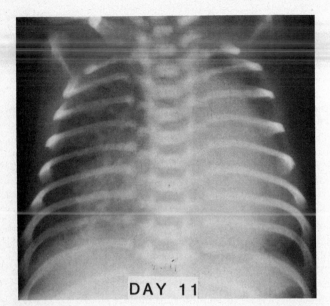

FIGURE 29–16 Chest roentgenogram in 11-day preterm infant with a large patent ductus arteriosus revealing cardiomegaly, pulmonary hypervascularity, and pulmonary edema. (From Higgins, C. B., et al.: Patent ductus arteriosus in preterm infants with idiopathic respiratory distress syndrome. Radiographic and echocardiographic evaluation. Radiology *124*:189, 1977.)

pulmonary edema (Fig. 29–16). Serial echocardiographic evaluations that demonstrate increases in left ventricular end-diastolic and left atrial dimensions, especially when correlated with the aforementioned radiographic signs, are highly accurate in detecting a large shunt (Fig. 29–17).[145,146] The clinical findings include bounding peripheral pulses, an infraclavicular and interscapular systolic murmur (occasionally a continuous murmur), precordial hyperactivity, hepatomegaly, and either multiple episodes of apnea and bradycardia or respirator dependency.

Management of the preterm infant with a patent ductus arteriosus varies, depending upon the magnitude of shunting and the severity of hyaline membrane disease, since the ductus may contribute importantly to mortality in the respiratory distress syndrome. Intervention in an asymptomatic infant with a small left-to-right shunt is unnecessary, since the patent ductus arteriosus will almost invariably undergo spontaneous closure and will not require late surgical ligation and division. Those infants who demonstrate unmistakable signs of a large ductal left-to-right shunt during the course of the respiratory distress syndrome are often unresponsive to medical measures to control congestive heart failure and require closure of the patent ductus arteriosus in order to survive. These infants are best managed within the first 2 to 7 days of life either by pharmacological inhibition of prostaglandin synthesis to constrict and close the ductus[136,139–143,147] or by surgical ligation.[27,148] Early intervention is advised in order to reduce the likelihood of bronchopulmonary dysplasia related to prolonged respirator and oxygen dependency. Less often, indications for pharmacological or surgical closure of the ductus consist of life-threatening episodes of apnea and bradycardia or a prolonged failure to gain weight and grow.

FULL-TERM INFANTS AND CHILDREN. In full-term newborns and older infants and children, patency of the ductus arteriosus occurs particularly in females and in the offspring of pregnancies complicated by first-trimester rubella. Although most frequent in isolated form, the anomaly may coexist with other malformations, particularly coarctation of the aorta, ventricular septal defect, pulmonic stenosis, and aortic stenosis. Flow across the ductus is determined by the pressure relationship between the aorta and the pulmonary artery and by the cross-sectional area and length of the ductus itself.[149] Most commonly, pulmonary pressures are normal, and a persistent gradient and shunt from aorta to pulmonary artery exist throughout the cardiac cycle. Physical examination reveals a char-

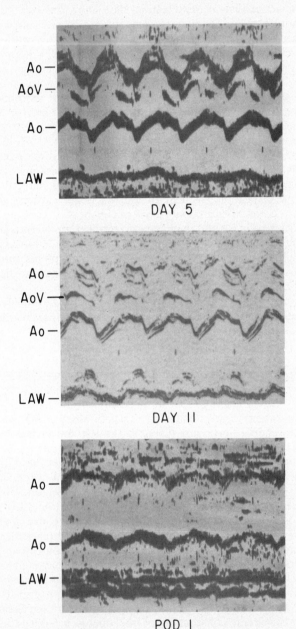

FIGURE 29–17 Serial echocardiograms in a preterm infant. On day 5, left atrial dimensions are normal but are increased on day 11, indicating the presence of a large left-to-right shunt across the ductus arteriosus. One day after ductus ligation (POD 1) left atrial dimensions have returned to normal. Ao = aorta, AoV = aortic valve, LAW = left atrial wall. (From Higgins, C. B., et al.: Patent ductus arteriosus in preterm infants with idiopathic respiratory distress syndrome. Radiographic and echocardiographic evaluation. Radiology *124*:189, 1977.)

acteristic thrill and a continuous "machinery" murmur with a late systolic accentuation at the upper left sternal border. The left atrium and left ventricle enlarge to accommodate the increased pulmonary venous return, and flow murmurs across the mitral and aortic valves may be detected. With significant left-to-right shunting, the runoff of blood through the ductus causes a widened systemic pulse pressure and bounding peripheral pulses. The hemodynamic abnormality is reflected electrocardiographically by left ventricular and occasionally left atrial hypertrophy, and radiologically by left atrial hypertrophy, and radiologically by left atrial and ventricular enlargement, and prominent ascending aorta and pulmonary artery, and pulmonary vascular engorgement. The clinical diagnosis may be difficult when the findings do not conform to the classic presentation.[150,151] As mentioned above, disappearance of the diastolic component of the murmur is common in premature infants because higher pulmonary arterial diastolic pressures exist at that age. In older patients both heart failure and pulmonary hypertension are associated with a reduction in the pressure gradient across the ductus arteriosus and result in atypical systolic murmurs. When severe pulmonary vascular obstructive disease results in reversal of flow through the ductus and preferential shunting of unoxygenated blood to the descending aorta, the toes, rather than the fingers, may show cyanosis and clubbing.

The full-term infant with patent ductus arteriosus may survive for a number of years, although occasionally a large defect results in heart failure and pulmonary edema early in life. The leading causes of death in older children are bacterial endocarditis and heart failure. Beyond the third decade severe pulmonary vascular obstruction has been known to cause aneurysmal dilatation, calcification, and rupture of the ductus.[150]

Cardiac catheterization is indicated when additional lesions or pulmonary hypertension is suspected, except in the preterm infant, in whom the risk of cardiac catheterization is high and the syndrome created by ductal patency can be recognized easily by noninvasive studies.[144,151] In the absence of severe pulmonary vascular disease with predominant left-to-right shunting the anatomical presence of a patent ductus is generally considered sufficient indication for operation.[150a] Ligation or division of the ductus carries a low risk, whether performed electively in the asymptomatic child or at any age if symptoms are present. The operative risk is reduced if heart failure can be compensated by medical measures before surgery. Operation should be deferred for several months in patients treated successfully for bacterial endarteritis because the ductus may remain somewhat edematous and friable. Rarely, when the infection will not subside with intensive antibiotic treatment, surgical ligation may be necessary to eradicate the infection.

Aorticopulmonary Septal Defect

Aorticopulmonary window or fenestration, partial truncus arteriosus, and aortic septal defect are other designations applied to this relatively uncommon anomaly. Septation of the aortopulmonary trunk occurs by fusion of the conotruncal ridges (see Fig. 29–4). The right and left sixth aortic arches, destined to become the pulmonary arteries, join the pulmonary artery to complete great artery development (see Fig. 29–5). Congenital defects between the ascending aorta and the pulmonary artery result from faulty development of this area during embryonic life. The typical aortopulmonary septal defect results because of incomplete fusion of the distal aortal-pulmonary septum.[152] Malalignment of the conotruncal ridges results in unequal partitioning of the aortopulmonary trunk, which may result in partial or complete fusion of the right pulmonary artery to the aorta. The usual defect consists of a communication between the aorta and pulmonary artery just above the semilunar valves. Persistent patency of the ductus arteriosus is an associated lesion in 10 to 15 per cent of cases. Less common accompanying cardiovascular lesions include ventricular septal defect, coarctation of the aorta, and right aortic arch. Aorticopulmonary septal defects are usually large and are accompanied by severe pulmonary arterial hypertension.

On *physical examination* the pulses are typically bounding, like those of a large patent ductus arteriosus. However, the murmur is rarely continuous, and a basal systolic murmur is most common.[153] Cardiomegaly is present, and pulmonary hypertension is reflected in a loud and palpable sound of pulmonary valve closure. Aorticopulmonary septal defect should be suspected whenever a large shunt into the pulmonary artery is demonstrated at catheterization.[153,154] Distinction from patent ductus and persistent truncus arteriosus is facilitated by selective angiocardiography with the injection of contrast material into the left ventricle and/or the root of the aorta (Fig. 29–18).[155] Although occasional patients may survive to adulthood with uncorrected aorticopulmonary septal defect, most will die during childhood unless surgical treatment is undertaken. Operative correction is indicated in children with large left-to-right shunts; total cardiopulmonary bypass is required, and the defect is closed usually via a transaortic approach with a prosthetic patch.[154–156,156a]

Persistent Truncus Arteriosus

Persistent truncus arteriosus is a rare but serious anomaly in which a single vessel forms the outlet of both ventri-

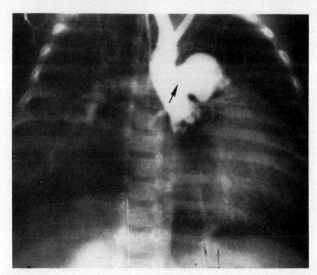

FIGURE 29–18 Aortic root injection of contrast material in the frontal view produces simultaneous opacification of aorta and pulmonary artery through a large aorticopulmonary septal defect (arrow). (Courtesy of Robert White, M.D.)

cles and gives rise to the systemic, pulmonary, and coronary arteries.[157,158] The defect results from failure of septation of the embryonic truncus by the infundibular truncal ridges (see Fig. 29–4). It is always accompanied by a ventricular septal defect and frequently by a right-sided aortic arch. The ventricular septal defect is due to the absence or underdevelopment of the distal portion of the pulmonary infundibulum. The truncal valve is usually tricuspid but is quadricuspid in approximately one third of patients and, rarely, bicuspid. Truncal valve regurgitation and truncal valve stenosis are each seen in 10 to 15 per cent of patients. There may be a single coronary artery, displacement of the coronary ostia (usually the left ostium posteriorly), or a single posterior descending coronary artery arising from the right coronary or, less often, from the left circumflex artery, especially in patients with a single coronary artery.[159]

Truncus malformations may be classified either anatomically according to the mode of origin of pulmonary vessels from the common trunk or from a functional point of view, based on the magnitude of blood flow to the lungs.[160] In the common type (type I) of truncus arteriosus malformation a partially separate pulmonary trunk of varying length exists because of the presence of an incompletely formed aorticopulmonary septum (Fig. 29–19). The pulmonary trunk is usually very short and gives rise to left and right pulmonary arteries. When the aorticopulmonary sep-

tum is absent, there is no discrete main pulmonary artery component, and both pulmonary artery branches arise directly from the truncus. In type II, each pulmonary artery arises separately but close to the other from the posterior aspect of the truncus. In type III, each pulmonary artery arises from the lateral aspect of the truncus. Less commonly, one pulmonary artery branch may be absent, with collateral arteries supplying the lung that does not receive a pulmonary artery branch from the truncus. Truncus arteriosus malformation should not be confused with "pseudotruncus arteriosus," which is the severe form of tetralogy of Fallot with pulmonary atresia in which the single aorta arises from the heart accompanied by a remnant of atretic pulmonary artery.

Pulmonary blood flow is governed by the size of the pulmonary arteries and the pulmonary vascular resistance. In infancy, pulmonary blood flow is usually excessive, since pulmonary vascular resistance is not greatly increased. Thus, despite an obligatory admixture of systemic and pulmonary venous blood in the common trunk, only minimal cyanosis is present. Rarely, pulmonary blood flow is restricted by hypoplastic or stenotic pulmonary arteries arising from the truncus. Pulmonary vascular obstruction does not appear to restrict pulmonary blood flow before 1 to 2 years of age.[161] Hence, the infant with truncus arteriosus usually presents with mild cyanosis coexisting with the cardiac findings of a large left-to-right shunt. Symptoms of heart failure and poor physical development usually appear in the first weeks or months of life. The most frequent physical findings include cardiomegaly, a systolic ejection sound accompanied by a thrill, a loud single second heart sound, a harsh systolic murmur, and a low-pitched mid-diastolic rumbling murmur and bounding pulses.

Truncal valve incompetence is suggested by the presence of a diastolic decrescendo murmur at the base of the heart.[162] The physical findings are quite different if pulmonary blood flow is restricted by either high pulmonary vascular resistance or pulmonary arterial stenosis: cyanosis is prominent, congestive failure is rare, and only a short systolic ejection may be audible accompanied occasionally by continuous murmurs posteriorly of bronchial collateral flow. Left ventricular hypertrophy alone or in combination with right ventricular hypertrophy is present electrocardiographically when a prominent left-to-right shunt exists; right ventricular hypertrophy is observed in patients with restricted pulmonary blood flow. The radiographic findings depend upon the hemodynamic circumstances. Gross cardiomegaly with left or combined ventricular enlargement, left atrial enlargement, and a small or absent main pulmonary artery segment with pulmonary vascular engorgement are the usual radiographic features. A right aortic arch is common (25 to 30 per cent of patients). When pulmonary blood flow is reduced, both heart size and pulmonary vascular markings are less prominent.

The *echocardiographic* features of truncus arteriosus include the detection of a large truncal root overriding the ventricular septum, an increase in the right ventricular dimension, and mitral valve–truncal root continuity.[163] The dimension of the left atrium determined echocardiographically provides a good index of pulmonary flow. Differentiation between truncus arteriosus and tetralogy of Fallot by ultrasound may be difficult unless pulmonic valve echoes are observed in the latter anomaly.[67] Diagnosis should be suspected at cardiac catheterization if the catheter fails to enter the central pulmonary arteries from the right ventricle. Selective angiocardiography and retrograde aortography are necessary to establish a precise diagnosis and to reveal the common trunk arising from the heart and the origin of the pulmonary arteries from the truncus.

The early fatal course as well as early development of pulmonary vascular obstructive disease in patients surviving infancy is responsible for the poor prognosis associated with truncus arteriosus. In infants and young children with

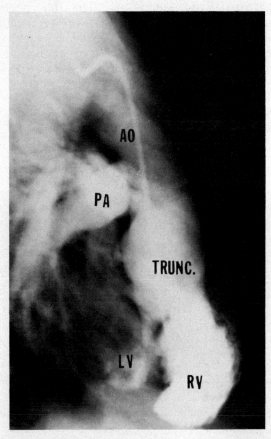

FIGURE 29–19   Right ventriculogram in the lateral view in a patient with type I truncus arteriosus. The contrast agent enters the left ventricle (LV) across a ventricular septal defect. The pulmonary artery (PA) arises directly from the persistent truncus arteriosus (TRUNC). AO = aorta; RV = right ventricle. (Courtesy of Robert White, M.D.)

large left-to-right shunts, surgical banding of one or both pulmonary arteries has been employed to reduce pulmonary flow.[164] Corrective operation is preferred before age 1 to 2 years if the patient is free of severe pulmonary vascular obstructive disease.[165-167,167a]

Operation consists of closure of the ventricular septal defect, leaving the aorta arising from the left ventricle; the pulmonary arteries are excised from their truncus origin and a valve-containing prosthetic conduit is used to establish continuity between the right ventricle and the pulmonary arteries. Truncal valve regurgitation significantly enhances the risk of corrective surgery, since valve replacement is associated with significantly increased surgical mortality. Patients with only one pulmonary artery are especially prone to early development of severe pulmonary vascular disease but otherwise are not at increased risk from surgery. With truncus arteriosus defects, the possible inequalities of pressure and flow between the two pulmonary arteries often make precise calculation of pulmonary resistance difficult.[161] Corrective operation may be performed in patients with at least one adequate pulmonary artery having low distal pressure or arteriolar resistance. Conversely, significant systemic arterial desaturation in a patient with two pulmonary arteries and with neither pulmonary artery stenosis nor a previous pulmonary artery band signifies that high pulmonary vascular resistance exists and that the condition is probably inoperable. It is not yet clear how often and at what age the conduit between the right ventricle and pulmonary artery must be replaced with a larger prosthesis either because of growth of the patient and/or obstruction caused by the new outflow tract.

CORONARY ARTERIOVENOUS FISTULA

Coronary arteriovenous fistula is an unusual anomaly that consists of a communication between one of the coronary arteries (rarely both) and an intracardiac chamber.[168] Connections between the coronary system and a cardiac chamber appear to represent persistence of embryonic intertrabecular spaces and sinusoids. The majority of these fistulas drain into the right ventricle, right atrium, or coronary sinus; fistulous communication to the pulmonary artery, left atrium, or left ventricle is much less frequent.[169] Most often the shunt through the fistula is of small magnitude, and myocardial blood flow is not compromised.[170] Potential complications include pulmonary hypertension and congestive heart failure if a large left-to-right shunt exists, bacterial endocarditis, rupture or thrombosis of the fistula or an associated arterial aneurysm, and myocardial ischemia distal to the fistula due to decreased coronary blood flow.

The majority of patients are asymptomatic and are referred because of a cardiac murmur that is loud, superficial, and continuous at the lower or midsternal border. The site of maximal intensity of the murmur is related to the site of drainage and is usually different from the second left intercostal space—the classic site of the continuous murmur of persistent ductus arteriosus—except when the fistula drains into the pulmonary artery or right ventricle. In the latter situation the murmur is louder in diastole than in systole because of compression of the fistula by contracting myocardium. The electrocardiogram and chest x-ray are quite often normal and rarely show selective chamber enlargement or myocardial ischemia.

Retrograde thoracic aortography or coronary arteriography can be employed to identify the size and anatomical features of the fistulous tract (Fig. 29–20), which may be closed by suture obliteration in most cases.[171] Indications for operation are not precise. In the presence of a large left-to-right shunt and symptoms of heart failure, the decision to operate is clearly justified. Most often the fistula is closed in asymptomatic patients in order to prevent future symptoms or complications. The risk of death or substantial morbidity following closure of a coronary artery–cardiac chamber fistula is quite low.

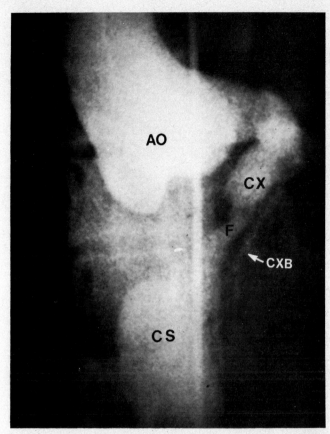

FIGURE 29–20 Coronary arteriovenous fistula draining into the coronary sinus in the frontal projection. AO = aorta, CX = circumflex coronary artery, CXB = circumflex coronary artery branch, F = fistula, CS = coronary sinus.

ANOMALOUS PULMONARY ORIGIN OF THE CORONARY ARTERY

This rare malformation occurs in approximately 0.4 per cent of patients with congenital cardiac anomalies. In almost all patients the left coronary artery originates from the posterior sinus of the pulmonary artery.[172-174]

Unusual cases have been reported in which the right coronary artery, or the entire coronary artery system, originates from the main pulmonary trunk.[172] Embryologically the distal coronary artery system is formed by 9 weeks from solid angioblastic buds that extend throughout the epicardium to form the major coronary artery branches. Proximally the coronary network forms a ring around the truncus arteriosus, joining with coronary buds from the primitive aortic sinuses as the truncus partitions to form the great arteries. The varieties of anomalous pulmonary origin of the coronary artery are the result of displacement in this proximal process.

During fetal life pulmonary artery pressure is slightly greater than aortic pressure, and perfusion of the left coronary artery is antegrade. After birth, when pulmonary artery pressure falls below aortic pressure, perfusion of the left coronary artery from the pulmonary artery ceases, and the direction of flow in the anomalous vessel reverses. Blood flows from the aorta to the right coronary artery, then through collateral channels to the left coronary artery, and finally to the pulmonary artery. In effect, the left coronary artery behaves as a fistulous communication between the aorta and pulmonary artery. If

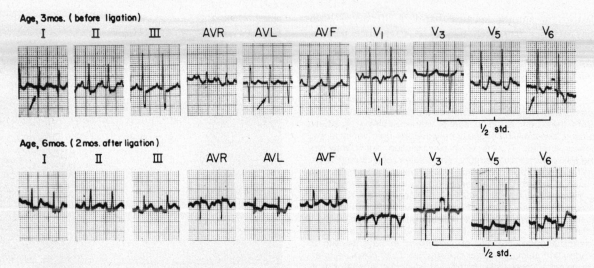

FIGURE 29–21   Typical electrocardiogram of an infant with anomalous left coronary artery before *(above)* and after *(below)* ligation of the anomalous left coronary artery. Arrows point to the abnormal Q waves. (Courtesy of Delores A. Danilowicz, M.D.)

adequate collateral channels exist or develop between the two coronary artery circulations, total myocardial perfusion through the right coronary artery increases. In 10 to 15 per cent of patients myocardial ischemia never develops because extensive intercoronary collaterals allow survival to adolescence or adulthood. In fact, if collateral blood flow is considerable, the patient may develop the clinical manifestations of a large arteriovenous shunt and a continuous or diastolic murmur. Older children or adults usually present with a continuous murmur or with mitral regurgitation resulting from dysfunction of ischemic or infarcted papillary muscles. In some instances the coronary anomaly is unsuspected until a previously well adolescent or adult experiences angina, heart failure, or sudden death.

By far the most common clinical presentation are those infants who suffer a myocardial infarction and develop congestive heart failure. The infant syndrome usually becomes manifest at age 2 to 4 months with angina-like symptoms that may occasionally be misinterpreted as colic. Feeding and defecation are often accompanied by dyspnea, irritability and crying, pallor, diaphoresis, and occasional loss of consciousness. The diagnosis of anomalous origin of the coronary artery is supported by the electrocardiographic demonstration of deep Q waves in association with ST-segment alterations and T-wave inversions in leads I, aV_1, V_5, and V_6 (Fig. 29–21). Chest roentgenograms show moderate to severe enlargement of the left atrium and ventricle. Aortography or coronary angiography is the definitive diagnostic procedure and demonstrates the retrograde drainage of the coronary vessel into the pulmonary artery (Fig. 29–22). It should be recognized that ventricular arrhythmias may complicate the course of hemodynamic study. Management of these infants depends, in part, upon the magnitude of shunting into the pulmonary artery, which may be determined by oximetry, indicator dilution curves, or angiography.

Medical treatment is indicated in all infants with myocardial infarction for congestive heart failure, arrhythmias, and cardiogenic shock. In patients with a small left-to-right shunt or no shunt at all, the prognosis is exceedingly poor with conservative management, justifying an attempt to reestablish a two coronary artery system. The operations that have been employed include reimplanting the left coronary artery into the aortic root, or anastomosis of the left coronary artery with the subclavian artery or with the aorta via a graft.[175,176] If clinical deterioration occurs in infants in whom a sizable left-to-right shunt exists into the pulmonary artery, simple ligation of the left coronary artery at its origin prevents retrograde flow and allows perfusion of the left ventricle with blood supplied through anastomoses with the right coronary artery. If medical management stabilizes the infant with significant intercoronary collaterals, operation should be postponed to allow the patient to grow, since increased size of the vessels

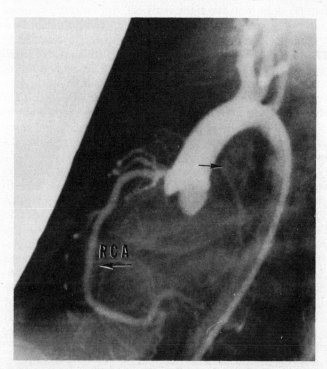

FIGURE 29–22   Lateral view of anomalous left coronary artery. Retrograde aortogram fills the right (RCA) and then the left coronary artery through collateral channels. The left coronary artery enters the main pulmonary artery (upper arrow). (Courtesy of Robert Freedom, M.D.)

enhances the likelihood of successful coronary arterial bypass surgery. The outcome of surgery and ultimate prognosis are influenced significantly by the degree of myocardial damage suffered preoperatively. In rare patients it is necessary to consider aneurysmectomy or mitral valve replacement.

AORTIC SINUS ANEURYSM AND FISTULA

Congenital aneurysm of an aortic sinus of Valsalva, particularly the right coronary sinus, is an uncommon anomaly occurring more often in males. The malformation consists of a separation, or lack of fusion, between the media of the aorta and the annulus fibrosis of the aortic valve.[177] The receiving chamber of the aorticocardiac fistula usually is the right ventricle, but occasionally, when the noncoronary cusp is involved, the fistula drains into the right atrium.

Five to 15 per cent of aneurysms originate in the posterior or noncoronary sinus; rarely is the left aortic sinus involved. Associated anomalies are common and include bicuspid aortic valve, ventricular septal defect, and coarctation of the aorta.

It is not clear whether the aneurysm itself is present at birth, although the deficiency in the aortic media would appear to be congenital. Reports in children are infrequent, since progressive aneurysmal dilatation of the weakened area develops but may not be recognized until the third or fourth decade of life when rupture into a cardiac chamber occurs.

The *unruptured aneurysm* generally does not produce a hemodynamic abnormality, although pressure on the intracardiac conduction system by an unruptured aneurysm may be a rare cause of complete atrioventricular block; myocardial ischemia may rarely be caused by coronary arterial compression.[177] Rupture often is of abrupt onset, causes chest pain, and creates continuous arteriovenous shunting and volume loading of both right and left heart chambers, which results in heart failure.[178-180] An additional complication is bacterial endocarditis, which may originate either on the edges of the aneurysm or on those areas in the right side of the heart that are traumatized by the jetlike stream of blood flowing through the fistula.

The presence of this anomaly should be suspected in a patient with a history of chest pain of recent onset, symptoms of diminished cardiac reserve, bounding pulses, and a loud superficial continuous murmur accentuated in diastole when the fistula opens into the right ventricle as well as a thrill along the right or left lower parasternal border. The *physical findings* may occasionally be difficult to distinguish from those produced by a coronary arteriovenous fistula. *Electrocardiography* shows biventricular hypertrophy, and chest roentgenography demonstrates generalized cardiomegaly. Two dimensional and pulsed Doppler *echocardiographic* studies may detect the wall of the aneuryms and disturbed flow within the aneurysm, respectively.[181,182] *Cardiac catheterization* reveals a left-to-right shunt at the ventricular or, less commonly, the atrial level; the diagnosis may be established definitively by retrograde thoracic aortography (Fig. 29–23). Preoperative medical management consists of measures to relieve cardiac failure and to treat coexistent arrhythmias or endocarditis, if present. At operation the aneurysm is closed and amputated, and the aortic wall is reunited with the heart, either by direct suture or with a prosthesis.[179,179a] Every effort should be made to preserve the aortic valve in children, since patch closure of the defect combined with prosthetic valve replacement greatly enhances the risk of operation in small patients.

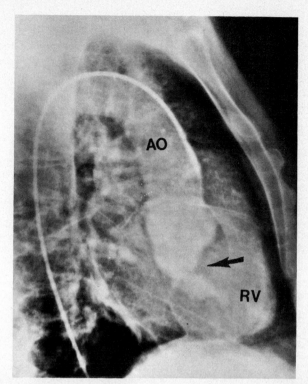

FIGURE 29–23 A retrograde aortogram shows the fistulous connection between the noncoronary sinus of Valsalva and the right ventricle (RV) (arrow). AO = aorta. (Courtesy of Robert White, M.D.)

VALVULAR AND VASCULAR LESIONS WITH OR WITHOUT RIGHT-TO-LEFT SHUNT

Aortic Arch Obstruction

The conventional anatomical and clinical division into pre- and postductal coarctation or infantile and adult types, respectively, is misleading, since the anatomical localization is inaccurate and the age-dependency of clinical presentation does not hold true (i.e., the adult type is seen often in the first weeks of life). A spectrum of anatomical lesions exists, causing obstruction of the aortic arch or proximal portion of the descending aorta. These range from a localized coarctation or constriction of the lumen, most commonly located just distal to the origin of the left subclavian artery and related closely to the attachment of the ductus arteriosus with the aorta, to diffuse narrowing or interruption of a portion of the aortic arch. In this chapter, aortic arch obstruction is divided into three types: (1) localized juxtaductal coarctation, (2) hypoplasia of the aortic isthmus, and (3) aortic arch interruption. *Pseudocoarctation* is a term used synonymously with "kinking," or "buckling," of the aorta, which is a subclinical form of localized juxtaductal coarctation of the aorta.[183]

Localized Juxtaductal Coarctation

MORPHOLOGY. This lesion consists of a localized shelflike thickening and infolding of the posterolateral aortic wall opposite the ductus arteriosus; the wall of the aorta into which the ductus or ligamentum arteriosum inserts is not involved.[184] Juxtaductal coarctation occurs two to five times more commonly in males than in females, and there is a high degree of association with gonadal dysgenesis (Turner's syndrome) and bicuspid aortic valve. Other common associated anomalies include ventricular septal defect and mitral stenosis or regurgitation. The most important extracardiac anomaly is aneurysm of the circle of Willis.

Juxtaductal coarctation is most likely related to an abnormality in the pattern of ductus arteriosus blood flow in utero, which, in turn, may be the result of associated intracardiac anomalies.[184-187] Thus, in fetal life, blood flow through the aortic isthmus constitutes only 12 to 17 per cent of the total cardiac output, while blood flow through the ductus arteriosus exceeds that across the aortic valve. The dorsal aortic wall directly opposite the ductus arteriosus will resemble morphologically the apex of a normal branch point of the aorta if ductal flow pathways in utero diverge, with some flow directed cephalad into the aortic isthmus and the remainder proceeding into the descending aorta. The aortic branch point is identical histologically to the posterior shelf of juxtaductal aortic coarctation. A divergence of ductal flow is fostered by the presence of lesions in the fetus that create an imbalance between left and right ventricular outputs, with right-sided flow predominating (e.g., bicuspid aortic valve, mitral valve anomaly). In the absence of an anomaly fostering augmented ductal flow, a branch point may be created by an alteration in the angle at which the ductus arteriosus meets the aorta, pointing the ductal stream directly against the posterior aortic wall rather than obliquely down into the descending aorta. Cardiac anomalies that cause augmented ascending aortic blood flow (e.g., pulmonic atresia or stenosis, tetralogy of Fallot) prevent development of a branch point and, indeed, are almost never seen in association with juxtaductal coarctation of the aorta.

During fetal life the posterior aortic shelf is not obstructive, since blood may pass readily from the ascending aorta to the descending aorta by traversing the anterior aortic segment and the aortic end of the ductus arteriosus. Postnatally, however, when the ductus undergoes obliteration at its aortic end, the shelflike projection of the posterior aortic wall unmasks the obstruction to aortic flow (Fig. 29–24). Following pharmacological interventions that dilate the ductus arteriosus (prostaglandin E₁ infusion) the pressure difference may be obliterated across the site of coarctation, since the fetal flow pattern is reestablished (Fig. 29–25).[59,138,188]

The *pathogenesis* of juxtaductal coarctation described above explains the prevalence of associated intracardiac anomalies that foster reduced ascending aortic and augmented ductus arteriosus flow in utero, and the absence of associated intracardiac anomalies in which the converse flow conditions exist in utero. The dependence of aortic obstruction on constriction of the ductus arteriosus postnatally explains the variable onset after birth of the clinical manifestations of coarctation, as well as the dramatic alleviation of obstruction produced pharmacologically by dilatation of the ductus arteriosus.

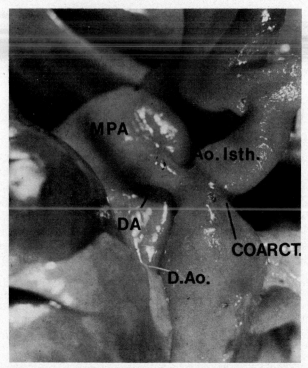

FIGURE 29–24 Juxtaductal coarctation (COARCT) unmasked by constriction of the ductus arteriosus (DA). MPA = main pulmonary artery; D.Ao. = descending aorta; Ao.Isth. = aortic isthmus. (Courtesy of Norman Talner, M.D.)

CLINICAL FINDINGS.   The manifestations of juxtaductal coarctation of the aorta depend upon the prominence of the posterolateral aortic shelf, which determines the intensity of obstruction, and on the rapidity with which obstruction develops. Rapid, severe obstruction in infancy is a prominent cause of left ventricular failure and systemic hypoperfusion. Substantial left-to-right shunting across a patent foramen ovale and pulmonary venous hypertension secondary to heart failure cause pulmonary arterial hypertension. Because little or no aortic obstruction existed during fetal life, the collateral circulation in the newborn period is often poorly developed. Characteristically in these infants, peripheral pulses are weak throughout

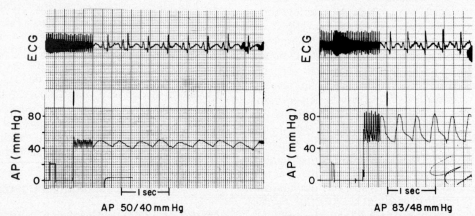

FIGURE 29–25 Abdominal aortic pressure tracing (AP) and electrocardiogram before (*left*) and after (*right*) intravenous infusion of prostaglandin E₁ in a newborn with coarctation of the aorta. The abdominal aortic pressure is low and damped distal to the coarctation (*left*) and rises dramatically when the ductus arteriosus is dilated with PGE₁ (*right*). Thus, dilatation of the ductus arteriosus has obliterated the pressure difference between the ascending and descending aorta by allowing blood to utilize the aortic end of the ductus to bypass the ridge of obstructing coarctation tissue. (Courtesy of Thomas Graham, Jr., M.D.)

the body until left ventricular function is improved with medical management; a significant pressure difference then develops between the arms and the legs, allowing detection of a pulse discrepancy. Cardiac murmurs are nonspecific in infancy and commonly are derived from associated lesions. The electrocardiogram shows right-axis deviation and right ventricular hypertrophy; the chest x-ray shows generalized cardiomegaly and pulmonary arterial and venous engorgement. Hemodynamic study allows delineation of the site and extent of aortic obstruction and the detection of associated cardiac malformations. Most infants with early-onset severe heart failure respond poorly to medical management, and surgical excision of the coarctation is often required.[189,190]

Aortic obstruction may develop slowly in infants in whom the posterolateral aortic shelf is not prominent at birth and in whom ductus arteriosus constriction is gradual. In these babies compensatory myocardial hypertrophy and an extensive collateral circulation have time to develop. If the obstruction does not intensify and cardiac failure does not occur by age 6 to 9 months, circulatory compensation is likely until adult life.

The majority of children with isolated juxtaductal coarctation are asymptomatic. Complaints of headache, cold extremities, and claudication with exercise may be noted, although attention is usually directed to the cardiovascular system by detection of a heart murmur or upper extremity hypertension on routine physical examination. Mechanical factors rather than those of renal origin play the primary role in the production of hypertension.[191] Absent, markedly diminished, or delayed pulsations in the femoral arteries and a low or unobtainable arterial pressure in the lower extremities with hypertension in the arms are the basic clues to the diagnosis. A midsystolic murmur over the anterior chest, back, and spinous processes is most frequent, becoming continuous if the lumen is narrowed sufficiently to result in a high-velocity jet across the lesion throughout the cardiac cycle. Additional systolic and continuous murmurs over the lateral thoracic wall may reflect increased flow through dilated and tortuous collateral vessels. *Electrocardiography* reveals left ventricular hypertrophy of varying degrees, depending on the height of arterial pressure above the obstruction and the patient's age. Combined with right ventricular hypertrophy, this usually implies a complicated lesion. *Chest roentgenograms* may show a dilated left subclavian artery high on the left mediastinal border and a dilated ascending aorta. Indentation of the aorta at the site of coarctation and pre- and poststenotic dilatation (the "3" sign) along the left paramediastinal shadow is almost pathognomonic. Poststenotic dilatation may also be detected by indentation of the barium-filled esophagus. Notching of the ribs, an important radiographic sign, is due to erosion by dilated collateral vessels, increases with age, and usually becomes apparent between the fourth and twelfth years of life. The aortic coarctation may be visualized directly by two-dimensional echocardiography from the suprasternal notch[34,67] and by digital subtraction and computer-assisted angiography.[192] Cardiac catheterization and aortography are indicated to localize accurately the site of obstruction, determine the length of the coarctation, and identify associated malformations (Fig. 29–26).

TREATMENT. *Surgical resection* and end-to-end anas-

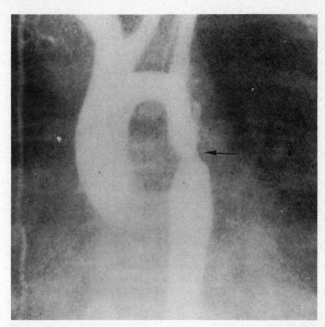

FIGURE 29–26 Retrograde aortogram demonstrates the discrete site of coarctation of the aorta (arrow) and post-stenotic dilatation of the descending aorta.

tomosis of uncomplicated juxtaductal coarctation of the aorta can be accomplished with excellent results in most patients;[192a] some surgeons prefer an on-lay patch across the site of obstruction or a subclavian patch angioplasty to widen the aortic lumen.[192b] In children who are asymptomatic it is preferable to delay surgery until age 4 to 6 years, at which time coarctation rarely recurs.[193] Paradoxical hypertension of short duration is often noted in the immediate postoperative period. A resetting of carotid baroreceptors and increased catecholamine secretion appear to be responsible for the initial phase of systemic hypertension with a later, second phase of prolonged elevation of systolic and particularly diastolic blood pressure related to activation of the renin-angiotensin system.[194,195] Occasionally, a necrotizing panarteritis of the small vessels of the gastrointestinal tract of uncertain cause complicates the course of recovery.

In those patients who survive the first two years of life, complications of juxtaductal coarctation are uncommon before the second or third decade. The chief hazards to patients with coarctation result from severe hypertension and include the development of cerebral aneurysms and hemorrhage, hypertensive encephalopathy, rupture of the aorta, left ventricular failure, and bacterial endocarditis. Systemic hypertension in the absence of residual coarctation has been observed in resting or exercise-stressed patients postoperatively and appears to be related to the duration of preoperative hypertension;[196–198] lifelong observation is desirable because of the late onset of hypertension in some postoperative patients.

HYPOPLASIA OF THE AORTIC ARCH

The aorta isthmus, the portion of aorta between the left subclavian artery and the ductus arteriosus, normally is narrowed in the fetus and newborn. The lumen of the aortic isthmus is approximately two-thirds that of the ascending and descending aorta until age 6 to 9 months, when the physiological narrowing disappears.[199] Pathological hypoplasia of the aortic arch is usually noted in the aortic isthmus and is referred to often as preductal or infantile coarctation of the aorta. Associated major cardiac malformations occur in virtually all such infants and include large ventricular septal defect, endocardial cushion defect, transposition of the great arteries, Taussig-Bing anomaly, and double-outlet right ventricle. Persistent patency of the ductus arteriosus commonly coexists, and right-to-left flow across the ductus arteriosus usually provides filling of the descending aorta. The adequacy of blood flow to the lower body depends upon the degree of aortic hypoplasia, the caliber of the ductus arteriosus, and the relationship between pulmonary and systemic vascular resistance. Substantial right-to-left shunting through a wide open ductus arteriosus minimizes the arterial blood pressure difference between the upper and lower body. Differential cyanosis of the toes and feet with normal color of the fingers and hands may be difficult to discern because intracardiac left-to-right shunting and pulmonary edema attenuate the differences in oxygen saturation in the ascending and descending aorta. Clinical deterioration is associated with ductal constriction or a fall in pulmonary vascular resistance. Moreover, the clinical presentation is often dictated by the hemodynamic effects of complex associated intracardiac malformations. Infants most often present with findings of a large left-to-right intracardiac shunt, pulmonary hypertension, and marked cardiac decompensation. Cardiac catheterization is required to evaluate the full extent of the intra- and extracardiac lesions.[200] Surgical repair of aortic arch hypoplasia must usually be accompanied by operative palliation or correction of associated intracardiac lesions. Aortic angioplasty incorporating the subclavian-aortic anastomosis, and a tubular prosthetic conduit are among the operative approaches to correct long segment narrowing. Recoarctation is common and often necessitates a second operation later in life to relieve anastomotic stenosis.

AORTIC ARCH INTERRUPTION

Aortic arch interruption is a rare and usually lethal anomaly; unless treated surgically almost all infants die within the first month of life.[201] Interruptions distal to the left subclavian artery (Type A) occur with approximately equal frequency to interruptions distal to the left common carotid artery (Type B); interruptions distal to the innominate artery (Type C) are extremely uncommon. The right subclavian artery is often of variable origin, arising frequently from the descending aortic segment distal to the interruption.[202] The clinical presentation resembles that seen in tubular hypoplasia or severe juxtaductal coarctation of the aorta with a patent ductus arteriosus. In almost all patients a ventricular septal defect and patent ductus arteriosus coexist with the arch interruption. Since the ductus arteriosus provides lower body blood flow, its spontaneous constriction results in profound clinical deterioration. The latter may be ameliorated temporarily by prostaglandin E$_1$ infusion.[59,188] Other complex intracardiac malformations, such as transposition of the great arteries, truncus arteriosus, and subaortic stenosis are common.[202,203] The major clinical problem is severe congestive heart failure as a consequence of volume overload of the left ventricle due to an associated intracardiac left-to-right shunt and of pressure overload imposed by systemic hypertension. Operation is rarely possible by direct anastomosis, and reconstitution usually necessitates a tubular synthetic graft or a direct anastomosis between the aorta and one of its major brachiocephalic vessels.[204,205]

AORTIC STENOSIS

Each of the specific congenital cardiovascular malformations that interfere with the ejection of blood from the left ventricle will be discussed separately. These malformations include congenital valvular aortic stenosis, the discrete as well as uncommon forms of congenital subaortic stenosis, and congenital narrowing of the supravalvular ascending aorta.

Valvular Aortic Stenosis
(See also page 1095)

MORPHOLOGY.   Congenital valvular aortic stenosis is a relatively common anomaly, estimated to occur in 3 to 6 per cent of patients with congenital cardiovascular defects. However, it must be appreciated that the true incidence of the malformation is probably grossly underestimated because the congenital bicuspid aortic valve may be undetected in early life, and becomes stenotic and of clinical significance only in adult life, at a time when it may be indistinguishable from the acquired forms of aortic stenosis. Congenital valvular aortic stenosis occurs much more frequently in males than in females, with the sex ratio approximating 4:1. Associated cardiovascular anomalies have been noted in as many as 20 per cent of patients.[206] Patent ductus arteriosus and coarctation of the aorta occur most frequently with valvular aortic stenosis; all three of these lesions may coexist.

The basic malformation consists of thickening of valve tissue with varying degrees of commissural fusion. Most commonly, the valve is bicuspid with a single, fused commissure and an eccentrically placed orifice. A third, incomplete, or rudimentary commissure may sometimes be apparent. Less commonly, the valve has three fused cusps with a stenotic central orifice. In some patients the stenotic aortic valve is unicuspid and dome-shaped with no or one lateral attachment to the aorta at the level of the orifice. In infants and young children with severe aortic stenosis the aortic valve ring may be relatively underdeveloped. This lesion forms a continuum with the hypoplastic left heart syndrome and the aortic atresia and hypoplasia complexes. Secondary calcification of the valve is extremely rare in childhood, but the dynamics of blood flow associated with the congenitally deformed aortic valve lead ultimately to thickening of the cusps and calcification in adult life. When the obstruction is hemodynamically significant, concentric hypertrophy of the left ventricular wall and dilatation of the ascending aorta occur.

HEMODYNAMICS.   The hemodynamic abnormalities produced by obstruction to left ventricular outflow are discussed on pages 1097 to 1099.[206a] A peak systolic gradient exceeding 75 mm Hg in association with a normal cardiac output or an effective aortic orifice less than 0.5 cm^2/m^2 body surface area is considered to reflect critical obstruction to left ventricular outflow.[206-208] The normal outflow orifice approximates 2.0 cm^2/m^2 body surface area; areas of 0.5 to 0.8 cm^2/m^2 signify moderate obstruction. When the area is larger than 0.8 cm^2/m^2, the obstruction is considered to be mild; when less than 0.4 cm^2/m^2, it is severe.

Generally, the resting cardiac output and stroke volume are within normal limits. During exercise, most children with critical stenosis show an elevation of the cardiac output and an associated elevation in the transvalvular pressure gradient.[209] When left ventricular failure occurs, the cardiac output decreases, and the left atrial, left ventricular end-diastolic, and pulmonary vascular pressures increase.

The blood supply to the myocardium may be compromised significantly in infants and children with aortic stenosis, despite normal patency of the coronary arteries.[210,211] Coronary blood flow and arterial oxygen content are critical determinants of oxygen supply to the myocardium. Since intramyocardial compressive forces are greatest in the subendocardium, blood flow to that region of left ventricle is entirely diastolic in the presence of elevated left ventricular systolic pressure. In patients with left ventricular outflow tract obstruction, coronary vasodilatation may give an inadequate response to an increase in the demands of the myocardium for oxygen at rest or with exercise. When subendocardial vessels are dilated maximally the coronary artery driving pressure and the duration of diastole determine the magnitude of subendocardial flow. When the duration of systolic ejection lengthens across the stenotic orifice, diastole is shortened, especially at high heart rates. Moreover, a reduction occurs in coronary driving pressure if left ventricular end-diastolic pressure is high or if aortic diastolic pressure is low, e.g., with aortic regurgitation or heart failure. In patients with severe aortic stenosis the redistribution of flow away from the subendocardium and the ischemia that results to that portion of ventricular muscle may be estimated by relating the diastolic pressure time index (DPTI) (i.e., the area between the aortic and left ventricular pressures in diastole) to the systolic pressure time index (SPTI) (a measure of myocardial oxygen demands) (Fig. 29–27). Inadequate subendocardial oxygen delivery has been shown to exist when the ratio [DPTI × arterial oxygen content/SPTI] falls below 10.[191]

INFANCY. Special comment concerning this malformation as it is seen in infants is warranted, in view of the unique problems presented by patients in this age group.[212] Fortunately, isolated aortic valvular stenosis seldom causes symptoms in infancy. Occasionally, however, this lesion may be responsible for profound and intractable heart failure. Despite normal coronary arterial anatomy, infarction of left ventricular papillary muscles may occur, resulting in an acquired form of mitral valvular regurgitation that intensifies the heart failure state. In addition, endocardial fibroelastosis may result from limited subendocardial oxygen delivery and myocardial degeneration may be significant.[213] The symptomatic infant with isolated valvular aortic stenosis is irritable, pale, and hypotensive and presents with tachycardia, cardiomegaly, and pulmonary congestion manifested by dyspnea, tachypnea, subcostal retractions, and diffuse rales. Cyanosis may be observed secondary to pulmonary venous desaturation. The systolic murmur in infants is often atypical; it is best heard at the

apex or along the lower left sternal border and may be confused with that caused by a ventricular septal defect. Occasionally, in infants with heart failure, the murmur may be absent or extremely soft, becoming louder when myocardial contractility is improved with digitalis and other medical measures. Frequently, the response to medical management of the infant with heart failure is poor.

The electrocardiographic findings may not be characteristic; left ventricular hypertrophy and/or strain as well as right atrial enlargement and right ventricular hypertrophy may be detected shortly after birth.[206,212] The latter signs of right heart involvement result from both pulmonary hypertension secondary to elevated left ventricular diastolic and left atrial pressures and from volume loading of the right ventricle due to left-to-right shunting across the foramen ovale. Survival past the early neonatal period does not preclude subsequent difficulties, and clinical deterioration may recur with the onset of physiological anemia.

Congenital aortic stenosis must be considered a medical emergency in the seriously ill newborn, and cardiac catheterization and angiocardiography may be indicated in the first 24 hours of life. Commonly, hemodynamic findings include left-to-right shunting at the atrial level, elevated left atrial and left ventricular end-diastolic pressures, and a small pressure drop across the aortic valve as a result of a markedly reduced cardiac output. Occasionally, right-to-left shunting across a patent ductus arteriosus is encountered. The presence of a normal or enlarged left ventricular cavity and normal of dilated ascending aorta allows distinction of aortic stenosis from the hypoplastic left heart syndrome angiographically. Because prolonged periods of stabilization are uncommon with medical therapy, early and definitive establishment of the diagnosis and prompt valvulotomy are usually justified. Poor myocardial performance resulting from endocardial fibroelastosis, subendocardial ischemia, and reduced left ventricular compliance, and inadequate relief of obstruction with or without significant aortic regurgitation are among the factors accounting for high operative mortality and morbidity.[214] Open repair under direct vision is the preferred type of operation.[215]

CHILDHOOD. Congenital aortic stenosis may be responsible for severe obstruction to left ventricular outflow in the absence of the clinical symptoms of diminished cardiac reserve that are so frequent in other forms of congenital heart disease.[216] Most children with congenital aortic stenosis grow and develop normally and are asymptomatic. Attention is usually called to these children when a murmur is detected on routine examination. When symptoms occur, those noted most commonly are fatigability, exertional dyspnea, angina pectoris, and syncope. Less often described are abdominal pain, profuse sweating, and epistaxis. Generally, the symptomatic child has critical stenosis. Sudden death poses a distinct threat to patients with severe obstruction.[55,207] Although the precise cause is poorly understood, ventricular arrhythmias, perhaps initiated by acute myocardial ischemia, are probably the most common inciting event. Speculation exists that an abrupt rise in intracavity left ventricular systolic pressure elicits a reflex hypotensive syncope that promotes acute ischemia and ventricular fibrillation.[217] Bacterial endocarditis occurs in approximately 4 per cent of patients with congenital valvular aortic stenosis.

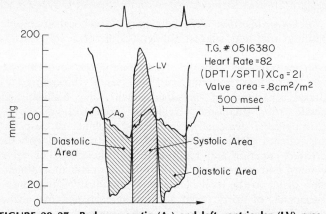

T.G. # 0516380
Heart Rate = 82
(DPTI/SPTI)XC$_a$ = 21
Valve area = .8cm^2/m^2
500 msec

FIGURE 29–27 Redrawn aortic (A$_o$) and left ventricular (LV) pressure curves used for calculation of the subendocardial flow index. The systolic pressure time index (SPTI) is the area under the LV curve during aortic ejection. The diastolic pressure time index (DPTI) is the area under the A$_o$ curve in the period when A$_o$ pressure is greater than the LV diastolic pressure. The ratio of DPTI × arterial oxygen content (C$_a$)/SPTI is proportional to the ratio of myocardial oxygen delivery to myocardial oxygen consumption.

DIAGNOSIS. *Physical Findings.* When the magnitude of obstruction is significant, a left ventricular lift is usually palpable, and a precordial systolic thrill is often palpated over the base of the heart with transmission to the jugular notch and along the carotid arteries; presystolic expansion is often palpable. Usually the obstruction is mild if neither a left ventricular lift nor a thrill is present.

Opening of the aortic valve produces a systolic aortic ejection sound that is typically present at the cardiac apex when the valve is mobile, particularly in patients with mild to moderate stenosis. A delay in closure of the stenotic aortic valve leads to a single or a closely split second heart sound, and paradoxical splitting may be present. Generally, a fourth heart sound is associated with severe obstruction. A loud, harsh, rhomboid-shaped systolic murmur starts after completion of left ventricular isometric contraction and is best heard at the base of the heart. The murmur, like the thrill, radiates to the suprasternal notch and carotid vessels as well as to the apex. An early diastolic blowing murmur of aortic regurgitation is present in some patients, but unless the valve leaflets have been eroded by bacterial endocarditis, the regurgitation is usually not hemodynamically significant; uncommonly, in patients with a congenitally bicuspid valve, aortic regurgitation may be severe and may predominate.

Electrocardiography and Vectorcardiography. There is a tendency for *electrocardiographic signs* of left ventricular hypertrophy to vary with the severity of obstruction, although a normal or near-normal electrocardiogram does not exclude severe aortic stenosis.[218] The presence of a left ventricular "strain pattern," consisting of left ventricular hypertrophy combined with ST-segment depressions and T-wave inversion in the left precordial leads, generally indicates that severe aortic stenosis is present (Fig. 29–28).

In patients under 10 years of age the *electrocardiogram* is a more reliable guide in indicating the severity of the stenosis than in older patients.[216] Findings in the younger age group that often accompany severe obstruction are T-wave vectors in the frontal plane to the left of $-40°$, widening of the angle between the mean QRS and T forces in the frontal plane in excess of $100°$, an S wave in V_1 greater than 16 mm, and an R wave in V_5 exceeding 20 mm. Nonetheless, it is important to recognize that these voltages may be excessive in patients who do not have severe stenosis. A good relationship appears to exist between exercise-induced electrocardiographic changes and the severity of obstruction; ischemic ST-segment changes have been observed in patients with normal resting cardiac indices and transvalvular pressure differences in excess of 50 mm Hg.[219,220]

The *vectorcardiogram* best shows the major influences of the left ventricular wall in the later phases of the QRS loop; left ventricular hypertrophy is reflected in the abnormal displacement of the mean spatial QRS vector in a posterior, superior, and leftward direction, maximal QRS forces exceeding 1.4 mm and QRS-T angle exceeding $60°$. Correlations have been reported between the severity of obstruction in patients with congenital aortic stenosis and the vectorcardiographic alterations[221] but have not been verified in other studies.[222] Infrequently, the vectorcardiogram may indicate the presence of severe aortic stenosis when the electrocardiogram does not.

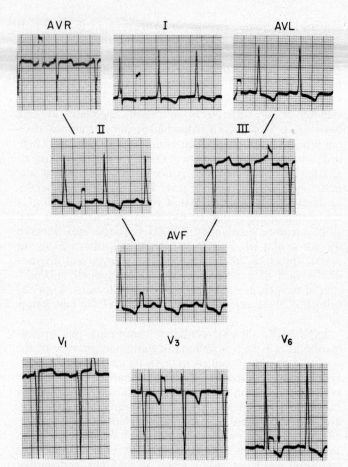

FIGURE 29–28 Congenital aortic stenosis. This tracing shows left ventricular hypertrophy and the typical left ventricular "strain" pattern (V_6, arrow). (Courtesy of Delores A. Danilowicz, M.D.)

Radiographically, overall heart size is normal or the degree of enlargement is slight in most children with congenital valvular aortic stenosis. Concentric left ventricular hypertrophy accompanies moderate or severe obstruction and is manifested by rounding of the cardiac apex in the frontal projection and posterior displacement in the lateral view.

Echocardiograms. The single-crystal echocardiographic findings that may suggest a diagnosis of aortic valve stenosis include multiple diastolic closure lines, or a single eccentrically placed diastolic closure line in the aortic lumen; left ventricular posterior wall and septal thickening; reduced separation of thickened aortic valve leaflets; and aortic root dilation.[223] Real-time cross-sectional echocardiography demonstrates impaired mobility of cusp tissue, altered phasic movement of the aortic valve with increased superior and reduced lateral excursions of valve echoes, and an increase in the internal aortic root dimension distal to the level of the valve annulus.[224] Direct measurements of aortic cusp separation corrected for aortic root diameter are likely to correlate with the severity of stenosis.

In patients without cardiac decompensation, a consistent relationship has been shown to exist between peak left ventricular systolic pressure and left ventricular wall thickness measured by ultrasound. A good correlation has been shown between the echocardiographically obtained end-

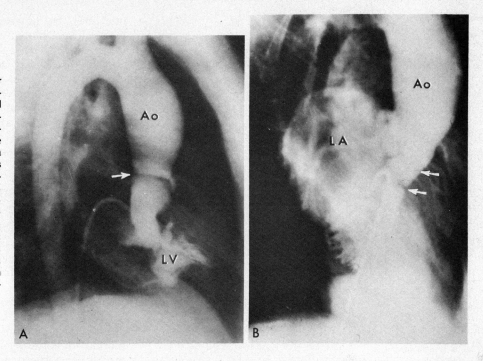

FIGURE 29-29 *A,* Left ventricular angiocardiogram obtained by the transseptal method in a patient with congenital valvular aortic stenosis. Ao = post-stenotic dilatation of the aorta; LV = left ventricle. Arrow denotes the thickened valve cusp. *B,* Selective angiocardiogram in a patient with discrete subvalvular stenosis (bottom arrow). Associated mitral regurgitation is evident from the reflux of contrast into an enlarged left atrium (LA). The aorta valve (top arrow) is normal, and the right coronary artery is visualized. (From Friedman, W. F., and Kirkpatrick, S. E.: Congenital aortic stenosis. *In* Moss, A. J., Adams, F. H., and Emmanouilides, G. C. (eds.): Heart Disease in Infants, Children and Adolescents. 2nd ed. Baltimore, Williams and Wilkins, 1977.)

systolic left ventricular posterior wall thickness–to–minor axis ratio. The relationship is expressed as left ventricular pressure (mm Hg) = 225 × systolic wall thickness/systolic internal diameter.[225] It would appear that end-diastolic dimensions may be even more accurate for predicting left ventricular peak systolic pressure by echocardiography. Using measurements of left ventricular end-diastolic posterior and septal wall thickness and left ventricular minor axis, a regression equation has been developed in which left ventricular systolic pressure (mm Hg) = 6 + 298 (h/r) ± 13.4, where $\bar{h}$ = mean of posterior and septal end-diastolic wall thickness at the equator and r = the end-diastolic minor semiaxis (half the end-diastolic minor axis).[226] Pulse Doppler echocardiography detects the altered and disturbed turbulence of flow and holds promise as a method to quantify the severity of obstruction.[227] The presence of aortic regurgitation may reduce the predictive accuracy of both these terminations.

Cardiac catheterization is more important for establishing the site and severity rather than the presence of aortic stenosis, since the malformation is usually diagnosed readily by clinical examination. Catheterization is indicated in any child with a clinical diagnosis of aortic stenosis in whom the clinical examination, roentgenogram, or resting or exercise electrocardiogram suggests the possibility of severe obstruction.[207] Even in the absence of such findings, hemodynamic study should be performed if symptoms exist that might be related to aortic stenosis. Moreover, in patients with mild or moderate obstruction, repeat left-sided heart catheterization should be carried out every 5 to 10 years because obstruction may progress.

The site and severity of obstruction are established at cardiac catheterization, and associated malformations are identified. Typically, the angiocardiographic features of valvular stenosis are thickening of the aortic cusps and of the left ventricular wall with slight or no dilatation of the left ventricular cavity, poststenotic dilatation of the ascending aorta, and occasionally a jet of contrast material entering the ascending aorta through a narrowed valve orifice that is central or eccentric (Fig. 29-29). The leaflets of the bicuspid valve are domed in systole; a central jet corresponds to the orifice of the stenotic valve. In contrast, the stenotic orifice of the unicommissural valve may be visualized by the systolic jet in contact with the posterior wall of the aorta, with leaflet tissue and valve motion seen only anteriorly.

Progression in the severity of obstruction differs in various studies (Fig. 29-30). Recent studies have shown that congenital aortic stenosis is frequently a progressive disorder, even early in life, in a significant fraction of patients presenting initially with mild obstruction.[228-236] Thus, clinical deterioration may be anticipated because of an intensification in the severity of stenosis rather than the development of significant aortic regurgitation. Progression of obstruction is usually the result of the increase in cardiac output that occurs concurrent with increased body growth. Less often, a decrease in the area of the orifice is an added factor in the intensification of obstruction. The onset of symptoms or changes in the phonocardiogram or graphic pulse tracings, chest roentgenograms, electrocardiograms, or vectorcardiograms cannot be depended upon to indicate progressive obstruction in the individual patient.

Management. The malformed aortic valve is a potential site of bacterial infection; antibiotic prophylaxis is recommended for all patients, regardless of the severity of obstruction. Strict avoidance of strenuous physical activity is advised if severe aortic stenosis is present. Participation in competitive sports should probably also be restricted in patients with milder degrees of obstruction. Digitalis should be administered to patients who have symptoms of diminished cardiac reserve and should also be considered in patients with left ventricular hypertrophy, even if they are not in heart failure.

The most important decision concerns the advisability of *surgical treatment.* Among the factors influencing the indi-

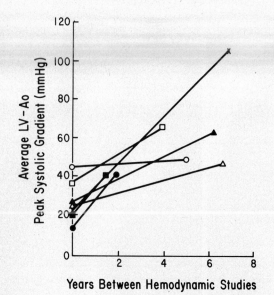

Years Between Hemodynamic Studies

REFERENCE	NUMBER OF PATIENTS	AVERAGE AGE (yrs.)	
		1st CATH	2nd CATH
■ HOHN et al.	4	6,10,10,45	N.A.
● BENTIVOGLIO et al.	1	27	29
□ EL-SAID et al.	18	7	11
○ HURWITZ	19	9	14
▲ FRIEDMAN et al.	9	6.8	13.1
△ COHEN et al.	15	8.5	15.1
X BANDY and VOGEL	1	5	12

FIGURE 29-30 Composite of serial hemodynamic studies from seven medical centers[228-234] showing the relationships between time and the left ventricular (LV)–aortic (Ao) pressure gradients in patients with congenital aortic stenosis. (From Friedman, W. F., et al.: Congenital aortic stenosis in adults. *In* Roberts, W. C. (ed.): Congenital Heart Disease in Adults. Philadelphia, F. A. Davis, 1979, p. 235.)

cations, techniques, and results of operation are the patient's age, the nature of the valvular deformity, and the experience of the surgical team.[207] The recommendation that operation is indicated depends more often on the presence of severe obstruction than on the symptoms described by the patient. At the present time, operation is advised for any child with critical stenosis (i.e., a peak systolic pressure gradient exceeding 75 mm Hg, measured in the basal state when the cardiac output is normal) or a calculated effective orifice less than 0.5 cm^2/m^2 body surface area. In the presence of clinical symptoms, a left ventricular strain pattern on the electrocardiogram, or an abnormal exercise electrocardiogram, operation may be recommended with less rigid regard to the hemodynamic assessment of the severity of stenosis. After severe stenosis has been established hemodynamically, the potential hazard of sudden death dictates that surgical treatment not be postponed unnecessarily. Operation is carried out under direct vision after institution of cardiopulmonary bypass; judicious incision of the fused commissures enlarges the valve orifice and does not result in significant aortic regurgitation. A mortality rate less than 2 percent can be expected when operation is performed by an experienced surgeon. Substantial relief of obstruction occurs in the majority of patients unless the valve ring is hypoplastic.[237]

Long-term follow-up studies have provided evidence that aortic valvulotomy is a safe and effective means of treatment with excellent relief of symptoms that were present preoperatively.[238,239] In some patients, aortic regurgita-

tion may be progressive and require prosthetic valve replacement. Moreover, following commissurotomy the valve leaflets remain somewhat deformed, and it is quite possible that further degenerative changes, including calcification, will lead to significant stenosis in later years.[240] Thus, prosthetic valve replacement may be required in a significant number of patients beyond the fifth decade of life. Since the valves are not rendered anatomically normal, antibiotic prophylaxis is indicated in all patients postoperatively, even if the systolic pressure gradient has been abolished completely.

DISCRETE SUBAORTIC STENOSIS

This malformation accounts for 8 to 10 per cent of all cases of congenital aortic stenosis and occurs twice as frequently in males as in females. The lesion consists of a membranous diaphragm or fibrous ring encircling the left ventricular outflow tract just beneath the base of the aortic valve.

Distinction of subvalvular from valvular aortic stenosis is extremely difficult by means of clinical findings alone.[206] A systolic ejection sound is rarely heard, and the diastolic murmur of aortic regurgitation is more common than it is in valvular aortic stenosis. Dilatation of the ascending aorta is common, but valvular calcification is not observed.

Echocardiography may be useful in the differentiation between valvular and subvalvular stenosis.[241,242] Using single-crystal methods, a fine, high-intensity echo in the left ventricular outflow tract may suggest the presence of a subaortic diaphragm. Multiple, thick echoes below the sinuses of Valsalva and from a level near the annular attachment of the anterior mitral leaflet have been observed with fibromuscular subaortic obstruction. Cross-sectional echo studies demonstrate persistent, prominent echoes in the subaortic left ventricle in both systole and diastole.[241] Most importantly, echocardiography also has the potential for identifying hypertrophic subaortic stenosis when it coexists with fixed subaortic stenosis and for differentiating between the two forms of obstruction.[243]

Definitive distinction between valvular and subvalvular obstruction is best provided by recording pressure tracings as a catheter is withdrawn across the outflow tract and valve or by localizing the site of obstruction with selective left ventricular angiocardiography (Fig. 29-29).

Mild degrees of aortic valvular regurgitation are commonly observed in patients with discrete subaortic stenosis and appear to be caused by thickening of the valve and impaired mobility of the cusps secondary to the trauma created by the high-velocity jet passing through the subaortic diaphragm. Further deformation of these abnormal valve cusps by the vegetations of bacterial endocarditis often results in severe aortic regurgitation.

Because of the likelihood of both progressive obstruction and aortic regurgitation, the presence of even mild or moderate subaortic stenosis warrants consideration of elective operation.[244,245] The risks of operation in patients with discrete subaortic stenosis and valvular aortic stenosis are essentially the same. Surgical correction is accomplished by excising the membrane or fibrous ridge. Operation may be expected to improve the hemodynamic state substantially; frequently it is totally curative.[246,247] In a small number of patients, secondary muscular hypertrophy of the outflow tract and a pressure gradient may persist following the operative relief of valvular or discrete subvalvular aortic stenosis.[248]

UNCOMMON FORMS OF SUBAORTIC STENOSIS.

In some patients, valvular and subvalvular aortic stenosis coexist, producing a tunnel-like narrowing of the left ventricular outflow tract.[249] Additional findings often include a small ascending aorta, hypoplasia of the aortic valve ring, and thickened valve leaflets. The subvalvular fibrous process usually extends onto the aortic valve cusps and almost always makes contact with the ventricular aspect of the anterior mitral leaflet at its base. The presence of "tunnel stenosis" may be suspected angiographically from the appearance of the outflow tract and the aortic root. Operative treatment is often complicated by the necessity for prosthetic replacement of the aortic valve as well as for enlarging the aortic annulus, proximal aorta, and left ventricular outlet tract. Recently, operation has been recommended utilizing a prosthetic, valve-containing conduit between the left ventricular apex and descending aorta.[250]

Various anatomical lesions other than a discrete membrane or ridge may produce subaortic stenosis.[206] Among these are abnormal adherence of the anterior leaflet of the mitral valve to the left septal surface, and the presence in the left ventricular outflow tract of accessory endocardial cushion tissue. In some patients with atrioventricular canal, the part of the ventricular septum that contributes to the wall of the left ventricular outflow tract is deficient, and the ventricular aspect of the anterior leaflet of the common atrioventricular valve is adherent to the posterior edge of the deficient septum, resulting in a narrow left ventricular outflow tract. Malalignment of the conoventricular septum, resulting in an inferior ventricular septal defect, produces a leftward superior deviation and insertion of the conal septum obstructing left ventricular outflow. In patients with single ventricle and an outflow chamber, the bulboventricular foramen serves as a potential site of aortic outflow obstruction. Additional, rarer causes of subaortic stenosis include redundant dysplastic left atrioventricular valve tissue in patients with congenitally corrected transposition of the great arteries and anomalous muscle bundles of the left ventricular outflow tract.[251,252] A muscular type of subaortic stenosis may result from a convergence of all the mitral chordae into one or two fused papillary muscles; a "parachute" deformity of the mitral valve is produced that is often seen in association with supravalvular stenosis of the left atrium and coarctation of the aorta. In some of these patients, discrete membranous subvalvular aortic obstruction has also been noted.[253]

In patients with ventricular septal defect, muscular subaortic stenosis has been shown to develop after surgical banding of the pulmonary artery, possibly as a result of hypertrophy of the conal septum or crista supraventricularis encroaching on the left ventricular outflow tract above the septal defect.

Subaortic muscular hypertrophy secondary to diffuse involvement of the myocardium by glycogen storage disease (Pompe's disease) is an extremely rare cause of obstruction to left ventricular outflow. A positive family history, symptoms of muscular weakness, heart failure in infancy, and the characteristic electrocardiographic findings of a short PR interval, high-voltage QRS and T waves, and left ventricular hypertrophy warrant skeletal muscle biopsy or fibroblast culture, permitting a premortem diagnosis.

The last relatively uncommon form of subaortic stenosis to be mentioned occurs infrequently in patients with congenitally corrected transposition of the great arteries in whom an anomalous muscle bundle in the subaortic area of the arterial ventricle obstructs outflow.

Supravalvular Aortic Stenosis

Supravalvular aortic stenosis is a congenital narrowing of the ascending aorta that may be localized or diffuse, originating at the superior margin of the sinuses of Valsalva just above the levels of the coronary arteries.

The clinical picture of supravalvular obstruction usually differs in major respects from that observed in the other forms of aortic stenosis. Chief among these differences is the association of supravalvular aortic stenosis with idiopathic infantile hypercalcemia, a disease that may be related to deranged vitamin D metabolism.[254-258] The designation "supravalvular aortic stenosis syndrome" or "Williams' syndrome" is applied to the distinctive clinical picture produced by coexistence of the cardiac and multiple system disorder. Additional manifestations of this syndrome include a peculiar "elfin" facies (Fig. 29–31), mental retardation, narrowing of peripheral systemic and pulmonary arteries, inguinal hernia, strabismus, and abnormalities of dental development. In some patients, moderate thickening of the aortic cusps and valvular pulmonary stenosis may occur in association with peripheral pulmonary artery stenosis. Rarely, patients have mitral valve abnormalities with prolapse and mitral regurgitation.

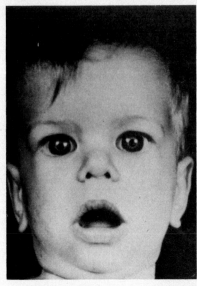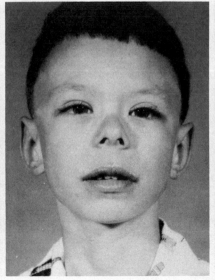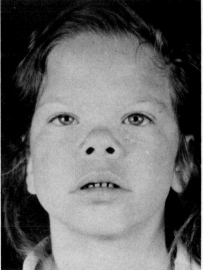

FIGURE 29–31 Typical elfin facies in three patients with supravalvular aortic stenosis. (From Friedman, W. F., and Kirkpatrick, S. E.: Congenital aortic stenosis. *In* Moss, A. J., Adams, F. H., and Emmanouilides, G. C. (eds.): Heart Disease in Infants, Children and Adolescents, 2nd ed. Baltimore, Williams and Wilkins, 1977.)

Experimental hypervitaminosis D produced in the pregnant rabbit has caused craniofacial abnormalities and malformations resembling those of supravalvular aortic stenosis in the offspring.[254-256] In humans, with one exception, chromosome studies have consistently revealed normal karyotypes. Most often supravalvular aortic stenosis is a feature of the distinctive syndrome described above. However, peripheral pulmonary artery stenosis and the aortic anomaly are also seen in familial and sporadic forms unassociated with the other features of the syndrome.[259] Genetic studies suggest that the familial anomaly is transmitted as an autosomal dominant with variable expression. Some family members may have supravalvular pulmonic stenosis either as an isolated lesion or in combination with the supravalvular aortic anomaly. Unlike the other forms of aortic stenosis, there appears to be no sex predilection.

Three anatomical types of supravalvular aortic stenosis are recognized, although some patients may have findings of more than one type. Most common is the hourglass type, in which marked thickening and disorganization of the aortic media produce a constricting annular ridge at the superior margin of the sinuses of Valsalva. The membranous type is the result of fibrous or fibromuscular semicircular diaphragm with a small central opening stretched across the lumen of the aorta. Uniform hypoplasia of the ascending aorta characterizes the hypoplastic type.

Because the coronary arteries arise proximal to the site of outflow obstruction in supravalvular aortic stenosis, they are subjected to the elevated pressure that exists within the left ventricle. These vessels are often dilated and tortuous, and premature coronary arteriosclerosis has been observed. Moreover, if the free edges of some or all of the aortic cusps adhere to the site of supravalvular stenosis, coronary artery inflow may be reduced. The formation of thoracic aortic aneurysms has been described in several patients.

Most often, patients with supravalvular aortic stenosis syndrome are mentally retarded and resemble one another in their facial features. The typical appearance is similar to the "elfin" facies observed in the severe form of idiopathic infantile hypercalcemia and is characterized by a high prominent forehead, epicanthal folds, underdeveloped bridge of the nose and mandible, overhanging upper lip, strabismus, and anomalies of dentition (Fig. 29–31). Recognition of this distinctive appearance, even in infancy, should alert the physician to the possibility of underlying multiple system disease. In addition, a positive family history in a patient with a normal appearance and clinical signs suggesting left ventricular outflow obstruction should lead to the suspicion of either supravalvular aortic stenosis or hypertrophic obstructive cardiomyopathy. Patients with supravalvular aortic obstruction appear to be subject to the same risks of unexpected sudden death and infective endocarditis as those with valvular aortic stenosis.

With few exceptions, the major *physical findings* resemble those observed in patients with valvular aortic stenosis. Among these exceptions are accentuation of aortic valve closure due to elevated pressure in the aorta proximal to the stenosis, an infrequent systolic ejection sound, and the especially prominent transmission of a thrill and murmur into the jugular notch and along the carotid vessels. Uncommonly, there is an early diastolic, decrescendo, blowing murmur of aortic regurgitation due to the fusion of one or more cusps to the area of stenosis. The narrowing of the peripheral pulmonary arteries that often coexists in these patients frequently produces a late systolic or continuous murmur that may help distinguish this anomaly from valvular aortic stenosis. This differentiation is reinforced by the frequent finding of a significant disparity between the arterial pressures in the upper extremities in supravalvular aortic stenosis; the systolic pressure in the right arm tends to be the higher of the two and occasionally exceeds that in the femoral arteries. The disparity in pulses may relate to the tendency of a jet stream to adhere to a vessel wall (Coanda effect) and selective streaming of blood into the innominate artery.[260,261]

Electrocardiography generally reveals left ventricular hypertrophy when obstruction is severe. However, biventricular, or even right ventricular, hypertrophy may be found if significant narrowing of peripheral pulmonary arteries coexists. In a number of patients without significant right-sided lesions the vectorcardiogram has shown displacement of the maximum transverse QRS loop rightward and posteriorly and a tendency for initial forces to be directed leftward, perhaps reflecting posterobasal left ventricular hypertrophy or a manifestation of left posterior hemiblock.[262] Radiographically, in contrast to valvular and discrete subvalvular aortic stenosis, poststenotic dilation of the ascending aorta is rarely seen. Usually the sinuses of Valsalva are dilated and ascending aorta and the aortic arch are of normal size or appear small. Retrograde aortic catheterization is the most valuable technique for localizing the site of obstruction to the supravalvular area and determining the degree of hemodynamic abnormality (Fig. 29–32).

The supravalvular aortic lumen may be widened by the insertion of an oval- or diamond-shaped fabric patch in those patients with a normal ascending aorta. If the aorta is hypoplastic, this operation merely displaces the pressure gradient distally without abolishing the obstruction. Under these circumstances, repair may require replacement or widening of the entire hypoplastic aorta with an appropriate prosthesis. Operation may be recommended when relatively little hypoplasia of the ascending aorta and arch

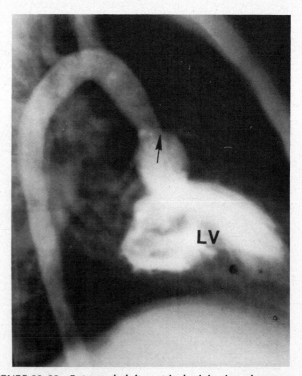

FIGURE 29–32 Retrograde left ventricular injection of contrast material in a patient with supravalvular aortic stenosis showing dilated sinuses of Valsalva and an aortic constriction just above the sinuses (arrow). **LV** = left ventricle.

exists and when the obstruction is discrete and severe, i.e., with a systolic gradient exceeding 75 mm Hg.

Hypoplastic Left Heart Syndrome

This designation is used to describe a group of closely related cardiac anomalies characterized by underdevelopment of the left cardiac chambers, atresia or stenosis of the aortic and/or the mitral orifices, and hypoplasia of the aorta.[263,264] These anomalies are an especially common cause of heart failure in the first week of life. The left atrium and ventricle often exhibit *endocardial fibroelastosis*. Pulmonary venous blood traverses a patent foramen ovale and a dilated and hypertrophied right ventricle acts as the systemic, as well as the pulmonary, ventricle; the systemic circulation receives blood via a patent ductus arteriosus (Fig. 29–33). The diagnosis should be considered in infants, particularly males, with the sudden onset of heart failure, systemic hypoperfusion, and nonspecific murmur. Electrocardiography frequently reveals right axis deviation, right atrial and ventricular enlargement, and ST and T-wave abnormalities in the left precordial leads. Chest roentgenography may show only slight enlargement shortly after birth, but with clinical deterioration there is marked cardiomegaly and increased pulmonary venous and arterial vascular markings.

The echocardiographic findings may be diagnostic and include a diminutive aortic root and left ventricular cavity and absence or poor visualization of aortic and mitral valve echoes, which, when seen, are of diminished amplitude and mobility.[265,266]

Medical therapy directed at cardiac decompensation,

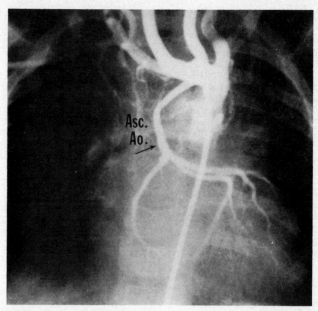

FIGURE 29–34 Retrograde aortogram showing marked hypoplasia of the ascending aorta (Asc. Ao.) (arrow) in an infant with hypoplastic left heart syndrome. (From Freedom, R. M., et al.: Aortic atresia with normal left ventricle: Distinctive angiocardiographic findings. Cath. Cardiovasc. Diag. *3*:283, 1977.)

hypoxemia, and metabolic acidemia rarely allows survival beyond the first days of life. Constriction of the patent ductus arteriosus and limited flow through a restrictive patent foramen ovale are the principal factors responsible for early death.[263,267] At present the anatomical lesions are not correctable (Fig. 29–34). Some centers are attempting staged surgical management in an effort to provide long-term palliation.[268,269] The first stage consists of creating an unobstructed communication between the right ventricle and aorta, usually with a prosthetic conduit connecting the pulmonary artery to the aorta; pulmonary blood flow and pressure are limited by a controlled opening in the conduit to the distal pulmonary artery. A large interatrial communication must also be assured in stage I. In stage II, an interatrial baffle is created to provide continuity between left atrium and tricuspid valve; the pulmonary arterial circulation is provided by anastomosis of the right atrium to the pulmonary arteries.

AORTIC REGURGITATION

Congenital aortic valve regurgitation is an extremely rare isolated congenital cardiac lesion.[270] Most often aortic regurgitation occurs in association with congenital valvular aortic stenosis in which the valve commissures are fused inhibiting cusp mobility, subvalvular aortic stenosis in which the aortic ring is dilated and the valve cusps are deformed, coarctation of the aorta when the aortic ring is dilated and the aortic valve is bicuspid, ventricular septal defect (see p. 965), and endocardial fibroelastosis.[271] Aortic valve regurgitation may also accompany aortic sinus aneurysm or be secondary to dilatation of the ascending aorta in patients with Marfan syndrome, cystic medial necrosis, or osteogenesis imperfecta in which the aortic lesions are manifestations of the underlying connective tissue disorder (Chap. 48).

Severe aortic regurgitation may also occur through channels other than the aortic valve.[272] Thus, aortico–left ventricular tunnel is a rare anomaly that must be distinguished from congenital aortic valve regurgitation, since the approach to management of the former does not usually include consideration for prosthetic valve replacement.

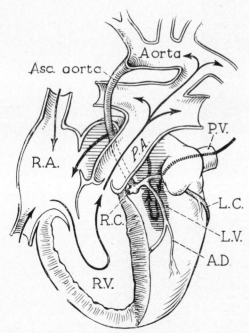

FIGURE 29–33 Hypoplastic left heart with aortic hypoplasia, aortic valve atresia, and a hypoplastic mitral valve and left ventricle. R.A. = right atrium; R.V. = right ventricle; R.C. = right coronary; P.A. = pulmonary artery; P.V. = pulmonary vein; L.C. = left coronary artery; L.V. = left ventricle; A.D. = anterior descending coronary artery. (From Neufeld, H. N., et al.: Diagnosis of aortic atresia by retrograde aortography. Circulation *25*:278, 1962, by permission of the American Heart Association, Inc.)

The aortico–left ventricular tunnel is an abnormal channel beginning in the ascending aorta above the right coronary orifice and ending in the left ventricle below the right aortic cusp. The channel usually passes behind the right ventricular infundibulum and through the ventricular septum.

Aortography is necessary to establish a precise diagnosis. In infants and children with congenital aortic valve insufficiency the severity of regurgitation increases with time, and valve replacement, rather than plication, is almost always necessary to correct the lesion. Operation should be deferred until symptoms and signs dictate its necessity.[273] Conversely, closure of an aortico–left ventricular communication is advisable before progressive dilation of the aortic annulus creates secondary changes in the aortic valve itself which may necessitate aortic valve replacement.

PULMONARY VEIN ATRESIA AND STENOSIS

Pulmonary vein atresia is a quite rare anomaly in which the pulmonary veins do not connect with the heart or with a major systemic vein.[274] The lesion is incompatible with life, but infants may survive for days, probably because communications exist between the pulmonary veins and the bronchial or esophageal veins that allow limited egress for pulmonary venous blood. Pulmonary vein stenosis may occur as a focal stenosis at the atrial junction or generalized hypoplasia of one or more pulmonary veins. There is an extremely high incidence of associated cardiac malformations, including atrial septal defect, tetralogy of Fallot, tricuspid and mitral atresia, and endocardial cushion defect. The severe pulmonary vein obstruction imposed by pulmonary vein abnormalities causes severe cyanosis, congestive cardiac failure, and early death. Focal stenosis of one or more pulmonary veins at the atrial junction, recognized on angiography, may be relieved surgically.

COR TRIATRIATUM

In this malformation failure of resorption of the common pulmonary vein results in a left atrium divided by an abnormal fibromuscular diaphragm into a posterosuperior chamber receiving the pulmonary veins and an anteroinferior chamber giving rise to the left atrial appendage and leading to the mitral orifice.[274,275] The communication between the divided atrial chambers may be large, small, or absent depending on the size of the opening(s) in the subdividing diaphragm, which determines the degree of obstruction to pulmonary venous return.[276] Elevations of both pulmonary venous pressure and pulmonary vascular resistance result in severe pulmonary artery hypertension. The diagnosis should be suspected at cardiac catheterization if the pulmonary arterial wedge pressure is higher than a simultaneous left atrial pressure. The diagnosis is established by visualizing the obstructing lesion angiographically (Fig. 29–35). Although rare, it is important to recognize the malformation because it may be easily correctable at operation.[276,277]

MITRAL STENOSIS

Anatomical types of mitral stenosis include the parachute deformity of the valve, in which shortened chordae tendineae converge and insert into a single large papillary muscle; thickened leaflets with shortening and fusion of the chordae tendineae; an anomalous arcade of obstructing papillary muscles; accessory mitral valve tissue; and a supravalvular circumferential ridge of connective tissue arising at the base of the atrial aspect of the mitral leaflets.[278,279] Associated cardiac defects are common, including endocardial fibroelastosis, coarctation of the aorta, patent ductus arteriosus, and left ventricular outflow tract ob-

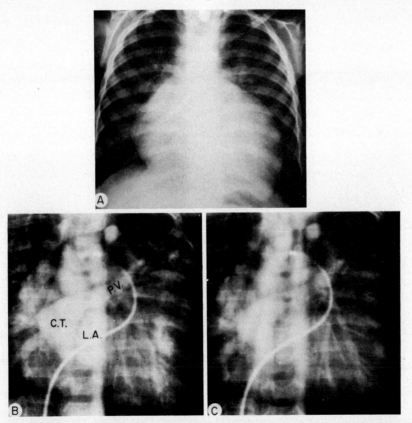

FIGURE 29–35   Chest roentgenogram (A) and levophase of pulmonary angiogram (B and C) in an infant with cor triatriatum (C.T.). The left atrium (L.A.) is divided by a radiolucent diaphragm; the upper chamber receives the pulmonary veins (P.V.). (Courtesy of Delores A. Danilowicz, M.D.)

struction. The clinical and hemodynamic consequences of isolated congenital mitral stenosis are similar to those of acquired mitral obstruction with modifications imposed by coexisting anomalies.[278,280,281] The prognosis is poor; symptoms attributable to pulmonary vein obstruction begin usually in infancy and the majority of patients expire before age one year.

MITRAL REGURGITATION

The syndrome of *mitral valve prolapse* is discussed on pages 1089 to 1094. This condition is generally quite benign in children. However, occasional difficulties exist with infective endocarditis, arrhythmias, atypical chest pain, and sudden death.

Isolated congenital mitral regurgitation of hemodynamic significance is an unusual lesion in infants and children. Most often, congenital malformations of the mitral valve producing insufficiency are encountered in association with endocardial cushion defect, congenitally corrected transposition of the great arteries, endocardial fibroelastosis, anomalous pulmonary origin of the coronary artery, congenital subaortic stenosis, hypertrophic obstructive cardiomyopathy, and coarctation of the aorta. Mitral valve dysfunction is also seen commonly in a variety of metabolic disorders (e.g., the mucopolysaccharidoses), primary and secondary cardiomyopathies, connective tissue disease (e.g., rheumatoid arthritis, Marfan syndrome, Ehlers-Danlos syndrome, pseudoxanthoma elasticum), and rheumatic and nonrheumatic inflammatory diseases of the myocardium[281] (see Chap. 48).

The various anatomical lesions that result in isolated congenital mitral regurgitation include prolapse of one or both mitral leaflets, cleft or perforated mitral leaflet, inadequate leaflet tissue, double orifice of the mitral valve, anomalous insertion of chordae tendineae (anomalous mitral arcade), redundant leaflet tissue, displacement inferiorly of the ring of the inferior leaflet into the left ventricle, and abnormal length of chordae tendineae.[282–288] The clinical and hemodynamic findings in patients with isolated congenital mitral incompetence resemble those observed in acquired mitral regurgitation. Mitral annuloplasty (which is preferred) or prosthetic valve replacement are procedures reserved for infants or children who are at least moderately symptomatic despite comprehensive medical management, often with repeated episodes of pulmonary infection, or cardiac failure with anorexia and retarded growth and development.[287,287a] Operative candidates are shown at hemodynamic and angiographic study to have pulmonary hypertension, a regurgitant fraction in excess of 50 per cent, and a marked increase in left ventricular end-diastolic volume.

PULMONARY ARTERIOVENOUS FISTULA

Abnormal development of the pulmonary arteries and veins in a common vascular complex is responsible for this rare congenital anomaly. A variable number of pulmonary arteries communicate directly with branches of the pulmonary veins; in some cases the fistula receives systemic arterial branches.[289] The majority of patients have an associated Weber-Osler-Rendu syndrome; additional associated problems include bronchiectasis and other malformations of the bronchial tree, and absence of the right lower lobe. Venoarterial shunting depends upon the extent of the fistulous communications and may result in cyanosis and secondary polycythemia. Patients with hereditary hemorrhagic telangiectasis are often anemic owing to repeated blood loss and may have less obvious cyanosis. Systolic and continuous murmurs are audible over areas of the fistula(s). Rounded opacities of variable size in one or both lungs on chest roentgenogram may suggest the presence of the lesion. Pulmonary angiography reveals the site and extent of the abnormal communication. Unless the lesions are widespread throughout both lungs, surgical treatment aimed at removing the lesions with preservation of healthy lung tissue is indicated to avoid the complications of massive hemorrhage, bacterial endocarditis, and rupture of arteriovenous aneurysms.

PERIPHERAL PULMONARY ARTERY STENOSIS

Stenosis of the pulmonary artery may be single or multiple and occur anywhere from the main pulmonary trunk to the smaller peripheral arterial branches. Associated defects are observed in the majority of patients and include pulmonic valvular stenosis, ventricular septal defect, tetralogy of Fallot, and supravalvular aortic stenosis.

The most important cause of significant pulmonary artery stenoses producing symptoms in the newborn is intrauterine rubella infection.[290] Diagnosis is facilitated in these infants by finding elevations of the IgM fraction and rubella antibody titer. Other cardiovascular malformations seen commonly in association with congenital rubella include patent ductus arteriosus, pulmonic valve stenosis, and atrial septal defect. Generalized systemic arterial stenotic lesions may also be a feature of the rubella embryopathy, often involving large and medium-sized vessels such as the aorta and coronary, cerebral, mesenteric, and renal arteries. Cardiovascular lesions are but one manifestation of intrauterine rubella infection, since cataracts, microphthalmia, deafness, thrombocytopenia, hepatitis, and blood dyscrasias are also common. Thus, the clinical picture in infants with rubella syndrome depends upon the severity of the cardiovascular lesions and the associated abnormalities of other organs and systems.

Obstruction within the pulmonary arterial tree may be classified into four types: (1) stenosis of the main pulmonary trunk or the main left or right branch; (2) narrowing at the bifurcation of the pulmonary artery, extending into both right and left branches; (3) multiple sites of peripheral branch stenosis; and (4) a combination of main and peripheral stenosis. Pulmonary artery obstruction may be produced by localized narrowing, diffuse constrictions, or rarely, by a membrane or diaphragm. Post-stenotic dilatation is usual when the stenosis is localized, but may be absent or minimal with elongated constriction. It should be recognized that a physiological branch pulmonary artery stenosis is often present in the normal newborn in whom both right and left main pulmonary arteries are small and arise almost perpendicular from a large main pulmonary artery.[291] The branch vessels increase in size with growth and become less angulated in their takeoff from the main pulmonary artery.

The degree of obstruction is the principal determinant of clinical severity; the type of obstruction determines the feasibility of direct surgical relief. The clinical features vary; most infants and children are asymptomatic.[292,293] An ejection systolic murmur at the upper left sternal border that is well transmitted to the axillae and back is most common. The presence of an ejection sound suggests that pulmonic valve stenosis coexists. The pulmonic component of the second heart sound may be slightly accentuated, but occasionally is extremely loud if multiple peripheral stenoses exist. A continuous murmur is audible, expecially in patients with main or branch stenosis, and particularly if an associated cardiovascular anomaly produces increased pulmonary blood flow. Electrocardiography shows right ventricular hypertrophy when obstruction is severe; left axis deviation with counterclockwise orientation of the frontal QRS vector is common in the rubella syndrome and when the lesion coexists with supravalvular

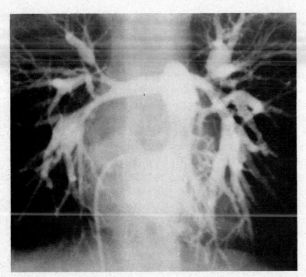

FIGURE 29–36 Right ventricular angiocardiogram showing multiple sites of peripheral pulmonic stenosis and post-stenotic dilatation of the peripheral pulmonic arteries.

aortic stenosis. Mild or moderate stenosis usually produces a normal chest roentgenogram; detectable differences in vascularity between regions of the lungs or dilated pulmonary artery segments are uncommon. When obstruction is bilateral and severe, right atrial and ventricular enlargement may be observed.

Diagnosis is confirmed by observing pressure gradients within the pulmonary arterial system at cardiac catheterization; selective pulmonary angiography defines the exact location, extent, and distribution of the lesion (Fig. 29–36). Mild to moderate unilateral or bilateral stenosis does not require surgical relief; numerous stenotic areas are not amenable to correction. Well-localized obstruction of severe degree in the main pulmonary artery or its major branches may be alleviated with a patch graft or bypassed with a tubular conduit. The natural history of peripheral pulmonary stenosis is not clear.[292] Obstruction may increase by discrepant growth between a stenotic area and normal portions of the pulmonary artery tree, or as a result of an increase in cardiac output, especially during adolescence. Rarely, hypertrophy is progressive of right ventricular infundibular muscle and results in hypercyanotic spells.

Pulmonic Stenosis with Intact Ventricular Septum

Valvular pulmonic stenosis, resulting from fusion of the valve cusps during mid to late intrauterine development, is the most common form of isolated right ventricular obstruction and occurs in approximately 7 per cent of patients with congenital heart disease. Hypertrophy of the septal and parietal bands narrowing the right ventricular infundibulum often accompanies the pulmonic valve lesion, especially if it is severe. Fused cusps of varying thickness and rigidity form a fibrous dome in the most severe forms. Pulmonic valve dysplasia, especially common in patients with Noonan's syndrome (p. 1614), produces obstruction in the absence of adherent leaflets because leaflets are thickened, rigid, and myxomatous and are limited in their lateral movement because of the presence of tissue pads within the pulmonic valve sinuses.[294,295]

INFANCY. The clinical presentation and course of circulation in the newborn with pulmonic stenosis depends on the severity of obstruction and the degree of development of the right ventricle and its outflow tract, the tricuspid valve, and the pulmonary arterial tree.[296-298] The greater the degree of pulmonic valve stenosis, the more closely the manifestations resemble those observed with pulmonary atresia and intact ventricular septum (see p. 988). Severe pulmonic stenosis is characterized by cyanosis due to right-to-left shunting through the foramen ovale, cardiomegaly, and diminished pulmonary blood flow in the absence of persistent patency of the ductus arteriosus. Hypoxemia and metabolic acidemia, rather than right ventricular failure, are the main clinical disturbances in the symptomatic infant. Distinction of these babies from those with tetralogy of Fallot or tricuspid or pulmonary atresia is usually possible, since infants with tetralogy generally do not have roentgenographic evidence of cardiomegaly; infants with tricuspid and pulmonary atresia show a preponderance of left ventricular forces by electrocardiography in contrast to the right ventricular hypertrophy observed usually with critical pulmonic stenosis in the absence of right ventricular hypoplasia. Cardiac catheterization and angiographic studies establish a precise diagnosis (Fig. 29–37). Pulmonary valvotomy is the operative procedure of choice, but a systemic-to-pulmonary arterial shunt may also be necessary in infants with underdevelopment of the right ventricular cavity.[296]

CHILDHOOD. The clinical profile of patients with valvular pulmonic stenosis beyond infancy is generally distinctive.[299] The severity of obstruction is the most important determinant of the clinical course. In the presence of a normal cardiac output a peak systolic transvalvular pressure gradient between 50 and 80 mm Hg or a peak systolic right ventricular pressure between 75 and 100 mm Hg is considered to be moderate stenosis; levels below and above that range are classified as mild and severe, respectively. Patients with mild pulmonic stenosis are generally asymptomatic and are discovered during routine examination. In patients with more significant obstruction the severity of stenosis may increase with time. Progression may be relative and reflect disproportionate physical growth of the patient, infundibular narrowing due to progressive hypertrophy of the right ventricular outflow tract, or fibrosis of the valve cusps. Symptoms, when present, vary from mild exertional dyspnea and mild cyanosis to signs and symptoms of heart failure depending upon the degree of obstruction and the level of myocardial compensation. Exertional fatigue, syncope, and chest pain are related to an inability to augment pulmonary blood flow during exercise in some patients with moderate or severe obstruction.

The severity of obstruction is often suggested by the physical findings. Right ventricular hypertrophy reduces compliance of that chamber and a forceful right atrial contraction is necessary to augment right ventricular filling. Prominent a-waves in the jugular venous pulse, a fourth heart sound, and occasionally, presystolic pulsations of the liver reflect a vigorous atrial contraction and suggest the presence of severe stenosis. Cardiomegaly and a right ventricular parasternal lift accompany moderate or severe obstruction. A systolic thrill is palpable along the upper left sternal border in all but the mildest forms of stenosis. The

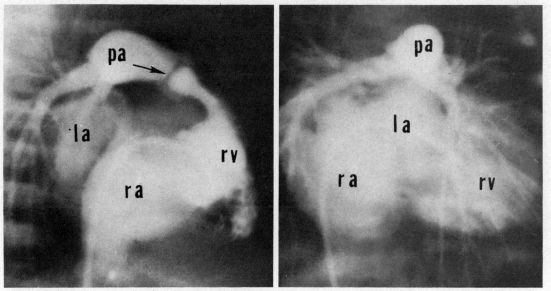

FIGURE 29–37 Right ventriculogram in an infant with critical pulmonic stenosis shows the thickened, nonmobile pulmonic valve (arrow) in the lateral projection (*left*). Both the lateral and frontal (*right*) projections show regurgitation of contrast material across the tricuspid valve into the right atrium (ra), with subsequent shunting across the foramen ovale to the left atrium (la). rv = right ventricle; pa = pulmonary artery. (Courtesy of Norman Talner, M.D.)

first heart sound is normal and is followed by a systolic ejection sound at the upper left sternal edge produced by sudden opening of the stenotic valve; an ejection sound is not heard in patients with pulmonic valve dysplasia. The ejection sound typically is louder during expiration; when it is inaudible or occurs less than 0.08 second from the onset of the Q wave on electrocardiogram, severe obstruction is suggested. Right ventricular ejection is prolonged in patients with moderate or severe stenosis and the sound of pulmonic valve closure is delayed and soft. The characteristic feature of valvular pulmonic stenosis on auscultation is a harsh, diamond-shaped systolic ejection murmur heard best at the upper left sternal border. The systolic murmur becomes louder and its crescendo occurs later in systole, obscuring the aortic component of the second sound with more severe degrees of valvular obstruction, since these patients have a greater prolongation of right ventricular systole. The holosystolic decrescendo murmur of tricuspid regurgitation may accompany severe pulmonic stenosis, especially in the presence of congestive heart failure. Cyanosis, reflecting venoarterial shunting through a patent foramen ovale, is absent with mild stenosis and infrequent with moderate obstruction. However, cyanosis may not be apparent in patients with severe obstruction if the atrial septum is intact.

Electro- and *vectorcardiography* may be helpful in assessing the degree of obstruction to right ventricular output.[300] In mild cases the electrocardiogram is often normal, whereas moderate and severe stenoses are associated with right axis deviation and right ventricular hypertrophy. A tall QR wave in the right precordial leads with T-wave inversion and ST-segment suppression (right ventricular "strain") reflects severe stenosis. When an rSR′ pattern is observed in lead V_1 (20 per cent of patients) generally lower right ventricular pressures are found than in patients with a pure R wave of equal amplitude. High amplitude P waves in leads II and V_1 indicating right atrial enlargement are associated with severe stenosis. The vectorcardiogram shows clockwise rotation of the QRS loop in the horizontal plane with a leftward anterior direction of initial forces, followed by a broad limb directed to the right anteriorly. Chest roentgenography in patients with mild or moderate pulmonic stenosis often shows a heart of normal size and normal pulmonary vascularity. Poststenotic dilatation of the main and left pulmonary arteries is often evident. Right atrial and right ventricular enlargement are observed in patients with severe obstruction and resultant right ventricular failure. The pulmonary vascularity may be reduced in patients with severe stenosis, right ventricular failure, and/or a venoarterial shunt at the atrial level. Echocardiography may be of limited value because of technical difficulties in imaging the pulmonic valve.[301] Complete opening of the pulmonic valve with atrial systole ("*a*" wave of a pulmonic valve echogram) may be seen with severe stenosis. Moreover, prolongation beyond 480 msec of the interval between the onset of the QRS complex of the electrocardiogram and the point of pulmonic valve cusp closure reflects the prolonged right ventricular ejection time associated with severe obstruction.

Cardiac catheterization and *angiocardiography* with right ventricular injection localizes the site of obstruction, evaluates its severity, and documents the coexistence of additional cardiac malformations (Fig. 29–38). The resting cardiac output is usually normal, even in cases of severe stenosis, and most children show the ability to increase cardiac output with exercise.[302,303] Right ventricular dysfunction occurs especially when venoarterial shunting is significant and produces systemic arterial desaturation.[304,305] In patients with critical stenosis, care must be taken during hemodynamic study that the cardiac catheter does not dangerously occlude the stenotic valve opening. The angiographic appearance of a typical valvular pulmonic stenosis differs from that of a dysplastic valve. The former is thickened and domes during systole, returning to a normal con-

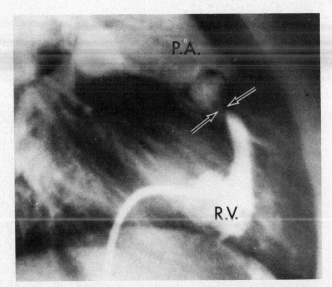

FIGURE 29–38 Lateral view of a right ventricular (R.V.) angiogram in a patient with severe pulmonic stenosis shows a thickened, domed pulmonic valve, below which exists marked hypertrophy of the right ventricular infundibulum (arrows). Post-stenotic dilatation of the pulmonary artery (P.A.) is evident.

figuration in diastole. Post-stenotic dilatation of the main pulmonary trunk and sometimes of the left pulmonary artery is observed often. The leaflets of the dysplastic valve are not fused anatomically, but are thickened and immobile, creating little change in the angiographic picture during the cardiac cycle. Moreover, a small annulus and narrow sinuses of Valsalva are common accompaniments of valve dysplasia. With either type of valve, systolic narrowing of the right ventricular infundibulum is usually associated with moderate or severe obstruction.

Mild and moderate pulmonic valve stenoses have a generally favorable course; uncommonly, progression occurs in the severity of obstruction.[306,307] Serial hemodynamic studies reveal unchanged pressure gradients over 4- to 8-year intervals in three fourths of patients. Equal percentages of the remainder have an increase or a decrease in the severity of obstruction; significant increases in the pressure gradient occur especially in children under age 4 years who have at least moderate obstruction at initial examination.

Surgical relief of moderate and severe degrees of pulmonic valve stenosis can be accomplished at extremely low risk.[308] The valve is approached through an incision in the pulmonary arterial trunk, and resection of infundibular muscle, if necessary, may be accomplished through the pulmonic valve. In patients with a dysplastic valve the thickened valve tissue is removed and a patch is often required to widen the annulus and proximal main pulmonary artery. In children with mild pulmonic valve stenosis prophylaxis against infective endocarditis is recommended; these patients need not restrict their physical activities.

PULMONIC ATRESIA WITH INTACT VENTRICULAR SEPTUM

This anomaly is an uncommon and serious cause of cyanosis in the neonatal period that may respond well to aggressive medical and surgical treatment.[309-311] In almost all infants the pulmonic valve is atretic; in the majority both the valve ring and the main pulmonary artery are hypoplastic. Occasionally, the right ventricular infundibulum may be atretic or extremely narrowed. The lesion is usually classified into two types: Type 1, with a diminutive right ventricular chamber, often with tricuspid stenosis, and Type 2, with a large right ventricle and frequently tricuspid regurgitation (Fig. 29–39).[312] In most infants the right ventricle is hypoplastic and sinusoidal communications exist between the right ventricular cavity and the coronary circulation, presumably kept open by the high right ventricular pressure.[313]

Since the pulmonic valve is imperforate and completely obstructed, systemic venous blood returning to the heart bypasses the right ventricle through an interatrial communication. Right ventricular output does not contribute to the effective cardiac output and is proportional to the magnitude of tricuspid regurgitation and the size and extent of the sinusoidal communications with the coronary arterial tree. The blood supply to the lungs is derived from the bronchial circulation and from flow through a persistently patent ductus arteriosus. The size and patency of the ductus arteriosus are critical determinants in postnatal survival; ductus closure results in death. Reduced pulmonary blood flow via a partially constricted ductus arteriosus results in profound hypoxemia, tissue hypoxia, and metabolic acidemia.

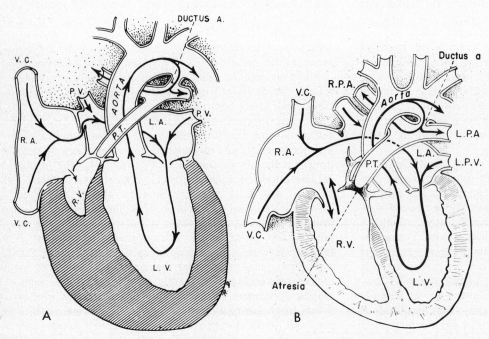

FIGURE 29–39 Pulmonic atresia with intact ventricular septum. With a competent tricuspid valve the right ventricular chamber is diminutive (*left panel*); significant tricuspid regurgitation is associated with a normal or large right ventricular cavity (*right panel*). V.C. = vena cava; R.A. = right atrium; R.V. = right ventricle; P.T. = pulmonary trunk; P.V. = pulmonary vein; L.A. = left atrium; L.V. = left ventricle; Ductus A. = ductus arteriosus; L.P.A. = left pulmonary artery; R.P.A. = right pulmonary artery; L.P.V. = left pulmonary vein. (From Edwards, J. E.: Congenital malformations of the heart and great vessels. *In* Gould, S. E. (ed.): Pathology of the Heart. 2nd ed. Springfield, Ill., Charles C Thomas, 1960.)

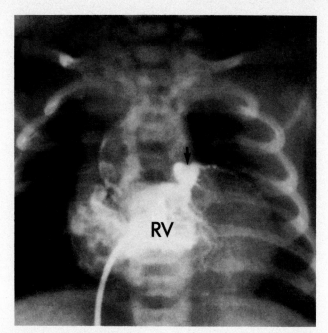

FIGURE 29–40 Right ventricular angiocardiogram in the frontal projection in a 1-day-old infant with an atretic pulmonic valve (arrow). The cavity of the right ventricle (RV) is small and eccentrically shaped. (Courtesy of Robert Freedom, M.D.)

The diagnosis is suggested by roentgenographic findings of pulmonary hypoperfusion and the electrocardiographic observation of a normal QRS frontal axis, absent of diminished right ventricular forces, and/or dominant left ventricular forces. In the minority of infants with marked tricuspid regurgitation, the right ventricle and right atrium are massively enlarged. The echocardiogram in the usual infant shows a small right ventricular cavity and diminutive or absent pulmonic valve echoes.[34,35] Only if tricuspid valve echoes are seen by ultrasound examination can tricuspid atresia be distinguished from pulmonic atresia.

Cardiac catheterization is performed usually on an emergency basis. Since survival depends upon patency of the ductus arteriosus, infusion of prostaglandin E_1 (0.05-0.1 μg/kg/min) intravenously may dramatically reverse clinical deterioration and improve arterial blood gases and pH.[59,60] The usual hemodynamic findings are right atrial and right ventricular hypertension, the latter often greater than systemic pressure, and a massive right-to-left interatrial shunt. Selective angiocardiography establishes the diagnosis and allows evaluation of the size of the right ventricular cavity and of the pulmonary arteries (Fig. 29–40). In the majority of infants with a diminutive right ventricle, balloon atrial septostomy followed by a systemic-pulmonary artery shunt provides palliation. The ultimate prognosis is bleak unless continuity can be established between the right ventricle and the pulmonary arteries by pulmonary valvotomy or prosthetic conduit at initial or second operation.[309] Decompression of the right ventricle permits that chamber to grow and both the tricuspid and pulmonary orifices to enlarge.[305] In some patients in whom systemic-pulmonary arterial shunt is not feasible for anatomical reasons, short-term palliation may be provided by formalin infiltration of the adventitia of the patent ductus arteriosus.[314]

INTRAVENTRICULAR RIGHT VENTRICULAR OBSTRUCTION

Infundibular pulmonic stenosis with an intact ventricular septum and the presence of anomalous muscle bundles are the principal causes of intraventricular right ventricular obstruction (Fig. 29–41).[315] Subpulmonic infundibular stenosis occurs usually at the proximal portion of the infundibulum and consists of a fibrous band at the junction of the right ventricular cavity and outflow tract. The clinical manifestations, course, and prognosis of patients with infundibular stenosis are similar to those with valvular stenosis, although the former diagnosis is suggested by the absence of a systolic ejection sound and a systolic murmur lower along the left sternal border. Withdrawal pressure tracings and selective right ventricular angiocardiography permit localization of the site of obstruction and assessment of its extent and severity. Surgical treatment consists of resection of the fibrotic narrowed area and hypertrophied muscle. Occasionally it may be necessary to widen the outflow tract with a pericardial or prosthetic patch.

A two-chambered right ventricle is formed by right ventricular obstruction due to anomalous muscle bundles; most of the patients have an associated ventricular septal defect.[316] Aberrant hypertrophied muscle bands traverse the right ventricular cavity, extending from its anterior wall to the crista supraventricularis and/or the portion of the adjacent interventricular septum. The anomalous pyramid-shaped muscle mass obstructs blood flow through the body of the right ventricle and produces a proximal high-pressure inflow chamber and a distal low-pressure

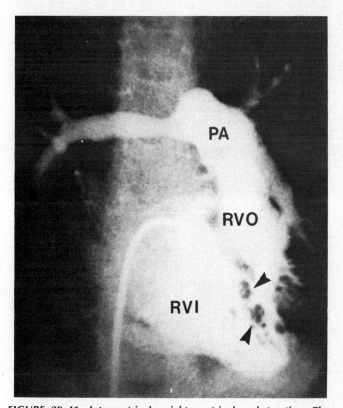

FIGURE 29–41 Intraventricular right ventricular obstruction. The right ventricular inflow (RVI) and outflow (RVO) tracts are separated by bands (arrows) creating intraventricular right ventricular obstruction. PA = pulmonary artery.

chamber. Thus, this type of obstruction is distinguishable from that in tetralogy of Fallot, in which hypertrophied infundibular muscle protrudes into but does not cross the cavity of the right ventricle.

The clinical, electrocardiographic, and chest roentgenographic findings resemble those observed in pulmonic valvular or subvalvular infundibular obstruction, although the systolic thrill and murmur may be displaced lower along the left sternal border. Progressive obstruction occurs in some patients.[317] Selective right ventricular angiocardiography is necessary for accurate diagnosis and reveals a filling defect in the midportion of the right ventricle which does not often change significantly with systole and diastole. The treatment for anomalous muscle bundles consists of surgical removal. In the absence of preoperative recognition of the anomaly, the surgeon should be alerted to the correct diagnosis by the presence of a dimple on the ordinarily smooth anterior surface of the right ventricle and/or the inability to view the tricuspid valve through a longitudinal ventriculotomy because of the presence of the abnormal muscle mass.

Tetralogy of Fallot

DEFINITION. The overall incidence of this anomaly approaches 10 per cent of all forms of congenital heart disease, and it is the most common cardiac malformation responsible for cyanosis after one year of age.[318] The four components of this malformation are (1) ventricular septal defect, (2) obstruction to right ventricular outflow, (3) overriding of the aorta, and (4) right ventricular hypertrophy. The basic anomaly is the result of an anterior deviation of the septal insertion of the infundibular ventricular septum from its usual location in the normal heart between the limbs of the trabecular septum. The interventricular defect usually is large, approximating the aortic orifice in size, and is located high in the septum just below the right cusp of the aortic valve, separated from the pulmonic valve by the crista supraventricularis.[319] The aortic root may be displaced anteriorly and straddle or override the septal defect, but, as in the normal heart, it lies to the right of the origin of the pulmonary artery. In the majority of cases no dextroposition of the aorta exists; the overriding aorta is a phenomenon secondary to the subaortic location of the ventricular septal defect.

HEMODYNAMICS. The degree of obstruction to pulmonary blood flow is the principal determinant of the clinical presentation. The site of obstruction is variable;[320] infundibular stenosis is the only major obstruction in approximately 50 per cent of patients and coexists with valvular obstruction in another 20 to 25 per cent (Fig. 29–42). Supravalvular and peripheral pulmonary arterial narrowing may be observed, and unilateral absence of a pulmonary artery (usually the left) is found in a small number of patients. Circulation to the abnormal lung is accomplished by bronchial and other collateral arteries.[321,322] Atresia of the pulmonic valve, infundibulum, or main pulmonary artery is referred to occasionally as "pseudotruncus arteriosus." True truncus arteriosus with absent pulmonary arteries (Type 4) differs from Fallot's tetralogy, in which pulmonary artery branches are present but are fed by a patent ductus arteriosus and/or bronchial arteries[323-326]

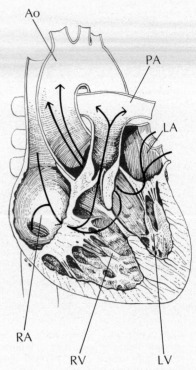

FIGURE 29–42 Tetralogy of Fallot with infundibular and valvular pulmonic stenosis. The arrows indicate direction of blood flow. A substantial right-to-left shunt exists across the ventricular septal defect. RA = right atrium; LA = left atrium; RV = right ventricle; LV = left ventricle; Ao = aorta; PA = pulmonary artery.

(see Fig. 29–47). A right-sided aortic knob, arch, and descending aorta occur in approximately 25 per cent of patients with tetralogy of Fallot. The coronary arteries may have surgically important variations:[327] the anterior descending artery may originate from the right coronary artery; a single right coronary artery may give off a left branch that courses anterior to the pulmonary trunk; a single left coronary artery may give off a right branch that crosses the infundibulum of the right ventricle. Enlargement of the infundibular branch of the right coronary artery often presents a problem with respect to a right ventriculotomy. Associated cardiac anomalies exist in approximately 40 per cent of patients. These include ostium secundum atrial septal defect, patent ductus arteriosus, left superior vena cava, and endocardial cushion defect. Associated extracardiac anomalies are present in 20 to 30 per cent of patients.

The relationship between the resistance to blood flow from the ventricles into the aorta and into the pulmonary vessels plays a major role in determining the hemodynamic and clinical picture. Thus, the severity of obstruction to right ventricular outflow is of fundamental significance. When right ventricular outflow tract obstruction is severe, the pulmonary blood flow is reduced markedly, and a large volume of unsaturated systemic venous blood is shunted from right to left across the ventricular septal defect. Severe cyanosis and polycythemia occur, and symptoms and sequelae of systemic hypoxemia are prominent. At the opposite end of the spectrum, the terms "acyanotic" or "pink" tetralogy of Fallot are often used to describe an interventricular communication and a milder degree of obstruction to right ventricular outflow with little or no venoarterial shunting. In many infants and children the obstruction to right ventricular outflow is mild but progressive, so that early in life pulmonary exceeds systemic blood flow, and the symptoms resemble those produced by a simple ventricular septal defect.

CLINICAL MANIFESTATIONS. Few children with tetralogy of Fallot remain asymptomatic or acyanotic. Most are cyanotic from birth or develop cyanosis before age one year.[47] In general, the earlier the onset of systemic hypoxemia, the more likely the possibility that severe pulmonary outflow tract stenosis or atresia exists. Dyspnea with exertion, clubbing, and polycythemia are common. When resting after exertion, children with tetralogy characteristically assume a squatting posture. The latter may be obvious even in infancy; many cyanotic infants prefer to lie in a knee-chest position. Spells of intense cyanosis related to a sudden increase in venoarterial shunting and a reduction in pulmonary blood flow have their onset most often between 2 and 9 months of age and constitute an important threat to survival.[44,46,328] The attacks are not restricted to patients with severe cyanosis; they are characterized by hyperpnea and increasing cyanosis that progresses to limpness and syncope and occasionally terminates in convulsions, a cerebrovascular accident, and death.

Physical examination reveals variable degrees of underdevelopment and cyanosis. Clubbing of the terminal digits may be prominent after the first year of life. The heart is not hyperactive or enlarged; a right ventricular impulse and systolic thrill are palpable often along the left sternal border. An early systolic ejection sound that is aortic in origin may be heard at the lower left sternal border and apex; the second heart sound is single, the pulmonic component rarely being audible. A systolic ejection murmur is produced by flow across the narrowed right ventricular infundibulum or pulmonic valve. The intensity and duration of the murmur vary inversely with the severity of obstruction—the opposite of the relationship that exists in patients with pulmonic stenosis and an intact ventricular septum. Polycythemia, decreased systemic vascular resistance, and increased obstruction to right ventricular outflow may all be responsible for a decrease in intensity of the murmur; with extreme outflow tract stenosis or pulmonic atresia and during an attack of paroxysmal hypoxemia, there may be no or only a very short, faint murmur.

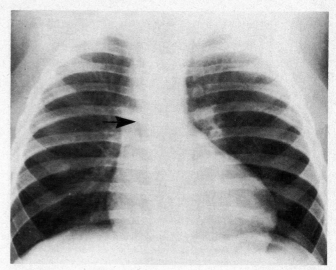

FIGURE 29-43 Chest roentgenogram in a patient with tetralogy of Fallot showing a small, boot-shaped heart, a right aortic arch (arrow), and diminished pulmonary vascular markings.

A continuous murmur faintly audible over the anterior or posterior chest reflects flow through enlarged bronchial collateral vessels. Occasionally, a loud continuous murmur of flow through a patent ductus arteriosus may be heard at the upper left sternal border.

LABORATORY EXAMINATION. The *electrocardiogram* ordinarily shows right ventricular and, less frequently, right atrial hypertrophy. In a patient with acyanotic tetralogy, combined ventricular hypertrophy may be noted initially, progressing to right ventricular hypertrophy as cyanosis develops. *Radiological* examination characteristically reveals a normal-sized, boot-shaped heart (coeur en sabot) with prominence of the right ventricle and a concavity in the region of the underdeveloped right ventricular outflow tract and main pulmonary artery (Fig. 29–43). The pulmonary vascular markings are typically diminished, and the aortic arch and knob may be on the right side; the ascending aorta is generally large. A uniform, diffuse, fine reticular pattern of vascular markings is noted in the presence of prominent collateral vessels. Single-crystal *echocardiographic* findings include aortic enlargement, aortic-septal discontinuity, and aortic overriding of the ventricular septum.[329] Saline contrast echocardiography after

(ECHOES ANT. TO MV & BEFORE E POINT)

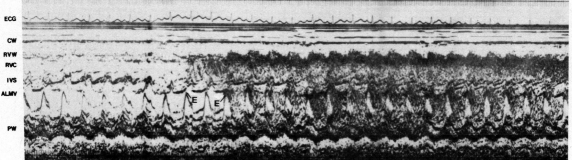

FIGURE 29-44 Saline contrast echocardiogram in a patient with tetralogy of Fallot showing the appearance of a cloud of echoes anterior to and before the E point of the mitral valve. ECG = electrocardiogram; CW = chest wall; RVW = right ventricular wall; RVC = right ventricular cavity; IVS = interventricular septum; ALMV = anterior leaflet mitral valve; PW = posterior wall. (Courtesy of Thomas DiSessa, M.D.)

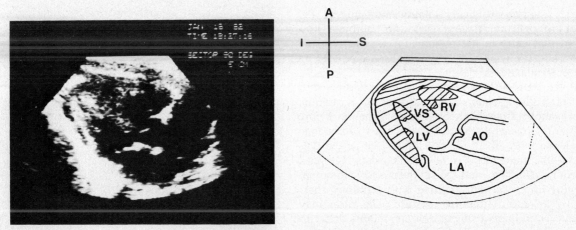

FIGURE 29–45   Two-dimensional echocardiogram of tetralogy of Fallot from the left parasternal long-axis view. The aorta (AO) is enlarged and overrides the ventricular septum (VS). Thus, the aorta originates from both the right ventricle (RV) and left ventricle (LV). A = anterior, I = inferior, P = posterior, S = superior. (Courtesy of Thomas DiSessa, M.D.)

intravenous injection shows filling of the left ventricle by a cloud of echoes anterior to the mitral valve and before the E point of the mitral valve, since left precedes right ventricular isovolumetric relaxation and right-to-left shunting occurs during that interval (Fig. 29–44).[330] Even two-dimensional echocardiographic distinction from truncus arteriosus may be difficult unless the pulmonic valve can be identified (Fig. 29–45). The demonstration of mitral-semilunar valve continuity helps distinguish tetralogy from double-outlet right ventricle with pulmonic stenosis, in which discontinuity of the mitral valve echo and the aortic cusp echo is a critical feature.[34,331]

Cardiac catheterization and selective *angiocardiography* (Fig. 29–46) are necessary to confirm the diagnosis; assess the magnitude of right-to-left shunting; evaluate the architecture of the right ventricular outflow tract, pulmonic valve, and annulus and the caliber of the main branches of the pulmonary arteries; and analyze the anatomy of the coronary arteries. *Axial cineangiography*, utilizing the sitting-up projection, greatly facilitates evaluation of the pulmonary outflow tract and arteries.[332] The preoperative assessment of tetralogy with pulmonic atresia must include delineation of the arterial supply to both lungs by selective

catheterization and visualization of bronchial collateral arteries with late serial filming; pulmonary arteries may be opacified only after the bronchial collateral arteries have cleared of contrast material (Fig. 29–47).[325,326] A patient with pulmonic atresia should not be ruled out as a candidate for surgical correction unless an inadequate pulmonary arterial supply to the lungs is demonstrated clearly. Rarely, injection of contrast through a catheter in the pulmonary venous capillary wedge position is required to assess the possibility that anatomical pulmonary arteries are present.[323] Computer-assisted axial tomography may visualize central pulmonary arteries when conventional angiography cannot.[324]

MANAGEMENT.   Among the factors that may complicate the management of patients with tetralogy are iron deficiency anemia, infective endocarditis, paradoxical embolism, polycythemia, coagulation disorders, and cerebral infarction or abscess. Paroxysmal hypercyanotic spells may respond quickly to oxygen, placing the child in the knee-chest position, and morphine. If the spell persists, metabolic acidosis will develop from prolonged anaerobic metabolism, and infusion of sodium bicarbonate may be necessary to interrupt the attack. Vasopressors, beta-ad-

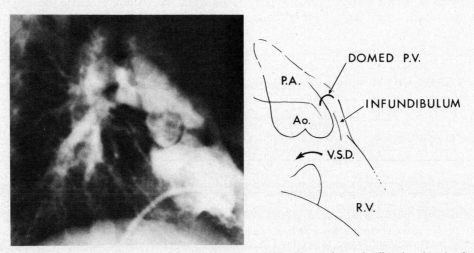

FIGURE 29–46   Lateral view of a right ventriculogram in a child with tetralogy of Fallot showing simultaneous opacification of the pulmonary artery (P.A.) and aorta (Ao.). P.V. = pulmonic valve; V.S.D. = ventricular septal defect; R.V. = right ventricle.

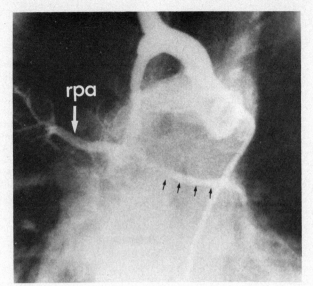

FIGURE 29–47 Selective systemic collateral bronchial arteriogram demonstrates "gull-wing" configuration of the hypoplastic right pulmonary artery (rpa) and left pulmonary artery (arrows) in a patient with tetralogy of Fallot and pulmonic atresia. (Courtesy of Robert Freedom, M.D.)

renergic receptor blockade, or general anesthesia may occasionally be necessary.

Total correction is advisable ultimately for almost all patients with tetralogy of Fallot. Early definitive repair, even in infancy, is currently advocated in most centers prepared properly for infant intracardiac surgery.[333-337] Successful early correction appears to avoid the consequences of progressive infundibular obstruction and acquired pulmonic atresia, delayed growth and development, and complications secondary to hypoxemia and polycythemia with bleeding tendencies. The size of the pulmonary arteries, rather than the age or size of the infant or child, is the most important determinant in assessing candidacy for primary repair; marked hypoplasia of the pulmonary arteries is a relative contraindication for early corrective operation. When the latter exists, a palliative operation designed to increase pulmonary blood flow is recommended and consists usually in the smallest infants of a systemic-pulmonary arterial anastomosis.[338-340,340a] A transventricular infundibulectomy or valvulotomy is an additional palliative procedure that may be considered. Total correction can then be carried out at a lower risk later in childhood or adolescence. The palliative procedures relieve hypoxemia due to diminished pulmonary blood flow and reduce the stimulus to polycythemia. Since pulmonary venous return is augmented, the left atrium and ventricle are stimulated to enlarge their capacity in anticipation of total correction. In the most severe forms of tetralogy of Fallot with pulmonic atresia, the goals of operation include establishment of nonstenotic continuity between the right ventricle and pulmonary arteries, closure of the intracardiac shunt(s), and interruption of surgically created shunts or major collateral arteries to the lungs.[341-343] When atresia is confined to the infundibulum or pulmonic valve, repair may be accomplished by infundibular resection and reconstruction of the outflow tract with a pericardial patch. If a long segment exists of pulmonary arterial atresia, a valve-containing conduit is inserted from the right ventricle to the distal pulmonary artery. The presence of a single pulmonary artery in the hilus of either lung is a prerequisite for repair of pulmonic atresia. A conduit may also be necessary in less severe forms of right ventricular outflow tract obstruction when an anomalous coronary artery crosses the right ventricular outflow tract.

A variety of complications are common in the postoperative period after palliative or corrective operation.[344] Mild-to-moderate left ventricular decompensation may be secondary to the sudden increase in pulmonary venous return; varying degrees of pulmonic valvular regurgitation increase right ventricular cavity size further.[345-347] Bleeding problems are seen frequently, especially in older polycythemic patients. Complete right bundle branch block or the pattern of left anterior hemiblock is seen often, but disabling dysrhythmias are infrequent.[348,349] Restricted pulmonary arterial flow is the greatest cause for early and late mortality and poor late results.[350,351] After convalescence from intracardiac repair, symptoms of hypoxemia and severe exercise intolerance are relieved even in the presence of some residual right ventricular outflow tract obstruction, pulmonic valve incompetence, and/or cardiomegaly.[352] However, cardiovascular performance at rest or during exercise may remain below normal, and major complications, such as trifascicular block, complete heart block, and sudden death may rarely occur many years after surgical treatment.[353-357,357a]

CONGENITAL ABSENCE OF THE PULMONIC VALVE

In the majority of cases of this rare malformation, the lesion is associated with a ventricular septal defect, a narrowed obstructive annulus of the pulmonic valve, and marked aneurysmal dilatation of the pulmonary arteries. The combination of anomalies is referred to often as tetralogy of Fallot with absent pulmonic valve. The obstructing lesion consists principally of underdeveloped, primitive valve tissue within a hypoplastic annulus; infundibular obstruction and the ventricular septal defect do not differ from classic tetralogy of Fallot. The massively dilated pulmonary arteries are often the major determinant of the clinical course, since they frequently result in upper airway obstruction and severe respiratory distress in infancy.[358,359] Post-stenotic pulmonary artery aneurysms develop in utero, and their size and location appear to be related to the magnitude of pulmonic regurgitation in fetal life, the orientation of the right ventricular infundibulum to the right or left, and the size of the ductus arteriosus.[359] It has been suggested that the aneurysmal dilatation is related pathogenetically to agenesis of the ductus arteriosus.[360]

The *clinical features* are often distinctive, with an early onset of severe respiratory distress due to tracheobronchial compression accompanied by a systolic ejection and a widely transmitted low-pitched, decrescendo diastolic murmur at the upper left sternal border. In the absence of pulmonary complications cyanosis is commonly mild. *Radiographically* the heart is moderately enlarged; hyperinflated lung fields are observed with large hilar densities representing the aneurysmally dilated pulmonary arteries. The *echocardiographic* features are similar to those seen in classic tetralogy of Fallot, but the marked right ventricular volume overload due to the pulmonic regurgitation results in paradoxical septal motion. Definitive diagnosis is established by cardiac catheterization and selective angiocardiography. Prognosis is related to the intensity of upper airway obstruction; pulmonary complications are the usual cause of death in infancy. If survival beyond infancy is accomplished the respiratory symptoms usually diminish, probably because of maturational changes in the structure of the tracheobronchial tree. The surgical approach in infancy is often unsatisfactory; a variety of procedures have been attempted, ranging from aneurysmorrhaphy to pulmonary artery suspension to transection and reanastomosis of pulmonary artery segments.[361,362] Also suggested are ligation of the main pulmonary artery and creation of a systemic-pulmonary shunt,[363] and primary repair of the ventricular septal defect with pulmonary arterial plication.[364] In older patients the stenotic annulus may be widened with a patch and the ventricular septal defect closed. It is rarely necessary to replace the pulmonic valve.

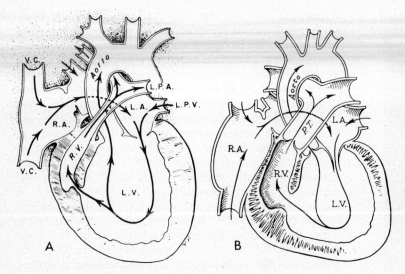

FIGURE 29–48 *A*, Tricuspid atresia with normally related great arteries, a small ventricular septal defect, diminutive right ventricular chamber, and narrowed outflow tract. *B*, An example of tricuspid atresia and complete transposition of the great arteries in which the left ventricular chamber is essentially a common ventricle, with the aorta arising from an infundibular component (R.V.) of the common ventricle. V.C. = vena cava; R.A. = right atrium; L.A. = left atrium; R.V. = right ventricle; L.V. = left ventricle; L.P.V. = left pulmonary vein; L.P.A. = left pulmonary artery. (From Edwards, J. E., and Burchell, H. B.: Congenital tricuspid atresia: Classification. Med. Clin. North Am. *33*: 1177, 1949.)

Tricuspid Atresia

This anomaly is characterized by absence of the tricuspid orifice, an interatrial communication, hypoplasia of the right ventricle, and the presence of a communication between the systemic and pulmonary circulations, usually a ventricular septal defect.[365,365a] Unequal division of the atrioventricular canal by fusion of the right-sided endocardial cushions has been proposed as the embryologic fault. Patients may be subdivided into those with normally related great arteries and those with D-transposition of the great arteries; further classification depends upon the presence of pulmonic stenosis or atresia and the absence or size of the ventricular septal defect (Fig. 29–48). Additional cardiovascular malformations are often present, especially in patients with D-transposition of the great arteries, and include persistent left superior vena cava, patent ductus arteriosus, coarctation of the aorta, and juxtaposition of the atrial appendages.

The association with other cardiac malformations determines whether or not pulmonary blood flow is decreased, normal, or increased and, therefore, the degree of systemic hypoxemia.[366,367] The clinical picture is dominated usually by symptoms resulting from greatly diminished pulmonary blood flow with severe cyanosis. Cyanosis results from an obligatory admixture of systemic and pulmonary venous blood in the left atrium and its intensity is dependent primarily upon the magnitude of pulmonary blood flow. Heart failure, rather than cyanosis, is the predominant problem in infants with torrential pulmonary blood flow, which results when D-transposition of the great arteries, a ventricular septal defect, and an unobstructed pulmonary outflow tract coexist. If the latter patients survive infancy, they are candidates for pulmonary vascular obstructive disease; a favorable response to pulmonary arterial banding is common early in life.

Clinical diagnosis is accurate in the vast majority of infants with tricuspid atresia and pulmonary hypoperfusion. The *electrocardiographic* findings of left-axis deviation, right atrial enlargement, and left ventricular hypertrophy in a cyanotic infant strongly suggest tricuspid atresia (Fig. 29–49).[368] *Echocardiography* reveals a small or absent right

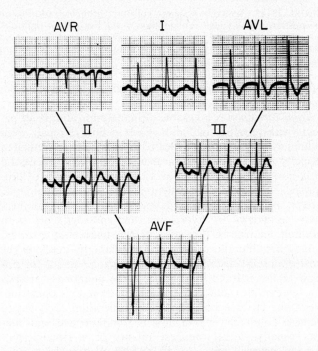

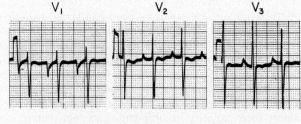

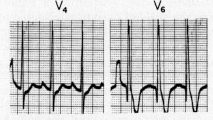

FIGURE 29–49 Tricuspid atresia. The electrocardiogram shows left-axis deviation and left atrial and ventricular enlargement. (Courtesy of Delores A. Danilowicz, M.D.)

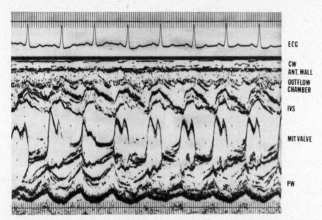

FIGURE 29–50 Echocardiogram in a patient with tricuspid atresia shows a diminutive right ventricular outflow chamber, absence of tricuspid valve echoes, and a large left ventricle with prominent mitral valve echoes. CW = chest wall; ANT. WALL = anterior wall; IVS = interventricular septum; MIT = mitral valve; PW = posterior wall. (Courtesy of Thomas DiSessa, M.D.)

right ventricle is not markedly hypoplastic, it may be utilized in the correction to generate forward flow into the pulmonary vascular bed. Also, if the right ventricle is not too hypoplastic, it may be used as a pumping chamber by anastomosis of the right atrial appendage to the right ventricle with the aid of a pericardial patch, leaving the outflow tract and pulmonic valve intact.[373,374] A previously existing systemic artery–to–pulmonary artery anastomosis must be closed, but a systemic vein–to–pulmonary artery anastomosis may be left in place. With appropriate palliative surgery in early life approximately half of patients survive to the second decade of life, when this operative approach may be considered. Candidates for these corrective procedures must have normal pulmonary vascular resistance and a mean pulmonary artery pressure less than 20 mm Hg, pulmonary arteries of adequate size, and good

ventricle, large left ventricle, and absent tricuspid valve echoes (Fig. 29–50); further, it may demonstrate the relationship of the great arteries unless pulmonic atresia is present.[34] Contrast and cross-sectional echocardiography reveal the abnormal low patterns and the atretic tricuspid orifice.[369] *Radiographically* there are diminished pulmonary vascular markings and a concavity in the region of the cardiac silhouette usually occupied by the main pulmonary artery. The right atrial shadow may be prominent unless left-sided juxtaposition of the atrial appendages exists, which produces a straight and flattened right heart border.

At *cardiac catheterization* the right ventricle cannot be entered directly from the right atrium. When the great arteries are related normally, pulmonary blood flow is found to be derived from shunting through a ventricular septal defect or via a patent ductus arteriosus; the latter and the bronchial collaterals are the source of pulmonary flow if the ventricular septum is intact.[370] In complete transposition the pulmonary artery fills directly from the left ventricle and the aorta indirectly through a ventricular septal defect and the hypoplastic right ventricle. Since complete admixture exists in the left atrium of pulmonary and systemic venous return, the degree of systemic arterial hypoxemia depends on the pulmonary: systemic flow ratio. Right atrial angiography does not opacify the right ventricle unless via a ventricular septal defect (Fig. 29–51). Selective left ventricular *angiography* permits identification of the hypoplastic right ventricle, the size and location of the ventricular septal defect, the type of pulmonary obstruction, the relationship between the great arteries, and the size of the distal pulmonary arterial tree.

Balloon atrial septostomy in those infants with a restrictive interatrial communication and palliative operations designed to increase pulmonary blood flow (systemic arterial– or venous–pulmonary artery anastomosis) are capable of producing clinical improvement of significant duration in patients with diminished blood flow.[371]

Functional correction of the anomaly has been accomplished by insertion of a prosthetic conduit between the right atrium and pulmonary artery and closure of the interatrial communication (Fontan procedure).[372,372a] If the

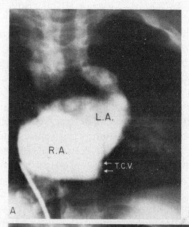

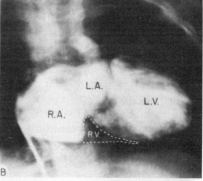

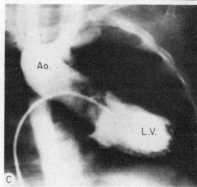

FIGURE 29–51 Right atrial angiogram in an infant with tricuspid atresia shows flow of contrast material from right atrium (R.A.) to left atrium (A), and then to left ventricle (L.V.) (B) and aorta (Ao.) (C). The tricuspid valve (T.C.V.) is atretic, and a radiolucency exists in the region of the right ventricle (R.V.).

left ventricular function.[375,376] The postoperative period is usually characterized by a superior vena cava syndrome with right heart failure, edema, ascites, and hepatomegaly.[377]

Ebstein's Anomaly of the Tricuspid Valve

This malformation is characterized by a downward displacement of the tricuspid valve into the right ventricle due to anomalous attachment of the tricuspid leaflets.[378] Tricuspid valve tissue is dysplastic and a variable portion of the septal and inferior cusps adhere to the right ventricular wall some distance away from the atrioventricular junction. The abnormally situated tricuspid orifice produces a portion of the right ventricle lying between the atrioventricular ring and the origin of the valve, which is continuous with the right atrial chamber. This proximal segment is "atrialized," and a distal, functionally small ventricular chamber exists. The degree of impairment of right ventricular function depends primarily on the extent to which the right ventricular inflow portion is atrialized and on the magnitude of tricuspid valve regurgitation.[379,380]

CLINICAL MANIFESTATIONS. These are variable because the spectrum of pathology varies widely and because of the presence of associated malformations. An interatrial communication consisting of a patent foramen ovale or an ostium secundum atrial septal defect is present in over half the cases. Other coexistent anomalies may include an ostium primum type of atrial septal defect, pulmonic stenosis or atresia, and ventricular septal defect alone or in combination with other lesions. The Ebstein's lesion is commonly observed in association with congenitally corrected transposition of the great arteries, in which the tricuspid valve guards the left atrioventricular orifice (p. 1003). The usual manifestations in infancy are cyanosis, a cardiac murmur, and severe congestive heart failure. The magnitude of tricuspid regurgitation in the neonate is enhanced because the pulmonary vascular resistance is normally high early in life (Fig. 29–52).[381,382] In this regard it may be difficult in some newborn infants with Ebstein's anomaly and massive tricuspid regurgitation to distinguish between organic pulmonic atresia and the presence of elevated perinatal pulmonary vascular resistance.[383] In such infants retrograde aortography is quite likely to fill the

pulmonary root and allow visualization of the pulmonic valve via a patent ductus arteriosus, serving to differentiate a normal from an abnormal pulmonary outflow tract. The tricuspid regurgitation in infants with Ebstein's anomaly may lessen substantially, and cyanosis may disappear early in life as pulmonary vascular resistance falls, only to recur at a later age when right ventricular dysfunction and/or paroxysmal arrhythmias develop. In some infants with Ebstein's malformation, cyanosis is intensified suddenly as the degree of pulmonary hypoperfusion is unmasked by spontaneous closure of a patent ductus arteriosus.

Beyond infancy the onset of symptoms is insidious; the most common complaints are exertional dyspnea, fatigue, and cyanosis. Approximately 25 per cent of patients suffer episodes of paroxysmal atrial tachycardia. A prominent systolic pulsation of the liver and a large v wave in the jugular venous pulse accompany the systolic thrill and murmur of tricuspid regurgitation. Wide splitting of the first and second heart sounds and prominent third and fourth heart sounds may produce a characteristically rhythmic auscultatory cadence with a triple, quadruple, or quintuple combination of sounds.

The *electrocardiographic abnormalities* commonly fall into two categories: those with a right bundle branch block pattern and those with the Wolff-Parkinson-White syndrome. The pattern in the latter is almost always type B, resembling left bundle branch block with predominant S waves in the right precordial leads. The presence of the Wolff-Parkinson-White pattern increases the risk of supraventricular paroxysmal tachycardia.[384,385] Most often the electrocardiogram shows giant P waves, a prolonged P-R interval, and prolonged terminal QRS depolarization, producing variable degrees of right bundle branch block. These distinctive findings help distinguish Ebstein's anomaly from other forms of right ventricular dysplasia whose presenting problem is often an arrhythmia.[386] *Roentgenographic* and fluoroscopic studies usually demonstrate an enlarged right atrium, a small right ventricle, and a pulmonary artery with reduced pulsations; the pulmonary vascularity may be reduced if a large right-to-left shunt is present.

The principal single-crystal *echocardiographic findings* observed in patients with this anomaly, as well as in those with other forms of right ventricular volume overload, are

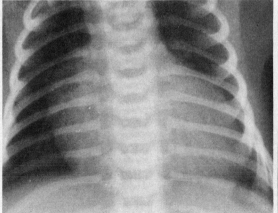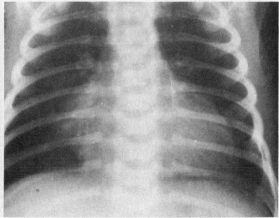

FIGURE 29–52 Chest roentgenograms in an infant with Ebstein's anomaly at ages 6 hours (*left*) and 2 weeks (*right*). The reduction in both overall heart size and right atrial prominence is a result of diminished tricuspid regurgitation as pulmonary vascular resistance falls postnatally. (Courtesy of Norman Talner, M.D.)

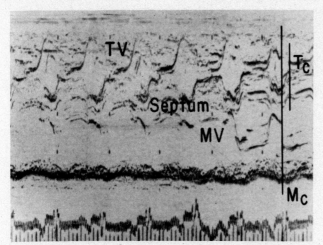

FIGURE 29-53 Echocardiogram in a child with Ebstein's anomally showing a delay in tricuspid valve (TV) closure (T$_c$) relative to mitral valve (MV) closure (M$_c$). (Courtesy of Thomas DiSessa, M.D.)

an increase in right ventricular dimension, paradoxical ventricular septal motion, an increase in tricuspid valve excursion, and an abnormal closing velocity of the tricuspid valve. More specific findings for Ebstein's anomaly include a delay in tricuspid valve closure relative to mitral closure and a decrease in the E-F slope of the tricuspid valve (Fig. 29-53), an abnormal anterior position of the tricuspid valve during diastole, and the detection of tricuspid valve echoes with more lateral placement of the transducer than usual.[387-389] Cross-sectional echocardiographic techniques are superior for observation of the inferior and leftward displacement of the tricuspid valve and simultaneously demonstrate the abnormal positional relation between the tricuspid and mitral valves. Moreover, the boundaries of the atrialized right ventricle may be defined by high-resolution cross-sectional methods.[390,391]

At *cardiac catheterization* the intracavitary electrocardiogram recorded just proximal to the tricuspid valve shows a right ventricular type of complex, while the pressure recorded is that of the right atrium (Fig. 29-54).[391] Usually a right-to-left atrial shunt is present. The hemodynamic findings depend upon the degree of tricuspid

regurgitation. The heart is unusually irritable and a high incidence of significant arrhythmias exists during catheterization. Selective right ventricular *angiocardiography* is the best means of showing the position of the displaced tricuspid valve, the size of the right ventricle, and the configuration of the outflow portion of the right ventricle (Fig. 29-55).

Ebstein's anomaly may be compatible with a relatively long and active life, with most patients surviving into the third decade.[379] In some disabled patients moderate improvement has resulted from anastomosis of the superior vena cava to the right pulmonary artery (the Glenn procedure) to divert systemic venous return from the right atrium and to increase pulmonary blood flow. Occasional benefit has resulted in older patients from prosthetic replacement of the tricuspid valve and closure of the atrial defect with or without ligation and marsupialization of the thin atrialized portion of the right ventricle.[392,393] It should be recognized, however, that patients with Ebstein's anomaly are poor surgical risks at all ages.

TRANSPOSITION COMPLEXES

The term *transposition* identifies a group of malformations that have in common abnormal relationships between the cardiac chambers and great arteries. In this chapter the term is employed to include both anomalous insertion of the pulmonary veins and cardiac malpositions.

Complete Transposition of the Great Arteries

ANATOMICAL FINDINGS. This is a common and potentially lethal form of heart disease in newborns and infants.[394] The malformation consists of the aorta arising from the morphological right ventricle and the pulmonary artery from the morphological left ventricle. With rare exceptions there is no fibrous continuity between the aortic and mitral valve.[395] Usually the origin of the aorta is to the right and anterior to, but may be lateral to, the main pulmonary artery. Thus, dextro or D-transposition is a term

FIGURE 29-54 With a catheter in the "atrialized" portion of the right ventricle (RV), the intracardiac electrocardiogram in a patient with Ebstein's anomaly continues to show a ventricular complex, while right atrial pressure (RA) is recorded at the same site. (Courtesy of Delores A. Danilowicz, M.D.)

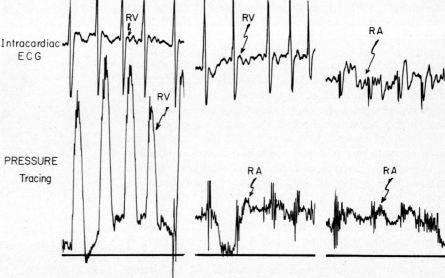

Intracardiac ECG

PRESSURE Tracing

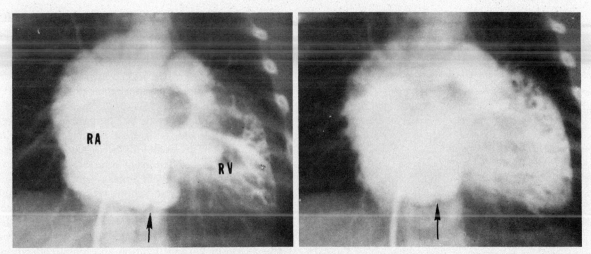

FIGURE 29–55   Right ventricular angiogram in an infant with Ebstein's anomaly shows the displaced tricuspid valve (arrows), tricuspid regurgitation, and a markedly enlarged right atrium (RA). RV = right ventricle. (Courtesy of Norman Talner, M.D.)

used interchangeably with complete transposition. The embryogenesis of complete transposition of the great arteries is controversial. There is consensus that the ventricular origins of the great arteries are reversed following development of a straight, rather than a spiral infundibulotruncal septum. Transposition appears to result from a transfer of the pulmonary artery, instead of the aorta, from the heart tube's outlet zone to the left ventricle. The latter may result from maldevelopment of the infundibulum, or a combination of both infundibulum maldevelopment and truncal malseptation; the former results if the subpulmonary, rather than the subaortic infundibulum, is absorbed.

The anatomical arrangement results in two separate and parallel circulations. Some communication between the two circulations must exist after birth in order to sustain life; otherwise, unoxygenated systemic venous blood is directed inappropriately to the systemic circulation and oxygenated pulmonary venous blood is directed to the pulmonary circulation. Almost all patients have an interatrial communication (Fig. 29–56). Two thirds have a patent ductus arteriosus, and about one third have an associated ventricular septal defect. Complete transposition occurs more frequently in the offspring of diabetic mothers and more often in males than in females. Without treatment, approximately 30 per cent of these infants die within the first week of life; 50 per cent within the first month; 70 per cent within 6 months; and 90 per cent within the first year.[394] Those who live beyond infancy have, as a general rule, either an isolated large atrial septal defect or a single ventricle, or ventricular septal defect and pulmonic stenosis. Current aggressive medical and surgical approaches to this group of patients have transformed the prognosis for an infant with this malformation from hopeless to hopeful.

The *clinical course* is determined by the degree of tissue hypoxia, the ability of each ventricle to sustain an increased workload in the presence of reduced coronary arterial oxygenation, the nature of the associated cardiovascular anomalies, and the anatomical and functional status of the pulmonary vascular bed.[396] A bidirectional shunt is always present, because continuous unidirectional shunting would result in a progressive depletion of the circulating

volume in either the pulmonary or the systemic vascular bed.

HEMODYNAMICS.   A major determinant of the systemic arterial oxygen saturation is the amount of blood exchanged between the two circulations by intercirculatory shunts. The net volume of blood passing left-to-right from the pulmonary to the systemic circulation represents the anatomical left-to-right shunt and is, in fact, the effective systemic blood flow (i.e., the amount of oxygenated pulmonary venous return reaching the systemic capillary bed). Conversely, the volume of blood passing right-to-left from the systemic to the pulmonary circulation constitutes the anatomical right-to-left shunt and is, in fact, the effective

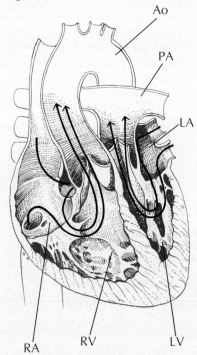

FIGURE 29–56 Complete transposition of the great arteries. Intercirculatory mixing occurs only at the atrial level. RA = right atrium; LA = left atrium; RV = right ventricle; LV = left ventricle; Ao = aorta; PA = pulmonary artery.

pulmonary blood flow (i.e., the net volume of unsaturated systemic venous return perfusing the pulmonary capillary bed). The net volume exchange between the two circulations per unit time is equal. The magnitude of the intercirculatory mixing volume is modified by the number of intercirculatory communications that exist, the presence of associated obstructive intra- and extracardiac anomalies, the extent of the bronchopulmonary circulation, and the relationships between pulmonary and systemic vascular resistance. For example, in the newborn with an intact ventricular septum and a constricted or closed patent ductus arteriosus, inadequate mixing through a small patent foramen ovale is often the cause of severe hypoxemia. If a large interatrial communication or a ventricular septal defect exists, systemic arterial oxygen saturation is influenced more importantly by the pulmonary–systemic blood flow relationship than by the adequacy of mixing; augmented pulmonary blood flow produces a higher systemic arterial saturation if the left ventricle can sustain a high-output state without the intervention of congestive heart failure and pulmonary edema. The systemic arterial oxygen saturation will be quite low, despite adequate intercirculatory mixing sites, if pulmonary blood flow is reduced by left ventricular outflow tract obstruction or increased pulmonary vascular resistance.

Infants with complete transposition of the great arteries are particularly susceptible to the early development of *pulmonary vascular obstructive disease.*[397–399] Severe morphological alterations develop in the pulmonary vascular bed by the age of 1 or 2 years in almost all patients with an associated large ventricular septal defect or large patent ductus arteriosus in the absence of obstruction to left ventricular outflow. Advanced pulmonary vascular disease is seen also within this same time frame in 5 to 10 per cent of patients without a patent ductus arteriosus and with an intact ventricular septum. Systemic arterial hypoxemia, increased pulmonary blood flow, and pulmonary hypertension contribute to the development of pulmonary vascular obstruction in these patients as they do in other forms of congenital heart disease. Among the additional factors implicated in the accelerated and more widespread pulmonary vascular obstruction found in patients with complete transposition is the presence of extensive bronchopulmonary anastomotic channels, which enter the pulmonary vascular bed proximal to the pulmonary capillary bed; thus, oxygen tension is reduced at the precapillary level, causing pulmonary vasoconstriction.[400] Beyond the early neonatal period many patients have an abnormal distribution pattern of pulmonary blood flow, with preferential flow to the right lung.[401] The asymmetrical distribution of pulmonary blood flow in these individuals results from an abnormal rightward inclination of the main pulmonary artery in the transposition malformation that favors flow from the main to the right pulmonary artery. Persistently increased pulmonary blood flow to the right lung would be expected to contribute to pulmonary vascular obstructive changes within the lung; in the left pulmonary vascular bed, thrombotic changes may occur because of the combination of reduced flow and polycythemia. Finally, it should be recognized that a prenatal alteration in pulmonary vascular smooth muscle may exist, since blood perfusing the fetal lungs in complete transposition of great

arteries has a higher than normal pO_2 and may serve to dilate pulmonary vessels in utero.[18] Postnatally such vessels may have an enhanced capacity to constrict in response to vasoactive stimuli and suffer anatomical, obliterative changes.[402]

CLINICAL FINDINGS. Average birthweight and size of infants born with complete transposition of the great arteries are greater than normal. The usual clinical manifestations are dyspnea and cyanosis from birth, progressive hypoxemia, and congestive heart failure. Early in postnatal life the clinical manifestations and course are influenced principally by the magnitude of intercirculatory mixing. The most severe cyanosis and hypoxemia are observed in infants with only a small patent foramen ovale or ductus arteriosus and an intact ventricular septum in whom mixing is inadequate, or in those infants with relatively reduced pulmonary blood flow because of left ventricular outflow tract obstruction.[403] With a large persistent patent ductus arteriosus or a large ventricular septal defect, cyanosis may be minimal and heart failure is the usual dominant problem after the first few weeks of life.[404] It should be recognized that a patent ductus arteriosus is present in about half of newborn infants with transposition, although it closes functionally and anatomically soon after birth in almost all cases. If the ductus arteriosus remains open, better mixing of the venous and arterial circulations is usually at the expense of pulmonary artery hypertension.

Cardiac murmurs are of little diagnostic significance and are absent or insignificant in approximately 30 to 50 per cent of infants with complete transposition of the great arteries and an intact ventricular septum. In infants with a large persistent patent ductus arteriosus, less than half exhibit physical signs typical of ductus arteriosus, such as continuous murmur, bounding pulses, or a prominent middiastolic rumble. Moreover, *differential cyanosis* due to reversed pulmonary-to-systemic shunting across the ductus arteriosus is difficult to detect because of generalized arterial desaturation. In those infants with a large ventricular septal defect, a pansystolic murmur emerges usually within the first 7 to 10 days of life. In newborns with transposition and severe pulmonic stenosis or atresia, the clinical findings are similar to those in the infant with tetralogy of Fallot.

The most usual *electrocardiographic findings* include right-axis deviation, right atrial enlargement, and right ventricular hypertrophy, reflecting that the right ventricle is the systemic pumping chamber. Combined ventricular hypertrophy may be present in those patients with a large ventricular septal defect and elevated pulmonary blood flow. Isolated left ventricular hypertrophy is encountered rarely in patients with a ventricular septal defect and a hypoplastic right ventricle, in many of whom the tricuspid valve is displaced abnormally and straddles a ventricular septal defect. In the first days of life the chest x-ray may appear normal, particularly in infants with an intact ventricular septum. Thereafter, roentgenographic findings are often highly suggestive of the diagnosis[405] and consist of (1) progressive cardiac enlargement in early infancy; (2) a characteristic oval or egg-shaped cardiac configuration in the anteroposterior view, and a narrow vascular pedicle created by superimposition of the aortic and pulmonary artery segments; and (3) increased pulmonary vascular

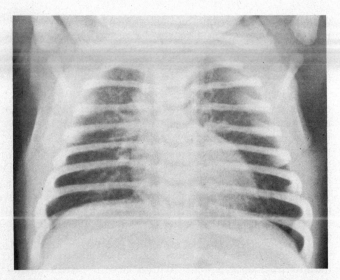

FIGURE 29–57 Chest roentgenogram in a 4-day-old infant with complete transposition of the great arteries showing an oval-shaped heart with a narrow base and increased pulmonary vascular markings.

markings (Fig. 29–57). A right aortic arch is seen in approximately 4 per cent of infants with an intact ventricular septum and 11 per cent of infants with a ventricular septal defect.

Echocardiography. Cross-sectional echocardiography is extremely useful in the diagnosis of complete transposition of the great arteries.[34,406] In the normal patient, single-crystal beams detect the anteriorly located pulmonary artery with angulation of the transducer placed in the left parasternal area laterally toward the left shoulder and outlines the posteriorly placed aorta when it is directed medially. Reversal of the anteroposterior relationship of the great arteries in complete transposition results in the ultrasound beam outlining the posteriorly placed pulmonary artery with superior and lateral beam angulation and the anterior vessel (aortic root) with medial beam direction. In many instances the single-echo beam simultaneously detects both outflow vessels, further identification of which may be established by analysis of the opening and closing times of the respective semilunar valves; the posterior pulmonic valve opens earlier and closes later than does the anterior aortic valve, since the duration of systole is longer in the left ventricle. In the presence of marked pulmonary arterial hypertension, semilunar valve closure intervals and systolic time intervals may not be helpful, since both valves may close simultaneously. Since the preejection period and the ejection time of each ventricle are in part related to distal vascular impedance, the ratio of left-to-right ventricular ejection time in patients with complete transposition approximates 1.2, in contrast to a normal value of 0.8. Similarly, the left/right ventricle preejection period in complete transposition averages 0.5, compared to 1.25 in normals.[407,408] Real-time, two-dimensional, cross-sectional echocardiography (Chap. 5) offers major advantages in the detection of transposition of the great arteries (Fig. 29–58). In sagittal cross sections the aorta is observed to ascend retrosternally in contrast to the normal posterior sweep of the pulmonary artery. With transverse short-axis cross-sectional imaging, the diagnosis is confirmed by demonstrating that the anterior great artery (the aorta) is to the right

of the posterior great artery (pulmonary) or that the two arteries are visualized side by side (Fig. 29–58). Moreover, from this plane the course of the two great arteries may be traced in order to delineate their ventricle of origin, demonstrating that the anterior rightward vessel (aorta) originates from the right ventricle and the posterior leftward vessel (pulmonary artery) originates from the left ventricle. Echocardiography may also assist in identifying associated defects. An enlarged left atrium and left ventricle suggest an associated ventricular septal defect or large patent ductus arteriosus. The nature of left ventricular outflow tract obstruction may be identified as a fixed obstruction caused by a fibromuscular ridge or as a dynamic obstruction caused by the apposition between a thickened interventricular septum and systolic anterior motion of the mitral valve.[409]

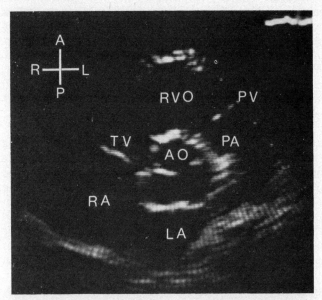

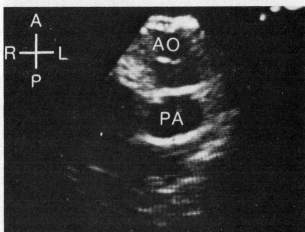

FIGURE 29–58 *Top,* A two-dimensional echocardiographic short-axis scan demonstrates normal great artery relationships. The right ventricular outflow tract (RVO) wraps around the aorta (AO) in a clockwise fashion. The pulmonic valve (PV) is to the left of the aortic valve. *Bottom,* Short-axis scan shows the abnormal great artery relationships in an infant with transposition of the great arteries. The aorta (AO) is directly anterior and slightly to the right of the pulmonary artery (PA). The clockwise partial encirclement of the aorta by the right ventricular outflow tract is no longer observed. A = anterior, L = left, P = posterior, R = right, LA = left atrium, RA = right atrium, TV = tricuspid valve.

Cardiac Catheterization and Angiocardiography.
These tests are usually performed on an emergency basis, especially in the newborn with poor mixing between the two circulations. The diagnostic portion of the cardiac catheterization allows confirmation of the anatomical derangement of the great arteries and establishes the presence of associated lesions; in the newborn it should always be accompanied by a palliative balloon atrial septostomy, which serves to enlarge the interatrial communication and improve oxygenation. Both the diagnostic and palliative procedures can be performed by percutaneous entry into the femoral vein, umbilical vein catheterization, or direct cutdown into the femoral or saphenous vein. The catheter passes easily across the foramen ovale into the left atrium and left ventricle and may be manipulated into the pulmonary artery by means of a flow-directed balloon-guided catheter or by manipulation of a standard catheter bent in the form of a J loop within the left ventricle, with the tip pointed posteriorly to the pulmonary artery.[394] When a large ventricular septal defect is present, a catheter can often be manipulated directly across it from the right ventricle into the pulmonary artery.

The major abnormal hemodynamic findings include right ventricular pressure at systemic levels and either a high or low left ventricular pressure, depending on pulmonary blood flow, pulmonary vascular resistance, and the presence or absence of left ventricular outflow tract obstructive lesions. Oxygen saturation in the aorta is lower than that in the pulmonary artery. Application of the Fick principle to the calculation of pulmonary and systemic blood flow in these patients is an important source of error. Assumed values of oxygen consumption are unreliable in the severely hypoxemic infant. Moreover, because systemic and particularly pulmonary arteriovenous oxygen differences may be quite reduced, small errors in oxygen saturation values result in large errors in flow calculations. Furthermore, because bronchial collaterals enter the pulmonary circuit at the precapillary level, a true mixed pulmonary artery saturation cannot be sampled; pulmonary blood flow is therefore overestimated when one uses a sample from the central pulmonary artery, and pulmonary vascular resistance values are often underestimated.

Selective ventricular angiography is diagnostic and demonstrates that the anteriorly placed aorta arises from the right ventricle and the posteriorly placed pulmonary artery in continuity with the mitral valve arises from the left ventricle (Fig. 29–59). The status of the ductus arteriosus and the site and size of a ventricular septal defect can be well visualized by angiography (Fig. 29–60). Interventricular defects posterior and inferior to the crista supraventricularis occur in approximately half of these patients; less often the defects are anterior and superior to the crista supraventricularis or are of the atrioventricular canal type.[395] A variety of lesions may be identified as the cause of left ventricular outflow tract obstruction, including ventricular septal hypertrophy with systolic anterior movement of the mitral valve, discrete or tunnel fibromuscular subpulmonic stenosis, valvular and supravalvular stenosis, and rarely, an aneurysm of the membranous ventricular septum or redundant tricuspid valve tissue protruding through a ventricular septal defect.

A number of coronary arterial patterns are seen in patients with complete transposition of the great arteries.[394]

In the majority, the left coronary artery originates in the left sinus and the right coronary artery originates in the posterior sinus, with single ostium above both the left and the posterior sinus. In almost 20 per cent of patients the left circumflex artery arises as a branch of the right coronary artery; a single coronary artery is present in approximately 6 per cent; in 3 to 4 per cent of patients either the right coronary and anterior descending arteries originate in the left sinus with the left circumflex originating in the posterior sinus, or two ostia are present above one sinus, one giving rise to the right and the other to the left coronary artery.

MANAGEMENT. *Medical treatment* is often of limited help but should be vigorous now that functional correction of the malformation has become a possibility. Conservative measures include the use of oxygen, digitalis, diuretics, iron (if an associated iron-deficiency anemia is present), and intravenous sodium bicarbonate for severe hypoxemic metabolic acidosis. The creation or enlargement of an interatrial communication is the simplest procedure for providing increased intracardiac mixing of systemic and pulmonary venous blood; preferably this is achieved by rupturing the valve of the foramen ovale by balloon catheter during transseptal catheterization of the left side of the heart (Rashkind's procedure). Surgical atrial septectomy is rarely required. The balloon should be inflated to a diameter of approximately 15 mm before pullback to the right atrium. Salutary results consist of a fall in left atrial pressure, equalization of mean left and right atrial pressures, and an increase in the systemic arterial oxygen saturation. When the foramen ovale is stretched by the balloon without accomplishing rupture of the septum primum valve of the fossa ovalis, the improvement in oxygenation is short-lived. Infusion intravenously of prostaglandin E_1 (0.05–0.1 mg/kg/min) has been shown to improve systemic oxygenation temporarily in the latter situation, presumably by dilating the ductus arteriosus and thereby facilitating intercirculatory mixing.[59] Although balloon atrial septotomy is usually successful in stabilizing the infant and allowing survival in the neonatal period, the initial rise in systemic arterial oxygen saturation to 65 to 75 per cent is often not sustained beyond 6 to 9 months of age.

Surgical Treatment. The development of *corrective operations* for infants born with transposition of the great arteries has greatly improved prognosis.[410–412] Intraatrial correction by the Mustard technique is accomplished by excision of the interatrial septum and creation of a new interatrial septum with a pericardial baffle diverting the systemic venous return into the left ventricle through the mitral valve and thence to the left ventricle and pulmonary artery, while the pulmonary venous blood is diverted through the tricuspid valve and right ventricle to the aorta.[412a] The Senning procedure is based upon a similar principle and consists of diversion of left pulmonary venous blood by a coronary sinus flap and rerouting of caval flow by the use of an atrial wall flap. In most major medical centers intraatrial corrective operation is performed at any age in patients with an intact ventricular septum who do not improve after balloon atrial septotomy. If palliative septostomy provides adequate relief of hypoxemia, the atrial rerouting operation is performed routinely in most infants with transposition of the great arteries and intact ventricular septum by 6 to 9 months of age with a surgical

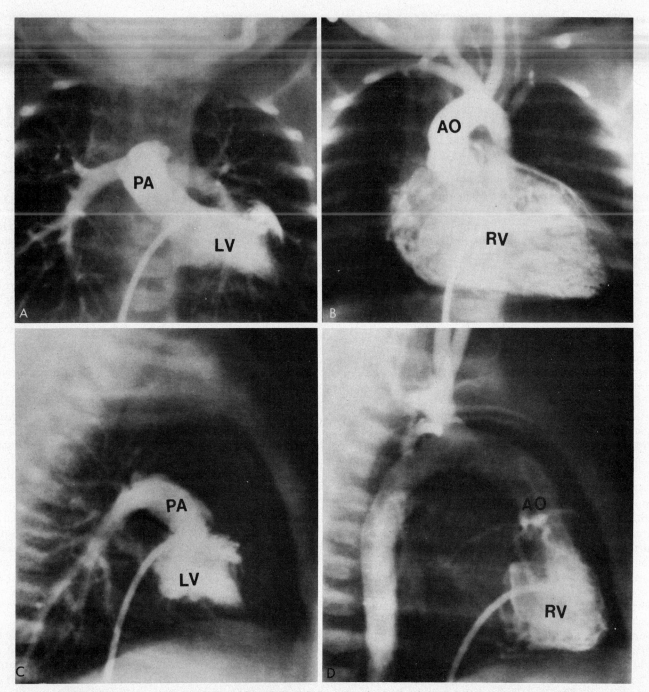

FIGURE 29–59   Frontal (*A* and *B*) and lateral (*C* and *D*) views of selective left (*A* and *C*) and right (*B* and *D*) ventricular angiograms in a patient with complete transposition of the great arteries and an intact ventricular septum. LV = left ventricle; PA = pulmonary artery; RV = right ventricle; AO = aorta. (Courtesy of Robert White, M.D.)

mortality less than 5 per cent. Clinical improvement is usually quite dramatic. In some patients postoperative complications are observed that are directly related to the intraatrial repair (shunts across the intraatrial patch and obstruction to either systemic or pulmonary venous return or both.[413,414] There is a high incidence of early and late postoperative dysrhythmias that are more likely to have their basis in injury to the sinoatrial node and/or its arterial supply than in disruption of internodal tracts or damage to the atrioventricular node.[415,416] Tricuspid regurgitation is a less common complication of operation and

may be related in some patients to a preexisting abnormality of the tricuspid valve,[417] whereas in most it is related to right ventricular dysfunction. Although the assessment of right ventricular contractility is difficult, it has been suggested that the right ventricular pump function is impaired prior to Mustard operation and does not return to normal following successful surgery.[418,419] It is not yet clear whether the right ventricle can perform as a systemic pumping chamber for the duration of a normal life span.[420]

In the unusual infant with an intact ventricular septum and a significant patent ductus arteriosus, an early intra-

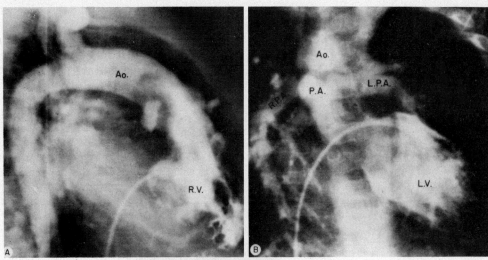

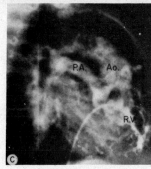

FIGURE 29–60 Lateral (*A* and *C*) and frontal (*B*) views of selective ventriculograms in a child with complete transposition of the great arteries and a ventricular septal defect (V.S.D.). Ao. = aorta; R.V. = right ventricle; P.A. = pulmonary artery; L.V. = left ventricle; R.P.A. = right pulmonary artery; L.P.A. = left pulmonary artery. (Courtesy of Delores A. Danilowicz, M.D.)

atrial corrective operation with closure of the ductus is indicated at 4 to 6 months of age to prevent the likely progression of pulmonary vascular disease.[404] Debate exists concerning the optimal management of patients with a large ventricular septal defect. In some centers pulmonary artery banding is advocated early in life, followed by definitive intracardiac repair at 1 to 2 years of age. Others favor a one-stage intraatrial repair with patch closure of the ventricular septal defect prior to age 6 months. Experience is accumulating with a one-stage operation designed to close the ventricular septal defect; transpose both coronary arteries to the posterior artery; and transsect, contrapose, and anastomose the aorta and pulmonary arteries (Jatene operation).[421,422] The arterial switch anatomical correction may be complicated by coronary ostial stenosis, acquired supravalvular aortic and/or pulmonary stenosis, and aortic incompetence. Infants with transposition of the great arteries plus a ventricular septal defect and left ventricular outflow tract obstruction may require a systemic–pulmonary artery anastomosis when a pronounced diminution in pulmonary blood flow exists. A later corrective procedure for these patients bypasses the left ventricular outflow obstruction and employs an intracardiac ventricular baffle connecting the left ventricle to the aorta and an extracardiac prosthetic conduit between the right ventricle and the distal end of a divided pulmonary artery (Rastelli procedure).[423] In patients with significant pulmonary vascular obstructive disease the risk of definitive repair (intraatrial baffle and closure of the ventricular septal defect) is great. In this group of patients a "palliative" Mustard procedure leaving the ventricular septal defect open often provides good, short-term, symptomatic improvement by

increasing arterial oxygen tension and reducing the stimulus to progressive polycythemia.[424]

Congenitally Corrected Transposition of the Great Arteries

This term is applied to two distinctly different anomalies, anatomically corrected transposition or malposition of the great arteries and physiologically corrected, levo- or L-transposition of the great arteries.

Morphology. Anatomically corrected malposition of the great arteries is a rare form of congenital heart disease in which the great arteries are abnormally related to each other and to the ventricles but arise, nonetheless, above the anatomically correct ventricles.[425,426] Because of this, the term *malposition*, rather than *transposition*, is preferable. The anomaly results from either leftward looping of the ventricular segment of the embryonic heart tube in the situs solitus heart, or rightward looping in the situs inversus heart. In this unusual malformation the aorta is to the left (levo- or L-malposition) and the pulmonary artery is to the right. When no other defect exists, the circulation proceeds normally. When an associated lesion prompts cardiac catheterization, diagnosis of the abnormal relationships between the great arteries may be made by biplane angiocardiography. Anomalies commonly associated with anatomically corrected malposition of the great arteries include ventricular septal defect, left juxtaposition of the atrial appendages, tricuspid atresia or stenosis, and valvular and subvalvular pulmonic stenosis.

Invariably, the term *congenitally corrected transposition* is applied to the patient in whom a functional correction of the circulation exists by virtue of the relationships between the ventricles and great arteries.[427,428] Corrected or L-transposition occurs when the primitive cardiac tube loops to the left, instead of to the right, during embryogenesis.[429] The anatomical right ventricle comes to lie on the left and receives oxygenated blood from the left atrium; this blood is ejected into an anteriorly placed, left-sided aorta. The anatomical left ventricle lies to the right and connects the right atrium to a posteriorly placed pulmonary artery. This arrangement of the great arteries and ventricles (in contrast to the uncorrected, complete, or D-transposition) permits functional correction, so that systemic venous blood passes into the pulmonary trunk while arterialized pulmonary venous blood flows into the aorta. In the heart with congenitally corrected transposition, the venae cavae and coronary sinus drain into a right atrium that is normal in position and structure. Venous blood flows from the right atrium, designated as the "venous atrium," across an atrioventricular valve that has the structure of a normal mitral valve and into the right-sided "venous ventricle." The venous ventricle, however, has the morphological characteristics of a normal left ventricle, i.e., its interior lining is trabeculated, it has no crista supraventricularis, and the atrioventricular valve is in continuity with the posteriorly placed semilunar valve. It ejects blood into the pulmonary trunk, which arises posterior to the ascending aorta. Oxygenated blood returns from the lungs to the left atrium, which is normal in position and structure; from here it flows into the left-sided "arterial ventricle" across an atrioventricular valve that has the structure of a normal tricuspid valve. The interior lining of the arterial ventricle has the morphological characteristics of a normal right ventricle (i.e., it has course trabeculations and a crista supraventricularis), and the tricuspid atrioventricular valve is not in continuity with the anteriorly placed semilunar valve. The arterial ventricle ejects blood into the aorta, which arises anterior to the pulmonary trunk. In addition to inversion of the cardiac ventricles, there is inversion of the conduction system and coronary arteries. Commonly associated anatomical lesions include atrial and/or ventricular septal defects; single ventricle with an outlet chamber with or without pulmonic stenosis; left atrioventricular valve regurgitation, usually because of an Ebstein's malformation of the left-sided tricuspid valve; ventricular septal defect and pulmonic stenosis; and dextrocardia.[430]

CLINICAL MANIFESTATIONS. The clinical presentation, course, and prognosis of patients with congenital functionally corrected transposition vary, depending on the nature and severity of the complicating intracardiac anomalies. Patients in whom corrected transposition exists as an isolated anomaly present no functional alterations and have no symptoms.

The physical findings in congenitally corrected transposition are those of the associated lesions with two exceptions: (1) a single accentuated second heart sound is usually present in the second left intercostal space, representing closure of the aortic valve lying lateral and anterior to the pulmonic valve; and (2) there is a high incidence of cardiac dysrhythmias. Because of the inversion of the heart's conduction system the electrocardiogram may provide important clues in the diagnosis. An abnormal direction of initial (septal) depolarization from right to left causes leftward, anterior, and superior orientation of the initial QRS forces and reversal of the precordial Q-wave pattern (Q waves are present in the right precordial leads and absent in the left [Fig. 29–61]).

LABORATORY EXAMINATION. In addition to inversion of the conduction system, the His bundle is elongated because of the greater distance between the atrioventricular node and the base of the ventricular septum.[432] The His bundle is located beneath the pulmonic valve in the position of mitral pulmonary continuity; thus, it is subject to significant excursions during mitral valve closure. This arrangement may be a causal factor in the arrhythmias and atrioventricular conduction disturbances commonly observed in these patients. First-degree atrioventricular (AV) block occurs in about 50 per cent, and complete AV block occurs in 10 to 15 per cent of patients. Other degrees of AV dissociation may be observed as well as paroxysmal supraventricular tachycardia and ventricular extrasystoles. In some patients, Kent bundle connections provide the anatomical substrate for preexcitation.[433] Roentgenographic examination characteristically reveals absence of the normal pulmonary artery segment and a smooth convexity of the left supracardiac border produced by the displaced ascending aorta (Fig. 29–62). The latter may be visualized by radionuclide scintillation scans of the central circulation.[434] The main pulmonary trunk is medially displaced and absent from the cardiac silhouette; the right pulmonary hilus is often prominent and elevated compared to the left, producing a right-sided "waterfall" appearance.

Real-time *cross-sectional echocardiography* may suggest the diagnosis of corrected transposition.[34,406] By tracing the great arteries back to their ventricles of origin in the short-axis plane, one would find that the anterior leftward great artery (the aorta) arises from the left-sided ventricle and is not in continuity with the left-sided atrioventricular valve. Because the ventricular septum lies in the anteroposterior plane parallel to the echo beam, it may not be visualized. In apical-basal, four-chamber echo views, the right and left ventricular morphology and the inverted atrioventricular valves may be ascertained correctly. The latter views may

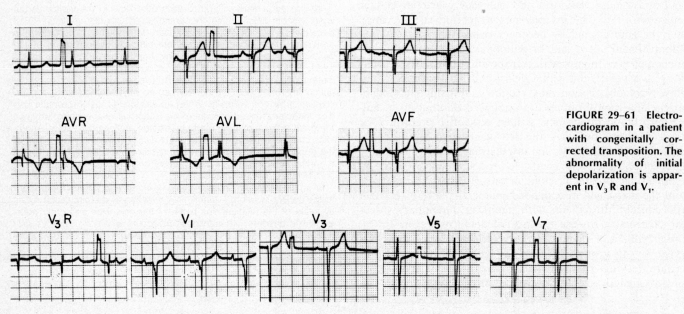

FIGURE 29–61 Electrocardiogram in a patient with congenitally corrected transposition. The abnormality of initial depolarization is apparent in V_3R and V_1.

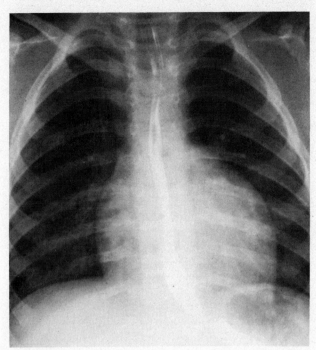

FIGURE 29-62 Chest roentgenogram in a child with congenitally corrected transposition of the great arteries. The smooth convexity of the left superior cardiac border is formed by the displaced ascending aorta. The main pulmonary artery is medially displaced and absent from the cardiac silhouette.

also allow detection of inferior displacement of the left-sided tricuspid valve when Ebstein's anomaly coexists.[34]

At *cardiac catheterization* the diagnosis should be suspected when the venous catheter enters a posterior and midline main pulmonary trunk. Retrograde arterial catheter passage establishes the typical position of the ascending aorta at the upper left cardiac border. Hemodynamic abnormalities depend upon the lesions associated with corrected transposition. Selective *angiocardiography* allows visualization of the transposed great arteries and morphological differentiation of the two ventricles (Fig. 29–63).[435] The ventricles tend to lie side by side, with the ventricular septum oriented in an anteroposterior direction. Selective aortography demonstrates the inverted coronary arterial pattern that is invariably present in corrected transposition. The competence of the left atrioventricular valve may be determined by injection of contrast material into the arterial ventricle.[436] When a left-sided Ebstein's malformation exists, the leaflets are displaced distal to the true valve annulus. The level of the annulus may be determined by visualization of the circumflex branch of the left coronary artery, which courses posteriorly in the AV groove.

Specific problems have attended operative repair of the lesions associated with congenitally corrected transposition, owing primarily to the course of the AV conduction system and the coronary arterial pattern.[437,438] Intraoperative electrophysiological mapping of the course of the conduction system has reduced, but not abolished, the risk of surgically induced heartblock. The AV bundle is located anteriorly and in relation to the anterolateral quadrant of the pulmonary outflow tract. Thus, when a ventricular septal defect is present, the bundle is usually related to the anterior and superior margins of the defect and lies beneath the pulmonic valve. In corrected transposition, the coronary arteries have a course appropriate to their ventricles, i.e., the anterior descending and circumflex arteries supply the morphological left ventricle, and the right coronary artery supplies the

morphological right ventricle. However, because the great arteries are transposed, the noncoronary sinus is the anterior sinus of the aortic valve. Occasionally, the inversion of the coronary arterial system may limit and preclude an incision into the venous ventricle, thereby interfering with exposure of intracardiac defects in the usual manner. The disadvantage in approaching intracardiac anomalies using an incision in the morphological right ventricle is that this is the systemic ventricle. Surgical risks are especially high in patients in whom significant regurgitation exists from the arterial ventricle to the arterial atrium.

Double-Outlet Right Ventricle

Other designations applied to this lesion include origin of both great arteries from the right ventricle, partial transposition, complete transposition of the aorta and levo-position of the pulmonary artery, complete dextroposition of the aorta, and the Taussig-Bing complex. An abnormal relationship exists in this malformation between the aorta and the pulmonary trunk, which both arise from the right ventricle.[439,440] The only outlet from the left ventricle is a ventricular septal defect. The anatomical classification of the various types of double-outlet right ventricle takes into account the location of the ventricular septal defect, the presence or absence of pulmonic stenosis, and whether or not dextro- or levo-malposition of the great arteries is present.[441] An increased incidence of the anomaly occurs in infants with the trisomy 18 syndrome. The most common associated anomalies are pulmonic stenosis, coarctation of the aorta, and patent ductus arteriosus. Less often associated are anomalous pulmonary venous connection, endocardial cushion defect, and atrial septal defect. The most common extracardiac malformations are asplenia and visceral heterotaxy.

The pathological features in most patients include side-by-side pulmonic and aortic valves and discontinuity between the mitral and aortic valves.[442] The latter exists because muscular infundibulum is usual beneath both semilunar valves. The ventricular septal defect may be remote from or related closely to one or both semilunar valves (Fig. 29–64).[443] When the interventricular defect is subpulmonic, with or without a straddling pulmonary trunk, the complex is designated "Taussig-Bing." In most patients the interventricular septal defect is below the crista supraventricularis and is subaortic in location. Least often the defect is either remote from both semilunar valves ("uncommitted") or underlies both ("doubly committed").

The *clinical and physiological picture* is determined by the size and location of the ventricular septal defect and the presence or absence of pulmonic stenosis. In the Taussig-Bing form of double-outlet right ventricle, the malformation resembles physiologically and clinically complete transposition with ventricular septal defect and pulmonary hypertension. When the ventricular septal defect is subaortic, the stream of blood from the left ventricle is directed preferentially to the aorta. Thus, there may be little or no detectable cyanosis, and these patients usually clinically resemble those with an isolated, large ventricular septal defect and pulmonary hypertension. The most important determinant of the natural history in both these types of double-outlet right ventricle is the progression of pulmonary vascular obstruction. In contrast, when there is pulmonary outflow tract obstruction, which is often severe and found commonly in those patients in whom the ventricular septal defect is subaortic, clinical findings are similar to those of cyanotic tetralogy of Fallot. In some patients, especially without pulmonic stenosis, the electrocardiogram shows a superiorly oriented counterclockwise frontal plane QRS loop in addition to right ventricular hypertrophy.[444] The pattern appears to result from relative hypoplasia of the anterosuperior left bundle and preferential activation of the posteroinferior left ventricular wall. Recent reports suggest that the presence of the latter electrocardiographic pattern in patients with double-outlet right ventricle should raise the possibility of a coexistent

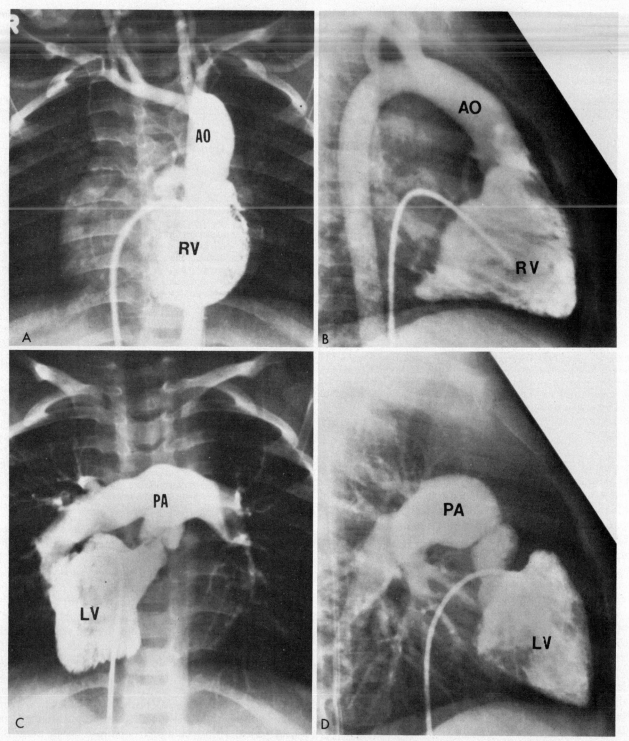

FIGURE 29-63   Congenitally corrected (levo-)transposition of the great arteries in a 4-year-old boy. *A*, Antero-posterior ventriculogram in left-sided ventricle with mesocardia. The morphological right ventricle (RV) is left-sided, indicating an L-ventricular loop (inverted ventricles in situs solitus). The aorta (AO) originates above the morphological right ventricle and is thus transposed and in the classic levo-transposition position. *B*, Lateral ventriculogram in left-sided ventricle (same frame as *A*). The aorta originates anteriorly above the morphological right ventricle (RV). *C*, Anteroposterior ventriculogram in right-sided morphological left ventricle (LV). The transposed pulmonary artery (PA) arises from this ventricle, and the ventricular septum appears intact. Pulmonic valve thickening is also evident. The aorta (A) is to the left of the pulmonary artery. Note that the ventricular septum in the L-ventricular loop is visualized best in the anteroposterior views. *D*, Lateral ventriculogram in right-sided ventricle (same frame as *C*). The pulmonary artery is posterior to the aorta, and supravalvular pulmonic narrowing is seen. (From Freedom, R. M., et al.: The differential diagnosis of levo-transposed or malposed aorta. An angiocardiographic study. Circulation *50*:1040, 1974, by permission of the American Heart Association, Inc.)

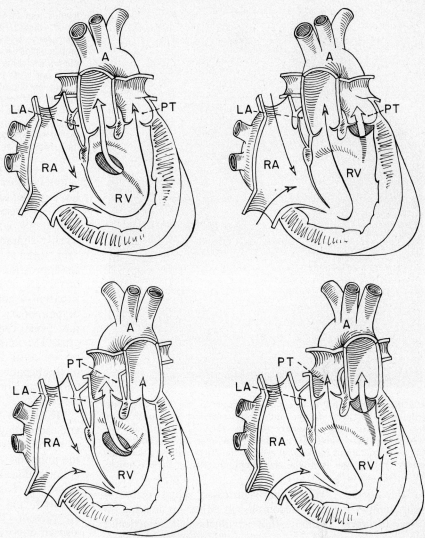

FIGURE 29–64 Double-outlet right ventricle (RV) with side-by-side relation of great arteries is illustrated in the top two panels. A subaortic ventricular septal defect (VSD) below the crista supraventricularis (*top left*) favors delivery of left ventricular blood to the aorta (A). Location of the VSD above the crista (*top right*) favors streaming to the pulmonary trunk (PT). When the great arteries are malposed (*bottom two panels*), streaming continues to depend on the relationship between a particular great artery and the VSD. The subcristal VSD (*bottom left*) favors delivery of left ventricular blood to the pulmonary trunk. The supracristal VSD depicted at the bottom right lies below the malpositioned aorta, which receives most of the left ventricular output. LA = left atrium; RA = right atrium; PT = pulmonary trunk. (From Sridaromont, S., et al.: Double outlet right ventricle: Hemodynamic and anatomic correlations. Am. J. Cardiol. *38*:85, 1976.)

endocardial cushion defect or abnormality of the mitral valve.[442] Two-dimensional *echocardiography* may reliably distinguish double-outlet right ventricle from other lesions causing cyanosis, such as tetralogy of Fallot and transposition of the great arteries. In the short-axis view, imaging is simultaneous with both great arteries in an anterior location; the ventricular septum is identified posteriorly. Atrioventricular valve–semilunar valve discontinuity and great artery relations are then defined by a variety of axial ultrasonic imaging views.[331,331a]

In each of the different types of double-outlet right ventricle, precise delineation of the malformation depends on careful angiocardiographic analysis. The diagnosis can be established with confidence when the angiographic findings include simultaneous opacification of both great vessels from the right ventricle, aortic and pulmonic valves at the same transverse level, and separation of the aortic valve from the aortic leaflet of the mitral valve by the crista supraventricularis (Fig. 29–65).[445] The position of the ventricular septal defect and the relationships between the great arteries must be defined in order to plan surgical procedures appropriately (Fig. 29–66).[446,447]

In double-outlet right ventricle with subaortic ventricular septal defect, repair is accomplished by creating an intraventicular baffle that conducts left ventricular blood

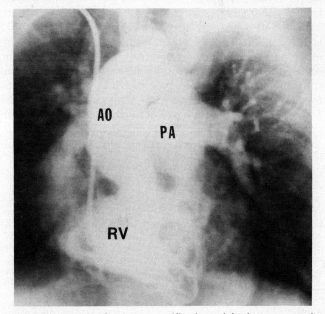

FIGURE 29–65 Simultaneous opacification of both great arteries from a right ventricular injection of contrast material in a patient with double-outlet right ventricle (RV). The aortic and pulmonic valves are at the same transverse level. AO = aorta; PA = pulmonary artery. (Courtesy of Robert White. M.D.)

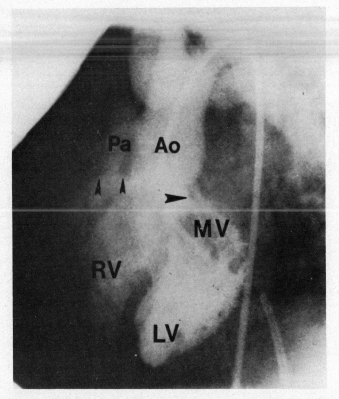

FIGURE 29–66 Left ventricular angiogram in the long-axis view from a patient with double outlet right ventricle, L-malposition of the aorta (Ao), and pulmonary stenosis. There is discontinuity between the mitral valve (MV) and the semilunar valve produced by the subaortic conus (horizontal arrow). The aorta and the pulmonary artery (Pa) emerge from the right ventricle. RV = right ventricle, LV = left ventricle.

to the aorta.[447a] When the ventricular septal defect is subpulmonic, repair is accomplished either by creating an intraventricular conduit that conducts left ventricular blood to the pulmonary arteries and performing the Mustard or Senning procedure, or by creating an intraventricular baffle directing left ventricular blood to the aorta and connecting the right ventricle to the pulmonary artery by use of a valve-containing conduit. When the ventricular septal defect is doubly committed, i.e., both subaortic and subpulmonic, operation consists of creating an intraventricular baffle that conducts left ventricular blood to the aorta. The type of double-outlet right ventricle in which the ventricular septal defect is remote and uncommitted to either semilunar orifice has rarely been repaired successfully.[446,448]

Double-Outlet Left Ventricle

One of the rarest cardiac anomalies consists of both great arteries arising from the morphological left ventricle. Usually, conal musculature or an infundibulum is absent or deficient beneath the orifices of both semilunar valves.[449,450] A broad spectrum of associated malformations exists. A ventricular septal defect and valvular or subvalvular pulmonic stenosis have been present in most patients. Angiocardiographic assessment of the spatial relations of the origins of the great arteries is essential to an accurate diagnosis and to evaluating the possibility of operative repair.[451]

Total Anomalous Pulmonary Venous Connection

This anomaly has been estimated to account for 1 to 3 per cent of all cases of congenital heart disease and 2 per cent of deaths there-

from in the first year of life.[452] The anomaly is the result of persistence during embryogenesis of communications between the pulmonary portion of the foregut plexus and the cardinal or umbilicovitelline system of veins, resulting in the connection of all the pulmonary veins either to the right atrium directly or to the systemic veins and their tributaries. Since all venous blood returns to the right atrium, an interatrial communication is an integral part of this malformation. Additional major cardiac malformations occur in about 30 per cent of patients.[453] Among these are common atrium, single ventricle, truncus arteriosus, and anomalies of the systemic veins. Extracardiac malformations, particularly of the alimentary, endocrine, and genitourinary systems, are present in 25 to 30 per cent of cases.

The *anatomical varieties* of total anomalous pulmonary venous connection may be subdivided depending upon the level of the abnormal drainage (Fig. 29–67). Table 29–9 provides average figures of the distribution of the sites of anomalous connection.[274] The anomalous connection is usually supradiaphragmatic and to the left brachiocephalic vein, right atrium, coronary sinus, or superior vena cava. In approximately 13 per cent, particularly in males, the distal site of connection is below the diaphragm. In this situation a common trunk originates from the confluence of pulmonary veins and descends in front of the esophagus, penetrating the diaphragm through the esophageal hiatus. The anomalous trunk then connects the portal vein or one of its tributaries, ductus venosus, or, rarely, to one of the hepatic veins. In rare cases various combinations of anomalous connection occur in which drainage is to multiple levels.

HEMODYNAMICS. The physiological consequences and, accordingly, the clinical picture depend upon the size of the interatrial communication and on the magnitude of the pulmonary vascular resistance.[453–455] When the interatrial communication is small, systemic blood flow is markedly limited. Right atrial and systemic venous pressures are elevated, and hepatic enlargement and peripheral edema are present. The size of the interatrial communication is also an important determinant in the development in utero and postnatally of the left atrium and left ventricle. Left atrial cavity size is usually somewhat reduced, whereas left ventricular volumes may be reduced or normal. The magnitude of pulmonary blood flow and therefore the ratio of oxygenated to unoxygenated blood that returns to the right atrium are a function of pulmonary vascular resistance. The arterial oxygen saturation, which ranges from markedly reduced to normal values, is inversely related to the pulmonary vascular resistance. In this regard, in most patients the principal determinant of pulmonary pressures and resistance is less related to augmented pulmonary blood flow and pulmonary arteriolar vascular obstruction

TABLE 29–9   SITE OF CONNECTION IN TOTAL ANOMALOUS PULMONARY VENOUS CONNECTION

1. Connection to right atrium	15%
2. Connection to common cardinal system	
a. (Right) superior vena cava	11%
b. Azygos vein	1%
3. Connection to left common cardinal system	
a. Left innominate vein	36%
b. Coronary sinus	16%
4. Connection to umbilicovitelline system	
a. Portal vein	6%
b. Ductus venosus	4%
c. Inferior vena cava	2%
d. Hepatic vein	1%
5. Multiple sites	7%
6. Unknown	1%

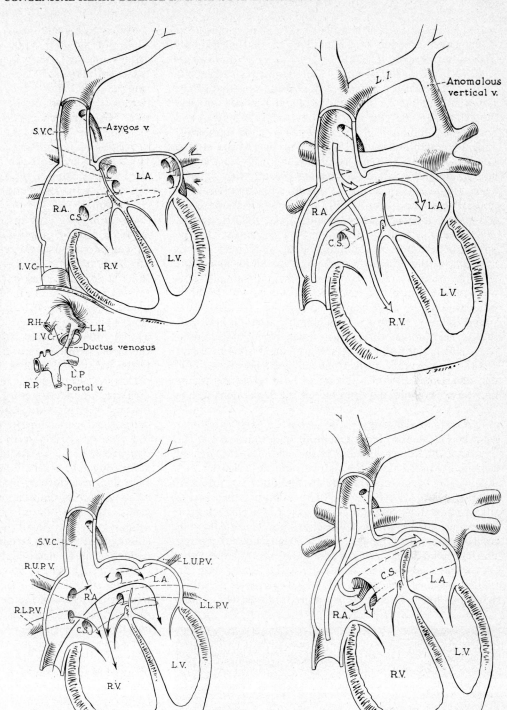

FIGURE 29–67 The normal venous drainage of the thorax and upper abdomen (*upper left*) is shown for reference purposes. The three most common types of total anomalous pulmonary venous connection are illustrated. These are connection to the right atrium (*upper right*), to the left innominate vein (*bottom left*), and to the coronary sinus (*bottom right*). S.V.C. = superior vena cava; I.V.C. = inferior vena cava; R.A. = right atrium; L.A. = left atrium; C.S. = coronary sinus; R.V. = right ventricle; L.V. = left ventricle; R.U.P.V. = right upper pulmonary veins; L.U.P.V. = left upper pulmonary veins; R.L.P.V. = right lower pulmonary veins; L.L.P.V. = left lower pulmonary veins; R.H. = right hepatic vein; L.H. = left hepatic vein; L.P.V. = left portal vein; R.P.V. = right portal vein; L.I. = left innominate vein. (From Wagenvoort, C. A., et al.: Pathology of the Pulmonary Vasculature. Springfield, Ill., Charles C Thomas, 1964.)

than to the presence and intensity of pulmonary venous obstruction.[456,457] Obstruction to pulmonary venous return and pulmonary venous hypertension are invariably present in patients with infradiaphragmatic anomalous pulmonary venous connection and in many with a supradiaphragmatic pathway. In the former type, pulmonary venous obstruction results from the length and narrowness of the common pulmonary venous trunk, compression at the esophageal hiatus of the diaphragm, constriction at the subdiaphragmatic site of insertion, or pulmonary venous return that must pass first through the portal-hepatic circulation before returning to the right atrium. When venous obstruction occurs in supradiaphragmatic types of drainage, constriction may exist at the entrance site of the anomalous veins into the systemic venous circulation, and/or the anomalous venous channel may be kinked or situated abnormally and compressed between the left pulmonary artery and left bronchus.[458,459] Occasionally the presence of a small, restrictive patent foramen ovale results in pulmonary venous obstruction. Pulmonary vascular obstructive disease is rare during infancy, although exceptions have been reported.[460,461] In patients without pulmonary venous obstruction the risk of developing the Eisenmenger reaction is comparable to that in patients with an atrial septal defect.

CLINICAL FINDINGS. The majority of patients with total anomalous pulmonary venous connection have symptoms during the first year of life, and 80 per cent will die before age one year if left untreated.[453,454] The few who remain asymptomatic have a relatively good prognosis; once the condition is detected, operation may be elected later in childhood.[457] Symptomatic infants with total anomalous pulmonary venous connection present with signs of heart failure and/or cyanosis. Infants with pulmonary venous obstruction present with the early onset of severe dyspnea, pulmonary edema, cyanosis, and right heart failure. Cardiac murmurs are often not prominent. In the unobstructed forms of total anomalous pulmonary venous connection the characteristic physical findings include right ventricular precordial overactivity and minimal cyanosis unless congestive heart failure intervenes. Multiple heart sounds are often audible, consisting of a first heart sound followed by an ejection sound; a fixed, widely split second heart sound with an accentuated pulmonic component; and a third and often a fourth heart sound. A soft systolic ejection murmur is usual along the left sternal border, and a mid-diastolic murmur of flow across the tricuspid valve is commonly audible at the lower left sternal border.

Laboratory Findings. The *electrocardiogram* shows right-axis deviation and right atrial and right ventricular hypertrophy. *Roentgenograms* of the chest reveal increased pulmonary blood flow; the right atrium and ventricle are dilated and hypertrophied, and the pulmonary artery segment is enlarged[463] (Fig. 29–68). In addition, the specific site of anomalous connection may result in a characteristic appearance of the cardiac silhouette. Thus, in patients with total anomalous pulmonary venous connection to the left brachiocephalic vein, the superior vena cava on the right, left brachiocephalic vein superiorly, and vertical vein on the left produce a cardiac shadow that resembles a "snowman" or "figure of eight." The upper right cardiac border

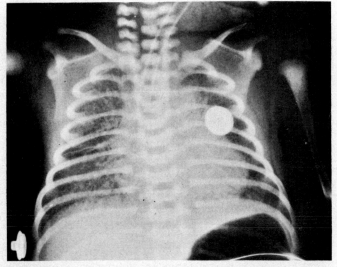

FIGURE 29–68 Chest roentgenogram in an infant with total anomalous pulmonary venous connection below the diaphragm shows normal overall heart size but diffuse pattern of pulmonary venous hypertension in both lung fields.

may be prominent when the anomalous connection is to the right superior vena cava. *Echocardiography* demonstrates marked enlargement of the right ventricle and a small left atrium.[462] Occasionally, an echo-free space representing the common pulmonary venous chamber may be seen to lie behind the left atrium on ultrasound examination.[35] Two-dimensional echocardiography allows a detailed assessment of the anatomy of pulmonary venous drainage. A combination of suprasternal, parasternal, and subcostal views is required to trace the course of anomalous pulmonary venous connections and visualize the level of entry of the anomalous venous channels into the systemic venous circulation.[464]

At *cardiac catheterization* those patients found to have systemic arterial saturations below 70 to 75 per cent and with pulmonary artery pressure at or above systemic levels are likely to have pulmonary venous obstruction. Variations in oxygen saturation in the systemic venous circulation may be helpful. In the subdiaphragmatic type, a step-up may not be apparent in inferior vena caval oxygen saturations obtained via femoral vein cannulation because of the contribution of highly oxygenated renal venous blood to the caval stream. In contrast, sampling of the hepatic or portal vein via a catheter inserted through the umbilical vein will yield diagnostically higher oxygen saturations, indicating anomalous return to those vessels. Selective pulmonary arteriography and *indicator dilution* studies at cardiac catheterization are especially helpful in determining the drainage pathways of the pulmonary veins. Indicator dye injected into the right ventricle or pulmonary artery takes longer to reach the peripheral arterial sampling site than does dye injected into the vena cava or right atrium. The contours of dilution curves obtained from a peripheral artery after injection into both the right atrium and a pulmonary vein are identical and show a large right-to-left shunt, while the left atrial curve is normal. If the cardiac catheter can be manipulated directly into the anomalous trunk through its site of connection, selective injection of contrast material into the common channel provides anatomical definition of the pulmonary venous tree. If the pulmonary veins cannot be entered directly, selective right and left main pulmonary artery injection of contrast material is often more helpful than is injection into a main pulmonary artery, since many infants have a persistent patent ductus arteriosus through which the contrast agent flows right to left. Moreover, the drainage from both lungs must be outlined clearly in order to exclude a mixed type of anomalous venous drainage. Pulmonary venous obstruction may be detected by noting a pressure difference between the pulmonary artery wedge pressure and the right atrium.

TREATMENT. Balloon atrial septotomy may provide dramatic palliation for the infant in whom the small size of an interatrial communication limits the amount of blood reaching the left side of the heart and systemic circulation. Unless pulmonary vascular disease is present, results of operation for total anomalous pulmonary venous connection in patients more than one year of age are generally good. The procedure consists of creating an anastomosis between the common pulmonary venous channel and left atrium and closing the atrial defect and the anomalous venous pathway.[464a] Improved results of operation in infancy may be anticipated if postoperative pulmonary venous hypertension can be averted by construction of a generally large anastomosis with or without enlargement of the left atrium.[460] Normal hemodynamics and cardiac function have been demonstrated after surgical correction.[465,466]

PARTIAL ANOMALOUS PULMONARY VENOUS CONNECTION

In this condition one or more of the pulmonary veins, but not all, are connected to the right atrium or to one or more of its venous tributaries. An atrial septal defect, particularly one of the sinus venosus type, commonly accompanies this anomaly; the usual connection involves the veins of the right upper and middle lobe and the superior vena cava.[274] Exclusive of atrial septal defects, major additional cardiac malformations occur in approximately 20 per cent of patients; these include ventricular septal defect, tetralogy of Fallot, and a variety of complex anomalies.

In the absence of associated anomalies, the physiological disturbance is determined by the number of anomalous veins and their site of connection, the presence and size of an atrial septal defect, and the state of the pulmonary vascular bed.[467] In the usual patient with isolated partial pulmonary venous connection, the hemodynamic state and physical findings are similar to those in atrial septal defect. Rarely, venous drainage of the right lung is into the inferior vena cava. This condition is often associated with hypoplasia of the right lung, dextroposition of the heart, pulmonary parenchymal abnormalities, and anomalous systemic supply to the lower lobe of the right lung from the abdominal aorta or its main branches.[468] This complex has been designated the "scimitar syndrome" because of the characteristic roentgenographic finding of a crescentlike shadow in the right lower lung field that is produced by the anomalous venous channel.

At *cardiac catheterization*, partial anomalous pulmonary venous connection to the coronary sinus, azygos vein, or superior vena cava may be identified by careful and frequent oximetry sampling. Oximetry is of limited value when the anomalous connection is to the inferior vena cava, because of both reduced flow through the right lung and the contribution to the vena caval stream of highly oxygenated blood from the renal veins. Selective angiography is most helpful the farther away from the right atrium the anomalous veins connect. Surgical repair offers definitive therapy at low risk if pulmonary vascular obliterative disease has not yet developed.

Malpositions of the Heart and Cardiac Apex

Positional anomalies of the heart refer to conditions in which the cardiac apex is located in the right side of the chest (dextrocardia) or is centrally located (mesocardia) or in which there is a normal location of the heart in the left side of the chest but abnormal position of the viscera (isolated levocardia). Commonly, such hearts are abnormal with respect to chamber localization and great artery attachments; associated complex intra- and extracardiac lesions are common.

Problems of terminology abound in the literature describing these complex cardiac anomalies, although sensible and uniform systems of classification are available.[469-473]

Defining the cardiac anatomy in instances of cardiac malposition requires a description of three cardiac segments—the visceroatrial situs, the ventricular loop, and the conotruncus (the atria, ventricles, and great arteries, respectively). In addition to defining positional interrelationships, the description of the malposed heart must also include the connections of the ventricles to the atria and great arteries as well as chamber identification, both morphologically and functionally.

In general, the determination of the body situs indicates the position of the atria. The visceral situs can usually be determined by the location of the stomach bubble and liver on a routine roentgenogram and of the inferior vena cava by means of the position of a cardiac catheter, or by means of a venous or radioisotope angiocardiogram. Situs solitus is the normal arrangement of viscera and atria, with the right atrium right-sided, and the left atrium left-sided. Situs solitus is further characterized by a trilobed right lung and eparterial bronchus (i.e., the right upper lobe bronchus that passes above the right pulmonary artery), a bilobed left lung and hyparterial bronchus (i.e., the left bronchus that passes below the left pulmonary artery), the major lobe of the liver on the right, a left-sided stomach and spleen, and right-sided venae cavae. Situs inversus is a mirror image of normal. Situs ambiguous or visceral heterotaxy refers to an anatomically uncertain or indeterminant body configuration. The latter is seen often in association with congenital asplenia, which resembles bilateral right-sidedness, and congenital polysplenia, which resembles bilateral left-sidedness.[470,471] Cardiac anomalies associated commonly with asplenia include anomalous systemic venous connection, atrial septal or complete endocardial cushion defect, common ventricle, transposition of the great arteries, severe pulmonic stenosis or atresia, and anomalous pulmonary venous connection. Polysplenia is associated commonly with absence of the hepatic portion of the inferior vena cava with azygos continuation, bilateral superior venae cavae, anomalous pulmonary venous connection, and atrial septal defect (either ostium secundum or endocardial cushion). Pulmonic stenosis and double-outlet right ventricle are each observed in approximately 25 per cent of cases. It is important to recognize these complex syndromes in order to distinguish them from forms of cyanotic heart disease that may be amenable to corrective surgical therapy. Diagnosis is suggested by a symmetrical liver shadow roentgenographically and, in asplenia, by the presence of Howell-Jolly and Heinz bodies in red blood cells demonstrated on blood smear, and it is confirmed by a negative or abnormal radioactive spleen scan.

Once the type of visceral situs is defined, it is necessary to describe the bulboventricular loop. Normally, the primitive cardiac tube bends to the right (D-loop), which brings the anatomical right ventricle to the right of the anatomical left ventricle. An L-loop brings the morphological right ventricle left-sided relative to the morphological left ventricle. The L-loop is normal in the presence of situs inversus, but in situs solitus it is synonymous with inverted ventricles.

The morphological features of each ventricle can be identified angiographically. The anatomical right ventricle is equipped with a tricuspid valve, is highly trabeculated, and contains the septal band of the single papillary muscle; its infundibulum lies anterior to and superiorly beyond the outlet of the left ventricle. The anatomical right ventricle generally connects with whichever of the two great arteries is the more anterior. The anatomical left ventricle is smooth-walled and contains an outlet that lies posterior to the right ventricular infundibulum; its entrance is guarded by a bicuspid mitral valve, the anterior leaflet of which is normally in continuity with elements of the semilunar valve at its outlet.

The great arteries are described in terms of their positional interrelationships and their ventricular connections. The ventricular attachments may be normal or may form the anomalies of double-outlet right or left ventricle or transposition. The arterial interrelationships are described as D (dextro), in which the ascending aorta sweeps toward the right and lies to the right of the main pulmonary artery; L (levo), in which the ascending aorta sweeps toward the left and lies to the left of the main pulmonary artery; or A (antero), which is the rare situation in which the aorta lies directly in front of the pulmonary artery. The D, L, and A descriptions of the aorticopulmonary artery interrelationships should not be confused with the D- or L-loop designation of the ventricular interrelationships.[471]

Employing segmental sets composed of descriptive units of visceroatrial situs/ventricular loop/great artery relationships greatly simplifies expression of the type of cardiac anatomy present in cardiac malposition.[469] For example, the normal heart in a patient with situs inversus and dextrocardia is referred to as inversus/L loop/L normal; complete transposition of the great arteries in a patient with situs inversus is referred to as inversus/L loop/L transposition; functionally corrected transposition in a patient with situs solitus is referred to as solitus/L loop/L transposition; dextrocardia and functionally corrected transposition is designated solitus/D loop/D transposition with dextrocardia.

After the cardiac chambers are diagnosed functionally (arterial and venous), the positional and morphological relationships are understood, and the presence of associated anomalies has been established, the principles of medical and surgical treatment apply to these cardiac malpositions as they do to normally located hearts.

Miscellaneous Conditions

CONGENITAL PERICARDIAL DEFECTS
(See also page 1517)

Isolated pericardial defects are rare. They occur most commonly in males and are usually left-sided, although they may be right-sided, diaphragmatic, or total.[474,475] The anomaly is produced by deficient formation of the pleuropericardial membrane, or, if diaphragmatic, defective formation of the septum transversum. Associated congenital anomalies of the heart and lungs occur in approximately 30 per cent of cases. Most patients with the isolated defect are asymptomatic. Nonspecific anterior chest pain may be the result of torsion of the great arteries due to absence of the stabilizing forces of the left pericardium.[474] With complete absence of the left pericardium[475] a conspicuous apical impulse may be noted shifted leftward to the anterior or midaxillary line. Electrocardiographic changes may be related to levo-position of the heart; a leftward displacement of the QRS transition in the precordial leads and vertical or right-axis deviation are usual. The diagnosis may be suggested by chest roentgenograms.[476] With a complete left pericardial absence, the heart is levo-posed, and

the aortic knob, pulmonary artery, and ventricles form three prominent left heart border convexities. A partial left pericardial defect may be suspected by varying degrees of prominence of the pulmonary artery and/or the left atrial appendage. Echocardiographic findings often mimic those observed in patients with right ventricular volume overload (enlarged right ventricle and abnormal ventricular septal motion), probably owing to the altered cardiac position and motion within the thorax.[477] The anomaly can be diagnosed definitively by inducing a left pneumothorax and observing air under the right pericardium when the patient is placed in the right lateral decubitus position, or preferably by angiocardiography.

Complete absence of the left pericardium requires no treatment. However, partial defects may impose serious risks, including herniation and strangulation of the ventricles or left atrial appendage with left-sided defects, or the possibility of a superior vena cava obstructive syndrome with right-sided defects. In the diaphragmatic type, cardiac compression by abdominal contents requires surgical repair. Partial left or right defects may be closed with a patch of mediastinal pleura.

SINGLE ATRIUM

Single or common atrium is a rare isolated defect. The anomaly consists of an absent atrial septum, usually with a cleft in the anteromedial leaflet of the mitral valve, and occasionally, with a cleft tricuspid valve as well. The lesion may be seen as one component of the Ellis–van Creveld syndrome (Table 29–2) or of the complex cardiac anomalies seen in patients with asplenia or polysplenia.

Single atrium may be suspected clinically by the presence of cardiac murmurs of an atrial septal defect and mitral regurgitation associated with mild cyanosis, roentgenographic evidence of cardiac enlargement and increased pulmonary blood flow, and electrocardiographic features of endocardial cushion defect.[478] Angiographically, the absence of the atrial septum produces a large, globular shaped, single atrial structure. Selective left ventricular angiocardiography shows the characteristic gooseneck appearance seen in the various forms of endocardial cushion defect. In the absence of pulmonary vascular obstructive disease surgical correction is indicated by means of a prosthetic patch.

SINGLE (COMMON) VENTRICLE

This rare anomaly consists of a single ventricular chamber that receives blood from two separate atrioventricular valves or a common atrioventricular valve[479,480] (Fig. 29–69). The latter situation is encountered especially in association with splenic anomalies. The definition excludes examples of tricuspid or mitral atresia.[481] Single ventricle is almost always accompanied by abnormal great artery positional relationships; the incidence of L-malposition of the great arteries is approximately equal to that of D-malposition.[482] Associated anomalies are common and include, in particular, pulmonic valvular or subvalvular stenosis, subaortic stenosis, total or partial anomalous pulmonary venous connection, and coarctation of the aorta.

Morphology.   In approximately 80 per cent of patients the single ventricle morphologically resembles a left ventricular chamber that is separated from an infundibular outlet chamber by a bulboventricular septum.[479] The infundibular chamber is considered to represent developmentally the outflow tract of the right ventricle. When the great arteries are malposed, the infundibulum lying anterior at the basal position of the single ventricle communicates with the aorta and may be in one of two positions: noninverted (D-malposition), when it is situated at the right basal aspect of the heart, or inverted (L-malposition), when it is located at the left base of the heart.[482] In the unusual situation in which the great arteries are related normally, the infundibulum communicates with the pulmonary trunk.[483] *Double-inlet left ventricle* is a term used synonymously to describe the most frequently encountered single ventricular chamber that has the anatomical characteristics of the left ventricle.[484] Less commonly the single ventricular chamber resembles a right ventricle (double-inlet right ventricle) or contains features suggestive of both or neither ventricle; the latter two situations have occasionally been designated common ventricle and single ventricle of the primitive type, respectively.[480]

Clinical Findings.   Depending upon the associated anomalies, the clinical presentation of single ventricle mimics other conditions in

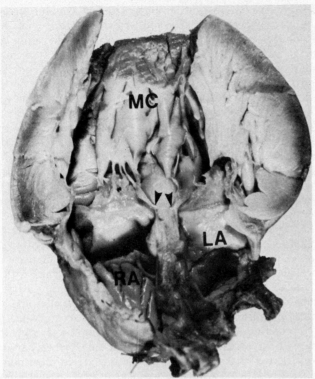

FIGURE 29–69 Anatomical specimen of a heart with a single ventricle cut in the same plane as an apical four-chamber echocardiogram view. A single main chamber (MC) is seen. Two atrioventricular valves enter the main chamber and attach to the crux of the heart at the same level (arrows). RA = right atrium, LA = left atrium. (Courtesy of Thomas DiSessa, M.D.)

which cyanosis and decreased (or increased) pulmonary blood flow coexist, e.g., tetralogy of Fallot or tricuspid atresia in the former instance, and complete transposition of the great arteries and double-outlet right ventricle in the latter.[485] The electrocardiogram in double-inlet left ventricle without inversion of the infundibulum (D-malposition) usually shows features of left ventricular hypertrophy. With infundibular inversion (L-malposition) the electrical forces are directed anteriorly and rightward, as they are in ventricular inversion without associated defects. In patients with the more primitive types of common or single ventricle there is a repetitious rS pattern in all the precordial electrocardiographic leads. Chest roentgenographic findings

resemble those observed in patients with complete (dextro-) transposition of the great arteries or functionally corrected (levo-) transposition of the great arteries without features distinctive for single ventricle.

In those patients in whom two separate atrioventricular valves communicate with the single ventricular chamber, echocardiography suggests the correct diagnosis when echoes are visualized from the two valves without an intervening interventricular septum.[486,487] In the absence of ventricular septal echoes when the two valves are not visualized simultaneously, they may be identified separately with a careful long-axis sweep of the ventricle. Occasionally, it is possible to detect the presence of a small outflow chamber anterior to the atrioventricular valves by using a high transducer position and pointing the echo beam in an inferomedial direction. The single ventricle with a single atrioventricular valve is suspected when the excursion of echoes from the single valve located posteriorly in the ventricular chamber is of large amplitude. Enhanced assessment of the atrioventricular valve(s) in patients with single ventricle is provided by saline contrast echocardiography.[488] In the presence of two atrioventricular valves, a peripheral or central venous injection of saline results in a cloud of echoes that appear in the tricuspid valve orifice during ventricular diastole and anterior to the mitral valve in the same cardiac cycle. The echo cloud appears within the ventricle during diastole after complete opening of the mitral valve (after the mitral valve E point). In most patients with a common atrioventricular valve, the cloud of echoes enters the ventricle during ventricular diastole, from behind the echoes of the only identifiable atrioventricular valve (Fig. 29–70). Occasionally, the contrast technique may identify the outflow chamber; the echo cloud appears initially in the common ventricular chamber during the rapid filling phase of ventricular diastole and arrives later in the outflow chamber during subsequent ventricular systole. Selective ventriculography is necessary to delineate with certainty the anatomical type of single ventricle and to diagnose the associated great artery interrelationships and the presence or absence of additional lesions (Fig. 29–71).

Attempts to partition the single ventricle with a Dacron or Teflon prosthetic patch have met with limited success as well as a high incidence of postoperative complete heart block, even with intraoperative electrophysiological mapping of the conduction system.[489–491] Creation of an atriopulmonary conduit (the Fontan procedure) and closure of the tricuspid orifice is a technique awaiting long-term evaluation.[492] Palliative procedures designed to either increase pulmonary blood flow (systemic-pulmonary anastomosis) or limit pulmonary blood flow (pulmonary artery banding) often allow survival to adolescence in patients with single ventricle.

VASCULAR RINGS

Morphology. The normal development of the aortic arch system was described on page 945 (see Fig. 29–5).

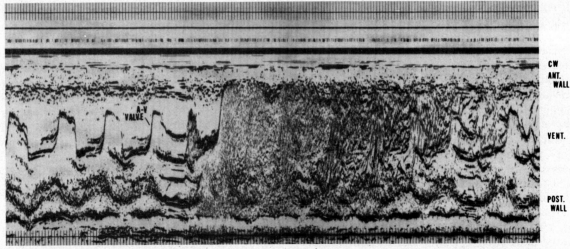

FIGURE 29–70 Saline contrast echocardiogram in a child with single ventricle and a common atrioventricular valve. The cloud of echoes enters the ventricle (VENT) during ventricular diastole from behind the echoes of the only identifiable AV valve. CW = chest wall; ANT. WALL = anterior wall; POST. WALL = posterior wall. (Courtesy of Thomas DiSessa, M.D.)

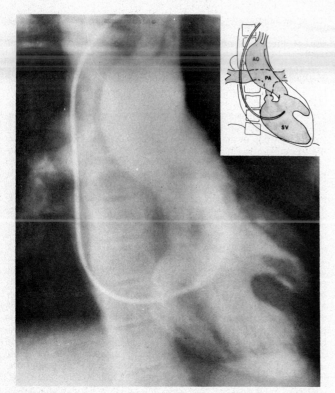

FIGURE 29–71 Selective ventriculogram in a child with single ventricle (SV). There is levo-malposition of the great arteries with the aorta (AO) communicating with a small outflow chamber. The pulmonary artery (PA) arises from a single ventricular chamber, which has the anatomical characteristics of a left ventricle. There is moderate pulmonic stenosis.

The term vascular ring is employed for those aortic arch or pulmonary artery malformations that exhibit an abnormal relationship with the esophagus and trachea, causing compression, dysphagia, and/or respiratory symptoms.[493] The most common and serious vascular ring is produced by a double aortic arch in which both the right and left fourth embryonic aortic arches persist. In the most common type of double aortic arch there is a left ligamentum arteriosum or ductus arteriosus, and both arches are patent, the right being larger than the left.[494] A right aortic arch with a left ductus or ligamentum arteriosum connecting the left pulmonary artery and the upper part of the descending aorta and with an anomalous right subclavian artery arising from the left descending aorta are additional important vascular ring arrangements.[495] The latter anomaly exists frequently in cases of tetralogy of Fallot and otherwise uncomplicated coarctation of the aorta. An unusual cause of tracheal compression is the "vascular sling" created by an anomalous left pulmonary artery that arises from a rightward, elongated pulmonary trunk and courses between the trachea and esophagus before it branches normally within the left lung.[496] This arrangement is commonly associated with other cardiac and extracardiac anomalies.

Clinical Findings.   The symptoms produced by vascular rings depend upon the tightness of anatomical constriction of the trachea and esophagus and consist principally of respiratory difficulties, cyanosis (associated especially with feeding), stridor, and dysphagia. The electrocardiogram is normal unless associated cardiovascular anomalies

are present. The barium esophagogram is a useful screening procedure. Prominent posterior indentation of the esophagus is observed in the common vascular ring arrangements, although the pulmonary artery "vascular sling" produces an anterior indentation. Unusual and rare aortic arch anomalies may create rings that impinge on the trachea but do not compress the esophagus and that will not be suspected by this simple radiographic procedure.[495] Selective contrast angiography is required to delineate the anatomy of the aorta and its branches or the course of the main pulmonary arteries.

Management.   The severity of symptoms and the anatomy of the malformation are the most important factors in determining treatment. Patients, particularly infants, with respiratory obstruction require prompt surgical intervention. Operative repair of the double aortic arch requires division of the minor arch (usually the left).[496a] A reported 20 to 30 per cent operative mortality is related, in part, to problems in postoperative respiratory care. Patients with a right aortic arch and a left ductus or ligamentum arteriosum require division of the ductus or ligamentum and/or ligation and division of the left subclavian artery, which is the posterior component of the ring. Operation is rarely indicated for patients with an aberrant right subclavian artery derived from a left aortic arch and left descending aorta. In patients with a pulmonary artery vascular sling, operation consists of detachment of the left pulmonary artery at its origin and anastomosis to the main pulmonary artery directly or via a conduit of its proximal end brought anterior to the trachea.[496,497]

Congenital Arrhythmias

Complete heart block and supraventricular tachycardia are the two most common and important congenital arrhythmias. The electrophysiological and electrocardiographic features of these arrhythmias are discussed elsewhere in the text (Chaps. 21 and 22).

CONGENITAL COMPLETE HEART BLOCK.   The atrioventricular node and the His bundle originate during fetal development as separate structures and later join together. Anatomical studies have shown the basic lesion in congenital complete heart block to consist of discontinuity between the atrial musculature and the AV node or the His bundle, if the AV node is absent. Occasionally, the anatomical interruption may be situated between the AV node and the main His bundle, or within the bundle itself.[498] No known etiology exists for the vast majority of cases of congenital heart block in infants who usually have otherwise anatomically normal hearts. However, fetal myocarditis, idiopathic hemorrhage and necrosis involving conduction tissue, and degeneration and fibrosis related in some instances to the transplacental passage of immune complexes from mothers with systemic lupus erythematosus are all entities capable of causing congenital heart block.[499–501] Less often, congenital heart block may be associated with various forms of congenital heart disease, the most common malformation being congenitally corrected transposition of the great arteries.

Detection of consistent fetal bradycardia (heart rate 40 to 80 beats/min) by auscultation or electronic monitoring allows anticipation of the correct diagnosis. The newborn, especially with a ventricular rate less than 50 beats/min and atrial rate in excess of 150 beats/min, is at highest risk; the presence of an associated cardiovascular anomaly greatly lessens the chances of survival.[501,502] Treatment is not required for the asymptomatic infant. Digitalization is recommended for the baby in congestive heart failure, irrespective of complete heart block.[503] Isoproterenol and other sympathomimetic drugs and atropine do not have permanent or beneficial effects. Congestive heart failure and Stokes-Adams attacks require pacemaker treatment at any age.[504] Initial management of the child in whom permanent epicardial pacemaker insertion is indicated usually involves preoperative insertion of a transvenous intracardiac electrode into the right ventricle in order to protect the patient from serious arrhythmias during the induction of anesthesia. A variety of problems may be anticipated after pacemaker implantation related to growth of the patient, which stresses the lead system; the fragility of the lead system in a physically active young patient; and the limited life span of the pulse generator. Patients with congenital complete heart block who survive infancy usually remain asymptomatic until late in childhood or adolescence.[501]

SUPRAVENTRICULAR TACHYCARDIA. Paroxysmal tachycardia of supraventricular origin may have its origin in utero or in the immediate postnatal period.[505-507] The most frequent arrhythmias producing symptoms are paroxysmal atrial tachycardia with or without ventricular preexcitation, atrial flutter, and junctional tachycardia. The arrhythmia may cause intrauterine cardiac failure; its detection and persistence prenatally should prompt consideration of administration of digitalis to the mother if amniocentesis indicates surfactant deficiency and fetal lung immaturity,[506] since early delivery is not indicated if the baby will have hyaline membrane disease, or cesarean section or induced labor if the fetus is close to term. No recognizable cause exists for the disorder in the vast majority of infants. The transplacental passage of long-acting thyroid-stimulating hormone (LATS) and immune gamma 2 globulin from hyperthyroid mothers, hypoglycemia, ventricular preexcitation pathways, and Ebstein's anomaly of the tricuspid valve are occasionally causative.[507,508] Symptoms produced by the tachyarrhythmia after birth are subtle and often go undetected until signs of heart failure have been present for 24 to 36 hours. Conversion to normal sinus rhythm is usually accomplished by administration of digitalis, direct-current cardioversion, or eliciting a diving reflex by covering the face with an ice-cold wet washcloth for 4 to 5 seconds.[509] Conversion should be followed by digitalization on a prophylactic basis. Common practice consists of digitalis treatment for 9 to 12 recurrence-free months followed by its abrupt cessation. Recurrence of tachycardia, particularly in those infants with ventricular preexcitation, is not uncommon; maintenance of normal rhythm may require the administration, alone or in combination, of digitalis, phenytoin sodium, verapamil, and propranolol.[510,511] The rate of recurrence falls substantially between ages 2 and 10 years, with a slight rise during adolescence. In general, the prognosis is excellent.

References

1. Mitchell, S. C., Korones, S. B., and Berendes, H. W.: Congenital heart disease in 56,109 births. Incidence and natural history. Circulation 43:323, 1971.
2. Roberts, W. C.: Anatomically isolated aortic valvular disease: The case against its being of rheumatic etiology. Am. J. Cardiol. 49:151, 1970.
3. Popp, R. L., Brown, O. R., Silverman, J. S., and Harrison, D. C.: Echocardiographic abnormalities in mitral valve prolapse syndrome. Circulation 49:428, 1974.
4. Fyler, D.C.: Report of the New England regional infant cardiac program. Pediatrics 65(Suppl.):375, 1980.
5. Fontana, R. S., and Edwards, J. E.: Congenital Cardiac Disease: A Review of 357 Cases Studied Pathologically. Philadelphia, W. B. Saunders Co., 1962.
6. Bankl, H.: Congenital malformations of the heart and great vessels: Synopsis of pathology, embryology and natural history. Baltimore-Munich, Urban and Schwarzenberg, 1977.
7. Greenwood, R. D., Rosenthal, R., Parisi, L., Fyler, D. C., and Nadas, A. S.: Extracardiac abnormalities in infants with congenital heart disease. Pediatrics 55:485, 1975.
8. Nora, J. J., Wolff, R.-R., and Miles, V. N.: Etiologic aspects of cardiovascular disease and pre-disposition detectable in the infant and child. In Friedman, W. F., Lesch, M., and Sonnenblick, E. H. (eds.): Neonatal Heart Disease. New York, Grune and Stratton, 1973, p. 279.
9. de la Cruz, M. V., Munoz-Castellanos, L., and Nadal-Ginard, S.: Extrinsic factors in the genesis of congenital heart disease. Br. Heart J. 33:203, 1971.
10. Wilson, J. G., and Warkeny, J.: Teratology: Principles and Techniques. Chicago, University of Chicago Press, 1965.
11. Ruttenberg, H. D.: Concerning the etiology of congenital cardiac disease. Am. Heart J. 84:437, 1972.
12. Ouelette, E. M., Rossett, H. L., Rossman, M. P., and Wiener, L.: Adverse effects on offspring of maternal alcohol abuse during pregnancy. N. Engl. J. Med. 297:528, 1977.
13. Noonan, J.: Twins, conjoined twins, and cardiac defects. Am. J. Dis. Child. 132:17, 1978.
13a.Corone, P., Bonaiti, C., Feingold, J., Fromont, S., and Berthet-Bondet, D.: Familial congenital heart disease: How are the various types related? Am. J. Cardiol. 51:942, 1983.
14. Nora, J. J., and Nora, A. H.: The evolution of specific genetic environmental counseling in congenital heart diseases. Circulation 57:205, 1978.
15. Anderson, R. H., and Ashley, G. T.: Anatomic development of the cardiovascular system. In Davies, J., and Dobbing, J. (eds.): Scientific Foundations of Paediatrics. London, Heinemann, 1974, p. 165.
16. Langman, J. and van Mierop, L. H. S.: Development of the cardiovascular system. In Moss, A. J., and Adams, F. H. (eds.): Heart Disease in Infants, Children and Adolescents. Baltimore, Williams and Wilkins, 1968, p. 3.
17. Los, J. A.: Embryology. In Watson, H. (ed.): Paediatric Cardiology. London, Lloyd Luke Ltd., 1968, p. 1.
18. Rudolph, A. M.: Congenital Diseases of the Heart. Chicago, Year Book Medical Publishers, 1974.
19. Rudolph, A. M., and Heymann, M. A.: Circulatory changes with growth in the fetal lamb. Circ. Res. 26:298, 1970.
20. Sheldon, C. A., Friedman, W. F., and Sybers, H. D.: Scanning electron microscopy of fetal and neonatal lamb cardiac cells. J. Molec. Cell. Cardiol. 8:853, 1976.
21. McPherson, R. A., Kramer, M. F., Covell, J. W., and Friedman, W. F.: A comparison of the active stiffness of fetal and adult cardiac muscle. Pediatr. Res. 10:660, 1976.
22. Friedman, W. F.: The intrinsic physiologic properties of the developing heart. Progr. Cardiovasc. Dis. 15:87, 1972.
23. Ingwall, J. S., Kramer, M. F., Woodman, D., and Friedman, W. F.: Maturation of energy metabolism in the lamb: Changes in myosin ATPase and creatine kinase activities. Pediatr. Res. 15:1128, 1981.
24. Friedman, W. F.: Neuropharmacologic studies of perinatal myocardium. Cardiovasc. Clin. 4:44, 1972.
25. Geis, W. P., Tatooles, C. J., Priola, D. V., and Friedman, W. F.: Factors influencing neurohumoral control of the heart and newborn. Am. J. Physiol. 228:1685, 1975.
26. Romero, T. E., and Friedman, W. F.: Limited left ventricular response to volume overload in the neonatal period. Pediatr. Res. 13:910, 1979.
27. Friedman, W. F., Fitzpatrick, K. M., Merritt, T. A., and Feldman, B. H.: The patent ductus arteriosus. Clin. Perinatol. 5:411, 1978.
28. Talner, N. S.: Heart failure. In Moss, A. J., Adams, F. H., and Emmanouilides, G. C. (eds.): Heart Disease in Infants, Children and Adolescents. 2nd ed. Baltimore, Williams and Wilkins, 1977, p. 660.
29. Lees, M. H., and Sunderland, C. O.: Heart disease in the newborn. In Moss, A. J., Adams, F. H., and Emmanouilides, G. C. (eds.): Heart Disease in Infants, Children and Adolescents. 2nd ed. Baltimore, Williams and Wilkins, 1977, p. 619.
30. Goldring, D., Hernandes, A., and Hartmann, A. F.: The critically ill child. Care of the infant in cardiac failure. Pediatrics 47:1056, 1971.
30a. Artman, M., Parrish, M. D., and Graham, T. P., Jr.: Congestive heart failure in childhood and adolescence: Recognition and management. Am. Heart J. 105:471, 1983.
31. Sahn, D. J., and Friedman, W. F.: Difficulties in distinguishing cardiac from pulmonary disease in the neonate. Pediatr. Clin. North Am. 20:293, 1973.
32. Stanger, P., Lucas, R. V., Jr., and Edwards, J. E.: Anatomic factors causing respiratory distress in acyanotic congenital cardiac disease: Special reference to bronchial obstruction. Pediatrics 43:760, 1969.
33. Hagan, A. D., Deely, W. J., Sahn, D. J., and Friedman, W. F.: Echocardiographic criteria for normal newborn infants. Circulation 48:1221, 1973.
34. Hagan, A. D., Di Sessa, T. G., Bloor, C., and Calleja, H. B.: Two-dimensional

echocardiography. *In* Clinical and Pathological Correlations in Adolescent and Adult Heart Disease. Boston, Little, Brown and Co., 1983.

35. Mercier, J. C., DiSessa, T. G., Jarmakani, J., and Friedman, W. F.: Two dimensional echocardiographic assessment of left ventricular volumes and ejection fraction. Circulation 65:962, 1982.

36. Williams, R. G., and Tucker, C. R.: Echocardiographic Diagnosis of Congenital Heart Disease. Boston, Little, Brown and Co., 1977.

37. Lister, G., and Talner, N. S.: Oxygen transport in congenital heart disease. *In* Engle, M. A. (ed.): Pediatric Cardiovascular Disease. Philadelphia, F. A. Davis, 1981, p. 129.

38. Rosenthal, A., Nathan, D. G., Marty, A. T., Button, L. N., Miettinen, O. S., and Nadas, A. S.: Acute hemodynamic effects of red cell volume reduction, polycythemia of cyanotic congenital heart disease. Circulation 42:297, 1970.

39. Voigt, G. C., and Wright, J. R.: Cyanotic congenital heart disease and sudden death. Am. Heart J. 87:773, 1974.

40. Fischbein, C. A., Rosenthal, A., Fischer, E. G., Nadas, A. S., and Welch, K.: Risk factors for brain abscess in patients with congenital heart disease. Am. J. Cardiol. 34:97, 1974.

41. Shaher, R. M., and Deuchard, D. C.: Hematogenous brain abscess in cyanotic congenital heart disease. Am. J. Med. 52:349, 1972.

42. Corrin, C.: Paradoxical embolism. Br. Heart J. 26:549, 1964.

43. Haroutunian, L. M., and Neill, C. A.: Pulmonary complications of congenital heart disease: Hemoptysis. Am. Heart J. 84:540, 1972.

44. Guntheroth, W. G., Morgan, B. C., and Mullens, G. L.: Physiologic studies of paroxysmal hyperpnea in cyanotic congenital heart disease. Circulation 31:1965.

45. Bonchek, L. I., Starr, A., Sunderland, C. O., and Menashe, V. D.: Natural history of tetralogy of Fallot in infancy. Circulation 48:392, 1973.

46. Talmer, N. S.: Congestive heart failure in the infant. Pediatr. Clin. North Am. 18:1011, 1971.

47. Rosenthal, A., and Castaneda, A. R.: Growth and development after cardiovascular surgery in infants and children. *In* Rosenthal, A., Sonnenblick, E. H., and Lesch, M. (eds.): Postoperative Congenital Heart Disease. New York, Grune and Stratton, 1975, p. 119.

48. Vogel, J. H. K.: Pulmonary hypertension. *In* Moss, A. J., Adams, F. H., and Emmanouilides, G. C. (eds.): Heart Disease in Infants, Children and Adolescents. 2nd ed. Baltimore, Williams and Wilkins, 1977, p. 629.

49. Heath, D., and Edwards, J. E.: The pathology of hypertensive pulmonary vascular disease. Circulation 18:533, 1958.

50. Levin, D. L., Rudolph, A. M., Heymann, M. A., and Phibbs, R. H.: Morphological development of the pulmonary vascular bed in the fetal lamb. Circulation 53:144, 1976.

51. Rabinovitch, M., and Reid, L. M.: Quantitative structural analysis of the pulmonary vascular bed in congenital heart defects. *In* Engle, M. A. (ed.): Pediatric Cardiovascular Disease. Philadelphia, F. A. Davis, 1981, p. 149.

52. Kaplan, E. L., and Taranta, A. V.: Infective Endocarditis. An American Heart Association Symposium. Dallas, The American Heart Association, Inc., 1977.

53. Durack, D. T.: Current practice in prevention of bacterial endocarditis. Br. Heart J. 37:478, 1975.

54. Kaplan, E. J.: Prevention of bacterial endocarditis. Circulation 56:139A, 1977.

55. Lambert, E. C., Menon, V. A., Wagner, H. R., and Vlad, P.: Sudden unexpected death from cardiovascular disease in children. Am. J. Cardiol. 34:89, 1974.

56. Nadas, A. S., Fyler, D. C., and Castaneda, A. R.: The critically ill infant with congenital heart disease. Mod. Conc. Cardiovasc. Dis. 42:53, 1973.

57. Rutkowski, M. M., Cohen, S. N., and Doyle, E. F.: Drug therapy of heart disease in pediatric patients. II. The treatment of congestive heart failure in infants and children with digitalis preparation. Am. Heart J. 86:270, 1973.

58. Cohen, S. N., Doyle, E. F., and Rutkowski, M. M.: Drug therapy of heart disease in pediatric patients. I. Congestive heart failure in infancy and concepts of developmental pharmacology. Am. Heart J. 86:133, 1973.

59. Freed, M. D., Hegmann, M. A., Lewis, A. B., Roehl, S. L., and Kensey, R. C.: Prostaglandin E₁ in infants with ductus arteriosus dependent congenital heart disease. Circulation 64:899, 1981.

60. Lewis, A. B., Freed, M. D., Hegmann, M. A., Roehl, S. L., and Kensey, R. C.: Side effects of therapy with prostaglandin E₁ in infants with critical congenital heart disease. Circulation 64:893, 1981.

61. Friedman, W. F., Kurlinski, J., Jacob, J., DiSessa, T. G., Gluck, L., Merritt, T. A., and Feldman, B. H.: Inhibition of prostaglandin and prostacyclin synthesis in clinical management of PDA. Semin. Perinatol. 4:125, 1980.

62. Benson, L. N., Bohn, D., Edwards, J. F., Fortune, R. L., Price, S. A., Williams, W. G., and Rowe, R. D.: Nitroglycerin therapy in children with low cardiac index after heart surgery. Cardiovasc. Med. 4:2, 1979.

63. Dillon, T. R., Janos, G. G., Meyer, R. A., Benzing, G., III, and Kaplan, S.: Vasodilator therapy for congestive heart failure. J. Pediatr. 96:623, 1980.

64. Kirkpatrick, S. E., Corrin, A., Higgins, C. B., and Nyhan, W. F.: Differential diagnosis of congenital heart disease in the newborn. West. J. Med. 128:127, 1978.

65. Friedman, W. F., Sahn, D. J., and Hirschklau, M. J.: A review: Newer, noninvasive cardiac diagnostic methods. Pediatr. Res. 11:190, 1977.

66. Kleinman, C. S., Donnerstein, R. L., Talner, N. S., and Hobbins, J. C.: Fetal echocardiography for evaluation of in utero congestive heart failure. N. Engl. J. Med. 306:568, 1982.

67. DiSessa, T. G., and Friedman, W. F.: Echocardiography in congenital heart disease. Cardiol. Clin. North Am. (*in press*)

68. Stanger, P., Heymann, M. A., Tarnoff, H., Hoffman, J. I. E., and Rudolph, A. M.: Complications of cardiac catheterization of neonates, infants and children. Circulation 50:595, 1974.

69. Hoffman, J. I. E., Rudolph, A. M., and Danilowicz, D.: Left to right atrial shunts in infants. Am. J. Cardiol. 38:68, 1972.

70. Hunt, C. E., and Lucas, R. V., Jr.: Symptomatic atrial septal defect in infancy. Circulation 42:1042, 1973.

71. Craig, R. J., and Seltzer, A.: Natural history and prognosis of atrial septal defect. Circulation 37:805, 1968.

72. Davea, J. E., Cheitlin, M. D., and Bedynek, J. L.: Sinus venosus atrial septal defect. Am. Heart J. 85:177, 1973.

73. Tanden, R., and Edwards, J. E.: Atrial septal defect in infancy. Common association with other anomalies. Circulation 49:1005, 1974.

74. Leachman, R. D., Cokkinos, D. V., and Cooley, D. A.: Association of ostium secundum atrial septal defects with mitral valve prolapse. Am. J. Cardiol. 38:167, 1976.

75. Levin, A. R., Spach, M. S., Boineau, J. P., Canent, R. V., Jr., Capp, M. P., and Jewett, P. H.: Atrial pressure flow dynamics and atrial septal defects (secundum type). Circulation 37:476, 1968.

76. O'Toole, J. D., Reddy, I., Curtiss, E. I., and Shaver, J. A.: The mechanism of splitting of the second heart sound in atrial septal defect. Circulation 41:1047, 1977.

77. Clark, E. B., and Kugler, J. D.: Preoperative secundum atrial septal defect with coexisting sinus node and atrioventricular node dysfunction. Circulation 65:976, 1982.

78. Taketa, R. M., Sahn, D. J., Simon, A. L., Pappelbaum, S. J., and Friedman, W. F.: Catheter positions in congenital cardiac malformations. Circulation 51:749, 1975.

79. Cohn, L. H., Morrow, A. G., and Braunwald, E.: Operative treatment of atrial septal defect: Clinical and hemodynamic assessments in 175 patients. Br. Heart J. 29:725, 1967.

80. Levin, A. R., Liebson, P. R., Ehlers, K. H., and Daimant, B.: Assessment of left ventricular function in atrial septal defect. Pediatr. Res. 9:894, 1975.

81. Ebstein, S. E., Beiser, G. D., Goldstein, R. E., Rosing, D. R., Redwood, D. R., and Morrow, A. G.: Hemodynamic abnormalities in response to mild and intense upright exercise following operative correction of an atrial septal defect or tetralogy of Fallot. Circulation 42:1065, 1973.

82. Ugarte, M., Enriques de Salamanca, F., and Quero, M.: Endocardial cushion defects and anatomical study of 54 specimens. Br. Heart J. 38:674, 1976.

83. Bharati, S., and Lev, M.: The spectrum of common atrioventricular orifice. Am. Heart J. 86:553, 1973.

84. Borkon, A. M., Pieroni, D. R., Varghese, P. J., Ho, C. S., and Rowe, R. D.: The superior QRS axis in ostium primum ASD. Am. Heart J. 92:15, 1975.

85. Goodman, D. J., Harrison, D. C., and Cannom, D. S.: Atrioventricular conduction in patients with incomplete endocardial cushion defect. Circulation 49:630, 1974.

86. Jacobsen, J. R., Gillette, P. C., Corbett, B. N., Rabinovitch, M., and McNamara, D. G.: Intracardiac electrography in endocardial cushion defects. Circulation 54:599, 1976.

87. Waldo, A. L., Kaiser, G. A., Bowman, F. O., Jr., and Malm, J. R.: Etiology of prolongation of the PR interval in patients with an endocardial cushion defect. Circulation 43:19, 1973.

88. Bierman, F. Z., and Williams, R. G.: Subxyphoid two-dimensional imaging of the interatrial septum in infants and neonates with congenital heart disease. Circulation 60:80, 1979.

89. Lange, L. W., Sahn, D. J., Allen, H. D., and Goldberg, S. J.: Subxyphoid cross-sectional echocardiography in infants and children with congenital heart disease. Circulation 59:513, 1979.

90. Baron, M. G.: Abnormalities of the mitral valve and endocardial cushion defect. Circulation 45:672, 1972.

91. Rastelli, G. C., Ongley, P. A., Kirklin, J. W., and McGoon, D. C.: Surgical repair of the complete former persistent common atrioventricular canal. J. Thorac. Cardiovasc. Surg. 55:299, 1968.

92. Elliott, L. P., Bargeron, L. M., Bream, P. R., Soto, B., and Curry, G. C.: Axial cineangiography in congenital heart disease. Circulation 46:1084, 1977.

93. Newfeld, E. A., Sher, M., Paul, M. H., and Nikaido, H.: Pulmonary vascular disease and complete atrioventricular canal defect. Am. J. Cardiol. 39:721, 1977.

94. Mair, D. D., and McGoon, D. C.: Surgical correction of atrioventricular canal during the first year of life. Am. J. Cardiol. 40:66, 1977.

95. Carpentier, A.: Surgical anatomy and management of the mitral component of atrioventricular canal defects. *In* Anderson, R. H., and Shinebourne, E. A. (eds.): Paediatric Cardiology. London, Churchill-Livingstone, 1978, p. 477.

96. Ebert, P. A., and Gordon, D. A.: Complete atrioventricular canal malformation: Further classification of the anatomy of the common leaflet and its relationship to the VSD in surgical correction. Ann. Thorac. Surg. 25:134, 1978.

97. McCabe, J. C., Engle, M. A., Gay, W. A., Jr., and Ebert, P. A.: Surgical treatment of endocardial cushion defect. Am. J. Cardiol. 39:72, 1977.

97a. Kawaguchi, A., Broda, J., Gingel, R., Roland, J-M., Pieroni, D., and Subramanian, S.: Surgical repair of complete atrioventricular canal. A new concept. J. Am. Coll. Cardiol. 1:651, 1983.

98. Friedman, W. F., Mehrizi, A., and Pusch, A. L.: Multiple muscular ventricular septal defects. Circulation 32:35, 1964.

99. Bloomfield, D. K.: Natural history of ventricular septal defect in patients surviving infancy. Circulation 29:914, 1964.

100. Keith, J. D., Rose, V., Collins, G., and Kidd, V. S. L.: Ventricular septal defect. Incidence, morbidity and mortality in various age groups. Br. Heart J. 33: 81, 1971.

101. Dickinson, D. F., Arnold, R., and Wilkinson, J. L.: Ventricular septal defects in children born in Liverpool. Evaluation of natural course and surgical implications in an unselected population. Br. Heart J. 46:47, 1981.

102. Collins, G., Calder, L., Rose, V., Kidd, L., and Keith, J. D.: Ventricular septal defect: Clinical and hemodynamic changes in the first five years of life. Am. Heart J. 84:695, 1972.

103. Hoffman, J. I. E.: Natural history of congenital heart disease. Circulation 37: 97, 1968.

104. Weidman, W. H., Blount, S. G., Jr., DuShane, J. W., Gersony, W. M., Hayes, C. J., and Nadas, A. S.: Clinical course in ventricular septal defect. Natural history study. Circulation 56 (Suppl.):I-56, 1977.

105. Lister, G., Hellenbrand, W. E., Kleinman, C. S., and Talner, N. S.: Physiologic effects of increasing hemoglobin concentration in left to right shunting in infants with ventricular septal defects. N. Engl. J. Med. 306:502, 1982.

106. Beekman, R. H., Rocchini, A. P., and Rosenthal, A.: Hemodynamic effects of hydralazine in infants with a large ventricular septal defect. Circulation 65:523, 1982.

107. Friedman, W. F., and Pitlick, P. T.: Ventricular septal defect in infancy — University of California, San Diego (Specialty Conference). West. J. Med. 120:295, 1974.

108. Alpert, B. S., Cook, D. H., Varghese, P. J., and Rowe, R. D.: Spontaneous closure of small ventricular septal defects: A ten-year follow-up. Pediatrics 63: 204, 1979.

109. Blumenthal, S., Griffiths, S. P., and Morgan, B. C.: Bacterial endocarditis in children with heart disease. (A review based on the literature and experience with 58 cases.) Pediatrics 26:993, 1960.

110. Kirklin, J. W.: Pulmonary artery banding in babies with large ventricular septal defect. Circulation 43:321, 1971.

111. Sigmann, J. M., Perry, B. L., Behrendt, M., Stern, A. M., Kirsh, M. M., and Sloan, H. E.: Ventricular septal defect: Results after repair in infancy. Am. J. Cardiol. 39:66, 1977.

112. Agosti, J., and Subramanian, S.: Corrective treatment of isolated ventricular septal defect in infancy. J. Pediatr. Surg. 10:785, 1975.

113. Dooley, K. J., Paresi-Buckley, L., Fyler, D. C., and Nadas, A. S.: Results of pulmonary arterial banding in infancy. Am. J. Cardiol. 36:484, 1975.

114. Sade, R. M., Williams, R. G., and Castaneda, A. R.: Corrective surgery for congenital cardiovascular defects in early infancy. Am. Heart J. 90:656, 1975.

115. Friedli, B., Kidd, B. S. L., Mustard, W. T., and Keith, J. D.: Ventricular septal defect with increased pulmonary vascular resistance. Am. J. Cardiol. 22: 403, 1974.

116. Hislop, A., Haworth, S. G., Shinebourne, E. A., and Reid, L.: Quantitative structural analysis of pulmonary vessels in isolated ventricular septal defect in infancy. Br. Heart J. 37:1014, 1975.

117. DuShane, J. W., and Kirklin, J. W.: Late results of the repair of ventricular septal defect on pulmonary vascular disease. In Kirklin, J. W. (ed.): Advances in Cardiovascular Surgery. New York, Grune and Stratton, 1973, p. 9.

118. Plauth, W. H., Braunwald, E., Rockhoff, S. D., Mason, D. T., and Morrow, A. G.: Ventricular septal defect and aortic regurgitation. Am. J. Med. 39:552, 1965.

119. Van Praagh, R., and McNamara, J. J.: Anatomic types of ventricular septal defect with aortic insufficiency: Diagnostic and surgical considerations. Am. Heart J. 75:604, 1968.

120. Sanfelippo, P. M., DuShane, J. W., McGoon, D. C., and Danielson, G. K.: Ventricular septal defects and aortic insufficiency: Surgical considerations and results of operation. Ann. Thorac. Surg. 17:213, 1974.

121. Trusler, G. A., Moes, C. A. F., and Kidd, B. S. L.: Repair of ventricular septal defect with aortic insufficiency. J. Thorac. Cardiovasc. Surg. 66:394, 1973.

122. Kawashima, Y., Danno, M., Shimizu, Y., Matsuda, H., Miyamoto, T., Fugita, T., Kozuka, T., and Manabe, H.: Ventricular septal defects associated with aortic insufficiency. Anatomic classification and method of operation. Circulation 47:1057, 1973.

123. Keane, J. F., Plauth, W. H., Jr., and Nadas, A. S.: Ventricular septal defect with aortic regurgitation. Natural history study. Circulation 56 (Suppl.):I-72, 1977.

124. Gersony, W. M., and Hayes, C. J.: Bacterial endocarditis in patients with pulmonary stenosis, aortic stenosis, or ventricular septal defect. Natural history study. Circulation 56 (Suppl.):I-84, 1977.

125. Sutherland, G. R., Godman, M. J., Smallhorn, J. F., Guiterras, P., Anderson, R. H., and Hunter, S.: Ventricular septal defect. Two-dimensional echocardiographic and morphological correlations. Br. Heart J. 47:316, 1982.

126. Elliott, L. P., Bargeron, L. M., Jr., Soto, B., and Bream, P. R.: Axial cineangiography in congenital heart disease. Radiol. Clin. North Am. 18:515, 1980.

127. Levin, A. E., Spach, M. S., Canent, R. V., Jr., Boano, J. P., Capp, M. P., Jain, V., and Barr, R. C.: Ventricular pressure flow dynamics in ventricular septal defect. Circulation 35:430, 1967.

127a. deLeval, M.: Ventricular septal defects. In Stark, J., and deLeval, M. (eds.): Surgery for Congenital Heart Defects, New York, Grune and Stratton, Inc., 1983, p. 271.

128. Godman, M. J., Roberts, N. K., and Izukawa, T.: Late postoperative conduction disturbances after repair of ventricular septal defect in tetralogy of Fallot. Circulation 49:214, 1974.

129. Okarama, E. O., Guller, B., Molony, J. D., and Weidman, W. H.: Etiology of right bundle-branch block pattern after surgical closure of ventricular-septal defects. Am. Heart J. 90:14, 1975.

130. Maron, B. J., Redwood, D. R., Hirschfield, J. W., Jr., Goldstein, R. E., Morrow, A. G., and Ebstein, S. E.: Postoperative assessment of patients with ventricular septal defect and pulmonary hypertension. Response to intense upright exercise. Circulation 48:864, 1973.

131. Jarmakani, A. M., Graham, T. P., Jr., and Canent, R. V.: Left ventricular contractile state of children with successfully corrected ventricular septal defect. Circulation (Suppl.) 46:102, 1972.

132. Graham, T. P., Jr., Atwood, G. F., Boucek, R. J., Jr., Cordell, D., and Boerth, R. C.: Right ventricular volume characteristics in ventricular septal defect. Circulation 54:800, 1976.

133. Heymann, M. A., and Rudolph, A. M.: Control of the ductus arteriosus. Physiol. Rev. 55:62, 1975.

134. Friedman, W. F., and Molony, D.: Prostaglandins and the perinatal period. Adv. Pediatr. 25:151, 1978.

135. Friedman, W. F., Printz, M. P., Skidgel, R. A., Benson, L. N., and Zednikova, M.: Prostaglandins and the ductus arteriosus. In Oates, J. A. (ed.): Prostaglandins and the Cardiovascular System, vol. 10: Samuelsson, B., and Paoletti, R. (eds.). Advances in Prostaglandin, Thromboxane and Leukotriene Research. New York, Raven Press, 1982, p. 277.

136. Mahony, L., Carnero, V., Brett, C., Heymann, M. A., and Clyman, R. I.: Prophylactic indomethacin therapy for patent ductus arteriosus in very low birth weight infants. N. Engl. J. Med. 306:506, 1982.

137. Gittenberger-DeGroot, A. C.: Persistent ductus arteriosus: Most probably a primary congenital malformation. Br. Heart J. 39:610, 1977.

138. Lange, P., Freed, M. D., Rosenthal, A., Castaneda, A. R., and Nadas, A. S.: The use of prostaglandin E in an infant with interruption of the aortic arch. J. Pediatr. 91:805, 1977.

139. Jones, R. W. A., and Pickering, D.: Persistent ductus arteriosus complicating the respiratory distress syndrome. Arch. Dis. Child. 52:274, 1977.

140. Friedman, W. F., Hirschklau, M. J., Printz, M. P., Pitlick, P. T., and Kirkpatrick, S. E.: Pharmacologic closure of patent ductus arteriosus in the premature infant. N. Engl. J. Med. 295:526, 1976.

141. Merritt, T. A., Gluck, L., Higgins, C., Friedman, W. F., and Nyhan, W. L.: Management of the premature infant with patent ductus arteriosus. West. J. Med. 128:212, 1978.

142. Jacob, J., Gluck, L., DiSessa, T. G., Kulovich, M., Kurlinski, J., Merritt, T., and Friedman, W. F.: The contribution of PDA in the neonate with severe RDS. J. Pediatr. 96:79–87, 1980.

143. Merritt, T. A., Harris, J. P., and Roghmann, K.: Early closure of the patent ductus arteriosus in very low birth weight infants: A controlled trial. J. Pediatr. 99:281, 1981.

144. Higgins, C. B., Rausch, J., Friedman, W. F., Hirschklau, M. J., Kirkpatrick, S. E., Goergen, T., and Reinke, R. T.: Patent ductus arteriosus in preterm infants with idiopathic respiratory distress syndrome. Radiographic and echocardiographic evaluation. Radiology 124:189, 1977.

145. Sahn, D. J., Vaucher, Y., Williams, D. E., Allen, H. D., Goldberg, S. E., and Friedman, W. F.: Echocardiographic detection of large left to right shunts and cardiomyopathies in infants and children. Am. J. Cardiol. 38:73, 1976.

146. Hirschklau, M. J., DiSessa, T. G., Higgins, C. B., and Friedman, W. F.: Echocardiographic pitfalls in the premature infant with large patent ductus arteriosus. J. Pediatr. 92:474, 1978.

147. Friedman, W. F., Heymann, M. A., and Rudolph, A. M.: Commentary: New thoughts on an old problem — patent ductus arteriosus in the premature infant. J. Pediatr. 90:338, 1977.

148. Eggert, L. D., Jung, A. J., McGough, E. C., and Ruttenberg, H. D.: Surgical treatment of patent ductus arteriosus in pre-term infants. Pediatr. Cardiol. 2: 15, 1982.

149. Jarmakani, M. M., Graham, T. P., Jr., Canent, R. V., Jr., Spach, M. S., and Capp, M. P.: Effect of site of shunt on left heart volume characteristics in children with ventricular septal defect and patent ductus arteriosus. Circulation 40: 411, 1969.

150. Berlind, S., Bojs, G., Korsgran, M., and Varnaukas, E.: Severe pulmonary hypertension accomapnying patent ductus arteriosus. Am. Heart J. 73:460, 1967.

151. Bessenger, F. B., Jr., Blieden, L. C., and Edwards, J. E.: Hypertensive pulmonary vascular disease associated with patent ductus arteriosus. Circulation 52: 157, 1975.

152. Neufeld, H. N., Lesser, R. G., Adams, P., Jr., Anderson, R. C., Lillehiei, C. W., and Edwards, J. E.: Aorticopulmonary septal defect. Am. J. Cardiol. 9:12, 1962.

153. Parker, B. M., Burford, T. H., Carlsson, E. C., and Buchner, E. F.: The diagnosis of aortico-pulmonary septal defect. Am. Heart J. 65:534, 1963.

154. Richardson, J. V., Doty, D. B., and Rossi, N. P.: The spectrum of anomalies of aorto-pulmonary septation. J. Thorac. Cardiovasc. Surg. 78:21, 1979.

155. Blieden, L. C., and Moller, J. H.: Aorticopulmonary septal defect. An experience in 17 patients. Br. Heart J. 36:630, 1974.

156. Doty, D. B., Richardson, J. V., Falkovsky, G. E., Gordanova, M. I., and Burakovsky, V. I.: Aorto-pulmonary septal defect: Hemodynamics, angiography and operation. Ann. Thorac. Surg. 32:244, 1981.

156a. Stark, J.: Aorto-pulmonary window. In Stark, J., and deLeval, M. (eds.): Surgery for Congenital Heart Defects, New York, Grune and Stratton, Inc., 1983, p. 483.

157. Van Praagh, R.: Classification of truncus arteriosus communis. Am. Heart J. 92: 129, 1976.

158. Crupi, G., Macartney, F. J., and Anderson, R. H.: Persistent truncus arteriosus: A study of 66 autopsy cases with special reference to definition and morphogenesis. Am. J. Cardiol. *40*:569, 1977.

159. Shrivastava, F., and Edwards, J. E.: Coronary arterial origin and persistent truncus arteriosus. Circulation *55*:551, 1977.

160. Calder, L., Van Praagh, R., Sears, W. P., Corwin, R., Levy, A., Keith, J. D., and Paul, M. H.: Truncus arteriosus communis. Am. Heart J. *92*:23, 1976.

161. Marceletti, C., McGoon, D. C., and Mair, D. D.: The natural history of truncus arteriosus. Circulation *54*:108, 1976.

162. Gelband, H., Van Meter, S., and Gersony, W. M.: Truncal valve abnormalities in infants with persistent truncus arteriosus. Circulation *45*:397, 1972.

163. Chung, K. J., Alexson, C. G., Manning, J. A., and Gramiak, R.: Echocardiography in truncus arteriosus. Circulation *48*:281, 1973.

164. McFall, R. C., Mair, D. D., Feldt, R. H., Ritter, D. G., and McGoon, D. C.: Truncus arteriosus and previous pulmonary arterial banding: Clinical and hemodynamic assessment. Am. J. Cardiol. *38*:626, 1976.

165. Turley, K. A., Tucker, W. Y., and Ebert, P. A.: The changing role of palliative procedures in the treatment of infants with congenital heart disease. J. Thorac. Cardiovasc. Surg. *79*:194, 1980.

166. Peetz, D., Spicer, R. L., Crowley, D. C., Sloan, H., and Behrendt, D. M.: Correction of truncus arteriosus in the neonate using a non-valved conduit. J. Thorac. Cardiovasc. Surg. *83*:743, 1982.

167. Wallace, R. B., Rastelli, G. C., Ongley, P. A., Titus, J. L., and McGoon, D. C.: Complete repair of truncus arteriosus defect. J. Thorac. Cardiovasc. Surg. *57*:95, 1969.

167a. deLeval, M.: Persistent truncus arteriosus. *In* Stark, J., and deLeval, M. (eds.): Surgery for Congenital Heart Defects, New York, Grune and Stratton, Inc., 1983, p. 417.

168. Morgan, J. R., Forker, A. D., O'Sullivan, M. J., and Fosburg, R. G.: Coronary arterial fistulas. Am. J. Cardiol. *34*:32, 1972.

169. Baim, D. S., Klein, H., and Silverman, J. F.: Bilateral coronary artery–pulmonary artery fistulas. Circulation *65*:810, 1982.

170. Liberthson, R. R., Sagar, K., Berkoben, J. P., Weintraub, R. M., and Levine, F. H.: Congenital coronary arteriovenous fistula. Circulation *59*:849, 1979.

171. Ruttenhouse, E. A., Doty, D. B., and Ehrenhaft, J. L.: Congenital coronary artery–cardiac chamber fistula. Review of operative management. Ann. Thorac. Surg. *20*:468, 1975.

172. Wesselhoeft, H., Fawcett, J. S., and Johnson, A. L.: Anomalous origin of the left coronary artery from the pulmonary trunk: Its clinical spectrum, pathology, and pathophysiology based on a review of 140 cases with 7 further cases. Circulation *38*:403, 1968.

173. Kimbris, D., Iskandrian, A. S., Segal, E. L., and Bemis, C. E.: Anomalous aortic origin of coronary arteries. Circulation *58*:606, 1978.

174. Askenazij, J., and Nadas, A. S.: Anomalous left coronary artery originating from the pulmonary artery. Circulation *51*:976, 1975.

175. Arciniegas, E., Farooki, Z. Q., Hakimi, M., and Green, E. W.: Management of anomalous left coronary artery from the pulmonary artery. Circulation *62* (Suppl. 1):180, 1980.

176. Stephenson, L. W., Edmunds, L. H., Jr., Friedman, S., Meijboon, E., Gewitz, M., and Weinberg, P.: Subclavian–left coronary artery anastomosis for anomalous origin of the left coronary artery from the pulmonary artery. Circulation *64* (Suppl. 2):130, 1981.

177. Fishbein, M. C., Obma, R., and Roberts, W. C.: Unruptured sinus of Valsalva aneurysm. Am. J. Cardiol. *35*:918, 1975.

178. Boutefeu, J. M., Morat, P. R., Hahn, C., and Hauf, E.: Aneurysms of the sinus of Valsalva. Report of seven cases in review of the literature. Am. J. Med. *65*:18, 1978.

179. Myer, J., Wukasch, D. C., Holman, G. L., and Cooley, D. A.: Aneurysm and fistula of the sinus of Valsalva. Clinical considerations and surgical treatment of 45 patients. Ann. Thorac. Surg. *19*:170, 1975.

179a. deLeval, M.: Congenital anomalies of sinuses of Valsalva and coronary arteries. *In* Stark, J., and deLeval, M. (eds.): Surgery for Congenital Heart Defects. New York, Grune and Stratton, Inc., 1983, p. 487.

180. Kakos, G. S., Kilman, J. W., Williams, T. E., and Hosier, D. M.: Diagnosis and management of sinus of Valsalva aneurysm in children. Ann. Thorac. Surg. *17*:474, 1974.

181. Engle, P. J., Held, J. S., Bel-Kahn, J. V. D., and Spitz, H.: Echocardiographic diagnosis of congenital sinus of Valsalva aneurysm. Circulation *63*:705, 1981.

182. Yokoi, K., Kambe, T., and Nishimura, K.: Ruptured aneurysm of the right sinus of Valsalva: Two post-Doppler echocardiographic studies. J. Clin. Ultrasound *9*:505, 1981.

183. Smyth, P. T., and Edwards, J. E.: Pseudocoarctation, kinking or buckling of the aorta. Circulation *46*:1027, 1972.

184. Hutchins, G. M.: Coarctation of the aorta explained as a branch point of the ductus arteriosus. Am. J. Pathol. *63*:203, 1971.

185. Rudolph, A. M., Heymann, M. A., and Spitznas, U.: Hemodynamic considerations of the development of narrowing of the aorta. Am. J. Cardiol. *30*:514, 1972.

186. Talner, N. S., and Berman, M. A.: Postnatal development of obstruction in coarctation of the aorta: Role of the ductus arteriosus. Pediatrics *56*:562, 1975.

187. Bruins, C.: Competition between aortic isthmus and ductus arteriosus; reciprocal influence of structure and flow. Eur. J. Cardiol. *8*:87, 1978.

188. Heymann, M. A., Berman, W., Jr., Rudolph, A. M., and Whitman, V.: Dilatation of the ductus arteriosus by prostaglandin E₁ in aortic arch abnormalities. Circulation *59*:169, 1979.

189. Connors, J. P., Hartmann, A. F., Jr., and Weldon, C. S.: Consideration in the surgical management of infantile coarctation of the aorta. Am. J. Cardiol. *36*: 489, 1975.

190. Fishman, N. H., Bronstein, N. H., Berman, W., Jr., Roe, B. B., Edmunds, L. H., Jr., Robinson, S. J., and Rudolph, A. M.: Surgical management of severe aortic coarctation/interrupted aortic arch in neonates. J. Thorac. Cardiovasc. Surg. *71*:35, 1976.

191. Rocchini, A. P., Rosenthal, A., Barger, A. C., Castaneda, A. R., and Nadas, A. S.: Pathogenesis of paradoxical hypertension after coarctation resection. Circulation *54*:382, 1976.

192. Godwin, G. D., Herfkens, R. J., Brundage, D. H., and Lipton, N. J.: Evaluation of coarctation of the aorta by computed tomography. J. Comput. Assist. Tomogr. *5*:153, 1981.

192a. Steele, P. M., Fuster, V., Weidman, W. H., Feldt, R., and McGoon, D. C.: Isolated coarctation of the aorta: Long-term operative results. J. Am. Coll. Cardiol. *1*:651, 1983.

192b. Hammon, J. W., Jr., Graham, T. P., Jr., Boucek, R. J., Jr., Parrish, M. D., and Bender, H. W.: Repair of coarctation of the aorta in infancy: Improved results with prostaglandin E₁ infusion and subclavian flap angioplasty. J. Am. Coll. Cardiol. *1*:663, 1983.

193. Beekman, R. H., Rocchini, A. P., Behrendt, D. M., and Rosenthal, A.: Re-operation for coarctation of the aorta. Am. J. Cardiol. *48*:1108, 1981.

194. Alpert, B. S., Bain, H. H., Balfe, J. W., Kidd, B. S. L., and Olley, P. M.: Role of the renin-angiotensin-aldosterone system in hypertensive children with coarctation of the aorta. Am. J. Cardiol. *43*:828, 1979.

195. Igler, F. O., Boerboom, L. E., Werner, P. H., Donegan, J. H., and Kampine, J. P.: Coarctation of the aorta and narrow receptor resetting. Circulation Res. *48*:365, 1981.

196. Nanton, M. A., and Olley, P. M.: Residual hypertension after coarctectomy in children. Am. J. Cardiol. *37*:769, 1976.

197. Maron, B. J., Humphries, J., Rowe, R. D., and Mellits, E. D.: Prognosis of surgically corrected coarctation of the aorta. Circulation *47*:119, 1973.

198. Freed, M. D., Rocchini, A., Rosenthal, A., Nadas, A. S., and Castaneda, A. R.: Exercise-induced hypertension after surgical repair of coarctation of the aorta. Am. J. Cardiol. *43*:253, 1979.

199. Van Woezik, E. V. M., Kline, H. W., and Krediet, P.: Normal internal calibers of ostia, great arteries and aortic isthmus in children. Br. Heart J. *39*:860, 1977.

200. Graham, T. P., Jr., Atwood, G. F., Boerth, R. C., Boucek, R. J., Jr., and Smith, C. W.: Right and left heart size and function in infants with symptomatic coarctation. Circulation *56*:641, 1977.

201. Trusler, G. A., and Freedom, R. M.: Surgical approach to the management of interruption of the aorta. *In* Godman, M. J., and Marquis, R. M. (eds.): Paediatric Cardiology, vol. 2. Edinburgh, Churchill-Livingstone, 1979, p. 268.

202. Dekker, A. O., Gittenberger-de-Groot, A. C., and Roozendaal, H.: The ductus arteriosus and associated cardiac anomalies in interruption of the aortic arch. Pediatr. Cardiol. *2*:185, 1982.

203. Jaffee, R. B.: Complete interruption of the aortic arch. II. Characteristic angiographic features with emphasis on collateral circulation to the descending aorta. Circulation *53*:161, 1976.

204. Moulton, A. L., and Bowman, F. O., Jr.: Primary definitive repair of type-B interrupted aortic arch, ventricular septal defect and patent ductus arteriosus. J. Thorac. Cardiovasc. Surg. *82*:501, 1981.

205. Sturm, J. T., van Heeckeren, P., and Borkart, G.: Surgical treatment of interrupted aortic arch in infancy with expanded polytetrafluoroethylene grafts. J. Thorac. Cardiovasc. Surg. *81*:245, 1981.

206. Friedman, W. F., and Benson, L. B.: Congenital aortic stenosis. *In* Adams, F. H., and Emmanouilides, G. C. (eds.): Moss' Heart Disease in Infants, Children and Adolescents. 3rd ed. Baltimore, Williams and Wilkins, 1983.

206a. Donner, R., Carabello, B. A., Black, I., and Spann, J. F.: Left ventricular wall stress in compensated aortic stenosis in children. Am. J. Cardiol. *51*:946, 1983.

207. Friedman, W. F., and Pappelbaum, S. J.: Indications for hemodynamic evaluation and surgery in congenital aortic stenosis. Pediatr. Clin. North Am. *18*: 1207, 1971.

208. Friedman, W. F.: Congenital aortic valve disease: Natural history, indications and results of surgery. *In* Morse, D., and Goldberg, H. (eds.): Important Topics in Congenital, Valvular, and Coronary Artery Disease. Mt. Kisco, N.Y., Futura Publishing Co., 1975, p. 43.

209. Cueto, L., and Moller, J. H.: Hemodynamics of exercise in children with isolated aortic valvular disease. Br. Heart J. *35*:93, 1973.

210. Buckberg, G., Eber, L., Herman, N., and Gorlin, R.: Ischemia in aortic stenosis: Hemodynamic prediction. Am. J. Cardiol. *35*:778, 1975.

211. Lewis, A. L., Heymann, M. A., Stanger, P., Hoffman, J. I. E., and Rudolph, A. M.: Evaluation of subendocardial ischemia in valvar aortic stenosis in children. Circulation *49*:978, 1974.

212. Lakier, J. B., Lewis, A. B., Heymann, M. A., Stanger, P., Hoffman, J. I. E., and Rudolph, A. M.: Isolated aortic stenosis of the neonate: Natural history and hemodynamic considerations. Circulation *50*:801, 1974.

213. Broderick, T. W., Higgins, C. B., and Friedman, W. F.: Critical aortic stenosis in neonates. Radiology *129*:393, 1978.

214. Keane, J. F., Bernhard, W. F., and Nadas, A. S.: Aortic stenosis surgery in infancy. Circulation *52*:1138, 1975.

215. Edmunds, L. H., Jr., Wagner, H. R., and Heymann, M. A.: Aortic valvulotomy in neonates. Circulation *61*:421, 1980.

216. Braunwald, E., Goldblatt, A., Aygen, M. M., Rockoff, S. D., and Morrow, A. G.: Congenital aortic stenosis. I. Clinical and hemodynamic findings in 100 patients. Circulation *27*:426, 1963.

217. Johnson, A. M.: Aortic stenosis, sudden death, and the left ventricular barore-ceptors, Br. Heart J. 33:1, 1971.
218. Wagner, H. R., Weidman, W. H., Ellison, R. C., and Miettinen, O. S.: Indirect assessment of severity in aortic stenosis. Natural history study. Circulation 56 (Suppl.):I-20, 1977.
219. Halloran, K. H.: A telemetered exercise electrocardiogram in congenital aortic stenosis. Pediatrics 47:31, 1971.
220. Chandramouli, B., Ehruka, D. A., And Lauer, R. M.: Exercise-induced electrocardiographic changes in children with congenital aortic stenosis. J. Pediatr. 87:725, 1975.
221. Gamboa, R., Hugenholtz, P. G., and Nadas, A. S.: Comparison of electrocardiograms in congenital arotic stenosis. Br. Heart J. 27:344, 1965.
222. Reeve, R., Kawamata, K., and Selzer, A.: Reliability of vectorcardiography in assessing the severity of congenital aortic stensos. Circulation 34:92, 1966.
223. Nanda, N. C., Gramiak, R., Shah, P. M. Steward, S., and DeWeese, J. A.: Echocardiography in the diagnosis of idiopathic hypertrophic subaortic stenosis coexisting with aortic valve disease. Circulation 50:752, 1974.
224. Williams, D. E., Sahn, D. J., and Friedman, W. F.: Cross-sectional echocardiographic localization of the sites of left ventricular outlfow tract obstruction. Am. J. Cardiol. 37:250, 1976.
225. Hagan, A. D., DiSessa, T. G., and Friedman, W. F.: Reliability of echocardiography in diagnosing and quantitating valvular aortic stenosis. J. Cardiovasc. Med. 5:391, 1980.
226. Aziz, K. U., van Grondelle, A., Paul, M. H., and Muster, A. J.: Echocardiographic assessment of the relation between left ventricular wall and cavity dimensions and peak systolic pressure in children with aortic stenosis. Am. J. Cardiol. 40:775, 1977.
227. Young, J. B., Quinones, M. A., Waggoner, A. D., and Miller, R. R.: Diagnosis and quantification of aortic stenosis with pulsed Doppler echocardiography. Am. J. Cardiol. 45:987, 1980.
228. Hohn, A. R., Van Praagh, S., Moore, A. A. D., Vlad, P., and Lambert, E. C.: Aortic stenosis. Circulation 31 (Suppl. III):4, 1965.
229. Bentivoglio, L. G., Sagarminaga, J., and Uricchio, J.: Congenital bicuspid aortic valve: A clinical and hemodynamic study. Br. Heart J. 22:321, 1960.
230. El-Said, G., Gallioto, F. J., Mullens, C. E., and McNamara, D. G.: Natural hemodynamic history of congenital aortic stenosis in childhood. Am. J. Cardiol. 30:6, 1972.
231. Hurwitz, R. A.: Aortic valve stenosis in childhood: Clinical and hemodynamic history. J. Pediatr. 82:228, 1973.
232. Friedman, W. F., Modlinger, J., and Morgan, J.: Serial hemodynamic observations in asymptomatic children with valvar aortic stenosis. Circulation 43:91, 1971.
233. Cohen, L. S., Friedman, W. F., and Braunwald, E.: Natural history of mild congenital aortic stenosis elucidated by serial hemodynamic studies. Am. J. Cardiol. 30:1, 1972.
234. Bandy, G. E., and Vogel, J. H. K.: Progressive congenital valvular aortic stenosis. Chest 60:189, 1971.
235. Friedman, W. F., Novak, V., and Johnson, A. D.: Congenital aortic stenosis in adults. In Roberts, W. C. (ed.): Congenital Heart Disease in Adults. Philadelphia, F. A. Davis, 1979, p. 235.
236. Wagner, H. R., Ellison, R. C., Keane, J. F., Humphries, J. O., and Nadas, A. S.: Clinical course in aortic stenosis. Natural history study. Circulation 56 (Suppl.):I-47, 1977.
237. Fisher, R. D., Mason, D. T., and Morrow, A. G.: Results of operative treatment in congenital aortic stenosis. J. Thorac. Cardiovasc. Surg. 59:218, 1970.
238. Sandor, E. G. S., Olley, P. M., Trusler, G. A., Williams, W. G., Rowe, R. D., and Morch, J. E.: Long-term follow-up with patients after valvotomy for congenital valvular aortic stenosis in children. J. Thorac. Cardiovasc. Surg. 80:171, 1980.
239. Conkle, D. M., Jones, M., and Morrow, A. G.: Treatment of congenital aortic stenosis: An evaluation of the late results of the aortic valvotomy. Arch. Surg. 107:649, 1973.
240. Presbitero, P., Sommerville, J., Chion, R. R., and Ross, D.: Open aortic valvotomy for congenital aortic stenosis. Last results. Br. Heart J. 47:26, 1982.
241. DiSessa, T. G., Hagan, A. D., Isabel-Jones, J. B., and Friedman, W. F.: Two-dimensional echocardiographic evaluation of discrete subaortic stenosis from the apical long axis view. Am. Heart J. 101:774, 1981.
242. Williams, D. E., Sahn, D. J., and Friedman, W. F.: Cross-sectional echocardiographic localization of the sites of left ventricular outflow tract obstruction. Am. J. Cardiol. 37:250, 1976.
243. Bloom, K. R., Meyer, R. A., Bove, K. E., and Kaplan, S.: The association of fixed and dynamic left ventricular outflow obstruction. Am. Heart J. 89:586, 1975.
244. Freedom, R. M., Dische, M. R., and Rowe, R. D.: Pathologic anatomy of subaortic stenosis and atresia in the first year of life. Am. J. Cardiol. 39:1035, 1977.
245. Newfeld, E. A., Muster, A. J., Paul, M. H., Idriss, F. S., and Riker, W. L.: Discrete subvalvular aortic stenosis in childhood. Am. J. Cardiol. 38:53, 1976.
246. Reis, R. L., Peterson, L. M., Mason, D. T., Simon, A. L., and Morrow, A. G.: Congenital fixed subvalvular aortic stenosis. An anatomical classification and correlations with operative results. Circulation 43(Suppl. I):I-11, 1971.
247. Champsaur, G., Trusler, G. A., and Mustard, W. T.: Congenital discrete subvalvar aortic stenosis. Surgical experience and long-term followup in 20 pediatric patients. Br. Heart J. 35:443, 1973.
248. Somerville, J., Stone, S., and Roth, D.: Fate of patients with fixed subaortic stenosis after surgical removal. Br. Heart J. 43:629, 1980.
249. Maron, B. J., Redwood, D. R., Roberts, W. C., Henry, W. L., Morrow, A. G., and Epstein, S. E.: Tunnel subaortic stenosis. Circulation 54:404, 1976.
250. Ergin, M. A., Cooper, R., LaCourte, M., Golinko, R., and Griepp, R. B.: Experience with left ventricular apicoaortic conduits for complicated left ventricular outflow obstruction in children and young adults. Ann. Thorac. Surg. 32:369, 1981.
251. Edwards, J. E.: Pathology of left ventricular outflow tract obstruction. Circulation 31:586, 1965.
252. Ferencz, C.: Atrioventricular defect of membranous septum: Left ventricular–right atrial communication of the malformed mitral valve simulating aortic stenosis. Bull. Johns Hopkins Hosp. 100:209, 1957.
253. Schon, J. D., Sellers, R. D., and Anderson, R. C.: The developmental complex of parachute mitral valve, supravalvular ring of left atrium, subaortic stenosis, and coarctation of aorta. Am. J. Cardiol. 11:714, 1963.
254. Friedman, W. F., and Roberts, W. C.: Vitamin D and the supravalvar aortic stenosis syndrome: The transplacental effects of vitamin D on the aorta of the rabbit. Circulation 34:77, 1966.
255. Friedman, W. F.: Vitamin D embryopathy. Adv. Teratol. 3:85, 1968.
256. Friedman, W. F., and Mills, L. F.: The relationship between vitamin D and the craniofacial and dental anomalies of the supravalvular aortic stenosis syndrome. Pediatrics 43:12, 1969.
257. Garcia, R. E., Friedman, W. F., Kaback, M. M., and Rowe, R. D.: Idiopathic hypercalcemia and supravalvular aortic stenosis: Documentation of a new syndrome. N. Engl. J. Med. 271:117, 1964.
258. Taylor, A. B., Stern, P. H., and Bell, N. H.: Abnormal regulation of circulating 25-hydroxy vitamin D in the William's syndrome. N. Engl. J. Med. 306:972, 1982.
259. Kahler, R. L., Braunwald, E., Plauth, W. H., Jr., and Morrow, A. G.: Familial congenital heart disease. Am. J. Med. 40:384, 1966.
260. French, J. W., and Guntheroth, W. G.: An explanation of asymmetric upper extremity blood pressure in supravalvular aortic stenosis: The Coanda effect. Circulation 42:31, 1970.
261. Goldstein, R. E., and Epstein, S. E.: Mechanism of elevated innominate artery pressures in supravalvular aortic stenosis. Circulation 42:23, 1970.
262. Gaum, W. E., Chou, T. C., and Kaplan, S.: The vectorcardiogram and electrocardiogram in supravalvular aortic stenosis and coarctation of the aorta. Am. Heart J. 84:620, 1972.
263. Noonan, J. A.: Hypoplastic left ventricle. In Moss, A. J., Adams, F. H., and Emmanouilides, G. C. (eds.): Heart Disease in Infants, Children and Adolescents. 2nd ed. Baltimore, Williams and Wilkins, 1977, p. 430.
264. Moodie, E. S., Gallen, W. J., and Friedberg, D. Z.: Congenital aortic atresia. Report of long survival and some speculations about surgical approaches. J. Thorac. Cardiovasc. Surg. 63:726, 1972.
265. Meyer, R. A., and Kaplan, S.: Echocardiography in the diagnosis of hypoplasia of the left to right ventricles in the neonate. Circulation 41:55, 1972.
266. Bass, J. L., Ben-Shaghar, G., and Edwards, J. E.: Comparison of M mode echocardiography and pathologic findings in the hypoplastic left heart syndrome. Am. J. Cardiol. 45:79, 1980.
267. Miller, G. A. H.: Aortic atresia: Diagnostic catheterization in the first week of life. Br. Heart J. 33:367, 1971.
268. Norwood, W. I., Lang, P., Castaneda, A. R., and Campbell, D. M.: Experience with operations for hypoplastic left heart syndrome. J. Thorac. Cardiovasc. Surg. 82:511, 1981.
269. Behrendt, D. M., and Rocchini, A.: An operation for hypoplastic left heart syndrome: Preliminary report. Ann. Thorac. Surg. 32:284, 1981.
270. Frahm, C. J., Braunwald, E., and Morrow, A. G.: Congenital aortic regurgitation. Am. J. Med. 31:63, 1961.
271. Carter, J. B., Sethi, S., Lee, G. B., and Edwards, J. E.: Prolapse of semilunar cusps as causes of aortic insufficiency. Circulation 43:922, 1971.
272. Somerville, J., English, T., and Ross, D. N.: Aortico-left ventricular tunnel. Clinical features and surgical management. Br. Heart J. 36:321, 1974.
273. Turley, K., Silverman, N. H., Teitel, D., Mavroudis, C., Snider, R., and Rudolph, A.: Repair of aortico–left ventricular tunnel in the neonate: Surgical, anatomic, and echocardiographic considerations. Circulation 65:1015, 1982.
274. Lucas, R. V., Jr., and Schmidt, R. E.: Anomalous venous connection, pulmonary and systemic. In Moss, A. J., Adams, F. H., and Emmanouilides, G. C., (eds.): Heart Disease in Infants, Children and Adolescents. 2nd ed. Baltimore, Williams and Wilkins, 1977, p. 437.
275. Marin-Garcia, J., Tandon, R., Lucas, R. V., Jr., and Edwards, J. E.: Cor triatriatum: Study of 20 cases. Am. J. Cardiol. 35:59, 1975.
276. Richardson, J. V., Doty, D. B., Siewers, R. D., and Zuberbuhler, J. R.: Cor triatriatum. J. Thorac. Cardiovasc. Surg. 81:232, 1981.
277. Jacobstein, M. D., and Hirschfeld, S. S.: Concealed left atrial membrane: Pitfalls in the diagnosis of cor triatriatum and supravalve mitral stenosing ring. Am. J. Cardiol. 49:780, 1982.
278. Macartney, F. J., Bain, H. H., Ionescu, M. I., Deverall, P. B., and Scott, O.: Angiocardiographic/pathologic correlations in congenital mitral valve anomalies. Eur. J. Cardiol. 4:191, 1976.
279. Ruckman, R. N., and Van Praagh, R.: Anatomic types of congenital mitral stenosis: Report of 49 autopsy cases with consideration of diagnosis and surgical implications. Am. J. Cardiol. 42:592, 1978.
280. Smallhorn, J., Tommasini, G., Deanfield, J., Douglas, J., and Macartney, F.: Congenital mitral stenosis. Anatomical and functional assessment by echocardiography. Br. Heart J. 45:527, 1981.
281. Perloff, J. K.: Evolving concepts of mitral valve prolapse. N. Engl. J. Med. 307:369, 1982.

282. Carney, E. K., Braunwald, E., Roberts, W. C., Aygen, M., and Morrow, A. G.: Congenital mitral regurgitation. Am. J. Med. 33:223, 1962.

283. Vlad, P.: Mitral valve anomalies in children. Circulation 33:465, 1971.

284. Ruschhaupt, D. G., Bharati, S., and Lev, M.: Mitral valve malformation of Ebstein type in absence of corrected transposition. Am. J. Cardiol. 38:109, 1976.

285. Sahn, D. J., Allen, H. D., Goldberg, S. J., and Friedman, W. F.: Mitral valve prolapse in children. Circulation 53:651, 1976.

286. Macartney, F. J., Bain, H. H., Ionescu, M. I., Deverall, P. B., and Scott, O.: Angiocardiographic/pathologic correlations in congenital mitral valve anomalies. Eur. J. Cardiol. 4:191, 1976.

287. Galioto, F. M., Jr., Midgley, F. M., Shapiro, S. R., Perry, L. W., and Scott, L. T.: Mitral valve replacement in infants and children. Pediatrics 67:230, 1981.

287a. Carpentier, A.: Congenital malformations of the mitral valve. In Stark, J., and deLeval, M. (eds.): Surgery for Congenital Heart Defects. New York, Grune and Stratton, Inc., 1983, p. 467.

288. Carpentier, A., Branchini, B., Cour, J. C., Asfaou, E., Villani, M., Deloche, A., Relland, J., D'Allaines, C., Blondeau, P., Piwnica, A., Parenzan, L., and Brom, G.: Congenital malformations of the mitral valve in children: Pathology and surgical treatment. J. Thorac. Cardiovasc. Surg. 72:854, 1976.

289. Dines, D. E., Arms, R. A., Bernatz, P. D., and Gomes, M. R.: Pulmonary arteriovenous fistulas. Mayo Clin. Proc. 49:460, 1974.

290. Venables, A. W.: The syndrome of pulmonary stenosis complicating maternal rubella. Br. Heart J. 27:49, 1965.

291. Danilowicz, D. A., Rudolph, A. M., Hoffman, J. I. E., and Heymann, M. A.: Physiologic pressure differences between main and branch pulmonary arteries in infants. Circulation 45:410, 1972.

292. Eldredge, W. J., Tingelstad, J. B., Robertson, L. W., Mauck, H. P., and McCue, C. M.: Observations on the natural history of pulmonary artery coarctation. Circulation 45:404, 1972.

293. Barrillon, A., Havy, G., Scebat, L., Baragan, J., and Gerbaux, A.: Congenital pressure gradients between main pulmonary artery and the primary branches. Br. Heart J. 36:669, 1974.

294. Koretzky, E., Moller, J. H., Korns, M. E., Schwartz, C. J., and Edwards, J. E.: Congenital pulmonary stenosis resulting from dysplasia of valve. Circulation 40:43, 1969.

295. Collins, E., and Turner, G.: The Noonan's syndrome—a review of the clinical and genetic features of 27 cases. J. Pediatr. 83:941, 1973.

296. Srinivasan, V., Konyer, A., Broda, J. J., and Subramanian, S.: Critical pulmonary stenosis in infants less than three months of age: A reappraisal of closed transventricular pulmonary valvotomy. Ann. Thorac. Surg. 34:46, 1982.

297. Danilowicz, D., Hoffman, J. I. E., and Rudolph, A. M.: Serial studies of pulmonary stenosis in infancy and childhood. Br. Heart J. 37:808, 1975.

298. Gersony, W. M., Bernhard, W. F., Nadas, A. S., and Gross, R. E.: Diagnosis and surgical treatment of infants with critical pulmonary outflow obstruction. Circulation 35:765, 1967.

299. Mody, M. R.: The natural history of uncomplicated valvular pulmonary stenosis. Am. Heart J. 90:317, 1975.

300. Ellison, R. C., and Miettinen, O. S.: Interpretation of rSR′ in pulmonic stenosis. Am. Heart J. 88:7, 1974.

301. LeBlanc, M. H., and Paquet, M.: Echocardiographic assessment of valvular pulmonary stenosis in children. Br. Heart J. 46:363, 1981.

302. Stone, F. M., Betthinger, F. B., Jr., Lucas, R. V., Jr., and Moller, J. H.: Pre- and postoperative rest and exercise hemodynamics in children with pulmonary stenosis. Circulation 49:1102, 1974.

303. Moller, J. H., Rao, S., and Lucas, R. V., Jr.: Exercise hemodynamics of pulmonary valvular stenosis: Study of 64 children. Circulation 46:1018, 1972.

304. Nazawa, M., Marks, R. A., Isabel-Jones, J., and Jarmakani, J. M.: Right and left ventricular volume characteristics in children with pulmonary stenosis and intact ventricular septum. Circulation 53:884, 1976.

305. Graham, T. P., Jr., Bender, H. W., Atwood, G. F., Page, D. L., and Fell, C. G. R.: Increase in right ventricular volume following valvulotomy for pulmonary atresia or stenosis with intact ventricular septum. Circulation 49 (Suppl.):II-69, 1974.

306. Neugent, E. W., Freedom, R. M., Nora, J. J., Ellison, R.C., Rowe, R. D., and Nadas, R. S.: Clinical course in pulmonary stenosis. Circulation 56 (Suppl.):I-38, 1977.

307. Wennevold, A., and Jacobsen, J. R.: Natural history of valvular pulmonary stenosis in children below the age of two years: Long-term follow-up with serial heart catheterizations. Eur. J. Cardiol. 8:371, 1978.

308. Finnigan, P., Ihenacho, H. N. C., Singh, S. O., and Abrams, L. D.: Hemo-dynamic studies at rest and during exercise in pulmonary stenosis after surgery. Br. Heart J. 36:913, 1974.

309. Trusler, G. A., Freedom, R. N., Patel, R., and Williams, W. G.: The surgical management of pulmonary atresia with intact ventricular septum. In Godman, M. J. and Marquis, R. N. (eds.): Paediatric Cardiology, vol. 2. Edinburgh, Churchill-Livingstone, 1979, p. 305.

310. Ellis, K., Casarella, W. J., Hayes, C. J., Gersony, W. M., Bowman, F. O., Jr., and Malm, J. R.: Pulmonary atresia with intact ventricular septum: New developments in diagnosis and treatment. Am. J. Roentgenol. 116:501, 1972.

311. Patel, R. G., Freedom, R. M., Moes, C. A. F., Bloom, K. R., Olley, P. M., Williams, W. B., Trusler, G. A., and Rowe, R. D.: Right ventricular volume determinations in 18 patients with pulmonary atresia and intact ventricular septum. Analysis of factors influencing right ventricular growth. Circulation 61: 428, 1980.

312. Zuberbuhler, J. R., and Anderson, R. H.: Morphological variations in pulmonary artresia with intact ventricular septum. Br. Heart J. 41:281, 1979.

313. Bharati, S., McAllister, H. A., Jr., Chiemmongkoltip, P., and Lev, M.: Con-genital pulmonary atresia with tricuspid insufficiency: Morphologic study. Am. J. Cardiol. 40:70, 1977.

314. Rudolph, A. M., Heymann, M. A., Fischman, N., and Lakier, J. B.: Formalin infiltration of the ductus arteriosus. N. Engl. J. Med. 299:1263, 1975.

315. Forster, J. W., and Humphreys, J. O.: Right ventricular anomalous muscle bundle: Clinical and laboratory presentation and natural history. Circulation 43:115, 1971.

316. Danilowicz, D., and Ishmael, R.: Anomalous right ventricular muscle bundle: Clinical pitfalls and extracardiac anomalies. Clin. Cardiol. 4:146, 1981.

317. Rowland, T. W., Rosenthal, A., and Castaneda, A. R.: Double chamber right ventricle: Experience in 17 cases. Am. Heart J. 89:455, 1975.

318. Engle, M. A.: Cyanotic congenital heart disease. Am. J. Cardiol. 37:283, 1976.

319. Kirklin, J. W., and Karp, R. B.: The tetralogy of Fallot: From a surgical viewpoint. Philadelphia, W. B. Saunders Co., 1970.

320. Rayo, B. N., Anderson, R. C., and Edwards, J. E.: Anatomic variations in tetralogy of Fallot. Am. Heart J. 81:361, 1971.

321. Faller, K., Haworth, S. G., Taylor, J. F. N., and Macartney, F. J.: Duplicate sources of pulmonary blood supply and pulmonary atresia with ventricular septal defect. Br. Heart J. 46:263, 1981.

322. Rabinovitch, M., DeLeon, V. H., Castaneda, A. R., and Reid, L.: Growth and development of the pulmonary vascular bed in patients with tetralogy of Fallot with or without pulmonary atresia. Circulation 64:1234, 1981.

323. Nihill, M. R., Mullins, C. E., and MacNamara, D. G.: Visualization of the pulmonary arteries in pseudo-truncus by pulmonary vein wedge angiography. Circulation 58:140, 1978.

324. Sondheimer, H. M., Oliphant, M., Schneider, B., Kavey, R. E. W., Blackman, M. S., and Parker, F. B.: Computerized axial tomography of the chest for visualization of absent pulmonary arteries. Circulation 65:1020, 1982.

325. Chesler, E., Matisonn, R., and Beck, W.: The assessment of the arterial supply to the lungs in pseudotruncus arteriosus and truncus arteriosus type IV in relation to surgical repair. Am. Heart J. 88:542, 1974.

326. McGoon, M. D., Fulton, R. E., Davis, G. D., Ritter, D. G., Neill, C. A., and White, R. I., Jr.: Systemic collateral and pulmonary artery stenosis in patients with congenital pulmonary valve atresia and ventricular septal defect. Circulation 56:474, 1977.

327. Fellows, K. E., Freed, M. D., Keane, J. F., Van Praagh, R., Bernard, W. R., and Castaneda, A. C.: Results of routine preoperative coronary angiography and tetralogy of Fallot. Circulation 51:561, 1977.

328. Morgan, B. C., Guntheroth, W. G., Blume, R. S., and Fyler, D. C.: A clinical profile of paroxysmal hyperpnea in cyanotic congenital heart disease. Circulation 31:66, 1965.

329. Morris, D. C., Felner, J. M., Schlant, R. C., and French, R. H.: Echocardiographic diagnosis of tetralogy of Fallot. Am. J. Cardiol. 36:908, 1975.

330. Seward, J. B., Tajik, A. J., Hagler, D. J., and Ritter, D. G.: Peripheral venous contrast echocardiography. Am. J. Cardiol. 39:202, 1977.

331. DiSessa, T. G., Hagan, A. D., Pope, C., and Friedman, W. F.: Two-dimensional echocardiographic characteristics of double outlet right ventricle. Am. J. Cardiol. 44:1146, 1979.

331a. Matina, D., van Doesburg, N. H., Fouron, J-C., Guerin, R., and Davignon, A.: Subxiphoid two-dimensional echocardiographic diagnosis of double-chamber right ventricle. Circulation 67:885, 1983.

332. Fellows, K. E., Smith, J., and Keane, J. S.: Preoperative angiocardiography in infants with tetrad of Fallot. Am. J. Cardiol. 47:1279, 1981.

333. Kirklin, J. W., Blackstone, E. H., Pacifico, A. D., Brown, R. N., and Bargeron, L. M.: Routine primary repair versus two stage repair of tetralogy of Fallot. Circulation 60:373, 1979.

334. Castaneda, A. R., Freed, M. D., Williams, R. G., and Norwood, W. I.: Repair of tetralogy of Fallot in infancy: Early and late results. J. Thorac. Cardiovasc. Surg. 74:372, 1977.

335. Sunderland, C. O., Matarazzo, R. G., Lees, M. H., Menashe, V. D., Bonchek, L. I., Rosenberg, J. A., and Starr, A.: Total correction of tetralogy of Fallot in infancy: Postoperative hemodynamic evaluation. Circulation 48:398, 1973.

336. Tucker, W. Y., Turley, K., Ullyot, D. J., and Ebert, P. A.: Management of symptomatic tetralogy of Fallot in the first year of life. J. Thorac. Cardiovasc. Surg. 78:490, 1979.

337. Garson, A., Jr., Gorry, G. A., McNamara, D. G., and Cooley, D. A.: The surgical decision in tetralogy of Fallot: Weighing risks and benefits with decision analysis. Am. J. Cardiol. 45:108, 1980.

338. Cole, R. B., Muster, A. J., Fixler, D. E., and Paul, M. H.: Long-term results of aortopulmonary anastomosis for tetralogy of Fallot. Circulation 43:263, 1971.

339. Roberts, W. C., Freisinger, G. C., Cohen, L. S., Mason, D. T., and Ross, R. S.: Acquired pulmonic atresia: Total obstruction to right ventricular outflow after systemic to pulmonary arterial anastomoses for cyanotic congenital cardiac disease. Am. J. Cardiol. 24:335, 1969.

340. Marbarger, J. P., Sandza, J. G., Hartmann, A. F., and Weldon, C. S.: Blalock-Taussig anastomosis: The preferred shunts in infants and newborns. Circulation 58(Suppl. 1):73, 1978.

340a. deLeval, M.: Systemic pulmonary and cavopulmonary shunts. In Stark, J., and deLeval, M. (eds.): Surgery for Congenital Heart Defects. New York, Grune and Stratton, Inc., 1983, p. 175.

341. Grinnell, V. S., Mehringer, C. M., Stanley, P., and Lurie, P. R.: Transaortic occlusion of collateral arteries to the lung by detachable valved balloons in the patient with tetralogy of Fallot. Circulation 65:1276, 1982.

342. Piehler, J. M., Danielson, G. K., McGoon, D. C., Wallace, R. V., and Mair, D. D.: Management of pulmonary atresia with ventricular septal defect and hypoplastic pulmonary arteries by right ventricular outflow construction. J. Thorac. Cardiovasc. Surg. 80:552, 1980.

343. Rocchini, A., Rosenthal, A., Keane, J. F., Castaneda, A. R., and Nadas, A. S.: Hemodynamics after surgical repair of right ventricle to pulmonary artery conduit. Circulation 54:951, 1976.

344. Richardson, J. P., and Clarke, C. P.: Tetralogy of Fallot. Risk factors associated with complete repair. Br. Heart J. 38:926, 1976.

345. Jarmakani, J. M., Nakazawa, M., Isabel-Jones, J., and Marx, R. A.: Right ventricular function in children with tetralogy of Fallot before and after aortic to pulmonary shunt. Circulation 53:556, 1976.

346. Graham, T. P., Jr., Cordell, D., Atwood, J. F., Bouseck, R. J., Jr., Boerth, R. C., Bender, H. W., Nelson, J. H., and Vaughn, W. K.: Right ventricular volume characteristics before and after palliative and reparative operations in tetralogy of Fallot. Circulation 54:417, 1976.

347. Borow, K. M., Green, L. H., Castaneda, A. R., and Keane, J. F.: Left ventricular function after repair of tetralogy of Fallot and its relationship to age at surgery. Circulation 61:1150, 1980.

348. Kavey, R. E. W., Blackman, M. S., and Sondheimer, H. M.: Incidence and severity of chronic ventricular dysrhythmias after repair of tetralogy of Fallot. Am. Heart J. 103:342, 1982.

349. Quattelbaum, P. G., Varghese, P. J., Neill, C. A., and Donahoo, J. S.: Sudden death among postoperative patients with tetralogy of Fallot. Circulation 54:289, 1976.

350. Pacifico, A. D., Kirklin, J. W., and Blackstone, E. H.: Surgical management of pulmonary stenosis in tetralogy of Fallot. J. Thorac. Cardiovasc. Surg. 74:382, 1977.

351. Garson, A., Jr., and McNamara, D. G.: Post-operative tetralogy of Fallot. In Engle, M. A. (ed.): Pediatric Cardiovascular Disease. Philadelphia, F. A. Davis, 1981, p. 407.

352. James, F. W., Kaplan, S., Schwartz, D. C., Chou, T. C., Sandker, M. J., and Naylor, V.: Response to exercise in patients after total correction of tetralogy of Fallot. Circulation 54:671, 1976.

353. Wessel, H. U., Cunningham, W. J., Paul, M. H., Muster, A. J., and Idriss, F. S.: Exercise performance in tetralogy of Fallot after intracardiac repair. J. Thorac. Cardiovasc. Surg. 80:582, 1980.

354. Yabek, S. M., Jarmakani, J. M., and Roberts, N.: Postoperative trifascicular block complicating tetralogy of Fallot repair. Pediatrics 58:236, 1976.

355. Niederhauser, H., Simonin, P., and Friedli, B.: Sinus node function and conduction system after complete repair of tetralogy of Fallot. Circulation 52:214, 1975.

356. Katz, N. M., Blackstone, E. H., Kirklin, J. W., Pacifico, A. D., and Bargeron, L. M.: Late survival and symptoms after repair of tetralogy of Fallot. Circulation 65:403, 1982.

357. Rocchini, A. P.: Hemodynamic abnormalities and response to supine exercise in patients after operative correction of tetrad of Fallot after early childhood. Am. J. Cardiol. 48:325, 1981.

357a. Tamer, D., Wolff, G. S., Ferrer, P., Pickoff, A. S., Casta, A., Mehta, A. V., Garcia, O., and Gelband, H.: Hemodynamics and intracardiac conduction after operative repair of tetralogy of Fallot. Am. J. Cardiol. 51:552, 1983.

358. Nasrallah, A., Williams, R. L., and Nouri, S.: Absent pulmonary valve and tetralogy of Fallot: Clinical and angiographic considerations with review of the literature. Cardiovasc. Dis. Bull. Texas Heart Inst. 1:392, 1974.

359. Lakier, J. B., Stanger, P., Heymann, M. A., Hoffman, J. I. E., and Rudolph, A. M.: Tetralogy of Fallot with absent pulmonary valve: Natural history and hemodynamic considerations. Circulation 50:167, 1974.

360. Emmanouilides, G. C., Thanopoulos, B., Siassi, B., and Fishbein, M.: Agenesis of ductus arteriosus associated with the syndrome of tetralogy of Fallot and absent pulmonary valve. Am. J. Cardiol. 37:403, 1976.

361. Stafford, E. G., Mair, D. D., McGoon, D. C., and Danielson, G. K.: Tetralogy of Fallot with absent pulmonary valve. Surgical considerations and results. Circulation 47(Suppl.):III-24, 1973.

362. Litwin, S. B., Rosenthal, A., and Fellows, K.: Surgical management of young infants with tetralogy of Fallot, absence of the pulmonary valve, and respiratory distress. J. Thorac. Cardiovasc. Surg. 65:552, 1973.

363. Byrne, J. P., Hawkins, J. A., Battiste, C. E., and Khoury, G. H.: Palliative procedures in tetralogy of Fallot in absent pulmonary valve: A new approach. Ann. Thorac. Surg. 33:499, 1982.

364. Dunnigan, A., Oldham, H. N., and Benson, D. W.: Absent pulmonary valve syndrome in infancy: Surgery reconsidered. Am. J. Cardiol. 48:117, 1981.

365. Anderson, R. H., Wilkerson, J. L., Gerlis, L. M., Smyth, A., and Becker, A. E.: Atresia of the right atrioventricular orifice. Br. Heart J. 39:414, 1977.

365a. Rao, P. S. (ed.): Tricuspid Atresia. Mt. Kisco, N.Y. Futura Publishing Co., Inc. 1982.

366. Dick, M., Fyler, D. C., and Nadas, A. S.: Tricuspid atresia, clinical course in 101 patients. Am. J. Cardiol. 36:327, 1975.

367. Sauer, U., and Hall, D.: Spontaneous closure or critical decrease in size of the ventricular septal in tricuspid atresia: Surgical implications. Herz. 5:369, 1980.

368. Bharati, S., and Lev, M.: Conduction system in tricuspid atresia with and without regular D-transposition. Circulation 56:423, 1977.

369. Koiwaya, Y., Watanabe, K., and Hirata, T.: Contrast two-dimensional echocardiography in diagnosis of tricuspid atresia. Am. Heart J. 101:507, 1981.

370. Williams, W. G., Rubis, L., Fowler, R. S., Rao, M., Trusler, G. A., and Mustard, W. T.: Tricuspid atresia: Results of treatment in 160 children. Am. J. Cardiol. 38:235, 1976.

371. Kyger, E. R., Reul, G. J., Jr., Sandiford, F. M., Wukash, E. C., Holman, G. L., and Cooley, D. A.: Surgical palliation of tricuspid atresia. Circulation 52:685, 1975.

372. Tatooles, C. J., Ardekani, R., Miller, R. A., and Serratto, M.: Operative repair of tricuspid atresia. Thorac. Surg. 6:499, 1976.

372a. Peterson, R. J., Franch, R. H., Fajman, W. A., and Jones, R. H.: Noninvasive

determination of exercise cardiac function following the Fontan operation. J. Am. Coll. Cardiol. 1:663, 1983.

373. Bjork, V. O., Olin, C. L., Bjarke, B. B., and Thoren, C. A.: Right atrial–right ventricular anastomosis for correction of tricuspid atresia. J. Thorac. Cardiovasc. Surg. 77:452, 1979.

374. Doty, B. D., Marvin, W. J., and Lauer, R. M.: Modified Fontan procedure. J. Thorac. Cardiovasc. Surg. 81:470, 1981.

375. LaCorte, M. A., Dick, M., Scheer, G., LaFarge, C. G., and Fyler, D. C.: Left ventricular function in tricuspid atresia. Circulation 52:996, 1975.

376. Shachar, G. B., Fuhrman, B. P., Wang, Y., Lucas, R. V., and Lock, J.: Rest and exercise hemodynamics after the Fontan procedure. Circulation 65:1043, 1982.

377. William, D. B., Kiernan, P. D., Schaff, H. V., and Danielson, G. K.: The hemodynamic response to dopamine and nitroprusside following right atrium–pulmonary artery bypass (Fontan procedure). Ann. Thorac. Surg. 34:51, 1982.

378. Ehren, B. L., Mills, M., and Lower, R. R.: Congenital tricuspid insufficiency: Definition and review. Chest 69:637, 1976.

379. Watson, H.: Natural history of Ebstein's anomaly of tricuspid valve in childhood and adolescence: An international cooperative study of 505 cases. Br. Heart J. 36:417, 1974.

380. Guiliani, E. R., Fuster, V., Brandenberg, R. O., and Mair, D. D.: Ebstein's anomaly: The clinical features and natural history of Ebstein's anomaly of the tricuspid valve. Mayo Clin. Proc. 54:163, 1979.

381. Bucciarelli, R. L., Nelson, R. M., Egan, E. A., Eitzman, D. Z., and Gessner, I. H.: Transient tricuspid insufficiency in the newborn: A form of myocardial dysfunction in stressed newborns. Pediatrics 59:330, 1977.

382. Boucek, R. J., Jr., Graham, T. P., Jr., Morgan, J. P., Atwood, G. F., and Boerth, R. C.: Spontaneous resolution of massive congenital tricuspid insufficiency. Circulation 54:795, 1976.

383. Freedom, R. M., Culham, J. A. G., Olley, P. M., Moes, C. A. F., and Rowe, R. D.: The differentiation of functional from organic pulmonary atresia: The role of aortography. Am. J. Cardiol. 41:914, 1978.

384. Kastor, J. A., Goldreier, B. N., Josephson, M. E., Perloff, J. K., Scharf, D. L., Manchester, J. H., Shelbourne, J. C., and Hirshfield, J. W., Jr.: Electrophysiologic characteristics of Ebstein's anomaly of the tricuspid valve. Circulation 52:987, 1975.

385. Lowe, K. G., Smith, D. E., Robertson, P. G. C., and Watson, H.: Scalar vector and intracardiac electrocardiograms in Ebstein's anomaly. Br. Heart J. 30:617, 1968.

386. Marcus, F. I., Fontaine, G. H., Frank, R., and Grosgogedt, Y.: Right ventricular dysplasia: A report of 24 adult cases. Circulation 65:384, 1982.

387. Gussenhoven, W. J., Spitaels, S.E.C., Bom, N., and Becker, A. E.: Echocardiographic criteria for Ebstein's anomaly of tricuspid valve. Br. Heart J. 43:31, 1980.

388. Farooki, Z. Q., Henry, G. J., and Green, E. W.: Echocardiographic spectrum of Ebstein's anomaly of tricuspid valve. Circulation 53:63, 1976.

389. Milner, S., Myer, R. A., Venables, A. W., Korfhagen, J., and Kaplan, S.: Mitral and tricuspid valve closure in congenital heart disease. Circulation 53:513, 1976.

390. Hirschklau, M. J., Sahn, D. J., Hagan, A. D., Williams, D. E., and Friedman, W. F.: Cross-sectional echocardiographic features of Ebstein's anomaly of the tricuspid valve. Am. J. Cardiol. 40:400, 1977.

391. Kerber, R. E., Markus, M. L., and Wolffson, P. M.: Demonstration of Ebstein's anomaly by simultaneous catheter tip localization of tricuspid valve and right coronary artery visualization: A new method. Chest 68:99, 1975.

392. Marcial-Barbero, M., Verginelli, G., Awad, M., Ferriera, S., Ebaid, M., and Zerbini, E. J.: Surgical treatment of Ebstein's anomaly. J. Thorac. Cardiovasc. Surg. 78:416, 1979.

393. Danielson, G. K., Maloney, J. D., and Devloo, R. A. E.: Surgical repair of Ebstein's anomaly. Mayo Clin. Proc. 54:185, 1979.

394. Paul, M. H.: D-Transposition of the great arteries. In Moss, A. J., Adams, F. H., and Emmanouilides, G. C. (eds.): Heart Disease in Infants, Children and Adolescents. 2nd ed. Baltimore, Williams and Wilkins, 1977, p. 301.

395. Thiene, G., Razzolini, R., and Dalla-Volta, S.: Aorto-pulmonary relationship, arterio-ventricular alignment, and ventricular septal defects in complete transposition of the great arteries. Eur. J. Cardiol. 4:13, 1976.

396. Mair, D. D., and Ritter, D. G.: Factors influencing systemic arterial oxygen saturation in complete transposition of the great arteries. Am. J. Cardiol. 31:742. 1973.

397. Lakier, J. B., Stanger, P., Heymann, M. A., Hoffman, J. I. E., and Rudolph, A. M.: Early onset of pulmonary vascular obstruction in patients with aorto-pulmonary transposition and intact ventricular septum. Circulation 51:875,1975.

398. Clarkson, P. M., Neutze, J. M., Wardill, J. C., and Barratt-Boyes, B. G.: The pulmonary vascular bed in patients with complete transposition of the great arteries. Circulation 53:539, 1976.

399. Newfeld, E. A., Paul, M. H., Muster, A. J., and Idriss, F. S.: Pulmonary vascular disease in complete transposition of the great arteries: A study of 200 patients. Am. J. Cardiol. 34:75, 1974.

400. Aziz, K. U., Paul, M. H., and Rowe, R. D.: Bronchopulmonary circulation in D-transposition of the great arteries: Possible role and genesis of accelerated pulmonary vascular disease. Am. J. Cardiol. 39:432, 1977.

401. Muster, A. J., Paul, M. H., Van Grondell, E. A., and Conway, J. J.: Asymmetric distribution of the pulmonary blood flow between the right and left lungs in D-transposition of the great arteries. Am. J. Cardiol. 38:352, 1976.

402. Dick, M., Heidelberger, K., Crowley, D., Rosenthal, A., and Hees, P.: Quantitative morphimetric analysis of the pulmonary arteries in two patients with D-transposition of the great arteries and persistence of the fetal circulation. Pediatr. Res. 15:1397, 1981.

403. Sansa, M., Tonkin, I. L., Bargeron, L. M., and Elliott, L. P.: Left ventricular outflow tract obstruction in transposition of the great arteries. Am. J. Cardiol. 44:88, 1979.

404. Waldman, J. D., Paul, M. H., Newfeld, E. A., Muster, A. J., and Idriss, F. S.: Transposition of the great arteries with intact ventricular septum and patent ductus arteriosus. Am. J. Cardiol. 39:232, 1977.

405. Tonkin, I. L., Kelley, M. J., Bream, P. R., and Elliott, L. P.: The frontal chest film as a method of suspecting transposition complexes. Circulation 53:1016, 1976.

406. Thompson, K., and Serwer, G. A.: Echocardiographic features of patients with and without residual defects after Mustard's procedure for transposition of the great vessels. Circulation 64:1032, 1981.

407. Hirschfeld, S., Meyer, R., Schwartz, D. C., Korthagen, J., and Kaplan, S.: Measurement of right and left ventricular systolic time intervals by echocardiography. Circulation 51:304, 1975.

408. Gutgesell, H. P.: Echocardiographic estimation of pulmonary artery pressure in transposition of the great arteries. Circulation 57:1151, 1978.

409. DiSessa, T. G., Childs, W., Ti, C. C., and Friedman, W. F.: Systolic anterior motion of the mitral valve in a one day old infant with transposition of the great vessels. J. Clin. Ultrasound 6:186, 1978.

410. Mahony, L., Turley, K., Ebert, P., and Heymann, M. A.: Long-term results after atrial repair of transposition of the great arteries in early infancy. Circulation 66:253, 1982.

411. Parenzan, L., Locatelli, C. T., Alfieri, O., and Giorgio, I.: The Senning operation for transposition of the great arteries. J. Thorac. Cardiovasc. Surg. 76:305, 1978.

412. Stark, J.: Surgical treatment of patients with transposition of the great arteries. Bull. Johns Hopkins Med. J. 140:181, 1977.

412a. Stark, J.: Concordant transpoition—Mustard operation. In Stark, J., and deLeval, M. (eds.): Surgery for Congenital Heart Defects. New York, Grune and Stratton, Inc., 1983, p. 331.

413. Gutgesell, H. P., Garson, A., and McNamara, D. G.: Prognosis for the newborn with transposition of the great arteries. Am. J. Cardiol. 44:96, 1979.

414. Graham, T. P., Jr.: Hemodynamic residua and sequelae following intra-atrial repair of transposition of the great arteries: A review. Pediatr. Cardiol. 2:203, 1982.

415. Arciniegas, E., Farooki, Z. Q., Hakimi, M., Perry, B. L., and Green, E. W.: Results of the Mustard operation for dextro-transposition of the great arteries. J. Thorac. Cardiovasc. Surg. 81:580, 1981.

416. Gillette, P. C., Kuglar, J. D., Garson, A., Jr., Gutgesell, H. P., Duff, D. F., and McNamara, D. G.: Mechanisms of cardiac arrhythmias after the Mustard operation for transposition of the great arteries. Am. J. Cardiol. 45:1225, 1980.

417. Huhta, J. C., Edwards, W. D., Danielson, G. K., and Feldt, R. H.: Abnormalities of the tricuspid valve in complete transposition of the great arteries with ventricular septal defect. J. Thorac. Cardiovasc. Surg. 83:569, 1982.

418. Borow, K. M., Keane, J. F., Castaneda, A. R., and Fried, M. D.: Systemic ventricular function in patients with tetralogy of Fallot, ventricular septal defect and transposition of the great arteries repaired during infancy. Circulation 64:878, 1981.

419. Graham, T. P., Jr., Atwood, G. F., Boucek, R. J., Jr., Boerth, R. C., and Bender, H. W., Jr.: Abnormalities of right ventricular function following Mustard operation for transposition of the great arteries. Circulation 52:678, 1975.

420. Benson, L. N., Bonet, J., Olley, P. M., Trusler, G., Rowe, R. D., and Morch, J.: Assessment of right ventricular function during supine bicycle exercise after Mustard's operation. Circulation 65:1052, 1982.

421. Freedom, R. M., Culham, J. A. G., Olley, P. M., Rowe, R. D., Williams, W. G., and Trusler, G. A.: Anatomic correction of transposition of the great arteries: Pre- and post-operative cardiac catheterization with angiocardiography in five patients. Circulation 63:905, 1981.

422. Yacoub, M. H., Berhard, A., Radley-Smith, R., Lange, P., Sievers, H., and Heintzen, P.: Supravalvular pulmonary stenosis after anatomic correction of transposition of the great arteries: Causes and prevention. Circulation 66 (Suppl. 1):193, 1982.

423. Moulton, A. L., deLeval, M. R., Macartney, F. J., Taylor, J. F. N., and Stark, J.: Rastelli procedure for transposition of the great arteries, ventricular septal defect, and left ventricular outflow tract obstruction. Early and late results in 41 patients. Br. Heart J. 45:20, 1981.

424. Mair, D. D., Ritter, D. G., Danielson, G. K., Wallace, R. B., and McGoon, D. C.: The palliative Mustard operation; rationale and results. Am. J. Cardiol. 37:762, 1976.

425. Van Praagh, R., Durnin, R. E., Jockin, H., Wagner, H. R., Korns, M., Garabedian, H., Endo, M., and Calder, A. L.: Anatomically corrected malposition of the great arteries. Circulation 51:20, 1975.

426. Kirklin, J. W., Pacifico, A. D., Bargeron, L. M., Jr., and Soto, B.: Cardiac repair and anatomically corrected malposition of the great arteries. Circulation 48:153, 1973.

427. Berry, W. B., Roberts, W. C., Morrow, A. G., and Braunwald, E.: Corrected transposition of the aorta and pulmonary trunk: Clinical, hemodynamic, and pathologic findings. Am. J. Med. 36:35, 1964.

428. Freedberg, D. Z., and Nadas, A. S.: Clinical profile of patients with congenital corrected transposition of the great arteries. N. Engl. J. Med. 282:1053, 1970.

429. Allwork, S. P., Bentall, H. H., Becker, A. E., Cameron, H., Gerlis, L. M., Wilkinson, J. L., and Anderson, R. H.: Congenitally corrected transposition of the great arteries. Morphologic study of 32 cases. Am. J. Cardiol. 38:910, 1976.

430. Bjarke, B. B., and Kidd, B. S. L.: Congenitally corrected transposition of the great arteries: A clinical study of 101 cases. Acta Paediatr. Scand. 65:153, 1976.

431. Victorika, B. E., Miller, B. L., and Gessner, H.: Electrocardiogram and vectorcardiogram and ventricular inversion (corrected transposition). Am. Heart J. 86:734, 1973.

432. Waldo, A. L., Pacifico, A. D., Bargeron, L. M., Jr., James, T. N., and Kirklin, J. W.: Electrophysiological delineation of specialized AV conduction system in patients with corrected transposition of the great vessels and ventricular septal defect. Circulation 52:435, 1975.

433. Bharati, B., Rosen, K., Steinfield, L., Miller, R. A., and Lev, M.: The anatomic substrate for pre-excitation in corrected transposition. Circulation 62:831, 1980.

434. Hagan, A. D., Friedman, W. F., Ashburn, W. L., and Alazraki, N.: Further applications of scintillation scanning techniques to the diagnosis and management of infants and children with congenital heart disease. Circulation 45:858, 1972.

435. Freedom, R. M., Harrington, D. P., and White, R. I., Jr.: The differential diagnosis of levotransposed or malposed aorta: An angiocardiographic study. Circulation 50:1040, 1974.

436. Henry, J. G., Gordon, S., and Timmis, G. C.: Corrected transposition of great vessels in Ebstein's anomaly of tricuspid valve. Br. Heart J. 41:249, 1979.

437. Marcelletti, C., Maloney, J. D., Ritter, D. G., Danielson, G. K., McGoon, D. C., and Wallace, R. B.: Corrected transposition in ventricular septal defect: Surgical experience. Ann. Surg. 191:751, 1980.

438. deLeval, M. R., Bastos, P., Stark, J., Taylor, J. F. N., Macartney, F. J., and Anderson, R. H.: Surgical technique to reduce the risk of heart block following closure of ventricular septal defect in atrioventricular discordance. J. Thorac. Cardiovase. Surg. 78:515, 1979.

439. Cameron, A. H., Acerete, F., Quero, M., and Castro, M. C.: Double outlet right ventricle. Study of 27 cases. Br. Heart J. 38:1124, 1976.

440. Sridaromont, S., Feldt, R. H., Ritter, D. G., Davis, G. D., and Edwards, J. E.: Double outlet right ventricle: Hemodynamic and anatomic correlations. Am. J. Cardiol. 38:85, 1976.

441. Van Praagh, R., Perez-Trevino, C., Reynolds, J. L., Moes, C. A. F., Keith, J. D., Roy, D. L., Belcort, C., Weinberg, P. M., and Parisi, L. F.: Double outlet right ventricle with subaortic ventricular septal defect and pulmonary stenosis. Am. J. Cardiol. 35:42, 1975.

442. Sondheimer, H. M., Freedom, R. M., and Olley, P. M.: Double outlet right ventricle: Clinical spectrum and prognosis. Am. J. Cardiol. 39:709, 1977.

443. Goor, A. A., and Edwards, J. E.: The spectrum of transposition of the great arteries with special reference to developmental anatomy of the conus. Circulation 48:406, 1973.

444. Goitein, K. J., Neches, W. H., Park, S. C., Matthews, R. A., Lennox, C. C., and Zuberbuhler, J. R.: Electrocardiogram in double chamber right ventricle. Am. J. Cardiol. 45:604, 1980.

445. Sridaromont, S., Ritter, D. G., Feldt, R. H., Davis, G. D., and Edwards, J. E.: Double outlet right ventricle: Anatomic and angiocardiographic correlations. Mayo Clin. Proc. 53:555, 1978.

446. Pitlick, P., French, J., Guthaner, D., Shumway, N., and Baum, D.: Results of intraventricular baffle procedure for ventricular septal defect in double outlet right ventricle or D-transposition of the great arteries. Am. J. Cardiol. 47:307, 1981.

447. Stewart, S.: Double outlet right ventricle. A collective review with a surgical viewpoint. J. Thorac. Cardiovasc. Surg. 71:355, 1976.

447a. Stark, J.: Double-outlet ventricles. In Stark, J., and deLeval, M. (eds.): Surgery for Congenital Heart Defects. New York, Grune and Stratton, 1983, p. 397.

448. Kirklin, J. K., and Castaneda, A. R.: Surgical correction of double-outlet right ventricle with non-committed ventricular septal defect. J. Thorac. Cardiovasc. Surg. 73:399, 1977.

449. Brandt, P. W. T., Calder, A. L., Barratt-Boyes, B. G., and Neutze, J. M.: Double outlet left ventricle: Morphology, cineangiographic diagnosis, and surgical treatment. Am. J. Cardiol. 38:897, 1976.

450. Van Praagh, R., and Weinberg, P. M.: Double outlet left ventricle. In Moss, A. J., Adams, F. H., and Emmanouilides, G. C. (eds.): Heart Disease in Infants, Children and Adolescents. 2nd ed. Baltimore, Williams and Wilkins, 1977, p. 367.

451. Murphy, E. A., Gillis, D. A., and Sridhara, K. S.: Intraventricular repair of double outlet left ventricle. Ann. Thor. Surg. 31:364, 1981.

452. Clarke, D. R., Stark, J., De Leval, M., Pincott, J. R., and Taylor, J. S. N.: Total anomalous pulmonary venous drainage in infancy. Br. Heart J. 39:436, 1977.

453. Gathman, G. E., and Nadas, A. S.: Total anomalous pulmonary venous connection: Clinical and physiologic observations in 75 pediatric patients. Circulation 42:143, 1970.

454. Gersony, W. M., Bowman, F. O., Jr., Steeg, C. N., Hayes, C. J., Jesse, M. J., and Malm, J. R.: Management of total anomalous pulmonary venous drainage in early infancy. Circulation 43(Suppl.):I-19, 1971.

455. Turley, K., Tucker, W. Y., Ullyot, D. J., and Ebert, P. A.: Total anomalous pulmonary venous connection in infancy. Influence of age and type of lesion. Am. J. Cardiol. 45:92, 1980.

456. Duff, D. N., Nyhill, M. R., and McNamara, D. G.: Infradiaphragmatic total anomalous pulmonary venous return. Review of clinical and pathological findings and results of operation in 28 cases. Br. Heart J. 39:619, 1977.

457. Jensen, J. B., and Blount, S. G., Jr.: Total anomalous pulmonary venous return: A review and report of the older surviving patient. Am. Heart J. 82:387, 1971.

458. Delisle, G., Endo, M., Calder, A. L., Zuberbuhler, J. R., Rochenmacher, S., Alday, L. E., Mangini, O., Van Praagh, S., and Van Praagh, R.: Total anomalous pulmonary venous connection: Report of 93 autopsy cases with emphasis on diagnostic and surgical considerations. Am. Heart J. 91:99, 1976.

459. Elliott, L. P., and Edwards, J. E.: The problem of pulmonary venous obstruction in total anomalous pulmonary venous connection to the left innominate vein. Circulation 25:913, 1962.

460. Byrun, C. J., Dick, M., Behrendt, D. M., and Rosenthal, A.: Repair of total anomalous pulmonary venous connection in patients younger than six months old: Late post-operative hemodynamic and electrophysiologic status. Circulation 66 (Suppl. 1):208, 1982.

461. Newfeld, E. A., Wilson, A., Paul, M. H., and Reisch, J. S.: Pulmonary vascular disease in total anomalous pulmonary venous drainage. Circulation 61:103, 1980.

462. Snider, A. R., Roge, C. L., Schiller, N. B., and Silverman, N.: Congenital left ventricular inflow obstruction evaluated by two-dimensional echocardiography. Circulation 61:848, 1980.

463. Haworth, S. G., Reid, L., and Simon, G.: Radiological features of the heart and lungs in total anomalous pulmonary venous return in early infancy. Clin. Radiol. 28:561, 1977.

464. Smallhorn, J. F., Sutherland, G. R., Tommasini, G., Hunter, S., Anderson, R. H., and Macartney, F. J.: Assessment of total anomalous pulmonary venous connection by two-dimensional echocardiography. Br. Heart J. 46:613, 1981.

464a. Stark, J.: Anomalies of the pulmonary venous return. In Stark, J., and deLeval, M. (eds.): Surgery for Congenital Heart Defects. 1983, Grune and Stratton, Inc., p. 235.

465. Matthew, R., Thilenius, O. G., Replogle, R. L., and Arcilla, R. A.: Cardiac function in total anomalous pulmonary venous return before and after surgery. Circulation 55:361, 1977.

466. Nakazawa, M., Jarmakani, J. M., Gyepes, M. T., Prochazka, J. V., Yabek, S. M., and Marks, R. A.: Pre- and postoperative ventricular function in infants and children with right ventricular volume overload. Circulation 55:479, 1977.

467. Healey, J. E.: An anatomic survey of anomalous pulmonary veins: Their clinical significance. J. Thorac. Cardiovasc. Surg. 23:433, 1952.

468. Kuiper-Oosterwal, C. H., and Moulaert, A.: The scimitar syndrome in infancy and childhood. Eur. J. Cardiol. 1:55, 1973.

469. Van Praagh, R.: Terminology of congenital heart disease: Glossary and commentary. Circulation 56:139, 1977.

470. Stanger, P., Rudolph, A. M., and Edwards, J. E.: Cardiac malpositions: An overview based on a study of 65 necropsy specimens. Circulation 56:159, 1977.

471. Van Praagh, R., Weinberg, P. M., and Van Praagh, S.: Malposition of the heart. In Moss, A. J., Adams, F. H., and Emmanouilides, G. (eds): Heart Disease in Infants, Children and Adolescents. 2nd ed. Baltimore, Williams and Wilkins, 1977, p. 394.

472. Shinebourne, E. A., Macartney, F. J., and Anderson, R. H.: Sequential chamber localization—Logical approach to diagnosis in congenital heart disease. Br. Heart J. 38:327, 1976.

473. de la Cruz, M. V., Berrazueta, J. R., Arteaga, M., Atti, E. F., and Soni, J.: Rules for diagnosis of arterioventricular discordance and spatial identification of ventricles. Crossed great arteries and transposition of the great arteries. Br. Heart J. 38:341, 1976.

474. Nasser, W. K.: Congenital absence of the left pericardium. Am. J. Cardiol. 26:466, 1970.

475. Morgan, J. R., Rogers, A. K., and Forker, A. D.: Congenital absence of the left pericardium: Clinical findings. Ann. Intern. Med. 74:370, 1971.

476. Pernot, C., Hoeffel, J. C., and Henry, M.: Radiologic patterns of congenital malformation of the pericardium. Radiol. Clin. (Basel) 44:505, 1975.

477. Payvandi, M. N., and Kerber, R. E.: Echocardiography in congenital and acquired absence of the pericardium. Circulation 53:86, 1976.

478. Rastelli G., Kirklin, J. W., and Titus, J. L.: Anatomic observations on complete form of persistent common atrioventricular canal with special reference to atrioventricular valves. Mayo Clin. Proc. 41:296, 1966.

479. Soto, B., Pacifico, A. D., and DiSciascio, G.: Univentricular heart: An angiographic study. Am. J. Cardiol. 49:787, 1982

480. Shimazaki, Y., Kawashima, Y., Mori, T., Matsuda, H., Kitamura, S., and Yokota, K.: Ventricular function of single ventricle after ventricular septation. Circulation 61:653, 1980.

481. Van Praagh, R., and Van Praagh, S.: What is a ventricle? The single ventricle trap. Pediatr. Cardiol. 2:79, 1982.

482. Ritter, D. G., Seward, J. B., Moodie, D., and Danielson, G. K.: Univentricular heart (common ventricle): Pre-operative diagnosis. Herz 4:198, 1979.

483. Marin-Garcia, J., Tandon, R., Moller, J. H., and Edwards, J. E.: Common (single) ventricle with normally related great arteries, with great vessels. Circulation 39:565, 1974.

484. Tandon, R., Becker, A. E., Moller, J. H., and Edwards, J. E.: Double inlet left ventricle. Straddling tricuspid valve. Br. Heart J. 36:747, 1974.

485. Macartney, F. J., Partridge, J. B., Scott, O., and Deverall, P. B.: Common or single ventricle: angiographic and hemodynamic study of 42 patients. Circulation 53:543, 1976.

486. Rigby, M. L., Anderson, R. H., Gibson, D., Jones, O. D. H., Joseph, M. C., and Shinebourne, E. A.: Two-dimensional echocardiographic categorization of the univentricular heart. Ventricular morphology, type, and mode of atrioventricular connection. Br. Heart J. 46:603, 1981.

487. Ritter, D. G.: Echocardiograms in common (single) ventricle: Angiographic, anatomic correlation. Am. J. Cardiol. 39:217, 1977.

488. Seward, J. B., Tajik, A. J., Haggler, D. J., and Ritter, D. G.: Contrast echocardiography in single or common ventricle. Circulation 55:513, 1977.

489. Danielson, G. K., McGoon, D. C., Maloney, J. D., and Ritter, G. D.: Surgical septation of univentricular heart with outlet chamber. Herz 4:262, 1979.

490. Krongrad, E., and Malm, J. R.: Intra-operative mapping in patients with univentricular heart. Herz 4:232, 1979.

491. Danielson, G. K., Giuliani, E. R., and Ritter, D. G.: Successful repair of common ventricles associated with complete atrioventricular canal. J. Thorac. Cardiovasc. Surg. 67:152, 1974.

492. Cabral, R. J. M., Miller, D. C., Oyer, P. E., Stinson, E., Reitz, E. A., and Shumway, N. E.: A surgical approach for single ventricle incorporating total right atrium–pulmonary artery diversion. J. Thorac. Cardiovasc. Surg. 79:202, 1980.

493. Eklof, O., Elstrom, G., Ericksson, B. O., Michaelsson, M., Stevenson, O., Soderlund, S., Thoren, C., and Wallgren, G.: Arterial anomalies causing compression of the trachea and/or the esophagus. Acta Paediatr. Scand. 60:81, 1971.

494. Shuford, W. H., Sybers, R. G., and Weens, H. S.: The angiographic features of double aortic arch. Am. J. Roentgenol. 116:126, 1972.

495. Park, C. D., Waldhausen, J. A., Friedman, S., Aberdeen, I., and Jamson, J.: Tracheal compression by the great arteries in the mediastinum: Report of 39 cases. Arch. Surg. 103:626, 1971.

496. Koopot, R., Nikaido, H., and Idriss, F. S.: Surgical management of anomalous left pulmonary artery causing tracheo-bronchial obstruction: Pulmonary artery sling. J. Thorac. Cardiovasc. Surg. 69:239, 1975.

496a. deLeval, M.: Vascular rings. Stark, J., and deLeval, M. (eds.): Surgery for Congenital Heart Defects, New York, Grune and Stratton, Inc., 1983, p. 227.

497. Said, R. M., Rosenthal, A., Fellows, K., and Castaneda, A. R.: Pulmonary artery sling. J. Thorac. Cardiovasc. Surg. 69:333, 1975.

498. Anderson, R. H., Wenick, A. C. G., Losekoot, T. G., and Becker, A. E.: Congenitally complete heart block. Circulation 56:90, 1977.

499. Chemeides, L., Truex, R. C., Vetter, V., Rashkind, W. J., Gallioto, F. M., and Noonan, J.: Association of maternal systemic lupus erythematosus with congenital complete heart block. N. Engl. J. Med. 297:1204, 1977.

500. McCue, C. M., Mantakas, M. E., Tingelstad, J. B., and Ruddy, S.: Congenital heart block in newborns of mothers with connective tissue disease. Circulation 56:82, 1977.

501. Michaelsson, M., and Engle, M. A.: Congenital complete heart block: An international study of the natural history. Cardiovasc. Clin. 4:85, 1972.

502. Scarpelli, E. M., and Rudolph, A. M.: The hemodynamics of congenital heart block. Progr. Cardiovasc. Dis. 6:327, 1964.

503. Thilenius, O. G., Chiemmongkoltip, P., Cassels, D. E., and Arcilla, R. A.: Hemodynamic studies in children with congenital atrioventricular block. Am. J. Cardiol. 30:13, 1972.

504. Benrey, J., Gillette, P. C., Nasraloah, A. T., and Hallman, G. L.: Permanent pacemaker implantation in infants, children, and adolescents. Circulation 53:245, 1976.

505. Kleinman, C. S., Donnerstein, R. L., DeVore, G. R., Jaffee, C. C., Lynch, D. C., Berkowitz, R. L., Talner, N. S., and Hobbins, J. C.: Fetal echocardiography for evaluation of in utero congestive heart failure. N. Engl. J. Med. 306:568, 1982.

506. Harrigan, J. T., Kangos, J. J., and Sikka, A.: Successful treatment of fetal congestive heart failure secondary to tachycardia. N. Engl. J. Med. 304:1527, 1981.

507. Radford, D. J., Izukawa, T., and Rowe, R. D.: Congenital paroxysmal atrial tachycardia. Arch. Dis. Child. 51:613, 1976.

508. Gillette, P. C.: The mechanisms of supraventricular tachycardia in children. Circulation 54:133, 1976.

509. Whitman, V., Friedman, Z., Berman, W., Jr., and Maisels, M. J.: Supraventricular tachycardia in newborn infants: An approach to therapy. J. Pediatr. 91:304, 1977.

510. Brechenmacher, C., Coumel, P., and James, T. N.: Intractable tachycardia in infancy. Circulation 53:377, 1976.

511. Porter, C. J., Gillette, P. C., Garson, A., Hesslein, P. S., Carpawich, P. P., and McNamara, D. G.: Effects of verapamil on supraventricular tachycardia. Am. J. Cardiol. 48:487, 1981.

30 CONGENITAL HEART DISEASE IN THE ADULT

by Kenneth M. Borow, M.D., Joseph S. Alpert, M.D., and Eugene Braunwald, M.D.

GENERAL PRINCIPLES

During the past 25 years our ability to diagnose and treat congenital heart disease has advanced rapidly. Until recently, the only patients to survive to adulthood were those with simple, uncomplicated defects. This is no longer the case. Palliative or corrective surgical procedures have been developed for almost all congenital cardiac anomalies, leading to an increase in the population of adult cardiac patients. As the effects of coronary atherosclerosis and systemic hypertension are superimposed upon cardiac malformations that have undergone varying degrees of surgical correction, the pathophysiology of congenital heart disease in the adult may become even more complicated. It is therefore of increasing importance that clinicians understand the anatomy, diagnostic approaches, and natural history of those congenital cardiac defects found most frequently in the adult population.

RELATIVE INCIDENCE IN ADULTS AND CHILDREN. The relative incidence of the various congenital heart lesions in adults differs from that in children. Complex congenital lesions are considerably more common in children than in adults. Ventricular septal defect is the most common cardiovascular malformation diagnosed in children, while stenosis of a congenital bicuspid aortic valve and atrial septal defect are the lesions most frequently found in adults. In infants the most common cardiac lesion producing cyanosis is transposition of the great arteries, while in the adult population it is tetralogy of Fallot.

Occasionally, congenital heart disease remains unde-

tected until the patient reaches adulthood. Two factors contribute to this delay in diagnosis: First, in children, a cardiovascular malformation may go unrecognized or may be mistaken for a functional murmur because of the subtle manner in which it expresses itself, the classic example being the small or moderate-sized isolated atrial septal defect. Second, medical attention may be inadequate, particularly for individuals who grow up in medically underserved areas, and as a consequence, cardiovascular anomalies of even moderate severity may go undetected.

GENETICS AND CONGENITAL HEART DISEASE (see also pages 942 and 1613). As an increasing number of individuals with congenital heart disease reach childbearing age, the need for detailed information regarding the etiology of such diseases becomes more apparent. Nora and Nora reported that the cause of congenital heart disease is predominantly genetic in 8 per cent of cases and predominantly environmental in 2 per cent. In the remaining 90 per cent, a complex interaction between genetic and environmental factors is thought to exist.[1] Not surprisingly, the greater the number of affected first-degree relatives with congenital heart disease within the family, the greater the risk of recurrence.[1-3] The recurrence risk is somewhat higher if the affected first-degree relative is a parent rather than a sibling. When two first-degree relatives are affected, the recurrence risk for the next child becomes two to three times as great compared to the case when only one first-degree relative is affected.[1-3] If one parent has a congenital cardiac defect, the chance of his offspring having the same lesion is approximately 2 to 4 per cent (Table 30–1). Surgical repair of a woman's congenital heart defect does not affect her risk of having affected children.[4]

TABLE 30–1 AFFECTED OFFSPRING, GIVEN ONE PARENT WITH A CONGENITAL HEART DEFECT

ANOMALY	AFFECTED OFFSPRING	
	Number	*%*
Ventricular septal defect	7/174	4.0
Persistent ductus arteriosus	6/139	4.3
Atrial septal defect	5/199	2.5
Tetralogy of Fallot	6/141	4.2
Pulmonic stenosis	4/111	3.6
Coarctation of the aorta	7/253	2.7
Aortic stenosis	4/103	3.9

Adapted from Nora, J. J., and Nora, A. H.: The evolution of specific genetic and environmental counseling in congenital heart disease. Circulation *57*:205, 1978. By permission of the American Heart Association, Inc.

Surgically Corrected Congenital Heart Defects

The adult with a surgically corrected congenital heart defect is now emerging as a new type of patient in cardiology practice.[5–7] Three categories of such patients exist: (1) asymptomatic individuals who have undergone complete repair of their defects, (2) asymptomatic or symptomatic patients with residual defects or complications despite surgical correction, and (3) symptomatic patients who had previously undergone palliative procedures.

The clinical course of asymptomatic patients in whom congenital cardiac malformations are totally corrected early in life appears to be a relatively stable one.[5] Many of these individuals are independent, socially well-adjusted, and free of anxiety concerning their cardiac condition. Patients who undergo correction of their defect in childhood are significantly less anxious in this regard than are those whose lesion is corrected during adult life.

Patients with residual defects or complications following repair may be asymptomatic or symptomatic.[5,8] Conditions frequently associated with altered hemodynamics postoperatively include: (1) ostium secundum atrial septal defect that has been closed, with residual mitral regurgitation due to associated mitral valve prolapse (p. 1089); (2) ventricular septal defect or tetralogy of Fallot with residual left-to-right shunt from a leak in the patch closing the septal defect; (3) congenital aortic stenosis with inadequate relief of the obstruction, restenosis of the valve, or significant aortic regurgitation; (4) persistent or recurrent systemic hypertension after coarctectomy; and (5) severe pulmonic regurgitation or residual right ventricular outflow tract obstruction after repair of pulmonic stenosis or tetralogy of Fallot. Such patients may remain asymptomatic or minimally symptomatic for many years. The ultimate effect of the residual cardiac abnormality depends on the specific lesion as well as its severity. Patients with residual cardiac abnormalities are, in general, less well adjusted socially and emotionally than are individuals without residual cardiac problems. Many of these patients have considerable difficulty obtaining life and health insurance policies and even employment.[9]

A modest number of patients who have undergone palliative procedures such as Blalock-Taussig, Potts, or Waterston systemic-to-pulmonary artery anastomoses survive to reach adult life.[10] The cardiac reserve of these patients is usually limited, often severely. Physically, such

individuals may be underdeveloped, with chest deformities such as pectus carinatum. Although these patients generally adapt to their condition, marked limitations in lifestyle are common. In some of these patients, complete correction is feasible during adult life, albeit at a higher risk than in childhood or adolescence; in others, the presence of irreversible changes in the pulmonary vascular bed or the complex nature of the malformation prohibits complete correction.

Taussig and associates have reviewed the long-term consequences of the Blalock-Taussig operation.[10] Their findings might be considered representative of those resulting from palliative procedures in patients with complex anomalies. One hundred and sixty-nine patients, mostly children, diagnosed clinically as having tetralogy of Fallot underwent a subclavian–pulmonary artery anastomosis only. At least 119 of these patients (70 per cent) were still alive and 62 (35 per cent) were not seriously disabled 20 to 28 years after their operation. Examination of the entire cohort of 685 patients originally treated with a Blalock-Taussig anastomosis for tetralogy of Fallot, including those without additional operation and those with subsequent palliative and corrective operative procedures, has revealed a vast improvement in their quality of life. Over 50 per cent of them have married and two-thirds of them have had children. Thirty-five per cent of the patients graduated from college and almost 70 per cent are earning substantial incomes. Approximately 70 per cent of these patients have repaid in taxes the cost to society of their medical treatment and rehabilitation.[10] However, a number of serious complications have also occurred. Infective endocarditis, most commonly due to streptococcus and staphylococcus, occurred 80 times in 71 of the patients. Sixteen (23 per cent) of these 71 affected patients died.

Over the past 25 years, more than 500,000 patients with functionally significant congenital cardiac malformations have attained adulthood.[9] The magnitude of this success is due primarily to the medical and surgical advances since the early 1960s.

ENDOCARDITIS PROPHYLAXIS (see also pages 951 and 1175). Surgical treatment may increase, decrease, or leave unchanged an individual's risk of endocarditis.[11,12] The incidence of postoperative endocarditis is so low in patients in whom a persistent ductus arteriosus or atrial septal defect has been closed that prophylaxis can be omitted. The risk of endocarditis after operation in persons with completely repaired ventricular septal defects and tetralogy of Fallot is also markedly reduced. On the other hand, patients with residual, hemodynamically insignificant left-to-right shunts following repair of a ventricular septal defect may be at even higher risk of endocarditis than they were preoperatively, despite the satisfactory physiological result. The risk of endocarditis also increases in patients who undergo prosthetic replacement of any valve or in whom a prosthetic conduit is inserted,[13] whereas the risk remains unchanged following aortic valvulotomy for congenital aortic stenosis or repair of coarctation of the aorta. Pulmonic stenosis carries a low risk of endocarditis both before and after valvulotomy. Because patients frequently feel so well after corrective and occasionally after palliative operations, it may be difficult to convince them of the importance of prophylactic antibiotics.

Pregnancy in Patients with Congenital Heart Disease (See also page 1769)

Most congenital cardiac malformations do not interfere with the *initiation* of pregnancy.[4,14-18] However, some of these parturients abort or give birth to premature, nonviable infants.[4] In a few cardiovascular malformations, pregnancy presents a definite danger to the mother. Among patients with severe pulmonary hypertension or marginally compensated cardiac failure, mortality is high during pregnancy. In women with small or moderate-sized left-to-right shunts (i.e., pulmonary-to-systemic flow ratios less than 2:1) and only modest pulmonary hypertension (i.e., pulmonary artery systolic pressure less than 50 mm Hg), pregnancy is generally well tolerated. In patients with larger left-to-right shunts, left ventricular failure may occur, while in those with more severe pulmonary hypertension, further elevation of pulmonary arterial pressure may occur during pregnancy.

In a review of the obstetrical experience of 28 women with unrepaired *coarctation of the aorta*, there was no maternal mortality and the spontaneous abortion rate was 25 per cent.[14] Most of the remaining pregnancies were uncomplicated, and the infants were normal. Because of the increased cardiac output associated with the second and third trimesters of pregnancy, parturients with unrepaired coarctation of the aorta may experience a significant increase in systolic arterial pressure, and antihypertensive therapy may be of some benefit. Nitroprusside infusion is often useful in treating acute elevations in blood pressure during delivery and the immediate postpartum period. In a small fraction of patients with coarctation of the aorta, aortic dissection or rupture occurs during pregnancy, but it is likely that in these cases intrinsic disease of the ascending aorta with cystic necrosis was present prior to pregnancy. Fortunately, this complication is so rare in women with unrepaired coarctation of the aorta followed in modern obstetrical practice that there seems to be little rationale for elective coarctectomy during pregnancy.[4,14] Rarely, the bacteremia that accompanies labor results in endocarditis or endarteritis in patients with coarctation.

Maternal and fetal mortality rates are high among patients with uncorrected *tetralogy of Fallot*. As is the case with other forms of cyanotic congenital heart disease, the infants tend to be small for their gestational age. Palliative surgical procedures carried out prior to pregnancy in these patients may decrease maternal and infant risk. Pregnancy after successful total correction of tetralogy of Fallot seems to pose little threat to either mother or child.[16] Patients with *congenital heart block* tolerate pregnancy without difficulty, although Stokes-Adams attacks have been reported to commence shortly after delivery.[17] Insertion of a temporary transvenous pacemaker may be helpful for maintaining stable hemodynamics at the time of delivery in women with marked bradycardia due to congenital heart block. In patients with permanent pacemakers inserted for either congenital or acquired complete heart block, improved hemodynamics may be achieved if the pacing rate is increased immediately prior to labor and delivery.

Pregnancy is contraindicated in women with severe *pulmonary vascular disease*.[18] If early termination of the pregnancy is not possible, close fetal and maternal monitoring as well as judicious medical care is required throughout the prenatal period. Maternal and fetal risk become maximal during labor and delivery. Uterine contractions, especially when associated with the application of forceps, may have an adverse effect on pulmonary and systemic hemodynamics.[19] Management of these patients should include inhalation of high concentrations of oxygen and epidural anesthesia. Serial arterial blood gas determinations may be useful in detecting changes in shunt flow associated with an acute increase in pulmonary vascular resistance or a sudden fall in systemic vascular resistance. Increased maternal risk extends at least several days into the immediate postpartum period.

SPECIFIC MALFORMATIONS

Valvular Aortic Stenosis
(See also pages 976 and 1095)

Congenital abnormalities of the aortic valve occur in 1 to 2 per cent of the general adult population. The most common cause of congenital valvular aortic stenosis is the bicuspid valve with peripheral fusion of the leaflets and diminished effective orifice size. A valve that is functionally normal early in life may become thickened, fibrotic, calcified, and stenotic during adulthood. Valvular aortic stenosis may be associated with coarctation of the aorta and, less frequently, ventricular septal defect or isolated pulmonic stenosis.[20]

In the young or middle-aged adult, isolated valvular aortic stenosis is usually congenital rather than rheumatic in origin.[21,22] By age 45, approximately 50 per cent of all bicuspid valves show some degree of stenosis.[20,23] The frequency and severity of valvular narrowing increase with age, in part reflecting progressive calcium deposition within the leaflets.[24] In many patients, the congenitally bicuspid aortic valve becomes regurgitant as well as stenotic. The noninfected congenitally bicuspid aortic valve is also an important cause of pure aortic regurgitation severe enough to require valve replacement.[25] All patients with congenital abnormalities of the aortic valve require antibiotic prophylaxis against infective endocarditis.

Pathophysiology. Left ventricular systolic hypertension acts as a stimulus for concentric hypertrophy (p. 1097). Left ventricular compliance is frequently decreased, resulting in elevations of left ventricular end-diastolic and left atrial mean pressures and symptoms of pulmonary congestion. Because of increased left ventricular muscle mass and high intracavity systolic pressure, left ventricular ischemia may occur even in the absence of significant coronary artery disease. In some patients with severe stenosis, cardiac output may not increase appropriately during exercise, reflecting severe mechanical obstruction at the valvular level and/or intrinsic abnormalities of the left ventricular contractile state. This can result in exercise-induced syncope or presyncope.

Symptoms. The major symptoms of congenital valvular aortic stenosis in the adult include angina pectoris, syncope, and congestive heart failure.[26] Sudden death during exercise can occur in patients with severe disease but is rarely the presenting event in a previously undiagnosed or asymptomatic adult.[27] Hemodynamic and clinical compensation are usual until middle age. However, from the time of onset of symptoms, the average survival in patients with unrepaired severe valvular aortic stenosis is less than five years.[26]

Physical Examination. The predominant physical finding in adults with congenital valvular aortic stenosis is a harsh systolic ejection murmur, loudest along the right upper sternal edge and radiating along the carotid arteries. In mild to moderate valvular aortic stenosis, an ejection click caused by abrupt cessation of movement of the thickened, doming leaflets is frequently present. In contrast to the click found in pulmonic stenosis, it does not vary in intensity with respiration. As the severity of the valvular aortic stenosis increases, the murmur becomes longer and louder and peaks later in systole. Examination of the carotid pulse demonstrates the characteristic findings of a delayed upstroke, low anacrotic shoulder, systolic shudder, and prolonged ejection time (see Figure 3–22, p. 56). The apical precordial impulse is often heaving and sustained, with a palpable atrial presystolic tap.

Noninvasive Studies. The *ECG* shows a variable degree of left ventricular hypertrophy. Approximately 75 per cent of adult patients with severe valvular aortic stenosis (left ventriculo-aortic pressure gradient greater than 75 mm Hg) exhibit left ventricular hypertrophy with strain. This finding is less common in patients with mild to moderate obstruction.

On *chest x-ray*, poststenotic dilatation of the ascending aorta (see Figure 6–52, p. 185) is common, but this finding does not correlate well with the severity of the obstruction. Calcification of the aortic valve becomes evident more frequently after the third decade of life. Overall heart size is usually normal until left ventricular failure occurs, although the left ventricle may be prominent in patients with only moderate obstruction (gradient of approximately 50 mm Hg) even without failure.

On *M-mode echocardiography*, the bicuspid aortic valve is often thickened, with an eccentric closure line reflecting the asymmetry of the valve leaflets (see Figure 5–48, p. 115). Rather than opening fully with ventricular systole, the leaflets frequently show a doming pattern. When this occurs, leaflet excursion seen on an M-mode study may not accurately reflect the severity of the stenosis. This problem can be solved in part by the use of two-dimensional echocardiography to demonstrate leaflet doming on the long-axis parasternal view and the presence of only two leaflets on the short-axis parasternal view[28] (Fig. 30–1). Pulsed Doppler echocardiography (p. 94) can also be useful in quantifying the severity of aortic stenosis and associated regurgitation.[29,30]

Surgical Treatment. The decision to operate for congenital valvular aortic stenosis in adults depends on multiple factors, including the magnitude and type of symptoms, the calculated aortic valve area at cardiac catheterization, and the state of left ventricular function.[27,31,31a] Our general criteria are a peak systolic ejection gradient exceeding 75 mm Hg in association with a normal forward cardiac output and an aortic valve area less than approximately 0.7 cm^2 (0.4 cm^2/m^2 body surface area). In patients with reduced forward cardiac output, the peak systolic ejection gradient may be low, reflecting underlying myocardial dysfunction or afterload mismatch. In such patients, calculation of the aortic valve area is vital for determining the hemodynamic significance of the left ventricular outflow tract obstruction. The young adult with severe valvular aortic stenosis but without calcification of the valve may be a candidate for aortic valvulotomy. However, residual or recurrent stenosis as well as valvular incompetence is a frequent complication of this procedure.[27,32,33] In the older patient, aortic valve replacement is often necessary owing to leaflet fibrosis and calcification.

Atrial Septal Defect (See also page 958)

This malformation frequently permits survival into middle age and beyond.[34,35] The diagnosis of atrial septal defect (ASD) may be difficult because the associated physical

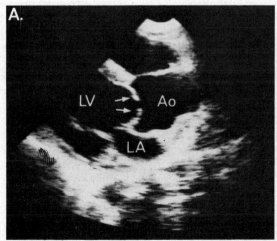
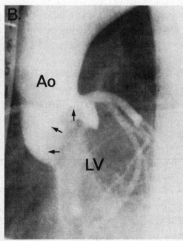

FIGURE 30–1 Echocardiographic and angiographic findings in a young adult with valvular aortic stenosis. *A,* Two-dimensional echocardiographic study with the transducer in the long-axis parasternal position demonstrating leaflet doming and thickening (arrows). *B,* Aortogram from the same patient showing doming of the aortic valve leaflets. The negative shadow in the proximal aortic root (Ao) is caused by a jet of nonpacified blood from the left ventricle (LV) as it exits through the stenotic aortic valve. LA = left atrium.

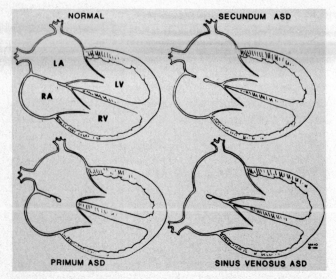

FIGURE 30–2 Normal atrial septum and anatomical sites of the three types of atrial septal defects (ASD) as visualized by the two-dimensional echocardiographic technique utilizing a subcostal position. (From Nasser, F. N., et al.: Diagnosis of sinus venosus atrial septal defect by two-dimensional echocardiography. Mayo Clin. Proc. *56*:571, 1981.)

findings may be subtle and the patient asymptomatic. Moreover, ASD may not be recognized in adults because of the presence of associated conditions, such as coronary artery disease or chronic obstructive pulmonary disease. One characteristic of ASD that sets it apart from many other significant congenital heart lesions is the prolonged period during which the patient remains asymptomatic or almost so. Serious limitation of exercise capacity may develop secondary to progressive pulmonary vascular disease, but this usually does not occur until the fourth or fifth decade of life.[34,34a] Three types of ASD are seen in adults: ostium secundum, ostium primum, and sinus venosus (Fig. 30–2). Ostium secundum ASD is by far the most common type.

PATHOPHYSIOLOGY. Blood flow through the ASD occurs primarily during late ventricular systole, early diastole, and atrial systole. The magnitude of the left-to-right shunt depends on the size of the defect, on the relationship between the compliance of the two ventricles, and indirectly on the relationship between pulmonary and systemic vascular resistance. The net effect in a patient with an uncomplicated ASD is volume overload of the right atrium and right ventricle with consequent enlargement of these chambers without dilatation of the left cardiac chambers. Some patients with ASD will have mild to modest elevations of pulmonary artery pressure on the basis of a high transpulmonary blood flow rather than elevated pulmonary vascular resistance.

The mechanism of heart failure in patients with ASD was first studied in 1956 by Dexter,[36] who noted that all four cardiac chambers are in communication during diastole. Ordinarily, a left-to-right shunt occurs at that time because the right ventricle offers less resistance to inflowing blood than does the left ventricle, despite equality of pressures in all four chambers. The right ventricle is more compliant than the left, so that when both atria and ventricles are in communication, blood follows the path of least resistance, i.e., into the more compliant right ventri-

cle. According to this concept, when a patient with ASD develops right ventricular hypertrophy as a consequence of a superimposed pressure overload from pulmonary hypertension, resistance to right ventricular filling is increased and the left-to-right shunt declines. As these processes continue, the right ventricle may become less compliant than the left, with resultant right-to-left shunting and the development of cyanosis.

Left ventricular failure in adults with ASD is usually the result of one or a combination of associated conditions that affect the left ventricle, such as ischemic heart disease, systemic hypertension, aortic valvular disease, or mitral regurgitation.[35-39] Left ventricular failure reduces chamber compliance, thus increasing the magnitude of the left-to-right shunt. If the right ventricle cannot accept an increase in the quantity of blood shunted from left to right, the diastolic pressures in all four cardiac chambers increase. As a consequence of the defect in the atrial septum, this increase in diastolic pressure produces systemic venous congestion. For these reasons, left ventricular failure in patients with ASD can elevate systemic venous pressure and result in the clinical signs usually associated with right heart failure.

The issue of whether left ventricular dysfunction occurs frequently in patients with uncomplicated ASD remains controversial. Older studies suggested that intrinsic abnormalities of left ventricular function do exist in some patients,[41] but these findings have been questioned.[38,40-42] Bonow et al. demonstrated that left ventricular ejection fraction at rest measured by radionuclide angiography was usually normal in adults with ASD without evidence of hemodynamically severe right or left ventricular failure. However, an abnormal response of the ejection fraction to exercise was common. Impairment of the left ventricular response to exercise resolved after operative closure of the defect. This study suggests that left ventricular dysfunction in patients with ASD may result from reversible mechanical factors related to right ventricular volume overload with abnormal displacement of the ventricular septum and perhaps compromise of left ventricular preload rather than to intrinsic, irreversible impairment of left ventricular contractility.

CLINICAL FINDINGS

Symptoms. Most patients over age 40 are symptomatic.[38,39] Dyspnea on exertion, fatigue, and symptoms secondary to supraventricular tachyarrhythmias are the most frequent complaints. Life expectancy is shortened in ASD, although many patients reach advanced years.[43,44] Even young adults who develop pulmonary hypertension usually survive beyond the age of 40 years. When patients succumb to ASD, the cause of death is usually right heart failure.[45] Other fatal complications include pulmonary embolism, in situ pulmonary thrombosis, bronchopulmonary infection, paradoxical embolism, brain abscess, and rupture of the pulmonary artery.

Pulmonary hypertension rarely occurs before age 20 in patients who reside at sea level; however, those who live at high altitudes may develop this complication earlier.[34] Patients with pulmonary hypertension usually complain of dyspnea and fatigue, effort cyanosis, and/or hemoptysis. Chest pain resembling angina may also occur.

CARDIAC DEFECT	Abnormal Q Waves or Myocardial Infarction Pattern	Biventricular Overload	Left Ventricular Pressure Overload	Left Ventricular Volume Overload	Right Ventricular Pressure Overload	Right Ventricular Volume Overload	Right Bundle Branch Block	Left Bundle Branch Block	Left Axis Deviation	Left Atrial Overload	Right Atrial Overload	Abnormal P-wave Orientation	Preexcitation Syndrome	Atrioventricular Block	Ventricular Arrhythmia	Supraventricular Tachycardia	Atrial Flutter/Fibrillation
Atrial septal defect (secundum)	0	0	0	0	+	+++	+	0	0	+	+	+	0	+	0	+	++
Prolapsed mitral valve syndrome	0	0	0	+	0	0	0	0	0	+	0	0	+	0	+	+	+
Aortic stenosis	++	0	++	0	0	0	0	+	+	+	0	0	0	+	++	0	0
Idiopathic hypertrophic subaortic stenosis	++	0	++	0	0	0	0	++	++	++	0	0	+	0	++	0	+
Pulmonary stenosis	0	0	0	0	++	+	0	0	0	0	+	0	0	0	0	0	0
Ventricular septal defect	0	++	0	++	0	0	0	0	+	+	++	0	0	0	0	0	++
Patent ductus arteriosus	0	+	0	++	0	0	0	0	+	++	0	0	0	0	0	0	0
Tetralogy of Fallot	0	0	0	0	++	0	+	0	+	0	+	0	0	0	+	0	+
Coarctation of aorta	0	+	++	0	0	0	0	0	0	+	+	0	0	0	0	0	+
Eisenmenger's syndrome	0	0	0	0	++	0	+	0	0	0	0	0	0	0	0	0	++
Atrial septal defect (primum)	0	++	0	+	0	++	+	0	+++	+	+	0	0	++	0	+	++
Corrected transposition*	+++	++	++	0	0	0	0	0	++	0	+++	0	++	+++	0	+++	+
Ebstein's anomaly	0	0	0	+	0	+	++	0	++	0	+++	0	+++	+	++	0	+
Tricuspid atresia	+	0	0	0	0	0	0	0	++	+	0	0	0	0	0	++	+
Congenital anomalies of coronary arteries	+++	0	++	+	0	0	0	+	+	0	+	0	0	0	++	0	0
Transposition of great arteries (postop)	0	0	0	0	+++	0	0	0	0	0	+	0	0	+	0	++	0

+++ = Almost always seen (characteristic of defect).

++ = Commonly seen with defect.

+ = Sometimes seen with defect (especially with associated defects or advancing age).

0 = Rarely seen with defect.

*The precordial QRS progression in corrected transposition may mimic left ventricular hypertrophy, usually with ST-segment abnormalities. True hypertrophy of the left-sided ventricle can occur in corrected transposition from associated left atrioventricular valvular regurgitation, ventricular septal defect, and so on.

From Ellison, R. C., and Sloss, L. J.: Electrocardiographic features of congenital heart disease in the adult. *In* Roberts, W. C. (ed.): Congenital Heart Disease in Adults. Philadelphia, F. A. Davis Co., 1979, p. 267.

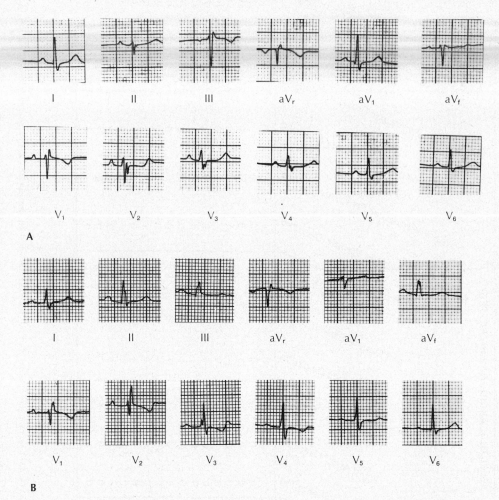

FIGURE 30–3 Representative 12-lead electrocardiograms (ECG) in adults with congenital heart disease. *A*, ECG of a 36-year-old woman with an ostium primum atrial septal defect, a large atrial left-to-right shunt with normal pulmonary pressures, and trivial mitral valve dysfunction. The P-R interval is upper normal. The P waves show evidence of mild right atrial overload in the precordial leads. There is a superior QRS axis and rather subtle evidence of volume-overload right ventricular hypertrophy ("incomplete right bundle branch block" pattern). *B*, ECG of a 52-year-old woman with a large left-to-right shunt via an ostium secundum atrial septal defect; pulmonary pressures are normal. The tracing shows borderline first-degree atrioventricular block and findings typical of volume-overload right ventricular hypertrophy. The P wave shows slight evidence of right atrial overload in the precordial leads, and the QRS axis is normal. *C*, ECG of a 21-year-old man with severe valvular pulmonic stenosis. Right ventricular peak systolic pressure is considerably higher than systemic levels. The P wave reflects right atrial overload, and the P-R interval is at the upper limit of normal. There is marked right-axis deviation and right ventricular hypertrophy with "strain." Left ventricular forces are not apparent. *D*, ECG of a 45-year-old man who presented with cyanosis and congestive heart failure of recent onset. Catheterization revealed a large persistent ductus arteriosus, pulmonary hypertension, and a bidirectional shunt. The tracing shows predominant right atrial and lesser left atrial overload. There is prolongation of the QRS complex with left anterior fascicular block and biventricular hypertrophy. (From Ellison, R. C., and Sloss, L. J.: Electrocardiographic features of congenital heart disease in the adult. *In* Roberts, W. C. (ed.): Congenital Heart Disease in Adults. Philadelphia, F. A. Davis Co., 1979, p. 119.)

Illustration continues on opposite page.

Physical Examination. Adults with ASD are usually normal in appearance, although a gracile habitus is relatively common. Occasionally the left precordium is prominent or even bulging. Cyanosis and digital clubbing may be seen in individuals with pulmonary hypertension and right-to-left shunts. Skeletal malformations characteristic of the autosomal dominant Holt-Oram syndrome may be present and consist of the inability to appose the thumb (which may have an accessory phalanx or be rudimentary) and a variety of other osseous changes involving the upper extremities (p. 1616).[46] The major differences in the cardiac examination between children and adults with ASD are that in the adult there is usually more marked widening of the two components of the second heart sound and the

mid-diastolic rumble due to increased flow across the tricuspid valve is less common.

Patients with severe pulmonary hypertension often have fourth heart sounds originating from the right ventricle and may also demonstrate murmurs of pulmonic and/or tricuspid regurgitation, a pulmonic ejection sound, and an accentuated pulmonic component of the second heart sound.[46a] There is an association between ostium secundum ASD and mitral valve prolapse,[39,47-49] and findings typical of both conditions are often found on physical examination. A murmur of clinically significant mitral regurgitation may be present in older patients with mitral valve abnormalities.

Electrocardiographic Findings (Table 30–2). Atrial

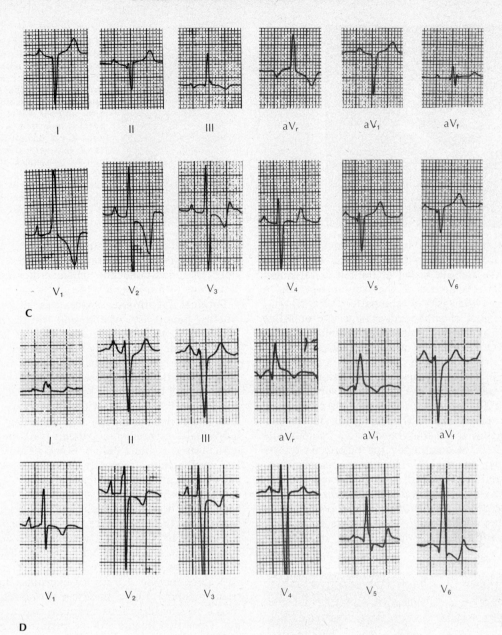

C

D

FIGURE 30–3 *Continued*

arrhythmias are more frequent in adults with ASD than in children.[43,44,50] Atrial fibrillation is the most common of these, followed by atrial flutter and paroxysmal atrial tachycardia. The P-R interval is often prolonged in adults, particularly in the elderly.[51,52] As pulmonary hypertension develops in adults with this malformation, the electrocardiogram reflects the development of right ventricular hypertrophy. Coexisting conditions, such as ischemic or hypertensive heart disease, which are common in adults, produce distinctive alterations that are superimposed on those already present on the ECG recording. Patients with ostium primum and secundum defects can frequently be distinguished electrocardiographically: The former usually have a normal QRS axis, while the latter usually manifest left-axis deviation (Fig. 30–3A and B).[52,53] Patients with sinus venosus atrial septal defects frequently have an ectopic atrial rhythm.

Roentgenographic Findings. The peripheral pulmonary vascular bed may be plethoric in adults with ASD and large left-to-right shunt (see Fig. 6–28, p. 166). With the development of pulmonary vascular obstruction, pulmonary hypertension and decreasing left-to-right shunting of blood, peripheral pulmonary vessels lose their prominence while the pulmonary trunk and central pulmonary arteries may increase in size. The pulmonary artery and its main branches may even become aneurysmal, with calcification of the vessel wall similar to that of the aortic wall in patients with systemic hypertension.

Echocardiographic Findings (see also page 120). The M-mode echocardiogram usually shows right ventricular dilatation, often associated with paradoxical or flattened movement of the ventricular septum. In the absence of mitral regurgitation, the left ventricle frequently appears decreased in size. This may reflect diminished left ventricular preload as well as an alteration in left ventricular geometry due to right ventricular dilatation.[41,54] Mitral valve prolapse may be present. Two-dimensional echocardiography can be useful in determining which anatomical type of ASD is present.[55,56] Visualization of the interatrial septum from the subcostal transducer position is particularly helpful for

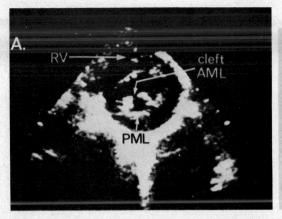

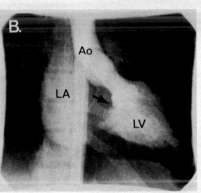

FIGURE 30–4 Studies from a 27-year-old patient with a primum atrial septal defect and cleft mitral valve. *A*, Two-dimensional echocardiographic study performed with the transducer in the short-axis parasternal position. The cleft in the anterior leaflet of the mitral valve (AML) is indicated (arrow). PML = posterior mitral leaflet; RV = right ventricle. *B*, Left ventriculogram showing the typical "gooseneck deformity" of the left ventricular (LV) outflow tract. The mitral valve cleft is indicated (arrow). Moderate mitral regurgitation is present. LA = left atrium; Ao = aorta.

distinguishing a secundum from a sinus venosus type of defect (Fig. 30–2). Patients with a primum ASD often have a cleft in the anterior leaflet of the mitral valve and abnormal chordal attachments to the septum, resulting in a characteristic two-dimensional echo pattern (Fig. 30–4).

Contrast injections of either indocyanine dye or saline into a peripheral arm vein can enhance the ability to diagnose an ASD.[57-60] In patients with a left-to-right shunt across the interatrial septum, a contrast-free area may be noted in the right atrium because of blood shunted from the left atrium washing out the "contrast" substance. In patients with right-to-left shunts, it is possible to visualize contrast echoes across the ASD (Fig. 30–5). In patients suspected of having a left-to-right shunt, a radionuclide scan can be helpful in quantifying the pulmonary-to-systemic blood flow ratio (p. 359).[61] It is not unreasonable to send a young adult patient with typical physical findings of an ASD to surgery without cardiac catheterization if (1) there is evidence of right ventricular volume overload, (2) the anterior leaflet of the mitral valve appears normal, (3) right-to-left shunting is not evident on two-dimensional

echocardiographic evaluation, (4) there is no electrocardiographic evidence of pulmonary hypertension, and (5) results of a radionuclide angiocardiographic study are consistent with a large left-to-right shunt.[62]

Surgical Treatment. Since it is impossible to predict whether pulmonary hypertension will develop in a patient with ASD, we recommend closure of defects (even in asymptomatic patients) for adults under 45 years of age with left-to-right shunts that result in a pulmonary-to-systemic blood flow ratio exceeding 1.5:1.0.[35,63,63a] Even elderly patients with large shunts have been shown to benefit from operation.[43,44,64] The risk of this procedure is very low (less than 1 per cent), although it is somewhat higher in older individuals, especially in patients with pulmonary hypertension and/or heart failure. Some residual right ventricular dysfunction frequently persists postoperatively in patients operated upon after the age of 40 years. Surgical correction is indicated in such patients as long as pulmonary blood flow substantially exceeds systemic blood flow (ratio > 2:1), unless severe left ventricular dysfunction is responsible for the shunt. In adults with ASD and moderate pulmonary hypertension, the net left-to-right shunt may be quite small; however, it may increase considerably with development of a myocardial infarction and left ventricular failure. Under these circumstances, closure of the defect may be hazardous and may lead to pulmonary edema. Operation should not be performed in patients with pulmonary-to-systemic blood flow ratios less than 1.5:1.0 who have severe pulmonary vascular obstructive disease (pulmonary-to-systemic resistance ratio ≥ 0.7:1.0).

Variants of Atrial Septal Defect

LUTEMBACHER'S SYNDROME. This term refers to the combination of ASD and mitral stenosis.[65] The latter is almost invariably rheumatic in origin. Lutembacher's syndrome is more common in adults than in children; only rarely does congenital mitral stenosis coexist with ASD.[65] Patients with this syndrome are invariably symptomatic, complaining of exertional dyspnea, fatigue, and palpitations. Orthopnea and paroxysmal nocturnal dyspnea are rare, and hemoptysis does not appear to occur. The ASD exerts a protective effect on the mitral stenosis by decompressing the left atrium and the pulmonary venous system, resulting in a large left-to-right shunt. Severe pulmonary congestion or edema does not occur in these patients unless the ASD is repaired without relief of the mitral stenosis.

The findings on *physical examination* suggest both le-

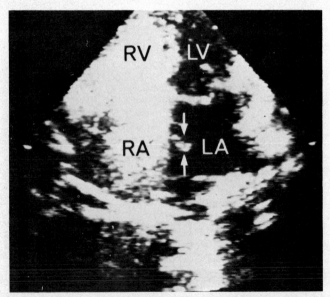

FIGURE 30–5 Two-dimensional echocardiographic study of a 53-year-old patient with a secundum atrial septal defect (ASD). Saline was injected into a peripheral arm vein, resulting in contrast echoes in the right atrium (RA) and right ventricle (RV). In addition, contrast echoes are seen crossing the ASD (arrows) into the left atrium (LA), confirming the presence of a right-to-left shunt at the atrial level. LV = left ventricle.

sions, i.e., a parasternal right ventricular heave and widely split second heart sound are uniformly present and a loud first heart sound and opening snap are also frequently heard. The *electrocardiogram* usually reveals right ventricular hypertrophy, while the chest roentgenogram shows pulmonary plethora and right atrial and ventricular enlargement. Elevated right atrial pressure with prominent *v* waves is a constant finding in patients with Lutembacher's syndrome.[65] The systemic flow index is usually low, while pulmonary blood flow is markedly elevated; thus, the pulmonary-to-systemic blood flow ratio is quite high.

PATENT FORAMEN OVALE. Patency of the foramen ovale is common,[66] with "pencil patent" foramina (0.6 to 1.0 cm in diameter) occurring in 6 per cent and "probe patent" foramina (0.2 to 0.5 cm in diameter) occurring in 29 to 35 per cent of adults at autopsy.[67] Patency of the foramen ovale produces no abnormality on physical examination, electrocardiogram, or chest roentgenogram.[66] Its presence may be deduced by means of a dilution curve obtained from injecting indicator dye into a systemic vein or the inferior vena cava and sampling from a systemic artery (p. 290) during a Valsalva maneuver; early appearance of the indicator dye is diagnostic of a right-to-left shunt. Contrast echocardiography can be used in a similar manner. This defect is significant only in that it is a potential route for paradoxical embolism.[66] Left-to-right shunts do not usually occur.

ANOMALOUS PULMONARY VENOUS DRAINAGE (see also page 1011). Partial anomalous pulmonary venous drainage occurs when one or more (but not all) of the pulmonary veins drain into the right atrium or systemic venous circulation rather than into the left atrium.[68–70] This malformation is often associated with an ASD of the sinus venosus type. When partial anomalous venous return is associated with ASD, the natural history, physical examination, electrocardiogram, and chest roentgenogram are usually indistinguishable from those for patients with isolated ASD. Patients with partial anomalous venous drainage and an *intact* atrial septum usually show respirophasic variation of the second heart sound and can thereby be distinguished from patients with associated ASD. Systolic flow murmurs across the pulmonary outflow tract and diastolic murmurs across the tricuspid orifice are common in patients with anomalous pulmonary venous return and an intact atrial septum. Electrocardiographic and roentgenographic findings are identical to those in patients with ASD. When the entire right lung drains into the inferior vena cava (the "scimitar syndrome"), the anomalous vein can sometimes be identified on the plain chest roentgenogram.

Identification of this anomaly may be difficult. Techniques that have been successful in establishing this diagnosis at the time of catheterization include differential indicator-dye dilution curves from the right and left main pulmonary arteries, careful probing of the atrial septum with a catheter, and pulmonary angiography and selective injection of contrast media into an anomalous pulmonary vein that has been entered by a catheter during cardiac catheterization.[68] Right heart pressures are usually normal. In most patients with anomalous pulmonary venous return and an intact atrial septum, the left-to-right shunt is usually modest in size (i.e., pulmonary-to-systemic blood flow ratio less than 2:1). Pulmonary hypertension rarely devel-

ops in these patients. Surgical correction consists of incorporating the site of drainage of the anomalous vein into the left atrium and closing the ASD, if it is present. Operation is usually indicated when the pulmonary-to-systemic blood flow ratio exceeds 1.5:1.0.[69]

Total anomalous pulmonary venous return (p. 1008) is rarely seen in adults.

Ventricular Septal Defect (See also page 963)

Ventricular septal defect (VSD) is the most common congenital malformation reported in infants and children. However, in adults, VSD is surpassed in frequency by ASD, a change that can be related to three factors: First —and most importantly—a significant number of VSD (even those with large left-to-right shunts) close spontaneously during infancy or childhood; occasionally, spontaneous closure occurs during adulthood.[71] Second, patients with VSD may die of heart failure early in life. Finally, many patients with VSD now undergo surgical closure of the defect during childhood.

Patients with moderate or large VSD without pulmonary vascular obstructive disease experience significant left-to-right shunting with volume overload of the left atrium and ventricle. Left ventricular hypertrophy is noted early in life. Although symptoms of left ventricular failure may develop in infants with VSD, left heart failure is generally *not* part of the natural history of this congenital defect in patients over 2 years of age unless aortic regurgitation or infective endocarditis supervene (see below).[71] Maron and coworkers,[72] and Lueker et al.[73] used exercise testing to evaluate postoperative cardiovascular function in adult patients with surgically closed VSD. In several patients they found normal hemodynamic measurements at rest but abnormal values with vigorous exercise, and they concluded that postoperative left ventricular function may be abnormal in patients who undergo closure of a large VSD at an older age. However, both studies assessed left ventricular function in patients whose defects were repaired during the 1960s when the myocardial preservation techniques used were inferior to those currently available. How much effect intraoperative myocardial ischemia had on postoperative left ventricular performance in these patients is unknown.

Recently, rest and exercise ventricular performance were compared using equilibrium gated radionuclide angiography in 34 patients (mean age 27 years) with hemodynamically documented VSD.[73a] The response of left ventricular ejection fraction to dynamic exercise was abnormal in patients who previously underwent surgical closure of VSD as well as in patients with residual defects. This again raises the issue of whether lifelong left ventricular volume overload may be detrimental to myocardial function.

Complications that accompany VSD in adult life include aortic regurgitation, infective endocarditis, pulmonary hypertension, infundibular pulmonic stenosis, and heart failure.[74]

Aortic regurgitation was noted in 5.5 per cent of all patients with a VSD followed in the Natural History Study of Congenital Heart Disease.[75] In most cases the VSD was either infracristal (membranous) or subpulmonic. No patient under 2 years of age had this combination of lesions, supporting the impression that the aortic regurgitation is an acquired problem. Of the 34 patients over 11 years of age with this combination of lesions, 20 (59 per cent) had aortic regurgitation of at least moderate severity, whereas most of the younger patients had mild disease, suggesting that the aortic regurgitation is frequently a progressive lesion. In another study, Corone et al.[74] noted the presence of aortic regurgitation in 6.3 per cent of 790 patients with VSD. In 15 to 20 per cent of these patients, aortic regurgitation developed as a consequence of infective endocarditis. A wide spectrum of hemodynamic abnormalities may be evident—from the abnormality seen with a large VSD with trivial aortic regurgitation to that of free regurgitation and a small VSD. If not operated upon during childhood, most patients with VSD and aortic regurgitation survive to adult life, at which time they usually develop left ventricular failure.

Infective endocarditis (Chap. 33) occurs in almost 4 per cent of patients with VSD,[71,74] most commonly by the third or fourth decade of life. Most often the infection occurs on the "jet" lesion, a traumatic endocardial deposit in the right ventricle that results from the impact of the high-velocity blood flow across a restricted defect (p. 1147). Risk of endocarditis may be higher in patients with associated aortic regurgitation,[74] and surgical closure of the VSD does not abolish this risk. However, the risk of endocarditis after spontaneous closure of a VSD is exceedingly low or nonexistent.

Progressive pulmonary vascular disease is one of the most feared complications in patients with VSD (Chap. 25).[4,76,77] Adults with pulmonary hypertension and a left-to-right shunt may develop progressively more severe obliterative pulmonary vascular disease, with eventual reversal of their shunt. Eisenmenger's complex (i.e., marked elevation of pulmonary vascular resistance with right-to-left shunting through the VSD), if it develops, usually appears before the end of the second or during the third decade of life.[74] Sudden death, hemoptysis, chest pain resembling angina, cerebral abscess, thrombosis, and paradoxical emboli are complications of VSD with pulmonary hypertension and right-to-left shunt.[78]

Infundibular pulmonic stenosis, which is gradually progressive, may develop in an occasional patient with isolated VSD. Left-to-right shunts may reverse in these patients when obstruction to right ventricular outflow becomes sufficiently severe.[74]

Left ventricular failure is usually common in patients with VSD, aortic regurgitation, and infective endocarditis. Undue fatigue is often the first manifestation of decompen-sation in a previously asymptomatic adult with a VSD. The prognosis with or without operation is distinctly poorer for patients who develop heart failure than for individuals without this complication.[74]

Electrocardiographic Findings.   In the adult with a small, uncomplicated VSD, the electrocardiogram is usually normal. When a large defect is present, left atrial and left ventricular enlargement occurs. Left ventricular hypertrophy, usually with a diastolic volume overload pattern, is present in uncomplicated, moderately large defects. The presence of right-axis deviation or a progressive rightward shift of the frontal plane QRS axis suggests right ventricular hypertrophy secondary to either acquired infundibular obstruction or pulmonary vascular disease.

Roentgenographic Findings.   The chest x-ray is usually normal in the adult patient with a small VSD. Large defects are characterized by increased pulmonary vascular markings in association with pulmonary arterial, left atrial, and left ventricular enlargement. With the development of pulmonary vascular obstructive disease, marked central pulmonary artery dilatation occurs with "pruning" of the peripheral arterial vessels.

Echocardiographic Findings.   The M-mode echocardiogram is generally not diagnostic of VSD, frequently showing only left atrial and left ventricular dilatation. Two-dimensional echocardiography can often provide a definitive diagnosis of VSD and can also demonstrate the position of the defect, chamber sizes, and ventricular shortening characteristics (Fig. 30–6).[79] Pulsed Doppler echocardiography can also be useful in localizing the position of VSD.[80]

Operative closure of VSD is usually reserved for adult patients with pulmonary-to-systemic blood flow ratios exceeding 1.5 to 1.0. The presence of even moderate levels of pulmonary hypertension accompanying a left-to-right shunt argues for prompt closure of the defect.[78] Ventricular conduction abnormalities usually involving the right bundle are common after repair of VSD.[81,82]

Ventricular Septal Defect With Obstruction to Right Ventricular Outflow (Tetralogy of Fallot) (See also page 990)

Several variations of VSD in association with right ventricular outflow tract obstruction occur. In classic tetralogy of Fallot, a large ventricular septal defect (malalignment type) is associated with infundibular and/or

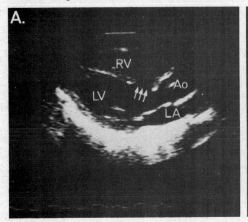

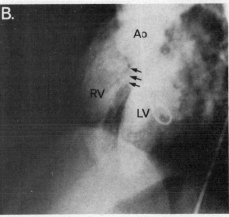

FIGURE   30–6 Two-dimensional echocardiogram (*A*) and cineangiogram (*B*) of a 34-year-old woman with a grade 3/6 holosystolic murmur, loudest along the left and right sternal borders. *A*, The long-axis parasternal view of the heart showed a high ventricular septal defect (VSD), probably in the membranous septum (arrows). *B*, The left ventriculogram confirmed the presence of a membranous VSD (arrows). The pulmonary-to-systemic flow ratio was 2.3 to 1.0; pulmonary artery pressures were mildly elevated. LV = left ventricle; LA = left atrium; RV = right ventricle; Ao = aorta.

valvular pulmonic stenosis.[83] In these patients right and left ventricular pressures are usually equalized. In the past, many adult patients diagnosed clinically as having "pink" or acyanotic tetralogy of Fallot had a high membranous VSD associated with hypertrophy of subinfundibular anomalous pulmonary bundles. These muscle bundles separated the right ventricle into a high-pressure proximal chamber and a low-pressure distal chamber (so-called double-chamber right ventricle).[84,84a] Many of these patients have right ventricular conduction abnormalities or subtle evidence of right ventricular hypertrophy on electrocardiogram.[85] In cases in which the VSD communicates with the low-pressure distal portion of the right ventricle, the physiology resembles that of a simple VSD rather than tetralogy of Fallot, and the patients remain acyanotic.

The pathophysiology of tetralogy of Fallot is determined by the severity of the right ventricular outflow tract obstruction, the size of the VSD, and the relationship between systemic vascular resistance and overall impedance to blood flow from the right ventricle. When the obstruction to right ventricular outflow is mild, the left-to-right shunt is predominant despite the equality of pressures in the two ventricles. The patient is acyanotic, the lung fields are plethoric, and there are usually two separate systolic murmurs, i.e., a holosystolic murmur resulting from the VSD and a midsystolic murmur secondary to the obstruction to right ventricular outflow. Cyanotic patients with severe obstruction to right ventricular outflow are usually recognized in childhood, at which time they frequently undergo surgical correction. Survival of patients with tetralogy of Fallot into adult life is related to the fact that the obstruction to right ventricular outflow is not severe and the pulmonary blood flow is relatively well maintained during infancy and childhood. Thus, adults with tetralogy of Fallot may give a history of cyanosis of delayed onset. This is related to the gradual and progressive development of obstruction to pulmonary outflow. Some patients will become noticeably cyanotic only under conditions of decreased systemic vascular resistance, i.e., exercise, sedation, fever, or general anesthesia. As the severity of the right ventricular outflow tract obstruction increases, the systolic ejection murmur, which is due to turbulent blood flow across the outflow tract, peaks earlier in systole and decreases in intensity. If the obstruction to right ventricular outflow is complete, a large obligatory right-to-left shunt occurs, the lungs are perfused through systemic collateral vessels, and there is severe cyanosis and usually no systolic murmur. Instead, there is a continuous murmur originating from bronchial collaterals. This variant of tetralogy of Fallot is termed *pseudotruncus arteriosus.*

Clinical Findings. Congestive heart failure is unusual in infants and children with tetralogy of Fallot. The VSD, which is usually large, allows decompression of the right ventricle, no matter how severe the stenosis, and prevents the right ventricular systolic pressure from exceeding that in the aorta. However, diminished cardiac reserve is not uncommon in adults with tetralogy of Fallot. Higgins and Mulder found exertional dyspnea and poor exercise tolerance in approximately one third of both cyanotic and acyanotic individuals with unoperated tetralogy of Fallot who survived into the third decade of life.[86] An occasional patient complains of orthopnea and/or paroxysmal nocturnal

dyspnea. Unfortunately, manifestations of heart failure may persist in adults even after surgical correction.[87] A recent study compared left ventricular function in patients with tetralogy of Fallot whose defects were repaired during infancy versus those repaired in late childhood or adolescence; left ventricular dysfunction was reported to be present only in patients with surgical correction after age 4 years.[88] An age-related comparison of the ultrastructural appearance of crista supraventricularis muscle resected at operative repair demonstrates that severe interstitial fibrosis, myofibrillar lysis, and other intracellular degenerative changes are common in adults but are absent from sam-

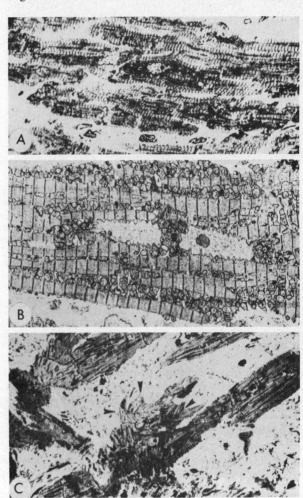

FIGURE 30–7 *A,* Light micrograph of crista supraventricularis muscle from a 2-year-old girl with tetralogy of Fallot. The cardiac muscle cells are mildly hypertrophied (up to 20 μ in diameter), cylindrical in shape, regular in orientation, and connected end-to-end. Cellular degeneration or interstitial fibrosis is not evident. Semithin (0.5 μ thick) section of Maraglas-embedded tissue stained with toluidine blue. ($\times$1,000, reduced by 18 per cent.) *B,* Electron micrograph of the same tissue. The cardiac muscle cell is binucleated and has a maximum diameter of 17 μ. Myofibrils and sarcomeres are intact, arranged in parallel, and separated by regularly arranged mitochondria. Occasional lipofuscin granules are present ($\times$4,450, reduced by 18 per cent). *C,* Light micrograph of area of marked interstitial fibrosis in crista supraventricularis from a 30-year-old woman with tetralogy of Fallot. The cardiac muscle cells are disorganized and show a loss of intercellular contacts. Myofibrils in the stellate-shaped cell (arrowheads) course irregularly at divergent angles. ($\times$ 400, reduced by 18 per cent.) (From Jones, M., and Ferrans, V. J.: Myocardial degeneration in congenital heart disease. Am. J. Cardiol. **39:**1051, 1977.)

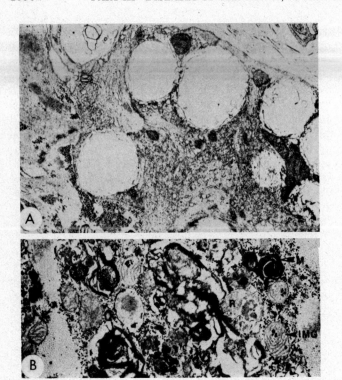

FIGURE 30–8 *A,* Electron micrograph of degenerated cardiac muscle cells from a 33-year-old man with tetralogy of Fallot. Normal myofibrillar structure has been completely lost, and the cells contain large lipid droplets, vesicles of sarcoplasmic reticulum, masses of Z-band material, glycogen particles, and actin filaments. Electron-dense lamellae are present at the periphery of the lipid droplets. (× 16,000, reduced by 18 per cent.) *B,* Portion of a muscle cell from a 36-year-old man with valvular and infundibular pulmonic stenosis and an atrial septal defect. The cell contains numerous myelin figures (M), residual bodies (R) of lysosomal origin, and deposits of intramitochondrial glycogen (IMG). Extramitochondrial glycogen and myofibrils are normal. (×27,000 reduced by 18 per cent.) (From Jones, M., and Ferrans, V. J.: Myocardial degeneration in congenital heart disease. Am. J. Cardiol. *39:*1051, 1977.)

ples obtained from children with tetralogy of Fallot (Figs. 30–7 and 30–8).[87] It is possible that such degenerative changes in the myocardium affect cardiac function adversely and are, in part, the cause of heart failure and arrhythmias in older patients with tetralogy of Fallot.

Adults with tetralogy complain frequently of severe headaches, dizziness, and episodes of exertional chest pain that resemble angina pectoris in character.[86] Their chronic hypoxemia stimulates release of increased amounts of erythropoietin, resulting in polycythemia. A hematocrit exceeding 65 per cent is associated with marked increases in blood viscosity and resistance to blood flow and substantially increases the possibility of intravascular thrombosis, thrombotic strokes, and paradoxical emboli. These patients are also at risk for brain abscesses and attacks of acute gouty arthritis, the latter resulting from a high turnover of erythrocyte nucleic acid and subsequent hyperuricemia. Women with unrepaired tetralogy of Fallot tolerate pregnancy poorly, and there is an increased incidence of fetal demise as well as of small-for-gestational-age babies.[89]

Laboratory Findings. The *electrocardiogram* is characterized by right-axis deviation, right ventricular hypertrophy, and, in older patients, a right ventricular conduction abnormality. By middle age, the patient with uncorrected tetralogy may develop atrial fibrillation or flutter.

The *roentgenographic* appearance of tetralogy of Fallot (Fig. 29–43, p. 991), which is classic for infants and children (i.e., a small, boot-shaped heart and pulmonary hypovascularity), is less typical in adults, who often have less distinctive cardiac silhouettes and normal-sized hearts on the posteroanterior chest roentgenogram; right ventricular enlargement is frequently but not invariably noted on the lateral view. Pulmonary vascularity is normal or even increased in almost half the adult patients, particularly those who are acyanotic.[86] Adults with tetralogy of Fallot usually have well-developed systemic-to-pulmonary collateral vessels that can be visualized during angiography and that may account for the long survival of some adults who do not undergo palliative or corrective surgical procedures for this defect.[86,90]

M-mode echocardiography (Fig. 24–44, p. 991) can be used to document the abnormal relationship between the aortic annulus and the interventricular septum. The VSD can occasionally be visualized as dropout of septal echoes. A *two-dimensional echocardiographic* examination gives information regarding the presence and degree of aortic overriding, the extent and location of the infundibular obstruction, the size of the pulmonic valve and main pulmonary artery, and the degree of right ventricular hypertrophy.

The major information to be obtained at *cardiac catheterization and angiography* includes the size of the pulmonary annulus and pulmonary arteries and the severity of right ventricular outflow tract obstruction. In patients with prior surgical systemic–to–pulmonary artery shunts, kinking of the pulmonary artery may have occurred at the anastomotic site, resulting in peripheral pulmonic stenosis. Angiography is also useful in locating collateral vessels, defining the coronary artery anatomy, and determining the significance of associated or acquired anomalies.

Surgical Treatment. Potential risks of palliative shunts include continued right-to-left shunting at the ventricular level with paradoxical emboli, endocarditis, and the development of pulmonary vascular obstructive disease. As a general rule, the adult patient with tetralogy of Fallot and a palliative shunt should undergo total operative repair. Total repair of tetralogy of Fallot can be undertaken in adults with a mortality rate comparable to that reported for children.[91,92,92a] Surgery usually consists of right infundibulectomy, pulmonary valvulotomy, patch closure of the ventricular septal defect with direction of the left ventricular outflow tract into the aorta, and a right ventricular outflow tract patch. Postoperative bleeding from extensive collateral vessels and impaired postoperative cardiac function may pose special problems in adults. Residual obstruction to right ventricular outflow and/or pulmonary regurgitation as well as VSD are the most common anatomical problems after repair.[91–94] Electrophysiological abnormalities include right bundle branch block; left anterior hemiblock; prolonged intra-atrial, AV nodal, and His-Purkinje conduction times; and complete heart block.[95–97] Several studies have shown a correlation between resting or exercise-induced ventricular arrhythmias, abnormal hemodynamics, and sudden death.[95–98] Ventricular ectopic activity may be a late developing phenomenon and may increase in severity with longer postoperative intervals.[98] Postoperative patients with tetralogy of Fallot who have ventricular arrhythmias should be treated aggressively with antiarrhythmic drugs.[96,98,98a]

Pulmonic Stenosis (See also page 986)

Pulmonic stenosis is among the more common congenital cardiac malformations in adults.[99] Prior to the development of surgical treatment, survival to age 50 and beyond was uncommon. However, even some infants with severe pulmonic stenosis have been known to survive into adult life without surgical correction. This undoubtedly reflects the tendency for the stenotic pulmonic valve orifice to enlarge somewhat as body size increases. On the other hand, a congenitally deformed pulmonic valve may become more fibrotic, thickened, and calcified in later adult life, thus reducing valve mobility and effective valve area. Also, the development of subvalvular muscular hypertrophy (i.e., infundibular stenosis), may occur and contributes further to the obstruction to right ventricular outflow. This occurs most often in older children and adults with valvular stenosis and can pose major difficulties in the early postoperative period unless resection of the infundibulum is carried out along with pulmonic valvulotomy.

Clinical Findings. Most adult patients with mild (right ventricular systolic pressure less than 75 mm Hg) to moderate (pressure between 75 and 100 mm Hg) pulmonic stenosis are asymptomatic. In adults with severe stenosis, dyspnea and fatigue secondary to an inadequate response of cardiac output to exercise are the most common symptoms.[100,101] Orthopnea does not occur in these patients, since their pulmonary venous pressure is normal; a small right-to-left shunt through a patent foramen ovale is common. Eventually, patients with more severe grades of pulmonic stenosis develop tricuspid regurgitation and frank right ventricular failure, which may ultimately become intractable and lead to death. Exertional syncope or lightheadedness occasionally occurs in patients with severe pulmonic stenosis, but sudden death is extremely rare.[100]

Chest pain resembling angina pectoris occasionally develops in children but is observed most frequently in adults with severe pulmonic stenosis in whom right ventricular oxygen requirements are greatly increased.[100,101] Patchy fibrosis of the hypertrophied right ventricle is a common finding in such patients at postmortem examination.

The physical findings, electrocardiogram (Fig. 30–3C), echocardiogram, and roentgenogram in adults are similar to those in children (p. 987). Calcification of the pulmonic valve, when present on roentgenography, is a sign of long-standing obstruction and is therefore usually seen only in adults.[101] With valvular calcification, the pulmonic ejection sound—an important auscultatory feature of mild or moderate pulmonic stenosis—disappears. It has been suggested that lung size, airway dimensions and conductance, and pulmonary diffusing capacity are reduced in adults with severe pulmonic stenosis.[102]

Treatment. It is generally agreed that symptomatic adults with pulmonic stenosis should undergo pulmonic valvulotomy.[4] Moreover, there is a consensus that when right ventricular systolic pressure at rest is less than 75 mm Hg, pulmonic stenosis is well tolerated, and such asymptomatic patients rarely if ever require surgical treatment.[100] More controversial is the question of whether asymptomatic adults with moderate or severe pulmonic stenosis (i.e., right ventricular systolic pressures exceeding 77 mm Hg) should undergo pulmonic valvulotomy. Johnson et al. reported two patients with severe pulmonic stenosis who were in their fifties.[100] These authors advised that surgical therapy be reserved for adults with symptomatic pulmonic stenosis. In general, since operative treatment by a skilled surgical team entails little risk, patients with right ventricular systolic pressures exceeding 75 mm Hg in the basal state should probably undergo surgery, regardless of symptoms.[103] Exercise capacity generally improves in symptomatic patients after successful surgery. When valvulotomy is performed, postoperative pulmonic regurgitation is common. Older patients, who seldom tolerate moderate or severe pulmonic regurgitation, may require pulmonic valve replacement.

PULMONARY ARTERY STENOSIS (see also page 985). Stenosis of the pulmonary artery (the main vessel or a branch, single or multiple) is commonly associated with other congenital malformations, including ASD and VSD, supravalvular aortic stenosis, persistent ductus arteriosus, tetralogy of Fallot, and the congenital rubella syndrome. Occasionally, the malformation occurs in an isolated form. Since pulmonary arterial stenosis is usually not lethal, an increasing number of patients with peripheral pulmonary artery stenosis are being recognized in adult life. The principal complication is right ventricular pressure overload. Poststenotic dilatation of peripheral pulmonary arterial branches occasionally leads to the formation of thin-walled aneurysms that can rupture and produce significant hemoptysis.[104,105] If the pulmonic valve is normal in these patients, pulmonic ejection sounds are absent, and splitting of the second heart sound is usually normal. The systolic murmurs are typically crescendo-decrescendo and are widely distributed over the thorax. Occasionally, stenosis in a pulmonary arterial branch gives rise to a continuous murmur. This occurs most frequently when moderate to severe pulmonary artery hypertension is present proximal to the area of narrowing and reflects the existence of a pressure gradient across the stenotic site throughout the cardiac cycle.

If stenosis of the pulmonary arterial branch is sufficiently close to the main pulmonary artery, and if there are no further peripheral branch stenoses, a graft can be constructed to bypass the obstruction from the main pulmonary artery to the branch distal to the stenosis. Alternatively, patch grafts may be placed to enlarge the lumen at sites of obstruction. If the area of peripheral pulmonary artery stenosis extends into the lung parenchyma, effective surgical repair may not be possible.[106]

Idiopathic Dilatation of the Pulmonary Artery

This malformation is characterized by congenital dilatation of the main pulmonary artery and its branches in the absence of any apparent anatomical or physiological cause. It may be the result of a defect in the normal development of the pulmonary arterial elastic tissue. Patients with this disorder are asymptomatic. *Physical examination* may reveal a palpable pulmonary arterial impulse in the second left intercostal space, a pulmonic ejection sound, and a midsystolic murmur heard best in the second left intercostal space. The second heart sound splits normally, although, on occasion, wide splitting is heard that varies normally with respiration. The *electrocardiogram* is normal; *roentgenograms* of the chest reveal a dilated pulmonary artery without cardiac chamber enlargement. Idiopathic dilatation of the pulmonary artery has no clinical significance, but this lesion must be distinguished from ASD and pulmonic stenosis.

Persistent Ductus Arteriosus
(See also page 967)

Persistent ductus arteriosus occurs three times more commonly in females than in males. The incidence of this condition is six times higher in individuals born at higher elevations than in those born at sea level. As is the case with other communications between the two sides of the heart, patients with persistent ductus arteriosus who continue to reside at higher elevations are also at increased risk of developing pulmonary vascular disease and reversed shunting. Although prior to widespread surgical correction of this malformation some patients with persistent ductus arteriosus survived to late adult life, few patients over the age of 40 years were encountered.[107] These statistics are analogous to those for VSD. Although late spontaneous closure of a persistent ductus arteriosus has been documented in patients in middle age, the number of instances of closure after infancy is far less than is the case for VSD. Rarely, delayed spontaneous closure of the ductus accompanies healing from an episode of ductal endarteritis.[108]

Three major complications may occur in adults with persistent ductus arteriosus: (1) ventricular dysfunction, (2) infective endarteritis, and (3) obliterative pulmonary vascular disease. Patients with small left-to-right shunts from a persistent ductus arteriosus rarely if ever develop heart failure or pulmonary vascular disease. However, they are at risk of developing infective endarteritis, usually occurring on the "jet lesion" that appears in the intima of the pulmonary artery opposite the orifice of the persistent ductus arteriosus. On occasion, endarteritis develops within the ductus itself. Patients with large left-to-right shunts may develop left ventricular failure, particularly during infancy and again after the age of 20 years.[108] However, survival to old age has been reported in the presence of persistent ductus arteriosus with a large shunt.[107] Right ventricular failure often occurs in patients with pulmonary vascular disease and reversed shunting.[109]

As is the case for VSD, pulmonary vascular disease in patients with persistent ductus arteriosus is either present from birth (in individuals who retain the high pulmonary vascular resistance of fetal life) or it develops gradually with time (in adolescence or early adult life).[108] A large left-to-right shunt with left ventricular failure and elevation of pulmonary venous pressure may accelerate the development of obliterative pulmonary vascular disease. Exertional dyspnea and/or fatigue occur commonly in patients with pulmonary vascular disease and are unusual in patients with normal or near normal pulmonary vascular resistance. Dilatation of the main pulmonary artery in patients with severe pulmonary vascular obstruction may compress the recurrent laryngeal nerve and cause hoarseness. Since most of the desaturated blood is shunted to the descending aorta, cyanosis and clubbing may be overlooked if the patient's feet are not inspected carefully (differential cyanosis). The fact that most of the right-to-left shunt is directed to the legs is primarily responsible for the complaint by some patients of marked leg fatigue in the absence of dyspnea. The continuous murmur of a persistent ductus disappears as pulmonary vascular resistance rises, often to be replaced by the early diastolic blowing murmur of pulmonic regurgitation (the Graham Steell murmur).

Paradoxical embolism occurs on occasion through a persistent ductus arteriosus with reversal of flow. Pulmonary hypertension secondary to pulmonary embolism may diminish or even reverse a previously present left-to-right shunt, thereby predisposing the patient to paradoxical embolism with the next embolic episode. Ductal aneurysms can occur in adults, and these may rupture or dissect with catastrophic outcome.[110]

Adults with normal pulmonary vascular resistance and moderate or large left-to-right shunts usually have electrocardiographic evidence of left ventricular hypertrophy, whereas those with pulmonary vascular disease exhibit right ventricular hypertrophy (Fig. 30–3*D*). Patients with large left-to-right shunts may develop atrial fibrillation. Calcification of the ductus arteriosus may occur in adults, and rarely calcification of the pulmonary arteries may develop when pulmonary hypertension has been present for many years. Pulsed Doppler echocardiography may be clinically useful in detecting pulmonary hypertension complicating persistent ductus arteriosus.[111]

Closure of a persistent ductus arteriosus in childhood is generally considered to be the simplest cardiothoracic surgical procedure currently performed.[4] In adult patients, ligation and/or division of a persistent ductus arteriosus may present a number of difficulties not present in children.[107] Since the ductus in older patients may be calcified and brittle as well as aneurysmally dilated, it can rupture during closure. The results of such a catastrophic event may be minimized by performing the procedure with cardiopulmonary bypass standby.

Porstmann and coworkers have developed a technique for closing a persistent ductus arteriosus using a femoral artery–to–femoral vein catheterization technique.[112] In this method, a small plug is guided into the ductus along a wire previously threaded from the aorta through the ductus into the right heart and down to the contralateral femoral vein. The technique has been employed successfully in over 200 patients in Germany and Japan, including patients at high risk because of pulmonary hypertension; it is particularly applicable to adults and older children.[112,113]

Coarctation of the Aorta
(See also pages 887 and 973)

Clinical Features. Coarctation of the aorta is one of the causes of surgically correctable hypertension. While it may cause left ventricular failure in infancy, adult patients with this anomaly are usually asymptomatic and are discovered during a search for the etiology of hypertension. Males with this malformation outnumber females by 2:1. Coarctation is particularly common in patients with Turner's syndrome (p. 973). It is commonly associated with other congenital malformations, including bicuspid aortic

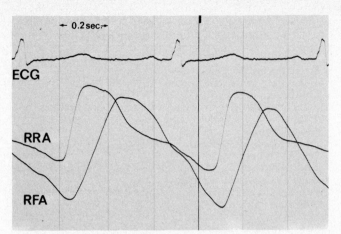

FIGURE 30-9 Simultaneously recorded right radial artery (RRA) and right femoral artery (RFA) pulses in a 20-year-old patient with coarctation of the aorta. The peak of the RFA is lower and occurred approximately 0.15 seconds after the peak of the RRA.

valve, persistent ductus arteriosus, ventricular septal defect, and mitral valve abnormalities.[114-116] Berry aneurysms of the circle of Willis, which are more common in patients with coarctation, are probably acquired rather than congenital abnormalities.[117]

These patients may complain of symptoms such as headache, intermittent claudication, and leg fatigue. They frequently seek medical attention because of symptoms associated with left ventricular failure, endarteritis, aortic rupture or dissection, or cerebral hemorrhage due to rupture of an aneurysm of the circle of Willis. Aortic rupture usually occurs in the ascending aorta or just distal to the coarctation in a poststenotic aortic aneurysm. Endocarditis occurs most commonly on an associated bicuspid valve; endarteritis of the coarctation is less common.[4,118] After the age of 40 years the incidence of congestive heart failure rises sharply.[117] In Campbell's review of 304 autopsied cases of unrepaired coarctation of the aorta, 25 per cent of the patients died before age 20 years, 50 per cent by age 32, 75 per cent by age 46, and 90 per cent by age 58. The mean age at death for patients with coarctation of the aorta was 34 years.[118]

The *diagnosis* of coarctation of the aorta in an adult patient can frequently be made on the basis of the physical examination.[62] There is hypertension, especially in the right arm, with systolic pressure rising more than diastolic. Lower extremity pulses are delayed or absent (Fig. 30-9). A systolic thrill in the suprasternal notch may be present.

Bounding carotid pulses reminiscent of aortic regurgitation often occur in individuals with isolated aortic coarctation, in part reflecting the patient's large pulse pressure proximal to the stenosis. In some cases, superficial collateral vessels, usually from the scapular arteries, may be palpated beneath the skin over the back. An apical fourth heart sound may be present. There is typically a grade II-III/VI systolic ejection murmur that is loudest over the left posterior thorax. The aortic component of the second heart sound is often increased in intensity due to the systolic hypertension. An ejection click best audible at the lower left sternal border is common and is associated with either a bicuspid aortic valve or dilatation of the ascending aorta.

Since it lies distal to the aortic coarctation, the renal vascular bed is perfused at a low pressure. This may explain the involvement of the renin-angiotensin system in the etiology of hypertension in patients with coarctation.[119] It is also of interest that patients with this anomaly have increased peripheral vascular resistance in the upper extremities but normal resistance in the lower extremities.[120-122] This difference continues to persist many years after corrective surgery has been performed,[121] and it may play a role in the etiology of hypertension in such patients.

Adults with coarctation of the aorta may demonstrate left ventricular hypertrophy or left bundle branch block on the *electrocardiogram*. Atrial fibrillation may be a late complication and is usually associated with congestive heart failure. On the chest roentgenogram, rib notching and left ventricular enlargement are almost universally present in adults with this malformation. *M-mode echocardiography* is useful in assessing associated lesions such as the presence of a bicuspid aortic valve. With two-dimensional echocardiography, using either a suprasternal or infraclavicular transducer position, the coarctation site can occasionally be visualized[123] (Fig. 30-10).

Treatment. In the adolescent or young adult patient with classic findings of coarctation of the aorta, the decision to perform surgery can be made without cardiac catheterization. In older patients and in patients with more complex problems, catheterization can define the severity of the coarctation, the anatomy of the arch vessels, the presence and extent of collateral vessels, and the significance of associated cardiac lesions.

Surgery for coarctation of the aorta in adults may not be curative in all cases.[123a] A paradoxical rise in blood pressure in the immediate postoperative period is common.[124,125] During the first 12 to 24 hours postoperatively, a rise in

FIGURE 30-10 *A*, Two-dimensional echocardiogram obtained using the infraclavicular transducer position. A discrete area of narrowing in the aorta can be seen just distal to the takeoff of the left subclavian artery (LSCA). *B*, Aortography confirmed a discrete coarctation of the aorta. Areas of pre- and poststenotic dilatation are present. Coarct = coarctation of the aorta; Ao arch = aortic arch; Desc Ao = descending aorta.

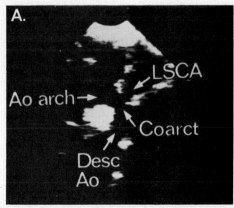

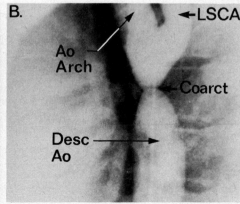

systolic pressure may occur, followed on the second or third day by a rise in diastolic pressure.[124] This hypertension that occurs within 24 hours of repair is associated with evidence of hyperactivity of the sympathetic nervous system, such as a decreased response to cold pressor stimuli[124] and markedly elevated plasma norepinephrine levels.[125] The paradoxical hypertension that occurs two to three days postoperatively is associated with a marked transient rise in plasma renin activity and is probably best treated with converting enzyme inhibitors or angiotensin II blocking agents.[124,126,127] Development of chronic persistent postoperative hypertension appears to be a function of age at the time of repair.

Optimal timing for surgery is one to five years of age. Even with early "correction," development of valvular stenosis or regurgitation secondary to a bicuspid aortic valve, residual stenosis at the coarctation site, or persistent hypertension at rest and particularly during exercise, despite apparently successful coarctectomy, may increase late mortality.[128]

OTHER FORMS OF CYANOTIC CONGENITAL HEART DISEASE

Cyanotic adults with congenital heart disease fall into two categories. The first includes patients with obligatory right-to-left shunts in whom cyanosis generally commences in infancy and often progresses (Table 30–3). Common examples are patients with tetralogy of Fallot or Ebstein's anomaly of the tricuspid valve. The number of patients with congenital tricuspid atresia (p. 994) who survive to adulthood is increasing due to successful palliative surgery

TABLE 30–3　CYANOTIC CONGENITAL HEART DISEASE IN ADULTS

I. Lesions Relatively Frequently Encountered
　A. Reduced pulmonary blood flow
　　1. Tetralogy of Fallot (pulmonic stenosis with ventricular septal defect)
　　2. Pulmonic atresia with ventricular septal defect
　　3. Pulmonic stenosis with atrial right-to-left shunt
　B. Increased pulmonary vascular resistance
　　1. Ventricular septal defect with Eisenmenger reaction
　　2. Patent ductus arteriosus with Eisenmenger reaction
　　3. Atrial septal defect with Eisenmenger reaction
II. Lesions Less Frequently Encountered
　A. Reduced pulmonary blood flow
　　1. Single ventricle with pulmonic stenosis or atresia
　　2. Tricuspid atresia with pulmonic stenosis or atresia or small ventricular septal defect
　　3. Transposition with pulmonic stenosis or atresia
　B. Increased pulmonary vascular resistance
　　1. Single ventricle with Eisenmenger reaction
　　2. Transposition with Eisenmenger reaction
　　3. Truncus arteriosus
　C. Ebstein's anomaly with atrial right-to-left shunt
III. Lesions Rarely Encountered
　A. Double-outlet right ventricle with or without pulmonic stenosis
　B. Congenital pulmonary arteriovenous fistula
　C. Congenital vena caval to left atrial communication
　D. Mitral atresia
　E. Double-outlet left ventricle
　F. Asplenia or polysplenia syndromes
　G. Total anomalous pulmonary venous return

From Graham, T. P., Jr., and Friesinger, G. C.: Complex cyanotic congenital heart disease in adults. *In* Roberts, W. C. (ed.): Congenital Heart Disease in Adults. Philadelphia, F. A. Davis Co., 1979, p. 383.

TABLE 30–4　CONGENITAL CARDIAC LESIONS THAT CAN BE COMPLICATED BY THE EISENMENGER REACTION

Aortic Shunts
　Patent ductus arteriosus
　Aorticopulmonary septal defect
　Truncus arteriosus
　Pulmonic atresia, ventricular septal defect, and large "bronchial" collateral vessels .
Ventricular Shunts
　Ventricular septal defect
　Single ventricle
　Transposition of the great arteries with ventricular septal defect
　Double-outlet right ventricle
　Tricuspid atresia and ventricular septal defect without pulmonic stenosis
　Mitral atresia and ventricular septal defect or single ventricle
　Atrioventricular canal
Atrial Shunts
　Atrial septal defect: secundum, primum, sinus venosus
　Common atrium
　Total anomalous pulmonary venous return
　Partial anomalous pulmonary venous return
　Transposition with atrial septal defect

From Graham, T. P., Jr.: The Eisenmenger reaction and its management. *In* Roberts, W. C. (ed.): Congenital Heart Disease in Adults. Philadelphia, F. A. Davis Co., 1979, p. 531.

during childhood and the development of a physiological repair using the Fontan procedure.[129–132] Rarely, patients with anomalies such as transposition of the great arteries, pulmonary atresia, truncus arteriosus, and single ventricle survive to adult life (Table 30–3).[133,134] In a few instances, surgical correction of these lesions during adult life has been successful.[135]

The second category includes patients in whom the right-to-left shunt occurs as a consequence of pulmonary vascular disease. While the term *Eisenmenger's complex* refers to VSD, pulmonary vascular disease, and right-to-left shunting of blood,[135,136] the term *Eisenmenger's syndrome* is used to describe any communication between the systemic and pulmonary circulation that produces pulmonary vascular disease of such severity that right-to-left shunting occurs (Table 30–4). Most of these patients become cyanotic in adolescence or early adult life; the cyanosis and disability are generally progressive. Significant clubbing and polycythemia are usually present in adults with Eisenmenger's syndrome.

Surgical intervention is generally contraindicated in patients with Eisenmenger's syndrome because elevated pulmonary vascular resistance persists or worsens after surgical closure of the defect[136,137]; frequently the result is severe right ventricular failure. Although the long-term outlook for patients with Eisenmenger's syndrome who are not operated upon is guarded because survival beyond the age of 50 years is unusual, it is often true that these patients may lead reasonably active and productive lives through early adulthood.

Death often occurs suddenly in these patients, although symptomatic arrhythmias do not usually pose a problem. Heart failure is a common complication of adults with Eisenmenger's syndrome, but it can usually be controlled by medical therapy and is not severely disabling. Although chest pain, syncopal attacks, and hemoptysis have been traditionally considered to be ominous prognostic signs, more recent studies have questioned this observation.

However, pregnancy is often life-threatening in patients with Eisenmenger's syndrome.[138]

EBSTEIN'S ANOMALY OF THE TRICUSPID VALVE
(See also page 996)

The principal abnormality of Ebstein's anomaly is downward displacement of a malformed tricuspid valve into an underdeveloped right ventricle with reduced pumping capacity.[139,140] The presence of a portion of the right ventricle between the atrioventricular groove and the downward displaced origin of the septal and posterior leaflets of the tricuspid valve results in a direct communication between the right atrium and the "atrialized" right ventricle. The degree of hemodynamic compromise to right ventricular function depends on the amount of right ventricular tissue above the tricuspid valve as well as the extent of adherence of the valve tissue to the right ventricular wall. The atrialized portion of the right ventricle is usually hypokinetic, contributing little to the ventricle's forward stroke volume. Tricuspid regurgitation, a problem frequently associated with Ebstein's anomaly, further compromises effective right ventricular output.[141] Many patients with Ebstein's anomaly have a concomitant interatrial communication (an atrial septal defect or patent foramen ovale) that allows right-to-left shunting of blood.

Cyanosis occurs in about three fourths of adult patients with this malformation and may appear or become worse with exercise, fatigue, or exposure to cold. In the other one fourth, right ventricular pumping capacity is almost normal. The severity of the anatomical abnormalities associated with Ebstein's anomaly is variable, with a considerable proportion of these patients surviving into adult life.[141,142] Patients with milder forms of Ebstein's anomaly may even have a normal life expectancy.[143]

Many patients remain asymptomatic until the third or fourth decade. Right ventricular failure, characterized by dyspnea, fatigue, weakness, and peripheral edema, usually marks the beginning of a downhill course for patients with Ebstein's anomaly; heart failure is the most common cause of death.[141,142] Syncope secondary to atrial and ventricular arrhythmias and precordial discomfort are also ominous signs. Palpitations are common, since patients with Ebstein's anomaly are prone to atrial and ventricular arrhythmias. Wolff-Parkinson-White syndrome (type B) occurs in 10 to 25 per cent of patients with this malformation.[141,144,145] Sudden death, presumably secondary to arrhythmias, occurs in as many as 20 per cent of adults with Ebstein's anomaly.[144] Paradoxical embolism and brain abscess are other common complications.

Two-dimensional echocardiography is useful in confirming the diagnosis of Ebstein's anomaly of the tricuspid valve as well as in assessing the significance of associated lesions (Fig. 30–11). Pulsed Doppler echocardiography is helpful in detecting tricuspid valvular regurgitation.[146]

Surgical treatment of Ebstein's anomaly has met with variable success. Operative approaches have included annuloplasty or replacement of the tricuspid valve, plication of the free wall of the atrialized portion of the right ventricle, right atrial reduction, and closure of the ASD.[147–150] If the right ventricle has sufficient capacity to accept the entire cardiac output, operative results may be salutary. If the right ventricle is diminutive and has a low compliance and pumping capacity, replacement of the tricuspid valve and closure of the interatrial communication result in severe, low-output right ventricular failure. Because of the rapid clinical deterioration that usually commences after the onset of right ventricular failure, surgical intervention should be considered for patients with this complication.

A.

B.

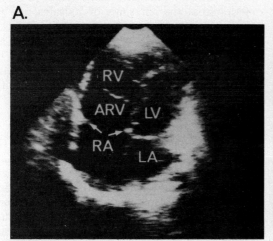
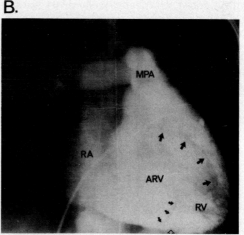

FIGURE 30–11 *A*, Systolic frame from a two-dimensional echocardiographic study obtained using the apical transducer position in a mildly cyanotic 25-year-old woman with a holosystolic murmur and multiple systolic clicks. Portions of the tricuspid valve are displaced downward into the right ventricle (RV). The arrows delineate the level of the atrioventricular (AV) groove. The portion of the RV between the AV groove and the downward displaced origin of the tricuspid valve leaflets is termed the "atrialized right ventricle" (ARV), an area that is hemodynamically right atrium (RA) but electrophysiologically RV. The true RA is enlarged. Both the left atrium (LA) and the left ventricle (LV) are decreased in size. Mitral valve prolapse is present. In other panels, right-to-left bowing of the interatrial septum was present, suggesting that the atrial septal defect was relatively small. Pulsed Doppler echocardiographic study confirmed the presence of tricuspid regurgitation. *B*, Right ventriculogram from the same patient demonstrating downward displacement of the large, sail-like anterior (straight solid arrows) and smaller posterior (curved solid arrows) leaflets of the tricuspid valve. A notch (open arrow) is apparent at the site of the anomalous insertion of the tricuspid valve. The RV is moderately hypoplastic. Pulmonic stenosis is not present. MPA = main pulmonary artery.

RIGHT VENTRICULAR DYSPLASIA

Right ventricular dysplasia is characterized by partial or total replacement of a portion of right ventricular musculature with fatty and fibrous tissue.[151-154] In its extreme, called *Uhl's anomaly*, there is apposition of endocardial and epicardial layers of the affected area.[155,156] Right ventricular dysplasia is more common in males and may be associated with mitral valve prolapse.[151] Adults with this lesion present frequently with palpitations or syncope. Ventricular tachycardia, usually with a left bundle branch block configuration, may be the predominant dysrhythmia. In a report of 24 patients with this condition, mean age at the time of hospitalization was 39 years.[151]

The cardiac examination in adults is often normal except for the right-sided fourth heart sound. Chest roentgenogram shows normal pulmonary blood flow with, at most, mild cardiomegaly. Two-dimensional echocardiography, which demonstrates right ventricular enlargement with normal left ventricular chamber size, can be helpful in distinguishing right ventricular dysplasia from other lesions such as Ebstein's anomaly of the tricuspid valve, atrial septal defect, anomalous pulmonary venous drainage, or congenital absence of the left pericardium.[151] At cardiac catheterization, angiography shows increased right ventricular size. In some cases, segmental motion abnormalities with systolic expansion of the infundibular area may be present.[151]

The pathogenesis and natural history of right ventricular dysplasia are unknown. Symptoms usually depend on the rate of the patient's tachyarrhythmia. Many patients with ventricular tachycardia respond to antiarrhythmic drug treatment; some require surgery, consisting of one or more ventricular incisions. The location of these incisions is based on the results of ventricular epicardial mapping performed during induced ventricular tachycardia as well as during either sinus or atrial paced rhythm.[151,152] Death resulting from ventricular fibrillation is infrequent.

CORONARY ARTERY ANOMALIES
AND CORONARY ARTERIOVENOUS FISTULA
(See also page 971)

Four anomalies involving the coronary circulation are of particular significance in adults: (1) origin of one coronary artery from the pulmonary artery; (2) origin of both coronary arteries from the right sinus of Valsalva; (3) origin of both coronary arteries from the left sinus of Valsalva; and (4) coronary arteriovenous fistula.

When *both coronary arteries originate from the pulmonary artery*, death usually occurs soon after birth.[157] Patients with origin of the right coronary artery from the pulmonary artery may be asymptomatic or minimally symptomatic as long as right ventricular oxygen demands remain normal. However, as might be anticipated, pulmonary hypertension of any etiology is tolerated poorly in such individuals. This anomaly has been noted as an incidental autopsy finding in patients dying of other causes.

Approximately 15 per cent of patients with anomalous origin of the left coronary artery from the pulmonary are able to reach adulthood largely because of effective intercoronary collaterals that reduce the hazards of myocardial ischemia.[157-161] These individuals may have a history of transient exertional chest pain and left ventricular failure. Other adults with this malformation complain of angina and left ventricular failure; they may present with mitral regurgitation or sudden death.[162,163] Adults may exhibit continuous or diastolic murmurs along either sternal border or at the base of the heart; these arise as a consequence of flow through the collaterals and through reversal of flow in the anomalous coronary artery. In addition, these patients frequently have murmurs of mitral regurgitation because of ischemic injury to papillary muscles. Surgical treatment consists of placement of a saphenous vein graft connecting the left coronary artery to the aorta and ligation of the pulmonary arterial ostium of the left coronary artery.[163-165] Alternatively, the anomalous left coronary artery may be reimplanted into the aorta[166] or the left subclavian artery may be anastomosed to the anomalous left coronary artery.[167]

Origin of both coronary arteries from the right or left sinus of Valsalva has been recognized with increasing frequency since the widespread employment of coronary arteriography.[168] This anomaly has been noted in a little over 1 per cent of a large number of patients who underwent coronary arteriography. Patients with origin of both coronary arteries from the right sinus of Valsalva are prone to sudden death.[169] Cheitlin et al. noted 9 unexplained sudden deaths among 33 patients (27 per cent) in whom both coronary arteries arose from the right sinus of Valsalva, and they suggested that the mechanism of death was acute myocardial ischemia.[169] The latter was considered to develop when increased cardiac output resulted in dilatation of the aorta and pulmonary artery, thereby stretching and narrowing the left coronary artery, the proximal portion of which was already narrowed because of the acute angle the vessel had to make in its leftward passage behind the pulmonary artery.

In patients with anomalous origin of both coronary arteries from the left sinus of Valsalva, the proximal right coronary artery may be compromised by a mechanism similar to that described for the left coronary artery when it arises from the right sinus of Valsalva. Chest pain, presumably angina pectoris, and one example of a subendocardial myocardial infarction have been noted in patients with this malformation.[169-172]

Congenital coronary arteriovenous fistulas occur between either the right or the left coronary artery and the right atrium, coronary sinus, or right ventricle. The right coronary artery is involved more frequently than the left, but both can be affected.[173] Hemodynamic disturbances consist of a left-to-right shunt of variable magnitude and myocardial ischemia. Most patients with this anomaly who are not operated upon survive to adulthood, although their life expectancy is usually reduced.[173] The majority of patients are asymptomatic until the fifth or sixth decade, when signs and symptoms of left ventricular failure occur secondary to the left-to-right shunt.[173,174] The development of heart failure is related to the magnitude and duration of the left-to-right shunt, which may increase as the fistula increases in size over a period of time. The continuous murmur characteristic of this anomaly may change to a systolic murmur in those adults who develop congestive heart failure with elevated right heart pressures. Adults with this malformation may demonstrate ischemic ST-segment changes in the precordial leads. Surgical closure of the fistula is indicated in patients with moderately large left-to-right shunts (pulmonary-to-systemic blood flow ratios exceeding 1.5:1.0); this procedure generally relieves manifestations of diminished cardiac reserve.[175]

CONGENITAL PULMONARY ARTERIOVENOUS FISTULAS
(See also page 985)

Pulmonary arteriovenous fistulas arise through abnormal development of pulmonary arteries and veins from a common vascular complex.[176] These fistulas usually involve the lower lobes or the right middle lobe; they can be solitary or multiple and of varying size.[177] The fistula replaces the normal capillary bed and usually consists of a tangle of tortuous vessels or several large and, on occasion, aneurysmal vascular trunks.[176] Pulmonary arteriovenous fistulas may coexist with systemic telangiectasias as part of the "Osler-Weber-Rendu" disease,[176] in which there are multiple small telangiectasias in the skin, oral and nasal mucosa, gastrointestinal tract, liver, central nervous system, and kidneys. The physiological consequences of pulmonary arteriovenous fistulas depend principally on the quantity of venous blood that is shunted into the systemic circulation; if this amount is sufficiently large, cyanosis can result. Usually only a modest increase in cardiac output occurs in contrast to the marked increase that may occur with a systemic arteriovenous fistula.[176,177]

Complications include rupture of the fistulous vessels, with resultant hemoptysis or hemothorax, paradoxical embolism, cerebral abscess, and infectious endarteritis.[176] Cardiac failure rarely if ever occurs in adults with this malformation. Pulmonary arteriovenous fistulas are usually discovered during routine chest roentgenography in asymptomatic individuals. A solitary fistula or multiple fistulas confined to one lobe can be treated by means of lobectomy; patients with fistulas in multiple lobes are usually not considered to be surgical candidates. Catheter embolization by mechanical occluding devices can also be employed in selected cases to obliterate a pulmonary arteriovenous fistula.[178]

Isolated varicose dilatation of one or more of the pulmonary veins without an arteriovenous communication is a rare malformation.[179] Hemoptysis is the principal complication.

CONGENITAL ANEURYSMS OF THE SINUS OF VALSALVA
(See also page 973)

Congenital absence of the media in the aortic wall behind a sinus of Valsalva may result in aneurysmal dilatation of the sinus,[180] which may enlarge over a period of years. Nonruptured aneurysms usually cause no cardiac dysfunction and are noted as incidental findings at autopsy,[181] but they may occasionally cause heart block as a result of compression of the atrioventricular conduction system. Rupture of an aneurysm of the sinus Valsalva occurs more commonly in males than in females.[182] This complication develops in adult life, generally between the ages of 18 and 30 years. When the fistula to a cardiac chamber produced by rupture of the aneurysm causes a large left-to-right shunt, patients often report the sudden onset of chest pain of epigastric discomfort and dyspnea. These symptoms may persist or may gradually resolve, even without specific therapy. A loud, continuous murmur accompanied by a thrill along the lower sternum is commonly found. The diagnosis is aided by both M-mode and two-dimensional echocardiography[183,184] and is established by aortography. Successful surgical obliteration of a ruptured aneurysm of the sinus of Valsalva results in dramatic relief of symptoms.[185]

CONGENITAL HEART BLOCK (See also page 1014)

Congenital heart block may be caused by a variety of lesions affecting the atrioventricular node or bundle of His.[186] Adults with congenital heart block without associated malformations may be asymptomatic for many years because of the presence of a stable accelerated junctional pacemaker under autonomic control, which allows for some increase in heart rate during exercise. This permits a reasonably normal hemodynamic response to exercise and other stresses.[187]

Hereditary congenital heart block, inherited as an autosomal dominant trait, has been noted in some families.[188] It is of considerable interest that mothers with systemic lupus erythematosus and other connective tissue diseases give birth to children with a surprisingly high incidence of congenital heart block. This observation suggests that environmental as well as genetic factors may be important in the etiology of this arrhythmia.[189,190] In general, patients with familial congenital heart block with wide QRS complexes and/or associated cardiac malformations have a poorer prognosis than do patients without these features. A number of serious complications have been noted in adults with congenital heart block, including malignant ventricular tachyarrhythmias (both with exercise testing and on Holter monitoring), Stokes-Adams attacks, and decreasing cardiac output.[17,191] Exercise stress testing and Holter monitoring should be carried out in these patients, since they may disclose an indication for antiarrhythmic therapy and/or permanent pacing, e.g., tachyarrhythmias, prolonged asystole, or marked ventricular slowing. Exercise intolerance secondary to bradycardia is also an indication for permanent pacing.

References

1. Nora, J. J., and Nora, A. H.: The evolution of specific genetic and environmental counseling in congenital heart disease. Circulation 57:205, 1978.
2. Smith, C.: Recurrence risks for multifactorial inheritance. Am. J. Hum. Genet. 23:578, 1971.
3. Czeizel, A., Pornoi, A., Peterffy, E., and Tarcal, E.: Study of children of parents operated on for congenital cardiovascular malformations. Br. Heart J. 47:290, 1982.
4. Whittemore, R., Hobbins, J. C., and Engle, M. A.: Pregnancy and its outcome in women with and without surgical treatment of congenital heart disease. Am. J. Cardiol. 50:641, 1982.
5. McNamara, D. G., and Latson, L. A.: Long-term followup of patients with malformations for which definitive surgical repair has been available for 25 years or more. Am. J. Cardiol. 50:560, 1982.
6. Graham, T. P.: Assessing the results of surgery for congenital heart disease — A continuing process. Circulation 65:1049, 1982.
7. Rashkind, W. J.: Historical aspects of surgery for congenital heart disease. J. Thorac. Cardiovasc. Surg. 84:619, 1982.
8. Graham, T. P.: Ventricular performance in adults after operation for congenital heart disease. Am. J. Cardiol. 50:612, 1982.
9. Manning, J. A.: Insurability and employability of young cardiac patients. In Engle, M. A.: Pediatric Cardiovascular Disease. Philadelphia, F. A. Davis, 1981, p. 117.
10. Taussig, H. B., Kallman, C. H., Nagel, D., Baumgardner, R., Momberger, N., and Kirk, H.: Long-time observations on the Blalock-Taussig operation. VIII. Twenty to 28-year followup on patients with a tetralogy of Fallot. Johns Hopkins Med. J. 137:13, 1975.
11. Johnson, D. H., Rosenthal, A., and Nadas, A. S.: A 40-year review of bacterial endocarditis in infancy and childhood. Circulation 41:581, 1975.
12. Johnson, C. M., and Rhodes, K. H.: Pediatric endocarditis. Mayo Clin. Proc. 57:86, 1982.

13. McGoon, D. C.: Long-term effects of prosthetic materials. Am. J. Cardiol. *50:* 621, 1982.

14. Deal, K., and Wooley, C. F.: Coarctation of the aorta and pregnancy. Ann. Intern. Med. *78:*706, 1973.

15. Blake, S., O'Neill, H., and MacDonald, D.: Haemodynamic effects of pregnancy in patients with heart failure. Br. Heart J. *47:*495, 1982.

16. Ralstin, J. H., and Dunn, M.: Pregnancies after surgical correction of tetralogy of Fallot. J.A.M.A. *235:*2627, 1976.

17. Reid, J. M., Coleman, E. N., and Doig, W.: Complete congenital heart block—Report of 35 cases. Br. Heart J. *48:*236, 1982.

18. Pirlo, A., and Herren, A. L.: Eisenmenger's syndrome and pregnancy. A case report and review of the literature. Anesth. Rev. *6:*9, 1979.

19. Midwall, J., Jaffin, H., Herman, M. V., and Kupersmith, J.: Shunt flow and pulmonary hemodynamics during labor and delivery in the Eisenmenger's syndrome. Am. J. Cardiol. *42:*299, 1978.

20. Roberts, W. C.: The congenitally bicuspid aortic valve. A study of 85 autopsy patients. Am. J. Cardiol. *26:*72, 1970.

21. Roberts, W. C.: The structure of the aortic valve in clinically isolated aortic stenosis—An autopsy study of 162 patients over 15 years of age. Circulation *42:*91, 1970.

22. Borow, K. M.: Congenital aortic stenosis in the adult. J. Cardiovasc. Med. (in press).

23. Fenoglio, J. J., McAllister, H. A., DeCastro, C. M., Davia, J. E., and Cheitlin, M. D.: Congenital bicuspid aortic valve after age 20. Am. J. Cardiol. *39:*164, 1977.

24. Wagner, S., and Selzer, A.: Patterns of progression of aortic stenosis—A longitudinal hemodynamic study. Circulation *65:*709, 1982.

25. Roberts, W. C., Morrow, A. G., McIntosh, C. L., Jones, M., and Epstein, S. E.: Congenitally bicuspid aortic valve causing severe, pure aortic regurgitation without superimposed infective endocarditis. Am. J. Cardiol. *47:*206, 1980.

26. Rappaport, E.: Natural history of aortic and mitral valve disease. Am. J. Cardiol. *35:*221, 1975.

27. Hossack, K. F., Heutze, J. M., Iowe, J. B., and Barratt-Boyes, B. G.: Congenital valvar aortic stenosis—Natural history and assessment of operation. Br. Heart J. *43:*561, 1980.

28. DeMaria, A. N., Bommer, W., Joye, J., Lee, G., Bouteller, J., and Mason, D. T.: Value and limitation of cross-sectional echocardiography of the aortic valve in the diagnosis and quantification of valvar aortic stenosis. Circulation *62:*304, 1980.

29. Young, J. B., Quinones, M. A., Waggoner, A. D., and Miller, R. R.: Diagnosis and quantification of aortic stenosis with pulsed Doppler echocardiography. Am. J. Cardiol. *45:*987, 1980.

30. Ciobanu, M., Abbasi, A. S., Allen, M., Herman, A., and Spellberg, R.: Pulsed Doppler echocardiography in the diagnosis and estimation of severity of aortic insufficiency. Am. J. Cardiol. *49:*339, 1982.

31. Friedman, W. F.: Indications for and results of surgery in congenital aortic stenosis. Adv. Cardiol. *17:*2, 1976.

31a. Stark, J., and deLeval, M. (eds.): Surgery for Congenital Heart Defects. New York, Grune and Stratton, Inc., 1983, p. 71–94.

32. Jones, M., Barnhart, G. R., and Morrow, A. G.: Late results after operation for left ventricular outflow tract obstruction. Am. J. Cardiol. *50:*569, 1982.

33. Prebiterc, P., Somerville, J., Revel-Chion, R., and Ross, D.: Open aortic valvotomy for congenital aortic stenosis—Late results. Br. Heart J. *47:*26, 1982.

34. Hamilton, W. T., Haffajee, C. I., Dalen, J. E., Dexter, L., and Nadas, A. S.: Atrial septal defect secundum: Clinical profile with physiologic correlates in children and adults. *In* Roberts, W. C. (ed.): Congenital Heart Disease in Adults. Philadelphia, F. A. Davis Co., 1979, p. 267.

34a. Konstam, M. A., Idoine, J., Wynne, J., Grossman, W., Cohn, L., Beck, J. R., Kozlowski, J., and Holman, B. L.: Right ventricular function in adults with pulmonary hypertension with and without atrial septal defect. Am. J. Cardiol. *51:*1144, 1983.

35. Breyer, R. H., Monson, D. O., Ruggie, N. T., Weinberg, M., and Najafi, H.: Atrial septal defect—Repair in patients over 35 years of age. J. Cardiovasc. Surg. *20:*583, 1979.

36. Dexter, L.: Atrial septal defect. Br. Heart J. *18:*209, 1956.

37. Popio, K. A., Gorlin, R., Teichholz, L. E., Cohn, P. F., Bechtel, D., and Herman, M. V.: Abnormalities of left ventricular function and geometry in adults with an atrial septal defect: Ventriculographic, hemodynamic and echocardiographic studies. Am. J. Cardiol. *36:*302, 1975.

38. Carabello, B. A., Gash, A., Mayers, D., and Spann, J. F.: Normal left ventricular systolic function in adults with atrial septal defect and left heart failure. Am. J. Cardiol. *49:*1868, 1982.

39. Liberthson, R. R., Boucher, C. A., Fallon, J. T., and Buckley, M. J.: Severe mitral regurgitation—A common occurrence in the aging patient with secundum atrial septal defect. Clin. Cardiol. *4:*229, 1981.

40. Bonow, R. O., Borer, J. S., Rosing, D. R., Bacharach, S. L., Green, M. V., and Kent, K. M.: Left ventricular functional reserve in adult patients with atrial septal defect: Pre- and postoperative studies. Circulation *63:*1315, 1981.

41. Hung, J., Uren, R. F., Richmond, D. R., and Kelly, D. T.: The mechanism of abnormal septal motion in atrial septal defect: Pre- and postoperative study of radionuclide ventriculography in adults. Circulation *63:*142, 1981.

42. Wanderman, K. L., Ovsyshcher, I., and Gueron, M.: Left ventricular performance in patients with atrial septal defect: Evaluation with noninvasive methods. Am. J. Cardiol. *41:*487, 1978.

43. Nasrallah, A. T., Hall, R. J., Garcia, E., Lechman, R. D., and Cooley, D. A.: Surgical repair of atrial septal defect in patients over 60 years of age: Long-term results. Circulation *53:*329, 1976.

44. St. John Sutton, M. G., Tajik, A. J., and McGoon, D. C.: Atrial septal defect in patients ages 60 years or older: Operative results and long-term postoperative followup. Circulation *64:*402, 1981.

45. Liberthson, R. R., Boucher, C. A., Strauss, H. W., Dinsmore, R. E., McKusick, K. A., and Pohost, G. M.: Right ventricular function in adult atrial septal defect—Preoperative and postoperative assessment and clinical implications. Am. J. Cardiol. *47:*56, 1981.

46. Moguilevsky, H. C., O'Reilly, M. V., Dizadji, H., and Shaffer, A. B.: Atrial septal defect associated with skeletal anomalies (Holt-Oram syndrome). Chest *57:*230, 1970.

46a. Fisher, J., Platia, E. V., Weiss, J. L., and Brinker, J. A.: Atrial septal defect in the adult: Clinical findings before and after surgery. Cardiovasc. Rev. Rep. *4:*396, 1983.

47. Pocock, W. A., and Barlow, J. B.: An association between the billowing posterior mitral leaflet syndrome and congenital heart disease, particularly atrial septal defect. Am. Heart J. *81:*720, 1971.

48. Nagata, S., Nimura, Y., Sakakibara, H., Beppu, S., Yung-Dae, P., Kawazoe, K., and Fujita, T.: Mitral valve lesion associated with secundum atrial septal defect—analysis by real time two dimensional echocardiography. Br. Heart J. *49:*51, 1983.

49. Schreiber, T. L., Feigenbaum, H., and Weyman, A. E.: Effect of atrial septal defect repair on left ventricular geometry and degree of mitral valve prolapse. Circulation *61:*888, 1980.

50. Kuzman, W. J., and Yuskis, A. S.: Atrial septal defects in the older patient simulating acquired valvular heart disease. Am. J. Cardiol. *15:*303, 1976.

51. Anderson, P. A. W., Rogers, M. C., Canent, R. V., Jr., and Spach, M. S.: Atrioventricular conduction in secundum atrial septal defects. Circulation *48:*27, 1973.

52. Ellison, R. C., and Sloss, L. J.: Electrocardiographic features of congenital heart disease in the adult. *In* Roberts, W. C. (ed.): Congenital Heart Disease in Adults. Philadelphia, F. A. Davis Co., 1979, p. 267.

53. Hynes, J. K., Tajik, A. J., Seward, J. B., Fuster, V., Ritter, D. G., Brandenburg, R. O., Puga, F. J., Danielson, G. K., and McGoon, D. C.: Partial atrioventricular canal defect in adults. Circulation *66:*284, 1982.

54. Weyman, A. E., Wann, S., Feigenbaum, H., and Dillon, J. C.: Mechanisms of abnormal septal motion in patients with right ventricular volume overload. Circulation *54:*179, 1976.

55. Nasser, F. N., Tajik, A. J., Seward, J. B., and Hagler, D. J.: Diagnosis of sinus venosus atrial septal defect by two-dimensional echocardiography. Mayo Clin. Proc. *56:*568, 1981.

56. Beppu, S., Nimura, Y., and Sakakibara, H.: Mitral cleft in ostium primum atrial septal defect assessed by cross-sectional echocardiography. Circulation *62:*1099, 1980.

57. Fraker, T. D., Harris, P. J., Behar, V. S., and Kisslo, J. A.: Detection and exclusion of interatrial shunts by two dimensional echocardiography and peripheral venous injection. Circulation *59:*379, 1979.

58. Bourdillon, P. D. V., Foale, R. A., and Rickards, A. F.: Identification of atrial septal defects by cross-sectional contrast echocardiography. Br. Heart J. *44:*401, 1980.

59. Gullace, G., Savoia, M. T., Ravizza, P., Knuppel, M., and Ranzi, C.: Detection of atrial septal defect with left-to-right shunt by inferior vena cava contrast echocardiography. Br. Heart J. *47:*445, 1982.

60. Valdes-Cruz, L. M., Pieroni, D. R., Jones, M., Roland, J. A., Shematek, J. P., Allen, H. D., Goldberg, S. J., and Sahn, D. J.: Residual shunting in the early postoperative period after closure of atrial septal defect. J. Thorac. Cardiovasc. Surg. *84:*73, 1982.

61. Botvinick, E. H., and Schiller, N.: The complementary role of M-mode echocardiography and scintigraphy in the evaluation of adults with suspected left-to-right shunts. Circulation *62:*1070, 1980.

62. Borow, K. M.: Under what circumstances can cardiac surgery be undertaken without catheterization? J. Cardiovasc. Med. *8:*84, 1983.

63. Anderson, M., Lyngborg, K., Moller I., and Wennwold, A.: The natural history of small atrial septal defects: Long-term followup with serial heart catheterizations. Am. Heart J. *92:*302, 1976.

63a. Steele, P. M., Fuster, V., Ritter, D. G., and McGoon, D. W.: Secundum atrial septal defect with pulmonary vascular obstructive disease: Long-term followup and prediction of outcome after surgical correction. J. Am. Coll. Cardiol. *1:*663, 1983.

64. Forfang, K., Simonsen S., Anderson, A., and Efskind, L.: Atrial septal defect of secundum type in the middle-aged. Am. Heart J. *94:*44, 1977.

65. Steinbrunn, W., Cohn, D. E., and Selzer, A.: Atrial septal defect associated with mitral stenosis: The Lutembacher syndrome revisited. Am. J. Med. *48:*295, 1970.

66. Meister, S. B., Grossman, W., Dexter, L., and Dalen, J. E.: Paradoxical embolism: Diagnosis during life. Am. J. Med. *53:*292, 1972.

67. Thompson, T., and Evans, W.: Paradoxical embolism. Quart. J. Med. *23:*135, 1930.

68. Alpert, J. S., Dexter, L., Vieweg, W. V. R., Haynes, F. W., and Dalen, J. E.: Anomalous pulmonary venous return with intact atrial septum: Diagnosis and pathophysiology. Circulation *56:*870, 1977.

69. Kalke, B. R., Carlson, R. G., Ferlic, R. M., Sellers, R. D., and Lillehei, C. W.: Partial anomalous pulmonary venous connection. Am. J. Cardiol. *20:*91, 1967.

70. Bauer, A., Korfer, R., and Bircks, W.: Left-to-right shunt of atrial level due to anomalous venous connection of the left lung. J. Thorac. Cardiovasc. Surg. *84:*626, 1982.

71. Weidman, W. H., DuShane, J. W., and Ellison, R. C.: Clinical course in adults with ventricular septal defect. Circulation 56:178, 1977.

72. Maron, B. J., Redwood, D. R., Hirshfeld, J. W., Jr., Goldstein, R. E., Morrow, A. G., and Epstein, S. E.: Postoperative assessment of patients with ventricular septal defect and pulmonary hypertension. Response to intense upright exercise. Circulation 48:864, 1973.

73. Lueker, R. D., Vogel, J. H. K., and Blount, S. G.: Cardiovascular abnormalities following surgery for left-to-right shunts. Circulation 40:785, 1969.

73a. Jablonsky, G., Hilton, J. D., Liu, P. P., March, J. E., Druck, M. N., Bar-Shlomo, B., and McLaughlin, P. R.: Rest and exercise ventricular function in adults with congenital ventricular septal defects. Am. J. Cardiol. 51:293, 1983.

74. Corone, P., Doyon, F., Gaudeau, S., Guerin, F., Vernant, P., Ducam, H., Rumeau-Rouquette, C., and Gaudeau, P.: Natural history of ventricular septal defect: A study involving 790 cases. Circulation 55:908, 1977.

75. Keane, J. F., Plauth, W. H., and Nadas, A. S.: Ventricular septal defect with aortic regurgitation. Circulation 56:172, 1977.

76. Friedman, W. F., and Heiferman, M. F.: Clinical problems of postoperative pulmonary vascular disease. Am. J. Cardiol. 50:631, 1982.

77. Rabinovitch, M., Castaneda, A. R., and Reid, L.: Lung biopsy with frozen section as a diagnostic and in patients with congenital heart defects. Am. J. Cardiol. 47:77, 1981.

78. Allan, H. D., Anderson, R. C., Noren, G. R., and Moller, J. H.: Postoperative followup of patients with ventricular septal defect. Circulation 50:465, 1974.

79. Sutherland, G. R., Godman, M. J., Smallhorn, J. F., Gutierras, P., Anderson, R. H., and Hunter, S.: Ventricular septal defects — Two-dimensional echocardiographic and morphological correlations. Br. Heart J. 47:316, 1982.

80. Stevenson, J. G., Kawabori, I., Dooley, T., and Guntheroth, W. G.: Diagnosis of ventricular septal defect by pulsed Doppler echocardiography. Circulation 58:322, 1978.

81. Blake, R. S., Chung, E. E., Wesley, H., and Hallidie-Smith, K. A.: Conduction defects, ventricular arrhythmias and late death after surgical closure of ventricular septal defect. Br. Heart J. 47:305, 1982.

82. Vetter, V. L., and Horowitz, L. N.: Electrophysiologic residua and sequelae of surgery for congenital heart defects. Am. J. Cardiol. 50:588, 1982.

83. Anderson, R. H., Allwork, S. P., Ho, S. Y., Lenox, C. C., and Zuberbuhler, J. R.: Surgical anatomy of tetralogy of Fallot. J. Thorac. Cardiovasc. Surg. 81:887, 1981.

84. Danilowicz, D., and Ishmael, R.: Anomalous right ventricular muscle bundle — Clinical pitfalls and extracardiac anomalies. Clin. Cardiol. 4:146, 1981.

84a. Matina, D., van Doesburg, N. H., Fouron, J., Guerin, R., and Davignon, A.: Subxiphoid two-dimensional echocardiographic diagnosis of double-chambered right ventricle. Circulation 67:885, 1983.

85. Goitein, K. J., Neches, W. H., Park, S. C., Mathews, R. A., Lenox, C. C., and Zuberbuhler, J. R.: Electrocardiogram in double chamber right ventricle. Am. J. Cardiol. 45:604, 1980.

86. Higgins, C. B., and Mulder, D. G.: Tetralogy of Fallot in the adult. Am. J. Med. 29:837, 1972.

87. Jones, M., and Ferrans, V. J.: Myocardial degeneration in congenital heart disease: Comparison of morphologic findings in young and old patients with congenital heart disease associated with muscular obstruction to right ventricular outflow. Am. J. Cardiol. 39:1051, 1977.

88. Borow, K. M., Green, L. H., Castaneda, A. R., and Keane, J. F.: Left ventricular function after repair of tetralogy of Fallot and its relationship to age at surgery. Circulation 61:1150, 1980.

89. Bertranou, E. G., Blackstone, E. H., Hazelrig, J. B., Turner, M. E., and Kirklin, J. W.: Life expectancy without surgery in tetralogy of Fallot. Am. J. Cardiol. 43:458, 1978.

90. Abraham, K. A., Cherian, G., Rao, V. D., Sukumar, I. P., Krishnaswami, S., and John, S.: Tetralogy of Fallot in adults: A report of 147 patients. Am. J. Med. 66:811, 1979.

91. Fuster, V., McGoon, D. C., Kennedy, M. A., Ritter, D. G., and Kirklin, J. W.: Long-term evaluation (12 to 22 years) of open heart surgery for tetralogy of Fallot. Am. J. Cardiol. 46:635, 1980.

92. Katz, N. M., Blackstone, E. H., Kirklin, J. W., Pacifico, A. D., and Bargeron, L. M.: Late survival and symptoms after repair of tetralogy of Fallot. Circulation 65:403, 1982.

92a. Hu, D. C., Seward, J. B., Puga, F. J., Fuster, V., and Tajik, A. J.: Total correction of tetralogy of Fallot at age 40 and older: Long-term followup. J. Am. Coll. Cardiol. 1:651, 1983.

93. Uretzky, G., Puga, F. J., Danielson, G. K., Hagler, D. J., and McGoon, D. C.: Reoperation after correction of tetralogy of Fallot. Circulation 66:I-202, 1982.

94. Ebert, P. A.: Second operation for pulmonary stenosis or insufficiency after repair of tetralogy of Fallot. Am. J. Cardiol. 50:637, 1982.

95. Deanfield, J. E., McKenna, W. J., Hallidie-Smith, K. A.: Detection of late arrhythmia and conduction disturbance after correction of tetralogy of Fallot. Br. Heart J. 44:248, 1980.

95a. Tamer, D., Wolff, G. S., Ferrer, P., Pickoff, A. S., Casta, A., Mehta, A. V., Garcia, O., and Gelband, H.: Hemodynamics and intracardiac conduction after operative repair of tetralogy of Fallot, Am. J. Cardiol. 51:552, 1983.

96. Gillette, P. C., Yeoman, M. A., Mullins, C. E., and McNamara, D. G.: Sudden death after repair of tetralogy of Fallot. Circulation 56:566, 1977.

97. Wessel, H. U., Bostanier, C. K., Paul, M. H., Berry, T. E., Cole, R. B., and Muster, A. J.: Prognostic significance of arrhythmia in tetralogy of Fallot after intracardiac repair. Am. J. Cardiol. 46:843, 1980.

98. Garson, A., Gillette, P. C., Gutgesell, H. P., and McNamara, D. G.: Stress-induced ventricular arrhythmia after repair of tetralogy of Fallot. Am. J. Cardiol. 46:1006, 1980.

98a. Deanfield, J. E., Ho, S., Anderson, R. H., McKenna, W. J., Allwork, S. P., and Hallidie-Smith, K. A.: Late sudden death after repair of tetralogy of Fallot — a clinicopathologic study. Circulation 67:626, 1983.

99. Hoffman, J. E., and Christianson, R.: Congenital heart disease in a cohort of 19,502 births with long-term followup. Am. J. Cardiol. 42:641, 1978.

100. Johnson, L. W., Grossman, W., Dalen, J. E., and Dexter, L.: Pulmonic stenosis in the adult: Long-term followup results. N. Engl. J. Med. 287:1159, 1972.

101. Covarrubias, E. A., Sheikh, M. U., Isner, J. M., Gomes, M., Hufnagel, C. A., and Roberts, W. C.: Calcific pulmonic stenosis in adulthood. Chest 75:399, 1979.

102. DeTroyer, A., Yernault, J. C., and Englert, M.: Lung hypoplasia in congenital pulmonary valve stenosis. Circulation 56:647, 1977.

103. Møller, I., Wennevold, A., and Lyngborg, K. E.: The natural history of pulmonary stenosis. Long-term followup with serial heart catheterizations. Cardiology 58:193, 1973.

104. Delaney, T. B., and Nadas, A. S.: Peripheral pulmonic stenosis. Am. J. Cardiol. 13:451, 1964.

105. Roberts, N., and Moes, C. A. F.: Supravalvular pulmonic stenosis. J. Pediart. 82:838, 1973.

106. Cohn, L. H., Sanders, J. H., Jr., and Collins, J. J., Jr.: Surgical treatment of congenital unilateral pulmonary arterial stenosis with contralateral pulmonary hypertension. Am. J. Cardiol. 38:257, 1976.

107. **John, S., Muralidharan, S., Mani, G. K., Krishnaswami, S., and Sukumar, I. P.: The adult ductus. J. Thorac. Cardiovasc. Surg. 82:314, 1981.**

108. Campbell, M.: Natural history of patent ductus arteriosus. Br. Heart J. 30:4, 1968.

109. Dexter, L.: Pulmonary vascular disease in acquired and congenital heart disease. Arch. Intern. Med. 139:922, 1979.

110. Borow, K. M., Hessel, S. J., and Sloss, L. J.: Fistulous aneurysm of ductus arteriosus. Br. Heart J. 45:467, 1981.

111. Stevenson, J. G., Kawabori, I., and Guntheroth, W. G.: Noninvasive detection of pulmonary hypertension in patent ductus arteriosus by pulsed Doppler echocardiography. Circulation 60:355, 1979.

112. Porstmann, W., Hieronymi, K., Wierny, L., and Warnke, H.: Nonsurgical closure of oversized patent ductus arteriosus with pulmonary hypertension: Report of a case. Circulation 50:376, 1974.

113. Sato, K., Fujino, M., Kozuka, T., Naito, Y., Kitamura, S., Nakano, S., Ohyama, C., and Kawashima, Y.: Transfemoral plug closure of patent ductus arteriosus. Experiences in 61 cases treated without thoracotomy. Circulation 51:337, 1975.

114. Serfas, D., and Borow, K. M.: Coarctation of the aorta. J. Cardiovasc. Med. (in press).

115. Rosenquist, G. C.: Congenital mitral valve disease associated with coarctation of the aorta. A spectrum that includes parachute deformity of the mitral valve. Circulation 49:985, 1974.

116. Rippe, J. M., Sloss, L. J., Angoff, G., and Alpert, J. S.: Mitral valve prolapse in adults with congenital heart disease. Am. Heart J. 97:561, 1979.

117. Liberthson, R. R., Pennington, D. G., Jacobs, M. L., and Dagget, W. M.: Coarctation of the aorta — Review of 234 patients and clarification of management problems. Am. J. Cardiol. 43:835, 1979.

118. Campbell, M.: Natural history of coarctation of the aorta. Circulation 41:1067, 1970.

119. Alpert, B. S., Bain, H. H., Balfe, J. W., Kidd, B. S. L., and Olley, P. M.: Role of the renin-angiotensin-aldosterone system in hypertensive children with coarctation of the aorta. Am. J. Cardiol. 43:828, 1979.

120. Samanek, M., Goetzova, J., Fiserova, J., and Skovranek, J.: Differences in muscle blood flow in upper and lower extremities of patients after correction of the aorta. Circulation 54:377, 1976.

121. Simon, A. B., and Zloto, A. E.: Coarctation of the aorta. Longitudinal assessment of operated patients. Circulation 50:456, 1974.

122. Shested, J., Baandrup, U., and Mikkelsen, E.: Different reactivity and structure of the prestenotic and poststenotic aorta in human coarctation — Implications for baroreceptor function. Circulation 65:1060, 1982.

123. Weyman, A. E., Caldwell, R. L., Hurwitz, R. A., Girod, D. A., Dillon, J. C., Feigenbaum, H., and Green, D.: Cross-sectional echocardiographic detection of aortic obstruction: Coarctation of the aorta. Circulation 57:498, 1978.

123a. Glancy, D. L., Morrow, A. G., Simon, A. L., and Roberts, W. C.: Juxtaductal aortic coarctation — analysis of 84 patients studied hemodynamically, angiographically, and morphologically after age 1 year. Am. J. Cardiol. 51:537, 1983.

124. Rocchini, A. P., Rosenthal, A., and Barger, C. A.: Pathogenesis of paradoxical hypertension after coarctation resection. Circulation 54:382, 1976.

125. Benedict, C. R., Grahame-Smith, D. G., and Fisher, A.: Changes in plasma catecholamine and dopamine beta-hydroxylase after corrective surgery for coarctation of the aorta. Circulation 57:598,1978.

126. Farrell, B. G., Parker, F. B., Poirier, R. A., Anderson, G., Streeter, D. H. P., and Blackman, M.: Angiotensin blockade in postoperative paradoxical hypertension of coarctation of the aorta. Surg. Forum 30:189, 1979.

127. Casta, A., Conti, V. R., Talabi, A., and Brouhard, B. H.: Effective use of captopril in postoperative paradoxical hypertension of coarctation of the aorta. Clin. Cardiol. 5:551, 1982.

128. Freed, M. D., Rocchini, A., and Rosenthal, A.: Exercise-induced hypertension after surgical repair of coarctation of the aorta. Am. J. Cardiol. 43:253, 1979.

129. Laks, H., Williams, H. G., Hellenbrand, W. E., Freedom, R. M., Talner, N. S., Rowe, R. D., and Trusler, G. A.: Results of right atrial to right ventricular

and right atrial to pulmonary artery conduits for complex congenital heart disease. Ann. Surg. *192*:382, 1980.

130. Patterson, W., Baxley, W. A., Karp, R. B., Soto, B., and Bargeron, L. L.: Tricuspid atresia in adults. Am. J. Cardiol. *49*:142, 1982.

131. Shackar, G. B., Fuhrnan, B. P., Wang, Y., Lucas, R. V., and Lock, J. E.: Rest and exercise hemodynamics after the Fontan procedure. Circulation *65*:1043, 1982.

132. Neveux, J. Y., Dreyfus, G., Leca, F., Marchand, M., and Bex, J. P.: Modified technique for correction of tricuspid atresia. J. Thorac. Cardiovasc. Surg. *82*:457, 1981.

133. Graham, T. P., Jr., and Friesinger, G. C.: Complex cyanotic congenital heart disease in adults. *In* Roberts, W. C. (ed.): Congenital Heart Disease in Adults. Philadelphia, F. A. Davis Co., 1979, p. 383.

134. Benson, L. N., Bonet, J., McLaughlin, P., Olley, P. M., Feiglin, D., Druck, M., Truoler, G., Rowe, R. D., and March, J.: Assessment of right ventricular function during supine bicycle exercise after Mustard's operation. Circulation *65*:1052, 1982.

135. Prusty, S., and Ross, D. N.: Adult cyanotic congenital heart disease. Thorax *30*:650, 1975.

136. Graham, T. P., Jr.: The Eisenmenger reaction and its management. *In* Roberts, W. C. (ed.): Congenital Heart Disease in Adults. Philadelphia, F. A. Davis Co., 1979, p. 531.

137. Brammell, H. L., Vogel, J. H. K., Pryor, R., and Blount, S. G., Jr.: The Eisenmenger syndrome: A clinical and physiologic reappraisal. Am. J. Cardiol. *28*:679, 1971.

138. Arias, F.: Maternal death in a patient with Eisenmenger's syndrome. Obstet. Gynecol. *50*:765, 1977.

139. Anderson, K. R., Zuberbuhler, J. R., Anderson, R. H., Becker, A. E., and Lie, J. T.: Morphologic spectrum of Ebstein's anomaly of the heart. Mayo Clin. Proc. *54*:174, 1979.

140. Anderson, K. R., and Lie, J. T.: Pathologic anatomy of Ebstein's anomaly of the heart revisited. Am. J. Cardiol. *41*:739, 1978.

141. Giuliani, E. R., Fuster, V., Brandenburg, R. O., and Mair, D. D.: Ebstein's anomaly: The clinical features and natural history of Ebstein's anomaly of the tricuspid valve. Mayo Clin. Proc. *54*:163, 1979.

142. Seward, J. B., Tajik, A. J., Feist, D. J., and Smith, H. C.: Ebstein's anomaly in an 85-year-old man. Mayo Clin. Proc. *54*:193, 1979.

143. Cabin, H. S., Wood, T. P., Smith, J. D., and Roberts, W. C.: Ebstein's anomaly in the elderly. Chest *80*:212, 1981.

144. Hansen, J. F., Leth, A., Dorph, S., and Wennevold, A.: The prognosis in Ebstein's disease of the heart—Long-term followup of 22 patients. Acta Med. Scand. *201*:331, 1977.

145. Watson, H.: Natural history of Ebstein's anomaly of tricuspid valve in childhood and adolescence. An international cooperative study of 505 cases. Br. Heart J. *36*:417, 1974.

146. Waggoner, A. D., Quinones, M. A., Young, J. B., Brandon, T. A., Shah, A. A., Verani, M. S., and Miller, R. R.: Pulsed Doppler echocardiographic detection of right-sided valve regurgitation. Am. J. Cardiol. *47*:279, 1981.

147. Bove, E. L., and Kirsh, M. M.: Valve replacement for Ebstein's anomaly of the tricuspid valve. J. Thorac. Cardiovasc. Surg. *78*:229, 1979.

148. Danielson, G. K., Maloney, J. D., and Devloo, R. A.: Surgical repair of Ebstein's anomaly. Mayo Clin. Proc. *54*:185, 1979.

149. Caralps, J. M., Aris, A., Bonnin, J. O., Solanes, H., and Torner, M.: Ebstein's anomaly: Surgical treatment with tricuspid valve replacement without right ventricular plication. Ann. Thorac. Surg. *31*:277, 1981.

150. Danielson, G. K., and Fuster, V.: Surgical repair of Ebstein's anomaly. Ann. Surg. *196*:499, 1982.

151. Marcus, F. I., Fontaine, G. H., Guiraudon, G., Frank, R., Laurenceau, J. L., Malergue, C., and Grosgogeat, Y.: Right ventricular dysplasia—A report of 24 adult cases. Circulation *65*:384, 1982.

152. Olsson, S. B., Edvardsson, N., Emanuelsson, H., and Enestrom, S.: A case of arrhythmogenic right ventricular dysplasia with ventricular fibrillation. Clin. Cardiol. *5*:591, 1982.

153. Frank, R., Fontaine, G., Vedel, J., Miolet, G., Sol, C., Guiraudon, G., Grosgogeat, Y. H.: Electrocardiologie de genetic case de dysplasie ventriculaire droite arythmogene. Arch. Mal Coeur *71*:963, 1978.

154. Vedel, J., Frank, R., Fontaine, G., Dobrinski, G., Guiraudon, G., Brocheriou C., and Grosgogeat, Y.: Tachycardies ventriculaires recidivantes et ventricule droit papyrace de l'adulte (à propos de deux observations anatomo-cliniques). Arch. Mal Coeur *71*:973, 1978.

155. Uhl, H. S.: A previously undescribed congenital malformation of the heart—Almost total absence of the myocardium of the right ventricle. Bull. Johns Hopkins Hosp. *91*:197, 1952.

156. Vecht, R. J., Carmichael, J. S., Gopal, R., and Phillip, G.: Uhl's anomaly. Br. Heart J. *41*:676, 1979.

157. Blake, H. A., Manion, W. C., Mattingly, T. W., and Baroldi, G.: Coronary artery anomalies. Circulation *30*:927, 1964.

158. Chaitman, B. R., Lesperance, J., Sahiel, J., and Bourassa, M. G.: Clinical, angiographic and hemodynamic findings in patients with anomalous origin of coronary arteries. Circulation *53*:122, 1976.

159. Wright, N. L., Baue, A. E., Baum, S., Blakemore, W. S., and Zinsser, H. F.: Coronary artery steal due to an anomalous left coronary artery origin from the pulmonary artery. J. Thorac. Cardiovasc. Surg. *54*:461, 1970.

160. Askenazi, J., and Nadas, A. S.: Anomalous left coronary artery originating from the pulmonary artery. Report on 15 cases. Circulation *51*:976, 1975.

161. Moodie, D. S., Cook, S. A., Gill, C. C., and Napoli, C. A.: Thallium-201 myocardial imaging in young adults with anomalous left coronary artery arising from the pulmonary artery. J. Nucl. Med. *21*:1076, 1980.

162. Harthorne, J. W., Scannell, J. A., and Dinsmore, R. E.: Anomalous origin of the left coronary artery: Remediable cause of sudden death in adults. N. Engl. J. Med. *275*:660, 1966.

163. Arciniegas, E., Farooki, Z. Q., Hakimi, M., and Green, E. W.: Management of anomalous left coronary artery from the pulmonary artery. Circulation *62* (Suppl.):I-180, 1980.

164. Stephenson, L. W., Edmunds, L. H., Freedman, S., Meyboom, E., Geurtz, M., and Weinberg, P.: Subclavian–left coronary artery anastomosis (Meyer operation) for anomalous origin of the left coronary artery from the pulmonary artery. Circulation *64*(Suppl.):II-130, 1981.

165. Wilson, C. L., Dlabal, P. W., and McGuire, S. A.: Surgical treatment of anomalous left coronary artery from pulmonary artery—Followup in teenagers and adults. Am. Heart J. *98*:440, 1979.

166. Grace, R. R., Angelini, P., and Cooley, D. A.: Aortic implantation of anomalous left coronary artery arising from pulmonary artery. Am. J. Cardiol. *39*:608, 1977.

167. Monro, J. L., Sharratt, G. P., and Conway, N.: Correction of anomalous origin of left coronary artery using left subclavian artery. Br. Heart J. *40*:79, 1978.

168. Kimbiris, D., Iskandrian, A. S., Segal, B. L., and Bemis, C. E.: Anomalous aortic origin of the coronary arteries. Circulation *58*:606, 1978.

169. Cheitlin, M. D., DeCastro, C. M., McAllister, H. A.: Sudden death as a complication of anomalous left coronary origin from the anterior sinus of Valsalva. A not-so-minor congenital anomaly. Circulation *50*:780, 1974.

170. Liberthson, R. R., Dinsmore, R. E., and Fallon, J. T.: Aberrant coronary artery origin from the aorta. Circulation *59*:748, 1979.

171. Liberthson, R. R., Zaman, L., Weyman, A., Kiger, R., Dinsmore, R. E., Leinbach, R. C., Strauss, H. W., and Buckley, M. J.: Aberrant origin of the left coronary artery from proximal right coronary artery. Diagnostic features and pre- and postoperative course. Clin. Cardiol. *5*:377, 1982.

172. Sharbaugh, A. H., and White, R. S.: Single coronary artery: Analysis of the anatomic variation, clinical importance and report of five cases. J.A.M.A. *230*:243, 1974.

173. Liberthson, R. R., Sagar, K., Berkoben, J. P., Weintraub, R. M., and Levine, F. H.: Congenital coronary arteriovenous fistula: Report of 13 patients, reviews of the literature and delineation of management. Circulation *59*:849, 1979.

174. Barnes, R. J., Cheung, A. C. S., and Wu, R. W. Y.: Coronary artery fistula. Br. Heart J. *31*:299, 1969.

175. Jaffe, R. B., Glancy, L., Epstein, S. E., Brown, B. G., and Morrow, A. G.: Coronary arterial–right heart fistulae: Long-term observations in seven patients. Circulation *47*:133, 1973.

176. Moyer, J. H., Glantz, G., and Brest, A. N.: Pulmonary arteriovenous fistulas. Am. J. Med. *32*:417, 1962.

177. Sahn, S. H., Bluth, I., and Schub, H.: Pulmonary arteriovenous fistula. Dis. Chest *44*:542, 1963.

178. Taylor, R. B., Cockerill, E. M., Manfredi, F., and Klatte, E. C.: Therapeutic embolization of the pulmonary artery in pulmonary arteriovenous fistula. Am. J. Med. *64*:360, 1978.

179. Nelson, W. P., Hall, R. J., and Garcia, E.: Varicosities of the pulmonary veins simulating arteriovenous fistulas. J.A.M.A. *195*:13, 1966.

180. Edwards, J. E., and Burchell, H. B.: Specimen exhibiting the essential lesion in aneurysm of the aortic sinus. Proc. Staff Meet. Mayo Clin. *31*:407, 1956.

181. Fishbein, M. C., Obma, R., and Roberts, W. C.: Unruptured sinus of Valsalva aneurysm. Am. J. Cardiol. *35*:918, 1975.

182. Kwittken, J., Christopoulos, P., Dua, N. K., and Bruno, M. S.: Congenital and acquired aortic sinus aneurysm. Arch. Intern. Med. *115*:684, 1965.

183. Matsumoto, M., Matsuo, H., Beppu, S., Yoshioka, Y., Kawashima, Y., Nimura, Y., and Abe, H.: Echocardiographic diagnosis of ruptured aneurysms of sinus of Valsalva: Report of two cases. Circulation *53*:382, 1976.

184. Engel, P. J., Held, J. S., Vander Bel Kahn, J., and Spitz, H.: Echocardiographic diagnosis of congenital sinus of Valsalva aneurysm with dissection of the interventricular septum. Circulation *63*:75, 1981.

185. Tanabe, T., Yokota, A., and Sugie, S.: Surgical treatment of aneurysms of the sinus of Valsalva. Ann. Thorac. Surg. *27*:133, 1979.

186. Ohkawa, S., Sugiura, M., Itoh, Y., Kitano, K., Hiraoka, K., Veda, K., and Murakami, M.: Electrophysiologic and histologic correlations in chronic complete atrioventricular block. Circulation *64*:215, 1981.

187. Corne, R. A., and Mathewson, F. A. L.: Congenital complete atrioventricular heart block: A 25-year followup study. Am. J. Cardiol. *29*:412, 1972.

188. Lynch, H. T., Mohiuddin, S., Moran, J., Kaplan, A., Sketch, M., Zencka, A., and Runco, V.: Hereditary progressive atrioventricular conduction defect. Am. J. Cardiol. *36*:297, 1975.

189. McCue, C. M., Mantakas, M. E., Tingelstad, J. B., and Ruddy, S.: Congenital heart block in newborns of mothers with connective tissue disease. Circulation *56*:82, 1977.

190. Chameides, L., Truex, R. C., Vetter, V., Rashkind, W. J., Galioto, F. M., Jr., and Noonan, J. A.: Association of maternal systemic lupus erythematosus with congenital complete heart block. N. Engl. J. Med. *297*:1204, 1977.

191. Winkler, R. B., Freed, M. D., and Nadas, A. S.: Exercise-induced ventricular ectopy in children and young adults with complete heart block. Am. Heart J. *99*:87, 1980.

31 ACQUIRED HEART DISEASE IN INFANCY AND CHILDHOOD

by William F. Friedman, M.D.

Since most of the topics discussed in this chapter are given more substantial coverage elsewhere in this text, the emphasis herein will be placed on features of acquired heart disease that are relatively unique to infancy and childhood, although the disease processes per se may not recognize age-related boundaries. Acute rheumatic fever and rheumatic heart disease have been excluded from this chapter, since these conditions are discussed extensively in Chapter 48. The hyperlipidemias are discussed in Chapters 35 and 47.

NONRHEUMATIC INFLAMMATORY DISEASE

Infective Myocarditis
(See also Chapter 41)

Infectious processes causing inflammatory disease of the heart may occur at any age, even during fetal life. Etiological agents include bacteria, viruses, fungi, protozoa, helminths, rickettsia, and spirochetes. As a general rule, very few of the generalized illnesses caused by these agents feature significant involvement of the heart. Myocardial involvement may be demonstrated histologically, but in most cases little or no expression of cardiac inflammation will be detected clinically. Important exceptions are infections due to certain viruses, diphtheria, and trypanosomes; these are discussed individually below.

Viral Myocarditis. Coxsackie B and rubella viruses are the most common causative agents in infective myocarditis of the newborn. The rubella embryopathy and its associated cardiovascular malformations are discussed on page 942. Active *rubella myocarditis* occurs in utero and may cause varying degrees of myocardial damage.[1] Invariably, however, other cardiovascular manifestations of the rubella syndrome dominate the clinical picture.

Coxsackie B typically causes outbreaks of epidemic myocarditis but may occur in the isolated infant in the newborn nursery, commonly with a fatal outcome.[2,3] The illness is of sudden onset and is characterized by fever, tachycardia, signs of systemic hypoperfusion, cyanosis, and occasionally cardiac failure. In some infants signs and symptoms of encephalomyelitis and hepatitis predominate. The diagnosis is suggested by electrocardiographic findings of atrial and/or ventricular arrhythmias, generalized ST-segment and T-wave changes, and low-voltage QRS complexes, accompanied by the appearance of marked generalized cardiomegaly and pulmonary vascular congestion on the chest roentgenogram. Echocardiography reveals dilatation of both ventricles and depressed indices of cardiac performance. Echocardiography is especially helpful in excluding congenital structural anomalies. The diagnosis is strongly suggested or confirmed when virus can be isolated from pericardial fluid, pharyngeal secretions, or feces, and elevations occur in type-specific–neutralizing, hemagglutination-inhibiting, or complement-fixing antibody.[4] Digitalis, diuretics, and general supportive measures are of limited benefit. Although increased sensitivity to the toxic effects of the glycosides is common, digitalis should be administered cautiously and continued until heart size is normal, since cardiac failure may recur when the drug is discontinued.

Numerous viral agents have been identified as a cause of myocarditis in childhood beyond infancy.[5–7] The most common are Coxsackie A and B (Fig. 31–1), influenza, adenovirus, and ECHO virus. Moreover, myocarditis, usually of mild degree, may be associated with the common viral infectious diseases of childhood, including mumps, measles, infectious mononucleosis, varicella, and variola. Although the diagnosis is generally one of exclusion, it may be

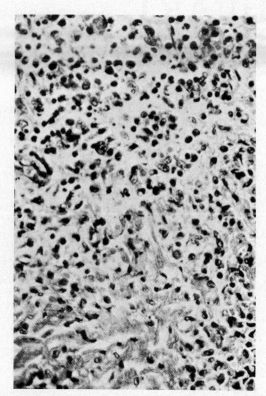

FIGURE 31–1   Photomicrograph of Coxsackie B₂ viral myocarditis. The major features are myocardial necrosis, edema, and heavy infiltrate of lymphocytes and large mononuclear cells. (× 400.) (From Gore, I., and Kline, I. K.: Pericarditis and myocarditis. *In* Gould, S. E. (ed.): Pathology of the Heart and Blood Vessels. 3rd ed. Springfield, Ill., Charles C Thomas, 1968, p. 740.)

suggested by the presence of cardiomegaly without significant murmurs, poor quality heart sounds, a gallop rhythm, an unexplained arrhythmia, and the electrocardiographic findings mentioned above. Important differential diagnostic possibilities include endocardial fibroelastosis, glycogen storage disease with cardiac involvement, anomalous pulmonary origin of a coronary artery, critical aortic stenosis in infancy, and coarctation of the aorta or hypoplastic left heart syndromes.

The vast majority of these children recover from the acute episode of myocarditis with little or no sequelae. On occasion patients may retain a permanent conduction defect or mild cardiac enlargement as a result of the acute illness. Rarely a child may progress from the acute episode to a chronic cardiomyopathy, characterized by signs of left ventricular dysfunction and mitral valve insufficiency. Unfortunately, there are no predictive criteria to identify the latter situation.[8]

Diphtheritic Myocarditis.   Diphtheria usually occurs in unimmunized children, especially in the western United States. Myocarditis results from the effect of the endotoxin on the heart rather than from cardiac invasion by the bacillus[9] (Fig. 31–2). Cardiac involvement occurs in approximately 10 per cent of affected patients and is the most common cause of death in this disease. Myocarditis is most reliably indicated by electrocardiographic changes, which range from ST-segment and T-wave changes to arrhythmias and conduction disturbances, including complete heart block.[10] Occasionally, the electrocardiographic

pattern of myocardial infarction may emerge. The electrocardiogram is a fair indicator of the extent of myocardial involvement and of prognosis. The latter is generally favorable if only ST-segment and T-wave changes are observed in the absence of conduction system disturbances. Right or left bundle branch block and complete atrioventricular block are associated with mortality rates of 50 to 80 per cent. The electrocardiographic findings may be accompanied by evidence of myocardial dysfunction and ventricular chamber dilatation on cardiac ultrasound.

Treatment for diphtheritic myocarditis is generally unsatisfactory. All patients should receive diphtheria antitoxin and intravenous penicillin after appropriate skin testing. Although corticosteroids have been used in the treatment of the myocardial problem, their value is debatable. Digitalis, diuretics, and antiarrhythmic medications are usually indicated. If the child recovers from the acute episode of diphtheritic myocarditis, the prognosis is quite good.

Myocarditis Due to Trypanosomal Infection.   Chagas' disease (p. 1438) is a chronic parasitosis caused by *Trypanosoma cruzi*, transmitted to humans by the bite of insects in the reduviid family. In the United States the disease is seen mostly in the southern states; endemic infection occurs in Latin America. Its most important clinical manifestation is a late-developing, chronic myocarditis and, much less frequently, an early acute myocarditis that is fatal in up to 10 per cent of cases.[11] In patients surviving the acute

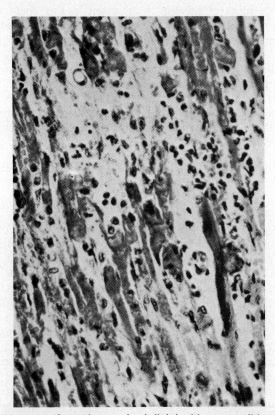

FIGURE 31–2   Photomicrograph of diphtheritic myocarditis. Prominent features are interstitial edema, hyaline degeneration of myocardial fibers, and cellular infiltrate consisting of lymphocytes, plasma cells, and histiocytes. (× 400.) (From Gore, I., and Kline, I. K.: Pericarditis and myocarditis. *In* Gould, S. E. (ed.): Pathology of the Heart and Blood Vessels. 3rd ed. Springfield, Ill., Charles C Thomas, 1968, p. 743.)

stage, cardiomyopathy may occur after an interval of 10 to 30 years.[12] Diagnosis of the acute illness is supported by findings of edema and adenitis in the region of the insect bite, associated with low-grade intermittent fever, sweating, muscular pain, and at times, diarrhea and vomiting; weeks or months later, cardiomegaly, gallop rhythm, and conduction disturbances may be noted. Xenodiagnosis (examination of the excreta of laboratory-bred insects fed on the patient) or complement-fixation tests provide confirmation.

Trypanosoma rhodesiense, which causes African sleeping sickness, may also produce myocardial hemorrhage, interstitial edema, mononuclear infiltration, and myocardial degeneration.[13] Cardiac involvement is usually relatively mild, and the clinical picture is dominated by evidence of encephalitis.

Infective Pericarditis

Numerous infectious agents may be responsible for infective pericarditis. Viral and tuberculous inflammatory pericardial disease is discussed in detail in Chapter 43. Of special concern in infancy and childhood is disease due to pyogenic bacteria.[14–16] Purulent pericarditis occurs most often in the first two decades of life and is especially common in children under 6 years of age. Acute bacterial pericarditis is usually fatal if misdiagnosed or improperly treated. The most common pathogens are *Staphylococcus aureus, Streptococcus pneumoniae, Hemophilus influenzae,* and *Neisseria meningitides.* Unusual organisms causing purulent pericarditis include *Escherichia coli, Pseudomonas, Salmonella, Klebsiella, Proteus,* and *Bacteroides. Hemophilus influenzae,* in particular, affects infants and young children, usually in association either with upper respiratory infection and croup or with lower respiratory pneumonia or bronchitis.

Presenting clinical signs and symptoms vary depending on the age of the patient, the responsible organism, and the site(s) of associated infection. The latter two require identification if therapy is to be effective. Fever, tachycardia, dyspnea, and chest pain are invariably present. Pericardial exudate resulting from the acute suppurative process commonly produces signs of life-threatening cardiac tamponade. Physical findings suggestive of purulent pericarditis include neck vein distention and hepatomegaly, pulsus paradoxicus, and/or systemic hypotension with a narrow pulse pressure, muffled and distant heart sounds, marked cardiomegaly, and a point of maximal cardiac impulse well within the area of percussed dullness. Although the presence of a pericardial friction rub points clearly to pericardial involvement, this sign occurs infrequently.

An enlarged, globular cardiac configuration on chest x-ray and electrocardiographic findings of diminished QRS amplitude and abnormalities of the ST segment (usually elevated) and T waves (often inverted) usually focus attention on the pericardium. Echocardiographic evaluation (p. 130) is superior to scintillation scanning in diagnostic reliability for establishing the diagnosis of pericardial effusion. Culture and examination of pericardial fluid obtained by pericardiocentesis are essential for diagnosis and treatment. Unless effective surgical drainage is combined with antibiotic treatment the mortality rate is high. Operation

should consist of creation of a subxiphoid pericardial window with placement of a drainage tube, or anterior pericardiectomy with tube drainage.[17] Early aggressive diagnosis and treatment reduce the risk of death substantially (10 to 20 per cent). Pericardial constriction is uncommon, but all patients should be followed carefully for this complication.

Postpericardiotomy Syndrome
(See also p. 1514)

In the first year after cardiac operation in which the pericardium is opened, and rarely in the second or third postoperative year, a febrile illness may occur, consisting of a pericardial and pleural inflammatory reaction with effusion and often with pulmonary parenchymal involvement. The illness occurs in approximately 25 per cent of children undergoing pericardiotomy and is usually self-limiting; infants undergoing open-heart surgery are affected rarely. It is characterized by fever; chest, neck, or shoulder pain that becomes worse with inspiration; anorexia; and laboratory findings of leukocytosis and an elevated erythrocyte sedimentation rate.[18] Recurrences are uncommon and usually mild. Physical, electrocardiographic, roentgenographic, and echocardiographic signs of pericardial involvement vary with the magnitude of the effusion. Cardiac tamponade, while not usual, occurs with sufficient frequency to warrant careful observation of the patient.

Viral infection and an autoimmume reaction have been implicated in the pathogenesis.[19] Serum antibodies and a rise in titer are found frequently against adenovirus, Coxsackie virus, and cytomegalovirus. Elevations in levels of heat-reactive antibody are common.

The syndrome must be distinguished from infective endocarditis and the postperfusion syndrome of atypical lymphocytosis and hepatomegaly, which occurs approximately 3 to 6 weeks after extracorporeal circulation and is caused by cytomegalovirus infection.[20]

Treatment of the postpericardiotomy syndrome depends upon the degree of patient discomfort and the magnitude of pericardial and/or pleural effusion. In some patients signs of cardiac tamponade will require pericardiocentesis.[21] Bed rest and salicylates or indomethacin lessen patient discomfort and diminish the production of pleural or pericardial fluid. Corticosteroids are indicated for severe illness and promptly relieve fever and symptoms. Antibiotics are not useful in treatment. Prolonged therapy is rarely necessary because of the self-limited nature of this postoperative complication.

PRIMARY CARDIOMYOPATHIES

Obstructive cardiomyopathies are discussed in Chapter 41. The important nonobstructive disorders in this category, of special concern in infants and children, are the familial and nonfamilial forms of endocardial fibroelastosis.[22–26]

ENDOCARDIAL FIBROELASTOSIS. Various designations have been applied to this condition, including endocardial sclerosis, fetal endocarditis, fetal endomyocardial fibrosis, and elastic tissue hyperplasia.[22] In recent years familial cases have been encountered more commonly than has the isolated form. The data provided by family studies fit neither an autosomal recessive nor a multifactorial mode of inheritance. Although the reasons are obscure, a marked reduction has been observed in the past decade of isolated, nonfamilial, endocardial fibroelastosis. No definite cause for this condition has been established, although a host of theories have been proposed; inadequate subendocardial blood flow and/or pre- or postnatal inflammation or infection are currently considered the most likely pathogenetic pathways.[8,24,25]

Pathologically, both primary and secondary forms of endocardial fibroelastosis (EFE) have been recognized.[26] In the *secondary* variety, focal areas of opaque fibroelastotic thickening of the mural endocardium or cardiac valves are observed in association with other types of cardiac malformations. Underlying cardiovascular anomalies are almost always obstructive lesions, particularly of the left side of the heart, and these create cardiac hypertrophy and an imbalance in the myocardial oxygen supply-demand relationship. Thus, secondary EFE occurs quite commonly in aortic stenosis, coarctation of the aorta, and hypoplastic left heart syndrome.

This discussion focuses on the *primary* form of EFE, which invariably involves the left ventricle and mitral and aortic valves without significant associated cardiac defects. Primary EFE commonly produces a marked dilatation of the left ventricle; rarely, a "contracted" type of primary EFE is observed, in which the left ventricle is relatively hypoplastic or normal in size. In the latter situation the right and left atrium and the right ventricle are markedly enlarged and hypertrophied, with minimal or no endocardial sclerosis. In the common, dilated type of primary EFE, microthrombi may be found adherent to the endocardium. The diffuse endocardial hyperplasia may be several millimeters thick (Fig. 31–3). The aortic and mitral valve leaflets are thickened and distorted; mitral regurgitation is especially common. The papillary muscles and chordae tendineae are involved in the fibroelastic process and are shortened and distorted.

Primary EFE is a disease of infancy; symptoms develop usually between 4 and 10 months of age, although rarely they may be present shortly after birth. Clinical features reflect left ventricular dysfunction and congestive heart failure.[27,28] Noted initially are fatigue and breathlessness during feeding, failure to thrive, irritability, pallor, increased sweating, peripheral cyanosis, cough, wheezing, or grunting. Symptoms are usually rapidly progressive. Examination of the infant reveals tachycardia, cardiomegaly, a gallop rhythm, and hepatosplenomegaly. Cardiac murmurs may be absent; approximately 40 per cent of infants have the characteristic apical systolic murmur of mitral regurgitation.

Chest roentgenography reveals marked, generalized cardiomegaly with normal or congested pulmonary vascular markings. A typical electrocardiographic finding is left ventricular hypertrophy with inverted T waves in the left precordial leads; less usual are tracings suggestive of myocardial infarction, varying degrees of atrioventricular block, or arrhythmias. Echocardiographic features include an increase in left atrial and left ventricular dimensions, reduced left ventricular septal and posterior wall motion, reduced ejection fraction, and abnormal mitral valve motion. The diagnosis of primary EFE is usually made easily by the characteristic clinical findings but is, nonetheless, one of exclusion. Differential diagnosis includes anomalous

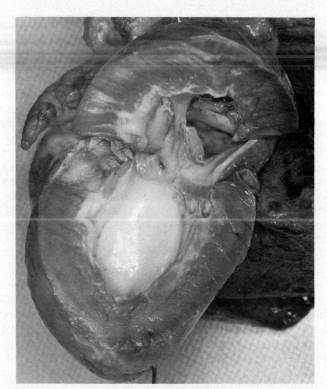

FIGURE 31–3 Diffuse left ventricular endocardial fibroelastosis. There is myocardial hypertrophy and obliteration of the papillary muscles as well as encroachment of the sclerotic subendocardial process onto the base of the aortic cusps. (From Tingelstaad, J. B., et al.: The electrocardiogram in the contracted type of primary endocardial fibroelastosis. Am. J. Cardiol. *27*:304, 1971.)

pulmonary origin of the left coronary artery, myocarditis, hypertrophic obstructive cardiomyopathy, anomalies causing left ventricular outflow tract obstruction, and glycogen storage disease of the heart. In general, the first four of these entities differ appreciably from fibroelastosis in their electrocardiographic or echocardiographic features; the skeletal muscle biopsy in glycogen storage disease is diagnostic.

Hemodynamic studies reveal evidence of left ventricular dysfunction.[29] This includes elevations in left ventricular end-diastolic and left atrial pressures, moderate pulmonary hypertension, widened arteriovenous oxygen differences, and reduced left ventricular stroke volume and cardiac output. Angiography usually demonstrates a markedly dilated left ventricle, a reduced ejection fraction, and varying degrees of mitral regurgitation. The configuration of the left ventricular chamber is usually globular or spherical; dyskinetic or akinetic patterns of contraction are uncommon. Endomyocardial catheter biopsy techniques (p. 297) are difficult to use in infants but, when employed, will show a diagnostic invasion of the endocardium and subendocardium by fibroelastic tissue.[30] The *contracted form* of primary EFE produces a clinical picture of left-sided obstructive disease, particularly if the mitral valve is small. Left atrial pressure is elevated, with pulmonary artery pressures at or near systemic arterial levels.

The optimal management of patients with primary EFE consists of early and prolonged treatment with digitalis. Glycoside therapy should be continued for many years after the disappearance of symptoms, since cessation of the drug may result in acute cardiac failure, even when the heart size has returned to normal. The results of pericardial poudrage and mitral valve replacement in seriously afflicted infants have been disappointing, and operative procedures are not recommended.

SECONDARY CARDIOMYOPATHIES

The designation "secondary" cardiomyopathy refers to intrinsic myocardial disease that is secondary to or associated with systemic disease or diseases of other organs or in other systems. Myocardial disease coexisting with collagen vascular disorders (Chap. 48), neuromuscular disorders (Chap. 50), neoplasms (Chap. 49), acute glomerulonephritis (Chap. 52), and thalassemia (Chap. 49) is discussed elsewhere in this text. Additional secondary cardiomyopathies of special interest to those caring for infants and children are those associated with glycogen storage disease, neonatal thyrotoxicosis, infantile beriberi, protein-calorie malnutrition, tropical endomyocardial fibrosis, and the mucocutaneous lymph node syndrome. Attention in this chapter will be directed to each of these latter disorders.

Glycogen Storage Disease and Infants of Diabetic Mothers

Glycogen storage disease is the result of a deficiency of one or more of the enzymes involved in the biosynthesis and degradation of glycogen.[31] The heart is involved in three of the eight types of glycogen storage disease—types II, III, and IV. Type III (Forbes' or Cori's disease) is a result of deficiency in the debranching enzyme amylo-1,6-glucosidase; type IV (Andersen's disease) is caused by a deficiency in the branching enzyme alpha-1,4 glucan-6 glucosyltransferase. Most cases of glycogen storage causing cardiomegaly occur in type II (Pompe's disease), which results from a deficiency of alpha-1,4-glucosidase (acid maltase), a lysosomal enzyme that hydrolyzes glycogen into glucose. This disease is a hereditary error of metabolism transmitted through a single recessive autosomal gene. Generalized glycogenosis takes place but occurs especially in heart, skeletal muscle, and liver. The glycogen within cardiac muscle cells is biochemically normal but is present in excessive amounts, both within lysosomes and free in the cytoplasm.[32] As a result, the heart enlarges, often to a marked degree, and congestive heart failure supervenes. Usually glycogen deposition within the myocardium is uniform, although occasionally the interventricular septum is especially involved, producing subpulmonic obstruction or a constellation of features indistinguishable from hypertrophic obstructive cardiomyopathy. Selective angiography has revealed a distinctive trabeculation of the left ventricle in some infants.[33]

Clinical signs of type II glycogen storage disease usually become prominent in the early neonatal period.[34] Characteristic symptoms include failure to thrive, progressive hypotonia, lethargy, and a weak cry. Prominent early features include nonspecific cardiac murmurs, cardiomegaly, signs of congestive heart failure, macroglossia, poor skeletal muscle tone, and weakness. The electrocardiogram shows extremely tall, broad QRS complexes with a short P-R interval (commonly less than 0.09 sec) (Fig. 31–4). The short P-R interval may be the result of facilitated atrioventricular conduction due to myocardial glycogen

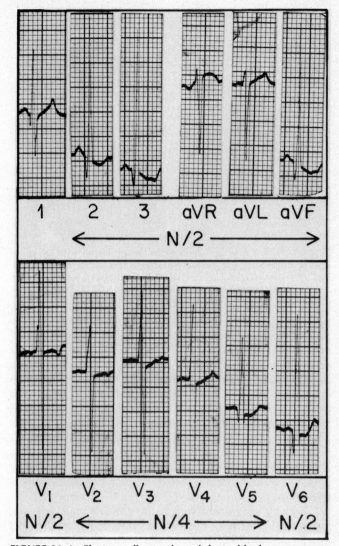

FIGURE 31–4 Electrocardiogram in an infant with glycogen storage disease showing a short PR interval and left ventricular hypertrophy.

deposition. Less often, deep Q waves are observed over the mid or left precordium as well as T-wave inversion and ST-segment elevation. Chest roentgenograms show an enlarged globular heart associated with pulmonary vascular congestion (Fig. 31–5). In rare patients with cardiac glycogenosis the cardiac murmur suggests left ventricular outflow tract obstruction and/or mitral regurgitation; the echocardiographic, hemodynamic, and angiographic features in this subgroup are indistinguishable from those in infants with hypertrophic obstructive cardiomyopathy. Diagnosis is confirmed by demonstrating the enzymatic deficiency in lymphocytes, skeletal muscle, or liver. Skeletal muscle biopsy reveals histological and histochemical evidence of glycogen deposition.

Cardiac glycogenosis may be confused with other entities that cause cardiac failure in the early months of life, including endocardial fibroelastosis, anomalous pulmonary origin of the left coronary artery, fixed and dynamic forms of left ventricular outflow tract obstruction, coarctation of the aorta, and myocarditis. The short P-R interval and the skeletal muscle hypotonia in glycogen storage disease help distinguish this disorder from *endocardial fibroelastosis.* Infants with an *aberrant left coronary artery* usually have a

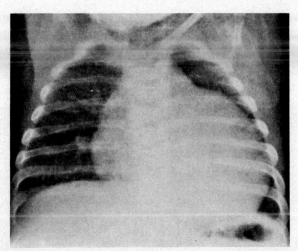

FIGURE 31–5 Chest roentgenogram of an infant with glycogen storage disease showing massive cardiomegaly and pulmonary edema. (From Taussig, H.: Congenital Malformations of the Heart. Vol. 2. 2nd ed. Commonwealth Fund, Harvard University, Boston, 1960, p. 901.)

distinctive electrocardiographic pattern of anterolateral myocardial infarction. In infants with *coarctation of the aorta* the pulse and blood pressure discrepancies between the upper and lower extremities point to the proper diagnosis (p. 975). *Myocarditis* is usually of abrupt onset in a previously healthy child and is not associated with marked hypotonia; the generally low-voltage electrocardiogram does not show the short P-R interval. Occasionally the skeletal muscle hypotonia and the macroglossia in infants with glycogen storage disease raise the possibilities of amyotonia congenita and cretinism or mongolism, respectively.

Cardiac glycogenosis leads to progressive impairment of myocardial function; Pompe's disease is uniformly fatal usually within the first year of life. Death is quite often the result of either cardiac failure or complications of respiratory management such as pneumonia or aspiration.

Infants born of diabetic mothers who are not afflicted with the enzyme disorder of glycogen storage disease occasionally display two basic forms of cardiomyopathy, both of which are usually transient.[34,35] It has been suggested that suboptimal metabolic control of maternal diabetes during pregnancy increases the incidence of these abnormalities.[36,37] In some of these infants, hypertrophy and hyperplasia of myocardial cells constitute a diffuse process, producing reversible signs and symptoms that resemble those of congestive cardiomyopathy. In other infants, the clinical findings are indistinguishable from hypertrophic obstructive cardiomyopathy. The natural history in this latter group has, in general, been one of gradual spontaneous regression of obstructive murmurs, cardiomegaly, and electrocardiographic and echocardiographic abnormalities typical of hypertrophic obstructive cardiomyopathy.

Neonatal Thyrotoxicosis

Long-acting thyroid-stimulating hormone, a 7S gamma$_2$ globulin, traverses the placental barrier and stimulates the fetal thyroid gland when maternal hyperthyroidism exists.[38] Infants are often born prematurely or are small for gestational age. Jitteriness and irritability are noted early. Cardiac findings include tachycardia, bounding pulses, systolic hypertension, and a precordial systolic murmur.[38–40] Frequently, congestive heart failure is present, and occasionally, the presenting finding is an episode of paroxysmal atrial tachycardia. A neonatal goiter may be observed, especially if the mother received iodine therapy during pregnancy.

Diagnosis should be anticipated whenever a history of hyperthyroidism exists in the mother. Neonatal thyrotoxicosis occurs in the offspring of about 1 to 2 per cent of these women. A maternal level of long-acting thyroid-stimulating hormone should be obtained before delivery in anticipation of the problem arising in the newborn infant, since high levels are often observed in both mother and offspring. A maternal level in excess of 300 per cent implies neonatal thyrotoxicosis, but a low value does not ensure that the newborn will not be affected. Thyroxine levels are increased in the newborn.

The infant who presents with heart failure may be treated with digitalis and propylthiouracil or carbamizole. However, the latter two drugs will not be completely effective for many weeks. Propranolol is usually the drug of choice. Supportive measures such as sedation and minimal manipulation may be helpful. Exchange transfusion or corticosteroid treatment is of no proven benefit.

Infants usually improve between the second and third months of life, although lack of attention to the problem or inadequate therapy may result in a fatal outcome.

Infantile Beriberi
(See also page 814)

Thiamine (vitamin B$_1$) deficiency occurs mainly in regions of southeast Asia, India, Brazil, and Africa, in which the dietary staple is polished rice or cassava. Thiamine functions as a coenzyme in decarboxylation of alpha-keto acids and in the utilization of pentose in the hexose monophosphate shunt. A reduction in myocardial energy production causes symptoms in the infant, usually between one and four months of age, who is breastfed by a thiamine-deficient mother.[41] Such infants are usually edematous, irritable, pale, and anorectic. Hoarseness or aphonia is common, owing to involvement of the recurrent laryngeal nerve; blepharoptosis occurs in one third of infants. Typically, cardiac involvement manifests as dilatation of the right ventricle and prominent signs of systemic venous congestion. Electrocardiographic findings are nonspecific, and radiological findings consist principally of right ventricular dilatation. Infantile beriberi may be rapidly fatal but responds quickly and well to administration of thiamine (25 to 50 mg intravenously initially, with reduction of the dose to 10 mg/day for several days, and then orally for several weeks). Dramatic amelioration occurs within a few days of the cardiac findings. Cure is complete with no known sequelae.

Protein-Calorie Malnutrition
(See also page 1742)

This is a major public health problem in underdeveloped areas of the tropics.[42,43] In infants, inadequate diet results in a state of emaciation termed "marasmus;" "kwashiorkor" is a designation applied to this syndrome in children beyond one year of age. The disease results from a deficiency of protein relative to calories, although the latter and other essential nutrients are often lacking as well. General muscle wasting, loss of subcutaneous fat, and atrophy of most organs, including the heart, are typical in marasmic infants. In both marasmus and kwashiorkor, thinning and atrophy of cardiac muscle fibers and interstitial edema or vacuolization of the myocardial fibers are noted.[44] As the condition progresses, listlessness becomes prominent. Cardiovascular collapse is precipitated easily in these infants by the stress of infection.

In both infancy and childhood the principal physical findings reflect systemic hypoperfusion and consist principally of hypothermia, hypotension, tachycardia, and low-amplitude peripheral pulsations. Peripheral edema is prominent, as are wasting of the skeletal musculature, exfoliative dermatitis, and gray or reddish discoloration of the hair. Changes seen on electrocardiogram and on radiographic examination are nonspecific.

Treatment should be directed at correcting fluid and electrolyte imbalance, eradication of infection, and management of such associated problems as anemia and parasitic infestation.[45] Care is required in the correction of dehydration or severe anemia, since volume overload of the heart is easily produced. Supplements of potassium and magnesium are often required, and because of deficiencies in these elements, digitalis should probably be avoided or used with extreme caution. If the infant or child survives the initial phase, a well-balanced diet will effect an impressive recovery over several months' duration.

Tropical Endomyocardial Fibrosis

Endomyocardial fibrosis is a rare, acquired, progressive disease, usually involving children and young adults from Africa, Southeast Asia, and South America. This cardiomyopathy of unknown etiology is characterized by focal, endocardial fibrosis of one or rarely both ventricles.[46] Conjecture exists as to whether or not tropical endomyocardial fibrosis, which is not associated with eosinophilia, and Löffler's endocarditis with eosinophilia (Chap. 41) are the same disorders described from tropical and temperate climates, respectively.[47] Endocardial fibrosis is located almost exclusively in the inflow tracts of the ventricles and commonly involves one or the other atrioventricular valve. Partial obliteration of either cardiac chamber results in reduced ventricular compliance with impairment of filling. The fibrotic process often involves the chordae tendineae, resulting in mitral and/or tricuspid regurgitation. Plaques of heaped-up fibrous tissue without elastic fibers are especially common within the left ventricle. Endocardial fibrosis involving the right ventricle may have to be differentiated from Ebstein's anomaly of the tricuspid valve (p. 996), and endomyocardial fibrosis involving the left ventricle may have to be differentiated from rheumatic mitral regurgitation.

When left ventricular disease predominates, the clinical findings often resemble those of mitral stenosis or regurgitation. When endocardial involvement of the right ventricle is more severe than that of the left ventricle, the patient usually presents with findings of markedly elevated systemic venous pressure and tricuspid regurgitation.

Treatment is supportive, and survival usually depends on the extent of endocardial and valvular involvement and is better when right ventricular disease predominates. Mean survival after the onset of symptoms is approximately 24 months. Specific treatment does not exist, and corticosteroid therapy has not proved efficacious. Surgical excision (decortication) of affected tissue, with prosthetic valve replacement has been associated with clinical improvement.[48,49] However, children most severely affected by this disease reside in regions of the tropics and subtropics where cardiac surgery is not readily available.

Mucocutaneous Lymph Node Syndrome

The mucocutaneous lymph node syndrome in infancy (Kawasaki's disease) has been accepted as a new syndrome by most Japanese pediatricians.[50] The clinical and pathological findings are strikingly similar to those of polyarteritis nodosa of infancy, and important questions and controversy exist about whether the two disorders are one and the same.[51,52] In excess of 18,000 cases have been reported and the disorder is being recognized with increasing frequency in North America and Europe.[53]

The syndrome is a febrile illness of children that occurs before the age of 10 and usually before the age of 2 years. Patients commonly present with fever and ocular and oral manifestations followed in 5 days by a rash and indurative edema of the hands and feet, with palmar and plantar erythema. Finally, after about 2 weeks, cutaneous desquamation occurs. Diagnostic criteria include (1) a fever lasting five days or more that is unresponsive to antibiotics; (2) bilateral congestion of the ocular conjunctiva; (3) peripheral limb changes that include an indurative peripheral edema and erythema of the palms and feet, followed later in the course of the illness by a membranous desquamation of the fingertips; (4) changes in the lips and mouth, including dry, erythematous, and fissured lips, injected oropharyngeal mucosa, and a strawberry tongue; and (5) a polymorphous exanthema of the trunk without crusts or vesicles. Diagnosis is accepted when the first criterion and at least three of the remainder are present.

In addition to the mucous membrane and cutaneous effects, multiple organ system involvement has been noted. Noncardiovascular complications of the illness include arthritis, cerebrospinal fluid pleocytosis, pulmonary infiltrates, and hydrops of the gallbladder. The illness is often accompanied by cervical adenopathy, diarrhea, leukocytosis with a predominance of neutrophils, thrombocytosis, sterile pyuria and proteinuria, elevated liver transaminases, an elevation in the erythrocyte sedimentation rate and alpha-2-globulin, and a positive C-reactive protein.

Based on pathologic data, progression of the disease may be divided into four stages.[54] In stage I, lasting 1 to 9 days, acute perivasculitis of the small arteries is evident and involves the vasa vasorum of the major coronary arteries. Pericarditis, interstitial myocarditis, and endocardial inflammation are also seen; these changes consist chiefly of neutrophilic, eosinophilic, and lymphocytic infiltrations. In stage II, of 12 to 25 days' duration, panvasculitis involves the major coronary arteries. It affects the intima, media, and adventitia and results in aneurysm and thrombus formation. In stage III, of 28 to 31 days' duration, granulating thrombi and marked intimal thickening cause partial

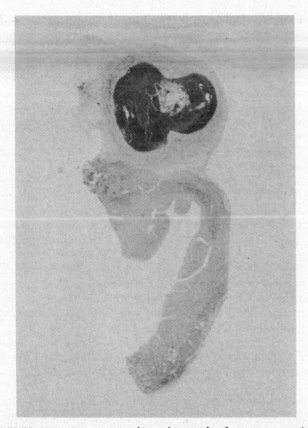

FIGURE 31-6 Low-power photomicrograph of a coronary artery aneurysm with recent occlusive thrombosis in a patient with mucocutaneous lymph node syndrome. (From Landing, B. H., and Larson, E. J.: Are infantile periarteritis nodosa with coronary artery involvement and fatal mucocutaneous lymph node syndrome the same? Comparison of 20 patients from North America with patients from Hawaii and Japan. Pediatrics *59*:651, 1977. Copyright American Academy of Pediatrics, 1977.)

or total occlusion of the major coronary arteries. Stage IV follows and may be of many years' duration, in which healing occurs, consisting of myocardial scarring, calcification, and recanalization of occluded arteries.

The syndrome has an associated mortality of 1 to 2 per cent, secondary to complications from coronary artery involvement, with a majority of deaths occurring in the third or fourth week of the illness.[55] Autopsy examination has almost uniformly demonstrated coronary arterial aneurysms, with occlusion due to thromboendarteritis (Fig. 31-6). Occasional findings include rupture of coronary arterial aneurysms, myocardial infarction, diffuse endocardial sclerosis, and aneurysms of peripheral arteries.

It appears that the disease has often been misdiagnosed in the United States as scarlet fever, Stevens-Johnson syndrome, Rocky Mountain spotted fever, rheumatoid arthritis, scleroderma, or lupus erythematosus.

Infants and children with this syndrome should be watched closely for signs of cardiac involvement. A significant number of patients show evidence of myocarditis or pericarditis, or both, in the early phases of the disease.[56,57] Electrocardiographic evidence of myocarditis with low voltage and nonspecific ST-T wave changes, are seen in 45 per cent of patients, echocardiographic evidence of poor left ventricular function in 25 per cent, pericardial effusion in 9 per cent, cardiomegaly on chest radiographs in 25 per cent, and a gallop rhythm in 12 percent. Aneurysms of the coronary arteries with narrowing, tortuosity, and obstruction are almost invariably present on aortography and coronary angiography[58,59] (Fig. 31-7). Excellent success has been achieved in visualizing these lesions with two-dimensional cross-sectional echocardiography (Fig. 31-8).[59,59a] Although the incidence of residual cardiac abnormalities following recovery from the acute illness phase is not known, estimates from 25 to 60 per cent have been

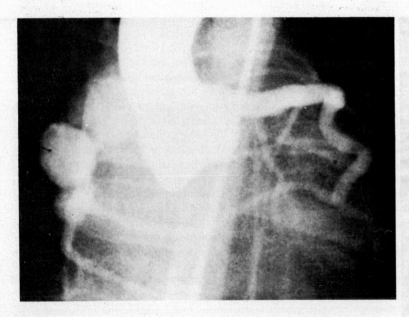

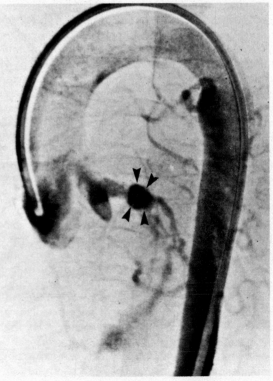

FIGURE 31-7 Aortic root cineangiograms from two patients with mucocutaneous lymph node syndrome. In the left panel, a dilated proximal left coronary artery is observed with collateral circulation and retrograde filling of the right coronary system, and three aneurysms of the right coronary artery. In the right panel, subtraction technique shows an aneurysm of the left coronary artery (arrowheads). (Courtesy of Dr. Thomas G. DiSessa.)

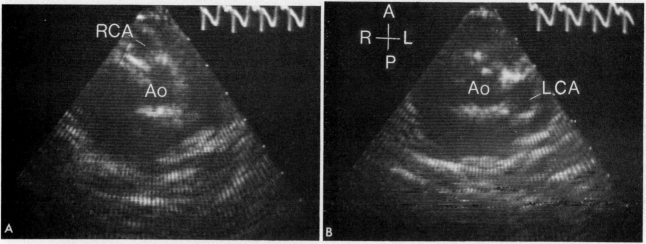

FIGURE 31-8 Short-axis cross-sectional echocardiographic views of aneurysms of the proximal right coronary artery (RCA) (*A*) and proximal left coronary artery (LCA) (*B*) in a 3-year-old boy with mucocutaneous lymph node syndrome. The right ventricular outflow tract is anterior (A) to the aorta (Ao) and the left atrium is posterior (P). R = right; L = left.

suggested.[60,61,61a] Associated findings may include compromise of left ventricular function secondary to the coronary arterial involvement and papillary muscle dysfunction with mital regurgitation. It has been suggested that corticosteroid therapy is detrimental during the acute illness. Salicylate treatment (30 mg/kg/day) is advisable for all patients in the acute phases of the illness. In patients who develop coronary arterial involvement, aspirin therapy is maintained indefinitely (5 to 10 mg/kg/day). In as many as 50 per cent of patients followed serially by means of coronary arteriography, it has been noted that the arterial aneurysms tend to regress.[61] Most children survive the acute phase of the illness, although the state of the coronary arteries in these survivors is usually not known. Two-dimensional echocardiography is indicated in all children with evidence of significant cardiac involvement; coronary angiography is suggested in those with proven coronary arterial aneurysm(s) or obstruction. The prognosis for these children should be guarded, and some may be candidates for coronary arterial bypass surgery.[61b,61c]

SYSTEMIC HYPERTENSION
(See also page 891)

Unfortunately, physicians usually consider hypertension a disease of adults and not of children. Thus, all too frequently, blood pressure is not recorded during the pediatric physical examination. It should be emphasized that elevations in systemic blood pressure may occur in as much as 2 per cent of the pediatric population, and that undetected or untreated hypertension may lead to unfortunate consequences.[62-64] Three points in particular require recognition:

1. Causes of hypertension in infants and children differ markedly from those in adults. Most children have secondary rather than essential forms of hypertension (Table 31-1), so that a premium should be placed on finding a remedial cause.

2. Offspring of hypertensive parents are known to have an increased susceptibility to blood pressure elevation (Chap. 47).

3. Children with elevated blood pressure require the same surveillance and treatment as do adults.

Accurate blood pressure measurements require cuffs of different sizes because of the variation in arm size from infancy through adolescence.[65] To measure blood pressure correctly, the inner rubber bag should be wide enough to cover two thirds of the length and three fourths of the circumference of the upper arm or thigh while leaving the antecubital or popliteal fossa free. A cuff that is too small is apt to produce spuriously high readings. In infants under age 2 years the flush technique may be used, although a Doppler instrument is preferred. Since disappearance of the Korotkoff sound may cause underestimation of the diastolic pressure, both muffling (the fourth Korotkoff sound) and the disappearance of the sound (the fifth Korotkoff sound) should be recorded. The fourth Korotkoff sound is the more accurate measure of diastolic pressure in most prepubertal children; beyond adolescence the fifth sound more closely reflects diastolic pressure.[67,68]

The normal ranges of blood pressure relative to age are illustrated in Figures 31-9 to 31-11 and serve as a guide in judging unsafe levels. Since considerable variation exists in most children's pressures, it should be recognized that a single blood pressure recording at, or higher than, the 90th percentile at a single point in time may not be an abnormal finding. In an apparently healthy child measurements should be repeated serially; further investigation is warranted if the blood pressure persists at or above the 95th percentile. In contrast, definite or severe hypertension, i.e., pressures well beyond the broad limits of normal, require prompt investigation and treatment.[69] Particularly urgent attention must be paid to those children whose systolic and diastolic pressures are remarkably high, i.e., equal to or greater than 180 and 110 mm Hg, respectively. Other findings identifying the patient at risk include localized neurological signs and/or local or generalized seizures; blurred vision or such eye ground changes as retinal hemorrhage, exudate, papilledema, or retinal arterial constriction; renal or abdominal pain; evidence of left ventricular hypertrophy or cardiac decompensation; renal dysfunction; palpation of an abdominal mass

TABLE 31–1   CONDITIONS ASSOCIATED WITH HYPERTENSION IN INFANTS AND CHILDREN

Congenital

Coarctation of the aorta
Gonadal dysgenesis (Turner's syndrome)
Rubella syndrome
Pseudoxanthoma elasticum (Ehlers-Danlos syndrome)
Ask-Upmark syndrome (segmental renal artery dysplasia)
Renal arterial abnormalities
Multiple systemic and pulmonary artery stenoses
Solitary renal cyst
Hydronephrosis

Genetic

Diabetes mellitus
Neurofibromatosis (von Recklinghausen's disease)
Adrenogenital syndrome
Pheochromocytoma
Polycystic kidney disease (infantile and adult forms)
Familial nephritis (Alport's syndrome)
Liddle's syndrome
Fabry's disease (angiokeratoma corporis diffusum)
Familial dysautonomia (Riley-Day syndrome)
Essential hypertension
Tuberous sclerosis with angiolipomas
Primary hyperparathyroidism
Porphyria

Pharmacological

Sympathomimetics: ephedrine, epinephrine, isoproterenol
Adrenal steroids
Heavy metals: mercury, lead
Licorice

Acquired, renal

Unilateral hydronephrosis
Unilateral pyelonephritis
Renal trauma
Renal tumors
Unilateral multicystic kidney
Unilateral ureteral occlusion
Renal artery stenosis
Renal arteritis
Fibromuscular dysplasia of the renal artery
Renal fistula
Renal artery aneurysm
Chronic pyelonephritis superimposed on abnormal kidneys
Nephritis: shunt nephritis, acute poststreptococcal disease, anaphylac-
    toid purpura, disseminated lupus erythematosus
Renal tuberculosis
Renal cortical necrosis: hemolytic uremic syndrome; sepsis
Renal vein thrombosis
Radiation nephritis
Postrenal transplantation

Acquired, other than renal

Hyperthyroidism
Retrosternal goiter
Guillain-Barré syndrome or poliomyelitis
Cerebral edema
Stevens-Johnson syndrome
Neuroblastoma
Hypercalcemia or hypernatremia
Adrenal adenoma or hyperplasia: primary aldosteronism or Cushing's
    syndrome
Hyperuricemic nephropathy
Burns

Modified from Lieberman, E.: Diagnostic evaluation of hypertensive children. Pediatr. Ann. *6*:390, 1977.

or enlargement of the kidneys; or auscultation of an abdominal bruit.

Evaluation of the asymptomatic child or adolescent with a blood pressure level above the 95th percentile on three or more occasions includes a careful history focusing on conditions or drugs known to be associated with or to predispose to high blood pressure. These include oral contraceptives (p. 873); use of corticosteroids; renal disease (p. 875); and symptoms suggesting aldosteronism (p. 883) i.e., spells, weakness, polyuria, muscle cramps or pheochromocytoma (p. 885); i.e., excessive sweating, palpitations. The

family history should be reviewed for eclampsia during the mother's pregnancy as well as any familial occurrence of hypertension, premature coronary artery disease, stroke, or renal failure.

Common *symptoms* in hypertensive children are headache, nausea and vomiting, loss of appetite, epistaxis, and palpitation. A dietary history should be obtained with an emphasis on sodium intake. The *physical examination* is directed at detecting conditions associated with secondary hypertension (Table 31–1) and finding evidence of target organ damage on funduscopic and cardiac examination. Typically, the physical findings in hypertensive disorders in children reflect the underlying cause of the elevated pressure; distinctive physical findings accompany many of the conditions listed in Table 31–1 (see also Chap. 26).

Laboratory studies are aimed primarily at identifying secondary causes of hypertension.[65] The minimal laboratory tests required are a urinalysis, complete blood count, blood urea nitrogen and/or creatinine, electrocardiogram, and chest roentgenogram. Since the most common cause of secondary hypertension in children is renal disease, evaluation often proceeds to include serum electrolytes, plasma renin activity with 24-hour urinary sodium excretion, rapid-sequence intravenous pyelogram, and isotopic or angiographic analysis of the kidneys and/or their blood supply. Fortunately, most identifiable causes of correctable hypertension in children and adolescents are associated with clinical findings that direct attention to a particular organ system (renal, endocrine, central nervous, and cardiovascular). Less often, hypertension may result from tumors (ganglioneuroma, pheochromocytoma, Wilms',[66] and neuroblastoma) or collagen vascular disease. Laboratory studies should be as specific as possible in order to avoid an unse-

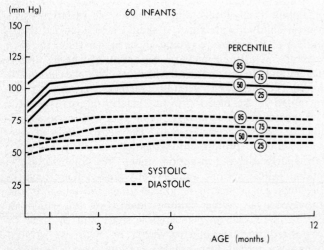

FIGURE 31–9   Percentile distributions of blood pressure in infancy. (From Levine, R. S., et al.: Tracking correlations of blood pressure levels in infancy. Pediatrics *61*:121, 1978. Copyright American Academy of Pediatrics, 1978.)

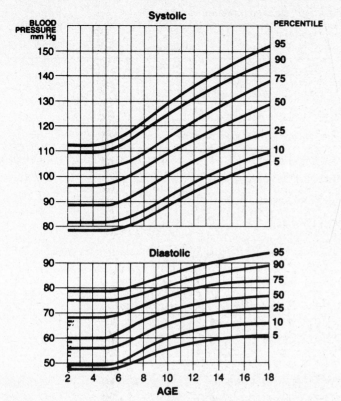

FIGURE 31–10 Percentile distribution of blood pressure in boys (right arm, seated). (From Blumenthal, S., et al.: Report of the task force on blood pressure control in children. Pediatrics *59* (Suppl.):797, 1977.)

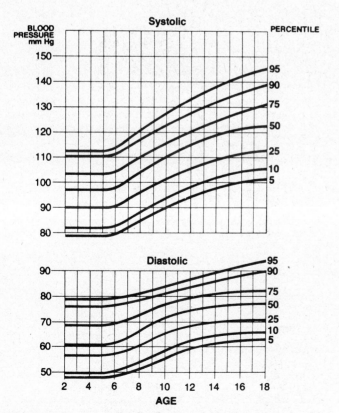

FIGURE 31–11 Percentile distribution of blood pressure in girls (right arm, seated). (From Blumenthal, S., et al.: Report of the task force on blood pressure control in children. Pediatrics *59* (Suppl.):797, 1977.)

lected analysis of every organ system theoretically associated with hypertension. In general, the younger the child and the higher the blood pressure elevation, the more vigorous the laboratory evaluation. It should be recognized that although essential hypertension is often a diagnosis by exclusion in prepubertal children, it is a viable diagnosis, particularly in adolescents.[69] In this author's opinion the need for extensive laboratory investigations has been overemphasized in children or adolescents with mild sustained elevations in blood pressure.

Asymptomatic children and adolescents with borderline or only mildly elevated blood pressure (<5 to 10 mm Hg beyond the 95th percentile values for age) may not require antihypertensive pharmacological agents but should receive counseling regarding weight control, salt abuse, and avoidance of agents with pressor effects (e.g., caffeine, some bronchoconstrictors, nicotine, etc.). These patients should be encouraged to be active physically, especially in exercises improving cardiovascular fitness. Isometric or static exercise, such as wrestling and weight lifting should be avoided, especially in children with evidence of left ventricular hypertrophy. If the latter exists or if these conservative measures do not result in normalization of blood pressure, treatment with antihypertensive drugs is indicated.

Drug therapy (Table 31–2) is aimed at prescribing the least complex regimen with the fewest side effects (see also Chap. 27). An oral thiazide diuretic is usually the initial drug of choice and may be combined with a potassium-sparing drug or with a dietary regimen that provides adequate potassium. If blood pressure control is not achieved, the beta-adrenergic blocking agent propranolol or methyldopa may be added to the regimen. Occasionally it is necessary to employ vasodilator agents such as hydralazine or minoxidil or the central sympathetic inhibitor clonidine in patient management.

Acute, life-threatening episodes of hypertension occur rarely and in a variety of clinical situations.[70] Encephalopathy is the most severe complication of an acute hypertensive crisis; its presence demands immediate lowering of the systemic arterial blood pressure. Diazoxide is the agent of choice as a first drug for the patient with encephalopathy. If diazoxide is ineffective, catecholamine-producing tumors must be suspected and consideration given to employing alpha-adrenergic blocking agents such as phentolamine or phenoxybenzamine. Sodium nitroprusside is generally considered the agent to be administered when all others have failed. If an etiology for sustained hypertension has been detected, medical and/or surgical treatment should be directed at the underlying disease process.

HYPERLIPIDEMIAS
(See also Chapters 35 and 47)

The importance of prevention of arteriosclerosis in childhood has only recently become generally accepted.[71,72] Hyperlipidemic children are likely to become hyperlipidemic adults and are therefore at greater risk of future atherosclerotic disease.[72,73] Although opinions vary about the feasibility of maintaining low serum lipid levels in normal children by dietary modification, a consensus exists that children whose serum cholesterol or triglyceride levels are beyond the 95th percentile for their age and sex should

TABLE 31-2   DRUGS COMMONLY USED IN PEDIATRIC CARDIOLOGY

DRUG	ROUTE OF ADMINISTRATION	DOSAGE
Acetaminophen (Tylenol)	PO or PR	<1 year 60 mg (q4h) 1 to 3 years 120 mg (q4h) >3 years 120 to 240 mg (q4h)
Acetylsalicylic acid (Aspirin)	PO or PR	30 to 100 mg/kg/day (q4h)
ε-Aminocaproic acid (Amicar)	IV	Total 100 mg/kg; ¼ total dose (q1h)
Aminophylline	PO, PR, or IV	12 mg/kg/day (q6h)
Ammonium chloride	PO	75 mg/kg/day (q6h)
Atropine	IV, SC, or PO	0.01 to 0.03 mg/kg (q4–6h)
Bicarbonate sodium	IV	1 to 2 mEq/kg/5 min
Bishydroxycoumarin (Dicumarol)	PO	Loading dose: 50 to 100 mg Maintenance dose: 10 to 50 mg/day (Regulate according to prothrombin times)
Bretylium	IV	5 mg/kg/dose over 10 minutes, then 50 to 100 μg/kg/min
Calcium chloride	IV	1 to 4 ml of 10% solution; for cardiac arrest, 10 mg/kg/dose
Calcium gluconate	IV PO	2 to 6 ml of 10% solution; for cardiac arrest, 10 mg/kg/dose 500 mg/kg/day (q6h)
Chlorothiazide (Diuril)	PO	20 to 40 mg/kg/day (q12h)
Chlorthalidone	PO	1 to 2 mg/kg/day (q12h)
Cholestyramine (Questran)	PO	250 to 1500 mg/kg/day (q6–12h)
Clofibrate (Atromid S)	PO	0.5 to 1.5 mg/day in divided doses
Clonidine (Catapres)	PO	0.002 to 0.008 mg/kg/day in divided doses
Codeine	PO	0.5 to 1.5 mg/kg/dose (q3h)
Dexamethasone (Decadron)	IV	0.2 to 0.4 mg/kg/dose (q6h) for cerebral edema
Diazoxide	IV	3 to 5 mg/kg/dose over 30 sec (q2–6h) (careful of severe hypotension)

Digitalis (Digoxin)		Loading dose:
		  Premature infants 0.030 mg/kg IV or IM
		  Term infants
		    Oral:
		      Up to 2 wk: 0.03 mg/kg
		      2 wk to 6 mo: 0.06 mg/kg
		      6 mo to 2 yr: 0.045 mg/kg
		      Beyond 2 yr: 0.03 mg/kg
		    Parenteral: 75% of oral dose
		Maintenance dose: ⅓ to ¼ of loading dose, given in two divided doses/24 hr

Dobutamine	IV	2 to 10 μg/kg/min
Dopamine	IV	1 gm in 250 ml D₅W; 2 to 20 μg/kg/min
Edrophonium chloride (Tensilon)	IV	0.05 to 0.2 mg/kg/dose
Ephedrine sulfate	IM or PO	0.8 to 1.6 mg/kg/day (q6h)
Epinephrine (Adrenalin)	IV	For cardiac arrest: single dose: 0.1 to 1.0 ml of 1:1000; 0.1 to 1.0 μg/min infusion
Ethacrynic acid (Edecrin)	IV	1.0 mg/kg/day
Ethylenediaminetetraacetic acid (EDTA) disodium salt	IV	20 mg/ml: 10 to 50 mg/kg (q12h)
Furosemide (Lasix)	IV or IM PO	1 to 2 mg/kg/dose 1 to 4 mg/kg/day

TABLE 31–2   DRUGS COMMONLY USED IN PEDIATRIC CARDIOLOGY (Continued)

DRUG	ROUTE OF ADMINISTRATION	DOSAGE
Glucagon	IV	0.05 to 0.10 mg/kg/hr
Glucose 50%	IV	1 mg/kg/dose
Glucose 50% + Insulin	IV	1 gm glucose/kg (50% solution) with insulin, 1 unit/3 gm glucose
Guanethidine sulfate (Ismelin)	PO	0.2 to 1.0 mg/kg/day (q6h)
Heparin	IV	100 units/kg (q4h)
Hydralazine hydrochloride (Apresoline)	IV PO	0.8 to 3.0 mg/kg/day (q4–6h) 0.75 to 7.5 mg/kg/day (q6–8h)
Hydrochlorothiazide	PO	1 to 3 mg/kg/day (q12h)
Hydrocortisone sodium succinate (Solu-Cortef)	IV	For shock: 50 to 75 mg/kg (q6h)
Indomethacin	IV	0.2 mg/kg/dose
Innovar (Fentanyl citrate & Droperidol)	IV	0.01 to 0.02 ml/kg
Isoproterenol hydrochloride (Isuprel hydrochloride)	IV	0.05 to 0.25 µg/kg/min
Lidocaine (Xylocaine hydrochloride)	IV	Single dose: 1 mg/kg; 20 to 50 µg/kg/min infusion
Magnesium sulfate, 3%	IV	For neonatal seizure: single dose: 2 to 6 ml
Mannitol	IV	For cerebral edema: 1 to 2 gm/kg Repeated doses: 250 mg/kg (q4h) For hemoglobinuria: single dose: 0.5 gm/kg; 5% solution infusion if necessary
Meperidine hydrochloride (Demerol)	IM or IV	1 mg/kg/dose (q3h)
Meralluride (Mercuhydrin)	IM	< 1 yr: single dose: 0.1 to 0.3 ml 1 to 5 yr: single dose: 0.3 to 0.7 ml > 5 yr: single dose: 1 ml
Mercaptomerin sodium (Thiomerin sodium)	IM	Same as Meralluride
Metaraminol (Aramine metaraminol bitartrate)	IV	Single dose: 0.1 mg/kg or 50 mg/500 ml; titrate to effect infusion
Methyldopa (Aldomet)	PO or IV	10 to 40 mg/kg/day (q6–8h)
Methylprednisolone (Solu-Medrol)	IV	For shock: 30 mg/kg/dose For cerebral edema: 4 to 5 mg/kg/dose
Minoxidil	PO	0.05 to 2.0 mg/kg/day
Morphine sulfate	SC	0.1 to 0.2 mg/kg/dose (q3h)
Naloxone hydrochloride (Narcan)	IM or IV	0.01 mg/kg/dose
Nitroprusside, sodium	IV	0.5 to 8.0 µg/kg/min initial rate; titrate to effect
Norepinephrine (Levophed bitartrate)	IV	0.1 to 1.0 µg/kg/min
Pentobarbital (Nembutal)	PO or IM	2 to 3 mg/kg/dose
Phenobarbital	PO or IM	3 to 5 mg/kg/day (q8h)
Phenoxybenzamine	IV	0.5 to 1.0 mg/kg
Phentolamine	IV	0.05 to 0.10 mg/kg

Table continues on following page

TABLE 31–2   DRUGS COMMONLY USED IN PEDIATRIC CARDIOLOGY (*Continued*)

DRUG	ROUTE OF ADMINISTRATION	DOSAGE
Phenylephrine (Neo-Synephrine hydrochloride)	IV	10 mg/100 ml D$_5$W; 1 to 10 μg/kg/min, titrate to effect
Phenytoin (Dilantin)	PO or IV	For seizures: 5 to 10 mg/kg/day (q8h) For arrhythmias: 1 to 5 mg/kg/5 min
Potassium chloride	PO IV	1 to 2 mEq/kg/day 0.5 mEq/kg/hr not to exceed 2 mEq/kg, as 40 to 80 mEq/l solution
Potassium gluconate (Kaon) and Potassium triplex	PO	1 to 2 mEq/kg/day
Procainamide hydrochloride (Pronestyl)	PO IM IV	40 to 60 mg/kg/day (q4–6h) 5 to 8 mg/kg (q6h) 1 mg/kg/dose over 5 min
Propranolol hydrochloride (Inderal)	PO IV IM	1.0 to 6.0 mg/kg/day (divide q6h) 0.01 to 0.15 mg/kg (q6–8h) 0.5 to 1.0 mg/kg (q4–6h)
Promethazine	PO	1 to 2 mg/kg/day (q6–8h)
Prostaglandin E$_1$	IV	0.1 μg/kg/min, reduce to 0.01 μg/kg/min to maintain effect
Protamine sulfate	IV	3 mg for every 200 units of heparin
Quinidine gluconate	PO IM or IV	10 to 30 mg/kg/day (q4–8h) 2 to 10 mg/kg/dose (q3–6h)
Quinidine sulfate	PO	3 to 12 mg/kg/dose (q3h)
Reserpine (Serpasil)	PO IM	0.01 to 0.02 mg/kg/day (q12h) 0.07 mg/kg (q12h)
Sodium polystyrene sulfonate (Kayexalate)	PR	1 gm/kg mixed with 70% sorbitol
Spironolactone	PO	1 to 3 mg/kg/day (q6–12h)
Succinylcholine chloride (Anectine chloride)	IM IV	2 mg/kg/dose 1 mg/kg/dose
Tolazoline (Prixoline)	IV	1 mg/kg/dose, then 1 to 3 mg/kg/hr
Triamterene	PO	2–4 mg/kg/day
Trimethaphan camsylate (Arfonad)	IV	50 mg in 100 ml D$_5$W, titrate to effect
Tris (Hydroxymethyl) aminomethane (THAM)	IV	(0.3M) weight (kg) × base deficit = dose in ml
Tubocurarine chloride (curare)	IM or IV	Initial dose: 0.3 to 0.5 mg/kg Subsequent dose: 0.1 mg/kg
Verapamil	IV	0.1 to 0.2 mg/kg/dose over 2 min
Vitamin K (Aquamephyton)	IM or IV	Single dose (neonate): 1 mg
Warfarin sodium crystalline (Coumadin)	PO or IM	Initial dose: 0.5 mg/kg Maintenance dose: 1 to 5 mg/day (Regulate according to prothrombin times)

TABLE 31–3 FASTING LIPID LEVELS IN SCHOOL CHILDREN

A. Cholesterol

		MALES					FEMALES		
Age	*5%*	*50%*	*95%*	*N*	*5%*	*50%*	*95%*	*N*
5	109	150	189	60	120	155	200	58
6	121	154	200	193	119	154	198	197
7	122	154	199	194	125	159	202	164
8	125	159	194	188	117	161	203	165
9	125	158	213	165	122	161	206	202
10	129	163	206	187	125	159	205	197
11	122	159	202	198	126	161	204	194
12	119	159	213	221	116	158	210	222
13	116	153	205	184	125	158	200	181
14	117	150	187	168	120	157	203	182
15	113	148	190	146	121	157	203	188
16	118	148	192	108	121	151	200	134
17	108	145	189	91	118	164	209	110

B. Triglyceride

		MALES					FEMALES		
Age	*5%*	*50%*	*95%*	*N*	*5%*	*50%*	*95%*	*N*
5	23	46	99	60	26	48	92	58
6	26	47	95	193	27	47	94	197
7	27	43	102	194	26	50	106	164
8	24	43	91	188	26	50	97	165
9	25	49	92	165	29	52	110	202
10	23	46	108	187	30	51	110	197
11	24	48	103	198	29	61	140	194
12	28	53	119	221	33	61	123	222
13	26	52	113	184	34	61	127	181
14	30	50	106	168	33	56	123	182
15	26	52	111	146	33	58	111	188
16	31	63	108	108	34	59	112	134
17	31	58	132	91	34	65	140	110

N = Number of children studied.

From Carter, G. A., et al.: Coronary heart disease risk factors: Identification and management. *In* Shen, J. T. (ed.): Clinical Practice of Adolescent Medicine. New York, Appleton-Century-Crofts, 1979.

be treated. Guidelines for abnormal levels in the first two decades of life are provided in Table 31–3.

Hyperlipidemia is defined as an increase in the plasma concentration of cholesterol or triglycerides, or both, above these normal values, but it should be recognized that the latter may be changed as a result of future studies. Diagnosis should be reserved for those children with elevated cholesterol or triglyceride levels on two or more separate determinations from venous blood samples after a 12-hour fast; the laboratory in which the tests are performed must be unquestionably accurate and reliable.

In the absence of mass screening programs or incorporation of this test as part of routine pediatric practice, serum lipid levels should be analyzed in all children from families with hyperlipidemia or with histories that include hypertension, myocardial infarction stroke, or peripheral vascular disease among parents or grandparents before age 50 years.[72,74,75] Differentiation is necessary between acquired hyperlipidemia and one of the familial, and presumably genetic, hyperlipidemias.

Homozygous familial hypercholesterolemia causes severe atherosclerosis of the coronary arteries and myocardial infarction in childhood; rarely it causes atherosclerosis of the aortic valve, leading to critical aortic stenosis that requires surgical treatment.[76]

References

1. Ainger, L. E., Lawyer, N. G., and Fitch, C. W.: Neonatal rubella myocarditis. Br. Heart J. *28*:691, 1966.
2. Ayuthya, T. S. N., Jayavasu, J., and Pongpanich, B.: Coxsackie group B virus in primary myocardial disease in infants and children. Am. Heart J. *88*:311, 1974.
3. Suckling, P. V., and Vogelpoel, L.: Coxsackie myocarditis of the newborn. Lancet *2*:421, 1970.
4. Lerner, A. M., and Wilson, F. M.: Virus myocardiopathy. Progr. Med. Virol. *15*:63, 1973.
5. Oda, T., Hamamoto, K. and Morinaga, H.: Clinical aspects of non-rheumatic myocarditis in children. Jap. Circ. J. *43*:443, 1979.
6. Wink, K., and Schmitz, H.: Cytomegalovirus myocarditis. Am. Heart J. *100*:667, 1980.
7. Arita, M., Ueno, Y., and Masuyama, Y.: Complete heart block in mumps myocarditis. Br. Heart J. *46*:342, 1981.
8. Noren, G. R., Kaplan, E. L., and Staley, N. A.: Non-rheumatic inflammatory cardiovascular disease. *In* Moss, A. J., Adams, F. H., and Emmanouilides, G. C. (eds.): Heart Disease in Infants, Children and Adolescents. Baltimore, Williams and Wilkins Co., 1977, p.p. 559–576.
9. Morgan, B. C.: Cardiac complications of diphtheria. Pediatrics *32*:549, 1963.
10. Srivastava, S. C., Puri, D. S., and Lumba, S. T.: An electrocardiographic study of myocarditis and diphtheria. J. Assoc. Phys. India *14*:365, 1966.
11. Prata, A.: Chagas' heart disease. Cardiologia *52*:79, 1968.
12. Rosenbaum, M. B.: Chagasic myocardiopathy. Progr. Cardiovasc. Dis. *7*:199, 1964.
13. Koten, J. W., and DeRaadt, P.: Myocarditis and *Trypanosoma rhodesiense* infections. Trans. R. Soc. Trop. Med. Hyg. *63*:485, 1969.
14. Gersony, W. M., and McCracken, G. H., Purulent pericarditis in infancy. Pediatrics *42*:24, 1967.
15. Okoroma, E. O., Terry, L. W., and Scott, L. T.: Acute bacterial pericarditis in children: Report of 25 cases. Am. Heart J. *90*:709, 1975.

16. VanReken, D., Strauss, A., Hernandez, A., and Feigin, R. D.: Infectious pericarditis in children. J. Pediatr. 85:165, 1974.

17. Lajos, T. Z., Black, H. E., Cooper, R. G., and Wanka, J.: Pericardial decompression. Ann. Thorac. Surg. 19:47, 1975.

18. Livelli, F. B., Johnson, R. A., McEnany, M. T., Block, P. C., and DeSanctis, R. W.: Unexplained in-hospital fever following cardiac surgery: Natural history, relationship to post-pericardiotomy syndrome, and a prospective study of therapy. N. Engl. J. Med. 57:968, 1978.

19. Engle, M. A., Ehlers, K. H., O'Laughlin, J. E., Linday, L. A., and Fried, R.: The post-pericardiotomy syndrome: Iatrogenic illness with immunologic and virologic components. In Engle, M. A. (ed.): Pediatric Cardiovascular Disease. Philadelphia, F. A. Davis, 1981, p. 381.

20. Paloheimo, J. A., Van Essen, R., Klemola, E., Kaarinen, L., and Siltanen, P.: Sub-clinical cytomegalovirus infections and cytomegalovirus mononucleosis after open heart surgery. Am. J. Cardiol. 22:624, 1968.

21. Shabetai, R.: Diagnosis and treatment of pericardial effusion. J. Cardiovasc. Med. 6:2, 1981.

22. Greenwood, R. D., Nadas, A. S., and Fyler, D. C.: The clinical course of primary myocardial disease in infants and children. Am. Heart J. 92:549, 1976.

23. Goodwin, J. F.: The frontiers of cardiomyopathy. Br. Heart J. 48:1, 1982.

24. Schryer, M. J. P., and Karnauchow, P. N.: Endocardial fibroelastosis: Etiologic and pathogenic considerations in children. Am. Heart J. 88:557, 1974.

25. Factor, S. M.: Endocardial fibroelastosis: Myocardial and vascular alterations associated with viral-like nuclear particles. Am. Heart J. 96:791, 1978.

26. Moller, J. N., Lucas, R. V., Adams, P., Anderson, R. C., Jorgens, J., and Edwards, J. R.: Endocardial fibroelastosis. A clinical and anatomic study of 47 patients with emphasis on its relationship to mitral insufficiency. Circulation 30:759, 1964.

27. Lambert, E. C., and Vlad, P.: Primary endomyocardial disease. Pediatr. Clin. North Am. 5:1057, 1958.

28. Sellers, F. J., Keith, J. D., and Manning, J. A.: The diagnosis of primary endocardial fibroelastosis. Circulation 29:49, 1964.

29. McLaughlin, T. G., Schiebler, G. L., and Krovetz, L. J.: Hemodynamic findings in children with endocardial fibroelastosis. Am. Heart J. 75:162, 1968.

30. Neustein, H. B., Lurie, P. R., and Fugita, M.: Endocardial fibroelastosis found on transvascular endomyocardial biopsy in children. Arch. Pathol. Lab. Med. 103:214, 1979.

31. Howell, R. R.: Glycogen storage diseases. In Stanbury, J. B., Wyngaarden, J. B., and Frederickson, D. S. (eds.): The Metabolic Basis of Inherited Disease, 3rd ed. New York, McGraw-Hill Book Co., 1972, pp. 149–173.

32. Bordiuk, J. N., Logato, M. J., Lovelace, R. E., and Blumenthal, S.: Pompe's disease: Electron myographic, electron microscopic and cardiovascular aspects. Arch. Neurol. (Chicago) 23:113, 1970.

33. Dickenson, E. F., Houlsby, W. T., and Wilkinson, J. L.: Unusual angiographic appearance of the left ventricle in two cases of Pompe's disease (glycogenosis type 2). Br. Heart J. 41:238, 1979.

34. Wolfe, R. R., and Way, G. L.: Cardiomyopathies in infants of diabetic mothers. Johns Hopkins Med. J. 140:177, 1977.

35. Gutgesell, H. P., Speer, M. E., and Rosenberg, H. S.: Characterization of the cardiomyopathy in infants with diabetic mothers. Circulation 51:441, 1980.

36. Miller, E., Hare, J. W., Cloherty, J. P., Dunn, P. J., Gleason, R. E., and Kitzmiller, J. L.: Elevated maternal hemoglobin A_{1C} in early pregnancy and major congenital anomalies in infants of diabetic mothers. N. Engl. J. Med. 304:1331, 1981.

37. Eriksson, U., Dahlstrom, E., Larsson, K. S., and Wellerstrom, C.: Increased incidence of congenital malformations in the offspring of diabetic rats and their prevention by maternal insulin therapy. Diabetics 31:1, 1982.

38. Whittemore, R., and Caddell, J. L.: Metabolic and nutritional diseases. In Moss, A. J., Adams, F. H., and Emmanouilides, G. C. (eds.): Heart Disease in Infants, Children and Adolescents. 2nd ed. Baltimore, Williams and Wilkins Co., 1977, pp. 579–602.

39. Sunshine, P., Kusumoto, H., and Kriss, J. P.: Survival time in circulating long-acting thyroid stimulator in neonatal thyrotoxicosis. Pediatrics 36:869, 1965.

40. Eason, E., Costom, B. and Papageorgiou, A. N.: Hypertension in neonatal thyrotoxicosis. J. Pediatr. 100:766, 1982.

41. Sanstead, H. H.: Clinical manifestations of certain vitamin deficiencies. In Goodhart, M. S., and Shils, M. E. (eds.): Modern Nutrition in Health and Disease. 5th ed. Philadelphia, Lea and Febiger, 1973, p. 593.

42. Sanstead, H. H.: Mineral metabolism and protein malnutrition. In Olson, R. E. (ed.): Protein Calorie Malnutrition. New York, Academic Press, 1975, p.213.

43. Cadell, J. L.: Diseases of the cardiovascular system. In Jelliffe, B. B. (ed.): Diseases of Children in the Subtropics and Tropics. London, Edward Arnold, Ltd., 1970, p. 398.

44. Nutter, D. O., Murray, T. G., Heymsfield, S. B., and Fuller, E. O.: The effect of chronic protein-calorie undernutrition in the rat on myocardial function and cardiac function. Circulation Res. 45:144, 1979.

45. Waterlow, J. C., and Alleyne, G. A. O.: Protein malnutrition in children: Advances in the last ten years. Adv. Protein Chem. 25:117, 1971.

46. Roberts, W. C., and Ferrans, V. J.: Pathological aspects of certain cardiomyopathies. Circ. Res. 34 (Suppl. II):II–128, 1974.

47. Roberts, W. C., Buja, L. M., and Ferrans, V. J.: Löffler's fibroplastic parietal endocarditis, eosinophilic leukemia, and Davies' endomyocardial fibrosis: The same disease at different stages? Pathol. Microbiol. (Basel) 35:90, 1970.

48. Lepley, D., Jr., Aris, A., Korns, M. E., Walker, J. A., and D'Cunha, R. M.: Endomyocardial fibrosis: A surgical approach. Ann. Thorac. Surg. 18:626, 1974.

49. Metras, D., Coulibaly, A. O., Schauvet, J., Ekra, A., Bertrand, E., and Castaneda, A. R.: Endomyocardial fibrosis. J. Thorac. Cardiovasc. Surg. 83:52, 1982.

50. Kawasaki, T., Kosaki, S., and Okawa, S.: A new infantile, acute febrile mucocutaneous lymph node syndrome prevailing in Japan. Pediatrics 54:71, 1974.

51. Tanaka, N., Sekimoto, K., and Naoe, S.: Kawasaki disease: Relationship with infantile periarteritis nodosa. Arch. Pathol. Lab. Med. 100:81, 1976.

52. Landing, B. H., and Larson, E. J.: Are infantile periarteritis nodosa with coronary artery involvement and fatal mucocutaneous lymph node syndrome the same? Comparison of 20 patients from North America with patients from Hawaii and Japan. Pediatrics 59:651, 1977.

53. DiSessa, T. G., Klitzner, T., Hiraishi, S., Welsh, M., and Kangarloo, H.: Cardiovascular effects of Kawasaki's disease. J. Cardiovasc. Med. 6:1159, 1981.

54. Hiraishi, S., Yashiro, K., Oguchi, K., and Nakazawa, K.: Clinical course of cardiovascular involvement in the mucocutaneous lymph node syndrome. Am. J. Cardiol. 47:323, 1981.

55. Kegel, S. M., Dorsey, T. J., Rowen, M., and Taylor, W. F.: Cardiac death in mucocutaneous lymph node syndrome. Am. J. Cardiol. 40:282, 1977.

56. Meade, R. H., and Brandt, L.: Manifestation of Kawasaki disease in New England outbreak of 1980. J. Pediatr. 100:558, 1982.

57. Onouchi, Z., Shimazu, S., Takamatsu, T., and Hamaoka, K.: Aneurysms of the coronary arteries in Kawasaki disease: An angiographic study of 30 cases. Circulation 66:6, 1982.

58. Chung, K., Brandt, L., Fulton, D. R., and Kreidberg, M. B.: Cardiac and coronary arterial involvement in infants and children with mucocutaneous lymph node syndrome. Am. J. Cardiol. 50:136, 1982.

59. Yoshida, H., Maeda, T., and Taniguchi, N.: Subcostal two-dimensional echocardiographic imaging of peripheral right coronary artery in Kawasaki disease. Circulation 65:956, 1982.

59a. Grenadier, E., Allen, H. D., Goldberg, S. J., Valdes-Cruz, L. M., Sahn, D. J., Lima, C. O., and Barron, J. V.: Left ventricular wall motion abnormalities in Kawasaki's disease. J. Am. Coll. Cardiol. 1:714, 1983.

60. Glanz, S., Bittner, S. J., Berman, M. A., Dolan, T. F., Jr., and Talner, N. S.: Regression of coronary artery aneurysms in infantile polyarteritis nodosa. N. Engl. J. Med. 294:939, 1976.

61. Kato, H., Ichinose, E., Matsunaga, S., Suzuki, K., and Rikatake, N.: Fate of coronary aneurysms in Kawasaki disease: Serial coronary angiography and long-term follow-up study. Am. J. Cardiol. 49:1758, 1982.

61a. Anderson, T., Meyer, R. A., and Kaplan, S.: Long term evaluation of cardiac size and function in patients with Kawasaki disease. J. Am. Coll. Cardiol. 1: 714, 1983.

61b. Suma, K., Takeuchi, Y., Shiroma, K., Tsuji, T., Inoue, K., Yoshikawa, T., Koyama, Y., Narumi, J., Asai, T., and Kusakawa, S.: Early and late postoperative studies in coronary arterial lesions resulting from Kawasaki's disease in children. J. Thorac. Cardiovasc. Surg. 84:224, 1982.

61c. Kitamura, S., Kawachi, K., Harima, R., Sakakibara, T., Hirose, H., and Kawashima, Y.: Surgery for coronary heart disease due to mucocutaneous lymph node syndrome (Kawasaki disease). Am. J. Cardiol. 51:444, 1983.

62. New, M. I., and Levine, L. S.: Hypertension in childhood and adolescence. Cardiovasc. Rev. 3:115, 1982.

63. Lieberman, E.: Diagnostic evaluation of hypertensive children. Pediatr. Ann. 6: 390, 1977.

64. McCrory, W. W.: What should blood pressure be in children? Pediatrics 70: 143, 1982.

65. Levine, R. S., Hennekens, C. H., Klein, B., Gourley, J., Briese, F. W., Hokanson, J., Gelband, H., and Jesse, M. J.: Tracking correlations of blood pressure levels in infancy. Pediatrics 61:1, 1978.

66. Luciani, J.-C., Baldet, P., Dumas, R., and Jean R.: Etude du systeme rénine-angiotensine dans deux cas de tumeur de Wilms avec hypertension artérielle sévère. Arch. Franç. Pédiatr. 36:230, 1979.

67. Berenson, G. S., Webber, L. S., and Voors, A. W.: Diagnosing hypertension in children. J. Cardiovasc. Med., 6:273, 1982.

68. Blumenthal, S., Epps, R. P., Heavenrich, R., Lauer, R. M., Lieberman, E., Mirkin, B., Mitchell, S. C., Naito, V. B., O'Hare, D., Smith, W. McF., Tarazi, R. C., and Upson, D.: Report of the task force on blood pressure control in children. Pediatrics 59 (Suppl.):797, 1977.

69. McLean, L. G.: Therapy of acute severe hypertension in children. J. A. M. A. 239:755, 1978.

70. Fleischmann, L. E.: Management of hypertensive crises in children. Pediatr. Ann. 6:410, 1977.

71. Lee, J., Lauer, R. M., and Clarke, W. R.: Coronary risk factors in children. In Engle, M. A., (ed.): Pediatric Cardiovascular Disease. Philadelphia, F. A. Davis, 1981, p. 1.

72. Schrott, H. G., Clark, W. R., Abrahams, P., Wiebe, D. A., and Lauer, R. M.: Coronary artery disease mortality in relatives of hypertriglyceridemic school children: The Muscatine study. Circulation 65:300, 1982.

73. Berwick, D. M., Cretin, S., and Keeler, E.: Cholesterol, children, and heart disease: An analysis of alternatives. Pediatrics 68:721, 1981.

74. Levy, R. I., and Rifkind, B. M.: Diagnosis and management of hyperlipoproteinemia in infants and children. Am. J. Cardiol. 31:547, 1973.

75. Neill, C. A., Ose, L., and Kwiterovich, P. O., Jr.: Hyperlipidemia: Clinical clues in the first two decades of life. Johns Hopkins Med. J. 140:171, 1977.

76. Forman, M. B., Kinsley, R. M., DuPlessis, J. P., Dansky, R., Milner, S., and Levin, S. E.: Surgical correction of combined supravalvular and valvular aortic stenosis in homozygous familial hypercholesterolemia. SA Med. J. 1:579, 1982.

32

VALVULAR HEART DISEASE

by Eugene Braunwald, M.D.

MITRAL STENOSIS

ETIOLOGY AND PATHOLOGY

The predominant cause of mitral stenosis is rheumatic fever[1] (p. 1647). Far less frequently, it is congenital, and this form is observed almost exclusively in infants and young children (p. 984). Rarely, mitral stenosis is a complication of malignant carcinoid (p. 1430), systemic lupus erythematosus,[1a] rheumatoid arthritis,[2] and the mucopolysaccharidoses of the Hunter-Hurley phenotype.[3] It has been suggested, though without proof, that many viruses, especially Coxsackie virus, may be responsible for chronic valvular heart disease.[4] Mitral stenosis, generally on a rheumatic basis, may be associated with atrial septal defect in Lutembacher's syndrome (p. 1032). Left atrial tumor, particularly myxoma (p. 1460); ball valve thrombus in the left atrium; and a congenital membrane in the left atrium, i.e., cor triatriatum (p. 984), may also obstruct left atrial outflow and therefore may simulate mitral stenosis. Although calcification of the mitral annulus usually causes mitral regurgitation (p. 1074), when subvalvular or intravalvular extension is extensive, mitral stenosis may result.[5]

Approximately 25 per cent of all patients with rheumatic heart disease have pure mitral stenosis, and an additional 40 per cent have combined mitral stenosis and regurgitation.[6] Two-thirds of all patients with rheumatic mitral stenosis are female.

Rheumatic fever results in four forms of fusion of the mitral valve apparatus leading to stenosis: (1) commissural, (2) cuspal, (3) chordal, and (4) combined.[3] Thickening of the commissures alone occurs in 30 per cent, of the cusps alone in 15 per cent, and of the chordae alone in 10 per cent; in the remainder, thickening of more than one of these structures is involved. Characteristically, mitral valve cusps fuse at their edges, and fusion of the chordae results in thickening and shortening of these structures. The stenotic mitral valve is typically funnel-shaped, and the orifice is frequently shaped like a "fish mouth" or buttonhole, with calcium deposits in the valve leaflets sometimes extending to involve the valve ring, which may become quite thick[7] (Figs. 32–1 and 48–5, p. 1647). The thickened leaflets may be so adherent and rigid that they cannot open or shut, reducing or rarely even abolishing the first heart sound (S_1) and leading to combined mitral stenosis and regurgitation.[8,9] There is a correlation between the severity of calcification and the transvalvular gradient.[10]

When rheumatic fever results exclusively or predominantly in contraction and fusion of the chordae tendineae, dominant mitral regurgitation results.

It probably takes a minimum of two years after the onset of acute rheumatic fever for severe mitral stenosis to develop, and most patients in temperate climates remain asymptomatic for at least a decade more.[11] Symptoms commence most commonly in the third or fourth decade, although mild mitral stenosis in the aged is becoming a more frequent finding. In the tropics, particularly in underdeveloped areas, the disease advances more rapidly, and severe mitral stenosis may be present in early adolescence.[12] The debate continues about whether the anatomical changes result from a smoldering rheumatic process or whether once the valve has been deformed by the initial episode, the constant trauma produced by the turbulent blood flow leads to progressive fibrosis, thickening, and calcification of the valve apparatus.[13]

Enlargement of the left atrium and resultant elevation of the left main stem bronchus, calcification of the left atrial wall, the development of mural thrombi, and obliterative changes in the pulmonary vascular bed (p. 830) may all result from chronic mitral stenosis.

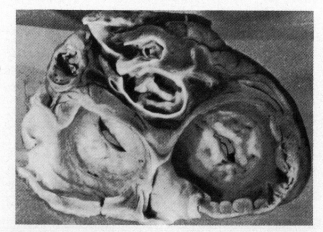

FIGURE 32–1   Severe mitral and tricuspid valve stenosis. The "buttonhole" orifice of the stenosed mitral valve (left) is well seen. Although partly hidden in this photograph, the anteromedial cusp (right) is, in fact, larger than the posterolateral cusp. The tricuspid valve (right) is thickened with commissural fusion. (From Oram, S.: Clinical Heart Disease. London, William Heinemann Medical Books, Ltd., 1971, p. 323.)

PATHOPHYSIOLOGY

In normal adults the mitral valve orifice is 4 to 6 cm². When the orifice is reduced to approximately 2 cm², which is considered mild mitral stenosis, blood can flow from the left atrium to the left ventricle only if propelled by an abnormal pressure gradient. When the mitral valve opening is reduced to 1 cm², which is considered critical mitral stenosis, a left atrioventricular pressure gradient of approximately 20 mm Hg (and therefore, in the presence of a normal left ventricular diastolic pressure, a mean left atrial pressure of approximately 25 mm Hg) is required to maintain normal cardiac output at rest (Figs. 32–2 and 32–3). The elevated left atrial pressure in turn raises pulmonary venous and capillary pressures, resulting in exertional dyspnea (p. 493). The first bouts of dyspnea in patients with mitral stenosis are usually precipitated by exercise, emotional stress, infection, or atrial fibrillation, all of which increase the rate of blood flow across the mitral orifice and result in further elevation of the left atrial pressure.[14,15]

In order to assess the severity of obstruction of the mitral valve (and, for that matter, of any valve), it is essential to measure both the transvalvular pressure gradient (Fig. 32–2) and the flow rate (Figure 9–8, p. 288). The latter depends not only on cardiac output but on heart rate as well. An increase in heart rate shortens diastole proportionately more than systole and diminishes the time available for flow across the mitral valve. Therefore, at any given level of cardiac output, tachycardia augments the transmitral valvular pressure gradient and elevates left atrial pressures further.[16] This explains the sudden development of dyspnea and pulmonary edema in previously asymptomatic patients who experience atrial fibrillation with a rapid ventricular rate[17,18] and the equally rapid improvement in these patients when the ventricular rate is slowed by means of cardiac glycosides and/or beta-adrenergic blocking agents, even when the cardiac output per minute remains constant. Hydraulic considerations dictate that at any given orifice size the transvalvular gradient is a function of the square of the transvalvular flow rate (p.

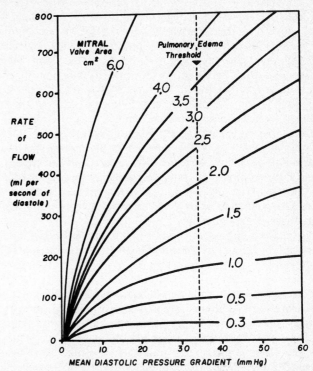

FIGURE 32–3 Chart illustrating the relation between mean diastolic gradient across the mitral valve and rate of flow across the mitral valve per second of diastole, as predicted by the Gorlin formula. Note that when the mitral valve area is 1.0 cm² or less, very little additional flow can be achieved by an increased pressure gradient. (Reproduced with permission from Wallace, A. G.: Pathophysiology of cardiovascular disease. *In* Smith, L. H., Jr., and Thier, S. O. [eds.]: Pathophysiology: The Biological Principles of Disease. The International Textbook of Medicine. Vol. 1. Philadelphia, W. B. Saunders Co., 1981, p. 1192.)

293 and Fig. 32–3).[19,20] Thus, a doubling of flow rate will quadruple the pressure gradient, so that a stress such as exercise in patients with moderate or severe stenosis will cause marked elevation of left atrial pressure.[21]

Atrial contraction augments the presystolic transmitral valvular gradient by approximately 30 per cent in patients with mitral stenosis. Withdrawal of atrial transport when atrial fibrillation develops decreases cardiac output by about 20 per cent. At any level of cardiac output, effective atrial contraction maintains lower levels of mean left atrial pressure than would be present in atrial fibrillation.[22] In addition, the more rapid ventricular rate that is common in atrial fibrillation raises the transvalvular pressure gradient. Thus, hemodynamic considerations indicate the desirability of maintaining sinus rhythm in patients with mitral stenosis.[17,23]

INTRACARDIAC AND INTRAVASCULAR PRESSURES

Left ventricular diastolic pressure is normal in patients with pure mitral stenosis; coexisting mitral regurgitation, aortic valve lesions, systemic hypertension, ischemic heart disease, or cardiomyopathy may all be responsible for elevations of left ventricular diastolic pressure. In approximately 85 per cent of patients with pure mitral stenosis, the end-diastolic volume is within the normal range, whereas it is reduced in the remainder.[24] In approximately one-third of patients the ejection fraction is below normal, most likely owing to chronic reduction in preload and per-

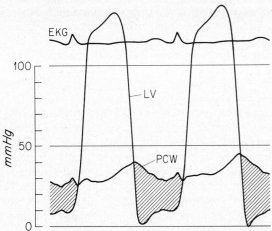

FIGURE 32–2 Pressure tracings from a 50-year-old woman with progressive fatigue and dyspnea on exertion and a history of childhood acute rheumatic fever. The pulmonary capillary wedge (PCW) pressure is elevated, and there is a mean gradient (cross-hatched area) of 22 mm Hg between pulmonary capillary wedge (PCW) and left ventricular (LV) pressures throughout diastole. The calculated mitral valve area was reduced to 0.8 cm².

haps to the extension of the scarring process from the mitral valve into the adjacent posterior basal myocardium[25] or to associated heart disease. The left ventricular mass is normal or slightly reduced.[26] Although it has long been postulated that persistent myocardial dysfunction,[27] perhaps caused by smoldering rheumatic myocarditis, may be responsible for the poor results following surgical treatment of some patients with pure mitral stenosis, the bulk of available evidence suggests that myocardial contractility is normal or only slightly impaired in the majority of patients.[28,29] Associated ischemic disease or rigidity of the mitral valve complex may be responsible for myocardial dysfunction. However, it is likely that preoperative myocardial dysfunction is only one of several reasons for unsatisfactory surgical results.[30]

In mitral stenosis and sinus rhythm, the *left atrial pressure pulse* often exhibits a prominent atrial contraction (*a*) wave and a gradual pressure decline after mitral valve opening (*y* descent); the mean left atrial pressure is elevated. In patients with mild to moderate mitral stenosis without elevation of pulmonary vascular resistance, pulmonary arterial pressure may be normal at rest and rises only during exercise. However, in patients with severe mitral stenosis and those in whom the pulmonary vascular resistance is significantly increased, pulmonary arterial pressure is elevated when the patient is at rest, and in cases of extreme elevation of the pulmonary vascular resistance it may exceed the systemic arterial pressure (Chap. 25). Further elevations of left atrial and pulmonary vascular pressures occur during exercise or tachycardia or both. With moderate elevation of pulmonary artery pressure, right ventricular performance is maintained.[31] An elevation of pulmonary arterial systolic pressure exceeding 70 mm Hg represents a serious impedance to emptying of the right ventricle, and when this level is exceeded in patients with rheumatic heart disease, right ventricular end-diastolic and right atrial pressures often rise.

The *clinical and hemodynamic features* of mitral stenosis of any given severity are dictated largely by the levels of cardiac output and pulmonary vascular resistance.[32] The response to a given degree of mitral obstruction may be characterized on one end of the hemodynamic spectrum by a normal cardiac output and a high left atrioventricular pressure gradient or, at the opposite end of the spectrum, by a markedly reduced cardiac output and low transvalvular pressure gradient. In some patients with moderately severe stenosis (mitral valve area = 1.0 to 1.5 cm²) cardiac output may be normal, not only at rest but during exertion as well. In these patients, marked elevation of left atrial and pulmonary capillary pressures leads to symptoms of severe pulmonary congestion. However, in the majority of patients with severe mitral stenosis, cardiac output is subnormal at rest and rises subnormally during exertion, thus reducing the pulmonary venous pressure and the severity of symptoms of pulmonary congestion more than would be the case if the output rose normally. In patients with severe stenosis (mitral valve area < 1.0 cm²), particularly when pulmonary vascular resistance is elevated, cardiac output is usually depressed at rest and fails to rise during exertion. These patients frequently have prominent symptoms secondary to a low cardiac output (p. 495).

Pulmonary hypertension in patients with mitral stenosis results from (1) passive backward transmission of the ele-

vated left atrial pressure; (2) arteriolar constriction, which presumably is triggered by left atrial and pulmonary venous hypertension (reactive pulmonary hypertension); and (3) organic obliterative changes in the pulmonary vascular bed, which may be considered to be a complication of longstanding and severe mitral stenosis (Chap. 25). In time, severe pulmonary hypertension results in right-sided failure and tricuspid and sometimes pulmonic regurgitation. However, it has been suggested that these changes in the pulmonary vascular bed may also be considered to exert a protective effect; the elevated precapillary resistance makes the development of symptoms of pulmonary congestion less likely by tending to prevent blood from surging into the pulmonary capillary bed and damming up behind the stenotic mitral valve, although this protection occurs at the expense of a decreased cardiac output.[33] Patients with severe mitral stenosis manifest a marked reduction in lung compliance, an increase in the work of breathing, and a redistribution of pulmonary blood flow from the bases to the apices (p. 1785).

The combination of mitral valve disease and atrial inflammation secondary to rheumatic carditis causes left atrial dilatation, fibrosis of the atrial wall, and disorganization of the atrial muscle bundles. The last leads to disparate conduction velocities and inhomogeneous refractory periods. Premature atrial activation due either to an automatic focus or to reentry may stimulate the left atrium during the vulnerable period and may thus precipitate a bout of atrial fibrillation. Chronic atrial fibrillation results in turn in diffuse atrophy of the muscle, which causes further inhomogeneity of refractoriness and conduction and leads to irreversible atrial fibrillation.[34]

CLINICAL MANIFESTATIONS
(Table 32–1)

History

The principal symptom of mitral stenosis is dyspnea, largely the result of reduced compliance of the lungs (p. 1785). Vital capacity is reduced, presumably owing to the presence of engorged pulmonary vessels and interstitial edema. Patients with critical obstruction to left ventricular inflow and dyspnea upon ordinary activity (functional Class III) generally have orthopnea and are at risk of experiencing attacks of frank pulmonary edema. The latter may be precipitated by effort, emotional stress, respiratory infection, fever, sexual intercourse, pregnancy,[35] or atrial fibrillation with a rapid ventricular rate or, indeed, by any condition that increases blood flow across the stenotic mitral valve, either by increasing total cardiac output or by reducing the time available for this flow of blood to occur. In patients with a markedly elevated pulmonary vascular resistance, right ventricular function is often impaired, and a rise in right ventricular output may be impossible. Therefore, they are less subject to sudden elevations of pulmonary capillary pressure and the accompanying attacks of pulmonary edema.[15,36]

Hemoptysis. Wood has differentiated between several kinds of *hemoptysis* complicating mitral stenosis.[15]

1. So-called pulmonary apoplexy, a sudden hemorrhage which, while often profuse, is rarely life-threatening.[37,38] This results from the rupture of thin-walled, dilated bronchial veins as a consequence of a sudden rise in left atrial

TABLE 32–1   DIAGNOSIS OF MITRAL VALVE DISEASE

	MITRAL STENOSIS	MITRAL REGURGITATION
Sex	Women > Men	Men > Women
Severity of rheumatic fever	Less severe	Often fulminating
Presystolic murmur	Present	Absent
First sound	Loud unless calcification	*Never loud*
Apical systolic murmur	Usually absent	Pansystolic or late
Mid-diastolic murmur	Long, not necessarily loud	*If present, short*
Opening snap of mitral valve	Present unless heavy calcification, pulmonary hypertension, or aortic regurgitation	Rarely present
Third sound	*Never present*	Commonly present and loud
Cardiac impulse	Tapping ("closing snap"); right ventricular type if pulmonary vascular resistance raised	Left ventricular type; right ventricular type if pulmonary vascular resistance raised
Radial pulse	Small volume	Small volume but collapsing
Systemic emboli	Common	Less common
Left atrial size	Enlarged but rarely aneurysmal	May be aneurysmal; systolic
Left ventricle	*Normal or poor filling,* aorta hypoplastic	*Enlarged, rapidly filling,* and hyperdynamic
Electrocardiogram	RVH if pulmonary vascular resistance raised	LVH; RVH if pulmonary vascular resistance raised
Hemodynamic data	a. LAP may be greatly raised	a. Less severely raised as a rule
	b. Gradient across valve in diastole	b. No gradient usually
	c. PVR may be severely raised	c. PVR not commonly greatly raised

RVH = right ventricular hypertrophy; LVH = left ventricular hypertrophy; LAP = left atrial pressure; PVR = pulmonary vascular resistance.
Modified from Oram, S.: Clinical Heart Disease. London, William Heinemann Medical Books, 1981, p. 335.

pressure. After several years of pulmonary venous hypertension, the walls of these veins thicken appreciably, and this form of hemoptysis tends to disappear.

2. Blood-stained sputum associated with attacks of nocturnal dyspnea.

3. Pink, frothy sputum characteristic of acute pulmonary edema due to rupture of alveolar capillaries.

4. Pulmonary infarction, a late complication of mitral stenosis associated with heart failure.

5. Blood-stained sputum complicating chronic bronchitis; the edematous bronchial mucosa in patients with chronic mitral stenosis increases the likelihood of chronic bronchitis, a common complication of mitral stenosis, particularly in Great Britain.

Chest Pain. A small fraction, perhaps 15 per cent, of patients with mitral stenosis experience chest discomfort that is indistinguishable from angina pectoris.[14,15] This symptom may be caused by right ventricular hypertension[39] or by coincidental coronary atherosclerosis, or it may be secondary to coronary obstruction caused by coronary embolization.[40] In many such patients, however, a satisfactory explanation cannot be uncovered even after complete hemodynamic and angiographic studies.

Thromboembolism. This is an important complication of mitral stenosis.[41,42] Prior to the development of surgical treatment, systemic embolism developed in at least 20 per cent of patients at some time during the course of their disease, and in the past as many as 10 to 15 per cent of this group died as a consequence. Before the era of anticoagulant therapy and surgical treatment, approximately one-fourth of all fatalities in patients with mitral valve disease were secondary to embolism. The tendency for embolization correlates inversely with cardiac output and directly with age and the size of the left atrial appendage; 80 per cent of patients in whom systemic emboli develop are in atrial fibrillation. When embolization occurs in patients in sinus rhythm, the possibility of underlying infective endocarditis should be considered. There is no simple correlation between the incidence of embolism on one hand and the size of the mitral orifice or the level of pulmonary vascular resistance on the other. Indeed, embolism

may be the first symptom of mitral stenosis and may occur in patients with mild mitral stenosis even prior to the development of dyspnea. Patients older than age 35 years and having atrial fibrillation, especially with a low cardiac output and dilation of the left atrial appendage, are at the highest risk from emboli and therefore should be considered for prophylactic anticoagulant treatment.

Since thrombi are found in the left atrium in only a minority of patients with a history of recent embolism at operation, it is likely that only fresh clots are discharged from the atria into the systemic circulation. Approximately half of all clinically apparent emboli are found in the cerebral vessels. Coronary embolism may lead to myocardial infarction or angina pectoris or both, and renal emboli may be responsible for the development of systemic hypertension. Emboli are recurrent and multiple in approximately 25 per cent of patients subject to this complication. Rarely, massive thrombosis develops in the left atrium, resulting in a pedunculated ball-valve thrombus, which may aggravate obstruction to left atrial outflow when a specific body position is assumed, or it may cause sudden death.[43]

Infective Endocarditis. This complication tends to occur less frequently on a rigid, thickened, calcified valve and is therefore more common in patients with mild than with severe mitral stenosis.

Other Symptoms. Compression of the left recurrent laryngeal nerve by a greatly dilated left atrium, enlarged tracheobronchial lymph nodes, and dilated pulmonary artery causes hoarseness (Ortner's syndrome).[44] A history of repeated hemoptysis is common in patients with pulmonary hemosiderosis, and longstanding elevation of pulmonary venous pressure is present in patients with pulmonary ossification. Systemic venous hypertension, hepatomegaly, edema, ascites, and hydrothorax are all signs of severe mitral stenosis with elevated pulmonary vascular resistance and right heart failure.

Physical Examination

Patients with severe mitral stenosis, a low cardiac output, and systemic vasoconstriction often exhibit the so-called mitral facies, characterized by pinkish-purple patches on the cheeks.[15] The *arterial pulse* is usually normal, but in patients in whom the stroke volume is reduced, the pulse may be small in volume. The *jugular venous pulse* usually exhibits a prominent *a* wave in patients with sinus rhythm and elevated pulmonary vascular resistance (Fig. 3–35, p. 63). In atrial fibrillation, the *x* descent of the jugular pulse disappears, and there is only one crest, a prominent *v* or *c-v* wave, per cardiac cycle and a slow *y* descent. *Palpation* of the cardiac apex usually reveals an inconspicuous left ventricle;[45] the presence of either a palpable presystolic expansion wave or an early diastolic rapid filling wave *excludes* significant mitral stenosis. The presence of a readily palpable, tapping first heart sound (S_1) suggests that the anterior mitral valve leaflet is pliable. When the patient is in the left lateral recumbent position, the low-pitched diastolic rumbling murmur of mitral stenosis is often palpable as a thrill at the apex. Often a right ventricular lift is palpable in the left parasternal region in patients with pulmonary hypertension. A markedly enlarged right ventricle may displace the left ventricle posteriorly and produce a prominent apex beat that can be confused with a left ventricular lift. A pulmonic closure sound (P_2) may be palpable in the second left intercostal space in patients with mitral stenosis and pulmonary hypertension.

AUSCULTATION. The auscultatory (and phonocardiographic) features of mitral stenosis (some of which are illustrated in Figures 3–14, p. 50, and Figures 32–4 and 32–5) include an accentuated S_1 with prolongation of the Q-S_1 interval (p. 43), correlating with the level of the left atrial pressure.[8] Accentuation of S_1 occurs when the mitral valve is flexible[46] and is due in part to the rapidity with which left ventricular pressure rises at the time of mitral valve closure as well as to the wide closing excursion of the valve leaflets. Marked calcification or thickening of the

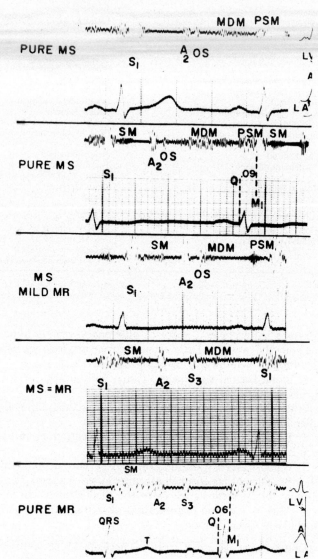

FIGURE 32–5 Representative phonocardiograms at the cardiac apex ranging from pure mitral stenosis (MS) to pure mitral regurgitation (MR), with illustrative left ventricular (LV) and left atrial (LA) pressure pulses at the two extremes. The first sound (S_1) gets progressively softer, the holosystolic murmur (SM) of mitral regurgitation becomes more prominent, the opening snap (OS) is replaced by a third heart sound (S_3), and the presystolic murmur (PSM) softens and vanishes, whereas the mid-diastolic murmur (MDM) shortens and finally disappears. (From Reichek, N., et al.: Clinical aspects of rheumatic valvular disease. *In* Sonnenblick, E. S., and Lesch, M. [eds.]: Valvular Heart Disease. New York, Grune and Stratton, 1974, p. 143, by permission of Grune and Stratton, Inc.)

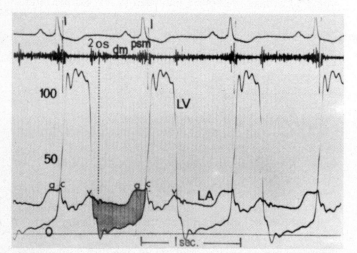

FIGURE 32–4 The auscultatory complex of mitral stenosis. An apical phonocardiogram demonstrates the accentuated first sound (1), opening snap (os), rumbling diastolic murmur (dm), and crescendo presystolic murmur (psm) in relation to simultaneous left ventricular (LV) and left atrial (LA) pressures. The first sound is coincident with the left atrial *c* wave, and the opening snap coincides with a notch (dotted line) on the downslope (*y* descent) of the left atrial *v* wave. The presystolic murmur exhibits a crescendo after the *a* wave peak, during a decline in the atrioventricular pressure gradient (shaded area). (Time lines = 0.04 sec.) (From Criley, J. M., et al.: Departures from the expected auscultatory events in mitral stenosis. *In* Likoff, W. [ed.]: Cardiovascular Clinics. Vol. 5, No. 2, Valvular Heart Disease. Philadelphia, F. A. Davis, 1973, p. 192.)

mitral valve leaflets or both reduce the amplitude of S_1, probably because of diminished movement of the leaflets. As pulmonary artery pressure rises, P_2 at first becomes accentuated and widely transmitted and can often be readily heard and recorded at both the mitral and the aortic areas. With further elevation of pulmonary artery pressure, splitting of S_2 narrows because of reduced compliance of the pulmonary vascular bed, which shortens the "hang-out interval" (p. 47). Finally, S_2 becomes single and accentuated. Other signs of pulmonary hypertension include a nonvalvular pulmonic ejection sound (See Figure 3–13, p. 49) that diminishes during inspiration, owing to dilatation of the pulmonary artery; the systolic murmur of tricuspid regurgitation; a Graham Steell murmur of pulmonic regurgitation; and an S_4 originating from the right ventricle.[47] An S_3 originating from the left ventricle is absent, unless significant mitral or aortic regurgitation coexists.

The *opening snap* (OS) of the mitral valve appears to be due to a sudden tensing of the valve leaflets by the chordae tendineae after the valve cusps have completed their opening excursion[48] and is best heard at the apex and with the diaphragm of the stethoscope.[49-52] It can usually be differentiated from P_2, since the OS occurs later, unless right bundle branch block is present. The mitral valve cannot be totally rigid if it produces an OS, which is usually accompanied by an accentuated S_1. Calcification confined to the top of the mitral valve does not preclude an OS, although calcification of the body and tip does.[53] In patients with combined mitral stenosis and regurgitation, the OS may be followed by an S_3. The mitral OS follows A_2 by 0.04 to 0.12 sec, and the A_2-OS interval varies inversely with left atrial pressure[51,52] (p. 49). Although a short A_2-OS interval is a reliable indicator of severe stenosis, the converse is not necessarily the case, since the time interval between the actual opening of the mitral valve and the OS can be prolonged in the presence of valvular calcification and tight stenosis.[48] The $(Q-S_1)$–$(A_2$-OS) correlates better with the height of the left atrial pressure than does either measurement alone.[49]

The diastolic murmur of mitral stenosis is a low-pitched, rumbling murmur, best heard at the apex and with the bell of the stethoscope. When this murmur is soft, it is limited to the apex, but when louder, it may radiate to the axilla or the lower left sternal area. Although the intensity of the diastolic murmur is not closely related to the severity of stenosis, the *duration* of the murmur is a guide to the severity of mitral narrowing, and in patients with combined mitral stenosis and regurgitation, a long diastolic murmur always signifies the presence of significant stenosis and, in general, persists for as long as the gradient across the mitral valve exceeds approximately 3 mm Hg. The murmur usually commences immediately after the mitral OS. In mild mitral stenosis, the murmur is brief but commences again in presystole. In severe stenosis, the murmur is holodiastolic, with presystolic accentuation.

Although a *presystolic murmur* is usually present in patients with sinus rhythm in whom transvalvular blood flow is accelerated by atrial contraction, such a murmur may also occur in patients with atrial fibrillation, in whom it results from the increased velocity of blood flow across a mitral valve orifice that begins to narrow after the onset of left ventricular contraction[54-56] (see Figure 4–18, p. 80). Since, in patients with atrial fibrillation, this murmur results from motion of the mitral valve leaflets, a flexible mitral valve is required for its generation; its absence in a patient with moderate or severe obstruction suggests either a rigid calcified valve or a markedly reduced cardiac output.

The *diastolic rumbling murmur* of mitral stenosis may be masked by the presence of obesity, pulmonary emphysema, and a low cardiac output with a low flow rate across the mitral valve. The rumble may be sharply localized and thus missed unless one uses palpation to detect the apex of the left ventricle and to pinpoint the area at which auscultation should be carried out. In so-called "silent" mitral stenosis, there is usually marked right ventricular enlargement, so that the right ventricle occupies the cardiac apex, and cardiac output is reduced, so that the murmur either is not audible at all or can be heard only in the mid- or posterior axillary line.[57] Auscultation of the murmur is facilitated by use of the bell of the stethoscope, placing the patient in the left lateral position and auscultating during expiration after a few sit-ups or other maneuvers described below.

Dynamic Auscultation. The diastolic murmur and OS of mitral stenosis are often reduced during inspiration and augmented during expiration[58]—the opposite of what occurs when these findings are secondary to tricuspid stenosis. During inspiration the A_2-OS interval widens, and three sequential sounds (A_2, P_2, and OS) are frequently audible. Sudden standing and the resultant reduction of venous return lower left atrial pressure and widen the A_2-OS interval[59]; this maneuver is useful in distinguishing an A_2-OS combination from a split S_2, which narrows. In contrast, A_2-OS is significantly narrowed during exercise.[60] The diastolic rumbling murmur of mitral stenosis is reduced during the strain of a Valsalva maneuver, and there is a delayed return to prestrain levels during the overshoot, six to eight beats after release. Amyl nitrite, coughing, isometric or isotonic exercise, and sudden squatting are all useful in accentuating a faint or equivocal murmur of mitral stenosis. Progressive narrowing of A_2-OS on serial examinations suggests an increase in the severity of stenosis, whereas widening of A_2-OS after mitral commissurotomy indicates that the severity of stenosis has been reduced significantly.

DIFFERENTIAL DIAGNOSIS. It is important to recognize that a variety of conditions other than mitral stenosis may exhibit auscultatory findings that can be confused with mitral stenosis, and these are summarized in Table 32–2. In addition to the findings listed in the table, the *Carey-Coombs* murmur of acute rheumatic fever (p. 1649) is a sign of active mitral valvulitis and can be confused with the murmur of mitral stenosis. It is a soft, early diastolic murmur, usually varies from day to day, and is higher pitched than the diastolic rumbling murmur of established mitral stenosis. In pure, severe *mitral regurgitation*—indeed, in any condition in which there is increased flow across a nonstenotic mitral valve—there may also be a loud, short, diastolic murmur following an S_3. *Left atrial myxoma* may produce auscultatory findings similar to those in rheumatic mitral valvular stenosis (p. 1460).

A *pansystolic murmur of tricuspid regurgitation* and an S_3 originating from the right ventricle may be audible in the fourth intercostal space in the left parasternal region in patients with severe mitral stenosis. These signs, secondary to pulmonary hypertension, may be confused with the findings of mitral regurgitation.[61] However, the inspiratory augmentation of the murmur and of the S_3 and the prominent v wave in the jugular venous pulse aid in establishing that the murmur originates from the tricuspid valve. A decrescendo diastolic murmur along the left sternal border in patients with mitral stenosis and pulmonary hypertension is usually due to aortic regurgitation and rarely represents a Graham Steell murmur of pulmonary regurgitation[62] (p. 1122); the latter, when present, characteristically increases during inspiration.

TABLE 32–2   CONDITIONS OTHER THAN MITRAL STENOSIS THAT MAY SIMULATE AUSCULTATORY FINDINGS IN MITRAL STENOSIS

AUSCULTATORY EVENT	CONDITION OTHER THAN MITRAL STENOSIS	EXPLANATION OF EVENT
Loud and snapping first sound	Hyperkinetic states	High left ventricular dP/dt at time of mitral closure
Early diastolic opening snap	Myxoma of left atrium	Tumor movement into ventricle
		Abrupt checking of tumor (tumor plop)
	Constrictive pericarditis	Checking of ventricular filling by pericardium
	Tricuspid stenosis	Stenotic valve
Diastolic rumbling murmur	Aortic regurgitation (Austin Flint murmur)	Preclosure of mitral valve
		(?) Regurgitant stream
		(?) Fluttering of mitral valve
	Dilated ventricle	Preclosure of mitral valve
	Myocarditis	(?) Centrifugal displacement of papillary muscles
	Cardiomyopathy	
	Hypertrophic, restrictive ventricle	Impaired filling of left ventricle
	Hypertrophic obstructive cardiomyopathy	(?) Impaired opening of mitral valve
	Aortic valve disease	
	Tricuspid stenosis	Narrow orifice
	Myxoma of left atrium	Narrow orifice
	Augmented atrioventricular flow	Preclosure of valve
	Mitral regurgitation	(?) Centrifugal displacement of papillary muscles
	Left-to-right shunts	
Crescendo presystolic murmur	Aortic regurgitation (Austin Flint murmur)	Preclosure of mitral valve opposing atrial systole
	Hypertrophic, restrictive ventricle	Summation of S_4 and S_1 may simulate presystolic murmur
	Tricuspid stenosis	Narrow orifice
	Myxoma of left atrium	Narrow orifice

Modified from Criley, J. M., et al.: Departures from the expected auscultatory events in mitral stenosis. *In* Likoff, W. (ed.): Cardiovascular Clinics. Vol. 5, No. 2, Valvular Heart Disease. Philadelphia, F. A. Davis, 1973, p. 213.

LABORATORY EXAMINATION

ELECTROCARDIOGRAM. The electrocardiogram and vectorcardiogram are relatively insensitive techniques for the detection of mild mitral stenosis, but they do show characteristic changes in patients with moderate or severe obstruction. Left atrial enlargement (P-wave duration in lead II > 0.12 sec, terminal negative P force in lead V_1 > .003 mv/sec, P-wave axis between +45 and −30 degrees) is a principal electrocardiographic feature of mitral stenosis (Fig. 7–11*A*, p. 208) and is found in 90 per cent of patients with significant mitral stenosis and sinus rhythm.[63,64] The electrocardiographic signs of left atrial enlargement correlate more closely with left atrial volume than with left atrial pressure[65] and often regress following successful valvulotomy.[15] When atrial fibrillation is present, the fibrillatory waves are coarse, i.e., greater than 0.1 mv in amplitude in V_1, also suggesting the presence of atrial enlargement.[66] The development of atrial fibrillation correlates with the preexistent electrocardiographic diagnosis of left atrial enlargement and is related to the size and the extent of fibrosis of the left atrial myocardium,[67] the duration of atriomegaly, and the age of the patient.[68]

Electrocardiographic evidence of right ventricular hypertrophy depends on the level of right ventricular systolic pressure; this finding is infrequent in patients with right ventricular systolic pressures less than 70 mm Hg.[63] However, approximately half of all patients with right ventricular systolic pressures between 70 and 100 mm Hg manifest the electrocardiographic criteria for right ventricular hypertrophy, including both a mean QRS axis that is greater than 80 degrees in the frontal plane and an R:S ratio greater than 1.0 in V_1.[69] In other patients with this degree of pulmonary hypertension, there is no frank evidence of

right ventricular hypertrophy, but the R:S ratio fails to increase from right to midprecordial leads. When right ventricular systolic pressures exceed 100 mm Hg, electrocardiographic evidence of right ventricular hypertrophy is found quite consistently. The mean QRS axis averages +150 degrees, and there is a Q-R morphology in the right precordial leads, accompanied by inverted or biphasic T waves.[70]

The *QRS axis in the frontal plane* often correlates with the severity of valve obstruction and with the level of pulmonary vascular resistance in pure mitral stenosis; thus, a mean frontal axis between 0 and +60 degrees suggests that the mitral valve area exceeds 1.3 cm², whereas an axis greater than 60 degrees generally indicates that the valve area is less than 1.3 cm². In patients in whom pulmonary vascular resistance is greater than 650 dynes-sec-cm⁻⁵, the mean axis usually exceeds +110 degrees.[69]

VECTORCARDIOGRAM. The characteristic *vectorcardiographic finding* in mitral stenosis is right ventricular hypertrophy Type C (Figure 7–17, p. 213) characterized by counterclockwise rotation in the horizontal plane and a terminal deflection directed to the right, posteriorly, and superiorly.[63,69–72] In other patients with mitral stenosis without frank right ventricular hypertrophy, QRS loops with posterior and rightward terminal appendages are evident without conduction delays.[63,69] There is vectorcardiographic evidence of right ventricular hypertrophy Type A (Figure 7–17, p. 213) in only 10 per cent of patients with mitral stenosis, but when present it indicates that both the hypertrophy and the stenosis are severe. Vectorcardiograms showing right ventricular hypertrophy Type B (Figure 7–17), are infrequent in mitral stenosis.

Rotation of the P loop in the frontal plane, with superior orientation of the terminal P forces and a wide angle between the initial and terminal P vectors, occurs in about one-fourth of patients with pure mitral stenosis and may be the only evidence of left atrial enlargement.[73] The terminal portion of the P loop is usually directed posteriorly and inferiorly, and the T loop is often directed leftward and posterosuperiorly and is discordant with respect to the QRS loop, resulting in a diphasic T wave with initial negativity and terminal positivity in lead V_1.[64]

RADIOLOGICAL FINDINGS (see also p. 163). Although the cardiac silhouette may be normal in the frontal projection, with the exception of an enlarged atrial appendage (Fig. 6–3*A*, p. 149), in patients with hemodynamically significant mitral stenosis, left atrial enlargement is almost invariably evident on the lateral and left anterior oblique views.[74,75] The size of the left atrium does *not* correlate with the severity of obstruction. However, extreme left atrial enlargement rarely occurs in pure mitral stenosis; when it is present, mitral regurgitation is usually severe. Enlargement of the pulmonary artery, right ventricle, and right atrium (as well as the left atrium) is commonly seen in severe mitral stenosis (Figure 6–2, p. 148, and Figure 6–13, p. 156). Occasionally, calcification of the mitral valve is evident on the chest roentgenogram (see Figure 6–9, p. 154), but, more commonly, fluoroscopy is required to detect valvular calcification.

Radiological changes in the lung fields (see Figure 6–26, p. 165) are useful in assessing the height of pulmonary venous pressure and thereby the severity of mitral stenosis. Interstitial edema, an indication of severe obstruction, is manifest as Kerley B lines (dense, short, horizontal lines most commonly seen in the costophrenic angles).[76] This finding is present in 30 per cent of patients with resting pulmonary artery wedge pressures below 20 mm Hg and in 70 per cent of patients with pressures exceeding 20 mm Hg. Severe, longstanding mitral obstruction often results in Kerley A lines (straight, dense lines up to 4 cm in length and running toward the hilum) as well as the findings of pulmonary hemosiderosis[77] and rarely of parenchymal ossification.

Angiograms exposed in the right and left anterior oblique projections afford the best views of the mitral valve.[78] Although, ideally, contrast medium should be injected into the left atrium, it is often possible to achieve good visualization of the left side of the heart by injecting a large volume of contrast medium into the main pulmonary artery. Such left atrial or pulmonary angiograms provide an assessment of left atrial size, may demonstrate thickening and reduced motion of the valve leaflets (Figure 6–54, p. 187), and may outline large intraluminal thrombi.[79] In most catheterization laboratories today, left cine ventriculography is the primary (and often the sole) angiographic procedure for assessment of mitral valve motion. Although this technique allows visualization of only the ventricular aspect of the leaflet in patients with pure mitral stenosis, it makes possible simultaneous assessment of left ventricular contractile function and of the subvalvular mitral apparatus.[80]

ECHOCARDIOGRAPHY (see also p. 109). Mitral stenosis can ordinarily be readily diagnosed by M-mode echocardiography (Figure 3–14, p. 50, and Figure 5–38, p. 110), but this technique does not allow a precise determination of its severity. Echoes of a thickened, calcified stenotic rheumatic valve demonstrate increased acoustic

impedance and fusion of the mitral valve leaflets and poor leaflet separation in diastole.[81,82] Normally, the posterior leaflet of the mitral valve moves posteriorly during early diastole, but in more than 90 per cent of patients with mitral stenosis, both leaflets move anteriorly at this time (Fig. 32–6). The E–F slope is reduced,[81–86] but this finding is not pathognomonic of mitral stenosis, since it may occur in other conditions in which left ventricular compliance and the velocity of left ventricular filling are reduced,[86] or in which there is substantial right ventricular pressure overload.[87] However, in these other conditions the posterior leaflet of the mitral valve moves normally, emphasizing the importance of recording the motion of this structure in order to establish the diagnosis of mitral stenosis by echocardiography.[81] Reduction of the E–F slope does not correlate with the severity of obstruction. However, the maximal diastolic separation of the anterior and posterior leaflets,[85] their rate of diastolic apposition,[82,86] and the slope of motion of the left ventricular posterior wall during diastole[87] appear to correlate more closely with the mitral valve area. The ratio $Q-C/A_2-E$ (where C and E represent mitral valve closure and opening, respectively, Q is the onset of the QRS complex, and A_2 the closure of the aortic valve) correlates well with the left atrial pressure.[88] Cross-

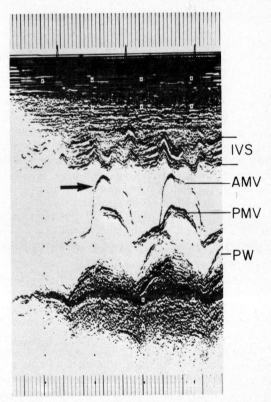

FIGURE 32–6 Mitral valve echogram in a patient with rheumatic mitral stenosis demonstrating limitation and concordance of motion of anterior (AMV) and posterior (PMV) leaflets, with thickening of the posterior leaflet typical of fibrosclerotic rheumatic mitral stenosis. Note that the PMV moves anteriorly (upward) during diastole. Also, there is a diminished E–F slope and slurring of the rapid and slow filling phases of mitral valve motion. The posterior wall (PW) of the left ventricle exhibits a continuous upward motion during diastole (i.e., diastolic filling), suggesting at least moderately severe mitral stenosis. In addition, high-frequency diastolic vibrations of the anterior leaflet (arrow) are noted, indicative of concomitant aortic regurgitation. (IVS = interventricular septum.)

sectional[81,84,89,90] echocardiography is more accurate than M-mode echocardiography in determining mitral orifice size (Figure 5–39, p. 110).

Other important echocardiographic findings in patients with pulmonary hypertension and mitral stenosis include a small or absent *a* wave in the pulmonic valve echogram (Figure 5–37, p. 109). The left atrium is usually enlarged, and the left ventricular cavity is normal or reduced in size. M-mode echocardiography is also useful in detecting mitral annular calcification, which may accompany mitral stenosis and in which a band of dense echoes is present in the region of the mitral annulus, in contrast to the thin and delicate echoes recorded from the normal mitral annulus. Two-dimensional echocardiography may be helpful in the preoperative recognition of left atrial thrombus,[91] although the demonstration of a thrombus by the finding of neovascularity on coronary arteriography is probably a more accurate technique.[92]

MANAGEMENT

Medical Treatment

Patients with rheumatic heart disease should receive penicillin prophylaxis for beta-hemolytic streptococcal infections, as outlined on p. 1655, and prophylaxis for bacterial endocarditis, as summarized on p. 1175. Adolescents and young adults should be advised to avoid physically strenuous occupations. Anemia and infections should be treated promptly and aggressively in patients with valvular heart disease.

In symptomatic patients with mitral valve disease, considerable improvement can be expected with oral diuretics and the restriction of sodium intake. Digitalis glycosides do not alter the hemodynamics and usually do not benefit patients with mitral stenosis and sinus rhythm[93] but are helpful in the treatment of right-sided heart failure. However, as pointed out below, cardiac glycosides are of greatest value in slowing the ventricular rate in patients with atrial fibrillation.

Measures designed to reduce pulmonary venous pressure, including sedation, assumption of the upright posture, and aggressive diuresis, are used to treat hemoptysis. If operation is not to be carried out, oral anticoagulants should be administered to patients with mitral stenosis who have suffered systemic emboli, as well as patients who are at high risk of embolization, i.e., those who are in atrial fibrillation, especially if they are older than 40 years and have a greatly enlarged left atrium.

Treatment of Arrhythmias. Frequent premature atrial contractions often presage atrial fibrillation, and the administration of antiarrhythmic drugs, as outlined on p. 700, may be effective in preventing this complication. However, once atrial fibrillation has developed, these agents may be ineffective in restoring sinus rhythm or even in maintaining sinus rhythm following electrical cardioversion, because of pathological changes that occur in the atrium secondary to the arrhythmia itself.[34] After electrical cardioversion, sinus rhythm can often be maintained with antiarrhythmic drugs in young patients with mild mitral stenosis without marked left atrial enlargement who have been in atrial fibrillation less than 6 months and who have been treated with adequate doses of quinidine. In any event, if elective cardioversion (pharmacological or electrical) is to be attempted in the patient with mitral stenosis and atrial fibrillation, a preparatory 3- to 4-week course of anticoagulation should be given to minimize the risk of systemic embolism when sinus rhythm has resumed. Immediate treatment of atrial fibrillation should be directed toward reducing the ventricular rate by means of digitalis and, if possible, toward reestablishing sinus rhythm by a combination of pharmacological treatment and cardioversion (p. 700). However, it must be appreciated that in 1 to 2 per cent of patients with mitral stenosis, systemic embolism develops following electrical or pharmacological cardioversion. Paroxysmal atrial fibrillation and repeated conversions, spontaneous or induced, carry the risk of embolization.[94] Following reversion to sinus rhythm, administration of quinidine or a similar antiarrhythmic agent should be continued indefinitely in order to diminish the likelihood of recurrent fibrillation. In patients who cannot be converted or maintained in sinus rhythm, the ventricular rate at rest should be maintained at approximately 60 to 65 beats/min with digitalis. If this is not possible, small doses of a beta blocker, such as propranolol (10 to 20 mg four times a day), may be added. Repeat cardioversion is not indicated if the patient has not sustained sinus rhythm while on adequate doses of quinidine.

In patients with rheumatic heart disease and heart failure and/or atrial fibrillation, anticoagulant therapy is helpful in preventing venous thrombosis and pulmonary embolism, in reducing the frequency of systemic embolism in patients who have experienced one or more previous embolic episodes, and in reducing the frequency of thromboembolism in patients with prosthetic heart valves. However, there is no firm evidence that anticoagulant therapy reduces the incidence of pulmonary or systemic embolism in patients in sinus rhythm in whom embolic episodes have not previously occurred and who are not in heart failure.

Natural History

The development of effective surgical treatment has obscured our understanding of the natural history of mitral stenosis and, for that matter, of all valvular lesions.[95] Although few meaningful data are available, it appears that after a latent period of 10 to 20 years following an attack of rheumatic fever during which the patient is asymptomatic, it takes approximately 5 to 10 years for most patients to progress from mild disability (i.e., early Class II) to total disability (i.e., Class IV). In the presurgical era, Olesen found 62 per cent 5-year and 38 per cent 10-year survival among patients in New York Heart Association functional Class III but only a 15 per cent 5-year survival rate in patients in Class IV.[96] Among asymptomatic medically treated patients (Class I) with mitral stenosis followed medically, 40 per cent had deteriorated or died within 10 years. Among mildly symptomatic patients (Class II), the comparable number was 80 per cent.[97] In medically treated patients with mitral stenosis or with combined mitral stenosis and regurgitation, Munoz et al. found a 45 per cent 5-year survival rate.[36] In a comparable group of patients subjected to mitral commissurotomy, the 5-year survival rate was substantially better. In an unselected mix of patients with mitral stenosis of varying severity, 80 per cent of the patients were alive after 5 years and 60 per cent after 10 years of medical treatment.[98]

Surgical Treatment

INDICATIONS FOR OPERATION. Patients with mitral stenosis who are asymptomatic or minimally symptomatic frequently remain so for years. However, once symptoms become more severe, the disease progresses relatively rapidly to death, and operation should therefore be carried out in patients with severe mitral stenosis (i.e., a mitral valve orifice size < 1.0 cm^2/m^2 body surface area [BSA]).

There has been considerable debate concerning the need for routine cardiac catheterization in determining whether operation is indicated.[99-101] Although a careful clinical evaluation and noninvasive assessment, particularly using two-dimensional echocardiography, can provide sufficient information to permit an informed decision in the majority of patients, the consequences of valvular surgery, particularly valve replacement, are so profound that I recommend routine preoperative catheterization and angiography in the majority of patients with mitral stenosis who are potential surgical candidates. These studies are particularly helpful in patients (1) with heart murmurs and other findings suggesting the presence of valve lesions in addition to mitral stenosis, (2) with associated chronic obstructive pulmonary disease, (3) in whom left atrial myxoma must be excluded, and (4) who are more than 45 years old and/or who have angina-like chest pain and in whom associated coronary artery disease must be excluded. Critical narrowing of one or more coronary vessels occurs in approximately one-fourth of all patients with severe mitral stenosis; it is more common in men over the age of 45 years who have angina and who have risk factors for coronary artery disease.[102,103] I believe that preoperative catheterization can usually be omitted in the young ($<$ 35 years) patient without angina who has typical symptoms and classic findings of pure mitral stenosis on physical examination and by noninvasive tests, including two-dimensional echocardiography.

Care of mildly symptomatic patients (Class II) must be individualized. If there are no obvious contraindications to operation, left- and right-heart catheterization should be performed to determine the size of the valve orifice. In general, surgery can be deferred in patients with mild stenosis (i.e., mitral valve orifice size > 1.0 cm^2/m^2 BSA), whereas it should be recommended for those with moderate or severe stenosis (i.e., mitral valve orifice size < 1.0 cm^2/m^2 BSA). However, this plan is subject to qualification. For instance, operation might well be deferred in a retired woman in her seventies with modest needs for elevated cardiac output and a mitral valve orifice of 0.8 cm^2/m^2 BSA, whereas a 25-year-old laborer whose family's economic well-being depends on his continued physical exertion might be an excellent candidate for operation, though the mitral valve orifice size is 1.2 cm^2/m^2 BSA.

Because of the high rate of recurrence, operation is also indicated in patients with mitral stenosis in whom systemic embolism has previously occurred, even if they are otherwise asymptomatic and even though there is no definitive evidence that the incidence of recurrent emboli will be significantly reduced. In these cases, anticoagulants should be administered up to the time of operation. Although the risk of operation is higher in patients with advanced disease characterized by severe pulmonary hypertension and right-sided heart failure, surviving patients nearly always show striking clinical and hemodynamic improvement, with a marked reduction in pulmonary vascular pressures. In the pregnant patient with mitral stenosis, operative treatment should be carried out only if serious pulmonary congestion occurs despite intensive medical treatment (p. 1777).

There is no evidence that surgical treatment improves the prognosis of patients with no or only slight functional impairment. Therefore, valvulotomy is *not* indicated in patients who are entirely asymptomatic, except in unusual circumstances. For example, I recently saw a 33-year-old woman with moderately severe mitral stenosis who had hemoptysis and pulmonary edema during the second trimester of a pregnancy at age 31. She then became asymptomatic but wishes to have another child. Hemodynamic study showed a pulmonary wedge pressure of 17 mm Hg and a mitral orifice area of 1.7 cm^2/m^2 BSA. Prophylactic mitral commissurotomy was undertaken in this patient, since it was virtually certain that another pregnancy would result in serious heart failure.

SURGICAL TECHNIQUES. Three basically different operative approaches are available for the treatment of rheumatic mitral stenosis:[104-112] (1) closed mitral commissurotomy; (2) open commissurotomy, i.e., commissurotomy carried out under direct vision with the aid of cardiopulmonary bypass; and (3) mitral valve replacement. *Closed mitral commissurotomy*, performed with the aid of a transventricular dilator, is generally preferred to simple transatrial finger fracture.[109,112] It is an effective operation, provided that mitral regurgitation, atrial thrombosis, or valvular calcification is not serious and that chordal fusion and shortening are not severe. Unfortunately, few patients satisfy all these criteria, and they are difficult to identify preoperatively. Therefore, if this procedure is carried out at all, it is with "pump standby"; if the surgeon is unable to achieve a satisfactory result, the patient is placed on cardiopulmonary bypass, and the commissurotomy is carried out under direct vision. This procedure is rarely used in the United States today, but is more popular in developing nations, where the expense of open-heart surgery is an important factor and where patients with mitral valve disease are younger.[113] In any event, echocardiography is useful in selecting suitable candidates without valvular calcification or dense fibrosis.[90,114]

Most surgeons prefer to carry out *direct-vision* or *open commissurotomy*.[115,116] Cardiopulmonary bypass is established, and in order to obtain a dry, quiet heart, body temperature is usually lowered, the heart is arrested, and the aorta is occluded intermittently (Chap. 55). Thrombi are removed from the atrium and its appendage, and the latter is often amputated in order to remove a potential source of postoperative emboli. The commissures are incised, and, when necessary, fused chordae are separated, the underlying papillary muscle is split, and the valves are debrided of calcium; mild or even moderate mitral regurgitation may be corrected with suture plication or annuloplasty. Left atrial and ventricular pressures are measured after bypass has been discontinued to confirm that the commissurotomy has, in fact, been effective.[107] In patients with atrial fibrillation, conversion to sinus rhythm is carried out at the completion of the operation.

The mortality rate after mitral commissurotomy, whether open or closed, ranges from 1 to 3 per cent, depending on the condition of the patient and the skill of the surgical team.[115] In general, open commissurotomy provides better hemodynamic relief of mitral valve obstruction than does the closed procedure,[117] and the risk of dislodging thrombi from the atrium or calcium from the mitral valve is also less.[115,116] However, it must be recognized that mitral commissurotomy, whether open or closed, is a palliative rather than a curative operation, and even when successful, it merely "turns the clock back." Thus, it does not result in a normal mitral valve but in one resembling the valve as it existed perhaps a decade earlier. Since the valve is not normal postoperatively, turbulent flow may persist in the paravalvular region, and this may well play a role in re-stenosis. These changes are analogous to the development of obstruction in a congenitally bicuspid aortic valve and are not usually the result of recurrent rheumatic fever.

Mitral Re-stenosis. This condition can be diagnosed with certainty only on the basis of three satisfactory hemodynamic investigations: a preoperative study; a second study following a satisfactory operation in which an increase in the size of the valvular orifice can be demonstrated; and a third one after the reappearance of symptoms, when a reduction in size relative to the earlier postoperative study is noted. Based on clinical grounds alone, the incidence of "re-stenosis" has been estimated to range widely, from 2 to 60 per cent;[118] approximately 10 per cent of patients who have undergone mitral commissurotomy require reoperation within 5 years, but that fraction increases to 60 per cent by 10 years.[119] However, the need for reoperation does not necessarily imply re-stenosis. More often, recurrent symptoms are due to an inadequate first operation, with residual stenosis; the presence or development of mitral regurgitation, either at operation or as a consequence of infective endocarditis; the progression of aortic valve disease; or the development of ischemic heart disease. In a study in which the size of the mitral valve orifice was estimated using cross-sectional echocardiography in 18 patients who had undergone successful mitral commissurotomy, no change in the mitral valve area occurred over a 10- to 14-year period in 13 patients, whereas in 5 (28 per cent) true re-stenosis developed.[119] Approximately 10 per cent of patients returning to the hospital with persistent or recurrent symptoms 6 years after operation have true re-stenosis.[120]

Thus, in properly selected patients, mitral commissurotomy results in a significant increase in the size of the mitral orifice and, at a low risk, favorably alters the clinical course of an otherwise progressive disease. Pulmonary artery pressure falls promptly and decisively when mitral obstruction is effectively relieved.[121–124] Some patients maintain clinical improvement for many (10 to 15) years of follow-up; indeed, fully one-fourth of the patients in functional Class III preoperatively maintain their improvement for 15 years.[33] When a second operation is required because of symptometic deterioration, the valve is often calcified and more seriously deformed than at the time of the first operation, and adequate reconstruction may not be possible. Accordingly, mitral valve replacement is then usually necessary. Also, in patients with combined mitral stenosis and regurgitation, and in those with extensive calcification involving the commissures of the valve, mitral replacement rather than commissurotomy is often required. The operative mortality following mitral valve replacement ranges from 5 to 8 per cent in most hospitals, and as described below (p. 1088), the long-term fate of the prosthetic valves is not yet clear; also, the hazards of lifelong anticoagulant treatment in patients with mechanical prostheses cannot be neglected. Therefore, in patients in whom preoperative evaluation suggests that valve replacement may be required, the threshold for operation should be higher than in patients believed to require commissurotomy alone.

MITRAL REGURGITATION

ETIOLOGY AND PATHOLOGY

The mitral valve apparatus involves the mitral annulus, the mitral leaflets per se, the chordae tendineae, and the papillary muscles. Abnormalities of any of these structures may cause mitral regurgitation (Table 32–3).[1,125–127] The mitral valve prolapse syndrome, an important cause of mitral regurgitation, is discussed in a separate section (p. 1089).

ABNORMALITIES OF VALVE LEAFLETS. Mitral regurgitation due to involvement of the valve leaflets occurs most commonly in chronic rheumatic heart disease and is more frequent in men than in women. It is a consequence of shortening, rigidity, deformity, and retraction of one or both cusps of the mitral valve as well as shortening and fusion of the chordae tendineae and papillary muscles.[128] Destruction of the mitral valve leaflets can also be a consequence of penetrating and nonpenetrating trauma (p. 1535) and of infective endocarditis (Chap. 33). Retraction of the mitral valve cusps during the healing phase of endocarditis can also cause mitral regurgitation.

ABNORMALITIES OF THE MITRAL ANNULUS

Dilatation. In a normal adult the mitral annulus measures approximately 10 cm in circumference. During systole, contraction of the surrounding left ventricular muscle causes the annulus to constrict, and this constriction contributes importantly to valve closure. Mitral regurgitation secondary to dilatation of the mitral annulus (Fig. 32–7) can occur in any form of heart disease characterized by severe dilatation of the left ventricle. It is often difficult to differentiate this secondary from the primary forms of mitral regurgitation (Table 32–4), but it is notable that regurgitation secondary to dilatation of the annulus is usually less severe than primary valvular regurgitation.

Calcification. Idiopathic calcification of the mitral annulus is one of the most common cardiac abnormalities

TABLE 32–3 CAUSES OF MITRAL REGURGITATION

I. *Disorders of the Mitral Valve Leaflets*
  A. Loss of contracture of valvular tissue
      Rheumatic fever
      Infection — bacterial, viral, fungal
      External and direct trauma
      Spontaneous rupture
      Systemic lupus erythematosus
      Methysergide-induced
  B. Incomplete or abnormal valvular development
      Anterior leaflet clefts with AV cushion defect
      Isolated clefts or perforations
      Absence of leaflets
      Redundancy of leaflets
      Congenital fusion of commissures
      Anomalous leaflet attachment
      Ebstein's malformation with corrected transposition
        of the great arteries
  C. Defects of the connective tissue
      Ehlers-Danlos syndrome
      Hurler's syndrome
      Marfan's syndrome
      Pseudoxanthoma elasticum
      Osteogenesis imperfecta
II. *Disorders of the Mitral Annulus*
  A. Calcification
      Degenerative
      Associated with coronary atherosclerosis, hypertension,
        and rheumatic heart disease
      Marfan's syndrome
  B. Destruction of the annulus fibrosus
      Bacterial valve ring abscesses
      Rheumatic fever
      Rheumatoid arthritis
  C. Dilatation of the annulus fibrosus
      Connective tissue disorder
      Left ventricular dilatation
  D. Disruption of ring of prosthetic valve
III. *Disorders of the Chordae Tendineae*
  A. Rupture of chordae tendineae
      Idiopathic
      Bacterial endocarditis
      Trauma
      Marfan's syndrome
      Ehlers-Danlos syndrome
      Rheumatic fever
      Myocardial infarction
      Hypertrophic obstructive cardiomyopathy

  B. Thickened or poorly defined chordae tendineae in association
      with
      Congenital mitral stenosis
      Congenital mitral regurgitation
      AV cushion defect
      Hypoplastic left heart syndrome
      Parachute mitral valve complex
      Supravalvular ring of left atrium
      Carcinoid syndrome
      Hurler's syndrome
  C. Elongated chordae tendineae
      Marfan's syndrome
      Ehlers-Danlos syndrome
      Idiopathic
  D. Arising from an unusual location in association with AV cushion
      defect
      Corrected transposition of great vessels
      Congenital mitral regurgitation
IV. *Disorders of the Papillary Muscles*
  A. Dysfunction or rupture of papillary muscle
      Myocardial infarction — ischemia, fibrosis, rupture
      Bacterial abscess
      Trauma
      Anomalous coronary artery
      Polyarteritis
      Aortic stenosis
      Syphilis
      Sarcoidosis
      Amyloidosis
      Mucocutaneous lymph node syndrome
      Myocardial disease
      Myocarditis
      Temporal disturbance of activation and contraction
  B. Malalignment
      Endocardial fibroelastosis
      Idiopathic hypereosinophilic syndrome
      Dilatation of the left ventricle
      Hypertrophic obstructive cardiomyopathy
      Massive left atrial enlargement
      Ventricular aneurysm
  C. Congenital abnormality in development
      Absent papillary muscle
      Congenital mitral stenosis
      Anomalous mitral arcade

Modified from Silverman, M. E., and Hurst, J. W.: The mitral complex: Clues to its afflictions. *In* Likoff, W. (ed.): Cardiovascular Clinics. Vol. 5, No. 2, Valvular Heart Disease. Philadelphia, F. A. Davis, 1973, pp. 37, 40, 45, and 48.

found at autopsy; in most hearts this degenerative change is of little functional consequence.[128,129] However, when severe it may be an important cause of mitral regurgitation in the elderly, and in contrast to rheumatic fever, this cause is more common in women than in men.[130] In addition to the idiopathic form, degenerative calcification of the mitral annulus is accelerated by systemic hypertension, aortic stenosis, and diabetes, as well as by an intrinsic defect in the fibrous skeleton of the heart, such as occurs in the Marfan and Hurler syndromes. In these two conditions, the mitral annulus not only is calcified but also is dilated, further contributing to mitral regurgitation. The incidence of mitral annular calcification is also increased in patients with hypertrophic obstructive cardiomyopathy[131] and in patients with chronic renal failure with secondary hyperparathyroidism.[132]

When annular calcification is severe, a rigid, curved bar or ring of calcium encircles the mitral orifice, and calcific spurs may project into the adjacent left ventricular myocardium;[133–136] the bulk of the calcium is located in the subvalvular region. The calcification may immobilize the

TABLE 32–4 PRIMARY AND SECONDARY FORMS OF CHRONIC MITRAL REGURGITATION

ANATOMIC OR HEMODYNAMIC FEATURE	PRIMARY	SECONDARY
Mitral valve	Mitral valve apparatus abnormal anatomically and functionally	Normal structural anatomy
Left ventricle	Enlarged	Markedly enlarged
Left atrium	Markedly enlarged	Enlarged
Pulmonary venous redistribution and pulmonary edema	Late in the course	Early
Left ventricular end-diastolic volume	Increased	Markedly increased
Left ventricular end-diastolic pressure	Normal until late in the course	Elevated early
Cardiac output	Normal, with decreases late in the course	Reduced early
Ejection fraction	Increased or normal (> 0.5)	Depressed (< 0.4)

Modified from Haffajee, C. I.: Chronic mitral regurgitation. *In* Dalen, J. E., and Alpert, J. S. (eds.): Valvular Heart Disease. Boston, Little, Brown, and Co., 1981, p. 97.

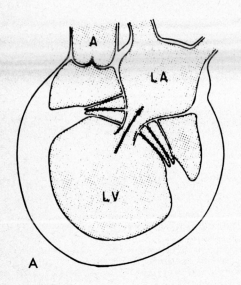
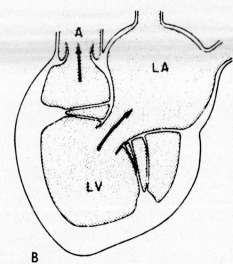

A   B

FIGURE 32–7 Proposed mechanism of regurgitation in left ventricular dilatation. The papillary muscles are displaced laterally and perhaps downward from the ring, permitting leaflet separation and regurgitation during early systole (*A*) and during ejection (*B*). (From Kremkau, E. L., et al.: Acquired, nonrheumatic mitral regurgitation: Clinical management with emphasis on evaluation of myocardial performance. Prog. Cardiovasc. Dis. *15*:414, 1973, by permission of Grune and Stratton, Inc.)

basal portion of the mitral leaflets, preventing their normal excursion in diastole and coaptation in systole and aggravating the mitral regurgitation that results from loss of the normal sphincteric action of the mitral ring. Rarely, when severe calcification encroaches on or protrudes into the mitral orifice, obstruction to left ventricular filling may occur. Calcification of the aortic valve cusps is an associated finding in approximately 50 per cent of patients with severe annular calcification, but this rarely causes aortic stenosis. In patients with severe regurgitation, calcium may invade the conduction system, leading to atrioventricular and/or intraventricular conduction defects.[126] Occasionally, calcific deposits extend into the coronary arteries. The annulus may also become thick and rigid as a consequence of rheumatic involvement, and when this process is severe, it also can interfere with valve closure.

ABNORMALITIES OF THE CHORDAE TENDINEAE. These are important causes of mitral regurgitation (Table 32–3).[137–139] The chordae may be congenitally abnormal, or they may rupture as a consequence of infective endocarditis, trauma, rheumatic fever, or myxomatous proliferation;[140] in most cases no cause for chordal rupture is apparent, other than increased mechanical strain.[141] Patients with idiopathic rupture of mitral chordae tendineae frequently exhibit pathological fibrosis of the papillary muscles, and it is possible that the dysfunction of the papillary muscles may have caused stretching and ultimately rupture of the chordae.[142] Chordal rupture may also result from acute left ventricular dilatation, regardless of etiology. Depending on the number and rate of chordal rupture, the resultant mitral regurgitation may be mild, moderate, or severe on the one hand or acute, subacute, or chronic on the other.

INVOLVEMENT OF THE PAPILLARY MUSCLES. Diseases of the left ventricular papillary muscles frequently cause mitral regurgitation (Table 32–3).[143] Since these muscles are perfused by the terminal portion of the coronary vascular bed,[144] they are particularly vulnerable to ischemia, and any disturbance in coronary perfusion may result in papillary muscle dysfunction (Fig. 32–8). When ischemia is transient, it results in temporary papillary muscle dysfunction and may cause transient episodes of mitral regurgitation during attacks of angina pectoris (p. 1339).

When ischemia is severe and persistent, as in acute myocardial infarction, it produces papillary muscle necrosis and permanent mitral regurgitation (Fig. 32–9). The posterior papillary muscle, which is supplied by the posterior descending branch of the right coronary artery, becomes

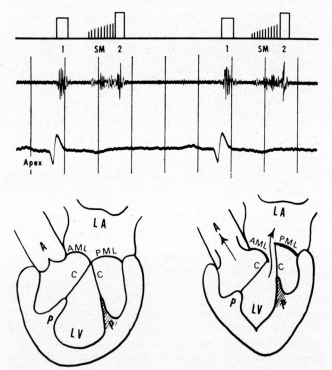

FIGURE 32–8 *Top,* Mitral regurgitation due to papillary muscle dysfunction. At the onset of systole (left), the anterior and posterior mitral valve leaflets (AML and PML) approximate. Later in systole (right), the anterior papillary muscle (P, nonhatched) contracts while the posterior papillary muscle (P, hatched) fails to contract because of ischemia or infarction. Part of the posterior leaflet is allowed to prolapse into the left atrium (LA) during systole, producing regurgitation. This process may involve either papillary muscle. C = chordae tendineae; LV = left ventricle; A = aorta.

Bottom, Late systolic murmur (SM) that developed in a patient following an inferior myocardial infarction and is probably due to weakening of the posterior papillary muscle with prolapse of the mitral leaflet into the atrium during late systole. (From Ravin, A., et al.: Auscultation of the Heart. 3rd ed. Chicago, Year Book Medical Publishers, 1977, p. 99.)

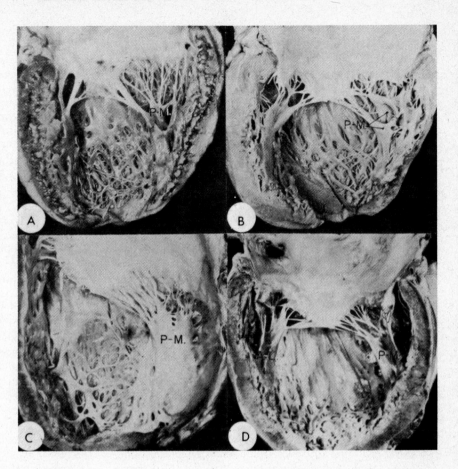

FIGURE 32–9 Myocardial infarction involving the papillary muscles. *A*, Light discoloration of the left ventricular wall in relation to the posteromedial (P-M) papillary muscle represents extensive acute myocardial infarction; the muscle was also infarcted but intact. *B*, Healed myocardial infarction of the distribution shown in *A*. In addition to thinning and scarring of the free wall of the left ventricle, atrophy of the posteromedial papillary muscle has resulted from healing of the infarction. *C*, Infarction of the inferior wall of the left ventricle with aneurysm formation. The endocardium over the infarct site is thickened. The related posteromedial papillary muscle is also involved in the process of infarction. *D*, Healed myocardial infarction of extensive nature in which both anterolateral (A-L) and posteromedial (P-M) papillary muscles are atrophic as the result of infarction and secondary scarring. (From Vlodaver, Z., and Edwards, J. E.: Mitral insufficiency in subjects 50 years of age or older. *In* Edwards, J. E. [ed.]: Clinical-Pathologic Correlations #2, Philadelphia, F. A. Davis, 1973, p. 158.)

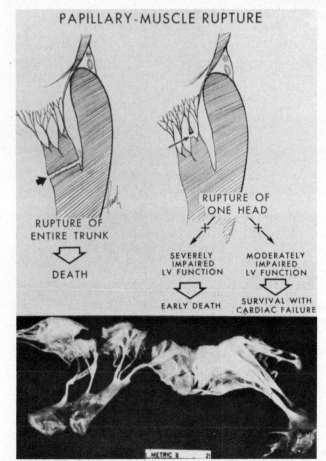

PAPILLARY-MUSCLE RUPTURE

RUPTURE OF ENTIRE TRUNK

DEATH

RUPTURE OF ONE HEAD

SEVERELY IMPAIRED LV FUNCTION

MODERATELY IMPAIRED LV FUNCTION

EARLY DEATH

SURVIVAL WITH CARDIAC FAILURE

ischemic and infarcted more frequently than does the anterolateral papillary muscle, which is supplied by diagonal branches of the left anterior descending coronary artery and often by marginal branches from the left circumflex artery as well. Ischemia of the papillary muscle is caused most commonly by coronary artery disease, but it may also occur in severe anemia, shock, coronary arteritis of any etiology, and anomalous left coronary artery. In pa-

FIGURE 32–10 *Top*, Diagrammatic representation of the types of, and possible consequences of, papillary muscle rupture during acute myocardial infarction. It is likely that rupture of the entire trunk (*left*) is incompatible with survival in any patient, since a major portion of the support to both valve leaflets is destroyed. With rupture of an apical head (*right*), survival would appear to depend on the extent to which left ventricular function has been impaired by the infarct. With severe impairment, the additional burden of even modest mitral regurgitation may be intolerable, and death will ensue. If the left ventricle is less severely compromised, survival is possible for weeks or months, but congestive heart failure will invariably develop.

Bottom, Rupture of a portion of one papillary muscle during acute myocardial infarction in a 51-year-old man who underwent mitral valve replacement 3 months after the onset of infarction. Preoperatively, pulmonary arterial pressure was 60/28 mm Hg (mean = 40); pulmonary arterial wedge pressure, mean = 28, v = 42; left ventricular pressure = 74/17 mm Hg; and cardiac index = 1.7 liters/min/sq meter. The excised mitral valve shows the ventricular aspects of the leaflets. The leaflets are normal, but the posteromedial papillary muscle is necrotic and fibrotic, and a portion of it is entwined in chordae tendineae at the margin of the anterior mitral leaflet. (From Roberts, W. C., et al.: Nonrheumatic valvular cardiac disease. A clinicopathologic survey of 27 different conditions causing valvular dysfunction. *In* Likoff, W. [ed.]: Cardiovascular Clinics. Vol. 5, No. 2, Valvular Heart Disease. Philadelphia, F. A. Davis, 1973, p. 395.)

tients with healed myocardial infarcts, mitral regurgitation is frequent and is caused by dyskinesis of the left ventricular myocardium at the base of a papillary muscle.[145]

Left ventricular dilatation of any cause, including ischemia, can alter the spatial relationships between the papillary muscles and the chordae tendineae and thereby result in mitral regurgitation (Fig. 32–7). Although *necrosis of a papillary muscle* is a frequent complication of myocardial infarction,[146] frank rupture of a papillary muscle is far less common. Total rupture of a papillary muscle is usually fatal because of extremely severe regurgitation, whereas rupture of one or two of the apical heads of a muscle, which results in a lesser degree of mitral regurgitation, makes survival possible, depending on the functional capacity of the left ventricle (Fig. 32–10).

Some degree of mitral regurgitation is found in approximately 30 per cent of those patients with coronary artery disease who are being considered for coronary bypass surgery[145] and is secondary to ischemic damage of the papillary muscles or dilatation of the mitral valve ring or both.[148,149] The incidence and severity of regurgitation vary inversely with the left ventricular ejection fraction and directly with the left ventricular end-diastolic pressure.

A variety of other disorders of papillary muscles may also be responsible for the development of mitral regurgitation (Table 32–3). These include congenital malposition; absence of one papillary muscle, resulting in the so-called parachute mitral valve syndrome (p. 1089); and involvement or infiltration of papillary muscles by a variety of processes, including abscesses, granulomas, neoplasms, amyloidosis and sarcoidosis.[126]

Other causes of mitral regurgitation, discussed in greater detail elsewhere, include a variety of congenital anomalies (p. 985), obstructive cardiomyopathy (p. 1409), prolapse of the mitral valve (p. 1089), trauma (p. 1535), and left atrial myxoma (p. 1466).

PATHOPHYSIOLOGY

Since the regurgitant mitral orifice is in parallel with the aortic valve, the resistance to ventricular emptying (left ventricular afterload) is reduced in mitral regurgitation. Consequently, as the left ventricle decompresses into the left atrium—both during isometric contraction and early during ejection—the left ventricular volume declines. Indeed, Eckberg et al. found that in patients with mitral regurgitation almost one-half the regurgitant volume is ejected into the left atrium before the aortic valve opens.[150]

The volume of mitral regurgitant flow depends on the size of the regurgitant orifice as well as on the pressure gradient between the left ventricle and left atrium;[151-153] both of these factors—orifice size and pressure gradient— are labile. Left ventricular systolic pressure and therefore the left ventricular–left atrial gradient are dependent on systemic vascular resistance and forward stroke volume,[151] and in patients in whom the mitral annulus is not calcific or rigid, the cross-sectional area of the mitral annulus may be altered by many interventions.[154] Thus, increases of both preload[155] and afterload and depressions of contractility increase left ventricular size and enlarge the mitral regurgitant orifice. In mitral regurgitation caused by conditions in which the mitral valve apparatus is not rigid, such as ven-

tricular dilatation due to ischemic heart disease, hypertensive heart disease or cardiomyopathy, dysfunction of papillary muscles, and rupture of chordae tendineae, the volume of regurgitant flow is influenced significantly by left ventricular dimensions, which in turn affect the regurgitant orifice. When ventricular size is reduced by treatment with cardiac glycosides, diuretics and particularly vasodilators, the volume of regurgitant flow may become diminished, as reflected in the height of the v wave in the left atrial pressure pulse (Figure 16–19, p. 540) and in the intensity and duration of the systolic murmur. Conversely, left ventricular dilatation may increase mitral regurgitation.

In experiments in which the acute effects of equally severe mitral and aortic regurgitation on the left ventricle were compared, left ventricular end-diastolic pressure, volume, and radius rose with both lesions, but far less so with mitral regurgitation.[156,157] Peak left ventricular wall tension rose markedly when aortic regurgitation was induced but either did not change greatly or actually declined with mitral regurgitation. According to Laplace's law (p. 431), myocardial wall tension is related to the product of intraventricular pressure and ventricular radius. Since mitral regurgitation reduces both late systolic ventricular pressure and radius, left ventricular wall tension declines markedly (and proportionately to a greater extent than left ventricular pressure), permitting the velocity of myocardial fiber shortening to increase.

At any given left ventricular end-diastolic and aortic systolic pressures, mitral regurgitation reduces the tension developed by the left ventricular myocardium. The reduced load on the ventricle allows a greater proportion of the contractile energy of the myocardium to be expended in shortening than in tension development and explains how the left ventricle can adapt to the load imposed by chronic mitral regurgitation. Thus, it appears to be the reduction in left ventricular tension in mitral regurgitation that allows the left ventricle to increase its total output and ultimately accounts for the finding that patients with mitral regurgitation can sustain large regurgitant volumes for prolonged periods while maintaining forward cardiac output at normal levels for many years. Although the left ventricle initially compensates for the development of acute mitral regurgitation, in part by emptying more completely,[151] as regurgitation persists or increases, the function of the left ventricle deteriorates, and left ventricular end-diastolic volume increases progressively (Fig. 32–11). This may enlarge the regurgitant orifice and thereby create a vicious cycle in which "mitral regurgitation begets more mitral regurgitation."

A large volume of mitral regurgitation induced experimentally produces increased myocardial oxygen consumption only slightly,[158] because myocardial fiber shortening, which is elevated in mitral regurgitation, is not as important a determinant of myocardial oxygen consumption[159] (p. 1238) as are the three major factors.[159] One of these, tension, may be reduced, whereas the other two, contractility and heart rate, are little affected in this condition. In addition, the duration of left ventricular systolic tension is reduced in mitral regurgitation. These experimental observations correlate with the low incidence of clinical manifestations of myocardial ischemia in patients with severe

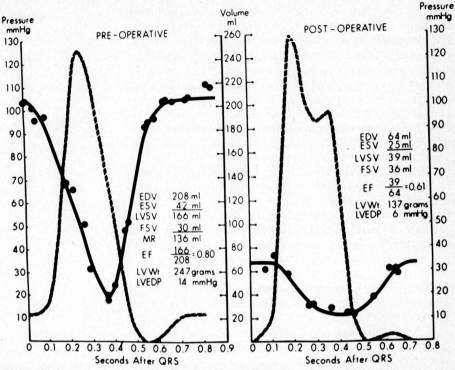

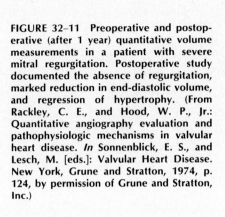

FIGURE 32–11 Preoperative and postoperative (after 1 year) quantitative volume measurements in a patient with severe mitral regurgitation. Postoperative study documented the absence of regurgitation, marked reduction in end-diastolic volume, and regression of hypertrophy. (From Rackley, C. E., and Hood, W. P., Jr.: Quantitative angiography evaluation and pathophysiologic mechanisms in valvular heart disease. *In* Sonnenblick, E. S., and Lesch, M. [eds.]: Valvular Heart Disease. New York, Grune and Stratton, 1974, p. 124, by permission of Grune and Stratton, Inc.)

mitral regurgitation, compared with that occurring in patients with aortic stenosis or regurgitation or both, in which myocardial oxygen demands are augmented.

In patients with chronic regurgitation, both left ventricular end-diastolic volume and mass are increased, with the degree of hypertrophy appropriate to the left ventricular dilatation, so that the ratio of left ventricular mass to end-diastolic volume is normal (Figure 13–7, p. 452).[26] In acute mitral regurgitation, on the other hand, the left ventricle dilates rapidly; and before the myocardium becomes hypertrophied, the ratio of left ventricular mass to end-diastolic volume is reduced, i.e., the left ventricle is thin-walled (Table 14–1, p. 474).

Patients with severe mitral regurgitation may actually exhibit small elevations in ejection phase indices of myocardial contractility (p. 480), such as ejection fraction, extent, and velocity of circumferential fiber shortening (VCF) when they are in the compensated state as a consequence of reduced afterload.[160,161] However, by the time patients become symptomatic,[162] peak and mean VCF have usually declined to normal levels. As mitral regurgitation persists, the tendency for a low impedance leak, which tends to increase myocardial shortening, is counteracted by the impairment of myocardial function characteristic of chronic overload. However, even in patients with overt heart failure secondary to valvular regurgitation, the ejection fraction and fractional fiber shortening may be only slightly reduced.[161,163] Therefore, *normal* values for the ejection phase indices of myocardial performance in patients with severe mitral regurgitation may actually reflect impaired myocardial function, whereas a moderately reduced value (e.g., an ejection fraction of 40 to 50 per cent) generally signifies severe, not moderate, impairment of contractility. An ejection fraction under 40 per cent in patients with marked mitral regurgitation represents advanced myocardial dysfunction; such patients are high operative risks and may not experience marked improvement follow-

ing mitral valve replacement, perhaps because of the increase in left ventricular afterload that occurs with abolition of the regurgitant leak.[164] In patients with chronic mitral regurgitation, there is often an increase in left ventricular compliance, so that ventricular end-diastolic volume may be increased with little or no elevation of end-diastolic pressure.[165]

End-systolic Volume. Preoperative myocardial contractility is an important determinant of the risk of cardiac failure in the perioperative period and of the level of left ventricular function postoperatively. Therefore, it is not surprising that end-systolic volume has emerged as a useful index for evaluating left ventricular function in patients with valvular regurgitation (p. 475). Indeed, this value was found to be more useful as a predictor of outcome than the ejection fraction, end-diastolic volume, or end-diastolic pressure.[166,167,167a] Patients with severe mitral regurgitation with a normal preoperative end-systolic volume (< 30 ml/m²) retained normal left ventricular function postoperatively, whereas marked enlargement of the end-systolic volume (> 90 ml/m²) signified a high perioperative mortality and residual left ventricular dysfunction. Patients with mitral regurgitation and modest enlargement of end-systolic volume (between 30 and 90 ml/m²) usually tolerate operation satisfactorily but may have reduced left ventricular function postoperatively. For any level of end-systolic volume, patients with mitral regurgitation have more severe left ventricular dysfunction than do patients with aortic regurgitation. This finding reflects the lower afterload in mitral regurgitation and correlates with the clinical observation that patients with mitral regurgitation have a less favorable response to surgical intervention than do those with aortic regurgitation.[168,169]

Effective (forward) *cardiac output* is usually depressed in seriously symptomatic patients, whereas total left ventricular output (the sum of forward and regurgitant flow, which can be measured by radionuclide ventriculography)[170] is usually elevated. The atrial contraction (*a*) wave in the left atrial pressure pulse is usually not as prominent in mitral regurgitation as in mitral stenosis, but the *v* wave is often much taller, since it is inscribed during ventricular systole, when the left atrium is filled with blood from the pulmonary veins as well as from the left ventricle (Fig. 32–12). During early diastole, as the distended left atrium suddenly empties, the *y* descent is particularly rapid. However, in patients with combined mitral stenosis and regurgitation, the *y* descent is gradual. Although a left atrioventricular pressure gradient persisting throughout diastole signifies the presence of significant associated mitral stenosis, a brief, early diastolic gradient may occur in patients with pure, severe regurgitation as a result of the torrential flow of blood across a normal-sized mitral orifice.

LEFT ATRIAL COMPLIANCE. The compliance of the left atrium (and pulmonary venous bed) is an important determinant of the hemodynamic and clinical picture in mitral regurgitation. Three major subgroups of patients with severe mitral regurgitation based on left atrial compliance have been identified[157,171,172] (Fig. 32–13) and are characterized as follows:

1. Normal or Reduced Compliance. There is little enlargement of the left atrium but marked elevation of the mean left atrial pressure, particularly of the *v* wave,[26,173,174] and pulmonary congestion is a prominent symptom. In most cases, severe mitral regurgitation has developed suddenly, as occurs with rupture of chordae tendineae, infarction of one of the heads of a papillary muscle, or perforation of a mitral leaflet as a consequence of trauma or endocarditis. Sinus rhythm is usually present; the left atrial wall frequently exhibits striking hypertrophy, is capable of contracting vigorously, and facilitates left ventricular filling. Thickening of the walls of the pulmonary veins and proliferative changes in the pulmonary arteries as well as marked elevation of pulmonary vascular resistance usually develop over the course of 6 to 12 months.

2. Markedly Increased Compliance. At the opposite end of the spectrum from patients in the first group are those with severe, longstanding mitral regurgitation with massive

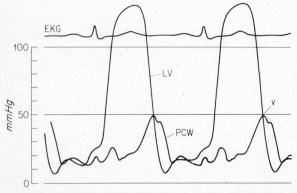

FIGURE 32–12 Pressure tracings from a 59-year-old man with shortness of breath on exertion, a loud systolic murmur, and evidence of ruptured chordae tendineae on echocardiogram. The pulmonary capillary wedge (PCW) pressure is elevated (mean = 25 mm Hg), with a markedly increased regurgitant (*v*) wave peaking at 50 mm Hg. In addition, left ventricular end-diastolic pressure is elevated to 27 mm Hg. These findings are consistent with severe mitral regurgitation.

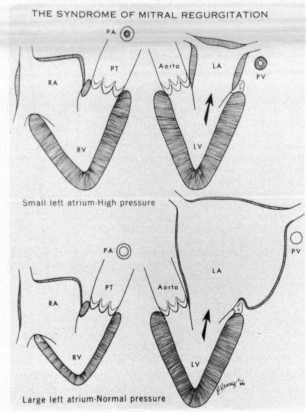

THE SYNDROME OF MITRAL REGURGITATION

Small left atrium-High pressure

Large left atrium-Normal pressure

FIGURE 32–13 Diagram depicting the two extremes of the spectrum in pure mitral regurgitation. When severe mitral regurgitation appears suddenly in individuals with previously normal or near-normal hearts, the left atrium (LA) is relatively small and the high pressure within it is reflected back into the pulmonary vessels and right ventricle (RV). The anatomical indicator of this latter physiological event is severe hypertrophy of the left atrial and right ventricular walls and marked intimal proliferation and medial hypertrophy of the pulmonary arteries (PA), arterioles, and veins (PV). At the other extreme, the left atrial cavity is of giant size and its wall is thin. It is thus able to "absorb" the left ventricular (LV) pressure without reflecting it back into the pulmonary vessels or right ventricle. As a consequence, pulmonary vessels remain normal, and the right ventricular wall does not thicken. PT = pulmonary trunk; RA = right atrium. (From Roberts, W. C., et al.: Nonrheumatic valvular cardiac disease. A clinicopathologic survey of 27 different conditions causing valvular dysfunction. *In* Likoff, W. [ed.]: Cardiovascular Clinics. Vol. 5, No. 2, Valvular Heart Disease. Philadelphia, F. A. Davis, 1973, p. 403.)

enlargement of the left atrium and normal or only slightly elevated left atrial pressure. The atrial wall contains only a small remnant of muscle surrounded by a great deal of fibrous tissue. Longstanding mitral regurgitation in these patients has altered the physical properties of the left atrial wall and thereby displaced the atrial pressure-volume curve, allowing a normal or almost normal pressure to exist in a greatly enlarged left atrium. Pulmonary artery pressure and pulmonary vascular resistance are normal or only slightly elevated at rest. Atrial fibrillation and a low cardiac output are almost invariably present.[171]

3. Moderately Increased Compliance. This, the most common subgroup, consists of patients between the ends of the spectrum represented by groups 1 and 2; these patients have severe chronic regurgitation and exhibit variable degrees of enlargement of the left atrium, associated with significant elevation of the left atrial pressure.

CLINICAL MANIFESTATIONS
(See Table 32–1, p. 1067)
History

The symptoms of patients with chronic mitral regurgitation are a function of the severity of regurgitation, its rate of progression, the level of pulmonary artery pressure, and the presence of associated valvular or coronary artery disease in patients with chronic rheumatic mitral regurgitation.[175] Since symptoms do not develop until the left ventricle fails, the time interval between the initial attack of rheumatic fever (when one has occurred) and the development of symptoms tends to be longer than in mitral stenosis and often exceeds two decades. The incidence of acute pulmonary edema is lower in chronic mitral regurgitation than in mitral stenosis, presumably because sudden surges in left atrial pressure are less frequent.[14] Similarly, although hemoptysis and systemic embolization do occur in mitral regurgitation, they are less common than in mitral stenosis. On the other hand, chronic weakness and fatigue secondary to a low cardiac output are more prominent.

Patients with mild mitral regurgitation may remain asymptomatic for their entire lives, and the majority of patients with mitral regurgitation of rheumatic origin have only mild disability, unless regurgitation progresses as a result of chronic rheumatic activity, infective endocarditis, or rupture of chordae tendineae.[176] The development of atrial fibrillation affects the course adversely but not as dramatically as it does in mitral stenosis, since rapid ventricular rate often caused by this arrhythmia does *not* elevate left atrial pressure as markedly in mitral regurgitation.

In patients with severe chronic mitral regurgitation with a greatly enlarged left atrium and with relatively mild left atrial hypertension (group 2 with increased left atrial compliance, described above), pulmonary vascular resistance does not usually rise. Instead, the major symptoms, i.e., fatigue and exhaustion, are related to a low cardiac output. In contrast, in patients with acute mitral regurgitation with a normal-sized left atrium (group 1 with normal or reduced left atrial compliance, described above), the left atrial pressure rises abruptly, possibly leading to pulmonary edema, marked elevation of pulmonary vascular resistance, and right-sided heart failure. The last, characterized by congestive hepatomegaly, ankle edema, and ascites, however, is also observed, both in patients with longstanding severe mitral regurgitation and in patients with acute regurgitation and elevated pulmonary vascular resistance. Angina pectoris is rare unless coronary artery disease coexists.

Natural History. This is variable and depends on a combination of the volume of regurgitation, the state of the myocardium, and the etiology of the underlying disorder. Asymptomatic patients with mild mitral regurgitation usually remain stable for many years;[177] severe regurgitation develops in only a small percentage of these, in some cases because of intervening infective endocarditis[176] or rupture of chordae tendineae. Regurgitation tends to progress more rapidly in patients with connective tissue diseases, such as Marfan's syndrome, than in those with chronic regurgitation on a rheumatic basis. In an unselected group of patients with mitral regurgitation who were treated medically, approximately 80 per cent survived 5 years after the

diagnosis had been established and almost 60 per cent survived 10 years;[98] patients with combined mitral stenosis and regurgitation had a poorer prognosis, with only 67 per cent surviving 5 years and 30 per cent surviving 10 years after the diagnosis. Munoz et al., in studying a group of patients with greater disability, found that medically treated patients with severe mitral regurgitation had a 5-year survival rate of only 45 per cent.[36] Among medically treated patients with mitral regurgitation, the arteriovenous oxygen difference and ventricular end-diastolic volume were significant (inverse) predictors of survival.[178]

Physical Examination

Palpation of the arterial pulse is helpful in differentiating aortic stenosis from mitral regurgitation, both of which may produce a prominent systolic murmur at the base of the heart; the carotid arterial upstroke is sharp in mitral regurgitation[179] and delayed in aortic stenosis; the volume of the pulse may be normal in both conditions or reduced in the presence of heart failure.

The cardiac impulse is brisk, hyperdynamic, and displaced to the left[14] (Fig. 3–28, p. 59), and a prominent left ventricular filling wave is frequently palpable in early diastole. A presystolic apical impulse is rarely palpable, except in patients with acute regurgitation. Systolic expansion of the enlarged left atrium may result in a late systolic thrust in the parasternal region, which may be confused with right ventricular enlargement (p. 30).[180] Rarely, a greatly enlarged left atrium may be palpable in the third left intercostal space during systole.[14]

AUSCULTATION. With severe, chronic mitral regurgitation due to defective valve cusps, S_1, produced by valve closure, is usually diminished. Wide splitting of S_2 is common and results from the shortening of left ventricular ejection and an earlier A_2 as a consequence of reduced resistance to left ventricular outflow. When pulmonary hypertension is present, P_2 is louder than A_2. The abnormal increase in the flow rate across the mitral orifice during the rapid filling phase is usually associated with an S_3, the auscultatory counterpart of a palpable rapid filling wave (Fig. 3–1, p. 41). A left ventricular S_3, i.e., one that is not augmented by inspiration, excludes predominant mitral stenosis (unless aortic regurgitation, ischemic heart disease, or another cause of an S_3 is present).

The *systolic murmur* is the most prominent physical finding in mitral regurgitation; it must be differentiated from the systolic murmur heard in aortic stenosis, tricuspid regurgitation, and ventricular septal defect (Table 32–5). In most cases of severe mitral regurgitation, the *systolic murmur* commences immediately after the soft S_1 (Fig. 32–5) and continues beyond and may obscure A_2 because of the persistence of the pressure difference between the left ventricle and left atrium (Fig. 4–2, p. 69). The holosystolic murmur of chronic mitral regurgitation is usually constant in intensity, blowing, high-pitched, and loudest at the apex (Fig. 4–11, p. 74) with radiation to the axilla and left infrascapular area; however, radiation toward the sternum or the aortic area may occur with abnormalities of the posterior leaflet. The murmur shows little change even in the presence of large beat-to-beat variations of left ventricular stroke volume, as occur in atrial fibrillation,[181] in contrast

TABLE 32–5 HELPFUL POINTS IN DIFFERENTIAL DIAGNOSIS OF MITRAL REGURGITATION, VENTRICULAR SEPTAL DEFECT, TRICUSPID REGURGITATION, AND AORTIC STENOSIS

PHYSICAL, ROENTGENOGRAPHIC, OR ELECTROCARDIOGRAPHIC FEATURE	MITRAL REGURGITATION	VENTRICULAR SEPTAL DEFECT	TRICUSPID REGURGITATION	AORTIC STENOSIS
Systolic murmur	Harsh and pansystolic	Harsh and pansystolic	Pansystolic	Ejection, crescendo-decrescendo
Primary location of murmur	Apex	Left sternal border	Left sternal border	Base of heart; occasionally apical
Radiation of murmur	Axilla; occasionally base and neck	Left precordium	Little	Carotids
Thrill	Occasionally present at apex	Usually present at left sternal border	Rare	Occasionally present at base
Murmur with inspiration	No change	No change	Increases	No change
Valsalva maneuver	May increase	Increases or no change	No change	Decreases
Venous pressure	Often normal	Slightly elevated with prominent *a* and *v* waves	Elevated, with very prominent *v* waves	Usually normal
Pulsatile liver	No	No	Yes	No
Pulmonary component of S₂	Normal; occasionally increased	Normal or loud; usually delayed	Usually increased	Normal
Apical impulse	Hyperkinetic; occasional heaving	Hyperkinetic	Weak or normal	Forceful and sustained
ECG	Left ventricular hypertrophy; left atrial hypertrophy	Biventricular hypertrophy	Right ventricular hypertrophy, occasional right atrial hypertrophy	Left ventricular hypertrophy with associated ST-T changes
Chest roentgenogram	Moderately enlarged heart, marked left atrial enlargement	Enlarged left and right ventricles	Enlarged right ventricle	Normal heart size or left ventricular hypertrophy

Reproduced with permission from Haffajee, C. I.: Chronic mitral regurgitation. *In* Dalen, J. E., and Alpert, J. S. (eds.): Valvular Heart Disease. Boston, Little, Brown and Co., 1981, p. 97.

to most midsystolic (ejection) murmurs, such as in aortic stenosis, which vary greatly in intensity with stroke volume and therefore with the duration of diastole.[182] There is little correlation between the intensity of the systolic murmur and the severity of mitral regurgitation. Indeed, in patients with severe mitral regurgitation due to left ventricular dilatation or paraprosthetic valvular regurgitation or in those who have marked emphysema, obesity, or chest deformity, the systolic murmur may be soft or even absent.[183]

Pansystolic and late systolic murmurs are both characteristic of mitral regurgitation. When the murmur is confined to late systole, the regurgitation is usually mild and may be secondary to prolapse of the mitral valve or papillary muscle dysfunction, conditions that cause late systolic regurgitation. These causes of mitral regurgitation are frequently associated with a normal S₁ because initial closure of the mitral valve cusps may be unimpaired. The systolic murmur is usually of no more than Grade 3/6 intensity, is a mid to late diamond-shaped murmur (Fig. 32–8), or exhibits late systolic accentuation and radiates more frequently to the lower left sternal border than to the axilla.[143] The murmur of papillary muscle dysfunction is particularly variable; it may become accentuated or holosystolic during acute myocardial ischemia and often disappears when ischemia is relieved.[184] The response of a mid- to late-systolic murmur to a number of maneuvers, as described on page 1091, helps to establish the diagnosis of prolapse of the mitral valve.

DYNAMIC AUSCULTATION. The holosystolic murmur of rheumatic mitral regurgitation shows little variation during respiration. However, sudden standing and amyl nitrite inhalation usually diminish the murmur (Table 32–6), whereas squatting and methoxamine or phenylephrine augment it. The murmur is reduced during the strain of the Valsalva maneuver and shows a left-sided response, i.e., a transient overshoot, six to eight beats following release. The murmur is usually intensified by isometric exercise, differentiating it from the systolic murmurs of valvular aortic stenosis and hypertrophic obstructive car-

TABLE 32–6 EFFECT OF VARIOUS INTERVENTIONS ON SYSTOLIC MURMURS

INTERVENTION	HYPERTROPHIC OBSTRUCTIVE CARDIOMYOPATHY	AORTIC STENOSIS	MITRAL REGURGITATION	MITRAL PROLAPSE
Valsalva	↑	↓	↓	↑ or ↓
Standing	↑	↑ or unchanged	↓	↑
Handgrip or squatting	↓	↓ or unchanged	↑	↓
Supine position with legs elevated	↓	↑ or unchanged	Unchanged	↓
Exercise	↑	↑ or unchanged	↓	↑
Amyl nitrite	↑↑	↑	↓	↑
Isoproterenol	↑↑	↑	↓	↑

↑↑ = Markedly increased.

Modified from Paraskos, J. A.: Combined valvular disease. *In* Dalen, J. E., and Alpert, J. S. (eds.): Valvular Heart Disease. Boston, Little, Brown and Co., 1981, p. 365.

diomyopathy, both of which are reduced by this intervention. The murmur of mitral regurgitation due to left ventricular dilatation decreases in intensity and duration with effective therapy with cardiac glycosides, diuretics, rest, and particularly vasodilators.

The holosystolic murmur of mitral regurgitation resembles that produced by a ventricular septal defect. However, the latter is usually loudest at the left sternal border rather than the apex and is often accompanied by a parasternal thrill. The murmur of mitral regurgitation may also be confused with that of tricuspid regurgitation, which is usually heard best along the left sternal border, is augmented during inspiration, and is accompanied by a prominent v wave and y descent in the jugular venous pulse.

When the chordae tendineae to the posterior leaflet of the mitral valve rupture, the regurgitant jet is often directed anteriorly, so that it impinges on the atrial septum adjacent to the aortic root and causes a systolic murmur most prominent at the base of the heart, which can be confused with that of aortic stenosis. The acoustic energy derived from the mitral regurgitant jet may be transmitted to the aorta by the impact of the jet on the portion of the left atrial wall adjacent to the aortic root.[185] On the other hand, when the chordae to the anterior leaflet rupture, the jet is usually directed to the posterior wall of the left atrium, and the murmur may be transmitted to the spine or even to the top of the head.[186] Because the v wave is markedly elevated in acute mitral regurgitation, the pressure gradient between the left ventricle and atrium declines at the end of systole, and the murmur may not be holosystolic but decrescendo, ending well before A_2 (Figure 4–16, p. 77). It is usually lower pitched and softer than the murmur of chronic mitral regurgitation. Pulmonary hypertension, common in acute mitral regurgitation, may increase the intensity of P_2 and the murmurs of pulmonary and tricuspid regurgitation, and right-sided S_4 may develop.

Patients with rheumatic disease of the mitral valve exhibit a spectrum of abnormalities, ranging from pure stenosis to pure regurgitation[187] (Fig. 32–5). The presence of an S_3, a rapid left ventricular filling wave and left ventricular impulse on palpation, and a soft S_1 all favor predominant regurgitation, whereas an accentuated S_1, a prominent OS with a short A_2-OS interval, and a soft short systolic murmur all point to predominant stenosis. Elucidation of the predominant valvular lesion may be complicated by the presence of a holosystolic murmur of tricuspid regurgitation in patients with pure mitral stenosis and pulmonary hypertension; this murmur, as has already been noted, may sometimes be heard at the apex when the right ventricle is greatly enlarged and may therefore be mistaken for the murmur of mitral regurgitation. Many patients with severe tricuspid regurgitation have a low cardiac output and an inaudible or barely audible diastolic murmur of mitral stenosis, further complicating the clinical diagnosis. An S_3 originating from the right ventricle in patients with mitral stenosis and pulmonary hypertension may falsely suggest the presence of mitral regurgitation. On the other hand, systolic expansion of the left atrium, as occurs in severe mitral regurgitation, often produces a late systolic parasternal expansion that may be confused with right ventricular hypertrophy and falsely attributed to mitral stenosis.

Laboratory Examination

ELECTROCARDIOGRAM AND VECTORCARDIO-GRAM. The principal *electrocardiographic* findings in patients with mitral regurgitation are left atrial enlargement and atrial fibrillation.[62,188,189] Electrocardiographic evidence of left ventricular enlargement occurs in about half the patients with severe mitral regurgitation. Approximately 15 per cent exhibit electrocardiographic evidence of right ventricular hypertrophy, a change which reflects the presence of pulmonary hypertension of sufficient severity to counterbalance not only the normally larger but actually hypertrophied left ventricle. The *vectorcardiogram* often shows left ventricular hypertrophy, with initial forces directed to the right and anteriorly, whereas the maximal QRS vector is directed to the left, posteriorly, and inferiorly, with an increased magnitude usually exceeding 2.0 mv; the T loop is usually discordant with respect to the QRS.[69-71] Vectorcardiographic evidence of combined right and left ventricular hypertrophy or right ventricular hypertrophy Type C, Figure 7–17, p. 213) is less common[63,190] and, as is the case for the electrocardiogram, reflects severe pulmonary hypertension.

RADIOLOGICAL FINDINGS (See also p. 163) Cardiomegaly with left ventricular, and particularly with left atrial, enlargement is a common finding in patients with chronic severe mitral regurgitation.[78,191] However, there is little correlation between left atrial size and pressure. Acute valvular regurgitation, even if severe, often does not increase overall cardiac size and may produce only mild left atrial enlargement despite marked elevation of left atrial pressure, as already noted. Changes in the lung fields are less prominent in mitral regurgitation than in mitral stenosis, but interstitial edema with Kerley B lines is frequently seen with acute regurgitation or with progressive left ventricular failure.

In patients with combined stenosis and regurgitation, overall cardiac enlargement and particularly left atrial dilatation are prominent findings. However, it is usually difficult to determine which lesion is predominant from the plain chest roentgenogram, since it may be difficult to distinguish between right and left ventricular enlargement. Predominant mitral stenosis is suggested by relatively mild cardiomegaly with significant changes in the lung fields, whereas predominant regurgitation is more likely when the heart is greatly enlarged and the changes in the lungs are relatively slight. When the left atrium is aneurysmally dilated, regurgitation is almost always the dominant lesion. Calcification of the mitral valve occurs in patients with stenosis, regurgitation, or mixed lesions.

Calcification of the mitral annulus, an important cause of mitral regurgitation in the elderly, is most prominent in the posterior third of the cardiac silhouette[78] and is best visualized on films exposed in the lateral or right anterior oblique projection, in which it appears as a dense, coarse, C-shaped opacity (Figure 6–24, p. 163).

The diagnosis of mitral regurgitation can be established by means of left *ventricular angiocardiography,*[192] the prompt appearance of contrast material in the left atrium following its injection into the left ventricle indicating the presence of mitral regurgitation. The injection should be rapid enough to permit left ventricular opacification but slow enough to avoid the development of premature ventricular contractions, which can induce spurious regurgitation.

The regurgitant volume can be determined from the difference between the total left ventricular stroke volume, estimated angiocardiographically, and the simultaneous measurement of the effective forward stroke volume by Fick's method. The results of such studies suggest that in patients with severe regurgitation, the regurgitant volume is of the same magnitude as, or may even exceed, the effective forward stroke volume.

Qualitative, but clinically useful estimates of the severity of regurgitation may be made by (cine)angiographic observation of the degree of opacification of the left atrium and pulmonary veins following the injection of contrast material into the left ventricle. Mitral regurgitation secondary to rheumatic heart disease is characterized angiographically by a central regurgitant jet and by thickened leaflets that exhibit reduced motion, whereas in regurgitation due to other causes, particularly dilatation of the mitral annulus or ruptured chordae and papillary muscles, the systolic jet may be eccentric, and the valves consist of thin filaments

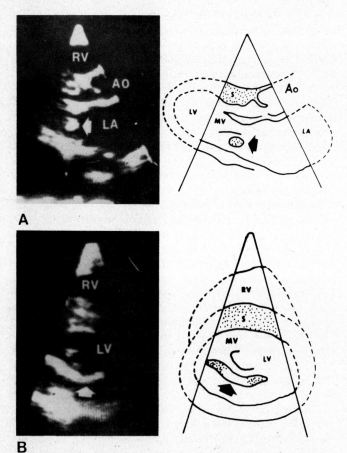

FIGURE 32–14   Long-axis (*A*) and short-axis (*B*) sector scans from a patient with mitral annular calcification (arrows). Atrioventricular junction in *A* was identified by the differing wall motion of the left atrium and the left ventricle, as seen on real-time recording and by location of the mitral valve. The extent of calcification can be appreciated only on the short-axis view. Ao = aorta; LA = left atrium; RV = right ventricle; LV = left ventricle; MV = mitral valve; S = interventricular septum. (Reproduced with permission from Kronzon, I., Mitchell, J., Shapiro, J., et al.: Two-dimensional echocardiography in mitral annulus calcification. Am. J. Radiol. *134*: 355, 1980.)

that display excessive motion.[170] The etiology of the regurgitation, e.g., prolapse of the mitral valve, and a flail leaflet are often distinguishable angiographically (Figure 32–8, p. 1094).

ECHOCARDIOGRAPHY (see also p. 111).   M-mode and two-dimensional echocardiography are more useful in determining the etiology than in estimating the severity of mitral regurgitation.[193,194] Severe mitral regurgitation results in enlargement of the left atrium and left ventricle,[195] with increased motion of both of these chambers. With acute mitral regurgitation, there may be little increase in the internal diameter of either of these chambers, but increased systolic motion is particularly prominent. The underlying cause of the regurgitation—e.g., rupture of chordae tendineae,[196] mitral valve prolapse (Figs. 5–41 to 5–43, p. 112; Fig. 32–14), flail leaflets (Figure 5–44, p. 113), and vegetations, Figure 5–45, p. 113)—can sometimes be determined, and the echocardiogram may also show calcification of the mitral annulus as a band of dense echoes between the mitral apparatus and the posterior wall of the heart (Fig. 32–14).[134,196a]

Two-dimensional echocardiography may be useful in the detection of significant mitral regurgitation by demonstrating failure of the leaflets to close,[197] and flail leaflets[198] and valvular prolapse may also be identified by this technique[199] (Figs. 5–42 and 5–43, p. 112). Pulsed Doppler echocardiography (Figure 5–12, p. 95) can reveal mitral regurgitant flow and may be useful in assessing its severity.[200,201,201a]

RADIOISOTOPE ANGIOGRAPHY.   Gated pool imaging or first-pass angiography may reveal an increased end-diastolic volume; the regurgitant fraction can be estimated from the ratio of left ventricular to right ventricular stroke volume;[167,202] in patients with mitral regurgitation and impaired left ventricular function, ejection fraction fails to rise normally during exercise.[203] Radionuclide angiograms are useful for interval follow-up of patients. Progressive increases in ventricular end-diastolic or endsystolic volumes often suggest that surgical treatment is necessary (see below).

MANAGEMENT

MEDICAL TREATMENT

This includes all the measures used in the treatment of heart failure, as outlined in Chapter 16. Digitalis glycosides clearly play a more important role in the management of mitral regurgitation than of mitral stenosis. Afterload reduction is also of conspicuous benefit in the management of mitral regurgitation—both the acute and the chronic forms.[204] By reducing the impedance to ejection into the aorta, the volume of blood regurgitating into the left atrium is reduced, causing left atrial pressure and, in particular, the elevated *v* wave, to decline (Figure 16–19, p. 540). In addition, decreasing left ventricular volume reduces the size of the mitral annulus and thereby the regurgitant orifice.[205] Afterload reduction with intravenous nitroprusside may be life-saving in acute mitral regurgitation due to rupture of the head of a papillary muscle occurring in the course of an acute myocardial infarction. It may permit stabilization of the patient's condition and thereby allow operation to be carried out with the patient in an optimal condition. When surgical treatment is contraindicated, chronic afterload reduction with oral hydralazine or prazosin may improve the clinical state for months or even years in patients with severe mitral regurgitation.

Antiarrhythmic therapy with quinidine or procainamide may be helpful in suppressing frequent atrial or ventricular premature contractions as well as in maintaining sinus rhythm following electrical or pharmacological conversion from atrial fibrillation. Appropriate prophylaxis to prevent infective endocarditis (p. 1175) is indicated.

Left-heart catheterization, selective left ventricular angiocardiography, and coronary arteriography are indicated in patients with significant functional disability despite optimal medical management. The objectives of these studies are to (1) confirm the presence of regurgitation and estimate its severity; (2) aid in the identification of patients with primary myocardial disease and relatively mild, functional mitral regurgitation secondary to ventricular dilatation who are not likely to benefit greatly from operation and in whom the operative risk is relatively high; (3) detect and assess the severity of any associated valve lesions; and (4) determine the presence and assess the extent of coronary artery disease.

SURGICAL TREATMENT

When operative treatment is under consideration, the chronic, often slowly progressive nature of the disease must be weighed against the immediate risks and long-term uncertainties attendant upon surgery. Surgical mortality depends on the patient's hemodynamic and clinical state, particularly the function of the left ventricle, the presence of associated conditions such as renal, hepatic, or pulmonary disease, as well as on the experience of the surgical team. It does not appear to depend significantly on which of the currently widely used tissue or mechanical valve prostheses is employed.

In selected patients with pure or predominant mitral regurgitation—i.e., patients who have severe noncalcific mitral regurgitation, a dilated mitral annulus, absence of severe subvalvular chordal thickening, and no major loss of leaflet substance—an annuloplasty, often using a rigid or semirigid prosthetic ring (i.e., a Carpentier ring),[206] direct suture repair of the valve (Fig. 32–15), or replacement of torn chordae tendineae has been successful. A relatively small number of surgeons, particularly in Europe, have reported a relatively low operative mortality rate, in the range of 5 per cent, with long-term clinical improvement in the majority of survivors.[207] The results of these "plastic" operations have, in general, been more favorable in children and adolescents with pliable valves and in patients with severe coronary artery disease and mitral regurgitation secondary to annular dilatation, papillary muscle dysfunction or rupture, or chordal rupture than in adults with primary valvular deformity and thickening.[208,209,209a] Most surgeons, however, particularly in the United States, have found that regurgitant valves are not amenable to direct repair in the majority of cases. Instead, mitral valve replacement has emerged as the principal surgical approach to pure mitral regurgitation or combined mitral stenosis and regurgitation.

Results. Mortality rates of 1 to 4 per cent in patients with predominant mitral stenosis and of 2 to 7 per cent in patients with pure or predominant regurgitation who undergo isolated mitral valve replacement operated upon electively in functional Class II or III are now common in

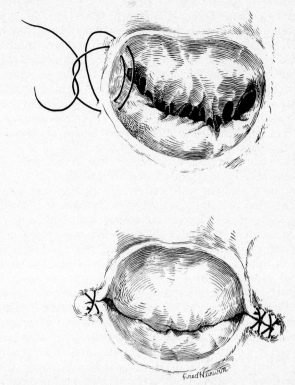

FIGURE 32–15 Commissural plication of the regurgitant mitral valve annulus. (From Starr, A., and Macmanus, Q.: Acquired valvular heart disease. *In* Efflet, D. B. [ed.]: Blades' Surgical Diseases of the Chest. 4th ed. St. Louis, The C. V. Mosby Co., 1978, p. 513.)

many centers.[210–213] Age per se is no barrier to successful surgery; mitral valve replacement can be carried out in patients more than 70 years of age with the same or only slightly higher risk as in younger patients,[214] if their general health status is adequate. Surgical treatment substantially improves survival in patients with symptomatic mitral regurgitation. Factors such as an age of less than 60 years, a preoperative New York Heart Association functional Class of II, a cardiac index exceeding 2.0 liters/min/m², a left ventricular end-diastolic pressure less than 12 mm Hg, and a normal ejection fraction all correlate with improved immediate as well as long-term survival. Patients with moderate impairment of the ejection fraction (30 to 50 per cent), in particular, exhibit improved survival following surgical compared with medical treatment.[178] In other series, only age and preoperative ejection fraction predicted long-term survival following mitral valve replacement.[213]

Emergency surgical treatment of acute left ventricular failure caused by acute mitral regurgitation due to myocardial infarction and rupture of the head of a papillary muscle, by trauma to the mitral valve, or by endocarditis is associated with a much higher mortality rate than is the elective surgical treatment of chronic mitral regurgitation. However, unless such patients with acute, severe endocarditis and heart failure are treated aggressively, a fatal outcome is almost certain. If, on the other hand, the condition of patients with mitral regurgitation secondary to acute infarction can be stabilized by medical treatment, it is preferable to defer operation until 4 to 6 weeks after infarction. Vasodilator treatment may be useful during this period. However, medical management should not be prolonged if multisystem (renal or pulmonary or both) failure occurs. Surgical mortality is also higher in patients with refractory heart failure (functional Class IV), in those in whom a previously implanted prosthetic valve must be replaced because of thromboembolism or valve dysfunction,[215] and in those with active infective endocarditis (of a natural or prosthetic valve). Despite the higher surgical risks, the efficacy of early operation has been established in patients with infective endocarditis complicated by medically uncontrollable congestive heart failure, recurrent emboli, or both[216,217] (p. 1171). Since fungal endocarditis responds poorly to medical management, it is now the practice to recommend valve replacement in these cases *before* the onset of heart failure or embolization.

In most patients with mitral regurgitation, the symptomatic state and thus the quality of life improve following valve replacement. Severe pulmonary hypertension is relieved almost uniformly,[121-124] and left ventricular end-diastolic volume and mass are reduced (Fig. 32–11). However, in contrast to patients with aortic or mitral stenosis, whose cardiac function and cardiac symptoms generally improve following operation, patients with mitral regurgitation who had marked left ventricular dysfunction preoperatively sometimes remain symptomatic following a technically satisfactory operation. Furthermore, long-term survival in patients with predominant mitral regurgitation who undergo mitral valve replacement may be poorer than in those with pure stenosis or mixed stenotic and regurgitant lesions, presumably because left ventricular dysfunction may be quite advanced and largely irreversible by the time patients with pure regurgitation become seriously symptomatic.[212,218] Since, as indicated earlier (p. 1084), mitral regurgitation reduces ventricular afterload, abolition of regurgitation raises afterload and thereby may interfere with left ventricular emptying, causing a reduction of the ejection fraction[165,213] and an increase of end-systolic volume; these hemodynamic changes may be particularly troublesome during the early postoperative period, when vasodilator treatment may be effective. However, even though it is clearly desirable to operate upon patients with mitral regurgitation before they develop marked left ventricular dysfunction, and despite these limitations of the results of surgical treatment in patients with severe left ventricular failure, operation is still indicated in the majority of these patients, since conservative therapy has little to offer.

The etiology of the mitral regurgitation also plays an important role in the outcome following surgical treatment. In patients in whom mitral dysfunction is secondary to ischemic heart disease, the 5-year survival rate is about 30 per cent, whereas in rheumatic mitral regurgitation it is much better, approximately 70 per cent. Furthermore, occlusive coronary artery disease coexisting with, but not the primary cause of mitral dysfunction is associated with decreased perioperative and long-term postoperative survival as well.[212] However, some improvement from mitral valve replacement can be expected even in patients with mitral regurgitation secondary to ischemic heart disease who are medically unresponsive and in congestive heart failure, as long as the cardiac index and ejection fraction exceed 1.5 liters/min/m[2] and 35 per cent, respectively. When left ventricular dysfunction is more severe, however, the risk of operative mortality becomes prohibitive.[219]

INDICATIONS FOR OPERATION. In view of the advances in surgical techniques, the reduction in operative mortality, the continuous improvement of artificial valves as well as the poor long-term results in many patients whose mitral regurgitation is corrected after a long history of heart failure, a more aggressive stance concerning the desirability of operation is in order. Only a few years ago many cardiologists, including the author, recommended operation for patients with chronic severe mitral regurgitation only if they were in functional Class III or IV,[220] i.e., with symptoms at rest or on ordinary activity despite intensive medical treatment; however, it is now my policy to recommend operation also for patients with severe mitral regurgitation who are in Class II, i.e., who become distinctly symptomatic only on heavy exertion, particularly if cardiomegaly and an elevated left ventricular end-systolic volume (> 30 ml/m[2] BSA) persist despite aggressive medical therapy. However, patients with mitral regurgitation who are asymptomatic or only mildly symptomatic are not considered to be candidates for surgical treatment at this time, since they may live for many years with little deterioration in their condition.

ARTIFICIAL CARDIAC VALVES
(see Table 32–7)

MECHANICAL PROSTHESES (Fig. 32–16). Two major types of artificial valves are currently available in models designed for both the atrioventricular (mitral and tricuspid) and the aortic positions—mechanical prostheses and tissue valves. The first series of successful replacements of the mitral and aortic valves was accomplished by Harken et al.[221] and Starr in 1960,[222] and at the present time, the *Starr-Edwards caged-ball valve*, in which the sewing ring and struts are cloth-covered to reduce the incidence of thromboembolism, is still widely used.[223,224] An alternative, the *Smeloff-Cutter valve*, has a double-cage design that is somewhat superior hydrodynamically, since the diameter of the valve orifice is equal to or slightly larger than the ball diameter, which is not the case for the Starr-Edwards valve.

Two types of tilting-disk valves are widely employed. The *Björk-Shiley valve* consists of a low-profile stellite valve housing covered with a Teflon fabric sewing ring. Its design allows an excellent ratio between the diameter of the valve orifice and tissue annulus. It contains a suspended tilting disk occluder made of pyrolytic carbon (Pyrolyte), which opens to an angle of 60 degrees, providing central laminar flow.[212,225] The *Lillehei-Kaster pivoting disk valve* consists of a titanium valve housing with a Teflon fabric sewing ring in which a pyrolite disk is suspended. In the open position, this disk swings to an angle of 80 degrees, providing a large central flow orifice.[226] A recently developed valve, the *St. Jude valve*, is made of pyrolytic carbon; two semicircular disks pivot between open and closed positions without the need for supporting struts. Although experience with this valve in patients dates back only to 1977, it appears to possess favorable flow characteristics and causes a lower transvalvular gradient at any outer diameter and cardiac output.[227]

All of these prosthetic valves have an excellent record of durability—up to 20 years in the case of the caged-ball valves. However, problems with thromboembolism persist despite the fact that the cloth covering of the sewing ring

TABLE 32-7 ADVANTAGES AND DISADVANTAGES OF COMMONLY USED PROSTHESES

TYPE	NAME-MODEL	ADVANTAGES	DISADVANTAGES
Caged ball (non–cloth-covered)	Starr-Edwards 1260, 6120 Smeloff-Cutter	1. Predictable performance 2. Abundant long-term experience 3. Inaudible	1. Thromboembolism 2. Anticoagulation 3. Bulky cage design
Caged ball (Cloth-covered)	Starr-Edwards 2400, 6400	1. Very low incidence of thrombo-embolism	1. Anticoagulation 2. Bulky cage design 3. Noise 4. Hemolysis 5. Poor hemodynamics in small sizes
Tilting disk	Björk-Shiley Lillehei-Kaster	1. Excellent hemodynamics 2. Very low profile 3. Durability	1. Anticoagulation 2. Thromboembolism 3. Noise
	St. Jude	1. Outstanding hemodynamics 2. Very low profile	1. Anticoagulation 2. Uncertainty about durability and actual incidence of thromboembolism
Porcine xenograft	Hancock Carpentier-Edwards	1. Very low incidence of thromboembolism 2. Central flow 3. No hemolysis 4. Inaudible 5. Anticoagulants usually unnecessary	1. Uncertain durability 2. Poor hemodynamic performance in small sizes (standard models)
Bovine pericardium	Ionescu-Shiley	1. Very low incidence of thrombo-embolism 2. Central flow 3. No hemolysis 4. Inaudible 5. Anticoagulants usually unnecessary 6. Excellent hemodynamics in aortic position	1. Uncertain durability 2. Gradients in mitral position

Reproduced with permission from Bonchek, L. E.: The basis for selecting a valve prosthesis. *In* McGoon, D. C. (ed.): Cardiovascular Clinics. Cardiac Surgery. Philadelphia, F. A. Davis Co., 1982, p. 103.

and struts has reduced the incidence of this complication considerably. Although the St. Jude valve results in a relatively low incidence of nonfatal emboli—possibly lower than that of the caged-ball valves[212,227]—the Björk-Shiley valve has been associated with massive thrombosis, despite anticoagulation; this uncommon, though potentially catastrophic, complication may be related to the limited excursion of the disk that results when a large valve is inserted into a relatively small ventricle.[228]

All prosthetic valves, regardless of design or placement (mitral, tricuspid, or aortic), require long-term anticoagulation because of the hazard of thromboembolism. Without anticoagulation the incidence of thromboembolism increases three- to sixfold;[229] the risk of thromboembolism is greatest in the first postoperative year. Anticoagulation with sodium warfarin should begin about 2 days after operation in order to achieve a prothrombin time in the range of 20 to 25 seconds (about twice the control value). This relatively conservative approach reduces the risk of anticoagulant hemorrhage, yet does not appear to be associated with a greater frequency of thromboembolism than a prothrombin time of 30 to 35 seconds. It must be recognized that the administration of warfarin carries its own morbidity and mortality, estimated at 0.2 and 2.2 per 100 patient-years, respectively,[229] and despite treatment with

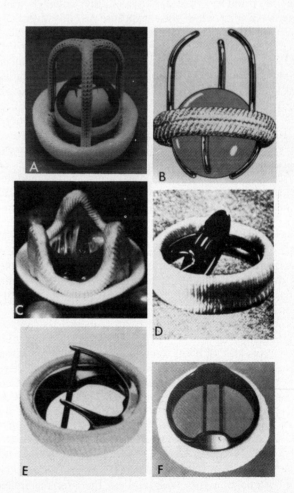

FIGURE 32-16 *A*, Model 2400 Starr-Edwards aortic prosthesis. The valve is totally cloth-covered, except for a thin track on the inside of the struts. *B*, Smeloff-Cutter. *C*, Hancock porcine bioprosthesis. *D*, Björk-Shiley. *E*, Lillehei-Kaster. *F*, St. Jude prosthesis with two semi-circular tilting leaflets. (*A* and *F* reproduced with permission from Bonchek, L. I.: Current status of cardiac valve replacement: Selection of a prosthesis and indications for operation. Am. Heart J. *101*: 96, 1981.)

anticoagulants, the incidence of thromboembolic complications is still about 0.2 (fatal) and 1 to 2 (nonfatal) per 100 patient-years.

Although their value has not been definitively established, in some centers acetylsalicylic acid, 0.6 gm twice daily, or dipyridamole, 25 to 50 mg three times daily,[229,229a] is also given to inhibit platelet aggregation.

TISSUE VALVES. Largely to overcome the complication of thromboembolism that is inherent in all prosthetic valves, considerable effort has been devoted to the development of nonthrombogenic tissue valves.[230] The first of these to be widely used were chemically sterilized homografts. Unfortunately, these exhibited a high incidence of breakdown within 3 years.[231] Fresh antibiotic-treated or frozen-irradiated homografts were then developed; these were somewhat more durable but also proved to have a significant late failure rate due to collagen dissolution of the valve cusp,[232] possibly representing a subtle form of rejection. The use of homograft valves has been restricted by continuing uncertainty about their durability, and difficulty of inserting unmounted grafts into the aortic position, and the problems inherent in their procurement.

To overcome these difficulties, *porcine heterografts* were developed and used clinically beginning in 1965. At first, these valves were sterilized with formalin, which dissolved the collagen cross linkages in the valve cusps and resulted in a high failure rate.[233] Carpentier et al. then developed the process of fixation and sterilization of porcine heterografts using a dilute solution of glutaraldehyde, which appears to promote the stability of the collagen cross linkages, so that after their exposure to this agent the valves become essentially inert collagen shells with little, if any, antigenicity.[234] The valves were then mounted on a semiflexible stent made of a stellite ring and flexible struts of polypropylene.[235] This form of the Hancock porcine bioprosthetic cardiac valve (Fig. 32–16) was the first quality-controlled, mass-produced tissue valve and has been widely used in the mitral, tricuspid, and aortic positions. The Carpentier-Edwards porcine valve is mounted on a stent made of Elgiloy—an alloy of spring steel. Heterologous (bovine) glutaraldehyde-fixed pericardium[236-238] has also been utilized for fabrication of cardiac valves mounted on a titanium frame. They have been employed successfully for more than 5 years with a record of durability, incidence of thromboembolism, and hemodynamic performance comparable to that of the porcine valves, although at this time the total experience with the latter is far greater than with all the other tissue valves combined. Homologous dura mater[239] has been used successfully in a similar manner, but there is little experience with this valve in the United States.

Tissue valves have succeeded in reducing the risk of thromboembolism.[211,229,240-243] The majority of the thromboembolic episodes with the xenograft in the mitral position occur in the first 6 to 12 postoperative weeks, and therefore it appears desirable to treat these patients with anticoagulants for this period of time.[243] Treatment is then gradually discontinued over a 2- to 10-week period[244] unless thrombogenic factors not related to the prosthesis persist, such as chronic atrial fibrillation,[244a] the finding of a clot in the atrium at operation, a markedly dilated left atrium, a calcified left atrial wall, or a postoperative thromboembolic event; with any of the aforementioned

conditions, anticoagulation is continued permanently. With this approach, the incidence of thromboembolic complications is extremely low, approximately 2 per 100 patient-years, comparable to that of anticoagulant-treated patients receiving the Björk-Shiley prostheses in the mitral position[243] over a 2-year follow-up period. The incidence of postoperative emboli following implantation of a porcine bioprosthesis into the mitral position is three times as high in patients with atrial fibrillation (despite anticoagulation) as in patients in sinus rhythm. It is unlikely that *any* replacement of the mitral valve can be associated with a thromboembolism rate much below 0.5 per cent per year, since some of the emboli in patients with longstanding mitral valve disease are derived from the left atrium rather than from the valve itself.[245] The incidence of embolization in patients who have experienced repeated emboli from a prosthetic mitral valve may be reduced by replacement with a tissue valve.

HEMODYNAMICS OF VALVE REPLACEMENTS. It must be recognized that all valve replacements—mechanical prostheses as well as tissue valves—have an effective in vitro orifice size that is smaller than a normal human valve.[246] After insertion, tissue ingrowth and endothelialization reduce the in vivo effective orifice size further,[247] and therefore most valve devices currently available must be considered to be at least mildly stenotic.[248] However, postoperative hemodynamic measurements of the rigid prostheses show reasonably good function, with effective valve orifice averaging 1.7 to 2.0 cm^2 and mitral valvular gradients of 4 to 8 mm Hg at rest. Although definitive comparisons have not been carried out, the cloth-covered Starr-Edwards valve appears to be intrinsically slightly more stenotic than the tilting-disk (Björk-Shiley or Lillehei-Kaster) valves; the St. Jude valve, in turn, may be slightly superior to the latter.[227] In hemodynamic studies, the recently modified porcine and the Ionescu bovine pericardial mitral valves behave in a fashion similar to that of an artificial prosthetic valve of the same diameter,[249,250] although subtle, late hemodynamic deterioration with the porcine bioprosthesis has been reported.[243] Serious hemodynamic obstruction of an artificial valve in the mitral position is quite uncommon, unless the valve is placed in a small left ventricular cavity or a small mitral annulus or unless the prosthesis chosen is too large.

SELECTION OF AN ARTIFICIAL VALVE. The characteristics of both tissue and prosthetic valves are almost evenly matched, and the choice between the two is difficult. It is important that the relative advantages and disadvantages of the various valves be explained to the patient, who should be a participant in the final decision. As indicated, there appear to be no significant differences insofar as hemodynamics are concerned, except that in patients with an unusually small left ventricular cavity or mitral annulus, the low-profile (tilting-disk) prosthetic, St. Jude, or tissue valve may be superior to the more bulky, caged-ball valve.[251] The hazard of thromboembolism, albeit lower than a decade ago, is still considerably higher with prosthetic than with tissue valves. Therefore, a tissue valve is preferred over a prosthesis in patients in whom anticoagulation is difficult to control or is especially hazardous—for example, in vigorous young adults whose vocations or avocations place them at particular risk for bleeding. Because of the uncertainties surrounding their long-term durability,[252,252a] I believe that a mechanical prosthetic valve is still the most desirable in patients under the age of 65 years without contraindications to anticoagulants. Patients with coexisting disease who are prone to hemorrhage or who are unwilling, unreliable, or unlikely to take anticoagulants on a regular basis or patients over the age of 65 years in whom the question of durability is less important and who are at a greater risk of hemorrhage while taking anticoagulants should receive a bioprosthesis. The high incidence of bioprosthetic valve failure in children and adolescents[253,254] and in patients on chronic hemodialysis[211] prohibits their use in these patients. In young adults (> 20 and < 35 years), the failure of bioprosthetic valves is somewhat higher than it is in older adults; this serves as a relative, not an absolute, contraindication in this age group.

Female patients with artificial mitral valves can tolerate the hemodynamic load of pregnancy well, but there is an increased risk of thromboembolism in such patients with prosthetic valves when anticoagulation is interrupted and an increased risk of fatal fetal hemorrhage in those in whom it is continued.[255] There may also be a risk of fetal malformation caused by the possible teratogenic effect of warfarin.[256] These problems represent powerful arguments for the use of tissue valves in all women of childbearing age.[257] In the case of a pregnant woman in whom a prosthetic valve is already in place, the risk to the fetus if the mother receives oral anticoagulants appears to be lower than is the risk to the mother if anticoagulants are discontinued.[258] It is therefore advisable in a pregnant patient with a prosthetic valve to use heparin during the first trimester and again after week 37 of gestation. Oral anticoagulants may be used in the interim period, provided that prothrombin times are monitored frequently. Anticoagulation with heparin should be discontinued with the onset of labor and then reinstituted 24 hours after uncomplicated delivery and continued until the desired effects of oral anticoagulation can be achieved.[256]

When noncardiac surgery is required in patients with prosthetic mitral valves who are receiving anticoagulants, the risk is minimal when the drug regimen is stopped 1 to 3 days preoperatively and for a similar period postoperatively. It may be desirable, however, to protect the patient with low molecular weight dextran during the perioperative period.

A distinct advantage of the rigid prostheses is their predictable performance and durability; some have now been in place and functioning successfully since 1961.[222] Although, with the exception of children and patients on chronic hemodialysis, the mechanical performance of the porcine xenograft preserved by glutaraldehyde has been excellent in the majority of patients for periods of up to 12 years[242,243] (at the time of this writing), there have been an increasing number of reports of valve breakdown after 5 years. Pathological changes in these valves include degeneration, deposition of fibrin on the inflow and outflow surfaces, inflammatory cell infiltrates, focal disruption of the fibrocollagenous structure, and ultimately calcification.[259-262] Although the fraction of all implanted valves that have failed to date has been very small (less than 1 per cent), these pathological observations indicate that the porcine bioprosthesis may not be totally inert in the human circulation, suggesting that replacement of the valve might ultimately become necessary in a significant, although as yet unknown, number of patients. The incidence of infection appears to be approximately equal with all available mechanical and tissue valves. Hemolysis is now rarely a serious problem, but when it does occur it is most conspicuous with the cloth-covered Starr-Edwards valve.

Artificial valves have characteristic auscultatory and phonocardiographic characteristics[263] (Figure 3–19, p. 52). Echocardiography, phonocardiography, and cineradiography[264] are extremely useful in the identification of artificial valve dysfunction.[265-267] Two-dimensional echocardiography is particularly promising in the follow-up of patients who demonstrate clinical deterioration in the postoperative period following porcine heterograft implantation. This technique may prove capable of distinguishing between failure of the bioprosthesis (abnormal structure or valve motion) and left ventricular dysfunction.[268,269]

THE MITRAL VALVE PROLAPSE SYNDROME

ETIOLOGY AND PATHOLOGY

The mitral valve prolapse (MVP) syndrome—which has been given many names, including the systolic click–murmur syndrome, Barlow's syndrome, billowing mitral valve syndrome, ballooning mitral cusp syndrome, floppy valve syndrome, and redundant cusp syndrome,[270-274]—is a common but variable clinical syndrome resulting from diverse pathogenic mechanisms of the mitral valve apparatus. The MVP syndrome has become recognized as one of the most prevalent cardiac valvular abnormalities, affecting as much as 5 to 10 per cent of the population.[275-277] It had been thought for many years that midsystolic clicks and late systolic murmurs, the auscultatory hallmarks of this syndrome, were of extracardiac origin. However, in 1961 it was postulated,[278] and 2 years later Barlow and associates demonstrated that these auscultatory findings are frequently associated with prolapse of the mitral valve, often with regurgitation.[279] Strong support for this formulation came from cineangiography and intracardiac phonocardiography and echocardiography.[274]

The many causes of or conditions associated with prolapse of mitral valves into the left atrium during ventricular systole are shown in Table 32–8. Prominent among these is myxomatous proliferation of the mitral valve, in which the spongiosa component of the valve, i.e., the middle layer of the leaflet composed of loose, myxomatous material, is unusually prominent[280,280a] and the quantity of acid mucopolysaccharide is increased secondary to a fundamental but as yet undefined abnormality of collagen metabolism.[281] The concordance between inadequate production of type III collagen with echocardiographic findings of MVP in patients with type IV Ehlers-Danlos syndrome suggests that this abnormality of collagen is responsible.[282] Mucopolysaccharide infiltration and fragmentation of valvular collagen are common findings.[283] A reduction of type III and AB collagen has also been found in a patient with MVP without the Ehlers-Danlos syndrome.[284]

TABLE 32–8   DOCUMENTED CONDITIONS CAUSING OR ASSOCIATED WITH MITRAL VALVE PROLAPSE OR NONEJECTION SYSTOLIC CLICK

DEFINITE OR PROBABLE CAUSE	PROBABLE ASSOCIATION
Marfan's syndrome	Congenital heart disease (atrial septal defect, ventricular septal defect, patent ductus arteriosus, complete absence of left pericardium, membranous subaortic stenosis, Ebstein's anomaly, and corrected transposition of great vessels)
Pseudoxanthoma elasticum	
Rheumatic endocarditis	
Occlusive coronary artery disease	
Congestive cardiomyopathy	
Hypertrophic obstructive cardiomyopathy	
Myocarditis	Turner's syndrome
Mitral valve surgery	Noonan's syndrome
Trauma	Congenital prolonged Q-T syndrome
Left atrial myxoma	Keratoconus
Polyarteritis nodosa	Hyperthyroidism
Left ventricular aneurysm	von Willebrand's syndrome
Ehler-Danlos syndrome	Chronic external progressive ophthalmoplegia
Relapsing polychondritis	
Lupus erythematosus	
Duchenne's muscular dystrophy	
Myotonia dystrophia	
Wolff-Parkinson-White syndrome	
Primary mitral valve prolapse	

Electron microscopy has shown haphazard arrangement, disruption, and fragmentation of collagen fibrils. In mild cases, the valvular myxoid stroma is enlarged on histological examination but the leaflets are grossly normal. However, with increasing quantities of myxoid stroma, the leaflets become grossly abnormal and redundant (Fig. 32–17) and prolapse;[128,285] the severity of mitral regurgitation depends on the extent of the prolapse. The cusps of the mitral valve, the chordae tendineae, and the annulus may all be affected by myxomatous proliferation. Degeneration of collagen within the central core of the chordae tendineae is primarily responsible for chordal rupture, which occurs commonly in this syndrome and may intensify the severity of mitral regurgitation,[286] although increased chordal tension resulting from the enlarged area of the valve cusps may play a contributory role. Myxomatous changes in the annulus may result in annular dilatation and calcification[286]—contributing to the severity of the mitral regurgitation. Myxomatous proliferation, although most commonly affecting the mitral valve, is not limited to this valve but has been described in the tricuspid, aortic, and pulmonic valves, particularly in patients with Marfan's syndrome, and may lead to regurgitation of these valves. Histological evidence of a left ventricular abnormality has been obtained on biopsy,[287] which has also revealed reductions in the ability of cardiac tissue to metabolize norepinephrine by means of monoamine oxidase.[288]

It has been proposed that the MVP syndrome exhibits a strong hereditary component,[289] transmitted as an autosomal dominant trait, and that some cases of this syndrome appearing without any other obvious disorders represent formes frustes of Marfan's syndrome.[290] Although myxomatous proliferation of the mitral valve is idiopathic in most patients, it occurs in association with a variety of connective tissue disorders, including Marfan's syndrome, Ehlers-Danlos syndrome,[291] osteogenesis imperfecta, pseudoxanthoma elasticum,[292] and periarteritis nodosa as well as with myotonic dystrophy,[293] Duchenne's muscular dystrophy,[294] cardiomyopathy,[295] von Willebrand's disease,[296] keratoconus,[297] hyperthyroidism[298] and congenital malformations such as Ebstein's anomaly of the tricuspid valve, atrial septal defect of the ostium secundum variety,[273,299–301] and the Holt-Oram syndrome (p. 1616). There appears to

be a high incidence of MVP in patients with asthenic habitus[302] and a variety of congenital thoracic deformities, including a straight back, a pectus excavatum, or a shallow chest.[303,304] The MVP syndrome may represent one manifestation of a number of systemic connective tissue disorders, and thoracic abnormalities may represent another manifestation of the same disorders; frequently they coexist. The mitral valve undergoes differentiation between day 35 and 42 of fetal life, at the same time as the vertebrae and thoracic cage undergo chondrification and ossification. It has been suggested that factors that influence fetal development during this period might affect both the mitral valve and the bony thorax.[304]

The MVP syndrome can coexist with rheumatic mitral stenosis,[305] and it may develop following mitral commissurotomy for mitral stenosis.[306] However, it is unlikely that rheumatic valvulitis, which is a proliferative process, causes extensive myxomatous degeneration of the mitral valve.

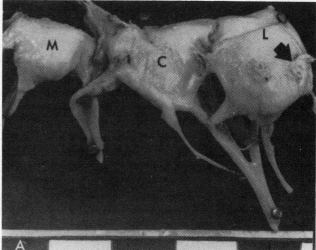

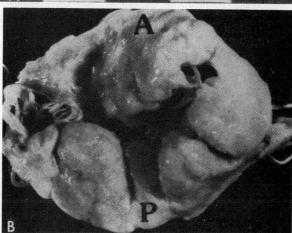

FIGURE 32–17   *A*, Floppy mitral valve excised from a 70-year-old woman with a 1-year history of retinal emboli and transient cerebral ischemic episodes. All three scallops of the posterior cusp are dome-shaped (M = medial; C = central; L = lateral). On the atrial surface of the lateral scallop are filiform processes, which, on section, contained platelet thrombi (arrow). *B*, The atrial view of a prolapsing mitral valve with redundant tissue. Note marked folding of the valve surface, more pronounced in the posterior cusp (P), exaggerating clear division of the valvular scallops. Widths of the anterior (A) and posterior cusps are almost equal, characteristic of severely myxomatous valve. (*A* reproduced with permission from Davies, M. J.: Pathology of Cardiac Valves. London, Butterworths, 1980. *B* from King, B. D., Clark, M. A., Baba, N., et al.: Circulation 66:288, 1982, by permisson of the American Heart Association, Inc.)

Rather it is more likely that the relationship between these two relatively common conditions is coincidental. In hypertrophic obstructive cardiomyopathy, prolapse of the posterior leaflet of the mitral valve may accompany the usual anterior displacement of the anterior mitral valve leaflet.[290,307]

Ischemic heart disease and MVP are both common disorders and coexist not infrequently; MVP may also occur secondary to papillary muscle dysfunction. In some patients, MVP has been documented to develop for the first time *following* myocardial infarction.[308] Since MVP has also been reported in patients who have suffered acute myocardial infarction despite normal coronary arteriograms,[309,310] it is possible that coronary artery emboli are responsible for the infarction in this syndrome (p. 1267). MVP may cause myocardial ischemia by increasing tension on the base of the involved muscle,[307] and it has also been proposed that coronary artery spasm occurs as a reflex response to prolapse of the posterior mitral leaflet and that the resultant ischemia may be responsible for angina or angina-like pain, myocardial infarction, arrhythmias, and sudden death in this syndrome.

CLINICAL MANIFESTATIONS

The clinical presentations of the MVP syndrome are diverse. The condition has been observed in patients of all ages and in both sexes. It is a common syndrome; indeed, prolapse of the mitral valve has been reported to occur in 6 per cent of healthy young women surveyed by echocardiography.[276] One series of 100 presumably healthy young women revealed that 17 had a midsystolic click or late systolic murmur or both and that 10 of these 17 had evidence of prolapse of the mitral valve on echocardiography.[277] Approximately 10 per cent of routine autopsies in a community hospital showed MVP.[273] About 20 per cent of patients who underwent mitral valve replacement had myxomatous proliferation of the valve on pathological examination.[311] Echocardiographic evidence of MVP has been found in more than 90 per cent of patients with Marfan's syndrome.[312] Indeed, MVP is now the most common cause of isolated regurgitation requiring mitral valve replacement.[313]

History

The overwhelming majority of patients with MVP are asymptomatic. In many cases, otherwise asymptomatic patients with MVP suffer from undue anxiety, perhaps precipitated by their having been informed of the presence of heart disease. Patients may complain of palpitations, chest discomfort, and, when mitral regurgitation is severe, symptoms of diminished cardiac reserve. Chest discomfort may be typical of angina, but most often is atypical in that it is prolonged, not clearly related to exertion, and punctuated by brief attacks of severe stabbing pain at the apex. The discomfort may be secondary to tension on papillary muscles and may be associated with abnormalities of wall motion or indentations of the wall of the left ventricle at the base of these muscles on angiography. It may be difficult to differentiate this discomfort from angina because of the coexistence of the MVP syndrome and true angina pectoris secondary to coronary artery disease.

Palpitations may be caused by arrhythmias. There may

be a history of sudden death in the family. Since prolapse of the mitral valve is sometimes associated with another form of heart disease, e.g., atrial septal defect, symptoms produced by the latter may predominate. It has been suggested that many of the symptoms are related to dysfunction of the autonomic nervous system, which occurs frequently in the MVP syndrome.[314,315] Patients with MVP have increased excretion of epinephrine and norepinephrine, presumably secondary to increased adrenergic tone, which may be responsible for many of the symptoms of the syndrome.[316,316a] Although many of the symptoms of MVP resemble those of neurocirculatory asthenia, the two conditions appear to be distinct and unrelated.[317]

Physical Examination

Palpation of the chest and of the carotid pulses reflects the severity of the existing mitral regurgitation (p. 1081). The physical findings unique to the MVP syndrome are detected by auscultation and can be corroborated by phonocardiography.[290] The most important is a systolic click at least 0.14 sec after S_1 (Figure 3–31, p. 61); this can be differentiated from a systolic ejection click, since it occurs distinctly *after* the beginning of the upstroke of the carotid pulse. Occasionally multiple mid- and late-systolic clicks are audible. They are most readily audible along the lower left sternal border and are believed to be produced by sudden tensing of the elongated chordae tendineae and of the prolapsing leaflets. The click is often, though not invariably, followed by a mid- to late-crescendo systolic murmur that continues to A_2. This murmur is similar to that produced by papillary muscle dysfunction, which is readily understandable, since both result from mid- to late-systolic mitral regurgitation. In general, the duration of the murmur is a function of the severity of the regurgitation, and when the murmur is confined to the latter portion of systole, regurgitation is usually not severe. However, as regurgitation becomes more severe, the murmur commences earlier and becomes holosystolic (Figure 4–17, p. 78). It is important to emphasize the variability of these findings. Some patients exhibit both a midsystolic click and a mid- to late-systolic murmur; others present with one or the other of these two findings; still others have only a click on one occasion and only a murmur on another, both on a third examination, and no abnormality at all on a fourth. A loud mitral component of S_1 at the apex in patients with nonrheumatic mitral regurgitation suggests holosystolic MVP.[318] Conditions other than MVP cause midsystolic clicks; these include extracardiac causes and atrial septal aneurysms.[319] MVP may also cause an early diastolic sound or murmur, best heard at the apex or left sternal border 70 to 110 msec following A_2, at a time when the prolapsed posterior leaflet returned from the left atrium.[320]

Dynamic Auscultation. The auscultatory and phonocardiographic findings are exquisitely sensitive to physiological and pharmacological interventions, and recognition of the changes induced by these interventions is of great value in the diagnosis of the MVP syndrome (Table 32–6).[290,321] The mitral valve begins to prolapse when the reduction of left ventricular volume during systole reaches a critical point at which the mitral valve leaflets no longer coapt; at this instant, the click occurs and the murmur commences.[322] Any maneuver that decreases left ventricular volume, such as a reduction of impedance to left ventricular outflow, a reduction in venous return, or an augmentation of contractility, will result in an earlier occurrence of prolapse during systole.[321] As a consequence, the click and onset of the murmur will move closer to S_1. When prolapse is severe or left ventricular size is markedly reduced or both, prolapse may begin with the onset of systole, and as a consequence, the click may not be audible and the murmur may be holosystolic. On the other hand, when left ventricular volume is increased by an increase in venous return, a reduction of myocardial contractility, bradycardia, or an increase in the impedance to left ventricular emptying, both the click and the onset of the murmur will be delayed. Indeed, if the left ventricle becomes extremely large, prolapse may not occur at all, and the abnormal auscultatory features may disappear entirely.

During the straining phase of the Valsalva maneuver, upon sudden standing,[323] and early during the inhalation of amyl nitrite,[324] cardiac size decreases, and both the click and the onset of the murmur occur earlier in systole. In contrast, a sudden change from the standing to the prone position, leg-raising, prompt squatting, maximal isometric exercise, and, to a lesser extent, expiration will delay the click and the onset of the murmur. During the overshoot phase of the Valsalva maneuver (i.e., six to eight cycles following release) and with prolongation of the R-R interval either following a premature contraction or in atrial fibrillation, the click and onset of the murmur are usually delayed, and the intensity of the murmur is reduced.

In general, when the onset of the murmur is delayed, both its duration and its intensity are diminished, reflecting a reduction in the severity of mitral regurgitation. With some maneuvers, however, there is a discrepancy between changes in the intensity and duration of the murmur. Following amyl nitrite inhalation, for example, the reduced left ventricular size results in an earlier click and longer murmur, but the lower left ventricular systolic pressure diminishes regurgitation and the intensity of the murmur. Conversely, phenylephrine and methoxamine delay the click and the onset of the murmur, but the larger volume of regurgitation consequent to the elevated left ventricular systolic pressure increases regurgitation and the intensity of the murmur. A psychological stress may increase the intensity of the click and exacerbate arrhythmias in MVP,[325] a finding that might explain the intermittency of the auscultatory findings and arrhythmias in these patients. In the diagnosis of the MVP syndrome, it is generally more helpful to determine the effect of interventions on the timing of the click and murmur than on the intensity of the latter.

There may be confusion between the systolic murmurs of hypertrophic obstructive cardiomyopathy (HOCM) and of MVP, particularly since midsystolic clicks and a late systolic murmur have been reported in HOCM[290] and since the murmur may increase in intensity and duration with standing and decrease with squatting in both conditions. However, the response to several interventions may be helpful in differentiating these two conditions. During the strain of the Valsalva maneuver, the murmur of HOCM increases in intensity[326] in contrast to that in the syndrome, which becomes longer but usually not louder. The murmur of HOCM becomes louder after amyl nitrite inhalation, whereas that of MVP does not. Following a premature beat, the murmur of HOCM increases in intensity and

duration, whereas that due to MVP usually remains unchanged or decreases.

LABORATORY EXAMINATION

Electrocardiography

Most commonly, the electrocardiogram is within normal limits in asymptomatic patients with typical auscultatory and echocardiographic findings. In a minority of asymptomatic patients and in many symptomatic patients, the electrocardiogram characteristically shows inverted or biphasic T waves and nonspecific ST-segment changes in leads II, III, and aV_f and occasionally in the anterolateral leads as well. The ST- and T-wave changes may become exaggerated during amyl nitrite inhalation and exercise. These electrocardiographic findings may be related to ischemia of the papillary muscles, or of the left ventricle at their bases, resulting from increased tension on these structures produced by the prolapsing valve. Alternatively, it is possible that the electrocardiographic abnormality reflects an underlying cardiomyopathy.

Arrhythmias. A spectrum of arrhythmias, including atrial and ventricular premature contractions and supraventricular and ventricular tachyarrhythmias[327-332,332a] as well as bradyarrhythmias due to sinus node dysfunction or varying degrees of atrioventricular block,[333] have been observed in the MVP syndrome. Indeed, this syndrome should be considered in patients with otherwise unexplained arrhythmias. The mechanism of the arrhythmias is not clear, but since diastolic depolarization of muscle fibers in the anterior mitral leaflet in response to stretch has been demonstrated experimentally,[334] the abnormal stretch of the prolapsed leaflet may be of pathogenetic significance. Wit et al. have shown that mitral valve leaflets contain atrium-like muscle fibers in continuity with left atrial myocardium, and it is possible that mechanical stimulation of these fibers generates slow-response action potentials and sustained rhythmic action that penetrates the cardiac chambers.[335,336] Although most of these arrhythmias are of little clinical importance, recurrent ventricular tachycardia, refractory to the usual agents, and even ventricular fibrillation have been reported. These serious ventricular arrhythmias are significantly more frequent in patients with ST-segment and T-wave abnormalities on the resting electrocardiogram.[337]

Paroxysmal supraventricular tachycardia is the most common sustained tachyarrhythmia in patients with the MVP syndrome and may be related to the high incidence of atrioventricular bypass trac this condition.[328] These bypass tracts are always left-sided and may be associated with the mitral valve abnormality. In the general population only 20 per cent of patients with paroxysmal supraventricular tachycardia have such bypass tracts, whereas the incidence in patients with MVP is three times as great. Conversely, there is evidence that there is a high incidence of MVP among patients with the Wolff-Parkinson-White syndrome.[338] However, the absence of electrocardiographic evidence of the Wolff-Parkinson-White syndrome should not be taken as evidence against the existence of bypass tracts in patients with the MVP syndrome who suffer attacks of supraventricular tachycardia. These considerations suggest that patients with the MVP syndrome who develop paroxysmal supraventricular tachycardia should be subjected to electrophysiological investigation. The outcome of such studies may be important, since digitalis or propranolol, which may be useful in reentry tachycardias, may be hazardous in the presence of antegrade conduction over an atrioventricular bypass tract. There is also an increased association between MVP and prolongation of the Q-T interval, and this association may play a role in the genesis of ventricular arrhythmias.[339,340]

The relation between the MVP syndrome and sudden death is not clear; Jeresaty collected 25 patients with MVP who died suddenly,[274] and Lucas and Edwards reported 14 such patients.[273] But these are "numerators without denominators," and when the high incidence of both conditions is considered, it is difficult to interpret the coincidence. Considering the frequency of both conditions, these numbers are not very impressive. Indeed, it is not clear how many of these instances of sudden death were in fact caused by or related to the MVP syndrome. The immediate cause of the sudden, unexpected death is probably a tachyarrhythmia,[274a] although complete heart block with prolonged asystole has also been reported in this syndrome and cannot be excluded.[341,342]

Echocardiography
(See also p. 111)

Echocardiography plays a key role in the diagnosis of MVP and has been most useful in the delineation of this syndrome (Figure 3–31, p. 61; Figure 4–17, p. 78; Figure 5–40, p. 111; and Figures 5–41 to 5–43, p. 112). The most common echocardiographic finding on M-mode echocardiography is abrupt posterior movement of the posterior leaflet or of both mitral leaflets in midsystole, resulting in a configuration on the M-mode echogram that has been likened to a "question mark turned approximately 90 degrees clockwise."[343] A second finding is pansystolic posterior prolapse of one or both leaflets, giving rise to a "U"- or "hammock"-shaped configuration in the C-D segment (Figure 5–41, p. 112) (the opposite of what is seen in hypertrophic obstructive cardiomyopathy, in which the anterior leaflet of the mitral valve moves toward the ventricular septum in midsystole). Rarely, there is a sudden posterior collapse of the anterior mitral leaflet as it approaches the prolapsing posterior leaflet in early systole.[290] All three of these echocardiographic patterns have in common the motion of the mitral valve posterior to the C-point. Although the systolic click usually occurs at the time of the abrupt posterior movement, there is considerable variability in the relationship between the auscultatory and echocardiographic events.

In studying patients with suspected prolapse of the mitral valve, it is important to direct the echo beam to the junction of the posterior walls of the left atrium and ventricle in order to visualize the posterior leaflet adequately. Since it is possible to establish a false-positive diagnosis from tracings obtained from the body of the leaflets, care must be taken to angulate the transducer in order to record valve motion from the free edge of the leaflet.[344] M-mode echocardiography has also missed MVP in some patients.[345] However, two-dimensional echocardiography, particularly the apical four-chamber view, has been proposed as the single best technique to define the syndrome (Figure 5–43, p. 112), which is present when the mitral valve leaf-

lets lie in the left atrium rather than in the left ventricle during systole.[346]

The echocardiographic findings of MVP have been reported to occur in a large number of first-degree relatives of patients with established MVP,[347] but the variability in physical findings in this syndrome, already commented upon, extends to the echocardiogram. Thus, some patients have a systolic click with or without a murmur and show no evidence of MVP on the echocardiogram. Conversely, the echocardiographic findings of MVP may be observed in patients without the click or murmur.[348] Others have both the typical echocardiographic and auscultatory features.

Two-dimensional echocardiography has also revealed prolapse of the tricuspid and aortic valves in approximately one-fifth of patients with MVP.[345,349] Conversely, however, prolapse of the tricuspid and aortic valves[350,351] occurs uncommonly in patients without prolapse of the mitral valve; the latter echocardiographic finding is usually not associated with any aortic regurgitation.

Stress Scintigraphy

The differential diagnosis between two common conditions—MVP associated with atypical chest pain and electrocardiographic abnormalities, and primary coronary artery disease associated with MVP—may be aided by myocardial scintigraphy using thallium-201 during exercise (p. 369). When findings are normal, i.e., when there is no evidence of exercise-induced regional myocardial ischemia, the diagnosis of MVP unrelated to ischemic heart disease is most likely.[352] However, the reverse is not always the case, since patients having MVP with or without associated coronary artery disease may exhibit myocardial perfusion defects—exercise-induced or following redistribution or both.[353]

Angiography

The configuration of the left ventriculogram during systole is helpful in the diagnosis of MVP.[354,355] The right anterior oblique projection is most useful for defining the posterior leaflet of the mitral valve and the left anterior oblique projection for studying the anterior leaflet. The most helpful sign is extension of the mitral leaflet tissue inferiorly and posteriorly to the point of attachment of the mitral leaflets to the annulus fibrosis[356] (Fig. 32–18). Angiography may also reveal scalloped edges of the leaflets, reflecting redundancy of tissue.

Other abnormalities noted on angiography include decreased contraction, dilatation, and calcification of the mitral annulus and poor contraction of the basal portion of the left ventricle.[357] There may be an indentation at the base of the posteromedial papillary muscle associated with prolapse of the posterior leaflet and resulting from abnormal traction on this muscle. With involvement of both papillary muscles, there may be an indentation of the anterior as well as the inferior wall of the left ventricle, giving the cardiac silhouette an "hourglass appearance." It has been proposed that these contraction abnormalities are primary, but the bulk of available evidence suggests that the left ventricular contraction abnormalities are secondary to redundancy of the mitral valve leaflets and transmission of the abnormal tension on these leaflets to the papillary muscles and underlying left ventricle. Patients with MVP

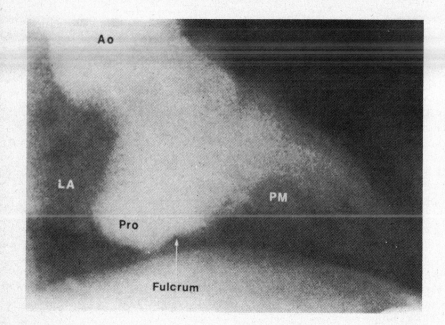

FIGURE 32–18 Systolic frame of left ventricular angiogram demonstrating prolapse (Pro) of the mitral valve. The posteromedial commissural scallop of the posterior mitral leaflet extends posteriorly and inferiorly to the fulcrum. PM = papillary muscle. (From Cohen, M. V., et al.: Angiographic-echocardiographic correlation in mitral valve prolapse. Am. Heart J. *97*:46, 1979.)

and little or no mitral regurgitation have normal left ventricular hemodynamics. An increased rate of circumferential fiber shortening may be observed in the presence of significant mitral regurgitation, as in patients with regurgitation of other etiologies.[357] Ejection fraction at rest determined by radionuclide angiography is normal in patients having MVP without associated mitral regurgitation. However, a subgroup of these patients do not exhibit a normal increase in ejection fraction during exercise, suggesting that a cardiomyopathic process may be responsible for the reduced cardiac reserve.[358]

Natural History

The outlook for MVP in children is excellent, a large majority remaining asymptomatic for many years without any change in clinical or laboratory manifestations.[359,360]

Progressive mitral regurgitation occurs in about 15 per cent of patients over a 10- to 15-year period; the incidence of this complication is significantly greater in patients with both murmurs and clicks than in those with an isolated click.[360] In many patients, rupture of chordae tendineae or infective endocarditis is responsible for the intensification of the mitral regurgitation.[273] When mitral regurgitation is severe, valve replacement may be required; indeed MVP is an important cause of pure mitral regurgitation in patients requiring mitral valve replacement.[313] Patients with the MVP syndrome are also at risk of developing infective endocarditis,[273,361,362] although the incidence appears to be extremely low in patients with only a midsystolic click. When encountered in the elderly, MVP is often a cause of heart failure.[363]

Acute hemiplegia, transient ischemic attacks, cerebellar infarcts, amaurosis fugax, and retinal arteriolar occlusions all appear to occur more frequently in patients with the MVP syndrome, suggesting that cerebral emboli are unusually common in this condition.[364–368] These neurological complications are often associated with shortened platelet survival[367] and platelet coagulant hyperactivity.[365] Loss of

endothelial continuity and tearing of the endocardium overlying the myxomatous valve may initiate platelet aggregation and the formation of mural platelet-fibrin complexes.[368a] The paroxysmal arrhythmias that occur in the MVP syndrome may contribute to the likelihood of embolization. Indeed, it is possible that cerebral embolization secondary to MVP may be a significant cause for unexplained strokes and other cerebral and retinal complications in young people with undetected cerebrovascular disease.[364,365] Similarly, myocardial infarction in patients with MVP and normal coronary arteries may be secondary to embolization.[368b]

Treatment

Asymptomatic patients (or those whose principal complaint is anxiety) with no arrhythmias evident on a routine extended electrocardiographic tracing and on prolonged auscultation, with normal ST segments and without evidence of serious mitral regurgitation should be reassured about the favorable prognosis but should have follow-up examinations every 2 or 3 years. Patients with a long systolic murmur may show progression of mitral regurgitation and should be examined more frequently, at intervals of approximately 12 months. Since infective endocarditis is a well-recognized complication of MVP,[273] *endocarditis prophylaxis* is advisable in patients with a typical systolic murmur and characteristic echocardiographic features. Although opinions on this point are not unanimous, prophylaxis is probably also advisable in patients with a midsystolic click without a systolic murmur, since bacterial endocarditis has been reported in such patients and it is well established that the systolic murmur may be intermittent or provoked.[273]

Patients with a history of palpitations, lightheadedness, dizziness, or syncope or those who have arrhythmias on clinical examination or on a routine electrocardiogram should undergo ambulatory (24-hour) electrocardiographic monitoring or treadmill exercise testing or both. Propranolol is the drug of choice for many ventricular arrhythmias, and either propranolol or phenytoin is useful in patients with prolongation of the Q-T interval. Aprindine (a drug not yet released for general use in the United States at this time) has resulted in a striking reduction in the number of premature ventricular extrasystoles and in the frequency and duration of ventricular tachycardia in patients with the MVP syndrome[369] and may be considered in patients who do not respond to other antiarrhythmic drugs. Stellate ganglion blockade followed by thoracic sympathectomy and even mitral valve replacement have been proposed for the treatment of refractory ventricular tachycardia; however, the results are insufficient to evaluate the effectiveness of these modes of therapy.

Beta-adrenergic blockade may be useful in the treatment of chest discomfort, both in patients with associated coronary artery disease and in those with normal coronary vessels in whom the symptoms may be due to regional ischemia secondary to MVP.[370] Nitrates should be used with caution, since the reduction of cardiac size induced by these drugs may intensify the prolapse and the resultant ischemia of the base of the papillary muscles.

Patients with symptoms of reduced functional cardiac reserve should be treated like other patients with severe mitral regurgitation (p. 1084), and those with severe regurgitation who are not responsive to medical management may require mitral valve replacement.[313] In patients with angina on effort and/or ischemic electrocardiographic changes and abnormalities on a thallium perfusion scan during exercise, coronary arteriography should be performed, and treatment should take into account the responsiveness of symptoms to medical management and the coronary anatomy, as outlined in Chapter 39. In patients with MVP who have had any of the aforementioned cerebral events and in whom no other etiology is apparent, anticoagulant therapy and/or drugs that interfere with platelet function, such as aspirin and dipyridamole, should be given.

Although this discussion has focused attention on complications of the MVP syndrome, it should not be forgotten that, on the whole, this is a benign condition and that the vast majority of patients with this syndrome remain asymptomatic for their entire lives and require, at most, observation every few years and reassurance.

AORTIC STENOSIS

ETIOLOGY AND PATHOLOGY

Obstruction to left ventricular outflow is localized most commonly at the aortic valve, discussed in this section. However, obstruction may also occur above the valve (supravalvular stenosis [p. 981]) or below the valve (discrete subvalvular aortic stenosis [p. 980]) or may be caused by hypertrophic obstructive cardiomyopathy (p. 1409). In an analysis of the hearts of 543 patients with valvular disease, Roberts found isolated aortic stenosis to be the most common lesion.[371] Valvular aortic stenosis without accompanying mitral valve disease is more common in men and very rarely occurs on a rheumatic basis but instead is usually either congenital or degenerative in origin[371-374] (Figs. 32–19 and 32–20).

CONGENITAL AORTIC STENOSIS (See also p.1026). Congenital malformations of the aortic valve may be unicuspid, bicuspid, or tricuspid or may be a dome-shaped diaphragm (Fig. 32–20).[128] *Unicuspid valves* produce severe obstruction in infancy[375] and are the most frequent malformations found in fatal valvular aortic stenosis in children under the age of 1 year.[376] Congenitally *bicuspid valves* may be stenotic with commissural fusion at birth, but more commonly they are not responsible for serious narrowing of the aortic orifice during childhood;[377-379] their abnormal architecture induces turbulent flow, which traumatizes the leaflets and ultimately leads to fibrosis, increased rigidity, and calcification of the leaflets and narrowing of the aortic orifice[380] (Fig. 32–21). Infective endocarditis may develop on a congenitally bicuspid valve, which then becomes regurgitant. Rarely, a congenitally bicuspid valve is purely regurgitant in the absence of antecedent infection. It should be emphasized that in a majority of cases, a bicuspid valve is not stenotic at birth and that the changes causing stenosis resemble those occurring in senile, degenerative calcific stenosis of a tricuspid aortic valve except

that in the congenitally bicuspid valve these changes occur several decades earlier.

A third form of a congenitally malformed valve is *tricuspid*, with the cusps of unequal size and some commissural fusion. Although many of these valves retain normal func-

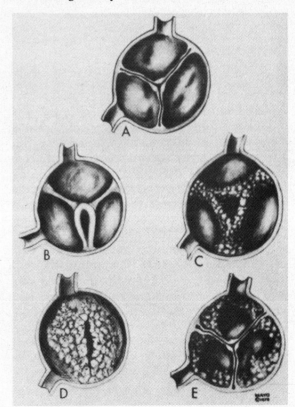

FIGURE 32–19 Types of aortic valve stenosis. *A*, Normal aortic valve. *B*, Congenital aortic stenosis. *C*, Rheumatic aortic stenosis. *D*, Calcific bicuspid aortic stenosis. *E*, Calcific senile aortic stenosis. (From Brandenburg, R. O., et al.: Valvular heart disease—When should the patient be referred? Pract. Cardiol. *5*:50, 1979.)

Congenital dome   Unicommissural

Rheumatic   Bicuspid calcific   Senile calcific

Mixed forms

FIGURE 32–20 Schematic representation of the types of aortic valve stenosis, viewed from above. (Reproduced with permission from Davies, M. J.: Pathology of Cardiac Valves. London, Butterworths, 1980.)

tion throughout life, it has been postulated that the turbulent flow produced by the mild congenital architectural abnormality may lead to fibrosis and ultimately to calcification and stenosis.[371] Tricuspid stenotic aortic valves in adults may be congenital, rheumatic, or degenerative in origin.

ACQUIRED AORTIC STENOSIS. *Rheumatic aortic stenosis* results from adhesions and fusion of the commissures and cusps and vascularization of the leaflets and the valve ring, leading to retraction and stiffening of the free borders of the cusps, with calcific nodules present on both surfaces and an orifice that is reduced to a small round or triangular opening. As a consequence, the rheumatic valve is often regurgitant as well as stenotic (Figs. 32–20, 32–21, and 32–22 and 48–5, p. 1647). The heart frequently exhibits other stigmata of rheumatic heart disease, especially mitral valve involvement. In *degenerative (senile) calcific aortic stenosis*, the cusps are immobilized by a deposit of calcium along their flexion lines at their bases. This common cause of aortic stenosis in adults appears to result from years of normal mechanical stress on the valve. Although degenerative calcification may extend in the direc-

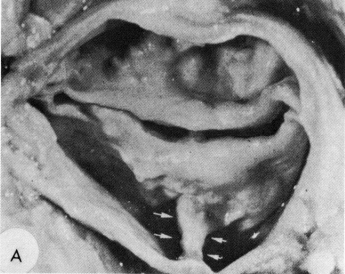
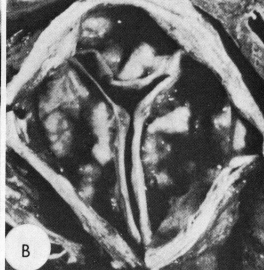
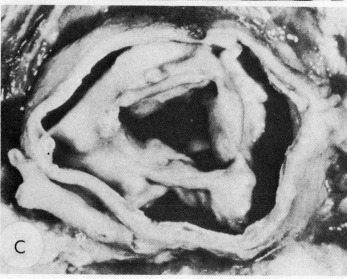

FIGURE 32–21 *A,* Calcified, stenotic, congenitally bicuspid aortic valve of a 59-year-old man. The cusps are situated anteriorly and posteriorly, with the commissures on the right and left, respectively. The valve has a raphe (white arrows) in the anterior cusp. Peak systolic gradient across the valve was 45 mm Hg, and the patient had complete heart block secondary to destruction of the atrioventricular bundle by calcium, which presumably had extended down from the aortic valvular cusps.

B, Stenotic tricuspid aortic valve in an 81-year-old man. Aortic stenosis in the elderly is characterized by calcific deposits on the aortic surfaces of the cusps and typically no or little commissural fusion.

C, Stenotic tricuspid aortic valve in a 55-year-old man. Each of the three commissures is fused, producing a triangular fixed central orifice that is both stenotic and incompetent. (From Roberts, W. C.: Valvular, subvalvular and supravalvular aortic stenosis: Morphologic features. *In* Edwards, J. E. [ed.]: Clinical-Pathologic Correlations #2. Philadelphia, F. A. Davis, 1973, pp. 100, 106, and 108.)

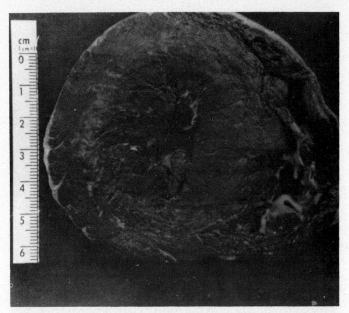

FIGURE 32–22 Heart from a man aged 62 years, who died suddenly with aortic valve stenosis (bicuspid calcific). The total heart weight was 610 gm. The left ventricular cavity is small, and the wall thickness is 3 cm. (Reproduced with permission from Davies, M. J.: Pathology of Cardiac Valves. London, Butterworths, 1980.)

tion of the cusps, no commissural fusion is present.[128] Degenerative "wear and tear" appears to be the most likely cause of this form of aortic stenosis, which is commonly accompanied by calcifications of the mitral annulus and coronary arteries but rarely by aortic regurgitation. The stenosis is produced by the calcific deposits that prevent the cusps from opening normally during systole (Fig. 32–21). In *atherosclerotic aortic valvular stenosis*, severe atherosclerosis involves the aorta and other major arteries; this form of aortic stenosis occurs most frequently in patients with severe hypercholesterolemia[381] and is observed in children with homozygous Type II hyperlipoproteinemia (p. 1630). *Rheumatoid involvement* of the valve is a rare cause of aortic stenosis and results in nodular thickening of the valve leaflets and involvement of the proximal part of the aorta (p. 1658). *Ochronosis* is another rare cause of aortic stenosis.[382]

Roberts studied hearts with aortic stenosis in patients between 15 and 65 years of age and found that almost 40 per cent were tricuspid. Since there was thickening of the mitral valve and a history of acute rheumatic fever in half of these cases, it is likely that the aortic stenosis was rheumatic in etiology; in the remainder it was either congenital or degenerative in origin. In 90 per cent of hearts examined at autopsy in patients with aortic stenosis who were older than 65 years, the valves were tricuspid, with nodular calcific deposits on the aortic aspects of the cusps, but without commissural fusion.[371]

Hemodynamically significant aortic stenosis leads to severe concentric left ventricular hypertrophy,[383] with heart weights as great as 1000 gm (Fig. 32–22). The interventricular septum often bulges into and encroaches on the right ventricular cavity. When left ventricular failure supervenes, the left ventricle dilates,[383] the left atrium enlarges, and changes secondary to backward failure occur in the pulmonary vascular bed, right side of the heart, and systemic venous bed.

Pathophysiology

The left ventricle responds to the sudden production of severe obstruction to outflow by dilatation and reduction of stroke volume. However, in adults with aortic stenosis, the obstruction usually develops and increases gradually over a prolonged period. In infants and children with congenital aortic stenosis, the valve orifice shows little change as the child grows, thereby intensifying obstruction quite gradually. Left ventricular function can be well maintained in experimentally produced, chronic, gradually developing subcoronary aortic stenosis.[384] Left ventricular output is maintained by the presence of left ventricular hypertrophy, which may sustain a large pressure gradient across the aortic valve for many years without a reduction in cardiac output, left ventricular dilatation, or the development of symptoms (Figs. 32–23 and 9–7, p. 288). A peak systolic pressure gradient exceeding 50 mm Hg in the presence of a normal cardiac output or an effective aortic orifice less than about 0.4 cm^2/m^2 of body surface area, i.e., less than approximately one-fourth of the normal orifice, is generally considered to represent critical obstruction to left ventricular outflow (Fig. 32–24).[385]

As contraction of the left ventricle becomes progressively more isometric, the left ventricular pressure pulse exhibits a rounded, rather than flattened, summit. The elevated left ventricular end-diastolic pressure, which is characteristic of severe aortic stenosis, does not necessarily signify the presence of left ventricular dilatation or failure but often reflects diminished compliance of the hypertrophied left ventricular wall; usually it results from both processes.

In patients with severe aortic stenosis, large *a* waves usually appear in the left atrial pressure pulse because of the combination of enhanced contraction of a hypertrophied left atrium and diminished left ventricular compliance. Atrial contraction plays a particularly important role in filling of the left ventricle in aortic stenosis.[23] It raises left ventricular end-diastolic pressure without producing a concomitant elevation of mean left atrial pressure.[386] This "booster pump" function of the left atrium prevents the pulmonary venous and capillary pressures from rising to levels that would produce pulmonary congestion, while at the same time maintaining left ventricular end-diastolic pressure at the elevated level necessary for effective left

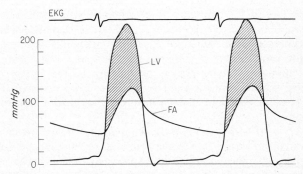

FIGURE 32–23 Pressure tracings from a 77-year-old man with a history of recent syncopal attacks. A mean pressure gradient of 90 mm Hg (cross-hatched area) between left ventricular (LV) pressure and arterial pressure measured at the right femoral artery (FA) is demonstrated. In addition, the arterial pressure curve has a markedly delayed upstroke with a reduced rate of rise. The calculated aortic valve area was narrowed to 0.5 cm^2.

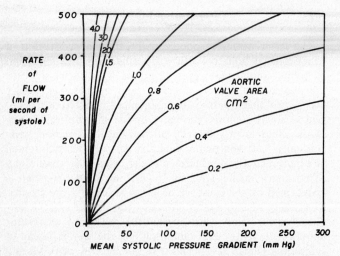

FIGURE 32–24 Chart illustrating the relation between mean systolic pressure gradient across the aortic valve and the rate of flow across the aortic valve per second of systole, as predicted by the Gorlin formula. Although the effective area of the aortic valve in the adult is about 2.6 to 3.5 cm², there is relatively little obstruction to blood flow until the area is markedly reduced. At the "critical" valve area, about 0.5 to 0.7 cm², relatively little further increase in flow is achieved, even with marked increases in mean systolic gradient. (Reproduced with permission from Wallace, A. G.: Pathophysiology of cardiovascular disease. *In* Smith, L. H., Jr., and Thier, S. O. [eds.]: Pathophysiology. The Biological Principles of Disease. Philadelphia, W. B. Saunders, 1981, p. 1200.)

ventricular contraction. Loss of appropriately timed, vigorous atrial contraction, as occurs in atrial fibrillation or atrioventricular dissociation, may result in rapid clinical deterioration in patients with severe aortic stenosis.

Although the *cardiac output* at rest is within normal limits in the majority of patients with severe aortic stenosis, it often fails to rise normally during exertion. Late in the course of the disease the cardiac output, stroke volume, and therefore the left ventricular–aortic pressure gradient all decline, whereas the mean left atrial, pulmonary capillary, pulmonary arterial, right ventricular systolic and diastolic, and right atrial pressures rise, sequentially. Aortic stenosis intensifies the severity of any existing mitral regurgitation by increasing the pressure gradient responsible for driving blood from the left ventricle to the left atrium. In addition, the dilatation of the left ventricle, which occurs late in the course of some patients with aortic valve disease, may produce mitral regurgitation, superimposing the hemodynamic changes associated with this lesion on those produced by aortic stenosis. Also, as a consequence of pulmonary hypertension or bulging of the hypertrophied septum into the right ventricular cavity or both, the *a* wave in the right atrial pressure pulse becomes prominent.

Left ventricular end-diastolic volume usually remains normal until quite late in the course of the disease, but left ventricular mass increases in response to the chronic pressure overload, resulting in an increase in the mass/volume ratio. However, the increase in mass may not be as great as that seen with aortic regurgitation or combined stenosis and regurgitation[26] (Table 14–1, p. 474).

In experimental animals, when the aorta is suddenly constricted, left ventricular pressure rises, and there is a large increase in wall stress, whereas both extent and ve-

locity of shortening decline. As pointed out in Chapter 13, the development of ventricular hypertrophy is one of the principal mechanisms by which the heart compensates for such an increased hemodynamic burden.[389a,389b] The increased systolic wall stress induced by aortic stenosis apparently leads to parallel replication of sarcomeres and concentric hypertrophy (Figure 13–7, p. 452), and the increase in left ventricular wall thickness is often sufficient to counterbalance the increased pressure, so that peak systolic wall tension returns to normal or remains so if the obstruction develops slowly[387] (Figure 13–8, p. 453). There is an inverse correlation between wall stress and ejection fraction in patients with aortic stenosis, suggesting that the depressed ejection fraction and velocity of fiber shortening that occur in some patients are a consequence of inadequate wall thickening,[388] resulting in "afterload mismatch."[389] Patients having aortic stenosis with compensated pressure overload as well as some with depressed left ventricular ejection fractions and overt congestive failure may have normal values for the rate of intraventricular stress ($d\sigma/dt$) and pressure (dp/dt) development.[390] In others, the lower ejection fraction is secondary to a depression of contractility (Fig. 13–9, p. 453); in the latter, the effectiveness of surgical treatment is reduced.[391] Thus, both altered contractility and increased afterload are operative in depressing left ventricular performance.[392]

From these considerations it is clear that in order to evaluate myocardial function in patients with aortic stenosis, it is critical to relate the ejection phase indices to the existing wall tension (p. 453).[393] Wall thickness is a critical determinant of ventricular performance in patients with aortic stenosis; inadequate hypertrophy, an intrinsic depression of myocardial contractility, or a combination of these two defects may lead to a depression of ventricular performance.

DIASTOLIC STIFFNESS. Although ventricular hypertrophy is a key compensatory mechanism, it presents an adverse pathophysiological consequence, i.e., greater intracavitary pressure is required for ventricular filling. Some patients with aortic stenosis manifest an increase in chamber stiffness due simply to an increase in muscle mass but with no alteration in muscle stiffness; others exhibit increases in muscle stiffness as well as in chamber stiffness, both of which contribute to the elevation of ventricular diastolic filling pressure at any level of ventricular diastolic volume.[394] Chamber stiffness may revert toward normal as hypertrophy regresses following relief of aortic stenosis, and at least in some patients muscle stiffness may also revert to normal; whether this occurs in all patients is not clear. It is not expected that this regression of stiffness would occur in patients with extensive myocardial fibrosis.

A variety of changes in the *myocardial ultrastructure* have been documented in patients with severe aortic stenosis. These include unusually large nuclei, loss of myofibrils, accumulation of mitochondria, the presence of large cytoplasmic areas devoid of contractile material, and the proliferation of fibroblasts and collagen fibers in the interstitial space.[395] The depression of cardiac function that occurs late in the course of the disease may well be related to these morphological alterations. In aortic stenosis, coronary blood flow at rest is elevated in absolute terms but is normal when corrected for myocardial mass.[396] There may be inadequate myocardial oxygenation in severe aortic stenosis, even in the absence of coronary artery disease. The hypertrophied left ventricular muscle mass, the elevated systolic pressure, and the prolongation of ejection all elevate myocardial oxygen requirements, and the abnormally elevated pressure compressing the coronary arteries exceeds the coronary perfusion pressure, thereby interfering with coronary blood flow.[397] Blood flow is also impaired by the elevation of left ventricular end-diastolic pressure, which lowers the diastolic aortic–left ventricular pressure (coronary perfusion pressure) gradient. Therefore, the subendocardium in severe aortic stenosis is susceptible to ischemia, and this underperfusion may be responsible for the development of myocardial ischemia.[396] Metabolic evidence of myocardial ischemia, i.e., lactate production, can be demonstrated when myocardial oxygen needs are stimulated by exercise or isoproterenol in patients with aortic stenosis, in both the presence and the absence of coronary arterial narrowing.

CLINICAL MANIFESTATIONS

History

In the natural history of adults with aortic stenosis, there is a long latent period during which there is gradually increasing obstruction and an increase in the burden on the myocardium while the patient remains asymptomatic. The cardinal symptoms of aortic stenosis, which commence most commonly in the sixth decade of life, are angina pectoris, syncope, and congestive heart failure.[399] However, in patients in whom the obstruction remains unrelieved, once these symptoms become manifest, the prognosis is poor; survival curves show that the interval from the onset of symptoms to the time of death is approximately 2 years in patients with heart failure, 3 years in those with syncope, and 5 years in those with angina.[400,401] *Angina* occurs in approximately two-thirds of patients with critical aortic stenosis (about half of whom have significant coronary artery obstruction)[398] and usually resembles that observed in patients with coronary artery disease, in that it is commonly precipitated by exertion and relieved by rest. It results from the combination of increased oxygen needs of the hypertrophied myocardium and reduction of oxygen delivery secondary to the excessive compression of coronary vessels.[396,402,403] Rarely, it results from calcium emboli entering the coronary vascular bed.[404] Angina may, of course, also result from coexisting coronary artery disease, and the absence of angina in a patient with aortic stenosis suggests that serious obstructive coronary artery disease is not present (p. 1338). *Syncope* is is usually orthostatic and is most commonly due to the reduced cerebral perfusion that occurs during exertion when arterial pressure declines consequent to systemic vasodilatation in the presence of a fixed cardiac output.[405] It may be preceded by premonitory symptoms and may be prolonged by arrhythmias.[406] Exertional hypotension may also be manifest as "graying out" spells or giddiness on effort. Syncope at rest may be due to transient ventricular fibrillation, from which the patient recovers spontaneously; transient atrial fibrillation with loss of the "atrial kick" and a precipitous decline in cardiac output; or transient

atrioventricular block due to extension of the calcification of the valve into the conduction system. *Exertional dyspnea* with orthopnea, paroxysmal nocturnal dyspnea, and pulmonary edema reflect varying degrees of pulmonary venous hypertension. These are late symptoms in aortic stenosis, and their presence for more than 5 years should suggest the possibility of associated mitral valvular disease. Gastrointestinal bleeding, idiopathic or due to angiodysplasia of the right colon or other vascular malformations, occurs more often than expected in patients with calcific aortic stenosis; it may cease after aortic valve replacement.[407,408] Infective endocarditis is a greater risk in younger patients with milder valvular deformity than in older patients with rock-like calcific aortic deformities. Cerebral emboli resulting in stroke or transient ischemic attacks may result from microthrombi on thickened bicuspid valves.[409] Calcific aortic stenosis may cause embolization of calcium to a variety of organs, including the heart, kidney, and brain. Abrupt loss of vision has been reported when calcific emboli occluded the central retinal artery.[410]

Since cardiac output is usually well maintained for many years in patients with severe aortic stenosis, marked fatigability, debilitation, peripheral cyanosis, and other manifestations of a low cardiac output are usually not prominent until quite late in the natural history of the disease. Atrial fibrillation, pulmonary hypertension, and systemic venous hypertension in patients with isolated aortic stenosis are often preterminal findings. Although aortic stenosis may be responsible for sudden death (p. 781), this usually occurs in patients who had previously been symptomatic.

Physical Examination
(Tables 32–9 and 32–10)

The arterial pulse characteristically rises slowly and is small and sustained (pulsus parvus et tardus) (p. 24).[411] In the advanced stage of the disease, systolic and pulse pressures are both reduced. However, in patients with mild stenosis with associated regurgitation and in older patients with an inelastic arterial bed, both systolic and pulse pressures may be normal or even increased. A systolic pressure exceeding 200 mm Hg is rare in patients with critical aortic stenosis.[411] The anacrotic notch and coarse systolic vibrations are felt most readily in the carotid arterial pulse, producing the so-called carotid shudder (Figures 3–22, p. 56, and 4–4, p. 70). Although pulsus alternans occurs commonly in aortic stenosis with left ventricular dysfunction[412] (Figure 3–26, p. 58), obstruction of the aortic valve may prevent it from being recognized by examination of the peripheral arterial pulse. The jugular venous pulse usually shows prominent *a* waves (Fig. 4–8, p. 73), reflecting reduced right ventricular compliance consequent to hypertrophy of the ventricular septum.[413] With pulmonary hypertension and secondary right ventricular failure and tricuspid regurgitation, *v* or *c-v* waves may be prominent.

The cardiac impulse is sustained with left ventricular failure; it becomes displaced inferiorly and laterally. Presystolic distention of the left ventricle, i.e., a prominent precordial *a* wave, is often both visible and palpable. A hyperdynamic left ventricle suggests concomitant aortic or mitral regurgitation. A systolic thrill is usually best appreciated when the patient leans forward in full expiration. It is felt most readily in the second left intercostal space on

TABLE 32-9   CONDITIONS FREQUENTLY CONFUSED WITH AORTIC STENOSIS

CONDITION	DISTINGUISHING FEATURES
Dilated aorta (hypertension, syphilis) with systolic murmur in second right intercostal space	No single or paradoxical S_2; A_2 normal or loud; murmur often short
Bruit arising in carotid or subclavian arteries (benign supraclavicular bruit, arterial occlusive disease)	Bruit louder in neck or supraclavicular fossae and may be obliterated by subclavian artery compression; bruit may be shorter; normal S_2
Pulmonic valvular stenosis	Murmur reaches A_2; more frequent systolic ejection click; P_2 faint and delayed; A_2 normal; right ventricular enlargement; occasional large jugular a wave
Severe aortic regurgitation	Widened pulse pressure; visible carotid pulse; A_2 may be normal
Minimal valvulitis or calcification	Normal A_2; normal respiratory motion of S_2; no left ventricular enlargement
Mitral regurgitation	Pansystolic or ejection murmur; normal respiratory variation of S_2; normal A_2; S_1 may be faint; S_3 gallop common if severe; aortic stenosis murmur often of grunting quality at cardiac apex; murmur usually well heard in left axilla, decreased by amyl nitrite inhalation (which increases murmur of aortic stenosis) and increased by administration of phenylephrine; no aortic valve calcification on fluoroscopy

From Fowler, N. O.: Aortic stenosis: Left ventricular outflow tract obstruction. *In* Fowler, N. O. (ed.): Cardiac Diagnosis and Treatment. 3rd ed. Hagerstown, Md., Harper and Row, 1980, p. 550.

either side of the sternum or in the suprasternal notch and is frequently transmitted along the carotid arteries.

Rarely, evidence of right ventricular failure with systemic venous congestion, hepatomegaly, and edema precedes left ventricular failure, probably owing to the so-called Bernheim effect, which results from the hypertrophied ventricular septum bulging into and encroaching on the right ventricular cavity and leads to impairment of right ventricular filling. In such cases, the jugular venous pressure is elevated and the *a* wave is prominent.

AUSCULTATION (Table 32–5). S_1 is normal or soft and S_4 is prominent, presumably because atrial contraction is vigorous and the mitral valve is partially closed during presystole.[414,415] S_2 may be single because calcification and immobility of the aortic valve make A_2 inaudible, because P_2 is buried in the prolonged aortic ejection murmur, or because prolongation of left ventricular systole makes A_2 coincide with P_2. Paradoxical splitting of S_2, which suggests associated left ventricular dysfunction, may also occur. With left ventricular failure and secondary pulmonary hypertension, P_2 may become accentuated. When the valve is rigid, A_2 may be inaudible, but when the valve is flexible, A_2 may be snapping and accentuated (Figure 3–22, p. 56).

An *aortic ejection sound* occurs simultaneously with the halting upward movement of the aortic valve. It is dependent on mobility of the valve cusps[416] and disappears when they become severely calcified. Thus, it is common in children with congenital aortic stenosis but rare in elderly adults with acquired calcific aortic stenosis and rigid valves. This sound occurs approximately 0.06 sec after the onset of S_1, has a frequency similar to S_1, and is heard most readily with the diaphragm of the stethoscope along the left sternal border, although it is often well transmitted to the apex, where it may be confused with S_1 (and the S_1 may be mistaken for an S_4). In contrast to a pulmonic ejection sound, aortic ejection sounds usually do not vary with respiration and usually occur later.

TABLE 32–10   COMPARISONS OF VALVULAR AORTIC STENOSIS, HYPERTROPHIC OBSTRUCTIVE CARDIOMYOPATHY, AND DISCRETE (CONGENITAL) SUBAORTIC STENOSIS

FEATURES	HYPERTROPHIC OBSTRUCTIVE CARDIOMYOPATHY	VALVULAR AORTIC STENOSIS	DISCRETE SUBAORTIC STENOSIS
Family history	Or familial	Extremely uncommon	Extremely uncommon
Symptoms	Dyspnea, angina, syncope	Dyspnea, angina, syncope	Dyspnea, angina, syncope
Arterial pulse	Quick upstroke, jerky; prominent tidal wave	Anacrotic	Normal or anacrotic
Cardiac impulse	Double thrust	Left ventricular	Left ventricular
Systolic ejection murmur	Maximal internal to apex beat; late onset	Maximal at aortic area (or apex)	Maximal at aortic area and apex; early onset
Reversed split of second heart sound	Rare	Common	Occasional
Systolic click	Occasional	Frequent unless calcified	Rare
Aortic valve closure	Audible	Audible unless heavily calcified	Inaudible
Aortic diastolic murmur	Rare	Not uncommon	Frequent
Mitral systolic murmur	Very common	Occasional	Common
Mitral diastolic murmur	Not uncommon	Not uncommon	Rare
Prominent *a* wave in jugular venous pulse	May be striking	Unimpressive unless pulmonary hypertension	Unimpressive
Atrial sound	Very common	Common	Common
Aortic valve calcification	Never seen	Very common after age 40	Absent
Left heart catheterization	Gradient across left ventricular outflow tract may be extremely variable or absent	Gradient constant across aortic valve	Subvalvular gradient
Dilatation of ascending aorta	Absent	Common	Common

From Cleland, W., et al.: Medical and Surgical Cardiology. Oxford, Blackwell Scientific Publications, 1969, p. 967.

The *midsystolic murmur* of aortic stenosis is heard best at the base of the heart but is often well transmitted along the carotid vessels and to the apex. Cessation of the murmur before A_2 is usually helpful in differentiating it from a pansystolic mitral murmur, but it may be falsely considered to be a pansystolic murmur because it may end with S_2, which represents pulmonic valve closure, A_2 being soft or even inaudible (Figures 3–22, p. 56, 4–1, p. 69, and 4–7, p. 72). In patients with calcified aortic valves, the murmur is harsh and rasping at the base, but high-frequency components selectively radiate to the apex (the so-called Gallavardin phenomenon), where it may actually be more prominent and where it may be mistaken for the murmur of mitral regurgitation. Frequently, there is a "quiet area" between the base and apex where the murmur is diminished in intensity, supporting the erroneous impression that the apical and basal murmurs have different origins. In general, the more severe the stenosis, the longer the duration of the murmur and the later in systole its peak intensity.[417]

In patients with degenerative or atherosclerotic aortic stenosis, there may be heavy valvular calcification, but obstruction may not be severe because the commissural fusion characteristic of congenital and rheumatic aortic stenosis is absent. The nonfused calcified cusps vibrate freely, resulting in a softer, more musical murmur, more prominent at the apex than the murmur of congenital or rheumatic aortic stenosis.[417] High-pitched decrescendo diastolic murmurs secondary to aortic regurgitation are common in many patients with dominant aortic stenosis.

Dynamic Auscultation (Table 32–6). The murmur of valvular aortic stenosis is augmented by the inhalation of amyl nitrite or with squatting or lying flat and is reduced in intensity during the Valsalva strain (which increases the murmur of hypertrophic obstructive cardiomyopathy or with vasopressors, moderate isometric exercise, or standing.[418] It varies in intensity from beat to beat when the duration of diastolic filling varies, as in atrial fibrillation or following a premature contraction, and this characteristic is helpful in differentiating aortic stenosis from mitral regurgitation, in which the murmur is usually unaffected (Figure 4–8, p. 70). An aortic diastolic murmur is frequently present in patients with valvular aortic stenosis. In hypertrophic obstructive cardiomyopathy, the murmur is delayed in onset and may continue up to A_2; the carotid artery characteristically rises sharply (Table 32–9) and is bisferiens. Palpation of the carotid pulse is also extremely helpful in differentiating between valvular aortic stenosis, on the one hand, and hypertrophic obstructive cardiomyopathy and mitral regurgitation, on the other, since the arterial pulse generally rises slowly in aortic stenosis but sharply in the other two conditions. However, confusion can arise in the young patient with congenital aortic stenosis, in whom sudden upward displacement ("doming") of the pliant aortic leaflet or leaflets with ventricular systole may result in a brisk initial upstroke in the carotid pulse, coincident with the systolic ejection click.

When the left ventricle fails in aortic stenosis and the cardiac output falls, the murmur becomes softer or disappears altogether, and the slowly rising pulse is more difficult to appreciate. Stated simply, the clinical picture changes to that of severe left ventricular failure with a low cardiac output and pulmonary edema. Thus, occult aortic stenosis may be a cause of intractable heart failure, and critical aortic stenosis should be actively sought in patients with severe heart failure of unknown cause, since operative treatment may be life-saving and may result in substantial clinical improvement.[419]

LABORATORY EXAMINATION

ELECTROCARDIOGRAM. The principal electrocardiographic change is left ventricular hypertrophy, which is found in approximately 85 per cent of patients with severe aortic stenosis[70] (Figure 7–14A, p. 210). The absence of left ventricular hypertrophy does not exclude the presence of critical aortic stenosis, and the relationship between the absolute voltages in precordial leads and the severity of obstruction, which is quite good in children with congenital aortic stenosis, is not as good in adults. T-wave inversion and ST-segment depressions in leads having upright QRS complexes are common. ST-segment depressions greater than 0.3 mv in patients with aortic stenosis suggest that severe ventricular hypertrophy is present. The progressive development of ST-segment and T-wave abnormalities suggests that hypertrophy has progressed. Occasionally, a "pseudoinfarction" pattern is present, characterized by a loss of r waves in the right precordial leads and an early vector directed posteriorly in the horizontal plane of the vectorcardiogram, simulating anteroseptal infarction.[420] A good correlation has been reported between the sum of the QRS amplitude in 12 leads and the height of the left ventricular systolic pressure.[421] There is evidence of left atrial enlargement in more than 80 per cent of patients with severe isolated aortic stenosis;[422] the principal manifestation is prominent late negativity of the P wave in V_1 rather than an increased duration in lead II, suggesting that hypertrophy rather than dilatation is present. Atrial fibrillation is an uncommon and late sign of pure aortic stenosis[423] and, when present in a patient who is not greatly disabled, should suggest the possibility of mitral valvular disease or ischemic heart disease.

The extension of calcific infiltrates from the aortic valve into the conduction system may cause various forms and degrees of atrioventricular and intraventricular block in 5 per cent of patients with calcific aortic stenosis;[424,425] almost 10 per cent of all instances of left anterior hemiblock are secondary to aortic valvular disease.[426]

Vectorcardiogram. In patients with severe aortic stenosis, the vectorcardiogram usually shows an increase in the maximal spatial voltage and counterclockwise inscription of the loop in the transverse plane, with the major forces in the left posterior quadrant. In the left sagittal plane, the QRS loop is usually directed posteriorly and superiorly.[427]

Graphic Recordings. The indirect carotid, jugular, and apical pulse tracings, systolic time intervals, and phonocardiographic findings in aortic stenosis are discussed in Chapters 3 and 4.

RADIOLOGICAL FINDINGS. Routine radiological examination may be entirely normal despite the presence of critical aortic stenosis. The heart is usually of normal size or slightly enlarged, with a rounding of the left ventricular border and apex (Figure 6–27, p. 165), unless regurgitation or left ventricular failure is present and causes substantial cardiomegaly.[428] Poststenotic dilatation of the ascending aorta is a common finding. Calcification of the aortic valve is found in almost all adults with hemodynamically significant aortic stenosis;[428a] it may have to be sought on fluoroscopy (or the echocardiogram) rather than on the roentgenogram. This is an important finding; indeed, the *absence* of calcium in the region of the aortic valve on careful fluoroscopic examination in a patient older than 35 years essentially rules out severe aortic stenosis. The converse is not true, however, and in patients over the age of 60 years, severe calcification of the aortic valve may occur with only mild obstruction. The left atrium may be slightly enlarged, and there may be radiological signs of pulmonary venous hypertension. However, when left atrial enlargement is marked, particularly if the atrial appendage is prominent, the presence of associated mitral valvular disease should be suspected.

Angiographic studies of the aortic valve are best performed by injecting contrast medium into the left ventricle and filming in the 30-degree right anterior oblique and 60-degree left anterior oblique projections. These examinations often make it possible to ascertain the number of cusps of the stenotic valve and to demonstrate doming of a thickened valve and a systolic jet. However, it must be appreciated that there is some hazard of the rapid injection of a large volume of contrast material into a high-pressure left ventricle.

ECHOCARDIOGRAPHY (see also p. 114). The normal range of opening of the aortic valve is 1.6 to 2.6 cm, and normally the aortic valve leaflets are barely visible in systole. In patients with severe aortic stenosis, thickened leaflets and a barely discernible aortic orifice in systole can often be recognized on the M-mode echocardiogram (Figure 5–47, p. 114). However, a reduced aortic valve opening may also be seen in other conditions, such as heart failure, in which there is decreased blood flow across the aortic valve. In patients with a bicuspid aortic valve, the valve cusps are asymmetrical, resulting in their eccentric position within the aortic root.[429] Dense, multiple echoes within the aortic root in the area of the aortic leaflets suggest valvular calcification and support the diagnosis of aortic stenosis. Systolic vibrations of the interventricular septum are common in congenital aortic stenosis.[430] Although M-mode echocardiography can be used to diagnose calcific aortic stenosis, detect marked elevations in left ventricular end-diastolic pressure by prolongation of the A-C interval (Figure 5–35, p. 107), detect dilatation of the aorta, and estimate the severity of left ventricular hypertrophy as well as assess left ventricular function,[431] it cannot establish the severity of obstruction directly; the ratio of left ventricular wall thickness to chamber radius at end diastole, however, correlates well with left ventricular systolic pressure.[432] Two-dimensional echocardiography may also be helpful in determining the severity of the stenosis, although the accuracy of this technique is limited in patients with an intermediate degree of obstruction (Figure 5–48, p. 115).[433–435]

MANAGEMENT
Medical Treatment

Patients with aortic stenosis should be apprised of the hazards of endocarditis, and the necessity for endocarditis prophylaxis should be explained (p. 1175). Patients who are asymptomatic should be advised to report the development of any symptoms to their physician. Those with known or suspected critical obstruction should be cautioned to avoid vigorous athletic and physical activity. However, such restrictions do not apply to patients with mild obstruction. It is important to recognize that with the passage of time there is a tendency for the obstruction to become progressively more severe in patients with aortic stenosis.[436] Thus, in children and young adults, mild aortic stenosis often progresses to severe obstruction in adulthood, and in adults, moderate stenosis may progress to severe obstruction in later life. Therefore, asymptomatic patients with aortic stenosis should be followed carefully; in doing so, it is essential to look for signs of possible progression.[437] Repeated clinical examinations and electrocardiographic and echocardiographic studies at intervals of 6 to 12 months are indicated in asymptomatic patients with significant aortic stenosis.

There is no need to use digitalis glycosides unless there is evidence of an increase in ventricular volume or a reduced ejection fraction on angiographic, echocardiographic, or radionuclide examination. Although diuretics are beneficial when there is abnormal accumulation of fluid, they must be used with caution, since hypovolemia may reduce the elevated left ventricular end-diastolic pressure, lower cardiac output, and produce orthostatic hypotension. Beta-adrenergic blockers can depress myocardial function and induce left ventricular failure and should be used only with great caution, if at all, in patients with aortic stenosis.

Atrial arrhythmias occur in less than 10 per cent of patients with severe aortic stenosis, perhaps because of the late occurrence of left atrial enlargement in this condition. When such an arrhythmia is observed in a patient with aortic stenosis, the possibility of associated mitral valve disease should be considered. In light of the adverse hemodynamic effects of loss of atrial booster pump function with atrial fibrillation in patients with aortic stenosis,[386] an effort should be made to prevent the development of this arrhythmia by means of pharmacological prophylaxis when premature atrial contractions are frequent. When atrial fibrillation does occur, the rapid ventricular rate may cause angina or electrocardiographic evidence of myocardial ischemia or both; in some cases, loss of the atrial "kick" and a sudden fall in cardiac output may cause serious hypotension. Therefore, this arrhythmia should be treated promptly (p. 700), and a search for previously unrecognized mitral valve disease should be undertaken.

Cardiac catheterization should be carried out in children in whom clinical examination and noninvasive tests suggest critical obstruction, regardless of whether or not symptoms are present. Adults considered to have severe aortic stenosis should have catheterization if any symptoms develop. The purpose of catheterization in patients with aortic stenosis is to localize the site and document the severity of the obstruction, to determine the state of left ventricular function, to ascertain the presence or absence of associated valvular disease, and, in patients with angina pectoris, to determine the status of the coronary circulation.[393]

Natural History

In contrast to mitral stenosis, which leads to symptoms almost immediately after its development, patients with severe aortic stenosis may be asymptomatic for many years despite the presence of severe obstruction. The systolic pressure gradient can exceed 150 mm Hg, and the peak left ventricular systolic pressure can reach approximately 300 mm Hg with relatively little increase in overall heart size on radiographic examination, with normal left ventricular end-diastolic and end-systolic volumes. Patients with severe chronic aortic stenosis tend to be free of cardiovascular symptoms until relatively late in the course of the disease. In Rapaport's series, 40 per cent of patients treated medically survived for 5 years and 20 per cent for 10 years after diagnosis.[98] In another series of patients with hemodynamically significant valvular aortic stenosis treated medically, the 5-year survival rate was 64 per cent. However, once patients with aortic stenosis become symptomatic with angina or syncope, the average survival is 2 to 3 years, whereas with congestive heart failure it is 1½ years[401] (Fig. 32–25). Sudden death, like syncope, in patients with severe aortic stenosis may be due to cerebral hypoperfusion followed by arrhythmia.[438,439] Among symptomatic patients with moderate or severe aortic stenosis not subjected to operation, mortality rates from onset of symptoms was approximately 25 per cent at 1 year and 50 per cent at 2 years; more than half of the deaths were sudden. Asymptomatic patients have an excellent prognosis without mortality.[440] The obstruction tends to progress more rapidly in patients with degenerative calcific disease than in those with congenital or rheumatic disease.[441]

Surgical Treatment

INDICATIONS FOR OPERATION. The most critical decision in the management of patients with aortic stenosis—indeed, of all patients with valvular heart disease—concerns the advisability and timing of surgical treatment. The indications for as well as the techniques and results of operation depend on the patient's age and the nature of the valvular deformity. In children and adolescents with noncalcific congenital aortic stenosis, who most commonly

have bicuspid aortic valves, simple commissural incision under direct vision usually leads to substantial hemodynamic improvement at a low risk, i.e., a mortality rate of less than 2 per cent (p. 980).[442] Therefore, this procedure is indicated not only in symptomatic patients but also in asymptomatic children and adolescents with critical aortic stenosis, i.e., a calculated effective orifice less than 0.4 cm^2/m^2 BSA. Despite the salutary hemodynamic results following this procedure, the valve is not rendered entirely normal anatomically, and the turbulent flow around it may lead to further deformation, calcification, the development of regurgitation, and re-stenosis after 10 to 20 years, probably requiring reoperation and valve replacement at some later date.

In most adults with calcific aortic stenosis, satisfactory valvular function *cannot* be restored, even by deliberate sculpturing procedures carried out under direct vision, and valve replacement will ultimately be necessary.[443] Replacement of the aortic valve should be carried out in patients with hemodynamic evidence of severe obstruction (aortic valve orifice < 0.75 cm^2 or < 0.4 cm^2/m^2 BSA) and symptoms believed to result from aortic stenosis as well as in asymptomatic patients with serious left ventricular dysfunction and progressive cardiomegaly. Although a prospective randomized controlled study has not been carried out, the long-term mortality in patients undergoing operation in the latter group appears to be lower than that in medically treated patients without operation.[444] As artificial valves and surgical skills continue to improve, it is likely that patients with severe aortic stenosis will become candidates for operation at earlier stages in the natural history of their disease. At the present time, the author does not recommend prophylactic replacement of a critically narrowed aortic valve in asymptomatic patients without evidence of progressive left ventricular dysfunction.

RESULTS. Successful replacement of the aortic valve has resulted in substantial clinical and hemodynamic improvement in patients with aortic stenosis, aortic regurgitation, or combined lesions.[445–453] In patients without frank left ventricular failure, the operative risk ranges from 5 to 10 per cent in most centers. Symptoms secondary to elevations of left atrial pressure and myocardial ischemia are relieved in virtually all patients. Hemodynamic results are equally impressive; elevated end-diastolic and end-systolic volumes show significant reductions. Ventricular performance returns to normal[454] more frequently in patients with aortic stenosis than in those with aortic regurgitation.[455] The increased left ventricular mass is reduced toward (but not quite to) normal within 18 months following aortic valve replacement in patients with aortic stenosis, regurgitation, or mixed lesions.[395,456]

When operation is carried out in patients with frank left ventricular failure or a depressed ejection fraction, the operative risk is higher, and the mortality ranges from 10 to 25 per cent, depending on the skill of the surgical team and the severity of depression of left ventricular function.[457] A depressed relation between ejection fraction and wall stress is a poor prognostic index (Figure 13–9, p. 453), as is a depressed level of dP/dt max at any given left ventricular end-diastolic pressure.[447] Furthermore, a number of factors are now recognized to exert an adverse effect on

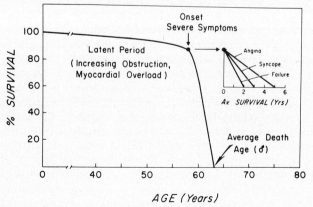

FIGURE 32–25 Natural history of aortic stenosis without operative treatment. (From Ross, J., Jr., and Braunwald, E.: Aortic stenosis. Circulation *38*(Suppl. 5):61, 1968, by permission of the American Heart Association, Inc.)

long-term survival; these include a history of acute myocardial infarction, heart failure, advanced functional disability, radiographic evidence of cardiac enlargement, elevations of left atrial and pulmonary artery pressures, and a depressed cardiac output,[444] as well as age and the presence of ventricular arrhythmias.[433] Obviously, it is desirable to perform surgery before these events occur, but even in the most desperate situations, such as cardiac arrest or pulmonary edema from aortic stenosis, emergency operation may be life-saving.[458] Certainly, in view of the extremely poor prognosis of such patients when they are treated medically, there is usually little choice but to advise immediate surgical treatment.[459] Many symptomatic patients with calcific aortic stenosis are elderly, and particular attention must be directed to the adequacy of their hepatic, renal, and pulmonary function. However, the results of aortic valve replacement are satisfactory in patients more than 70 years of age, and if the patient's general condition permits, age, per se, should not be considered a contraindication to operation.[460] In patients with aortic stenosis and obstructive coronary artery disease, aortic valve replacement and myocardial revascularization should be performed together.[461,462] Although the risk of aortic valve surgery is increased by the association of coronary artery disease, the operative mortality in patients undergoing the combined procedure is not necessarily higher than that of isolated aortic valve replacement in this group.[463] The ability to avoid serious myocardial ischemia in the perioperative period is a major factor that has served to reduce operative mortality. After the patient has been placed on cardiopulmonary bypass, the heart is protected by means of hypothermic cardiac arrest alone or combined with cardioplegia. The calcified valve must be removed with great care to avoid embolization of calcified fragments into the systemic circulation.

Characteristics of Artificial Valves
(Fig. 32–16)

The general issues surrounding replacement of the aortic valve are similar to those already discussed in relation to mitral valve replacement (p. 1086), with a number of qualifications: (1) thromboembolic complications are less common following replacement of the aortic than of the mitral valve, which may be related, in part, to the fact that after operation, patients with aortic valvular disease are rarely left with enlarged, fibrillating atria, where clots readily form; (2) the aortic annulus is smaller than the mitral annulus, increasing the likelihood of stenosis of the artificial valve; and (3) the hydraulic stress placed on the aortic valve is greater than that placed on the mitral valve, which *may* lead to a somewhat higher risk of valve dysfunction.

MECHANICAL PROSTHESES. As is the case for prosthetic mitral valves, the Starr-Edwards caged-ball valve is the "benchmark" in aortic valve replacement. Model No. 1260 now has a record of durability extending back to 1965;[464] the addition of a cloth covering has decreased the incidence of thromboembolism[465] but has increased the likelihood of valve dysfunction. Tilting-disk valves (Björk-Shiley and Lillehei-Kaster) in the aortic valve position have resulted in a low incidence of thromboembolism, but just as in the mitral valve position, total thrombosis of these valves has been reported in a few instances.[210,214,466] The overall embolic rate for prosthetic aortic valve replacement in patients treated with anticoagulants ranges from 1 to 5 per 100 patient-years, with fatal emboli occurring in approximately 0.2 per 100 patient-years.[229]

Since the Starr-Edwards caged-ball valve intrudes on the diameter of the ascending aorta, obstruction may be produced not only by the orifice of the prosthetic valve itself but also by encroachment of the valve on the lumen of the aortic annulus. To avoid this obstruction, patching with a prosthetic gusset may be required. The Smeloff-Cutter double-caged valve[467] provides a slightly more effective orifice-to-diameter ratio than that provided by the Starr-Edwards prosthesis. The Björk-Shiley, Lillehei-Kaster, and St. Jude disk valves employ semicentral or central flow rather than the circumferential flow of the ball valves, improve the effective orifice area, and do not obstruct the aorta above the annulus. These valves therefore result in larger effective orifice areas, at any annulus diameter, than do the caged-ball valves. They are preferable to the Starr-Edwards and Smeloff-Cutter valves in patients with unusually small aortic annuli. All these valves, including the Magovern-Cromie sutureless caged-ball valve,[468] have excellent records of durability. Experience with the St. Jude valve suggests that it has a larger effective orifice for any size of aortic orifice, and it may therefore prove to be the prosthetic valve of choice in patients with a small aortic root.[227,451]

TISSUE VALVES. As is the case when they are placed in the mitral position (p. 1088), homografts that are sterilized by a variety of techniques and used to replace the aortic valve initially had a relatively high incidence of breakdown, but this problem has been largely corrected; procurement and preparation still present problems, and with some exceptions[446] their use has been largely abandoned. The glutaraldehyde-treated porcine heterograft has a good record of durability.[211–213,469] However, this valve is slightly stenotic, because of a residual bar of right ventricular muscle on the inferior aspect of the right coronary cusp, which becomes increasingly obstructive as the diameter of the valve is reduced. Indeed, significant transvalvular gradients have been documented in the 21 and 23 mm sizes of the conventional Hancock porcine aortic valve.[470] The heterograft has been modified by replacing the muscular cusp with a nonmuscular cusp from a second porcine aortic valve. This appears to reduce the obstruction[212,449,450,471] and places the ratio of the effective orifice-to-annulus diameter in the same range as that of the prosthetic valves, which are most favorable from a hemodynamic point of view. The Ionescu-Shiley bovine pericardial bioprosthesis has excellent hemodynamic characteristics in the aortic position.[238] The porcine heterograft in the aortic valve position is associated with a low incidence of thromboembolism (1 per 100 patient-years) without anticoagulant treatment, in contrast to the higher incidence of thromboembolism with prosthetic valves despite the use of anticoagulants. Thus, the incidence of thromboembolism in patients not treated with anticoagulants is comparable to the incidence of complications due simply to anticoagulant therapy.

SELECTION OF AN ARTIFICIAL VALVE. In choosing a replacement for the aortic valve, one must relate the patient's specific anatomical factors, age, and clinical features to the durability, thromboembolic potential, and hemodynamic properties of the replacement valve. If durability is the principal concern, as in a relatively young (< 45 years) patient, the Starr-Edwards and Smeloff-Cutter valves have the best records of performance. However, the Björk-Shiley and Lillehei-Kaster valves also appear to be extremely promising in this regard, since they have been in use for 13 years. There is least experience with the St. Jude valve (6 years at this writing) but it, too, looks promising. The porcine heterografts also have a good durability record (more than 11 years at the time of this writing), but as already discussed (p. 1089), reports of valve deterioration are beginning to appear, and there is some concern about their long-term durability, particularly in children and young adults.

Thromboembolic complications are markedly reduced with all tissue valves, and the need for long-term anticoagulation, which presents its own risks, is thereby obviated. Therefore, in patients for whom long-term anticoagulation is contraindicated or difficult or in whom the threat of bleeding is unusually high, a tissue valve is indicated. Since the question of their durability has not been answered, but since anticoagulants present a greater hazard in the elderly, tissue valves may be most appropriate in patients over the age of 65 years. In patients with small aortic annuli, the caged-ball valves are inappropriate. The small-diameter, tilting-disk, and the St. Jude valves result in less

obstruction, although the modified Hancock porcine heterograft and the Ionescu-bovine pericardial heterograft may prove to be as effective hemodynamically.

As has already been pointed out (p. 1086), all valve replacements, when functioning in vivo, must be considered to be intrinsically stenotic. This problem may be most serious in patients with aortic stenosis, in whom the annulus into which the prosthesis is inserted is usually smaller than in patients with regurgitation, and the surgeon may be forced to select an artificial valve of relatively small size. As a consequence, aortic valve replacement may not abolish obstruction but merely convert severe to mild or moderate obstruction. When the smaller models of the porcine xenograft or mechanical prosthesis are placed into the aortic position, effective orifice areas of about 1.0 to 1.3 cm^2 are common. In such patients, peak transvalvular gradients as high as 40 mm Hg during exercise have been recorded,[470] and it is possible that the poor late results observed in a minority of patients may be the delayed effects of moderate stenosis of the prosthesis. In patients who do not exhibit clinical improvement postoperatively, it is important to evaluate both prosthetic and left ventricular function. This can be accomplished by means of right- and eft-heart catheterization, left ventricular angiocardiography, and cross-sectional echocardiography. Rarely, reoperation to correct a malfunctioning artificial valve is necessary.

AORTIC REGURGITATION

ETIOLOGY AND PATHOLOGY

Aortic regurgitation may be caused by primary disease of either the aortic valve leaflets or the wall of the aortic root or both (Table 32–11).

VALVULAR DISEASE. *Rheumatic fever* is a common cause of primary disease of the valve leading to regurgitation.[3,472] The cusps become infiltrated with fibrous tissues and retract, a process that prevents cusp apposition during diastole and that usually leads to regurgitation into the left ventricle through a defect in the center of the valve. Often the associated fusion of the commissures may also restrict the opening of the valve, resulting in combined aortic stenosis and regurgitation (Fig. 32–26*B*); some mitral valve involvement is common. Other primary valvular causes of aortic regurgitation include *infective endocarditis* (Chap. 33), in which the infection may destroy the valve or cause a perforation of a leaflet, or the vegetations may interfere with proper coaptation of the cusps. *Trauma* (p. 1564) resulting in a tear of the ascending aorta and loss of commissural support can cause prolapse of an aortic cusp. Although the most common complication of a *bicuspid valve* is stenosis in adult life, the larger of the two cusps of a congenitally *bicuspid valve* may prolapse[473] and cause regurgitation in childhood; more commonly, progressive regurgitation of a congenitally bicuspid valve develops in the third and fourth decades[474,475] (as may the aortic cusps in patients with Marfan's syndrome, Ehlers-Danlos syndrome, cystic medionecrosis of the aorta, myxomatous proliferation of the aortic valve, and related diseases of connective tissue). Less common causes of aortic regurgitation include rupture of a congenitally fenes-

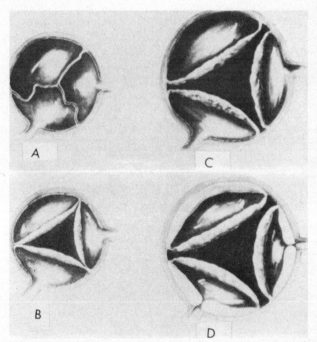

FIGURE 32–26 Variations in the aortic valve. *A*, The normal valve. *B*, Shortening of the cusps characteristic of rheumatic aortic regurgitation. The caliber of the aorta is normal. *C*, Dilatation of the aorta, as occurs in syphilitic aortitis and other conditions in which dilatation is responsible for aortic regurgitation. The main feature results from bowing of the leaflets. Commissural separation is illustrated and may also be present. *D*, In addition to the features shown in *C*, there is atherosclerosis of the aorta, as occurs in syphilitic aortitis, with consequent coronary ostial narrowing. (From Roberts, W. C.: Valvular, subvalvular and supravalvular aortic stenosis: Morphologic features. In Edwards, J. E. [ed.]: Clinical-Pathologic Correlations #2. Philadelphia, F. A. Davis, 1973, p. 133.)

TABLE 32–11   MECHANISMS OF AORTIC REGURGITATION

1. Cusp abnormality	Perforation	Bacterial endocarditis
	Reduction in area	Rheumatic disease Rheumatoid disease Ankylosing spondylitis
2. Aortic root distortion (aortitis)		Ankylosing spondylitis Nonspecific urethritis Nonspecific aortitis Rheumatoid disease Syphilis
3. Loss of commissural support		Fallot-type VSD Dissection tears of aorta
	Aortitis (inflammatory)	Syphilis All other aortitis
4. Aortic root dilatation		
	"Aortopathy" (non-inflammatory)	Marfan Familial Idiopathic Ehlers-Danlos Pseudoxanthoma elasticum

Reproduced with permission from Davies, M. J.: Pathology of Cardiac Valves. London, Butterworths, 1980.

trated valve[476] in the presence of hypertension,[477] systemic lupus erythematosus,[477,478] rheumatoid arthritis,[479] ankylosing spondylitis,[480] and Whipple's disease.[480a] Isolated congenital aortic regurgitation is an uncommon lesion on necropsy studies, but when present, it is usually associated with a bicuspid valve.[481]

AORTIC ROOT DISEASE. A variety of diseases produce aortic regurgitation by causing marked dilatation of the ascending aorta (Fig. 32–26C). These conditions, discussed in detail in Chapter 45, include annuloaortic ectasia, cystic medionecrosis of the aorta (either isolated or associated with classic Marfan's syndrome), osteogenesis imperfecta, syphilitic aortitis, ankylosing spondylitis, Behçet's disease,[481a] psoriatic arthritis, arthritis associated with

ulcerative colitis, relapsing polychondritis, Reiter's syndrome, giant cell arteritis, and systemic hypertension.[482–490]

Table 32–12 presents a comparison of the findings in four important conditions in which dilation of the aorta causes aortic regurgitation. In each of these, the aortic annulus may become greatly dilated, the aortic leaflets separate, and aortic regurgitation may ensue. Dissection of the diseased aortic wall may occur and may aggravate the aortic regurgitation. Dilatation of the aortic root may also have secondary effects on the aortic valve, since it results in tension and bowing of the individual cusps, which may thicken, retract, and become too short to close the aortic orifice. This leads to intensification of the aortic regurgita-

Table 32–12   CARDIOVASCULAR MANIFESTATIONS OF CONDITIONS CAUSING AORTIC REGURGITATION

	SYPHILIS	ANKYLOSING SPONDYLITIS	RHEUMATOID ARTHRITIS	MARFAN'S SYNDROME
Average age	50	45	70	30
Predominant sex	Men	Men	Women	Men
Aortic regurgitation	+ + + +	+ + + +	+	+ + + +
Mitral regurgitation	0	+ +	+	+ + +
Conduction disturbances	+	+ + + +	+ +	+
Serology (STS)	+	0	0	0
Morphology of aorta				
Thickened adventitia	+ + + +	+ + + +	+	+
Degenerated media	+ + +	+ + +	0	+ + + +
Intimal proliferation	+ + +	+ + +	0	+
Vasa vasorum abnormal	+ + + +	+ + + +	0	0
Calcium	+ +	+	0	0
Aneurysms	+ + +	0	0	+ + +
Rupture	+	0	0	+
Dissection	0	0	0	+
Limited to sinuses	0	+	0	0
Morphology of aortic valve				
Cusp thickening				
Diffuse	0	+	0	0
Focal	+	0	+	+
Cusp calcification	0	0	0	0
Shortening	0	+	0	0
Commissural abnormality	+	+	0	0

From Roberts, W. C., et al.: Nonrheumatic valvular cardiac disease: A clinicopathologic survey of 27 different conditions causing valvular dysfunction. In Likoff, W. (ed.): Cardiovascular Clinics. Vol. 5, No. 2, Valvular Heart Disease. Philadelphia, F. A. Davis, 1973, p. 424.

tion, which increases left ventricular stroke volume, further dilating the ascending aorta and thus leading to a vicious cycle.

Aortic regurgitation, regardless of its etiology, produces dilatation and hypertrophy of the left ventricle, dilatation of the mitral valve ring, and sometimes hypertrophy and dilatation of the left atrium. Endocardial pockets frequently develop in the left ventricular cavity at sites of impact of the regurgitant jet.

PATHOPHYSIOLOGY

In contrast to mitral regurgitation, in which a fraction of the left ventricular stroke volume is delivered into the low-pressure left atrium, in aortic regurgitation the entire left ventricular stroke volume is ejected into a high-pressure chamber, i.e., the aorta (although the low aortic diastolic pressure does facilitate ventricular emptying during early systole). Whereas in mitral regurgitation the reduction of wall tension (i.e., reduced afterload) allows more complete systolic emptying (p. 1078), in aortic regurgitation the increase in left ventricular end-diastolic volume provides major hemodynamic compensation.[383,489,491,491a,491b,491c]

Severe aortic regurgitation may occur with a normal effective forward stroke volume and a normal ejection fraction (total [forward plus regurgitant] stroke volume/end-diastolic volume), together with an elevated left ventricular end-diastolic pressure and volume (Figs. 32–27 and 32–28). In accord with Laplace's law (p. 431), left ventricular dilatation increases the left ventricular systolic tension required to develop any level of systolic pressure. The increased wall stress leads to replication of sarcomeres in series, elongation of fibers, and sufficient wall thickening to maintain systolic wall stress at normal levels; the ratio of ventricular wall thickness to cavity radius remains normal.[492] This contrasts with the events in aortic stenosis, i.e., replication of sarcomeres in parallel (p. 452) and an increased ratio of wall thickness to cavity radius (p. 454).

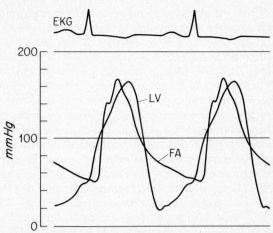

FIGURE 32–27 Pressure curves obtained from a 63-year-old man with symptoms of left ventricular failure and a loud decrescendo diastolic murmur. The femoral arterial (FA) pressure tracing demonstrates a widened pulse pressure of 115 mm Hg and equalization with left ventricular (LV) pressure late in diastole. The LV pressure curve exhibits a steady pressure increase throughout diastole, culminating in a markedly elevated end-diastolic pressure of 45 mm Hg. These findings are indicative of severe aortic regurgitation.

In aortic regurgitation, left ventricular mass is usually greatly elevated (Fig. 32–28), often to levels even higher than in isolated aortic stenosis[383] and sometimes exceeding 1000 gm.

Patients with severe chronic aortic regurgitation have the largest end-diastolic volumes of any form of heart disease[26] (Fig. 32–28) (resulting in the so-called *cor bovinum*), but end-diastolic pressure is not uniformly elevated (i.e., left ventricular compliance often becomes increased), and there is a wide scatter in the relationship between end-diastolic volume and end-diastolic pressure.[383] In the more severe cases of aortic regurgitation, the regurgitant flow may exceed 20 liters/min, so that the total left ventricular output approaches 30 liters/min,[26] a level that can be achieved only by a trained endurance runner during maximal exer-

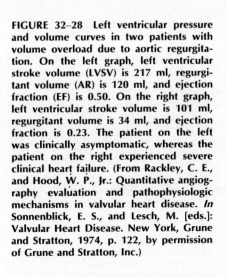

FIGURE 32–28 Left ventricular pressure and volume curves in two patients with volume overload due to aortic regurgitation. On the left graph, left ventricular stroke volume (LVSV) is 217 ml, regurgitant volume (AR) is 120 ml, and ejection fraction (EF) is 0.50. On the right graph, left ventricular stroke volume is 101 ml, regurgitant volume is 34 ml, and ejection fraction is 0.23. The patient on the left was clinically asymptomatic, whereas the patient on the right experienced severe clinical heart failure. (From Rackley, C. E., and Hood, W. P., Jr.: Quantitative angiography evaluation and pathophysiologic mechanisms in valvular heart disease. *In* Sonnenblick, E. S., and Lesch, M. [eds.]: Valvular Heart Disease. New York, Grune and Stratton, 1974, p. 122, by permission of Grune and Stratton, Inc.)

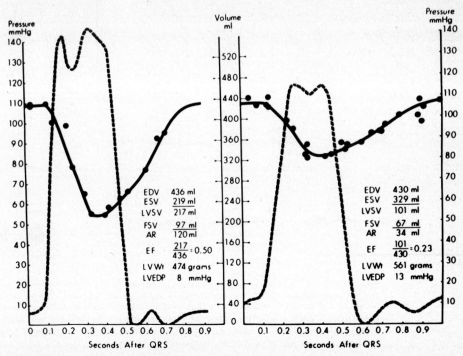

cise. Thus, the adaptive response to chronic and gradually increasing aortic regurgitation permits the ventricle to function as an effective low-compliance pump, handling large end-diastolic and stroke volumes, often with little increase in filling pressure. During exercise, peripheral vascular resistance declines, and with an increase in heart rate, diastole shortens and the regurgitation per beat decreases,[493,494] facilitating an increment in effective forward cardiac output without substantial increases in end-diastolic volume and pressure. As left ventricular function deteriorates, the end-diastolic volume increases without further elevation of the aortic regurgitant volume; the ejection fraction and forward stroke volume decline, and ventricular emptying is impaired, i.e., end-systolic volume increases (Fig. 32–28). Many of these changes precede the development of symptoms. In advanced stages there may be considerable elevation of the left atrial, pulmonary artery wedge, pulmonary arterial, right ventricular, and right atrial pressures and lowering of the effective cardiac output, even at rest.

As is the case for mitral regurgitation (p. 1079), the end-systolic volume is a sensitive index of myocardial function in patients with aortic regurgitation and correlates with operative mortality and postoperative left ventricular dysfunction.[166] Both the immediate and the long-term results are excellent in patients with normal left ventricular end-systolic volumes (< 30 ml/m^2), poor in patients in whom this index is elevated (> 90 ml/m^2), and variable in patients with intermediate values. In general, however, for any given preoperative level of impairment of left ventricular function, the outlook for left ventricular function in the

postoperative period is better in patients with aortic than with mitral regurgitation.

When *acute* aortic regurgitation is induced experimentally, preload, wall tension, and myocardial oxygen consumption all rise substantially,[158,491] a situation contrasting with that produced by acutely induced mitral regurgitation (p. 1078). In patients with chronic severe aortic regurgitation, myocardial oxygen requirements are also augmented by the increase in left ventricular mass. Since the major portion of coronary blood flow occurs during diastole, when arterial pressure is lower than normal, coronary perfusion pressure is reduced.[495] The result—a combination of increased oxygen demand and reduced supply—sets the stage for the development of myocardial ischemia, especially during exercise.[496] The heightened activity of the adrenergic nervous system as a compensatory mechanism in patients with chronic aortic regurgitation is reflected in an abnormal increase in plasma catecholamine content during exercise, accompanied by a reduction in cardiac norepinephrine stores.[497] Symptomatic patients with severe chronic aortic regurgitation generally exhibit a depression of the relations between end-systolic pressure and stress and end-systolic volume. This depression of myocardial function, combined with the increased demands placed on the left ventricle, augments left ventricular end-diastolic volume and ultimately pressure, causing symptoms of pulmonary congestion.[498] Symptomatic patients with aortic regurgitation demonstrate a failure of the normal decline in end-systolic volume or rise in ejection fraction during exercise, as determined by radionuclide angiography.[499] However,

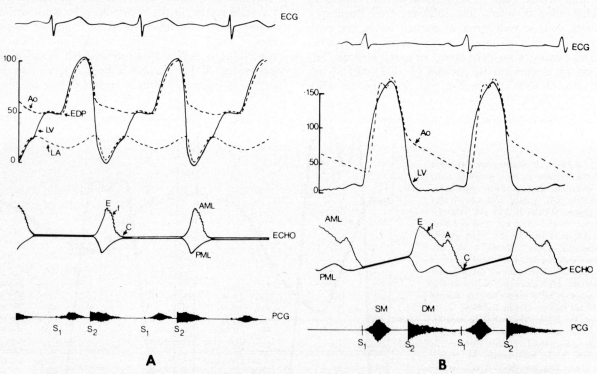

FIGURE 32–29 Schematic representations contrasting the hemodynamic, echocardiographic (ECHO), and phonocardiographic (PCG) manifestations of acute severe (*A*) and chronic severe (*B*) aortic regurgitation. Ao = aorta; LV = left ventricle; LA = left atrium; EDP = end-diastolic pressure; f = flutter of anterior mitral valve leaflet; AML = anterior mitral valve leaflet; PML = posterior mitral leaflet; SM = systolic murmur; DM = diastolic murmur; C = closure point of mitral valve. (From Morganroth, J. et al.: Acute severe aortic regurgitation. Ann. Intern. Med. *87*:225, 1977.)

Table 32–13 DIFFERENCES BETWEEN ACUTE AND CHRONIC SEVERE AORTIC REGURGITATION

CLINICAL FEATURES	*Acute*	*Chronic*
Congestive heart failure	Early and sudden	Late and insidious
Arterial pulse		
Rate per minute	Increased	Normal
Rate of rise	Normal	Increased
Systolic pressure	Normal to decreased	Increased
Diastolic pressure	Normal to decreased	Decreased
Pulse pressure	Near normal	Increased
Contour of peak	Single	Bisferiens
Pulsus alternans	Common	Uncommon
Left ventricular (LV) impulse	Nearly normal to moderately displaced, not hyperdynamic	Displaced hyperdynamic
Auscultation		
S_1	Soft to absent	Normal
Aortic component of S_2	Soft	Normal or decreased
Pulmonic component of S_2	Normal or increased	Normal
S_3	Common	Uncommon
S_4	Consistently absent	Usually absent
Aortic systolic murmur	Grade 3 or less	Grade 3 or more
Aortic regurgitant murmur	Short, medium-pitched	Long, high-pitched
Austin Flint	Mid-diastolic	Presystolic, mid-diastolic, or both
Peripheral arterial auscultatory signs	Absent	Present
Electrocardiogram	Normal LV voltage with minor repolarization abnormalities	Increased LV voltage with major repolarization abnormalities
Chest roentgenogram		
Left ventricle	Normal to moderately increased	Markedly increased
Aortic root and arch	Usually normal	Prominent
Pulmonary venous vascularity	Increased	Normal

HEMODYNAMIC FEATURES	*Acute*	*Chronic (Without Left Ventricular Failure)*
Left ventricular (LV) compliance	Normal	Normal or increased
Regurgitant volume	Increased	Increased
LV end-diastolic pressure	Markedly increased	Normal or increased
LV ejection velocity	Not significantly increased	Markedly increased
Aortic systolic pressure	Not increased	Increased
Aortic diastolic pressure	Normal to decreased	Markedly decreased
Systemic arterial pulse pressure	Slightly to moderately increased	Markedly increased
Ejection fraction	Normal or decreased	Normal
Effective stroke volume	Decreased	Normal
Effective cardiac output	Decreased	Usually normal
Heart rate	Increased	Normal
Peripheral vascular resistance	Usually increased	Normal

ECHOCARDIOGRAPHIC FEATURES	*Acute*	*Chronic*
Mitral valve		
Closure point	Premature	Normal
Opening point	Delayed	Normal
E–F slope	Decreased	Normal
Fluttering	Usually present	Usually present
Left ventricle		
Internal dimension (end diastole)	Normal	Increased
Septal and free wall thickness	Normal	Normal
Septal and free wall motion	Normal	Increased
Left ventricular mass	Normal	Increased

From Morganroth, J., et al.: Acute severe aortic regurgitation. Ann. Intern. Med. *87*:224, 228, and 230, 1977.

abnormal left ventricular function can be discerned even in subgroups of asymptomatic patients with normal ejection fractions; this dysfunction is reflected in failure of the normal increase in ejection fraction during exercise[500,501] or a depressed end-systolic pressure-volume relation.[501] These techniques are likely to prove of great value in the identification of those patients with severe chronic aortic regurgitation, who, although asymptomatic or almost so, are at greater risk of developing left ventricular failure and therefore are candidates for consideration of surgical treatment.

ACUTE AORTIC REGURGITATION (Table 32–13). In contrast to the pathophysiological events in chronic aortic regurgitation described above, in which the left ventricle has had the opportunity to adapt to the increased load, in *acute* regurgitation (caused most commonly by infective endocarditis, aortic dissection, and trauma) the regurgitant blood fills a ventricle of normal size that cannot accommodate the combined large regurgitant volume and inflow from the left atrium. Since total stroke volume cannot rise markedly, forward stroke volume declines, left ventricular diastolic pressure rises rapidly to high levels,[489] and the left ventricle operates on a less compliant (steep) portion of its pressure-volume curve (Figure 12–12, p. 428).[491]

The hemodynamic findings in acute aortic regurgitation contrast with those in chronic aortic regurgitation.[502] For a similarly severe degree of aortic regurgitation, the patient with acute regurgitation has a much smaller aortic pulse pressure and effective forward cardiac output, a smaller left ventricular chamber size, and a higher heart rate than the patient with chronic aortic regurgitation. In addition, as left ventricular pressure rises rapidly above left atrial pressure during early diastole, the mitral valve closes prematurely in diastole (Fig. 32–29).[488,502,503] This protects the pulmonary venous bed from backward transmission of the greatly elevated end-diastolic pressure. Premature closure of the mitral valve, together with the tachycardia that shortens diastole, reduces the time interval during which the mitral valve is open.[503] Left ventricular and aortic systolic pressures exhibit little change. Since aortic diastolic pressure cannot decline below the elevated left ventricular end-diastolic pressure, the systemic arterial pulse pressure widens relatively little.

CLINICAL MANIFESTATIONS

History

In patients with *chronic*, severe aortic regurgitation, there is a long period during which the left ventricle gradually undergoes enlargement while the patient remains asymptomatic or almost so.[504–506] Symptoms of reduced cardiac reserve or myocardial ischemia develop, most often in the fourth or fifth decades and usually only after considerable cardiomegaly and myocardial dysfunction have occurred. When symptoms do develop, exertional dyspnea, orthopnea, and paroxysmal nocturnal dyspnea are the principal complaints. Syncope is rare, and although angina pectoris is less frequent than in patients with aortic stenosis, nocturnal angina, often accompanied by diaphoresis, which occurs when the heart rate slows and arterial diastolic pressure falls to extremely low levels, may be particularly troublesome; these episodes may be accompanied by abdominal discomfort, presumably caused by splanchnic ischemia. Patients with severe aortic regurgitation often complain of an uncomfortable awareness of the heart beat, especially on lying down, and disagreeable thoracic pain due to pounding of the heart against the chest wall. Tachycardia, occurring with emotional stress or exertion, may produce palpitations and head pounding; premature ventricular contractions are particularly distressing because of the great heave of the volume-loaded left ventricle during the postpremature beat. These complaints may be present for many years before symptoms of left ventricular dysfunction develop.

In light of the limited ability of the left ventricle to tolerate *acute* regurgitation, patients with this valvular lesion often develop sudden clinical manifestations of cardiovascular collapse, with weakness, severe dyspnea, and hypotension; angina is uncommon (Table 32–12).[502,502a]

Physical Examination

In patients with chronic severe aortic regurgitation, the head frequently bobs with each heartbeat (*de Musset's sign*),[507] and the pulses are of the waterhammer or collapsing type with abrupt distention and quick collapse (*Corrigan's pulse*). This pulse is readily visible in the carotid arteries and can be best appreciated by palpation of the radial artery with the patient's arm elevated. A bisferiens pulse may be present (Figure 3–24, p. 57) and is more readily recognized in the brachial and femoral than in the carotid arteries. A variety of auscultatory findings provide confirmation of a wide pulse pressure. *Traube's sign* refers to booming systolic and diastolic sounds heard over the femoral artery, *Müller's sign* consists of systolic pulsations of the uvula, and *Duroziez's sign* consists of a systolic murmur heard over the femoral artery when it is compressed proximally and a diastolic murmur when it is compressed distally. Capillary pulsations, i.e., *Quincke's sign*, can be detected by pressing a glass slide on the patient's lip or by transmitting a light through the patient's fingertips.

Systolic arterial pressure is elevated, and diastolic pressure is abnormally low. *Hill's sign* refers to popliteal cuff systolic pressure exceeding brachial cuff pressure by more than 60 mm Hg. Korotkoff sounds often persist to zero even though intraarterial pressure rarely falls below 30 mm Hg. The point of change in intensity of the Korotkoff sounds, i.e., the muffling of these sounds in phase IV, correlates with the diastolic pressure. As heart failure supervenes, peripheral vasoconstriction may occur and arterial diastolic pressure may rise. However, this finding should not be interpreted as a reduction in the severity of the aortic regurgitation.

The apical impulse is diffuse and hyperdynamic and is displaced laterally and inferiorly; there may be systolic retraction over the parasternal region (see Figure 2–6, p. 27). A rapid ventricular filling wave is often palpable at the apex, as is a systolic thrill at the base of the heart or suprasternal notch and over the carotid arteries, resulting from the augmented stroke volume. In many patients, a carotid shudder is palpable or may be recorded.[508]

AUSCULTATION. In *chronic* severe aortic regurgitation, a soft S_1 and prolongation of the P-R interval are frequently present. A_2 is soft or absent, and P_2 may be obscured by the early diastolic murmur.[509] Thus, S_2 is variable; it may be absent or single or exhibit narrow or paradoxical splitting. A systolic ejection sound, presumably related to abrupt distention of the aorta by the augmented stroke volume, is frequently audible. An S_3 gallop correlates with an increased left ventricular end-systolic volume and has been suggested as a sign useful in considering patients with severe regurgitation for surgical treatment (Fig. 32–30).[510]

The aortic regurgitant murmur is one of high frequency that begins immediately after A_2 (see Figures 3–24, p. 57, and 4–22 and 4–23, p. 82). It may be distinguished from the murmur of pulmonic regurgitation (p. 1122) by its earlier onset, i.e., immediately after A_2 rather than after P_2, and often by the presence of a widened pulse pressure. The murmur is heard best through the diaphragm of the stethoscope while the patient is sitting up and leaning forward, with the breath held in deep expiration. In severe aortic regurgitation, the murmur reaches an early peak and then has a dominant decrescendo pattern throughout diastole.

The severity of the regurgitation correlates better with the *duration* than with the *intensity* of the murmur. In mild aortic regurgitation, the murmur may be limited to

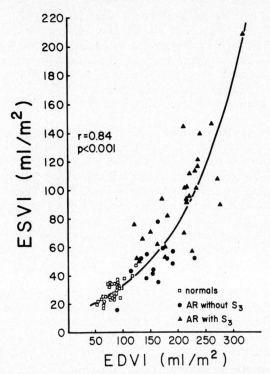

FIGURE 32–30 Exponential curvilinear relationship between the end-diastolic and end-systolic volume index (EDVI and ESVI, respectively) in 31 normal subjects and 42 patients with aortic regurgitation (AR). The latter group consists of 28 patients with and 14 without an S_3 gallop. Note higher values for EDVI and ESVI in patients with than without an S_3. (From Abdulla, A. M., Frank, M. J., Erdin, R. A., Jr., and Canedo, M. I.: Circulation 64:464, 1981, by permission of the American Heart Association, Inc.)

the early phase of diastole and is typically high-pitched; in moderately severe and severe regurgitation, the murmur is holodiastolic and may have a rough quality. When the murmur is musical ("cooing dove" murmur), it usually signifies eversion or perforation of an aortic cusp. In severe aortic regurgitation and left ventricular decompensation, equilibration of aortic and left ventricular diastolic pressures in late diastole abolish this component of the regurgitant murmur. The murmur is best heard along the left sternal border in the third and fourth intercostal spaces when regurgitation is due to primary valvular disease, but it is often more readily audible along the right sternal border when it is due mainly to dilatation of the ascending aorta.[511] Murmurs in the latter position may be overlooked if auscultation along the right sternal border is not carried out routinely.

A mid- and late-diastolic apical rumble, the *Austin Flint murmur,* is common in severe aortic regurgitation and may occur in the presence of a normal mitral valve (Figures 4–22, p. 82, and 32–31). This murmur appears to be created by rapid antegrade flow across a mitral orifice[494] that may be being narrowed by the rapidly rising left ventricular diastolic pressure caused by severe aortic reflux.[512,513] The Austin Flint murmur may be difficult to differentiate from that due to mitral stenosis, but the presence of an opening snap and a loud S_1 in mitral stenosis and the absence of these findings in aortic regurgitation are helpful clues. As the left ventricular end-diastolic pressure rises, the Austin Flint murmur commences and terminates earlier, and in

acute aortic regurgitation with premature diastolic closure of the mitral valve, the presystolic portion of the Austin Flint murmur is eliminated. A short, midsystolic murmur, grades 1 to 4/6, related to the increased ejection rate and stroke volume, may be audible at the base of the heart and transmitted to the carotid vessels. It may be higher pitched and less rasping than the murmur of aortic stenosis but is often accompanied by a thrill.

Dynamic Auscultation. The diastolic murmur of aortic regurgitation may be accentuated when the patient sits up and leans forward or by any intervention that raises the arterial pressure, such as infusion of a vasopressor drug, squatting, or isometric exercise; it is reduced by interventions that lower the systolic pressure, such as amyl nitrite inhalation and the strain of the Valsalva maneuver.[514] The Austin Flint murmur, like the murmur of aortic regurgitation, is augmented by isometric exercise and vasopressors and is reduced by amyl nitrite inhalation (Fig. 32–31).[514]

ACUTE AORTIC REGURGITATION. These patients often appear gravely ill, with tachycardia, severe peripheral vasoconstriction and cyanosis, and sometimes pulmonary congestion and edema (Table 32–13).[502,502a] The peripheral signs of aortic regurgitation are often not impressive and certainly not as dramatic as in patients with chronic aortic regurgitation.[503] Duroziez's murmur, pistol shot sounds over the peripheral arteries, and bisferiens pulses are absent. The arterial pulse may exhibit pulsus alternans. The normal pulse pressure may lead to serious underestimation of the severity of the valvular lesion. The left

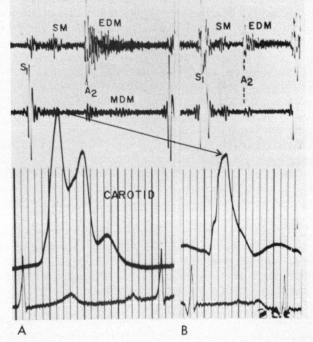

FIGURE 32–31 Response of the Austin Flint mid-diastolic murmur (MDM) to inhalation of amyl nitrite. *A,* Control tracing showing the midsystolic murmur (SM) of rapid flow, the early diastolic murmur (EDM) of aortic regurgitation, and the mid-diastolic murmur (MDM) of Austin Flint. Note the bisferiens carotid pulse. *B,* Test tracing showing loss of the bisferiens pulse as aortic regurgitation diminishes, together with a decrease in intensity of the early diastolic murmur and disappearance of the mid-diastolic Austin Flint murmur. (From Reichek, N., et al.: Clinical aspects of rheumatic valvular disease. Prog. Cardiovasc. Dis. 15:521, 1973, by permission of Grune and Stratton.)

ventricular impulse is normal or nearly so, and the rocking motion of the chest characteristic of chronic aortic regurgitation is not apparent. S_1 may be soft or absent because of premature closure of the mitral valve.[515] Instead, the sound of mitral valve closure is heard occasionally in mid diastole. However, closure of the mitral valve may be incomplete, and diastolic mitral regurgitation may occur.[516] Evidence of pulmonary hypertension, with an accentuated P_2 and an S_3 and S_4, is frequently present. The early diastolic murmur of acute aortic regurgitation is lower pitched and shorter than that of chronic aortic regurgitation, since as left ventricular end-diastolic pressure rises, the pressure gradient between the aorta and the left ventricle is rapidly reduced. The Austin Flint murmur, if present, is brief and ceases when left ventricular pressure exceeds left atrial pressure in diastole.

LABORATORY EXAMINATION

ELECTROCARDIOGRAM. *Chronic* aortic regurgitation results in left axis deviation and a pattern of left ventricular diastolic volume overload, characterized by an increase in initial forces (prominent Q waves in leads I, aV_1, and V_3 to V_6) and a relatively small r wave in V_1. With the passage of time, these initial forces diminish, but the total QRS amplitude increases. The T waves may be tall and upright in left precordial leads early in the course, but more commonly they are inverted, with ST-segment depressions.[517,518] Left intraventricular conduction defects occur late in the course. When aortic regurgitation is caused by an inflammatory process, P-R prolongation may result. In *acute* aortic regurgitation, the electrocardiogram may (Figure 7-14B, p. 210) or may not show left ventricular hypertrophy, despite the presence of left ventricular failure, depending upon the severity and duration of the regurgitation. However, nonspecific ST-segment and T-wave changes are common.

RADIOLOGICAL FINDINGS (p. 164). Cardiac size is a function of the duration and severity of regurgitation and the state of left ventricular function. In *acute* aortic regurgitation, there may be little cardiac enlargement, but marked enlargement is a common finding in *chronic* regurgitation. Typically, the left ventricle enlarges in an inferior and leftward direction, causing a significant increase in the long axis (Figure 6-4A, p. 150) but sometimes little or no increase in the transverse diameter of the heart. Calcification of the aortic valve is uncommon in patients with pure aortic regurgitation but is often present in patients with combined stenosis and regurgitation. As is the case with aortic stenosis, the presence of distinct left atrial enlargement in the absence of heart failure should suggest the possibility of mitral valve disease. Dilatation of the ascending aorta is more marked than in aortic stenosis and may involve the entire aortic arch, including the aortic knob. Severe, aneurysmal dilatation of the aorta should suggest that aortic root disease (e.g., Marfan's syndrome, cystic medionecrosis, or annuloaortic ectasia) is responsible for the aortic regurgitation.

For angiographic assessment of aortic regurgitation, contrast material should be injected rapidly (i.e., 25 to 35

ml/sec) into the aortic root, and filming should be carried out in the right and left anterior oblique projections. Opacification may be improved by filming during a Valsalva maneuver. In acute aortic regurgitation, there is only a slight increase in ventricular end-diastolic volume, but with the passage of time both the end-diastolic volume and the thickness of the ventricular wall increase, often in parallel.

ECHOCARDIOGRAM (p. 114). The severity of regurgitation is reflected in increased motion of the septum and posterior wall. In *chronic aortic regurgitation,* the left ventricular end-diastolic diameter and extent of systolic shortening are both augmented[519] (Fig. 32-32). There is increased motion of the interventricular septum and posterior left ventricular wall in compensated patients, but shortening is normal or reduced in patients with left ventricular failure. Serial studies may detect early changes in left ventricular function, as reflected in increased end-diastolic and end-systolic diameters and reduced fractional shortening, which may be of assistance in selecting the optimal time for surgical intervention. Dilatation of the aortic root may point to an aortic root rather than a valvular origin of the reflux (Fig. 32-33). Increased thickness of the interventricular septum and the posterior wall of the left ventricle and an increase in the diameter of the left atrium may be detected.[520]

In *acute aortic regurgitation* (Table 32-13 and Fig. 32-29), the echocardiogram reveals a reduction in amplitude of the opening movement of the mitral valve, premature closure (see Figure 5-34, p. 106) and delayed opening of the mitral valve,[521] and a reduction in the E-F slope, indicating that the left ventricle is operating on the steep portion of its pressure-volume curve. Left ventricular end-

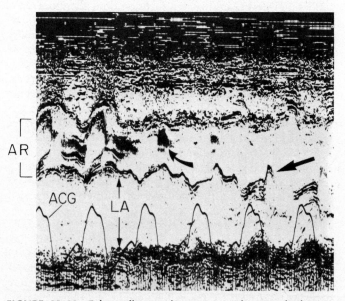

FIGURE 32-32 Echocardiogram in severe aortic regurgitation. A markedly dilated aortic root (AR) is apparent on the left, appearing anterior to a slightly enlarged left atrium (LA). The left ventricle (at the right of the tracing) is dilated and demonstrates vigorous symmetrical contractile motion of the posterior wall and interventricular septum. Projecting anterior to the mitral valve is an abnormal diastolic echo (curved arrow) suggestive of a partially disrupted aortic valve cusp prolapsing into the left ventricular outflow tract. ACG = apexcardiogram.

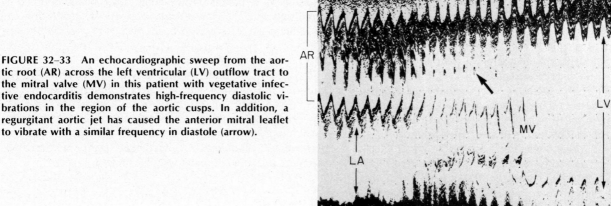

FIGURE 32–33   An echocardiographic sweep from the aortic root (AR) across the left ventricular (LV) outflow tract to the mitral valve (MV) in this patient with vegetative infective endocarditis demonstrates high-frequency diastolic vibrations in the region of the aortic cusps. In addition, a regurgitant aortic jet has caused the anterior mitral leaflet to vibrate with a similar frequency in diastole (arrow).

diastolic dimensions are not markedly increased, and fractional shortening is normal. This contrasts with the findings in chronic aortic regurgitation, in which end-diastolic dimensions and wall motion are increased. Occasionally, with equilibration of aortic and left ventricular pressures in diastole, premature opening of the aortic valve may be detected.[522] Sometimes the echocardiogram may identify the cause of acute regurgitation by revealing echoes due to a partially disrupted aortic valve cusp (Fig. 32–32), vegetations of infective endocarditis (Fig. 32–33), or aneurysmal dilatation of the aortic root. Rarely, in patients with regurgitation due to a flail aortic valve leaflet, its fluttering may be recognized.

High-frequency, diastolic fluttering of the anterior leaflet of the mitral valve during diastole (Figs. 32–34 and 5–34, p. 106) is an important echocardiographic finding in both acute and chronic aortic regurgitation;[523] it does not occur, however, when the mitral valve is rigid. This sensitive sign, which, unlike the Austin Flint rumble, occurs even in mild aortic regurgitation, results from the movement imparted to the anterior leaflet of the mitral valve by the jet of blood regurgitating from the aorta.

Two-dimensional echocardiography is extremely useful in determining the etiology of aortic regurgitation[524] (Fig. 32–35). In patients with severe reflux, short-axis views charac-teristically display an abnormal indentation of the mitral valve in early diastole caused by the regurgitant jet.[525]

Echocardiography has also proved useful in assessing left ventricular function in order to allow appropriate selection of patients for operation (see below).

RADIONUCLIDE TECHNIQUES.   Radionuclide angiography, by allowing determination of the regurgitant fraction and of the left ventricular/right ventricular stroke volume ratio, provides an accurate noninvasive quantitation of aortic regurgitation.[526,526a] As indicated above, these techniques are of value in the assessment of left ventricular function in patients with aortic regurgitation.[499–501]

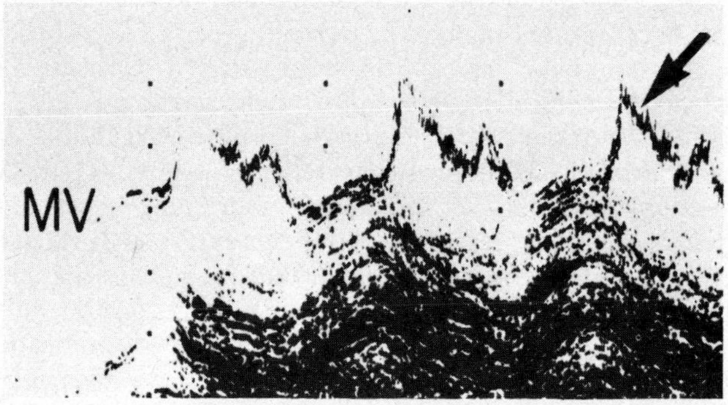

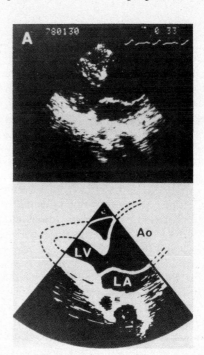

FIGURE 32–35   Panel A, Long-axis view of the aortic root (Ao) in end systole by two-dimensional echocardiography. The unusually dilated aortic root is visualized. (Reproduced with permission from Imaizumi, T., Orita, Y., Koiwaya, Y., et al.: Utility of two-dimensional echocardiography in the differential diagnosis of the etiology of aortic regurgitation. Am. Heart J. *103*:887, 1982.)

FIGURE 32–34   Echocardiogram in aortic regurgitation. High-frequency diastolic vibrations (arrow) of the anterior mitral valve leaflet (MV) are typical of aortic regurgitation.

MANAGEMENT

ACUTE AORTIC REGURGITATION. Since early death due to left ventricular failure is frequent in patients with severe *acute aortic regurgitation* despite intensive medical management, prompt surgical intervention is indicated. Even a normal ventricle cannot sustain the burden of acute severe volume overload, and therefore the risk of *acute* regurgitation is much greater than that of chronic aortic regurgitation.[502,503] In patients with severe regurgitation secondary to active infective endocarditis, operation may be deferred to allow 10 days to 2 weeks of intensive antibiotic therapy if the patient remains hemodynamically stable.[527] However, valve replacement should be undertaken at the earliest sign of hemodynamic instability or immediately upon completion of a 2-week course of antibiotics when acute, severe regurgitation has developed. The cautious use of vasodilators may be helpful in stabilizing the patient's condition but is no substitute for prompt surgery in the patient with pulmonary edema, severe pulmonary congestion, and/or an obvious low forward cardiac output state.

NATURAL HISTORY. Management of patients with *chronic aortic regurgitation* must take into account the natural history of the lesion.[528] Severe or moderately severe chronic aortic regurgitation is associated with a generally favorable prognosis for many years. Approximately 75 per cent of patients survive for 5 years and 50 per cent for 10 years after diagnosis.[98] However, as is the case for aortic stenosis, once the patient becomes symptomatic, the condition often deteriorates rapidly. Without surgical treatment, death usually occurs within 4 years after the development of angina and within 2 years after the onset of heart failure.[529,530]

Medical Treatment

Although there is no unanimity of opinion on this subject, the author believes that cardiac glycosides should be employed in patients with severe aortic regurgitation and left ventricular dilatation even in the absence of symptoms. If present, systemic arterial diastolic hypertension should be treated, since it increases the regurgitant flow; however, drugs that impair left ventricular function, such as propranolol, should be avoided. Atrial fibrillation and bradyarrhythmias are poorly tolerated and should be prevented if possible. Since these and other cardiac arrhythmias and infections are poorly tolerated in patients with free aortic regurgitation, such complications must be treated promptly and vigorously. Even though nitroglycerin and other nitrates are not as helpful in relieving anginal pain as they are in patients with coronary artery disease or aortic stenosis, they are worth a trial when this symptom occurs. Patients with aortic regurgitation secondary to syphilitic aortitis (p. 1562) should receive a full course of penicillin therapy. Although patients with left ventricular failure secondary to aortic regurgitation require surgical treatment, they also respond, at least temporarily, to treatment with digitalis glycosides, salt restriction, and diuretics. The response to vasodilator therapy is often impressive (see Figure 16–20, p. 541). Hemodynamic studies have shown beneficial effects of intravenous hydralazine,[531,532] sublingual nifedipine,[533] and oral prazosin.[533b] This form of therapy may be particularly helpful in stabilizing patients

with acute lesions or those with decompensated chronic regurgitation who are awaiting operation. Preliminary observations on the long-term effects of therapy suggest that the initial hemodynamic improvement may be maintained in some patients.[531] If the severity of aortic regurgitation can be reduced on a long-term basis, then it is possible that regression of left ventricular changes and alteration of the natural history might occur.

Asymptomatic patients with severe *chronic* aortic regurgitation and normal left ventricular function should be examined at intervals of approximately 6 months. In addition to clinical examination, x-ray, and electrocardiogram, serial noninvasive assessments of left ventricular size and performance should be carried out using echocardiography or radionuclide angiography or both.

Surgical Treatment

INDICATIONS FOR OPERATION. There is general agreement that operative correction is indicated in patients with severe *chronic* aortic regurgitation who have become symptomatic. Irreversible changes in left ventricular function are present in a subset of such patients; even after successful surgical correction of aortic regurgitation, this subset of patients may develop congestive heart failure or have persistent cardiomegaly as well as depressed left ventricular function.[533–540] Postoperative left ventricular function is usually excellent in patients who are asymptomatic and have normal systolic function preoperatively.[538] Therefore, in order to minimize the risk of postoperative dysfunction, every effort should be made to operate on the patient before serious left ventricular dysfunction occurs.[535–540] Although quantitative biplane ventriculography is the most precise method for assessing left ventricular performance, it cannot be readily employed in serial fashion. Instead, serial echocardiograms, or radionuclide ventriculograms or both should be obtained to detect changes in left ventricular size and function. These examinations can provide valuable information concerning progressive deterioration in left ventricular function at rest. Radionuclide angiography, in particular (p. 362), is a safe, simple, and noninvasive method that allows repeated evaluation of ejection fraction and end-systolic volume at rest and during exercise.[499–501]

In some asymptomatic patients with chronic severe aortic regurgitation in whom both left ventricular end-diastolic pressure and ejection fraction are normal at rest, the ejection fraction measured by radionuclide angiography during exercise or the end-systolic pressure–volume relation or both are subnormal, indicating early left ventricular dysfunction. This approach provides a sensitive and potentially clinically useful index of the functional state of the left ventricle in patients with aortic regurgitation. M-mode echocardiographic measurement of end-systolic dimensions exceeding 55 mm,[536,538,539] shortening of left ventricular diameter less than 30 per cent,[535] and elevated levels of end-diastolic radius/wall thickness ratios and end-systolic stress[533,533a] all correlate with poor postoperative left ventricular function. By providing an early indication of diminished left ventricular functional reserve, these techniques help to identify patients who, while still asymptomatic, require surgical intervention.

OPERATIVE PROCEDURES. The surgical treatment of aortic regurgitation and of combined aortic stenosis and regurgitation is valve replacement. Since the aortic annulus in patients with severe aortic regurgitation is usually not as narrow as it is in patients with aortic stenosis, a larger artificial valve can be inserted, and postoperative obstruction to left ventricular outflow is not a problem, as it may be in some patients with stenosis. Occasionally, when a leaflet has been torn from its attachments to the aortic annulus by trauma, surgical repair may be possible. In patients in whom aortic regurgitation is due to aneurysmal dilatation of the annulus and the ascending aorta, regurgitation may occasionally be reduced or eliminated by narrowing the annulus or by excising a portion of the aorta. More often, effective treatment in these patients requires replacement of the aortic valve and excision of the aneurysmal portion of the aorta and its replacement with a graft, sometimes with reimplantation of the coronary arteries. This more extensive procedure is associated with a higher operative risk than is aortic valve replacement alone.

Aortic valve replacement is discussed on page 1103. In general, results in patients with aortic regurgitation are similar to those in patients with aortic stenosis, with a large fraction of patients exhibiting striking clinical improvement. Reductions in heart size and in left ventricular diastolic volume and mass occur in the majority of patients.[541,541a,541b] However, as already indicated, the extent of improvement in left ventricular function may not be as salutary as in patients with aortic stenosis,[534-540] perhaps reflecting the fact that ventricular dysfunction is more advanced in patients with aortic regurgitation by the time they become symptomatic and are referred for surgical treatment.[541c,541d] As is the case for aortic stenosis, the operative risk of aortic valve replacement in patients with aortic regurgitation depends on the general condition of the patient, the state of left ventricular function,[541,542] and the skill of the surgical team; the mortality rate ranges from 5 to 10 per cent in most medical centers. A late mortality of approximately 5 per cent per year is observed in survivors in whom cardiac enlargement was marked and left ventricular dysfunction was prolonged preoperatively. By extending the indications for operation to symptomatic patients with normal left ventricular function as well as to asymptomatic patients with early left ventricular dysfunction, it is likely that both early and late results will improve. It is likely that with the continued improvement of surgical techniques and results, it will become possible to extend the recommendation for operative treatment to asymptomatic patients with severe regurgitation and normal or nearly normal cardiac function. However, the risk of operation and the uncertainties of function of artificial valves suggests that the time for such a policy has not yet arrived.[543]

DISEASES OF THE TRICUSPID AND PULMONIC VALVES

TRICUSPID STENOSIS

Etiology and Pathology

Tricuspid stenosis is almost always rheumatic in origin. Other causes of obstruction to right atrial emptying are unusual and include tricuspid atresia (p. 994), right atrial tumors (which may produce a clinical picture suggesting rapidly progressive tricuspid stenosis [p. 1459]), and the carcinoid syndrome (which usually produces tricuspid regurgitation [p. 1430] but which may occasionally produce stenosis). Rarely, obstruction to right ventricular inflow can be due to pericardial constriction, extracardiac tumors, and vegetations.

Rheumatic tricuspid stenosis almost never occurs as an isolated lesion but generally accompanies mitral valve disease;[544-547] in many patients the aortic valve is also involved. Tricuspid stenosis is present at autopsy in 14 per cent of patients with rheumatic heart disease but is of clinical significance in only about 5 per cent.[548]

Organic tricuspid valve disease is more common in India than in North America or Western Europe and has been reported to occur in the hearts of more than one-third of patients with rheumatic heart disease studied at autopsy in that country.[549] The anatomical changes of rheumatic tricuspid stenosis resemble those of mitral stenosis (Fig. 32–1), with fusion and shortening of the chordae tendineae and fusion of the leaflets at their edges producing a diaphragm with a fixed central aperture.[128] As is the case for mitral stenosis, tricuspid stenosis is more common in women and, in the United States, is seen most commonly in persons between the ages of 20 and 60 years. Again, as in mitral valve disease, stenosis, regurgitation, or some combination of the two may exist.

The right atrium is often greatly dilated, and its walls are thickened. There may be evidence of severe passive congestion, with enlargement of the liver and spleen.

Pathophysiology

A diastolic pressure gradient between the right atrium and ventricle—the hemodynamic expression of tricuspid stenosis—is augmented when the transvalvular blood flow increases during exercise or inspiration and is reduced when flow declines during expiration. A mean diastolic pressure gradient exceeding 5 mm Hg is usually sufficient to elevate mean right atrial pressure to levels that result in systemic venous congestion and, unless sodium intake has been restricted or diuretics have been given, is associated with jugular venous distention, ascites, and edema.

In patients with sinus rhythm, the right atrial *a* wave may be extremely tall (Fig. 32–36) and may even approach the level of the right ventricular systolic pressure. Resting cardiac output is usually markedly reduced and fails to rise during exercise, accounting for the normal or only slightly elevated left atrial, pulmonary arterial, and right ventricular systolic pressures, despite the presence of accompanying mitral valve disease.

A small mean diastolic pressure gradient across the tricuspid valve as low as 2 mm Hg is sufficient to establish the diagnosis of tricuspid stenosis. Therefore, whenever this diagnosis is suspected, right atrial and ventricular

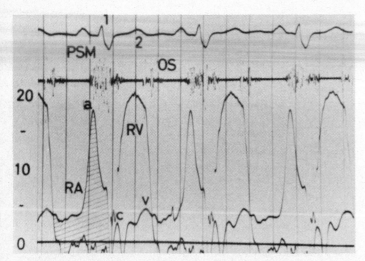

FIGURE 32-36 Phonocardiogram and right heart pressures in a patient with tricuspid stenosis. The giant right atrial *a* wave (a) nearly equals right ventricular (RV) systolic pressure and produces a large diastolic gradient (shaded area). A presystolic murmur (PSM), loud first heart sound (1), and early diastolic opening snap (OS) simulate the findings in mitral stenosis. (Time lines = 0.2 sec.) (From Criley, J. M., et al.: Departures from the expected auscultatory events in mitral stenosis. *In* Likoff, W. [ed.]: Valvular Heart Disease. Philadelphia, F. A. Davis, 1973, p. 214.)

pressures should be recorded simultaneously, using two catheters or a single catheter with a double lumen, with one lumen opening on either side of the tricuspid valve. The effects of respiration on any pressure difference should be examined.

Clinical Manifestations

HISTORY. The low cardiac output characteristic of tricuspid stenosis causes fatigue, and patients often complain of discomfort due to hepatomegaly, swelling of the abdomen, and anasarca. These symptoms, which are secondary to an elevated systemic venous pressure, are out of proportion to the degree of dyspnea.[546] Some patients complain of a fluttering discomfort in the neck, caused by giant *a* waves in the jugular venous pulse. Despite the coexistence of mitral stenosis, the symptoms characteristic of this valve lesion, i.e., hemoptysis, paroxysmal nocturnal dyspnea, and acute pulmonary edema, are usually absent. Indeed, the absence of the symptoms of pulmonary congestion in a patient with obvious mitral stenosis should suggest the possibility of tricuspid stenosis.

PHYSICAL EXAMINATION. Because of the high frequency with which mitral stenosis occurs in patients with tricuspid stenosis, the diagnosis of tricuspid stenosis is commonly overlooked, since the physical findings are attributed to mitral stenosis, and therefore a high index of suspicion is required to detect the tricuspid valve lesion. In the presence of sinus rhythm (which is surprisingly common), the *a* wave in the jugular venous pulse is tall, sharp, and flicking and on first impression may be confused with an arterial pulsation; a presystolic hepatic pulsation is often palpable. The *y* descent is slow and barely appreciable, indicating the absence of normal rapid, early right ventricular filling. The lung fields are clear, and despite engorgement of the neck veins and the presence of ascites and anasarca, the patient is normally comfortable while lying

flat. A parasternal (right ventricular) lift is inconspicuous, and pulmonic valve closure is not palpable, but occasionally the pulsations of a greatly enlarged right atrium may be felt to the right of the sternum. Thus, on inspection and palpation the combination of a prominent *a* wave in the jugular venous pulse in a patient with mitral stenosis without the clinical signs of pulmonary hypertension or right ventricular enlargement should suggest the diagnosis of tricuspid stenosis. This suspicion is strengthened when a diastolic thrill of tricuspid stenosis is felt at the lower left sternal edge, particularly during inspiration.[14]

The auscultatory findings of mitral stenosis are usually prominent and often overshadow the more subtle signs of tricuspid stenosis. A tricuspid valvular opening snap (OS) may be audible but is often difficult to distinguish from a mitral OS. However, the tricuspid OS usually follows the mitral OS, and is localized to the lower left sternal border, whereas the mitral OS is usually most prominent at the apex and is more widely distributed. The diastolic murmur of tricuspid stenosis is commonly heard best along the lower left parasternal border in the fourth intercostal space and is usually softer, higher pitched, and shorter in duration than the murmur of mitral stenosis. The presystolic component has a scratchy quality, commences earlier (0.06 sec after the P wave in tricuspid stenosis compared with 0.12 in mitral stenosis), and has a crescendo-decrescendo configuration, diminishing before S_1. The diastolic murmur and OS of tricuspid stenosis are both augmented by inspiration, the Mueller maneuver, assumption of the right lateral decubitus position, leg-raising, inhalation of amyl nitrite, prompt squatting, and both isotonic and isometric exercise. They are reduced during expiration or the strain of the Valsalva maneuver and return to control levels immediately (i.e., within two to three beats) after Valsalva release.

Laboratory Examination

ELECTROCARDIOGRAM. In the absence of atrial fibrillation, tricuspid stenosis is suggested by the presence of electrocardiographic evidence of right atrial enlargement disproportionate to the degree of right ventricular hypertrophy. The P-wave amplitude in leads II and V_1 exceeds 0.25 mv (p. 207), and there may be depression of the P-R segment resulting from increased magnitude of the atrial T wave. Since most patients with tricuspid stenosis have mitral valve disease, the electrocardiographic signs of biatrial enlargement (p. 208) with abnormally tall, broad P waves in leads II, III, and aV_f and prominent positive and negative deflections in V_1 are commonly found. Right atrial dilatation may rotate the ventricular septum and affect QRS morphology in a manner so that the large volume of the right atrium between the exploring electrode and the ventricles reduces the amplitude of the QRS complex in lead V_1 (which often has a Q wave), whereas the QRS complex is much taller in V_2.[64]

RADIOLOGICAL FINDINGS. The key radiological findings in tricuspid stenosis are marked cardiomegaly, with conspicuous enlargement of the right atrium (i.e., prominence of the right heart border), which extends into a dilated superior vena cava and azygos vein, but without dilatation of the pulmonary artery. The vascular changes

EKG

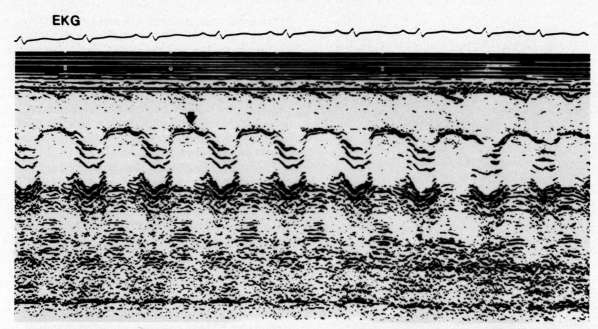

FIGURE 32–37 M-mode echocardiogram of a patient with carcinoid involvement of the tricuspid valve. The flat E–F slope (arrow) is consistent with tricuspid stenosis. (Reproduced with permission from Strickman, N. E., et al.: Carcinoid heart disease: A clinicial, pathologic and therapeutic update. *In* Harvey, W. P., et al. (eds.): Current Problems in Cardiology. Copyright © 1982 by Year Book Medical Publishers, Inc., Chicago.)

in the lungs characteristic of mitral valve disease may be masked, with little or no interstitial edema or vascular redistribution.

Angiography carried out following injection of contrast material into the right atrium and filming in the 30-degree right anterior oblique projection is useful for evaluating the appearance of the tricuspid valve. Thickening and decreased mobility of the leaflets, a jet through the constricted orifice, and thickening of the right atrial wall are characteristic findings.

ECHOCARDIOGRAM (see also p. 115). Although the motion of the normal tricuspid valve is similar to that of the normal mitral valve, it is more difficult to image. The changes in the echocardiogram in tricuspid stenosis resemble those observed in mitral stenosis. Thus, there is a reduction in the E–F slope of the anterior leaflet and usually paradoxical motion of the septal leaflet in diastole (Fig. 32–37).[550,550a] Calcification and thickening of the tricuspid valve often results in multiple and disorganized echoes. In the presence of elevated right ventricular end-diastolic pressure, there is prolongation of the A-C interval, and the time difference between the electrocardiographic P-R interval and the echocardiographic A-C interval is abbreviated. Two-dimensional echocardiography is useful in estimating the size of the tricuspid orifice.[551,552]

Management

Although the fundamental approach to the management of severe tricuspid stenosis is surgical treatment, intensive sodium restriction and diuretic therapy may diminish the symptoms secondary to the accumulation of excess salt and water. A prolonged preparatory period of diuresis may diminish hepatic congestion and thereby improve hepatic function sufficiently to diminish the risks of subsequent operation.

Surgical treatment of tricuspid stenosis should be carried out at the time of mitral commissurotomy or valve replacement in patients with tricuspid stenosis in whom mean diastolic pressure gradients exceed 5 mm Hg and tricuspid orifices are less than approximately 2.0 cm². Since tricuspid stenosis is almost always accompanied by significant tricuspid regurgitation, simple finger fracture valvulotomy often does not result in significant hemodynamic improvement but may merely substitute severe regurgitation for stenosis. However, open commissurotomy in which the stenotic tricuspid valve is converted into a functionally bicuspid one may result in substantial improvement. The commissures between the anterior and septal leaflets and between the posterior and septal leaflets are opened; it is not advisable to open the commissure between the anterior and posterior leaflets for fear of producing severe regurgitation.[208] If open commissurotomy does not restore reasonably normal valve function, the tricuspid valve may have to be replaced.[553,553a] A tissue valve such as a porcine heterograft (p. 1087) is generally preferred to a mechanical prosthesis in the tricuspid valve position.

TRICUSPID REGURGITATION

Etiology and Pathology

The most common cause of tricuspid regurgitation is not intrinsic involvement of the valve itself but *dilatation of the right ventricle* and of the tricuspid annulus, which may be complications of right ventricular failure of any cause (Fig. 32–38). Functional tricuspid regurgitation is observed in patients with right ventricular hypertension secondary to any form of cardiac and pulmonary vascular disease, most commonly mitral valve disease, right ventricular infarction,[554,555] congenital heart disease (e.g., pulmonic stenosis and pulmonary hypertension secondary to Eisenmenger's syndrome), primary pulmonary hypertension, and

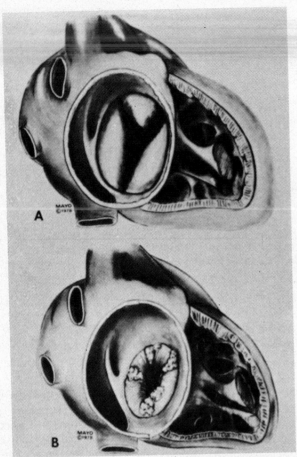

FIGURE 32–38 Types of tricuspid incompetence. *A*, Functional tricuspid incompetence secondary to dilatation of the right ventricle. *B*, Organic rheumatic tricuspid incompetence. (From Brandenburg, R. O., et al.: Valvular heart disease—When should the patient be referred? Pract. Cardiol. *5*:50, 1979.)

cor pulmonale. Severe tricuspid regurgitation has been reported to be the presenting manifestation in thyrotoxicosis.[556] In infants, tricuspid regurgitation may complicate right ventricular failure secondary to neonatal pulmonary diseases and pulmonary hypertension with persistence of the fetal pulmonary circulation.[557] In all these cases, tricuspid regurgitation reflects the presence of, and in turn aggravates, severe right ventricular failure. All of these forms of functional regurgitation may diminish or disappear as the right ventricle decreases in size. Tricuspid regurgitation can also occur as a consequence of dilatation of the annulus in Marfan's syndrome, in which it is not associated with right ventricular dilatation secondary to pulmonary hypertension.

A variety of disease processes can affect the tricuspid valve apparatus *directly* and lead to regurgitation. Thus, organic tricuspid regurgitation may occur on a congenital basis, as a part of Ebstein's anomaly (p. 996), common atrioventricular canal, when the tricuspid valve is involved in the formation of an aneurysm of the ventricular septum,[558] or as an isolated congenital lesion.[438] Rheumatic fever may attack the tricuspid valve directly, and when it does so, it usually leads to both regurgitation and stenosis (Fig. 32–38*B*). Infarction, rupture, or ischemia of the papillary muscles of the right ventricle in coronary artery disease[554,555] and in perinatal asphyxia[555] is an important cause

of tricuspid regurgitation. Tricuspid regurgitation associated with prolapse of the tricuspid valve resulting from myxomatous changes in the valve and chordae tendineae usually, but not always, accompanies prolapse of the mitral valve[559] and may be associated with atrial septal defect.[560] Other causes include trauma[561] (p. 1535), infective endocarditis (Chap. 33),[562] particularly staphylococcal endocarditis in drug addicts, and surgical excision that has been necessary in patients with infective endocarditis unresponsive to medical management.[563,564]

Tricuspid regurgitation can occur as part of the *carcinoid syndrome* (p. 1430), which leads to focal or diffuse deposits of fibrous tissue on the endocardium of the valvular cusps and cardiac chambers and on the intima of the great veins and coronary sinus. The white, fibrous carcinoid plaques are most extensive on the right side of the heart, where they are usually deposited on the ventricular surfaces of the tricuspid valve and cause the cusps to adhere to the underlying right ventricular wall, thereby producing tricuspid regurgitation.[565–568] In addition, deposition of the fibrous tissue on the right atrial endocardium reduces its compliance.[569] Less common causes of tricuspid regurgitation include cardiac tumors, particularly right atrial myxoma (p. 1459); endomyocardial fibrosis (p. 1428); and, rarely, constrictive pericarditis. Tricuspid regurgitation may also occur rarely as an isolated congenital lesion.[570]

Clinical Manifestations

HISTORY. In the absence of pulmonary hypertension, tricuspid regurgitation is generally well tolerated. However, when pulmonary hypertension and tricuspid regurgitation coexist, cardiac output declines, and the manifestations of right-sided heart failure, become intensified. Thus, the symptoms of tricuspid regurgitation result from a reduced cardiac output and from ascites, painful congestive hepatomegaly, and massive edema. Occasionally, patients complain of throbbing pulsations in the neck due to jugular venous distention, which intensify on effort.[14] In the many patients with tricuspid regurgitation who have mitral valve disease, the symptoms of the latter predominate. Symptoms of pulmonary congestion may abate as tricuspid regurgitation develops, but they are replaced by weakness, fatigue, and other manifestations of a depressed cardiac output.

PHYSICAL EXAMINATION (Figures 3–32, p. 62, 3–37, p. 64, and 4–13, p. 75). Evidence of weight loss, cachexia, cyanosis, and jaundice is often present on inspection. Atrial fibrillation is common. There is jugular venous distention, the normal x and x^1 descents disappear, and a prominent systolic ("s") wave, i.e., a c-v wave, is apparent. The descent of this wave, the y descent, is sharp and becomes the most prominent event in the venous pulse, unless there is coexisting tricuspid stenosis. The right ventricular impulse is hyperdynamic and thrusting in quality. Occasionally, a right atrial systolic impulse may be observed or palpated along the right lower sternal edge.[14] In patients with combined mitral valve disease and tricuspid regurgitation, a relatively quiet zone may be present between the apex and the left sternal edge. Systolic pulsations of an enlarged tender liver are commonly present initially (see Figure 15–5, p. 497), but in chronic tricuspid regurgitation with congestive cirrhosis, the liver may be firm and nontender. Ascites and edema are frequent.

Auscultation (Table 32–5). This usually reveals an S_3 originating from the right ventricle, i.e., one which is accentuated by inspiration; when tricuspid regurgitation is associated with pulmonary hypertension, P_2 is accentuated as well. The pansystolic murmur of tricuspid regurgitation is high-pitched and loudest in the fourth intercostal space in the parasternal region but occasionally in the subxiphoid area. When tricuspid regurgitation is mild, the murmur may be short. With acute tricuspid regurgitation, due to infective endocarditis or trauma, the murmur is usually of low intensity and limited to the first half of systole. When the right ventricle is greatly dilated and occupies the anterior surface of the heart, the murmur may be most prominent at the apex and difficult to distinguish from that produced by mitral regurgitation; this may also occur in tricuspid regurgitation secondary to Ebstein's malformation.

The response of the murmur to respiration and other maneuvers is of considerable aid in establishing the diagnosis of tricuspid regurgitation. It is usually augmented during inspiration.[14,571,572] (Rivero-Carvello's sign), but when the failing ventricle can no longer increase its stroke volume, the inspiratory augmentation is lost. Under these circumstances, respiratory variation may be elicited by standing and thereby reducing venous return. The murmur also increases during inspiration, the Mueller maneuver (forced inspiration against a closed glottis), exercise, leg-raising, and amyl nitrite inhalation as well as after a prolonged diastole, and it demonstrates an immediate overshoot after release of the Valsalva strain. It is reduced in intensity and duration in the standing position and during the strain of the Valsalva maneuver. Rarely, tricuspid regurgitation is silent except for the selective appearance of a soft systolic murmur during inspiration.[573]

Increased atrioventricular flow may cause a short early diastolic flow rumble in the left parasternal region following S_3 (see Figure 3–37, p. 64).

Laboratory Examination

Radiological Findings. Marked cardiomegaly secondary to the condition responsible for the dilatation of the right ventricle is usually evident. The right atrium is prominent (Figures 6–2, p. 148). Evidence of elevated right atrial pressure may include distention of the azygos vein and the presence of pleural effusion. Ascites with upward displacement of the diaphragm may be present. Rarely, with prolonged elevation of right ventricular pressure, the tricuspid ring may calcify. The findings of pulmonary arterial and venous hypertension are common. Fluoroscopy may reveal systolic pulsation of the right atrium.

Electrocardiogram. This is usually nonspecific and characteristic of the lesion causing tricuspid regurgitation. Incomplete right bundle-branch block, Q waves in lead V_1 (Figure 7–12, p. 209), and atrial fibrillation are commonly found.

Echocardiogram (see also p. 116). The right ventricle is usually dilated, and there is evidence of right ventricular diastolic overload, with paradoxical motion of the ventricular septum similar to that in atrial septal defect.[574] Exaggerated motion and delayed closure of the tricuspid valve are evident in patients with Ebstein's anomaly. In patients with tricuspid regurgitation secondary to right ventricular dilatation and pulmonary hypertension, the pulmonic valve echogram shows a diminished or absent a deflection (Figure 5–37, p. 109). *Prolapse of the tricuspid valve* may be evident on M-mode echocardiography,[575] and simultaneous echocardiographic studies of the tricuspid valve and phonocardiography may reveal a nonejection systolic click that occurs at the onset of prolapse, originating from the right side of the heart, since it is delayed during inspiration. Two-dimensional echocardiography is particularly useful in the diagnosis of tricuspid prolapse; it reveals the leaflet or leaflets lying above the tricuspid valve ring, i.e., in the right atrium, in systole.[559,576] Cross-sectional echocardiography also allows measurement of right atrial size (which is always increased in the presence of moderate or severe tricuspid regurgitation) as well as detection of paradoxical motion of the ventricular septum.[444]

Contrast echocardiography involving rapid injection of saline or indocyanine green dye into an antecubital vein during two-dimensional echocardiography (p. 95) is both sensitive and specific for tricuspid regurgitation.[577] The injection produces microcavities that are readily visible on echocardiography and normally travel as a bolus through the circulation. In tricuspid regurgitation, these microcavities can be seen to travel back and forth across the tricuspid orifice and to pass into the inferior vena cava and hepatic veins during systole (Fig. 32–39).[578] Tricuspid regurgitation secondary to carcinoid heart disease shows thickened, retracted valve leaflets,[567,568] whereas that due to endocarditis may reveal vegetations on the valve.[562]

HEMODYNAMIC AND ANGIOGRAPHIC FINDINGS. The right atrial and right ventricular end-diastolic pressures are characteristically elevated in tricuspid regurgitation, whether the condition is due to organic disease of the tricuspid valve or is secondary to right ventricular systolic overload (e.g., pulmonary hypertension and pulmonic stenosis). The right atrial pressure tracing reveals absence of the x descent, a prominent v or c-v wave ("ventricularization" of the atrial pressure); thus the right atrial pressure pulse increasingly resembles the right ventricular pressure pulse as the severity of tricuspid regurgitation increases (Fig. 32–40).[579,580] A rise or no change in right atrial pressure on deep inspiration, rather than the usual fall, is characteristic of tricuspid regurgitation.[571] Pulmonary artery (or right ventricular) systolic pressure may offer a rough guide as to whether the tricuspid regurgitation is primary (disease of the valve or its supporting structures) or secondary. Pulmonary artery or right ventricular systolic pressure less than 40 mm Hg favors a primary etiology, whereas when the systolic pressure is greater than 60 mm Hg, the tricuspid regurgitation could be primary or secondary to right ventricular dilatation and failure. In some cases of tricuspid regurgitation, abnormalities in the right atrial pressure contour may be mild or absent. A more sensitive and precise tool for assessing tricuspid regurgitation is the indicator dilution technique.[581] Injection of indicator substance (e.g., indocyanine green) into the right ventricle with sampling in both the right atrium and a peripheral artery allows detection of the "early appearance" of indicator in the right atrium as well as quantitation of the relative magnitudes of forward versus regurgitant flows (Fig. 32–41).

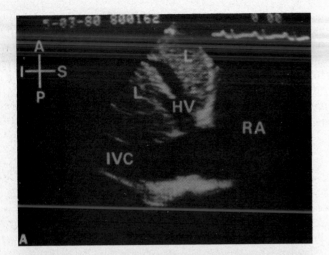

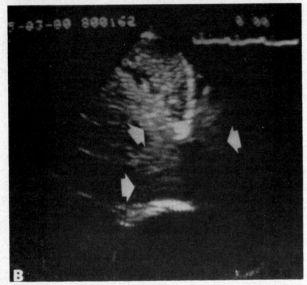

FIGURE 32–39   Stop-frame photographs from a subcostal two-dimensional echocardiographic study of the inferior vena cava (IVC) and right atrium (RA) before (*A*) and immediately after (*B*) upper extremity injection of 5 per cent dextrose in water. The IVC and hepatic vein (HV) filled with contrast (arrows) in this patient with tricuspid regurgitation that was later confirmed by intraoperative right atrial palpation. L = liver; A = anterior; P = posterior; I = inferior; S = superior. (From Meltzer, R. A., van Hoogenhuyze, D., Serruys, P. W., et al.: Diagnosis of tricuspid regurgitation by contrast echocardiography. Circulation *63*:1093, 1981, by permission of the American Heart Association, Inc.)

The role of *angiography* in the diagnosis and quantitation of tricuspid regurgitation has been controversial.[581,582] A modification of previous angiographic techniques has been introduced in which a special, preformed catheter is positioned in the right ventricle, and angiography is carried out at low injection rates;[583] or a special balloon catheter is employed to minimize the induction of extrasystoles which can cause spurious regurgitation.[584] Diagnosis and quantitative assessment of tricuspid regurgitation can be aided in many instances by right ventriculography, but the fact that the catheter must be positioned across the tricuspid valve cannot exclude the possibility of a false-positive diagnosis of tricuspid regurgitation.

Management

Tricuspid regurgitation in the absence of pulmonary hypertension usually does not require surgical treatment. Indeed, both patients and experimental animals tolerate total excision of the tricuspid valve, as long as right ventricular systolic pressure is normal.[563,564] *Surgical treatment* of acquired regurgitation secondary to pulmonary hypertension was greatly improved when Carpentier and his associates pointed out that the portion of the tricuspid annulus supported by the free ventricular wall participates in annular dilatation to a greater extent than does that portion of the annulus supported by the interventricular septum. They introduced the concept of suturing the annulus to a nondeformable prosthetic ring of appropriate dimensions.[585] That portion of the annular circumference supported by the free ventricular wall may be shortened by a plicating suture.[586,587]

In patients with tricuspid regurgitation associated with mitral valve disease and pulmonary hypertension, the severity of the regurgitation should be assessed by palpation of the valve at the time of mitral commissurotomy or valve replacement. Patients with mild tricuspid regurgitation usually do not require surgical treatment; pulmonary vascular pressures decline following successful mitral valve surgery, and the mild tricuspid regurgitation tends to disappear. Excellent results have also been reported in patients with moderate tricuspid regurgitation with the use of a tricuspid annuloplasty,[585–587] often utilizing a Carpentier ring[588] (Fig. 32–42). However, management of severe regurgitation is more controversial. It is not clear whether severe tricuspid regurgitation should be treated by an-

FIGURE 32–40   Appearance of right atrial (RA) pressure contour in patients with severe tricuspid regurgitation (TR), moderate TR, and no TR (normal). Note the regurgitant systolic (S) wave that blends with the normal filling (V) wave in severe TR. The resultant RA pressure waveform resembles a right ventricular (RV) pressure recording. (From Grossman, W. [ed.]: Cardiac Catheterization and Angiography. 2nd ed. Philadelphia, Lea and Febiger, 1980.)

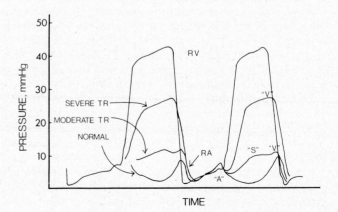

nuloplasty or valve replacement, but most surgeons now prefer the latter approach.[589,590]

Organic disease of the tricuspid valve responsible for tricuspid regurgitation usually requires valve replacement. The risk of thrombosis of valvular prostheses is greater in the tricuspid than in the mitral position, presumably because pressure and flow rates are lower in the right side of the heart. For this reason, the artificial valve of choice for the tricuspid position at present is the glutaraldehyde-preserved porcine heterograft. Anticoagulants are not required, and a durability of up to 10 years has been established. Tricuspid valve replacement has also been employed successfully in the treatment of severe tricuspid regurgitation in patients with carcinoid heart disease[565] and cardiogenic shock with right ventricular infarction.[590]

In treating the difficult problem of tricuspid valve endocarditis in heroin addicts, it has been noted that total excision of the tricuspid valve *without immediate replacement* can be tolerated. When antibiotic therapy is unsuccessful, valvular replacement frequently results in reinfection or continued infection. To manage this difficult problem, all

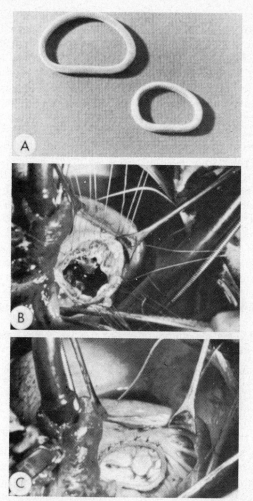

FIGURE 32–42 *A*, Carpentier rings. *B*, Ring being sutured into place. *C*, Completion of Carpentier ring annuloplasty. (From Starr, A.: Acquired disease of the tricuspid valve. *In* Sabiston, D. C., Jr., and Spencer, F. C. [eds.]: Gibbon's Surgery of the Chest. Philadelphia, W. B. Saunders Co., 1976, p. 1182.)

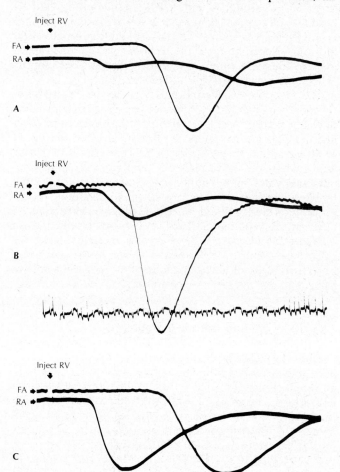

FIGURE 32–41 Indicator dilution curves after injection in the right ventricle (RV), with sampling from the right atrium (RA) and femoral artery (FA). The appearance of dye in the right atrium earlier than in the femoral artery indicates the presence of tricuspid regurgitation. Patient with mild (*A*), moderate (*B*), and severe (*C*) tricuspid regurgitation. For convenience, all curves are recorded at 5 mm/sec paper speed. (From Hansing, C. E., and Rowe, G. G.: Tricuspid insufficiency. A study of hemodynamics and pathogenesis. Circulation *45*:794, 1972, by permission of the American Heart Association, Inc.)

diseased valvular tissue should be excised to eradicate the endocarditis, and antibiotic treatment can be continued. Most patients tolerate loss of the tricuspid valve without great difficulty. However, if medical management does not control the tricuspid regurgitation and the infection has been controlled, an artificial valve can be inserted.[564]

PULMONIC VALVE DISEASE

ETIOLOGY AND PATHOLOGY. The congenital form is the most common cause of *pulmonic stenosis.* Its manifestations in children are discussed on page 986 and in adults on page 1037. *Rheumatic* inflammation of the pulmonic valve is usually associated with involvement of other valves and rarely leads to serious deformity. However, a high incidence of significant pulmonic valve involvement secondary to rheumatic fever has been reported in Mexico City, perhaps related to the pulmonary hypertension that occurs at high altitudes and the resultant greater stress on the pulmonic valve.[591] *Carcinoid* plaques, similar to those involving the tricuspid valve (p. 1430), are often present in the outflow tract of the right ventricle in patients with malignant carcinoid and result in construction of the pulmonic valve ring, retraction and fusion of the valve cusps, and obstruction to right ventricular outflow.[566] Obstruction in the region of the pulmonic valve may be extrinsic to the valve apparatus and may be produced by cardiac tumors or aneurysm of the sinus of Valsalva.[592]

By far the most common cause of *pulmonic regurgitation* is dilatation of the valve ring secondary to pulmonary hypertension (of any etiology) or to dilatation of the pulmonary artery, either idiopathic[593,594] or consequent to a connective tissue disorder such as Marfan's syndrome.[595] Less frequently it results from a variety of lesions directly affecting the pulmonic valve. These include congenital malformations, such as absent, malformed, fenestrated, or supernumerary leaflets.[126] These anomalies may occur as isolated lesions but more often are associated with other congenital anomalies, particularly tetralogy of Fallot, ventricular septal defect, and pulmonic valvular stenosis.[596-603] Pulmonic regurgitation may occur as a consequence of infective endocarditis[604] or following surgical correction of valvular or subvalvular stenosis or surgical removal of the valve for treatment of endocarditis; less common causes include carcinoid syndrome, rheumatic involvement,[591] injury produced by a pulmonary artery flow-directed catheter,[605] and syphilis.[593]

Clinical Manifestations

Like tricuspid regurgitation, isolated pulmonic regurgitation may be tolerated for many years without difficulty unless it complicates or is complicated by pulmonary hypertension, in which case it is usually accompanied by and aggravates right ventricular failure. In most patients the clinical manifestations of the primary disease are severe and usually overshadow the pulmonic regurgitation, which often results only in incidental auscultatory findings. *Physical examination* reveals a hyperdynamic right ventricle, producing palpable systolic pulsations in the left parasternal area and an enlarged pulmonary artery that often results in palpable systolic pulsations in the second left intercostal space; sometimes systolic and diastolic thrills are felt in the same area. A tap reflecting pulmonic valve closure is usually easily palpable in the second left intercostal space in patients with pulmonary hypertension and secondary pulmonic regurgitation.

AUSCULTATION. In patients with congenital absence of the pulmonic valve, P_2 is not audible, but this sound is accentuated in patients with pulmonic regurgitation secondary to pulmonary hypertension, particularly when the dilated pulmonary artery is near the chest wall. There may be wide splitting of S_2 due to prolongation of right ventricular ejection accompanying the augmented stroke volume.[606] A nonvalvular systolic ejection click due to the sudden expansion of the pulmonary artery by the augmented right ventricular stroke volume frequently initiates a midsystolic ejection murmur, most prominent in the second left intercostal space. An S_3 and S_4 originating from the right ventricle are often audible, most readily in the fourth intercostal space at the left parasternal area, and are augmented by inspiration.

In the absence of pulmonary hypertension, the diastolic murmur of pulmonic regurgitation is low-pitched and is usually heard best at the third and fourth left intercostal spaces adjacent to the sternum (Figure 4–24, p. 83). The murmur commences when the pulmonary artery and right ventricular pressures diverge, approximately 0.04 sec after P_2. It is diamond-shaped in configuration and brief, reaching a peak intensity when the gradient between these pressures is maximal and ending with equilibration of the pressures.[607] The murmur becomes louder during inspiration and following inhalation of amyl nitrite.

When pulmonary artery systolic pressure exceeds approximately 70 mm Hg, dilatation of the pulmonic annulus results in a regurgitant jet of high velocity that is responsible for the so-called Graham Steell murmur of pulmonic regurgitation. This murmur is a high-pitched, blowing decrescendo murmur beginning immediately after P_2 and is most prominent in the left parasternal region in the second to fourth intercostal spaces (see Figure 4–24, p. 83). Thus, although it resembles the murmur of aortic regurgitation, it is usually accompanied by the findings of severe pulmonary hypertension, i.e., an accentuated P_2 or fused S_2, an ejection sound, and a systolic murmur of tricuspid regurgitation. Sometimes a low-frequency presystolic murmur is present, i.e., a right-sided Austin Flint murmur originating from the tricuspid valve that is analogous to the more common left-sided Austin Flint murmur originating from the mitral valve[608] (p. 1111).

The Graham Steell murmur of pulmonic regurgitation secondary to pulmonary hypertension usually increases in intensity with inspiration, exhibits little change after amyl nitrite inhalation or vasopressors, is diminished during the Valsalva strain, and returns to baseline intensity almost immediately after release of the Valsalva strain. This murmur resembles and may be confused with the diastolic blowing murmur of aortic regurgitation. However, indicator dilution studies[609] and retrograde thoracic aortography[610] have established that a diastolic blowing murmur along the left sternal border in patients with rheumatic heart disease and pulmonary hypertension—even in the absence of peripheral signs of aortic regurgitation—is usually due to aortic and not pulmonic regurgitation.

Laboratory Examination

ELECTROCARDIOGRAM. In the absence of pulmonary hypertension, pulmonic regurgitation often results in an electrocardiogram that reflects right ventricular diastolic overload, i.e., an rSr' (or rsR') configuration in the right precordial leads. Pulmonic regurgitation secondary to pulmonary hypertension is usually associated with electrocardiographic evidence of right ventricular hypertrophy.

RADIOLOGICAL FINDINGS. Both the pulmonary artery and the right ventricle are usually enlarged,[611] but these signs are nonspecific. Fluoroscopy may demonstrate pronounced pulsation of the main pulmonary artery. Pulmonic regurgitation can be diagnosed by observing opacification of the right ventricle following injection of contrast material into the main pulmonary artery (Figure 32–43). The diagnosis is supported by noting superimposition of the pulmonary artery and right ventricular pressure curves during mid and late diastole. Indicator dilution techniques

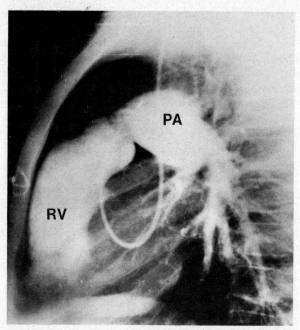

FIGURE 32–43 Pulmonic valvular regurgitation. Contrast medium has been injected into the main pulmonary artery (PA) and regurgitates back into an enlarged right ventricle (RV). (From Carlsson, E., et al.: The radiological diagnosis of cardiac valvar insufficiencies. Circulation 55:921, 1977, by permission of the American Heart Association, Inc.)

with injections into the pulmonary artery and sampling from the right ventricle,[612] as well as intracardiac phonocardiography,[593,613] can also be helpful in establishing the diagnosis in mild cases.

ECHOCARDIOGRAM. This shows right ventricular dilatation and, in patients with pulmonary hypertension, right ventricular hypertrophy as well. Diastolic fluttering of the tricuspid valve leaflets, similar to that of the mitral valve leaflets in aortic regurgitation, is often noted. Abnormal motion of the septum characteristic of volume overload of the right ventricle in diastole may be evident. The motion of the pulmonic valve may point to the etiology of the pulmonic regurgitation.[614] Absence of *a* waves and systolic notching of the posterior leaflet suggest pulmonary hypertension; large *a* waves indicate pulmonic stenosis. The pulsed Doppler technique is extremely accurate in detecting pulmonary regurgitation. Abnormal Doppler signals in the right ventricular outflow tract whose velocity is sustained throughout diastole are observed in patients in whom dilatation of the valve ring (functional regurgitation) is the cause. When the velocity falls during diastole, the pulmonary artery pressure is normal, and the regurgitation is caused by an abnormality of the valve itself.[614]

Management

Pulmonic regurgitation *per se* is seldom severe enough to require specific treatment. Cardiac glycosides are useful in the management of right ventricular dilatation or failure. Treatment of the primary condition responsible for the pulmonary hypertension, such as surgical treatment of mitral valvular disease, often ameliorates the pulmonic regurgitation. Surgical treatment of primary pulmonic regurgitation directed specifically at the pulmonic valve is required only occasionally because of intractable right heart failure, and in this case valve replacement may be carried out.[601]

MULTIVALVULAR DISEASE

Multivalvular involvement is common, particularly in patients with rheumatic heart disease, and a variety of clinical and hemodynamic syndromes can be produced by different combinations of valvular abnormalities. Development of pulmonic and tricuspid regurgitation secondary to dilatation of the pulmonic valve ring and tricuspid annulus, respectively, and as a consequence of disease involving the mitral or aortic valve or both, has already been discussed (pp. 1117 and 1121), as has the combination of *organic* tricuspid and mitral valvular disease (p. 1117). As a general rule, clinical manifestations produced by the more proximal (upstream) of two valvular lesions, i.e., the mitral valve in patients with combined mitral and aortic valvular disease and the tricuspid valve in patients with combined tricuspid and mitral valvular disease, are more prominent than those produced by the distal lesion.

It is important to recognize multivalvular involvement preoperatively, since failure to correct all significant valvular disease at the time of operation increases mortality considerably. In patients with multivalvular disease, the relative severity of each lesion may be difficult to estimate by clinical examination and noninvasive techniques, because one lesion may mask the manifestations of the other. For this reason, patients suspected of multivalvular in-

volvement and in whom surgical treatment is under consideration should undergo (in addition to careful clinical examination and noninvasive work-up, with emphasis on two-dimensional echocardiography), right- and left-heart catheterization and angiography. If there is any question concerning the presence of significant aortic stenosis in patients undergoing an operation on the mitral valve, the aortic valve should be inspected, since overlooking this condition can lead to a high perioperative mortality. Similarly, it is useful to palpate the tricuspid valve at the time of operation on the mitral valve.

Mitral Stenosis and Aortic Regurgitation

Approximately two-thirds of patients with severe mitral stenosis have an early blowing diastolic murmur along the left sternal border with a normal pulse pressure; in 90 per cent of these patients the murmur is due to aortic regurgitation and is usually of little clinical importance. However, approximately 10 per cent of patients with mitral stenosis have severe rheumatic aortic regurgitation,[505] which can usually be recognized by the peripheral signs of a widened pulse pressure, left ventricular dilatation and increased wall motion on echocardiography, and signs of left ventricular enlargement on radiological and electrocardiographic examinations.

On clinical examination of patients with obvious aortic regurgitation, errors may be made in that mitral stenosis may be missed or, conversely, may be falsely diagnosed. An accentuated S_1 and an opening snap in a patient with aortic regurgitation should suggest the possibility of mitral valvular disease. On the other hand, an Austin Flint murmur may be considered to be a mitral diastolic rumbling murmur of mitral stenosis. These two murmurs may be distinguished at the bedside by means of amyl nitrite inhalation, which diminishes the Austin Flint murmur (Fig. 32–31, p. 1111) but augments the murmur of mitral stenosis (p. 1069); isometric handgrip and squatting augment the diastolic murmur of aortic regurgitation and the Austin Flint murmur. Echocardiography is of decisive value in the detection of both lesions.

Mitral Stenosis and Aortic Stenosis

When mitral and aortic stenosis coexist, the mitral obstruction masks many of the clinical manifestations of aortic stenosis. The cardiac output tends to be reduced further than in patients with isolated aortic stenosis, and the atrial booster pump mechanism, so important in filling the ventricle in aortic stenosis (p. 1097), has little impact when mitral stenosis is present. The reduction in cardiac output lowers both the transaortic valvular pressure gradient and the left ventricular systolic pressure, diminishes the incidence of angina, and retards the development of aortic calcification and left ventricular hypertrophy.[615,616] On the other hand, clinical manifestations associated with mitral stenosis, such as pulmonary congestion and hemoptysis, atrial fibrillation, and systemic embolization, occur more frequently than in patients with isolated aortic stenosis. On physical examination, presystolic distention of the left ventricle and an S_4, common in pure aortic stenosis, are usually not present. The midsystolic murmur may be reduced in intensity and duration because of the reduced stroke volume. The *electrocardiogram* may fail to demonstrate left ventricular hypertrophy, but left atrial enlargement is common in patients in sinus rhythm. The *chest roentgenogram* is usually typical of mitral stenosis except for calcium in the region of the aortic valve. The two-dimensional *echocardiogram* is of the greatest value because stenosis of both valves may be evident. The indirect *carotid pulse* tracing reveals a delayed upstroke.

It is vital to recognize the presence of hemodynamically significant aortic valvular disease (stenosis and/or regurgitation) preoperatively in patients who are to undergo surgical correction of mitral stenosis, since isolated mitral valvulotomy may be hazardous in such patients; this operation can impose a sudden hemodynamic load on the left ventricle that may lead to acute pulmonary edema.

Aortic Stenosis and Mitral Regurgitation

The combination of severe aortic stenosis and mitral regurgitation is hazardous but fortunately relatively uncommon. Obstruction to left ventricular outflow, on the one hand, augments the volume of mitral regurgitant flow,[151] whereas the presence of mitral regurgitation, on the other, diminishes the ventricular preload necessary for mainte-

nance of the left ventricular stroke volume in aortic stenosis. The result is reduced cardiac output and marked left atrial and pulmonary venous hypertension. The physical findings may be confusing because the delayed arterial pulse of aortic stenosis may be counteracted by the sharp upstroke of mitral regurgitation, and it may be difficult to recognize two distinct systolic murmurs. On echocardiography the left ventricle is usually larger than in pure aortic stenosis.

Aortic Regurgitation and Mitral Regurgitation

In this relatively frequent combination[617] the clinical features of aortic regurgitation usually predominate, and it may be difficult to determine whether the mitral regurgitation is due to organic involvement of this valve or dilatation of the mitral valve ring secondary to left ventricular enlargement. This combination of lesions also occurs as a consequence of dilatation of the mitral and aortic annuli in connective tissue diseases such as Marfan's syndrome. When both valvular leaks are severe, this combination of lesions is poorly tolerated. The normal mitral valve ordinarily serves as a "backup" to the aortic valve, and premature (diastolic) closure of the mitral valve limits the volume of reflux that occurs in patients with acute aortic regurgitation.[489] With combined regurgitant lesions, regardless of the etiology of the mitral lesion, blood may reflux from the aorta through both chambers of the left heart into the pulmonary veins. Physical and laboratory examination will usually show evidence of both lesions.

When mitral regurgitation occurs in patients with aortic valvular disease (stenosis and/or regurgitation) secondary to left ventricular dilatation, it often regresses following aortic valve replacement. If severe, it may be corrected by annuloplasty at the time of aortic valve replacement; replacement of an intrinsically normal mitral valve with regurgitation due to a dilated annulus is neither necessary nor advisable.

Surgical Treatment of Multivalvular Disease

DOUBLE VALVE REPLACEMENT. Combined aortic and mitral valve replacement is usually associated with a higher risk and poorer survival than is replacement of one of these two valves.[618,619] Thus, in one representative series, operative mortality was 10.8 per cent for mitral valve replacement, 9.0 per cent for aortic valve replacement, and 18.6 per cent for combined mitral and aortic valve replacement; the 5-year survival was 71 per cent for mitral valve replacement, 70 per cent for aortic valve replacement, and 47 per cent for combined mitral and aortic valve replacement.[620] Some surgeons, however, have reported no increased mortality or lower survival in patients undergoing double compared with single valve replacement.[621]

TRIPLE VALVE REPLACEMENT. Hemodynamically significant disease involving the mitral, aortic, and tricuspid valves is uncommon. Patients with these lesions often present in advanced heart failure with marked cardiomegaly, and surgical correction of all three valvular lesions is imperative. Attempts to shorten the duration of operation by leaving one severely impaired valve in place after a double valve replacement are usually unsatisfactory.[208] However, triple valve replacement is a long and complex operation that has been reported to be associated with a mortality rate of 18 per cent in patients in functional Class III and 40 per cent in Class IV.[622] However, even this high risk must often be accepted because of the otherwise dismal prognosis in these patients.

Patients who survive triple valve replacement usually show substantial clinical improvement in the early postoperative period,[623,624] and postoperative catheterization studies show marked reductions in pulmonary arterial and capillary pressures.[625] However, some patients succumb to arrhythmias[624a] or congestive heart failure in the late postoperative period despite normally functioning prostheses. The cause of cardiac failure in this situation is not known, but it has been speculated that it may be related to intraoperative myocardial ischemia, microemboli from the multiple prostheses, or continued subclinical episodes of rheumatic myocarditis.[621]

References

MITRAL STENOSIS

1. Roberts, W. C.: Morphologic features of the normal and abnormal mitral valve. Am. J. Cardiol. *51*:1005, 1983.
1a. Evans, D. T. P., and Sloman, J. G.: Mitral stenosis and mitral incompetence due to Libman-Sacks endocarditis and mitral valve replacement. Aust. N.Z. J. Med. *11*:526, 1981.
2. Roberts, W. C., Kehoe, J. A., Carpenter, D. F., and Golden, A.: Cardiac valvular lesions in rheumatoid arthritis. Arch. Intern. Med. *122*:121, 1968.
3. Johnson, G. L., Vine, D. L., Cottrill, C. M., and Noonan, J. A.: Echocardiographic mitral valve deformity in the mucopolysaccharidoses. Pediatrics *67*:401, 1981.
4. Chandy, K. G., John, T. J., and Cherian, G.: Coxsackieviruses and chronic valvular heart disease. Am. Heart J. *100*:578, 1980.
5. Osterberger, L. E., Goldstein, S., Khaja, F., and Lakier, J. B.: Functional mitral stenosis in patients with massive annular calcification. Circulation *64*:472, 1981.
6. Kumar, A., Sinha, M., and Sinha, D. N. P.: Chronic rheumatic heart diseases in Rancho. Angiology *33*:141, 1982.
7. Rusted, I. E., Schiefly, C. H., and Eduardo, J. E.: Studies of the mitral valve. II. Certain anatomic features of the mitral valve and associated structures in mitral stenosis. Circulation *14*:398, 1956.
8. Wells, B.: The assessment of mitral stenosis by phonocardiography. Br. Heart J. *16*:261, 1954.
9. Craige, E.: Phonocardiographic studies in mitral stenosis. N. Engl. J. Med. *257*:650, 1957.
10. Lachman, A. S., and Roberts, W. C.: Calcific deposits in stenotic mitral valves. Circulation *57*:808, 1978.
11. Bowe, J. C., Bland, F., Sprague, H. B., and White, P. D.: Course of mitral stenosis without surgery: ten and twenty year perspectives. Ann. Intern. Med. *52*:741, 1960.
12. Tendon, R., Potti, S., Mathur, V. S., and Ray, S. B.: Critical mitral stenosis in children. Indian Pediatr. *9*:171, 1972.
13. Selzer, A., and Cohn, K. E.: Natural history of mitral stenosis: A review. Circulation *45*:878, 1972.
14. Reichek, N., Shelburne, J. C., and Perloff, J. R.: Clinical aspects of rheumatic valvular disease. Prog. Cardiovasc. Dis. *15*:491, 1973.
15. Wood, P.: An appreciation of mitral stenosis. Br. Med. J. *1*:1051 and 1113, 1954.
16. Arandi, D. T., and Carleton, R. A.: The deleterious role of tachycardia in mitral stenosis. Circulation *36*:511, 1967.
17. Mitchell, J. H., and Shapiro, W.: Atrial function and the hemodynamic consequences of atrial fibrillation in man. Am. J. Cardiol. *23*:556, 1969.
18. Selzer, A.: Effects of atrial fibrillation upon the circulation in patients with mitral stenosis. Am. Heart J. *59*:518, 1960.
19. Gorlin, R., and Gorlin, S. G.: Hydraulic formula for calculation of the area of stenotic mitral valve, other cardiac valves and central circulatory shunts. Am. Heart J. *41*:1, 1951.
20. Cohen, M. V., and Gorlin, R.: Modified orifice equation for the calculation of mitral valve area. Am. Heart J. *84*:839, 1972.
21. Nakhjavan, F. K., Katz, M. R., Maranhao, V., and Goldberg, H.: Analysis of influence of catecholamine and tachycardia during supine exercise in patients with mitral stenosis and sinus rhythm. Br. Heart J. *31*:753, 1969.
22. Thompson, M. E., Shaver, J. A., and Leon, D. T.: Effect of tachycardia on atrial transport in mitral stenosis. Am. Heart J. *94*:297, 1977.
23. Stott, D. K., Marpole, D. G. F., Bristow, J. D., Kloster, F. E., and Griswold, H. E.: The role of left atrial transport in aortic and mitral stenosis. Circulation *41*:1031, 1970.

24. Kennedy, J. W., Yarnall, S. R., Murray, J. A., et al.: Quantitative angiocardiography. IV. Relationships of left atrial and ventricular pressure and volume in mitral valve disease. Circulation *41*:817, 1970.
25. Heller, S. J., and Carleton, R. A.: Abnormal left ventricular contraction in patients with mitral stenosis. Circulation *42*:1099, 1970.
26. Dodge, H. T., Kennedy, J. W., and Petersen, J. L.: Quantitative angiographic methods in the evaluation of valvular heart disease. Prog. Cardiovasc. Dis. *16*:1, 1973.
27. Harvey, R. M., Ferrer, M. I., Samet, P., Bader, R. A., Bader, M. E., Cournand, A., and Richards, D. W.: Mechanical and myocardial factors in rheumatic heart disease in mitral stenosis. Circulation *11*:531, 1955.
28. Bolen, J. L., Lopes, M. G., Harrison, D. C., and Alderman, E. L.: Analysis of left ventricular function in response to afterload changes in patients with mitral stenosis. Circulation *52*:894, 1975.
29. Ahmed, S. S., Regan, T. J., Fiore, J. J., and Levinson, G. E.: The state of the left ventricular myocardium in mitral stenosis. Am. Heart J. *94*:28, 1977.
30. Selzer, A., and Cohn, K. E.: The "myocardial factor" in valvular heart disease. *In* Likoff, W. (ed.): Cardiovascular Clinics. Vol. 5, No. 2, Valvular Heart Disease. Philadelphia, F. A. Davis, 1973, p. 171.
31. Wroblewski, E., Spann, J. F., and Bove, A. A.: Right ventricular performance in mitral stenosis. Am. J. Cardiol. *47*:51, 1981.
32. Hugenholtz, P. G., Ryan, T. J., Stein, S. W., and Abelmann, W. H.: The spectrum of pure mitral stenosis. Hemodynamic studies in relation to clinical disability. Am. J. Cardiol. *10*:773, 1962.
33. Dalen, J. E., and Alpert, J. S.: Valvular Heart Disease. Boston, Little, Brown and Co., 1981, 473 pp.
34. Noble, R. J., and Fisch, C.: Factors in the genesis of atrial fibrillation in rheumatic valvular disease. *In* Likoff, W. (ed.): Cardiovascular Clinics. Vol. 5, No. 2, Valvular Heart Disease. Philadelphia, F. A. Davis, 1973, p. 97.
35. Ueland, K.: Rheumatic heart disease and pregnancy. *In* Elkayam, U., and Gleicher, N. (eds.): Cardiac Problems in Pregnancy. New York, Alan R. Liss, 1982, p. 80.
36. Munoz, S., Gallardo, J., Diaz-Gorrin, J. R., and Medina, O.: Influence of surgery on the natural history of rheumatic mitral and aortic valve disease. Am. J. Cardiol. *35*:234, 1975.
37. Diamond, M. A., and Genovese, P. D.: Life-threatening hemoptysis in mitral stenosis: Emergency mitral valve replacement resulting in rapid sustained cessation of pulmonary bleeding. J.A.M.A. *215*:441, 1971.
38. Schwartz, R., Meyerson, R. M., Lawrence, L. T., and Nichols, H. T.: Mitral stenosis, massive pulmonary hemorrhage and emergency valve replacement. N. Engl. J. Med. *275*:755, 1966.
39. Ross, R. S.: Right ventricular hypertension as a cause of precordial pain. Am. Heart J. *61*:134, 1961.
40. Baxter, R. H., Reid, J. M., McGuiness, J. B., and Stevenson, J. G.: Relation of angina to coronary artery disease in mitral and aortic valve disease. Br. Heart J. *40*:918, 1978.
41. Nielson, G. H., Galea, E. G., and Hossack, K. F.: Thromboembolic complications of mitral valve disease. Aust. N. Z. J. Med. *8*:372, 1978.
42. Daley, R., Mattingly, T. W., Holt, C. L., Bland, E. F., and White, P. D.: Systemic arterial embolism in rheumatic heart disease. Am. Heart J. *42*:566, 1951.
43. Lie, J. T., and Entman, M. L.: "Hole-in-one" sudden death: Mitral stenosis and left atrial thrombus. Am. Heart J. *91*:798, 1976.
44. Sharma, N. G. K., Kapoor, C. P., Mahambre, L., and Borkar, M. P.: Ortner's syndrome. J. Indian Med. Assoc. *60*:427, 1973.
45. Mounsey, P.: Inspection and palpation of the cardiac impulse. Prog. Cardiovasc. Dis. *10*:187, 1967.
46. McCall, B. W., and Price, J. L.: Movement of mitral valve cusps in relation to first heart sound and opening snap in patients with mitral stenosis. Br. Heart J. *29*:417, 1967.
47. Perloff, J. K.: Auscultatory and phonocardiographic manifestations of pulmonary hypertension. Prog. Cardiovasc. Dis. *9*:303, 1967.
48. Kalmanson, D., Veyrat, C., Bernier, A., Witchitz, S., and Chiche, P.: Opening snap and isovolumic relaxation period in relation to mitral valve flow in patients with mitral stenosis: Significance of the A_2-OS interval. Br. Heart J. *38*:135, 1976.
49. Craige, E.: Phonocardiographic studies in mitral stenosis. N. Engl. J. Med. *257*:650, 1957.
50. Mounsey, P.: The opening snap of mitral stenosis. Br. Heart J. *15*:135, 1953.
51. Yigitbasi, O., Nalbantgil, I., Birand, A., and Terek, A.: O-I/II A-OS formula for predicting left atrial pressure in mitral stenosis. Br. Heart J. *32*:547, 1970.
52. Ebringer, R., Pitt, A., and Anderson, S. T.: Haemodynamic factors influencing opening snap interval in mitral stenosis. Br. Heart J. *32*:350, 1970.
53. Chandraratna, P. A. N., Aronow, W. S., and Lurie, M.: Cross-sectional echocardiographic observations on the mechanism of preservation of the opening snap in calcific mitral stenosis. Chest *78*:822, 1980.
54. Criley, J. M., Chambers, R. D., Blaufuss, A. H., and Friedman, N. J.: Mitral stenosis: Mechanico-acoustical events. *In* Leon, D. F., and Shaver, J. A. (eds.): Physiological Principles of Heart Sounds and Murmurs. New York, American Heart Association Monograph No. 46, 1975, pp. 149–159.
55. Toutouzas, P., Koidakis, A., Velimezis, A., and Avgoustakis, D.: Mechanisms of diastolic rumble and presystolic murmur in mitral stenosis. Br. Heart J. *36*:1096, 1974.
56. Tavel, M. E., and Bonner, A. J., Jr.: Presystolic murmur in atrial fibrillation: Fact or fiction? Circulation *54*:167, 1976.
57. Harvey, W. P.: Silent valvular heart disease. *In* Likoff, W. (ed.): Cardio-

vascular Clinics. Vol. 5, No. 2, Valvular Heart Disease. Philadelphia, F. A. Davis, 1973, p. 77.

58. Delman, A. J., and Stein, E.: Rheumatic mitral stenosis. In Dynamic Cardiac Auscultation and Phonocardiography. Philadelphia, W. B. Saunders Co., 1979, p. 849.

59. Surawicz, B.: Effect of respiration and upright position on the interval between the two components of the second heart sound and that between the second sound and mitral opening snap. Circulation 16:422, 1957.

60. Delman, A. J., Gordon, G. M., Stein, E., and Escher, D. J. W.: The second sound–mitral opening snap (A2-OS) interval during exercise in the evaluation of mitral stenosis. Circulation 33:399, 1966.

61. Aravanis, C., and Michaelides, G.: Tricuspid insufficiency masquerading as mitral insufficiency in patients with severe mitral stenosis. Am. J. Cardiol. 20: 417, 1967.

62. McArthur, J. D., Sukumar, I. P., Munis, S. C., Krishnaswami, S., and Cherian, G.: Reassessment of Graham Steell murmur using platinum electrode technique. Br. Heart J. 36:1023, 1974.

63. Cooksey, J. D., Dunn, M., and Massie, E.: Clinical Vectorcardiography and Electrocardiography. 2nd ed. Chicago, Year Book Medical Publishers, 1977, p. 272.

64. Rios, J. C., and Goo, W.: Electrocardiographic correlates of rheumatic valvular disease. In Likoff, W. (ed.): Cardiovascular Clinics, Vol. 5, No. 2, Valvular Heart Disease. Philadelphia, F. A. Davis, 1973, p. 248.

65. Kasser, I., and Kennedy, J. W.: The relationship of increased left atrial volume and pressure to abnormal P waves on the electrocardiogram. Circulation 39: 339, 1969.

66. Mounsey, P.: The atrial electrocardiogram as a guide to prognosis after mitral valvulotomy. Br. Heart J. 21:1611, 1961.

67. Bailey, G. W., Braniff, B. A., Hancock, E. W., and Cohn, K. E.: Relationship of left atrial pathology to atrial fibrillation in mitral valvular disease. Ann. Intern. Med. 69:13, 1968.

68. Probst, P., Goldschlager, N., and Selzer, A.: Left atrial size and atrial fibrillation in mitral stenosis: Factors influencing their relationship. Circulation 48:1282, 1973.

69. Cueto, J., Toshima, J., Armyo, G., Tuna, N., and Lillehei, C. W.: Vectorcardiographic studies in acquired valvular disease with reference to the diagnosis of right ventricular hypertrophy. Circulation 33:588, 1967.

70. Taymor, R. C., Hoffman, I., and Henry, E.: The Frank vectorcardiogram in mitral stenosis. Circulation 30:865, 1964.

71. Walston, A., Harley, A., and Pipberger, H. V.: Computer analysis of the orthogonal electrocardiogram and vectorcardiogram in mitral stenosis. Circulation 50:472, 1974.

72. Donoso, E., Jick, S., Braunwald, E., Lamelas, M., and Grishman, A.: The spatial vectorcardiogram in mitral valve disease. Am. Heart J. 53:760, 1957.

73. Gooch, A. S., Calatayud, J. B., Gorman, P. A., Saunders, J. L., and Caceres, C. A.: Leftward shift of the terminal P forces in the ECG associated with left atrial enlargement. Am. Heart J. 71:727, 1966.

74. Chen, J. T. T., Behar, V. S., Morris, J. J., Jr., McIntosh, H. D., and Lester, R. G.: Correlation of roentgen findings with hemodynamic data in pure mitral stenosis. Am. J. Roentgenol. Radium Ther. Nucl. Med. 102:280, 1968.

75. Amplatz, K.: The roentgenographic diagnosis of mitral and aortic valvular disease. Am. Heart J. 64:556, 1962.

76. Melhem, R. E., Dunbar, J. D., and Booth, R. W.: "B" lines of Kerley and left atrial size in mitral valve disease: Their correlation with mean left atrial pressure as measured by left atrial puncture. Radiology 76:65, 1961.

77. Fleischner, F. G., and Reiner, L.: Linear x-ray shadows in acquired pulmonary hemosiderosis and congestion. N. Engl. J. Med. 250:900, 1954.

78. Van Houten, F. X., Adams, D. F., and Abrams, H. C.: Radiology of valvular heart disease. In Sonnenblick, E. H., and Lesch, M. (eds.): Valvular Heart Disease. New York, Grune and Stratton, 1974, p. 1.

79. Parker, B. M., Friedenberg, M. J., Templeton, A. W., and Burford, T. H.: Preoperative angiocardiographic diagnosis of left atrial thrombi in mitral stenosis. N. Engl. J. Med. 273:136, 1965.

80. Akius, C. W., Kirklin, J. K., Block, P. C., Buckley, M. J., and Austen, W. G.: Preoperative evaluation of subvalvular fibrosis in mitral stenosis. A predictive factor in conservative vs. replacement surgical therapy. Circulation 60(Suppl. I):71–76, 1978.

81. Parisi, A. F., and Tow, D. C.: Noninvasive Approaches to Cardiovascular Diagnosis. New York, Appleton-Century-Crofts, 1979, p. 113.

82. Thuillez, C., Theroux, P., Bourassa, M., Blanchard, M., Peronneau, P., Guermonprez, J.-L., Diebold, B., and Waters, D. D.: Pulsed Doppler echocardiographic study of mitral stenosis. Circulation 61:381, 1980.

83. Henry, W. L., and Kastl, D. G.: Echocardiographic evaluation of patients with mitral stenosis. Am. J. Med. 62:813, 1977.

84. Wann, L. S., Weyman, A. E., Feigenbaum, H., Dillon, J. C., Johnston, K. W., and Eggleton, R. C.: Determination of mitral valve area by cross-sectional echocardiography. Ann. Intern. Med. 88:337, 1978.

85. Fisher, M. L., Parisi, A. F., Plotnick, G. D., DeFelice, C. E., Carliner, N. H., and Fortuin, N. J.: Assessment of severity of mitral stenosis by echocardiographic leaflet separation. Arch. Intern. Med. 139:402, 1979.

86. Shiu, M. F., Crowther, A., Jenkins, B. S., and Webb-Peploe, M. M.: Echocardiographic and exercise evaluation of results of mitral valvotomy operations. Br. Heart J. 41:139, 1979.

87. Wise, J. R., Jr.: Echocardiographic evaluation of mitral stenosis using diastolic posterior left ventricular wall motion. Circulation 61:1037, 1980.

88. Palomo, A. R., Quinones, M. A., Waggoner, A. D., Kumpuris, A. G., and

89. Miller, R. R.: Echo-phonocardiographic determination of left atrial and left ventricular filling pressures with and without mitral stenosis. Circulation 61:1043, 1980.

89. Motro, M., Schneeweiss, A., Lehrer, E., Rath, S., and Neufeld, H. N.: Correlation between cardiac catheterization and echocardiography in assessing the severity of mitral stenosis. Int. J. Cardiol. 1:25, 1981.

90. Naito, M., Morganroth, J., Mardelli, T. J., Chen, C. C., and Dreifus, L. S.: Rheumatic mitral stenosis: Cross-sectional echocardiographic analysis. Am. Heart J. 100:34, 1980.

91. Schweizer, P., Bardos, P., Erbel, R., Meyer, J., Merx, W., Messmer, B. J., and Effert, S.: Detection of left atrial thrombi by echocardiography. Br. Heart J. 45:148, 1981.

92. Colman, T., de Ubago, J. L. M., and Figueroa, A.: Coronary arteriography and atrial thrombosis in mitral valve disease. Am. J. Cardiol. 47:973, 1981.

93. Beiser, G. D., Epstein, S. E., Stampfer, M., Robinson, B., and Braunwald, E.: Studies on digitalis. XVIII. Effects of ouabain on the hemodynamic response to exercise in patients with mitral stenosis in normal sinus rhythm. N. Engl. J. Med. 278:131, 1968.

94. Levine, H. J.: Which atrial fibrillation patients should be on chronic anticoagulation? J. Cardiovasc. Med. 6:483, 1981.

95. Kloster, F. E., and Morris, C. D.: Natural history of valvular heart disease. Circulation 65:1283, 1982.

96. Olesen, K. H.: The natural history of 271 patients with mitral stenosis under medical treatment. Br. Heart J. 24:349, 1962.

97. Rowe, J. C., Bland, E. F., Sprague, H. B., and White, P. D.: The course of mitral stenosis without surgery: Ten- and twenty-year perspectives. Ann. Intern. Med. 52:741, 1960.

98. Rapaport, E.: Natural history of aortic and mitral valve disease. Am. J. Cardiol. 35:221, 1975.

99. Sutton, M. J. St. J., Oldershaw, P., Sacchetti, R., Paneth, M., Lennox, S. C., Gibson, R. V., and Gibson, D. G.: Valve replacement without preoperative cardiac catheterization. N. Engl. J. Med. 305:1233, 1981.

100. Brandenburg, R. O.: No more routine catheterization for valvular heart disease? N. Engl. J. Med. 305:1277, 1981.

101. O'Rourke, R. A.: Preoperative cardiac catheterization. Its need in most patients with valvular heart disease. J.A.M.A. 248:745, 1982.

102. Chun, P. K. C., Gertz, E., Davia, J. E., and Cheitlin, M. D.: Coronary atherosclerosis in mitral stenosis. Chest 81:36, 1982.

103. Ramsdale, D. R., Faragher, E. B., Bennett, D. H., Bray, C. L., Ward, C., and Beton, D. C.: Preoperative prediction of significant coronary artery disease in patients with valvular heart disease. Br. Med. J. 284:223, 1982.

104. Cohn, L. H., and Collins, J. J., Jr.: Surgical treatment of mitral stenosis. A medical milestone. N. Engl. J. Med. 289:1035, 1973.

105. Gobel, F. L., Andrew, D. J., Witherspoon, J. M., Lillehei, R. C., Castaneda, A., and Wang, Y.: The hemodynamic results of instrumental and digital valvotomy in patients with mitral stenosis. Circulation 39:317, 1969.

106. Appelbaum, A., Kouchoukos, N. T., Blackstone, E. H., and Kirklin, J. W.: Early risks of open heart surgery for mitral valve disease. Am. J. Cardiol. 37:201, 1976.

107. Mullin, E. M., Jr., Glancy, D. L., Higgs, L. M., Epstein, S. E., and Morrow, A. G.: Current results of operation for mitral stenosis: Clinical and hemodynamic assessments in 124 consecutive patients treated by closed commissurotomy, open commissurotomy or valve replacement. Circulation 46:298, 1972.

108. Ellis, L. B., Harken, D. E., and Black, H.: A clinical study of 1,000 consecutive cases of mitral stenosis two to nine years after mitral valvuloplasty. Circulation 19:803, 1959.

109. Logan, A., and Turner, R.: Surgical treatment of mitral stenosis with particular reference to the transventricular approach with a mechanical dilator. Lancet 2:874, 1959.

110. Cohn, P. F.: Mitral valve surgery. Circulation 63:965, 1981.

111. Bryant, L. R., and Trinkle, J. K.: Mitral valvotomy in the valve replacement era. Ann. Surg. 173:1024, 1971.

112. Olinger, G. N., Rios, F. W., and Maloney, J. F., Jr.: Closed valvulotomy for calcific mitral stenosis. J. Thorac. Cardiovasc. Surg. 62:357, 1971.

113. Commerford, P. J., Hastie, T., and Beck, W.: Closed mitral valvotomy: Actuarial analysis of results in 654 patients over 12 years and analysis of preoperative predictors of long-term survival. Ann. Thorac. Surg. 33:473, 1982.

114. Dernevik, L., Brorsson, L., Wallentin, I., and William-Olsson, G.: Improved results of closed commissurotomy for mitral stenosis using ultrasonocardiography as selection ground. Acta Med. Scand. 210:283, 1981.

115. Gross, R. I., Cunningham, J. N., Jr., Snively, S. L., Catinella, F. P., Nathan, I. M., Adams, P. X., and Spencer, F. C.: Long-term results of open radical mitral commissurotomy: Ten year followup study of 202 patients. Am. J. Cardiol. 47:821, 1981.

116. Smith, W. M., Neutze, J. M., Barratt-Boyes, B. G., and Lowe, J. B.: Open mitral valvotomy. Effect of preoperative factors on result. J. Thorac. Cardiovasc. Surg. 82:738, 1981.

117. Aryanpur, I., Shakibi, J., Yazdanyar, A., Mehranpur, M., Paydar, M., Azar, H., Motlagh, F. A., Tarbiat, S., and Siassi, B.: Closed versus open mitral commissurotomy in children with rheumatic mitral stenosis. J. Thorac. Cardiovasc. Surg. 76:223, 1978.

118. Aora, R., Khalilullah, M., Gupta, M. P., and Padmavati, S.: Mitral restenosis. Incidence and epidemiology. Indian Heart J. 30:265, 1978.

119. Heger, J. J., Wann, L. S., Weyman, A. E., Dillon, J. C., and Feigenbaum, H.:

Long-term changes in mitral valve area after successful mitral commissurotomy. Circulation *59*:443, 1979.

120. Higgs, L. M., Glancy, D. L., O'Brien, K. P., Epstein, S. E., and Morrow, A. G.: Mitral restenosis: An uncommon cause of recurrent symptoms following mitral commissurotomy. Am. J. Cardiol. *26*:34, 1970.

121. Ward, C., and Hancock, B. W.: Extreme pulmonary hypertension caused by mitral valve disease. Natural history and results of surgery. Br. Heart J. *37*:74, 1975.

122. Braunwald, E., Braunwald, N. S., Ross, J., Jr., and Morrow, A. G.: Effects of mitral valve replacement on the pulmonary vascular dynamics of patients with pulmonary hypertension. N. Engl. J. Med. *273*:509, 1965.

123. Dalen, J. E., Matloff, J. M., Evans, G. L., Hoppin, F. G., Jr., Bhardwaj, P., Harken, D. E., and Dexter, L.: Early reduction of pulmonary vascular resistance after mitral valve replacement. N. Engl. J. Med. *277*:387, 1967.

124. Zener, J. C., Hancock, E. W., Shumway, N. E., and Harrison, D. C.: Regression of extreme pulmonary hypertension after mitral valve surgery. Am. J. Cardiol. *30*:820, 1972.

MITRAL REGURGITATION

125. Silverman, M. E., and Hurst, J. W.: The mitral complex: Clues to its afflictions. *In* Likoff, W. (ed.): Cardiovascular Clinics. Vol. 5, No. 2, Valvular Heart Disease. Philadelphia, F. A. Davis, 1973, p. 36.

126. Roberts, W. C., Dangel, J. C., and Bulkley, B. H.: Nonrheumatic valvular cardiac disease: A clinicopathologic survey of 27 different conditions causing valvular dysfunction. *In* Likoff, W. (ed.): Cardiovascular Clinics. Vol. 5, No. 2, Valvular Heart Disease. Philadelphia, F. A. Davis, 1973, p. 334.

127. Perloff, J. D., and Roberts, W. C.: The mitral apparatus. Functional anatomy of mitral regurgitation. Circulation *46*:227, 1972.

128. Davies, M. J.: Pathology of Cardiac Valves. London, Butterworths, 1980.

129. Bloor, C. M.: Valvular heart disease in the elderly. J. Am. Geriatr. Soc. *30* :466, 1982.

130. Korn, D., DeSanctis, R. W., and Sell, S.: Massive calcification of the mitral annulus. N. Engl. J. Med. *267*:900, 1962.

131. Wanderman, K. L., and Margulis, G.: Coexistence of hypertrophic obstructive cardiomyopathy and mitral annular calcification: Proposed etiologic relationship. Isr. J. Med. Sci. *15*:422, 1979.

132. DePace, N. L., Rohrer, A. H., Kotler, M. N., Brezin, J. H., and Parry, W. R.: Rapidly progressive, massive mitral annular calcification. Occurrence in a patient with chronic renal failure. Arch. Intern. Med. *141*:166, 1981.

133. Papa, L. A., Raniolo, J., and Schiff, S.: Mitral anular calcification: Clinical and echocardiographic findings. J.A.O.A. *81*:471, 1982.

134. Zanolla, L., Marino, P., Nicolosi, G. L., Peranzoni, P. F., and Poppi, A.: Two-dimensional echocardiographic evaluation of mitral valve calcification. Sensitivity and specificity. Chest *82*:154, 1982.

135. Mellino, M., Salcedo, E. E., Lever, H. M., Vasudevan, G., and Kramer, J. R.: Echographic-quantified severity of mitral anulus calcification: Prognostic correlation to related hemodynamic, valvular, rhythm, and conduction abnormalities. Am. Heart J. *103*:222, 1982.

136. Kronzon, I., Mitchell, J., Shapiro, J., Winer, H. E., and Newman, P.: Two-dimensional echocardiography in mitral annulus calcification. Am. J. Roentgenog. *134*:355, 1980.

137. Scott-Jupp, W., Barnett, N. L., Gallagher, P. J., Monro, J. L., and Ross, J. K.: Ultrastructural changes in spontaneous rupture of mitral chordae tendineae. J. Pathol. *133*:185, 1981.

138. Selzer, A., Kelly, J. J., Jr., Vannitamby, M., Walker, P., Gerbode, F., and Kerth, W. J.: The syndrome of mitral insufficiency due to isolated rupture of the chordae tendineae. Am. J. Med. *43*:822, 1967.

139. Luther, R. R., and Meyers, S. N.: Acute mitral insufficiency secondary to ruptured chordae tendineae. Arch. Intern. Med. *134*:568, 1974.

140. Caulfield, J. B., Page, D. L., Kastor, J. A., and Sanders, C. A.: Dissolution of connective tissue in ruptured chordae tendineae. Circulation *40*:57, 1969.

141. Godley, R. W., Wann, L. S., Rogers, E. W., Feigenbaum, H., and Weyman, A. E.: Incomplete mitral leaflet closure in patients with papillary muscle dysfunction. Circulation *63*:565, 1981.

142. Gallagher, P. J., Caves, P. K., and Stinson, E. B.: Pathological changes in spontaneous rupture of chordae tendineae. Ann. Cir. Gynaecol. *66*:135, 1977.

143. Burch, G. E., DePasquale, N. P., and Phillips, J. H.: The syndrome of papillary muscle dysfunction. Am. Heart J. *75*:399, 1968.

144. Estes, E. H., Jr., Dalton, F. M., Entman, M. L., et al.: The anatomy and blood supply of the papillary muscle of the left ventricle. Am. Heart J. *71*:356, 1966.

145. Gahl, K., Sutton, R., Pearson, M., Caspari, P., Lairet, A., and McDonald, L.: Mitral regurgitation in coronary heart disease. Br. Heart J. *39*:13, 1977.

146. Becker, A. E., and Anderson, R. H.: Mitral insufficiency complicating acute myocardial infarction. Eur. J. Cardiol. *2*:351, 1975.

147. Morrow, A. G., Cohen, L. S., Roberts, W. C., Braunwald, N. S., and Braunwald, E.: Severe mitral regurgitation following acute myocardial infarction and ruptured papillary muscle. Hemodynamic findings and results of operative treatment in four patients. Circulation *37*(Suppl. II):124, 1968.

148. Bulkley, B. H., and Roberts, W. C.: Dilatation of the mitral annulus. Am. J. Med. *59*:457, 1975.

149. Balu, V., Hershowitz, S., Masud, A. R. Z., Bhayana, J. N., and Dean, D. C.: Mitral regurgitation in coronary artery disease. Chest *81*:550, 1982.

150. Eckberg, D. L., Gault, J. H., Bouchard, R. L., Karliner, J. S., and Ross, J., Jr.: Mechanics of left ventricular contraction in chronic severe mitral regurgitation. Circulation *47*:1252, 1973.

151. Braunwald, E., Welch, G. H., Jr., and Sarnoff, S. J.: Hemodynamic effects of quantitatively varied experimental mitral regurgitation. Circ. Res. *5*:539, 1957.

152. Selzer, A., and Katayama, F.: Mitral regurgitation: Clinical patterns, pathophysiology and natural history. Medicine (Baltimore) *51*:337, 1972.

153. Pierpont, G. L., and Talley, R. C.: Pathophysiology of valvar heart disease. Arch. Intern. Med. *142*:998, 1982.

154. Yellin, E. L., Yoran, C., Sonnenblick, E. H., Gabbay, S., and Frater, R. W. M.: Dynamic changes in the canine mitral regurgitant orifice area during ventricular ejection. Circ. Res. *45*:677, 1979.

155. Yoran, C., Yellin, E. L., Becker, R. M., Gabbay, S., Frater, R. W. M., and Sonnenblick, E. H.: Dynamic aspects of acute mitral regurgitation: Effects of ventricular volume, pressure and contractility on the effective regurgitant orifice area. Circulation *60*:170, 1979.

156. Urschel, C. W., Covell, J. W., Sonnenblick, E. H., Ross, J., Jr., and Braunwald, E.: Myocardial mechanics in aortic and mitral valvular regurgitation: The concept of instantaneous impedance as a determinant of the performance of the intact heart. J. Clin. Invest. *47*:867, 1968.

157. Braunwald, E.: Mitral regurgitation: Physiological, clinical and surgical considerations. N. Engl. J. Med. *281*:425, 1969.

158. Urschel, C. W., Covell, J. W., Graham, T. P., Clancy, R. L., Ross, J., Jr., Sonnenblick, E. H., and Braunwald, E.: Effects of acute valvular regurgitation on the oxygen consumption of the canine heart. Circ. Res. *23*:33, 1968.

159. Braunwald, E.: Control of myocardial oxygen consumption: Physiologic and clinical considerations. Am. J. Cardiol. *27*:416, 1971.

160. Sasayama, S., Takahashi, M., Osakada, G., Hirose, K., Hamashima, H., Nishimura, E., and Kawai, C.: Dynamic geometry of the left atrium and left ventricle in acute mitral regurgitation. Circulation *60*:177, 1979.

161. Ross, J., Jr.: Left ventricular function and the timing of surgical treatment in valvular heart disease. Ann. Intern. Med. *94*:498, 1981.

162. Ronan, J. A., Jr., Steelman, R. B., DeLeon, A. C., Jr., Waters, T. J., Perloff, J. K., and Harvey, W. P.: The clinical diagnosis of acute severe mitral insufficiency. Am. J. Cardiol. *27*:284, 1971.

163. Vokonas, P. S., Gorlin, R., Cohn, P. F., Herman, M. V., and Sonnenblick, E. H.: Dynamic geometry of the left ventricle in mitral regurgitation. Circulation *48*:786, 1973.

164. Osbakken, M. D., Bove, A. A., and Spann, J. F.: Left ventricular regional wall motion and velocity of shortening in chronic mitral and aortic regurgitation. Am. J. Cardiol. *47*:1055, 1981.

165. Wong, C. Y. H., and Spotnitz, H. M.: Systolic and diastolic properties of the human left ventricle during valve replacement for chronic mitral regurgitation. Am. J. Cardiol. *47*:40, 1981.

166. Borow, K., Green, L. H., Mann, T., Sloss, L. J., Braunwald, E., Collins, J. J., Cohn, L., and Grossman, W.: End-systolic volume as a predictor of postoperative left ventricular performance in volume overload from valvular regurgitation. Am. J. Med. *68*:655, 1980.

167. Boucher, C. A., Bingham, J. B., Osbakken, M. D., Okada, R. D., Strauss, W. H., Block, P. C., Levine, F. H., Phillips, H. R., and Pohost, G. M.: Early changes in left ventricular size and function after correction of left ventricular volume overload. Am. J. Cardiol. *47*:991, 1981.

167a.Zile, M. R., Gaasch, W. H., Carroll, J. D., and Levine, H. J.: Chronic mitral regurgitation: Predictive value of preoperative echocardiographic indices of LV function and wall stress. J. Am. Coll. Cardiol. *1*:625, 1983 (Abstr.).

168. Peterson, C. R., Herr, R., Crisera, R. V., Starr, A., Bristow, D., and Griswold, H. E.: The failure of hemodynamic improvement after valve replacement surgery. Ann. Intern. Med. *66*:1, 1967.

169. Barnhorst, D. A., Oxman, H. A., Connolly, D. C., Pluth, J. R., Danielson, G. K., Wallace, R. B., and McGoon, D. C.: Long-term followup of isolated replacement of the aortic or mitral valve with the Starr-Edwards prosthesis. Am. J. Cardiol. *35*:228, 1975.

170. Konstam, M. A., Wynne, J., Holman, B. L., Brown, E. J., Neil, J. M., and Kozlowski, J.: Use of equilibrium (gated) radionuclide ventriculography to quantitate left ventricular output in patients with and without left-sided valvular regurgitation. Circulation *64*:578, 1981.

171. Braunwald, E., and Awe, W. C.: The syndrome of severe mitral regurgitation with normal left atrial pressure. Circulation *27*:29, 1963.

172. Roberts, W. C., Braunwald, E., and Morrow, A. G.: Acute severe mitral regurgitation secondary to ruptured chordae tendineae. Clinical, hemodynamic and pathologic considerations. Circulation *33*:58, 1966.

173. Cohen, L. S., Mason, D. T., and Braunwald, E.: Significance of an atrial gallop sound in mitral regurgitation: A clue to the diagnosis of ruptured chordae tendineae. Circulation *35*:112, 1966.

174. Kennedy, J. W., Baxley, W., and Dodge, H. T.: Hemodynamics of acute ruptured chordae tendineae. Circulation *34*:142, 1966.

175. Fowler, N. O.: Cardiac Diagnosis and Treatment. Hagerstown, Md., Harper and Row, 1980, pp. 541–546.

176. Allen, H., Harris, A., and Leatham, A.: Significance and prognosis of an isolated late systolic murmur. Br. Heart J. *36*:525, 1974.

177. Leatham, A., and Brigden, W.: Mild mitral regurgitation and the mitral prolapse fiasco. Am. Heart J. *99*:659, 1980.

178. Hammermeister, K. E., Fisher, L., Kennedy, J. W., Samuels, S., and Dodge, H. T.: Prediction of late survival in patients with mitral valve disease from clinical, hemodynamic, and quantitative angiographic variables. Circulation *57*:341, 1978.

179. Elkins, R. C., Morrow, A. G., Vasko, J. S., and Braunwald, E.: The effects of mitral regurgitation on the pattern of instantaneous aortic blood flow. Clinical and experimental observations. Circulation 36:45, 1967.

180. Basta, L. L., Wolfson, P., Eckberg, D. L., and Abboud, F. M.: The value of left parasternal impulse recordings in the assessment of mitral regurgitation. Circulation 48:1055, 1973.

181. Perloff, J. K., and Harvey, W. P.: Auscultatory and phonocardiographic manifestations of pure mitral regurgitation. Prog. Cardiovasc. Dis. 5:172, 1962.

182. Karliner, J. S., O'Rourke, R. A., Kearney, D. J., and Shabetai, R.: Haemodynamic explanation of why the murmur of mitral regurgitation is independent of cycle length. Br. Heart J. 35:397, 1973.

183. Aravanis, C.: Silent mitral insufficiency. Am. Heart J. 70:620, 1965.

184. Dusall, J. C., Pryor, R., and Blount, S. G.: Systolic murmur following myocardial infarction. Am. Heart J. 87:577, 1974.

185. Antman, E. M., Angoff, G. H., and Sloss, J. J.: Demonstration of the mechanism by which mitral regurgitation mimics aortic stenosis. Am. J. Cardiol. 42:1044, 1978.

186. Merendino, K. A., and Hessel, E. A.: The murmur on top of the head in acquired mitral insufficiency. J.A.M.A. 199:392, 1967.

187. Perloff, J. K.: Combined mitral stenosis and regurgitation: An auscultatory evaluation of their relative significance. In Segal, B., and Likoff, W. S. (eds.): The Theory and Practice of Auscultation. Philadelphia, F. A. Davis, 1964, p. 448.

188. Bentoviglio, L. G., Uricchio, J. F., Waldow, A., Likoff, W., and Goldberg, H.: An electrocardiographic analysis of mitral regurgitation. Circulation 18:572, 1956.

189. Morris, J. J., Estes, E. H., Whalen, R. E., Thompson, H. K., and McIntosh, H. D.: P wave analysis in valvular heart disease. Circulation 29:242, 1964.

190. Hamer, J.: The vectorcardiogram in mitral valve disease. Br. Heart J. 32:149, 1970.

191. Priest, E. A., Finlayson, J. K., and Short, D. S.: The x-ray manifestations in the heart and lungs of mitral regurgitation. Prog. Cardiovasc. Dis. 5:219, 1962.

192. Wexler, L., Silverman, J. F., DeBusk, R. F., and Harrison, D. C.: Angiographic features of rheumatic and nonrheumatic mitral regurgitation. Circulation 44:1080, 1971.

193. Mourant, A. J., Weaver, J., and Johnston, K.: Echocardiographic findings in rheumatic mitral valve disease with chordal rupture. J. Clin. Ultrasound 10:79, 1982.

194. Kotler, M. N., Mintz, G. S., Parry, W. R., and Segal, B. L.: M-mode and two-dimensional echocardiography in mitral and aortic regurgitation: Pre- and postoperative evaluation of volume overload of the left ventricle. Am. J. Cardiol. 46:1144, 1980.

195. Burgess, J., Clark, R., and Kamigaki, M.: Echocardiographic findings in different types of mitral regurgitation. Circulation 48:97, 1973.

196. Sweatman, T., Selzer, A., Kamageki, M., and Cohn, K.: Echocardiographic diagnosis of mitral regurgitation due to ruptured chordae tendineae. Circulation 46:580, 1972.

196a. Nair, C. K., Aronow, W. S., Sketch, M. H., Mohiuddin, S. M., Pagano, T., Esterbrooks, D. J., and Hee, T. T.: Clinicial and echocardiographic characteristics of patients with mitral annular clacification. Am. J. Cardiol. 51:992, 1983.

197. Wann, L. S., Feigenbaum, H., Weyman, A. E., and Dillon, J. C.: Cross-sectional echocardiographic detection of rheumatic mitral regurgitation. Am. J. Cardiol. 41:1258, 1978.

198. Child, J. S., Skorton, D. J., Taylor, R. D., Krivokapich, J., Abbasi, A. S., Wong, M., and Shah, P. D.: M-mode and cross-sectional echocardiographic features of flail posterior mitral leaflets. Am. J. Cardiol. 44:1383, 1979.

199. Mintz, G. S., Kotler, M. N., Segal, B. L., and Parry, W. R.: Two-dimensional echocardiographic recognition of ruptured chordae tendineae. Circulation 57:244, 1978.

200. Abbasi, A. S., Allen, M. W., DeCristofaro, D., and Ungar, I.: Detection and estimation of the degree of mitral regurgitation by range-gated pulsed Doppler echocardiography. Circulation 61:143, 1980.

201. Pearlman, A. S.: Assessing valvular regurgitation by pulsed Doppler echocardiography. J Cardiovasc. Med. 6:251, 1981.

201a. Patel, A. K., Rowe, G. G., Thomsen, J. H., Dhanani, S. P., Kosolcharoen, P. and Lyle, L.E.W.: Detection and estimation of rheumatic mitral regurgitation in the presence of mitral stenosis by pulsed Doppler echocardiography. Am. J. Cardiol. 51:986, 1983.

202. Thompson, R., Ross, I., and Elmes, R.: Quantification of valvular regurgitation by cardiac gated pool imaging. Br. Heart J. 46:629, 1981.

203. Boucher, C. A., Okada, R. D., and Pohost, G. M.: Current status of radionuclide imaging in valvular heart disease. Am. J. Cardiol. 46:1153, 1980.

204. Greenberg, B. H., Massie, B. M., Brundage, B. H., Botvinick, E. H., Parmley, W. W., and Chatterjee, K.: Beneficial effects of hydralazine in severe mitral regurgitation. Circulation 58:273, 1978.

205. Yoran, C., Yellin, E. L., Becker, R. M., Gabbay, S., Frater, R. W. M., and Sonnenblick, E. H.: Mechanism of reduction of mitral regurgitation with vasodilator therapy. Am. J. Cardiol. 43:773, 1979.

206. Chopra, P. S., Rowe, G. G., Young, W. P., Loring, L. L., Hamann, R. C., and Kahn, D. R.: Carpentier ring annuloplasty in severe noncalcific mitral insufficiency. Arch. Surg. 112:1469, 1977.

207. Kay, J. H., Zubiate, P., Mendez, M. A., Vanstrom, N., and Yokoyama, T.: Mitral valve repair for significant mitral insufficiency. Am. Heart J. 96:253, 1978.

208. Spencer, F. C.: Acquired heart disease. In Schwartz, S. I., Shires, G. T., Spencer, F. C., and Storer, E. H. (eds.): Principles of Surgery. 2nd ed. New York, McGraw-Hill Book Co., 1979, p. 813.

209. Kay, J. H., Zubiate, P., Mendez, M. A., Vanstrom, N., Yokoyama, T., and Gharavi, M. A.: Surgical treatment of mitral insufficiency secondary to coronary artery disease. J. Thorac. Cardiovasc. Surg. 79:12, 1980.

209a. Radley-Smith, R., and Yacoub, M. H.: Evaluation of long term results of valve conserving operations for severe mitral regurgitation in children. J. Am. Coll. Cardio. 1:587, 1983 (Abstr.).

210. Dalby, A. J., Firth, B. G., and Forman, R.: Preoperative factors affecting the outcome of isolated mitral valve replacement: A 10 year review. Am. J. Cardiol. 47:826, 1981.

211. Cohn, L. H., Mudge, G. H., Pratter, F., and Collins, J. J., Jr.: Five- to eight-year followup of patients undergoing porcine heart-valve replacement. N. Engl. J. Med. 304:258, 1981.

212. Bonchek, L. I.: Current status of cardiac valve replacement: Selection of a prosthesis and indications for operation. Am. Heart J. 101:96, 1981.

213. Phillips, H. R., Levine, F. H., Carter, J. E., Boucher, C. A., Osbakken, M. D., Okada, R. D., Akins, C. W., Daggett, W. M., Buckley, M. J., and Pohost, G. M.: Mitral valve replacement for isolated mitral regurgitation: Analysis of clinical course and late postoperative left ventricular ejection fraction. Am. J. Cardiol. 48:647, 1981.

214. Jamieson, W. R. E., Thompson, D. M., and Munro, A. I.: Cardiac valve replacement in elderly patients. Can. Med. Assoc. J. 123:628, 1980.

215. Cohn, L. H., Koster, J. K., VandeVanter, S., and Collins, J. J.: The in-hospital risk of rereplacement of dysfunctional mitral and aortic valves. Circulation 66 (Suppl. I):I-153, 1982.

216. Levitsky, S., Mammana, R. B., Silverman, N. A., Weber, F., Hiro, S., and Wright, R. N.: Acute endocarditis in drug addicts: Surgical treatment for gram-negative sepsis. Circulation 66(Suppl. I):I-135, 1982.

217. Dinubile, M. J.: Surgery in active endocarditis. Ann. Intern. Med. 96:650, 1982.

218. Schuler, G., Peterson, K. L., Johnson, A., Francis, G., Dennish, G., Utley, J. R., Dailey, P. O., Ashburn, W., and Ross, J., Jr.: Temporal response of left ventricular performance to mitral valve surgery. Circulation 59:1218, 1979.

219. Gann, D., Colin, C., Hildner, F. J., Samet, P., Yahr, W. Z., Byrd, C., and Greenberg, J. J.: Mitral valve replacement in medically unresponsive congestive heart failure due to papillary muscle dysfunction. Circulation 56(Suppl. II):101, 1977.

220. Fowler, N. O., and VanDerBel-Kahn, J. M.: Indications for surgical replacement of the mitral valve. With particular reference to common and uncommon causes of mitral regurgitation. Am. J. Cardiol. 44:148, 1979.

221. Harken, D. E., Soroff, M. S., and Taylor, M. C.: Partial and complete prostheses in aortic insufficiency. J. Thorac. Cardiovasc. Surg. 40:744, 1960.

222. Starr, A., and Edwards, M. L.: Mitral replacement: Clinical experience with a ball-valve prosthesis. Ann. Surg. 154:726, 1961.

223. Teply, J. F., Grunkemeier, G. L., Sutherland, H. D'A., Lambert, L. E., Johnson, V. A., and Starr, A.: The ultimate prognosis after valve replacement: An assessment at twenty years. Ann. Thorac. Surg. 32:111, 1981.

224. Fuster, V., Pumphrey, C. W., McGoon, M. D., Chesebro, J. H., Pluth, J. R., and McGoon, D. C.: Systemic thromboembolism in mitral and aortic Starr-Edwards prostheses: A 10- to 19-year followup. Circulation 66(Suppl. I):I-157, 1982.

225. Björk, V. O.: A new tilting disc valve prosthesis. Scand. J. Thorac. Cardiovasc. Surg. 3:1, 1969.

226. Zwart, H. H. J., Hicks, G., Schuster, B., Nathan, M., Tabrah, F., Wenzke, F., Ahmed, T., and DeWall, R. A.: Clinical experience with the Lillehei-Kaster valve prosthesis. Ann. Thorac. Surg. 28:158, 1979.

227. Nicoloff, D. M., Emery, R. W., Arom, K. V., Northrup, W. F., Jorgensen, C. R., Wang, Y., and Lindsay, W. G.: Clinical and hemodynamic results with the St. Jude medical cardiac valve prosthesis. A three-year experience. J. Thorac. Cardiovasc. Surg. 82:674, 1981.

228. Copans, H., Lakier, J. B., Kinsley, R. H., Colsen, P. R., Fritz, V. U., and Barlow, J. B.: Thrombosed Björk-Shiley mitral prostheses. Circulation 61:169, 1980.

229. Edmunds, L. H., Jr.: Thromboembolic complications of current cardiac valvular prostheses. Ann. Thorac. Surg. 34:96, 1981.

229a. Shattel, L.F.B.: The prevention of prosthetic valve thromboembolism. Uses and limitations of anti-platelet drugs. Int. J. Cardiol. 3:87, 1983.

230. Ionescu, M. I.: Tissue Heart Valves. London, Butterworths, 1979.

231. Ross, D. N.: Homograft replacement of the aortic valve. Lancet 2:487, 1962.

232. Barrett-Boyes, B. G., Roche, A. H. G., and Whitlock, R. M. L.: Six-year review of results of freehand aortic valve replacement using an antibiotic sterilized homograft valve. Circulation 55:353, 1977.

233. Buch, S., Kosek, J. C., and Angell, W. W.: Deterioration of formalin-treated aortic heterografts. J. Thorac. Cardiovasc. Surg. 69:673, 1970.

234. Carpentier, A., Lemaigre, G., and Robert, L.: Biological factors affecting long-term results of valvular heterografts. J. Thorac. Cardiovasc. Surg. 58:467,1969.

235. Reis, R. L., Hancock, W. D., Yarbrough, J. W., et al.: The flexible stent: A new concept in the fabrication of tissue heart valve prostheses. J. Thorac. Cardiovasc. Surg. 62:683, 1971.

236. Ionescu, M. I., Tandon, A. P., Mary, D. A. S., et al.: Heart valve replacement with the Ionescu-Shiley pericardial xenograft. J. Thorac. Cardiovasc. Surg. 73:31, 1977.

237. Becker, R. M., Sandor, L., Tindel, M., and Frater, R. W. M.: Medium-term followup of the Ionescu-Shiley heterograft valve. Ann. Thorac. Surg. 32:120, 1981.

238. Silverton, N. P., Tandon, A. P., and Ionescu, M. I.: Mitral valve replacement without long term anticoagulation using the Ionescu-Shiley pericardial xenograft. J. Am. Coll. Cardiol. 1:700, 1983.

239. Puig, L. B., Verginelli, G., Iryia, K., et al.: Homologous dura mater cardiac valves. J. Thorac Cardiovasc. Surg. 69:722, 1975.

240. Reitz, B. A., Stinson, E. B., Griepp, R. B., and Shumway, N. E.: Tissue valve replacement of prosthetic heart valves with thromboembolism. Am. J. Cardiol. 41:512, 1978.

241. Cevese, P. G., Gallucci, V., Morea, M., Volta, S. D., Fasoli, G., and Casarotto, D.: Heart valve replacement with the Hancock Bioprosthesis. Analysis of long-term results. Circulation 56(Suppl. II):111, 1976.

242. Oyer, P. E., Stinson, E. B., Reitz, B. A., Miller, D. C., Rossiter, S. J., and Shumway, N. E.: Long-term evaluation of the porcine xenograft bioprosthesis. J. Thorac. Cardiovasc. Surg. 78:343, 1979.

243. DiSesa, V. J., Collins, J. J., Jr., and Cohn, L. H.: Mitral valve replacement with the porcine bioprosthesis. In Ionescu, M. I., and Cohn, L. H. (eds.): The Mitral Valve. London, Butterworths, 1983 (in press).

244. Angell, W. W., Angell, J. D., Sywak, A., and Kosek, J. C.: The tissue valve as a superior cardiac valve replacement. Surgery 82:875, 1977.

244a. Janusz, M. T., Jamieson, W. R. E., Burr, L. H., Miyagishima, R. T., and Tyers, F. O.: Thromboembolic risks and role of anticoagulants in patients in chronic atrial fibrillation following mitral valve replacement with porcine bioprostheses. J. Am. Coll. Cardiol. 1:587, 1983.

245. Hetzer, R., Hill, J. D., Kerth, W. J., Ansbro, J., Adappa, M. G., Rodvien, R., Kamm, B., and Gerbode, F.: Thromboembolic complications after mitral valve replacement with Hancock xenograft. J. Thorac. Cardiovasc. Surg. 75:651, 1978.

246. Ubago, J. L., Figueroa, A., Colman, T., Ochoteco, A., and Duran, C. G.: Hemodynamic factors that affect calculated orifice areas in the mitral Hancock xenograft valve. Circulation 61:388, 1980.

247. Rahimtoola, S.: The problem of valve prosthesis—patient mismatch. Circulation 58:20, 1978.

248. Holen, J., H ie, J., and Semb, B.: Obstructive characteristics of Björk-Shiley, Hancock, and Lillehei-Kaster prosthetic mitral valves in the immediate postoperative period. Acta Med. Scand. 204:5, 1978.

249. Hannah, H., and Reis, R. L.: Current status of porcine heterograft prostheses. Circulation 54(Suppl. III):27, 1976.

250. Luri, A. J., Miller, R. R., Maxwell, K. S., Grehl, T. M., Vismara, L. A., Hurley, E. J., and Mason, D. T.: Hemodynamic assessment of the glutaraldehyde-preserved porcine heterograft in the aortic and mitral positions. Circulation 56 (Suppl. II):104, 1977.

251. Roberts, W. C.: Complications of cardiac valve replacement: Characteristic abnormalities of prostheses pertaining to any specific site. Am. Heart J. 103:113, 1982.

252. Kirklin, J. W.: The replacement of cardiac valves. N. Engl. J. Med. 304:291, 1981.

252a. Schoen, F. J., Collins, J. J., Jr., and Cohn, L. W.: Long-term failure rate and morphologic correlations in porcine bioprosthetic heart valves. Am. J. Cardiol. 51:957, 1983.

253. Miller, D. C., Stinson, E. B., Oyer, P. E., Billingham, M. E., Pitlick, P. T., Reitz, B. A., Jamieson, S. W., Baumgartner, W. A., and Shumway, N. E.: The durability of porcine xenograft valves and conduits in children. Circulation 66 (Suppl. I): I–172, 1982.

254. Attie, F., Kuri, J., Zanoniani, C., Renteria, V., Buendia, A., Ovseyevitz, J., Lopez-Soriano, F., Garcia-Cornejo, M., and Martinez-Rios, M. A.: Mitral valve replacement in children with rheumatic heart disease. Circulation 64:812, 1981.

255. Taguchi, K.: Pregnancy in patients with a prosthetic heart valve. Surg. Gynecol. Obstet. 145:206, 1977. Managing pregnant patients with a heart valve prosthesis. Contemp. Ob. Gyn. 11:82, 1978.

256. Harrison, E. C., Roschke, J., Ferenczi, G., and Mitani, G. H.: Managing Pregnant Patients with a heart valve prosthesis. Contemp. Obstet. Gynecol. 11:82, 1978.

257. Oakley, C., and Doherty, P.: Pregnancy in patients after valve replacement. Br. Heart J. 38:1140, 1976.

258. Limet, R., and Grondin, C. M.: Cardiac valve prostheses, anticoagulation and pregnancy. Ann. Thorac. Surg. 23:337, 1977.

259. Spray, T. L., and Roberts, W. C.: Structural changes in porcine xenografts used as substitute cardiac valves. Gross and histologic observations in 51 glutaraldehyde-preserved Hancock valves in 41 patients. Am. J. Cardiol. 40:319, 1977.

260. Fishbein, M. C., Gissen, S. A., Collins, J. J., Jr., Barsamian, E. M., and Cohn, L. H.: Pathologic findings after cardiac valve replacement with glutaraldehyde-fixed porcine valves. Am. J. Cardiol. 40:331, 1977.

261. Rose, A. G., Forman, R., and Bowen, R. M.: Calcification of glutaraldehyde-fixed porcine xenograft. Thorax 33:111, 1978.

262. Thandroyen et al.: Severe calcification of glutaraldehyde preserved porcine xenografts. Am. J. Cardiol. 45:1980.

263. Smith, N. D., Raizada, V., and Abrams, J.: Auscultation of the normally functioning prosthetic valve. Ann. Intern. Med. 95:594, 1981.

264. Cunha, C. L. P., Giuliani, E. R., Callahan, J. A., and Pluth, J. R.: Echophonocardiographic findings in patients with prosthetic heart valve malfunction. Mayo Clin. Proc. 55:231, 1980.

265. Stein, P. D., Sabbah, H. N., Lakier, J. B., Magilligan, D. J., Jr., and Goldstein, S.: Frequency of the first heart sound in the assessment of stiffening of mitral bioprosthetic valves. Circulation 63:200, 1981.

266. Morris, D. C.: Management of patients with prosthetic heart valves. Curr. Probl. Cardiol. 7: Aug., 1982.

267. Griffiths, B. E., Charles, R., and Coulshed, N.: Echophonocardiography in diagnosis of mitral paravalvular regurgitation with Bjork-Shiley prosthetic valve. Br. Heart J. 43:325, 1980.

268. Schapira, J. N., Martin, R. P., Fowles, R. E., Rakowski, H., Stinson, E. B., French, J. W., Shumway, N. E., and Popp, R. O.: Two-dimensional echocardiographic assessment of patients with bioprosthetic valves. Am. J. Cardiol. 43:510, 1979.

269. Alam, M., Madrazo, A. C., Magilligan, D. J., and Goldstein, S.: M-mode and two dimensional echocardiographic features of porcine valve dysfunction. Am. J. Cardiol. 43:502, 1979.

MITRAL VALVE PROLAPSE

270. Cheitlin, M. D.: Mitral valve prolapse. Circulation 59:610, 1979.

271. Abrams, J.: Mitral valve prolapse: A plea for unanimity. Am. Heart J. 92:413, 1976.

272. Barlow, J. B., and Pocock, W. A.: Mitral valve prolapse, the specific billowing mitral leaflet syndrome, or an insignificant non-ejection systolic click. Am. Heart J. 97:277, 1979.

273. Lucas, R. V., and Edwards, J. E.: The floppy mitral valve. Curr. Probl. Cardiol. 7: July, 1982.

274. Jeresaty, R. M.: Mitral Valve Prolapse. New York, Raven Press, 1979, 251 pp.

274a. Chesler, E., King, R. A., and Edwards, J. E.: The myxomatous mitral valve and sudden death. Circulation 67:632, 1983.

275. Devereaux, R. B., Perloff, J. K., Reichek, N., and Josephson, M. D.: Mitral valve prolapse. Circulation 54:3, 1976.

276. Procacci, P. M., Savran, S. V., Schreiter, S. L., and Bryson, A. L.: Prevalence of clinical mitral valve prolapse in 1,169 young women. N. Engl. J. Med. 294:1086, 1976.

277. Markiewicz, W., Stoner, J., London, E., Hunt, S. A., and Popp, R. L.: Mitral valve prolapse in one hundred presumably healthy young females. Circulation 53:464, 1976.

278. Reid, J. V.: Mid-systolic clicks. S. Afr. Med. J. 35:353, 1961.

279. Barlow, J. B., and Pocock, W. A., Marchand, P., and Denny, M.: The significance of the late systolic murmurs. Am. Heart J. 66:443, 1963.

280. Olsen, E. G. J., and Al-Rufaie, H. K.: The floppy mitral valve. Study on pathogenesis. Br. Heart J. 44:674, 1980.

280a. Pyeritz, R. E., and Wappel, M. A.: Mitral valve dysfunction in the Marfan syndrome. Am. J. Med. 74:797, 1983.

281. Davies, M. J., Moore, B. P., and Braimbridge, M. V.: The floppy mitral valve. Study of incidence, pathology and complications in surgical, necropsy and forensic material. Br. Heart J. 40:368, 1978.

282. Jaffe, A. S., Geltman, E. M., Rodey, G. E., and Uitto, J.: Mitral valve prolapse: A consistent manifestation of Type IV Ehlers-Danlos syndrome. The pathogenetic role of the abnormal production of Type III collagen. Circulation 64:121, 1981.

283. King, B. D., Clark, M. A., Baba, N., Kilman, J. W., and Wooley, C. F.: "Myxomatous" mitral valves: Collagen dissolution as the primary defect. Circulation 66:288, 1982.

284. Hammer, D., Leier, C. V., Baba, N., Vasko, J. S., Wooley, C. F., and Pinnell, S. R.: Altered collagen composition in a prolapsing mitral valve with ruptured chordae tendineae. Am. J. Med. 67:863, 1979.

285. Gravanis, M. B., and Campbell, W. G., Jr.: The syndrome of prolapse of the mitral valve. Arch. Pathol. Lab. Med. 106:369, 1982.

286. Child, J. S., Cabeen, W. R., Jr., and Roberts, N. K.: Mitral valve prolapse complicated by ruptured chordae tendineae. West. J. Med. 129:160, 1978.

287. Malcolm, A. D., Chayen, J., Cankovic-Darracott, S., Jenkins, B. S., and Webb-Peploe, M. M.: Biopsy evidence of left ventricular myocardial abnormality in patients with mitral leaflet prolapse and chest pain. Lancet 1:1052, 1979.

288. Malcolm, A. D.: Myocardial mysteries surrounding mitral leaflet prolapse. Am. Heart J. 100:265, 1980.

289. Rizzon, P., Biasco, G., Brindicei, G., and Mauro, F.: Familial syndrome of midsystolic click and late systolic murmur. Br. Heart J. 35:245, 1973.

290. O'Rourke, R. A., and Crawford, M. H.: The systolic click-murmur syndrome: Clinical recognition and management. Curr. Probl. Cardiol. 1:1–60, 1976.

291. Cabeen, W. R., Jr., Reza, M. J., Kovick, R. B., and Stern, M. S.: Mitral valve prolapse and conduction defects in Ehlers-Danlos syndrome. Arch. Intern. Med. 137:1227, 1977.

292. Lebwohl, M. G., Distefano, D., Prioleau, P. G., Uram, M., Yannuzzi, L. A., and Fleischmajer, R.: Pseudoxanthoma elasticum and mitral valve prolapse. N. Engl. J. Med. 307:228, 1982.

293. Strasberg, B., Kanakis, C., Dhingra, R. C., and Rosen, K. M.: Myotonia dystrophica and mitral valve prolapse. Chest 78:845, 1980.

294. Sanyal, S. K., Johnson, W. W., Dische, M. R., Pitner, S. E., and Beard, C.: Dystrophic degeneration of papillary muscle and ventricular myocardium. A basic for mitral valve prolapse in Duchenne's muscular dystrophy. Circulation 62:430, 1980.

295. Mason, J. W., Koch, F. H., Billingham, M. E., and Winkle, R. A.: Cardiac biopsy evidence for a cardiomyopathy associated with symptomatic mitral valve prolapse. Am. J. Cardiol. 42:557, 1978.

296. Pickering, N. J., Brody, J. I., and Barrett, M. J.: Von Willebrand syndrome and mitral valve prolapse. Linked mesenchymal dysplasias. N. Engl. J. Med. 305:131, 1981.

297. Beardsley, T. L., and Foulks, G. N.: An association of keratoconus and mitral valve prolapse. Ophthalmology 89:35, 1982.

298. Channick, B. J., Adlin, E. V., Marks, A. D., et al.: Hyperthyroidism and mitral valve prolapse. N. Engl. J. Med. 305:497, 1981.

299. Jeresaty, R. M.: Mitral valve prolapse–click syndrome in atrial septal defect. Chest 67:132, 1975.

300. Somerville, J., Kaku, S., and Saravalli, O.: Prolapsed mitral cusps in atrial septal defect. An erroneous radiological interpretation. Br. Heart J. 40:58, 1978.

301. Rippe, J. M., Sloss, J. J., Angoff, G., and Alpert, J. S.: Mitral valve prolapse in adults with congenital heart disease. Am. Heart J. 97:561, 1979.

302. Zema, M. J., Chiaramida, S., DeFilipp, G. J., Goldman, M. A., and Pizzarello, R. A.: Somatotype and idiopathic mitral valve prolapse. Cathet. Cardiovasc. Diagn. 8:105, 1982.

303. Udoshi, M. B., Shah, A., Fisher, V. J., and Dolgin, M.: Incidence of mitral valve prolapse in subjects with thoracic skeletal abnormalities—A prospective study. Am. Heart J. 97:303, 1979.

304. Bon Tempo, C. P., Ronan, J. A., Jr., de Leon, A. C., Jr., and Twigg, H. L.: Radiographic appearance of the thorax in systolic click-late systolic murmur syndrome. Am. J. Cardiol. 36:27, 1975.

305. Weinrauch, L. A., McDonald, D. G., DeSilva, R. A., Hawkins, E. T., Leland, O. S., and Shubrooks, S. J., Jr.,: Mitral valve prolapse in rheumatic mitral stenosis. Chest 72:752, 1977.

306. Gottdiener, J. S., Sherber, H. S., and Harvey, W. P.: Mid-systolic click and mitral valve prolapse following mitral commissurotomy. Am. J. Med. 64:295, 1978.

307. Barlow, J. B., Pocock, W. A., and Obel, I. W. P.: Mitral valve prolapse: Primary, secondary, both or neither? Am. Heart J. 102:140, 1981.

308. Crawford, M. H.: Mitral valve prolapse due to coronary artery disease. Am. J. Med. 62:447, 1977.

309. Chesler, E., Matisonn, R. E., Lakier, J. B., Pocock, W. A., Obel, I. W. P., and Barlow, J. B.: Acute myocardial infarction with normal coronary arteries. A possible manifestation of the billowing mitral leaflet syndrome. Circulation 54:203, 1976.

310. Imaizumi, T., Chandraratna, P. A. N., Whayne, T. F., Jr., Schechter, E., and Bhatia, S. K.: Transmural myocardial infarction. With the prolapsing mitral-leaflet syndrome and normal coronary arteries. Arch. Intern. Med. 138:1354, 1978.

311. Tutassaura, H., Gerein, A. N., and Miyagishima, R. T.: Mucoid degeneration of the mitral valve. Clinical review, surgical management and results. Am. J. Surg. 132:276, 1976.

312. Brown, O. R., DeMots, H., Kloster, F. E., Roberts, A., Menashe, V. D., and Beals, R. K.: Aortic root dilatation and mitral valve prolapse in Marfan's syndrome. Circulation 52:651, 1975.

313. Guy, F. C., MacDonald, R. P. R., Fraser, D. B., and Smith, E. R.: Mitral valve prolapse as a cause of hemodynamically important mitral regurgitation. Can. J. Surg. 23:166, 1980.

314. Goghlan, H. C., Phares, P., Cowley, M., Copley, D., and James, T. N.: Dysautonomia in mitral valve prolapse. Am. J. Med. 67:236, 1979.

315. Gaffney, F. A., Karlsson, E. S., Campbell, W., Schutte, J. E., Nixon, J. V., Willerson, J. T., and Blomqvist, C. G.: Autonomic dysfunction in women with mitral valve prolapse syndrome. Circulation 59:894, 1979.

316. Boudoulas, H., Reynolds, J. C., Mazzaferri, E., and Wooley, C. F.: Metabolic studies in mitral valve prolapse syndrome. A neuroendocrine-cardiovascular process. Circulation 61:1200, 1980.

316a.Puddu, P. E., Pasternac, A., Tubau, J. F., Krol, R., Farley, L., and de Champlain, J.: QT Interval prolongation and increased plasma catecholamine levels in patients with mitral valve prolapse. Am. Heart J. 105:422, 1983.

317. Leor, R., and Markiewicz, W.: Neurocirculatory asthenia and mitral valve prolapse—Two unrelated entities? Isr. J. Med. Sci. 17:1137, 1981.

318. Tei, C., Shah, P. M., Cherian, G., Wong, M., and Ormiston, J. A.: The correlates of an abnormal first heart sound in mitral valve prolapse syndromes. N. Engl. J. Med. 307:334, 1982.

319. Alexander, M. D., Bloom, K. R., Hart, P., D'Silva, F., and Murgo, J. P.: Atrial septal aneurysm: A cause of midsystolic click. Report of a case and review of the literature. Circulation 63:1186, 1981.

320. Wei, J. Y., and Fortuin, N. J.: Diastolic sounds and murmurs associated with mitral valve prolapse. Circulation 63:559, 1981.

321. Delman, A. J., and Stein, E.: Mitral valve prolapse. In Dynamic Cardiac Auscultation and Phonocardiography. Philadelphia, W. B. Saunders Co., 1979, p. 888.

322. Liedtke, A. J., Gault, J. H., Leaman, D. M., and Blumenthal, M. S.: Geometry of left ventricular contraction in the systolic click syndrome. Circulation 47:27, 1973.

323. Towne, W. D., Patel, R., Cruz, J., Kramer, N., and Chawla, K. K.: Effects of gravitational stresses on mitral valve prolapse. I. Changes in auscultatory findings produced by progressive passive head-up tilt. Br. Heart J. 40:482, 1978.

324. Winkle, R. A., Goodman, D. J., and Popp, R. L.: Simultaneous echocardiographic-phonocardiographic recordings at rest and during amyl nitrite administration in patients with mitral valve prolapse. Circulation 51:522, 1975.

325. Combs, R. L., Shah, P. M., Klorman, R. S., and Klorman, R.: Effects of induced psychological stress on click and rhythm in mitral valve prolapse. Am. Heart J. 99:714, 1980.

326. Braunwald, E., Oldham, H. N., Jr., Ross, J., Jr., Linhart, J. W., Mason, D. T., and Fort, L., III: The circulatory response of patients with idiopathic hypertrophic subaortic stenosis to nitroglycerin and to the Valsalva maneuver. Circulation 29:422, 1964.

327. Swartz, M. H., Teichholz, L. E., and Donoso, E.: Mitral valve prolapse. A review of associated arrhythmias. Am. J. Med. 62:377, 1977.

328. Josephson, M. E., Horowitz, L. N., and Kastor, J. A.: Proximal supraventricular tachycardia in patients with mitral valve prolapse. Circulation 57:111, 1978.

329. Wei, J. Y., Bulkley, B. H., Schaeffer, A. H., Greene, H. L., and Reid, P. R.: Mitral valve prolapse syndrome and recurrent ventricular tachyarrhythmias. Ann. Intern. Med. 89:6, 1978.

330. Bharati, S., Granston, A. S., Liebson, P. R., Loeb, H. S., Rosen, K. M., and Lev, M.: The conduction system in mitral valve prolapse syndrome with sudden death. Am. Heart J. 101:667, 1981.

331. Ritchie, J. L., Hammermeister, K. E., and Kennedy, J. W.: Refractory ventricular tachycardia and fibrillation in a patient with prolapsing mitral leaflet syndrome: Successful control with overdrive pacing. Am. J. Cardiol. 37:314, 1976.

332. Winkle, R. A., Lopes, M. G., Popp, R. L., and Hancock, E. W.: Life-threatening arrhythmias with mitral valve prolapse syndrome. Am. J. Med. 60:961, 1976.

332a.Hochreiter, C., Kramer, H. M., Kligfield, P., Kramer-Fox, R., Devereaux, R. B., and Borer, J. S.: Arrhythmias in mitral valve prolapse. Effect of additional mitral regurgitation. J. Am. Coll. Cardiol. 1:607, 1983 (Abstr.).

333. Gelfand, M. L., and Kloth, H.: Bradyarrhythmia in mitral valve prolapse treated with a pacemaker. Bull. N. Y. Acad. Med. 54:889, 1978.

334. Wit, A. L., Fenoglio, J. J., Wagner, B. M., and Bassett, A. L.: Electrophysiological properties of cardiac muscle in the anterior mitral valve leaflet and the adjacent atrium in the dog. Possible implications for the genesis of atrial dysrhythmias. Circ. Res. 32:731, 1973.

335. Perloff, J. K.: Evolving concepts of mitral valve prolapse. N. Engl. J. Med. 307:369, 1982.

336. Wit, A. L., Fenoglio, J. J., Hordof, A. J., and Reemtsma, K.: Ultrastructure and transmembrane potentials of cardiac muscle in the human anterior mitral valve leaflet. Circulation 59:1283, 1979.

337. Campbell, R. W. F., Godman, M. G., Fiddler, G. I., Marquis, R., and Julian, D. G.: Ventricular arrhythmias in syndrome of balloon deformity of mitral valve. Definition of possible high risk group. Br. Heart J. 38:1053, 1976.

338. Gallagher, J. J., Gilbert, M., and Svenson, R. H.: Wolff-Parkinson-White syndrome. The problem, evaluation and surgical correction. Circulation 57:767, 1975.

339. Bekheit, S. G., Ali, A. A., Deglin, S. M., and Jain, A. C.: Analysis of QT interval in patients with idiopathic mitral valve prolapse. Chest 81:620, 1982.

340. Jeresaty, R. M.: Sudden death in the mitral valve prolapse–click syndrome. Am. J. Cardiol. 37:317, 1976.

341. Woodley, D., Chambers, W., Starke, H., Dzindzio, B., and Forker, A. D.: Intermittent complete atrioventricular block masquerading as epilepsy in the mitral valve prolapse syndrome. Chest 72:369, 1977.

342. Leichtman, D., Nelson, R., Gobel, F. L., Alexander, C. S., and Cohn, J. N.: Bradycardia with mitral valve prolapse. A potential mechanism of sudden death. Ann. Intern. Med. 85:453, 1976.

343. Popp, R. L., Brown, O. R., Silverman, J. F., and Harrison, D. C.: Echocardiographic abnormalities in the mitral valve prolapse syndrome. Circulation 49:428, 1974.

344. Weiss, A. N., Mimbs, J. W., Ludbrook, P. A., and Sobel, B. E.: Echocardiographic detection of mitral valve prolapse. Circulation 52:1091, 1975.

345. Morganroth, J., Jones, R. H., Chen, C. C., and Naito, M.: Two-dimensional echocardiography in mitral, aortic and tricuspid valve prolapse. The clinical problem, cardiac nuclear imaging considerations and a proposed standard for diagnosis. Am. J. Cardiol. 46:1164, 1980.

346. Morganroth, J., Mardelli, T. J., Naito, M., and Chen, C. C.: Apical cross-sectional echocardiography. Standard for the diagnosis of idiopathic mitral valve prolapse syndrome. Chest 79:23, 1981.

347. Sahn, D. J., Wood, J., Allen, H. D., Peoples, W., and Goldberg, S. J.: Echocardiographic spectrum of mitral valve motion in children with and without mitral valve prolapse: The nature of false positive diagnosis. Am. J. Cardiol. 39:422, 1977.

348. DeMaria, A. N., Neumann, A., Lee, G., and Mason, D. T.: Echocardiographic identification of the mitral valve prolapse syndrome. Am. J. Med. 62:819,1977.

349. Ogawa, S., Hayashi, J., Sasaki, H., Tani, M., Akaishi, M., Mitamura, H., Sano, M., Hoshino, T., Handa, S., and Nakamura, Y.: Evaluation of combined valvular prolapse syndrome of two-dimensional echocardiography. Circulation 65:174, 1982.

350. Gooch, A. S., Maranhao, V., Scampardonis, G., Cha, S. D., and Yang, S. S.: Prolapse of both mitral and tricuspid leaflets in systolic murmur–click syndrome. N. Engl. J. Med. 287:1218, 1972.

351. Rodger, J. C., and Morley, P.: Abnormal aortic valve echoes in mitral prolapse. Echocardiographic features of floppy aortic valve. Br. Heart. J. 47:337, 1982.

352. Klein, G. J., Kostuk, W. J., Boughner, D. R., and Chamberlain, M. J.: Stress myocardial imaging in mitral leaflet prolapse syndrome. Am. J. Cardiol. 42:746, 1978.

353. Butman, S., Chandraratna, P. A. N., Milne, N., Olson, H., Lyons, K., and Aronow, W. S.: Stress myocardial imaging in patients with mitral valve prolapse: Evidence of a perfusion abnormality. Cathet. Cardiovasc. Diagn. 8:243, 1982.

354. Scampardonis, G., Yang, S. S., Maranhao, V., Goldberg, H., and Booch, A. S.: Left ventricular abnormalities in prolapsed mitral leaflet syndrome. Review of eighty-seven cases. Circulation 48:287, 1973.

355. Ranganathan, N., Silver, M. D., Robinson, T. I., and Wilson, J. K.: Idiopathic prolapse mitral leaflet syndrome. Angiographic-clinical correlations. Circulation 54:707, 1976.

356. Cohen, M. V., Shah, P. K., and Spindola-Franco, H.: Angiographic-echocardiographic correlation of mitral valve prolapse. Am. Heart J. 97:43, 1979.

357. Cipriano, P. R., Kline, S. A., and Baltaxe, H. A.: An angiographic assessment of left ventricular function in isolated mitral valvular prolapse. Invest. Radiol. 15:293, 1980.

358. Gottdiener, J. S., Borer, J. S., Bacharach, S. L., Green, M. V., and Epstein, S. E.: Left ventricular function in mitral valve prolapse: Assessment with radionuclide cineangiography. Am. J. Cardiol. 47:7, 1981.

359. Bisset, G. S., III, Schwartz, D. C., Meyer, R. A., James, F. W., and Kaplan, S.: Clinical spectrum and long-term followup of isolated mitral valve prolapse in 119 children. Circulation 62:423, 1980.

360. Bisset, G. S., III: Mitral valve prolapse in children. Primary Cardiol. 8:71, 1982.

361. Mills, P., Rose, J., Hollingsworth, J., Amara, I., and Craige, E.: Long-term prognosis of mitral valve prolapse. N. Engl. J. Med. 297:13, 1977.

362. Corrigall, D., and Popp, R.: Mitral valve prolapse and infective endocarditis. Am. J. Med. 63:215, 1977.

363. Tresch, D. D., Siegel, R., Keelan, M. H., Jr., Gross, C. M., and Brooks, H. L.: Mitral valve prolapse in the elderly. J. Am. Geriatr. Soc. 27:421, 1979.

364. Barnett, H. J. M., Boughner, D. R., Taylor, D. W., Cooper, P. E., Kostuk, W. J., and Nichol, P. M.: Further evidence relating mitral-valve prolapse to cerebral ischemic events. N. Engl. J. Med. 302:139, 1980.

365. Caltrider, N. D., Irvine, A. R., Kline, H. J., and Rosenblatt, A.: Retinal emboli in patients with mitral valve prolapse. Am. J. Ophthalmol. 90:534, 1980.

366. Walsh, P. N., Kansu, T. A., Corbett, J. J., Savino, P. J., Goldburgh, W. P., and Schatz, N. J.: Platelets, thromboembolism and mitral valve prolapse. Circulation 63:552, 1981.

367. Hanson, M. R., Conomy, J. P., and Hodgman, J. R.: Brain events associated with mitral valve prolapse. Stroke 11:499, 1980.

368. Cheitlin, M. D.: Thromboembolic studies in the patient with the prolapsed mitral valve. Has Salome dropped another veil? Circulation 60:46, 1979.

368a. Schnee, M. A., and Bucal, A. A.: Fatal embolism in mitral valve prolapse. Chest 83:285, 1983.

368b. Makino, H., and Al-Sadir, J.: Myocardial infarction in patients with mitral valve prolapse and normal coronary arteries. J. Am. Coll. Cardiol. 1:661, 1983.

369. Troup, P. J., and Zipes, D. P.: Aprindine treatment of recurrent ventricular tachycardia in patients with mitral valve prolapse. Am. Heart J. 97:322, 1979.

370. Winkle, R. A., and Harrison, D.: Propranolol for patients with mitral valve prolapse. Am. Heart J. 93:422, 1977.

AORTIC STENOSIS

371. Roberts, W. C.: Valvular, subvalvular and supravalvular aortic stenosis. Morphologic features. Cardiovasc. Clin. 5:97, 1973.

372. Roberts, W. C.: Anatomically isolated aortic valvular disease. The case against its being of rheumatic origin. Am. J. Med. 49:151, 1970.

373. Roberts, W. C.: The congenitally bicuspid aortic valve. A study of 85 autopsy cases. Am. J. Cardiol. 26:72, 1970.

374. Roberts, W. C., Perloff, J. K., and Constantino, T.: Severe valvular aortic stenosis in patients over 65 years of age. A clinicopathologic study. Am. J. Cardiol. 27:497, 1971.

375. Roberts, W. C., and Morrow, A. G.: Congenital aortic stenosis produced by a unicommissural valve. Br. Heart J. 27:505, 1965.

376. Moller, J. H., Nakib, A., Elliott, R. S., and Edwards, J. E.: Symptomatic congenital aortic stenosis in the first year of life. J. Pediatr. 67:728, 1966.

377. Fenoglio, J. J., Jr., McAllister, H. A., Jr., DeCastro, C. M., Davis, J. E., and Cheitlin, M. D.: Congenital bicuspid aortic valve after age 20. Am. J. Cardiol. 29:164, 1977.

378. Mills, P., Leech, G., Davies, M., and Leatham, A.: The natural history of a non-stenotic bicuspid aortic valve. Br. Heart J. 40:951, 1978.

379. Emanuel, R., Withers, R., O'Brien, K., Ross, P., and Feizi, O.: Congenitally bicuspid aortic valves. Clinicogenetic study of 41 families. Br. Heart J. 40:1402, 1978.

380. Braunwald, E., Goldblatt, A., Aygen, M. M., Rockoff, S. D., and Morrow, A. G.: Congenital aortic stenosis: Clinical and hemodynamic findings in 100 patients. Circulation 27:426, 1963.

381. Narang, N. K., Andrew, A. M. R., Chaudhury, H. R., and Gaba, B. S.: Aortic stenosis due to familial hypercholesterolemic xanthomatosis. A case report with brief review of literature. Indian Heart J. 30:189, 1978.

382. Gould, L., Reddy, C. V. R., DePalma, D., DeMartino, A., and Kalish, P. E.: Cardiac manifestations of ochronosis. J. Thorac. Cardiovasc. Surg. 72:788, 1976.

383. Kennedy, J. W., Twiss, R. D., Blackmon, J. R., et al.: Quantitative angiocardiography. III. Relationships of left ventricular pressure volume and mass in aortic valve disease. Circulation 38:838, 1968.

384. Carabello, B. A., Mee, R., Collins, J. J., Jr., Kloner, R. A., Levin, D., and Grossman, W.: Contractile function in chronic gradually developing subcoronary aortic stenosis. Am. J. Physiol. 240:H80, 1981.

385. Morrow, A. G., Roberts, W. C., Ross, J., Jr., Fisher, D. R., Behrendt, D. M., Mason, D. T., and Braunwald, E.: Clinical staff conference. Obstruction to left ventricular outflow. Current concepts of management and operative treatment. Ann. Intern. Med. 69:1255, 1968.

386. Braunwald, E., and Frahm, C. J.: Studies on Starling's law of the heart. IV. Observations on the hemodynamic functions of the left atrium in man. Circulation 24:633, 1961.

387. Sasayama, S., Ross, J., Jr., Franklin, D., Bloor, C. M., Bishop, S., and Dilley, R. B.: Adaptations of the left ventricle to chronic pressure overload. Circ. Res. 38:172, 1976.

388. Gunther, S., and Grossman, W.: Determinants of ventricular function in pressure overload hypertrophy in man. Circulation 59:679, 1979.

389. Ross, J., Jr.: Afterload mismatch and preload reserve: A conceptual framework for the analysis of ventricular function. Prog. Cardiovasc. Dis. 18:255, 1976.

389a. Donner, R., Carabello, B. A., Black, I., and Spann, J. F.: Left ventricular wall stress in compensated aortic stenosis in children. Am. J. Cardiol. 51:946, 1983.

389b. DePace, N. L., Ren, J-F., Iskandrian, A. S., Kotler, M. N., Hakki, A-H., and Segal, B. L.: Correlation of echocardiographic wall stress and left ventricular pressure and function in aortic stenosis. Circulation 67:854, 1983.

390. Fifer, M. A., Gunther, S., Grossman, W., Mirsky, I., Carabello, B., and Barry, W. H.: Myocardial contractile function in aortic stenosis as determined from the rate of stress development during isovolumic systole. Am. J. Cardiol. 44:1318, 1979.

391. Carabello, B. A., Green, L. H., Grossman, W., Cohn, L. H., Koster, J. K., and Collins, J. J., Jr.: Hemodynamic determinants of prognosis of aortic valve replacement in critical aortic stenosis and advanced congestive heart failure. Circulation 62:42, 1980.

392. Huber, D., Grimm, J., Koch, R., and Krayenbuehl, H. P.: Determinants of ejection performance in aortic stenosis. Circulation 64:126, 1981.

393. Johnson, A. D., Engler, R. L., LeWinter, M., Karliner, J., Peterson, K., Tauji, I. J., and Daily, P. O.: The medical and surgical management of patients with aortic valve disease. A Symposium. West. J. Med. 126:460, 1977.

394. Peterson, K. J., Tsuji, J., Johnson, A., DiDonna, J., and LeWinter, M.: Diastolic left ventricular pressure-volume and stress-strain relations in patients with valvular aortic stenosis and left ventricular hypertrophy. Circulation 58:77, 1978.

395. Schwarz, F., Flameng, W., Schaper, J., Langebartels, F., Sesto, M., Hehrlein, F., and Schlepper, M.: Myocardial structure and function in patients with aortic valve disease and their relation to postoperative results. Am. J. Cardiol. 41:661, 1978.

396. Bertrand, M. E., LaBlanche, J. M., Tilmant, P. Y., Thieuleux, F. P., Delforge, M. R., and Carre, A. G.: Coronary sinus blood flow at rest and during isometric exercise in patients with aortic valve disease. Mechanism of angina pectoris in presence of normal coronary arteries. Am. J. Cardiol. 47:199, 1981.

397. Vinten-Johansen, J., and Weiss, H. R.: Oxygen consumption in subepicardial and subendocardial regions of the canine left ventricle—The effect of experimental acute valvular aortic stenosis. Circ. Res. 46:139, 1980.

398. Hakki, A.-H., Kimbiris, D., Iskandrian, A. S., Segal, B. L., Mintz, G. S., and Bemis, C. E.: Angina pectoris and coronary artery disease in patients with severe aortic valvular disease. Am. Heart J. 100:441, 1980.

399. Contratto, A. W., and Levine, S. A.: Aortic stenosis with special reference to angina pectoris and syncope. Ann. Intern. Med. 10:1636, 1936.

400. Ross, J., Jr., and Braunwald, E.: The influence of corrective operations on the natural history of aortic stenosis. Circulation 37(Suppl. V):61, 1968.

401. Frank, S., Johnson, A., and Ross, J., Jr.,: Natural history of valvular aortic stenosis. Br. Heart J. 35:41, 1973.

402. Fallen, E. L., Elliott, W. C., and Gorlin, R.: Mechanisms of angina in aortic stenosis. Circulation 36:480, 1967.

403. Storstein, O., and Enge, I.: Angina pectoris in aortic valvular disease and its relation to coronary pathology. Acta Med. Scand. 205:275, 1979.

404. Holley, K. E., Bahn, R. C., McGoon, D. C., and Mankin, H. T.: Spontaneous calcific embolization associated with calcific aortic stenosis. Circulation 27:197, 1963.

405. Flamm, M. D., Braiff, B. A., Kimball, R., and Hancock, E. W.: Mechanism of effort syncope in aortic stenosis. Circulation 36(Suppl. II):109, 1967.

406. Schwartz, L. S., Goldfischer, J., Sprague, G. J., and Schwartz, S. P.: Syncope and sudden death in aortic stenosis. Am. J. Cardiol. 23:647, 1969.

407. Shoenfeld, Y., Eldar, M., Bedazovsky, B., Levy, M. J., and Pinkhas, J.: Aortic stenosis associated with gastrointestinal bleeding. A survey of 612 patients. Am. Heart J. 100:179, 1980.

408. Love, J. W.: The syndrome of calcific aortic stenosis and gastrointestinal bleeding: Resolution following aortic valve replacement. J. Thorac. Cardiovasc. Surg. 83:779, 1982.

409. Pleet, A. B., Massey, E. W., and Vengrow, M. E.: TIA, stroke, and the bicuspid aortic valve. Neurology 31:1540, 1981.

410. Brockmeier, L. B., Adolph, R. J., Gustin, B. W., Holmes, J. C., and Sacks, J. G.: Calcium emboli to the retinal artery in calcific aortic stenosis. Am. Heart J. 101:32, 1981.

411. Wood, P.: Aortic stenosis. Am. J. Cardiol. 1:553, 1958.

412. Cooper, T., Braunwald, E., and Morrow, A. G.: Pulsus alternans in aortic stenosis: Hemodynamic observations in 50 patients studied by left heart catheterization. Circulation 18:64, 1958.

413. Perloff, J. K.: Clinical recognition of aortic stenosis. The physical signs and

differential diagnosis of the various forms of obstruction to left ventricular outflow. Prog. Cardiovasc. Dis. *10*:323, 1968.

414. Goldblatt, A., Aygen, M. M., and Braunwald, E.: Hemodynamic-phonocardiographic correlations of the fourth heart sound in aortic stenosis. Circulation *26*: 92, 1962.

415. Caulfield, W. H., deLeon, A. C., Perloff, J. K., and Steelman, R. B.: The clinical significance of the fourth heart sound in aortic stenosis. Am. J. Cardiol. *28*:179, 1971.

416. Hancock, E. W.: The ejection sound in aortic stenosis. Am. J. Med. *40*:569, 1966.

417. Morton, B. C.: Natural history and management of chronic aortic valve disease. Can. Med. Assoc. J. *126*:477, 1982.

418. Delman, A. J., and Stein, E.: Valvular aortic stenosis. *In* Dynamic Cardiac Auscultation and Phonocardiography. Philadelphia, W. B. Saunders Co., 1979, p. 795.

419. Morgan, D. J. R., and Hall, R. J. C.: Occult aortic stenosis as cause of intractable heart failure. Br. Med. J. *1*:784, 1979.

420. Kini, P. M., Eddelman, E. E., and Pipberger, H. V.: Electrocardiographic differentiation between left ventricular hypertrophy and anterior myocardial infarction. Circulation *42*:875, 1970.

421. Siegel, R. J., and Roberts, W. C.: Electrocardiographic observations in severe aortic valve stenosis: Correlative necropsy study to clinical, hemodynamic, and ECG variables demonstrating relation of 12-lead QRS amplitude to peak systolic transaortic pressure gradient. Am. Heart J. *103*:210, 1982.

422. Gooch, A. S., Calatayud, J. B., Rogers, P. A., and Garman, P. A.: Analysis of the P wave in severe aortic stenosis. Dis. Chest *49*:459, 1966.

423. Myler, R. K., and Sanders, C. A.: Aortic valve disease and atrial fibrillation: Report of 122 patients with electrocardiographic, radiographic and hemodynamic observations. Arch. Intern. Med. *121*:530, 1968.

424. Thompsom, R., Mitchell, A., Ahmed, M., Towers, M., and Yacoub, M.: Conduction defects in aortic valve disease. Am. Heart J. *98*:3, 1979.

425. Dhingra, R. C., Amat-y-Leon, F., Pietras, R. J., Wyndham, C., Deedwania, P. C., Wu, D., Denes, P., and Rosen, K. M.: Sites of conduction disease in aortic stenosis. Significance of valve gradient and calcification. Ann. Intern. Med. *87*: 275, 1977.

426. Rosenbaum, M., Elizari, M., and Lazari, J.: Los Hemibloques. Buenos Aires, Paidos, 1968, p. 363.

427. Bell, H., Pugh, D., and Dunn, M.: Vectorcardiographic evolution of left ventricular hypertrophy. Br. Heart J. *30*:70, 1968.

428. Klatte, E. C., Tampas, J. P., Campbell, J. A., and Lurie, P. R.: The roentgenographic manifestations of aortic stenosis and aortic valvular insufficiency. Am. J. Roentgenol. Radium Ther. Nucl. Med. *88*:57, 1962.

428a. Siegel, R. J., Maurer, G., Nivatpumin, T., and Shah, P. K.: Accurate non-invasive assessment of critical aortic valve stenosis in the elderly. J. Am. Coll. Cardiol. *1*:639, 1983.

429. Nanda, N. C., Gramiak, R., Manning, J., Mahoney, E. B., Lipchik, E. O., and DeWeese, J. A.: Echocardiographic recognition of the congenital bicuspid aortic valve. Circulation *49*:870, 1974.

430. Vukas, M., Wallentin, I., and Hjalmarson, A.: Analysis of systolic vibrations of interventricular septum in patients with aortic valvular stenosis. Acta Med. Scand. *210*:397, 1981.

431. McDonald, I. G.: Echocardiographic assessment of left ventricular function in aortic valve disease. Circulation *53*:860, 1976.

432. Reichek, N., and Devereaux, R. B.: Reliable estimation of peak left ventricular systolic pressure by M-mode echographic–determined end-diastolic relative wall thickness: Identification of severe valvular aortic stenosis in adult patients. Am. Heart J. *103*:202, 1982.

433. DeMaria, A. N., Bommer, W., Joye, J., Lee, G., Bouteller, J., and Mason, D. T.: Value and limitations of cross-sectional echocardiography of the aortic valve in the diagnosis and quantification of valvular aortic stenosis. Circulation *62*:304, 1980.

434. Godley, R. W., Green, D., Dillon, J. C., Rogers, E. W., Feigenbaum, H., and Weyman, A. E.: Reliability of two-dimensional echocardiography in assessing the severity of valvular aortic stenosis. Chest *79*:657, 1981.

435. Weyman, A. E.: Cross-sectional echocardiographic assessment of aortic obstruction. Acta Med. Scand. (Suppl. 627):120, 1979.

436. Cohen, L. S., Friedman, W. F., and Braunwald, E.: Natural history of mild congenital aortic stenosis elucidated by serial hemodynamic studies. Am. J. Cardiol. *30*:1, 1972.

437. Cheitlin, M. D., Gertz, E. W., Brundage, B. H., Carlson, C. J., Quash, J. A., and Bode, R. S., Jr.: Rate of progression of severity of valvular aortic stenosis in the adult. Am. Heart J. *98*:689, 1979.

438. Hammarsten, J. F.: Syncope in aortic stenosis. Arch. Intern. Med. *87*:274, 1951.

439. Morrow, A. G., Goldblatt, A., and Braunwald, E.: Congenital aortic stenosis. II. Surgical treatment and the results of operation. Circulation *27*:450, 1963.

440. Chizner, M. A., Pearle, D. L., and deLeon, A. C., Jr.: The natural history of aortic stenosis in adults. Am. Heart J. *99*:419, 1980.

441. Wagner, S., and Selzer, A.: Patterns of progression of aortic stenosis: A longitudinal hemodynamic study. Circulation *65*:709, 1982.

442. Spencer, F. C.: Congenital heart disease. *In* Schwartz, S. I., Shires, G. T., Spencer, F. C., and Storer, E. H. (eds.): Principles of Surgery. 2nd ed. New York, McGraw-Hill Book Co., 1979, p. 755.

443. Henry, W. L., Bonow, R. O., Borer, J. S., Kent, K. M., Ware, J. H., Redwood, D. R., Itscoitz, S. B., McIntosh, C. L., Morrow, A. G., and Epstein, S.

E.: Evaluation of aortic valve replacement in patients with valvular aortic stenosis. Circulation *61*:814, 1980.

444. Copeland, J. G., Griepp, R. B., Stinson, E. B., and Shumway, N. E.: Long-term followup after isolated aortic valve replacement. J. Thorac. Cardiovasc. Surg. *74*:875, 1977.

445. Krayenbuehl, H. P., Turina, M., Hess, O. M., Rothlin, M., and Senning, A.: Pre- and postoperative left ventricular contractile function in patients with aortic valve disease. Br. Heart J. *41*:204, 1979.

446. Rahimtoola, S. H.: Outcome of aortic valve surgery. Circulation *60*:1191, 1979.

447. Mirsky, I., Henschke, C., Hess, O. M., and Krayenbuehl, H. P.: Prediction of postoperative performance in aortic valve disease. Am. J. Cardiol. *48*:295, 1981.

448. Khanna, S. K., Ross, J. K., and Monro, J. L.: Homograft aortic valve replacement: Seven years' experience with antibiotic-treated valves. Thorax *36*: 330, 1981.

449. Rossiter, S. J., Miller, D. C., Stinson, E. B., Oyer, P. E., Reitz, B. A., Moreno-Cabral, R. J., Mace, J. G., Robert, E. W., Tsagaris, T. J., Sutton, R. B., Alderman, E. L., and Shumway, N. E.: Hemodynamic and clinical comparison of the Hancock modified orifice and standard orifice bioprostheses in the aortic position. J. Thorac. Cardiovasc. Surg. *80*:54, 1980.

450. DiSesa, V. J., Collins, J. J., Jr., and Cohn, L. H.: Valve replacement in the small annulus aorta: Performance of the Hancock modified-orifice bioprosthesis. *In* Cohn, L. H., and Gallucci, V.: Cardiac Bioprostheses. New York, Yorke Medical Books, 1982, p. 552.

451. Gill, C. C., King, H. C., Lytle, B. W., Cosgrove, D. M., Golding, L. A. R., and Loop, F. D.: Early clinical evaluation of aortic valve replacement with the St. Jude medical valve in patients with a small aortic root. Circulation *66* (Suppl. I):I–147, 1982.

452. Cheung, D., Flemma, R. J., Mullen, D. C., Lepley, D., Jr., Anderson, A. J., and Weirauch, E.: Ten-year followup in aortic valve replacement using the Björk-Shiley prosthesis. Ann. Thorac. Surg. *32*:138, 1981.

453. Acar, J., Ducimetiere, P., Cadilhac, M., Jallut, H., and Vahanian, A.: Prognosis of surgically treated chronic aortic valve disease. Predictive indicators of early postoperative risk and long-term survival, based on 439 cases. J. Thorac. Cardiovasc. Surg. *82*:114, 1981.

454. Croke, R. P., Pifarre, R., Sullivan, H., Gunnar, R., and Loeb, H.: Reversal of advanced left ventricular dysfunction following aortic valve replacement for aortic stenosis. Ann. Thorac. Surg. *24*:38, 1977.

455. Pantely, G., Morton, M., and Rahimtoola, S. H.: Effects of successful, uncomplicated valve replacement on ventricular hypertrophy, volume and performance in aortic stenosis and in aortic incompetence. J. Thorac. Cardiovasc. Surg. *75*:383, 1978.

456. Kennedy, J. W., Doces, J., and Stewart, D. K.: Left ventricular function before and following aortic valve replacement. Circulation *56*:944, 1977.

457. O'Tolle, J. D., Geiser, E. A., Reddy, S., Curtiss, E. I., and Landfair, R. M.: Effect of preoperative ejection fraction on survival and hemodynamic improvement following aortic valve replacement. Circulation *58*:1175, 1978.

458. Sanders, J. H., Jr., Cohn, L. H., Dalen, J. E., and Collins, J. J., Jr.: Emergency aortic valve replacement. Am. J. Surg. *135*:495, 1976.

459. Smith, N., McAnulty, J. H., and Rahimtoola, S. H.: Severe aortic stenosis with impaired left ventricular function and clinical heart failure: Results of valve replacement. Circulation *58*:255, 1978.

460. Kay, P. H., and Paneth, M.: Aortic valve replacement in the over seventy age group. J. Cardiovasc. Surg. *22*:312, 1981.

461. Richardson, J. V., Kouchoukos, N. T., Wright, J. O., and Karp, R. B.: Combined aortic valve replacement and myocardial revascularization: Results in 220 patients. Circulation *59*:75, 1979.

462. Kirklin, J. W., and Kouchoukos, N. T.: Aortic valve replacement without myocardial revascularization. Circulation *63*:252, 1981.

463. MacManus, Q., Grunkemeier, G., Lambert, L., Dietl, C., and Starr, A.: Aortic valve replacement and aorto-coronary bypass surgery. Results with perfusion of proximal and distal coronary arteries. J. Thorac. Cardiovasc. Surg. *75*:865, 1978.

464. Starr, A., Pierie, U. R., Raible, D. A., et al.: Cardiac valve replacement. Experience with the durability of silicone rubber. Circulation *34*(Suppl. I):1, 1966.

465. Bonchek, L. I., and Starr, A.: Ball valve prostheses: Current appraisal of late results. Am. J. Cardiol. *35*:843, 1975.

466. Yoganathan, A. P., Corcoran, W. H., Harrison, E. C., and Carl, J. R.: The Björk-Shiley aortic prosthesis: Flow characteristics, thrombus formation and tissue overgrowth. Circulation *58*:70, 1978.

467. Sarma, R., Roschke, E. J., Harrison, E. C., Edmiston, W. A., and Lau, F. Y. K.: Clinical experience with the Smeloff-Cutter aortic valve prosthesis: An 8-year followup study. Am. J. Cardiol. *40*:338, 1977.

468. Magovern, G. J., Liebler, G. A., Cushing, W. J., Park, S. G., and Burkholder, J. A.: A thirteen-year review of the Magovern-Cromie aortic valve. J. Thorac. Cardiovasc. Surg. *73*:64, 1977.

469. Stinson, E. B., Griepp, R. B., Oyer, P. E., and Shumway, N. E.: Long-term experience with porcine aortic valve xenografts. J. Thorac. Cardiovasc. Surg. *73*:54, 1977.

470. Morris, D. C., King, S. B., III, Douglas, J. S., Jr., Wickliffe, C. W., and Jones, E. L.: Hemodynamic results of aortic valvular replacement with the porcine xenograft valve. Circulation *56*:841, 1977.

471. Wright, J. T. M.: A pulsatile flow study comparing the Hancock porcine xenograft aortic valve prostheses models 242 and 250. Med. Instrum. *11*:114, 1977.

AORTIC REGURGITATION

472. Stapleton, J. F., and Harvey, W. P.: A clinical analysis of aortic incompetence. Postgrad. Med. 46:156, 1969.
473. Carter, J. B., Sethi, S., Lee, G. B., and Edward, J. E.: Prolapse of semilunar cusps as causes of aortic insufficiency. Circulation 43:922, 1971.
474. Frahm, C. J., Braunwald, E., and Morrow, A. G.: Congenital aortic regurgitation. Clinical and hemodynamic findings in four patients. Am. J. Med. 31:63, 1961.
475. Roberts, W. C., Morrow, A. G., McIntosh, C. L., Jones, M., and Epstein, S. E.: Congenitally bicuspid aortic valve causing severe, pure aortic regurgitation without superimposed infective endocarditis. Am. J. Cardiol. 47:206, 1981.
476. Morain, S. V., Casanegra, P., Maturana, G., and Dubernet, J.: Spontaneous rupture of a fenestrated aortic valve. Surgical treatment. J. Thorac. Cardiovasc. Surg. 73:716, 1977.
477. Puchner, T. C., Huston, J. H., and Hellmuth, G. A.: Aortic valve insufficiency in arterial hypertension. Am. J. Cardiol. 5:758, 1960.
478. Thandroyen, F. T., Matisonn, R. E., and Weir, E. K.: Severe aortic incompetence caused by systemic lupus erythematosus. S.A. Med. J. 54:166, 1978.
479. Devlin, A. B., Goldstraw, P., and Caves, P. K.: Aortic valve replacement in rheumatoid aortic incompetence. Thorax 33:612, 1978.
480. Schilder, D. P., Harvey, W. P., and Hufnagel, C. A.: Rheumatoid spondylitis and aortic insufficiency. N. Engl. J. Med. 255:11, 1956.
480a. Bostwick, D. G., Bensch, K. G., Burke, J. S., Billingham, M. E., Miller, D. C., Smith, J. C., and Keren, D. F.: Whipple's disease presenting as aortic insufficiency. N. Engl. J. Med. 305:995, 1981.
481. Darvill, F. R., Jr.: Aortic insufficiency of unusual etiology. J.A.M.A. 184:753, 1963.
481a. Rae, S. A., Vandenburg, M., and Scholtz, C. L.: Aortic regurgitation and false aneurysm formation in Behçet's disease. Postgrad. Med. J. 56:438, 1980.
482. Emanuel, R., Ng, R. A. L., Marcomichelakis, J., Moores, E. C., Jefferson, K. E., Macfaul, P. A., and Withers, R.: Formes frustes of Marfan's syndrome presenting with severe aortic regurgitation. Clinicogenetic study of 18 families. Br. Heart J. 39:190, 1977.
483. Roberts, W. C., Hollingsworth, J. F., Bulkley, B. H., Jaffe, R. B., Epstein, S. E., and Stinson, E. B.: Combined mitral and aortic regurgitation in ankylosing spondylitis: Angiographic and anatomic features. Am. J. Med. 56:237, 1974.
484. Reid, G. D., Patterson, M. W. H., Patterson, A. C., and Cooperberg, P. L.: Aortic insufficiency in association with juvenile ankylosing spondylitis. J. Pediatr. 95:78, 1979.
485. Paulus, H. E., Pearson, C. M., and Pitts, W., Jr.: Aortic insufficiency in five patients with Reiter's syndrome: A detailed clinical and pathologic study. Am. J. Med. 53:464, 1972.
486. Hollingworth, P., Hall, P. J., Knight, S. C., and Newman, R.: Lone aortic regurgitation, sacroiliitis, and HLA B27: Case history and frequency of association. Br. Heart J. 42:229, 1979.
487. Heppner, R. L., Babitt, H. I., Bianchine, J. W., and Warbasse, J. R.: Aortic regurgitation and aneurysm of sinus of Valsalva associated with osteogenesis imperfecta. Am. J. Cardiol. 31:654, 1973.
488. Waller, B. F., Zoltick, J. M., Rosen, J. H., Katz, N. M., Gomes, M. N., Fletcher, R. D., Wallace, R. B., and Roberts, W. C.: Severe aortic regurgitation from systemic hypertension (without aortic dissection) requiring aortic valve replacement. Analysis of four patients. Am. J. Cardiol. 49:473, 1982.
489. Welch, G. H., Jr., Braunwald, E., and Sarnoff, S. J.: Hemodynamic effects of quantitatively varied experimental aortic regurgitation. Circ. Res. 5:546, 1957.
490. Soorae, A. S., McKeown, F., and Cleland, J.: Aortic valve replacement for severe aortic regurgitation caused by idiopathic giant cell aortitis. Thorax 35:60, 1980.
491. Belenkie, I., and Rademaker, A.: Acute and chronic changes after aortic valve damage in the intact dog. Am. J. Physiol. 241:H95, 1981.
491a. Iskandrian, A. S., Hakki, A-H., Manno, B., Amenta, A., and Kane, S. A.: Left ventricular function in chronic aortic regurgitation. J. Am. Coll. Cardiol. 1:1374, 1983.
491b. Boucher, C. A., Wilson, R. A., Kanarek, D. J., Hutter, A. M., Jr., Okada, R. D., Liberthson, R. R., Strauss, H. W., and Pohost, G. M.: Exercise testing in asymptomatic or minimally symptomatic aortic regurgitation: Relationship of left ventricular ejection fraction to left ventricular filling pressure during exercise. Circulation 67:1091, 1983.
491c. Johnson, L. L., Powers, E. R., Tzall, W. R., Feder, J., Sciacca, R. R., and Cannon, P. J.: Left ventricular volume and ejection fraction response to exercise in aortic regurgitation. Am. J. Cardiol. 51:1379, 1983.
492. Grossman, W., Jones, D., and McLaurin, L.: Wall stress and patterns of hypertrophy in the human left ventricle. J. Clin. Invest. 56:56, 1975.
493. Judge, T. P., Kennedy, J. W., Bennett, L. J., Willis, R. E., Murray, J. A., and Blackman, J. R.: Quantitative hemodynamic effects of heart rate on aortic regurgitation. Circulation 44:355, 1971.
494. Laniado, S., Yellin, E. L., Yoran, C., Strom, J., Hori, M., Gabbay, S., Terdiman, R., and Frater, R. W. M.: Physiologic mechanism in aortic insufficiency. I. The effect of changing heart rate on flow dynamics. II. Determinants of Austin Flint murmur. Circulation 66:226, 1982.
495. Falsetti, H. L., Carroll, R. J., and Cramer, J. A.: Total and regional myocardial blood flow in aortic regurgitation. Am. Heart J. 97:485, 1979.
496. Uhl, G. S., Boucher, C. A., Oliveros, R. A., and Murgo, J. P.: Exercise-induced myocardial oxygen supply-demand imbalance in asymptomatic or mildly symptomatic aortic regurgitation. Chest 80:686, 1981.
497. Maurer, W., Ablasser, A., Tschada, R., Hausen, M., Saggau, W., and Kubler, W.: Myocardial catecholamine metabolism in patients with chronic aortic regurgitation. Circulation 66(Suppl. I):I-139, 1982.
498. Osbakken, M., Bove, A. A., and Spann, J. F.: Left ventricular function in chronic aortic regurgitation with reference to end-systolic pressure, volume and stress relations. Am. J. Cardiol. 47:193, 1981.
499. Dehmer, G. J., Firth, E. G., Hillis, L. D., Corbett, J. R., Lewis, S. E., Parkey, R. W., and Willerson, J. T.: Alterations in left ventricular volumes and ejection fraction at rest and during exercise in patients with aortic regurgitation. Am. J. Cardiol. 48:17, 1981.
500. Lewis, S. M., Riba, A. L., Berger, H. J., Davies, R. A., Wackers, F. J. T., Alexander, J., Sands, M. J., Cohen, L. S., and Zaret, B. L.: Radionuclide angiographic exercise left ventricular performance in chronic aortic regurgitation: Relationship to resting echographic ventricular dimensions and systolic wall stress index. Am. Heart J. 103:498, 1982.
501. Schuler, G., Olshausen, K. V., Schwarz, F., Mehmel, H., Hofmann, M., Hermann, H.-J., Lange, D., and Kubler, W.: Noninvasive assessment of myocardial contractility in asymptomatic patients with severe aortic regurgitation and normal left ventricular ejection fraction at rest. Am. J. Cardiol. 50:45, 1982.
502. Morganroth, J., Perloff, J. K., Zeldis, S. M., and Dunkman, W. B.: Acute severe aortic regurgitation. Pathophysiology, clinical recognition and management. Ann. Intern. Med. 82:223, 1977.
502a. Perlofff, J. K.: Acute severe aortic regurgitation: Recognition and management. J. Cardiovasc. Med. 8:209, 1983.
503. Mann, T., McLaurin, L. P., Grossman, W., and Craige, E.: Assessing the hemodynamic severity of acute aortic regurgitation due to infective endocarditis. N. Engl. J. Med. 293:108, 1975.
504. Spagnuolo, M., Kloth, H., Taranta, A., Doyle, E., and Pasternack, B.: Natural history of rheumatic aortic regurgitation: Criteria predictive of death, congestive heart failure and angina in young patients. Circulation 44:368, 1971.
505. Segal, J., Harvey, W. P., and Hufnagel, C. A.: Clinical study of one hundred cases of severe aortic insufficiency. Am. J. Med. 21:200, 1956.
506. Bland, E. F., and Wheeler, E. O.: Severe aortic regurgitation in young people. A long-term perspective with reference to prognosis. N. Engl. J. Med. 256:667, 1957.
507. Sapira, J. D.: Quincke, deMusset, Duroziez and Hill: Some aortic regurgitations. South. Med. J. 74:459, 1981.
508. Alpert, J. S., Vieweg, W. V. R., and Hagan, A. D.: Incidence and morphology of carotid shudders in aortic valve disease. Am. Heart J. 92:435, 1976.
509. Sabbah, H. N., Khaja, F., Anbe, D. T., and Stein, P. D.: The aortic closure sound in pure aortic insufficiency. Circulation 56:859, 1977.
510. Abdulla, A. M., Frank, M. J., Erdin, R. A., Jr., and Canedo, M. I.: Clinical significance and hemodynamic correlates of the third heart sound gallop in aortic regurgitation. A guide to optimal timing of cardiac catheterization. Circulation 64:464, 1981.
511. Harvey, W. P., Corrado, M. A., and Perloff, J. K.: "Right-sided" murmurs of aortic insufficiency. Am. J. Med. Sci. 245:53, 1963.
512. Fortuin, N. J., and Craige, E.: On the mechanism of the Austin Flint murmur. Circulation 45:558, 1972.
513. O'Brien, K. P., and Cohen, L. S.: Hemodynamic and phonocardiographic correlates of the Austin Flint murmur. Am. Heart J. 77:603, 1969.
514. Delman, A. J., and Stein, E.: Aortic regurgitation. In Dynamic Cardiac Auscultation and Phonocardiography. Philadelphia, W. B. Saunders Co. 1979, pp. 811-824.
515. Spring, D. A., Folts, J. D., Young, W. P., and Rowe, G. G.: Premature closure of the mitral and tricuspid valves. Circulation 45:663, 1972.
516. Wong, M.: Diastolic mitral regurgitation. Hemodynamic and angiographic correlation. Br. Heart J. 31:468, 1969.
517. Perloff, J. K., and Singer, D.: Electrocardiogram of free aortic insufficiency. Circulation 26:786, 1962.
518. Estes, E. H.: Left ventricular hypertrophy in acquired heart disease: A comparison of the vectorcardiogram in aortic stenosis and aortic insufficiency. In Hoffman, I. (ed.): Vectorcardiography. Amsterdam, North Holland Publishing Co., 1976.
519. Paoloni, H. J., Wilcken, D. E. L., and Dadd, M. J.: The role of echocardiography in the assessment of chronic aortic regurgitation. Aust. N.Z.J. Med. 7:491, 1977.
520. Abdulla, A. M., Frank, M. J., Canedo, M. I., and Stefadouros, M. A.: Limitations of echocardiography in the assessment of left ventricular size and function in aortic regurgitation. Circulation 61:148, 1980.
521. Pridie, R. B., Benham, R., and Oakley, C. M.: Echocardiography of the mitral valve in aortic valve disease. Br. Heart J. 33:296, 1971.
522. Weaver, W. F., Wilson, C. S., Rourke, T., and Caudill, C. C.: Mid-diastolic aortic valve opening in severe acute aortic regurgitation. Circulation 55:112, 1977.
523. Winsberg, F., Gabor, G. E., Hernberg, J. G., et al.: Fluttering of the mitral valve in aortic insufficiency. Circulation 41:225, 1970.
524. Imaizumi, T., Orita, Y., Koiwaya, Y., Hirata, T., and Nakamura, M.: Utility of two-dimensional echocardiography in the differential diagnosis of the etiology of aortic regurgitation. Am. Heart J. 103:887, 1982.
525. Rowe, D. W., Pechacek, L. W., DeCastro, C. M., Garcia, E., and Hall, R. J.: Initial diastolic indentation of the mitral valve in aortic insufficiency. J. Clin. Ultrasound 10:53, 1982.
526. Manyari, D. E., Nolewajka, A. J., and Kostuk, W. J.: Quantitative assessment

of aortic valvular insufficiency by radionuclide angiography. Chest *81*:170, 1982.

526a.Steingart, R. M., Yee, C., Weinstein, L., and Scheuer, J.: Radio-nuclide ventriculographic study of adaptations to exercise in aortic regurgitation. Am. J. Cardiol. *51*:483, 1983.

527. Utley, J. R., Mills, J., and Roe, B. B.: The role of valve replacement in the treatment of fungal endocarditis. J. Thorac. Cardiovasc. Surg. *69*:255, 1975.

528. Goldschlager, N., Pfeifer, J., Cohn, K., Pepper, R., and Selzer, A.: The natural history of aortic regurgitation. A clinical and hemodynamic study. Am. J. Med. *54*:577, 1973.

529. Dexter, L.: Evaluation of the results of cardiac surgery. *In* Jones, A. M. (ed.): Modern Trends in Cardiology. Vol. 2. New York, Appleton-Century-Crofts, 1969, p. 311.

530. Massell, B. F., Ameccua, F. J., and Czohiczer, G.: Prognosis of patients with pure or predominant aortic regurgitation in the absence of surgery. Circulation *34*(Suppl. II):164, 1966.

531. Greenberg, B. H.: Aortic insufficiency: Vasodilator therapy. Primary Cardiol. *8*: 35, 1982.

532. Greenberg, B. H., DeMots, H., Murphy, E., and Rahimtoola, S. H.: Mechanism for improved cardiac performance with arteriolar dilators in aortic insufficiency. Circulation *63*:263, 1981.

533. Fioretti, P., Benussi, B., Scardi, S., Klugmann, S., Brower, R. W., and Camerini, F.: Afterload reduction with nifedipine in aortic insufficiency. Am. J. Cardiol. *49*:1728, 1982.

533a.Gaasch, W. H., Carroll, J. D., Levine, H. J., and Criscitiello, M. G.: Chronic aortic regurgitation: Prognostic value of left ventricular end-systolic dimensions and end-diastolic radius/thickness ratio. J. Am. Coll. Cardiol. *3*:775, 1983.

533b.Jebavy, P., Koudelkova, E., and Henzlova, M.: Unloading effects of prazosin in patients with chronic aortic regurgitation. Am. Heart J. *105*:567, 1983.

534. Kumpuris, A. G., Quinones, M. A., Waggoner, A. D., Kanon, D. J., Nelson, J. G., and Miller, R. R.: Importance of preoperative hypertrophy, wall stress and end-systolic dimension as echocardiographic predictors of normalization of left ventricular dilatation after valve replacement in chronic aortic insufficiency. Am. J. Cardiol. *49*:1091, 1982.

535. Cunha, C. L. P., Giuliani, E. R., Fuster, V. Seward, J. B., Brandenburg, R. O., and McGoon, D. C.: Preoperative M-mode echocardiography as a predictor of surgical results in chronic aortic insufficiency. J. Thorac. Cardiovasc. Surg. *79*: 256, 1980.

536. Henry, W. L., Bonow, R. O., Rosing, D. R., and Epstein, S. E.: Observations on the optimum time for operative intervention for aortic regurgitation. II. Serial echocardiographic evaluation of asymptomatic patients. Circulation *61*: 484, 1980.

537. Toussaint, C., Cribier, A., Cazor, J. L., Soyer, R., and Letac, B.: Hemodynamic and angiographic evaluation of aortic regurgitation 8 and 27 months after aortic valve replacement. Circulation *64*:456, 1981.

538. Bonow, R. O., Rosing, D. R., Kent K. M., and Epstein, S. E.: Timing of operation for chronic aortic regurgitation. Am. J. Cardiol. *50*:325, 1982.

539. Henry, W. L., Bonow, R. O., Borer, J. S., Ware, J. H., Kent, K. M., Redwood, D. R., McIntosh, C. L., Morrow, A. G., and Epstein, S. E.: Observations on the optimum time for operative intervention for aortic regurgitation. I. Evaluation of the results of aortic valve replacement in symptomatic patients. Circulation *61*:471, 1980.

540. O'Rourke, R. A., and Crawford, M. H.: Timing of valve replacement in patients with chronic aortic regurgitation (Editorial). Circulation *61*:493, 1980.

541. Gaasch, W. H., Andrias, C. W., and Levine, H. J.: Chronic aortic regurgitation. The effect of aortic valve replacement on left ventricular volume, mass and function. Circulation *58*:825, 1978.

541a.Carroll, J. D., Gaasch, W. H., Naimi, S., and Levine, H. J.: Regression of myocardial hypertrophy: Electrocardiographic-echocardiographic correlations after aortic valve replacement in patients with chronic aortic regurgitation. Circulation *65*:980, 1982.

541b.Bonow, R. O., Rosing, D. R., Maron, B. J., Jones, M., McIntosh, C. L., and Epstein, S. E.: Reversal of left ventricular dysfunction after valve replacement in patients with aortic regurgitation. Influence of duration of preoperative left ventricular dysfunction. J. Am. Coll. Cardiol. *1*:639, 1983 (Abstr.).

541c.Pomar, J. L., Garcia-Dorado, D., Almazan, A., Betriu, A., Chaitman, B. R., and Pelletier, C.: Determinants of clinical status following valve replacement for pure aortic regurgitation. J. Am. Coll. Cardiol. *1*:586, 1983 (Abstr.).

541d.Carroll, J. D., Gaasch, W. H., Zile, M. R., and Levine, H. J.: Serial changes in left ventricular function after correction of chronic aortic regurgitation. Dependence on early changes in preload and subsequent regression of hypertrophy. Am. J. Cardiol. *51*:476, 1983.

542. Thompson, R., Ahmed, M., Seabra-Gomes, R., Ilsley, C., Rickards, A., Towers, M., and Yacoub, M.: Influence of preoperative left ventricular function on results of homograft replacement of the aortic valve for aortic regurgitation. J. Thorac. Cardiovasc. Surg. *77*:411, 1979.

543. Rahimtoola, S. H.: Valve replacement should *not* be performed in all asymptomatic patients with severe aortic incompetence. J. Thorac. Cardiovasc. Surg. *79*:163, 1980.

TRICUSPID AND PULMONIC VALVE DISEASE

544. Smith, J. A., and Levine, S. A.: Clinical features of tricuspid stenosis. Am. Heart. J. *23*:739, 1942.

545. Morgan, J. R., Forker, A. D., Coates, J. R., and Myers, W. S.: Isolated tricuspid stenosis. Circulation *44*:729, 1971.

546. Perloff, J. K., and Harvey, W. P.: The clinical recognition of tricuspid stenosis. Circulation *22*:346, 1960.

547. Killip, T., and Lukas, D. S.: Tricuspid stenosis. Clinical features in twelve cases. Am. J. Med. *24*:836, 1958.

548. Kitchin, A., and Turner, R.: Diagnosis and treatment of tricuspid stenosis. Br. Heart J. *26*:354, 1964.

549. Mahapatra, R. K., Agarwal, J. B., and Wasir, H. S.: Rheumatic tricuspid stenosis. Indian Heart J. *30*:138, 1978.

550. Joyner, C. R., Hey, B. E., Jr., Johnson, J., and Reid, J. M.: Reflected ultrasound in the diagnosis of tricuspid stenosis. Am. J. Cardiol. *19*:66, 1967.

550a.Daniels, S. J., Mintz, G. S., and Kotler, M. N.: Rheumatic tricuspid valve disease. Two-dimensional echocardiographic, hemodynamic, and angiographic correlations. Am. J. Cardio. *51*:492, 1983.

551. Mardelli, T. J., Morganroth, J., Chen, C. C., Naito, M., and Vergel, J.: Tricuspid valve prolapse diagnosed by cross-sectional echocardiography. Chest *79*: 201, 1981.

552. Veyrat, C., Kalmanson, D., Farjon, M., Manin, J. P., and Abitbol, G.: Noninvasive diagnosis and assessment of tricuspid regurgitation and stenosis using one and two dimensional echo-pulsed Doppler. Br. Heart J. *47*:596, 1982.

553. Péterffy, A., Jonasson, R., and Henze, A.: Haemdynamic changes after tricuspid valve surgery. Scand J. Thorac. Cardiovasc. Surg. *15*:161, 1981.

553a.Throburn, C. W., Morgan, J. J., Shanahan, M. X., and Chang, V. P.: Long-term results of tricuspid valve replacement and the problem of prosthetic valve thrombosis. Am. J. Cardiol. *51*:1128, 1983.

554. Zone, D. D., and Botti, R. E.: Right ventricular infarction with tricuspid insufficiency and chronic right heart failure. Am. J. Cardiol. *37*:445, 1976.

555. McAllister, R. G., Jr., Friesinger, G. C., and Sinclair-Smith, B. C.: Tricuspid regurgitation following inferior myocardial infarction. Arch. Intern. Med. *136*: 95, 1976.

556. Dougherty, M. J., and Craige, E.: Apathetic hyperthyroidism presenting as tricuspid regurgitation. Chest *63*:767, 1973.

557. Nelson, R. M., Bucciarelli, R. L., Eitzman, D. V., Egan, E. A., II, and Gessner, I. H.: Serum creatine phosphokinase MB fraction in newborns with transient tricuspid insufficiency. N. Engl. J. Med. *298*:146, 1978.

558. Esaghpour, E., Kawai, N., and Linhart, J. W.: Tricuspid insufficiency associated with aneurysm of the ventricular septum. Pediatrics *61*:586, 1978.

559. Chen, C. C., Morganroth, J., Mardelli, J. T., and Naito, M.: Tricuspid regurgitation in tricuspid valve prolapse demonstrated with contrast cross-sectional echocardiography. Am. J. Cardiol. *46*:983, 1980.

560. Chandraratna, P. A. N., Littman, B. B., and Wilson, D.: The association between atrial septal defect and prolapse of the tricuspid valve. An echocardiographic study. Chest *73*:839, 1978.

561. Bardy, G. H., Talano, J. V., Meyers, S., and Lesch, M.: Acquired cyanotic heart disease secondary to traumatic tricuspid regurgitation. Am. J. Cardiol. *44*:1401, 1979.

562. Ginzton, L. E., Siegel, R. J., and Criley, J. M.: Natural history of tricuspid valve endocarditis: A two-dimensional echocardiographic study. Am. J. Cardiol. *49*:1853, 1982.

563. Arbulu, A., and Asfaw, I.: Tricuspid valvulectomy without prosthetic replacement. Ten years of clinical experience. J. Thorac. Cardiovasc. Surg. *82*: 684, 1981.

564. Sethia, B., and Williams, B. T.: Tricuspid valve excision without replacement in a case of endocarditis secondary to drug abuse. Br. Heart J. *40*:579, 1978.

565. Gutierrez, F. R., McKnight, R. C., Jaffe, A. S., Ludbrook, P. A., Biello, D., and Weldon, C. S.: Double porcine valve replacement in carcinoid heart disease. Chest *81*:101, 1982.

566. Lie, J. T.: Carcinoid tumors, carcinoid syndrome, and carcinoid heart disease. Primary Cardiol. *8*:163, 1982.

567. Come, P. C., Come, S. E., Hawley, C. R., Gwon, N., and Riley, M. F.: Echocardiographic manifestations of carcinoid heart disease. J. Clin. Ultrasound *10*:233, 1982.

568. Baker, B. J., McNee, V. D., Scovil, J. A., Bass, K. M., Watson, J. W., and Bissett, J. K.: Tricuspid insufficiency in carcinoid heart disease: An echocardiographic description. Am. Heart J. *101*:107, 1981.

569. Roberts, W. C., and Sjoerdsma, A.: The cardiac disease associated with the carcinoid syndrome (carcinoid heart disease). Am. J. Med. *36*:5, 1964.

570. Pernot, C., Hoeffel, J. C., Henry, M., and Piwurca, A.: Case report of congenital tricuspid insufficiency. Cathet. Cardiovasc. Diagn. *4*:71, 1978.

571. Lingamneni, R., Cha, S. D., Maranhao, V., Booch, A. S., and Goldberg, H.: Tricuspid regurgitation: Clinical and angiographic assessment. Cathet. Cardiovasc. Diagn. *5*:7, 1979.

572. Cha, S. D., Gooch, A. S., and Maranhao, V.: Intracardiac phonocardiography in tricuspid regurgitation: Relation to clinical and angiographic findings. Am. J. Cardiol. *48*:578, 1981.

573. Sepulveda, G., and Lukas, D. S.: The diagnosis of tricuspid insufficiency: Clinical features in 60 cases with associated mitral valve disease. Circulation *11*: 552, 1955.

574. Seides, S. F., DeJoseph, R. L., Brown, A. E., and Damato, A. N.: Echocardiographic findings in isolated, surgically created tricuspid insufficiency. Am. J. Cardiol. *35*:679, 1975.

575. Chandraratna, P. A., Lopez, J. M., Fernandez, J. J., and Cohen, L. S.: Echocardiographic detection of tricuspid valve prolapse. Circulation *51*:823, 1975.

576. Lieppe, W., Behar, V. S., Scallion, R., and Kisslo, J. A.: Detection of tricuspid regurgitation with two-dimensional echocardiography and peripheral vein injections. Circulation 57:128, 1978.

577. Meltzer, R. S., van Hoogenhuyze, D., Serruys, P. W., Haalebos, M. M. P., Hugenholtz, P. G., and Roelandt, J.: Diagnosis of tricuspid regurgitation by contrast echocardiography. Circulation 63:1093, 1981.

578. Tei, C., Shah, P. M., and Ormiston, J. A.: Assessment of tricuspid regurgitation by directional analysis of right atrial systolic linear reflux echoes with contrast M-mode echocardiography. Am. Heart J. 103:1025, 1982.

579. McCord, M. C., and Blount, S. G., Jr.: The hemodynamic pattern in tricuspid valve disease. Am. Heart J. 44:671, 1952.

580. Rubeiz, G. A., Nassar, M. E., and Dagher, I. K.: Study of the right atrial pressure pulse in functional tricuspid regurgitation and normal sinus rhythm. Circulation 30:190, 1964.

581. Hansing, C. E., and Rowe, G. G.: Tricuspid insufficiency. A study of hemodynamics and pathogenesis. Circulation 45:793, 1972.

582. Pepino, C. J., Nichols, W. W., and Selby, J. H.: Diagnostic tests for tricuspid insufficiency: How good? Cathet. Cardiovasc. Diagn. 5:1, 1979.

583. Lingameni, R., Cha, S. D., Maranhao, V., Gooch, A. S. and Goldberg, H.: Tricuspid regurgitation: Clinical and angiographic assessment. Cathet. Cardiovasc. Diagn. 5:7, 1979.

584. Ubago, J. L., Figueroa, A., Colman, T., Ochoteco, A., Rodriguez, M., and Duran, C. M. G.: Right ventriculography as a valid method for the diagnosis of tricuspid insufficiency. Cathet. Cardiovasc. Diagn. 7:433, 1981.

585. Carpentier, A., Deloche, A., and Dauptain, J.: A new reconstructive operation for correction of mitral and tricuspid insufficiency. J. Thorac. Cardiovasc. Surg. 61:1, 1971.

586. Peterffy, A., Jonasson, R., Szamosi, A., and Henze, A.: Comparison of Kay's and DeVega's annuloplasty in surgical treatment of tricuspid incompetence. Clinical and haemodynamic results in 62 patients. Scand. J. Thorac. Cardiovasc. Surg. 14:249, 1980.

587. Duran, C. M. G., Pomar, J. L., Colman, T., Figueroa, A., Revuelta, J. M., and Ubago, J. L.: Is tricuspid valve repair necessary? J. Thorac. Cardiovasc. Surg. 80:849, 1980.

588. Carpentier, A., Deloche, A., Hanania, G., Furman, J., Sellier, P., Piwnica, A., and Dubost, C.: Surgical management of acquired tricuspid valve disease. J. Thorac. Cardiovasc. Surg. 67:53, 1974.

589. Breyer, R. H., McClenathan, J. H., Michaelis, L. L., McIntosh, C. L., and Morrow, A. G.: Tricuspid regurgitation. A comparison of nonoperative management, tricuspid annuloplasty, and tricuspid valve replacement. J. Thorac. Cardiovasc. Surg. 72:867, 1976.

590. Korr, K. S., Levinson, H., Bough, E. W., Gheorghiade, M., Stone, J., McEnany, M. T., and Shulman, N. R.: Tricuspid valve replacement for cardiogenic shock after acute right ventricular infarction. J.A.M.A. 244:1958, 1980.

591. Vela, J. E., Conteras, R., and Sosa, F. R.: Rheumatic pulmonary valve disease. Am. J. Cardiol. 23:12, 1969.

592. Seymour, J., Emaneul, R., and Patterson, N.: Acquired pulmonary stenosis. Br. Heart J. 30:776, 1968.

593. Runco, V., and Levin, H. S.: The spectrum of pulmonic regurgitation. In Physiologic Principles of Heart Sounds and Murmurs. American Heart Association Monograph No. 46, 1975, p. 175.

594. Brayshaw, J. R., and Perloff, J. K.: Congenital pulmonary insufficiency complicating idiopathic dilatation of the pulmonary artery. Am. J. Cardiol. 10:282, 1962.

595. Childers, R. W., and McCrea, P. C.: Absence of the pulmonary valve. A case occurring in the Marfan's syndrome. Circulation 29:598, 1964.

596. Hamby, R. I., and Gulotta, S. J.: Pulmonic valvular insufficiency: Etiology, recognition and management. Am. Heart J. 74:110, 1967.

597. Harris, B. C., Shaver, J. A., Kroetz, F. W., and Leonard, J. J.: Congenital pulmonary valvular insufficiency complicating tetralogy of Fallot. Intracardiac sound and pressure correlates. Am. J. Cardiol. 23:864, 1969.

598. Holmes, J. C., Fowler, N. O., and Kaplan, S.: Pulmonary valvular insufficiency. Am. J. Med. 44:851, 1968.

599. Osman, M. Z., Meng, C. C. L., and Girdany, B. R.: Congenital absence of the pulmonary valve: Report of eight cases with review of the literature. Am. J. Roentgenol. 106:58, 1969.

600. Layton, C. A., McDonald, A., McDonald, L., Towers, M., Weaver, J., and Yacoub, M.: The syndrome of absent pulmonary valve. Total correction with aortic valvular homografts. J. Thorac. Cardiovasc. Surg. 63:800, 1972.

601. Emery, R. W., Landes, R. G., Moller, J. H., and Nicoloff, D. M.: Pulmonary valve replacement with a porcine aortic heterograft. Ann. Thorac. Surg. 27:148, 1979.

602. Hurwitz, L. E., and Roberts, W. C.: Quadricuspid semilunar valve. Am. J. Cardiol. 31:623, 1973.

603. Collins, N. P., Braunwald, E., and Morrow, A. G.: Isolated congenital pulmonic valvular regurgitation. Am. J. Med. 28:159, 1960.

604. Levin, H. S., Runca, V., Wooley, C. F., and Ryan, J. M.: Pulmonic regurgitation following staphylococcal endocarditis. An intracardiac phonocardiographic study. Circulation 30:411, 1964.

605. O'Toole, J. D., Wurtzbacher, J. J., Wearner, N. E., and Jain, A. C.: Pulmonary valve injury and insufficiency during pulmonary-artery catheterization. N. Engl. J. Med. 301:1167, 1979.

606. Jacoby, W. J., Tucker, D. H., and Sumner, R. G.: The second heart sound in congenital pulmonary valvular insufficiency. Am. Heart J. 69:603, 1965.

607. Bousvaros, G. A., and Deuchar, D. C.: The murmur of pulmonary regurgitation which is not associated with pulmonary hypertension. Lancet 2:962, 1961.

608. Green, E. W., Agruss, N. S., and Adolph, R. J.: Right-sided Austin Flint murmur. Documentation by intracardiac phonocardiography, echocardiography and postmortem findings. Am. J. Cardiol. 32:370, 1973.

609. Braunwald, E., and Morrow, A. G.: A method for detection and estimation of aortic regurgitant flow in man. Circulation 17:505, 1958.

610. Runco, V., Molnar, W., Meckstroth, C. V., and Ryan, J. M.: The Graham Steell murmur versus aortic regurgitation in rheumatic heart disease. Results of aortic valvulography. Am. J. Med. 31:71, 1961.

611. Pernot, C., Hoeffel, J. C., Henry, M., Worms, A. M., Stehlin, H., and Louis, J. P.: Radiological patterns of congenital absence of the pulmonary valve in infants. Radiology 102:619, 1972.

612. Collins, N. P., Braunwald, E., and Morrow, A. G.: Detection of pulmonic and tricuspid valvular regurgitation by means of indicator solutions. Circulation 20:561, 1959.

613. Levin, H. S., Runco, V., Wooley, C. F., and Ryan, J. M.: Intracardiac phonocardiography in organic pulmonic insufficiency. Circulation 24:980, 1961.

614. Miyatake, K., Okamoto, M., Kinoshita, N., Matsuhisa, M., Nagata, S., Beppu, S., Park, Y.-D., Sakakibara, H., and Nimura, Y.: Pulmonary regurgitation studied with the ultrasonic pulsed Doppler technique. Circulation 65:969, 1982.

MULTIVALVULAR DISEASE

615. Honey, M.: Clinical and hemodynamic observations on combined mitral and aortic stenosis. Br. Heart J. 23:545, 1961.

616. Schattenberg, T. T., Titus, J. L., and Parkin, T. W.: Clinical findings in acquired aortic valve stenosis. Effect of disease of other valves. Am. Heart J. 73:322, 1967.

617. Melvin, D. B., Tecklenberg, P. L., Hollingsworth, J. F., Levine, F. H., Glancy, D. L., Epstein, S. E., and Morrow, A. G.: Computer-based analysis of preoperative and postoperative prognostic factors in 100 patients with combined aortic and mitral valve replacement. Circulation 48(Suppl. III):58, 1973.

618. Nitter-Hauge, S., Frøysaker, T., Enge, I., and Rostad, H.: Clinical and haemodynamic observations after combined aortic and mitral valve replacement with the Björk-Shiley tilting disc valve prosthesis: Early and late results in 25 patients. Scand. J. Thorac. Cardiovasc. Surg. 13:25, 1979.

619. Baxley, W. A., and Soto, B.: Hemodynamic evaluation of patients with combined mitral and aortic prostheses. Am. J. Cardiol. 45:42, 1980.

620. Isom, O. W., Spencer, F. C., Glassman, E., Teiko, P., Boyd, A. D., Cunningham, J. N., and Reed, G. E.: Long-term results in 1375 patients undergoing valve replacement with the Starr-Edwards cloth-covered steel ball prosthesis. Ann. Surg. 186:310,1977.

621. Cohn, L. H., Koster, J. K., Mee, R. B. B., and Collins, J. J., Jr.: Long-term followup of the Hancock bioprosthetic heart valve. A 6-year review. Circulation 60(Suppl. II):93, 1979.

622. Stephenson, L. W., Kouchoukos, N. T., and Kirlin, J. W.: Triple valve replacement: An analysis of eight years' experience. Ann. Thorac. Surg. 23:327, 1977.

623. MacManus, Q., Grunkemeier, G., and Starr, A.: Late results of triple valve replacement: A 14-year review. Ann. Thorac. Surg. 25:402, 1978.

624. Péterffy, A., Jonasson, R., and Björk, V. O.: Ten years' experience of surgical management of triple valve disease. Early and late results in thirty-four consecutive cases. Scand. J. Thorac. Cardiovasc. Surg. 13:191, 1979.

624a. Vatterott, P. J., Gersh, B. J., Fuster, V., Schaff, H. V., Danielson, G. K., Pluth, J. R., and McGoon, D. C.: Long-term followup (2–20 years) of patients with triple valve replacement. J. Am. Coll. Cardiol. 1:586, 1983 (Abstr.).

625. Rhodes, G. R., McIntosh, C. L., Redwood, D. R., Itscoitz, S. B., and Epstein, S. E.: Clinical and hemodynamic results following triple valve replacement: Mechanical vs. procine xenograft prostheses. Circulation 56(Suppl. II):122, 1977.

33 INFECTIVE ENDOCARDITIS

by Louis Weinstein, M.D., Ph.D.

HISTORY

Probably the first description of endocarditis was recorded by Lazare Riviere in 1646.[1] His patient sought his attention because of "palpitation of the heart." Riviere "found the pulse, small, irregular, with every variety of irregularity." The patient developed severe dyspnea and edema of the legs, gradually became more ill, produced bloody sputum, and died. The following findings were noted at autopsy: "In the left ventricle of the heart, round carunculae were found like the substance of the lungs, the larger of which resembled a cluster of hazel nuts and filled up the opening of the aorta."

In 1883, Eichorst published the first clinical classification of the different forms of endocarditis.[1] He defined the different presentations of the disease as *acute* (septic), *subacute* (endocarditis verrucosa), and *chronic* (endocarditis retrahens). With the possible exception of the last, this classification remains standard. In his Gulstonian lectures in 1885,[2] Osler pointed out that about 75 per cent of patients who developed bacterial endocarditis had underlying damage to the cardiac valves. He described the clinical and pathological features of the disease in detail and commented that "micrococci are constant elements in the vegetations." Interest in subacute bacterial endocarditis among physicians in the United States was stimulated by the publication of the classic paper of Libman and Celler in 1910.[3] They reported their observations in 43 cases of the disease and presented detailed descriptions of the causative organisms.

No effective means of treatment were available, however. Sulfonamides were used to treat bacterial endocarditis after their introduction in 1937, but results were poor; only 4 to 6 per cent of patients were said to have been cured.[4,5] These drugs probably played a much more important role in reducing the risk of valvular infections by controlling extracardiac disease produced by the pneumococcus, *Strep-tococcus pyogenes*, gonococcus, and bacteremia caused by sensitive organisms.

A new era in the natural history of infective endocarditis began in 1943 and 1944 with the reports by Florey and Florey[6] and Loewe et al.[7] of the successful cure of the subacute form of the disease with penicillin. As more and more antimicrobial agents have become available over the ensuing years, it has become possible to treat a broader variety of etiologically different types of infective endocarditis effectively. In more recent years a number of other features—microbiological, immunological, and therapeutic—have altered the course and management of this disease. Among these are the increasingly frequent involvement of unusual organisms, the increase in infections of the right side of the heart (related primarily to the wide use of intravenously administered illicit drugs such as heroin), the longer life spans of patients, a striking change in the types of cardiac disease on which valvular infection is superimposed, and a striking increase in and knowledge of the immunological phenomena that contribute to complications of infective endocarditis. An important new aspect of this disease has been the development of and increasing experience with cardiac surgery, which may be responsible for valvular infections (prosthesis) or be the critical maneuver in the cure of the infection (both natural and prosthetic valves) or which may be responsible for the management of potential complications such as intractable congestive failure or intracardiac complications such as abscesses, aneurysms, and the like.

The incidence of infective endocarditis in the United States in 1936 was reported by Hedley to have been 4000 to 5000 cases, or 4.2 per 100,000 of the population.[8] Approximately 70 per cent of all cases were of the subacute variety. These data in the preantibiotic era are comparable to the experience in Great Britain, where an annual average of 964 cases of bacterial endocarditis was reported in the years 1924 to 1944.[9]

Kaye and his colleagues noted a marked decrease in the incidence of infective endocarditis.[10] They suggested that the factors responsible for this were (a) widespread use of antibiotics in all types of infections, (b) chemoprophylaxis for patients with rheumatic or congenital heart disease, and (c) the tendency to refer patients with valvular infections to "referral" teaching hospitals. A fall in the number of cases admitted to large municipal hospitals has been reported by Finland[11] and Afremow.[12] However, Cherubin and Neu noted no change in the incidence of the disease over a period of 30 years (1938 to 1967).[13] In contrast, Lerner and Weinstein suggested that there has been a definite *increase* in the frequency of this disease over the past 25 years.[14] When the increase in the number of factors proven to predispose to the development of infective endocarditis is considered, it seems likely to this author that the incidence of the disease has increased and continues to do so. Thus, although there is still some controversy concerning the present incidence of infective endocarditis, there is general agreement that there has been a change in its distributions at various levels.

Though involving primarily young adults in the preantibiotic era, the disease now affects chiefly older individuals, as emphasized by analysis of data obtained from study at necropsy. Thus, the mean age of patients with subacute bacterial endocarditis has increased from 32 years of age in the 1930's and 1940's [16] to 40 to 42 years in the 1950's[17,18] and to 50 to 54 years in the 1960's.[15-20] Endocarditis remains an uncommon disease in the first decade of life but is becoming increasingly common in the 60- to 80-year age group.[14] Endocarditis affecting infants under the age of two years is usually of the acute variety and attacks normal valves, with a predilection for the tricuspid valve. There is a striking difference in the sex distribution of infective endocarditis. A male-female ratio of 2 to 1 was noted by Lerner and Weinstein.[14] However, in patients 51 to 60 years of age, this ratio increased to 9:1.

The etiological agents responsible for all types of bacterial endocarditis have changed since the advent of penicillin therapy. The number of acute cases due to pneumococcus, gonococcus, meningococcus, and group A hemolytic streptococci decreased strikingly in the first decade of antibiotic therapy; there was a relative, but not absolute, increase in nonhemolytic streptococcal cases. In the second decade of the antibiotic era, an increase in cases due to *Staphylococcus aureus* became apparent.[14a]

MICROBIOLOGY OF ENDOCARDITIS

Infective endocarditis has usually been classified primarily as acute or subacute according to the nature of the responsible organism. Thus, when *Staphylococcus aureus, Streptococcus pneumoniae, Neisseria meningitidis, Neisseria gonorrhoeae, Strep. pyogenes,* and *Hemophilus influenzae* are the causative agents, the endocarditis is considered acute. In contrast, when viridans streptococcus or *Staph. epidermidis* is recovered from the blood, the infection is called subacute. This clinical differentiation remains important because the presenting manifestations, the duration of the course, the nature of the complications, and the final outcome differ greatly, even when appropriate antimicrobial therapy and other therapeutic modalities are applied. It has become clear, however, that there is an appreciable number of instances in which no relation to the invading organism exists. For this reason, Lerner and Weinstein suggested that the designations *acute* and *subacute* be abolished, because disease that is originally acute may be converted to subacute status by appropriate therapy, while subacute disease may suddenly become life-threatening when serious complications develop.[14] In addition, they and others[21-23] have studied patients with valvular infections caused by *Staph. aureus* with a consistently subacute course as well as other patients infected with *Streptococcus viridans* in whom clinical behavior was entirely acute; this has been true especially in some instances of enterococcal disease.

The microbiology of infective endocarditis is summarized in Table 33–1.

MICROBIOLOGY OF INFECTIONS OF PROSTHETIC VALVES

Infections of prosthetic valves have involved a large number of microbes, some of which have been associated only with this kind of disease. The bulk of microorganisms responsible for invasion of cardiac prostheses is, however, the same as those that cause infection of natural valves. For example, *Staph. aureus, Staph. epidermidis,* various streptococci, *Hemophilus, Brucella,* and *Candida* are known to invade prosthetic as well as natural valves. Among those that have been involved primarily in infection of valvular prostheses are gram-negative bacteria such as *Serratia, Acinetobacter calcoaceticus, Pseudomonas cepacia, Ps. aeruginosa, Ps. multophilia, Flavobacterium, Bacteroides, Edwardsiella tarda,* and *Eikenella corrodens.* Gram-positive organisms that invade prosthetic rather than natural valves include groups B, D, and K streptococci. *Staph. epidermidis* affects patients with prostheses more often than it does those who have not had valves replaced, and it is the most frequent cause of disease early after operation. When prosthetic infection occurs late, both staphylococci and streptococci are commonly involved; however, *Staph. epidermidis* is much more common than *Staph. aureus* in necropsied cases. Most instances of endocarditis due to *Propionibacterium acnes, Bacteroides,* and *Eikenella corrodens* have occurred in individuals with cardiac prostheses.

Valvular disease caused by the atypical mycobacteria *Mycobacterium chelonei* and *M. gordonae* has been observed only when cardiac bioprostheses (porcine valves [Table 33–1]) have been present.

The recent striking increase in the incidence of endocarditis caused by yeasts and fungi is attributable almost entirely to the presence of valvular prostheses, to the increased number of patients addicted to drugs administered intravenously, and to long-term antimicrobial therapy. The organisms most commonly involved are *Candida, Aspergillus,* and *Histoplasma.* Among the species of *Candida* recovered from infected prostheses have been *albicans, parapsilosis, tropicalis, stellatoidea,* and *krusei* (Table 33–1).

An appreciable number of infections involving prosthetic valves—especially those caused by unusual bacteria, yeasts, and fungi—are probably superinfections induced by antimicrobial chemoprophylaxis or therapy. Organisms may also be introduced into the bloodstream during intravenous injection of drugs in addicted persons.

Cumulative experience indicates that aortic valve prostheses are more frequently infected than prostheses replacing other valves. One study of prosthetic endocarditis demonstrated infection in 3 per cent of patients in whom the aortic valve was replaced versus 1 per cent of those with mitral valve prostheses.[111] Infection of combined mitral and aortic valve prostheses is not uncommon. Complications of infected prostheses include ruptured mycotic aneurysms, ruptured aorta, ruptured aneurysm of the sinus of Valsalva, perivalvular abscess, myocardial abscess, pericardio-mediastinal fistula, abscess of the atrioventricular ring, and thrombosis of the prosthesis.

TABLE 33–1   MICROBIOLOGY OF ENDOCARDITIS

<table>
<tr><td colspan="2" align="center">GRAM-POSITIVE COCCI</td></tr>
<tr><td>Streptococcus viridans</td><td>Responsible for 50% of all cases of endocarditis, 70% of subacute disease. Three instances of progressive, invasive disease.[24] Predisposing factors: trauma; dental manipulations (extractions, flossing, gingivectomy, periapical abscess, Water-Pik). May produce disease in edentulous patients.[25] Usually produces subacute disease, rarely acute.</td></tr>
<tr><td>Enterococcus</td><td>Member of group D streptococci. May produce α, β, or γ hemolysis. Species: Strep. liquefaciens, Strep. zymogenes, Strep. faecalis, Strep. faecium, Strep. durans. Source of organisms: GU and GI tracts and oral cavity. Causes 3–17% of cases of endocarditis. Course of the disease acute or subacute.</td></tr>
<tr><td>Streptococcus bovis</td><td>Member of group D, but not an enterococcus. Responsible for about 50% of cases caused by group D streptococci.[26] Fails to grow in medium containing 6.5% saline. Sensitive to penicillin G. Survival rate higher than with enterococcus. High degree of association of endocarditis with cancer of the colon, Crohn's disease, ulcerative colitis.[27–30]</td></tr>
<tr><td>Peptostreptococcus</td><td>Anaerobe—causes 3–8.5% of cases.[17] Requires culture under anaerobic conditions (thioglycollate broth). Produces mostly subacute disease, occasionally acute.</td></tr>
<tr><td>Streptococcus pyogenes
(group A, "beta-hemolytic")</td><td>Currently an uncommon cause of endocarditis, probably because of high rate of successful treatment of pharyngitis, cellulitis, and other extracardiac foci of infection. Although organism usually produces "beta-hemolysis," some strains may be alpha-hemolytic on surface of blood agar. Clinical course of valvular infection is acute. May produce intracardiac complications, e.g., rupture of valve leaflets.</td></tr>
<tr><td>Streptococcus pneumoniae</td><td>Frequency of endocarditis decreasing because of highly successful therapy of pneumonia and other extracardiac infections caused by this organism. Current incidence about 5 to 6%.[31] Disease is usually acute. High frequency of destructive intracardiac complications. Increased risk of valvular infection in patients with multilobar pulmonary involvement and bacteremia.</td></tr>
<tr><td>Other Species of Streptococci</td><td>Strep. mutans.[32] Group G.[33] Group C—uncommon, acute disease, with destruction of valves.[34] Organism may be "tolerant" to penicillin G.[35] Strep. constellatus—only one case reported.[36] Group B[37]—involves mitral valve most commonly; next is aortic valve. Groups D, G, and K.[38] Group L.[39]</td></tr>
<tr><td>Nutritionally-Deficient Streptococci ("satelliting" streptococci)</td><td>Uncommon. Require pyridoxine for growth. Thioglycollate broth plus pyridoxine is good medium. Colonies group around colonies of Staph. aureus (satelliting). Grow in ordinary broth, but cannot be subcultured from these or agar.[40]</td></tr>
<tr><td>Staphylococcus aureus</td><td>Commonest organism producing acute endocarditis. Predisposing factors: cardiac surgery, intravenous abuse of drugs, infections of the skin, osteomyelitis, peripheral sepsis, rheumatic carditis (rare). No underlying cardiac disease in 50 to 60% of cases. No murmurs in presence of endocarditis in about 1/3 of patients. High frequency of intracardiac complications: rupture of valvular leaflets, septal abscesses, aneurysm of sinus of Valsalva, myocardial abscesses. Disseminated extracardiac infections common. Proved staphylococcal bacteremia in absence of evidence of endocarditis is associated with risk of valvular infection in 30 to 65% of cases.[41] Most strains are resistant to penicillin G. Treatment with a penicillinase-resistant penicillin or an active cephalosporin is required. Some strains are "methicillin-resistant" ("tolerant") and fail to be killed by penicillins and cephalosporins. Replacement of infected valve with a prosthesis is often required. Average fatality rate about 50%.</td></tr>
<tr><td>Staphylococcus epidermidis ("albus")</td><td>Incidence has increased over the past 25 years. Occasionally involves normal valves; most patients have underlying valvular disease. Common in "main-line" drug addicts. Thought to be commonest organism infecting prosthetic valves. Produces subacute and chronic endocarditis. High incidence of recurrence after "appropriate" antimicrobial therapy. May require replacement of involved valve. Organism variably sensitive to antibiotics. Fatality rate high.[42]</td></tr>
<tr><td colspan="2" align="center">GRAM-POSITIVE BACILLI</td></tr>
<tr><td>Erysipelothrix insidiosa</td><td>Acquired from fish, birds, cats. May involve normal heart. Disease is acute. Fatality rate 50%.[43]</td></tr>
<tr><td>Lactobacillus</td><td>Dental procedures predisposing factor. May be no underlying cardiac disease.[44,45]</td></tr>
<tr><td>Listeria monocytogenes</td><td>Rare. Involves natural and prosthetic valves. High incidence of systemic embolization.[46]</td></tr>
<tr><td>Corynebacteria</td><td>Aerobic diphtheroids and anaerobic Propionibacterium acnes. Uncommon cause of endocarditis.[47,48]</td></tr>
<tr><td>Corynebacterium diphtheriae</td><td>Rare cause of endocarditis. Only 8 cases (1944–1980). Not all strains produce toxin. Increased susceptibility with congenital heart disease.[49,50]</td></tr>
<tr><td>Bacillus cereus</td><td>Only two reported cases. Has involved only prosthetic valves.[51]</td></tr>
<tr><td>Bacillus subtilis</td><td>Only one reported case. Drug addict—right heart involved.[52]</td></tr>
<tr><td>Rothia dentocariosa</td><td>Only two reported cases of endocarditis. Produces subacute disease.[53,54]</td></tr>
<tr><td colspan="2" align="center">GRAM-NEGATIVE COCCI</td></tr>
<tr><td>Neisseria gonorrhoeae</td><td>Caused 10 to 14% of cases in preantibiotic era[55]; now uncommon. Not always related to genital infection. Aortic and mitral valves involved most often. High incidence of infection of right heart. Arthritis in 50% of cases. No underlying heart disease in most patients. One patient with prolapsed mitral valve described.[56] Frequent intra- and extracardiac complications requiring surgery. Recent increase in number of penicillin-resistant strains.</td></tr>
<tr><td>Neisseria meningitidis</td><td>Rare. Always secondary to bacteremia, with or without meningitis. Acute endocarditis.</td></tr>
<tr><td>Other Gram-negative Cocci</td><td>N. flava, N. catarrhalis, N. pharyngis, N. mucosa,[14] Megasphaera elsdenii (anaerobe).[57]</td></tr>
<tr><td colspan="2" align="center">GRAM-NEGATIVE BACILLI</td></tr>
<tr><td>Escherichia coli</td><td>Responsible for about 3 to 10% of endocarditis. For a recent detailed review, see Ref. 58. Murmur not always present. Mitral valve most often involved.[59]</td></tr>
<tr><td>Enterobacter</td><td>Uncommon. Manipulation of genitourinary tract predisposing factor is 50% of cases.[60]</td></tr>
<tr><td>Klebsiella pneumoniae</td><td>Very rare. Preceding infection of urinary tract.[61]</td></tr>
<tr><td>Proteus</td><td>Rare. Both indole-positive and indole-negative strains involved. Infection of urinary tract predisposing factor.[62]</td></tr>
<tr><td>Pseudomonas aeruginosa</td><td>Most common in drug addicts. In nonaddicted, occurs most often during therapy of another infection (superinfection). Emboli produce necrosis of walls of blood vessels. Tricuspid valve commonly involved. Infection of more than one valve not rare.[63,64]</td></tr>
<tr><td>Other Species of Pseudomonas</td><td>Ps. multophilia,[65] Ps. cepacia.[66]</td></tr>
<tr><td>Salmonella</td><td>Uncommon cause of endocarditis. Most patients over 50 years old. Underlying cardiac disease in most instances. Course often acute. GI tract source of organism in <50% of patients. Fatality rate high, even when treated.[67]</td></tr>
<tr><td>Hemophilus</td><td>Responsible for about 0.5% of cases of endocarditis. Three species involved: H. influenzae,[68] H. parainfluenzae,[69] and H. aphrophilus.[70] High frequency of embolization with H. parainfluenzae.</td></tr>
</table>

TABLE 33–1   MICROBIOLOGY OF ENDOCARDITIS *(Continued)*

Brucella	Rare. Species involved: *Br. abortus, Br. suis, Br. melitensis.* Underlying heart disease in most cases. Mitral valve most often involved. Occasionally acute. Bulky vegetations.[71]
Pasteurella	Rare. Usual source is animal bite or scratch. Cats and dogs carry organism. Three species: *P. multocida* (commonest),[72] *P. pneumotropica, P. hemolytica.*
Acinetobacter	May involve normal heart. Acute or subacute disease. Cardiac failure and embolization in > 50% of cases. Fatality rate 50–75%.[73]
Serratia	75% of cases in drug addicts. Infection of prosthetic valves common. Subacute course commonest. Large emboli in most instances. Fatality rate about 70%.[74]
Campylobacter (Vibrio)	One species, *fetus.* May involve normal heart. Dental manipulation a predisposing factor. Aortic valve usually affected.[75]
Streptobacillus moniliformis	Rare. Endocarditis occurs during course of rat bite fever.[76]
Cardiobacterium hominis	Uncommon. Organism present in pharynx of 70% of normal people. Usually involves abnormal valves. Course subacute. Emboli in 50% of cases.[77]
Actinobacillus actinomycetemcomitans	Most common in middle-aged and older men. Normal valves involved in 2/3 of cases. Course subacute. Organism grows slowly.[78]
Flavobacterium	Only one case reported. Ulceration of aortic valve.[79]
Edwardsiella tarda	Single case report.[80]
Citrobacter diversus	Single case.[81]

YEASTS AND FUNGI

Yeasts	Species of *Candida* involved: *C. albicans, C. parapsilosis, C. guilliermondii, C. krusei, C. stellatoidea, C. tropicalis* (commonest cause in drug addicts). One third of cases follow cardiac surgery. 20% related to superinfection. Course subacute. Emboli in 50% of patients—occlude large arteries. Blood cultures negative in 75% of cases.[82-84] *Torulopsis glabrata.*[85]
Histoplasma capsulatum	Uncommon. Most cases in eastern U.S., Ohio, and Mississippi Valley. Involves natural and prosthetic valves. Embolus to large artery may be first sign. Cultures of blood usually negative.[86]
Aspergillus	Various species involved. All cases in debilitated or immunocompromised patients or those treated with antibiotics. Prosthetic valves most commonly involved. Infection or mural endocardium common. Blood cultures rarely positive.[87]
Other Yeasts and Fungi	*Penicillium, Phialophora, Hormodendrum, Paecilomyces, Curvilacea, Saccharomyces, Mucor, Torulopsis glabrata, Trichosporon cutaneum, Cryptococcus, Rhodotorula.*[88-90]

OTHER ORGANISMS

Mycobacterium chelonei	Porcine bioprostheses involved. Organisms cultured from the valves prior to insertion.[91]
Mycobacterium gordonae	An atypical mycobacterium—one instance of infection of a prosthetic valve.[92]
Mycobacterium tuberculosis	Usually involves only natural valves as a complication of disseminated tuberculosis.[93] Infection of homograft valves reported.[94]
Coxiella burnetii (Q fever)	All cases of endocarditis have occurred in the course of Q fever. Very few reported from the United States; all others in Australia and New Zealand. Duration of Q fever before development of endocarditis—1 to 20 years. Diagnosis made by detection of rising titer of phase-1 complement-fixing antibody.[95]
Actinomyces israelii (bovis)	Infection by this organism very rare.[96] Both natural and prosthetic valves involved.
Nocardia israelii	Very rare.[97] Both natural and prosthetic valves involved.
Bacteroides	Several species involved. Only 11 reported cases. Usually subacute but may be acute. Infects both prosthetic and natural valves.[98,99]
Fusobacterium	Only 10 reported cases. May be fulminant.[98]
Chlamydia psittaci	Infection not proved by isolation of the organism. Contact with birds important. Diagnosis made by staining endocardial biopsies with fluorescein-labeled specific antibody.[100]
Chlamydia trachomatis	Infection or aortic valve in one case; complicated by pericarditis.[101]
Cell Wall–Deficient Organisms	Possible but not proved cause of endocarditis. Thought to be responsible for fever persisting despite appropriate therapy. Commonest in drug addicts and in patients undergoing cardiac surgery.[102,103]
Polymicrobial Infection	Incidence from 1 in 250 to 1 in 10.[104,105] More than 2 organisms in some cases.[14] Mostly mixtures of gram-positive cocci, or these with gram-negative rods or yeast.
Virus	Indirect evidence. One case of serologically proved coxsackievirus B endocarditis.[106]

ENDOCARDITIS ASSOCIATED WITH DRUG ADDICTION

Staph. aureus	Incidence higher than in nonaddicted patients. Right side of heart involved more often. Commonest organism.[107]
Streptococci	*Strep. viridans, Strep. faecalis,* enterococcus.[108]
Other Bacteria	Various species of *Pseudomonas,* aerobic and anaerobic diphtheroids. *Staph. epidermidis, Hemophilus, Strep. pneumoniae,* anaerobes and gram-negative organisms.[109,110]
Yeasts and Fungi	*Histoplasma, Saccharomyces, Paecilomyces, Mucor, Cryptococcus, Candida, Aspergillus.* 5% of patients.[105]
Polymicrobial Infection	Reported to range from 1 case in 250 up to as high as 5%. Mixtures of different streptococci, other gram-positive cocci with gram-negative rods, gram-negative bacilli, and/or yeasts and fungi.[104,105]

PATHOLOGY OF ENDOCARDITIS

Vegetations are common to all types of infective endocarditis and are situated most frequently on the valvular leaflets and less often on the endocardium of the ventricles or of the left atrium (McCallum's patch of rheumatic carditis) and on pulmonary or other arteries. When fresh, the vegetations are pink, red, yellow, or green but change to gray as they heal. These lesions are usually larger and much more friable than those of rheumatic fever; small particles are easily broken off and become disseminated in the blood stream as emboli. The largest vegetations develop in the course of fungal infections of the valves; emboli that arise from these are large enough to occlude large arteries, a distinguishing characteristic of this type of endocarditis (Fig. 33–1). Occasionally, the vegetations formed during infection by *Staph. aureus* are larger than those associated with alpha-streptococci. In some instances of infection of prosthetic valves and, less often, when staphylococci or some gram-negative organisms are involved, valvular lesions may be of such a size that they obstruct the valve orifice, sharply reduce cardiac output, and lead to congestive heart failure.

Infective endocarditis involves the left side of the heart much more frequently than the right, affecting the mitral, aortic, or both valves, in that order.[112] Disease of the pul-

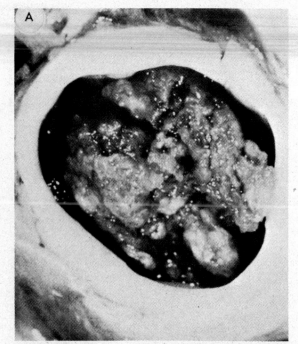

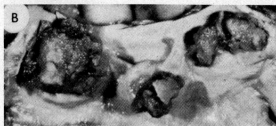

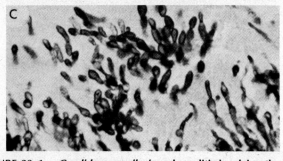

FIGURE 33–1   *Candida parapsilosis* endocarditis involving the aortic valve led to an embolus to the left anterior descending coronary artery with a large transmural acute myocardial infarct two months before death. *A,* Aortic valve viewed from above. The large vegetations appear to obstruct the valve orifice. *B,* Opened valve showing vegetations on each cusp. *C,* Photomicrograph of vegetation showing pseudomycelia of *C. parapsilosis.* (Methenamine silver stain.) (From Roberts, W. C., and Buchbinder, N. A.: Healed left-sided infective endocarditis. A clinicopathological study of 59 patients. Am. J. Cardiol. *40:*876, 1976.)

monic and tricuspid valves is relatively uncommon; however, the latter has increased over the past 15 years with the rise in drug addiction. Although much more common in acute than in subacute valvular infections, vegetations on the mitral valve may extend along the chordae tendineae to the apex of the papillary muscles. This may lead to rupture of these structures, especially in acute infections. Rupture is rare in subacute endocarditis unless the infection has remained untreated for a prolonged period. This is also the case when aortic valvular vegetations spread by

contiguity along the ventricular endocardium or when ulcerated lesions appear on the ventricular surface of the anterior mitral cusp.

Necrosis of the affected valve may lead to aneurysms and/or perforation of the cusps. This occurs most often in acute infective endocarditis, especially that caused by *Staph. aureus,* but only rarely in subacute valvular infections. In addition to aneurysms of the sinus of Valsalva, these lesions, when present at the base of the aorta, may extend into the pericardial space between the aorta and pulmonary artery and produce a hemorrhagic, pyogenic, or fibrinous pericarditis (Fig. 33–2). The infectious process may invade the interventricular septum. Septal perforation may follow when endocarditis is acute.

Arnett and Roberts have described both the gross and histological abnormalities in the active and healed stages of various types of infective endocarditis.[113] In a study of 45 cases of *active left-sided endocarditis,* as well as a review of autopsy reports, Buchbinder and Roberts[114] noted that myocardial lesions were present in 88 to 100 per cent of cases. Evidence of bacterial endocarditis involving previously normal valves was found in as many as 42 per cent of patients. Heart failure due to valvular dysfunction occurred in 59 to 74 per cent of patients studied at autopsy. Papillary muscle necrosis that did not lead to mitral regurgitation was present in 58 per cent. Pericarditis produced by direct extension of inflammation into the pericardium was noted in 8 per cent of patients. Of 31 individuals with infection of the aortic valve, 12 had ring abscesses, an indication of severe destruction of valvular cusps.

Studies of the gross pathology of *healed left-sided endocarditis* revealed that half had anatomical lesions readily attributable to healed infective endocarditis.[115] Unequivocal residua of valvular infection were more common in purely incompetent than in stenotic or mixed valvular disease. Half of the patients had either cuspal perforation, probably secondary to ring abscesses, ruptured chordae tendineae, or aneurysms. The most common organism was alpha-streptococcus. The mitral or aortic valve, or both, were either stenotic or purely incompetent. Patients with valvular perforations and ruptured chordae tendineae usually had pure regurgitation. Three individuals with ring abscesses

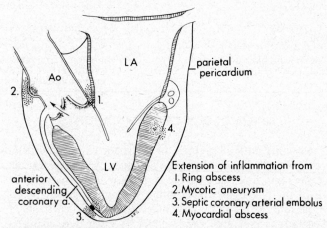

FIGURE 33–2   Schematic portrayal of the pathogenesis of pericarditis in infective endocarditis. Ao = aorta; LV = left ventricle; LA = left atrium. (From Roberts, W. C., and Buchbinder, N. A.: Healed left-sided infective endocarditis. A clinicopathological study of 59 patients. Am. J. Cardiol. *40:*876, 1976.)

had competent valves. All of the stenotic valves were diffusely fibrotic; most contained calcific deposits. Diffuse or focal fibrosis was present in incompetent valves. Autopsy findings suggested that the left-sided valves had been anatomically normal in 15 per cent of patients prior to the development of endocarditis. Forty-one per cent of patients had underlying rheumatic heart disease and 29 per cent had a congenital cardiac lesion.

The pathoanatomy of right-sided bacterial endocarditis in 12 patients was reported by Roberts and Buchbinder.[116] Bacteria were present on the tricuspid or pulmonary valve in 7 cases. Among the lesions observed were ruptured chordae tendineae, necrosis of the papillary muscles, and suppurative or nonsuppurative myocarditis. In 9 of 12 patients the vegetations in the right side of the heart did not extend to involve the basal attachments of the leaflets to the annuli. Mural lesions were observed in 3 cases; in 2, they were present on the right ventricular endocardium.

Pathology of Prosthetic Valve Endocarditis. Excellent studies of the gross pathology of endocarditis involving *prosthetic valves* have been recorded by Arnett and Roberts[117] and Anderson et al.[118] The former studied 22 necropsied patients with infections of rigid-frame valvular prostheses replacing aortic valves in 15 and mitral valves in 7 cases (Fig. 33–3). Endocarditis developed within two months after operation in 8, and 2 months or longer postoperatively in 14 patients. The organism recovered most often was located behind the site of attachment of the prosthesis to the valve ring. It spread to adjacent structures in 13 patients, 11 of whom had aortic prostheses. In most cases, the prosthetic valve was detached. Conduction defects, including left bundle branch or complete block, were present in 7 individuals. These were observed most often when aortic prostheses were present, suggesting that conduction abnormalities were related to the presence of abscess or necrosis in the upper area of the interventricular septum.

Among 22 patients with endocarditis involving valvular prostheses studied by Anderson et al. at autopsy, 95 per cent had cardiac hypertrophy and 73 per cent had dilated left ventricles.[118] Dysfunction of the prosthesis was present in 17 per cent and was due to ulceration of a cusp, paravalvular leak, entrapment of the poppet by a thrombus, perforation of a ring abscess into the right ventricle, or mitral stenosis (most common). Fifty-seven per cent of patients experienced infection of the aortic annulus, while involvement of the mitral annulus was observed in 43 per cent. Fibrinous or purulent pericarditis, aortic stenosis due to exuberant vegetations, and embolic myocarditis (abscess and focal necrosis) were also noted. In no instance did infection of a prosthesis spread to the other valves. In two persons with first-degree block, the atrioventricular node was extensively involved by the inflammatory process that had extended from an abscess of the aortic ring; the bundle of His was intact. Among the extracardiac findings were peripheral (85 per cent), splenic (59 per cent), renal (50 per cent), and cerebral (45 per cent) emboli.

The pathological features of infected *Hancock porcine bioprostheses* have been described by Bartolloti et al.[119] (Fig. 33–4). The vegetations were friable, small to massive, and present on the inflow surface of the valve. Infected cusps were torn, frayed, or perforated. Ring abscess or valvular calcification was uncommon. Among the histological findings were deposition of fibrin on the inflow surface of the valve and breakdown of collagen. Moderate to marked subendothelial inflammation was present in some instances. Macrophages, neutrophils, and clusters of bacteria within the tissue of the cusps were noted in all cases. Granulomas were present when fungi were involved. The following features that distinguish endocarditis involving porcine valves from that of infection of rigid-frame prostheses have been pointed out by Ferrans et al.[120]: (a) infection can involve the porcine valve itself as well as fibrin, organized thrombi, and fibrous tissue of the patient, and

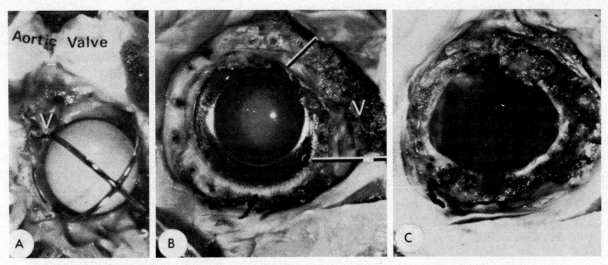

FIGURE 33–3 Prosthetic mitral valve endocarditis caused by *Staphylococcus epidermidis*. The infection appeared 10 years after replacement of both mitral and tricuspid valves. At necropsy, only the mitral prosthesis was infected. *A,* Infected mitral valve prosthesis viewed from the left ventricle. Vegetative material (V) is present on the prosthetic annulus just below the aortic valve. *B,* Prosthesis as viewed from the left atrium showing vegetations (V) at the junction of the prosthetic and natural valve annuli. *C,* Same view after removal of the prosthesis, showing even greater extension of the infection at the site of attachment of the prosthesis. (From Arnett, E. N., and Roberts, W. C.: Prosthetic valve endocarditis. Clinicopathological analysis of 22 necropsy patients with comparison of observations in 74 necropsy patients with active infective endocarditis involving natural left-sided cardiac valves. Am. J. Cardiol. *38:*281, 1976.)

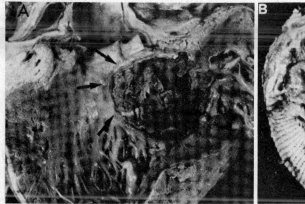
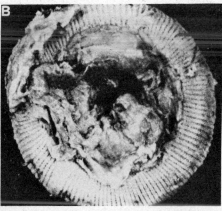
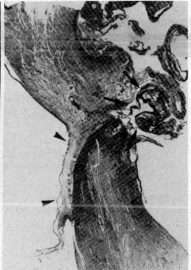

FIGURE 33–4   A 41-year-old man had undergone mitral valve replacement with a Hancock porcine bioprosthesis. One month later the clinical signs of endocarditis with mitral regurgitation developed. Blood cultures grew *Enterobacter cloacae*. The patient died of sepsis 2 months after operation. *A*, Mitral orifice viewed from the left ventricle; the device was removed before the photograph was taken. Despite the presence of abundant vegetations, mitral insufficiency was found. This dysfunction was caused by prosthetic detachment owing to a ring abscess (arrows). *B*, Atrial view of the explanted heterograft with moderate thrombotic vegetations. *C*, Histological examination of the conducting tissue revealed a spared atrioventricular node (arrowheads) and bundle and an extensive ring abscess (arrows) on the left side of the central fibrous body. (Elastic van Gieson stain, orig. mag. × 3.) (From Bortolotti, U., et al.: Pathological study of infective endocarditis on Hancock porcine bioprostheses. J. Thorac. Cardiovasc. Surg. *81*:934, 1981. Reproduced with permission.)

destroy the valve; (b) ring abscesses are uncommon; (c) perforation of cusps does not occur; (d) valvular stenosis is common; and (e) paravalvular leaks are uncommon.

Histological Changes. Histological abnormalities of subacute infective endocarditis were described by Libman and Friedberg. They noted that the vegetations consisted essentially of platelet-fibrin thrombi containing colonies of bacteria on and below the surface and suggested that the

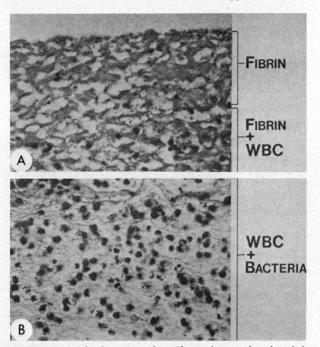

FIGURE 33–5   Infective vegetation. Photomicrographs of an infective vegetation. *A*, Note fibrin and a few leukocytes near the surface. *B*, Deeper, toward the base in the vegetation, are numerous leukocytes and stainable bacteria. Note the lack of vascular channels. (From Applefeld, M. M., and Woodward, T. E.: Infective endocarditis: A clinical overview. *In* Harvey, W. P., et al. (eds.): Current Problems in Cardiology. Vol. 2, No. 5. Copyright © 1977 by Year Book Medical Publishers, Inc., Chicago. Reproduced with permission of the publishers and courtesy of Dr. William C. Roberts.)

thrombus was derived from the inflamed valve that had undergone destructive change (Fig. 33–5). The inflammatory reaction consisted chiefly of mononuclear cells, lymphocytes, and histiocytes; very few polymorphonuclear cells were present. Not uncommonly, giant cells containing phagocytized bacteria were present. The cusp underlying the vegetation was the site of a destructive process that was either localized or extended to both surfaces. Healing was an early and prominent feature. At this stage, most of the bacteria had disappeared. In addition to inflammatory cells, the cusp contained numerous capillaries and fibroblasts. When healing was prolonged, the vegetations became calcified.

The myocardium may show a variety of lesions. These are usually diffuse or localized collections of lymphocytes and mononuclear cells and are the so-called Bracht-Wachter lesions that replace the muscle itself. Diffuse or localized collections of polymorphonuclear cells, with or without myocardial necrosis or miliary abscesses, are observed occasionally. Gross suppuration is absent. Muscle fibers may show degenerative changes, often with small scars in various stages of healing. The small coronary branches show swelling and proliferation of the endothelial cells of capillaries and arterioles, arteriolitis, or necrosis of the media or adventitia; perivascular cellular infiltrates and scars may be present. A large branch of a coronary artery may contain an embolus or reveal a mycotic aneurysm.

Among the lesions noted in cases of right-sided endocarditis have been myocardial abscesses containing colonies of bacteria, septic emboli (extramural or intramural) in one or more coronary arteries, foci of necrosis in the ventricular wall or papillary muscles, calcification of individual myocardial fibers, and acute pneumonia with pulmonary infarcts or abscesses.[116] The histopathological findings observed during necropsy of patients with left-sided infective endocarditis were foci of myocardial fibrosis in the ventricular papillary muscles, ventricular free wall, or both.[115] In about 20 per cent of cases, there was greater than 75 per cent cross-sectional narrowing of coronary arterial lumina.

The microanatomy of acute bacterial endocarditis is entirely different from that of the subacute form of the disease. In the former, the histological picture is of a rapidly progressive destructive lesion, with no features that indicate any attempt at healing, such as the presence of fibroblasts or organization. In untreated cases, the fibrin-platelet thrombus contains only polymorphonuclear leukocytes and large numbers of bacteria. The affected underlying valve is the site of necrosis. These features satisfy the criteria for the term *ulcerative endocarditis* that has been applied to this type of disease and explain the predisposition to tearing of the valvular leaflets, rupture of papillary muscles and chordae tendineae, the formation of aneurysms, and the frequency of intracardiac spread of infection — common complications of this type of disease.

Portals of Entry and Predisposing Factors

The most important factor predisposing to infection of cardiac valves is invasion of the bloodstream by any of the organisms suspected to be involved in this disease. The bacteremias or fungemias that initiate infective endocarditis may be persistent or transient, may arise in the course of a variety of manipulations in patients without a predisposing infected site, or may be a consequence of spread into the circulation from an area of established infection.

Transient Bacteremias. It is remarkable that transient bacteremias occur following various types of manipulation of areas in which organisms are normally present, such as the mouth, upper airway, skin, external genital tract, and intestine. An excellent review of transient bacteremia has been published recently by Everett and Hirschman,[121] a summary of which is presented here:

The reported incidence of transient bacteremia associated with extraction of teeth has varied from 18 to 85 per cent. The organisms are most commonly streptococci, usually of the alpha type, but occasionally enterococci. They are rarely present in the blood for longer than 15 to 20 minutes, but this may be prolonged when multiple teeth are removed; the number of bacteria in the blood is small and ranges from as few as 5 to as many as 50 to 60 per ml. In addition to streptococci, "diphtheroids," *Staph. epidermidis*, and anaerobic members of the normal oral microflora have also been recovered. Peterson and Peacock noted transient bacteremia in 35 per cent of 101 youngsters who had nondiseased primary teeth removed, in 53 per cent of those in whom diseased primary and permanent teeth were extracted, and in 61 per cent undergoing removal of healthy permanent teeth.[122] Among dental procedures other than extraction associated with transient bacteremia are rocking of teeth, chewing of paraffin or hard candy, scaling of gums, brushing of teeth, periodontal operations, dental prophylaxis, use of unwaxed dental floss, and employment of oral irrigation devices (Water-Pik). It must be emphasized that infective endocarditis may occur in edentulous individuals.[123]

Tonsilloadenoidectomy is the procedure involving the airway most commonly associated with bacteremia; from 28 to 38 per cent of patients subjected to this operation experience transient bacterial invasion of the bloodstream. Other manipulations in this area that may lead to bacteremia are bronchoscopy (the rigid but not the fiberoptic instrument), orotracheal intubation, and nasal operations. Among the organisms present in the circulation have been *Staph. aureus*, streptococci, *Hemophilus* species, *Strep. pneumoniae*, and *Staph. epidermidis*. A recent study of nasotracheal suctioning by LeFrock et al. demonstrated bacteremia lasting up to 15 minutes[124] in 17.6 per cent of 68 patients who underwent this procedure.

Barium enema may be accompanied by transient bacteremia. LeFrock and his associates reported that in 11.4 per cent of patients who underwent this study, bacteria appeared transiently in the blood.[125] In another study LeFrock and his colleagues noted that 10 per cent of patients who underwent sigmoidoscopy had transient bacteremia; viridans streptococci were present in 90 per cent of these.[126] Shull et al. carried out fiberoptic gastroscopy in 50 patients; after the procedure, 4 exhibited bacteremia that lasted from 5 to 30 minutes.[127] This incidence is lower than that following sigmoidoscopy, presumably because of the diameter and greater flexibility of the fiberoptic colonoscope.[128] Transient bacteremia also occurs with percutaneous biopsy of the liver.[129]

A large variety of urological procedures have resulted in transient bacterial invasion of the blood[130] with incidence as follows: internal urethrotomy, 75 per cent; urethral dilatation of external urethrotomy, 85.9 per cent; transurethral prostatectomy, 12.3 per cent in general, but 10.8 per cent when urine was sterile and 57.5 per cent when organisms were present in the urine; removal of indwelling catheter from patients with infected urine, 26.3 per cent; retropubic prostatectomy, 7.4 to 12.8 per cent when urine has been sterile and 82.4 per cent when bacteriuria has been a problem; cystoscopy, 0 to 17 per cent; urethral catheterization, 8 per cent. Gram-negative bacilli are the commonest transient intruders.

Most studies of transient bacteremia from various gynecological procedures have produced negative results. Invasion of the bloodstream does not occur during parturition. However, a recent study has indicated that about 85 per cent of patients who underwent a suction abortion experienced transient bacteremia; the bacteria were present only intermittently in some; in others, the bacteremia persisted for as long as one hour after the abortion was completed. In a few instances, organisms were recovered from the blood following only bimanual pelvic examination.[131]

Cirrhosis. Snyder et al. reported that infective endocarditis[132] among patients admitted to the hospital was 3.4 times more frequent when cirrhosis was present than when it was absent.

Drug Addiction and Surgery. Addiction to the intravenous use of drugs has become an increasingly important factor predisposing to the development of infective endocarditis. This is also true of cardiac surgery, especially the insertion of prosthetic valves; the appearance of a paravalvular leak, probably because it produces hemodynamic abnormalities, favors the deposition of platelet-fibrin thrombi on which organisms may be implanted. Prolonged use of polyethylene catheters or any type of "long line" is associated with an increased risk of endocarditis related to either colonization of the tip of the catheter or entry of organisms at the site where the tube enters the skin.

Burns. Burned patients appear to be more susceptible to infective endocarditis. In the study by Baskin et al., the infection involved the right side of the heart in 18 patients, the left in 9, and both sides in 8.[133] The disease was acute in 22 and subacute in 13. Murmurs were detectable in only two instances. The commonest organism present on the valves was *Staph. aureus* (77 per cent).

Pacemakers. An uncommon source of infection of the heart is the transvenous cardiac pacemaker.[134] Sustained staphylococcal bacteremia (at least 12 hours) may develop 2 weeks to 10 months after insertion of the apparatus. About 5 to 6 per cent of cases of endocarditis have been associated with infection in the subcutaneous pocket into which the pacemaker is inserted. Of seven cases reported up to 1975, the tricuspid valve was infected in four, the mitral endocardium of the left atrium in two, and the right ventricle in one. Myocardial abscess resulting from contamination of the wire is even less common.

Other Predisposing Factors. A number of other infectious and noninfectious predisposing factors have been reported by Garvey and Neu.[135] Among these are neoplastic disease, nonmalignant hematological disorders, "collagen-vascular" disease, diabetes mellitus, chronic active viral hepatitis, preexisting renal failure, treatment with corticosteroids (50 per cent of patients), antitumor chemotherapy and radiation (20 per cent of cases), perinephric abscess, obstruction of the common bile duct, perforation of the bowel (*Clostridium perfringens* endocarditis), and infections of sternal wounds produced in the course of cardiac surgery.

Hyperalimentation is also associated with an increased risk of fungal endocarditis.

Extracardiac Foci of Infection. Foci of infection *outside* the heart may serve as sources of bacteremia that lead to the development of endocarditis. Among such lesions are mild to severe infections of the skin ("pimple," boils), especially if they are mishandled by squeezing or inappropriate surgical incision. The organism most often responsible for disease in this situation is *Staph. aureus*. Pneumonia, particularly that caused by *Strep. pneumoniae*, was a relatively common predisposing factor in the preantibiotic era. Disease of the lung caused by *Strep. pyogenes* and other highly invasive organisms such as *H. influenzae* may also serve as a source of bacteremia and subsequent infective endocarditis.

Among other extracardiac lesions are acute hematogenous osteomyelitis, acute pyelonephritis, meningococcemia with or without meningitis, brucellosis, Q fever, rat-bite fever, and a variety of immunosuppressive disorders including the vasculitides when they are complicated by bacteremia, and superinfection by bacteria or fungi induced by therapy with antibiotics. Garvey and Neu[135] and Rosen and Armstrong [136] have noted that a significant number of the patients with infections of normal valves were immunosuppressed because of major underlying disease or treatment with corticosteroids or radiation. These individuals were older, and involvement of the right side of the heart was more likely than in those who were immunologically competent. They were also more susceptible to invasion of the valves by gram-negative bacilli and fungi. In about one-third of cases, the presence of infective endocarditis was not suspected during life. The fatality rate was 57 per cent in this group and only 28 per cent in patients who were without immunological abnormalities.

Infective endocarditis is a subtle and often lethal complication of *hemodialysis*.[137] The source of the organisms has been infection or manipulation of access sites and dental procedures, most commonly involving *Staph. aureus*. The incidence of infection is lower in patients with arteriovenous fistulas than in those with arteriovenous cannulas. Although *Pseudomonas aeruginosa* is a frequent cause of infection of access sites, it produces endocarditis uncommonly. Cure of the cardiac infection requires, in addition to antimicrobial therapy, removal of the shunt.

A rare predisposing factor in the pathogenesis of infective endocarditis is penetration of the heart by a foreign body.[138] Cardiac catheterization may rarely be associated with a transient bacteremia that leads to the development of infective endocarditis.

UNDERLYING HEART DISEASE

RHEUMATIC HEART DISEASE. Although chronic rheumatic heart disease was the underlying lesion in from 80 to 90 per cent of cases of subacute bacterial endocarditis for many years,[18] this has not been so since antimicrobial agents have become available. This may be related to the decreased incidence of acute rheumatic fever and to the highly successful prevention of recurrences of the disease. At present, only about 40 to 60 per cent of instances of infective endocarditis are superimposed on preexisting rheumatic heart disease.[14] The long-held concept that patients with pure mitral stenosis, atrial fibrillation, and congestive heart failure were at extremely low risk of developing endocarditis does not appear to be as important as it was in the past.

Uncommonly, both acute or subacute bacterial endocarditis and acute rheumatic carditis may be present simultaneously. The differential diagnosis of acute rheumatic fever and infective endocarditis may, in some instances, be diffi-

cult because (1) blood cultures may occasionally be positive in the former and negative in the latter, (2) both conditions feature fever and leukocytosis, and (3) petechiae may be present in both. Blood cultures should be obtained in patients in whom fever persists despite treatment with adequate doses of salicylate. If four or more cultures yield an organism, the possibility of superimposed infective endocarditis must be seriously considered and appropriate antimicrobial therapy instituted.

CONGENITAL HEART DISEASE. Although probably more frequently the basis for endocarditis in children, congenital heart disease is also important in adults. Gelfman and Levine[139] reported in 1942 that endocarditis occurred in about 6.5 per cent of 453 youngsters over the age of 2 years with congenital heart disease studied at necropsy; the incidence has been recorded to be as high as 16 per cent.[140,141] In patients younger than 2 years, valvular infection is less commonly superimposed on anatomical defects of the heart. In the first weeks or months of life, this disease is usually a complication of an episode of overwhelming sepsis; murmurs are usually absent, diagnosis is difficult, and the fatality rate is inordinately high.

Patent ductus arteriosus, ventricular septal defect, and tetralogy of Fallot are the congenital lesions most commonly associated with infective endocarditis[142]; aortic or pulmonic stenosis is less frequent. The frequency of infection in patients with ventricular septal defect (Fig. 33–6) has been estimated to be 1 in 470 patient years, or 2.1 per 100 cases in 10 years.[143] When ventricular septal defect and aortic regurgitation coexist, the incidence of endocarditis increases to about 24 per cent. In patients with the tetralo-

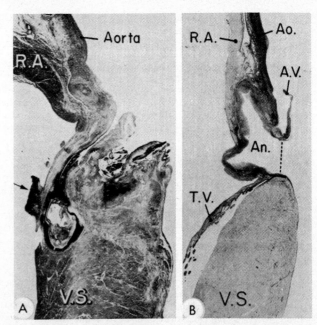

FIGURE 33–6   Photomicrographs of longitudinal sections of ventricular septum (V.S.) at two levels. *A*, Section showing extension of the infective process through the entire thickness of the muscular V.S. A small vegetation (arrow) is apparent on the endocardium of the right side of the heart. R.A. = right atrium. *B*, Section includes aneurysm (An.) of membranous portion of V.S. The dashed line represents the normal site of the ventricular septum. T.V. = tricuspid valve leaflet; A.V. = aortic valve cusp; Ao. = aorta. (From Roberts, W. C., and Buchbinder, N. A.: Healed left-sided infective endocarditis. A clinicopathological study of 59 patients. Am. J. Cardiol. **40:** 876, 1976.)

gy of Fallot in whom an anastomosis has been created between the systemic and pulmonary circulations, infective endocarditis occurs more frequently than in any other form of congenital heart disease. The aortic valve may, at times, become infected in patients with the tetralogy of Fallot or pulmonary atresia. The aortic root and descending aorta are larger than normal, and the aortic abnormalities induce turbulence of blood flow in the aortic root, which may produce sufficient trauma to the normal endocardium to cause deposition of a platelet-fibrin thrombus, the focus for bacterial invasion,[144] and aortic regurgitation may ensue.

Atrial septal defects are rarely infected, probably because of the absence of large interatrial pressure gradients.[143] However, endocarditis involving the mitral valve has occurred in patients with ostium primum defects. Two other congenital cardiac lesions that predispose to the development of valvular infection are bicuspid aortic valves and coarctation of the aorta. Endocarditis tends to develop most frequently in congenital lesions that produce significant pressure gradients.[145] In cases of coarctation of the aorta the infectious process is usually situated on the poststenotic side and on an accompanying bicuspid aortic valve.[146] The pulmonic valve is most often involved when the tetralogy of Fallot is present.[144] The left pulmonary artery in the area of the ductal orifice is the site most often infected in patients with patent ductus arteriosus.

ATHEROSCLEROSIS AND CALCIFICATION. Kerr suggested that, as the population aged, atherosclerotic heart disease would probably become a significant lesion predisposing to the development of infective endocarditis.[19] It has since become clear that certain factors associated with aging play an important role in the pathogenesis of this infection and account for the increase in the incidence of bacterial disease of the heart in the older age group. Atheromatous deposits on the aortic valve have been noted at autopsy in 25 per cent of patients over 40 years of age who have succumbed to endocarditis. The incidence of valvular atheromas, excrescences, and nodules increases progressively with age; these lesions are most prominent in areas where the change in pressure and turbulence of flow are greatest, such as the left side of the heart, in general, and the aortic valve, in particular.[147] Watanakunakorn has described five older patients with calcification of the mitral valve annulus (p. 1074) who developed endocarditis.[148] The organisms involved were gram-negative cocci and *Staph. aureus.* He pointed out that (a) murmurs may not be present, (b) significant narrowing of the mitral orifice was absent, and (c) vegetations were most commonly present on the *posterior* leaflet of the mitral valve. An analysis of the frequency of calcification of the valves in a population without endocarditis showed that about 5 per cent of uninfected persons between 50 and 70 years of age have calcified mitral valves. In those older than 90 years, the incidence of calcification of the valves is about 60 per cent.

HYPERTROPHIC OBSTRUCTIVE CARDIOMYOPATHY. The incidence of infective endocarditis in patients with this condition is usually considered to be in the range of 5 to 10 per cent, but in one recent report was as high as 50 per cent.[149] Wang and his associates have reported that the aortic valve is infected most often, followed by the mitral valve alone or both valves simultaneously.[150] They suggested that the infectious process originates on the ventricular aspect of the anterior portion of the anterior mitral leaflet. This area is frequently thickened and becomes susceptible to bacterial invasion as a result of the trauma produced by the abutting action of the anterior mitral leaflet against the thickened septum (p. 1411). Infection may then extend to the chordae tendineae and produce tears. In 10 patients with discrete membranous subaortic stenosis and endocarditis, the infection was noted to involve the aortic valve in all, the aorta above the aortic valve in 6, the mitral valve in 4, and the membranous ridge in 3. The high incidence of endocarditis of the aortic valve and wall in this condition compared to valvular infection in hypertrophic cardiomyopathy suggested that there is a more prominent jet stream in discrete membranous stenosis than in hypertrophic cardiomyopathy, and that this causes more damage to the aortic leaflets and wall. Aortic regurgitation is also a more common complication of endocarditis in the discrete, membranous form than in hypertrophic obstructive cardiomyopathy. Infection of the aortic wall has not been reported with hypertrophic obstructive cardiomyopathy but is common in the membranous type of disease and may be complicated by mycotic aneurysms, which may rupture.

MARFAN SYNDROME AND MITRAL VALVE PROLAPSE. Up until 1974, 21 cases of infective endocarditis occurring in patients with the *Marfan syndrome* (p. 1665) had been reported.[151] The mitral valve is infected most often. Although the aortic valve is commonly abnormal in this disease, it is rarely the site of infection. The *mitral valve prolapse syndrome* (p. 1089) has been identified as a predisposing condition in the development of infective endocarditis.[152,152a] *Staph. aureus* is commonly involved; in some instances, alpha-streptococci and enterococci have been recovered from the blood.[153]

CARDIAC SURGERY. Cardiac surgery represents an iatrogenic type of underlying heart disease that predisposes to the development of infective endocarditis. Before 1957, about 1 per cent of patients subjected to operations on the heart developed infection. During the next 10 years, the incidence of this complication rose considerably, especially in cases in which valvular prostheses were implanted. The incidence of endocarditis complicating placement of Starr-Edwards valves has been recorded to be as high as 10 per cent.[154,155] However, as experience with cardiac surgery has increased, the frequency of infection has fallen to 3 to 3.5 per cent with valve replacement and to about 1 per cent with other types of operation on the heart. Stein et al. pointed out that the type of surgical procedure played a role in determining the incidence of endocarditis.[156] They noted infection in only 0.6 per cent of patients undergoing closed-heart operations, in 0.9 per cent of those undergoing open cardiac procedures, and in 3.3 per cent of those in whom prosthetic valves were placed. Infected suture material appears to be an important contributing factor. Decrease in the effectiveness of removal of organisms from the bloodstream by phagocytosis, which has been shown to be impaired by use of cardiopulmonary bypass, may also play an important role in increasing susceptibility to valvular infection.

Several studies have indicated that *infection of prosthetic valves* may occur at various times after operation.[157] Most reports divide the cases into early or late. "Early" has been defined as within one to three weeks and "late" as longer than one, two, or three months. It has been suggested that evidence of infection in the first one or two weeks postoperatively usually indicates extracardiac infection, and that the later fever develops, the more likely prosthetic valvular endocarditis is present.[158] Although this is true in many instances, there are a number of cases in which fever developing in the first few days after operation has been found to be the first manifestation of infection of the prosthesis.[159] In sharp contrast are the occasional cases in which endocarditis does not appear until five or more years after the device has been implanted (Fig. 33–3). A study by Wilson et al. indicated that, in a group of 45 patients, infection of the prosthesis became apparent within two months in 36 per cent, while in the remaining 64 per cent, the disease did not become manifest until more than two months after operation.[157] In early cases, the commonest organisms were *Staph. aureus* (44 per cent) and gram-negative bacilli (38 per cent); in late cases, *Strep. viridans* and gram-negative bacilli were commonest. In a similar study of 38 patients by Dismukes et al., 50 per cent of patients developed infection in less than 60 days (early) and the other 50 per cent after 60 days (late).[38] Again, *Staph. aureus* was most frequently involved in the early and streptococci in the late episodes. A study of 122 cases of postcardiotomy endocarditis by Starkebaum et al. indicated that the disease appeared within two weeks in 27 per cent[160]; 70 per cent occurred with 2 months. "The findings were consistent with the hypothesis that the incubation period of postcardiotomy endocarditis is short."

Certain types of cardiac surgery impose a higher risk of infective endocarditis than does the implantation of a prosthesis. Kaplan et al. have reported that 8 per cent of patients with tetralogy of Fallot developed endocarditis following the Pott's procedure (i.e., aortopulmonary shunt). Intracardiac infection also appears to be increased in patients operated on for tricuspid atresia.[161] The highest risk of infective endocarditis is associated with operative procedures on patients with transposition of the great arteries. Valvular infections have not been a notable complication in coronary bypass operations.

Among the conditions predisposing to invasion of prosthetic valves by organisms in the *early* postoperative period are infected surgical wounds in the chest and urinary catheters. Sources of infection include contamination of blood by the oxygenator and of the blood used to prime the pump; the connecting tubes on the large venous and arterial cannulas; direct contamination by hands, instruments, or room air; reactivation of latent infection in patients with episodes of endocarditis prior to placement of the prosthetic valve; and contamination of the prosthesis. Predisposing conditions in the convalescent period include bacteremia from sites of infection in the chest wound or at the cannulation site, infected pleural fluid, postoperative pneumonia, tracheostomy, contaminated indwelling catheters, and superinfections related to prophylaxis or therapy with antimicrobial agents. Other conditions predisposing to *late* endocarditis are infections of the urinary tract, dental procedures, disease of the upper airway, ingrown toenails, use of the nasal cautery and pilonidal cyst. The primary factor involved in both early and late convalescence is bacteremia resulting from dental, dermatological, gastrointestinal, and genitourinary procedures or minor surgical operations. In addition to these, Dismukes et al. reported that cystoscopy, excision of a carbuncle, uterine dilatation and curettage, paravalvular leaks that developed immediately postoperatively, and preexisting endocarditis (same organism) predisposed to infection of the prosthetic valves.[38]

There is an increasing number of instances of infective endocarditis involving otherwise *normal valves*, particularly in cases of the acute disease. For example, 40 to 60 per cent of patients with infections caused by *Staph. aureus* have previously normal cardiac valves. This is also true in an appreciable number of instances in which *Strep. pyogenes, Strep. pneumoniae, N. meningitidis*, and *N. gonorrhoeae* are involved. In recent years, endocarditis affecting normal valves has occurred more frequently because of the increase in the number of individuals using intravenous illicit drugs.

Seven cases of bacterial endocarditis following penetration of the heart by *foreign bodies* have been recorded.[138]

MYOCARDIAL INFARCTION. Infective endocarditis may occur as a complication of myocardial infarction.[162] The location of the infection is determined by the site of necrosis of the muscle, and the predisposing factor is the development of a platelet-fibrin clot over the infarcted area. The infection may be situated on the left side of the septum in cases of anteroseptal infarction or on the endocardium over the site of damage in the left ventricle. In addition, development of an *aneurysm* in which a clot forms provides a potential area of invasion for organisms.

NONVALVULAR INFECTIVE ENDOCARDITIS. Nonvalvular infective endocarditis may occur in *ventricular septal defect* (Fig. 33–6). Although the tricuspid valve may be infected occasionally, three other sites are involved more commonly. One is the point of impact of the jet stream on the right ventricular endocardium; the resulting injury leads to the formation of a small platelet-fibrin thrombus on which bacteria may be implanted. Infection may also develop on the right side of the septal opening; the Venturi effect created by the flow of blood from an area of high (left ventricle) to one of lower pressure (right ventricle) leads to the deposition of a clot around the opening on the right side of the septum. Much less common is infection of the left ventricular side of the defect. The risk of infection is reduced when the septal opening is large, because this does not produce an interventricular pressure gradient.

A rare form of nonvalvular infection of the heart is infected *atrial myxoma*. A patient described by Graham et al. is one of four similar cases, three of which had *Staph. aureus* infections.[163] Embolization to the central nervous system occurred in every instance. Infection of an atrial myxoma by *Histoplasma capsulatum* has been described.[164]

Single or multiple *myocardial abscesses* may develop in the course of bacteremias unrelated to valvular infection. *Staph. aureus* and *N. meningitidis* are among the organisms involved. Several instances of subacute bacterial endocarditis in patients with *rheumatic valvular disease* in which the infection did not involve any of the affected valves have been noted. In these cases, the infectious process was superimposed on McCallum's patch, an area of endocardial injury in the left atrium induced by the acute rheumatic process.

TABLE 33–2   LOCI OF LESIONS IN ENDOCARDITIS

CONDITION	HIGH-PRSSURE SOURCE	ORIFICE	LOW-PRESSURE SINK	LOCATION OF LESIONS	SATELLITE LESIONS
Coarctation of aorta	Central aorta	Coarctation	Distal aorta	Downstream wall	Lateral wall of aorta peripheral to stenotic lesion
Patent ductus arteriosus	Aorta	Ductus	Pulmonary artery	Pulmonary artery	Pulmonic valve
Arteriovenous fistula	Artery	Fistula	Vein	Fistula and vein	
Ventricular septal defect	Left ventricle	Defect	Right ventricle	Right ventricular surface defect	Pulmonary artery
Aortic regurgitation	Aorta	Closed aortic valves	Left ventricle	Ventricular surface aortic valve	Mitral chordae
Mitral regurgitation	Left ventricle	Closed mitral valves	Left atrium	Atrial surface mitral valve	Atrium
Pulmonic regurgitation	Pulmonary artery	Closed pulmonic valves	Right ventricle	Ventricular surface pulmonic valve	
Tricuspid regurgitation	Right ventricle	Closed tricuspid valves	Right atrium	Atrial surface tricuspid valve	

Adapted from Rodbard, S.: Blood velocity and endocarditis. Circulation *27*:18, 1963, by permission of the American Heart Association, Inc.

PATHOGENESIS

Subacute Endocarditis

Since Osler's[2] classic description of endocarditis, many investigators have tried to explain the fact that infected endocardial vegetations consistently occur in the same location. Four mechanisms are responsible for the initiation and localization of the *subacute* infection: (1) a previously damaged cardiac valve or a hemodynamic situation in which damage results from a jet effect, produced by blood flowing from a zone of high to one of relatively low pressure, as in mitral regurgitation or ventricular septal defect (Table 33–2); (2) a sterile platelet-fibrin thrombus; (3) bacteremia, often transient; and (4) a high titer of agglutinating antibody against the infecting organism.

THE JET AND VENTURI EFFECTS. Of 1024 patients with infective endocarditis studied by Lepeschkin at autopsy, mitral valves were involved in 86 per cent, aortic valves in 55 per cent, tricuspid valves in 19.6 per cent, and pulmonic valves in 1.1 per cent.[165] By correlating the impact of pressure on these valves with the frequency of involvement of the corresponding valves, Lepeschkin presented a strong argument for *mechanical stress* as a critical factor in the evolution of endocarditis. By injecting a bacterial aerosol into the air stream passing through an agar Venturi tube, Rodbard elegantly demonstrated how high pressure drives an infected fluid into a low-pressure sink to establish a characteristic pattern of colony distribution; a collar of maximal deposition consistently appeared in the low-pressure sink immediately beyond the orifice (Fig. 33–7).[145] This model helps to explain the distribution of lesions often complicating various cardiac valvular and septal defects (Table 33–2). The early observation that in infective endocarditis the atrial side of the valve and adjacent segment of atrium are characteristically involved in patients with mitral regurgitation is also explained; a Venturi effect is produced when blood is driven from a high-pressure source (the left ventricle) through an orifice (the nearly closed but regurgitant mitral valve) into a low-pressure sink (the atrium). A jet effect on the atrial wall establishes the other site of potential involvement, McCallum's patch (Fig. 33–8).

The sites of aortic valvular infection are established in a similar way. Some degree of aortic regurgitation is crucial. The high-pressure source is the aorta, and the low-pressure sink is the left ventricle. Vegetations are typically found on the ventricular surface of the aortic leaflets. Satellite lesions, which may be found on the chordae tendineae, are the result of a high-velocity regurgitant stream from an incompetent aortic valve—a situation analogous to the jet effect in mitral regurgitation. In a ventricular septal defect with a small orifice and left-to-right shunt, a Venturi effect often leads to the development of lesions around the orifice on the right ventricular side of the opening. Secondary lesions may be present on the right ventricular wall opposite the defect, the site of impact of the jet. Similar hemodynamic relations in tricuspid regurgitation, arteriovenous fistula, coarctation of the aorta, and patent ductus arteriosus can be used, in each instance, to predict the location of the endothelial lesions. Table 33–2 presents the distribution of endocardial infections in common cardiovascular disorders.

Attenuation of the jet and Venturi effects is seen in congestive heart failure and atrial fibrillation and helps to ex-

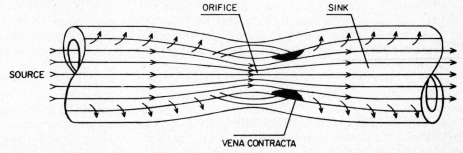

FIGURE 33–7   Venturi model of high-pressure source driving a bacterial aerosol into a low-pressure sink. Characteristic distribution of bacterial colonies is shown at the vena contracta. (From Rodbard, S.: Blood velocity in endocarditis. Circulation *27*:18, 1963, by permission of the American Heart Association, Inc.)

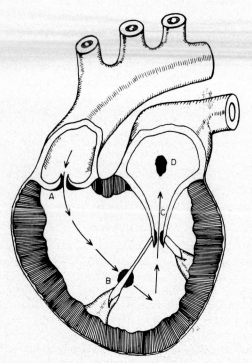

FIGURE 33–8   High-velocity streams in mitral and aortic regurgitation and sites of endocarditis lesions. Arrow at left indicates a high arterial pressure that generates regurgitant flow from aorta to ventricle. The vena contracta and endocarditic lesions appear at the ventricular surface of the aortic valve (A). The stream through the incompetent aortic valve may produce lesions on the chordae tendineae of the aortic leaf of the mitral valve (B). If the mitral valves cannot seat properly during ventricular systole, the regurgitant stream (arrow at right) will pass to the sink of the left atrium, and the endocarditic lesion will tend to become engrafted on the atrial surface of the mitral valve (C). The atrial endocardium in line with the regurgitant stream may produce a fibrous area, MacCallum's patch (D), which may become another site of endocarditic lesions. (Adapted from Rodbard, S.: Blood velocity in endocarditis. Circulation *27*:18, 1963, by permission of the American Heart Association, Inc.)

plain the long recognized infrequency of infective endocarditis in these settings.[166] Likewise, defects with surface areas large enough to abolish a gradient and those in which smaller volumes minimize the gradient are not associated with endocarditis. These findings probably explain the rarity of endocarditis in isolated atrial septal defects and the greater threat of infection in small than in large ventricular septal defects. The lesion responsible for the initiation of endocarditis is occasionally too small to produce enough turbulence to create an audible murmur.

THE PLATELET-FIBRIN THROMBUS. Turbulence and the jet effect traumatize the endothelial surface and initiate a series of events that may lead to the establishment of an infected focus. Collagen is exposed, and platelet deposition occurs in a manner analogous to the formation of the primary platelet plug of normal hemostasis after vascular injury. Central to these events is the role of the sterile platelet-fibrin thrombus, or so-called nonbacterial thrombotic endocarditis. The nonspecific nature of the sterile platelet-fibrin thrombus is emphasized by the fact that it can be produced as a result of numerous types of stress or injury.

BACTEREMIA AND AGGLUTINATING ANTIBODIES. As already pointed out (p. 1143), transient

bacteremias occur frequently in normal persons. They are usually without clinical importance, even when sterile platelet-fibrin thrombi are situated on the cardiac valves. In most cases, the failure of implantation of organisms on such sites is related to the small number and low invasive capability of circulating organisms. A major factor, probably involved in initiating subacute valvular infection because it permits large numbers of bacteria to adhere to the sterile platelet-fibrin thrombus, is *circulating antibody*, especially agglutinins. By clumping the organisms, the antibody produces an inoculum large enough to induce bacterial multiplication and infection—a phenomenon much more important in the pathogenesis of subacute than of acute endocarditis.

Evidence of the importance of antibody may be found in studies of the development of endocarditis in horses[167] undergoing immunization with pneumococci. Infected vegetations appeared late in the course of immunization, coincidentally with the highest titers of antibody. The exact mechanism by which pathogens ultimately adhere to the platelet-fibrin thrombus is unknown. One possibility is that the platelet-covered lesion somehow provides a favorable surface.

Acute Endocarditis

The pathoanatomical mechanisms involved in the development of acute bacterial endocarditis are quite different from those in the subacute form. In 50 to 60 per cent of acute cases, previously *normal* valves are the sites of infection. It appears, therefore, that the presence of a sterile platelet-fibrin thrombus is unnecessary in the pathogenesis of this form of the valvulitis. Because the organisms responsible for the acute infection (*Staph. aureus, Strep. pneumoniae, N. meningitidis* or *gonorrhoeae, Strep. pyogenes,* and *H. influenzae*) are highly invasive, only small numbers are required to establish infection. Thus, the critical requirement in the pathogenesis of acute endocarditis is bacteremia caused by an invasive organism. It should be pointed out, however, that acute infective endocarditis may also occur in patients with underlying acquired or congenital valvular damage and that, in these patients, sterile platelet-fibrin thrombi may develop and facilitate infection just as is the case in subacute endocarditis.

The exact mechanism by which pathogenic bacteria invade normal valve leaflets has now been determined. Recent studies have indicated that specific properties of various bacteria determine their ability to adhere to the surface of cardiac valves. Gould et al.[168] and Holmes and Ramirez[169] examined the capacity of a number of organisms to adhere to canine and human valvular leaflets in vitro. The degree of adherence was found to vary with the type of organism studied, being highest with enterococci and *Staph. aureus,* followed by viridans streptococci, *Staph. epidermidis,* and *P. aeruginosa* and lowest with *Escherichia coli* and *Klebsiella pneumoniae.* These data are of potentially great clinical importance because they probably explain the relative frequency with which certain bacteria, especially *Staph. aureus,* invade previously normal valves. Of equal clinical interest is the demonstration of the poor adherence of *E. coli* and *K. pneumoniae,* which may very well account for the low incidence of endocarditis caused by these organisms, despite the well-known high frequency with which they produce bacteremia.

In subacute bacterial endocarditis, the inducing bacteremia frequently originates not from an infectious process but from trauma to areas where the causative organisms normally reside as components of the indigenous flora, such as the teeth, urogenital tract, or intestine. In acute endocarditis, the inducing bacteremia originates in an active infection, usually at a site remote from the heart, such as the skin, lungs, or genitourinary tract. In an appreciable number of instances, however, there is no demonstrable portal of entry of the organisms into the bloodstream; this may be the case when *Staph. aureus* is the causative agent.

CLINICAL MANIFESTATIONS

Four mechanisms may be involved in the clinical manifestations of infective endocarditis: (1) the infectious process on the involved valve, (2) embolization, (3) metastatic infection, and (4) deposition of abnormal globulins and circulating immune complexes at various sites remote from the heart. All these are not present in every patient, and there are also striking qualitative and quantitative differences in their roles in the acute and subacute forms of the disease.[170]

Modes of Onset

SUBACUTE ENDOCARDITIS

Incubation Period. The exact "incubation period" of subacute infective endocarditis is very difficult to define. However, an extensive review of the literature by Starkebaum et al.,[160] based on a study of the time elapsing between exposure to a situation that might induce transient bacteremia and the development of the first manifestations of valvular infection, suggested that the median "incubation period" is about one week. Symptoms appeared within two weeks in about 84 per cent of the patients. Thus, the "incubation period" of subacute bacterial endocarditis is often shorter than realized. Procedures carried out more than two weeks before onset of symptoms are not likely to be causally related.

Manifestations of Infection. In many instances, the onset of subacute infective endocarditis is characterized by the *general manifestations of infection* without any signs or symptoms suggesting disease of the heart or any other organ. Common complaints include persistent low-grade fever, lassitude, anorexia, fatigue, loss of weight, sleepiness, and a grippe-like syndrome. Libman and Friedberg pointed out that this infection may simulate a number of disorders that suggest involvement of extracardiac sites, as follows: (a) headache, generalized pain, malaise, and respiratory symptoms resembling influenza; (b) fever, cough, loss of weight, weakness, pain in the chest, and even hemoptysis, suggesting the possibility of tuberculosis; (c) elevated temperature and arthralgia or arthritis suggestive of acute rheumatic fever; (d) diarrhea, fever, headache, and drowsiness, symptoms similar to those of typhoid fever; (e) intermittent chills and fever, resembling malaria (common in persons who are treated with salicylates intermittently to control fever and who experience rigor as the temperature begins to rise); (f) dyspnea, precordial discomfort, palpitation, and, at times, peripheral edema (frequently in patients in whom valvular infection has been present for weeks or months and in whom congestive heart failure finally develops); (g) fever and pain in the right upper abdomen consistent with hepatic or subdiaphragmatic infection; (h) fever, abdominal pain, and urinary symptoms with or without hematuria; (i) a clinical picture suggesting carcinoma of the stomach, characterized by vomiting, postprandial distress, and anorexia, or a syndrome suggestive of appendicitis.[171]

Development of Complications. Other modes of onset of subacute infective endocarditis are related to the development of complications of the disease that often appear before therapy is initiated, especially when the infection has not been treated for weeks or months. Some of these are embolic, some are due to progressive involvement of the valve, while others result from the development and activity of immunological disorders.[172]

Embolic Complications. Manifestations of this type of onset include (a) *sudden occlusion of the middle cerebral artery* leading to hemiplegia; (b) a clinical picture of *acute meningitis*, in which the spinal fluid is sterile but contains an increased number of cells, concentration of protein and a normal sugar content; (c) manifestations consistent with diffuse encephalitis; (d) sudden development of pain in either the right of left upper abdominal quadrant due to gross infarction of either the kidney or the spleen; (e) hematuria without pain, caused by small, multiple infarcts of the kidney, interstitial nephritis, or diffuse proliferative glomerulonephritis; (f) unilateral blindness of acute onset caused by embolic occlusion of the retinal artery; and (g) myocardial infarction caused by embolic occlusion of one of the coronary arteries. The first manifestation of endocarditis involving the right side of the heart, particularly the tricuspid valve, may be the development of "pneumonia" which is actually an embolic pulmonary infarct. The appearance of multiple areas of infiltration in the lungs in a patient with fever and a murmur should alert the physician immediately to the possibility of infection of the right side of the heart.

Progressive Involvement of the Valves. The modes of onset related to continued activity of the infectious process on the affected valve in untreated persons are a change in the character of a murmur and the development of progressive cardiac failure due to valvular dysfunction induced by slow destruction and fibrosis of the involved valve.

Immunological Disorders. An increasing number of patients with infective endocarditis in whom the diagnosis is delayed for weeks or months may have, as the first manifestation suggesting the possibility of subacute disease, findings related to the development of immunological phenomena. Some individuals may first come to medical attention because of the weakness, anorexia, and anemia associated with renal failure due to interstitial nephritis or proliferative glomerulonephritis resulting from the deposition of immune complexes in the kidney. Others may complain of arthralgias or arthritis probably related to the presence of the same type of complexes in the synovia. An occasional patient may complain of increasing difficulty with "palpitations." This may be immunological in origin, as suggested by the presence of Bracht-Wächter bodies in the myocardium, or may be the result of spread of infection from the valve to the conducting system in the interventricular septum. That the initial presentation of subacute endocarditis may be related to the development of immunological reactions is supported by the observation that the Osler node and probably the Roth spot may be, in part, due to vasculitis (see below).

Lumbar Pain. Persistent pain in the lumbar area has become an increasingly common early complaint of patients with subacute endocarditis. This is not due to vertebral osteomyelitis, as evidenced by failure to demonstrate any changes in the vertebral bodies over months of radiographic examination, and by the rapid disappearance of the pain after effective antimicrobial therapy is initiated.

Prosthetic Valvular Infections. The onset of infection involving prosthetic valves is often difficult to recognize because there may be no signs or symptoms, with the exception of fever, that clearly indicate the presence of this disease.

Drug Users. The mode of onset of infective endocarditis in persons who use illicit drugs intravenously is not sufficiently suggestive to permit a diagnosis; however, two features may indicate the presence of valvular infection in these patients. In those in whom the tricuspid valve is involved, the appearance of repeated episodes of pulmonary infarction is suggestive of the diagnosis. In persons with fungal infection of the mitral or aortic valves, the first manifestation may be embolic occlusion of a major artery, most often in one of the legs, because of the large size of the vegetations characteristic of this type of disease. In these cases, diagnosis is often established by embolectomy and isolation of the organism from the clot.

ACUTE ENDOCARDITIS

The mode of onset of acute infective endocarditis is distinctly different from that of the subacute form. Patients are usually previously well and become ill rapidly, with manifestations of severe infection. There are usually no signs indicating the presence of valvular disease in the early stage. Unlike subacute endocarditis, complications related directly to the rapidly advancing destructive process occur commonly within a week or less after infection and are often reflected by the rapid development of heart failure, especially when the aortic valve is involved. Because the thrombi on the affected valve are moderately large and soft, embolization is often the first manifestation of the disease, and patients may first be seen by a physician because of multiple petechiae or purpuric lesions of the skin, acute onset of neurological signs, or, if the infection involves the right side of the heart, "pneumonia" or single or multiple abscesses of the lung.

Signs and Symptoms

Elevation of the temperature is by far the most common sign of infective endocarditis; it has been reported in 100 per cent of cases by some investigators. However, the type and course of the fever are variable; normal or subnormal temperatures may be present in from 3 to 15 per cent of cases.[173] Absence of fever is not uncommon in elderly individuals with the subacute form of infection. This may be so because, with increasing age, basal (96.7°F or 36°C) and maximal (98.6°F or 37°C) daily temperatures tend to become lower than in young individuals. It is probably for

this reason that older patients with subacute infective endocarditis have "normal" temperatures. The writer has seen a number of cases of this disease in patients in their 70's who have been thought to be free of fever. However, when the course of the daily temperatures is charted over a period, variations ranging from 96.8°F (36°C) in the early morning to 98.6°F (37°C) in the late afternoon are noted, representing fever in such individuals. Absence of an elevated temperature should not preclude obtaining blood cultures when other signs and symptoms suggest endocarditis.

Other conditions in which fever may be absent in the face of subacute endocarditis are massive intracerebral or subarachnoid hemorrhage, cardiac failure, uremia, and administration of antimicrobial drugs in doses sufficient to decrease elevated temperatures but inadequate to eradicate the valvular infection. Repeated short courses of antimicrobial therapy, interspersed with periods during which treatment is withheld in patients with undiagnosed endocarditis, produce a characteristic pattern of repetitive episodes of remission and relapse of fever; this course should alert physicians to the possibility of the disease in any patient in whom a murmur is audible. With few exceptions, the maximal daily temperature of patients with acute infective endocarditis is higher (102 to 104°F or 39 to 40°C) than when the disease is subacute. Shaking chills are strikingly infrequent in the subacute infection unless salicylates are administered at inappropriate intervals; rigor will usually appear as the antipyretic activity disappears and the temperature begins to increase. In sharp contrast, patients with the acute form of infective endocarditis frequently experience high-grade fever in the range of 102 to 104°F (39 to 40°C) or higher early in the disease; shaking chills are common even when salicylates are not given.

Cardiac Murmurs

It was accepted dogma for many years that absence of a murmur ruled out the possibility of infective endocarditis, especially the subacute form of the disease. However, it is now apparent that up to 10 per cent of patients with subacute bacterial endocarditis do not have a detectable murmur when they first come to medical attention. In most instances, a murmur appears at some time during the period of treatment; less frequently, a murmur may not be detected until two to three months after therapy has been discontinued; in a rare patient, a murmur may never appear, even many years after cure of the infection.

Murmurs are not present in about one-third of patients with acute valvular infections involving the left side of the heart.[172,174] One of 167 patients with subacute and 7 of 54 patients with acute endocarditis were reported by Pankey to be free of murmurs.[175] He noted that changes in the character of the murmur occurred in 16.7 per cent of the subacute cases. This has not been the experience of this writer, who, in studies of more than 900 patients with subacute valvular infections, has found changing murmurs to be very uncommon. A change in a murmur occurs much more frequently in patients with acute valvular infections. One-third of cases of endocarditis of the right side of the heart, especially the tricuspid valve, and all with infection of the mural endocardium are free of murmurs. Basal systolic murmurs, caused either by the flow of blood from the left ventricle into a widened tortuous aorta or by atherosclerotic changes in the aortic valve, often pose a problem in the diagnosis of infective endocarditis, especially the subacute form, since the physician detects no change in the character of the murmur, the presence of which he may have been aware of for a long time. It must be stressed that, in older patients with unexplained fever who are known to have had a murmur for many years, the possibility of subtle bacterial endocarditis must always be entertained, even in the occasional instance in which blood cultures are negative. With respect to infective endocarditis, *no murmur can be considered "innocent."* Personal experience has taught that the discovery of a so-called "flow" or systolic "ejection" murmur that remains unchanged over long periods of observation has resulted in failure to consider the possibility of valvular infection.

Anemia is a universal feature of both acute and subacute infective endocarditis; *pallor* of the skin and mucous membranes is common. Libman and Friedberg called attention to rare patients who exhibited erythema of the nose and surrounding skin, especially the cheeks, bearing a slight resemblance to the facial lesion in systemic lupus erythematosus.[21]

Characteristic Diagnostic Lesions ("Peripheral Stigmata")

Five lesions involving the skin and its appendages and the eye have, for many years, been considered the classic peripheral manifestations of subacute bacterial endocarditis: *petechiae, subungual hemorrhages, Osler nodes, Janeway lesions,* and *Roth spots.* Because of the long course of the active disease in the pre-antibiotic era, these peripheral lesions were much more common than now, when effective antibiotic therapy usually rapidly brings the disease under control.[173] There has been a decrease in the incidence of *petechiae,* especially in the subacute form of the disease, from about 85 per cent before antimicrobial agents were available to 19 to 40 per cent at present.[14,17,19,172,174] Libman and Friedberg pointed out that petechiae with pale centers are of greater diagnostic importance than those with yellow centers.[171] These lesions are often present in the conjunctivae and are detectable, in some cases, only when the upper eyelids are everted. They also tend to occur most prominently on the skin on the dorsa of the hands and feet but are also commonly seen on the anterior chest and abdominal wall, oral and pharyngeal mucosa, and soft palate. Purpuric lesions develop occasionally and are rarely associated with thrombocytopenia. The presence of petechiae is not always diagnostic of infective endocarditis, since these lesions develop in patients with various types of hematological disorders (especially when the number of circulating platelets is markedly reduced), systemic lupus erythematosus, scurvy, renal insufficiency, bacteremia without endocarditis (staphylococcal, streptococcal, meningococcal, and gonococcal), atrial myxoma, and verrucous endocardiosis ("marantic endocarditis"). Over 50 per cent of patients who undergo cardiopulmonary bypass develop conjunctival petechiae in the immediate postoperative period, in the absence of infection, presumably owing to fat microemboli.[176] Because these persons are especially susceptible to valvular infection, physicians must be aware of this "false-positive" sign.

Subungual ("splinter") hemorrhages are uncommon in patients with bacterial endocarditis. At present they are observed more frequently in general hospital populations than in individuals with valvular infections[177] and are often related to advanced age and trauma. The characteristic features of a splinter hemorrhage are its linear form and the fact that its distal end does not reach the anterior edge of the nail bed; the latter distinguishes this lesion from a true splinter. The number of fingers involved is variable and ranges from a single nail bed with only one hemorrhage to several fingers, each of which contains several "splinters." In some cases, the toes may be involved, either alone or together with the fingers. In trichinosis, subungual hemorrhages are very common, and each nail bed contains numerous lesions.

Osler nodes are small, raised, nodular, red to purple, painful, tender lesions that are present most often in the pulp spaces of the terminal phalanges of the fingers. They may also be present on the back of the toes, soles of the feet, and the thenar and hypothenar eminences. They are less common on the sides of the fingers, the forearms, and the ears and rarely occur on the trunk. The most characteristic feature of these lesions is their tenderness. At times, patients can anticipate the development of Osler nodes because of an antecedent peculiar, local "sensation" or pain at a site in which the lesion later appears. They may be fleeting in some cases and disappear within a few hours after they have developed; however, they usually persist for four to five days but remain tender for only two to three days and rarely become necrotic. Although almost completely restricted to the subacute type of endocarditis, Osler nodes are present rarely in the acute form of valvular infection. There has been a striking decrease in the incidence of Osler nodes over the past 30 years.

Janeway lesions are small (1 to 4 mm in diameter), irregular, flat, erythematous, nontender, painless macules present most often on the thenar and hypothenar eminences of the hands and the soles of the feet of patients with subacute infective endocarditis. They appear less often on the tips of the fingers and plantar surfaces of the toes; rarely, they take the form of a diffuse macular erythematous rash over the extremities and trunk. The lesions on the hands and feet blanch with pressure and with elevation of the extremities. When present in cases of acute valvular infection, the lesions tend to be purple in color and hemorrhagic.

Clubbing of fingers and/or toes was present in virtually all patients with subacute bacterial endocarditis 25 to 30 years ago but is now quite uncommon.

Ocular signs are occasionally present in patients with infective endocarditis, especially the subacute type. In addition to the conjunctival petechiae, these lesions may also appear in the sclera and in the retina, where they are circular or flame-shaped. The *Roth spot,* as first described, is located in the retina and has the appearance of a "cotton-wool" exudate; it consists of aggregations of cytoid bodies.[178] Histological study of these lesions has shown them to be composed of perivascular collections of lymphocytes in the nerve layer of the retina that may or may not be surrounded by edema and hemorrhage. Because the association of these lesions with infective endocarditis was first recognized by Litten,[179] they are referred to as "Litten's sign" in the French literature. The boat-shaped hemorrhage in the retina, erroneously called a Roth spot, was first described by Doherty and Trubek, who attributed it to recurrent crops of petechiae.[180] They noted that these lesions often appeared over a period of only a few hours. Both the cytoid bodies and hemorrhagic spots have decreased in incidence over the years and are now present in less than 5 per cent of cases. Round white spots are occasionally present in the retina; they are noted more often in the acute than in the subacute form of the disease. Optic neuritis occurs occasionally.

Splenomegaly is still a relatively frequent sign in patients with endocarditis but is not as common as in the preantibiotic era, when it occurred in 80 to 90 per cent of cases. The spleen may be only slightly enlarged and barely palpable; in the acute form of the disease it may be large, soft, painful, and tender.

A number of other signs and symptoms, some of which are uncommon or rare, may be present in infective endocarditis. Among these are pericardial friction rub, manifestations of congestive heart failure, cardiac arrhythmias of various types, hematuria (in the absence of renal infarction), cough that may occur early and be very distressing, hoarseness, arthritis, and pain and tenderness of the long bones and of the sternum (especially when anemia is severe).

BACTERIA-FREE STAGE

The "bacteria-free stage" of endocarditis, first described by Libman in 1913,[181] is now very rare as a result of early diagnosis and treatment of the disease. However, this syndrome is still seen, albeit uncommonly, in patients in whom the disease remains unsuspected and untreated for months. The outstanding features of this form of valvular infection include congestive heart failure, diaphoresis, pain in the joints, swelling of the legs, and severe pain in the thighs. Fever is absent in most cases but develops when embolism occurs. Organisms are usually not present in the embolus. Although all patients have lesions of the mitral or aortic valves, new murmurs do not develop; in fact, they may disappear. The kidney is usually involved; macroscopic hematuria is common, even in the absence of infarction. Renal insufficiency is frequent and is the cause of death in about one third of cases. Anemia is universal. The white blood count is usually low, and granulocytopenia may develop. The spleen is enlarged to such an extent that it dominates the clinical picture. Petechiae are much less common than in the active stage of the disease, but purpuric lesions are more frequent. Osler nodes are uncommon. Two of the most frequent signs of the bacteria-free stage of endocarditis are marked tenderness of the sternum and a striking brown pigmentation of the face and back of the hands.

The criteria for the diagnosis of this syndrome are absence of manifestations indicating active valvular infection, during which bacteremia may have been present; negative blood cultures but organisms still present in the vegetations; renal insufficiency; severe progressive anemia; embolic phenomena; striking splenomegaly; brown pigmentation of the face; and absence of fever. Patients with this syndrome have survived for as long as three years and usually die from renal insufficiency or congestive heart failure.

COMPLICATIONS

Cardiac Complications

HEART FAILURE.   Congestive heart failure resulting from acute aortic regurgitation is currently the leading cause of death from infective endocarditis. This may occur over a varying period of time in untreated cases of the subacute form of the disease. In sharp contrast, cardiac failure may appear with startling rapidity in acute endocarditis when the aortic valve is infected and may become so severe within a week after the onset of infection that replacement of the valve becomes an emergency procedure. In a review of 144 cases of infective endocarditis, Mills et al. noted congestive failure in 55 per cent.[182] Eighty per cent of those with failure had regurgitant aortic valves and/or enterococcal infection. Cardiac decompensation occurred in about 50 per cent of patients with mitral valve regurgitation and in less than 20 per cent of those with congenital heart disease or infection of the tricuspid valve. Nearly 95 per cent of patients who experienced cardiac failure within six months after the onset of endocarditis had premonitory manifestations within one month after infection. Heart failure seldom developed de novo after six months. The organisms involved were (in order of frequency) enterococcus, *Strep. pneumoniae, Staph. aureus,* and *Strep. viridans.* Review of collected studies of congestive heart failure complicating infective endocarditis indicates an incidence ranging from 15 to 65 per cent. Aortic or mitral valve regurgitation may develop as early as one month after infection and nearly always within six months; in some instances, it may not occur until as long as one year after the appearance of endocarditis. Although it had been suggested that myocarditis is the basis of cardiac failure, it now seems clear that the primary cause is valvular destruction.

Another complication responsible for heart failure, said to be common in patients with severe aortic regurgitation, is the impact of the jet stream created by the regurgitant aortic valve on the mitral valve, leading to the development of a secondary lesion that varies in character from erosion to perforation of a cusp; the regurgitant stream may occasionally cause rupture of the chordae tendineae.[183] Severe involvement of the mitral valve accentuates the left ventricular overload imposed by the aortic regurgitation and markedly exaggerates the heart failure.

Hemodynamically important valvular stenosis may result from infective endocarditis when the vegetations are unusually large, as in fungal infection, and obstruct the flow of blood to and from the left ventricle.[184,185] One of the reasons for the development of congestive heart failure in patients with the Starr-Edwards prosthesis is progressive obstruction of the valvular outlet during the course of infection; this is most common when the invading organism is *Candida* or *Aspergillus,* because of the characteristically large vegetations. The hemodynamic changes in aortic regurgitation produced by infective endocarditis have been evaluated by Mann and his colleagues.[186] They noted that the mean pulse pressure, left ventricular end-diastolic volume, and stroke volume were significantly smaller in patients who developed aortic regurgitation acutely than in those with the chronic condition (p. 1111).

OTHER CARDIAC COMPLICATIONS. A number of intracardiac complications related directly to the valvular involvement may develop in the course of infective endocarditis and are much more common in the acute than in the subacute form of the disease.[170,172] Some, but not all, are associated with rapid or progressive congestive heart failure, a change in the character of an existing murmur, or the appearance of a murmur not previously detected. Some of the complications result from disruption of the valves and their supporting structures (Fig. 33–9). Among these are fenestration or tears of a leaflet, detachment of one or more areas of a valve from its annulus, and rupture of the chordae tendineae or papillary muscles. Another group of intracardiac complications includes the formation of fistulas, aneurysms (particularly of the sinus of Valsalva) that often involve the fibrous atrioventricular body, perforation of valve cusps, septal and other abscesses, and acute pericarditis with cardiac tamponade. In studies correlating anatomical and electrocardiographic abnormalities in 24 patients with aortic valve endocarditis, Roberts and Somerville found prolonged P-R intervals unrelated to digitalis therapy in 18 and atrioventricular dissociation in 4.[187] In 4 of 6 with prolonged P-R intervals and in 3 of 4 with normal conduction and left bundle branch block, aneurysms had invaded the interventricular septum; 4 out of 6 patients with prolonged conduction died suddenly.

Abscesses. One of the most serious intracardiac complications of bacterial endocarditis is the development of abscesses (Fig. 33–10) that are thought to be present in about 20 per cent of patients who succumb to valvular infections.[188,189] Abscesses tend to occur most often when *Staph. aureus* and enterococci are involved and are rare when infection is caused by *Strep. viridans*. Multiple myocardial abscesses may be present, especially when coagulase-positive staphylococci cause the disease and when antimicrobial therapy is not instituted until relatively late in the course of infection. A single large abscess may be present and rupture into the pericardial sac, causing rapid

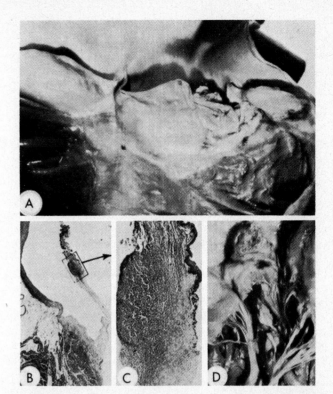

FIGURE 33–9 *Staphylococcus aureus* endocarditis involving pulmonic (*A, B,* and *C*) and mitral (*D*) valves. The vegetation on the pulmonic valve caused tearing of one leaflet. *B,* Histological section through portion of pulmonic valve cusp. *C,* Higher power view of a portion of the infected cusp shown in *B.* (From Roberts, W. C., and Buchbinder, N. A.: Right-sided valvular infective endocarditis. Am. J. Med. *53*:7, 1972.)

death from the resulting pyohemopericardium (Fig. 33–2). Septal abscesses are not uncommon in patients with acute staphylococcal endocarditis. In some instances, these completely destroy the involved area and produce a left-to-right shunt.

Abscesses of the interventricular septum secondary to in-

FIGURE 33–10 Pneumococcal endocarditis involving tricuspid (*A*) and aortic (*B*) valves. The vegetation on the tricuspid valve is small, whereas the vegetations on the aortic valve are large and cause extensive destruction of the cusps. *C,* Histological section of a portion of the tricuspid leaflet showing abscess formation. (From Roberts, W. C., and Buchbinder, N. A.: Right-sided valvular infective endocarditis. Am. J. Med. *53*:7, 1972.)

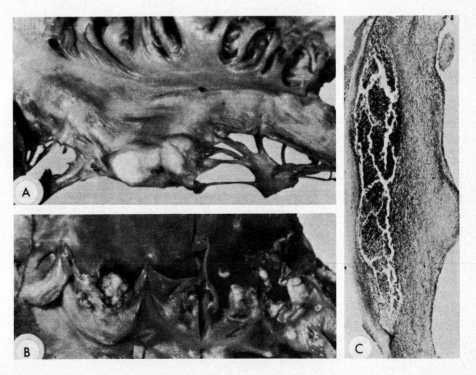

fection of the mitral valve are usually located in the lower part of the septum. The presence of this complication may be suspected on the basis of serial changes in the electrocardiogram, consisting of a gradual increase in atrioventricular conduction time and eventually left bundle branch block; the right bundle is much less frequently involved. Recognition of this entity during life is of great importance because surgical removal of the abscess and its replacement by a patch may be life-saving. A much more serious threat, because it is less often manageable surgically and is usually not suspected clinically, is an abscess involving the upper end of the septum that develops as a result of contiguous spread from an acutely infected aortic valve. In these cases, the electrocardiographic changes are not as characteristic as in the lower septal lesions; the diagnosis is usually overlooked. However, the appearance of various types of arrhythmias, including varying degrees of heart block, especially complete block, should alert the physician to the possibility of this type of abscess. Surgical removal is required for cure.

A specific type of *intracardiac abscess* involving the valvular ring has been described by Arnett and Roberts in 27 patients who succumbed to infective endocarditis.[190] The aortic annulus was involved most often, and abscess of the atrioventricular ring was observed in a few instances. This complication was not related to the age or sex of the patients, the status of the valves prior to the development of endocarditis, the nature of the infecting organism, or treatment with antimicrobial agents. The following criteria were found to be of value in the diagnosis of abscesses of valvular rings: (a) infection of the aortic valve, (b) recent appearance of regurgitation, (c) the presence of pericarditis, (d) a high degree of atrioventricular block (complete in five cases and Mobitz type II in one case), and (e) short duration of symptoms followed by the rapid development of severe disability and death.

Pericarditis. This is a rare complication of the subacute type of infective endocarditis and is not the result of bacterial invasion of the pericardial space in the vast majority of cases. It probably represents an immunological reaction, possibly deposition of immune complexes, in most instances. In contrast, the pericarditis that occasionally complicates the acute type of valvular infection is often purulent and results from hematogenous deposition of organisms in the pericardial space or from rupture of a myocardial abscess into the sac (Fig. 33–2). Other causes of pericarditis in patients with infective endocarditis include erosion of a mycotic aneurysm of the sinus of Valsalva, extension of infection from the aortic valve into the pericardial wedge between the root of the aorta and the pulmonary artery, uremia, and reactivation of rheumatic fever during the course of endocarditis.

Myocarditis. Although its pathogenesis is unclear at the moment, many observers consider myocarditis one of the important complications of infective endocarditis.[191,192] Whether it is the result of ischemic damage secondary to occlusion of the coronary arteries by emboli, damage produced by bacterial toxins, myocardial invasion by organisms, or the activity of immune complexes, or whether it may have a variety of causes, is as yet undetermined. The typical lesions associated with the myocarditis are the so-called Bracht-Wächter bodies (see earlier). Diffuse collections of lymphocytes or localized of diffuse aggregations of

polymorphonuclear leukocytes, with or without myocardial necrosis or miliary abscesses, are occasionally present. The myocardium may show areas of degeneration. Proliferation of the cells of capillaries and arterioles, arteriolitis or necrosis of the media or adventitia, and perivascular cellular infiltrations are detectable in some cases.

EMBOLIZATION. Next to complications involving the heart itself, arterial embolization is the most common potentially serious complication of infective endocarditis; its incidence has decreased over the past 30 years. Emboli were clinically detected in 70 to 97 per cent of patients in the preantibiotic era but are now found in only 15 to 35 per cent.[9,14,17,19,193] The most common sites are the spleen, kidneys, coronary vessels, and brain, although almost every tissue and organ may be involved. Splenic emboli have been discovered at autopsy in 44 per cent of cases but are suspected only rarely during life. Renal infarcts have been detected in as many as 56 per cent of patients studied at necropsy but are recognized clinically less often.[15] Bell has reported embolic glomerular lesions in the kidneys of 52 per cent of patients with subacute and in 7 per cent with acute bacterial endocarditis.[194] Myocardial infarction, often undetected by electrocardiography, has been found in 40 to 60 per cent of autopsied patients with valvular infections and is due to embolization of the coronary arterial bed. When the aortic valve is infected, infarction of the myocardium often leads to the development of congestive heart failure.[9,195–197] Major cerebral emboli have been observed in almost one third of patients with endocarditis at autopsy.[170]

The middle cerebral artery and its branches are most frequently involved, and hemiplegia is the most frequent consequence.[170,198] Jochman's dictum, "In hemiplegia in young adults or children always think of subacute bacterial endocarditis," is as applicable today as when it was first stated in 1914.[199] Three per cent of all emboli to the brain arise from infections of the cardiac valves.[200] Embolic occlusion of cerebral vessels may be the presenting sign of endocarditis. The clinical manifestations resulting from this are discussed below. Embolization of the vascular supply of the spinal cord is rare; it usually produces girdle pain and paraplegia.[201] Weakness, peripheral neuropathy, nerve tenderness, sensory disturbances, and localized pain may develop when emboli invade supplying peripheral nerves.[202–204]

Unilateral blindness due to embolization of the retinal artery, infarction of the retina with formation of a hole, and mononeuropathy may complicate valvular infections.[205]

It is important to emphasize that embolic occlusion of large arteries (e.g., the femoral) is rare when bacteria cause endocarditis; the most likely cause is fungal valvular disease or atrial myxoma. Large vegetations may also be present in an occasional case caused by *Staph. aureus*. It is well known that embolic phenomena may occur weeks to months after the infectious process on the valve has been eradicated. Most likely this is related to the fact that as long as six months may be required before the vegetations on the affected valve become completely covered by endothelium.

Metastatic Infections

In the acute infection, especially that due to *Staph. aureus*, an abscess develops at every site at which an embolus is deposited. In most patients who succumb to staphylococcal endocarditis, abscesses are present in almost every organ and tissue. If such lesions are not present at other sites, they are practically always detected in the kidneys and myocardium; the abscesses are usually small. The clinical course of staphylococcal endocarditis complicated by multiple diffuse abscesses may often be sufficiently characteristic to be diagnostic. The distinguishing features are (a) defervescence early during antimicrobial therapy; (b) return of fever either during treatment or after it has been discontinued; (c) failure to respond to the drug given initially or to the administration of another "effective" agent; and (d) negative blood cultures. If organisms are recovered from the blood, they are frequently still sensitive to the drug employed at the beginning of treatment.

In sharp contrast to this, metastatic infection following deposition of emboli in the course of subacute endocarditis, particularly that caused by *Strep. viridans*, is distinctly rare, probably because the number of organisms in the embolus is small, the bacteria have a low invasive capability, and most patients with this type of infection have high titers of specific bactericidal antibody that, in the presence of normal serum levels of complement, rapidly kills the few streptococci that are deposited. Thus, although infarction of the myocardium, brain, kidneys, and spleen develop in patients with subacute endocarditis, abscesses in these organs—suppurative myocarditis, pyogenic meningitis, splenic abscess, or pyelonephritis—are very rare. However, a sterile meningitis, with the biochemical and cellular characteristics of so-called aseptic meningitis, or a syndrome consistent with diffuse encephalitis with an abnormal or normal cerebrospinal fluid may occur in the subacute type of valvular infection and provide the first clue to the diagnosis, especially in cases in which an audible murmur is not present.

MYCOTIC ANEURYSMS. Mycotic aneurysms are a major complication of infective endocarditis. Although they have probably not decreased in incidence over the years, as indicated by the results of studies of autopsied cases, they are now detected clinically less often and are not as frequently fatal as they were in the past. They have been reported to occur in about 2.5 per cent of patients with valvular infections[206] and constitute 2.5 to 6.2 per cent of *all* aneurysms involving the brain. These lesions usually develop during the active phase of the infectious process but may not become manifest for months to years after it has been eradicated. They are most common when relatively noninvasive organisms such as *Strep. viridans* are involved and are less frequent when *Staph. aureus* is the causative agent. Several mechanisms may be involved in their pathogenesis. Among these are injury produced by deposition of immune complexes in the arterial wall, embolic occlusion of the vasa vasorum and sterile infarction of a blood vessel (usually in subacute endocarditis), and direct invasion by organisms or deposition of bacteria-laden emboli followed by infarction and the formation of an abscess in the vascular wall (common in acute infections). When mycotic aneurysms develop in the course of endocarditis due to *Staph. aureus*, there is a high incidence of rupture at the area of involvement of the blood vessel. Although any artery may be the site of an aneurysm, the vessels most often involved are those in the brain; the sinuses of Valsalva; ligated ductus arteriosus; the abdominal aorta

and its branches; and the coronary and pulmonary arteries.[15,207] The development of aneurysms is usually silent; clinical manifestations appear usually after the lesions have started to leak slowly or rupture and produce gross hemorrhages. When present in the brain, their pressure effects may produce headache or cranial nerve palsies. Areas in which mycotic aneurysms pose the greatest threat to life are the brain, abdominal aorta, the superior mesenteric, splenic, and coronary arteries, and ligated ductus arteriosus.

Neurological Complications

Neurological complications are some of the most life-threatening complications of infective endocarditis in both treated and untreated patients. The reported incidence of these phenomena has ranged from 9 to 80 per cent, with an average of about 15 to 30 per cent. They have been classified into three groups: (1) vascular phenomena due to embolization, (2) rupture of mycotic aneurysms, and (3) acute meningitis or meningocerebritis. Ziment[208] grouped the neurological manifestations of endocarditis on the basis of their etiology as follows:

Toxic—headache, impaired concentration, drowsiness, insomnia, vertigo, and irritability.

Psychiatric—neurosis, psychosis, confusion, disorientation, emotional instability, delirium, auditory and visual disturbances, apathy, and altered personality.

Cerebrovascular—hemi-, di-, para-, or quadriplegia, sensory and motor aphasia, aphonia, stupor, and coma.

Meningoencephalitis—acute brain syndrome.

Cranial nerves—visual disturbances, palsies of various cranial nerves, pseudobulbar palsy, and sensory impairment.

Dyskinesia—tremor, ataxia, parkinsonism, seizures, chorea, hemifacial dyskinesia, hiccupping, and myoclonus.

Spinal cord or peripheral nerves—girdle pain, weakness, paraplegia, paresis, sensory disturbances, myalgia, and peripheral neuropathy.

The brain may be the site of embolic abscesses in about 1 per cent of cases of subacute and in about 25 per cent of patients with acute infective endocarditis. Subdural empyema has also occurred. Ziment noted that encephalomalacia and endarteritis due to vasculitis of the cerebral arteries may be present. Petechiae and purpuric lesions may develop in the brain; they appear mostly in the white matter adjacent to the lateral ventricles but also in the gray matter along the aqueduct and in the corpus callosum. Meningeal or cerebral edema is present in some cases but usually produces no signs or symptoms. In addition to embolic retinal arterial occlusion, multiple retinal and conjunctival hemorrhages may develop. Other ocular complications of infective endocarditis are papilledema, iridocyclitis, panophthalmitis (usually in acute endocarditis), nystagmus, conjugate deviation of the eyes, and paresis of the third cranial nerves.

A study of the neurological complications observed in 281 cases of infective endocarditis admitted to the Massachusetts General Hospital has been reported by Pruitt et al.[209] Eighty-four patients (39 per cent) experienced neurological dysfunction during the course of the disease. The sex distribution of the cases was even; ages ranged from 3 months to 89 years, with most patients older than 50 years. The fatality rate was 58 per cent in those with manifestations of nervous system disorders, but only 20 per cent in persons with no neurological abnormalities. It was noted that neurological complications were most common with valvular infections caused by *Staph. aureus*, followed by streptococci, *Strep. pneumoniae*, and *Enterobacter*. Disturbances in function of the nervous system were noted in 79 of 84 patients with underlying cardiac valvular disease but in none with nonvalvular congenital heart disease.

Embolic cerebral infarction is the commonest neurological complication of infective endocarditis. It occurs in 6 to 31 per cent of patients with this disease and is associated more often with infection of the mitral than of the aortic valve. The infarctions are both macroscopic and microscopic. Emboli are present in other organs simultaneously with those in the brain in about half of cases. Cerebral infarction tends to occur within 2 weeks after the onset of valvular infection when highly invasive organisms such as *Staph. aureus*, enterococci, and *E. coli* are involved; staphylococci are responsible for about 70 per cent of these. When other bacteria, principally streptococci, produce the disease, cerebral infarctions develop in a biphasic manner and occur either 2 to 4 weeks or 1 to 3 months after the onset of the endocarditis. The fatality rate of cerebral infarction complicating infective endocarditis ranges from 17 to 81 per cent in patients who experience embolic strokes; approximately three fourths die within one year after onset of their valvular infection.[209]

Mycotic aneurysms of cerebral arteries are present in 2 to 10 per cent of patients with infective endocarditis and account for 2.5 to 6.2 per cent of all intracranial aneurysms.[209] A study of 85 cases of endocarditis in which the presence of cerebral mycotic aneurysms was demonstrated by angiography, indicated a fatality rate of 80 per cent in cases in which the lesions ruptured, and 30 per cent in those in which it remained intact; the overall death rate was 46 per cent.[210] Multiple aneurysms were present in 15 patients (17.6 per cent); in three, the second aneurysm did not appear until after treatment of the first. Angiographic examination showed that single aneurysms tended to be peripheral to the first bifurcation of a major intracranial artery; 20 of the lesions were at or proximal to that point. Sixty-five per cent of the aneurysms ruptured spontaneously; they disappeared in 10 cases.

Cerebral abscesses were noted at necropsy in 9 of the 218 patients (4.1 per cent); these lesions were not detected during life. In 8 cases, the abscesses were microscopic (< 1 cm³). In 6 cases, multiple microabscesses in the brain associated with similar lesions in other organs.

Neurological dysfunction of various types has been noted to be the presenting manifestation in a large number of cases of infective endocarditis.[209] Evidence of a major cerebral embolic episode involving mainly the middle cerebral arteries was the commonest problem that brought individuals to medical attention. Other manifestations included focal and/or generalized seizures (11 per cent), signs of cerebral embolus and hemorrhage, personality change, weakness of the lower extremities, subdural hemorrhage, and cortical blindness and obtundation without a focal defect. Among the disturbances of the nervous system developing after admission to the hospital were those listed above as well as multiple cerebral microemboli, microscopic brain

abscesses, visual disturbances, cranial or peripheral neuropathy, mycotic aneurysms, cerebral infarcts in the "watershed areas" due to hypotension, and psychiatric disturbances.

Cerebrospinal fluid has been normal in 28 per cent of the patients with neurological manifestations.[209] Polymorphonuclear leukocytes were predominant in cases caused by *Staph. aureus*, gram-negative bacilli, and *Strep. pneumoniae*. In the other instances, the meningitis was considered aseptic; these were associated, in most instances, with valvular disease produced by relatively avirulent bacteria such as *Strep. viridans*. Thirteen per cent of the patients had hemorrhagic cerebrospinal fluid.

MUSCULOSKELETAL SYSTEM.   Churchill, Geraci, and Hunder noted involvement of the musculoskeletal system in 44 per cent of patients with infective endocarditis.[211] In 27 per cent, symptoms and signs of dysfunction of the muscles or joints were the first or among the first complaints. The commonest manifestation was arthralgia. The shoulder joint was most commonly involved, followed, in descending order of frequency, by the knees, hips, wrists, ankles, and metatarsophalangeal and metacarpophalangeal joints. Multiple joints were affected in some cases. Objective evidence of arthritis was present in about one third of the cases. The ankle was most often involved, followed by the knees, wrists, sternoclavicular joints, elbows, metatarsophalangeal and metacarpophalangeal joints, and shoulder, hip, and acromioclavicular joints. Migrating polyarthritis was present in some instances. Pain in the lumbar area of the back, diffuse myalgias, and synovitis were also noted. Acute arthritis or arthralgia is present in 33 per cent of cases of gonococcal and 50 per cent of meningococcal endocarditis.

Renal Involvement

Involvement of the kidney is relatively common in patients with either acute or subacute infective endocarditis. Five types of renal lesions may develop.[212,213] Two are caused by embolization. While large bland infarcts of the kidney, associated with gross hematuria, were quite common 25 to 30 years ago, they now occur only infrequently.[174] However, multiple small infarcts are a relatively frequent finding at autopsy. One or more large abscesses or, more often, multiple microabscesses are commonly present in the kidneys of patients who die from acute valvular infections caused by *Staph. aureus*. The other lesions are all the result of immunological reactions and include interstitial nephritis and either acute or chronic proliferative glomerulonephritis. The acute form of the latter has been reported by Bell in 64 per cent of patients with subacute and 28 per cent of those with acute infective endocarditis.[194]

Immunological Phenomena

Immunoglobulins.   Specific agglutinating, complement-fixing, and bactericidal antibodies and cryoglobulins are present in the serum of patients with infective endocarditis, especially the subacute form. *Hypergammaglobulinemia* has been demonstrated by Cordeiro et al.,[214] who noted an early increase in 19S and 7S globulins followed by a rise in alpha₂ globulin. Immunoglobulins with specific affinities for the renal glomerular basement membrane, vascular walls, and myocardium of normal individuals were present. In patients with subacute endocarditis, gamma globulin was fixed in the sarcolemma and myofibrils of the myocardium; in the walls of blood vessels, especially in the intima and subintima; and in the basal layer of the glomeruli of the kidney.

The first report of the presence of *rheumatoid factor* in the blood of patients with subacute infective endocarditis was that of Williams and Kunkel.[215] They demonstrated positive latex fixation reactions in about 50 per cent of cases of the subacute type of endocardial infection, with high titers in most instances. The reactive factor was 19S globulin. With successful treatment, titers of circulating rheumatoid factor fell rapidly; even when very high, they reached zero within about 2 months after therapy was initiated. The latex fixation test is positive in about 50 per cent of patients with valvular infections present for 6 or more weeks. In addition to the duration of disease, the degree of elevation of serum levels of gamma G immunoglobulin is an important factor in determining positivity of this test. Other immunological abnormalities detected in some patients with infective endocarditis are antinuclear antibody and depression of total hemolytic complement as well as both C_3 and C_4.[216]

Sheagren et al. have reported that elevated titers of rheumatoid factor may also develop in patients with acute infective endocarditis.[217] They noted that 13 (24 per cent) of 55 parenteral drug users with valvular infections caused by *Staph. aureus* had circulating antibody of this type at some point in the course of their disease.

The presence of *circulating immune complexes* has been demonstrated by Bayer and his colleagues in 97 per cent of patients with infective endocarditis.[218] Blood levels of the complexes were greater than 12 $\mu g/ml$ in all instances and were significantly higher than in patients with sepsis without endocarditis. Circulating immune complexes were correlated with long duration of valvular infection, extravascular manifestations of the disease, and hypocomplementemia. In general, the complexes disappeared from the circulation within 6 weeks following successful antimicrobial or surgical treatment; this was concurrent with the resolution of extravascular signs, eradication of the bacteria from the bloodstream, and an increase in serum concentration of complement. In some patients, the concentration of the complexes in the blood did not fall until the infected valve was removed surgically.

Two studies have defined the type of endocardial disease associated with circulating immune complexes (IC). McKenzie and his colleagues[219] detected IC in 75 per cent of patients with valvular infections. This correlated with a subacute course and associated cutaneous vasculitis, glomerulonephritis, involvement of joints, and tissue deposits of immunoglobulins and complement. There was no correlation of IC with acute endocarditis, major embolic phenomena, Osler's nodes, Janeway lesions, or clinical evidence of renal disease. Serial determinations of IC were found to be important in monitoring the activity of the disease in patients whose blood cultures were negative, and in those with continued extravalvular manifestations of activity of the disease. Assessment of IC was of value in evaluating the need for replacement of valves. Kauffman et al.[220] studied four types of cases: endocarditis, septicemia without endocardial disease, endocardial lesions with nonseptic fever, and uncomplicated preexisting endocardial defects. IC was positive in 63 per cent of patients with endocarditis on admission. It occurred in 7 to 12 per cent of the others. The incidence of positive IC was higher when preexisting endocardial lesions were present, when endocarditis was caused by nonvirulent organisms, and when valvular infection had been present for more than 4 weeks. No differences were detected between left- and right-sided endocarditis. The levels of IC were higher when renal involvement was present. Higher mean peak levels were not detected when petechiae, subungual hemorrhages, Osler's nodes, Janeway lesions, or embolization developed.

Immunological phenomena play a critical role throughout the course of subacute infective endocarditis. A prime factor involved in the pathogenesis of this syndrome is the gradual development of *specific agglutinating antibody* as a result of repeated episodes of transient bacteremia over a period of years. It is believed that this finally stimulates development of a sufficient level of agglutinin to cause conglutination of the small number of organisms present in a transient bacteremia and leads to deposition of a bacterial inoculum

of sufficient size to initiate infection in the sterile platelet-fibrin clot. Until a high concentration of this antibody develops in the circulation over a period of years, usually as a result of multiple intrusions of organisms (most often *Strep. viridans*) infection does not occur, because the bacteria are few in number, have low invasive capability, remain in the bloodstream for a short time (usually no more than 5 to 10 minutes), and are rapidly eliminated by effective humoral and cellular clearing mechanisms. In the absence of technical problems (discussed below), blood cultures are negative in patients with valvular infection as a result of another immunological factor—specific bactericidal antibody.

Clinical Manifestations of Immunological Origin. Several of the manifestations present during the early stage of subacute bacterial endocarditis are probably immunological in origin. *Roth spots* resemble the cytoid bodies that may appear in systemic lupus erythematosus and other vasculitides. *Janeway lesions* may represent an immunological reaction.[216] It has also been postulated that the pathology of *Osler nodes* is strongly suggestive of an Arthus reaction. Howard has demonstrated a perivasculitis in many tiny vessels in the malpighian layers, without evidence of emboli or bacteria in these lesions.[221] Alpert et al.[222] have isolated *Staph. aureus* and *Candida* from these lesions and have suggested, as did Kerr,[15,19] that Osler nodes "are in all probability caused by minute emboli." The arthralgias of infective endocarditis are now also thought to be caused by deposition of immune complexes in the synovia; however, this has not been proved.

Among other clinical manifestations of infective endocarditis that may be related to disposition of immune complexes are sterile pericarditis, dermal vasculitis, deposition of immunoglobulin in blood vessels of normal skin, and leukocytoclastic angiitis of skin (purpuric lesions).[223,224] The best proved example of the operation of immunological reactions in the pathogenesis of complications of both acute and subacute valvular infection is acute, subacute, and chronic proliferative glomerulonephritis. These have been demonstrated in endocarditis caused by viridans streptococci as well as *Staph. aureus*.[225,226] Gutman and his associates noted discrete deposits of fibrin containing IgG and complement in the basement membrane and/or in the mesangial region of the glomeruli. Antibody eluted from the kidney of a patient with subacute endocarditis who died of renal failure was shown by Levy and Hong to combine specifically with the bacteria cultured from the blood.[227] The elute also contained antiglomerular antibody and activated complement in the destroyed basement membrane. Lumpy-bumpy glomerular fluorescence, when stained for IgG and $\beta_1 C$, has been demonstrated in patients with subacute endocarditis.[228]

ENDOCARDITIS INVOLVING THE RIGHT SIDE OF THE HEART

Infective endocarditis involving the right side of the heart occurs in about 5 per cent of cases[229,230] (Figs. 33–9 and 33–10), but there has been a sharp increase in this type of cardiac disease in recent years. This is, for the most part, due to infection of the tricuspid valve in users of illicit drugs. Many of these infections are caused by *Staph. aureus, Pseudomonas*, yeasts, and fungi.

Two thirds of the cases of right-sided endocarditis studied at the Mayo Clinic were acute, with prominent pulmonary manifestations; murmurs, splenomegaly, or multiple cutaneous and renal abscesses were present in about one third of cases.[229] Blood cultures were usually positive. *Staph. aureus* was isolated in half the cases; *Strep. pneumoniae, N. gonorrhoeae,* streptococci *(viridans, faecalis, and pyogenes),* and gram-negative bacilli have also been recovered. Hearts with congenital malformations or normal ones are most often involved. Infections of skin wounds, respiratory tract *(Strep. pneumoniae),* and urethra; prostatic massage; dental sepsis; normal parturition; septic abortion; and narcotic addiction are among the reported pathogenetic factors.[229,230] In 80 per cent of the cases with tricuspid valve involvement a murmur was not heard, and the diagnosis was not suspected during life.[229] Renal involvement, most commonly abscesses or diffuse pyelonephritis, was detected in 65 per cent of patients. Glomerular and tubular hemorrhage and focal embolic glomerulonephritis have also been noted. In congenital lesions with exclusive or predominant left-to-right shunts, defects of the interventricular septum, or patent ductus arteriosus complicated by endocarditis, emboli are deposited almost exclusively in the lungs early in the course of the disease and may produce hemoptysis, pleurisy, or pneumonia;[231] peripheral embolization may occur later.

Myocarditis is one of the complications of endocarditis involving the right side of the heart. Histologically, this consists of small foci of perivascular collections of polymorphonuclear leukocytes or diffuse infiltrates with the same type of cell or miliary abscesses. The lungs are the primary site for the deposition of emboli, resulting in the development of single or multiple *pulmonary infarcts.* If the infecting organisms are relatively avirulent (e.g., *Strep. viridans*), the infarcted areas will only rarely be infected. In contrast, when a highly invasive bacterium such as *Staph. aureus* is the causative agent, the infarcts are almost always infected and are rapidly converted to abscesses. Other pulmonary complications include pneumonia, thrombosis, and septic arteritis of the branches of the pulmonary artery. Among the *renal complications* of endocarditis involving the right side of the heart are suppurative nephritis, focal or diffuse proliferative glomerular nephritis, or tubular hemorrhages.

The sequential appearance of repeated episodes of "pneumonia" (infarcts of the lung) followed by hepatomegaly, often associated with a mild degree of jaundice, and finally the development of progressive renal failure in patients with persistent fever, should raise the possibility of infection of the right heart, even in the absence of a murmur. Blood cultures are frequently negative when relatively noninvasive organisms are involved. However, when infectious process is caused by *Staph. aureus,* blood culture is often positive *after* the development of infected pulmonary infarcts, which become the source of bacteria entering the systemic circulation. Causes of death in untreated persons with involvement of the right heart, and even in some who receive appropriate therapy, are multiple pulmonary infarcts and abscesses, cardiac failure, and post-operative hemorrhages in patients subjected to surgery for patent ductus arteriosus.

INFECTIVE ENDOCARDITIS IN CHILDREN
(See also p. 951)

Kerr noted that only about 2 to 3 per cent of cases of infective endocarditis occur during the first decade of life.[15]

Only 5 cases in over 400 instances of valvular infection were noted by Cates and Christie.[9] The subacute form of the disease has been identified in babies as young as 8 and 10 months of age,[15] and mycotic endocarditis has been observed in a 7-week-old premature infant. Although bacterial endocarditis is exceedingly uncommon in neonates, a recent report[141] has described three babies (one aged 7 weeks and two only 7 hours old) who died of infective endocarditis. The diagnosis was made only at autopsy. The tricuspid valve was involved in two and the mitral valve in one of the neonates. The responsible bacteria were *Staph. epidermidis* in one, *E. coli* in another; no organisms were recovered from the third baby. All the infants had had catheters inserted into the umbilical or other veins.

An analysis by Zakrzewski and Keith of 50 cases of infective endocarditis in children has indicated that underlying rheumatic heart disease is a very uncommon predisposing factor[232]; the commonest one appears to be the tetralogy of Fallot, followed in order of frequency by aortic stenosis, patent ductus arteriosus, and pulmonic stenosis. There is a striking difference in the factors that predispose to valvular infection in children and adults. In children, these include severe burns, osteomyelitis, asthma, bronchitis, infection of the urinary tract, otitis media, thrombophlebitis, pneumonia, pansinusitis, diarrhea, dermatitis, circumcision, and acute rheumatic fever.

A difference in the frequency of specific organisms responsible for endocarditis in children was noted by Zakrzewski and Keith in a comparison of cases studied from 1952 to 1961 and those observed between 1958 and 1962.[232] *Staph. aureus* was responsible for 37 per cent and *Strep. viridans* for 32 per cent in the first period; in the latter one, *Staph. aureus* and *epidermidis* caused 72 per cent, while *Strep. viridans* was involved in about 20 per cent; the marked increase in staphylococcal valvular disease is undoubtedly related to the greater frequency of cardiac surgery.

Infective endocarditis in infants less than 2 years of age, most of whom were only a few weeks or months old, was characterized by a number of features that distinguish it from that involving older children[143]; all cases were of the acute type and involved more than one valve. Congenital heart disease was present in only 8 per cent. About 60 per cent had infection of the mitral valve; the tricuspid valve was affected in 32 per cent, the aortic valve in 17 per cent, and the pulmonic valve in 6.5 per cent. Embolic phenomena were present in only 18 per cent. In every instance, there was evidence of disease at extracardiac sites. Among these were infections of the skin, enteritis, empyema, osteomyelitis, and tuberculosis. Diagnosis of endocarditis in these infants was usually made post mortem. Valvular infections in older children were caused most commonly by *Staph. aureus*; next most frequent were *Strep. viridans* and *Staph. epidermidis*; together, these three organisms were responsible for 80 per cent of the cases. Other bacteria involved included *Pseudomonas, E. coli, H. influenzae,* and *K. pneumoniae*; enterococci rarely caused the disease. Although before 1958 rheumatic heart disease was the underlying lesion in 50 per cent of the older children, in the following years this disorder was rarely a predisposing factor. Osler nodes were not observed in any of these children.

An extensive review of 149 instances of bacterial endocarditis in 141 children studied at the Children's Hospital Medical Center in Boston during the period 1933 to 1972 has been presented by Johnson, Rosenthal, and Nadas.[233] Six of the patients had two and one had three episodes of the disease. Predisposing factors, in order of frequency, included infected extracardiac foci (urinary tract infection, meningitis, and osteomyelitis), dental manipulation, cardiac surgery, catheterization, and orthopedic and otolaryngological surgical procedures. The commonest underlying types of heart disease were congenital (118 cases) and rheumatic (14 cases). There were no significant disorders of the heart in 17 patients. The most frequent underlying lesion was the tetralogy of Fallot; the others, in order of incidence, were ventricular septal defects, aortic stenosis, rheumatic heart disease, patent ductus arteriosus, and transposition of the great arteries. Blood cultures were sterile in 19 children. Presenting clinical manifestations consisted of fever (87 per cent), splenomegaly (65 per cent), petechiae (42 per cent), and heart failure (34 per cent). In 21 per cent, heart murmurs were present and underwent changes during the course of the disease. The most frequent complication was congestive heart failure; others included central nervous system disorders, pulmonary emboli, and aortic regurgitation.

A study of 33 autopsies of patients who had endocarditis during the first decade of life disclosed that rheumatic rather than congenital heart disease was the commonest underlying cardiac lesion. The left side of the heart was involved more often than the right; peripheral septic foci and pneumonia were the most frequent sources of infection.[234]

Fifty children (aged 6 months to 16 years) with endocarditis were studied at the Mayo Clinic over a 30-year period.[140] Thirty-seven had congenital heart disease, 4 had a history of rheumatic carditis, 17 had undergone cardiac surgery, 8 had had some type of instrumentation or noncardiac surgical procedure within 2 weeks before developing valvular infection, and 11 had an obvious extracardiac bacterial infection. A cardiac murmur was present in all but one. Microscopic hematuria, neurologic deficits, or other embolic phenomena and abnormal funduscopic findings were present in some patients. Staph. aureus was the most common infecting organism. Viridans streptococci were next most common. The rest were produced by other gram-positive organisms or gram-negative bacilli. The fatality rate was significantly higher in younger children. Older ones had a better outcome, as did those (any age) with viridans streptococcal infection. The results of this study indicated that pediatric endocarditis occurs primarily in children with congenital heart disease. The mortality is high, despite antibiotic therapy. The findings of persistent unexplained fever and bacteremia in a child with congenital heart disease should suggest the presence of endocarditis.

PROSTHETIC VALVE ENDOCARDITIS

The clinical features of infection of prosthetic valves are, for the most part, the same as those that characterize endocarditis involving natural valves. Infection of the surgical wound in the sternum, or sternal osteomyelitis, is a common predisposing factor. Variations in the period of time elapsing between operation and the onset of prosthetic infection were discussed earlier (p. 1146). The develop-

ment of fever associated with or following detection of a new murmur suggestive of a paravalvular leak suggests the presence of endocarditis.

Several complications are peculiar to prosthetic valvular endocarditis. One is associated primarily with the presence of a ball-type prosthesis, especially the Starr-Edwards valve (Fig. 33–3), and consists of the gradual development of congestive heart failure due to progressive obstruction of the outlet of the valve by growth of bacteria or, more commonly, yeasts or fungi. Another complication of endocarditis of prosthetic valves, shared by patients addicted to intravenously administered drugs, is an increased incidence of embolization of large arteries due to the greater frequency of fungal colonization and infection. Persistent elevation of temperature in patients with valvular prostheses, in the absence of either a change in an existing murmur or the development of a new one, together with sterile cultures of blood, is highly suggestive of an abscess in the annulus, frequently at the site of one or more of the sutures anchoring the prosthesis. Rarely, diffuse invasion of the annulus may lead to almost complete tearing away of the prosthesis. Synthetic materials used to close septal defects may also become infected. The clinical features of endocarditis associated with this last condition are not specific, and the complications that develop do not specifically suggest infection of the synthetic materials.

ENDOCARDITIS DURING PREGNANCY AND THE PUERPERIUM

Libman and Friedberg pointed out that bacterial endocarditis may occur during pregnancy or shortly after childbirth.[171] They suggested that, in the presence of pelvic inflammatory disease, a transient bacteremia occurring during labor and delivery might be followed by subacute endocarditis in women with underlying cardiac disease. If the uterus becomes infected during the puerperium (puerperal sepsis), especially when the infection is exogenous in origin, the endocarditis may be of the acute type, because of the high frequency with which Strep. pyogenes is the responsible organism. When endocarditis develops as a complication of endogenous puerperal sepsis, it is likely to be subacute and caused by relatively noninvasive organisms such as Strep. viridans. Although there is currently no evidence that the fetus is infected during the course of endocarditis occurring during pregnancy, it is entirely possible that this may occur if the infective organism is highly pathogenic. When the disease is caused by Staph. aureus, Strep. pyogenes, Strep. pneumoniae, N. gonorrhoeae, or H. influenzae, especially if bacteremia is present, fetal infection may develop and lead to the death of the baby or spontaneous abortion.

RELAPSE AND RECURRENCE OF INFECTIVE ENDOCARDITIS

Early or intercurrent relapses are defined as the development of manifestations of infection together with positive blood cultures that appear during or shortly after (< 3 months) completion of treatment with antimicrobial agents. Among the factors responsible are (a) superinfection (by an organism different from the one initially present) often associated with the use of "broad-spectrum" antibiotics; (b) spread, via the circulation, of a drug-resistant bacterium or fungus from an extracardiac site such as a colonized intravenous catheter, suppurative thrombophlebitis, or infection of the urinary tract; (c) the development of resistance of the organism initially responsible for the disease; and (d) the appearance of "cell wall–deficient" organisms ("persisters"), especially when drugs that inhibit the synthesis of the bacterial cell wall (penicillins, cephalosporins) are administered. This last factor has been suggested, but its importance in intercurrent relapses remains to be proved.

A syndrome that appears to be an early relapse but is actually due to an intra- or extracardiac complication occurs occasionally in patients with endocarditis caused by *Staph. aureus.* As pointed out above (p. 1155), the development of abscesses in one or more other organs is usually accompanied by a return of fever and bacteremia after a period of what appears to be a satisfactory therapeutic response; however, this is not due to relapse of infection in the affected valve.

Late relapse is defined as return of all the features of active endocarditis three to six months after antimicrobial treatment has led to apparent "cure" of the infection. The causative agent of the relapse may be different from the one initially responsible for the valvular disease. In some instances, however, it is identical to the one originally recovered from the blood. Late relapse is relatively common in patients with endocarditis caused by yeasts or fungi. The reasons for this are (a) relative insensitivity of the organism to the drug used for treatment, (b) failure of the antifungal agent to penetrate the valvular lesion to a depth great enough to eradicate all the organisms, and (c) spread of the infection to sites in the heart contiguous to the affected valve. Late relapses are also quite common when endocarditis involves prosthetic valves, and the causative agent is often the one initially involved. However, in some instances, the initial bacterial infection may be followed, either during treatment or within six months by invasion of the prosthesis by a fungus or yeast, especially when combined "broad-spectrum" antimicrobial therapy is given.

Recurrent Endocarditis. This is defined as the reappearance of all the cardinal manifestations of infective endocarditis and positive blood cultures later than six months after cure of the initial episode. It may be caused by the same organism that produced the first episode but is often due to a different bacterium or fungus. A mechanism that may be responsible for recurrent endocarditis has been suggested by Cordeiro and Pimental.[235] They noted that bacteria frequently persist in healed valvular lesions for longer than 10 months after a clinical "cure" had been accomplished by means of appropriate chemotherapy and compared this situation with "inactive" tuberculosis. The incidence of recurrent endocarditis has been reported to range from 2 to 4 per cent;[19] however, higher frequencies have been recorded when the period of follow-up study has been long. Morgan and Bland noted second episodes in 8.5 per cent of their patients.[20] Patients with prosthetic valves may experience recurrent infections over a period of months or years. This writer has studied one patient who experienced a mixture of five relapses and recurrences. The first involved a natural valve; the others were infections of various types of valvular prostheses, each of

which was removed. A different organism was responsible for each of the episodes.

Recurrent endocarditis was noted by Welton and his associates in 18 of 58 patients (31 per cent). In addition to drug abuse, prior heart disease and periodontitis were each related to recurrence. Patients with two or more of these three risk factors were more likely to have a recurrence than those with only one risk factor, and the fatality rate was higher with recurrences than with initial episodes of endocarditis.[235]

LABORATORY FINDINGS

Elevation of erythrocyte sedimentation rate is the most common and almost universal abnormal laboratory finding in infective endocarditis.[14] *Anemia* is present in from 50 to 80 per cent of patients with this disease when they first come to medical attention. In those with subacute infection, the loss of hemoglobin is gradual and may reach strikingly low levels when the process is prolonged. In the acute form, the anemia may progress with striking rapidity and become pronounced within one to two weeks after onset. In both instances, the characteristics of the anemia are those observed in all types of infection. In rare instances, an acute hemolytic process may develop in both acute and subacute endocarditis.

In subacute infective endocarditis the *white blood count*, in most instances, does not exceed 7,000 to 8,000/mm^3. However, in almost all cases, there is a shift to the left, and a varying percentage of immature forms is the rule. In contrast, leukocytosis, with white blood counts ranging from 15,000 to 20,000/mm^3 or higher, is usual when the acute disease is present; there is usually a shift to the left. It must be stressed, however, that a normal white blood count and even leukopenia may be present in the acute infection.

Hyperstimulation of the reticuloendothelial system, as evidenced by an *increase in the number of plasma cells in the bone marrow*, is common in subacute endocarditis. In rare cases, the number of these cells in the marrow is so great that a diagnosis of multiple myeloma or disseminated tuberculosis is suspected. Large lymphocytic cells—histiocytes—are detectable in the capillary blood in 15 to 25 per cent of the subacute cases. These are usually not present in the peripheral blood but are demonstrable in blood obtained from the tip of a finger or the lobe of the ear.

Although *thrombocytopenia* due to disseminated intravascular coagulation occurs as a rare complication of acute bacterial endocarditis, this may appear as an infrequent, isolated finding in both the subacute and acute types of valvular infection. The presence of some types of immunological abnormalities in both acute and subacute endocarditis is an important finding that may be helpful in diagnosis (p. 1149).

The *urine* is normal in uncomplicated cases of infective endocarditis. In some instances, *proteinuria* may be the only abnormality and is often related to the presence of fever. Red blood cells in the urine usually indicate renal infarction. *Hematuria, red blood cell casts,* and *proteinuria* suggest acute proliferative glomerulonephritis.

Unless patients have problems with water loss through sweating or vomiting or develop glomerulonephritis, renal infarcts, or interstitial nephritis, BUN, creatinine, and serum electrolyte levels are normal. In the early stages of bacteremia and endocarditis due to gram-negative organisms, alkalosis may develop; this appears to be due to hyperventilation induced, in an unknown manner, by stimulation of the respiratory center and loss of CO_2.

DIAGNOSIS

CLINICAL FEATURES. The characteristic features, especially of the subacute form of infective endocarditis, have undergone such remarkable changes over the past 30 years that if present-day physicians relied on the clinical diagnostic criteria established in the years preceding 1950, the disease would not be suspected in 90 per cent or more of the cases.[14,22,82,174] Thus, as already pointed out, Osler nodes, Janeway lesions, and Roth spots have become quite uncommon. Even subungual hemorrhages and petechiae are seen only occasionally.

The most striking feature of "modern" infective endocarditis is the increasing frequency with which *cardiac murmurs are absent* in both acute and subacute forms of the disease. Fifty years ago, the absence of a murmur was considered to rule out subacute endocarditis. It has now become apparent that an increasing number of patients with this type of infection have no detectable murmur when first seen; the diagnosis is usually suspected on the basis of multiple positive blood cultures, in the absence of any other source of infection and, quite often, the development of an embolic complication. In most of these individuals, a murmur develops during the course of treatment; in a few, it does not become detectable until two to three months after cure is accomplished and is not related to recurrence of the infection; in a rare instance, a murmur may never develop. The increased number of patients who do not have murmurs when they first come to medical attention is due, in part, to the higher frequency of acute endocarditis involving the left side of the heart and acute or subacute infection of the tricuspid valve. These forms of endocarditis are characterized by absence of a murmur in about one third of cases early in the course of the disease. In most, a murmur usually appears at some time during or after treatment.

Most physicians are still under the impression that a change in the character of the murmur is common in infective endocarditis and that this is a diagnostic feature of the disease. This is rarely the case in subacute valvular infection. It is, however, fairly common in patients in whom the process is acute, especially when it is caused by *Staph. aureus.* The cause of the change is practically always destruction of the valve and its supporting structures. Very common in patients with staphylococcal endocarditis involving the aortic valve is the sudden appearance of a loud diastolic blowing murmur related to the development of aortic regurgitation. Less common, but also responsible for a change in murmur in the acute disease, is rupture of the chordae tendineae or papillary muscles or separation of a leaflet of the valve from the annulus. In patients with prosthetic valves, the appearance of a murmur or a change in one already present is often associated with a paravalvular leak that may or may not be induced by infection.

One of the most difficult diagnostic problems is presented by the older patient known to have had a grade 2 or 3 basal systolic murmur for years, who develops fever, whose blood culture may or may not be positive, and who presents with none of the peripheral manifestations of infective endocarditis. This type of murmur is usually caused by calcific, degenerative changes in the aortic valve or may be due only to the widening and tortuosity of the aorta associated with aging. Often the diagnosis of valvular infection is not considered seriously in such individuals, especially when blood cultures are negative. A similar problem is encountered with younger patients in whom a grade 2 "ejection" or "flow" murmur is considered "innocent," whereas, in fact, it represents a valvular abnormality on which either acute or subacute infection may become superimposed.

The availability of effective antimicrobial agents has resulted in an important diagnostic problem, which, if not appreciated, may lead to potentially life-threatening complications of subacute infective endocarditis. Typically, the patient seeks medical attention because of fever. Despite detection of a murmur, blood cultures are not carried out, but oral therapy with an antibiotic is initiated. In the individual with valvular infection caused by an organism susceptible to the drug administered, defervescence often occurs within 4 to 5 days. However, when the fever is a manifestation of endocarditis, it usually returns in about 7 to 10 days after treatment has been discontinued. This usually leads to another visit to the physician, who often makes a diagnosis of "viral infection" and reinstitutes treatment with the antibiotic that had previously reduced the elevated temperature. Such short periods of exposure to one or more antimicrobial agents may be repeated several times before it becomes apparent that the patient is becoming increasingly ill, or until an embolic episode, heart failure, or some other complication develops, when the patient is finally hospitalized, blood samples are cultured, and the diagnosis is established. It must be emphasized that each recurrence of fever, because it represents the recrudescence of the valvular infection, adds to the valvular damage. This course of events in a patient with fever and cardiac murmur is so highly suggestive of infective endocarditis that a full course of antimicrobial therapy with bactericidal agents should be instituted even when multiple blood cultures prove to be sterile.

BLOOD CULTURES. The sine qua non for the diagnosis of infective endocarditis is recovery of the causative organism from the blood.

Whether or not bacteria or other infectious agents are grown depends on a number of factors, some of which are technical and some of which involve specific clinical and immunological phenomena.[236] It is now clear that the bacteremia of endocarditis is qualitatively continuous but quantitatively discontinuous, i.e., organisms are probably always present but their numbers vary considerably. This is illustrated by the study of Beeson et al.,[239] who showed that only about 3 per cent of blood cultures of patients with subacute valvular infections contained more than 100 organisms/ml. Only 2 of 19 blood cultures were found to be positive by Mallen et al.[238] The incidence of positive blood cultures, as recorded by various observers, has varied considerably. Werner and his colleagues obtained positive cultures in 95 per cent of 789 cultures in 206 patients.[239] The first culture of the blood of individuals with streptococcal endocarditis was positive in 95 per cent of the cases; one of the first two cultures yielded the causative agent in 98 per cent. When infection was caused by organisms other than streptococcus, positive cultures were obtained in only 82 per cent. The bacteremia was commonly of "low magnitude"; only 17 per cent of the blood samples contained more than 100 organisms/ml. Others have reported an incidence of positive blood cultures ranging from 53 to 74 per cent.[240,241] Belli and Waisbren noted that the organism responsible for the valvular infection could be isolated from one of the three initial blood cultures in only 82 per cent of their patients.[241] Differences in the colony counts in blood collected from different arterial and venous sites were noted by Beeson and his coworkers.[237] In general, mixed venous blood entering the heart contained about 35 per cent fewer colonies than did arterial blood. Despite this, a number of other observers have noted no advantage in culture of arterial over venous blood in establishing the presence of clinically significant bacteremia in cases of infective endocarditis.

A unique approach in determining the site of infection in patients with valvular infection caused by *Pseudomonas* has been recorded by Pazan and his colleagues,[242] who catheterized the left brachial artery, right atrium, right pulmonary artery, right ventricle, superior vena caval–right atrial junction, pulmonary artery, and ascending aorta; blood obtained from each of these sites was cultured quantitatively. The largest number of organisms was recovered during "pull-back" from the pulmonary artery. There was no consistent "step-up" over the mitral valve. There was a "step-up" in the number of bacteria between the superior and inferior vena cava and the right atrium. This suggested infection and regurgitation of the tricuspid valve, which was confirmed by dye dilution curves, phonocardiography, and angiography.

In a rare instance, culture of bone marrow may identify the organism responsible for endocarditis when the blood is sterile. It must be emphasized, however, that a single positive culture is not diagnostic; instead, a minimum of three, all of which yield the same agent, is required before a causal relation between the recovered bacterium and the disease can be considered suggestive. This is also true for positive cultures of the urine in the absence of bacteremia; in the uncommon case in which this occurs, there are usually no sedimentary abnormalities indicating infection of the urinary tract.

In patients with fungal endocarditis, especially when the causative agent is *Aspergillus* blood cultures are frequently negative. However, the fungus responsible for the valvular infection may often be recovered from an embolus that lodges in a large artery—a relatively frequent occurrence in this type of disease.

Cultures of the blood of patients with infective endocarditis have been reported to be sterile in from 2.5 to 65 per cent.[243] A number of factors are responsible for this. Some are technical in nature, while others involve the type of disease, the kind of patient affected, the characteristics of the organism responsible for the infection, and the use of antimicrobial agents.

Renal insufficiency has been common in persons with negative cultures of blood. These cases are identical to the "bacteria-free stage" of the disease described by Libman in which organisms, although absent from the blood, are still present on the infected valves.[21] Lerner and Weinstein confirmed the relation between renal failure and negative blood cultures.[14] However, later studies have indicated that the important factor involved in the sterility of the blood is the duration of untreated disease and that specific bactericidal antibody is responsible for the absence of organisms. Although bacteria are still present in the vegetations, they are rapidly eradicated by this antibody when they enter the circulation.

An analysis of 1500 cases of infective endocarditis by Cannady and Sandford showed that cultures of the blood were sterile in from 2.5 to 31 per cent.[243] They pointed out that among the factors involved in this were mural endocarditis, bacteria with special growth requirements, and nonbacterial organisms such as *Coxiella burnetii* and *Chlamydia*.

Negative Cultures. One of the increasingly important reasons for the greater frequency of negative blood cultures in patients with infective endocarditis is treatment with one or more antimicrobial agents before the diagnosis is established.[244-246] As short a period of exposure to an antibiotic as two days may make it impossible to retrieve organisms from the blood, despite the fact that they are still present on the vegetations. It is difficult to indicate how long a period is required after therapy has been discontinued before blood cultures will again become positive. This

does not depend entirely on the time required for the antimicrobial agent to be excreted for three reasons: (1) animal studies in which fibrin clots were used as models of the basic lesion of endocarditis—the sterile platelet-fibrin thrombus—have shown that all antimicrobial agents persist in a mass of fibrin for as long as 12 or more hours after they are no longer detectable in the blood[247,248]; (2) some antibiotics persist in the circulation for fairly long periods; and (3) exposure to an antibacterial drug may completely eradicate the organisms lying on the surface of the platelet-fibrin thrombus but may fail to kill all those buried in the fibrin mass, which, when therapy is discontinued, require a varying time to resume multiplication until they reach the surface of the lesion, from which they are shed into the bloodstream. The longer the exposure to drug, the greater the time required for this to occur.

It is impossible to state categorically, in any patient, how long it would take for blood rendered sterile by an antimicrobial agent to yield organisms after cessation of treatment. In some instances, especially when the period of treatment has been only two to three days, cultures may become positive 48 hours after the drug has been withdrawn. In contrast, when an antiinfective compound has been administered for longer periods, cultures may not become positive until a week or more after its use has been discontinued. Because of this, patients who are suspected on clinical grounds of having infective endocarditis and who have been treated must no longer receive the drug. Culturing of the blood should be initiated 24 to 48 hours after therapy has been withdrawn. If results are negative, cultures should be repeated until 7 to 10 days have elapsed. If the blood is still sterile at that time, a factor other than the antimicrobial therapy, the presence of an unusual organism, or a diagnosis other than infective endocarditis should be considered. When subacute bacterial endocarditis is present, there is no real danger in delaying therapy for as long as a week, since (1) if, as in the bulk of instances, fever is absent, the patient has already been partially treated, and (2) early death is not related to the infectious process but rather to a potentially lethal embolic episode—an unpredictable event that is not prevented by the most effective antimicrobial therapy. This is not true in most cases of acute endocarditis, in which a delay of 24 to 48 hours in initiating treatment may be seriously life-threatening.

In a number of cases, technical factors, including the use of inadequate quantities of blood or medium, improper timing of the culture, too small a number of specimens, and inappropriate incubation, are responsible for failure to recover the causative agent from patients with infective endocarditis. Because the number of organisms in the blood is small and variable, the optimal quantity drawn should be no less than 10 ml, in order to furnish an inoculum adequate to initiate bacterial growth. Many patients, especially those who have had the subacute form of the disease, have low to moderate concentrations of antibody or have received treatment with minimal doses of an orally administered antibiotic; therefore, the quantity of medium into which a single specimen of blood is innoculated should be 100 ml. The optimal ratio of blood to medium is about 1:10. This may dilute the quantity of circulating antibody or antibiotic sufficiently to inhibit antibacterial activity. Clearly the quantity of blood drawn cannot always be 10 ml, particularly since several cultures are required to establish the diagnosis; this presents the greatest problem in young children. In this case, the ratio of blood to medium should still be at least 1:10. It must be stressed, however, that the quantity of blood obtained should be maximum for a given clinical situation.

Techniques. There has been considerable discussion concerning the optimal time for drawing blood and the number of cultures required to establish the presence of endocarditis. A single positive culture is of no diagnostic value because, regardless of the nature of the organism recovered, it may represent contamination. The minimal number of cultures of the blood required to establish the presence of infective endocarditis has been reported by Belli and Waisbren to be five.[241] Probably the best time for obtaining a blood culture is two hours before the temperature begins to rise. This is based on the well-established observation that this is the period required for bacterial endotoxin to stimulate the production of endogenous pyrogen by neutrophilic leukocytes and macrophages. However, this is not always practical. The writer uses the following approach to timing and number of blood cultures: Temperature is monitored, from a normal level, every hour until about 1°F of fever is present. At this point, a specimen of blood is drawn every 5 to 10 minutes until six samples have been obtained. In most instances, three or more of these will be positive; a similar approach the following day usually yields the same results. If the first six cultures are all negative, all succeeding sets of the same number are usually also sterile.

All blood obtained must be cultured aerobically and anaerobically. Because about 10 per cent of cases of infective endocarditis are caused by microaerophilic streptococci and a small number are caused by strict anaerobes such as *Peptostreptococcus, Peptococcus,* or *Bacteroides*, it is imperative that the blood be incubated anaerobically. Some organisms, e.g., *N. gonorrhoeae, N. meningitidis,* and *Brucella abortus,* grow best in an atmosphere of 5 to 10 per cent CO_2. The presence of *H. influenzae* in the blood will be overlooked unless Levinthal liquid medium or chocolate agar is used for culture. If cell wall–deficient organisms are suspected, culture of the blood in an osmotically stable medium is required; on repeated subculture, these bacteria may revert to the parent cell wall–containing form. A series of negative blood cultures in patients with a clinical picture highly suggestive of infective endocarditis should suggest the possibility that nutritionally variant strains of streptococci may be involved. These organisms grow in the initial culture of blood in liquid media. Although their presence in the broth can be demonstrated on Gram stain, they fail to multiply when subcultured on solid media, unless this is supplemented with thiol compounds (cysteine or thioglycollate broth). These are also known as "satelliting" streptococci because, if a streak of *Staph. aureus* is placed on the agar, the organisms grow in close proximity to the area in which the staphylococcus grows. Another type of streptococcus responsible for an occasional instance of subacute valvular infection requires pyridoxine for growth. The optimal solution to the problem of negative blood cultures in cases in which nutritionally fastidious and all other streptococci as well as most of the other bacteria may be involved is the use of a medium containing cysteine and pyridoxine. It should be emphasized that *Pseudomonas* will not grow in unvented bottles. Special media or tissue cultures are required to identify *Coxiella burnetii* and *Chlamydia,* rare causes of endocarditis. The use of a medium containing broth and soft agar (Castaneda principle) increases the yield of fungi.

Inappropriate periods of incubation may be responsible for "negative" blood cultures when some organisms are involved. Although most bacteria grow in cultures of blood within a few days to a week, some require a considerably longer period. Cultures for *Brucella* may not become positive until after four to six weeks of incubation.

Growth of many common organisms may be delayed for a week or longer in cases in which antibiotics have been administered. Most of the fungi involved in endocarditis grow slowly and may multiply more rapidly when incubated at room temperature than at 37°C. *Aspergillus* frequently cannot be recovered from cultures until they have been incubated for as long as 20 days. In most cases, these organisms cannot be recovered from the blood, no matter how long the period of incubation.

Serological Tests. A positive serological test may be of value in establishing the diagnosis of infective endocarditis. Examples of this are *Coxiella burnetii, Chlamydia, Brucella, Cryptococcus,* and *Candida.*

The importance of serological tests for teichoic acid in establishing the diagnosis of valvular infection caused by *Staph. aureus* has been demonstrated.[249]

Concomitant elevation of IgG and IgM antibody levels has been demonstrated by Wheat et al.[250] in 50 per cent of patients with endocarditis or complicated bacteremia. These antibodies were detected in only about 5 per cent of cases of other types of staphylococcal infections, and in about 3 per cent of normal persons. Studies of antibody to bacterial peptidoglycan in the serum of patients with endocarditis or bacteremia due to *Staph. aureus* have been carried out by Zeiger et al.[251] Patients treated with beta-lactam antibiotics had higher antigen-binding levels than healthy individuals or those receiving exclusively vancomycin. Serological studies in patients with candidal endocarditis have indicated that persisting or rising levels of precipitating or agglutinating antibodies, or both, whether or not associated with candidemia, signal invasion of prosthetic valves by the organism.[252] Although humoral antibodies to *Candida* increase after operations on the heart in some patients, even in the absence of clinical evidence of endocarditis, serial immunological studies are of value in patients with clinical manifestations of valvular infection by *Candida*, especially in patients whose blood cultures fail to grow the yeast.[253] Scheld et al.,[254] using an experimental model of candidal endocarditis in rabbits, found the enzyme-linked immunoabsorbent assay (ELISA) was much more sensitive than culturing of blood or determination of fever. This assay is more highly specific and more sensitive than the currently available techniques for demonstrating antibodies for *Candida.*

SCINTILLATION SCANNING. Scanning of the heart with gallium-67 appears to be of diagnostic value in some instances of bacterial endocarditis. Scintillation scanning of the precordial region 2 to 7 days after the intravenous administration of 3 mc of the radionuclide has been reported to yield positive results in seven individuals, three of which were confirmed by postmortem imaging at autopsy.[255] The scans were negative at 48 hours and positive from 3 to 8 days following injection. Fifteen patients without endocarditis, who served as controls, showed no uptake of the isotope in the region of the myocardium 48 hours or more after it was injected. A ventricular abscess in a patient was first suspected on the basis of a positive gallium-67 scan[256]; the disadvantages of this approach to the diagnosis of infective endocarditis are an insufficient degree of resolution to indicate the site of infection, the length of time (48 hours) required for localization of the radionuclide, and a 40 per cent incidence of false-negative results.[257]

ELECTROCARDIOGRAPHY. Changes in the electrocardiogram are not diagnostic in uncomplicated infective endocarditis. However, as pointed out earlier (p. 1153), this approach is helpful in that incomplete or complete heart block, bundle branch block, and premature ventricular contractions are associated with septal abscesses or myocarditis. The anatomical relation of the noncoronary cusp of the aortic valve and the mitral annulus to the conduction apparatus has been considered responsible for the development of abnormalities of conduction and is of some value in localizing the site of the lesion. Miller and Casey have expressed the importance of obtaining serial electrocardiograms in patients with the diagnosis of infective endocarditis: "Electrocardiographic evidence of an infarction or heart block is associated with a poor prognosis. New conduction defects indicate abscess or aneurysm formation and may suggest the need for surgical intervention."[257]

RADIOGRAPHY. Radiological findings in patients with endocarditis involving the left side of the heart are usually not impressive until destruction of the affected valve is so far advanced that congestive failure develops.[258] There are no diagnostic radiographic abnormalities in cases in which the right side of the heart is involved until pulmonary infarction, with or without infection, develops.

Echocardiography (See also page 116)

Echocardiography provides another approach to the diagnosis of infective endocarditis and some of its intracardiac complications. An increasing number of studies have pointed out the limits of this diagnostic technique, as well as the features that permit recognition of the specific valve involved and the characteristics of specific complications.[259]

The value of echocardiography in staphylococcal infection of the aortic valve has been reported by Fox and his colleagues.[260] "Shaggy" echoes were recorded from the aortic leaflets in diastole as well as irregular diastolic densities in the left ventricular outflow tract, suggesting that the infection caused flailing of the aortic leaflets. Echocardiographic detection of flail aortic leaflets and premature closure of the mitral valve indicated the need for immediate replacement of the aortic valve.

Of 14 patients with endocarditis involving the aortic valve studied by Berger et al.,[261] 12 had vegetations demonstrated by two-dimensional echocardiography; in the others, the presence of the disease was identified anatomically. This technique was found to be superior to the M-mode in determining the size, shape, and movement of the vegetations. The echocardiographic (two-dimensional) characteristics of aortic valvular endocarditis were noted to include (a) globular, polypoid masses, (b) elongated lesions with chaotic movement, and (c) a cord-like structure. Serial echocardiography carried out after completion of antimicrobial therapy in seven patients disclosed no change in the vegetations in five and complete disappearance in two. The authors made the following important statement: "In those patients with negative two-dimensional echocardiograms, the vegetations were 3 mm in diameter or less at surgery or autopsy. Vegetations that were visualized on two-dimensional echocardiography were found to be at least 5 mm in diameter at the time of operation." Two echocardiographic features characteristic of aortic valvular endocarditis are (a) thick, uneven cusp echoes that may be present only in systole or diastole or, less commonly, in both, and (b) normal systolic excursion of all cusps, regardless of their involvement in the disease.

Echocardiography has also been found to be of value in identification of abscesses of various valvular ring abscesses. Using both M-mode and two-dimensional techniques in a patient with a suspected mitral ring abscess, Nakamura et al.[262] observed a round, dense, echo mass between the posterior mitral leaflet and the posterior wall of the left ventricle. The diagnosis was confirmed at surgery.

They pointed out that the two-dimensional procedure was superior to the M-mode. The diagnosis of an aortic root abscess, the presence of which was not suspected clinically, was established only by two-dimensional echocardiography by Wong and his colleagues.[263] They noted an abscess cavity and a vegetation posterior and lateral to the root that deformed the left atrial cavity. The lesion was confirmed by cardiac catheterization and at surgery.

Scanlan et al.[264] expressed the same opinion and emphasized that wide-angle two-dimensional echocardiography was the only noninvasive technique of value in direct visualization of ring abscesses complicating infection of the aortic valve. The presence of the abscesses was identified by the demonstration of an echo-free cavity in the tissues around the valve. The lesions extended into the perivalvular space, the left ventricular myocardium, and the myocardium or contiguous fibrous structures.

An extensive study by Andy and his colleagues of the efficacy of echocardiography in the detection of infective endocarditis and its complications, especially in relation to involvement of specific valves, indicated that vegetations on the tricuspid valve, as visualized by echocardiography, were always larger than those on the mitral valve.[265] No patients with tricuspid regurgitation demonstrated torn cusps. Wide-angle two-dimensional echocardiograms were found by Berger and his colleagues[266] to be superior to the M-mode technique in identifying endocarditis involving the tricuspid and pulmonic valves. The use of multiple transducer positions led to better visualization of the valves. Studies carried out after the completion of antimicrobial therapy in seven patients showed that the vegetations were unchanged in three, decreased in mass in the same number, and had disappeared in one.

Two-dimensional echocardiography has also been noted to be useful in establishing the diagnosis of isolated pulmonic valve endocarditis[267] and in demonstrating infection in cases of intraventricular septal defect.

Since size is critical to detection of the valvular vegetations in patients with infective endocarditis, echocardiography might be expected to give positive results more often when infections are caused by fungi because of the characteristically large valvular lesions. The features of aortic valvular disease caused by *Candida parapsilosis* have been described by Gomes and his associates[268] and include clusters of abnormal echoes visible intermittently in the aortic root; thickening of the valve leaflets, with abnormal "shaggy" echoes in both systole and diastole; and normal excursion of the leaflets except when damage is extensive.

Eighty-seven patients with clinical evidence of infective endocarditis studied by Stewart et al.[269] were divided into two groups on the basis of positive and negative echocardiography (M-mode and two-dimensional). The individuals in whom one or more vegetations were demonstrated by the noninvasive technique were found to be at a higher risk of developing complications (emboli, congestive cardiac failure, and need for surgery) than those in whom echocardiography demonstrated no vegetations. The authors stressed the important point that "although the detection of vegetations by echocardiography in patients with clinical syndrome of endocarditis clearly identifies a subgroup at risk of complications, decisions regarding clinical management made solely on the basis of the presence or absence of vegetative lesions are hazardous. Management of such patients must continue to be based on the clinical integration of multiple factors."

The effectiveness of M-mode and two-dimensional echocardiography in detecting masses in patients suspected, on clinical grounds, of having endocarditis was studied by Martin et al.[270] No individual without evidence of valvular infection had any echocardiographic abnormalities. Of 36 confirmed cases of endocarditis studied by the M-mode technique, 5 (14 per cent) had a demonstrable mass; in 12 there was a nonspecific abnormality, and in 19 no mass was detected. When two-dimensional echocardiography was used, the frequency with which a mass was found increased to 81 per cent; this technique was found to be more useful in cases in which a mass was present on a prosthetic mitral or aortic valve.

Hickey and his colleagues[271] have reported that "M-mode echocardiography can reliably detect vegetations in patients with bacterial endocarditis even in the presence of pre-existing valvular lesions, and may permit the identification of a subset of high risk patients who may need early surgery." Those in whom vegetations were not detected echocardiographically appeared to be less likely to develop serious complications than those in whom valvular deposits were demonstrable. In contrast, Markiewicz et al.[272] suggested that caution must be exercised in the interpretation of findings of "vegetations" by echocardiography in cases in which preexisting valvular disease is present.

An interesting study of the value of echocardiography in the diagnosis of endocarditis in 11 patients with negative blood cultures in whom the presence of the disease was established during cardiac surgery was carried out by Rubenson et al.[273] Both natural (5 cases) and prosthetic valves (6 cases) were involved. Valvular masses were identified by echocardiography in 8 cases. The other three had prosthetic aortic valves that showed the diastolic mitral valve vibration characteristic of aortic regurgitation. In 3 instances, the illness was poorly defined clinically. The authors emphasize the point that, in these individuals, echocardiography was a prime factor in identifying the presence of endocarditis.

Dillon et al.[274] have suggested that initial and serial echocardiographic studies carried out over the course of treatment not only play an important role in diagnosis but are also of value in evaluation of the size of vegetations and the state of valvular function while antimicrobial therapy is being administered. Strom et al.[275] have reported the results of an interesting study of the correlation between the findings demonstrated by echocardiography and those identified at the time of cardiac surgery. Only 84 per cent of 32 valves thought to be involved when examined echocardiographically before operation were found to carry vegetations at the time of surgery. The presence of a myocardial abscess, suspected in five patients on the basis of the findings present during the noninvasive studies, was proved in only one during cardiac surgery.

As discussed above, one of the important points to remember about the use of echocardiography in the diagnosis of infective endocarditis is related to the size of the vegetations on the affected valve. Clearly the larger the lesions, the more likely their presence is to be detected by echocardiography. Thus, this technique produces positive results in fungal valvular infections most often because, as a rule, the vegetations are large. The technique is of less value, but still useful, in acute endocarditis caused by Staph. aureus, in which endocardial lesions are often of moderate size. The primary difficulty of echocardiographic diagnosis arises in patients with the subacute form of the disease, because of the very small size of the vegetations associated with infection by viridans streptococci and other relatively avirulent organisms.

In addition to the demonstration of vegetative lesions, echocardiography is of great value in determining hemodynamic abnormalities related to the complications associated with valvular infections (Chap. 5).

MANAGEMENT OF INFECTIVE ENDOCARDITIS

Prior to the antibiotic era, attempts to treat infective endocarditis were relatively unsuccessful. For the most part, physicians were limited to observation and study of the "natural history" of this almost invariably fatal disease.

The development of highly potent antimicrobial agents followed by refinements of and advances in the techniques of cardiac surgery have so altered this heretofore "hopeless" situation that today young physicians are often perplexed when defervescence fails to occur within 24 to 48 hours after initiation of treatment, and older physicians are upset by a fatal outcome when, not long ago, they were amazed if their patients recovered.

Antimicrobial Therapy

Although penicillin—the first antibiotic effective in the management of infective endocarditis—still remains the agent of choice in the majority of cases, the increasing involvement of uncommon bacterial species and fungi in the pathogenesis of the disease has posed difficult and, at times, insurmountable therapeutic problems and underscores the need for careful application of sensitive microbiological techniques not only to isolate all organisms involved but also to identify them and evaluate their susceptibility to a wide range of antimicrobial agents.

Selection of Drugs. The choice of specific antimicrobial therapy for infective endocarditis depends strictly on the nature of the organism recovered from the blood and its susceptibility to various drugs. Usually treatment need not be immediate in the subacute form of infection, since most of these patients have been ill for several weeks to as long as 3 or more months before the diagnosis is established. Therefore, a delay in instituting treatment of two or three days until definitive microbiological data become available is of little or no prognostic importance. If death occurs before therapy is begun in such cases, it is most often due, not to the infectious process, but rather to one of its sequelae, such as rupture of a mycotic aneurysm or embolic occlusion of a coronary artery—complications not prevented by chemotherapy.

In sharp contrast to this, it is imperative that there be no delay in treatment in acute bacterial endocarditis, especially when it involves a highly destructive organism such as Staph. aureus, because of the rapidity with which valve leaflets, papillary muscles, or chordae tendineae may rupture or myocardial and/or septal abscesses may develop. In the absence of bacteriological evidence, the etiology of acute endocarditis may, at times, be suspected on the basis of the circumstances in which it developed. For example, a staphylococcal skin infection in a patient with endocarditis should implicate this organism as the cause of the valvular infection. Examination of stained smears of petechial lesions or of the "buffy coat" of the peripheral blood may reveal the causative organism one or two days before results of blood cultures are available. Despite the urgent need for treatment in these cases, administration of antimicrobial agents should be withheld until sufficient blood cultures have been obtained, a procedure that usually involves a delay of no more than one hour. If the clinical features of the disease are mild, if the duration of manifestations has been short, or if there is no demonstrable primary extracardiac focus of infection, it may be safe to wait 24 hours, the time usually required to recover the causative organism. However, chemotherapy must be started before the results of sensitivity tests become available; if these tests indicate that a drug other than the one being given is preferable, the appropriate agent should be substituted.

Antibacterial Effectiveness. It is very important that, in addition to its antimicrobial activity, the agent selected pose minimal risk of untoward effects, be administered by a route acceptable to the patient, and present no problems with respect to the physiological, biochemical, and anatomical characteristics of the host.[276] In general, bactericidal drugs appear to be more effective than bacteriostatic ones not only in eradicating the valvular infection but also in reducing the risk of relapse after therapy has been completed.

To determine the effectiveness of chemotherapy, it is often helpful to measure the antibacterial activity of the patient's serum against the organism recovered from the blood. This is readily accomplished by adding a standard inoculum from an overnight culture of the organism to serial, twofold dilutions of serum obtained at various intervals after administration of a dose of antibiotics.[277] Inhibition of bacterial growth, both bacteriostatic and bactericidal, by dilutions of 1:8, 1:16, or higher usually indicates a potentially favorable therapeutic response.[278] Although this is standard practice in the treatment of infective endocarditis, its importance in evaluating the response to treatment has been questioned on the basis of experiments demonstrating that the quantity of antibiotic penetrating a fibrin clot and the duration of antibacterial activity depend on only two factors: the peak serum concentration and the degree of protein-binding of the drug.[243,248] Thus, it is clear that antibacterial effects usually persist at the site of infection for many hours after they are no longer demonstrable in the blood. In addition, it has been reported that in some instances, there may be no correlation between serum antibacterial activity and therapeutic outcome.[279]

Dosage Considerations. Despite the fact that antimicrobial agents have been used for more than 30 years in the treatment of infective endocarditis, no firm data are available concerning the proper daily dose of any of these drugs. Regimens vary greatly and depend on the experience of the physician. Thus, doses of penicillin ranging from as low as 4 to 6 million units to as high as 20 to 30 million units per day have been administered to patients with subacute disease when the responsible agent has been a highly susceptible strain of alpha-streptococcus or other organism. Unfortunately there is no proof that either of these extremes of dosage is necessary or ideal. For this reason, the doses of antibiotics recommended below for the management of valvular infections are necessarily based on published experiences and are perforce empirical.

In terms of generating the highest levels and longest duration of antimicrobial activity, Barza et al. have shown that the bolus injection of an antibiotic is more effective than is a constant intravenous infusion.[280] Although the question of what constitutes an optimal interval between doses in the management of infective endocarditis still remains unsettled, experimental data obtained from studies of the penetration and persistence of antimicrobial activity in fibrin, combined with 35 years of experience treating both acute and subacute infective endocarditis, have convinced this author that an interval of 6 hours between doses of a parenterally administered drug is effective in most adults; it is possible that this might be extended in

older individuals, because of decreased renal tubular secretory function; however, in children, a shorter interval (3 to 4 hours) between doses may be required to maintain effective concentrations of drug in the infected platelet-fibrin thrombus, because of the high level of tubular secretory function that leads to rapid urinary excretion of penicillins and cephalosporins.

Duration of Therapy. The duration of therapy required to cure infective endocarditis is, for the most part, empirical and therefore often controversial. Although many physicians continue treatment for only 4 weeks, there is an increasing tendency to extend this to 6 weeks despite the lack of statistically significant evidence that this leads to a higher percentage of cures or reduces the incidence of relapse in most cases, especially when the organisms are highly susceptible to the antibiotic used. It remains to be proved whether 6 weeks of exposure to an antibiotic is required when the infection is caused by uncommon bacterial species, by strains less sensitive to antimicrobial agents, or by fungi. The observation that the risk of superinfection is directly related to the length of time over which an antibiotic is administered, especially when the drug used has a "broad spectrum" of activity,[281] suggests that there may actually be some danger in prolonging therapy beyond 4 weeks. Attempts have also been made to limit the duration of treatment to 2 weeks in patients with subacute bacterial endocarditis caused by such noninvasive organisms as *Strep. viridans*.[282] Although cure has been reported in some instances, this approach can not yet be recommended until considerably more data regarding rate of cure and risk of relapse become available.

Routes of Administration. Most physicians experienced in the treatment of subacute infective endocarditis recommend parenteral administration of antibiotics, usually by the intravenous route. However, in a number of cases, successful treatment of this disease with oral penicillin has been reported. The stimulus for this approach has been the desire to avoid the pain of intramuscular or intravenous injection and to eliminate such complications as thrombophlebitis and sterile or infected abscesses in muscle. Antimicrobial agents that have been administered orally include buffered penicillin G and phenoxymethylpenicillin (penicillin V).[282-285] In many instances, oral treatment with one of the penicillins has been combined with the intramuscular injection of streptomycin. Therapy with this regimen has also been continued for only 2 weeks in a number of cases.[282] While high rates of cure have been reported by several investigators,[282-285] relapses have occurred in a relatively small number of cases. This type of therapy must be restricted to patients with *subacute* bacterial endocarditis caused by organisms that are highly susceptible to the antibiotic used; it has no place and is extremely dangerous in treatment of the acute type of valvular infections. Although Burman et al.[286] have recently reported a cure of refractory staphylococcal endocarditis with rifampin and erythromycin, it must be pointed out that this approach is potentially dangerous and should not be used except in the most unusual circumstances.

A recent review by Phillips and Watson of oral therapy for infective endocarditis points out that "despite much discussion, no final conclusion has been reached about the optimum duration of oral treatment."[287] Short courses (2 weeks) have been reported to be effective, while some investigators have recommended therapy for as long as 6 or more weeks. Despite the reports of success with oral antibiotics, many physicians prefer to treat this disease parenterally. The following objections to oral administration have been raised.[288]

1. Large groups of patients treated with parenteral antibiotics have experienced no relapses, an important consideration, since each recrudescence of valvular infection not only adds an increment of permanent damage to an already functionally poor valve but also presents a risk of death.

2. Orally administered antibiotics may be irregularly absorbed, especially in patients who are quite ill; this necessitates constant monitoring of blood levels of the antibiotic, a technique not available in most "routine" diagnostic microbiological laboratories.

3. Patients may fail to take each dose of drug unless under the continuous watchful eye of the physician or nurse.

4. Gastrointestinal irritation leading to nausea, vomiting, and diarrhea is associated with the oral use of antibiotics in some persons.

5. The risk of superinfections, even rapidly fatal ones, is not eliminated when antibiotics are taken orally.

Although 4 weeks of intravenous or intramuscular injection of an antimicrobial agent causes discomfort in most individuals, vast clinical experience has indicated that, with proper attention and encouragement from the physician, almost all patients accept this form of treatment with minimal complaint.

Problems of Therapy. A fairly common therapeutic problem arises when the clinical picture is highly suggestive of subacute bacterial endocarditis but the blood cultures are repeatedly sterile. Because of the high fatality rate when the disease is not treated, therapy is usually based on experience and clinical judgment. Initially therapy should be directed at possible enterococcal infection, as discussed below (p.1169). Cannady and Sandford[243] have made the following suggestions regarding therapy of patients with suspected endocarditis when blood cultures have failed to yield an organism: If there is no satisfactory response after 2 weeks of empirical treatment, administration should be continued for an additional 14 days, during which cultures and serological tests may indicate the presence of infection caused by fungi, *Chlamydia, Rickettsia,* or *Brucella.* If all these studies are negative, treatment should be discontinued and the patient reevaluated. These investigators also point out that the most difficult problem involves the compromised host who has received many antibiotic regimens or the patient with a prosthetic heart valve. The latter may have fungal endocarditis and may well be a candidate for empirical therapy with amphotericin B, but surgical removal of the infected valve may be necessary to cure the disease.

It must be emphasized that these suggestions apply only to individuals with the *subacute* form of valvular infection. There is no place for delay in the management of the acute disease, which progresses rapidly and leads to potentially lethal intra- and extracardiac complications. Negative cultures of the blood are rarely, if ever, a problem in acute infections involving the left side of the heart. In endocarditis involving the right side of the heart, organisms may not be recovered from the peripheral circulation until pulmonary infarction and infection occur, after which cultures of the blood become positive. However, if embolization to the lungs does not occur and the blood remains sterile, therapy must be undertaken as soon as possible and should be directed against organisms known to be most often responsible for this kind of disease, especially coagulase-positive staphylococcus. When the enterococcus may be the causative agent, the use of a penicillinase-resistant penicillin plus an aminoglycoside is recommended; an optimal choice is nafcillin or oxacillin (12 gm/day, in divided doses) plus gentamicin or tobramycin (80 mg every 8 hours).

ANTICOAGULANTS

The use of anticoagulants in patients with infective endocarditis has been and remains controversial.[289] It is clear that anticoagulants are of no benefit in the management of valvular infections because these drugs do not prevent separation of small fragments from the valvular thrombus and the vegetations do not increase in size if antimicrobial therapy is effective. Anticoagulation may cause bleeding at the site of deposition of an embolus. It is this author's view that when a condition such as phlebothrombosis of the extremities or pelvis results in pulmonary embolism, with or without infarction, and requires anticoagulation with heparin or coumadin, the presence of infective endocarditis does not absolutely contraindicate the use of these drugs. When embolization from the infected valve occurs, the situation must be reevaluated relative to the risks of hemorrhage at the sites where emboli have been deposited and of a fatal pulmonary infarct; anticoagulation is very likely to be of no value in this situation. When the phlebothrombosis involves the extremities or pelvis, the issue can be resolved by surgical occlusion of the vena cava. That anticoagulation was of no danger in patients with subacute endocarditis was suggested by Loewe et al., who treated all their patients with heparin and penicillin.[7]

TREATMENT OF ENDOCARDITIS CAUSED BY SPECIFIC ORGANISMS (Table 33–3)

Gram-Positive Cocci

STREPTOCOCCI. Of the organisms responsible for subacute infective endocarditis, *Streptococcus viridans* is the commonest. Although the majority of these bacteria are highly sensitive to penicillin G, it must be emphasized that all strains in this group do not constitute a single species, and all are not susceptible to this antibiotic. Among these are enterococci as well as vitamin B_6 (pyridoxal hydrochloride)–dependent streptococci.

Treatment of streptococcal (viridans) endocarditis with a combination of penicillin and streptomycin or gentamicin has been recommended on the basis of in vitro synergy of the drugs.[290] However, this author's experience with over 900 cases given penicillin alone does not support this recommendation; all the patients survived, and none relapsed over the six months following discontinuation of treatment. Two recent reports have confirmed this experience.[291,292]

For patients sensitized to penicillin, several approaches are available: one involves desensitization to this drug—a

TABLE 33-3   CHEMOTHERAPY OF INFECTIVE ENDOCARDITIS

Symbols:

AMB = Amphotericin B	ETH = Ethambutol	SM = Streptomycin
AMK = Amikacin	FC = 5-Fluorocytosine	SN/TMP = Sulfamethoxazole plus trimethoprim
AMP = Ampicillin	GM = Gentamicin	TBM = Tobramycin
CARB = Carbenicillin	INH = Isoniazid	TC = Tetracycline
CFM = Cefamandole	KN = Kanamycin	TIC = Ticarcillin
CFX = Cefoxitin	MNZ = Metronidazole	VC = Vancomycin
CL = Clindamycin	NF = Nafcillin	
CM = Chloramphenicol	OX = Oxacillin	Third Generation Cephalosporins = They may eventually
CP = Cephalothin	PCN = Penicillin G	prove valuable in the therapy of infective endocarditis, but
CY = Cycloserine	RF = Rifampin	current experience with them is too limited to evaluate
EM = Erythromycin	RST = Results of Sensivity Tests	them effectively.

	DRUG		
ORGANISM	*1st Choice*	*2nd Choice*	*3rd Choice*
Alpha-streptococcus	PCN	CP	AMP
Strep. bovis	PCN	CP	AMP
Pyridoxine-dependent streptococci	PCN + GM or TBM	PCN + SM	—
Enterococcus	PCN + GM, TBM, or SM	AMP	VC
Other streptococci	RST	—	—
Strep. pneumoniae	PCN[1]	CP	EM
Peptostreptococcus	PCN[2]	RST	RST
Staph. aureus	PCN,[2,3] CP, OX	NF	EM
Methicillin-resistant *Staph. aureus*	VC	RST	—
Staph. epidermidis	RST	—	—
Micrococcus	RST	—	—
Aerobic diphtheroids	PCN[3]	PCN + GM	EM
Listeria monocytogenes	PCN	EM	CP
Lactobacillus acidophilus	PCN + SM	RST	—
Lactobacillus plantarum	PCN	CP	RST
Bacillus subtilis	RST	—	—
Bacillus cereus	EM	GM, TBM	TC, CL, or CM
Nocardia israelii	SM + SN/TMP	AMP + SN/TMP	TC + CY or SN/TMP
Escherichia coli	CP	AMP	GM or TBM
Klebsiella pneumoniae	CP	GM, TBM	CM + SM
Enterobacter species	RST	—	—
Proteus mirabilis	AMP	CP	PCN
Pseudomonas aeruginosa	TMB + CARB or TIC	GM + CARB or TIC	AMK
Pseudomonas cepacia	SN/TMP + KN	RST	—
Serratia marcescens	AMK	SN/TMP	RST
Vibrio fetus	CM	EM	RST
Hemophilus influenzae	AMP[3,4]	CFM	CM
Hemophilus parainfluenzae	AMP	CM	GM, CP, or CARB
Hemophilus aprophilus	CM	GM	PCN, CP, or RF
Cardiobacterium hominis	PCN	RST	—
Brucella—all types	TC + SM	CM + SM	RF
Salmonella—all species	RST[5]	—	—
Pasteurella multicoda	PCN	TC	—
Acinetobacter	SN/TMP	KN or TBM	GM
Actinobacillus actinomycetemcomitans	AMP + GM	AMP + SM	RST
Flavobacterium	RF	CL	SN/TMP or VC
Streptobacillus moniliformis	PCN	EM	CP
Neisseria meningitidis	PCN	EM	CM
Neisseria gonorrhoeae	PCN[6]	CFX sh,14,15 EM	
Nonpathogenic *Neisseria*	RST	—	—
Bacteroides fragilis	CL + CARB or TIC	CARB or TIC	MNZ
Bacteroides melaninogenicus	PCN	CARB	RST
Propionibacterium acnes	EM	PCN[7]	RST
Mycobacterium tuberculosis	INH + ETH + SM[8]	ETH + RF + SM[8]	RST
Mycobacterium chelonei	INH + ETH + RF[9]	RST	—
Yeasts and Fungi	AMB + FC[10]	—	—
Chlamydia trachomatis or *psittaci*	TC	CM	—
Coxiella burnetii (Q fever)	TC	CM	—

[1] Rare strains of the pneumococcus are resistant to penicillin.

[2] May require as much as 40 to 80 million units of penicillin G per day.

[3] Only if organism is sensitive to penicillin.

[4] Increasing number of strains are resistant to ampicillin.

[5] Ampicillin and chloramphenicol are the most effective agents; some strains are resistant to one or both of these agents. Infection caused by *Salmonella typhi* has been shown to respond favorably to large doses of sulfamethoxazole/trimethoprim in some cases.

[6] Some strains are totally resistant to penicillin G.

[7] Many strains are resistant to penicillin G.

[8] One gm of streptomycin daily for one month followed by 1 gm every Monday and Thursday for two months, and then discontinued.

[9] The combination of isoniazid plus rifampin produces hepatoxicity more often then does either drug alone.

[10] Before 5-fluorocytosine is given, organism must be examined for sensivity to the drug.

simple and minimally dangerous procedure that is often not necessary because of the availability of other effective antimicrobial agents. An adequate substitute for penicillin G in these cases is intravenous cephalothin, 2 gm every 4 hours. (The risk of cross-reactivity between these agents has been less than 1 per cent in the experience of this author.) Another cephalosporin, cefazolin, has been reported by Quinn et al. to be effective in the treatment of staphylococcal endocarditis.[293] However, relapses have been noted when this antibiotic has been used.[294] Vancomycin (2 gm/day) has been reported to be effective in some instances of this type of endocarditis.[295] Most strains of *Strep. viridans* susceptible to penicillin are sensitive to erythromycin, 1 gm given intravenously every 6 hours. In endocarditis caused by alpha-streptococci, clindamycin is thought to be a "third-line" drug for use in patients who have previously had a serious reaction to both penicillins and cephalosporins,[296] because relapse has occurred after therapy was discontinued.

Since the first report that treatment of enterococcal endocarditis with penicillin plus streptomycin was more effective than the use of either agent alone,[297] a considerable body of information has accumulated concerning the mechanism by which these antibiotics act synergistically. Moellering and his colleagues have demonstrated that drugs that inhibit the synthesis of bacterial cell walls (penicillins, cephalosporins, vancomycin, cycloserine, bacitracin) allow entry of aminoglycosides (streptomycin, gentamicin, tobramycin, amikacin) into the cell, resulting in death of the organisms.[298,299] Failure to achieve synergism against the enterococcus can be correlated with resistance to the aminoglycoside being used[299]; and a therapeutic effect can be produced by substitution of another aminoglycoside.[300] Thus, if the organism is resistant to 2000 μg/ml of streptomycin, the addition of this compound will not, in most instances, yield synergistic activity. It must be emphasized that, although usually synergistic in vitro, the combination of cephalothin plus streptomycin or gentamicin is therapeutically ineffective.

A number or regimens have been found to be of value in the management of endocarditis caused by enterococci. Among these are penicillin G (20 million units intravenously every 6 hours) plus streptomycin (0.5 gm intramuscularly every 12 hours) or gentamicin or tobramycin (3 to 5 mg/kg in three equally divided doses at 8-hour intervals). A combination that has proved to be more effective than penicillin plus an aminoglycoside in vitro is nafcillin plus gentamicin or tobramycin; the intravenous dose of nafcillin is 1 gm every 3 hours or 2 gm every 4 hours. Some strains of enterococci are quite sensitive to ampicillin; the dose of this drug for subacute endocarditis is 8 to 12 gm/day, in three or four equally divided and spaced intravenous injections, together with gentamicin or tobramycin. In patients sensitized to penicillins, the administration of 4 gm/day of erythromycin (1 gm intravenously every 6 hours) has proved to be highly effective when the organism is sensitive to this dosage. Vancomycin (0.5 gm every 6 hours) has been reported to be effective in the management of this type of disease.[295] Rather than resort to the use of other antibiotics, some have preferred to desensitize penicillin-sensitive individuals and then administer this agent together with an aminoglycoside or vancomycin.

Optimal therapy of infections caused by vitamin B$_6$–dependent streptococci has been found to be a combination of penicillin G and streptomycin.[301] Doses should be in the same range as those used for the therapy of disease caused by the enterococcus.

Strep. bovis is highly sensitive to penicillin G.[302] Therapy for endocarditis caused by this organism is the same as that for disease caused by alpha-streptococci sensitive to this antibiotic. Valvular infection produced by *Peptostreptococcus* (anaerobic streptococcus) responds well to the administration of penicillin G. However, these organisms are generally relatively insensitive to this drug, and disease caused by them requires the use of "massive" doses of the order of 15 to 20 million units every 6 hours intravenously. Because this quantity may produce seizures and cardiac arrhythmia with death, the following precautions must be taken: The dose must be reduced in the presence of any degree of renal insufficiency, because this is associated with decreased excretion of the drug and accumulation in the brain to levels that may be epileptogenic. In addition, because the commercially available penicillin is the potassium salt (1 million units of penicillin contains about 1.5 mEq/liter of K$^+$), potentially lethal hyperkalemia may develop. Patients with either localized or generalized disease of the brain may develop jacksonian epilepsy or generalized convulsions. The plasma level of sodium must be kept within normal limits, since hyponatremia increases the susceptibility to convulsions.[303,304]

STAPHYLOCOCCI. Despite the use of antimicrobial agents effective against *Staph. aureus* in vitro, the clinical results of therapy of endocarditis caused by this organism are relatively poor, when compared to subacute disease produced by alpha-streptococci. In patients not sensitized to penicillins, this group of agents is first choice. However, because about 15 per cent of infections caused by *Staph. aureus* that occur outside hospitals and over 90 per cent that develop during hospitalization are caused by penicillin-resistant strains, initial therapy must consist of a penicillinase-resistant drug such as nafcillin, oxacillin, or cephalothin. The minimal dose of these agents should be 12 gm/day (2 gm every 4 hours intravenously). If in vitro studies indicate that the organism isolated from the blood is susceptible to penicillin G, therapy with this agent may be substituted. The dose of this drug is empirical; this author recommends 20 to 30 million units given intravenously in four equally divided and spaced doses per day. Failure to respond raises the question of a methicillin-resistant" or tolerant" strain (p. 1171). Some of these organisms are tolerant" not only to the penicillins but also to the cephalosporins. Vancomycin is useful in many of these cases.

The fatality rate from staphylococcal endocarditis in 25 patients treated with a single antibiotic (penicillin G, methicillin, nafcillin, cephalothin, or vancomycin) was noted to be 40 per cent. It was identical in 15 individuals who received combined therapy (nafcillin plus gentamicin, penicillin plus gentamicin, or methicillin plus gentamicin).[305] A recent prospective study has indicated that treatment with a single effective antibiotic (a penicillinase-resistant penicillin or a cephalosporin) is curative, and that the addition of an aminoglycoside does not increase the rate of cure.[306]

A number of other approaches to the management of

valvular infections caused by *Staph. aureus* have been employed, especially in patients sensitized to the penicillins. Despite some variability in results,[307] vancomycin (0.5 gm every 6 hours intravenously) should be considered a potentially effective alternative in patients with staphylococcal endocarditis sensitized to penicillins and cephalosporins. This drug is clearly the agent of choice for infection by strains of *Staph. aureus*, which are resistant to practically all the antimicrobial compounds currently available, and for patients highly sensitized to the penicillins and cephalosporins. Clindamycin has been found to be ineffective in the therapy of staphylococcal endocarditis in patients sensitized to penicillin,[296] and the results with cefazolin are equivocal.[293,296]

The results of the therapy of endocarditis caused by coagulase-positive staphylococci are not as good as those reported in cases of the disease produced by streptococci, regardless of the antibiotic employed. A varying fatality rate, in excess of that of alpha-streptococcal infection, has characterized the treatment of staphylococcal infection. This is largely related to the intracardiac complications described earlier (p. 1153).

In the author's experience, even large doses of the most active antimicrobial drugs fail to cure the infection in patients in whom a large number of abscesses develop either before or after therapy has been initiated. An important determinant of the eventual outcome of this disease is failure to institute treatment early in the course of the disease; a delay of as little as 4 to 5 days may increase the risk of a fatal outcome.

Despite the low invasive capacity of *Staph. epidermidis*, the prognosis for recovery from endocarditis produced by this organism is generally poor, even when patients are treated with an antibiotic that is considered to be sensitive to it on the basis of in vitro study. A common course of events in this type of valvular infection is relapse after discontinuation of treatment. This may occur several times, in spite of repeated administration of an effective drug, and may finally lead to congestive failure. At this point, replacement of the affected valve with a prosthesis is indicated.

Yeasts and Fungi

Over a decade of use has demonstrated the effectiveness of amphotericin B in the management of infections caused by a large variety of yeasts and fungi. Therapy with this agent has been beneficial in histoplasmosis, cryptococcosis, and candidiasis. However, experience indicates that the treatment of fungal infections of the heart presents a number of problems that are unique to this organ, and are quite different from those encountered when this kind of disease involves other organs. Although sporadic reports have suggested that candidal endocarditis has been eradicated by administration of amphotericin B alone, the diagnosis in these cases has been based largely on the demonstration of candidemia, a finding not always diagnostic of cardiac or systemic disease.[308,309]

The relatively poor results of chemotherapy of fungal infections of cardiac valves has prompted consideration of adjunct therapy, i.e., surgical removal of the infected site. In 1961, Kaye and his colleagues reported an instance of candidal endocarditis resistant to amphotericin B that was ultimately cured by débridement of an infected tricuspid valve.[310] Experience since then has emphasized the intolerably high frequency of primary drug failure and underscores the need for surgical intervention in infections not only of natural valves but especially of prosthetic valves.[311] It must be pointed out, however, that not even this combined therapeutic approach results in an acceptable rate of cure. When the diagnosis of fungal endocarditis is established, treatment with amphotericin B must be initiated promptly. After about a week of administration of the antibiotic, it is best to remove the infected valve, replace it with a prosthesis, and continue chemotherapy for at least 6 to 8 weeks. When this fails, it has been the practice in some instances to replace the prosthetic valve with a new one. However, even this has failed to eradicate the disease in many cases.

Another approach to this problem has been suggested recently. In individuals in whom endocarditis is limited to the tricuspid valve, total valvulectomy without prosthetic replacement has been carried out.[312] Patients apparently get along fairly well following operation. Administration of amphotericin B was continued for a number of weeks until there was a clinical impression of eradication of the infectious process. A prosthesis was then inserted, and treatment continued. It must be emphasized that, of all types of endocarditis, the prognosis for recovery is poorest in those due to yeasts and fungi.

Several regimens have been recommended for intravenous therapy with amphotericin B.[313,314] One involves administration of 0.25 mg/kg the first day, followed by an increase of 0.25 mg/kg each day until a dose of 1 mg/kg/day is reached. This is continued until the completion of therapy. In severe infections, such as is the case in fungal endocarditis, the daily dose may be increased to 1.5 mg/kg/day. Another approach involves the administration of 1 mg the first day and 5 mg the second day, followed by daily increases of 5 to 10 mg until 1 mg/kg/day is being administered. The sclerosing activity of the drug and the immediate unpleasant side effects associated with its administration have prompted the use of a regimen designed to minimize the frequency and possibly the intensity of these reactions. This involves the intravenous infusion of 1.5 mg/kg every other day[313]; the individual daily dose must not exceed 90 mg. This procedure appears to be pharmacologically sound. Peak serum levels are usually higher with treatment on alternate days.

Because of lack of precise information, choice of the period over which amphotericin is given is empirical but is commonly 6 to 8 weeks. In some instances, this has been extended. It may be necessary to administer a second or even third course of the antibiotic, if relapse follows discontinuation of therapy.

A compound of potential value in the management of fungal diseases is 5-fluorocytosine, a drug that can be administered orally. In most instances, this agent is being used, together with amphotericin B, for the treatment of fungal endocarditis when the responsible organism is susceptible to both drugs. This combination is of no value if the organism is resistant to 5-fluorocytosine. In some instances in which the organism is susceptible, the latter has been given alone for varying periods of time, often many months, after "cure" has been accomplished by combined therapy.

When given orally, 5-fluorocytosine is well absorbed from the gastrointestinal tract and reaches clinically effective concentrations.[315-317] Blood levels may be 'cidal for some strains of *Candida* but only 'static for others.[317] The dose of the drug is 50 to 150 mg/kg given at 6-hour intervals; this must be reduced in the presence of renal insufficiency. The most frequent side effects are hepatotoxicity and depression of the bone marrow, which are usually reversible when the drug is discontinued. Nausea and vomiting are fairly common.

Assessment of cure of fungal endocarditis should be made with caution because symptoms of the disease may remain suppressed for long periods.[318] A more accurate view of this situation is that it is "stabilized." Patients should be followed from the time chemotherapy is discontinued, because relapse may occur as long as 2 years after completing treatment. Blood cultures are usually negative. Antibodies to *Candida* may be absent in the presence of infection, and their detection does not identify an active infectious process, because precipitins to *Candida* are present in 40 per cent of individuals who undergo cardiac surgery and are not infected, as well as in those in whom there has been an apparent cure.[253]

Surgical Therapy

Despite the emphasis on the medical management of infective endocarditis over the past 40 years, it must be pointed out that the first spontaneous cure of an infection of the cardiovascular system was accomplished by Touroff and Vessell in 1940 when they ligated an infected patent ductus arteriosus.[319] After a hiatus of many years, during which the prognosis of endocarditis changed from almost complete hopelessness to a high expectancy of recovery as more and more highly effective antimicrobial agents became available, surgical approaches have again become the ultimate therapeutic modality in patients in whom all other forms of treatment have been unsuccessful. However, as is often the case with progress in medicine, the development of new methods of management, while solving one set of problems, has frequently created new ones that are often more difficult to solve than the ones they replace. This is unquestionably the case in the surgical treatment of infective endocarditis. On the one hand, successful surgical manipulation of the uninfected heart has been responsible for an appreciable increment in the incidence of cardiovascular infections (p. 1141). On the other hand, while it is often the final successful approach to the eradication of valvular infections, surgical intervention raises difficult questions in relation not only to its advisability and indications but also, once such a course has been accepted as necessary, to the time when it should be undertaken.[319a]

One of the most critical and unquestioned indications for surgical intervention in cases of infective endocarditis is the development of intractable cardiac failure due to disruption of valve leaflets or their supporting structures. It must be pointed out, however, that the mere appearance of even severe decompensation of the heart does not always necessitate surgical therapy. In some instances this condition may be well controlled by medical management alone. However, when all conventional measures have failed, or decompensation progresses despite intensive treatment of heart failure, surgical repair should be undertaken without

delay; temporizing may lead to failure, even when the surgical manipulation itself has been entirely successful. The role of intractable congestive failure in death from infective endocarditis is emphasized by the fact that this is the most common cause of fatality in this disease. Involvement of the aortic valve is most often the cause of this problem,[320-322] but severe mitral regurgitation, although less common, has also required replacement of the damaged valve with a prosthesis.[323,324] It has become increasingly clear that the *presence of active infection is not a contraindication to cardiac surgery* in patients whose valves and their supporting structures have been severely injured or destroyed by infection.[325,326]

A study of ten patients with acute aortic valve regurgitation requiring urgent valvular replacement led Wise and his colleagues to distinguish two syndromes—acute and chronic.[327] In their opinion, only the acute form required immediate surgical intervention. The clinical features that indicated the presence of this syndrome (p. 1111) were (a) diastole of shorter duration than systole, (b) low cardiac output, (c) soft murmurs, (d) lack of appreciable enlargement of the left ventricle on radiographic or electrocardiographic study, and (e) diminished intensity of the first heart sound secondary to high left ventricular diastolic pressure. Although an important degree of aortic regurgitation can usually be detected on physical examination, determination of the significance of mitral valve incompetence in the course of infective endocarditis may require cardiac catheterization.

The fatality rate in emergency aortic valve replacement has been reported to be about 33 per cent but it is probably declining[320-322]; it is far less when it is carried out electively.[320] The necessity of surgical intervention in patients with perforation of the aortic valve leading to regurgitation during the course of endocarditis is emphasized by a report of eight patients in whom operation was not carried out and all of whom died; of seven individuals with the same lesion who underwent repair of the perforation or replacement of the valve, only three succumbed.[328] Griffin et al. have stressed the need for immediate insertion of a prosthesis when severe cardiac failure complicates valvular infections.[329] They also suggested that this procedure be performed early in patients with mild decompensation of the heart because of a significant risk of sudden death from embolic myocardial infarction or the development of potentially lethal arrhythmias.

INDICATIONS. The following are the important indications for cardiac surgery in patients with infective endocarditis: (1) *Congestive failure* that does not respond to intensive medical management. Active infection is not a contraindication. (2) *No response of the infectious process* on the involved valve despite appropriate, intensive antimicrobial therapy for about one week. An additional benefit in this situation is removal of the bulk of the bacterial load. (3) *Repeated embolic occlusions*, especially when vital areas such as brain, eyes, coronary arteries, and kidneys are involved. In this situation, the problem that arises involves a decision as to when surgery should be performed. Should this be after the first, second, third, or more embolic episode? There are no data that indicate the answer to this question. (4) *Presence of a septal abscess.* (5) *Relapse of infection* (3 months or less after "cure"). It is this writer's practice to treat the first relapse over the same length of time as the original infection. A second relapse should prompt serious consideration of removal of the affected valve. (6) *Recurrence of endocarditis* (> 6 months after "cure") involving the valve initially affected or a different one. If it is the same valve, management involves the same approach as that used for the first *relapse*. If the recurrence involves a different valve, treatment is the same as for an initial episode. (7) Endocarditis involving aneurysms of sinus of Valsalva or atrioventricular junctional tissues. (8) *Fungal endocarditis*; replacement by a prosthesis after 7 to 10 days of antifungal therapy.

PROSTHETIC VALVE INFECTION. Infection superimposed on prosthetic valves or on "patches" inserted into previously uninfected hearts poses difficult problems in management. While chemotherapy based on the sensitivity of the responsible organism is effective in a small number of cases, especially those in which the diagnosis is made and treatment is instituted early, medical management alone often fails to eradicate the disease.[330-333] The development of bacteremia following insertion of a prosthetic valve poses a dilemma difficult to resolve because its cause may be extracardiac as well as intracardiac. A study has suggested criteria that may be helpful in indicating the site of the infectious process from which organisms have invaded the bloodstream: (a) if the interval between operation and the detection of organisms in the circulation is less than 25 days, it is more likely that the infection is extracardiac; (b) a longer period is suggestive of an intracardiac infection; (c) the appearance of new murmurs suggests the possibility that bacteria have colonized the prosthesis; and (d) detectable extracardiac sources of bacteremia (e.g., sternal infection, the presence of indwelling venous or urinary tract catheters, suppurative phlebitis or pneumonia) suggest, but do not prove, that the prosthetic valve is not the source of the organisms.[158] It must be emphasized, however, that none of these criteria, singly or together, always distinguishes extra- from intracardiac infections.[159] This author recommends no more than one attempt at eradication of the infection by medical means. If this fails, antimicrobial agents are given for about one week, the infected valve is removed and replaced by a prosthesis, and treatment is continued for 3 to 4 weeks after surgery.

In a study of 12 cases of infection involving prosthetic valves, Block et al.[334] applied two criteria to separate their patients: (a) at least two blood cultures must contain the same organism, and (b) other clinical findings of bacterial endocarditis must be present, on the basis of which they characterized cases as "early" (infection occurring within 60 days of operation) and "late" (infections occurring after 60 days). Five of the seven patients with "early" disease (71 per cent) died. "Late" disease was less severe and was generally related to dental procedures or other manipulations for which chemoprophylaxis had not been given. One of the five patients (20 per cent) in this category succumbed. The results of this study were thought to indicate that vigorous antimicrobial therapy of infection of prosthetic valves should make reoperation unnecessary, in some instances. Another study of the natural history of infective endocarditis following insertion of prostheses into the heart has indicated that antibiotic therapy alone may be effective in eradicating disease that develops 6 months or more after operation.[335] In instances in which infection

of the prosthesis appeared within two months of its insertion, 40 per cent died before chemotherapy was instituted; the others survived following replacement of the prosthesis and treatment with vancomycin. It was suggested that the prognosis of prosthetic valvular infection that occurs later than 6 months after operation is the same as that for endocarditis involving a natural valve. These conclusions differ from the experience of Sande et al. who noted a 100 per cent fatality rate in patients treated with antibiotics for infectious processes involving cardiac prostheses.[158]

Wilson et al. have indicated that replacement of cardiac valves may be carried out successfully in patients with active infective endocarditis even when blood cultures are positive in the immediate preoperative period.[336] The hemodynamic status of these patients is the factor that determines the time when the valve should be replaced. The activity of the infection or the duration of antimicrobial therapy prior to surgery is of little or no importance in the decision to insert a prosthesis. In individuals with myocardial or aortic abscesses in whom conventional aortic valve replacement is not possible, a radical surgical procedure may be necessary. Richardson and his colleagues have reported that heart failure and annular and myocardial abscesses—present most often with staphylococcal and fungal endocarditis—were the primary cause of death in infection involving natural as well as prosthetic valves.[337] Operation significantly improved survival in cases with moderate or severe cardiac decompensation, in infection of natural valves when moderate or severe heart failure was present, and in patients with staphylococcal infection of prosthetic valves.

Rapaport[338] made the following editorial comments concerning the data analyzed by Richardson and his colleagues[337]:

It is important to point out that the conclusions reached by Richardson et al. regarding the indications for surgery in staphylococcal native valve endocarditis are not applicable to tricuspid valve involvement. Tricuspid valve endocarditis has a surprisingly good prognosis when managed medically. There is increasing recognition that patients with native valve endocarditis who develop significant hemodynamic impairment manifested by moderate to severe cardiac decompensation are best managed surgically with immediate operation in view of the 50 to 89 per cent mortality rate under these circumstances otherwise. Surgery can be accomplished successfully even when the infection is rampant. . . . It would seem more prudent to recommend that all patients with native valve endocarditis due to *Staphylococcus aureus* who do not have evidence of moderate or severe cardiac failure should be initially managed medically with appropriate antibiotics. This may prove to be adequate.

If this fails, and especially if hemodynamic difficulties develop, surgical removal of the affected valve is indicated.

Endocarditis involving the right side of the heart often presents a special problem with respect to the need for surgical treatment. It has been suggested that excision of the tricuspid valve may be the therapy of choice when there is failure to respond to antimicrobial agents. It is now clear that the prognosis for cure of infection involving this valve, when it is caused by *Pseudomonas* and other gram-negative bacteria, fungi, and other organisms, is dramatically improved by surgical removal of the valve and not replacing it with a prosthesis.[339-341] With normal pulmonary artery pressure, cardiac output can be maintained for at least limited periods in the absence of the tricuspid valve.

Taking all available information into account, it is the general opinion that tricuspid valvulectomy without prosthetic replacement should be reserved for patients in whom the disease is due to an antibiotic-resistant organism. It has also been suggested that the procedure should be carried out only after 6 weeks of antimicrobial therapy have failed to result in a cure.[312] In some instances, a prosthesis has been inserted many months after treatment and has not led to recurrence of endocarditis.

Sixty-one of the patients with bacterial or candidal tricuspid endocarditis whose involved valves were removed and not replaced by a prosthesis have been restudied by Arbulu and Asfaw 10 years later.[342] Four patients (6 per cent) died during the first 30 days postoperatively, and two died 44 and 60 days after surgery. Five patients died "late"; three deaths were not related to the operation, while two patients succumbed after another episode of endocarditis. Most striking was the observation that, even as long as 10 years after the tricuspid valve was removed, there were no differences in the clinical status in the 11 individuals in whom a prosthetic valve was inserted at some time, and those who continued without a tricuspid valve over this period. The authors concluded that "tricuspid valvulectomy without prosthetic replacement is the method of choice in the treatment of patients with right-sided, intractable infective endocarditis. Prosthetic valve insertion, at a second operation, is indicated only when medical treatment has failed to control the hemodynamic alterations."

Complications resulting from the insertion of prosthetic valves in patients with endocarditis include paravalvular leaks, congestive heart failure, complete heart block, systemic arterial emboli, and valvular obstruction; these are often associated with the preoperative presence of annular and myocardial abscesses. Infective endocarditis may recur after insertion of a cardiac prosthesis; the incidence ranges from 1 to 4 per cent.[343] It often becomes apparent within two months of the original operation, and seems to be related to inadequate débridement, occult sources of infection from preoperative septic emboli, and the characteristics of the original organism.[343] Retained local infection, preexisting peripheral abscesses, and virulent bacteria limit the effectiveness of valve replacement in these patients. It is well known that endocarditis involving a prosthetic valve may appear months to years after operation.

PROGNOSIS

Despite the availability of effective antibiotics and the increasing effectiveness of surgical treatment, the mortality and morbidity of infective endocarditis are still significant. The overall five-year survival has been reported to range from 47 to 90 per cent; of the patients who live, about 15 to 24 per cent are incapacitated by heart failure or the sequelae of embolization.[20,344,345] Factors that are prominent in determining the ultimate outcome are age, type of organism, duration of illness before institution of therapy, site and extent of valvular involvement, presence of renal insufficiency, congestive heart failure, and complications such as embolization, mycotic aneurysms, superinfections,

myocarditis, and myocardial abscess. Pearce and Guze suggested that all electrocardiographic abnormalities except left ventricular hypertrophy and P mitrale as well as severe alcoholism and/or portal cirrhosis are associated with a poor prognosis for recovery from infective endocarditis.[346]

The fatality rate of infective endocarditis increases with age.[347] Valvular infections are more likely to develop during the course of neoplastic disease or disorders or the urinary and gastrointestinal tracts in older patients; the manifestations of these other conditions often overshadow the endocarditis and result in dangerous delay of therapy.[182] The fatality rate within the first 30 days of illness was found by NcNeill et al. to be the same for both sexes.[348] However, fewer men (48 per cent) than women (58 per cent) lived for 6 months. The annual death rate during the first 4 years after treatment was found to be 7 per cent.

Endocarditis due to Staph. aureus, enterococci, gram-negative bacteria, and fungi is associated with an appreciably higher death rate than when it is caused by alpha-streptococci. The prognosis for survival is best when Strep. viridans is involved and is worst when Staph. epidermidis and Staph. aureus, yeasts, and fungi cause the disease.[348] The fatality rate of endocarditis caused by Candida is about 80 per cent when patients are treated by either medical or surgical methods alone. However, when these therapeutic modalities are combined, the risk of death is reduced to 20 per cent, especially when the involved valve is replaced by a prosthesis within a few days after the diagnosis of candidal endocarditis is established.

Delay in diagnosis with late initiation of therapy results in a relatively poor prognosis in subacute endocarditis. All patients treated within two weeks of onset of the disease recover. The survival rate falls appreciably when therapy is delayed longer than eight weeks and when complications (embolic phenomena, heart failure, and central nervous system involvement) develop. Lerner and Weinstein observed that, of the patients with the subacute disease treated within two weeks after the onset of symptoms, 90 per cent survived; only 74 per cent were cured when therapy was withheld for longer than eight weeks.[14]

Studies that suggest that the prognosis for patients with infection of the aortic valve is poorer than for those with disease of the mitral valve have not considered contributing factors (such as age, sex, nature of the underlying cardiac lesion, organism, and delay in therapy). For example, the mitral valve is more likely to be infected than the aortic in females with rheumatic heart disease; the opposite is true in males.[9] Highly invasive organisms such as staphylococci, pneumococci, and Strep. pyogenes tend to invade aortic valves and the right side of the heart more often than microaerophilic and viridans streptococci or enterococci, and not uncommonly affect otherwise normal valves. Infective endocarditis due to highly virulent organisms occurs frequently in males, especially older ones with arteriosclerotic valvular changes. Although these factors predispose to involvement of the aortic valve, they pose an increased risk of death in themselves.

Perforated valves, torn cusps, or ruptured chordae tendineae—lesions heralded by the appearance of new murmurs, aortic regurgitation, or rapidly developing heart failure—often precede a fatal issue. Although these complications are relatively common in acute infective endocarditis, they have also been observed occasionally in patients with the subacute type of disease.[14]

Cardiac decompensation increases the incidence of failure of antimicrobial therapy and of early and late death. Lerner and Weinstein reported that 6 months after completion of treatment, the survival rate was four times greater in patients with normal than in those with abnormal cardiac function.[14] This has also been observed by others.[345,349] That this problem has become more prominent since the advent of effective chemotherapy is substantiated by experiences at the Philadelphia General Hospital between 1933 and 1938 and 1950 and 1960.[350] Uncontrolled infection was responsible for 64 per cent and heart failure for 6 per cent of the deaths in the preantibiotic era; cardiac decompensation occurred in 61 per cent of the fatal cases—a tenfold increase—in the later period.

Several observers have noted that *myocarditis* is common and is probably an important factor in determining the prognosis of endocarditis.[192,351,352] The presence of myocardial abscesses involving either the septum or walls of the ventricles increases the risk of death. However, if these are recognized early and are removed surgically, the prognosis improves.

Although the presence of *myocardial infarction* is seldom detected during life, it is a relatively common autopsy finding.[9,353-355] Coronary occlusions, even those of minor degree, but especially when multiple, threaten the prognosis not only because they are, in themselves, potentially lethal but also because they may provoke cardiac decompensation.[9] Jackson and Allison have presented strong evidence in support of the role of myocardial infarction in the congestive heart failure that occurs in infective endocarditis; they found the incidence of embolic coronary lesions to be much higher than that of dynamic aortic regurgitation (with or without perforation or rupture of a valve) in persons dying of heart failure.[356]

The development of *renal dysfunction* during or after recovery from infective endocarditis is an ominous prognostic sign, especially if heart failure is also present. It has been suggested that "severe renal damage, particularly proliferative glomerulonephritis, may prove fatal, in spite of penicillin therapy."[9] About 5 to 10 per cent of the deaths in treated endocarditis are associated with renal failure.[9,20] Many observers have documented the finding that even severe uremia may be reversed by intensive antimicrobial therapy.

When *embolic phenomena* supervene, the prognosis for survival depends greatly on the site at which the emboli are deposited, the time in the course of the disease when they develop, and whether or not they produce suppuration.[20,172] Thus, embolization of the coronary arteries or vital areas of the brain and lung (if cardiac failure is present) is a considerably greater threat to survival than involvement of other organs. Systemic emboli have been found in 60 and 45 per cent, respectively, of fatal cases of acute and subacute endocarditis studied at the Massachusetts General Hospital.[20] Cerebral vessels were involved in over 60 per cent. Embolization may occur longer than 6 months after successful treatment of the cardiac infection but is rarely fatal at that time.[345,352,357,358]

Mycotic aneurysms often begin to develop in the early stages of infective endocarditis but may not rupture until many weeks or months after apparent recovery.[9,19] The degree of danger with which they are associated depends on their location; tears do not mean inevitable death. Pearce and Guze noted that, when cerebral emboli and mycotic aneurysms are not immediately fatal, the prognosis for recovery is good.[346] Of 20 patients with mycotic aneurysms studied by Cates and Christie, 17 died; the cerebral vessels were involved in all but one of the fatal cases.[9] Aneurysms of the sinus of Valsalva are said to occur in 10 to 15 per cent.[20,175] In addition to the cerebral arteries, which are the commonest and most dangerous sites, aneurysms have been found in the abdominal aorta, superior mesenteric artery, sinus of Valsalva, mitral valve, splenic artery, ligated ductus arteriosus, and coronary arteries.[146,359-362] Karchmer[363] has pointed out that improvement in the prognosis of infective endocarditis rests on "anticipating complications, recognizing them as they occur, and referring patients promptly to a major medical center when an operation is essential."

PROSTHETIC VALVULAR INFECTIONS. The prognosis in infection of prosthetic valves is determined, in general, by the same factors that influence the outcome in patients with endocarditis involving natural valves. In addition, it is also dependent on whether complications develop, such as obstruction of the valvular outlet (Starr-Edwards valve), paravalvular leaks, or separation of the prosthesis to a degree that causes congestive heart failure or severe bleeding as a result of improper control with anticoagulants. The fatality rate in infections that developed when a previously infected natural valve was replaced with a prosthesis was found to be 28 per cent by Boyd et al.[364] and was 90 per cent in patients treated for 4 to 6 weeks without control of the infection or surgical intervention. In those with uncontrolled disease who were operated upon within 10 days, the survival rate was 83 per cent. A review of the literature indicated that the average fatality rate in individuals with infected intracardiac prostheses was about 70 per cent.[365] It is clear from these and other recorded experiences that early recognition of infection of prosthetic valves and prompt medical and surgical treatment greatly improve the possibility of survival.[366]

Young and his co-workers studied 163 episodes of infective endocarditis in which 32 cardiac operations were performed during the active stage of the disease.[367] Cardiac failure was the primary reason for surgical intervention in 88 per cent. *Staphylococcus* and enterococcus were the organisms most often involved. Postoperative complications were rare. There were no instances of continued infection, prosthetic dehiscence, or advanced heart block; one patient developed a paravalvular leak and another a systemic embolus. Eleven individuals were moribund prior to surgery. The authors emphasized that there is a "high medical and surgical mortality in patients with IE and that delayed operative intervention may be a major causative factor resulting in a high surgical mortality." They also pointed out that these experiences "justify an aggressive surgical approach in patients with valve dysfunction and heart failure." Kaplan[368] studied 63 patients who had been subjected to cardiac surgery before developing infective endocarditis. Fifty-five per cent had had a prosthetic valve inserted; most of these had underlying rheumatic heart disease. Most of the patients studied had congenital heart disease with systemic artery–to–pulmonary artery shunts. In this group, the highest risk of developing endocardial infection was in those who were cyanotic and had palliative pulmonary artery–to–systemic artery shunts. In discussing the prognosis of infective endocarditis, Scalia et al.[369] stressed the point that early surgical intervention affects favorably the prognosis, especially in cases of isolated aortic valve involvement." In a study of the prognosis of endocarditis involving prosthetic valves in 48 patients studied between 1962 and 1978, Masur and Johnson[370] indentified a fatality rate of 69 per cent, with 20 per cent of the deaths associated with embolization to the central nervous system. A fatal outcome that exceeded 75 per cent was noted when the aortic valve was involved, when a nonstreptococcal organism was the causative agent, when new or increased regurgitant murmurs developed, and when significant congestive failure supervened. The fatality rate was lowest when the prosthesis was invaded by streptococci (29 per cent) and when a mitral valve had been replaced (47 per cent). Cohn and his colleagues have reported that, of 128 patients who underwent porcine heart-valve replacement (aortic 47, mitral 62, combined mitral-aortic 19), only 5 (4 per cent) developed infective endocarditis over the following 5 to 8 years.[371]

PREVENTION

Although there are still no statistically valid data to establish the effectiveness of chemoprophylaxis in infective endocarditis, anecdotal experiences are sufficient to support it. In general, all individuals known to have disease of the heart, particularly that involving the valves, should be considered candidates for prophylaxis. This includes patients with congenital heart disease (excluding uncomplicated secundum atrial septal defect and ligated and divided patent ductus arteriosus), acquired lesions (rheumatic, atherosclerotic, calcific), prolapsing mitral valve with regurgitation ("click murmur"), hypertrophic obstructive cardiomyopathy, calcified mitral annulus, and an intracardiac prosthesis or "patch," or those who, after a previous episode of valvular infection, are subjected to dental manipulations (extraction, deep scaling, and gingivectomy) or surgery involving the respiratory, gastrointestinal, urinary, or genital tracts.

The value of prophylaxis is uncertain in procedures that may be associated with a transient bacteremia associated with an indwelling vascular catheter, transvenous pacemakers, arteriovenous shunts, ventriculoatrial shunts, barium enema, sigmoidoscopy, colonoscopy, and biopsy of the liver. Available evidence does not prove its necessity in these situations. Nevertheless, some physicians recommend chemoprophylaxis, despite the probably very small risk of the development of endocarditis. Kaye[372] has made the comment that optimal antimicrobial prophylaxis administered to patients undergoing various procedures known to be associated with transient bacteremia could be expected to prevent only a few cases of endocarditis.

Selection of appropriate prophylactic antibiotics requires knowledge both of the organisms most likely to invade the blood during procedures producing transient bacteremia and of those most often responsible for infection of cardiac valves. For example, the bacteria present in the blood after dental manipulation or operations on the upper respiratory tract are, for the most part, *Strep. viridans*; however, enterococci or staphylococci may also invade the circulation. Transient bacteremia associated with procedures involving the urinary, gastrointestinal, and genital tracts are usually characterized by the presence of various species of streptococci, gram-negative bacteria, and occasionally *Bacteroides*. *Staph. aureus* is a common culprit in cardiac surgery involving extracorporeal circulation. When incision and drainage of an abscess or débridement of contaminated tissue is carried out, the choice of the prophylactic agent is based on the type of organism recovered from the infected site.

Prophylaxis

A variety of approaches to prophylaxis have been recommended for patients undergoing dental manipulation or operations on the upper respiratory tract. One involves the administration of 250 mg of phenoxymethyl penicillin (penicillin V) orally three or four times a day for 2 days before, the day of, and for 2 days after surgery. In addition, a dose of 600,000 or 1.2 million units of procaine penicillin G is given intramuscularly on the day of operation. An alternate program recommends the intramuscular injection of 1 million units of penicillin G one hour before and one hour after surgical manipulation. It has been suggested by some that patients receive a daily injection of the same dose of antibiotic for 2 days after operation. This author prefers to use erythromycin because, in his experience, this drug is active against most strains of *Strep. viridans*, enterococcus, and penicillin-sensitive or penicillin-resistant *Staph. aureus*. This program involves the administration of 1 gm of erythromycin orally one hour before the procedure and 0.5 gm one hour after the surgery, followed by 0.5 gm every 6 hours for a total of four doses. Another regimen employed by others, especially for patients sensitized to penicillin, involves the administration of 0.5 gm of erythromycin every 6 hours for 2 days before, on the day of, and for 2 days after dental surgery. In the author's opinion, this program is excessive prophylaxis for a transient bacteremia that persists, as a rule, no longer than 20 minutes.

AMERICAN HEART ASSOCIATION GUIDELINES. A committee of the American Heart Association has made a number of recommendations for chemoprophylaxis in patients with underlying cardiac disease (Table 29–5, p. 952).[373] They have pointed out that "since there have been no controlled clinical trials, adequate data for comparing various methods for prevention of endocarditis in man are not available." Its recommendations are as follows: For all dental procedures associated with bleeding or surgery or instrumentation of the upper respiratory tract, two regimens are suggested. The first involves the intramuscular injection of 1 million units of penicillin G mixed with 600,000 units of procaine penicillin G 30 to 60 minutes prior to the procedure. This is followed by 500 mg of phenoxymethyl penicillin (penicillin V) orally every 6 hours for 8 doses. The regimen for children is the same, but the dose of penicillin is reduced to 30,000 units/kg and that of procaine penicillin is unchanged; the oral dose of penicillin V is reduced to 250 mg every 6 hours for eight doses. The second involves only oral administration of antibiotics. Adults are given 2 gm of penicillin V orally 30 to 60 minutes before the procedure and 500 mg of the same drug every 6 hours for eight doses postoperatively. The same regimen is used for children over 60 pounds in weight; for those under 60 pounds, the preoperative dose of penicillin V is 1 gm and the postoperative dose is 250 mg at the same interval and number of doses as for adults. A third recommended regimen includes the same doses of the various penicillins, as described above for parenteral prophylaxis, with the addition of 1 gm of streptomycin (20 mg/kg for children) postoperatively. The following programs are recommended for patients allergic to penicillin: Adults, 1 gm of vancomycin intravenously 30 to 60 minutes preoperatively followed by 500 mg of erythromycin orally every 6 hours for eight doses. The doses of vancomycin and erythromycin for children are reduced to 20 mg/kg and 10 mg/kg, respectively.

The American Heart Association's recommendations for

prophylaxis for surgery or instrumentation of the genito-urinary and gastrointestinal tracts are as follows: Adults are given 2 million units of penicillin G or 1 gm of ampicillin plus gentamicin (1.5 mg/kg but no more than 80 mg) intramuscularly or intravenously *or* 1 gm of streptomycin 30 to 60 minutes prior to the procedure. When gentamicin is used, a similar dose of this drug plus penicillin or ampicillin is given every 8 hours for two doses. When streptomycin has been given prior to the procedure, a similar dose is given together with penicillin every 12 hours for two doses. The program for children is similar, but the doses of penicillin G, ampicillin, gentamicin, and streptomycin are reduced to 30,000 units/kg, 50 mg/kg, 2 mg/kg, and 20 mg/kg, respectively. Adults sensitive to penicillin are given 1 gm of vancomycin intramuscularly preoperatively. Although this may not be necessary, a second course of these drugs may be given 12 hours after operation. The dose of both vancomycin and streptomycin for children sensitized to penicillin is 20 mg/kg.

Dismukes[374] has reported the results of a review of published data indicating the level of risk of transient bacteremia associated with procedures involving the airway, gastrointestinal tract, and urologic manipulation. On the basis of the frequency and four types of organisms recovered from the blood stream, he recommended specific antimicrobial prophylaxis for procedures involving various organ systems. The data in the paper differ, in some respects, from those presented by the American Heart Association,[373] which, as both he and others have pointed out, are based on the results of animal studies.

Keys[375] has suggested chemoprophylactic procedures that represent a modification of those recommended by the American Heart Association,[373] which he says are "inconvenient, painful and expensive" and "may not be enforced in actual practice." He also emphasizes the point with which this author (L.W.) (with the exception of the word "secure") fully agrees, that "although experimental studies in animals have provided a secure foundation for our concepts of antimicrobial prophylaxis, carefully conducted clinical trials of various programs are urgently needed." In commenting about chemoprophylaxis in patients susceptible to the risk of transient bacteremia in the course of dental manipulation, Oakley and Somerville[376] made the statement that "it is a sobering thought that a rise in the standard of oral hygiene in this country would probably help more than any other measure to reduce the incidence of streptococcal infective endocarditis. If we can accomplish this and prophylaxis, too, then endocarditis should become a rare disease."

Despite specific recommendations for antimicrobial prophylaxis in patients with underlying heart disease subjected to procedures associated with transient bacteremia, the problem remains unsolved because of a lack of acceptable data to support it. The present state of the art has best been defined by Schadelin[377] in the following statement: "Prophylactic antibiotic coverage of all interventions with a high risk of bacteremia is accepted practice in patients with valvular heart disease. A true cost-benefit ratio, however, has not been possible to demonstrate due to the low risk involved in these procedures and, therefore, the current recommendations rely on experimental work with animals. Full application of these findings in patients is difficult and even so incapable of preventing the majority of cases of infective endocarditis."

Prophylaxis for Surgery. The effectiveness of the chemoprophylaxis for "open-heart" surgery has been studied by a number of investigators. One report has indicated no difference in the incidence of infection when penicillin G, methicillin, or a placebo was administered.[378] A similar observation has been made in patients given penicillin G plus streptomycin, oxacillin, or a placebo prophylactically.[379] A study comparing methicillin and cephalothin demonstrated that none of 492 persons receiving the cephalosporin but 11 of 129 given methicillin developed endocarditis.[380] Other investigations comparing cephalothin with cloxacillin and gentamicin given before, during, and after operation have failed to show any significant reduction in the risk of prosthetic infection.[379] A recent prospective double-blind study involving 200 patients in whom prosthetic valves were implanted and who were given cephalothin for 2 or 6 days produced no convincing evidence that the longer period of prophylaxis had an advantage over the shorter one.[380]

Infective endocarditis that develops early in the postoperative period is often caused by *Staph. aureus* or *Staph. epidermidis*. Organisms less frequently responsible are streptococci, gram-negative bacteria, and fungi. Because there is no chemoprophylactic program that will protect against invasion by all organisms, prudence suggests that it be directed primarily against the staphylococcus. For this reason, the antibiotics used most frequently have been oxacillin, nafcillin, or cephalothin, the latter protecting against invasion not only by staphylococci but also by common gram-negative bacilli such as *E. coli*, *Proteus mirabilis*, and *K. pneumoniae*. An acceptable regimen for these antibiotics is 2 gm intravenously 2 hours before operation, 1 gm intraoperatively, and 1 gm every 4 hours for no more than 2 to 3 days in order to minimize the risk of superinfection. The author prefers cephalothin because of its activity against most staphylococci and streptococci as well as against the common gram-negative bacteria. Vancomycin, 1 gm intravenously 2 hours before surgery followed by the same dose every 12 hours for 2 days, may be used in persons sensitized to the penicillins or cephalosporins.

A prophylactic program for patients with underlying cardiac disease who undergo surgical or other manipulation of the genitourinary or gastrointestinal tract must include drugs that inhibit multiplication of many gram-positive and gram-negative bacteria. The program recommended by the American Heart Association, although not supported by data, proving its efficacy, may be used.[373] This involves administration of 1 gm of ampicillin plus 1.5 mg/kg of gentamicin intramuscularly or intravenously 30 to 60 minutes prior to the procedure. The same doses of the antibiotics are repeated 8 and 16 hours after operation.

All individuals with cardiac diseases known to predispose to endocarditis who have active extracardiac infections and who must undergo some type of surgical procedure should be treated before an operation is performed. The drugs selected are those to which the causative organism is sensitive, and conventional therapeutic doses should be administered. It may be necessary only to bring the infectious process under control when there is an urgent need for surgery; whenever possible, however, it is probably best to eradicate the infection completely before the surgical procedure is undertaken.

It must be emphasized that the chemoprophylactic programs currently used to prevent recurrences of rheumatic fever may not eliminate the risk of the development of infective endocarditis. For this reason, all patients on such programs who are subjected to manipulations of the oral cavity or upper respiratory, urinary, or gastrointestinal tracts must receive additional prophylaxis, as described above.

References

1. Major, R. H.: Notes on the history of endocarditis. Bull. Hist. Med. *17*:351, 1945.
2. Osler, W.: Malignant endocarditis. Gulstonian Lectures. Lancet *1*:459, 1885.
3. Libman, E., and Celler, H. L.: The etiology of subacute infective endocarditis. Am. J. Med. Sci. *140*:516, 1910.
4. Lichtman, S. S.: Treatment of subacute bacterial endocarditis: Current results. Ann. Intern. Med. *19*:787, 1943.
5. Kelson, S. R.: Observations on the treatment of subacute bacterial (streptococcal) endocarditis since 1939. Ann. Intern. Med. *22*:75, 1945.
6. Florey, M. E., and Florey, H. W.: General and local administration of penicillin. Lancet *1*:387, 1943.
7. Loewe, L., Rosenblatt, P., Greene, H. J., and Russel, M.: Combined penicillin and heparin therapy of subacute bacterial endocarditis. J.A.M.A. *124*:144, 1944.
8. Hedley, O. F.: Rheumatic heart disease in Philadelphia hospitals. III. Fatal rheumatic heart disease and subacute bacterial endocarditis. Pub. Health Rep. *55*:1707, 1940.

9. Cates, J. E., and Christie, R. V.: Subacute bacterial endocarditis. A review of 442 patients treated in 14 centres appointed by the Penicillin Trials Committee of the Medical Research Council. Q. J. Med. 20:93, 1951.

10. Kaye, D., McCormack, R. C., and Hook, E. W.: Bacterial endocarditis: Changing pattern since introduction of penicillin therapy. Antimicrob. Agents Chemother. 3:37, 1961.

11. Finland, M., and Barnes, M. W.: Changing etiology of bacterial endocarditis in the antibacterial era: Experiences at Boston City Hospital 1933–1965. Ann. Intern. Med. 72:341, 1970.

12. Afremow, M. L.: Review of 202 cases of bacterial endocarditis. III. Med. J. 107:67, 1955.

13. Cherubin, C. E., and Neu, H. C.: Infective endocarditis at the Presbyterian Hospital in New York City from 1938–1967. Am. J. Med. 51:83, 1971.

14. Lerner, P. I., and Weinstein, L.: Infective endocarditis in the antibiotic era. N. Engl. J. Med. 274:199, 259, 323, 387, 1966.

14a. Brandenburg, R. O., Guiliani, E. R., Wilson, W. R., and Geraci, J. E.: Infective endocarditis –A 25-year overview of diagnosis and therapy. J. Am. Coll. Cardiol. 1:280, 1983.

15. Kerr, A., Jr.: Bacterial endocarditis—revisited. Mod. Con. Cardiovasc. Dis. 33:831, 1964.

16. Hamburger, M.: Acute and subacute bacterial endocarditis. Arch. Intern. Med. 112:1, 1963.

17. Wedgwood, J.: Early diagnosis of subacute bacterial endocarditis. Lancet 2:1058, 1955.

18. Kelson, S. R., and White, P. D.: Notes on 250 cases of subacute bacterial (streptococcal) endocarditis studied and treated between 1927 and 1939. Ann. Intern. Med. 22:40, 1940.

19. Kerr, A., Jr.: Subacute bacterial endocarditis. In Pullen, R. L. (ed.): Springfield, Ill., Charles C Thomas, 1955. (No. 274, Am. Lecture Series, Monograph of Bannerstone Division of Am. Lectures in Internal Medicine.)

20. Morgan, W. L., and Bland, E. F.: Bacterial endocarditis in antibiotic era. Circulation 19:753, 1959.

MICROBIOLOGY AND PATHOLOGY

21. Libman, E., and Friedberg, C. K.: Subacute Bacterial Endocarditis. New York, Oxford University Press, 1941.

22. Uwaydah, M. M., and Weinberg, A. N.: Bacterial endocarditis—a changing pattern. N. Engl. J. Med. 273:1231, 1965.

23. Kaye, D., McCormack, R. C., and Hook, E. W.: Bacterial endocarditis: The changing patterns since introduction of penicillin therapy. In Antimicrobial Agents and Chemotherapy. American Society of Microbiology. Washington, D.C., 1961, pp. 37–46.

24. Hosea S. H.: Virulent Streptococcus viridans bacterial endocarditis. Am. Heart J., 101:174, 1981.

25. Cameron, I. W.: Subacute bacterial endocarditis in an edentulous patient: A case report. Br. Dent. J. 130:404, 1971.

26. Moellering, R. C., Jr., Watson, B. K., and Kunz, L. J.: Endocarditis due to group D streptococci. Comparison of disease caused by Streptococcus bovis with that produced by enterococci. Am. J. Med. 57:239, 1974.

27. Keusch, G. T.: Opportunistic infections in colon carcinoma. Am. J. Clin. Nutr. 27:1481, 1974.

28. Klein, R. S., Recco, R. A., Catalano, M. T., Edberg, S. C., Casey, J. I., and Steigbigel, N. H.: Association of Streptococcus bovis with carcinoma of the colon. N. Engl. J. Med. 297:800, 1977.

29. Rose, D. F., Richman, H., and Localio, S. A.: Bacterial endocarditis associated with colorectal carcinoma. Ann. Surg. 179:190, 1974.

30. Reid, T. M. S.: Group D streptococcal endocarditis. Scott. Med. J. 22:13, 1977.

31. Wilson, L. M.: Etiology of bacterial endocarditis: Before and since introduction of antibiotics. Ann. Intern. Med. 58:946, 1963.

32. Harder, E. J., Wilkowske, C. J., Washington, J. A., III, and Geraci, J. E.: Streptococcus mutans endocarditis. Ann. Intern. Med. 80:364, 1974.

33. Bouza, E., Meyer, R. A., and Busch, D. F.: Group G streptococcal endocarditis. Am. J. Clin. Pathol. 70:108, 1978.

34. Davies, M. K., Ireland, M. A., and Clarke, D. B.: Infective endocarditis from group C streptococci causing stenosis of both the aortic and mitral valves. Thorax 36:69–71, 1981.

35. Portnoy, D., Wink, I., Richards, G. K., and Blanc, M. Z.: Bacterial endocarditis due to a penicillin-tolerant group C streptococcus. CMA J. 122:69–75, 1980.

36. Levin, R. M., Pulliam, L., Mondry, C., Levy, D., Hadley, W. K., and Grossman, M.: Penicillin-resistant Streptococcus constellatus as a cause of endocarditis. Am. J. Dis. Child. 136:42–45, 1982.

37. Eickoff, T. C., Klein, J. O., Daly, A. K., Ingall, D., and Finland, M.: Neonatal sepsis and other infections due to group B beta-hemolytic streptococci. N. Engl. J. Med. 271:1221, 1974.

38. Dismukes, W. E., Karchmer, A. W., Buckley, M. J., Austen, W. G., and Swartz, M. N.: Prosthetic valve endocarditis. Circulation 48:365, 1973.

39. Bevanger, L., and Stamnes, T. I.: Group L streptococci as the cause of bacteraemia and endocarditis. Acta Pathol. Microbiol. Scand. 87:301–302, 1979.

40. Roberts, K. B., and Sidlak, M. J.: Satellite streptococci: A major cause of "negative" blood cultures in bacterial endocarditis? J.A.M.A. 241:2293, 1979.

41. Wilson, R., and Hamburger, M.: Fifteen years' experience with staphylococcus septicemia in large city hospital: Analysis of fifty-five cases in Cincinnati General Hospital 1940–1954. Am. J. Med. 22:437, 1957.

42. Keys, T. F., and Hewitt, W. L.: Endocarditis due to micrococci and Staphylococcus epidermidis. Arch. Intern. Med. 132:216, 1973.

43. Simberkoff, M. S., and Rahal, J. J., Jr.: Acute and subacute endocarditis due to Erysipelothrix rhusiopathiae. Am. J. Med. Sci. 266:53, 1978.

44. Axelrod, J., Keusch, G. T., Bottone, E., Cohen, S. M., and Hirschman, S. Z.: Endocarditis caused by Lactobacillus plantarum. Ann. Intern. Med. 78:33, 1973.

45. Dupont, B., and Lapreste, C. L.: Maladie d'Osler à lactobacille. Nouv. Presse Med. 6:3627, 1977.

46. Bayer, A. S., Chow, A. N., and Guze, L. B.: Listeria monocytogenes endocarditis: Report of a case and review of the literature. Am. J. Med. Sci. 273:319, 1977.

47. Kaplan, K., and Weinstein, L.: Diphtheroid infections in man. Ann. Intern. Med. 70:919, 1969.

48. Murray, B. E., Karchmer, A. W., and Moellering, R. C., Jr.: Diphtheroid prosthetic valve endocarditis. A study of clinical features and infecting organisms. Am. J. Med. 69:838–848, 1980.

49. Gaurd, R. W.: Non-toxigenic Corynebacterium diphtheriae causing subacute bacterial endocarditis. Pathology 11:533, 1979.

50. Love, J. W., Medina, D., Anderson, S., and Braniff, B.: Infective endocarditis due to Corynebacterium diphtheriae: Report of a case and review of the literature. Johns Hopkins Med. J. 148:41, 1981.

51. Block, C. S., Levy, M. L., and Fritz, V. U.: Bacillus cereus endocarditis. A case report. S. Afr. Med. J. 53:556, 1978.

52. Reller, L. B.: Endocarditis caused by Bacillus subtilis. Am. J. Clin. Pathol. 60:714, 1973.

53. Schafer, F. J., Wing, E. J., and Norden, C. W.: Infectious endocarditis caused by Rothia dentocariosa. Ann. Intern. Med. 91:747, 1979.

54. Pape, J., Singer, C., Kiehn, T. E., Lee, B. J., and Armstrong, D.: Infective endocarditis caused by Rothia dentocariosa. Ann. Intern. Med. 91:746, 1979.

55. Thayer, W. S.: Bacterial or infective endocarditis. Edinburgh Med. J. 38:237–265, 207–334, 1931.

56. Sugar, A. M., Utsinger, P. D., and Santoro, J.: Gonococcal endocarditis in a patient with mitral valve prolapse. Study of host immunology and organism characteristics. Am. J. Med. Sci. 283:165–168, 1982.

57. Brancaccio, M., and Legendre, G. G.: Megasphaera elsdenii endocarditis. J. Clin. Microbiol. 10:72–74, 1979.

58. Cohen, P. S., Maguire, J. H., and Weinstein, L.: Infective endocarditis caused by gram-negative bacteria: A review of the literature, 1945–1977. Prog. Cardiovasc. Dis. 22:205–242, 1980.

59. Hansing, C. E., Allen, V. D., and Cherry, J. D.: Escherichia coli endocarditis: A review of the literature and a case study. Arch. Intern. Med. 120:472–477, 1967.

60. Carruthers, M. M.: Endocarditis due to enteric bacilli other than Salmonellae: Case reports and literature review. Am. J. Med. Sci. 273:203, 1977.

61. Satterwhite, T. K., McGee, Z. A., Schaffner, W., et al.: Infection of an avulsed papillary muscle tip stimulating bacterial endocarditis. Am. Heart J. 86:107–111, 1973.

62. Rosen, P., and Armstrong, D.: Infective endocarditis in patients treated for malignant neoplastic disease (a postmortem study). Am. J. Clin. Pathol. 59:241–250, 1978.

63. Carruthers, M. M., and Kanokvechayant, R.: Pseudomonas aeruginosa endocarditis: Report of a case, with review of the literature. Am. J. Med. 55:811, 1973.

64. Reyes, M. P., Palutke, W. A., Wylin, R. F., Lerner, A. M., Arbulu, A. M., Pursel, S. E., and Schatz, I. J.: Pseudomonas endocarditis in the Detroit Medical Center, 1969–1973. Medicine 52:173, 1973.

65. Yu, V. L., Rumans, L. W., Wing, E. J., et al.: Pseudomonas maltophilia causing heroin-associated infective endocarditis. Arch. Intern. Med. 138:1667–1671, 1978.

66. Noriega, E. R., Rubinstein, E., Simberkoff, M. S., et al.: Subacute and acute endocarditis due to Pseudomonas cepacia in heroin addicts. Am. J. Med. 59:29–36, 1975.

67. Rubin, R. H., and Weinstein, L.: Salmonenosis. Microbiologic Pathologic and Clinical Features. New York, Stratton Intercontinental Medical Book Corporation, 1977.

68. Emmerson, A. M., Perinpanayagam, R. M., and Barnado, D. E.: Haemophilus endocarditis. Postgrad. Med. J. 57:117–119, 1981.

69. Jemsek, J. G., Greenberg, S. B., Gentry, L. O., Welton, D. E., and Mattox, K. L.: Haemophilus parainfluenzae endocarditis: Two cases and review of the literature in the past decade. Am. J. Med. 66:51, 1979.

70. Root, T. E., Silva, E. A., Edwards, L. D., and Topp, J. H.: Hemophilus aphrophilus endocarditis with a probable dental focus of infection. Chest 80:109, 1981.

71. Golden, B., Layman, T. E., Koontz, F. P., et al.: Brucella suis endocarditis. S. Med. J. 63:392–395, 1970.

72. Lehmann, V., Knutsen, S. B., Ragnhildstveit, E., et al.: Endocarditis caused by Pasteurella multocida. Scand. J. Infect. Dis. 9:247–248, 1977.

73. Block, P. C., Desanctis, R. W., Weinberg, A. W., et al.: Prosthetic valve endocarditis. J. Thorac. Cardiovasc. Surg. 60:541–548, 1970.

74. Mills, J., and Drew, D.: Serratia marcescens endocarditis. A regional illness associated with intravenous drug use. Ann. Intern. Med. 84:29, 1976.

75. Schmidt, J., Chmel, H., Kaminski, Z., and Sen, P.: The clinical spectrum of Campylobacter fetus infections: Report of five cases and review of the literature. Q. J. Med. 49:431, 1980.

76. McCormack, R. C., Kaye, D., and Hook, E. W.: Endocarditis due to Strepto-

bacillus moniliformis. A report of two cases and review of the literature. J. Am. Med. Assoc. *200*:183, 1967.

77. Weiner, M., and Werthamer, S.: *Cardiobacterium hominis* endocarditis — Characterization of the unusual organisms and review of the literature. Am. J. Clin. Pathol. *63*:131, 1975.

78. Geraci, J. E., Wilson, W. R., and Washington, J. A., III: Infective endocarditis caused by *Actinobacillus actinomycetemcomitans.* Mayo Clin. Proc. *55*:415, 1980.

79. Schiff, J., Suter, L. S., Gourley, R. D., et al.: *Flavobacterium* infection as a cause of bacterial endocarditis: Report of a case, bacteriological studies and review of the literature. Ann. Intern. Med. *55*:499, 1961.

80. LeFrock, L. J., Klainer, A. S., and Zuckerman, K.: *Edwardsiella tarda* bacteremia. S. Med. J. *69*:188, 1976.

81. McCullough, D., Menzies, R., and Corhere, B. M.: Endocarditis due to *Citrobacter diversus* developing resistance to cephalothin. N. Z. Med. J. *85*:182, 1977.

82. Walsh et al.: Fungal infections of the heart: Analysis of 51 autopsied patients. Am. J. Cardiol. *45*:357, 1980.

83. Parker, J. C.: The potentially lethal problem of cardiac candidosis. Am. J. Clin. Pathol. *73*:356, 1980.

84. Brandstetter, R. D., and Brause, B. D.: *Candida parapsilosis* endocarditis. Recovery of the causative organism from an addict's own syringe. J.A.M.A. *243*:1073, 1980.

85. Hollway, H. D., Keipper, V., and Kaiser, A. B.: *Torulopsis glabrata* endocarditis. J.A.M.A. *140*:2088, 1980.

86. Hartley, R. A., Remsberg, J. R. S., and Sinaly, N. P.: *Histoplasma* endocarditis: Case report and review of the literature. Arch. Intern. Med. *119*:527, 1967.

87. Baret, R. J., Prince, A. S., and Neu, H. C.: *Aspergillus* endocarditis in children: Case report and review of the literature. Pediatrics *68*:73, 1981.

88. Gaynes, R. P., Gardner, P., and Causey, W.: Prosthetic valve endocarditis caused by *Histoplasma capsulatum.* Arch. Intern. Med. *141*:1533, 1981.

89. Del Rossi, A. J., Morse, D., Spagna, P. M., and Lemole, G. M.: Succesful management of *Penicillium* endocarditis. J. Thorac. Cardiovasc. Surg. *80*:945, 1980.

90. Arnold, A. G., Gribbin, B., DeLeval, M., Macartney, F., and Slack, M.: *Trichosporon capitatum* causing recurrent fungal endocarditis Thorax *36*:478, 1981.

91. Tyras, D. H., Kaiser, G. C., Barnes, H. B., Laskowski, L. F., and Marr, J. J.: Atypical mycobacteria and the xenograft valve. J. Thorac. Cardiovasc. Surg. *75*:331, 1978.

92. Lohr, D. C., Goeken, J. A., Doty, D. B., and Donta, S.: *Mycobacterium gordonae* infection of a prosthetic valve. J.A.M.A. *239*:1528, 1978.

93. Baker, R. D.: Endocardial tuberculosis. Arch. Pathol. *19*:621, 1935.

94. Anyanwu, C. H., Nassau, E., and Yacoub, M.: Miliary tuberculosis following homograft valve replacement. Thorax *31*:101, 1976.

95. Tobin, M. J., Cahill, N., Gearty, G., Maurer, B., Blake, S., Daly, K., and Hone, R.: Q fever endocarditis. Am. J. Med. *72*:396, 1982.

96. Waters, E. W., Romansky, M. J., Johnson, A. C., and Conway, S. J.: *Actinomyces bovis* endocarditis: An uncommon and complex problem. *In* Sylvester, J. C. (ed.): Antimicrobial Agents and Chemotherapy — 1962. Proceedings of the Second Interscience Conference on Antimicrobial Agents and Chemotherapy. American Society of Microbiology, 1963, p. 517.

97. Vlachakis, N. D., Gazes, P. C., and Hairston, P.: Nocardial endocarditis following mitral valve replacement. Chest *63*:276, 1975.

98. Nastro, I. J., and Finegold, S. M.: Endocarditis due to anaerobic gram-negative bacilli. Am. J. Med. *54*:482, 1973.

99. Fredericka, D. N.: Endocarditis and brain abscess due to *Bacteroides oralis.* J. Infect. Dis. *145*:918, 1982.

100. Jones, R. B., Priest, J. B., and Kuo, C. C.: Subacute chlamydial endocarditis. J.A.M.A. *247*:655, 1982.

101. Van der Bel-Kahn, J. M., Watanakunakorn, C., Menefee, N. G., Long, H. D., and Dicter, R.: *Chlamydia trachomatis* endocarditis. Am. Heart J. *95*:627, 1978.

102. Mattman, L. H., and Mattman, P. E.: L-forms of *Streptococcus fecalis* in septicemia. Arch. Intern. Med. *115*:315, 1965.

103. Piepkorn, M. W., and Reichenbach, D. D.: Infective endocarditis associated with cell wall–deficient bacteria. Electron microscopic findings in four cases. Hum. Pathol. *9*:163, 1978.

104. Dale, A. J., and Geraci, J. E.: Mixed cardiac valvular infections: Report of case and review of literature. Proc. Staff Meet. Mayo Clin. *36*:288, 1965.

105. Saravolatz, L. D., Burch, K. H., Quinn, E. L., et al.: Polymicrobial infective endocarditis. Am. Heart J. *95*:163, 1978.

106. Bharucha, P. E., and Nair, K. G.: Coxsackie B₁ endocarditis. Clin. Pediatr. *14*:188, 1975.

107. Sklaver, A. R., Hoffman, T. A., and Greenman, R. I.: Staphylococcal endocarditis in addicts. South. Med. J. *71*:638, 1978.

108. Reiner, N. E., Gopalakrishna, K. V., and Lerner, P. I.: Enterococcal endocarditis in heroin addicts. J.A.M.A. *235*:1861, 1976.

109. Dreyer, N. P., and Fields, B. N.: Heroin–associated infective endocarditis. Ann. Intern. Med. *78*:699, 1973.

110. Rosenblatt, J. E., Dahlgran, J. G., Fishback, R. S., and Talky, F. P.: Gram-negative bacterial endocarditis in narcotic addicts. Calif. Med. *118*:1, 1973.

111. Bailey, I. K., and Richards, J. G.: Infective endocarditis in a Sydney teaching hospital — 1962–1971. Aust. N. Z. Med. *5*:413, 1975.

112. Pankey, G. A.: The prevention and treatment of bacterial endocarditis. Am. Heart J. *98*:102, 1979.

113. Arnett, E. N., and Roberts, W. C.: Acute infective endocarditis: A clinicopathologic analysis of 137 necropsy patients. Curr. Probl. Cardiol. *1*:3, 1976.

114. Buchbinder, N. A., and Roberts, W. C.: Left-sided valvular active endocarditis. Am. J. Med. *53*:20, 1972.

115. Roberts, W. C., and Buchbinder, N. A.: Healed left-sided infective endocarditis. A clinicopathological study of 59 patients. Am. J. Cardiol. *40*:876, 1976.

116. Roberts, W. C., and Buchbinder, N. A.: Right-sided valvular infective endocarditis. Am. J. Med. *53*:7, 1972.

117. Arnett, E. N., and Roberts, W. C.: Prosthetic valve endocarditis. Clinicopathological analysis of 22 necropsy patients with comparison of observations in 74 necropsy patients with active infective endocarditis involving natural left-sided cardiac valves. Am. J. Cardiol. *38*:281, 1976.

118. Anderson, D. J., Buckley, B. H., and Hutchins, G. M.: A clinicopathologic study of prosthetic valve endocarditis in 22 patients: Morphologic basis for diagnosis and therapy. Am. Heart J. *94*:325, 1977.

119. Bortolotti, U., Thiene, G., Milano, A., Panizzon, G., Valente, M., and Gallucci, V.: Pathological study of infective endocarditis on Hancock porcine bioprostheses. J. Thorac. Cardiovasc. Surg. *81*:934–942, 1981.

120. Ferrans, V. J., Boyce, S. W., Billingham, M. E., Spray, T. L., and Roberts, W. C.: Infection of glutaraldehyde-preserved porcine valve heterografts. Am. J. Cardiol. *43*:1123–1135, 1979.

121. Everett, E. D., and Hirschman, J. V.: Transient bacteremia and endocarditis: A review. Medicine *56*:61, 1977.

122. Peterson, L. J., and Peacock, R.: The incidence of bacteremia in pediatric patients following tooth extraction. Circulation *53*:676, 1976.

123. Goodman, J. S., Kolhouse, J. F., and Koenig, M. G.: Recurrent endocarditis due to *Streptococcus viridans* in an edentulous" man. South. Med. J. *66*:352, 1973.

124. LeFrock, J. L., Klainer, A. S., Wu, W. H., and Turndorf, H.: Transient bacteremia associated with nasotracheal suctioning. J.A.M.A. *236*:1610, 1977.

125. LeFrock, J. L., Ellis, C. A., Klainer, A., and Weinstein, L.: Transient bacteremia associated with barium enema. Arch. Intern. Med. *135*:835, 1975.

126. LeFrock, J. L., Ellis, C. A., Turchik, J. B., and Weinstein, L.: Transient bacteremia associated with sigmoidoscopy. N. Engl. J. Med. *289*:469, 1973.

127. Shull, H. J., Green, B. M., Allen, S. R., Dunn, G. D., and Schenker, S.: Bacteremia with upper gastrointestinal endoscopy. Ann. Intern. Med. *83*:212, 1975.

128. Rafoth, A. J., Sorenson, R. M., and Bond, J. H.: Bacteremia following colonoscopy. Gastrointest. Endosc. *22*:32, 1975.

129. LeFrock, J. L., Ellis, C. A., Turchik, J. B., Zawacki, J. K., and Weinstein, L.: Transient bacteremia associated with percutaneous liver biopsy. J. Inf. Dis. *131* (Suppl.):104, 1975.

130. Sullivan, N. M., Sutter, V. L., Mims, M. M., Marsh, V. H., and Finegold, S. M.: Clinical aspects of bacteremia after manipulation of the genitourinary tract. J. Inf. Dis. *127*:49, 1973.

131. Ritvo, R., Monroe, P., and Andriole, V. T.: Transient bacteremia due to suction abortion. Implications for SBE prophylaxis. Yale J. Biol. Med. *50*:471, 1977.

132. Snyder, N., Atterbury, C. E., Correia, J. P., and Conn, H. F.: Increased concurrence of cirrhosis and bacterial endocarditis. Gastroenterology *73*:1107, 1977.

133. Baskin, T. W., Rosenthal, A., and Pruitt, B. A., Jr.: Acute bacterial endocarditis: A silent source of sepsis in the burn patient. Ann. Surg. *184*:618, 1976.

134. Lemire, G. G., Morin, J. E., and Dobell, A. R. C.: Pacemaker infections: A 12-year review. Can. J. Surg. *18*:181–184, 1975.

135. Garvey, G. J., and Neu, H. C.: Infective endocarditis — an envolving disease. A review of endocarditis at the Columbia-Presbyterian Medical Center, 1968–1973. Medicine *57*:105, 1978.

136. Rosen, P., and Armstrong, D.: Infective endocarditis in patients treated for malignant neoplastic disease. Am. J. Clin. Pathol. *60*:241, 1973.

137. Cross, A. S., and Steigbigel, R. T.: Infective endocarditis and access site infections in patients on hemodialysis. Medicine *55*:453, 1976.

138. Markowitz, S. M., Szentpetery, S., Lower, R. R., and Duma, R. J.: Endocarditis due to accidental penetrating foreign bodies. Am. J. Med. *60*:571, 1976.

UNDERLYING HEART DISEASE AND PATHOGENESIS

139. Gelfman, R., and Levine, S. A.: The incidence of acute and subacute bacterial endocarditis in congenital heart disease. Am. J. Med. Sci. *204*:324, 1942.

140. Johnson, C. M., and Rhodes, H. K.: Pediatric endocarditis. Mayo Clin. Proc. *57*:86–94, 1982.

141. McGuinness, G. A., Schieken, R. M., and Maguire, G. F.: Endocarditis in the newborn. Am. J. Dis. Child. *134*:577–580, 1980.

142. Shah, P., Singh, W. S. A., Rose, V., and Keith, J. D.: Incidence of bacterial endocarditis in ventricular septal defects. Circulation *34*:127, 1966.

143. Hallidie-Smith, K. A., Olsen, E. G. J., Oakley, C. M., Goodwin, J. F., and Cleland, W. P.: Ventricular septal defect and aortic regurgitation. Thorax *24*:257, 1969.

144. Blumenthal, S., Griffiths, S. P., and Morgan, B. C.: Bacterial endocarditis in children with heart disease. Pediatrics *26*:933, 1960.

145. Rodbard, S.: Blood velocity and endocarditis. Circulation *27*:18, 1963.

146. Glenn, F., Stewart, H. J., Engle, M. A., Lukas, D. S., Artusio, J., Steinberg, I. S., and Holswade, G. R.: Coarctation of aorta complicated by bacterial endocarditis and an aneurysm of the sinus of Valsalva. Circulation *17*:432, 1958.

147. Korn, D., DeSanctis, R. W., and Sell, S.: Massive calcification of the mitral annulus: a clinicopathologic study of fourteen cases. N. Engl. J. Med. 267:900, 1962.

148. Watanakunakorn, C.: Staphylococcus aureus endocarditis on the calcified mitral annulus fibrosus. Am. J. Med. Sci. 266:219, 1973.

149. Chagnac, A., Rudniki, C., and Loebel, H.: Infectious endocarditis in idiopathic hypertrophic subaortic stenosis. Report of three cases and review of the literature. Chest 81:346–349, 1982.

150. Wang, K., Gobel, F. L., and Gleason, D. F.: Bacterial endocarditis in idiopathic hypertrophic subacute stenosis. Am. Heart J. 89:359, 1975.

151. Soman, V. R., Breton, G., Hershkowitz, M., and Mark, H.: Bacterial endocarditis of mitral valve in Marfan's syndrome. Br. Heart J. 36:1247, 1974.

152. Lachman, A. S., Branwell-Jones, D. M., Lakier, J. B., Pocock, W. A., and Barlow, J. B.: Infective endocarditis in the billowing mitral leaflet syndrome. Br. Heart J. 37:326, 1975.

152a. Clemens, J. E., Horowitz, R. I., Jaff ee, C. C., Feinstein, A. R., and Stanton, B. F.: A controlled evaluation of the risk of bacterial endocarditis in persons with mitral valve prolapse. N. Engl. J. Med. 307:776, 1982.

153. Nolan, C. M., Kane, J. J., and Grunow, W. A.: Infective endocarditis and mitral prolapse. A comparison with other types of endocarditis. Arch. Intern. Med. 141:447–450, 1981.

154. Amoury, R. A., Bowman, F. O., Jr., and Malm, J. R.: Endocarditis associated with intracardiac prostheses. J. Thorac. Cardiovasc. Surg. 51:36, 1966.

155. Yeh, T. J., Anabtani, I. N., Cornett, V. E., White, A., Stern, W. H., and Ellison, R. G.: Bacterial endocarditis following open-heart surgery. Ann. Thorac. Surg. 3:29, 1967.

156. Stein, P. D., Harken, D. E., and Dexter, L.: The nature and prevention of prosthetic valve endocarditis. Am. Heart J. 71:393, 1966.

157. Wilson, W. R., Jaumun, P. M., Danielson, G. K., Giuliani, E. R., Washington, J. A., III, and Geraci, J. E.: Prosthetic valve endocarditis. Ann. Intern. Med. 82:751, 1975.

158. Sande, M. A., Johnson, W. D., Jr., Hook, E. W., and Kaye, D.: Sustained bacteremia in patients with prosthetic valves. N. Engl. J. Med. 286:1067, 1972.

159. Weinstein, L.: Infected prosthetic valves: A diagnostic and therepeutic dilemma. N. Engl. J. Med. 286:1108, 1972.

160. Starkebaum, M., Durack, D., and Beeson, P.: The "incubation period" of subacute bacterial endocarditis. Yale J. Biol. Med. 50:49–58, 1977.

161. Kaplan, E., Helmsworth, J. A., Ahearn, E. N., Benzing, G., III, Daoud, G., and Schwartz, D. C.: Results of palliative procedures for tetralogy of Fallot in infants and young children. Ann. Thorac. Surg. 5:489, 1968.

162. Persuad, V.: Two unusual cases of mural endocarditis with a review of the literature. Am. J. Clin. Pathol. 53:832, 1970.

163. Graham, H. V., von Hartitzch, B., and Medina, J. R.: Infected atrial myxoma. Am. J. Cardiol. 38:658, 1976.

164. Rogers, E. W., Weyman, A. E., Nobel, R. J., and Burns, S. C.: Left atrial myxoma infected with Histoplasma capsulatum. Am. J. Med. 64:683, 1978.

165. Lepeschkin, E.: On the relation between the site of valvular involvement in endocarditis and the blood pressure resting on the valve. Am. J. Med. Sci. 224:318, 1952.

166. Allen, A. C.: Mechanism of localization of vegetations of bacterial endocarditis. Arch. Pathol. 27:399, 1939.

167. Wadsworth, A. B.: A study of the endocardial lesions developing during pneumococcus infection in horses. J. Med. Res. 34:279, 1919.

168. Gould, K., Ramirez-Ronda, C. H., Holmes, R. K., and Sanford, J. P.: Adherence of bacteria to heart valves in vitro. J. Clin. Invest. 56:1364, 1975.

169. Holmes, R. K., and Ramirez-Ronda, C. H.: Adherence of bacteria to the endothelium of heart valves. Infective Endocarditis, an American Heart Association Monograph. No. 52, 1977, pp. 12–13.

CLINICAL MANIFESTATIONS

170. Weinstein, L., and Schlesinger, J. J.: Pathoanatomic, pathophysiologic and clinical correlations in endocarditis. N. Engl. J. Med. 291:832, 1122, 1974.

171. Libman, E., and Friedberg, C. K.: Subacute Bacterial Endocarditis. 2nd ed. New York, Oxford University Press, 1948.

172. Weinstein, L., and Rubin, R. H.: Infective endocarditis—1973. Progr. Cardiovasc. Dis. 16:239, 1973.

173. Weinstein, L.: Infective endocarditis: Past, present and future. J. R. Coll. Phys. Lond. 6:161, 1972.

174. Weinstein, L.: Modern infective endocarditis. J.A.M.A. 233:260, 1975.

175. Pankey, G. A.: Acute bacterial endocarditis at University of Minnesota Hospitals, 1939–1959. Am. Heart J. 64:583, 1962.

176. Willerson, J. T., Moellering, R. C., Jr., Buckley, M. J., and Austen, W. G.: Conjunctival petechiae after open-heart surgery. N. Engl. J. Med. 284:539, 1971.

177. Kilpatrick, Z. M., Greenberg, P. A., and Sanford, J. P.: Splinter hemorrhages—their clinical significance. Arch. Intern. Med. 115:730, 1965.

178. Roth, M.: Ueber Netzhautaffectionen bei Wundfiebern. Dtsch. Z. Chir. 1:471, 1872.

179. Litten, M.: Ueber akute maligne Endocarditis und die dabei vorkommender Retinalveränderungen. Charit. Ann. 3:137, 1878.

180. Doherty, W. B., and Trubek, M.: Significant hemorrhagic retinal lesions in bacterial endocarditis (Roth's spots). J.A.M.A. 97:308, 1931.

181. Libman, E.: The clinical features of cases of subacute bacterial endocarditis that have spontaneously become bacteria-free. Am. J. Med. Sci. 146:625, 1913.

182. Mills, J., Utley, J., and Abbott, J.: Heart failure in infective endocarditis: Predisposing factors, course and treatment. Chest 66:151, 1974.

183. Gonzalez-Lavin, L., Lise, M., and Ross, D.: The importance of the "jet lesion" in bacterial endocarditis involving the left heart: Surgical considerations. J. Thorac. Cardiovasc. Surg. 59:185, 1970.

184. Roberts, W. C., Ewy, G. A., Glancy, D. L., and Marcus, F. I.: Valvular stenosis produced by active infective endocarditis. Circulation 36:449, 1967.

185. Sacks, P. V., Lakier, J. B., and Barlow, J. B.: Severe aortic stenosis produced by bacterial endocarditis. Br. Med. J. 3:97, 1969.

186. Mann, T., McLaurin, L., Grossman, W., and Graige, E. E.: Assessing the hemodynamic severity of acute regurgitation due to infective endocarditis. N. Engl. J. Med. 293:108, 1975.

187. Roberts, N. K., and Somerville, J.: Pathological significance of electrocardiographic changes in aortic valve endocarditis. Br. Heart J. 31:395, 1969.

188. Gopalakrishna, K. V., Kwan, K., and Shah, A.: Metastatic myocardial abscess due to group F streptococci. Am. J. Med. Sci. 274:329, 1977.

189. Kim, H-S., Weilbacher, D. G., Lie, J. T., and Titus, J. L.: Myocardial abscesses. Am. J. Clin. Pathol. 70:18, 1978.

190. Arnett, E. N., and Roberts, W. C.: Valve ring abscess in active infective endocarditis. Frequency, location and clues to clinical diagnosis from the study of 95 necropsy patients. Circulation 54:140, 1976.

191. Perry, E. L., Fleming, R. G., and Edwards, J. E.: Myocardial lesions in subacute bacterial endocarditis. Ann. Intern. Med. 36:126, 1952.

192. Blankenhorn, M. A., and Gall, E. A.: Myocarditis and myocardiosis: Clinicopathologic appraisal. Circulation 13:217, 1956.

193. Vogler, W. R., and Dorney, E. R.: Bacterial endocarditis in congenital heart disease. Am. Heart J. 64:198, 1962.

194. Bell, E. T.: Glomerular lesions associated with endocarditis. Am. J. Pathol. 8:639, 1932.

195. Pfeifer, J. F., Lipton, M. J., Oury, J. H., Angell, W. W., and Hulgren, H. N.: Acute coronary embolism complicating bacterial endocarditis: Operative treatment. Am. J. Cardiol. 37:920, 1976.

196. Menzies, C. J. G.: Coronary embolism with infarction in bacterial endocarditis. Br. Heart J. 23:464, 1961.

197. Brunson, J. G.: Coronary embolism in bacterial endocarditis. Am. J. Pathol. 29:689, 1953.

198. Horder, T. J.: Infective endocarditis: With an analysis of 150 cases and with special reference to the chronic form of the disease. Q. J. Med. 2:289, 1909.

199. Jochman, G.: Lehrbuch der Infektionskrankheiten für Ärtze und Studierende. Berlin, Julius Springer, 1914, pp. 144–148.

200. McDevitt, E.: Treatment of cerebral embolism. Mod. Treat. 2:52, 1965.

201. Harrington, A. W.: Embolism of the spinal cord. Glasgow Med. J. 103:28, 1925.

202. Harrison, M. J. G., and Hampton, J. R.: Neurological presentation of bacterial endocarditis. Br. Med. J. 2:148, 1967.

203. Kernohan, J. W., Woltman, H. W., and Barnes, A. R.: Involvement of the nervous system associated with endocarditis: Neuropsychiatric and neuropathological observations in forty-two cases of fatal outcome. Arch. Neurol. Psych. 42:789, 1939.

204. Jones, H. R., Jr., and Siekert, R. G.: Embolic mononeuropathy and bacterial endocarditis. Arch. Neurol. 19:535, 1968.

205. Schocket, S., and Braver, D.: Cilioretinal artery occlusion in a patient with suspected bacterial endocarditis. South. Med. J. 63:1, 1970.

206. Roach, M. R., and Drake, C. G.: Ruptured cerebral aneurysms caused by microorganisms. N. Engl. J. Med. 273:240, 1963.

207. Kauffman, S. L., Lynfield, J., and Hennigar, G. R.: Mycotic aneurysms of the intrapulmonary arteries. Circulation 35:90, 1967.

208. Ziment, I.: Nervous system complications in bacterial endocarditis. Am. J. Med. 47:593, 1969.

209. Pruitt, A. A., Rubin, R. H., Karchmer, A. W., and Duncan, G. W.: Neurologic complications of bacterial endocarditis. Medicine 57:329, 1978.

210. Bohmfalk, G. L., Story, J. L., Wissinger, J. P., and Brown, W. E.: Bacterial intracranial aneurysm. J. Neurosurg. 48:369, 1978.

211. Churchill, M. A., Geraci, J. E., and Hunder, G. G.: Musculoskeletal manifestations of bacterial endocarditis. Ann. Intern. Med. 87:754, 1977.

212. Baehr, G.: Renal complications of endocarditis. Trans. Assoc. Am. Phys. 46:87, 1931.

213. Villarreal, H., and Sokoloff, L.: The occurrence of renal insufficiency in subacute bacterial endocarditis. Am. J. Med. Sci. 220:655, 1950.

214. Cordeiro, A., Costa, H., and Lagenha, F.: Editorial. Immunologic phase of subacute bacterial endocarditis. A new concept and general considerations. Am. J. Cardiol. 16:477, 1965.

215. Williams, R. C., and Kunkel, H. G.: Rheumatoid factor, complement and conglutinin aberrations in patients with subacute bacterial endocarditis, J. Clin. Invest. 41:666, 1962.

216. Williams, R. C.: Bacterial endocarditis—an analysis of immunopathology of infective endocarditis. An American Heart Association Symposium (No. 52) 1977, pp. 20–23.

217. Sheagren, J. N., Tuazon, C., Griffin, C., and Padmore, N.: Rheumatoid factor in acute bacterial endocarditis. Arthritis Rheum. 19:887, 1976.

218. Bayer, A. S., Theofilopoulos, A. N., Eisenberg, R., Dixon, F. J., and Guze, J. B.: Circulating immune complexes in infective endocarditis. N. Engl. J. Med. 295:1500, 1976.

219. McKenzie, P. E., Hawke, D., Woodroffe, A. J., Thompson, A. J., Seymour, A. E., and Clarkson, A. R.: Serum and tissue immune complexes in infective endocarditis. J. Clin. Lab. Immunol., 4:125–132, 1980.

220. Kauffman, R. H., Thompson, J., Valentijn, R. M., et al.: The clinical implications and the pathogenetic significance of circulating immune complexes in infective endocarditis. Am. J. Med. 71:17–25, 1981.

221. Howard, E. J.: Osler's nodes. Am. Heart J. 59:633, 1960.

222. Alpert, J. S., Krous, H. F., Dalen, J. E., O'Rourke, R. A., and Bloor, C. M.: Pathogenesis of Osler's nodes. Ann. Intern. Med. 85:471, 1976.

223. Davis, J. A., Weisman, M. H., and Dail, D. H.: Vascular disease in infective endocarditis: Report of immune-mediated events in skin and brain. Arch. Intern. Med. 138:480, 1978.

224. Rubenfeld, S., and Kyung-Whan, M.: Leucocytoclastic angiitis in subacute bacterial endocarditis. Arch. Dermatol. 113:1073, 1977.

225. Tu, W. H., Shearn, M. A., and Lee, J. C.: Acute diffuse glomerulonephritis in acute staphylococcal endocarditis. Ann. Intern. Med. 71:335, 1969.

226. Gutman, R. A., Striker, G. E., Gilliland, B. C., and Cutler, R. E.: The immune complex glomerulonephritis of bacterial endocarditis. Medicine 51:1, 1972.

227. Levy, R. L., and Hong, R.: The immune nature of subacute bacterial endocarditis (SBE) nephritis. Am. J. Med. 64:645, 1973.

228. Keslin, M. H., Messner, R. P., and Williams, R. C., Jr.: Glomerulonephritis with subacute bacterial endocarditis. Arch. Intern. Med. 132:578, 1973.

229. Bain, R. C., Edwards, J. E., Scheiffey, C. H., and Geraci, J. E.: Right-sided bacterial endocarditis and endarteritis: Clinical and pathologic study. Am. J. Med. 24:98, 1958.

230. Bashour, F. A., and Winchell, C. P.: Right-sided bacterial endocarditis. Am. J. Med. Sci. 240:411, 1960.

231. Altschule, M. D.: Subacute bacterial endocarditis of the right heart. Med. Sci. 15:50, 1964.

232. Zakrzewski, T., and Keith, J.: Bacterial endocarditis in infants and children. J. Pediatr. 67:1179, 1965.

233. Johnson, D. H., Rosenthal, A., and Nadas, A. S.: A forty-year review of bacterial endocarditis in infancy and childhood. Circulation 51:581, 1975.

234. Mendelsohn, G., and Hutchins, G. M.: Infective endocarditis during the first decade of life. Am. J. Dis. Child. 133:619, 1979.

235. Welton, D. E., Young, J. B., Gentry, W. O., Raizner, A. E., Alexander, J. K., Chahine, R. A., and Miller, R. R.: Recurrent infective endocarditis. Am. J. Med. 66:932, 1979.

236. Pankey, G. A.: The prevention and treatment of bacterial endocarditis. Am. Heart J. 98:102, 1979.

237. Beeson, P. B., Brannon, E. S., and Warren, J. V.: Observations on the sites of removal of bacteria from the blood in patients with bacterial endocarditis. J. Exp. Med. 81:9, 1945.

238. Mallen, M. S., Hube, E. L., and Brenes, M.: Comparative study of blood cultures made from artery, vein and bone marrow in patients with subacute bacterial endocarditis. Am. Heart J. 33:692, 1947.

239. Werner, A. S., Cobbs, C. G., Kaye, D., and Hook, E. W.: Studies on the bacteremia of bacterial endocarditis. J.A.M.A. 202:127, 1967.

240. Kelson, S. E., and White, P. D.: Notes on 250 cases of subacute bacterial (streptococcal) endocarditis studied and treated between 1927 and 1929. Ann. Intern. Med. 22:40, 1945.

241. Belli, J., and Waisbren, B. A.: The number of blood cultures necessary to diagnose most cases of bacterial endocarditis. Am. J. Med. Sci. 232:284, 1956.

242. Pazan, G. J., Person, K. L., Guff, F. W., Shaver, J. A., and Ho, M.: Determination of site of infection in endocarditis. Ann. Intern. Med. 82:746, 1975.

243. Cannady, P. B., Jr., and Sandford, J. P.: Negative blood cultures in infective endocarditis: A review. South. Med. J. 69:1420, 1976.

244. Pesanti, E. L., and Smith, I. M.: Infective endocarditis with negative blood cultures. An analysis of 52 cases. Am. J. Med. 66:43, 1979.

245. Pazin, G. J., Saul, S., and Thompson, M. E.: Blood culture positivity. Suppression by outpatient antibiotic therapy in patients with bacterial endocarditis. Arch. Intern. Med. 142:263, 1982.

246. Van Scoy, R. E.: Culture-negative endocarditis. Mayo Clin. Proc. 57:149, 1982.

247. Weinstein, L., Daikos, G., and Perrin, T. S.: Studies on the relationship of tissue fluid and blood levels of penicillin. J. Lab. Clin. Med. 38:715, 1951.

248. Barza, M., Samuelson, T., and Weinstein, L.: Penetration of antibiotics into fabrin loci in vivo: II. Comparison of nine antibiotics: Effect of dose and degree of protein binding. J. Inf. Dis. 129:66, 1974.

249. Nagel, J. G., Tuazon, C. U., Cardella, T. A., and Sheagren, J. N.: Teichoic acid serologic diagnosis of staphylococcal endocarditis. Use of gel diffusion and counterimmunoelectrophoretic methods. Ann. Intern. Med. 82:13, 1975.

250. Wheat, L. J., Kohler, R. B., Tabarah, Z. A., and White, A.: IgM antibody response to staphylococcal infection. J. Infect. Dis. 144:307, 1981.

251. Zeiger, A. R., Tuazon, C. U., and Sheagren, J. N.: Antibody levels to bacterial peptidoglycan in human sera during the time course of endocarditis and bacteremic infections caused by Staphylococcus aureus. Infect. Immun. 33 (Suppl.):795, 1981.

252. Seelig, M. S., Speth, C. P., Kozinn, P. J., Taschdjian, C. L., Toni, E. F., and Goldberg, P.: Patterns of Candida endocarditis following cardiac surgery: Importance of early diagnosis and therapy (an analysis of 91 cases). Progr. Cardiovasc. Dis. 17:125, 1974.

253. Parsons, E. R., and Nassau, E.: Candida serology in open-heart surgery. J. Med. Microbiol. 7:415, 1974.

254. Scheld, W. M., Brown, R. S., Jr., Harding, S. A., and Sande, M. A.: Detection of circulating antigen in experimental Candida albicans endocarditis by an enzyme-linked immunoabsorbent assay. J. Clin. Microbiol. 12:679, 1980.

255. Wiseman, J., Rouleau, J., Rigo, P., Strauss, H. W., and Pitt, B.: Gallium-67 myocardial imaging for the detection of bacterial endocarditis. Radiology, 120:135, 1976.

256. Spies, S. M., Myers, S. M., Barresi, V., Grais, I. M., and DeBoer, A.: A case of myocardial abscess evaluated by radionuclide techniques: A case report. J. Nucl. Med. 18:1089, 1977.

257. Miller, M. H., and Casey, J. I.: Infective endocarditis: New diagnostic techniques. Am. Heart J. 96:123, 1978.

258. Ellis, K., Jaffe, C., Malm, J. R., and Bowman, F. O., Jr.: Infective endocarditis: Roentgenographic considerations. Radiol. Clin. North Am. 11:415, 1973.

259. Stewart, J. A., Silimperi, D., Harris, P., Wise, N. K., Fraker, T. D., Jr., and Kisslo, J. A.: Echocardiographic documentation of vegetative lesions in infective endocarditis: Clinical implications. Circulation 61:374, 1980.

260. Fox, S., Kotler, M. N., Segal, B. L., and Parry, W.: Echocardiographic diagnosis of acute aortic valve endocarditis. Arch. Intern. Med. 137:85, 1977.

261. Berger, M., Gallerstein, P. E., Benhuri, P., Balla, R., and Goldberg, E.: Evaluation of aortic valve endocarditis by two-dimensional echocardiography. Chest 80:61, 1981.

262. Nakamura, K., Suzuki, S., Satomi, G., Hayashi, H., and Hirosawa, K.: Detection of mitral ring abscess by two-dimensional echocardiography. Circulation 65:816, 1982.

263. Wong, A. M., Oldershaw, P., and Gibson, D. G.: Echocardiographic demonstration of aortic root abscess after infective endocarditis. Br. Heart J. 46:584, 1981.

264. Scanlan, J. G., Seward, J. B., and Tajik, A. J.: Valve ring abscess in infective endocarditis: Visualization with wide-angle two-dimensional echocardiography. Am. J. Cardiol. 49:1794, 1982.

265. Andy, J. J., Sheikh, M. U., Nayab, A., Barores, B. O., Fox, L. M., Curry, C. L., and Roberts, W. C.: Echocardiographic observations on opiate addicts with infective endocarditis. Am. J. Cardiol. 40:17, 1977.

266. Berger, M., Delfin, L. A., Helveh, M., and Goldberg, E.: Two-dimensional echocardiographic findings in right-sided infective endocarditis. Circulation 61:855, 1980.

267. Dander, B., Richetti, B., and Poppi, B.: Echocardiographic diagnosis of isolated pulmonary valve endocarditis. Br. Heart J. 47:298, 1982.

268. Gomes, J. A., Calderon, J., Lajam, F., Sakurai, H., Friedman, H. S., and Tatz, J. S.: Echocardiographic detection of fungal vegetations in Candida parapsilosis endocarditis. Am. J. Med. 61:273, 1976.

269. Stewart, J. A., Silimperi, D., Harris, P., Wise, N. K., Fraker, T. D., and Kisslo, J. A.: Echocardiographic documentation of vegetative lesions in infective endocarditis: Clinical implications. Circulation 61:374, 1980.

270. Martin, R. P., Meltzer, R. S., Louria, B., Stinson, B., Stinson, E. B., Makowski, H., and Popp, R. L.: Clinical utility of two-dimensional echocardiography in infective endocarditis. Am. J. Cardiol. 46:379, 1980.

271. Hickey, A. J., Wolfers, J., and Wilcken, D. E. L.: Reliability and clinical relevance of detection of vegetations by echocardiography in bacterial endocarditis. Br. Heart J. 46:624, 1981.

272. Markiewicz, W., Peled, B., Alroy, G., Pollack, S., Brook, G., Rapoport, J., and Kerner, H.: Echocardiography in infective endocarditis. Lack of specificity in patients with valvular pathology. Eur. J. Cardiol. 10:247, 1979.

273. Rubenson, D. A., Tucker, C. R., Stinson, E. B., London, E. J., Oyer, P., Moreno-Cabral, R., and Popp, R. L.: The use of echocardiography in diagnosing culture-negative endocarditis. Circulation 64:641, 1981.

274. Dillon, T., Meyer, R. A., Korfhagen, J. C., Kaplan, S., and Chung, K. J.: Management of infective endocarditis using endocardiography. J. Pediatr. 96:552, 1980.

275. Strom, J., Becker, R., Davis, R., Matsomoto, M., Frishman, W., Sonnenblick, E. H., and Frater, R. W. M.: Echocardiographic and surgical correlations in bacterial endocarditis. Circulation 62:164, 1980.

MANAGEMENT

276. Weinstein, L., and Dalton, A. C.: Host determinants of response to antimicrobial agents. N. Engl. J. Med. 279:467, 524, 580, 1968.

277. Schlichter, J. G., MacLean, H., and Milzer, A.: Effective penicillin therapy in subacute bacterial endocarditis and other chronic infections. Am. J. Med. Sci. 217:600, 1949.

278. Hall, B., and Dowling, H. F.: Negative blood cultures in bacterial endocarditis: A decade's experience. Med. Clin. North Am. 50:159, 1966.

279. Cooper, R., and Mills, J.: Serratia endocarditis. A follow-up report. Arch. Intern. Med. 140:199, 1980.

280. Barza, M., Brusch, J., Bergeron, M. G., and Weinstein, L.: Penetration of antibiotics into fibrin loci in vivo. III. Intermittent versus continuous infusion and effect of probenecid. J. Inf. Dis. 129:73, 1974.

281. Weinstein, L., Goldfield, M., and Chang, T-W.: Infections occurring during chemotherapy: A study of their frequency, type and predisposing factors. N. Engl. J. Med. 251:247, 1954.

282. Tan, J. S., Kaplan, S., Terhune, C. A., Jr., and Hamburger, M.: Successful two-week treatment schedule for penicillin-susceptible Streptococcus viridans endocarditis. Lancet 2:1340, 1971.

283. Walker, W. F., and Hamburger, M.: Penicillin-sensitive streptococcal endocarditis. Arch. Intern. Med. 100:359, 1957.

284. Goodman, S., Berry, R. H., Benjamin, J. E., Schiro, H. S., and Hamburger, M.: Subacute bacterial endocarditis treated with oral penicillin. Arch. Intern. Med. 104:625, 1959.

285. Hamburger, M., Kaplan, S., and Walker, W. F.: Subacute bacterial endocarditis caused by penicillin-sensitive streptococci. J.A.M.A. 175:554, 1961.
286. Burman, N. D., Joffe, H. S., and Watson, C.: Oral antibiotic cure of staphylococcal endocarditis. Postgrad. Med. J. 49:920, 1973.
287. Phillips, B., and Watson, G. H.: Oral treatment of subacute bacterial endocarditis in children. Arch. Dis. Child. 52:235, 1977.
288. Weinstein, L., and Schlesinger, J.: Treatment of infective endocarditis — 1973. Progr. Cardiovasc. Dis. 6:275, 1973.
289. Kanis, J. A.: The use of anticoagulants in bacterial endocarditis. Postgrad. Med. J. 50:312, 1974.
290. Wolfe, J. C., and Johnson, W. D.: Penicillin-sensitive streptococcal endocarditis. In vitro and clinical observations on penicillin-streptomycin therapy. Ann. Intern. Med. 81:178, 1974.
291. Karchmer, A. W., Moellering, R. C., Jr., Maki, D. G., and Swartz, M. N.: Single-antibiotic therapy for streptococcal endocarditis. J.A.M.A. 241:1801, 1979.
292. Malacoff, R. F., Frank, E., and Andriole, V. T.: Streptococcal endocarditis (nonenterococcal, non-group A). J.A.M.A. 241:1807, 1979.
293. Quinn, E. L., Pohlod, D., Madhaven, T., Burch, K., Fisher, E., and Cox, F.: Clinical experience with cefazolin and other cephalosporins in bacterial endocarditis. J. Inf. Dis. 128 (Suppl.):S386, 1973.
294. Bryant, R. E., and Alford, R. H.: Unsuccessful treatment of staphylococcal endocarditis with cefazolin. J.A.M.A. 237:569, 1977.
295. Geraci, J. E., and Wilson, W. R.: Vancomycin therapy for infective endocarditis. Rev. Infect. Dis. 3:S250, 1981.
296. Hinthom, D. R., Baker, L. H., Romig, D. A., Voth, D. W., and Liu, C.: Endocarditis treated with clindamycin: Relapse and liver dysfunction. South. Med. J. 70:823, 1977.
297. Hunter, T. H.: Use of streptomycin in the treatment of bacterial endocarditis. Am. J. Med. 2:436, 1974.
298. Moellering, R. C., Jr., and Weinberg, A. N.: Studies on antibiotic synergism against enterococci. J. Clin. Invest. 50:2580, 1971.
299. Standiford, H. D., de Maine, J. B., and Kirby, W. M. M.: Antibiotic synergism of enterococci. Arch. Intern. Med. 126:255, 1970.
300. Moellering, R. C., Jr., Wennersten, C., and Weinberg, A. N.: Synergy of penicillin and gentamicin against enterococci. J. Infect. Dis. 124 (Suppl.):207, 1971.
301. Carey, R. A., Brause, B. D., and Roberts, R. B.: Antimicrobial therapy of vitamin B_6-dependent streptococcal endocarditis. Arch. Intern. Med. 87:150, 1977.
302. Thornsberry, C., Baker, C. N., and Facklain, R. R.: Antibiotic susceptibility of Streptococcus bovis and other group D causing endocarditis. Antimicrob. Agents Chemother. 5:228, 1974.
303. Weinstein, L., Lerner, P. I., and Chew, W. H.: Clinical and bacteriologic studies of the effect of massive doses of penicillin G on infections caused by gram-negative bacilli. N. Engl. J. Med. 271:525, 1964.
304. Smith, H., Lerner, P. I., and Weinstein, L.: Neurotoxicity and "massive" intravenous therapy with penicillin. Arch. Intern. Med. 120:47, 1967.
305. Watanakunakorn, C., and Baird, I. M.: Prognostic factors in Staphylococcus aureus endocarditis and results of therapy with penicillin and gentamicin. Am. J. Med. Sci. 273:133, 1977.
306. Abrams, B., Sklaver, A., Hoffman, T., and Greenman, R.: Single or combination therapy of staphylococcal endocarditis in intravenous drug abusers. Ann. Intern. Med. 90:789, 1979.
307. Gopal, V., Bisno, A. L., and Silverblatt, F. J.: Failure of vancomycin treatment in Staphylococcus aureus endocarditis. J.A.M.A. 236:1604, 1976.
308. Menda, K. B., and Gorbach, S. L.: Favorable experience with bacterial endocarditis in heroin addicts. Ann. Intern. Med. 78:25, 1973.
309. Mayrer, A. R., Brown, A., Weintraub, R. A., Ragni, M., and Postic, B.: Successful medical therapy for endocarditis due to Candida parapsilosis. Chest 73:546, 1978.
310. Kay, J. H., Bernstein, S., Feinstein, D., and Biddle, M.: Surgical cure of Candida albicans endocarditis with open heart surgery. N. Engl. J. Med. 264:907, 1961.
311. Kay, J. H., Bernstein, S., Tsuji, H. K., Redington, J. V., Milgram, M., and Brem, T.: Surgical treatment of Candida endocarditis. J.A.M.A. 203:621, 1968.
312. Arbulu, A., Thomas, N. W., and Wilson, R. F.: Valvulectomy without prosthetic replacement. A life-saving operation for tricuspid Pseudomonas endocarditis. J. Thorac. Cardiovasc. Surg. 64:103, 1972.
313. Bindschadler, D. D., and Bennett, J. E.: A pharmacologic guide to the clinical use of amphotericin B. J. Inf. Dis. 120:427, 1969.
314. Drutz, D. J., Spickard, A., Rogers, D. E., and Koenig, M. G.: Treatment of disseminated mycotic infections: A new approach to amphotericin B therapy. Am. J. Med. 45:405, 1968.
315. Fass, R. J., and Perkins, R. L.: 5-Fluorocytosine in the treatment of cryptococcal and Candida mycoses. Ann. Intern. Med. 74:535, 1971.
316. Vandevelde, A. G., Mauceri, A. A., and Johnson, J. E., III: 5-Fluorocytosine in the treatment of mycotic infections. Ann. Intern. Med. 77:43, 1972.
317. Record, C. O., Skinner, J. M., Sleight, P., and Speller, D. C. E.: Candida endocarditis treated with 5-fluorocytosine. Br. Med. J. 1:262, 1971.
318. Galgiani, J. N., and Stevens, D. A.: Fungal endocarditis: Need for guidelines in evaluating therapy. J. Thorac. Cardiovasc. Surg. 73:293, 1977.
319. Touroff, A. S. W., and Vessell, H.: Subacute Streptococcus viridans endarteritis complicating patent ductus arteriosus. J.A.M.A. 115:1270, 1940.
319a. Croft, C.H., Woodward, W., Elliott, A., Commerford, P. J., Barnard, C. N., and Beck, W.: Analysis of surgical versus medical therapy in active complicated native valve infective endocarditis Am. J. Cardiol. 51:1650, 1983.

320. Hancock, E. W., Shumway, N. E., and Remington, J. S.: Valve replacement in active bacterial endocarditis. J. Infect. Dis. 123:106, 1971.
321. Kaiser, G. C., Williams, V. L., Thurmann, M., and Hanlon, C. R.: Valve replacement in cases of aortic insufficiency due to active endocarditis. J. Thorac. Cardiovasc. Surg. 54:491, 1967.
322. Wise, J. R., Jr., Cleland, W. P., Halldie-Smith, K. A., Bentall, H. H., Goodwin, J. F., and Oakley, C. M.: Urgent aortic-valve replacement for acute aortic regurgitation due to infective endocarditis. Lancet 2:115, 1971.
323. Robicsek, F., Payne, R. B., Daugherty, H. K., and Sanger, P. W.: Bacterial endocarditis of the mitral valve treated by excision and replacement. Ann. Surg. 166:854, 1967.
324. Khonsari, S., Bahabozurgui, S., Cook, W. A., and Frater, R. W. M.: Urgent open-heart surgery for endocarditis of mitral valve. N.Y. State J. Med. 71:2650, 1971.
325. Jung, J. Y., Saab, S. B., and Almond, C. H.: The case for early surgical treatment of left-sided primary infective endocarditis. A collective review. J. Thorac. Cardiovasc. Surg. 70:509, 1975.
326. Stinson, E. B., Griepp, R. B., Vosti, K., Copeland, J. G., and Shumway, N. E.: Operation treatment of active endocarditis. J. Thorac. Cardiovasc. Surg. 71:659, 1976.
327. Wise, J. R., Jr., Cleland, W. P., Haldie-Smith, K. A., et al.: Urgent aortic-valve replacement for acute regurgitation due to infective endocarditis. Lancet 2:115, 1971.
328. Fowler, N. O., Hamgurger, M. H., and Bove, K. E.: Aortic valve perforation. Am. J. Med. 42:539, 1967.
329. Griffin, F. M., Jr., Jones, G., and Cobbs, C. G.: Aortic insufficiency in bacterial endocarditis. Ann. Intern. Med. 76:23, 1972.
330. Robinson, M. J., Greenberg, J. J., Korn, M., and Rywlin, A. M.: Infective endocarditis at autopsy: 1965–1969. Am. J. Med. 52:492, 1972.
331. Walker, S. R., Shumway, N. E., and Merigan, T. C.: Man agement of infected cardiac valve prostheses. J.A.M.A. 208:531, 1969.
332. Watanakunakorn, C., and Hamburger, M.: Staphylococcus epidermidis endocarditis complicating a Starr-Edwards prosthesis: A therapeutic dilemma. Arch. Intern. Med. 126:1014, 1970.
333. Okies, J. E., Viroslav, J., and Williams, T. W., Jr.: Endocarditis after cardiac valve replacement. Chest 59:198, 1971.
334. Block, P. C., DeSanctis, R. W., Weinberg, A. N., and Austen, W. G.: Prosthetic valve endocarditis. J. Thorac. Cardiovasc. Surg. 60:540, 1970.
335. Dorney, E. R., and King, S. R.: Bacterial endocarditis following prosthetic valve surgery: Early and late occurrence. Circulation 41 (Suppl. 3):150, 1970.
336. Wilson, W. R., Danielson, G. K., Givliani, E. R., Washington, J. A., III, Jaumin, P. M., and Geraci, J. E.: Valve replacement in patients with active infective endocarditis. Circulation 58:585, 1978.
337. Richardson, J. V., Karp, R. B., Kirklin, J. W., and Dismukes, W. E.: Treatment of infective endocarditis: A 10-year comparative analysis. Circulation 58:589, 1978.
338. Rapaport, E.: Editorial. The changing role of surgery in the management of infective endocarditis. Circulation 58:598, 1978.
339. Simberkoff, M. S., Isom, W., Smithivast, T., Noriega, E. R., and Rahal, J. J., Jr.: Two-stage tricuspid valve replacement for mixed bacterial endocarditis. Arch. Intern. Med. 133:212, 1974.
340. Robin, E., Thoms, N. W., Arbulu, A., Ganguly, S. N., and Magnisalis, K.: Hemodynamic consequences of total removal of the tricuspid valve without prosthetic replacement. Am. J. Cardiol. 35:481, 1975.
341. Sethia, B., and Williams, B. T.: Tricuspid valve excision without replacement in a case of endocarditis secondary to drug abuse. Br. Heart J. 40:579, 1978.
342. Arbulu, A., and Asfaw, I.: Tricuspid valvulectomy with prosthetic replacement. J. Thorac. Cardiovasc. Surg. 82:684, 1981.
343. Bogart, D. B., Hodges, G. R., Lewis, H. D., Jr., and Fixley, M. S.: Prosthetic valve endocarditis: Reviewing the problem. Postgrad. Med. 62:119, 1977.

PROGNOSIS

344. Wallach, J. B., Glass, M., Lakash, L., and Angrist, A. A.: Bacterial endocarditis in aged. Ann. Intern. Med. 42:1206, 1955.
345. Bunn, P., and Lunn, J.: Late follow up of 64 patients with subacute bacterial endocarditis treated with penicillin. Am. J. Med. Sci. 243:549, 1962.
346. Pearce, M. L., and Guze, L. B.: Some factors affecting prognosis in bacterial endocarditis, Ann. Intern. Med. 55:270, 1961.
347. Cummings, V., Furman, S., Dunset, M., and Rubin, I. L.: Subacute bacterial endocarditis in older age group. J.A.M.A. 172:137, 1960.
348. McNeill, K. M., Strong, J. E., Jr., and Lockwood, W. R.: Bacterial endocarditis: An analysis of factors affecting long-term survival. Am. Heart J. 95:448, 1978.
349. Wedgwood, J.: Prognosis in subacute bacterial endocarditis. Lancet 2:922, 1957.
350. Robinson, M. J., and Ruedy, J.: Sequelae of bacterial endocarditis. Am. J. Med. 32:922, 1962.
351. Guze, L. B., and Pearce, M. L.: Hospital-acquired bacterial endocarditis. Arch. Intern. Med. 112:56, 1963.
352. Zeman, F. D.: Subacute bacterial endocarditis in aged. Am. Heart J. 29:661, 1945.
353. Menzies, C. J.: Coronary embolism with infarction in bacterial endocarditis. Br. Heart J. 23:464, 1961.

354. Marietta, J. S.: Acute bacterial endocarditis and coronary embolism. Texas State J. Med. 56:426, 1960.
355. Brunson, J. G.: Coronary embolism in bacterial endocarditis. Am. J. Pathol. 29:689, 1953.
356. Jackson, J. F., and Allison, F., Jr.: Bacterial endocarditis. South. Med. J. 54:1331, 1961.
357. Priest, W. S., and Smith, J. M.: Effect of healed subacute bacterial endocarditis on cardiac dynamics. Arch. Intern. Med. 95:646, 1955.
358. Mendelson, C. E., Cahue, A., Katz, L. N., and Brams, W. A.: Long-term outlook for healed subacute bacterial endocarditis. J.A.M.A. 160:437, 1956.
359. Hoffman, F. G., and Robinson, J. J.: Aneurysm of mitral valve associated with bacterial endocarditis. Am. Heart J. 63:826, 1962.
360. Blum, L.: Development of current concept of mycotic aneurysm. N.Y. State J. Med. 64:1317, 1964.
361. Poblacion, D., McKenty, J., and Campbell, M.: Mycotic aneurysm of the superior mesenteric artery complicating subacute bacterial endocarditis: Successful resection. Canad. Med. Assoc. J. 90:744, 1964.
362. Case Records of the Massachusetts General Hospital (Case 43371). N. Engl. J. Med. 257:515, 1957.
363. Karchmer, A. W.: Active infective endocarditis: When to operate. J. Cardiovasc. Med. 6:1015, 1981.
364. Boyd, A. A., Spencer, F. C., Isom, O. W., Cunningham, J. N., Reed, G. E., Acinapura, A. J., and Tice, D. A.: Infective endocarditis: An analysis of 54 surgically treated patients. J. Thorac. Cardiovasc. Surg. 73:23, 1977.
365. Sandza, J. G., Clark, R. E., Ferguson, T. B., Connors, J. P., and Weldon, C. S.: Replacement of prosthetic heart valves. J. Thorac. Cardiovasc. Surg. 74:864, 1977.
366. Utley, J. R., Mills, J., and Roe, B. B.: The role of valve replacement in the treatment of fungal endocarditis. J. Thorac. Surg. 69:255, 1975.
367. Young, J. B., Welton, D. E., Raizner, A. E., et al.: Surgery in infective endocarditis. Circulation 60 (Suppl. I):177, 1979.
368. Kaplan, E. L., Rich, H., Gersony, W., and Manning, J.: A collaborative study of infective endocarditis in the 1970's. Emphasis on infections in patients who have undergone cardiovascular surgery. Circulation 59:327, 1979.
369. Scalia, D., Bortolotti, U., Milano, A., Stritoni, P., Panizzon, G., Valfre, C., Mazzucco, A., and Gallucci, V.: Surgical treatment of infectious endocarditis in the active phase. Experience in 40 cases. G. Ital. Cardiol. 11:643, 1981.
370. Masur, H., and Johnson, W. D., Jr.: Prosthetic valve endocarditis. J. Thorac. Cardiovasc. Surg. 80:31, 1980.
371. Cohn, L. H., Mudge, G. H., Pratter, F., and Collins, J. J., Jr.: Five to eight-year follow-up of patients undergoing porcine heart-valve replacement. N. Engl. J. Med. 304:258, 1981.
372. Kaye, D. (ed.): Prophylaxis of Endocarditis. Baltimore, University Park Press, 1976, p. 245.
373. Kaplan, E. L., Anthony, B. F., Bisno, A., Durack, D., Houser, H., Millard, H. D., Sanford, J., Shulman, S. T., Stillerman, M., Taranta, A., and Wenger, N.: Prevention of bacterial endocarditis. Circulation 56:139A, 1977.
374. Dismukes, W. E.: Who needs endocarditis prophylaxis? J. Cardiovasc Med. 6: 347, 1981.
375. Keys, T. F.: Antimicrobial prophylaxis for patients with congenital or valvular heart disease. Mayo Clin. Proc., 57:171, 1982.
376. Oakley, C., and Somerville, W.: Prevention of infective endocarditis. Br. Heart J. 45:233, 1981.
377. Schadelin, J.: Praktische probleme der endokarditis prophylaxe. Schweiz. Med. Wochenschr. 111:646, 1981.
378. Fekety, F. R., Cluff, L. E., Sabiston, D. C., Seidl, L. F., Smith, J. W., and Thoburn, R.: A study of antibiotic prophylaxis in cardiac surgery, J. Thorac. Cardiovasc. Surg. 57:757, 1969.
379. Goodman, J. S., Schaffner, W., Collins, H. A., Battersky, E. J., and Koenig, M. G.: Infection after cardiovascular surgery. Clinical study including examination of antimicrobial prophylaxis. N. Engl. J. Med. 278:117, 1968.
380. Myerowitz, P. D., Caswell, K., Lindsay, W. G., and Demetre, M. N.: Antibiotic prophylaxis for open heart surgery. J. Thorac. Cardiovasc. Surg. 73:625, 1977.
381. Hill, D. G., and Yates, A. K.: Prophylactic antibiotics in open heart surgery, N.Z. Med. J. 81:414, 1975.
382. Goldman, D. A., Hopkins, C. C., Karchmer, A. W., Abel, R. M., McEnany, M. T., Akins, C., Buckley, M. J., and Moellering, R. C., Jr.: Cephalothin prophylaxis in cardiac valve surgery. J. Thorac. Cardiovasc. Surg. 73:470, 1977.

34

PRINCIPLES OF THE PATHOGENESIS OF ATHEROSCLEROSIS

by Robert W. Wissler, Ph.D., M.D.

The purpose of this chapter is to provide an understanding of the pathological processes that lead to progressive atherosclerotic plaques in the coronary arteries. In addition, it is hoped that it will furnish information of value in the clinician's attempts to prevent the development of clinically important plaques, retard their progression, and perhaps make possible their regression. It also presents some of the increasing evidence indicating that plaque formation is not only a largely preventable pathological process but also a substantially reversible one. The process has been found to be multifaceted in its origins as well as in its anatomical, biochemical, and pathophysiological manifestations.[1,2] An attempt will also be made to elucidate the relationship between coronary atherosclerotic plaques and the development of ischemic heart disease, including classic acute myocardial infarction, sudden death (usually as a result of acute-onset ventricular fibrillation), and chronic angina pectoris.

Atherosclerosis is a special type of thickening and hardening of the medium-sized and large arteries that accounts for a large proportion of heart attacks and cases of ischemic heart disease.[3] It also accounts for many strokes (those due to cerebral ischemia and infarction), numerous instances of peripheral vascular disease, and most aneurysms of the lower abdominal aorta, which can rupture and cause sudden fatal hemorrhage.

A geographically unevenly distributed pathological condition, atherosclerosis manifests itself as a progressive process, resulting in clinical disease in groups making up only about one-fourth of the world's total population. It is largely limited to the more industrialized countries, especially in the temperate zones of North America, Europe, and the Soviet Union. It is rare to find a high rate of heart attacks due to atherosclerosis in Asia (including China, Japan, India, and most of Southeast Asia), much of the Near East, Africa, or South and Central America. Many epidemiological and geographical pathological studies spanning the last half century have linked the remarkable contrast in clinical heart attack rate and mortality to the level of serum cholesterol in these populations and, in turn, to life styles, in particular, dietary habits.[4-6] Additional risk factors considered in these and many other studies include the incidence of hypertension, cigarette smoking, and diabetes as well as the effects of factors generally beyond control, such as sex, age, hemodynamic forces, and genetic mechanisms. Hardness of water consumed, a sedentary life style, and emotional stress have also been surveyed repeatedly and offer interesting correlations which may help us understand the factors influencing the response of the arterial wall to injury.[7] In Chapter 35 the environmental "risk factors" for the development of atherosclerosis are considered in detail, and in Chapter 47 the genetic aspects of lipoprotein metabolism as they pertain to atherosclerosis are explained.

In this chapter, the major emphasis is on the arterial wall. Its pathophysiological response to the many alterations in constituents, both cellular and fluid, will be considered. Salient aspects of the dynamics of blood flow which appear to be important in the initiation, progression, and regression of the advanced atherosclerotic plaque, particularly in coronary arteries, will be presented.

In arteries of all sizes, the transected wall shows three major microscopic layers: the intima, the media, and the adventitia.[8]

INTIMA. The major constituents of the normally thin intima are endothelium, basement membrane, an occasional smooth muscle myointimal cell, a few collagen and/or elastic fibers, and an infrequent blood-derived mononuclear cell.[9] In arteries where it is prominent, the intimal elastic membrane or lamina (IEM or IEL) defines the limit of the intima. The multilayered cushion of myointimal cells formed in arteries at all ages in many species, including human, may be a pathological finding.[10] It is not clear whether these cushions predispose toward or protect against atherosclerosis.[11] It is likely that hemodynamic stimulation can lead to fibrous lesions (diffuse intimal thickening) and hence to atheromatous lesions when the blood lipids are elevated.[12]

The arterial endothelium probably both admits and discharges macromolecules of the size of low-density lipoproteins (LDL) (p. 1211).[13] Their concentration in the lymph from the arterial wall has been found to be about one-tenth that in the bloodstream.[14,15] Although most plasma proteins can enter the artery in this concentration,[16] lipoproteins and fibrinogen are particularly likely to accumulate in the intima.[17]

"Large pore" transendothelial vesicle chains allow entrance into the arterial wall.[13,18] Additional quantitative study is needed to determine the effect on this transverse channel of dilatation of arteries or increased tension on arterial wall.[19] Other risk factors may also be important in altering endothelial permeability.[1,20]

Another factor suspected of being involved in controlling endothelial permeability is the glycocalyx—the thin, fuzzy layer of complex carbohydrate on the luminal side of the endothelial cell that localizes ruthenium red dye or lectins, such as concanavalin-A. This layer is remarkably thin in those areas of the artery prone to the development of atherosclerotic plaques and at sites where plaques develop in some experimental animals.[21,22]

MEDIA.   The media of the mammalian artery—both the large elastic artery, such as the aorta, or the medium-sized muscular artery, such as the coronary artery—is formed by multiple layers of smooth muscle cells (SMC), usually two cells wide, separated by a prominent elastic membrane.[9] Each of these recurring structures, which contain an elastic membrane in the center and a SMC on each side, is called a "lamellar unit." In a given species, the number of these units in each artery appears to be highly predictable relative to the size of the animal and many other factors.[1,23,24] The apparent interstitial "space" between the cells and the regularly recurring elastic membranes contain variable quantities of collagen, elastin, and glycosaminoglycans.

At present, both circumstantial evidence and careful in

vitro studies of the arterial SMC indicate that it can synthesize collagen, elastin, and glycosaminoglycans.[25–29] These multiple cell products, which appear prominent when the SMC reacts to certain pathological stimuli, led us a number of years ago to dub it the "malfunctional medial mesenchymal cell." At that time we suggested that it should be considered the most prominent and important cell in the process of atherogenesis (Fig. 34–1).[25] No new evidence has come to light to revise this assumption, but it must be borne in mind that the blood-derived monocyte (or macrophage) is probably present, at least in small numbers, in most atheromatous lesions. These cells, as well as platelets, can exert a strong influence on the atherosclerotic process during various stages of development and regression of the plaque.[2,30–32]

Significant new observations about the functional anatomy of the artery are being reported with increasing frequency.[33] It now appears likely that relationships between cells, collagen, and elastin in the media are orderly and beautifully designed, permitting the strength and relative inflexibility of collagen to interact in the best possible way with elastin.[34] This yields a highly functional vessel that can adapt to varying demands and pathophysiological conditions.[24,33] The SMC probably acts as the major monitor of this adaptability, since it can vary its synthesis of the various fiber proteins and matrix carbohydrates in response to different physical and chemical stimuli.

ADVENTITIA.   The adventitia of the artery is important to arterial function. Its mainly collagenous structure provides the major mechanical support when the media is badly weakened owing to advanced atherosclerosis. It is also important because it provides the media of larger arteries with much of its nutrition by means of the vasa vasorum, as well as with lymphatic drainage and innervation of the arteries. The predominant cell of the adventitia is the fibroblast.

Penetrating branches of the vasa vasorum, terminating at about the twenty-ninth lamellar unit of the media, are consistently found in large arteries of large mammals and humans.[23,24] This finding may help to explain the more severe atherosclerosis usually observed in the abdominal aor-

THE SMOOTH MUSCLE CELL FROM THE ARTERIAL MEDIA IS
STIMULATED BY LDL OR VLDL TO TAKE UP LIPID, PROLIFERATE, MIGRATE
AND ("TRANSFORM" ?)

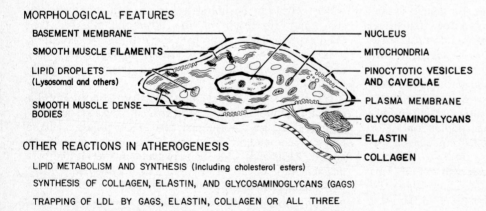

MORPHOLOGICAL FEATURES

BASEMENT MEMBRANE

SMOOTH MUSCLE FILAMENTS

LIPID DROPLETS
(Lysosomal and others)

SMOOTH MUSCLE DENSE
BODIES

NUCLEUS

MITOCHONDRIA

PINOCYTOTIC VESICLES
AND CAVEOLAE

PLASMA MEMBRANE

GLYCOSAMINOGLYCANS

ELASTIN

COLLAGEN

OTHER REACTIONS IN ATHEROGENESIS

LIPID METABOLISM AND SYNTHESIS (Including cholesterol esters)

SYNTHESIS OF COLLAGEN, ELASTIN, AND GLYCOSAMINOGLYCANS (GAGS)

TRAPPING OF LDL BY GAGS, ELASTIN, COLLAGEN OR ALL THREE

INJURY OR NECROSIS OF THESE CELLS AS THE PLAQUE PROGRESSES

DECREASED SMOOTH MUSCLE MYOSIN SYNTHESIS, ESPECIALLY AS
THE CELLS ACCUMULATE MORE LIPID DROPLETS (?)

FIGURE 34–1 The major morphological features of the "multifunctional medial mesenchymal cell," the principal cell type involved in atherogenesis, along with a listing of some of its functions that are particularly important in atherosclerosis. (Modified from Wissler, R. W., et al.: Abnormalities of the arterial wall and its metabolism in atherogenesis. Prog. Cardiovasc. Dis. *18*:5, 1976, by permission of Grune and Stratton.)

ta of *Homo sapiens*. Wolinsky and Glagov have suggested that the absence of penetrating vasa vasorum in the human abdominal aorta and the unusual physical stresses to which this part of the artery is exposed may make it particularly vulnerable to atherogenesis.

MAJOR FEATURES OF ATHEROSCLEROTIC LESIONS

Human atherosclerosis produces its effects largely in the medium-sized muscular arteries (such as the coronary, carotid, basilar, and vertebral). It also affects arteries supplying the lower extremities and the larger arteries (such as the aorta and iliac). It should not be confused with many of the minor intimal and medial forms of *arterio*sclerosis, which rarely produce clinical effects, or with the clinically important forms of sclerosis of small arteries (arteriolosclerosis) that often appear in hypertension and diabetes (Fig. 34–2).

The feature that sets *athero*sclerosis apart from other forms of arteriosclerosis is the lipid, which in the advanced plaque is often represented by a central necrotic core that is rich in cholesterol esters and is often accompanied by visible cholesterol crystals. This part of the lesion, which on gross examination is usually soft and grumous, is responsible for the name of the disease process, derived from the Greek stem "athera," meaning gruel or porridge.

LOCALIZATION. The distribution of atherosclerotic plaques in the arterial tree of human subjects follows certain patterns (Fig. 34–3). In general, the abdominal aorta, for reasons just discussed, is much more extensively involved than is the thoracic aorta, and aortic lesions tend to be much more prominent near ostia of major branches.[24] Renal arteries are usually spared from stenosing plaques, except at their ostia;[35] coronary arteries show the most intense atherosclerotic involvement within the first 6 cm.[36] The severity of involvement of the coronary artery is, on the average, less than that of the abdominal aorta in most age groups and is somewhat more severe and extensive than that of the adjacent thoracic aorta, from which these arteries are derived—a phenomenon that may be related to the peculiarities of blood flow in the coronary artery.[37] Other interesting aspects of plaque distribution are beyond

I. **Large artery or medium artery.**

  A. **Primarily Intimal**

    1. **Atherosclerosis**

    2. **Fibrosclerosis**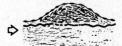

    3. **Myxofibrosclerosis**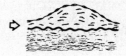

  B. **Medial**

    1. **Mönckeberg's sclerosis**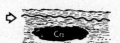

II. **Small artery or arteriole.**

  A. **Hyaline (intimal)**

  B. **Proliferative (intimal)**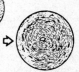

  C. **Hyperplastic (proliferative) medial**

FIGURE 34–2 A classification of arteriosclerosis represented diagrammatically to contrast the features of atherosclerosis with other commonly observed forms of arteriosclerosis. *Fibrosclerosis* is used to describe the commonly observed benign collagen-rich intimal thickenings that show little or no lipid or necrosis. *Myxofibrosclerosis* is a term we have used to describe lipid-poor lesions that are rich in glycosaminoglycans. They are frequently observed in large arteries of patients with diabetes and in arteries distal to a point of severe stenosis or mechanical occlusion.

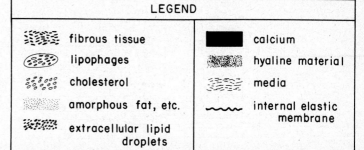

LEGEND			
fibrous tissue		calcium	
lipophages		hyaline material	
cholesterol		media	
amorphous fat, etc.		internal elastic membrane	
extracellular lipid droplets			

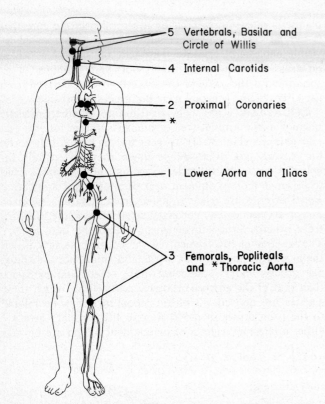

5   Vertebrals, Basilar and Circle of Willis

4   Internal Carotids

2   Proximal Coronaries

*

1   Lower Aorta and Iliacs

3   Femorals, Popliteals and *Thoracic Aorta

FIGURE 34–3   Sites of predilection for clinically significant atherosclerosis, in usual rank order. Substantial exceptions can occur, often without an obvious reason.

the scope of this discussion; most can be explained by variations due to hemodynamic forces or by localized conditions of the architecture of the arterial wall.[24]

COMPONENTS.   As has already been suggested, the major components of the atherosclerotic plaque are its cells, mostly arterial SMC, and its lipid, much of which is

extracellular (Fig. 34–4A). The relative proportions of these two major components, along with the fibrous proteins and complex carbohydrate products of the SMC, vary greatly from plaque to plaque. These proportions also vary during the sequence of development or regression of a given plaque. Unfortunately, however, at our present stage of technology, it is virtually impossible to quantitate these major components in the human plaque at any specific time, short of surgical removal or examination at autopsy.

CLINICAL EFFECTS.   The clinical effects of advanced plaques of most medium-sized arteries, which include the main coronary vessels, are due to either their space-occupying characteristics, which lead to stenosis, or their thrombogenic qualities, which often appear related to fracture or rupture of the fibrous cap and the resulting ulceration of the plaque surface (Fig. 34–4B). This frequently results in an obstructing thrombus, which in a major coronary artery can—and often does—form over a well-developed atheromatous plaque and lead to acute sudden coronary occlusion and myocardial infarction.

It has recently been proposed that the eccentric, largely intimal, advanced atheromatous plaque found in most muscular arteries may have quite different functional effects relative to stenosis, thrombosis, spasm, and susceptibility to regression than do the rather rare concentric, transmural plaques which are sometimes observed.[38,39]

The major clinical effects of plaques in the aorta (and sometimes in the iliac arteries) are usually not the result of their space-occupying features. They are much more likely to be caused by thinning of the media beneath the plaques, weakening of the wall, aneurysm formation and rupture, or formation of a mural thrombus over ulcerated areas, with embolization to more distal radicles of the arterial system.

The composition and clinical consequences of the plaque are not necessarily functions of how long it has been in the

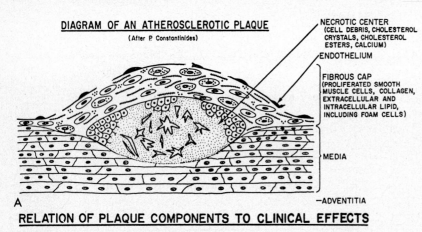

DIAGRAM OF AN ATHEROSCLEROTIC PLAQUE
(After P Constantinides)

NECROTIC CENTER (CELL DEBRIS, CHOLESTEROL CRYSTALS, CHOLESTEROL ESTERS, CALCIUM)

ENDOTHELIUM

FIBROUS CAP (PROLIFERATED SMOOTH MUSCLE CELLS, COLLAGEN, EXTRACELLULAR AND INTRACELLULAR LIPID, INCLUDING FOAM CELLS)

MEDIA

A   —ADVENTITIA

FIGURE 34–4   *A*, Major components of the advanced (clinically important) atherosclerotic plaque. *B*, Characteristics of the advanced plaque that account for its clinical effects in medium-sized (muscular) arteries. (Modified from Wissler, R. W., and Vesselinovitch, D.: Animal models of regression. *In* Schettler, G., et al. (eds.): Atherosclerosis IV. Berlin, Springer-Verlag, 1977, p. 377.)

RELATION OF PLAQUE COMPONENTS TO CLINICAL EFFECTS

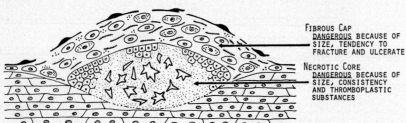

FIBROUS CAP
DANGEROUS BECAUSE OF SIZE, TENDENCY TO FRACTURE AND ULCERATE

NECROTIC CORE
DANGEROUS BECAUSE OF SIZE, CONSISTENCY AND THROMBOPLASTIC SUBSTANCES

B

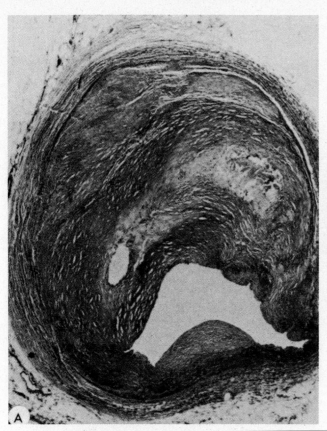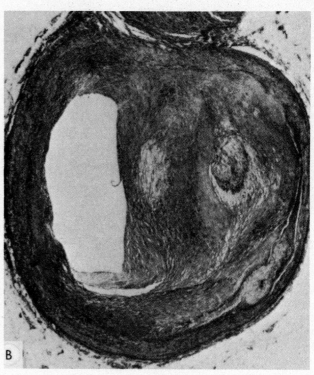

FIGURE 34–5 *A,* An advanced plaque in the coronary artery of a 29-year-old woman with heterozygous familial hypercholesterolemia (Type II disease) who died with ischemic heart disease. *B,* Plaque in severe coronary artery atherosclerosis in 71-year-old man who died suddenly of left ventricular free-wall rupture. Note the resemblance in principal components (necrotic core and fibrous cap) to the severe atherosclerosis in *A.* (From Roberts, W. C.: The coronary arteries in coronary heart disease: Morphologic observations. Pathobiol. Annu. *5:*249, 1975.)

process of formation. In fact, the few well-illustrated reports of plaques in relatively young individuals who are victims of fatal heart attacks and who have displayed severe, genetically controlled elevations in LDL levels show the same lesion components in about the same proportions as those plaques which usually occur in older individuals (Fig. 34–5).[40,41]

THEORIES OF PATHOGENESIS

Historically, pathologists who have studied the mechanisms by which the atherosclerotic plaque develops have approached the problem from two points of view. One of these, often believed to have been proposed by Virchow, holds that a principal factor in the progression of the plaque is the increased passage and accumulation of plasma constituents from the arterial lumen into the arterial intima, i.e., a type of low-grade inflammatory edema (insudation). The second, often associated with Rokitansky, specifies that small mural thrombi on areas of arterial intimal injury (hemodynamic and otherwise) occur early in atherogenesis (encrustation) and that the organization of these thrombi by SMC as well as their gradual growth plays a definitive role in the progression of the plaque.

The two concepts described differ principally in that the latter, the encrustation formulation, attributes much more weight to the environmental factors which cause arterial endothelial injury and trigger thrombus formation of the

type frequently seen in arteries, i.e., thrombi of the "white" (platelet, fibrin, and leukocyte) variety. These encrusted white thrombi are thought by some to form much of the space-occupying substance of the developing plaque. According to this hypothesis, the lipid in the plaque is a more or less passive and secondary product of the spongelike action of the thrombus and the breakdown of platelets and leukocytes.

The insudation theory, on the other hand, more easily accommodates the role of elevated levels of serum lipoproteins in carrying cholesterol into the artery wall. It has gradually become the predominant theory within the scientific community, especially in the United States.

In general, all theories of pathogenesis of atherosclerosis support the notion that plaque development begins rather early in life, with the process then continuing over a period of many years (Fig. 34–6).[42] There are indications of periods of quiescence and even regression interspersed with periods of progression, until the disease reaches a point at which it becomes clinically important.[43]

Insudation and Encrustation

ROLE OF SERUM CHOLESTEROL. The emergence of the insudation theory is the result of two major developments: one positive and one negative. The positive one is the accumulation of consistent evidence indicating that a sustained elevation in the level of serum cholesterol

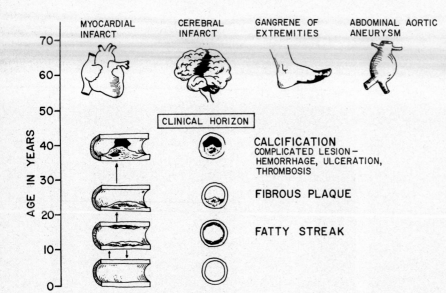

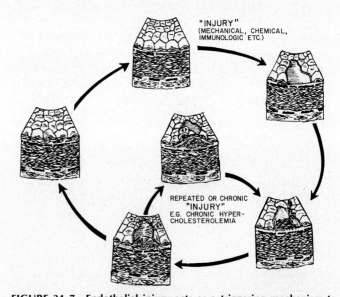

FIGURE 34–6 The natural history of atherosclerosis. Plaques usually develop slowly and insidiously over many years, and they generally progress from a fatty streak to a fibrous plaque and then to a complicated plaque that is likely to lead to clinical effects. Not shown is the concept that this pathological process can probably be accelerated by arterial endothelial injury. In addition, the degree of elevation of either blood pressure or levels of serum cholesterol may help to determine the severity of endothelial injury. (Modified from McGill, H. C., Jr., et al.: Natural history of human atherosclerotic lesions. *In* Sandler, M., and Bourne, G. H. (eds.): Atherosclerosis and Its Origin. New York, Academic Press, 1963, p. 42.)

leads to classic progressive atherosclerotic lesions. This elevation may be endogenously induced as a result of genetic factors or of metabolic disease such as "lipoid" nephrosis and hypothyroidism, or it may be exogenously produced by the long-term effects of a high-fat, high-cholesterol diet. However, the inverse of this relationship appears to be equally true, i.e., if the serum cholesterol is maintained at a low level in human subjects and in most species of mammals, then atherosclerosis is a rare development. The evidence supporting these relationships comes from many types of studies: epidemiological, geographical, and pathological (autopsy) studies of the natural history of the plaque. In fact, no population has been identified in which progressive atherosclerosis develops if the serum cholesterol level is low. These relationships are also supported by clinicopathological studies, experimental animal studies and, more recently, investigations in cell biology and molecular pathology.[1,2,44] These results, in general, reinforce each other and provide strong evidence that the significant class of substances accumulating in the arterial intima in excessive amounts during insudation comprises cholesterol-rich lipoproteins. If these macromolecules are derived from serum having an elevated cholesterol content, the influx tends to support the eventual development of a progressive, and ultimately an advanced, atherosclerotic plaque of the type that leads to clinical manifestations, including ischemic heart disease.[1]

ENDOTHELIAL DAMAGE AND PLATELET ADHESION. Pathologists who have studied the natural history of human atherosclerosis generally support the concept of organization of thrombi over advanced plaques as a mechanism of plaque growth. On the other hand, they have failed to find evidence of sufficient encrustation to support organization of arterial mural thrombi as a major pathogenetic mechanism for early atherogenesis.[36] This negative reaction to the classic encrustation theory is supported by the recent experimental evidence that clearly shows that even extensive endothelial damage to normal arteries following balloon catheterization or other intima-destroying experimental manipulations does not support the development of a progressive mural thrombus and does not lead to a typical atheromatous plaque.[45,46] As will be considered later, platelets do accumulate along with some fibrin and leukocytes, and some SMC proliferation does occur under these conditions. However, unless sustained hypercholesterolemia is present, these proliferative lesions tend to regress and heal, and the arterial intima is restored nearly to normal (Fig. 34–7).[2,47]

Much more work needs to be done, but in general it now appears likely that these two previously divergent theories are in the process of combining into a unified concept for the pathogenesis of atherosclerosis, which proposes that the insudation of hyperlipidemic serum, with its cholesterol-rich low-density lipoprotein fractions, is an

FIGURE 34–7 Endothelial injury acts as a triggering mechanism to promote the sticking and spreading of platelets. This in turn releases the "platelet factor" that stimulates migration of arterial smooth muscle cells from the arterial media and proliferation of these cells in the intima and media. The process is represented as being almost completely reversible when only one episode of endothelial damage occurs; it is progressive when repeated or continuous endothelial injury occurs, as is likely with elevation of serum low-density lipoprotein or other chronic endothelial injuries. (Slightly modified from Ross, R., and Glomset, J. A.: The pathogenesis of atherosclerosis. N. Engl. J. Med. *295*:420, 1976, reprinted by permission of the New England Journal of Medicine.)

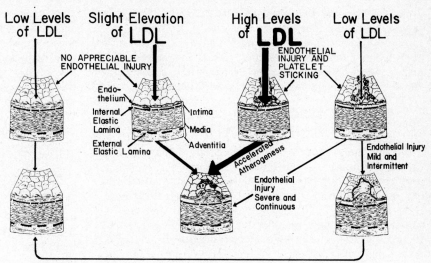

FIGURE 34–8 Several of the pathways of inter-action between elevated levels of low-density li-poprotein and arterial endothelial injury to produce a progressive atherosclerotic plaque. Although in extreme instances of continuous and severe endothelial damage, progressive plaque formation can occur even when the low-density lipoprotein levels are low (*extreme right*), this does not negate the protective effect of low lev-els of low-density lipoproteins if the endotheli-um is not being damaged severely (*extreme left*) or is damaged slightly and not very often. (Mod-ified from Ross, R., and Glomset, J. A.: The pathogenesis of atherosclerosis. N. Engl. J. Med. *295*:420, 1976, reprinted by permission of the New England Journal of Medicine.)

important element in atherogenesis and, under most condi-tions, is the *predominant* factor in determining whether or not progressive plaques develop. It also suggests that en-dothelial injury often plays a major part in accelerating atherogenesis because it results in encrustation of platelets and monocytes, which in turn expose the intimal and me-dial arterial SMC to the peptides that stimulate cell prolif-eration (liberated by these cell fragments and cells). This element of endothelial dysfunction may also help deter-mine where plaques develop most frequently and promi-nently. It helps to explain the occasional exceptional or paradoxical case in which severe, clinically important ath-erosclerotic plaques develop in young people who do not seem to have sufficiently elevated lipoproteins or other risk factors commonly recognized, such as cigarette smoking or untreated hypertension (Fig. 34–8).

Another reason for including *arterial endothelial damage and platelet sticking* in theories of atherogenesis is the in-creasing evidence that hypercholesterolemia itself leads to increased endothelial permeability and endothelial damage, thus creating a "vicious cycle" that can sustain and aug-ment endothelial injury from some other cause and lead to progressive plaque formation.[48–51] Furthermore, it now ap-pears that one mechanism by which cigarette smoking and hypertension act as risk factors at the cellular level is by means of the endothelial dysfunction they produce.[52–55]

The Initial Lesion

One of the current problems in explaining the morpho-genesis of the atherosclerotic process is the emerging doubt whether or not the classic grossly evident "fatty streak" is the precursor lesion in the histogenetic sequence of athero-sclerosis. There has long been some controversy about this slightly raised, poorly defined yellow streak in which most of the lipid can be seen on microscopic examination to be within cells of the intima and inner media. First, it is com-monly seen in infants and young children in virtually all the populations of the world, whether or not progressive atherosclerosis develops in that population. To some ex-tent, this is true in many other species of mammals also—

even though few of them are likely to develop progressive atherosclerosis unless other measures are taken. Further-more, Mitchell and Schwartz have presented evidence from autopsies indicating that the locations of aortic fatty streaks in young individuals did not coincide with those of the progressive and advanced plaques in the aortas of older persons.[56] More recently, Smith et al. and others, as a result of extensive biochemical and immunochemical studies, have also questioned the role of the fatty streak, as usually defined and described, in the process of atherogen-esis.[16,57–61]

It is evident that this problem needs further study. A preliminary study of young Americans who succumbed to sudden accidental death has recently been extended. It has been shown that "fatty streaks" include a variety of lesions that differ considerably in their staining characteristics.[62] Even though all are yellow, poorly demarcated, and only slightly raised in the formalin-fixed state, some contain most of the stainable lipid within the cytoplasm of the myointimal cells, whereas in others most of the lipid is in extracellular pools; in many, it occurs in both locations. Many reveal stainable lipid in and around the in situ medi-al cells of the inner media, and occasionally the positive staining of fat with oil red O is limited to the more or less intact internal elastic lamella. Of particular interest in this study has been the finding that most of the stainable lipid is extracellular and that few foam cells are seen in these aortic fatty streaks from accidental death victims in the 15 to 35 age group studied.[63]

More definitive postmortem studies are planned to as-certain whether any of these or other variable features of fatty streaks can be correlated with known major risk fac-tors. Assessment of risk factors can be obtained from ret-rospective investigation of the history of accidental sudden death victims in their late teens, twenties, or early thirties when much of the evidence indicates that rapid progres-sion of atherosclerosis in the human aorta is most likely to occur.

Smith and coworkers have suggested that the lesions most likely to progress are those identified as "gelatinous," owing to their appearance in unfixed specimens. They have presented evidence that these lesions are especially rich in extracellular lipid and contain relatively large amounts of LDL apoprotein B and fibrinogen and a relatively large quantity of cholesterol linoleate. This is in contrast to a high proportion of cholesterol oleate in the classic fatty streak, where the stainable lipid is mostly intracellular.[59,60]

THE EMERGING PATHOBIOLOGY OF ATHEROGENESIS

During the past 25 years, utilizing the methodology of the cellular and molecular biologist, a number of investigators have provided results that have added substantially to our understanding of atherosclerosis and its pathogenesis (Fig. 34–9).[1,2,30,64,65] The results have indicated that atherogenesis is a complex disorder which involves several cell types, especially the arterial medial smooth muscle cells, endothelial cells, and macrophages, as well as the interaction of two major processes, namely, lipid (cholesterol ester) accumulation and cell proliferation. Without both of these processes, it is clear that progressive atherosclerosis of clinical significance will not develop. Many of these seminal discoveries during this period of rapid progress have come from studies of human plaques at various stages of development through the use of transmission electron microscopy and chemical (biochemical and physicochemical) and histochemical, as well as immunohistochemical, approaches.

THE INTERACTION OF ARTERIAL CELLS AND LIPOPROTEINS

Beginning in the early 1960's, a number of ultrastructural studies revealed that the predominant cells in the hu-

man atherosclerotic plaque are modified medial SMC's, the features of which are diagrammed in Figure 34–1.[25,66–69] It was proposed that these cells accumulated as a result of migration and proliferation from the inner media. Classic fibroblasts, believed previously to be the dominant cells of the plaque, were not generally identified, although some cells of the human lesion were admittedly difficult to identify. A few had ultrastructural features associated with blood-derived leukocytes, including lymphocytes, granulocytes, and monocytes; many of the last-named were filled with lipid droplets. From the outset there was some doubt—and still is—about whether most of the lipid-filled "foam" cells, which generally make up a small proportion of the cells of the human plaque, are derived from blood monocytes or whether they are mostly modified SMC's which have lost some of their mature features as a reaction to the large quantities of lipid which they had imbibed. This important question needs further study using improved and more definitive cell markers for these types of cells.

These ultrastructural studies of the human plaque have indeed been embellished by a few immunohistochemical studies which utilized fluorescein or horseradish peroxidase–labeled antibody to smooth muscle myosin to indicate that most plaque cells resemble arterial medial SMC's immunohistochemically.[64,70,71] The Campbells from Melbourne have made very good use of both ultrastructural studies and immunohistochemistry as well as in vitro approaches to establish the concept of phenotypic modulation.[72–75] Their astute observations have helped to illuminate some of the structural and functional changes from normal medial cells displayed by plaque SMC.

The other key advance of the 1960's which has helped

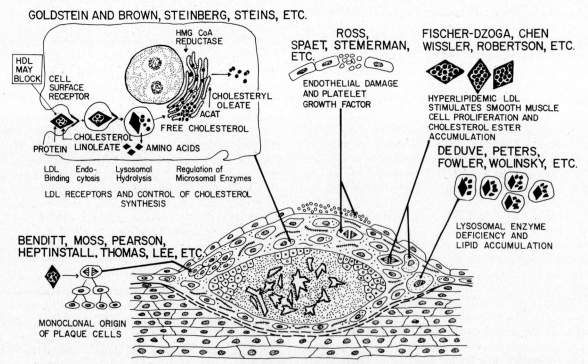

FIGURE 34–9 Some of the major recent developments in understanding a few of the cellular pathobiological reactions that appear to be important in the pathogenesis (and regression) of the atherosclerotic plaque. (Modified from Wissler, R. W.: Coronary atherosclerosis and ischemic heart disease. *In* Zülch, K. J., et al. (eds.): Brain and Heart Infarct. Berlin, Springer-Verlag, 1977, p. 206.)

TABLE 34–1 NEW RELATIONSHIPS OF LIPOPROTEIN FRACTIONS TO ATHEROGENESIS

CURRENT LIPOPROTEIN DESIGNATIONS	PREDOMINANT APO PROTEIN (S)	FUNCTIONS AND PRESUMED FUNCTIONS IN ATHEROGENESIS
Chylomicrons	Apo B 240 Apo E	May furnish cholesterol and triglycerides for atherogenesis at the arterial cell surface due to action of lipoprotein lipase (LPL) (Zilversmit) and via other remnants (Mahley, Getz)
VLDL	Apo B 335, Apo E Apo C-1 to C-III	Very little evidence of atherogenic effect except via LPL activity
Broad-beta VLDL	Apo B 240 Apo E	Highly atherogenic remnant particles derived from chylomicrons in subjects (especially dogs) fed a high-cholesterol, high-fat ration (Mahley)
H-LDL*† LDL I†	Apo B 335	Perhaps the most consistently atherogenic fraction in human species (FH) and lipogenic and mitogenic in other primates (Fless, Scanu, Fischer-Dzoga); when altered by endothelial cells or by malondialdehyde, it is avidly taken up by macrophages in vitro (Scanu, Rudel)
LDL II†		May support build up of cholesterol in arterial SMC
LDL III†	Apo B 335	Little direct evidence of atherogenicity with the exception of mitogenic effect of particle after neuraminidase treatment (Fless, Scanu, et al.)
LDL IV†		Probably identical with LPa; epidemiological evidence supports atherogenicity
HDL_C	Apo E	Probably especially important in cholesterol excretion
HDL₁	Apo A-I Apo A-II	High-affinity receptors for hepatic apo E may help in cholesterol excretion
HDL₂	Apo E Apo A-I Apo A-II Apo C	Serum level correlated with protection against atherosclerosis in numerous species, including humans Precursor to HDL₁
HDL₃	Apo A-I Apo A-II Apo C	Precursor to HDL₂, but the level is not predictive

*LDL from hyperlipidemic serum (enlarged cholesterol-rich particle).
†LDL fractions as designated by Fless and Scanu.

to foster the modern era of atherosclerosis research was the demonstration by numerous methods that most of the cholesterol and cholesterol esters in human plaques at various stages of development was probably derived from low-density lipoprotein (LDL) or very low-density lipoprotein (VLDL) that gained entrance to the intima and the inner media from the bloodstream (Fig. 34–9).[76–81] As modern work on the pathogenesis of atherosclerosis has progressed, it has become increasingly evident that in addition to LDL from hyperlipidemic serum, several other lipoprotein fractions may be important in depositing cholesterol and cholesterol esters in the artery. Those receiving most attention are listed in Table 34–1. It has now become clear that the LDL particles are not a homogeneous family and that the large, cholesterol-rich LDL from hyperlipidemic serum (H-LDL) may have a number of important features which distinguish it from LDL derived from subjects with normal basal levels of LDL.[82,83] Furthermore, recent work by Fless and Scanu using rhesus monkeys has yielded important new evidence of heterogeneity of LDL. They have utilized single-spin, gradient-density centrifugation to produce LDL I, II, III, and IV, each of which appears to have distinctive qualities.[84–86] Some of those fractions most relevant to atherogenesis will be discussed later.

As the interactions between various cells and lipoproteins are studied further, it has become evident that LDL which is altered in the test tube or by platelet[87] or endothelial cell[88] action also has distinguishing features which de-

crease its avidity for apo B receptors on the smooth muscle cells and increase its binding and internalization for macrophages.[31,89] Furthermore, as more is understood about the artery wall lipases, a new concept has been developed by Zilversmit[90] which relates VLDL and chylomicron metabolism to atherogenesis. It has also become clear from the work of Mahley and coworkers that broad β-VLDL resulting from hyperresponses to an atherogenic ration may have a definitive role in promoting progressive atherogenesis in certain species, such as the dog.[91]

All of these new discoveries and new concepts must be evaluated in relation to the established body of evidence indicating that in the human atheromatous lesion the major apoprotein of LDL (apo B) can regularly be identified by immunohistochemical means, both intracellularly and extracellularly. Furthermore, apo B appears to be the only apoprotein which increases as the plaque develops in size and severity from the early, nonelevated lesion, in which lipid stained with oil red O is barely discernible, to the most advanced lesions with large, necrotic, lipid-rich cores surrounded by "foam" cells and overlaid by a thick, fibrous cap (see Fig. 34–4A).[76–81]

ROLE OF PLATELETS AND ENDOTHELIAL DAMAGE

During the 1970's, another aspect of the pathogenesis of atherosclerosis began to receive attention. Using "balloon catheter" injury as an experimental method to produce denudation of the arterial intima and modern pathobiological methods to study cells, Ross and coworkers discovered that sticking of platelets to the damaged arterial intimal surfaces and disintegration of platelets were important contributors to the development of arterial SMC proliferation.[74-76] These studies followed the work of Mustard and coworkers, who pioneered the elucidation of the platelet-endothelial phenomena that occur on the arterial intimal surface, where atherosclerosis is likely to develop.[92] They, along with others, have in more recent studies demonstrated that some of the risk factors for atherogenesis lead to an increased tendency for platelets to agglutinate and to be consumed rapidly.[93-100]

Ross recognized that platelets liberate a potent peptide (or peptides) that promotes proliferation of arterial SMC's in vitro.[2,32,47,101] This observation was combined with important in vivo studies which demonstrated that factors which inhibit platelet sticking, spreading, and disintegration over areas of damaged arterial endothelium also inhibit SMC proliferation in these areas. These studies led Ross, Harker, and Glomset to utilize nonhuman primate experimental models and to coordinate these findings with observations in human subjects with metabolic disorders, especially homocystinemia, and with their in vitro study of the proliferative response of arterial SMC in tissue culture.[2,32,47,101-104] These investigators have proposed that the proliferative response of the SMC's in atherosclerotic plaques that develop over injured arterial intima is mainly due to the "platelet factor," which appears to be liberated from adherent and disintegrating platelets (Fig. 34–7). This work by the Seattle group has been reviewed in light of other observations that support the importance of endothelial injury in some cases of human atherosclerosis and in some types of experimental plaque formation.[2,32]

Recent advances in the understanding of the platelet-derived growth factor have included the purification of this active peptide[105-107] and the demonstration that it supports SMC migration as well as proliferation,[108] that it interacts with mesenchymal cells to increase pinocytosis,[109] and that it binds specifically with a receptor on the surface of cells it stimulates.[110,111]

One of the paradoxes about endothelial injury and atherogenesis which is the subject of intensive investigation is the observation first reported by Minick, Stemerman, and Insull.[112] They found that the most severe rabbit atherogenesis did not occur in the balloon catheter–denuded areas which were carpeted by platelets, but rather in the areas where endothelial cells had recently grown over the denuded areas. Further study has indicated that, in part at least, this increased atherogenesis in the reendothelialized areas may be correlated with the increased binding of lipoprotein lipid by proteoglycans associated with this newly covered area,[113] and that these areas are prone to increased cholesterol synthesis and decreased hydrolysis.[114]

The recognition that arterial endothelial damage is important in some cases of atherogenesis has additional implications which support the role of LDL in atherogenesis. One of the weaknesses of the so-called "lipid theory" of the pathogenesis of atherosclerosis has been the occasional exceptional case, in which advanced atherosclerosis with clinical effects occurs at an early age and in the absence of major risk factors (hypercholesterolemia, hypertension, and cigarette smoking). It now appears that a number of these exceptional or paradoxical cases may fall into a specific category, represented diagrammatically in the right-hand portion of Figure 34–8. If accelerated and advanced plaque formation can occur even when LDL (cholesterol) levels are low, while arterial endothelial injury is *severe* and *sustained* or *repeated frequently*, this would offer a rational explanation for a number of clinical reports and recent experimental results.[115-119] Recognition of the importance of arterial endothelial injury in the absence of hypercholesterolemia, cigarette smoking, and hypertension should encourage the search for better clinical tests to help the practicing physician detect and correct endothelial injury as a major risk factor when it is a predominant part of atherogenesis or when it is an important adjunct of hypercholesterolemia (Table 34–2).[120] Thus far, platelet survival time seems to be the best available laboratory test for measuring severe endothelial damage.[102] Unfortunately, this is a rather cumbersome invasive procedure that requires the removal of blood, separation of the patient's own

TABLE 34–2   FACTORS WHICH HAVE BEEN SHOWN TO INJURE ARTERIAL ENDOTHELIUM AND TO PRODUCE INCREASED PERMEABILITY TO MACROMOLECULES, INCLUDING LIPOPROTEINS

SUBSTANCE OR PHYSICAL CONDITION	MECHANISM INVOLVED	CLINICAL CONDITION
Hemodynamic forces; tension, stretching, shearing, eddy currents	Separation or damage to endothelial cells, increased permeability, platelet sticking, stimulation of smooth muscle cell proliferation	Hypertension
Angiotensin II	"Trap-door" effect	Hypertension
Carbon monoxide or decreased O_2 saturation	Destruction of endothelial cells	Cigarette smoking
Catecholamines (epinephrine, norepinephrine, serotonin, bradykinin)	Hypercontraction, swelling and loss of endothelial cells, platelet agglutination	Stress, cigarette smoking
Metabolic products	Endothelial cell damage	Homocystinemia, uremia, and so on
Endotoxins and other similar bacterial products	Endothelial cell destruction, platelet sticking	Acute bacterial infections
Ag-Ab complexes, immunological defects	Platelet agglutination	Serum sickness, transplant rejection, immune complex diseases, lupus erythematosus
Virus diseases	Endothelial cell infection and necrosis	Viremias
Mechanical trauma to endothelium	Platelet sticking, increased local permeability	Catheter injury
Hyperlipidemia with increase in circulating lipoproteins (cholesterol, triglycerides, phospholipids) and free fatty acids	Platelet agglutination in areas of usually hemodynamic damage, over "fatty streaks"	Chronic nutritional imbalance (high-fat and high-cholesterol diets), familial hypercholesterolemia, diabetes, nephrosis, hypothyroidism

FIGURE 34–10 This diagram indicates the probable interactions between the two major pathogenetic mechanisms proposed for atherogenesis. The steps involved according to the endothelial injury formulation are on the left, and those for the lipid-cholesterol formulation are on the right. The interactions are numbered as follows: (1) LDL in high concentrations induces endothelial injury; (2) endothelial injury increases influx of LDL; (3) hyperlipoproteinemia stimulates platelet aggregation; (4) high LDL levels stimulate proliferation of arterial SMC which are in the stationary phase; and (5) SMC-produced extracellular matrix binds and traps LDL molecules, which in turn may permit increased cellular uptake of LDL. (From Steinberg, D.: Metabolism of lipoproteins at the cellular level in relation to atherogenesis. *In* Miller, N. E., and Lewis, B. (eds.): Lipoproteins, Atherosclerosis and Coronary Heart Disease. Amsterdam, Elsevier, 1981, p. 31.)

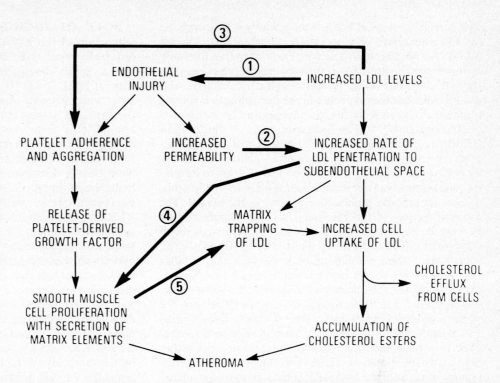

platelets, and labeling of these platelets with an appropriate radioactive isotope. A simpler but reliable noninvasive procedure, such as radioimmunoassay for circulating platelet factor 4, may ultimately be useful to detect widespread endothelial damage and platelet sticking in the absence of other risk factors.[121]

As the concepts of lipoprotein insudation and arterial endothelial injury advance and become more clearly understood, it becomes increasingly evident that we are dealing with strongly interacting pathogenetic mechanisms. These interactions have been recently summarized in a highly useful diagrammatic form by Steinberg.[122] He has indicated (Fig. 34–10) the ways in which elevated levels of LDL (or β-VLDL) and the various forms of endothelial injury may interact to support the progression of the atherosclerotic plaque. In the last analysis, it now seems likely that both of these pathological processes may be active in plaque formation.

ROLE OF MACROPHAGES

Another area of study which has had a recent upsurge, relative to the pathobiology and pathogenesis of atherosclerosis, is the evaluation of the role of the macrophages in the developing atherosclerotic lesion. This is not a new area of interest, since the proposal of a special function for the blood-derived macrophage in certain well-defined experimental atheromatous lesions has existed for many years.[123] Because of the evidence which, in general, indicates that the fibroblast and the arterial SMC have, under most circumstances, limited capacities for lipid accumulation, there has been a general trend to search for a "scavenger cell" of another type which could correspond to the appearance of the limited number of foam cells in most human atherosclerotic lesions.

The macrophage fulfills this role, since it has a very large capacity to take up and store altered low-density[89] or diet-induced β-VLDL lipoproteins.[31] Furthermore, it has

been demonstrated that LDL can be altered in several ways to a suitable form to be inbibed by macrophages which might be active during atherogenesis. These include malondialdehyde alterations of LDL by platelets,[87] conversion of LDL to a special form by endothelial cells,[88] and the formation of quantities of β-VLDL by cholesterol and fat feeding.[91] The macrophage and its functions are complex, and at the present time, although no one doubts its role as a scavenger, it is difficult to be certain whether its scavenger function is more likely to inhibit lesion progression by removing lipid as well as furnishing collagenases and elastases, or whether it is a major force in producing more lipid accumulation and SMC proliferation by depositing altered LDL lipid (by means of foam cell death) and secreting a growth factor or factors which stimulate arterial SMC proliferation. Unfortunately, none of these functions has been well documented in human atherosclerotic lesions.

IN VITRO STUDIES

Recently, some of the most promising and most exciting developments in the investigation of the pathogenesis of atherosclerosis have come from the use of in vitro as well as microdissection methods to study the pathobiology of cells of the arterial wall.[1,64,120,124] A variety of methods have been utilized in these studies, ranging from the biochemical and cell kinetic investigations of small fragments of arterial media or atherosclerotic plaques derived from humans or animals, to the study and growth of cells from explants of arterial media or subcultures of these outgrowths, to the study of dispersed cells or homogenates from small, carefully selected, microdissected samples of human or animal lesions.

Each of these approaches has yielded valuable new insights into the atherosclerotic process, but none is more surprising or innovative than the reports of Benditt and coworkers. These investigators found that many foci of

SMC's from plaques of black women who are heterozygotic for the isoenzymes of glucose-6-phosphate dehydrogenase (G-6-PD) and whose mesenchymal cells therefore normally contain equal quantities of these two isoenzymes, usually showed only one form of this enzyme.[125-128] This corresponds with findings reported in similar subjects involving benign tumors such as fibroleiomyoma in the uterus and other neoplasms.[129-131] This finding of isoenzymatically similar cells is interesting because it suggests that these collections of cells in the atherosclerotic plaque are either monoclonal or monotypic in origin. The analogy to neoplasia raises important questions about the nature of the stimuli that initiate the proliferative process in the plaque. The essential aspects of this discovery have been confirmed by Pearson et al. and by Thomas et al.[132-135] Although much more work needs to be done, the studies by Thomas et al. suggest that these collections of isoenzymatically similar cells arise rather late in plaque formation and that, in general, most of the atherosclerotic plaques in the aorta of any one individual are likely to contain clumps of cells of the same isoenzymic type. Both these findings, if confirmed and extended, tend to support a "natural selection" mechanism to explain the origin of these monotypic cells rather than a somatic mutation. There is no doubt that this painstaking effort and the rationale behind it have stimulated further research into the fundamental nature of the processes controlling cell proliferation in the atherosclerotic plaque.

Other significant recent findings have come from the investigations by Goldstein and Brown at the University of Texas, using in vitro techniques.[31,89,91,136-138] These scientists have discovered the defective control mechanisms in the mesenchymal cells of patients suffering from familial hypercholesterolemia. They have established the importance of receptors to apo B on the surfaces of peripheral cells as well as their role in regulating cholesteryl ingress into the cell and the rates at which cholesterol ester is hydrolyzed and free cholesterol is esterified. This fascinating series of studies and the genetic principles involved are reviewed in Chapter 47.

Mahley et al. have extended this approach to the study of the enhanced avidity of arginine-rich apoproteins (Apo E) for receptors on mesenchymal and some parenchymal cells.[139] This too, appears to be only an initial step in discovering the pathobiology of plaque formation using in vitro methods, since clearly it is necessary to extend these studies to include the quantitative variations that occur in the more or less normal mesenchymal cells of most individuals who acquire this disease process. Furthermore, much is still to be learned about the alternate routes by which cholesterol gains entrance to the cytoplasm of arterial SMC when apolipoprotein receptors are absent. The Mahley group, combined with Goldstein, Brown, and others,[138] has gone far to clarify the genetic aspects of familial dysbetalipoproteinemia (i.e., type 3 hyperlipoproteinemia). Mahley and his colleagues have provided a clear-cut view of the comparative pathology of atherogenesis in a number of species. Specifically, they have documented the importance of β-VLDL in atherogenesis and demonstrated that SMC really can develop into foam cells in the dog.[139] The mechanisms of egress—short of cell death—of excess cholesterol and cholesteryl ester from the cells of the atherosclerotic lesion are an almost untouched area of research.

ROLE OF HIGH-DENSITY LIPOPROTEIN. The interaction of the high-density lipoprotein (HDL) fraction (especially some of its components) with arterial SMC's is also a rapidly developing field of investigation. It appears that rat HDL apo C-III (or human HDL apo A-I), particularly when present with certain phospholipids, facilitates the egress of substantial quantities of cholesterol and cholesterol ester from the cytoplasm of cultured lipid-laden SMC's.[140-143] Scanu, Byrne, and Milhovilovic have recently reviewed this complex area.[144] Innerarity, Pitas, and Mahley have clearly demonstrated a modulating effect of canine high-density lipoproteins rich in apo E on the cholesteryl ester synthesis in macrophages usually stimulated by β-VLDL.[145] These studies of cultured cells are supported by a substantial amount of epidemiological work and some work with experimental animals.[146-149] They have led to the hypothesis that the HDL fraction, which is relatively poor in cholesterol and rich in phospholipid, acts as a protective molecule that can transport cholesterol from peripheral tissues back to the liver, where, if conditions are favorable, it may be excreted rather than re-utilized in the production of more LDL.[150,151] Knowledge of HDL contribution to cholesterol excretion has been substantially increased recently by the discovery of the hepatic apo E receptor and its relationship to apo B, E hepatic receptor.[152]

One of the most interesting new aspects of research to confirm the protective effect of a relatively high level of HDL in the circulation is the positive correlation between regular physical exercise, such as that recommended to strengthen the cardiorespiratory system, and the favorable ratio between HDL and LDL that seems to accompany this type of activity.[153-155] This phenomenon has now been demonstrated clearly in nonhuman primates.[156] So far, the reasons for this correlation at the cellular or basic biochemical level are not clear, but this appears to be a rich field for further study and may ultimately provide a more compelling justification for regular, vigorous exercise to prevent atherogenesis.

We have already described the work of Ross and colleagues relative to the emerging pathobiology of arterial SMC proliferation in vitro as part of their study of the role of endothelial injury and "platelet factor" in the development of the atherosclerotic plaque.[101-104] Ross' observations[2,32] play a prominent role in a number of studies yielding new findings about endogenous factors in the mammal that may exert important influences on the proliferation of mesenchymal cells in health and disease.[157] Knowledge in this fast-changing field will be substantially advanced when the mechanism of action and the interrelationships of these potent stimulators of cell proliferation are better defined.

EFFECT OF LDL ON SMOOTH MUSCLE CELLS. Apparently quite separate from the platelet, macrophage, and endothelial cell factors and equally incompletely understood is the SMC proliferation–stimulating effect of LDL obtained from hyperlipidemic rhesus monkey or rabbit serum, first reported from our laboratory in 1968.[158] This effect is apparently due to a narrow fraction of LDL, not present in normal serum (H-LDL) and over a wide range is not dose dependent on LDL cholesterol concentration.[159-161] It apparently is also not related to the type of food fat fed, even though the latter may affect plaque cell proliferation in vivo.[162]

This growth-stimulating effect of LDL from hyperlipidemic monkey serum is distinct from and additive to the effects of the platelet factor.[163,164] Chen et al. have also demonstrated similar effects using LDL from hyperlipidemic rabbit serum and subcultures from rabbit aortic medial cells.[165,166] Robertson has reported that subcultures of human arterial SMC exposed to LDL from hyperlipidemic human serum are stimulated to increased mitotic activity and increased incorporation of ^{3}H thymidine.[167,168] Serum and LDL from homozygous type II patients have been tested on stationary outgrowths from aortic media explants of rhesus monkeys.

Myasnikov et al., in the Soviet Union, demonstrated as early as 1966 the cell growth–stimulating effect of hyperlipidemic serum from patients with atherosclerosis.[169] This followed their earlier demonstration of similar effects with rabbit hyperlipidemic serum and aortic cells.[170]

Estradiol and HDL from normal serum block the mitosis-stimulating effect of LDL from hyperlipidemic serum.[171,172] This general effect of LDL from hyperlipidemic serum on arterial SMC proliferation has recently been clarified somewhat by the work of Fless and Scanu.[85,86] They have found that it is possible to identify and isolate fractions of rhesus monkey LDL, which they have designated LDL I, II, III, and IV. LDL I, usually present in rather small amounts in normal monkey serum, will stimulate quiescent arterial SMC to proliferate. It is similar to, but probably not identical with, the predominant LDL fraction (H-LDL), which is elevated in hyperlipidemic rhesus monkey serum. LDL II, III, and IV have no such cell proliferation stimulatory effect in their native form, but LDL III from normal monkey serum becomes active when it is suitably treated with sialidase from *Clostridium perfringens*. These recently reported results make it possible to study the entire question of the mechanism of stimulation of arterial SMC proliferation by LDL from hyperlipidemic serum under carefully controlled conditions.

Stimulatory effects of serum from diabetic animals and humans, first demonstrated by Ledet,[173-178] and from untreated hypertensive animals, reported by Fischer-Dzoga and Pick and others,[179-184] are other possible mechanisms by which risk factors increase arterial SMC proliferation. These observed effects do not seem to be related to proliferation stimulated by insulin or glucose content of the serum. Further work is indicated to determine whether these serum factors are major contributors to the hyperplasia of arterial smooth muscle cells.

Some effects of various types of lipoproteins on the lipid and cholesterol metabolism of subcultures of arterial smooth muscle cells have been described in detail in Chapter 47. Studies by Chen et al., by Bates and Wissler, and more recently by St. Clair et al.[185-191] indicate that the LDL from hyperlipidemic serum is able to promote accumulation of cholesteryl esters in arterial smooth muscle cells. This may be due to qualitative differences between LDL from hyperlipidemic serum and normolipidemic serum, to an HDL/LDL imbalance, or to some other mechanism. This phenomenon supports the importance of elevated LDL levels in atherogenesis.

In vitro studies using cultured endothelial cells and other modern cell biological studies promise to yield important data.[192-195] They have been used to investigate antihemophilic and von Willebrand factors and to develop knowledge about the metabolism of endothelium as it relates to atherosclerosis.[13,195-200] Since synthesis and deposition of extracellular products of the arterial SMC, such as collagen, elastin, and glycosaminoglycans, may be influenced by the same factors as are atherosclerotic plaques, further study is needed.[25,27-29]

Factors that allow egress of lipid from these cells are also important in determining the extent of necrosis and ulceration. The elegant in vitro systems now available will continue to be applied to further investigation of the mechanisms of lipid accumulation, cell proliferation, cell necrosis, synthesis of fiber proteins, and lipid egress, all of which are important in atherosclerosis research.

EXPERIMENTAL MODELS OF ATHEROSCLEROSIS

The inaccessibility of tissues and the gradual development of the disease process over decades in humans, as well as the difficulties of conducting controlled studies of large groups of free-living people, make reliable animal models of atherosclerosis relevant and especially valuable. Experimental counterparts of the human disease process are becoming much more highly developed, and their similarities to, as well as their differences from, the lesions in people are becoming better documented. Animal models are thus making a growing contribution to an understanding of the pathogenesis or the regression of atheromatous lesions.[123,201-205]

Although all of the commonly used animal models have contributed valuable information, some are much more useful for the study of advanced disease.[201] The swine and the macaque monkey models appear to provide a much closer approximation to the clinically demonstrable disease process than do some of the older models. Although the dog has generally been reported to be relatively resistant to diet-induced disease, it has been possible to produce advanced disease and to study successfully the regression of canine lesions subsequent to induction of severe hypercholesterolemia by means of an atherogenic ration and thyroid suppression.[206,207] Recently, the dog has proved to be valuable in the study of atherogenicity of hydrogenated coconut oil.[208,209] Using either of these means of induction, Mahley et al. have demonstrated that the development of significant atherosclerosis in the dog correlates well with hypercholesterolemias which have unusually high levels of cholesterol-rich and apo B–rich lipoproteins with a density of 1.006 gm/ml or below (so called broad-beta or beta-rich VLDL).[210]

Studies of the Monkey

The rhesus monkey (*Macaca mulatta*) has been the most frequently utilized species of the nonhuman primate models, since it has virtually no spontaneous atheromatous disease but develops progressive atherosclerosis with "clinical" complications soon after being fed a mixed and well-balanced commercial monkey ration supplemented with saturated fat and cholesterol (Fig. 34–11).[30,202,204,211-219]

Ingestion of Coconut Oil. In pioneering studies, Taylor et al. showed that rhesus monkeys developed lesions which were essentially similar to human plaques in distribution and in plaque components.[11,220-226] Unlike in nonprimate models, there appeared to be little small artery involvement, little loading of the reticuloendothelial system (RES), and relatively little monocyte-derived foam cell lesion component. Subsequently, studies in this laboratory showed that substitution in the ration of coconut oil for part of the butterfat augmented the process.[64,123,211,227]

In studies with the cebus monkey, we have observed that coconut oil is more effective than butterfat in inducing an elevation of serum LDL levels. The atherosclerotic lesions produced by it seem to exhibit more cell proliferation, a larger necrotic center, and more evidence of irritation or low-grade inflammation of the artery wall, based on mononuclear cell infiltrates in the adventitia.[211,228] Since coconut oil is increasingly used often as a "hidden" ingredient labeled only as "vegetable fat," the special atherogenicity of this food fat is a cause for concern.[208-211,229]

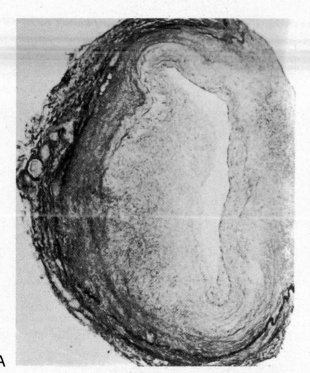

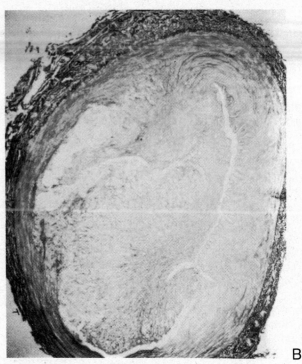

A

B

FIGURE 34–11   These photomicrographs depict muscular arteries of rhesus monkeys fed an atherogenic ration for 17 months. *A,* This severely atherosclerotic left circumflex coronary artery shows an eccentric plaque composed of both extracellular and intracellular lipid and rather extensive fibrosis of the proliferated arterial cells that make up most of the lesions. Little evidence of a necrotic core is seen in this section (Verhoeff-van Gieson stain). *B,* This carotid artery reveals a thick, eccentric plaque showing extensive fibrosis and a relatively large necrotic atheromatous area beneath it (Verhoeff-van Gieson stain). (From Armstrong, M. L.: Regression of atherosclerosis. *In* Paoletti, R., and Gotto, A. M., Jr. (eds.): Atherosclerosis Reviews. Vol. 1. New York, Raven Press, 1976, p. 137.)

Ingestion of Peanut Oil.   Peanut oil, even though rich in polyunsaturated fat, has repeatedly been shown to be highly atherogenic in rat, rabbit, and swine as well as in rhesus monkey.[230-234] Since these studies have involved peanut oil as the sole food fat in a cholesterol-rich ration, the results are difficult to apply to humans, who usually consume a variety of food fats. Furthermore, when human populations consume peanut oil as a major food fat, they usually consume little cholesterol. Experimental lesions linked to peanut oil ingestion show abundant proliferation of smooth muscle cells and tend to be especially rich in collagen and elastin and to have smaller necrotic centers than do lesions resulting from ingestion of butterfat or corn oil. The paradoxically severe peanut oil lesions may be the result of behenic and arachidic acids, the arrangement of fatty acids on the triglyceride molecules, and the disturbance of the intracellular metabolism of the artery wall when lipoproteins of these fatty acids are involved in developing lesions.[230,234-238]

Monkeys fed a peanut oil–enriched ration with large quantities of cholesterol also show more extensive ultrastructural endothelial damage than do animals fed other food fats in an otherwise similar ration.[239]

These effects of coconut oil and peanut oil make it likely that some of the variations in human atherosclerotic lesions are due to the predominant food fats included in the foods of people consuming high-fat, cholesterol-rich diets.[30]

Reversal of Atherosclerosis

The extensive use of the rhesus monkey for lesion regression studies has helped significantly to establish the potential for regression or reversal of the atheromatous plaque under many experimental conditions.[215,240-245] For the purposes of this discussion, the terms "regression" and "reversal" are used interchangeably to indicate a substantial reduction in the "space-occupying" nature of atheromatous lesions as well as in the danger they pose to the health and well-being of the individual.

Experimental and Human Plaque Regression.   Considerable circumstantial, epidemiological, and autopsy evidence prior to 1970

suggested that the clinical effects and severity of human atherosclerosis might be at least partially reversible.[246-249] Although attempts were made to reverse atheromatous lesions induced in animals under experimental conditions, and some of these studies yielded promising results,[242,245,250-252] many (in particular, those in the rabbit) demonstrated an *increase* in severity of the lesions when the animals were shifted to a therapeutic regimen consisting of a low-cholesterol, low-fat ration.[201,203] In retrospect, it appears likely that these failures were related to the complication of severe cholesterol storage disease that the rabbit frequently develops.[123] This unresponsiveness of the rabbit to a low-cholesterol, low-fat therapeutic diet has now been studied further, and three recent reports indicate that advanced atheromatous changes can be reversed by increasing the ambient oxygen supply to the arterial wall in the presence of cholestyramine and/or estradiol therapy or by adding Mg EDTA to the diet.[253-255]

Recently, regression has been studied effectively in accelerated and severe lesions in swine produced by a combination of endothelial injury in the aorta due to balloon catheterization and an atherogenic (high-cholesterol, high-fat) ration.[251,256] These studies have supplemented the usual histopathological, morphometric, and chemical evidence of regression with measurements of the DNA synthetic activity and measurements of the numbers of smooth muscle cells during atherogenesis and following longstanding regression. They have also provided the first preliminary evidence that the amount of calcium in these lesions decreases during regression.

Changes in the Lesion During Regression.   In general, all the studies reported so far in the rhesus monkey and in swine have shown substantial agreement and have indicated that as a result of regression periods lasting 12 to 40 months, during which serum cholesterol returns to baseline levels, the lesions appear to become much smaller, contain much less visible lipid, and show remarkable decreases in cholesterol and cholesterol esters.[242,243,250-252,257,258] The lesions also show substantial remodeling of the fiber proteins along with chemical evidence of an absolute decrease in collagen and elastin after about 18 months.[243,259,260] The decreases in fiber proteins in these plaques are much more evident if the results are expressed in

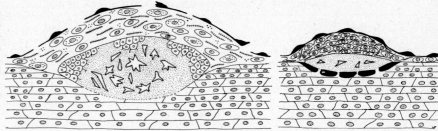

FIGURE 34-12 Changes reported to occur during regression of advanced atheromatous lesions in rhesus monkey and swine models. The plaques become substantially smaller, and both the fibrous cap and the components of the necrotic center decrease in size. Intracellular lipid virtually disappears, and extracellular lipid decreases. The collagen and elastic condense and remodel themselves to fit the smaller lesion, and the endothelial damage heals.

content per anatomical unit and *not* in terms of milligrams per gram of dry weight.[261]

Furthermore, it appears that the lipid-rich necrotic centers of advanced atheromas decrease or disappear.[242,243,249,256,257] In studies reported from this laboratory, the small quantities of stainable lipid that remain in even the most prominent of the regressed plaques are confined largely to the internal elastic membrane, and almost no intracellular lipid is present.[243] It is apparent that these substantial reductions in cells, necrotic centers, and cholesterol, in addition to the remodeling and condensation of fiber proteins, cause both the space-occupying and the thrombogenic properties of these plaques to diminish (Fig. 34-12). These features and the tendency of regressing plaques to show endothelial healing[262] make it probable that the clinical effects of the lesions will be greatly mitigated. More recent reports have indicated that many of these beneficial effects may be achieved even if the serum cholesterol is not restored to the lowest level possible for the species being studied.[244,247,258,263]

Cholestyramine and Regression. We have reported the preliminary results of a series of experiments that considered the effects of cholestyramine, a bile acid–sequestering resin, with or without a low-cholesterol, low-fat diet.[247,263-265] Cholestyramine administered with an atherogenic ration results in regression of plaques in monkeys when the serum cholesterol is not restored to baseline levels. On the other hand, the resin therapy appears to have little additional effect on decreasing the incidence or severity of coronary involvement over that produced by a low-fat, low-cholesterol regimen. Perhaps a major mechanism by which cholestyramine therapy induces regression may be related to its effects on increasing hepatic apo B receptors.[266] Obviously, a better understanding of the cellular and metabolic mechanisms by which regression takes place is needed—a goal that seems to be attainable by study of the available animal models of atherosclerosis.

Current studies on human patients utilizing measurements of functional parameters or quantitative measurements of plaques viewed by means of sequential arteriography after institution of cholesterol-lowering therapy have yielded promising evidence of retardation of the progression or regression of plaques.[267-275] Other reviews of the regression of atherosclerosis in patients have appeared recently.[276,277] Furthermore, at least two recent prospective studies in which relatively large decreases in serum cholesterol have been documented have also shown definite decreases in heart attack rates and mortality from atherosclerosis of the coronary artery.[278,279]

Potential for Prevention

Atherosclerosis, as we learn more about its pathogenesis and cellular pathobiology, would appear to be a largely preventable disease process. The utilization of improved animal models should help us attain this goal. Nutritional elements are being discovered and evaluated at the lesion level, several of which appear to have great promise for prevention of plaques and/or retardation of their progression.

Among these elements are alfalfa seed saponins, as studied and reported by Malinow and coworkers;[280,281] calcium blockers in general, including agents such as lanthanum and ethane hydroxydiphosphate (EHDP), as investigated by Kramsch and coworkers;[282,283] and soybean-derived products.[284,285] Each of these has been shown to have very powerful preventive effects on the development of atherosclerosis and in some instances on regression of atherosclerosis in animals even when administered with rations which induce progressive lesions.

More recently, Connor and coworkers have demonstrated large decreases in blood triglyceride levels and in some instances remarkable

drops in serum cholesterol levels when fish oils containing large proportions of omega (ω)-3 fatty acids are added to the diets of normal subjects[286] or patients who have genetically induced hyperlipidemia.[287,288] This is done by the simple expedient of adding fish oil to the diet, often in the form of table-prepared fish. This nutritional approach of supplementing the diet with oils rich in omega-3 fatty acids (especially eicosa pentaenoic acid) also has been demonstrated to produce very favorable effects on platelet aggregation and lengthened bleeding time. These new clinical studies are strongly supported by nutritional work in many species of experimental animals and offer great promise for future studies of prevention and retardation of human atherosclerotic plaques. It would appear that we are nearing the time when the experimental model best suited to the problem of prevention can be selected with considerable confidence and assurance of success.

SUMMARY AND RECOMMENDATIONS

The results of the studies summarized here delineate how the major risk factors for atherosclerosis—both those recognized and those still emerging—may function at the cellular level (Table 34-3). The application of modern knowledge from cellular pathobiology and chemical pathology to explain atherogenesis and the prevention and/or regression of the plaque has increased the usefulness of observations derived from epidemiologists, clinicians, and experimental pathologists. It also forms the basis for developing a rational method to control the disease process by interrupting the pathogenetic progression at the molecular and cell component level (Fig. 34-13). In fact, it is evident that simply lowering serum cholesterol to minimum levels—which in many populations of the world appears to be somewhat less than 150 mg/100 ml—will be likely to reverse many of the pathological mechanisms diagrammed in Figure 34-7. Arterial endothelial damage may prove to be a major mechanism by which hypertension and cigarette smoking combine with very low-density hyperlipoproteinemia to increase the rate of progression of atherosclerosis. These risk factors may be reversible if hypertension is controlled or cigarette smoking is discontinued (see Table 34-3).[289-291]

Unfortunately, our knowledge of atherosclerosis related to diabetes is not as far advanced. Some methods of treatment may actually increase the rate of progression of atherosclerosis in this disease process.[292,293] Evidence is emerging that a regular exercise program may help to remove excess cholesterol from peripheral tissues, including the arterial wall,[153-155] providing justification for some of the older epidemiological data as well as supporting common-sense views proposing that this is an effective means of protecting the heart and arteries.[294]

New leads supported by a growing body of clinical evidence indicate that the diabetic patient may benefit from nutritional measures which include supplements of oat

TABLE 34-3   PROBABLE MECHANISMS OF ACTION OF RISK FACTORS AT THE CELLULAR LEVEL

Hypercholesterolemia (Whether due to high-cholesterol-calorie-saturated fat *diet** or metabolically induced,* including inherited types	Increased levels of circulating low-density lipoproteins (LDL) damage endothelium and carry cholesterol into artery wall, especially if high-density lipoprotein (HDL) levels are low; lipid (cholesterol) is "trapped," accumulates in smooth muscle cells, or is bound to their extracellular products; leads to cell proliferation and/or necrosis, increased collagen formation, and so on
Hypertension	Increased endothelial permeability to LDL *due to* 1. Increased artery wall tension 2. "Trap-door effect" of and endothelial damage from angiotensin 3. Platelet sticking (norepinephrine-induced?) with release of vasoactive amines 4. Especially bad when added to hypercholesterolemia 5. Serum "factor" stimulates arterial smooth muscle cell (SMC) proliferation
Cigarette smoking	*Damage to cells of artery wall due* to 1. Circulating CO 2. Platelet agglutination (norepinephrine-induced?) 3. ↑lipid mobilization (norepinephrine-induced?), leading to hyperlipemia and increased lipid in artery wall
Diabetes	CHO-induced hyperlipemia (VLDL) along with an increase of glycosaminoglycans in the intima that binds lipoproteins; factors in the serum of diabetics that are not related to lipoproteins, insulin, or sugar stimulate arterial smooth muscle cell (SMC) proliferation
Sedentary living and obesity	Appear to increase the tendency toward elevated serum LDL with relatively low serum levels of HDL, increased incidence of diabetes and hypertension, poor cardiac reserve, and increased work for the heart

*May also stimulate platelet sticking and clotting tendency so that superimposed thrombosis is more likely to occur.

bran along with its naturally occurring gums and fibers.[295] We must also be alert to the existence of unrecognized risk factors that may produce chronic and substantial damage to the arterial endothelium.

The current spectrum of promising interventions in the process of atherosclerosis is presented in Figure 34-13. The natural history of the development of lesions during an individual's lifetime offers an opportunity at almost all ages for prevention or treatment. The major problem for the general public, for public health professional personnel and officers, and for the practicing physician is still the early detection of risk factors before the catastrophic and life-threatening effects of severe atherosclerosis ensue.

Here, too, the advancement of knowledge is swift and promising. For many years, the absence of coronary thrombi in most people who died suddenly with advanced coronary atherosclerosis presented a dilemma.[296–298] Now it appears that there are actually two or more pathogenic mechanisms in acute heart attacks, although, in almost all cases, both should be regarded as results of severe coro-

nary atherosclerosis.[299–301] One is the classic development of *thrombosis of the coronary artery and transmural myocardial infarction,* which usually does not lead to sudden death and which benefits from prompt medical attention and hospitalization. In this instance, attempts are made to limit the size of the infarct, and modern coronary care is provided.[302]

The second is the *sudden onset of ventricular fibrillation* at home, at work, or in the community as a result of electrical instability of cardiac rhythm triggered by mechanisms that are not always clear (Chap. 23). These victims will die suddenly unless promptly rescued by individuals trained in cardiopulmonary resuscitation (CPR). This must be followed by prompt attention from trained emergency medical care teams equipped with modern defibrillation and life-support devices and medication. We now know that many of these victims are not likely to develop electrocardiographic or enzymatic evidence of myocardial infarction if resuscitation and defibrillation are successful.[303] However, this type of heart attack tends to recur, and

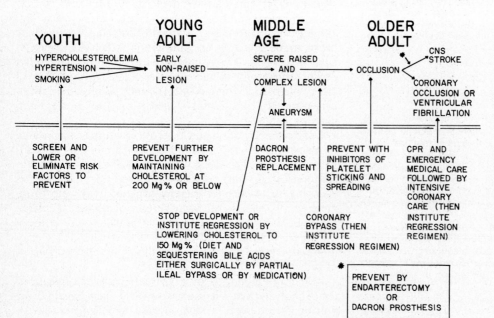

FIGURE 34-13 A spectrum of the available methods of intervention in human atherosclerosis, beginning early in life with an emphasis on prevention and later employing measures designed to retard or reverse the development of progressive plaques. As clinical effects of lesions develop, therapy should be designed to prolong life and facilitate regression of the plaques. (Modified from Wissler, R. W., and Vesselinovitch, D.: Regression of atherosclerosis in experimental animals and man. Verh. Dtsch. Ges. Inn. Med. (Munich) *81*:857, 1975.)

these patients should be considered to be prone to the serious effects of atherosclerosis. They not only should be protected from subsequent episodes of ventricular fibrillation by means of the most reliable and effective medications available but also should undergo therapy to slow the progress of the lesion, which, it is hoped, will in some instances result in regression of the underlying disease.

Chronic angina is another clinical effect of atherosclerosis that does not always seem to fit into the commonly accepted concept of risk factors leading to lipid-filled plaques, which, in turn, lead to coronary thrombosis and finally myocardial infarction. For one thing, females show a propensity for angina, and, in addition, these patients appear to have a lower rate of myocardial infarction than would be expected in individuals with severe atherosclerosis without angina.[304] Are the coronary atherosclerotic lesions different in these patients with chronically recurring angina than in those who develop acute myocardial infarction? Is there greater involvement of the small artery? Does this type of heart disease have a different set of risk factors that are more endogenously determined, such as coronary arterial spasm? Recent observations point to the role of spasm near areas of especially severe coronary atherosclerosis possibly triggered by products released by adherent platelets in these highly damaged and diseased areas.[305-307] The spasms demonstrated angiographically in these studies have correlated well with the onset of symptoms of angina.

In general, it appears that the atherosclerosis in patients with angina is qualitatively similar to that in other patients but may be more diffuse in distribution and more fibrous in character. Also, the small coronary radicles are not involved in most patients. We have not learned to identify other risk factors for the syndrome, if indeed, any exist. We therefore have much to learn about this manifestation of atherosclerosis.

Patients who have had a myocardial infarction or who have undergone coronary bypass surgery, endarterectomy, or balloon arterioplasty must have skillful and diligent medical management with emphasis on removing all recognizable risk factors. The areas of severe disease, the junctions with grafts, and the areas of arterial manipulation are particularly vulnerable to progression of the atherosclerotic process. In those especially vulnerable patients who already have evidence of advanced atherosclerosis, it is important that every effort be made to retard or to produce regression of the atherogenic process.

Acknowledgments

The author is grateful to Gertrud Friedman, Gwen Matthews, and Denise Wooten for their diligent and skillful work in helping to prepare this revision. He also wishes to acknowledge the help of Mr. Gordon Bowie in preparing much of the accompanying illustrative material. Many colleagues and coworkers have also helped greatly in the studies in this laboratory which have sustained our interest in the pathogenesis of atherosclerosis and have helped us to contribute in a modest way to the concepts of pathogenesis and regression herein described. Special recognition is extended to Draga Vesselinovitch, Sandra Bates, Jayme Borensztajn, Robert Chen, Katti Fischer-Dzoga, Robin Fraser, Godfrey Getz, Seymour Glagov, Masako Mitsumata, Ruth Pick, Leon Resnekov, Arthur Rubenstein, Angelo Scanu, Thomas Schaffner, Yoji Yoshida, and Christopher Zarins, as well as to our technical and scientific associates, Manuela Bekermeier, Blanche Berger, Tim Bridenstine, Gabrielle Chassagne, Laurence Frazier, Laura Harris, Randolph Hughes, and Rose Jones.

The studies in this laboratory referred to and summarized in this chapter were supported in part by funds from U.S. Public Health Service grants HL 15062, HL 17648, HL 12308, and HL 6894 as well as the Cardiovascular Research Foundation of The University of Chicago.

References

1. Wissler, R. W., Vesselinovitch, D., and Getz, G. J.: Abnormalities of the arterial wall and its metabolism in atherogenesis. Prog. Cardiovasc. Dis. 18:341, 1976.
2. Ross, R., and Glomset, J. A.: The pathogenesis of atherosclerosis. N. Engl. J. Med. 295:369, 420, 1976.
3. Arteriosclerosis, 1981. Report of the Working Group on Arteriosclerosis of the National Heart, Lung and Blood Institute. Vol. 1, DHHS–NIH Publication No. 81–2034, Washington, 1981.
4. Stamler, J.: Diet-related risk factors for human atherosclerosis: Hyperlipidemia, hypertension, hyperglycemia—Current status. In Sirtori, C., Ricci, G., and Gorini, G. (eds.): Diet and Atherosclerosis. (Adv. Exp. Med. Biol., Vol. 60.) New York, Plenum Press, 1975, p. 125.
5. Keys, A.: Coronary heart disease—The global picture. Atherosclerosis 22:149, 1975.
6. Intersociety Commission for Heart Disease Resources Report: Primary prevention of the atherosclerotic diseases. Circulation 62:A–55, 1970.
7. Kuller, L. H.: Epidemiology of cardiovascular diseases: Current perspectives Am. J. Epidemiol. 104:425, 1976.
8. Meyer, W. W., Walsh, S. Z., and Lind, J.: Functional morphology of arteries during fetal and post-natal development. In Schwartz, C. J., Werthessen, N. T., and Wolf, S. (eds.): Structure and Function of the Circulation. Vol. I. New York, Plenum Press, 1980, p. 95.
9. Hess, R., and Staubli, W.: Ultrastructure of vascular changes. In Schettler, F. G., and Boyd, G. S. (eds.): Atherosclerosis: Pathology, Physiology, Aetiology, Diagnosis and Clinical Management. Amsterdam, Elsevier Publishing Co., 1969, p. 49.
10. McGill, H. C.: The lesion. In Schettler, G., and Weizel, A. (eds.): Atherosclerosis III. Berlin, Springer-Verlag, 1974, p. 27.
11. Taylor, C. B., Trueheart, R. E., and Cox, G. E.: Atherosclerosis in rhesus monkeys. III. The role of increased thickness of arterial walls in atherogenesis. Arch. Pathol. 76:14, 1963.
12. Zarins, C. K., Bomberger, R. A., and Glagov, S.: Local effects of stenoses: Increased flow velocity inhibits atherogenesis. Circulation 64:II–221, 1981.
13. Gimbrone, M. A., Jr.: Vascular endothelium and atherosclerosis. In Moore, S. (ed.): Vascular Injury and Atherosclerosis. New York, Marcel Dekker, 1981, p. 25.
14. Reichl, D., Simons, L. A., Myant, N. B., Pflug, J. J., and Mills, G. L.: The lipids and lipoproteins of human peripheral lymph with observations on the transport of cholesterol from plasma and tissues into lymph. Clin. Sci. Mol. Med. 45:313, 1973.
15. Scott, P. J., and Hurley, P. J.: The distribution of radio-iodinated serum albumin and low density lipoprotein in tissues and the arterial wall. Atherosclerosis 11:77, 1970.
16. Smith, E. B., and Slater, R. W.: Relationship between low density lipoprotein in aortic intima and serum lipid levels. Lancet 1:463, 1972.
17. Day, C. E., and Levy, R. S.: Control of the precipitation reaction between low density lipoproteins and polyions. Artery 1:150, 1975.
18. Stein, O., Stein, Y., and Eisenberg, S.: Radioautographic study of the transport of ^{125}I-labeled serum lipoproteins in rat aorta. Z. Zellforsch Mikrosk. Anta. 138:223, 1973.
19. Esterly, J., and Glagov, S.: Altered permeability of the renal artery of the hypertensive rat: An electron microscopic study. Am. J. Pathol. 43:619, 1963.
20. Wissler, R. W.: Progression and regression of atherosclerotic lesions. In Chandler, A. B., Eurenius, K., McMillan, G. C., Nelson, C. B., Schwartz, C. J., and Wessler, S. (eds.): The Thrombotic Process in Atherogenesis. New York, Plenum Press, 1978, p. 77.
21. Gerrity, R., Richardson, M., Somer, J. B., Bell, F. P., and Schwartz, C. J.: Endothelial cell morphology in areas of in vivo Evans Blue uptake in the aorta of young pigs. Am. J. Pathol. 89:313, 1977.
22. Weber, G., Fabbrini, P., and Resi, L.: On the presence of a concanavallin-A reactive coat over the endothelial aortic surface and its modifications during early experimental cholesterol atherogenesis in rabbits. Virchows Arch. Abt. A. Path. Anat. 259:299, 1973.
23. Wolinsky, H., and Glagov, S.: Comparison of abdominal and thoracic aortic medial structure in mammals. Deviation of man from the usual pattern. Circ. Res. 25:677, 1969.
24. Glagov, S.: Hemodynamic risk factors: Mechanical stress, mural architecture, medial nutrition and the vulnerability of arteries to atherosclerosis. In Wissler, R. W., and Geer, J. C. (eds.): The Pathogenesis of Atherosclerosis. Baltimore, The Williams and Wilkins Co., 1972, p. 164.
25. Wissler, R. W.: The arterial medial cell, smooth muscle or multifunctional mesenchyme? J. Atheros. Res. 8:201, 1968.
26. Fischer-Dzoga, K., Jones, R. M., Vesselinovitch, D., and Wissler, R. W.: Ultrastructural and immunohistochemical studies of primary cultures of aortic medial cells. Exp. Mol. Pathol. 18:162, 1973.

27. Ross, R., and Klebanoff, S. J.: The smooth muscle cell. I. In vivo synthesis of connective tissue proteins. J. Cell Biol. 50:159, 1971.

28. Ross, R.: The smooth muscle cell. II. Growth of smooth muscle in culture and formation of elastic fibers. J. Cell Biol. 50:172, 1971.

29. Wight, T. N., and Ross, R.: Proteoglycans in primate arteries. II. Synthesis and secretion of glycosaminoglycans by arterial smooth muscle cells in culture. J. Cell Biol. 67:675, 1975.

30. Wissler, R. W.: Atherosclerosis: Its pathogenesis in perspective. In Homberger, F. (ed.): Comparative Pathology of the Heart. (Advances in Cardiology, Vol. 13.) Basel, Karger, 1974, p.10.

31. Goldstein, J. L., Ho, Y. K., Brown, M. S., Innerarity, T. L., and Mahley, R. W.: Cholesteryl ester accumulation in macrophages resulting from receptor-mediated uptake and degradation of hypercholesterolemic canine β-very low density lipoproteins. J. Biol. Chem. 255:1839, 1980.

32. Ross, R.: Atherosclerosis: A problem of the biology of arterial wall cells and their interactions with blood components. Arteriosclerosis 1:293, 1981.

33. Clark, J. M., and Glagov, S.: Structural integration of the arterial wall. I. Relationships and attachments of medial smooth muscle cells in normally distended and hyperdistended aortas. Lab. Invest. 40:587, 1979.

34. Glagov, S.: Relation of structure to function in arterial walls. Artery 5:295, 1979.

35. Glagov, S., and Ozoa, A.: Significance of the relatively low incidence of atherosclerosis in the pulmonary, renal and mesenteric arteries. Ann. N.Y. Acad. Sci. 149:940, 1968.

36. Strong, J. P., Eggen, D. A., and Oalmann, M. C.: The natural history, geographic pathology, and epidemiology of atherosclerosis. In Wissler, R. W., and Geer, J. C. (eds.): The Pathogenesis of Atherosclerosis. Baltimore, The Williams and Wilkins Co., 1972, p. 20.

37. Glagov, S., Rowley, D. A., Cramer, D. B., and Page, R. G.: Heart rate during 24 hours of usual activity for 100 normal men. J. Appl. Physiol. 29:799, 1970.

38. Wissler, R. W., and Vesselinovitch, D.: Atherosclerosis—Relationship to coronary blood flow. Sixth Triennial Australian National Heart Foundation Conference on Physiology and Pathology of Coronary Heart Disease, Canberra, Australia, February 1982. Am. J. Cardiol. (in press).

39. Wissler, R. W., and Vesselinovitch, D.: New concepts of factors involved in the natural history and regression of atherosclerosis. First World Vascular Day and 7th International Symposium of the International Society for Angiography and Angiology, Berlin, West Germany. Periodica Angiologica, 1982.

40. Roberts, W. C.: The status of the coronary arteries in fatal ischemic heart disease. Cardiovasc. Clin. 7:1, 1975.

41. Roberts, W. C.: The coronary arteries in coronary heart disease: Morphologic observations. Pathobiol. Ann. 5:249, 1975.

42. McGill, H. C., Jr., Geer, J. C., and Strong, J. P.: Natural history of human atherosclerotic lesions. In Sandler, M., and Bourne, G. H. (eds.): Atherosclerosis and its origin. New York, Academic Press, 1963, p. 42.

43. Constantinides, P.: Experimental Atherosclerosis. Amsterdam, Elsevier Publishing Co., 1965.

44. Brown, M. S., Kovanen, P. T., and Goldstein, J. L.: Regulation of plasma cholesterol by lipoprotein receptors. Science 212:628, 1981.

45. Stemerman, M. B., and Ross, R.: Experimental atherosclerosis I. Fibrous plaque formation in primates, an electron microscopic study. J. Exp. Med. 136:769, 1972.

46. Bjorkerud, S., and Bondjers, G.: Repair responses and tissue lipid after experimental injury to the artery. Ann. N.Y. Acad. Sci. 275:180, 1976.

47. Ross, R.: Atherosclerosis and the arterial smooth muscle cell. Science 180:1332, 1973.

48. Getz, G. S., Wissler, R. W., Hughes, R. H., Graber, C., and Tantraj, S.: Metabolism of lipids in the atherosclerotic rhesus monkey aorta. Proc. Inst. Med. Chicago 27:106, 1968.

49. Adams, C. M., Morgan, R. S., and Bayliss, O. B.: The differential entry of 123I-albumin into mildly and severely atheromatous rabbit aortas. Atherosclerosis 11:119, 1970.

50. Ross, R., and Harker, L.: Hyperlipidemia and atherosclerosis. Science 193:1094, 1976.

51. Stemerman, M. B.: Effects of moderate hypercholesterolemia on rabbit endothelium. Arteriosclerosis 1:25, 1981.

52. Wanstrup, J., Kjeldsen, K., and Astrup, P.: Acceleration of spontaneous intimal-subintimal changes in rabbit aorta by prolonged moderate carbon monoxide exposure. Acta Pathol. Microbiol. Scand. 75:353, 1969.

53. Kjeldsen, K., Astrup, P., and Wanstrup, J.: Ultrastructural intimal changes in the rabbit aorta after a moderate carbon monoxide exposure. Atherosclerosis 16:67, 1972.

54. Robertson, A. L., Jr., and Khairallah, P. A.: Arterial endothelial permeability and vascular disease: The "trap-door" effect. Exp. Mol. Pathol. 18:241, 1973.

55. Schwartz, S. M.: Assessment of angiotensin endothelial injury by incident light microscopy. Fed. Proc. 35:208, 1976.

56. Mitchell, J. R. A., and Schwartz, C. J.: Arterial Disease. Oxford, Blackwell Scientific Publishers, 1965.

57. Smith, E. B., Slater, R. S., and Chu, P. K.: The lipids in raised fatty and fibrous lesions in human aorta. A comparison of changes at different stages of development. J. Atheros. Res. 8:399, 1968.

58. Smith, E. B., Slater, R. S., and Crothers, D. C.: Quantitative interrelationships between plasma constituents and normal and atherosclerotic human intimal tissue. In Schettler, G., and Weizel, A. (eds.): Atherosclerosis III. Berlin, Springer-Verlag, 1974, p. 96.

59. Smith, E. B., and Slater, R. S.: Lipids and low density lipoproteins in intima

in relation to its morphological characteristics. In Atherogenesis: Initiating Factors (Ciba Found. Symp. No. 12). Amsterdam, Elsevier Publishing Co., 1973, p. 39.

60. Smith, E. B.: Molecular interactions in human atherosclerotic plaques. Am. J. Pathol. 86:665, 1977.

61. Panganamala, R. V., Geer, J. C., Sharma, H. A., and Cornwell, D. G.: The gross and histologic appearance and the lipid composition of normal intima and lesions from human coronary arteries and aorta. Atherosclerosis 20:93, 1974.

62. Wissler, R. W., McAllister, H. A., Jr., and Vesselinovitch, D.: A histopathological study of the fatty streak in aortas and coronary arteries of young American military personnel. Am. J. Pathol. 78:64a, 1975.

63. Yang, C., Schaffner, T., and Wissler, R. W.: Enzyme histochemical and histopathological features of human atherosclerotic plaques in young Americans. Unpublished observations.

64. Wissler, R. W.: Development of the atherosclerotic plaque. In Braunwald, E. (ed.): The Myocardium: Failure and Infarction. New York, HP Publishing Co., 1974, p. 155.

65. Getz, G. S., Vesselinovitch, D., and Wissler, R. W.: A dynamic pathology of atherosclerosis. Am. J. Med. 46:657, 1969.

66. Haust, M. D., More, R. H., and Movat, H. Z.: The role of the smooth muscle cell in the fibrogenesis of atherosclerosis. Am. J. Pathol. 37:377, 1960.

67. Geer, J. C., McGill, H. C., Jr., and Strong, J. P.: Fine structure of human atherosclerotic lesions. Am. J. Pathol. 38:263, 1961.

68. McGill, H. C., and Geer, J. C.: The human lesion, fine structure. In Jones, R. J. (ed.): Evolution of the Atherosclerotic Plaque. Chicago, University of Chicago Press, 1963, p. 65.

69. Geer, J. C., and Haust, M. D.: Smooth Muscle Cells in Atherosclerosis. (Monographs on Atherosclerosis, Vol. 2.) Basel, Karger, 1972.

70. Knieriem, H. J., Kao, V. C., and Wissler, R. W.: Actinomyosin and myosin and the deposition of lipids and serum lipoproteins. Arch. Pathol. 84:118, 1967.

71. Becker, C. G., and Murphy, G. E.: Demonstration of contractile protein in endothelium and cells of the heart valves, endocardium, intima, arteriosclerotic plaques, and Aschoff bodies of rheumatic heart disease. Am. J. Pathol. 55:1, 1969.

72. Chamley, J. H., Groschel-Stewart, U., Campbell, R. G., and Burnstock, G.: Distinction between smooth muscle, fibroblasts and endothelial cells in culture by the use of fluoresceinated antibodies against smooth muscle actin. Cell Tissue Res. 177:445, 1977.

73. Campbell, G. R., Uehara, Y., Mark, G., and Burnstock, G.: Fine structure of smooth muscle cells grown in tissue culture. J. Cell Biol. 49:21, 1971.

74. Chamley-Campbell, J., Campbell, G. R., and Ross, R.: The smooth muscle cell in culture. Physiol. Rev. 59:1, 1979.

75. Campbell, G. R., Chamley-Campbell, J. H., and Burnstock, G.: Differentiation and phenotypic modulation of arterial smooth muscle cells. In Schwartz, C. J., Werthessen, N. T., and Wolf, S. (eds.): Structure and Function of the Circulation. (Vol. III) New York, Plenum Press, 1981, p. 357.

76. Hanig, M., Shainoff, J. R., and Lowry, A. D.: Flotational lipoproteins extracted from human atherosclerotic aortas. Science 124:176, 1956.

77. Gero, S., Gergely, J., Jakab, L., Szekely, J., and Virac, S.: Comparative immunoelectrophoretic studies on homogenates of aorta, pulmonary arteries and inferior vena cava of atherosclerotic individuals. J. Atheros. Res. 1:88, 1961.

78. Tracy, R. E., Merchant, E. B., and Kao, V.: On the antigenic identity of human serum beta and alpha-w lipoproteins and their identification in aortic intima. Circ. Res. 9:472, 1961.

79. Watts, H. F.: Role of lipoproteins in the formation of atherosclerotic lesions. In Jones, R. J. (ed.): Evolution of the Atherosclerotic Plaque. Chicago, University of Chicago Press, 1963, p. 117.

80. Kao, V. C. Y., and Wissler, R. W.: A study of the immunohistochemical localization of serum lipoproteins and other plasma proteins in human atherosclerotic lesions. Exp. Mol. Pathol. 4:465, 1965.

81. Hollander, W., Kramsch, D. M., and Inoue, G.: The metabolism of cholesterol, lipoproteins and acid mucopolysaccharides in normal and atherosclerotic vessels. In Miras, C. H., Howard, A. N., and Paoletti, R. (eds.): Progress in Biochemical Pharmacology. (Vol. 4.) Basel, Karger, 1968, p. 270.

82. Fless, G., Wissler, R. W., and Scanu, A. M.: Study of abnormal plasma low density lipoprotein in rhesus monkeys with diet-induced hyperlipidemia. Biochemistry 15:5799, 1976.

83. Rudel, L. L., Pitts, L. L., II, and Nelson, C. A.: Characterization of plasma low density lipoproteins of nonhuman primates fed dietary cholesterol. J. Lip. Res. 18:211, 1977.

84. Fless, G., and Scanu, A. M.: Isolation and characterization of the three major low density lipoproteins from normolipidemic rhesus monkeys (Macaca mulatta). J. Biol. Chem. 254:8653, 1979.

85. Fless, G. M., Kirchhausen, T., Fischer-Dzoga, K., Wissler, R. W., and Scanu, A. M.: Relationship between the properties of apo B containing low-density lipoproteins (LDL) of normolipidemic rhesus monkey and their mitogenic action on arterial smooth muscle cells grown in vitro. In Gotto, A. M., Jr., Smith, L. C., and Allen, B. (eds.): Proceedings of the 5th International Symposium on Atherosclerosis. New York, Springer Verlag, 1980, p. 607.

86. Fless, G. M., Kirchhausen, T., Fischer-Dzoga, K., Wissler, R. W., and Scanu, A. M.: Serum low density lipoproteins with mitogenic effect on cultured aortic smooth muscle cells. Atherosclerosis 41:171, 1982.

87. Fogelman, A. M., Shechter, I., Seager, J., Hokom, M., Child, J. S., and Edwards, P. A.: Malondialdehyde alterations of low density lipoprotein leads to

cholesteryl ester accumulation in human monocyte-macrophages. Proc. Natl. Acad. Sci. USA 77:2214, 1980.

88. Henriksen, T., Mahoney, E. M., and Steinberg, D.: Enhanced macrophage degradation of low density lipoprotein previously incubated with cultured endothelial cells: Recognition by receptors for acetylated low density lipoproteins. Proc. Natl. Acad. Sci. USA 78:6499, 1981.

89. Goldstein, J. L., Ho, Y. K., Basu, S. K., and Brown, M. S.: A binding site on macrophages that mediates the uptake and degradation of acetylated low-density lipoprotein producing massive cholesterol deposition. Proc. Natl. Acad. Sci. 76:333, 1979.

90. Zilversmit, D. B.: Atherogenesis: A postprandial phenomenon. Circulation 60:473, 1979.

91. Mahley, R. W., Innerarity, T. L., Brown, M. S., Ho, Y. K., and Goldstein, J. L.: Cholesteryl ester synthesis in macrophages: Stimulation by β-very low density lipoproteins from cholesterol-fed animals of several species. J. Lipid Res. 21:970, 1980.

92. Mustard, J. F., Packham, M. A., and Kinlough-Rathbone, R. L.: Platelets, atherosclerosis and clinical complications. In Moore, S. (ed.): Vascular Injury and Atherosclerosis. New York, Marcel Dekker, 1981, p. 79.

93. Mustard, J. F.: Increased activity of the clotting mechanism during alimentary lipemia: Its significance with regard to thrombosis and atherosclerosis. Can. Med. Assoc. J. 77:308, 1957.

94. Murphy, E. A., and Mustard, J. F.: Coagulation tests and platelet economy in atherosclerotic and control subjects. Circulation 25:114, 1962.

95. Farbiszewski, R., and Worowski, K.: Enhancement of platelet aggregation and adhesiveness by beta lipoprotein. J. Atheros. Res. 8:988, 1968.

96. Carvalho, A. C. A., Colman, R. W., and Lees, R. S.: Platelet function in hyperlipoproteinemia. N. Engl. J. Med. 290:434, 1974.

97. Nordøy, A., and Rødset, J. M.: Platelet function and platelet phospholipids in patients with hyperlipoproteinemia. Acta Med. Scand. 189:385, 1971.

98. Sullivan, J. M., Heinle, R. A., and Gorlin, R.: Studies of platelet adhesiveness, glucose tolerance and serum lipoprotein patterns in patients with coronary artery disease. Am. J. Med. Sci. 264:475, 1972.

99. Nordøy, A., and Rødset, J. M.: The influence of dietary fats on platelets in man. Acta Med. Scand. 190:27, 1971.

100. Mustard, J. F., and Murphy, E. A.: Effect of smoking on blood coagulation and platelet survival in man. Br. Med. J. 1:846, 1963.

101. Ross, R., Glomset, J., Kariya, B., and Harker, L.: A platelet-dependent serum factor that stimulates the proliferation of arterial smooth muscle cells in vitro. Proc. Natl. Acad. Sci. USA 71:1207, 1974.

102. Harker, L. A., Slichter, S. J., Scott, C. R., and Ross, R.: Homocystinemia: Vascular injury and arterial thrombosis. N. Engl. J. Med. 291:537, 1974.

103. Harker, L. A., Ross, R., Schlicter, S. J., and Scott, C. R.: Homocystine-induced arteriosclerosis. The role of endothelial cell injury and platelet response in its genesis. J. Clin. Invest. 58:731, 1976.

104. Harker, L. A., Ross, R., and Glomset, J.: Role of the platelet in atherogenesis. Ann. N.Y. Acad. Sci. 275:321, 1976.

105. Antoniades, H. N., Scher, C. D., and Stiles, C. D.: Purification of human platelet-derived growth factor. Proc. Natl. Acad. Sci. 76:1809, 1979.

106. Heldin, C. H., Westermark, B., and Wasteson, A.: Platelet derived growth factor. Isolation by a large scale procedure and analysis by subunit composition. Biochem J. 193:907, 1981.

107. Raines, E. W., and Ross, R.: Platelet-derived growth factor. I. High yield purification and evidence for multiple forms. J. Biol. Chem. 257:5154, 1982.

108. Grotendorst, G. R., Seppa, H., Kleinman, H. K., and Martin, G. R.: Attachment of smooth muscle cells to collagen and their migration toward platelet-derived growth factor. Proc. Natl. Acad. Sci. 78:3669, 1981.

109. Davies, P. F., and Ross, R.: Mediation of pinocytosis in cultured arterial smooth muscle and endothelial cells by platelet-derived growth factor. J. Cell Biol. 79:663, 1978.

110. Bowen-Pope, D. F., and Russell, R.: Platelet-derived growth factor. II. Specific binding to cultured cells. J. Biol. Chem. 257:5161, 1982.

111. Glenn, K., Bowen-Pope, D. F., and Ross, R.: Platelet-derived growth factor. III. Identification of a platelet-derived growth factor receptor by affinity labeling. J. Biol. Chem. 257:5172, 1982.

112. Minick, C. R., Stemerman, M. B., and Insull, W., Jr.: Role of endothelium and hypercholesterolemia in intimal thickening and lipid accumulation. Am. J. Pathol. 95:131, 1979.

113. Falcone, D. J., Hajjar, D. P., and Minick, C. R.: Enhancement of cholesterol and cholesteryl ester accumulation in re-endothelialized aorta. Am. J. Pathol. 99:81, 1980.

114. Hajjar, D. P., Falcone, D. J., Fowler, S., and Minick, C.: Endothelium modifies the altered metabolism of the injured aortic wall. Am. J. Pathol. 102:28, 1981.

115. Jensen, G., and Sigurd, B.: Systemic lupus erythematosus and acute myocardial infarction. Chest 64:653, 1973.

116. Tsakraklides, V. G., Glieden, L. C., and Edwards, J. E.: Coronary atherosclerosis and myocardial infarction associated with systemic lupus erythematosus. Am. Heart J. 87:637, 1974.

117. Bulkley, B. H., and Roberts, W. C.: The heart in systemic lupus erythematosus and the changes induced in it by corticosteroid therapy. Am. J. Med. 58:243, 1975.

118. More, S.: Thromboatherosclerosis in normolipemic rabbits: A result of continued endothelial damage. Lab. Invest. 29:478, 1973.

119. Friedman, R. J., Moore, S., and Singal, D. P.: Repeated endothelial injury and induction of atherosclerosis in normolipemic rabbits by human serum. Lab. Invest. 32:404, 1975.

120. Wissler, R. W.: Coronary atherosclerosis and ischemic heart disease. In Zülch, K. J., Kaufman, W., Hossmann, K. A., and Hossman, V. (eds.): Brain and Heart Infarct. Berlin, Springer-Verlag. 1977, p. 206.

121. Kaplan, K. L., and Owen, J.: Plasma levels of beta-thromboglobulin and platelet factor 4 as indices of platelet activation in vivo. Blood 57:199, 1981.

122. Steinberg, D.: Metabolism of lipoproteins at the cellular level in relation to atherogenesis. In Miller, N. E., and Lewis, B. (eds.): Lipoproteins, Atherosclerosis and Coronary Heart Disease. Amsterdam, Elsevier Publishing Co., 1981, p. 31.

123. Wissler, R. W., and Vesselinovitch, D.: Experimental models of human atherosclerosis. Ann. N.Y. Acad. Sci. 149:907, 1968.

124. Wissler, R. W.: The emerging cellular pathobiology of atherosclerosis. Artery 5:409, 1979.

125. Benditt, E. P., and Benditt, J. M.: Evidence for a monoclonal origin of human atherosclerotic plaques. Proc. Nat. Acad. Sci. USA 70:1753, 1973.

126. Benditt, E. P.: Implications of the monoclonal character of human atherosclerotic plaques. Am. J. Pathol. 86:693, 1977.

127. Benditt, E. P.: The origin of atherosclerosis. Sci. Am. 236:74, 1977.

128. Benditt, E. P., and Gown, A. M.: Atheroma: The artery wall and the environment. Int. Rev. Exp. Pathol. 21:56, 1980.

129. Lindner, D., and Gartler, S. M.: Glucose-6-phosphate dehydrogenase mosaicism: Utilization as a cell marker in the study of leiomyomas. Science 150:67, 1965.

130. Fialkow, P. J.: Use of genetic markers to study cellular origin and development of tumors in human females. Adv. Cancer Res. 15:191, 1972.

131. Fialkow, P. J.: The origin and development of human tumors studied with cell markers. N. Engl. J. Med. 291:26, 1974.

132. Pearson, T. A., Wang, A., and Solex, K.: Clonal characteristics of fibrous plaques and fatty streaks from human aortas. Am. J. Pathol. 81:379, 1975.

133. Pearson, T. A., Kramer, E. D., Solez, K., and Heptinstall, R. H.: The human atherosclerotic plaque. Am. J. Pathol. 86:657, 1977.

134. Thomas, W. A., Janakidevi, K., Florentin, R. A., and Reiner, J. M.: The reversibility of the human atherosclerotic plaque. In Hauss, W. H., Wissler, R. W., and Lehmann, R. (eds.): International Symposium: State of Prevention and Therapy in Human Arteriosclerosis and in Animal Models. Opladen. Westdeutscher Verlag. Vol. 63:1978, p. 73.

135. Thomas, W. A., Reiner, J. M., Florentin, R. A., Janakidevi, K., and Lee, K. J.: Arterial smooth muscle cells in atherogenesis: Births, deaths and clonal phenomena. In Schettler, G., Goto, G., Hata, Y., and Klose, G. (eds.): Atherosclerosis IV. Berlin, Springer-Verlag, 1977, p. 16.

136. Goldstein, J. L., and Brown, M. S.: The low density lipoprotein pathway and its relation to atherosclerosis, Ann. Rev. Biochem. 46:897, 1977.

137. Goldstein, J. L., and Brown, M. S.: Familial hypercholesterolemia—Pathogenesis of receptor disease. Johns Hopkins Med. J. 143:8, 1978.

138. Schneider, W. T., Kovanen, P. T., Brown, M. S., Goldstein, J. L., Utermann, G., Weber, W., Havel, R. J., Kotite, L., Kane, J., Innerarity, T. L., and Mahley, R. W.: Familial dysbetalipoproteinemia. Abnormal binding of mutant apoprotein E to low density lipoprotein receptors of human fibroblasts and membranes from liver and adrenal of rats, rabbits, and cows. J. Clin. Invest. 68:1075, 1981.

139. Mahley, R. W.: Atherogenic hyperlipoproteinemia. The cellular and molecular biology of plasma lipoproteins altered by dietary fat and cholesterol. Med. Clin. North Am. 66:375, 1982.

140. Jackson, R. L., Stein, O., Gotto, A. N., and Stein, Y.: A comparative study on the removal of cellular lipids from Landschütz ascites cells by human plasma apolipoproteins. J. Biol. Chem. 250:7204, 1975.

141. Stein, Y., Glange, M. C., Fainaru, M., and Stein, O.: The removal of cholesterol from aortic smooth muscle cells in culture and Landschütz ascites cells by fractions of human high-density lipoproteins. Biochim. Biophys. Acta 380:106, 1975.

142. Stein, O., Vanderhoek, J., and Stein, Y.: Cholesterol content and sterol synthesis in human skin fibroblasts and rat aortic smooth muscle cells exposed to lipoprotein-depleted serum and high density apolipoprotein/phospholipid mixtures. Biochim. Biophys. Acta 431:347, 1976.

143. Stein, Y., and Stein, O.: Interaction between serum lipoproteins and cellular components of the arterial wall. In Scanu, A. M., Wissler, R. W., and Getz, G. S. (eds.): The Biochemistry of Atherosclerosis. New York, Marcel Dekker, 1979, p. 313.

144. Scanu, A. M., Byrne, R. E., and Mihovilovic, M.: Functional roles of plasma high density lipoproteins. CRC Crit. Rev. Biochem. 13:109, 1982.

145. Innerarity, T. L., Pitas, R. E., and Mahley, R. W.: Modulating effects of canine high density lipoproteins on cholesteryl ester synthesis induced by β-very low density lipoproteins in macrophages. Arteriosclerosis 2:114, 1982.

146. Miller, G. J., and Miller, N. E.: Plasma-high-density-lipoprotein concentration and development of ischaemic heart disease. Lancet 1:16, 1975.

147. Castelli, W. P., Doyle, J. T., Gordon, T., Hames, C., Hulley, S. B., Kagan, A., McGee, D., Vicic, W. J., and Zukel, W. J.: HDL cholesterol levels (HDLC) in coronary heart disease (CHD)—Cooperative lipoprotein phenotyping study. Circulation 52(Suppl. II):97, 1975.

148. Miller, N. W., Weinstein, D. B., and Steinberg, D.: Uptake and degradation of high density lipoprotein—Comparison of fibroblasts from normal subjects and from homozygous familial hypercholesterolemic subjects. J. Lipid Res. 19:644, 1978.

149. Hayes, K. C., Hojnacki, J. L., and Nicolosi, R. J.: High density lipoproteins in nonhuman primates. In Day, C. E., and Levy, R. S. (eds.): High Density Lipoproteins. New York, Plenum Press, 1981.

150. Carew, T. E., Koschinsky, T., Hayes, S. B., and Steinberg, D.: A mechanism by which high density lipoproteins may slow the atherogenic process. Lancet *1*: 1315, 1976.

151. Miller, N. W., Nestel, P. J., and Clifton-Bligh, P.: Relationships between plasma lipoprotein cholesterol concentrations and the pool size and metabolism of cholesterol in man. Atherosclerosis 23:535, 1976.

152. Mahley, R. W., Hui, D. Y., Innerarity, T. L., and Weisgraber, K. H.: Two independent lipoprotein receptors on hepatic membranes of the dog, swine, and man: The apo-B, E and apo-E receptors. J. Clin. Invest. *68*:1197, 1981.

153. Krauss, R. M., Lindgren, F. T., Wood, P. D., Haskell, W. L., Albers, J. J., and Cheung, M. C.: Differential increases in plasma high density lipoprotein subfractions and apolipoproteins (APO-LP) in runners. Circulation *56*(Suppl. III):100, 1977.

154. Wood, P. D., Haskell, W. L., Klein, H., Lewis, S., Stern, M. P., and Farquhar, J. W.: The distribution of plasma lipoproteins in middle-aged male runners. Metabolism 25:1249, 1976.

155. Erkelens, D. W., Albers, J. J., Hazzard, W. R., Frederick, R. C., and Bierman, E. L.: Moderate exercise increases high density lipoprotein cholesterol in myocardial infarction survivors. Clin. Res. 26:158a, 1978.

156. Kramsch, D., Aspen, A. J., Abramowitz B. M., Kreimendahl, T., and Hood, W. B., Jr.: Reduction of coronary atherosclerosis by moderate conditioning exercise in monkeys on an atherogenic diet. N. Engl. J. Med. 305:1485, 1981.

157. Wissler, R. W., Fischer-Dzoga, K., Bates, S. R., and Chen, R. M.: Arterial smooth muscle cells in tissue culture. *In* Schwartz, C. J., Werthessen, N. T., and Wolf, S. (eds.): Structure and Function of the Circulation, (Vol. III.) New York, Plenum Press, 1981, p. 427.

158. Kao, V. C. Y., Wissler, R. W., and Dzoga, K.: The influence of hyperlipemic serum on the growth of medial smooth muscle cells on Rhesus monkey aorta in vitro. Circulation *38*(Suppl. VI):12, 1968.

159. Fischer-Dzoga, K., Wissler, R. W., and Scanu, A. M.: The lipoproteins and arterial smooth muscle cells: cellular proliferation and morphology. *In* Manning, G. W., and Haust, M. D. (eds.): Atherosclerosis: Metabolic, Morphologic and Clinical Aspects (Advances in Experimental Medicine and Biology Vol. 82). New York, Plenum Press, 1977, p. 915.

160. Fischer-Dzoga, K., Chen, R., and Wissler, R. W.: Effects of serum lipoproteins on the morphology, growth and metabolism of arterial smooth muscle cells. *In* Wagner, W. D., and Clarkson, T. B. (eds.): Arterial Mesenchyme and Arteriosclerosis. New York, Plenum Press, 1974, p. 299.

161. Fischer-Dzoga, K., and Wissler, R. W.: Stimulation of proliferation in stationary primary cultures of monkey aortic smooth muscle cell. II. Effect of varying concentrations of hyperlipemic serum and low density lipoproteins of varying dietary fat origins. Atherosclerosis 24:515, 1976.

162. Fischer-Dzoga, K., Fraser, R., and Wissler, R. W.: Stimulation of proliferation in stationary primary cultures of monkey and rabbit aortic smooth muscle cells. I. Effects of lipoprotein fractions of hyperlipemic serum and lymph. Exp. Mol. Pathol. 24:346, 1976.

163. Fischer-Dzoga, K., and Wissler, R. W.: Response of arterial smooth muscle cells to hyperlipemia. *In* Schettler, G., Goto, Y., Hata, Y., and Klose, G. (eds.): Atherosclerosis IV. Berlin, Springer-Verlag, 1977, p. 624.

164. Fischer-Dzoga, K., Kuo, Y.-F., and Wissler, R. W.: The proliferative effect of platelets and hyperlipidemic serum on stationary primary cultures. Atherosclerosis 47:35, 1983.

165. Chen, R. M., Getz, G. S., Fischer-Dzoga, K., and Wissler, R. W.: The role of hyperlipidemic serum on the proliferation and necrosis of aortic medial cells in vitro. Exp. Mol. Pathol. 26:359, 1977.

166. Chen, R. M., Fischer-Dzoga, K., and Wissler, R. W.: Influence of lysosomal enzyme stability in hyperlipemic serum-induced metabolic changes of monkey aortic medial cells. *In* Schettler, G., Goto, Y., Hata, Y., and Klose, G. (eds.): Atherosclerosis IV. Berlin, Springer-Verlag, 1977, p. 649.

167. Robertson, A. L., Jr.: The artery and process of arteriosclerosis. Pathogenesis. *In* Wolf, S., (ed.): Advances in Experimental Medicine and Biology. Vol. 16A. New York, Plenum Press, 1971, p. 229.

168. Robertson, A. L.: Functional characterization of arterial cells involved in spontaneous atheroma. *In* Schettler, G., and Weizel, A. (eds.): Atherosclerosis III. Berlin, Springer-Verlag, 1974, p. 175.

169. Myasnikov, A. L., Block, Y. E., and Pavlov, V. M.: Influence of lipemic serums of patients with atherosclerosis on tissue cultures of adult human aortas. J. Atheros. Res. 6:224, 1966.

170. Myasnikov, A. L., and Block, Y. E.: Influence of some factors in lipoidosis and cell proliferation in aorta tissue cultures of adult rabbits. J. Atheros. Res. 5:33, 1965.

171. Fischer-Dzoga, K., Vesselinovitch, D., and Wissler, R. W.: The effect of estrogen on the rabbit aortic medial tissue culture cells. Am. J. Pathol. 74:52a, 1974.

172. Yoshida, Y., Fischer-Dzoga, K., and Wissler, R. W.: Effects of normolipemic HDL on proliferation of monkey aortic smooth muscle cells induced by hyperlipemic LDL. Circulation *56*(Suppl. III):100, 1977.

173. Ledet, T., Fischer-Dzoga, K., and Wissler, R. W.: Diabetic macroangiopathy: in vitro study of the proliferation of the aortic smooth muscle cells. Am. J. Pathol. 74:50a, 1974.

174. Ledet, T., Fischer-Dzoga, K., and Wissler, R. W.: Growth of rabbit aortic smooth muscle cells cultured in media containing diabetic and hyperlipemic serum. Diabetes 25:207, 1976.

175. Ledet, T.: Diabetic cardiomyopathy: Quantitative histological studies of the heart from young juvenile diabetics. Acta Pathol. Microbiol. Scand. (Sect. A) 84:421, 1976.

176. Ledet, T.: Growth hormone stimulating the growth of arterial medial cells in vitro: absence of effect of insulin. Diabetes 25:1011, 1976.

177. Ledet, T.: Growth of rabbit aortic smooth muscle cells in serum from patients with juvenile diabetes. Acta Pathol. Microbiol. Scand. (Sect. A) 84:508, 1976.

178. Ledet, T.: Growth hormone antiserum suppresses the growth effect of diabetic serum. Studies of rabbit aortic medial cell cultures. Diabetes 26:798, 1977.

179. Fischer-Dzoga, K., Pick, R., and Kuo, Y.: In vitro response of aortic smooth muscle cells to serum of hypertensive monkeys. Circulation *56*(Suppl. III):100, 1977.

180. Belfiore, F., Napoli, E., Lo Vecchio, L., and Rabuazzo, A. M.: Serum acid phosphatase activity in diabetes mellitus. Am. J. Med. Sci. 266:139, 1973.

181. Wolinsky, H., Goldfischer, S., Schiller, B., and Kasak, L. E.: Lysosomes in aortic smooth muscle cells: effects of hypertension. Am. J. Pathol. 73:727, 1973.

182. Wolinsky, H., Goldfischer, S., Schiller, B., and Kasak, L. E.: Modification of the effects of hypertension on lysosomes and connective tissue in the rat aorta. Circ. Res. 34:233, 1974.

183. Wolinsky, H., Goldfischer, S., Daly, M. M., Kasak, L. E., and Coltoff-Schiller, B.: Arterial lysosomes and connective tissue in primate atherosclerosis and hypertension. Circ. Res. 36:553, 1975.

184. Fushimi, H., and Tarui, S.: Beta-glycosidases and diabetic microangiopathy. I. Decreases of beta-glycosidase activities in diabetic rat kidney. J. Biochem. 79:265, 1976.

185. Chen, R.: Effects of Hyperlipemic Rabbit Serum and its Lipoproteins on Proliferation and Lipid Metabolism of Rabbit Aortic Medial Cells In Vitro. Doctoral Thesis, The University of Chicago, 1973.

186. Chen, R. M., and Fischer-Dzoga, K.: Effect of hyperlipemic serum lipoproteins on the lipid accumulation and cholesterol flux of rabbit aortic medial cells. Atherosclerosis 28:339, 1977.

187. Chen, R. M., Getz, G. S., Fischer-Dzoga, K., and Wissler, R. W.: Effect of hyperlipemic serum and its lipoproteins on the lipid metabolism of rabbit aortic medial cells in vitro. Unpublished observation.

188. Chen, R. M., and Yang, F. P.: Effect of Metformin on the metabolism of rabbit aortic cells in vitro. Fed. Proc. 37:934, 1978.

189. Bates, S. R.: Effect of hyperlipemic serum on cholesterol accumulation in monkey aortic medial cells. Fed. Proc. 35:208, 1976.

190. Bates, S. R., and Wissler, R. W.: Effect of hyperlipemic serum on cholesterol accumulation in monkey aortic medial cells. Biochim. Biophys. Acta 450:78, 1976.

191. St. Clair, R. W., Smith, B. P., and Wood, L. L.: Stimulation of cholesterol esterification in rhesus monkey arterial smooth muscle cells. Circ. Res. 40:166, 1977.

192. Jaffe, E. A., Nachman, R. L., Becker, C. G., and Minick, C. R.: Culture of human endothelial cells derived from umbilical veins. Identification by morphological and immunological criteria. J. Clin. Invest. 52:2745, 1973.

193. Thorgeirsson, G., and Robertson, A. L., Jr.: The vascular endothelium — Pathobiologic significance. Am. J. Pathol. 93:803, 1978.

194. Schwartz, S. M., Gajdusek, C., and Owens, G. K.: Vessel wall growth control. *In* Nossel, H., and Vogel, H. J. (eds.): Pathobiology of the Endothelial Cell. New York, Academic Press, 1982, p. 63.

195. Gimbrone, M. A., Jr.: Culture of vascular endothelium. Progr. Hemost. Thromb. 3:1, 1976.

196. Jaffe, E. A., Hoyer, L. W., and Nachman, R. L.: Synthesis of antihemophilic factor antigen by cultured human endothelial cells. J. Clin. Invest. 52:2757, 1973.

197. Jaffe, E. A., Hoyer, L. W., and Nachman, R. L.: Synthesis of von Willebrand factor by cultured human endothelial cells. Proc. Nat. Acad. Sci. USA 71:1906, 1974.

198. Jagannathan, S. N., Connor, W. E., and Lewis, L. J.: Cholesterol metabolism in human endothelial cells in culture. *In* Manning, G. W., and Haust, M. D. (eds.): Atherosclerosis: Metabolic, Morphologic and Clinical Aspects. New York, Plenum Press, 1977, p. 244.

199. Booyse, F. M., Quarfoot, A. J., Bell, S., Fass, D. N., Lewis, J. C., Mann, K. G., and Bowie, E. J. W.: Cultured aortic endothelial cells from pigs with von Willebrand disease: in vitro model for studying the molecular defect(s) of the disease. Proc. Nat. Acad. Sci. USA 74:5702, 1977.

200. Gimbrone, M. A., Jr., and Alexander, R. W.: Prostaglandin production by vascular endothelial and smooth muscle cells in culture. *In* Silver, M. J., et al. (eds.): Prostaglandins in Hematology. New York, Spectrum, 1977, p. 121.

201. Wissler, R. W., and Vesselinovitch, D.: Differences between human and animal atherosclerosis. *In* Schettler, G., and Weizel, A. (eds.): Atherosclerosis III. Berlin, Springer-Verlag, 1974, p. 319.

202. Wissler, R. W., and Vesselinovitch, D.: Atherosclerosis in nonhuman primates. *In* Brandley, C. A., Corneliu, C. E., and Simpson, C. F. (eds.): Advances in Veterinary Science and Comparative Medicine. Vol. 21. (Cardiovascular Pathophysiology). New York, Academic Press, 1977, p. 351.

203. Wissler, R. W., and Vesselinovitch, D.: Animal models of regression. *In* Schettler, G., Goto, Y., Hata, Y., and Klose, G. (eds.): Atherosclerosis IV. Berlin, Springer-Verlag, 1977, p. 377.

204. Strong, J. P.: Atherosclerosis in Primates. (Prim. Med. Vol. 9.) Basel, Karger, 1976.

205. Gresham, G. A.: Primate Atherosclerosis. (Monogr. Atheros. Vol. 7.) Basel, Karger, 1976.

206. Bevans, M., Davidson, J. D., and Kendall, F. F.: Regression of lesions in canine arteriosclerosis. Arch. Pathol. 51:288, 1951.

207. Mahley, R. W., Innerarity, T. L., Weisgraber, K. H., and Fry, D. L.: Canine

hyperlipoproteinemia and atherosclerosis. Accumulation of lipid by aortic medial cells in vivo and in vitro. Am. J. Pathol. 87:205, 1977.

208. Lazzarini-Robertson, A., Butkus, A., Ehrhart, L. A., and Lewis, L. A.: Experimental arteriosclerosis in dogs. Evaluation of anatomopathological findings. Atherosclerosis 15:307, 1972.

209. McCullagh, K. G., and Ehrhart, L. A.: Increased arterial collagen synthesis in experimental canine atherosclerosis. Atherosclerosis 19:13, 1974.

210. Mahley, R. W., Weisgraber, K. H., and Innerarity, T.: Canine lipoproteins and atherosclerosis. II. Characterization of the plasma lipoproteins associated with atherogenic and nonatherogenic hyperlipidemia. Circ. Res. 35:722, 1974.

211. Wissler, R. W.: Recent progress in studies of experimental primate atherosclerosis. In Miras, C. J., Howard, A. N., and Paoletti, R. (eds.): Progress in Biochemical Pharmacology. Vol. 4. Basel, Karger, 1968, p. 378.

212. Scott, R. F., Morrison, E. S., Jarmolych, J., Nam, S. C., Kroms, M., and Coulston, F.: Experimental atherosclerosis in rhesus monkeys. I. Gross and light microscopy features and lipid values in serum and aorta. Exp. Mol. Pathol. 7:11, 1967.

213. Scott, R. F., Jones, R., Daoud, A. S., Zumbo, O., Coulston, F., and Thomas, W. A.: Experimental atherosclerosis in rhesus monkeys. II. Cellular elements of proliferative lesions and possible role of cytoplasmic degeneration in pathogenesis as studied by electron microscopy. Exp. Mol. Pathol. 7:34, 1967.

214. Armstrong, M. L., Connor, W. E., and Warner, E. D.: Tissue cholesterol concentration in the hypercholesterolemic rhesus monkey. Arch. Pathol. 87:81, 1969.

215. Tucker, C. F., Catsulis, C., Strong, J. P., and Eggen, D. A.: Regression of early cholesterol-induced aortic lesions in rhesus monkeys. Am. J. Pathol. 65:493, 1972.

216. Armstrong, M. L., and Warner, E. D.: Morphology and distribution of diet-induced atherosclerosis in rhesus monkeys. Arch. Pathol. 92:295, 1971.

217. Manning, P. J., Clarkson, T. B., and Lofland, H. B.: Cholesterol absorption, turnover, and excretion rates in hypercholesterolemic rhesus monkeys. Exp. Mol. Pathol. 14:75, 1971.

218. Manning, P. J., and Clarkson, T. B.: Development, distributions and lipid content of diet-induced atherosclerotic lesions of rhesus monkeys. Exp. Mol. Pathol. 17:38, 1972.

219. Eggen, D. A.: Cholesterol metabolism in rhesus monkey, squirrel monkey and baboon. J. Lipid Res. 15:139, 1974.

220. Taylor, C. B., Cox, G. E., Counts, M., and Yogi, N.: Fatal myocardial infarction in the rhesus monkey with diet-induced hypercholesterolemia. Am. J. Pathol. 35:674, 1959.

221. Taylor, C. B., Cox, G. E., Manalo-Estrella, P., Southworth, J., Patton, D. E., and Cathcart, C.: Atherosclerosis in rhesus monkeys. II. Arterial lesions associated with hypercholesteremia induced by dietary fat and cholesterol. Arch. Pathol. 74:16, 1962.

222. Taylor, C. B., Trueheart, R. E., and Cox, G. E.: Atherosclerosis in rhesus monkeys. III. The role of increased thickness of arterial walls in atherogenesis. Arch. Pathol. 76:14, 1963.

223. Cox, G. E., Trueheart, R. W., Kaplan, J., and Taylor, C. B.: Atherosclerosis in rhesus monkeys. IV. Repair of arterial injury—an important secondary atherogenic factor. Arch. Pathol. 76:166, 1963.

224. Taylor, C. B., Manalo-Estrella, P., and Cox, G. E.: Atherosclerosis in rhesus monkeys. V. Marked diet-induced hypercholesteremia with xanthomatosis and severe atherosclerosis. Arch. Pathol. 76:239, 1963.

225. Taylor, C. B., Patton, D. E., and Cox, G. E.: Atherosclerosis in rhesus monkeys. VI. Fatal myocardial infarction in a monkey fed fat and cholesterol. Arch. Pathol. 76:404, 1963.

226. Taylor, C. B.: Experimentally induced arteriosclerosis in nonhuman primates . In Roberts, J. C., Jr., and Straus, R. (eds.): Comparative Atherosclerosis. New York, Harper and Row, 1965, p. 215.

227. Vesselinovitch, D., Wissler, R. W., Schaffner, T. J., and Borensztajn, J.: The effects of various diets on atherogenesis in rhesus monkeys. Atherosclerosis 35:189, 1980.

228. Wissler, R. W., Frazier, L. W., Hughes, R. H., and Rasmussen, R. A.: Atherogenesis in the cebus monkey. I. A comparison of three food fats under controlled dietary conditions. Arch. Pathol. 74:312, 1962.

229. Malmros, H., and Sternby, N. H.: Induction of atherosclerosis in dogs by a thiouracil-free semi-synthetic diet containing cholesterol and hydrogenated coconut oil. In Miras, C. J., Howard, A. N., and Paoletti, R. (eds.): Progress in Biochemical Pharmacology. Vol. 4. Basel, Karger, 1968, p. 482.

230. Vesselinovitch, D., Getz, G. J., Hughes, R. H., and Wissler, R. W.: Atherosclerosis in the rhesus monkey fed three food fats. Atherosclerosis 20:303, 1974.

231. Gresham, G. A., and Howard, A. N.: The independent production of atherosclerosis and thrombosis in the rat. Br. J. Exp. Pathol. 41:395, 1960.

232. Imai, H., Lee, K. T., Pastori, S., Panlilio, E., Florentin, R., and Thomas, W. A.: Atherosclerosis in rabbits. Architectural and subcellular alterations of smooth muscle cells of aortas in response to hyperlipemia. Exp. Mol. Pathol. 5:273, 1966.

233. Florentin, R. A., and Nam, S. C.: Dietary-induced atherosclerosis in miniature swine. Exp. Mol. Pathol. 8:263, 1968.

234. Kritchevsky, D., Tepper, S. A., Vesselinovitch, D., and Wissler, R. W.: Cholesterol vehicle in experimental atherosclerosis. Part 11. Peanut oil. Atherosclerosis 14:53, 1971.

235. Kritchevsky, D., Tepper, S. A., Vesselinovitch, D., and Wissler, R. W.: Cholesterol vehicle in experimental atherosclerosis. Part 13. Randomized peanut oil. Atherosclerosis 17:225, 1973.

236. Kritchevsky, D., Muher, J. J., Marai, L., and Kuskis, A.: Aglycerol structure of peanut oils of different atherogenic potential. Lipids 12:775, 1977.

237. Kritchevsky, D., Tepper, S. A., Kim, H. K., Story, J. A., Vesselinovitch, D., and Wissler, R. W.: Experimental atherosclerosis in rabbits fed cholesterol-free diets. 5. Comparison of peanut, corn, butter and coconut oils. Exp. Mol. Pathol. 24:375, 1976.

238. Kritchevsky, D., Tepper, S. A., Scott, D. A., Klurfeld, D. M., Vesselinovitch, D., and Wissler, R. W.: Cholesterol vehicle in experimental atherosclerosis. 18. Comparison of North American, African and South American Peanut Oils. Atherosclerosis 38:291, 1981.

239. Jones, R. M., Hughes, R., Vesselinovitch, D., and Wissler, R. W.: Ultrastructural changes in the aortas of rhesus monkeys fed large quantities of food fats for short periods. Fed. Proc. 31:273, 1972.

240. Stary, H. C.: Cell proliferation and ultrastructural changes in regressing atherosclerotic lesions after reduction of serum cholesterol. In Schettler, G., and Weizel, A. (eds.): Atherosclerosis III. Berlin, Springer-Verlag, 1974, p. 187.

241. Strong, J. P.: Reversibility of fatty streaks in rhesus monkey. Primates Med. 9: 300, 1976.

242. Armstrong, M. L., Warner, F. D., and Connor, W. E.: Regression of coronary atheromatosis in rhesus monkeys. Circ. Res. 27:59, 1970.

243. Vesselinovitch, D., Wissler, R. W., Hughes, R., and Borensztajn, J.: Reversal of advanced atherosclerosis in rhesus monkeys. I. Light microscopic studies. Atherosclerosis 23:155, 1976.

244. Bond, M. G., Bullock, B. C., Clarkson, T. B., and Lehner, N. D.: The effect of plasma cholesterol concentrations on "regression" of primate atherosclerosis. Am. J. Pathol. 82:69a, 1976.

245. Armstrong, M. L.: Regression of atherosclerosis. In Paoletti, R., and Gotto, A. M., Jr. (eds.): Atherosclerosis Reviews. Vol. 1. New York, Raven Press, 1976, p. 137.

246. Katz, L. N., Stamler, J., and Pick, R.: Nutrition and Atherosclerosis. Philadelphia. Lea and Febiger, 1958.

247. Wissler, R. W., and Vesselinovitch, D.: Studies of regression of advanced atherosclerosis in experimental animals and man. In Atherogenesis (Proceedings of the 1st International Symposium). Ann. N.Y. Acad. Sci. 275: 363, 1976.

248. Vartiainen, T., and Kanerva, K.: Arteriosclerosis and wartime. Ann. Med. Intern. Fenn. 36:748, 1947.

249. Wilens, S. L.: The resorption of arterial atheromatous deposits in wasting disease. Am. J. Pathol. 23:793, 1947.

250. Vesselinovitch, D., and Wissler, R. W.: Comparison of primates and rabbits as animal models in experimental atherosclerosis. In Manning, G. W., and Haust, M. D. (eds.): Atherosclerosis: Metabolic, Morphologic and Clinical Aspects. (Advances in Experimental Medicine and Biology, Vol. 82.) New York, Plenum Press, 1977, p. 614.

251. Fritz, K. E., Augustyn, J. M., Jarmolych, J., Daoud, A. S., and Lee, K. T.: Regression of advanced atherosclerosis of swine (Chemical studies). Arch. Pathol. Lab. Med. 100:380, 1976.

252. Armstrong, M. L., and Megan, M. B.: Lipid depletion in atheromatous coronary arteries in rhesus monkeys after regression diets. Circ. Res. 30:675, 1972.

253. Wartman, A., Lampe, T. L., McCann, D. S., and Boyle, A. J.: Plaque reversal with MgEDTA in experimental atherosclerosis: Elastin and collagen metabolism. J. Atheros. Res. 7:331, 1967.

254. Kjeldsen, K., Astrup, P., and Wanstrup, J.: Reversal of rabbit atheromatosis by hyperoxia. J. Atheros. Res. 10:173, 1969.

255. Vesselinovitch, D., Wissler, R. W., Fischer-Dzoga, K., Hughes, R., and DuBien, L.: Regression of atherosclerosis in rabbits. I. Treatment with low fat diet, hyperoxia and hypolipidemic agents. Atherosclerosis 19:259, 1974.

256. Daoud, A. S., Jarmolych, J., Augustyn, J. M., Fritz, K. E., Singh, J. K., and Lee, K. T.: Regression of advanced atherosclerosis in swine. Arch. Pathol. Lab. Med. 100:372, 1976.

257. Vesselinovitch, D., Wissler, R. W., and Schaffner, T.: Quantitation of lesions during progression and regression of atherosclerosis in rhesus monkeys. In Naito, H. (ed.): Nutrition and Heart Disease. New York, S.P. Medical and Scientific Books, 1982, p. 121.

258. Vesselinovitch, D., and Wissler, R. W.: Correlation of types of induced lesions with regression of coronary atherosclerosis in two species of macaques. In Noseda, G., Fragiacomo, C., Fumagalli, R., and Paoletti, R. (eds.): Lipoproteins and Coronary Atherosclerosis. Amsterdam, Elsevier Publishing Co., 1982, p. 401.

259. Armstrong, M. L., and Megan, M. B.: Arterial fibrous proteins in cynomolgus monkeys after atherogenic and regression diets. Circ. Res. 36:256, 1975.

260. Armstrong, M. L.: Connective tissue in regression. In Paoletti, R., and Gotto, A. M. (eds.): Atherosclerosis Reviews. Vol. 3. New York, Raven Press, 1978 p. 147.

261. Armstrong, M. L.: Connective tissue changes in regression. In Schettler, G., Goto, Y., Hata, Y., and Klose, G. (eds.): Atherosclerosis IV. Berlin, Springer-Verlag, 1977, p. 405.

262. Weber, G., Fabbrini, P., Resi, L., Jones, R., Vesselinovitch, D., and Wissler, R. W.: Regression of arteriosclerotic lesions in rhesus monkey aortas after regression diet: Scanning and transmission electron microscope observations of the endothelium. Atherosclerosis 26:535, 1977.

263. Wissler, R. W., and Vesselinovitch, D.: The combined effects of cholestyramine and probucol on regression of atherosclerosis in rhesus monkey aortas. J. Appl. Pathol., July, 1983.

264. Wissler, R. W.: Current status of regression studies. In Paoletti, R., and

Gotto, A. M. (eds.): Atherosclerosis Reviews. Vol. 3. New York, Raven Press, 1978, p. 213.

265. Borensztajn, J., Foreman, K., Wissler, R. W., von Zutphen, H., Vesselinovitch, D., and Hughes, R.: Egress of aortic cholesterol and cholesterol ester during regression of atherosclerosis in rhesus monkeys. Circulation 52(Suppl. II):269, 1975.

266. Slater, H. R., Packard, C. J., Bicker, S., and Shepherd, J.: Effects of cholestyramine on receptor-mediated plasma clearance and tissue uptake of human low density lipoproteins in the rabbit. J. Biol. Chem. 255:10210, 1980.

267. Zelis, R., Mason, D. T., Braunwald, E., and Levy, R. I.: Effects of hyperlipoproteinemias and their treatment on the peripheral circulation. J. Clin. Invest. 49:1007, 1970.

268. Buchwald, H. L., Moore, R. B., and Varco, R. L.: Surgical treatment of hyperlipidemia. III. Clinical status of the partial ileal bypass operation. Circulation 49(Suppl. I):22, 1974.

269. Baltaxe, H. A., Amplatz, K., Varco, R. L., and Buchwald, H.: Coronary arteriography in hypercholesterolemic patients. Am. J. Roentgenol. Radium Ther. Nucl. Med. 105:784, 1969.

270. Knight, L., Scheibel, R., Amplatz, K., Varco, R. L., and Buchwald, H.: Radiographic appraisal of the Minnesota partial ileal bypass study. Surg. Forum 23:141, 1972.

271. Blankenhorn, D. H., Brooks, S., II., Selzer, R. H., Crawford, D. W., and Chin, H. P.: Assessment of atherosclerosis from angiographic images. Proc. Soc. Exp. Biol. Med. 145:1298, 1974.

272. Crawford, D. W., Beckenbach, E. S., Blankenhorn, D. H., Selzer, R. H., and Brooks, S. H.: Grading of coronary atherosclerosis: Comparison of a modified IAP visual grading method and a new quantitative angiographic technique. Atherosclerosis 19:231, 1974.

273. Blankenhorn, D. H.: Studies of regression/progression of atherosclerosis in man. In Manning, G. W., and Haust, M. D. (eds.): Atherosclerosis: Metabolic, Morphologic and Clinical Aspects. (Advances in Experimental Medicine and Biology, Vol. 82.) New York, Plenum Press, 1977, p. 453.

274. Buchwald, H., Moore, R. B., and Varco, R. L.: The partial ileal bypass operation in treatment of hyperlipemias. In Kritchevsky, D., Paoletti, R., and Holmes, W. (eds.): Lipids, Lipoproteins and Drugs. (Advances in Experimental Medicine and Biology, Vol 63.) New York, Plenum Press, 1975, p. 221.

275. Barndt, R., Jr., Blankenhorn, D. H., Crawford, D. W., and Brooks, S. H.: Regression and progression of early femoral atherosclerosis in treated hyperlipoproteinemic patients. Ann. Intern. Med. 86:139, 1977.

276. Malinow, M. R.: Regression of atherosclerosis in humans: Fact or myth? Circulation 64:1, 1981.

277. Blankenhorn, D. H.: Discussion, Chapter 23. In Bond, W. G., and Insull, W., Jr. (eds.): Clinical Diagnosis of atherosclerosis. Quantitative Methods of Evaluation. Mock, M. B.: Review of clinical studies on the quantification and progression of atherosclerosis. New York, Springer-Verlag, 1983.

278. Dorr, A. E., Gundersen, K. Schneider, J. C., Spencer, T. W., and Martin, W. B.: Colestipol hydrochloride in hypercholesterolemic patients: effect on serum cholesterol and mortality. J. Chron. Dis. 31:5, 1978.

279. Turpeinen, D.: Effect of cholesterol-lowering diet on mortality from coronary heart disease and other causes. Circulation 59:1, 1979.

280. Malinow, M. R., McLaughlin, P., Naito, H. K., Lewis, L. A., and McNulty, W. P.: Effect of alfalfa meal on shrinkage (regression) of atherosclerotic plaques during cholesterol feeding in monkeys. Atherosclerosis 30:27, 1978.

281. Malinow, M. R., McLaughlin, P., Papworth, L., Stafford, C., Kohler, G. O., Livingston, A. L., and Cheeke, P. R.: Effect of alfalfa saponins on intestinal cholesterol absorption in rats. Am. J. Clin. Nutr. 30:2061, 1977.

282. Kramsch, D. M., Chan, C. T., Aspen, A. J., and Wells, H.: Prevention and therapy of induced atherosclerosis in rabbits and monkeys by anticalcemic drugs regardless of serum cholesterol levels. In Hauss, W. H., Wissler, R. W., and Lehmann, R. (eds.): International Symposium: State of Prevention and Therapy in Human Arteriosclerosis and in Animal Models. Opladen, Westdeutscher Verlag, Vol. 63, 1978, p. 153.

283. Kramsch, D. M., Aspen, A. J., and Apstein, C. S.: Suppression of experimental atherosclerosis by the Ca^{++}-antagonist lanthanum. J. Clin. Invest. 65:967, 1980.

284. Kim, D. N., Lee, K. T., Reiner, J. M., and Thomas, W. A.: Effect of a soy protein product on serum and tissue cholesterol concentrations in swine fed high-fat, high-cholesterol diets. Exp. Mol. Pathol. 29:385, 1978.

285. Hamilton, R. M. G., and Carroll, K. K.: Plasma cholesterol levels in rabbits fed low fat, low cholesterol diets. Effects of dietary proteins, carbohydrates and fiber from different sources. Atherosclerosis 24:47, 1976.

286. Harris, W. S., Connor, W. E., and McMurry, M. P.: The comparative reductions of the plasma lipids and lipoproteins by dietary polyunsaturated fats: Salmon oil versus vegetable oil. Metabolism 32:179, 1983.

287. Harris, W. S., and Connor, W. E.: The effects of salmon oil upon plasma lipids, lipoproteins, and triglyceride clearance. Trans. Assoc. Am. Physicians 43:148, 1980.

288. Goodnight, S. J., Jr., Harris, W. S., Connor, W. E., and Illingworth, D. R.: Polyunsaturated fatty acids, hyperlipidemia, and thrombosis. Arteriosclerosis 2:87, 1982.

289. Veterans Administration Cooperative Study Group on Antihypertensive Agents: Effects of treatment on morbidity in hypertension. J.A.M.A. 213:1143, 1970.

290. Hypertension Detection and Follow-up Program Cooperative Group. Five-year findings of the Hypertension Detection and Follow-up Program. I. Reduction in mortality of persons with high blood pressure, including mild hypertension. J.A.M.A. 242:2562, 1979.

291. Rogot, E.: Smoking and mortality among U.S. veterans. J. Chron. Dis. 27:189, 1974.

292. The University Group Diabetes Program: A study of the effects of hypoglycemic agents on vascular complications in patients with adult-onset diabetes. I. Design, method and baseline results. Diabetes 19(Suppl. II):747, 1970.

293. Stamler, J.: Atherosclerotic coronary heart disease. In Sussman, K. E., and Metz, R. J. S. (eds.): Diabetes Mellitus. 4th ed. New York, American Diabetes Association, 1975, p. 229.

294. Morris, J. N., Heady, J. A., Raffle, P. A. B., Roberts, C. G., and Parks, J. W.: Coronary heart disease and physical activity of work. Lancet 2:1054, 1111, 1953.

295. Kirby, R. W., Anderson, J. W., Sieling, B., Rees, E. D., Chen, W. L., Miller, R. W., and Kay, R. M.: Oat-bran intake selectively lowers serum low-density lipoprotein cholesterol concentrations of hypercholesterolemic men. Am. J. Clin. Nutr. 34:824, 1981.

296. Spain, D. M., Bradess, V. A., Matero, A., and Taiter, R.: Sudden death due to coronary atherosclerotic heart disease. J.A.M.A. 207:1347, 1969.

297. Friedman, M., Manwaring, J. H., Rosenman, R. H., Donlon, G., Ortega, P., and Grube, S. M.: Instantaneous and sudden deaths. Clinical and pathological differentiation in coronary artery disease. J.A.M.A. 225:1319, 1973.

298. Miller, R. D., Burchell, H. B., and Edwards, J. E.: Myocardial infarction with and without coronary occlusion. Arch. Intern. Med. 88:597, 1951.

299. Schwartz, C. J., and Gerrity, R. G.: The anatomic pathology of sudden unexpected cardiac death. Circulation 52(Suppl. III):78, 1975.

300. Wissler, R. W.: Current concepts of coronary thrombosis as related to atherosclerosis in myocardial infarction. In Manning, G. W., and Haust, M. D. (eds.): Atherosclerosis: Metabolic, Morphologic and Clinical Aspects. (Advances in Experimental Medicine and Biology, Vol. 82.) New York, Plenum Press, 1977, p. 86.

301. Buja, L. M., Hillis, L. D., Petty, C. S., and Willerson, J. T.: The role of coronary arterial spasm in ischemic heart disease. Arch. Pathol. Lab Med. 105:221, 1981.

302. Chandler, A. B., Chapman, I., Erhardt, L. R., Roberts, W. C., Schwartz, C. J., Sinapius, D., Spain, D. M., Sherry, S., Ness, P. M., and Simon, T. L.: Coronary thrombosis in myocardial infarction. Report of a workshop on the role of coronary thrombosis in the pathogenesis of acute myocardial infarction. Am. J. Cardiol. 34:823, 1974.

303. Baum, R. S., Alvarez, H., III, and Cobb, L. A.: Survival after resuscitation from out-of-hospital ventricular fibrillation. Circulation 50:1231, 1974.

304. Gorlin, R.: Coronary Artery Disease. Philadelphia, W. B. Saunders Co., 1976.

305. Maseri, A., L'Abbate, A., Baroldi, G., Chierchia, S., Marzilli, M., Ballestra, A. M., Severi, S., Parodi, O., Biagini, A., Distante, A., and Pesola, A.: Coronary vasospasm as a possible cause of myocardial infarction. A conclusion derived from the study of "preinfarction" angina. N. Engl. J. Med. 299:1271, 1978.

306. Maseri, A., Severi, S., De Nes, M., L'Abbate, A., Chierchia, S., Marzilli, M., Ballestra, A. M., Parodi, O., Biagini, A., and Distante, A.: "Variant" angina: One aspect of a continuous spectrum of vasospastic myocardial ischemia. Pathogenetic mechanisms, estimated incidence and clinical and coronary arteriographic findings in 138 patients. Am. J. Cardiol. 42:1019, 1978.

307. Kligfield, P.: New concepts in ischemic heart disease: The role of coronary artery spasm. New York, Science and Medicine Publishing Co., 1979.

35

RISK FACTORS FOR CORONARY ARTERY DISEASE AND THEIR MANAGEMENT

by Robert I. Levy, M.D., and Manning Feinleib, M.D., Dr. P.H.

During the past half century, epidemiologists and vital statisticians have observed wide variations in the rate of occurrence of coronary artery disease (CAD) in regard to time, place, and person. CAD and its major clinical manifestation, myocardial infarction, was a medical rarity prior to the First World War.[1] This was due in part to the fact that myocardial infarction was only first described in 1912. During the 1920's and 1930's, it was recognized with increasing frequency as being a common problem among white men in urban areas of North America and Europe, particularly among the more affluent. By 1940, CAD was the leading cause of death in the United States and several other countries, and its frequency continued to increase through the 1950's.

In the late 1940's and early 1950's, several studies of free-living populations were begun to discern the factors associated with the occurrence of CAD and how the disease evolves and terminates in a total population. Clinical impressions were soon confirmed—CAD did not occur randomly in the population. Its rate of occurrence varied greatly according to such demographical factors as age, race, and sex. Personal attributes detectable by simple medical examination—high serum cholesterol, high blood pressure, hyperglycemia, and obesity—were found to increase the frequency of the disease. Personal habits which the patient could easily recognize himself—cigarette smoking, lack of exercise, and nutritional habits—were also investigated. More recently, some specific environmental hazards—carbon disulfide and oral contraceptives—have been associated with increased occurrence of CAD. Underlying these factors, familial and genetic effects are believed to play an inceptive role, in concert with their complex interrelationships with social and psychological factors.

EPIDEMIOLOGICAL STUDIES

Epidemiologists have used a variety of strategies to study the precursors of CAD, but two have been paramount: (1) comparison of CAD rates and associated characteristics of large population groups, such as differences between countries, racial groups, religious groups, or occupations; and (2) studies of characteristics of individuals and the relation of the development of CAD in these individuals to these characteristics. The first strategy is usually based on disease rates derived from vital statistics on mortality and from relatively crude data on group characteristics, e.g., diet. Data on vital statistics are prone to many uncertainties: varying fashions in the certification of causes of death; lack of standardization of evidence to be used in establishing diagnoses; and incompleteness of reporting. Yet these data, being based on large numbers, can document major differences in the death rates from CAD in different populations. More detailed clinical and autopsy studies have generally confirmed the major trends established by data on vital statistics.[2,3] Certain trends in vital statistics can be accounted for by deliberate changes in the manner of classifying data on death certificates, such as the major change introduced with the eighth revision of the International Classification of Diseases in the manner of coding hypertension.[4] This resulted in an apparent sharp rise in the death rates from CAD (or Ischemic Heart Disease, as it is officially designated in the ICD) from 1967 to 1968 and a compensating sharp decline in deaths attributed to hypertension.

The limitations of data on the relevant characteristics of populations are also legion, and only gross estimates of incidence can be obtained for such important factors as diet, cigarette smoking, or quality of medical care. Furthermore, large populations differ from one another in multiple unmeasurable characteristics that may play important roles in determining the overall rates of occurrence of CAD. Thus, comparisons between populations must be considered circumspectly; they may, however, suggest important clues for further research, corroborate broad hypotheses, or be useful for didactic purposes.

As observations and hypotheses regarding the occurrence and etiology of CAD accumulated during the 1920's and 1930's, the need to use a more organized and better controlled approach to studying its precursors and natural history became evident. Long-term prospective, population-based studies of individuals were considered the optimal strategy to acquire the necessary data. It was recognized that representative samples of several thousand persons would be needed; that these people would have to be examined while they were ostensibly healthy (i.e., before clinically overt CAD had become manifest); that carefully standardized examination procedures, questionnaires, and laboratory methods were required; and that diligent and careful surveillance of the entire group must be maintained for many years. With this general approach, numerous epidemiological studies involving tens of thousands of people have been undertaken in a variety of populations during the last three decades.

The Framingham Heart Study is perhaps the best known of these,[5] but major contributions have been made by many others, including those in the National Cooperative Pooling Project,[6,7] the Tecumseh Study,[8] the Western Collaborative Group Study,[9] the Seven Countries Study,[10] the Evans County Study,[11] the Puerto Rico Study,[12] the Ni-Hon-San Study of Japanese Men,[13] the Göteborg Study,[14] and the Paris Study.[15]

These prospective epidemiological studies started out by examining several thousand men who were free from clinical evidence of heart disease. (The Framingham, Tecumseh, and Evans County studies are among the few that studied women.) Each study attempted to include representative samples of populations defined by location or occupation. Considering the difficulties of such undertakings, all achieved satisfactorily high rates of cooperation. Each participant was examined for a variety of characteristics, including weight, blood pressure, blood composition, smoking habits, and electrocardiographical evidence of CAD. In some studies, many other variables were investigated, such as diet, exercise, behavioral characteristics, and social factors. Each study then followed the participants for several years, using repeated examinations and other surveillance procedures to document all deaths and all new cardiovascular disease developing in the cohorts.

Despite the large size and careful design of these studies, they cannot be considered to be formal scientific experiments. The variation in baseline characteristics occurred naturally, without any manipulation by the investigators, and was beyond their control and ken. There was no element of randomization in determining who had a high level and who had a low level of a particular trait. At best, these were "natural experiments" rather than controlled experiments. Because the factors, largely unknown, that may have led to the particular distribution of characteristics in the subjects might also be related to the occurrence of disease through other independent pathways, clear-cut causal relationships cannot be established by such studies.

Well-designed scientific experiments of causal hypotheses generally require, at the minimum, manipulation of the level of the causal factor (exposure) and random allocation of exposure to the participants in the study. This type of design is the one employed currently in the various prophylactic trials and intervention studies conducted by the National Heart, Lung, and Blood Institute to test various components of the "risk factor hypothesis." The hypothesis, therefore, must be considered to be resting on naturally occurring associations between traits and disease states, rather than being the outcome of controlled experimentation. Thus, we prefer to speak of the various traits studied in these epidemiological studies as "risk factors" or "predictors of disease," rather than as causes or etiological factors in the disease process. Although this may appear academic and overly cautious in view of the volume of evidence that has accumulated for some risk factors, it will serve to remind us that firm experimental confirmation is not yet available.

DEMOGRAPHICAL VARIATIONS IN FREQUENCY OF CAD

The frequency of occurrence of CAD and its mortality are known to vary according to the characteristics of person, place, and time. Comparison of mortality data based on age and sex for different places and over several decades provides insight into the evolution of CAD as the major health problem of most developed countries during the last 50 years.

In describing the demographical features of the occurrence of CAD, it would be desirable to have data for mortality (deaths from CAD) as well as morbidity (nonfatal CAD events). However, when dealing with national populations, only mortality data derived from routine death certificates are usually available. Morbidity data must be derived from special surveys (such as the Household Interview Survey), examinations (such as the Health and Nutrition Examination Survey), or searches of records (such as the Hospital Discharge Survey).[16-18]

When comparing mortality data for different subgroups of a population, one may first consider the absolute number of deaths from a specified cause occurring during a stated time period. Since the number of deaths obviously depends on the size of the population, its age structure, and other characteristics of the group, however, vital statisticians use various calculated rates to take these factors into account. The crude death rate for a specified cause is the absolute number of deaths from the specified cause during a year, divided by the size of the population at midyear. Thus, during 1979, there were a total of 551,365 deaths attributed to CAD in the United States. The estimated midyear population was 224,567,000, yielding a crude mortality rate for CAD of 245.5 per 100,000.[19] One may calculate mortality rates for specific subgroups of the population if one knows the numerator (the number of deaths in the specific subgroup from the cause of interest) and the denominator (the size of the specific subgroup). Thus, Table 35–1 shows the age-, sex-, and race-specific mortality rates from CAD in the U.S. from 1950 to 1977.

Occasionally, it may be necessary to compare mortality rates for populations of diverse age and sex distributions, e.g., in comparing the trends in the mortality rates of different countries or in one country at different points in time. To do this, vital statisticians commonly employ adjusted mortality rates or standardized ones. These are weighted averages of the age- and sex-specific mortality rates, using a standard, albeit arbitrary, set of weightings. Most commonly, a specified historical distribution of population is used as the standard weight, e.g., the 1940 distribution of population in the U.S. These standardized rates are also shown in Table 35–1.

Age.   The mortality of CAD shows a striking relationship to age in each sex and race group. Although quite rare in younger white women, the disease is aready a ma-

TABLE 35–1   ISCHEMIC HEART DISEASE DEATH RATES PER 100,000 POPULATION IN THE UNITED STATES

WHITE

	Men				Women			
AGE GROUP	1950*	1960*	1968†	1977†	1950*	1960*	1968†	1977†
35–44	77.5	86.0	87.6	59.8	13.2	12.7	16.3	11.1
45–54	323.1	352.5	350.0	266.9	66.6	61.9	72.8	56.5
55–64	812.9	901.3	945.2	715.1	267.5	277.6	283.7	216.9
65–74	1608.2	1909.2	2119.3	1642.8	838.9	916.3	998.3	704.8
Age-adjusted	259.5	305.3	336.5	264.7	120.6	137.8	160.8	119.0

NONWHITE

	Men				Women			
AGE GROUP	1950*	1960*	1968†	1977†	1950*	1960*	1968†	1977†
35–44	74.3	87.8	134.9	91.3	48.1	46.7	68.6	36.6
45–54	254.2	297.0	419.4	315.9	165.7	168.0	222.9	144.7
55–64	554.1	723.7	998.1	786.3	366.7	482.3	623.6	423.0
65–74	943.1	1340.2	1920.2	1435.5	656.8	807.0	1362.1	945.8
Age-adjusted	164.0	219.5	316.9	245.3	112.6	145.8	213.2	152.3

*7th Revision ICD Code 420.
†8th Revision ICD Code 410–413.
Crude comparability ratio $\frac{8th}{7th}$ = 1.1457.

jor cause of death for men aged 35 to 44 years. The mortality of CAD rapidly increases, so that by age 55 to 64, 35 per cent of all deaths among men are due to this single cause.

Sex. As shown in Table 35–1, the male mortality rates from CAD are much higher than those for females, for both whites and nonwhites. The ratios of the mortality rates of men to those of women are much higher for whites than nonwhites, however, and in both groups are higher at the younger ages than at older ages. Thus, among whites, in 1979, the male mortality rate from CAD was 5.2 times greater than in females at ages 35 to 44 and was 2.4 times as great at ages 65 to 74, whereas among nonwhites the respective ratios were 2.8 and 1.6. As an approximation, the female rates lag behind the male rates by about 10 years among whites and by about 7 years among nonwhites.

Race. The differences in the mortality of CAD between whites and nonwhites have not been wholly consistent during the last 30 years. Nonwhite men tended to have lower rates than white men prior to 1968, but since then they have had higher rates up to the age of 65. Nonwhite women have tended to have higher rates than white women throughout this period.

Among specific ethnic groups in the United States, Japanese men in Hawaii and California and men in Puerto Rico have been found to have about half the amount of CAD as Caucasians.[20]

Geography. Mortality rates from CAD vary both between different countries and within countries. Figure 35–1 shows the mortality rates in the United States. Marked regional differences can be noted. High mortality rates occur in those states along the southeastern Atlantic Coast and in the industrialized states of the Midwest and Northeast. The lowest rates are found in the Great Plains and mountain states. These rather clear regional differences have not been adequately explained, although some relationships have been found with ecological factors. Climatic variables have also been implicated to some degree: Extremes of temperature and snowfall have been related to increased

mortality rates.[21] Altitude, either directly or via other factors, may play a role; areas at highest altitudes tend to have lower rates of CAD.[22]

A positive association has been reported between the *hardness of drinking water* and local mortality rates from heart disease in the U.S., Great Britain, and Canada, but inconsistent relationships have been found with the content of trace elements in the water.[23–25] One constituent of water in particular that has been studied extensively is artificial fluoride. In a study of all U.S. cities with more than 25,000 people between 1945 and 1969, no association was found between the introduction of artificial fluoride to the water supply and changes in mortality of heart disease.[26]

International differences in mortality of CAD are also striking (Table 35–2). It should be noted, however, that reliable data are lacking for most of the countries of Asia, Africa, and Latin America. It is believed that CAD is uncommon in most nonindustrialized countries, so that it is safe to assume, on the basis of the data available, that there is at least a 10-fold variation in the international rates of death from CAD. As with the regional differences within the United States, these international differences have not been satisfactorily explained. Comparative autopsy studies and standardized investigations in different countries show that these differences are not simply artifacts of varying practices in death certification.[2,3,10,26] It might be speculated that these differences can be accounted for by genetic factors. Thus, one is struck by the finding that after Finland, the next seven countries with highest mortality from CAD are the major English-speaking countries of the world. However, studies of migrants and of people of similar ethnic backgrounds in different countries point to *environmental* factors as being of major importance.[13,27,28] Furthermore, there have been marked changes in mortality rates from CAD over time that cannot be explained by sudden changes in the genetic structure of the populations.[29,30,31]

The mortality from CAD in Japan and the experience of the Japanese in different areas of the world provide interesting material for speculation about the possible roles of

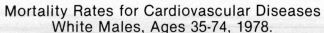

Mortality Rates for Cardiovascular Diseases
White Males, Ages 35-74, 1978.

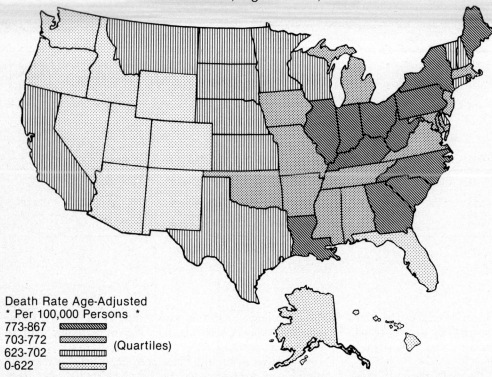

FIGURE 35–1   Mortality rates for cardiovascular diseases, white males, ages 35 to 74, 1978.

Death Rate Age-Adjusted
* Per 100,000 Persons *
773-867
703-772   (Quartiles)
623-702
0-622

genetics and environment. The low CAD rates in Japan, even after some allowance for differences in death certification, indicate that industrialization need not be automatically associated with high rates of heart disease. However, Japanese in Hawaii and California have almost twice the rate of CAD as do Japanese in Japan, but still only about half the CAD rate of U.S. Caucasians. Thus, the experience of Japanese in the United States indicates that although environmental factors may play a major role, they cannot account for all the differences between certain groups.[13,20,32]

Time Trends. Table 35–1 also shows that mortality rates from CAD have varied over time. After a general increase in mortality rates for all age-sex-race groups in the U.S. through the 1950's, there was a leveling off of the rates for most subgroups through the 1960's. Since 1968, however, there has been a steady and dramatic decline in the death rate for each subgroup. The U.S. adjusted mor-

TABLE 35–2   DEATH RATES FOR CORONARY HEART DISEASE AND ALL CAUSES IN 1977 FOR SELECTED COUNTRIES: MEN, AGES 55 TO 64*

Country	CORONARY HEART DISEASE		ALL CAUSES	
	1977	Per cent Change 1969–1977	1977	Per cent Change 1969–1977
Finland	996.9**	−3.8	2398.6**	−12.3
Northern Ireland	925.0	+11.4	2199.1	−0.1
Scotland	899.8	−0.3	2265.1	−8.5
Australia	730.9	−20.2	1815.6	−15.1
New Zealand	766.6†	−10.0	1887.2†	−6.4
U.S.A. (White)	715.1	−22.2	1848.9	−16.1
England and Wales	710.8	+0.3	1877.4	−13.2
Canada	697.0**	−5.6	1834.4**	−1.5
Israel	513.0	−24.5	1518.5	−8.5
Norway	570.5	−9.1	1466.3	−9.7
Denmark	578.2	+7.0	1613.6	−3.2
Sweden	563.6	+15.8	1411.8	−1.9
Netherlands	519.8	+2.4	1584.9	−7.9
German Federal Republic	462.5	−0.4	1806.6	−17.0
Hungary	477.3††	+11.4	2125.0††	+8.1
Austria	442.8	+0.3	1857.5	−15.5
Italy	326.6††	+6.1	1804.4††	−7.6
Switzerland	321.1	+5.9	1460.0	−15.9
Japan	94.8	−22.4	1284.8	−25.6

*Per 100,000 population.
**Rates for 1975.
†Rates for 1976.
†† Rates for 1974.

tality rate from CAD has fallen 26.5 per cent from 1968 to 1978 (Fig. 35–2). In most other countries, CAD rates are continuing to increase or are showing considerably smaller declines. The reasons for the decline in the U.S. are still speculative, but there is some evidence that much of it can be associated with changes in habits and life styles that may decrease the average person's risk for CAD.[30-36]

ATHEROSCLEROTIC RISK FACTORS

In order to uncover individual characteristics that are related to the occurrence of CAD, it is necessary to turn from studies of vital statistics to studies of individual people. Epidemiological studies of free-living populations followed for many years have identified specific characteristics of people and some personal habits that are strongly related to the chance of developing CAD. These bodily characteristics and personal habits have been called "risk factors" for CAD.

An example of the relationship between risk factors and the chance of developing disease is given in Figure 35–3. This figure is based on data from the Framingham Heart Study, but its main features have been confirmed in virtually all the studies cited previously.[37-40] Figure 35–3 shows the probability of developing CAD in 8 years according to sex and age. For each sex, three risk categories are shown, as defined by four characteristics of the individual: systolic blood pressure, serum cholesterol level, cigarette smoking, and evidence of glucose intolerance. The wide differences in the chances of developing CAD among these risk categories is a measure of our ability to identify, while they are still healthy, those men and women who are most prone to develop clinical disease.

Figure 35–3 shows the combined effects of all four risk

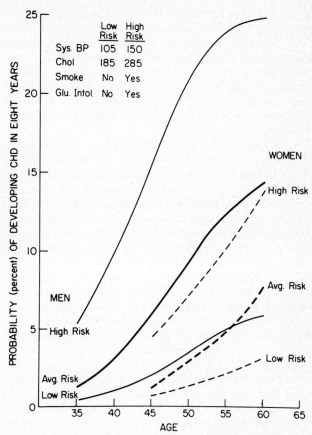

FIGURE 35–3   Probability of developing CAD in eight years according to age, sex, and risk category (The Framingham Heart Study).

factors for CAD, determined by using a multivariate logistic regression model (discussed later). Similar analyses have been done for each factor separately. These show that each of the four risk factors indicated makes a separate and significant contribution to the risk of developing CAD. Following is a brief discussion of each of the major risk factors taken individually and then a consideration of their cumulative effects.

Blood Lipids (See also p. 1628)

Among the numerous recognized risk factors for the development of atherosclerosis, one of the best documented is the association between blood lipids and CAD.[6] The evidence of the association between serum cholesterol level and CAD is extensive and unequivocal.[41-44] It is derived from a variety of sources, including (1) production of atherosclerotic lesions in animals by use of hypercholesterolemia-inducing diets; (2) the nature and dynamics of the human atherosclerotic plaque (see Chapter 34); (3) the occurrence of hyperlipidemia in groups of subjects with clinically manifested atherosclerotic disease; (4) the study of genetic hyperlipidemias associated with premature CAD; and (5) epidemiological studies of populations with differing serum cholesterol levels. Although triglyceride levels have been associated with CAD in several cross-sectional studies, prospective studies remain inconclusive in their indictment of serum triglycerides as a coronary risk factor.[45-47] In sharp contrast, evidence from several prospective studies clearly establishes that in an otherwise healthy population, the risk

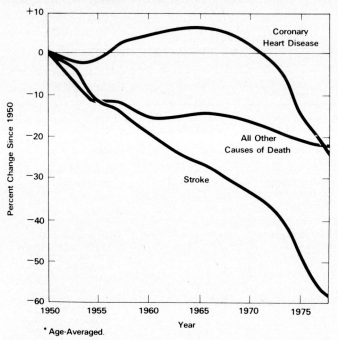

FIGURE 35–2   Per cent change in death rates since 1950 for CAD, stroke, and all other causes, ages 35 to 74, United States, 1950 to 1978. (From Levy, R. I.: Declining mortality in coronary heart disease. Arteriosclerosis 7:312, 1981.)

of CAD is directly related to the concentration of plasma cholesterol.[10,48,49] The accuracy of predicting the risk of CAD according to cholesterol concentrations is, however, greater in the young (younger than age 65) than in the elderly. One of the most important results of these studies is the demonstration that subjects with the highest cholesterol levels are at a greater risk of developing CAD, but even those with the lowest levels are not completely immune to the disease.[50]

As indicated later in this discussion, it has become evident that even more information can be obtained by measuring the plasma cholesterol in terms of the units of lipid transport—the lipoproteins—than by simply calculating total cholesterol. Until long-term data in relation to specific levels of lipoprotein accumulate, however, definition of cardiovascular risk must be based on the evidence relating to total cholesterol obtained during the past three decades.

The continuous relationship between cholesterol levels and the incidence of CAD is of the utmost importance. When considering CAD risk, there is little justification for using the gaussian distribution to define "normal" levels. It must be appreciated that the higher the cholesterol level, the greater the need for concern; but no single level of plasma cholesterol separates those at risk from those who are not.

It is important for the clinician to realize that for differential diagnosis and effective treatment of disorders of lipid transport associated with marked elevations of cholesterol or triglycerides, or both, systems currently exist that use arbitrary limits (usually the 90th or 95th percentile) of cholesterol, low-density lipoprotein, and triglycerides. A clear distinction should exist between these arbitrary limits used to define "types" of hyperlipoproteinemia and the concept of cholesterol as a risk factor.

TRANSLATING HYPERCHOLESTEROLEMIA INTO HYPERLIPOPROTEINEMIA. The major plasma

lipids, including cholesterol and triglyceride, do not circulate freely in solution in the blood but rather are transported in the form of lipoprotein complexes (Table 35–3).[51] The major lipoprotein families—chylomicrons, very low-density lipoproteins (VLDL), low-density lipoproteins (LDL), and high-density lipoproteins (HDL)—are usually conveniently classified in terms of physicochemical properties such as density or electrophoretic mobility.[52] Sufficient elevation in the concentration of any of the lipoprotein families can result in hypercholesterolemia. Similarly, hypertriglyceridemia can result from increased concentrations of chylomicrons, VLDL, or IDL (intermediate-density lipoproteins) alone or in various combinations.

Plasma concentrations of LDL correlate closely with plasma concentrations of cholesterol, as would be expected, since 60 to 75 per cent of the total plasma cholesterol is normally transported in this lipoprotein. They thus have more or less the same predictive capability.

HDL, which normally accounts for 20 to 25 per cent of the total plasma cholesterol, is also a potent risk factor for CAD. Whereas LDL cholesterol is directly related to risk, however, HDL shows an indirect relationship. In spite of numerous studies in the past that demonstrated this inverse relationship between HDL and atherosclerosis, HDL is only now becoming part of a standard coronary risk profile. Gordon et al. have shown that in both men and women older than the age of 50 years, HDL cholesterol has the strongest relationship to CAD.[53] They suggest that HDL should be integrated into the risk profile for CAD, together with LDL and VLDL, and that this inclusion would greatly improve our ability to predict CAD.

THE LIPOPROTEINS

Chylomicrons. Chylomicrons are composed primarily of triglycerides and originate from exogenous dietary fat in the intestine. Seventy to 100 gm of dietary fat are trans-

TABLE 35–3   BIOCHEMICAL AND CLINICAL FEATURES OF LIPOPROTEINS

FAMILY	ORIGIN	FUNCTION	CATABOLISM	PLASMA APPEARANCE	CLINICAL FEATURES OF ELEVATED LEVEL
Chylomicrons	Intestine, from dietary fat	Transport of dietary fat	Lipoprotein lipase at tissue sites; chylomicron remnant cleared by liver	Creamy supernate; clear infranate	Eruptive xanthoma; lipemia retinalis; organomegaly; pancreatitis
VLDL	Liver and small bowel, from carbohydrates, free fatty acids, medium-chain triglycerides	Transport of endogenus triglycerides	Complex; probably requires lipoprotein lipase for degradation	Turbid serum	Glucose intolerance; hyperuricemia
IDL	VLDL	Unknown	Unclear; degradation to LDL	Turbid serum	Glucose intolerance; hyperuricemia; premature atherosclerosis; tuboeruptive, tendinous, and palmar planar xanthoma
LDL	VLDL; IDL (? alternative source)	Unknown	Primary site and removal unclear	Clear	Premature atherosclerosis; corneal arcus; tendinous and tuberous xanthoma; xanthelasma
HDL	? Intestine ? Liver	? Facilitates cholesterol ester and triglyceride metabolism	? Liver	Clear	No associated abnormality

ported from the intestine to sites of utilization and storage each day. Chylomicrons are usually absent in plasma after 12 to 14 hours of fasting. Their presence in fasting plasma should always be considered abnormal. When present, these large particles produce turbidity and, upon standing in a cold test tube 24 to 40 hours, will rise as a creamy layer to the top of the tube. When chylomicronemia is present, the cholesterol/triglyceride ratio in the plasma can be as high as 1:20. Even marked chylomicronemia has not been associated with premature CAD.

Very Low-Density Lipoproteins (VLDL). VLDL are composed primarily of triglyceride, derived endogenously from the liver and small intestine. The cholesterol/triglyceride ratio in this class of lipoproteins is normally about 1:5. Between 15 and 25 gm of VLDL glyceride are released into the bloodstream daily. Diets high in carbohydrate will invariably increase triglyceride levels, at least transiently. Other factors that contribute to the lability of VLDL triglyceride levels include changes in weight, alcohol intake, stress, and exercise.

Although sustained elevation of VLDL has sometimes been associated with premature atherosclerosis, epidemiological evidence of the relationship of plasma triglycerides to CAD is less clear.[47,54-59] One of the difficulties is in distinguishing an elevated level of triglycerides as a separate risk factor from the hypertension, obesity, and glucose intolerance that often accompany it.

Intermediate-Density Lipoproteins (IDL). Intermediate-density lipoproteins are essentially a transitional form in the catabolism of VLDL to LDL. Their average cholesterol content is 30 per cent, and the triglyceride content is 40 per cent. There is evidence that IDL may be identical in form to the abnormal lipoprotein that characterizes Type III hyperlipoproteinemia, but further confirmation of this is needed. In Type III hyperlipoproteinemia, excess levels of IDL-like particles are associated with premature coronary and peripheral vessel disease.[59]

Low-Density Lipoproteins (LDL). It is now known that LDL are the product of the intravascular metabolism of the glyceride-rich lipoprotein, VLDL.[60,61] One of the major functions of VLDL is to transport glyceride through the plasma. It is then catabolized rapidly to an intermediate form (IDL) and ultimately to LDL. Thus, subjects with increased LDL in the plasma are accumulating the remnants of the metabolism of VLDL. The increase may be due either to overproduction of VLDL (which is uncommon) or to a defective clearance of LDL.

LDL as a molecule is approximately 50 per cent cholesterol by weight. Thus, a patient with an elevated level of LDL will usually have an increased level of cholesterol. The other lipoproteins—chylomicrons, VLDL, and HDL—also contain cholesterol, but in lesser amounts than LDL. The major reason for measuring LDL is that this lipoprotein has been most directly associated with CAD.[54,63] In a population with "normal" levels of LDL, a comparison of levels below 119 mg/dl with levels above 150 mg/dl (equivalent to a plasma cholesterol level of approximately 230 mg/dl) reveals a clear difference in the rates of cardiovascular events.[64] Subjects with high levels of LDL more often have CAD, measured as either overt heart attacks or other events, such as angina. Thus, even in a normal population, the higher levels of LDL carry a greater risk of vascular disease.

High-density Lipoproteins (HDL). Exciting recent findings have focused attention on the high-density lipoproteins. The role of HDL in lipid transport is unclear. It may serve to remove cholesterol from tissues or, alternatively, to accept it during VLDL metabolism in vivo. Unlike the atherogenic LDL, HDL has been *inversely* associated with CAD risk.[65-67] Moreover, the negative correlation between HDL cholesterol and CAD is independent of other risk factors.[53,64,67] Earlier reports that healthy men have higher levels of HDL than men with CAD were largely ignored, inexplicably, until a 1975 review of the evidence thrust HDL into the forefront of lipoprotein research.[65] Mounting epidemiological findings support the tempting hypothesis that increased concentrations of HDL may be a protective factor in the development of vascular disease. The cause and effect of the inverse relationship between HDL and CAD remains unclear, however. Levels of HDL have been correlated positively with exercise and moderate ingestion of alcohol and inversely related to obesity, smoking, poor control of diabetes, and the use of progestin-containing contraceptives.[68,69] The results of a recent study show that the prevalence of CAD at HDL levels of 30 mg/dl was *double* that at 60 mg/dl.[66] Mean values of HDL cholesterol were lower in subjects with CAD. *These findings provide a cogent reason to determine whether elevated cholesterol levels are due to increases in LDL or HDL.* Familial excesses of HDL or deficiencies of LDL have been associated with decreased risk of CAD.[70]

DISTRIBUTION OF PLASMA LIPIDS AND LIPOPROTEINS. The variability in plasma lipids and lipoproteins precludes the establishment of universally acceptable limits. What may be considered normal for one population group may not necessarily be applicable to another. Even within a country, these "normal" limits may vary from one region to another and are markedly age- and sex-dependent.

The relative contribution of genetic and environmental factors to the distribution curve for concentration of cholesterol cannot be assessed with certainty in any population. However, studies of families and twins have shown that genetic components (including polygenic effects as well as the mutant allele responsible for familial hypercholesterolemia) may account for as much as 40 per cent of the total variability. On the other hand, environmental factors, although not clearly understood, also markedly influence the variability in the distribution of concentrations of cholesterol between populations. For example, immigrants who come to the U.S. from countries where the mean level of cholesterol is low usually acquire the high levels characteristic of North America. Nutritional factors have important effects upon the metabolism of lipids and probably play a dominant role in the pathogenesis of the mild hypercholesterolemia so commonly found in Western populations.

The Lipid Research Clinics (LRC) Program recently completed a series of surveys that have yielded data of interest to both epidemiologists and clinicians. These surveys were conducted to determine the prevalence of hyperlipidemias and the distribution of various levels of lipids and lipoproteins in 11 North American populations.[71,72] The resulting data are of particular interest because of the size and diversity of the populations studied: Triglyceride and cholesterol levels were determined for more than 70,000 in-

TABLE 35–4 TOTAL PLASMA CHOLESTEROL (mg/dl) IN 11 FREE-LIVING NORTH AMERICAN WHITE POPULATIONS*

	MALES (n = 3580)			FEMALES (n = 3413)		
		Percentiles			Percentiles	
AGE	Mean ± SEM	10TH	90TH	Mean ± SEM	10TH	90TH
5–9	155.3 ± 1.8	131	183	164.0 ± 1.8	135	189
10–14	160.9 ± 1.5	132	191	160.1 ± 1.5	131	191
15–19	153.1 ± 1.4	123	183	159.5 ± 1.6	126	198
20–24	162.2 ± 2.5	126	197	170.3 ± 2.5	132	220
25–29	178.7 ± 2.1	137	223	179.5 ± 1.7	142	217
30–34	193.1 ± 1.8	152	237	179.2 ± 1.7	141	215
35–39	200.6 ± 1.9	157	248	189.6 ± 2.1	149	233
40–44	205.2 ± 1.9	161	251	197.5 ± 1.9	156	241
45–49	213.4 ± 1.9	171	258	206.2 ± 2.0	162	256
50–54	213.2 ± 1.9	168	263	217.3 ± 2.4	171	267
55–59	215.0 ± 2.2	172	260	228.7 ± 2.4	182	278
60–64	216.6 ± 3.3	170	262	232.2 ± 3.7	186	282
65–69	221.0 ± 3.8	174	275	234.1 ± 4.0	179	282
70+	210.3 ± 3.4	160	253	224.5 ± 2.8	181	268

*From Lipid Research Clinics Population Studies Data Book. Vol. 1. The Prevalence Study. Washington, D.C., U.S. Department of Health and Human Services, Public Health Service. NIH Publ. No. 80-1527, 1980.

TABLE 35–5 PLASMA TRIGLYCERIDES (mg/dl) IN 11 FREE-LIVING NORTH AMERICAN WHITE POPULATIONS*

	MALES (n = 3580)			FEMALES (n = 3413)		
		Percentiles			Percentiles	
AGE	Mean ± SEM	10TH	90TH	Mean ± SEM	10TH	90TH
5–9	51.9 ± 1.7	34	70	63.8 ± 2.5	37	103
10–14	63.4 ± 1.6	37	94	72.0 ± 1.7	44	104
15–19	78.2 ± 2.4	43	125	72.8 ± 1.9	40	112
20–24	89.3 ± 3.7	50	146	87.3 ± 2.9	42	135
25–29	104.2 ± 4.2	51	171	87.4 ± 2.8	45	137
30–34	122.1 ± 3.7	57	214	86.0 ± 2.8	45	140
35–39	140.8 ± 5.5	58	250	98.3 ± 3.2	47	170
40–44	152.4 ± 6.9	69	252	98.1 ± 2.6	51	161
45–49	143.4 ± 5.9	65	218	112.5 ± 3.4	55	180
50–54	153.4 ± 5.5	75	244	116.0 ± 3.4	58	190
55–59	134.3 ± 4.2	70	210	133.1 ± 4.8	65	229
60–64	130.6 ± 8.7	65	193	132.1 ± 9.1	66	210
65–69	138.6 ± 11.1	61	227	136.5 ± 6.8	64	221
70+	132.8 ± 7.2	71	202	128.3 ± 6.5	68	189

*From Lipid Research Clinics Population Studies Data Book. Vol. 1. The Prevalence Study. Washington, D.C., U.S. Department of Health and Human Services, Public Health Service. NIH Publ. No. 80-1527, 1980.

TABLE 35–6 PLASMA LDL CHOLESTEROL (mg/dl) IN 11 FREE-LIVING NORTH AMERICAN WHITE POPULATIONS*

	MALES (n = 3540)			FEMALES (n = 3413)		
		Percentiles			Percentiles	
AGE	Mean ± SEM	10TH	90TH	Mean ± SEM	10TH	90TH
5–9	92.5 ± 1.8	69	117	100.4 ± 2.1	73	125
10–14	96.8 ± 1.4	73	123	97.4 ± 1.3	73	126
15–19	94.4 ± 1.3	68	123	95.7 ± 1.5	66	129
20–24	103.3 ± 2.4	73	138	103.7 ± 2.2	65	141
25–29	116.7 ± 1.9	75	157	110.2 ± 1.6	75	148
30–34	126.4 ± 1.6	88	166	111.3 ± 1.5	77	146
35–39	133.2 ± 1.7	92	176	119.7 ± 2.0	81	161
40–44	135.6 ± 1.6	98	173	125.1 ± 1.8	84	165
45–49	143.7 ± 1.8	106	185	129.4 ± 1.9	89	173
50–54	142.3 ± 1.7	102	185	138.1 ± 2.3	94	186
55–59	145.8 ± 2.1	103	191	146.1 ± 2.4	97	199
60–64	146.3 ± 3.1	106	188	152.0 ± 3.6	105	191
65–69	150.4 ± 3.5	104	199	153.8 ± 4.1	99	205
70+	142.9 ± 2.9	100	182	148.6 ± 2.7	108	189

*From Lipid Research Clinics Population Studies Data Book. Vol. 1. The Prevalence Study. Washington, D.C., U.S. Department of Health and Human Services, Public Health Service. NIH Publ. No. 80-1527, 1980.

dividuals, and lipoprotein determinations were done for approximately 25 per cent of that group. Although the populations studied were not necessarily statistically representative of the entire North American population, they were well-defined, diverse target groups that (1) spanned a range of ethnic, geographical, socioeconomic, occupational, and age groups; and (2) were studied according to highly standardized procedures. Tables 35–4 to 35–7 give the means and selected percentiles of the distributions of plasma lipids and lipoproteins determined in the LRC Study.[73]

THE EVALUATION OF HYPERLIPOPROTEINEMIA

The lack of specificity of hypercholesterolemia and hypertriglyceridemia makes their translation into hyperlipoproteinemia useful for both differential diagnosis and treatment. Five patterns (types) of hyperlipoproteinemia have been described (Table 35–8).[51,54,74] Each is a "shorthand" or jargon term that describes which lipoproteins are increased in the plasma. Since all the lipoprotein families have a relatively fixed composition, and since two of them refract light and produce turbidity, defining hyperlipoproteinemia usually only requires a look at the standing plasma (after storage overnight at 4°C) and an accurate and precise measurement of cholesterol and triglyceride levels (see Table 35–3). Hyperchylomicronemia can be differentiated from increased VLDL (both of which produce hypertriglyceridemia) by noting the appearance of the plasma. A creamy layer over a clear infranatant is generally diagnostic of Type I. In cases of hyperbetalipoproteinemia (Type IIA), the cholesterol level is elevated, and the plasma is clear. Turbid plasma may be observed in Types IIB, III, IV, and V. There may be a separate creamy layer of chylomicrons in Types III and V.

Sometimes, additional procedures such as ultracentrifugation or the determination of concentrations of HDL (or both) may be necessary to establish the type of lipoprotein. Electrophoresis is not usually necessary for the translation of hyperlipidemia into hyperlipoproteinemia. Frequently, the type of lipoprotein can be related to the patient's history and the clinical features of the disease.

TABLE 35–7 PLASMA HDL CHOLESTEROL (mg/dl) IN 11 FREE-LIVING NORTH AMERICAN WHITE POPULATIONS*

	MALES (n = 3573)			FEMALES (n = 3407)		
		Percentiles			Percentiles	
AGE	Mean ± SEM	10TH	90TH	Mean ± SEM	10TH	90TH
5–9	55.8 ± 1.0	43	70	53.2 ± 1.0	38	67
10–14	54.9 ± 0.7	40	71	52.2 ± 0.7	40	64
15–19	46.1 ± 0.6	34	59	52.3 ± 0.7	38	68
20–24	45.4 ± 1.0	32	57	53.3 ± 1.0	37	72
25–29	44.7 ± 0.7	32	58	56.0 ± 0.8	39	74
30–34	45.5 ± 0.6	32	59	56.0 ± 0.7	40	73
35–39	43.5 ± 0.6	31	58	55.0 ± 0.8	38	75
40–44	44.2 ± 0.6	31	60	57.8 ± 0.9	39	79
45–49	45.5 ± 0.6	33	60	59.4 ± 1.0	41	82
50–54	44.1 ± 0.6	31	58	62.0 ± 1.0	41	84
55–59	47.6 ± 0.9	31	54	62.2 ± 1.1	41	85
60–64	51.5 ± 1.3	34	69	63.8 ± 1.4	44	87
65–69	51.1 ± 1.5	33	74	63.3 ± 1.8	38	85
70+	50.5 ± 1.7	33	70	60.7 ± 1.4	38	82

*From Lipid Research Clinics Population Studies Data Book. Vol. 1. The Prevalence Study. Washington, D.C., U.S. Department of Health and Human Services, Public Health Service. NIH Publ. No. 80-1527, 1980.

TABLE 35–8   TYPES OF HYPERLIPOPROTEINEMIA

	FEATURES	SECONDARY CAUSES
Type I	Increased chylomicrons	Insulinopenic diabetes mellitus Dysglobulinemia Lupus erythematosus
Type IIA	Increased LDL	Nephrotic syndrome Hypothyroidism
Type IIB	Increased LDL and VLDL	Obstructive liver disease Porphyria Multiple myeloma
Type III	Increased IDL	Hypothyroidism Dysgammaglobulinemia
Type IV	Increased VLDL	Diabetes mellitus Nephrotic syndrome Pregnancy Hormone use Glycogen storage disease Alcoholism Gaucher disease Niemann-Pick disease
Type V	Increased chylomicrons and VLDL	Insulinopenic diabetes mellitus Nephrotic syndrome Alcoholism Myeloma Idiopathic hypercalcemia

Simple quantitative techniques can determine whether an elevated cholesterol level is due to an increased amount of LDL or to other lipoproteins. In the absence of chylomicrons, only three forms of lipoproteins are present in the plasma—VLDL, LDL, and HDL. Since VLDL is the primary triglyceride-carrying form in the fasting patient, one can approximate its concentration by dividing the amount of plasma triglyceride by 5 (based on the triglyceride/cholesterol ratio of VLDL).[75] HDL cholesterol can be measured directly with a very simple precipitation technique.[76] LDL may be calculated by using a formula based on cholesterol (C) and triglyceride (TG) values:

$$C - LDL = total\ C - [TG/5 + (C - HDL)].$$

A few facts must be remembered for measurement of lipid or lipoprotein levels to be most useful:

1. Reliable measurements of plasma lipids are not routinely obtained in many laboratories. Results from laboratories that employ convenience techniques, or even multiphasic automated procedures, are often imprecise and inaccurate. Many large automated laboratories are employing techniques that yield values 10 to 40 per cent higher than those obtained with the standard Abel-Kendall procedure for determining cholesterol. The particular method being used must be known, and allowance must be made for any systematic difference in accuracy that occurs in comparison with the standard procedure.

2. The concentrations of lipids and lipoproteins increase with age. A value for cholesterol that is acceptable in a person 40 to 50 years old might be alarmingly high in a 10-year-old child. Hyperlipoproteinemia of one type or another is usually somewhat arbitrarily defined in terms of the level of a lipid or lipoprotein. The diagnosis of Type II or hyperbetalipoproteinemia, for example, requires the finding of an age-adjusted level of LDL cholesterol that is greater than the 95th percentile. Hyperprebetalipoproteinemia (Type IV) requires a value for plasma triglyceride that is greater than the 95th percentile as well as the ab-

sence of chylomicrons. It must be appreciated, however, that the presence of a level of LDL cholesterol or triglyceride lower than the cut-off points used to define hyperlipoproteinemia does not indicate absence of risk. As already noted, a continuous relationship has been shown between the level of plasma (and LDL) cholesterol and the risk of occurrence of atherosclerotic events.

3. Chylomicrons normally appear in the blood 2 to 10 hours after a meal; thus, a fasting specimen (12 to 16 hours after eating) is necessary to exclude this potentially confounding influence.

4. Concentrations of lipoproteins are under dynamic metabolic control and are easily affected by diet, illness, drugs, and weight gain and loss. The level of lipoproteins in the blood changes dramatically immediately after a myocardial infarction, and these fluctuations continue about 6 weeks. The levels of plasma cholesterol and LDL may fall as much as 60 per cent in the first few days.

5. Samples should be obtained from patients in a steady state who are on a regular diet. If the results are abnormal, at least two confirmatory samples should be obtained before therapy is recommended.

6. To conclude a diagnostic work-up of hyperlipoproteinemia, possible secondary causes must be ruled out (Fig. 35–4).[51,54] Dietary excess may be a causal factor. Consumption of large quantities of eggs, butter, milk, cheese, and organ meat will increase levels of LDL. Other factors that can raise levels of lipid include hypothyroidism, nephrotic syndrome, multiple myeloma, porphyria, liver disease, and alcoholism. If these disorders are ruled out, and primary hyperlipoproteinemia is diagnosed, family screening should be performed to uncover possible genetic transmission as well as to detect others at risk for CAD.

TYPING HYPERLIPOPROTEINEMIA

As already noted, equal degrees of hypercholesterolemia and hypertriglyceridemia may result from elevation of the levels of different lipoproteins. By identifying the specific lipoprotein that is abnormal, one can assume a more rational approach to diagnosis and management. There are two equally important questions to be considered: "How much cholesterol or triglyceride is present in the plasma," and "How are these lipids distributed in the lipoproteins?"

Studies of the lipoprotein apoproteins, i.e., the protein moieties to which the lipids are bound, have helped clarify the role of lipoproteins in the transport of lipids. Quantification of the apolipoproteins is rapidly becoming a practical immunochemical technique which promises to facilitate the diagnosis of hyperlipoproteinemia and, potentially, the assessment of the risk of developing CAD.[77]

In 1967, a system for classification of the hyperlipoproteinemias was introduced. It was adopted by the WHO in 1971, with minor modifications. Two main shortcomings were soon detected in the everyday use of this system: (1) Its value in genetic analysis is limited; and (2) elaborate techniques and equipment, not readily available in every clinical laboratory, are required to define some types specifically and to distinguish between types. Nevertheless, judicious application of this typing system in the classification of patients with clearly elevated levels of plasma lipids can greatly clarify diagnosis and rationalize the therapeutic approach.

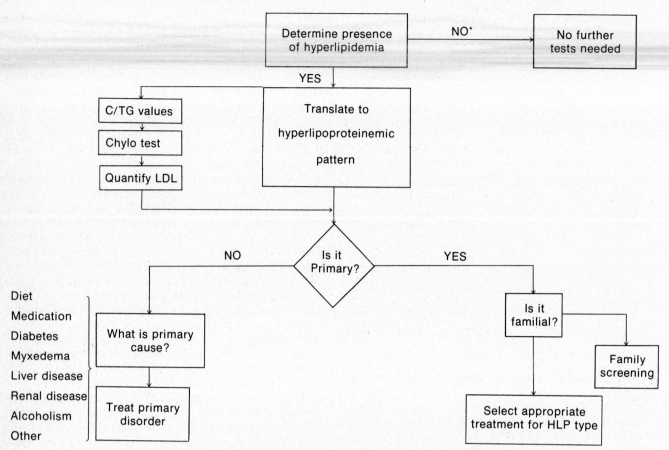

FIGURE 35–4   Schema used in diagnosis of hyperlipoproteinemia.

It should be realized that the "types" of hyperlipoproteinemia are not disease entities but are, instead, groups of disorders that affect similarly the concentrations of plasma lipids and lipoproteins and result in similar patterns of lipoproteins (see Table 35–8). Therefore, classifying a patient as being one of the hyperlipoproteinemic types is not making a clinical diagnosis per se, but rather it is defining a lipoprotein pattern that may result from different underlying disorders.

A clear distinction must be made between *primary* and *secondary* hyperlipoproteinemia in the patient who has elevated levels of plasma lipids and lipoproteins, since this distinction has important therapeutic and prognostic consequences. Treatment of secondary hyperlipoproteinemias is usually aimed at the underlying cause, and the abnormal pattern of lipoproteins resolves when the basic disorder is corrected. The prognosis for the patient with secondary hyperlipoproteinemia clearly depends on the prognosis associated with the basic disease.

Table 35–8 details some of the major causes of secondary hyperlipoproteinemias and delineates the association between the hyperlipoproteinemic patterns and these disorders. Observation of heterogeneity within the primary disorders portends a new classification system based on the specific underlying biochemical defects.

Type I.[78] Familial Type I hyperlipoproteinemia is transmitted as a recessive trait and is characterized by excess levels of chylomicrons in fasting plasma (measured 14 hours or more following a meal).[78] The excess of chylomicrons observed in Type I can also be secondary to insulinopenic diabetes, dysglobulinemia, or lupus erythematosus. The pattern results from the body's inability to clear exogenous triglyceride from the plasma. Patients with Type I have a deficient amount of the enzyme lipoprotein lipase, which originates in the adipose cell and muscle and is involved in the catabolism of circulating triglycerides. An identical clinical syndrome has been described in a family lacking apolipoprotein CII, the apoprotein catalyst involved in the intravascular hydrolysis of triglyceride by lipoprotein lipase.[79,80]

Primary Type I hyperlipoproteinemia often occurs in childhood with recurrent bouts of abdominal pain. Other clinical features include pancreatitis, eruptive xanthomas, hepatosplenomegaly, and lipemia retinalis. Despite a marked increase in the level of triglyceride and, sometimes, cholesterol, this pattern has *not* been associated with an increased risk of developing vascular disease.

Type II.[78] Type II (hyperbetalipoproteinemia) is characterized by elevated levels of LDL, either alone (Type IIA) or associated with increased VLDL (Type IIB).[78] The level of cholesterol generally ranges from 300 to 600 mg/dl. In its most common primary form, the disorder is diagnosable at birth. (Levels of LDL are elevated.) Primary Type II is often familial and is inherited most commonly as an autosomal dominant trait, so that there is a 50 per cent chance that each sibling and child of a victim will be affected. Since Type II is associated with a high risk of developing premature vascular disease, sampling of all first-degree relatives of patients found to have primary hyperbetalipoproteinemia is always indicated.[63] Hypercholesterolemia may also be secondary to dietary excess, obstructive liver disease, hypothyroidism, nephrosis, porphyria, myxedema, or multiple myeloma. Clinical features of familial Type II (familial hypercholesterolemia) sometimes include tendon xanthomas at the elbows, extensor surfaces of the hands, and the Achilles tendons; premature corneal arcus (arcus in a Caucasian younger than age 55); and xanthelasma. Tuberous xanthomas may also occur, but these are less frequent. They may develop in late adolescence or adulthood in patients with heterozygous forms of the disease. In a study of more than 1000 relatives of 116 kindred affected with primary Type II, the probability of developing fatal or nonfatal CAD by age 40 in heterozygous Type II men was 16 per cent; by age 60, the risk rose to 56 per cent (Fig. 35-5).[63] In women, the risk lagged by more than a decade but was found to increase with age. In the more severe homozygous case, xanthomas can be observed at birth or in early childhood, accompanied by pronounced elevation of LDL. CAD develops early and progresses rapidly, and patients rarely survive to adulthood.

Accumulating evidence suggests that primary hyperbetalipoproteinemia is heterogeneous and represents a multiplicity of disorders. In addition to familial hypercholesterolemia (just described), there is also familial combined hyperlipoproteinemia, in which parents and siblings may have increased levels of LDL accompanied by excesses of other lipoprotein fractions (p. 1634).

In recent years, the basic defect in familial hypercholesterolemia has been partially elucidated. Brown and Goldstein have shown that fibroblasts and lymphocytes from patients with familial hypercholesterolemia have a defective receptor-mediated uptake of LDL (p. 1629).[81] Homozygous patients are divided into three major groups, according to the type of defect in function of the receptors: (1) those with receptor-negative cells unable to bind LDL with high affinity; (2) those with receptor-defective cells that bind LDL with a strength of only about 10 per cent of normal; and (3) those with a defect in internalization (i.e., LDL is bound normally to cells but is not internalized into them). The homozygous state is characterized by a lack of functional receptors for LDL. In heterozygous patients with familial hypercholesterolemia, the values for degradation of LDL are about halfway between those of normal persons and homozygous patients with familial hypercholesterolemia. It should be noted, however, that no routine receptor assay for clinical laboratory use is yet available.

Type III.[78]   Like Type II, Type III is associated with an increased risk of developing premature vascular disease.[78] Patients with this disorder manifest, at a relatively young age, an increased incidence of intermittent claudication, angina pectoris, myocardial infarction, or other evidence of atherosclerosis.[54]

Type III is an uncommon disorder characterized by an increased concentration of IDL. This lipoprotein, not seen in normal fasting plasma, has flotation properties that overlap with VLDL but, on paper electrophoresis, migrates as a broad band with beta mobility. Neither of these diagnostic criteria, however, has proved specific enough when used alone for diagnosis without first ascertaining the associated clinical findings. A chemical method of diagnosis based on a detailed description of the clinical and biochemical features of Type III has been proposed.[82,83] More recently, a diagnostic assay for apolipoprotein E (one of the seven known lipoprotein apoproteins) has also been proposed, but its usefulness remains to be demonstrated.[84,85]

Clinically, primary Type III can be recognized by the discovery of unusual orange-yellow deposits in the palmar creases. Tuboeruptive xanthomas are also common. Peripheral vascular disease is as prevalent as CAD, but in men it is much more common and occurs earlier than in women.[83] Type III patients are exquisitely sensitive to caloric balance, dietary carbohydrate, estrogens, and clofibrate. Primary Type III is a fascinating disorder of lipid transport that responds readily to therapy.

Type IV.[78]   The distinguishing abnormality in lipoproteins in Type IV is an increased accumulation of VLDL, always accompanied by hypertriglyceridemia. The level of cholesterol is generally normal.[78] The pattern is a very common one, but diagnosis of the familial form or forms is complicated because of the influence that diet, stress, intake of alcohol, environmental factors, and fluctuations in body weight have on levels of triglycerides.

Type IV is often associated with glucose intolerance. Obesity and hyperuricemia are often present, and eruptive xanthomas occasionally occur in patients with severely increased levels of VLDL. Familial Type IV usually does not manifest itself until adulthood and is frequently secondary to other disorders, particularly diabetes mellitus. It is also found frequently in women between the ages of 20 and 50 years who are using oral contraceptives.[86]

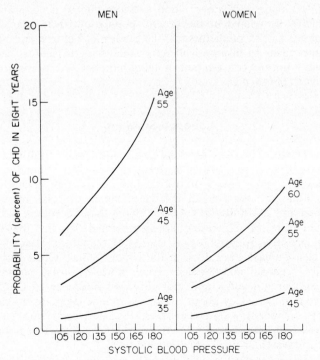

FIGURE 35-5   Cumulative probability by decade of developing fatal or nonfatal CAD. (From Stone, N. J., et al.: Coronary artery disease in 116 kindred with familial Type II hyperlipoproteinemia. Circulation 49:482, 1974, by permission of the American Heart Association, Inc.)

Although primary Type IV has been observed in a high proportion of young subjects with CAD, this has been counterbalanced by the greater prevalence of Type IV among clinically "normal" adults as well.[47,57,87,88] A further difficulty in clarifying the association between Type IV and CAD is separating the risk resulting from excess VLDL from the often concomitant risk factors of obesity, glucose intolerance, and elevated blood pressure.

Type V.[78] Type V is a mixed pattern of chylomicronemia and increased levels of VLDL.[78] Levels of triglyceride in the plasma are grossly elevated, ranging from 1000 to 6000 mg. The clinical features of the disorder are the same as in Type I, except that they do not manifest themselves until adulthood. The glucose intolerance and hyperuricemia associated with Type IV are common in Type V and are more acute. Excess intake of alcohol can also aggravate the disorder. Type V is a relatively uncommon pattern and may be secondary to insulinopenic diabetes mellitus, nephrosis, myeloma, or alcoholism.

A descriptive analysis of a population of primary Type V subjects confirmed the distinctiveness of this lipoprotein abnormality.[89] A high incidence of hyperuricemia, diabetes, pancreatitis, and xanthomatosis was found among the 32 propositi studied, but less striking excesses were found among affected relatives: Evaluation of the 32 families failed to provide any evidence of excessive CAD.

Blood Pressure
(See also Chap. 26)

Elevated blood pressure, either systolic or diastolic, is predictive of an increased risk of developing CAD.[90] Both systolic and diastolic blood pressure have a continuous, unimodal distribution in the population when measured under usual office conditions. Although there is some skewing of the distribution toward high values, there is no evidence of bimodality. Thus, although the level of blood pressure appears to have a major genetic determination,[91,92] it occurs as a continuously distributed trait with no clear cut-off points to differentiate qualitatively distinct entities. Furthermore, the curve of the risk of morbidity and mortality from CAD, as well as the risk of other atherosclerotic diseases, shows a smooth, direct relationship to the levels of blood pressure over the entire range of values. As with the concentration of plasma cholesterol, there is no cut-off point at which risk suddenly changes from low to high values.

Blood pressure is often subject to marked changes, not only over the years but also within the span of a few minutes. Posture, exercise, emotional stress, ambient temperature, and a variety of other factors affect blood pressure. A major contribution of the prospective epidemiological studies was the confirmation that casual measurements of blood pressures, obtained under usual office conditions, were potent predictors of the risk of developing CAD.[90] The gradient of risk as it relates to blood pressure is illustrated in Figure 35–6. As an individual predictor, blood pressure has been found to be more reliable than the level of cholesterol or cigarette smoking. Although blood pressure normally tends to rise with age, elevated blood pressure is still a risk factor in the elderly. The common notion that elderly people tolerate hypertension better than

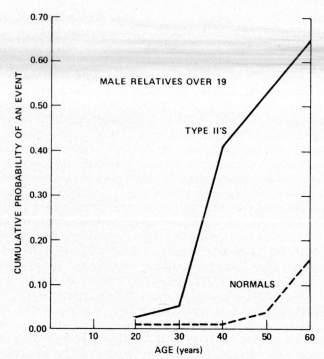

FIGURE 35–6   Probability of developing CAD within 8 years according to systolic blood pressure levels in persons with cholesterol levels measuring 235 mg/dl who are nonsmokers and have normal glucose tolerance.

younger ones has little basis in the epidemiological data. Furthermore, the relationship between blood pressure and the risk of developing CAD is as strong in women as it is in men.[90]

In several studies, systolic blood pressure has been found to be a better predictor of the risk of developing CAD than is diastolic blood pressure. Since the two are highly correlated in the general population, their relative merits as risk predictors may be academic. Yet it would be imprudent to dismiss isolated systolic hypertension as being a normal concomitant of aging, unrelated to the risk of developing CAD.

Tobacco Smoking

Tobacco smoking has long been considered a health hazard that is particularly harmful to the lungs. Numerous investigations have demonstrated, however, that cigarette smoking is also a major risk factor for myocardial infarction and death due to CAD.[93–98] More than 12 million person-years of experience are represented by the major prospective epidemiological studies of the effects of smoking that have been done in the United States, Great Britain, Canada, and Sweden. Total mortality, total cardiovascular mortality, and mortality and incidence of CAD were increased by about 1.6 times in male cigarette smokers compared with nonsmokers. Pipe and cigar smokers, however, were found to have only slight increases in total cardiovascular deaths and morbidity.[93]

Most prospective studies with sufficient data tend to show that the risk of developing CAD is directly related to the number of cigarettes smoked per day (Table 35–9). Furthermore, and of major importance for the prevention

TABLE 35–9 RELATIVE RISK OF CAD AND CIGARETTE SMOKING IN MEN

	Number of Cigarettes Smoked Per Day			
	None	*< 20*	*20*	*> 20*
Framingham Heart Study[5]				
Ages 45–54	1.00	1.29	1.67	2.15
55–64	1.00	1.15	1.32	1.51
65–74	1.00	1.12	1.24	1.39
Western Collaborative Group Study[9]				
Ages 39–49	1.00	1.29	1.56	1.95
50–59	1.00	1.33	1.77	2.35

of CAD, those who discontinue smoking assume a lesser risk than those who continue to smoke.[99,100] For CAD, as opposed to lung cancer and emphysema, the excess risk in ex-smokers seems to decline within a year or two of discontinuation of the habit but tends to remain slightly greater than the risk assumed by nonsmokers.[43,101] Discontinuation of the smoking habit may be followed by a slight increase in weight and uric acid levels but has no discernible effect on other CAD risk factors.[102] Although the ex-smokers in these epidemiological studies are a self-selected group, the improvement in their mortality rates is not due to differences in baseline risk factors from those in persons who continue to smoke.[103] Switching to filter cigarettes does not seem to offer any protection against the subsequent risk of CAD.[104] Unfortunately, the few randomized trials on smoking intervention that have been reported to date have not been consistent. Some failed to show any marked improvement in CAD rates among the smokers who have stopped, whereas the Multiple Risk Factor Intervention Trial showed that high-risk men who discontinue this habit had a marked reduction in morality.[105,106,106a]

A few other questions have arisen about the consistency of the data relating cigarette smoking to the development of CAD. There is some indication from the Framingham Study that the harmful effects of cigarettes may diminish as one gets older (see Table 35–9).[100,101] However, other studies, such as the Western Collaborative Group Study, show no decrease in the effect of smoking with age.[107]

The relationship of cigarette smoking to development of CAD among women is somewhat more complex. In relation to myocardial infarction, women show about the same gradient of risk correlated with the amount of smoking as do men.[108,109] Because of the smaller number of cases available for study, however, these gradients do not usually achieve the high level of statistical significance that they do for men. The effects in women are further obscured by the inconsistent relationship found between cigarette smoking and the occurrence of angina pectoris.[101,107,110,111] Since the most frequent manifestation of CAD in women is angina, the total rates of occurrence of CAD in women fail to show a relationship to cigarette smoking.[108]

Nevertheless, the overwhelming evidence supports a strong and definite relationship between cigarette smoking and CAD. A variety of mechanisms have been suggested for the adverse effects of cigarette smoking on the heart and blood vessels. The results of each of the hypothesized mechanisms could also be reversed upon discontinuation of the smoking habit. Among these mechanisms is the effect of nicotine and carbon monoxide upon the heart, the coronary arteries, and the blood. Specific changes include increased myocardial demand for oxygen, induced by nicotine; interference with oxygen supply by carboxyhemoglobin; increased adhesiveness of platelets; and lowering of the threshold for ventricular fibrillation. Cigarette smoking has also been found to be associated with decreased levels of HDL cholesterol, compared with those in nonsmokers and ex-smokers.[68,112]

Abnormal Glucose Tolerance

Clinically overt diabetes mellitus has long been recognized as a precursor of vascular disease, and this association has been confirmed in prospective epidemiological studies.[113–118] These studies have also shown that hyperglycemia and glucose intolerance, as measured from levels of blood sugar obtained 1 hour after administration of a standardized oral glucose load, or even as indicated by high casually measured levels of blood sugar, are associated with increased risk of developing CAD.[116–118] Men with glucose intolerance have about a 50 per cent greater chance of developing CAD than men with no evidence of glucose intolerance, whereas in women the risk is more than doubled—virtually eliminating the differential in rates of CAD between men and women.[59,108] Although early-onset diabetes appears to be primarily involved in mortality from renal disease, adult-onset diabetes is associated with death from CAD.[119] In adults, both insulin-dependent and non–insulin-dependent diabetics appear to be at increased risk for development of CAD.[116,118,120]

In the Coronary Drug Project, in which the effects of several lipid-lowering agents on mortality and coronary conditions in men who had previously suffered a myocardial infarction were studied, the prognostic importance of the level of plasma glucose was examined.[121] It was found that a high fasting level of glucose is a significant predictor of subsequent risk of myocardial infarction even after adjustment for many other risk factors and concomitant variables is made.

The mechanism associating hyperglycemia and increased risk of CAD is obscure, although several aspects have been investigated.[113] Hyperlipidemia, particularly hypertriglyceridemia, is often linked with diabetes.[122] Both hyperlipidemia and hyperglycemia tend to be associated with obesity and thereby indirectly with hypertension. A variety of interrelationships between glucose intolerance and levels of insulin have been observed, which may suggest several mechanisms related to the initiation or promotion of atherosclerosis. They involve the real or potential effects of insulin or glucose or both on the synthesis and/or catabolism of cellular and extracellular elements in the arterial wall. Still other associations have been noted between hyperglycemia and the increased adhesiveness of platelets and other abnormalities of coagulation. Thus, several complex mechanisms may be involved, separately or in concert.

The relationship between the methods for control of hyperglycemia and the risk of developing CAD is exceedingly confused and controversial at the present time. The University Group Diabetes Program has investigated the effects of several oral hypoglycemic agents and of two regimens of insulin usage on the vascular complications in patients with adult-onset diabetes.[123,124] When compared with the placebo group, no significant benefits were found for any of the treatment modalities. There has been considerable controversy over these results, but it would appear that no current regimen used to control hyperglycemia has an appreciable effect on the atherosclerotic complications of diabetes.[113,125]

Other Risk Factors

GOUT. Gouty arthritis has been associated with a doubling of the risk of developing CAD.[126] There also appears to be a moderate association between CAD and level of uric acid in the absence of clinical gout.[127] However, elevated levels of uric acid tend also to be associated with higher levels of blood pressure, elevated levels of serum cholesterol and triglyceride, and obesity.[128] These may reflect interrelated metabolic processes.

MENOPAUSE AND ORAL CONTRACEPTIVES. The marked difference in risk between women and men has already been noted. Undoubtedly, part of this difference can be attributed to hormonal factors, but the relationship of the risk of developing CAD to specific hormones has not yet been established. Among women, however, both the menopause and the use of oral contraceptive agents appear to be related to an increased risk of developing CAD. Women in their 40's and 50's who have undergone menopause have been found to have three times the incidence of CAD as do women of these ages who are still menstruating.[129] Although menopause is associated with changes in other risk factors as well, these do not account entirely for the increased risk of developing CAD.

The use of oral contraceptive drugs has recently been suspected of having a marked influence on the occurrence of CAD in premenopausal women.[130–133] The risk of myocardial infarction in young women using oral contraceptives who already have associated adverse risk factors, particularly hypertension and diabetes, is greatly enhanced. In some studies, women who smoked cigarettes and who also used oral contraceptives were at extremely high risk, pointing to a strong interaction between the effects of both these hazards.[134] Oral contraceptives also tend to produce an increase in blood pressure (p. 873) and an alteration of serum levels of lipoproteins[135] as well as disturbances in clotting and enhancement of thromboembolic changes. Oral contraceptives containing high doses of progestin tend to lower levels of HDL cholesterol, whereas those containing high doses of estrogen tend to raise levels of HDL.[69]

The effect of estrogens on the risk of developing CAD is a somewhat controversial issue. In postmenopausal women, exogenous estrogens had no discernible effect on the risk of developing CAD in most studies[136–138] but did lower risk in some.[139] Stilbestrol used in men for the treatment of prostatic cancer, conjugated equine estrogens given to men in the Coronary Drug Project to lower levels of serum cholesterol, and noncontraceptive estrogens used by young women, however, all tended to *increase* the risk of developing CAD.[140–143]

VASECTOMY. Recent experimental work in two species of monkeys found that arteries of vasectomized animals developed more severe atherosclerotic plaques than did the vessels of control animals.[144] This effect seemed to be independent of plasma lipid levels, and it was postulated that the mechanism responsible involved endothelial damage from circulatory antibodies to sperm antigens. Studies of vasectomized men, however, have failed to show any increased risk of CAD in these men compared with nonvasectomized men matched for a variety of risk factors.[145,145a] Neither is there any consistent evidence at present for a significant excess of sex hormone concentrations in men with CAD.[146]

OBESITY. Although obesity has long been known to predispose to CAD,[147] its *independent effect* has been questioned,[148,149] since several studies have shown that the relationship of CAD to obesity is virtually entirely accounted for by the relationship of obesity to other risk factors.[59,150] However, when populations are followed for many years, obesity has been found to be a risk factor for CAD independent of its association with other risk factors.[151,151a]

There has been little agreement regarding how to define or measure obesity in epidemiological studies.[149] Measurement of body fat requires elaborate techniques (e.g., total body immersion to estimate body density) and is not adaptable to population studies.[152] Measurement of the thickness of the subcutaneous fat at several body sites has been recommended but has not been employed uniformly. Thus, measurements of overweight rather than of obesity or fatness have generally been employed. Whatever criterion for overweight is used, it tends to confound weight due to muscular development (e.g., as found in football players) with that due to fat accumulation. Two general criteria of overweight have been used: (1) relative weight, as determined by distribution of weight according to height, such as the Metropolitan Life Insurance Company standards or the Framingham Relative Weight based on median weight for each inch of height[153]; and (2) indices derived from the mathematical relationship between height and weight.[154] Of the latter, the body mass index (weight divided by the square of height) has been found to be most useful as a measure of relative obesity.

Overweight has been found in many studies to be highly associated with hypertension, glucose intolerance, and adverse lipid profiles.[56] Furthermore, in both metabolic ward and epidemiological studies, a direct cause-and-effect relationship has been found between change in weight and an alteration of these risk factors.[68,155,156] Therefore, it should not be surprising that when obesity is considered in combination with these traits as a predictor of the incidence of CAD, its effects as an independent contributor are overshadowed by the possibly more direct influence of the other risk factors,[59,150] and its independent contribution to CAD risk requires many years of follow-up to detect.[151] Nevertheless, although the association between obesity and the risk of developing CAD may operate through the effects of obesity on other characteristics, the role of obesity as a risk variable should not be denigrated. Furthermore, recent studies have found that obesity may indeed be an independent contributor in populations with low levels of other risk factors, e.g., Japanese men in Hawaii, and in younger individuals.[157,158]

PHYSICAL ACTIVITY. The evidence of a beneficial effect of physical activity on the development of CAD is gradually accumulating, although controversial aspects still exist.[159–167,167a] Despite the problems inherent in self-selection of physically active jobs and leisure activities, documentation of quantitative levels of physical activity, and adjustment for variations of other risk factors, the bulk of evidence supports the hypothesis that regular physical exercise may have a protective effect on developing CAD. However, there is little agreement regarding whether moderate amounts of exercise will suffice (threshold model) or whether more strenuous and prolonged exercise is needed to obtain any benefit. There is also no agreement about whether exercise improves myocardial function and coronary circulation directly or whether its protective effect acts through the alteration of other risk factors.[168-171]

TYPE OF PERSONALITY BEHAVIOR (See also p. 1826). In the late 1950's, Friedman and Rosenman put forward the concept of a behavior pattern which they called Type A and which they believed was related to the occurrence of CAD.[9,172] In the past 20 years, many investigators have confirmed in varying degrees the existence of a "coronary-prone behavior pattern."[173-175] Rosenman has described the Type A behavior pattern as follows.[176]

We conceive of the Type A behavior pattern as being a particular action-emotion complex that is possessed and exhibited by an individual who is engaged in a relatively chronic and excessive struggle to obtain an unlimited number of things from the environment in the shortest period of time and/or against the opposing efforts of other persons or things in the same environment. This chronic struggle might consist of attempts to achieve or to do more and more in less and less time or other conflicts with one or more persons. Since the Type A subject rarely despairs of losing the chronic struggle, such individuals sharply differ from those with fear or anxiety or other simple neurotic states. Type A's exhibit enhanced personality traits of aggressiveness, ambitiousness and competitiveness. They are often preoccupied with deadlines and are work-oriented. In this interplay, Type A's exhibit chronic impatience and usually a strong sense of time urgency. The converse Type B individual is mainly free of such enhanced personality traits and generally feels no pressing conflict with either time or other persons and is therefore free of any habitual sense of time urgency.

The 20th century environment that is associated with the CHD incidence has generally encouraged Type A behavior because it appears to offer special rewards to those who can perform rapidly and aggressively. Moreover, with increasing urbanization and technological progress as well as increasing population density, our civilization presents unique new challenges never experienced by earlier and less time-conscious generations. Type A behavior does not stem solely from individual personality but emerges when certain challenges or conditions of the milieu arise to elicit this complex of responses in susceptible individuals.[176]

The Western Collaborative Group Study, after 8.5 years of follow-up of 3154 men who had been characterized as having the Type A pattern of behavior, found that Type A men had twice the risk of developing CAD as did Type B men.[9] Similar risks have recently been found for Type A women.[174,177] Personality type appears to act independently of such risk factors as high blood pressure, smoking, and high cholesterol levels.[178] The severity of atherosclerotic involvement of coronary vessels observed angiographically is positively associated with Type A behavior.[178]

Other Psychological and Social Risk Factors. Jenkins has presented comprehensive reviews of the evidence supporting psychological and social risk factors for coronary disease.[180] For some factors, the evidence is highly suggestive, whereas for others the evidence is weak or inconsistent. Sociological indices such as socioeconomic status, occupation, religious affiliation, education, and marital status have been widely studied, but conflicting results have been obtained. Social mobility and incongruity of status (defined as the simultaneous possession of the identifying markings of different social classes) have been suspected to be related to the incidence of CAD. Recent studies, however, have tended to add to the confusion rather than to clarify matters. It would seem that these sociological concepts are more complex than they first appeared, at least with respect to their association with CAD.

A family of symptoms and behavior referred to as "anxiety" and "neuroticism" is, according to a variety of studies, related to CAD.[180] Studies comparing patients having CAD with patients suffering from other diseases failed to discriminate whether the anxiety preceded the CAD or resulted from it. Yet many of these studies, and the few with prospective data, tend to show that anxiety, depression, irritability, and sleeplessness—which may reflect "emotional drain"—are related to CAD.

Problems, dissatisfaction, and stress associated with life changes have been difficult to study. The available evidence is not consistent, although some of the reported relationships are provocative. For example, social support systems seem to protect the individual from the health hazards associated with stressful life situations, a fact that gives hope of developing more effective coping behavior for dealing with life's stresses.[32] The possible adverse effects of retirement and stressful job situations upon risk of CAD have recently been highlighted.[181,182] Much more research is needed in this area.

FAMILY HISTORY. Familial and genetic factors may play an important role in the determination of some major risk factors—in particular, hypertension, glucose intolerance, and levels of lipoprotein.[183] It is also clear that some risk factors have their onset in childhood.[184] It appears that there may be a familial or genetic predisposition toward CAD per se that is independent of the other known risk factors.[185,185a]

DIETARY CHOLESTEROL AND SATURATED FAT. Striking correlations have been found between average intake of fat and average levels of serum cholesterol in epidemiological studies comparing Western and non-Western populations. In the Seven Countries Study, the relationship of diet to the level of serum cholesterol was studied in men between the ages of 40 and 59.[10,186] A direct correlation was found between the intake of saturated fat, on the one hand, and the incidence of CAD and hypercholesterolemia, on the other. The populations of Greece and Yugoslavia derive an average of 30 per cent of total calories from fat, compared with 40 per cent in the American diet. These differences in fat intake were interpreted as being major factors in the three- to fivefold difference between these countries in the incidence of CAD. Another study that reported direct correlations between intake of fat and levels of serum cholesterol compared Japanese men living in Japan with those in Hawaii and California.[187] The mean percentage of calories derived from fat ranged from 15 per cent in Japan to 36.7 per cent in California. Serum cholesterol levels were lowest in Japan (180 mg/dl), higher in Hawaii (218 mg/dl), and highest in California (225 mg/dl). Data from studies of Seventh-Day Adventists show that those adhering to a vegetarian diet have one-third the mortality rate from CAD of nonvegetarians, but whether or not this difference is mediated through differences in serum lipid levels is not yet clear.[188]

It is interesting that a clear correlation is lacking when individuals *within* populations are studied. In Framingham, no correlation was found between individual diets, levels of serum cholesterol measured concomitantly, and subsequent risk of developing CAD.[189] An analysis of the association between daily dietary intake and levels of serum lipids in the Tecumseh population did not exclude the existence of a relationship between dietary cholesterol and the amount of serum cholesterol, although obesity was found to be more highly correlated with lipid levels than were specific dietary factors.[190] In contrast, the 20-year follow-up report of the Western Electric Study has revealed highly correlated results between diet score (intake of dietary cholesterol, saturated fat, and polyunsaturated fatty acids) and serum cholesterol levels, and between change in diet score and change in serum cholesterol levels and has demonstrated a positive prospective association between mean baseline diet score and 19-year risk of death from CAD.[191] Forthcoming data from the Lipid Research Clinics (LRC) prevalence studies should clarify further the association between individual dietary habits and levels of plasma cholesterol. A preliminary report from the LRC program indicates a significant fall (5 to 10 per cent) in the level of cholesterol in the U.S. population in the last decade.[192] This finding is consistent with U.S. Department of Agriculture reports of declining consumption of butter and other animal fats and oils and the increased use of vegetable oils.

The evidence from other types of studies is also illuminating. Numerous metabolic ward investigations involving controlled dietary manipulation show a strong and direct correlation between dietary and serum lipids. Mean levels of serum cholesterol responded predictably to the intake of saturated and polyunsaturated fat and dietary cholesterol.[193-195] Innumerable animal studies performed over the past 60 years provide further evidence that cholesterol-feeding diets raise levels of serum cholesterol, leading to atherosclerosis. The disease will regress following termination of the diet, however.[196]

Concentrations of LDL are directly related to the ingestion of dietary saturated fats and cholesterol, whereas polyunsaturated fats have been shown to depress levels of LDL.

Carbohydrate Consumption. A change in the American diet consisting of the consumption of large amounts of sucrose and glucose and smaller amounts of fiber and more purified foods has been incriminated as a causal factor in the development of CAD, hyperlipidemia, obesity, and diabetes mellitus. The evidence from a number of sources suggests an association but does not yet prove causality.

The average per capita consumption of sugar in the U.S. is 50 kg per year. Epidemiological correlations suggest that this factor may be involved in the mortality rates for CAD, but there is no conclusive proof, and opinions are divided.[197] Evidence from animal studies does not suggest a correlation between the consumption of dietary sucrose or carbohydrates and the development of atherosclerosis.

Studies involving feeding of carbohydrates generally show that a short-term increase in the consumption of dietary carbohydrates provokes a marked rise in the level of plasma triglycerides.[198,199] This induction of hypertriglyceridemia has been shown to be transitory, however; in general, its effects on serum lipids are confusing, owing in part to inadequate experimental designs.

Moreover, there are divergent views regarding which type of carbohydrate is the most hypertriglyceridemic. Studies also show that most population groups with a low incidence of CAD derive 65 to 85 per cent of their total energy from whole grain and potatoes. Current studies of the effects of fiber on the metabolism of lipids show clear indications of changes in the absorption of carbohydrate and lipid.[200,201] At the present time, the evidence is far from conclusive, and further work is needed to separate fact from hypothesis.

Salt Intake. (See also Chap. 26) Studies have shown that diets high in sodium can produce hypertension in genetically predisposed animals. The role of sodium in the etiology of hypertension in humans, however, has not been established. Some epidemiological studies have suggested a strong association between sodium and the prevalence of hypertension, but other factors such as intake of potassium, body weight, and physical activity complicate the assessment of this association.[202,203]

In the treatment of hypertension, restriction of sodium is beneficial for some patients, but a recent study has shown that weight reduction may be more important.[204] Although it is unknown whether or not limiting the intake of salt will prevent hypertension, it would be prudent to recommend restraint in the consumption of sodium. Specifically, this would include avoiding overly salted prepared foods, refraining from adding salt to cooked foods, reducing the amount of sodium added to baby foods, and cooking with small amounts of salt.

Alcohol Consumption. The evidence relating daily consumption of alcohol to the development of CAD is conflicting. A number of recent studies report negative associations and suggest a possible preventive result from moderate daily intake of alcohol.[205-209] Other investigators have found either a positive association or no apparent overall association.[210-212]

The effect of the consumption of alcohol on lipid transport is well known, but the emphasis of earlier studies was principally on its effect on triglycerides. The Cooperative Lipoprotein Phenotyping Study and the LRC Prevalence Study have reported significant positive associations between alcohol intake and HDL cholesterol levels.[213,214] Alcohol intake has also been reported to be positively associated with blood pressure.[207,209]

Coffee Ingestion. Although large doses of caffeine have been associated with distinct cardiovascular changes (tachycardia, arrhythmias, and extrasystoles), there is no definitive proof that the ingestion of coffee increases the risk of cardiovascular disease. Evidence from both case control and prospective studies is conflicting.[215-217] Although the data on caffeine as an independent risk factor for CAD are mixed, they do suggest that coffee plays a role in association with other existing factors, such as hypertension.

Trace Metals. Ecologic studies comparing different regions or communities have demonstrated an inverse relationship between the hardness of drinking water and local cardiovascular mortality rates.[23,218] ("The harder the water, the softer the arteries.") Hardness of water is not a specific chemical element but is a complex characteristic measured by titration with a chelating agent. Efforts to identify specific chemical components that are related to mortality from CAD have produced conflicting results. Protective effects have been attributed to magnesium, chromium, selenium, and zinc, whereas harmful effects have been suspected for cadmium, manganese, and lead. At the present time, it cannot be recommended that the hardness or trace metal content of drinking water be altered in an effort to decrease the incidence of CAD.

Miscellaneous Risk Factors. A variety of other factors have been suspected as being related to the occurrence of CAD, and some have received corroboration from one or two studies. Vital capacity was found to have an inverse relation to CAD in the Framingham Study.[108] Blood groups have been investigated in several populations.[219,220] There have been some consistent findings that Type O individuals are at lesser risk than those with Type A blood. Although coagulation factors play a role in the formation of thrombi and in the atherosclerotic process, there is scant evidence linking clotting abnormalities to the risk of developing CAD, other than the previously mentioned association between CAD and contraceptive pills.[221] It has been speculated that increased blood viscosity may play a role in the development of thrombotic processes and may exacerbate the potential for development of ischemia.[222] This might explain the associations reported between elevated hematocrit and risk of CAD.[223] Increased severity of atherosclerosis in patients with nephrotic syndrome or in those undergoing long-term dialysis has not been consistently found.[224-227]

The role of immunological factors is obscure. There has been some discussion that autoimmune thyroiditis may be a risk factor.[228] On the other hand, patients with rheumatoid arthritis tend to have a lower incidence of CAD, which has been attributed by some to aspirin therapy and its inhibition of the aggregation of platelets.[229] Another uncommon but apparently strong risk factor is post-radiation treatment for mediastinal tumors.[230] Another factor about which there is some speculation is ear-lobe creases.[231]

Environmental Factors. Evidence regarding the impact of environmental factors on cardiovascular disease is inconclusive.[232] Water softness, trace metals, carbon monoxide, noise exposure, and physical and psychosocial stress have been associated with cardiovascular effects, but the available data are inadequate and inconsistent.

Only in the case of two industrial chemicals, carbon disulfide and aliphatic nitrates, has the association been established. Studies of the effects of cold snaps and snowstorms on the incidence of ischemic heart disease have failed to show any association in relation to either age or preexisting heart disease.[233,234] In most studies of external environmental effects, it has proved difficult to separate these risk factors from other concomitant conditions that vary from place to place.

Undoubtedly, other risk factors exist. Several studies comparing the incidence of heart disease in different groups have shown that the currently known risk factors cannot explain all the differences that have been found. For example, the male-female differences are not accounted for. Differences between Japanese and Puerto Rican men compared with Caucasian men cannot be attributed to variations in smoking, blood pressure, or levels of cholesterol.[20] Thus, the search for additional risk factors or for new relationships among existing ones must continue.

Multivariate Risk Functions For CAD

The preceding discussion clearly indicates that many attributes of individuals are related to their risk of developing CAD. It has also been stated that most risk factors make independent contributions to the prediction of the risk; i.e., they supply additional information beyond that provided by a knowledge of the other risk factors possessed by the individual. In order to describe the cumulative effect of numerous factors acting simultaneously and in order to assess the relative contribution of each factor, statisticians have explored several multivariate methods of describing these relationships. An initial approach was to divide each risk factor into two or three levels (e.g., hypertensive-normotensive) and to subclassify the study population into several subgroups on the basis of the combined levels of three or four risk factors. Although this method is feasible when only a few risk factors are involved—and is a desirable method for studying specific interactions—it is readily apparent that as the number of subgroups increases geometrically, the number of observations in any one subgroup can become quite small.

Other approaches included discriminant function analysis and multiple regression techniques. A linear multiple regression function for predicting the risk of disease (P = probability of developing disease in a stated period of time) from a knowledge of the levels of several risk factors $(X_1, X_2, \ldots, X_k)$ takes the following form:

$$P = \beta_0 + \beta_1 X_1 + \beta_2 X_2 + \ldots + \beta_k X_k$$

where the betas are appropriate coefficients to be estimated from the data set. This states that risk is a weighted sum of the values of the individual risk factors. Two deficiencies of this model soon became apparent. (1) For some individuals, the estimated value of P could be negative, and for others it could be greater than 1. (Since P is an estimate of probability, it should always lie between 0 and 1.) (2) A linear relationship did not adequately describe the curvilinear relationship that existed for some of the risk factors.

An improved model was developed in which the logarithm of the odds of developing disease (log P/1 − P) was used as the dependent variable. This has been called the "multiple logistical model." An example is given in Figure 35–2, with six curves defined by sex and three specified levels (designated high, low, and average) for each of four risk factors. The six curves then allow for the independent effect of variation in age. The curvilinear estimates of risk are apparent, and these must lie between 0 and 1.

Another explicit numerical example of the multivariate approach to risk is given in Table 35–10. This shows the probability of developing CAD in 8 years for both 45-year-old men and 65-year-old men according to five other risk factors: systolic blood pressure, total serum cholesterol, cigarette smoking, evidence of glucose intolerance, and electrocardiographic evidence of left ventricular hypertrophy. Similar tables for men of other ages and for women have also been published.[37,235] Approximate estimates for these groups can be obtained from Table 35–10 by interpolating between the ages shown, or, for women, by using estimates for men 10 years younger. These tables emphasize that the risk of developing CAD is a continuous graded function of the level of the risk factors of blood pressure and cholesterol. This probably also applies to the other risk factors, but we do not have appropriate scales or sufficient data for glucose intolerance and left ventricular hypertrophy (on the electrocardiogram). These gradients of risk hold for other populations, although the absolute levels may differ.[38-40] This latter point suggests that other risk factors which are not included in the tables also contribute to the likelihood of developing disease. One factor that has recently been introduced into the quantitative risk model is the Type A pattern of behavior.[9] One would increase the probabilities shown in Table 35–10 by 20 per cent for a Type A individual and decrease them by 20 per cent for a Type B person.

Two other observations should be made about the use of these tables. Although these estimates have been confirmed in studies of other groups, new functions will have to be estimated as new or additional risk factors are introduced to allow for a possible overlap of effects or for interactions. Thus, for example, use of data on levels of specific lipoproteins may modify or even eliminate the importance of total cholesterol in the risk function.[66] In addition, data on certain risk factors in the model produce similar information. For example, knowledge of diastolic blood pressure does not enhance the ability of a model to predict the occurrence of disease if systolic blood pressure is already contained in the equation. Likewise, indices of obesity do not seem to make any significant contribution to the model, presumably because the effects of obesity operate through its associations with the other included risk factors.

Thus, the multivariate risk function is a useful concept for quantifying the combined effect of a group of interrelated risk factors. It emphasizes that risk must be assessed as a multifactorial phenomenon with a continuous gradient of response. With currently available data, it is possible to identify, for each age group, the 10 per cent at greatest risk (among whom a quarter to a third of all new cases of CAD will occur). This provides relatively powerful predictive ability for use in screening programs and for advising individual patients.

MANAGEMENT OF RISK FACTORS

Having identified the patient who is at relatively high risk of developing CAD because of the presence of adverse risk factors, the physician must consider possible approaches to the management of these risk factors. There is no doubt that many can be changed, but the question of whether modification of these risk factors will reduce the

TABLE 35–10   PROBABILITY OF DEVELOPING CORONARY ARTERY DISEASE IN 8 YEARS*

45-YEAR-OLD MAN†

	Does Not Smoke Cigarettes							Smokes Cigarettes					
	SBP 105	*120*	*135*	*150*	*165*	*180*		*SBP 105*	*120*	*135*	*150*	*165*	*180*
					LVH—ECG Negative								
Glucose intolerance absent	CHOL							CHOL					
	185	20	24	29	35	42	51	185	32	39	46	56	67	81
	210	25	30	36	44	53	64	210	40	48	58	69	83	99
	235	31	38	45	55	66	79	235	50	60	72	86	103	122
	260	39	47	56	68	81	97	260	62	74	89	106	126	149
	285	48	58	70	84	100	119	285	76	92	109	130	153	181
	310	60	72	87	104	123	146	310	94	113	134	158	186	217

	SBP 105	*120*	*135*	*150*	*165*	*180*	*SBP 105*	*120*	*135*	*150*	*165*	*180*
Glucose intolerance present	CHOL						CHOL					
185	25	30	36	44	53	64	40	48	58	69	83	99
210	31	38	45	55	66	79	50	60	72	86	102	122
235	39	47	56	68	81	97	62	74	89	106	126	149
260	48	58	70	84	100	119	76	91	109	130	153	181
285	60	72	87	103	123	146	94	112	134	158	186	217
310	75	89	107	127	150	177	116	138	163	191	223	259

LVH—ECG Positive

	SBP 105	*120*	*135*	*150*	*165*	*180*	*SBP 105*	*120*	*135*	*150*	*165*	*180*
Glucose intolerance absent	CHOL						CHOL					
185	41	50	60	72	86	102	65	78	93	111	132	157
210	51	62	74	89	106	126	81	96	115	136	161	189
235	64	76	91	109	130	153	100	118	141	166	195	227
260	79	94	112	134	158	186	122	145	171	200	234	270
285	97	116	138	163	191	223	149	176	206	240	277	318
310	120	142	167	196	229	266	181	212	246	284	326	370

	SBP 105	*120*	*135*	*150*	*165*	*180*	*SBP 105*	*120*	*135*	*150*	*165*	*180*
Glucose intolerance present	CHOL						CHOL					
185	51	62	74	88	105	126	81	96	115	136	161	189
210	64	76	91	109	129	153	99	118	140	166	195	227
235	79	94	112	133	158	186	122	145	171	200	233	270
260	97	116	137	162	191	223	149	176	206	240	277	318
285	119	142	167	196	229	265	181	211	246	284	325	370
310	146	172	202	235	272	313	217	252	291	333	378	425

*Sixteen-year follow-up of the Framingham Study. Probability is shown in thousandths.

†Men aged 45 years have an average systolic blood pressure of 131 mm Hg and an average serum cholesterol of 235 mg/dl. Sixty-seven per cent smoke cigarettes, 1.3 per cent have definite LVH according to electrocardiographic findings, and 3.8 per cent have glucose intolerance. At these average values, the probability of developing coronary heart disease in 8 years is 60/1000.

Table continues on opposite page.

incidence of CAD is still under a great deal of scientific investigation. The evidence is strongest that curtailment of cigarette smoking is associated with a fairly rapid decline in the incidence of heart attacks, to levels approaching those associated with people who have never smoked.[83,95-106] There is fairly strong evidence that effective treatment of moderate and high degrees of hypertension will result in lower mortality, particularly from strokes and congestive heart failure. Recently, the efficacy of treating even mild hypertension has been demonstrated, suggesting benefit for both cerebrovascular disease and CAD.[236,237] There is still less certitude about the effects of modifying adverse levels of cholesterol, and this, too, is under intense study.[106,238] The management strategies recommended in the next section are based on recent assessments by several panels of experts of the available evidence and of current theories on the pathogenesis of atherosclerosis. As the results of the ongoing studies of interventions accumulate, more specific strategies may be developed.

In the management of the high-risk patient, the active participation of the patient and his family may be even more important than the role of the physician. It is well recognized that changing established life styles is difficult, but new techniques have appeared to guide the physician in helping the patient to help himself.[239] The physician should not hesitate to call on trained professionals and paraprofessionals who are knowledgeable about the techniques of behavior modification used for health maintenance. This may be particularly important in the management of obesity and the cigarette habit, as described further on.

Adverse risk factors may be managed with respect to the natural history of the disease process. Three phases may be defined: (1) efforts to prevent the occurrence of adverse risk factors; (2) management of established adverse risk factors before the occurrence of clinically manifest CAD; and (3) management of risk factors after CAD develops. Phase 1, the primary prevention of adverse risk factors, generally must start early in life, preferably in childhood, if it is to be effective in preventing or delaying the atherosclerotic process. Phase 3 is usually referred to as secondary prevention of subsequent coronary events. In secondary prevention the patient has already developed CAD, and the risk factors just described play a smaller role in determining the patient's progress than they do before the occurrence of manifest disease. In the Coronary Drug Project, an analysis of the factors influencing prognosis after recovery from myocardial infarction indicates that the major determinants of long-term survival are the state of the myocardium and its functional ability.[240] The traditional risk factors, particularly the level of serum cholesterol, did demonstrate some predictive ability in this

TABLE 35–10   PROBABILITY OF DEVELOPING CORONARY ARTERY DISEASE IN 8 YEARS* Continued

65-Year-old Man**

| | | Does Not Smoke Cigarettes | | | | | | | Smokes Cigarettes | | | | | |

LVH—ECG Negative

		SBP 105	120	135	150	165	180		SBP 105	120	135	150	165	180
	CHOL							CHOL						
Glucose	185	67	80	96	115	136	151	185	105	124	147	174	204	237
intolerance	210	69	83	99	118	140	165	210	107	128	151	178	209	243
absent	235	71	85	102	121	143	169	235	111	131	155	183	214	249
	260	73	88	104	124	147	174	260	114	135	159	187	219	254
	285	75	90	107	128	151	178	285	117	139	164	192	224	260
	310	77	93	110	131	155	183	310	120	142	168	197	230	266
		SBP 105	120	135	150	165	180		SBP 105	120	135	150	165	180
	CHOL							CHOL						
Glucose	185	83	99	118	140	165	194	185	128	152	179	209	243	281
intolerance	210	85	102	121	144	169	199	210	132	156	183	214	249	287
present	235	88	105	125	148	174	204	235	135	160	188	220	255	294
	260	90	108	128	151	178	209	260	139	164	193	225	261	300
	285	93	111	131	155	183	214	285	143	168	197	230	267	307
	310	95	114	135	160	188	219	310	146	173	202	236	273	314

LVH—ECG Positive

		SBP 105	120	135	150	165	180		SBP 105	120	135	150	165	180
	CHOL							CHOL						
Glucose	185	132	156	184	215	250	288	185	198	231	268	308	351	397
intolerance	210	136	160	188	220	256	295	210	203	237	274	314	358	404
absent	235	139	164	193	226	262	301	235	208	242	280	321	365	412
	260	143	169	198	231	268	308	260	213	248	286	328	373	419
	285	147	173	203	237	274	314	285	219	254	293	335	380	427
	310	151	178	208	242	280	321	310	224	260	299	342	387	435
		SBP 105	120	135	150	165	180		SBP 105	120	135	150	165	180
	CHOL							CHOL						
Glucose	185	161	189	221	256	295	337	185	237	274	315	359	405	453
intolerance	210	165	193	226	262	302	344	210	243	281	322	366	412	461
present	235	169	198	231	268	308	351	235	248	287	329	373	420	468
	260	173	203	237	274	315	359	260	254	293	335	380	428	476
	285	178	208	243	280	322	366	285	260	300	342	388	435	484
	310	183	214	248	287	328	373	310	266	306	349	395	443	491

**Men aged 65 years have an average systolic blood pressure of 143 mm Hg and an average serum cholesterol of 236 mg/dl. Forty-five per cent smoke cigarettes, 7.9 per cent have definite LVH according to electrocardiographic findings, and 9.6 per cent have glucose intolerance. At these average values, the probability of developing coronary heart disease in 8 years is 145/1000.

From Gordon, T., Sorlie, P., and Kannel, W. B.: Coronary heart disease, atherothrombotic brain infarction, intermittent claudication—a multivariate analysis of some factors related to their incidence: Framingham Study, 16-year followup. *In* Kannel, W. B., and Gordon, T. (eds.): The Framingham Study. An Epidemiological Investigation of Cardiovascular Disease. Section 27, 1971.

group of approximately 2800 post–myocardial infarction patients, but their relatively minor role indicates that it is unlikely that much benefit from intervention aimed at traditional risk factors will be demonstrated in patients with preexisting myocardial damage. In these patients, the extent of damage to the heart will be the most decisive factor affecting prognosis.

It matters little whether we refer to Phase 2 as primary prevention of clinical disease, as most do, or as secondary prevention of the effects of established risk factors, as others prefer. From either point of view, it is clear that intervention aimed at adverse risk factors would appear to have the most beneficial effect if done before the occurrence of CAD. Again, however, the ability of modification of risk factors to arrest or reverse the atherosclerotic process and thereby decrease the morbidity in high-risk patients has not been fully established. In fact, the recently completed Multiple Risk Factor Intervention Trial, involving 12,866 high-risk men aged 35 to 57 years, failed to demonstrate a mortality benefit over a 6-year period from a special intervention program consisting of stepped-care treatment for hypertension, counseling for cigarette smoking, and dietary advice for lowering blood cholesterol levels.[106a] It is uncertain whether this is because risk factor intervention does not affect coronary heart disease mortality or more likely because the current secular trends in coronary heart dis-

ease mortality and risk factor changes in the control group or an unfavorable response in a subgroup with hypertension and an abnormal electrocardiogram at baseline prevented demonstration of a positive response.

Evidence for the Reversibility of the Atherosclerotic Process
(See also p. 1196)

The notion that atherosclerosis is a reversible process that might be affected by a reduced intake of dietary fat was first suggested in the 1920's. Obtaining experimental proof of this hypothesis has been problematic, however. Most direct evidence for the regression of atherosclerosis comes from animal studies that cannot be duplicated in humans, but that do offer encouraging results for further investigation.[241]

In a study by Armstrong et al. of four groups of nonhuman primates, one group was maintained on a low-cholesterol chow, whereas the three other groups were fed a high-cholesterol, high-fat human chow.[242] One of the three high-fat diet groups was sacrificed after 12 months, and extensive coronary arteriosclerosis was found in these monkeys (measured by amounts of luminal narrowing, internal thickening, and lipid in the vessels). The other two high-fat groups were changed to (1) a low-fat, low-cholesterol chow, and (2) a diet high in unsaturated fat and low in cholesterol. When both groups were sacrificed 1 year later, not only had the progression of the vascular disease been arrested, but actual evidence of regression throughout the coronary system was found as well.

Other animal studies have focused on the fate of the arterial connective tissue in regression.[243,244] The change in the protein content of plaques is less well established at present.

The evidence of the reversibility of the atherosclerotic process in humans is more ambiguous, owing in part to the difficulties in *collecting* this type of evidence. Perhaps the main problem is determining the extent and degree of atherosclerosis in living humans. If one relies on secondary prevention trials of lipid lowering, it is necessary for asymptomatic arteriosclerosis first to become symptomatic —a process that may take many years. As the data from the Coronary Drug Project show, an enormous number of subjects must sustain a sufficient number of coronary events before the efficacy of the lowering of cholesterol can be assessed meaningfully. Primary prevention data are still limited, although the results of current studies such as the Lipid Research Clinics' Coronary Primary Prevention Trial should prove enlightening.

For the data on regression in humans that *are* available at present, there are often problems of interpretation.[245-247] Thus, in the case of Starzl's patient with homozygous Type II hyperlipoproteinemia who received a portacaval shunt, regression of atherosclerotic lesions was found to have accompanied the reduction of plasma cholesterol, but the patient died suddenly from advanced myocardial disease.

Two caveats must be remembered in attempting to relate the evidence from animal studies to that from studies of humans. First, the human atherosclerotic lesion develops differently from the experimentally induced atherosclerosis in animals. Consequently, the finding of regression in animals cannot be generalized in toto to humans. Second, atherosclerosis in humans may be due to a multiplicity of causes and not just to hypercholesterolemia, as is the experimental atherosclerosis induced in animals. Future studies will need to focus on the interaction of other cardiovascular risk factors in the reversal of the atherosclerotic process.

Intervention in Childhood

From the previous discussion, it should be apparent that the most effective measures for the management of adverse risk factors will be aimed at the prevention of their occurrence. This will probably require one to start early in childhood to establish good health habits and a life style that avoids adverse risk factors. Although there is much to be learned about the onset of high blood pressure and elevated levels of cholesterol in youth, there are certain risk factors that might be avoided at an early age. It is usually easier to establish good habits early than to change them later. Intervention for obesity, lack of exercise, and cigarette smoking can begin in childhood. Proper nutrition in childhood without the intake of excess calories, engaging in vigorous but nonviolent sports, and prevention of ciga-

rette smoking are likely to decrease greatly the rates of coronary artery disease in adulthood.

More active management may be considered for some children. Thus, children in families with a strong history of premature CAD or with markedly adverse risk factors may be considered for fuller evaluation and periodic follow-up. In the absence of any direct evidence for the efficacy of intervention aimed at risk factors during childhood, the individual physician must exercise careful judgment in recommending long-term therapy that may possibly have side effects or may produce undue anxiety.

General Nutritional Guidelines

A few prudent nutritional guidelines should now become evident. Each is founded on good nutritional practices that promise to help develop and maintain health and promote optimal nutrition. As detailed later in this chapter, some of these guidelines become *rules* when dealing with subjects obviously at risk, i.e., with hyperlipoproteinemia, hypertension, diabetes, or obesity, or a combination of these factors.

1. Avoidance of weight gain and overt obesity is a lifelong task that requires cognizance of the fact that caloric intake does count and that caloric balance must be individualized to meet demands for energy. Maintenance of ideal weight should be the starting point of any prudent diet.

2. In the United States today, our diet is characterized by the ingestion of 40 to 45 per cent of calories as fat, much of it saturated and of animal origin, containing 400 to 700 mg of cholesterol per day. Moderate reduction of the amount of fat, especially of saturated fat, coupled with a prudent decrease in intake of cholesterol, can lower the average American's blood level of cholesterol (and LDL) by 5 to 15 per cent. These reductions can usually be achieved simply by avoiding or limiting the intake of foods high in saturated fat and cholesterol and by replacing them, when necessary, with complex carbohydrates and polyunsaturated vegetable fats and oils.

Intake of cholesterol may be curbed by avoiding excessive consumption of foods rich in cholesterol, e.g., liver and other organ meats, shrimp (limit to once or twice monthly), and egg yolks (limit to 3 per week).

Intake of saturated fat may be controlled by decreasing the amount of animal fat, e.g., butter, whole milk, cheese, heavily marbled (usually more expensive grade) meats, cold cuts and sausage, vegetable fats so hydrogenated that they become as saturated as animal fats, and most "nondairy" products (such as nondairy sour cream containing highly saturated coconut oil).

Polyunsaturated fats may be substituted for saturated fats at the table and in most recipes. These sources provide the vegetable oils: corn, cottonseed, soybean, safflower, sunflower, and walnut. The liquids on the grocery shelf labeled "vegetable oil" are usually soybean oil or a mixture of soybean and cottonseed oil. It is important to note that the commercial use of vegetable oil often involves coconut oil, especially in nondairy and bakery items such as frostings and crackers. Advising the patient to read nutritional labels on food products prior to purchase is important.

Although it has not yet been proved in humans that reduction of the intake of cholesterol will reduce cardiovascular risk, there is little likelihood that such dietary changes will do harm. Such measures will indeed lower the level of plasma cholesterol. In fact, over the past 10 years, a 4 to 8 per cent average fall in blood levels of cholesterol in Americans of all ages is temporarily associated with a decrease in fat, especially saturated fat and cholesterol, in the diet.[33,62,248,249]

More specific nutritional guidelines have been released by the Senate Select Committee on Nutrition.[250] How rigidly these should be followed must depend for the moment on each individual physician's index of suspicion and certitude in regard to the relationship of diet to cardiovascular disease. These guidelines include a decrease in the intake of fat to less than 30 per cent of calories (and only 10 per cent of the fat should be saturated), reduction to ideal body weight, reduction of intake of salt (and avoidance of salt-rich foods such as processed items, soups, and cheeses), reduction of consumption of cholesterol to less than 300 mg/day, and an increase in the intake of dietary carbohydrates (not refined) to 50 to 60 per cent of calories.

Management of Hyperlipoproteinemia

Hyperlipoproteinemia can be effectively controlled with dietary manipulation and a variety of powerful hypolipidemic drugs. The first objective of treatment is to lower elevated levels of lipoproteins to or as near the normal range as possible.[251,252,252a] Treatment of hyperlipoproteinemia is based on the selection of diet or drug therapy, or both, aimed at either decreasing production or increasing removal of the lipoprotein fractions that are elevated.

DIET THERAPY. A dietary prescription for hyperlipoproteinemia must be formulated on an individual basis and is partly dependent on the clinical situation. In America today, mild to moderate hypercholesterolemia (increased levels of LDL) is frequently related to dietary habits (ingestion of excess amounts of cholesterol and saturated fats). Excessive consumption of any food with an associated weight gain may lead to hypertriglyceridemia through an increase in the level of VLDL; this is particularly true in individuals with already elevated levels of triglycerides. Even moderate weight reduction in hypertriglyceridemic overweight patients usually leads to lower levels of VLDL. Common sense dictates that the first step in the evaluation and management of hyperlipoproteinemia is a careful dietary history and detailed dietary instruction, ideally provided by a dietitian. In many patients with primary hyperlipoproteinemia, the levels of plasma lipids will return to normal if a dietary regimen is followed. The recommended dietary guidelines for the treatment of hyperlipoproteinemia are outlined in Table 35–11.[253]

Increased Number of Chylomicrons. Since chylomicrons are derived from dietary fat, their plasma concentration can be lowered effectively by decreasing the intake of fat from the usual 70 to 120 gm per day to 25 gm per day, supplemented by medium-chain triglycerides. Both saturated and unsaturated long-chain fatty acids must be restricted in the diet. Such treatment results within days in clearing of the lipemia, with associated correction of the hyperlipidemia, cessation of the abdominal attacks, and regression of eruptive xanthomas and hepatosplenomegaly. Maintenance of sufficiently low levels of triglyceride will prevent recurrence of abdominal pain. There is no effective drug for the treatment of Type I.

Correction of the combined chylomicronemia and increase in VLDL found in Type V is often achieved by reduction to ideal weight, followed by a maintenance

TABLE 35–11 DIETS FOR TYPES I–V HYPERLIPOPROTEINEMIA

	TYPE I	TYPE IIA	TYPE IIB AND TYPE III	TYPE IV	TYPE V
Diet Prescription	Low fat, 25–35 gm	Low cholesterol, polyunsaturated fat increased	Low cholesterol Approximately: 20% cal Protein 40% cal Fat 40% cal CHO	Controlled CHO (approximately 45% of calories) Moderately restricted cholesterol	Restricted fat, 30% of calories Controlled CHO, 50% of calories Moderately restricted cholesterol
Calories	Not restricted	Not restricted	Achieve and maintain "ideal" weight, i.e., reduction diet if necessary	Achieve and maintain ideal" weight, i.e., reduction diet if necessary	Achieve and maintain ideal" weight, i.e. reduction diet if necessary
Protein	Total protein intake is not limited	Total protein intake is not limited	High protein	Not limited other than control of patient's weight	High protein
Fat	Restricted to 25–35 gm Kind of fat not important	Saturated fat intake limited Polyunsaturated fat intake increased	Controlled to 40% calories (polyunsaturated fats recommended in preference to saturated fats)	Not limited other than control of patient's weight (polyunsaturated fats recommended in preference to saturated fats)	Restricted to 30% of calories (polyunsaturated fats recommended in preference to saturated fats)
Cholesterol	Not restricted	As low as possible; the only source of cholesterol is the meat in the diet	Less than 300 mg— the only source of cholesterol is the meat in the diet	Moderately restricted to 300–500 mg	Moderately restricted to 300–500 mg
Carbohydrate	Not limited	Not limited	Controlled—concentrated sweets are restricted	Controlled— concentrated sweets are restricted	Controlled—concentrated sweets are restricted
Alcohol	Not recommended	May be used with discretion	Limited to 2 servings (substituted for carbohydrate)	Limited to 2 servings (substituted for carbohydrate)	Not recommended

regimen in which intake of both fat and carbohydrate is restricted. Alcohol is strictly forbidden, for it can grossly exacerbate the hypertriglyceridemia seen in Type V.

Increased Levels of VLDL. Increased levels of VLDL are associated with factors such as obesity, stress, glucose intolerance, and hyperinsulinemia. In the majority of patients, weight reduction and achievement of ideal weight will be sufficient to control excess VLDL. Further decreases may be attained by reducing the intake of the precursors of VLDL triglyceride, namely, carbohydrates and alcohol. Cholesterol is moderately restricted (300 to 500 mg per day), and polyunsaturated fats are preferred.

Increased Levels of IDL. As with increased levels of VLDL, weight reduction is the most important step in controlling excess IDL. Maintenance of ideal weight through a balanced diet containing protein, fat, and carbohydrates in the proportions of 20:40:40 is recommended. Cholesterol is restricted to less than 300 mg per day, and the P/S ratio* is raised to 2:1.

Increased Levels of LDL. An effective means of lowering the high level of LDL in Type II patients is a low-cholesterol (< 300 mg per day), high P/S (2:1) diet. Strict adherence, as in metabolic wards, usually reduces total levels of plasma cholesterol and LDL by 15 to 25 per cent. In the free-living population, reductions of 10 to 20 per cent are often observed. The dietary changes enhance the rate of clearance of LDL from the bloodstream. No direct relationship exists between changes in body weight and LDL.

Multiple Increases in Lipoproteins. When more than one lipoprotein is increased, the above recommendations for the treatment of elevations of individual lipoproteins are additive. For example, in patients with increased levels

*Polyunsaturated/saturated ratio.

of VLDL and LDL (Type IIB), the former may be controlled with caloric restriction, and the latter with a diet low in cholesterol and high in polyunsaturated fats.

DRUG THERAPY. A number of potent hypolipidemic drugs are available for the treatment of hyperlipoproteinemia.[254–257,257a] Because of the heterogeneity of the disorders, no one drug is effective in controlling all lipoprotein increases. All have side effects, and patients should be carefully monitored for potential drug toxicity.[258]

The currently available drugs can control hyperlipoproteinemia by one of two mechanisms: (1) decreasing production of lipoproteins or (2) increasing clearance of lipoproteins. Clofibrate and nicotinic acid belong to the former category, whereas cholestyramine, colestipol, dextrothyroxine, and possibly probucol are in the latter group (Table 35–12).

Nicotinic Acid. Nicotinic acid is primarily indicated in states characterized by increased levels of VLDL. It is also useful in decreasing IDL and LDL, and increasing levels of HDL. The initial dose is 100 mg orally three times a day, with increases of 300 mg/day every 4 to 7 days until the maintenance dose of 3 to 9 gm per day is reached.

Side effects include cutaneous flushing and pruritus in the vast majority of patients. These effects usually decrease rapidly after the first few days of administration of the medication, even when dosage is greatly increased. Other transient effects include nausea, vomiting, and diarrhea. More serious side effects are abnormal liver function tests, abnormal glucose tolerance, and hyperuricemia. Nicotinic acid should therefore be used with extreme caution, if at all, in patients with liver disease, diabetes mellitus, or gout.

Clofibrate. Clofibrate has been especially useful in states characterized by increased levels of VLDL and IDL. It has limited value in controlling increases in LDL and sometimes, in fact, increases levels of LDL. It is prepared

TABLE 35–12 APPROVED HYPOLIPIDEMIC AGENTS

	To Decrease Lipoprotein Synthesis	Enhanced Intravascular Lipoprotein Catabolism		To Increase Lipoprotein Catabolism		
	Nicotinic Acid	*Clofibrate*	*Gemfibrozil*	*Colestipol Cholestyramine*	*D-Thyroxine*	*Probucol*
Primary indication	↑ VLDL; ↑ IDL (Types III, IV, and V)	↑ IDL (Type III)	↑ VLDL (Types IV and V)	↑ LDL (Type II)	↑ LDL (Type II)	↑ LDL (Type II)
Other indications	↑ LDL (Type II)	↑ VLDL (Types IV and V)	? ↑ IDL (Type III)		↑ IDL (Type III)	
Initial dose	100 mg t.i.d.	1 gm b.i.d.		8 gm b.i.d.	2 mg q.i.d.	250 mg b.i.d.
Maintenance dose	1–3 gm t.i.d.	1 gm b.i.d.	600 mg b.i.d.	8–16 gm b.i.d.	4–8 mg q.d.	500 mg b.i.d.
Major side effects	Flushing Pruritus Nausea Diarrhea	Nausea Diarrhea	Nausea GI discomfort	Constipation Nausea	Mild hypermetabolism ↑ Angina and cardiac irritability in patients with heart disease	Diarrhea Nausea
Other side effects	Glucose intolerance Hyperuricemia Hepatotoxicity	Myositis Ventricular ectopy Abnormal liver function tests Cholelithiasis	? ↑ Glucose intolerance ? Cholelithiasis	Hyperchloremic acidosis Biliary tract calcification Steatorrhea	Glucose intolerance Neutropenia	?
Drug interactions	↑ Vasodilatation by ganglioplegic antihypertensive agents	↑ Hypoprothrombinemic effect of warfarin sodium	Potentiates effect of anticoagulants	↓ Absorption of phenylbutazone, thiazides, tetracycline, phenobarbital, thyroid, digitalis, and warfarin sodium	↑ Hypoprothrombinemic effect of warfarin	?

in 500-mg capsules and is administered orally in a total dose of 1.5 to 2 gm per day, in two divided doses.

The drug has not usually produced serious side effects. However, in the Coronary Drug Project, the drug was associated with a twofold increase in cholelithiasis and a significant increase in arrhythmias, new angina, thromboembolism, and intermittent claudication in patients who had had a myocardial infarction.[258] In a recently completed primary prevention trial, treatment with clofibrate was associated with an increase in overall mortality, although a significant decline in suspected and proven myocardial infarction was noted.[259]

Cholestyramine. Cholestyramine is a highly effective bile acid sequestrant that is indicated for the treatment of states characterized by excess LDL. It may actually increase levels of VLDL and IDL in subjects with excesses of these lipoproteins. It is manufactured as a powder and is taken orally mixed with a liquid such as fruit juice or lemonade. The initial dose is 16 gm per day, given in two to four divided doses at meals. This may be raised by 4 to 8 gm every 2 to 3 weeks until a maximum dose of 32 gm per day is reached.

The most frequent side effects involve the gastrointestinal system, but these usually respond to a reduction in dosage.

Colestipol. Colestipol is a bile acid sequestrant whose effect on plasma cholesterol is similar to that of cholestyramine. It is indicated for treatment of the same states as cholestyramine.[261]

Colestipol is available in water-insoluble beads. The usual dose is 4 to 5 gm three times per day, although doses up to 10 gm three times per day have been used.

D-Thyroxine. D-Thyroxine is indicated for controlling increased levels of LDL. However, because it has been associated with serious potential cardiotoxic effects in patients with CAD, its role as a primary hypolipidemic agent must be considered limited. The initial dose is 2 mg per day orally, increased by 1 to 2 mg per month to a maintenance dose of 4 to 8 mg per day.

The drug was withdrawn from the Coronary Drug Project because of excess morbidity and mortality in patients with symptoms or signs of CAD who were in the D-thyroxine treatment group.[260]

Probucol and Gemfibrozil. Probucol has only recently been approved by the Food and Drug Administration for use in patients with hyperlipidemia.[262–264] Its mechanism of action is unclear. Experience with the drug is limited, so that its potential usefulness and side effects are not well defined. Serious side effects have thus far been few. In a dosage of 500 mg b.i.d., the drug appears to be most effective in subjects with mild to moderate elevations of LDL. The potential value of probucol in the prevention or control of CAD is limited by its consistent reduction of HDL levels greater or equal to its reduction of LDL concentrations.[264] In this regard, *gemfibrozil*, the most recently approved lipid-lowering drug, apparently increases levels of HDL while lowering concentrations of VLDL and LDL.[265] As with probucol, experience with this new drug is limited, and its mechanisms of action and potential usefulness are still unclear.

Combination Chemotherapy. The combination of hypolipidemic agents that act by alternate mechanisms has proved highly effective in some cases. For example, cholestyramine and nicotinic acid can function synergistically to reduce extremely high levels of LDL in Type II homozygotes and in some heterozygotes. Other combinations of drugs are still being investigated. Since all hypolipidemic agents have side effects, and the efficacy of their use in the control of cardiovascular disease is still uncertain, combination hypolipidemic therapy should usually be instituted with caution.[266]

OTHER THERAPY. *Partial ileal bypass* can significantly lower levels of LDL.[267] As with the bile acid sequestrants, levels of VLDL and IDL either are unaffected or may increase. The use of the bypass procedure for Type II subjects with or greatly at risk for CAD has been recommended by some. At present, the authors recommend it only for high-risk subjects with the heterozygous form of primary Type II who are unable to follow other therapies of their own accord (e.g., drug therapy). In the Type II homozygote, ileal bypass has not proved effective.[268]

Portacaval shunt dramatically lowered levels of LDL in one subject with homozygous Type II hyperlipoproteinemia, with an associated disappearance of angina and coronary atherosclerosis. Its use in other homozygous Type II subjects has been much less dramatic, however, usually lowering levels of LDL by only 10 to 20 per cent.[269]

Recently, *plasma exchange* on a monthly basis has been used with some effectiveness in controlling the levels of LDL and decreasing xanthomatosis and possibly coronary artery disease in homozygous Type II individuals.[270]

When to Treat

Dietary advice aimed at normalizing body weight and reducing levels of plasma lipids should be offered to any individual with a total plasma cholesterol greater than 240 mg per 100 ml. All patients with strong family histories (CAD, stroke, or arteriosclerotic peripheral vascular disease) should receive dietary advice, even though their levels of plasma lipids may be only moderately elevated. Therapeutic goals should be a level of cholesterol less than 220 mg per 100 ml and a value for triglycerides below 250 mg per 100 ml.

Since all the currently available lipid-lowering drugs have unproven efficacy but proven side effects, the use of drugs should usually be considered only after at least 6 months of unrelenting effort by the physician and dietitian has failed to achieve therapeutic goals. Even then, it should be considered only for the following groups: (1) patients with clinically manifest CAD; (2) patients with strong family histories of CAD, hyperlipidemia, or both; and (3) patients with one or more of the other established risk factors besides the hyperlipidemia, e.g., hypertension, diabetes, or cigarette smoking.

Management of Hypertension
(See also Chap. 27)

The logistic risk model described previously indicates that the risk of developing CAD is related to blood pressure in a continuous graded manner. As shown in Figure 35–6, the higher the blood pressure, the greater the risk. There is no discrete level of blood pressure that marks a discontinuous transition from low risk to high risk. Furthermore, levels of blood pressure are distributed in a smooth, continuous, unimodal curve in the general population.[271] Despite these observations, it has become rather firmly entrenched in medical thinking that there are operational cut-off points that can define an optimal strategy for managing elevated blood pressure. The strategy described here is that recommended by the National Committee on Detection, Evaluation, and Treatment of High Blood Pressure.[272]

As stated previously, approximately 40 per cent of the adult population in the United States meets the usual criterion for having hypertension, i.e., mean blood pressure on two occasions of greater than 140/90 mm Hg. Although the level of blood pressure has been found to be associated with a number of personal characteristics (family history, obesity, renal disease, sex, and race), there is little that our present state of knowledge can contribute to the primary prevention of hypertension per se. If we therefore concede that hypertension represents a disease state already in process, we must rely on secondary prevention to abort its progression and prevent its sequelae. The key modalities of secondary prevention in this case are early detection and effective treatment.

Every adult should have his blood pressure measured at least annually by a competent and properly trained observer. The Joint National Committee recommends that all adults (age 18 and older) with diastolic pressures 95 mm Hg or greater on initial measurement should be remeasured within 3 months. A diagnosis of hypertension is confirmed when this average of multiple measurements on at least two subsequent visits is 90 mm Hg or greater. The efficacy of a systematic antihypertensive treatment program in reducing mortality of persons with high blood pressure has been clearly demonstrated by the Hypertension Detection and Follow-up Program.[236] In this community-based, randomized clinical trial involving 10,940 persons with high blood pressure, 5-year mortality from all causes was 17 per cent lower for the group receiving a systematic stepped-care program than for the group referred to usual community medical therapy. Even among those with diastolic blood pressure between 90 to 104 mm Hg at entry into the study, mortality was 20 per cent lower among those receiving the stepped-care regimen. It therefore seems likely that systematic management of "mild" hypertension, as outlined in Chapter 27, has great potential for reducing overall mortality. Details of the stepped-care approach are given in Chapter 27.

Changing Cigarette Smoking Habits

Cigarette smoking has definitely been implicated as a major contributor to cardiovascular mortality and morbidity.[95,96,273] Cigarette smokers have a risk that is 60 per cent or more higher than that of nonsmokers in respect to total mortality, cardiovascular mortality, and coronary artery disease mortality and incidence.[93,95–97] There is also massive evidence that in ex-smokers and cigarette smokers who switch to cigars or pipes, risk is lowered to about the level of those who never smoked.[93,99,100]

Two limitations of the evidence, however, must be con-

ceded. In persons older than the age of 65, cigarette smoking has not shown up as a major risk factor for coronary artery disease, although it is still a major contributor to morbidity from lung cancer and chronic bronchitis and emphysema.[95,96] The second anomaly is the lack of a consistent relationship between cigarette smoking and angina pectoris.[101,107,110,111] This issue has been used to obscure the definite and consistent relationship between cigarette smoking and other forms of atherosclerotic disease and mortality.

Since the appearance of the Surgeon General's report in 1964, there have been marked changes in the cigarette smoking habits of Americans. By 1975, the proportion of men smoking cigarettes had declined by 25 per cent, from 53 per cent in 1964 to 39 per cent in 1975.[274] The number of pounds of cigarette tobacco consumed per capita had declined by 19 per cent, although the number of cigarettes sold per capita remained essentially constant. This is true because of the increased use of filter-tip cigarettes, which contain less tobacco than regular cigarettes.

Despite the widespread warning that cigarette smoking is a health hazard, and despite the vigorous public health campaigns to educate the general population about the harmful effects of smoking, many people continue to smoke. Teenaged boys continue to assume the habit as frequently now as they did in 1964, whereas teenaged girls and younger women smoked considerably more in the 1970's than their peers did in the 1960's. Many public health activists are urging legislative measures to curb cigarette smoking, including prohibition of smoking in many public areas and segregation of smokers from nonsmokers in planes and restaurants. Indeed, such rulings are already in effect in many areas.

As a group, physicians have shown a much greater decline in cigarette smoking than has the general population.[275] Thus, many physicians are able to serve as appropriate role models for patients who wish to discontinue smoking. However, simply informing patients of the ill effects of smoking and advising them to quit will not influence many who have been enjoying the habit for years. The physician who shows genuine concern about and understanding of his patient's smoking problem, who spends time with the patient to explain that cessation of smoking will have beneficial effects, and who offers helpful, practical advice and reinforcement may achieve considerable success.[273,276]

The American Heart Association Ad Hoc Committee on Cigarette Smoking and Cardiovascular Diseases has made some practical recommendations for actively encouraging the elimination of cigarette smoking.[273] The Committee advises the following:

1. Do not allow patients or nurses in physicians' offices to smoke.
2. Always raise the question of smoking in connection with the finding of vascular or pulmonary disease and in general health examinations.
3. Locate and refer patients to smoking cessation clinics when necessary.
4. Obtain help from the family in the endeavors to cease smoking.
5. Check on compliance with advice periodically.

Management of Obesity

Although obesity has not been established firmly as an independent risk factor for CAD (p. 1218), it has long been associated with the development of vascular disease. As such, it represents a major health problem for 30 to 50 per cent of the adult population of the United States.[277] The management of obesity poses a formidable challenge, however, and studies have shown that although obesity is preventable, it is almost incurable. Regardless of the weight-reducing method used, most people will fail to lose weight or to maintain weight loss for any length of time. The rates of recidivism are high, with most obese patients regaining the weight they lost within 1 to 6 years.

The procedures for the management of obesity that are most widely accepted by the medical community include: (1) diet, (2) exercise, (3) behavior modification, (4) surgical intervention, (5) pharmacological intervention, and (6) psychotherapy. Of these, behavior modification appears to hold the most promise because it deals directly with the cause of obesity, namely, eating behavior, and focuses on changing eating habits permanently so that weight loss may be maintained on a long-term basis.[278]

One of the difficulties in weight reduction lies in the creation of a negative caloric balance, that is, expending more energy than is being ingested. The vast majority of sources agree that the creation of a negative energy balance is the only reliable way to lose weight.[279,280] This can be achieved through reduction of caloric intake or increasing the caloric expenditure, or a combination of both. The results of numerous studies evaluating the effects of diet combined with exercise versus diet alone show that significantly more weight is lost by the group following both restricted caloric intake and regular exercise.[281,282] However, without concomitant behavioral changes, the attrition rate in clinical treatment programs is discouragingly high, as are the chances of recidivism.

The difficulties in weight reduction have helped popularize a number of recent diets based on the premise that weight can be lost by changing the composition of the diet without reducing the quantity of food consumed. Diets such as the high protein, high-fat, or low-carbohydrate plans are some of the most popular, but the evidence shows that these diets may have serious side effects and can be dangerous. Moreover, weight is frequently regained rapidly once the diet is terminated. Medical authorities agree that a good reducing diet should do the following:

1. Provide for adequate basic nutrition.
2. Create the desired degree of negative caloric balance.
3. Adapt as closely as possible to the tastes of the individual dieter.
4. Be palatable, socially acceptable, easy to obtain, and inexpensive.
5. Protect the dieter from hunger, satisfy his need for food, and result in a minimum of fatigue.
6. Help create new eating habits that can contribute to the maintenance of a lower body weight, once it is achieved.

None of the existing methods for treatment of obesity assures success, partly because treatment programs often fail to reinforce new eating habits and neglect the long-term maintenance of weight. Thus, alterations in diet and exercise should be viewed within the context of overall behavioral modification.

Exercise

There is a growing enthusiasm in Americans for various forms of leisure-time physical activity. The direct evidence for a protective effect of physical activity in regard to development of CAD is still rather weak. Judging from the recent public enthusiasm for jogging, cycling, tennis, and similar activities, however, many people believe that this is a pleasant way to achieve better health and improve the "quality of life."

Most individuals with sedentary occupations will probably benefit from a regular program of moderate exercise. Paul Dudley White was a vocal advocate of regular exercise in the form of bicycle riding and walking. Modern enthusiasts have urged more vigorous pursuits such as jogging and running. It is not possible at the current state of knowledge to formulate with any scientific basis an exercise program that will be optimal for most people.[163]

The physician should be prepared to urge all who wish to embark on exercise programs to do so, but only after observing a few obvious precautions. It has been recommended that anyone older than the age of 35 who has not engaged in regular exercise for a number of years should undergo a medical examination before starting an exercise program. The examination would include evaluation of the heart and lungs, a resting electrocardiogram, and assessment of the coronary risk factors. Many also advocate a treadmill exercise test. Those with evidence of possible CAD should be encouraged to engage in a carefully graded exercise program, but they should be warned not to increase their activity too rapidly.

A gradual increase in the level of physical activity over a period of weeks or even months is probably desirable for all who have previously been sedentary. The use of proper equipment for the chosen activity will help to prevent muscle, bone, and joint problems. Patients should be advised to consult a reliable book concerning appropriate equipment, warm-up exercises, and training methods. In general, the patient can avoid many of the acute aches and pains that often afflict the novice sports enthusiast by not overdoing it too early.

Psychosocial Tension

The recognition that psychosocial factors may play a role in the induction of CAD has only recently begun to receive support from epidemiological studies. Most clinicians have probably had occasion to warn a patient to "take it easy or you'll have a heart attack." This is usually accompanied by advice to relax more, slow down a little, take a vacation, or develop a new hobby. Such advice is clearly intended to help the anxious, overworked, harried patient to change a life style that the physician believes to be associated with an increased risk of developing acute CAD. Since psychosocial tension may arise from a wide variety of stressful interactions and can be handled differently by different individuals, it is impossible to give specific advice for its management.

A few patterns have been sufficiently well defined, however, and evidence of their association with CAD has begun to appear, so that some help may be offered the high-risk patient. It should be borne in mind that no studies have yet been done that demonstrate that modification of these patterns will reduce the risk of heart disease.

Epidemiological studies have shown that the Type A behavior is a predictor of increased risk of developing CAD.[173] It is this type of behavior that generates the admonition to "take it easy." Friedman and Rosenman have provided some guidelines that may be useful for some patients.[172] These include techniques for providing positive reinforcement of non-Type A behavior and suggestions for avoiding situations that elicit Type A behavior. In one prospective study on a group of postinfarction patients, it was shown that advice and counseling designed to diminish the intensity of Type A behavior reduced the rate of reinfarction.[283]

More general indices of psychosocial tension that have been related to incidence of CAD, such as status incongruity, lack of peer support systems, and geographical and cultural mobility, have not yet yielded clues for effective intervention strategies. To the extent that these situations are accompanied by depression, anxiety, or other psychological manifestations, the sympathetic physician should provide appropriate counseling.

Acknowledgment

The authors wish to acknowledge with gratitude Ms. Irene Kuraeff for her diligent and skillful work in helping to prepare this chapter.

References

1. White, P. D.: Perspectives. Prog. Cardiovasc. Dis. 14:250–255, 1971.
2. McGill, H. D., Jr. (ed.): Geographic Pathology of Atherosclerosis. Baltimore, The Williams and Wilkins Co., 1968.
3. Puffer, R. R., and Griffith, G. W.: Patterns of urban mortality. Report of the Inter-American Investigation of Mortality. Pan American Health Organization Scientific Publ. No. 151, 1967.
4. Klebba, A. J., and Dolman, A. B.: Comparability of mortality statistics for the seventh and eighth revision of the International Classification of Diseases. United States. Vital and Health Statistics: Series 2, No. 66. Washington, D. C., DHEW Publ. No. (HRA) 76-1340, 1976.
5. Kannel, W. B., McGee, D., and Gordon, T.: A general cardiovascular risk profile: The Framingham Study. Am. J. Cardiol. 38:46, 1976.
6. Inter-society Commission for Heart Disease Resources: Primary prevention of the atherosclerotic diseases. Circulation 42:A55, 1970.
7. Stamler, J., and Epstein, F. H.: Coronary heart disease: Risk factors as guides to preventive action. Prev. Med. 1:27, 1972.
8. Epstein, F. H., Napier, J. A., Block, W. D., Hayner, N. S., Higgins, M. P., Johnson, B. C., Keller, J. B., Mitzner, H. L., Montoye, H. J., Ostrander, L. D., and Ullman, B. M.: The Tecumseh Study. Design, progress and prospectives. Arch. Environ. Health 21:402, 1970.
9. Rosenman, R. H., Brand, R. J., Sholtz, R. I., and Friedman, M.: Multivariate prediction of coronary heart disease during 8.5 year follow-up in the Western Collaborative Group Study. Am. J. Cardiol. 37:903, 1976.
10. Keys, A.: Coronary heart disease in seven countries. Circulation 41(Suppl. 1):I-1–I-211, 1970.
11. Hames, C. J.: Evans County cardiovascular and cerebrovascular epidemiologic study—Introduction. Arch. Intern. Med. 128:833, 1971.
12. Garcia-Palmieri, M. R., Costas, R., Jr., Cruz-Vidal, M., Cortes-Alicea, M., Colon, A. A., Feliberti, M., Ayala, A. M., Patterne, D., Subrino, R., Torres, R., and Nazario, E.: Risk factors and prevalence of coronary heart disease in Puerto Rico. Circulation 42:541, 1970.
13. Marmot, M. G., Syme, S. L., Kagan, A., Kato, H., Cohen, J. B., and Belsky, J.: Epidemiologic studies of coronary heart disease and stroke in Japanese men living in Japan, Hawaii and California: Prevalence of coronary and hypertensive heart disease and associated risk factors. Am. J. Epidemiol. 102:514, 1975.
14. Tibblin, G., Wilhelmsen, L., and Werko, L.: Risk factors for myocardial infarction and death due to ischemic heart disease and other causes. Am. J. Cardiol. 35:514, 1975.
15. Ducimetiere, P., Richard, J. L., Cambien, F., Rakotovao, R., and Claude, J.

R.: Coronary heart disease in middle-aged Frenchmen. Comparisons between Paris Prospectives Study, Seven Countries Study, and Pooling Project. Lancet 1:1346, 1980.
16. Health Interview Survey Procedure. Vital and Health Statistics. Series 1, No. 11. Washington, D. C., DHEW Publ. No. (HSM) 73-1311, 1957–1974.
17. Plan and Operation of the Health and Nutrition Examination Survey (United States). Vital and Health Statistics: Series 1, No. 10. Washington, D. C., DHEW Publ. No. (HSM) 73-1310, 1971–1973.
18. Uniform Hospital Abstract: Minimum basic data set. A report of the United States National Committee on Vital and Health Statistics. Vital and Health Statistics: Series 4, No. 14, Washington, D.C., DHEW Publ. No. (HSM) 73-1451, 1973.
19. Monthly Vital Statistics Report. National Center for Health Statistics, Washington, D. C., Vol. 31, No. 6, September 30, 1982.
20. Gordon, T., Garcia-Palmieri, M. R., Kagan, A., Kannel, W. B., and Schiffman, J.: Differences in coronary heart disease in Framingham, Honolulu and Puerto Rico. J. Chronic Dis. 27:329, 1974.
21. Rogot, E., and Padgett, S. J.: Associations of coronary and stroke mortality with temperature and snowfall in selected areas of the United States, 1962–1966. Am. J. Epidemiol. 103:565, 1976.
22. Fabsitz, R., and Feinleib, M.: Geographic patterns in county mortality rates from cardiovascular diseases. Am. J. Epidemiol. 111:325, 1980.
23. Comstock, G. W.: Water hardness and cardiovascular diseases. Am. J. Epidermiol. 110:375, 1979.
24. Sharrett, A. R.: Water hardness and cardiovascular disease. Circulation 63:247A, 1980.
25. Masisoni, R., Pisa, Z., and Clayton, D.: Myocardial infarction and water hardness in the WHO myocardial infarction registry network. Bull. WHO 57:291, 1979.
26. Rogot, E., Sharrett, A. R., Feinleib, M., and Fabsitz, R. R.: Trends in urban mortality in relation to fluoridation status. Am. J. Epidemiol. 106:104, 1978.
27. Reid, D. D., Cornfield, J., Markush, R. E., Seigal, D., Pederson, E., and Haenzel, W.: Studies of disease among migrants and native populations in Great Britain, Norway and the United States. III. Prevalence of cardio-respiratory symptoms among migrants and native born in the United States. Nat. Cancer Inst. Monogr. 19:321, 1966.
28. Medalie, J. H., Kahn, H. A., Neufeld, H. N., Riss, E., Goldbourt, U., Perlstein, T., and Oron, D.: Myocardial infarction over a five-year period. I. Prevalence, incidence and mortality experience. J. Chronic Dis. 24:63, 1973.
29. Anderson, T. W.: Mortality from ischemic heart disease. Changes in middle-aged men since 1900. J.A.M.A. 224:336, 1973.
30. Levy, R. I.: Declining mortality in coronary heart disease. Arteriosclerosis 1:312, 1981.
31. Patrick, C. H., Palesch, Y. Y., Feinleib, M., and Brody, J. A.: Sex differences in declining cohort death rates from heart disease. Am. J. Public Health 72:161, 1982.
32. Marmot, M. G., and Syme, S. L.: Acculturation and coronary heart disease in Japanese-Americans. Am. J. Epidemiol. 104:225, 1976.
33. Havlik, R. J., and Feinleib, M.: Proceedings of the Conference on the Decline in Coronary Heart Disease Mortality. U.S. Department of Health, Education, and Welfare, NIH Publ. No. 79-1610, 1979, p. 399.
34. Feinleib, M., Havlik, R. J., and Thom, T. J.: The changing pattern of ischemic heart disease. J. Cardiovasc. Med. 7:139, 1982.
35. Strong, J. P., and Guzman, M. A.: Decrease in coronary atherosclerosis in New Orleans. Lab. Invest. 43:297, 1980.
36. Dwyer, T., and Netzel, B. S.: A comparison of trends of coronary heart disease mortality in Australia, U.S.A. and England and Wales with reference to three major risk factors—hypertension, cigarette smoking and diet. Int. J. Epidemiol. 9:65, 1980.
37. Gordon, T., Sorlie, P., and Kannel, W. B.: The Framingham Study. An Epidemiological Investigation of Cardiovascular Disease. Section 27. Coronary Heart Disease, Antherothrombotic Brain Infarction, Intermittent Claudication—A Multivariate Analysis of Some Factors Related to their Incidence: Framingham Study, 16-Year Follow-up. Washington, D.C., U.S. Government Printing Office, 1971.
38. McGee, and Gordon, T.: The results of the Framingham Study applied to four other U.S.-based epidemiologic studies of cardiovascular disease. The Framingham Study—Section 31. Washington, D.C., DHEW Publication No. (NIH) 76-1083, 1976.
39. Brand, R. J., Rosenman, R. H., Sholtz, R. I., and Friedman, M.: Multivariate prediction of coronary heart disease in the Western Collaborative Group Study compared to the findings of the Framingham Study. Circulation 53:348, 1976.
40. Keys, A., Aravanis, C., Blackburn, H., Buchem, F. S. P., Buzina, R., Djordjevic, B. S., Fidanza, F., Karvonen, M. J., Menotti, A., Puddu, V., and Taylor, H. L.: Probability of middle-aged men developing coronary heart disease in 5 years. Circulation 45:815, 1972.
41. Arteriosclerosis 1981. Report of the Working Group on Arteriosclerosis of the National Heart, Lung, and Blood Institute. Vols. 1 and 2. Washington, D.C., U.S. Department of Health and Human Services, Public Health Service, NIH Publ. No. 81–2034 and 82–2035, 1981 and 1982.
42. Dawber, T. R., Kannel, W. B., Revotskie, N., and Kagan, A.: The epidemiology of coronary heart disease. The Framingham enquiry. Proc. Roy. Soc. Med. 551:265, 1962.
43. Stamler, J.: Diet, serum lipids, and coronary heart disease: The epidemiologic evidence. In Levy, R. I., Rifkind, B. M., Dennis, B. H., and Ernst. N. (eds.):

Nutrition, Lipids, and Coronary Heart Disease—A Global View. New York, Raven Press, 1979.

44. Kannel, W. B., Castelli, W. P., and Gordon, T.: Cholesterol in the prediction of atherosclerotic disease. New perspectives based on the Framingham Study. Ann. Intern. Med. 90:85, 1979.
45. Albrink, M. M., Meigs, J. W., and Man, E. B.: Serum lipids, hypertension and coronary artery disease. Am. J. Med. 31:4, 1961.
46. Carlson, L. A.: Serum lipids in men with myocardial infarction. Acta Med. Scand. 167:399, 1960.
47. Hulley, S. B., Rosenman, R. H., Bawol, R. D., and Brand, R. J.: Epidemiology as a guide to clinical decisions. N. Engl. J. Med. 307:1383, 1980.
48. Kannel, W. B., Castelli, W. P., Gordon, T., and McNamara, P.: Serum cholesterol, lipoproteins and the risk of coronary heart disease. The Framingham Study. Ann. Intern. Med. 74:1, 1971.
49. Kinch, S. H., Doyle, J. T., and Hilleboe, H. E.: Risk factors in ischaemic heart disease. Am. J. Public Health 53:438, 1963.
50. Stamler, J.: Lifestyles, major risk factors, proof and public policy. Circulation 58:3, 1978.
51. Fredrickson, D. S., Levy, R. I., and Lees, R. S.: Fat transport in lipoproteins —an integrated approach to mechanisms and disorders. N. Engl. J. Med. 276:32, 1967.
52. Hatch, F. T., and Lees, R. S.: Practical methods for plasma lipoprotein analysis. Adv. Lipid Res. 6:1, 1968.
53. Gordon, T., Castelli, W. P., Hjortland, M., Kannel, W. B., and Dawber, T.: High density lipoprotein as a protective factor against coronary artery disease: The Framington Study. Am. J. Med. 62:707, 1977.
54. Fredrickson, D. S., and Levy, R. I.: Familial hyperlipoproteinemia. In Stanbury, J. B., Wyngaarden, J. B., and Fredrickson, D. S. (eds.): The Metabolic Basis of Inherited Disease. 3rd ed. New York, McGraw-Hill Book Co., 1972.
55. Brown, D. F., Kinch, S. H., and Doyle, J. T.: Serum triglycerides in health and in ischemic heart disease. N. Engl. J. Med. 273:947, 1965.
56. Levy, R. I., and Glueck, C. J.: Hypertriglyceridemia, diabetes mellitus and coronary vessel disease. Arch. Intern. Med. 123:220, 1969.
57. Heinle, R. A., Levy, R. I., Fredrickson, D. S., and Gorlin, R.: Lipid and carbohydrate abnormalities in patients with angiographically documented coronary artery disease. Am. J. Cardiol. 24:178, 1969.
58. Carlson, L. A., and Bottiger, L. D.: Ischemic heart disease in relation to fasting values of plasma triglycerides and cholesterol. Lancet 1:865, 1972.
59. Tatami, R., Mabuchi, H., Veda, K., Veda, R., Haba, T., Kametani, T., Ito, S., Koizumi, J. U., Ohta, M., Miyamoto, S., Nakayama, A., Kanaya, H., Oiwake, H., Genda, A., and Takeda, R.: Intermediate-density lipoprotein and cholesterol-rich very low density lipoprotein in angiographically determined coronary artery disease. Circulation 64:1174, 1981.
60. Levy, R. I., Bilheimer, D. W., and Eisenberg, S.: The structure and metabolism of chylomicrons and very low density lipoproteins (VLDL). In Smellie, R. M. S. (ed.): Plasma Lipoproteins. New York, Academic Press, 1971.
61. Havel, R. J.: Mechanisms of hyperlipoproteinemia. Adv. Exp. Med. Biol. 26:57, 1972.
62. Levy, R. I.: Cholesterol, lipoproteins, apoproteins, and heart disease: Present status and future prospects. Clin. Chem. 27:653, 1981.
63. Stone, N. J., Levy, R. I., Fredrickson, D. S., and Verter, J.: Coronary artery disease in 116 kindred with familial type II hyperlipoproteinemia. Circulation 49:476, 1974.
64. Rhoads, G. C., Gulbrandsen, C. L., and Kagan, A.: Serum lipoproteins and coronary heart disease in a population of Hawaii Japanese men. N. Engl. J. Med. 294:293, 1976.
65. Miller, G. J., and Miller, N. E.: Plasma high density lipoprotein concentration and development of ischemic heart disease. Lancet 1:16, 1975.
66. Castelli, W. P., Doyle, J. T., Gordon, T., Haines, C. G., Hjortland, M., Hulley, S. B., Kagan, A., and Zukel, W. J.: HDL cholesterol and other lipids in coronary heart disease. The Cooperative Lipoprotein Phenotyping Study. Circulation 55:767, 1977.
67. Miller, N. E., Thelle, D. S., Forde, O. H., and Mjos, O. D.: The Tromso Heart-Study. High density lipoprotein and coronary heart disease: A prospective case-control study. Lancet 1:965, 1977.
68. Tyroler, H. A. (ed.): Epidemiology of plasma high-density lipoprotein cholesterol levels. The Lipid Research Clinics Program Prevalence Study. Circulation 62(Suppl.):4, 1980, 1.
69. Bradley, D. D., Wingred, J., Petitti, D. B., Krauss, R. M., and Ramcharan, S.: Serum high-density-lipoprotein cholesterol in women using oral contraceptives, estrogens and progestins. N. Engl. J. Med. 299:17–20, 1978.
70. Glueck, C. J., Gartside, P., Fallat, R. W., Sielski, J., and Steiner, P. M.: Longevity syndromes: Familial hypobeta and familial hyperalpha lipoproteinemia. J. Lab. Clin. Med. 88:941, 1976.
71. Lipid Research Clinics (LRC) Program Epidemiology Committee: Plasma lipid distributions in 11 North American populations: The Lipid Research Clinics Program Prevalence Study. Circulation 60:427, 1979.
72. Rifkind, B. M., Tamir, I., Heiss, G., Wallace, R. B., and Tyroler, H. A.: Distribution of high-density and other lipoproteins in selected Lipid Research Clinics Prevalence Study populations: A brief survey. Lipids 14:105, 1979.
73. Lipid Research Clinics Population Studies Data Book. Vol. 1. The Prevalence Study. Washington, D.C., U.S. Department of Health and Human Services, Public Health Service. NIH Publ. No. 80-1527, 1980.
74. WHO Bulletin. Classification of hyperlipidemias and hyperlipoproteinemias. Circulation 45:501, 1972.
75. Friedewald, W. T., Levy, R. I., and Fredrickson, D. S.: Estimation of the concentration of low-density lipoprotein cholesterol in plasma, without use of the preparative ultracentrifuge. Clin. Chem. 18:499, 1972.
76. Lipid Research Clinics Program. Manual of Laboratory Operations, Vol. 1, Washington, D.C., DHEW Publ. No. (NIH) 75-628, 1974.
77. Schaefer, E. J., Eisenberg, S., and Levy, R. I.: Lipoprotein apoprotein metabolism. J. Lipid Res. 19:667, 1978.
78. Rifkind, B. M., and Levy, R. I. (eds.): Hyperlipidemia: Diagnosis and Therapy. New York, Grune and Stratton, 1977.
79. Breckenridge, W. C., Little, J. A., Steiner, G., Chow, A., and Poapst, M.: Hypertriglyceridemia associated with deficiency of apolipoprotein C-II. N. Engl. J. Med. 298:1265, 1978.
80. Cox, D. W., Breckenridge, W. C., and Little, J. A.: Inheritance of apolipoprotein C-II deficiency with hypertriglyceridemia and pancreatitis. N. Engl. J. Med. 299:1421, 1978.
81. Brown, M. S., and Goldstein, J. L.: Familial hypercholesterolemia: A genetic defect in the low-density lipoprotein receptor. N. Engl. J. Med. 294(25):1386, 1976.
82. Fredrickson, D. S., Morganroth, J., and Levy, R. I.: Type III hyperlipoproteinemia: An analysis of two contemporary definitions. Ann. Intern. Med. 82:150, 1975.
83. Morganroth, J., Levy, R. I., and Fredrickson, D. S.: The biochemical, clinical and genetic features of Type III hyperlipoproteinemia. Ann. Intern. Med. 82:158, 1975.
84. Kushwaha, R. S., Hazzard, W. R., Wahl, P. W., and Hoover, J. J.: Type III hyperlipoproteinemia: Diagnosis in whole plasma by apolipoprotein-E immunoassay. Ann. Intern. Med. 86:509, 1977.
85. Ghiselli, G., Gascon, P., and Brewer, H. B., Jr.: Type III hyperlipoproteinemia associated with apolipoprotein E deficiency (letter). Science 214:1239, 1980.
86. Wallace, R. B., Hoover, J., Sandler, D., and Rifkind, B. M.: Altered plasmalipids associated with oral contraceptive or estrogen consumption. Lancet 2:11, 1977.
87. Goldstein, J. L., Hazzard, W. R., Schrott, H. G., Bierman, E. L., and Motulsky, A. G.: Hyperlipidemia in coronary heart disease. I. Lipid levels in 500 survivors of myocardial infarction. J. Clin. Invest. 52:1533, 1973.
88. Wood, P. D., Stern, M. P., Silvers, A., Reaven, G. M., and Von der Groeben, J.: Prevalence of plasma lipoprotein abnormalities in a free-living population of the Central Valley, California. Circulation 45:114, 1972.
89. Greenberg, B. H., Blackwelder, W. C., and Levy, R. I.: Primary Type V hyperlipoproteinemia. A descriptive study of 32 families. Ann. Intern. Med. 87:526, 1977.
90. Kannel, W. B.: Role of blood pressure in cardiovascular disease: The Framingham Study. Angiology 26:1, 1975.
91. Feinleib, M., Garrison, R., Borhani, N., Rosenman, R., and Christian, J.: Studies of hypertension in twins. In Paul, O. (ed.): Epidemiology and Control of Hypertension. Miami, Symposia Specialists, 1975, pp. 3–20.
92. Feinleib, M.: Genetics and familial aggregation of blood pressure. In Onesti, G., and Klimt, C. (eds.): Hypertension Determinants. Complications and Intervention. The Fifth Hahnemann International Symposium on Hypertension. New York, Grune and Stratton, 1979, pp. 35–48.
93. Feinleib, M., and Williams, R. R.: Relative risks of myocardial infarction, cardiovascular disease and peripheral vascular disease by type of smoking. Proc. Third World Conf. Smoking and Health 1:243, 1976.
94. Aronow, W. S.: Effect of cigarette smoking and of carbon monoxide on coronary heart disease. Chest 70:514, 1976.
95. The Health Consequences of Smoking. Washington, D.C., U.S. Public Health Service, 1973.
96. The Health Consequences of Smoking. Washington, D.C., U.S. Public Health Service, 1971.
97. Wilhelmsson, C., Vedin, J. A., Elmfeldt, D., Tibblin, G., and Wilhelmsen, L.: Smoking and myocardial infarction. Lancet 1:415, 1975.
98. Report of the Surgeon General: Smoking and Health. U.S. Department of Health, Education and Welfare, Public Health Service Publ. No. 79-50066, 1979.
99. Rogot, E.: Smoking and general mortality among U.S. veterans, 1954–1969. Washington, D.C., DHEW Publ. No. (NIH) 74-544, 1974.
100. Gordon, T., Kannel, W. B., McGee, D., and Dawber, T. R.: Death and coronary attacks in men after giving up cigarette smoking. A report from the Framingham study. Lancet 2:1345, 1974.
101. Doyle, J. T., Dawber, T. R., Kannel, W. B., Kinch, S. H., and Kahn, H. A.: The relationship of cigarette smoking to coronary heart disease. The second report of the combined experience of the Albany, N.Y., and Framingham, Mass. studies. J.A.M.A. 190:886, 1964.
102. Friedman, G. D., and Siegelaub, A. B.: Changes after quitting cigarette smoking. Circulation 61:716, 1980.
103. Friedman, G. D., Petitti, D. B., Bawol, R. D., and Siegelaub, A. B.: Mortality in cigarette smokers and quitters. Effect of base-line differences. N. Engl. J. Med. 304:1407, 1981.
104. Castelli, W. P., Garrison, R. J., Dawber, T. R., McNamara, P. M., Feinleib, M., and Kannel, W. B.: The filter cigarette and coronary heart disease: The Framingham Study. Lancet 2:109, 1981.
105. Rose, G., and Hamilton, P. J. S.: A randomised controlled trial of the effect on middle-aged men of advice to stop smoking. J. Epidemiol. Community Health 32:275, 1978.
106. Hjermann, I., Velve-Byre, K., Holme, I., and Leren, P.: Effect of diet and

smoking intervention on the incidence of coronary heart disease. Report from the Oslo Study Group of a randomised trial in healthy men. Lancet 2:1303, 1981.

106a. Multiple Risk Factor Intervention Trial Research Group: Multiple Risk Factor Intervention Trial. Risk factor changes and mortality results. J.A.M.A. 248: 1465, 1982.

107. Jenkins, C. D., Rosenman, R. H., and Zyzanski, S. J.: Cigarette smoking: Its relationship to coronary heart disease and related risk factors in the Western Collaborative Group Study. Circulation 38:1140, 1968.

108. Shurtleff, D.: Some characteristics related to the incidence of cardiovascular disease and death: The Framingham Study, 18-year follow-up. Washington, D.C., DHEW Publ. No. (NIH) 74-599, Section No. 30, 1974.

109. Slone, D., Shapiro, S., Rosenberg, L., Kaufman, D. W., Hartz, S. C., Rossi, A. C., Stolley, P. D., and Miettinen, O. S.: Relation of cigarette smoking to myocardial infarction in young women. N. Engl. J. Med. 298:1273–1276, 1978.

110. Shapiro, S., Weinblatt, E., Frank, C. W., and Sager, S. V.: Incidence of coronary heart disease in a population insured for medical care (HIP): Myocardial infarction, angina pectoris, and possible myocardial infarction. Am. J. Public Health 59(Suppl.):1, 1969.

111. Mulcahy, R., and Hickey, N.: Cigarette smoking habits of patients with coronary heart disease. Br. Heart J. 28:404, 1966.

112. Garrison, R. J., Kannel, W. B., Feinleib, M., Castelli, W. P., McNamara, P. M., and Padgett, S. J.: Cigarette Smoking and HDL cholesterol. The Framingham Offspring Study. Atherosclerosis 30:17, 1978.

113. Ostrander, L. D., and Epstein, F. H.: Diabetes, hyperglycemia and atherosclerosis: New research directions. In Fajans, S. (ed.): Diabetes Mellitus. Washington, D.C., DHEW Publ. No. (NIH) 76-854, 1976.

114. Sharkey, T. P.: Diabetes mellitus—present problems and new research. The heart and vascular disease. J. Am. Diet. Assoc. 58:336, 1971.

115. Report of the National Commission on Diabetes. Washington, D.C., DHEW Publ. No. (NIH) 76-1022, 1975.

116. Garcia, M. J., McNamara, P. M., Gordon, T., and Kannel, W. B.: Morbidity and mortality of diabetes in the Framingham population. Sixteen year follow-up study. Diabetes 23:105, 1976.

117. Ostrander, L. D., Jr., Block, W. D., Lamphiear, D. E., and Epstein, F. H.: Altered carbohydrate and lipid metabolism and coronary heart disease among men in Tecumseh, Michigan. In Camerini-Davalos, R. A., and Cole, H. S. (eds.): Vascular and Neurological Changes in Early Diabetes. New York, Academic Press, 1973, p. 73.

118. Fuller, J. N., Shipley, M. J., Rose, G., Jarrett, R. J., and Keen, N.: Coronary heart disease risk and impaired glucose tolerance. The Whitehall Study. Lancet 1:1373, 1980.

119. Knowles, H. C., Jr.: Magnitude of the renal failure problem in diabetic patients. Kidney International, Vol. 6, No. 4, Suppl. 1. New York, Springer-Verlag, 1974.

120. Vigorita, V. J., Moore, G. W., and Hutchins, G. N.: Absence of correlation between coronary arterial atherosclerosis and severity or duration of diabetes mellitus of adult onset. Am. J. Cardiol. 46:535, 1980.

121. Coronary Drug Project Research Group, Baltimore: The prognostic importance of plasma glucose levels and the use of oral hypoglycemic drugs after myocardial infarction in men. Diabetes 26:453, 1977.

122. Sosenko, J. N., Breslow, J. L., Niettinen, O. S., and Gabbay, K. N.: Hyperglycemia and plasma lipid levels. A prospective study of young insulin-dependent diabetic patients. N. Engl. J. Med. 302:650, 1980.

123. University Group Diabetes Program: A study of the effects of hypoglycemic agents on vascular complications in patients with adult-onset diabetes. II. Mortality results. Diabetes 19(Suppl. 2):785, 1970.

124. Knatterud, G. L., Klimt, C. R., Levin, M. E., Jacobson, M. E., and Goldner, M. G.: Effects of hypoglycemic agents in vascular complications in patients with adult-onset diabetes. VII. Mortality and selected nonfatal events with insulin treatment. J.A.M.A. 240:37, 1978.

125. Carlstrom, S.: Treatment with sulphonylurea drugs and cardiovascular disease. Proc. Ninth Congr. Int. Diabetes Federation. Amsterdam, Excerpta Medica, 1977, pp. 426–433.

126. Hall, A. P.: Correlations among hyperuricemia, hypercholesterolemia, coronary disease and hypertension. Arthritis Rheum. 8:846, 1965.

127. Fessel, W. J.: High uric acid as an indicator of cardiovascular disease: Independence from obesity. Am. J. Med. 68:401, 1980.

128. Persky, V. W., Dyer, A. R., Idris-Soven, E., Stamler, J., Shekelle, K. B., Schoenberger, J. A., Berkson, D. M., and Lindberg, H. A.: Uric acid: a risk factor for coronary heart disease? Circulation 59:969, 1979.

129. Kannel, W. B., Hjortland, M. C., McNamara, P. M., and Gordon, T.: Menopause and risk of cardiovascular disease: The Framingham Study. Ann. Intern. Med. 85:447, 1976.

130. Mann, J. I., and Inman, W. H. W.: Oral contraceptives and death from myocardial infarction. Br. Med. J. 2:245, 1975.

131. Jick, H., Dinan, B., and Rothman, K. J.: Oral contraceptives and nonfatal myocardial infarction. J.A.M.A. 239:1403, 1978.

132. Layde, P. M., Beral, V., and Kay, C. R.: Further analysis of mortality in oral contraceptive users. Royal College of General Practitioners' Oral Contraception Study. Lancet 1:549, 1981.

133. Slone, D., Shapiro, S., Kaufman, D. W., Rosenberg, L., Niettinen, O. S., and Stolley, P. D.: Risk of myocardial infarction in relation to current and discontinued use of oral contraceptives. N. Engl. J. Med. 305:420, 1981.

134. Vessey, M. P., McPherson, K., and Yeates, D.: Mortality in oral contraceptive users. Lancet 1:549, 1981.

135. Wallace, R. B., Hoover, J., Barrett-Conner, E., Rifkind, B. M., Hunninghake, D. B., Mackenthun, A., and Heiss, G.: Altered plasma lipid and lipoprotein levels associated with oral contraceptive and estrogen use. Lancet 2:111, 1979.

136. Rosenberg, L., Armstrong, B., and Jick, H.: Myocardial infarction and estrogen therapy in post-menopausal women. N. Engl. J. Med. 294:1256, 1976.

137. Pfeffer, R. I., Whipple, G. H., Kurosaki, T. T., and Chapman, J. M.: Coronary risk and estrogen use in post-menopausal women. Am. J. Epidemiol. 107:479, 1978.

138. Barrett-Conner, E., Brown, W. V., Turner, J., Austin, M., and Criqui, M.: Heart disease risk factors and hormone use in postmenopausal women. J.A.M.A. 241:2167, 1979.

139. Ross, R. K., Paganini-Hill, A., Mack, T. M., Arthur, N., and Henderson, B. E.: Menopausal oestrogen therapy and protection from death from ischaemic heart disease. Lancet 1:858, 1981.

140. Byar, D. P.: The Veterans Administration Cooperative Urological Research Group's studies on cancer of the prostate. Cancer 32:1126, 1973.

141. The Coronary Drug Project Research Group: The Coronary Drug Project. Initial findings leading to modification of its research protocol. J.A.M.A. 226:652, 1973.

142. The Coronary Drug Project Research Group: The Coronary Drug Project. Findings leading to discontinuation of the 2.5 mg/day estrogen group. J.A.M.A. 226:652, 1973.

143. Jick, H., Dinan, B., and Rothman, K. J.: Noncontraceptive estrogens and nonfatal myocardial infarction. J.A.M.A. 239:1407, 1978.

144. Clarkson, T. B., and Alexander, N. J.: Does vasectomy increase the risk of atherosclerosis? J. Cardiovasc. Med. 5:999, 1980.

145. Walker, A. M., Jick, H., Hunter, J. R., Danford, A., Watkins, R. N., Alhadeff, L., and Rothman, K. J.: Vasectomy and non-fatal myocardial infarction. Lancet 1:13, 1981.

145a. Goldacre, M. J., Holford, T. R., and Vessey, M. P.: Cardiovascular disease and vasectomy. Findings from two epidemiologic studies. N. Engl. J. Med. 308: 805, 1983.

146. Heller, R. F., Jacobs, H. S., Vermeulen, A., and Deslypere, J. P.: Androgens, oestrogens, and coronary heart disease. Br. Med. J. 282:438, 1981.

147. Lew, E. A., and Garfinkel, L.: Variations in mortality by weight among 750,000 men and women. J. Chronic Dis. 32:563, 1979.

148. Keys, A.: Coronary heart disease—the global picture. Atherosclerosis 22:149, 1975.

149. Keys, A.: Overweight and the risk of heart attack and sudden death. In Bray, G. A. (ed.): Obesity in Perspective. Vol. 2, Part 2. Washington, D. C., DHEW Publ. No. (NIH) 75-708, 1976, p. 215.

150. Gordon, T., and Kannel, W. B.: Obesity and cardiovascular disease: The Framingham Study. Clin. Endocrinol. Metab. 5:367, 1976.

151. Hubert, N., Feinleib, M., McNamara, P. M., and Castelli, W. P.: Obesity as an independent risk factor for cardiovascular disease in Framingham. Presented at the Twenty-Second Annual Cardiovascular Epidemiology Meeting, March 1982, San Antonio, Texas.

151a. Hubert, H. B., Feinleib, M., McNamara, P. M., and Castelli, W. P.: Obesity as an independent risk factor for cardiovascular disease. A 26-year follow-up of participants in the Framingham Heart Study. Circulation 67:968, 1983.

152. Grande, F.: Assessment of body fat in man. In Bray, G. A. (ed.): Obesity in Perspective. Vol. 2, Part 2. Washington, D.C., DHEW Publ. No. (NIH) 76-852, 1976, pp. 189–203.

153. Bray, G. A. (ed.): Standard for definitions of overweight and obesity. In Bray, G. A. (ed.): Obesity in Perspective. Vol. 1, Part 1, Chap. 2. Washington, D.C., DHEW Publ. No. (NIH) 75-708, 1976, p. 7.

154. Keys, A., Fidanza, F., Karvonen, M. J., Kimura, N., and Taylor, H. L.: Indices of relative weight and obesity. J. Chronic Dis. 25:322, 1972.

155. Ashley, F. W., and Kannel, W. B.: Relation of weight change to changes in atherogenic traits: The Framingham Study. J. Chronic Dis. 27:103, 1974.

156. Streja, D. A., Boyko, E., and Rabkin, S. W.: Changes in plasma high-density lipoprotein cholesterol concentration after weight reduction in grossly obese subjects. Br. Med. J. 281:770, 1980.

157. Kagan, A., Gordon, T., Rhoads, G. G., and Schiffman, J. C.: Some factors related to coronary heart disease incidence in Honolulu Japanese men: The Honolulu Heart Study. Int. J. Epidemiol. 4:271, 1975.

158. Rabkin, S. W., Mathewson, F. A. L., and Hsu, P.: Relation of body weight to development of ischemic heart disease in a cohort of young North American men after a 26 year observation period: The Manitoba Study. Am. J. Cardiol. 39:452, 1977.

159. Paffenbarger, R. S., and Hale, W. E.: Work activity and coronary heart mortality. N. Engl. J. Med. 292:545, 1975.

160. Paffenbarger, R. S., Hale, W. E., Brand, R. J., and Hyde, R. T.: Work-energy level, personal characteristics and fatal heart attack: A birth cohort effect. Am. J. Epidemiol. 105:200, 1977.

161. Cooper, K. H., Pollock, M. L., Martin, R. P., White, S. R., Linnerud, A. L., and Jackson, A.: Physical fitness levels vs. selected coronary risk factors. A cross-sectional study. J.A.M.A. 236:166, 1976.

162. Hickey, N., Mulcahy, R., Bourke, G. J., Graham, J., and Wilson-Davis, K.: Study of coronary risk factors related to physical activity in 15,171 men. Br. Med. J. 3:507, 1975.

163. Fox, S. M., and Naughton, J. P.: Physical activity and the prevention of coronary heart disease. Prev. Med. 1:92, 1972.

164. Wyndham, C. H.: The role of physical activity in the prevention of ischemic heart disease. S. Afr. Med. J. 36:7, 1979.

165. Siegel, A. J., Hennekens, C. H., Rosner, B., and Karlson, L. K.: Paternal his-

tory of coronary-heart disease reported by marathon runners. N. Engl. J. Med. 301:90, 1979.

166. Noakes, T. D., Opie, C. H., Rose, A. G., and Kleynhans, P. H. T.: Autopsy-proved coronary atherosclerosis in marathon runners. N. Engl. J. Med. 301:86, 1979.

167. Morris, J. N., Everitt, M. G., Pollard, R., Chave, S. P. W., and Semmence, A. M.: Vigorous exercise in leisure-time: Protection against coronary heart disease. Lancet 2:1207, 1980.

167a. Gibbons, L. W., Blair, S. N., Cooper, K. H., and Smith, M: Association between coronary heart disease risk factors and physical fitness in healthy adult women. Circulation 67:977, 1983.

168. Wood, P. D., and Haskell, W. L.: The effect of exercise on plasma high density lipoproteins. Lipids 14:417, 1979.

169. Hartung, G. H., Foreyt, J. P., Mitchell, R. E., Vlasek, I., and Gotto, A. M., Jr.: Relation of diet to high-density-lipoprotein cholesterol in middle-aged marathon runners, joggers, and inactive men. N. Engl. J. Med. 302:357, 1980.

170. Soman, V. R., Koivisto, V. A., Deibert, D., Felig, P., and DeFronzo, R. A.: Increased insulin sensitivity and insulin binding to monocytes after physical training. N. Engl. J. Med. 301:1200, 1979.

171. Williams, R. S., Logue, E. E., Lewis, J. L., Barton, T., Stead, N. W., Wallace, A. G., and Pizzo, S. V.: Physical conditioning augments the fibrinolytic response to venous occlusion in healthy adults. N. Engl. J. Med. 302:987, 1980.

172. Friedman, H., and Rosenman, R. H.: Type A Behavior and Your Heart. New York, Alfred A. Knopf, 1974.

173. Dembroski, T. M., Feinleib, M., Haynes, S. G., Shields, J. L., and Weiss, S. M. (eds.): Proceedings of the forum on coronary-prone behavior. Washington, D. C., DHEW Publ. No. (NIH) 78-1451, 1978.

174. Haynes, S. G., Feinleib, M., and Kannel, W. B.: The relationship of psychosocial factors to coronary heart disease in the Framingham Study. III. Eight-year incidence of coronary heart disease. Am. J. Epidemiol. 111:37, 1980.

175. Review Panel on Coronary-Prone Behavior and Coronary Heart Disease. Coronary-prone behavior and coronary heart disease: A critical review. Circulation 63:1199, 1981.

176. Rosenman, R. H.: History and definition of the Type A coronary-prone behavior pattern. In Dembroski, T. M., Feinleib, M., Haynes, S. G., Shields, J. L., and Weiss, S. M. (eds.): Proceedings of the forum on coronary-prone behavior. Washington, D.C., DHEW Publ. No. (NIH) 78-1451, 1978, p. 13.

177. Haynes, S. G., Feinleib, M., Levine, S., Scotch, N., and Kannel, W. B.: The relationship of psychosocial factors to coronary heart disease in the Framingham Study. II. Prevalence of coronary heart disease. Am. J. Epidemiol. 107:384, 1978.

178. Haynes, S. G., and Feinleib, M.: Type A behavior and the incidence of coronary heart disease in the Framingham Heart Study. Adv. Cardiol. 29:85, 1982.

179. Frank, K. A., Heller, S. S., Kornfeld, D. S., Sporn, A. A., and Weiss, M. B.: Type A behavior pattern and coronary angiographic findings. J.A.M.A. 240:761, 1978.

180. Jenkins, C. D.: Recent evidence supporting psychologic and social risk factors for coronary disease. N. Engl. J. Med. 294:987, 1976.

181. Casscells, W., Hennekens, C. H., Evans, D., Rosener, B., DeSilva, R. A., Lown, B., Davies, J. E., and Jesse, M. J.: Retirement and coronary mortality. Lancet 1:1288, 1980.

182. Haynes, S. G., and Feinleib, M.: Women, work and coronary heart disease: Prospective findings from the Framingham Heart Study. Am. J. Public Health 70:133, 1980.

183. Report from the National Heart and Lung Institute Task Force on Genetic Factors in Atherosclerotic Disease. Washington, D.C., DHEW Publ. No. (NIH) 76-922, 1976.

184. Lee, J., Lauer, R. M., and Clarke, W. R.: Coronary risk factors in children. In Engle, M. E. (ed.): Pediatric Cardiovascular Disease, Philadelphia, F.A. Davis, 1981.

185. Snowden, D. B., McNamara, P. M., Garrison, R. J., Feinleib, M., Kannel, W. B., and Epstein, F. H.: Predicting coronary heart disease in siblings—a multivariate assessment: The Framingham Heart Study. Am. J. Epidemiol. 115:217, 1982.

185a. Neufeld, H. N., and Goldbourt, U.: Coronary heart disease: Genetic aspects. Circulation 67:943, 1983.

186. The diet and all-cause death rate in the Seven Countries Study. Lancet 2:58, 1981.

187. Kato, H., Tillotson, J., Nichaman, M., Rhoads, G., and Hamilton, H.: Epidemiologic studies of coronary heart disease and stroke in Japanese men living in Japan, Hawaii, and California: Serum lipids and diet. Am. J. Epidemiol. 97:372, 1973.

188. Phillips, R. L., Lemon, F. R., Beeson, L., and Kuzman, J. W.: Coronary heart disease mortality among Seventh-Day Adventists with differing dietary habits: A preliminary report. Am. J. Clin. Nutr. 31:S191, 1978.

189. The Framingham Study. An Epidemiological Investigation of Cardiovascular Disease. Section 23. The Framingham Diet Study: Diet and the regulation of serum cholesterol. Washington, D.C., U.S. Government Printing Office, 1970.

190. Nichols, A. B., Ravenscroft, C., Lamphiear, D. E., and Ostrander, L. D., Jr.: Daily nutritional intake and serum lipid levels. The Tecumseh Study. Am. J. Clin. Nutr. 29:1384, 1976.

191. Shekelle, R. B., Shryock, A. M., Paul, O., Lepper, M., Stamler, J., Liu, S., and Raynor, W. J.: Diet, serum cholesterol, and death from coronary heart disease. The Western Electric Study. N. Engl. J. Med. 304:65, 1981.

192. NIH release first data from Lipid Research Clinic Program. J. Am. Oil Chemists' Soc. 54:717A, 1977.

193. Ahrens, E. H., Jr., Insull, W., Blomstrand, R., Hirsch, J., Tsaltas, T. T., and Peterson, M. L.: The influence of dietary fats on serum-lipid levels in man. Lancet 1:943, 1957.

194. Keys, A., Anderson, J. T., and Grande, F.: Serum cholesterol response to changes in the diet. Metabolism 4:747, 1965.

195. Mattson, F. H., Erickson, B. A., and Kligman, A. M.: Effect of dietary cholesterol on serum cholesterol in man. Am. J. Clin. Nutr. 25:589, 1972.

196. Kuller, L. H.: Epidemiology of cardiovascular disease: Current perspectives. Am. J. Epidemiol. 104:425, 1976.

197. Connor, W. E., and Connor, S. E.: Sucrose and carbohydrate. In Present Knowledge in Nutrition. 4th ed. New York, Nutrition Foundation, Inc., 1976, p. 33.

198. Bierman, E. L., and Porte, D., Jr.: Carbohydrate intolerance and lipidemia. Ann. Intern. Med. 68:926, 1968.

199. Glueck, C. J., Levy, R. I., and Fredrickson, D. S.: Immunoreactive insulin, glucose tolerance and carbohydrate inducibility in types II, III, and IV hyperlipoproteinemia. Diabetes 18:739, 1969.

200. Jenkins, D. J. A., Leeds, A. R., Gassull, M. A., Cochet, B., and Alberti, K. G.: Decrease in postprandial insulin and glucose concentrations by guar and pectin. Ann. Intern. Med. 86:20, 1977.

201. Kritchevsky, D.: Dietary fiber and other dietary factors in hypercholesterolemia. Am. J. Clin. Nutr. 30:979, 1977.

202. Report of the Hypertension Task Force. Vol. 8. Current Research and Recommendations from the Task Force Subgroups on (1) Renin-Angiotensin-Aldosterone; (2) Salt and Water. U.S. DHEW, Public Health Service, NIH Publ. No. 79-1630, 1979.

203. Page, L. B.: Epidemiologic evidence on etiology of human hypertension and its possible prevention. Am. Heart J. 91:527, 1976.

204. Reisin, E., Abel, R., Modan, M., Silverberg, D. S., Eliahou, H. E., and Modan, B.: Effect of weight loss without salt restriction and the reduction of blood pressure in overweight hypertensive patients. N. Engl. J. Med. 298:1, 1978.

205. Shurtleff, D.: Some characteristics related to the incidence of cardiovascular disease and death: Framingham Study, 16-year follow-up. In Kannel, W. B., and Gordon, T. (eds.): The Framingham Study, Section 26, Washington, D.C., U.S. Government Printing Office, 1970.

206. Yano, K., Rhoads, G. G., and Kagan, A.: Coffee, alcohol and risk of coronary heart disease among Japanese men living in Hawaii. N. Engl. J. Med. 297:405, 1977.

207. Hennekens, C. H., Willett, W., Rosner, B., Cole, D. S., and Mayrent, S. L.: Effects of beer, wine, and liquor in coronary deaths. J.A.M.A. 242:1973, 1979.

208. Marmot, M. G., Rose, G., Shipley, M. J., and Thomas, B. J.: Alcohol and mortality: A U-shaped curve. Lancet 1:580, 1981.

209. Kozarevic, D., McGee, D., Vojrodic, N., Racic, Z., Dawber, T. R., Gordon, T., and Zukel, W.: Frequency of alcohol consumption and morbidity and mortality: The Yugoslavia Cardiovascular Disease Study. Lancet 1:613, 1980.

210. Wilhelmsen, L., Wedel, H., and Tibblin, G.: Multivariate analysis of risk factors for coronary heart disease. Circulation 48:950, 1973.

211. Stason, W. B., Neff, R. K., Miettinen, O. S., and Jick, H.: Alcohol consumption and nonfatal myocardial infarction. Am. J. Epidemiol. 104:603, 1976.

212. Dyer, A. R., Stamler, J., Paul, O., Berkson, D. M., Lepper, M. N., McKean, H., Shekelle, R. B., Lindburg, H. A., and Garside, D.: Alcohol consumption, cardiovascular risk factors and mortality in two Chicago epidemiologic studies. Circulation 56:1067, 1977.

213. Castelli, W. P., Gordon, T., Hjortland, M. C., Kagan, A., Doyle, J. T., Hames, C. G., Hulley, S. B., and Zukel, W.: Alcohol and blood lipids. The Cooperative Lipoprotein Phenotyping Study. Lancet 2:154, 1977.

214. Gordon, T., Ernst, N., Fisher, M., and Rifkind, B. M.: Alcohol and high-density lipoprotein cholesterol. Circulation 64(Suppl III):III–63, 1981.

215. Dawber, T. R., Kannel, W. B., and Gordon, T.: Coffee and cardiovascular disease: Observations from the Framingham Study. N. Engl. J. Med. 291:871, 1974.

216. Boston Collaborative Drug Surveillance Program: Coffee drinking and acute myocardial infarction. Lancet 2:1278, 1972.

217. Jick, H., Miettinen, O. S., Neff, R. K., Shapiro, S., Heinonen, O. P., and Slone, D.: Coffee and myocardial infarction. N. Engl. J. Med. 289:63, 1973.

218. Crawford, M. D., Clayton, D. G., Stanley, F., and Shaper, A. G.: An epidemiological study of sudden death in hard and soft water areas. J. Chronic Dis. 30:69, 1977.

219. Medalie, J. H., Levene, C., Papier, L., Goldbourt, U., Dreyfuss, F., Oron, D., Neufeld, H., and Riss, E.: Blood groups, myocardial infarction, and angina pectoris among 10,000 adult males. N. Engl. J. Med. 285:1348, 1971.

220. Garrison, R. J., Havlik, R. J., Harris, R. B., Feinleib, M., Kannel, W. B., and Padgett, S. J.: ABO blood group and cardiovascular disease. The Framingham Study. Atherosclerosis 25:311, 1976.

221. Meade, T. W., North, W. R. S., Chakrabarti, R., Stirling, Y., Haines, A. P., Thompson, S. G., and Brozovic, M.: Haemostatic function and cardiovascular death: Early results of a prospective study. Lancet 1:1050, 1980.

222. Dintenfass, L.: Viscosity factors in hypertensive and cardiovascular disease. Cardiovasc. Med. 2:337, 1977.

223. Sorlie, P. D., Garcia-Palmieri, M. R., Costas, R., Jr., and Havlik, R. J.: Hematocrit and risk of coronary heart disease: The Puerto Rico Heart Health Program. Am. Heart J. 101:456, 1981.

224. Curry, R. C., Jr., and Roberts, W. C.: Status of the coronary arteries in the nephrotic syndrome. Analysis of 20 necropsy patients aged 15 to 35 years

to determine if coronary atherosclerosis is accelerated. Am. J. Med. 63:183, 1977.

225. Wass, V. J., Jarrett, R. J., Chilvers, C., and Cameron, J. S.: Does the nephrotic syndrome increase the risk of cardiovascular disease? Lancet 2:664, 1979.

226. Lundsgaard-Hansen, P.: Intensive plasmapheresis as a risk factor for arteriosclerotic cardiovascular disease? Vox Sang. 33:1, 1977.

227. Nicholls, A. J., Gatto, G. R. D., Edward, N., Engeset, J., and Macleod, M.: Accelerated atherosclerosis in long-term dialysis and renal-transplant patients: Fact or fiction? Lancet 1:276, 1980.

228. Editorial: Thyroiditis, autoimmunity, and coronary risk factors. Lancet 2:173, 1977.

229. Davis, R. F., and Engleman, E. G.: Incidence of myocardial infarction in patients with rheumatoid arthritis. Arthritis Rheum. 17:527, 1974.

230. Rodgers, D. L.: Precocious myocardial infarction after radiation treatment for Hodgkin's disease. Chest 70:675, 1976.

231. Doering, C., Ruhsenberger, C., and Phillips, D. S.: Ear-lobe creases and heart disease. J. Am. Geriatr. Soc. 25:183, 1977.

232. Report of the American Heart Association Task Force on Environment and the Cardiovascular System (W. R. Harlan, Chairman). Impact of the Environment on Cardiovascular Disease. Circulation 63:244A, 1981.

233. Anderson, T. W., and Rochard, C.: Cold snaps, snowfall and sudden death from ischemic heart disease. Can. Med. Assoc. J. 121:1580, 1979.

234. Glass, R. I., Wiesenthal, A. M., Zack, M. M., and Preston, M.: Risk factors for myocardial infarction associated with the Chicago snowstorm of January 13–15, 1979. J.A.M.A. 245:164, 1981.

235. Coronary Risk Handbook. Estimating risk of coronary heart disease in daily practice. New York, American Heart Association, 1973.

236. Five-year findings of the Hypertension Detection and Follow-up Program: I. Reduction in mortality of persons with high blood pressure, including mild hypertension. J.A.M.A. 242:2562, 1979.

237. Report of the Management Committee. The Australian therapeutic trial in mild hypertension. Lancet 1:1261, 1980.

238. Lipid Research Clinics Program: The Coronary Primary Prevention Trial: Design and implementation. J. Chronic Dis. 32:609, 1979.

239. Pomerleau, O., Bass, F., and Crown, V.: Role of behavior modification in preventive medicine. N. Engl. J. Med. 292:1277, 1975.

240. The Coronary Drug Project Research Group: The Coronary Drug Project: Factors influencing long-term prognosis after recovery from myocardial infarction. Three-year findings of the Coronary Drug Project. J. Chronic Dis. 27:267, 1974.

241. Clarkson, T. B., Lehner, D. M., Wagner, W. D., St. Clair, R. W., Bond, M. G., and Bullock, B. C.: A study of atherosclerosis regression in Macaca mulatta. I. Design of experiment and lesion induction. Exp. Mol. Pathol. 30:360, 1979.

242. Armstrong, M. L., Warner, E. D., and Connor, W. E.: Regression of coronary atheromatosis in rhesus monkeys. Circ. Res. 25:59, 1970.

243. Armstrong, M. L., and Megan, M. B.: Arterial fibrous proteins in cynomolgus monkeys after atherogenic and regression diets. Circ. Res. 36:256, 1975.

244. Vesselinovitch, D., Wissler, R. W., Hughes, R., and Borensztajn, J.: Reversal of advanced atherosclerosis in rhesus monkeys. Atherosclerosis 23:155, 1976.

245. Starzl, T. E., Chase, H. P., Putnam, C. W., and Nora, J. J.: Follow-up of patient with portacaval shunt for the treatment of hyperlipidaemia. Lancet 2:714, 1974.

246. Starzl, T. E., Chase, H. P., Putnam, C. W., Nora, J. J., Fennell, R. H., Jr., and Porter, K. A.: Portacaval shunt in hyperlipidaemia. Lancet 2:1263, 1974.

247. Barndt, R., Jr., Blankenhorn, D. H., Crawford, D. W., and Brooks, S. H.: Regression and progression of early femoral atherosclerosis in treated hyperlipoproteinemic patients. Ann. Intern. Med. 86:139, 1977.

248. Glueck, C. J., Mattson, F., and Bierman, E. L.: Sounding boards: Diet and coronary heart disease: Another view. N. Engl. J. Med. 298:1471, 1978.

249. Status Report: Current Findings of the Lipid Research Clinics Program. Press conference given at NIH, Bethesda, Maryland, July 13, 1977. (Also cited in Clinical Trends in Cardiology, Vol. 7, No. 1, p. 1, 1977.)

250. Select Committee on Nutrition and Human Needs, United States Senate: Dietary Goals for the United States. 2nd ed. Washington, D.C., U.S. Government Printing Office, 1977.

251. Levy, R. I., and Rifkind, B. M.: Lipid-lowering drugs and hyperlipidemia. Drugs 6:12, 1973.

252. Levy, R. I., Fredrickson, D. S., Shulman, R., Bilheimer, D. W., Breslow, J. L., Stone, N. J., Lux, S. E., Sloan, H. R., Krauss, R. M., and Herbert, P. N.: Dietary and drug treatment of primary hyperlipoproteinemia. Ann. Intern. Med. 77:267, 1972.

252a.Heath, G. W., Ehasni, A. A., Hagberg, J. M., Hinderliter, J. M., and Goldberg, A. P.: Exercise training improves lipoprotein lipid profiles in patients with coronary artery disease. Am. Heart J. 105:889, 1983.

253. Fredrickson, D. S., Levy, R. I., Bonnell, M., and Ernst, N.: Dietary Management of Hyperlipoproteinemia. Washington, D.C., DHEW Publ. No. (NIH) 75-110, 1974.

254. Gotto, A. M., Jr.: Drug treatment of hyperlipidemia. Mod. Med. February 15, 1978, p. 92.

255. Levy, R. I.: Drugs used in the treatment of hyperlipoproteinemia. In Goodman, A. G. (ed.): Goodman and Gilman's The Pharmacological Basis of Therapeutics. 6th ed. New York, Macmillan, 1980, pp. 834–847.

256. Levy, R. I.: Hyperlipoproteinemia and its management. J. Cardiovasc. Med. 5:435, 1980.

257. Kane, J. P., Malloy, M. J., Tun, P., Phillips, N. R., Freedman, D. D., Williams, M. L., Rowe, J. S., and Havel, R. J.: Normalization of low-density-lipoprotein levels in heterozygous familial hypercholesterolemia with a combined drug regimen. N. Engl. J. Med. 304:251, 1981.

257a.Mabuchi, H., Sakai, T., Sakai, Y., Yoshimura, A., Watanabe, A., Wakasugi, T., Koizumi, J., and Takeda, R.: Reduction of serum cholesterol in heterozygous patients and familial hypercholesterolemia. Additive effects of compactin and cholestyramine. N. Engl. J. Med. 308:609, 1983.

258. The Coronary Drug Project: Clofibrate and niacin in coronary heart disease. J.A.M.A. 213:360, 1975.

259. Report from the Committee of Principal Investigators: A cooperative trial in the primary prevention of ischaemic heart disease using clofibrate. Br. Heart J. 40:1069, 1978.

260. Kuo, P. T., Hayase, K., Kostis, J. B., and Moreyra, A. E.: Use of combined diet and colestipol in long-term (7–7½ years) treatment of patients with type II hyperlipoproteinemia. Circulation 59:199, 1979.

261. The Coronary Drug Project: Findings leading to further modifications of its protocol with respect to dextrothyroxine. J.A.M.A. 220:996, 1972.

262. The Medical Letter on Drugs and Therapeutics: Probucol for hypercholesterolemia. Vol. 19, No. 10, May 20, 1977.

263. Heel, R. C., Brogden, R. N., Speight, T. M., and Avery, G. S.: Probucol: A review of its pharmacological properties and therapeutic use in patients with hypercholesterolemia. Drugs 15:409, 1978.

264. Simons, L. A., Balasubramanian, S., and Beins, D. M.: Metabolic studies with probucol in hypercholesterolaemia. Atherosclerosis 40:299, 1981.

265. Royal Society of Medicine: Gemfibrozil: A new lipid-lowering agent. Proc. R. Soc. Med. 69(Suppl. 2):1, 1976.

266. Levy, R. I., and Rifkind, B. M.: Lipid lowering drugs and hyperlipidaemia. In Avery, G. S. (ed.): Cardiovascular Drugs, Vol. 1: Antiarrhythmic, Antihypertensive and Lipid Lowering Drugs. Sydney, Australia, ADIS Press Australasia Pty., Ltd., 1977, p. 1.

267. Buchwald, H., Moore, R. B., and Varco, R. L.: Surgical treatment of hyperlipidemia. Circulation 49(v29 Suppl. 1):1, 1974.

268. Thompson, G. R., and Gotto, A. M.: Ileal bypass in the treatment of hyperlipoproteinemia. Lancet 2:35, 1973.

269. Starzl, T. E., Putnam, C. W., and Koep, L. J.: Portacaval shunt and hyperlipidemia. Arch. Surg. 113:71, 1978.

270. Thompson, G. R., Myant, N. B., Kilpatrick, D., Oakley, C. M., Raphael, M. J., and Steiner, R. E.: Assessment of long-term plasma exchange for familial hypercholesterolaemia. Br. Heart J. 43:680, 1980.

271. Pickering, G.: High Blood Pressure. New York, Grune and Stratton, 1968.

272. Hypertension Detection and Follow-up Program Cooperative Group: Five-year findings of the Hypertension Detection and Follow-up Program. J.A.M.A. 242:2562, 1979.

273. Kannel, W. B., Doyle, J. T., Fredrickson, D. T., and Harlan, W. R.: Report of the Ad Hoc Committee on Cigarette Smoking and Cardiovascular Diseases for Health Professionals. Circulation 57:406A, 1978.

274. Adult use of tobacco — 1975. Atlanta, Georgia. Center for Disease Control, Bureau of Health Education, June, 1976.

275. Statistical Abstract of the United States, 1975, p. 751.

276. Hymowitz, N.: The practicing physician and smoking cessation. J. Med. Soc. N.J. 74:139, 1977.

277. Bray, G. A. (ed.): Obesity in America. Washington, D.C., DHEW Publ. No. (NIH) 79-359, 1979.

278. Stuart, R. B.: Behavioral control of overeating: A status report. In Bray, G. (ed.): Obesity in Perspective. Washington, D.C., DHEW Publ. No. 75-708, 1973.

279. Young, C. M.: Dietary treatment of obesity. In Bray, G. (ed.): Obesity in Perspective. Washington, D.C., DHEW Publ. No. 75-708, 1973.

280. Hashim, S. A., and Porikos, K.: Food intake behavior in man: Implications for treatment of obesity. Clin. Endocrinol. Metab. 5:503, 1976.

281. Hursch, L. M.: Exercise in weight reduction. Nebr. Med. J. 61:158, 1976.

282. Bjorntorp, P.: Exercise in the treatment of obesity. Clin. Endocrinol. Metab. 5:431, 1976.

283. Friedman, M., Thorensen, G. B., Gill, J. J., et al.: Recurrent Coronary Prevention Project Study: Methods, baseline results and preliminary findings. Circulation 66:83, 1982.

36
CORONARY BLOOD FLOW AND MYOCARDIAL ISCHEMIA

by Eugene Braunwald, M.D., and Burton E. Sobel, M.D.

Hypoxia, or *hypoxemia,* is a state of reduced oxygen supply to tissue despite adequate perfusion; *anoxia* is the absence of oxygen supply despite adequate perfusion; *ischemia* is the condition of oxygen deprivation accompanied by inadequate removal of metabolites consequent to reduced perfusion. Although clinical manifestations of coronary insufficiency generally reflect the effects of ischemia, under selected experimental and clinical conditions, deprivation of oxygen can be separated from reduced washout of metabolites. For example, in isolated hearts perfused at high flow rates with media equilibrated with a gas mixture poor in oxygen, anoxia without ischemia results, since washout of metabolites is not hindered. An analogous situation is seen in patients with cyanotic congenital heart disease, as well as in those with cor pulmonale and marked hypoxemia but with a normal coronary circulation. In contrast, the reduction of regional myocardial perfusion in the presence of hyperbaric oxygen may produce localized ischemia with limitation of the removal of metabolites, without concomitant impairment of oxygen delivery to cuffs of cells surrounding myocardial capillaries.

Neither ischemia nor hypoxia can be defined in absolute terms, since the blood flow and quantity of oxygen required to support myocardium under one set of conditions will not necessarily pertain under another. In man, blood flow of 60 to 90 ml/min per 100 gm of myocardium is generally required under basal physiological conditions. On the other hand, when the mechanical activity of the heart and its metabolic requirements are markedly reduced, myocardial viability may be maintained by perfusion at much lower rates, approximately 10 to 20 ml/min per 100 gm, or even with complete interruption of perfu-

sion for periods of up to 100 minutes. Examples of conditions that reduce oxygen needs include ventricular fibrillation, asystole, cardiopulmonary bypass, and hypothermia with or without cardiopulmonary bypass. Another example of lowered cardiac oxygen needs occurs following the administration of nitroglycerin and other nitrates, which reduce the preload and afterload, and of beta-adrenergic blockers, which lower heart rate and contractility. This reduction of oxygen needs is perhaps the *principal* mechanism by which these agents relieve anginal pain (p. 1349).

The importance of defining ischemia in *relative* rather than absolute terms is underscored by the use of a variety of stress tests to detect or assess the severity of coronary artery disease. Whether the endpoint is angina, deviation of the ST-segment on the electrocardiogram (Chap. 8), relative diminution of accumulation of ^{201}Tl in myocardial "perfusion images," regional wall motion disorders or diminution of ejection fraction detectable with gated blood pool images (Chap. 11), the underlying principle is the same. Induction of stress by exercise, atrial pacing, hand grip, or any other means leads to a transitory disparity in the balance between oxygen supply and demand. Although this balance may be adequate under conditions of rest, the disparity becomes manifest when stress is imposed.

CONTROL OF MYOCARDIAL OXYGEN CONSUMPTION

The heart is an aerobic organ; that is, it relies almost exclusively on the oxidation of substrates for the generation of energy, and it can develop only a small oxygen debt.

1235

Therefore, in a steady state, determination of the heart's $\dot{V}O_2$ provides an accurate measure of its total metabolism.

It has been known for many years that the total metabolism of the arrested, quiescent heart is only a small fraction of that of the working organ. The $\dot{V}O_2$ of the beating canine heart ranges from 8 to 15 ml/min per 100 gm, while the $\dot{V}O_2$ of the noncontracting heart is approximately 1.5 ml/min per 100 gm.[1,2] This quantity of oxygen is required for those physiological metabolic processes not directly associated with contraction. Increases in the frequency of depolarization in the noncontracting heart are accompanied by only very small increases of $M\dot{V}O_2$. Indeed, the quantity of oxygen required for electrical activation of the heart is approximately only 0.5 per cent of the total oxygen consumed by the normal working heart; thus, the oxygen cost of electrical depolarization is trivial in relation to the cost of contractile activity.[3]

In 1915 Evans and Matsuoka concluded from studies on the Starling heart-lung preparation that "there is a relation between the tension set up on contraction and the metabolism of the contractile tissue."[4] Subsequently, experimental techniques for regulating the external performance of the heart improved enormously. In 1955, in a systematic investigation of the relative effects of aortic pressure, stroke volume, and heart rate on $M\dot{V}O_2$, it became apparent that it is not possible to estimate the energy needs of the myocardium simply from the external work produced by the heart when work is calculated in the classic manner as the product of developed pressure and stroke volume. As a corollary, it was shown that myocardial efficiency, i.e., the ratio of the work performed to the oxygen consumed, varies widely depending on the hemodynamic conditions.[5,6] These investigations suggested that the tension-time index, i.e., the area under the left ventricular pressure curve, is an important determinant of the $M\dot{V}O_2$ (Fig. 36–1). Subsequently, it was emphasized that the tension in the wall of the

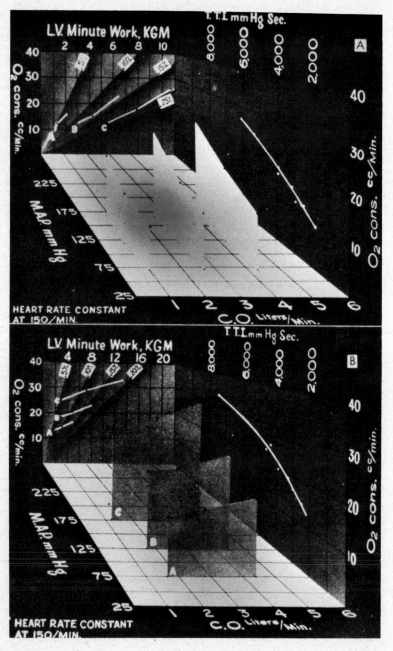

FIGURE 36–1 Summary of the interrelationships between various hemodynamic variables and myocardial oxygen consumption. In both top and bottom panels, the *base grids* show the experimental conditions, cardiac output (C.O.), and aortic pressure (M.A.P.) at which each determination of oxygen consumption was made. The height above the base grid of each experimental point represents its oxygen consumption. The *rear grids* show the plot of left ventricular minute work against myocardial oxygen consumption. The shaded lines on the rear grid labeled with percentage figures are isoefficiency lines. The *right grids* show the relation between the tension-time index (T.T.I.) in mm Hg-sec and myocardial oxygen consumption.

A, Three pressure runs at low, medium, and high levels of cardiac output. Note the negligible change in external efficiency as aortic pressure is increased within any given run. *B*, Three flow runs at low, medium, and high mean levels of aortic pressure. Note the increase in external efficiency within the course of any given flow run. (From Sarnoff, S. J., Braunwald, E., Welch, G. H., Jr., Case, R. B., Stainsby, W. N., and Macruz, R.: Hemodynamic determinants of oxygen consumption of the heart with special reference to the tension-time index. Am. J. Physiol. *192*:148, 1958.)

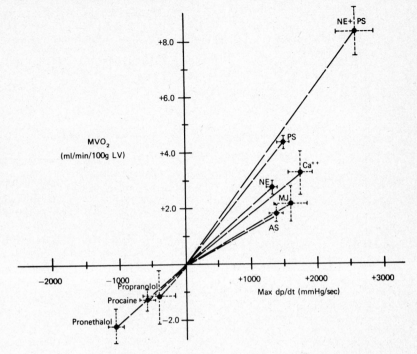

FIGURE 36–2 Relation between changes in maximal intraventricular dP/dt and myocardial oxygen consumption ($M\dot{V}O_2$). Each point represents the average of a series of experiments ± SE. AS = acetylstrophanthidin; MJ = noncatecholamine nonglycoside positive inotropic agent; Ca++ = calcium; NE = norepinephrine; PS = paired electrical stimulation. (From Braunwald, E.: Control of myocardial oxygen consumption: Physiologic and clinical considerations. Am. J. Cardiol. *27*:416, 1971.)

ventricle is a direct function of the radius and the intraventricular pressure and is inversely related to ventricular wall thickness. Also, tension in the myocardial wall is a more definitive determinant of myocardial energy utilization than is developed pressure.[7] Later studies demonstrated that velocity of myocardial contraction—a reflection of the heart's contractile state—is an additional, important determinant of $M\dot{V}O_2$ (Fig. 36–2).[8]

Recent reexamination of the determinants of $M\dot{V}O_2$ has emphasized that it correlates closely with the left ventricular systolic pressure-volume area, which consists of the sum of the area within the systolic pressure-volume loop, i.e., the external mechanical work, and the end-systolic elastic potential energy in the ventricular wall.[9,10] Rooke and Feigl have provided impressive evidence that $M\dot{V}O_2$ is also influenced by stroke volume (and therefore stroke work), although less so than by pressure development.[2] They have also provided an experimental basis for the use of the systolic pressure-rate product (plus an estimate of the oxygen consumption of the noncontracting heart) as a clinically useful index of $M\dot{V}O_2$. These observations are consistent with Fenn's classic observations on skeletal muscle which showed that the energy release (a variable related to $\dot{V}O_2$) is proportional to the sum of tension development and external work of the muscle.[11,12] Thus, both skeletal muscle and myocardium have the capacity to adjust their energy costs to external conditions imposed *after* stimulation.

EFFECT OF INOTROPIC AGENTS. The effect on $M\dot{V}O_2$ of positive inotropic stimuli, such as cardiac glycosides or catecholamines, is the end result of their influence on two major determinants of $M\dot{V}O_2$ which change in opposite directions: tension, which declines as a consequence of a reduction in heart size, and myocardial contractility, which is augmented. In the failing, dilated ventricle, the increased contractility reduces the left ventricular end-diastolic pressure and volume. On the basis of the Laplace relation (p. 431), this reduction in ventricular volume leads

to a decline in intramyocardial tension, which tends to reduce $M\dot{V}O_2$. However, the decrease in $M\dot{V}O_2$ that might be expected to result from falling tension in the ventricular wall is offset by the increase in contractility, which tends to augment $M\dot{V}O_2$. The net result of these opposing effects is to produce no change, a small increase, or a small decrease in $M\dot{V}O_2$. Thus, the change in $M\dot{V}O_2$ that follows a stimulation of contractility depends on the extent to which intramyocardial tension is reduced in relation to the extent to which the contractile state is augmented.[13] In the absence of heart failure, drugs that stimulate myocardial contractility elevate $\dot{V}O_2$, since heart size and, therefore, wall tension are not reduced and do not offset the effect on metabolism of the stimulation of contractility.

The conclusion that myocardial contractility is an important determinant of $M\dot{V}O_2$ is supported by observations on the effects of reducing contractility. Thus, in animal experiments reductions in contractility and in the velocity of contraction produced by cardiac depressant drugs, including propranolol, and procainamide, were shown to reduce $M\dot{V}O_2$ when wall tension was held constant, or almost so.[14]

The results of experiments in which the relative effects on $M\dot{V}O_2$ of changes in tension development and in myocardial contractility were assessed in the same heart are summarized in Figure 36–3.[15] The three diagonal parallel lines are $M\dot{V}O_2$ isopleths, showing the levels of tension and V_{max} associated with 20, 40, and 60 μ liters/beat per 100 gm, respectively. The reciprocal relation between tension and velocity is evident. A given level of $M\dot{V}O_2$ can be achieved with a relatively high level of V_{max} and low peak developed tension, or a low level of V_{max} and a relatively high level of tension. The broken lines near the center of the figure illustrate the increases in peak developed tension and V_{max} required to increase $M\dot{V}O_2$ by 50 per cent. Such an increase could be achieved either by increasing V_{max} at a constant developed tension, as shown by the vertical arrow, or by increasing peak developed tension at a constant V_{max}, as shown by the horizontal arrow. From these stud-

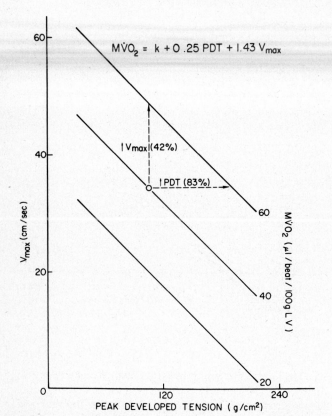

FIGURE 36–3 $M\dot{V}O_2$ isopleths as a function of V_{max} and peak developed tension (PDT). Isopleths were calculated from the equation at the top of the figure, which was derived by multiple regression analysis of a series of experiments in dogs. Broken lines indicate the effect on $M\dot{V}O_2$ of hypothetical increases in PDT at a constant V_{max} (horizontal lines) and in V_{max} at a constant PDT (vertical line). (From Graham, T. P., Jr., Covell, J. W., Sonnenblick, E. H., Ross, J., Jr., and Braunwald, E.: Control of myocardial oxygen consumption: Relative influence of contractile state and tension development. J. Clin. Invest. 47:375, 1968.)

ies it was concluded that the quantitative effects on $M\dot{V}O_2$ of changes in contractility and tension development are both substantial and of the same order of magnitude.

It is important to emphasize that in these experiments heart rate was purposely held constant, since heart rate itself is an important determinant of $M\dot{V}O_2$. An augmentation of rate elevates the level of $M\dot{V}O_2$ per minute by

TABLE 36–1   DETERMINANTS OF MYOCARDIAL OXYGEN CONSUMPTION

1. Tension development
2. Contractile state
3. Heart rate
4. Shortening against a load (Fenn effect)
5. Maintenance of cell viability in basal state
6. Depolarization
7. Activation
8. Maintenance of active state
9. Direct metabolic effect of catecholamines
10. Fatty acid uptake

increasing the frequency of tension development per unit of time, as well as by increasing contractility.[5,16]

Although the exact costs of maintenance of the active state of the myocardium have not yet been clearly defined, they are likely to be relatively low. In studies on isolated papillary muscles, $\dot{V}O_2$ was found to be a function of the tension that is developed and the velocity of shortening of the unloaded muscle. Shortening against a load requires oxygen above and beyond that required for the development of tension. Almost the entire increase in $M\dot{V}O_2$ produced by the administration of catecholamines results from the increased contractile activity produced, rather than from a direct stimulating effect of the catecholamines on myocardial metabolism. Severe valvular regurgitation does not increase myocardial consumption significantly when myocardial tension is held constant because of the low oxygen cost of the additional muscle shortening associated with valvular regurgitation[5,17] (Table 36–1). $M\dot{V}O_2$ is influenced also by the substrate utilized. Specifically, it varies directly with the fraction of energy derived from the metabolism of fatty acids, which in turn varies directly with the arterial concentration of fatty acids and inversely with that of glucose and insulin.[18]

REGULATION OF CORONARY BLOOD FLOW (Fig. 36–4)

ANATOMICAL FACTORS.   Coronary blood flow is influenced by anatomical, hydraulic, mechanical, and metabolic factors.[6,19,20,20a] During diastole, when the aortic valve is closed, aortic diastolic pressure is transmitted without impediment through the dilated sinuses of Valsal-

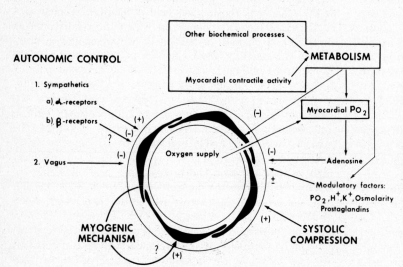

FIGURE 36–4 Schematic representation of principal factors influencing coronary blood flow. (+) = factors that reduce arteriolar lumen by compression or by contraction of vascular smooth muscle (ring of four overlapping cells). (−) = factors that relax vascular smooth muscle. Force exerted by blood pressure to stretch the vessel is not shown. Note that metabolic factors can act either via adenosine or other metabolites or by some direct effect on the vessel wall. (From Berne, R. M., and Rubio, R.: Coronary circulation. In Berne, R. M., Sperelakis, N., and Geiger, S. R. (eds.): Handbook of Physiology. Section 2, The Cardiovascular System. Bethesda, Md., American Physiological Society, 1979, p. 897.)

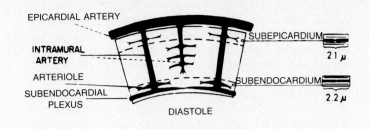

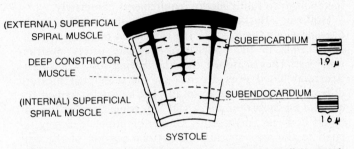

FIGURE 36–5 Cross-section of the left ventricular wall in systole and diastole. Factors involved in the susceptibility of the subendocardium to the development of ischemia include the greater dependence of this region on diastolic perfusion and the greater degree of shortening, and therefore of energy expenditure, of this region during systole. (From Bell, J. R., and Fox, A. C.: Pathogenesis of subendocardial ischemia. Am. J. Med. Sci. 268:2, 1974.)

va to the ostia themselves. The sinuses then act as miniature reservoirs, facilitating maintenance of relatively uniform coronary inflow through diastole.[21] Both the left and right coronary arteries course across the epicardial surface of the heart. Major vessels and their branches give rise to smaller penetrating vessels approximately at right angles (Fig. 36–5).[22] The dense capillary network of about 4000 capillaries/sq mm cross-section of the heart[23] is not uniformly patent, since precapillary sphincters appear to serve a regulatory function,[24] depending on the flow needs of the myocardium.

Anastomotic connections without an intervening capillary bed exist between portions of the same coronary artery and between different coronary arteries. The distribution and extent of these collateral vessels differ markedly between species, as well as among different individuals of the same species. In canine hearts, an extensive epicardial network of collateral vessels is common, but epicardial collateral vessels are not prominent in porcine hearts. In human hearts, the distribution and extent of collateral vessels are quite variable.[25] Under physiological conditions, such vessels are generally less than 40 μ in diameter and appear to have little or no functional role. However, when myocardial perfusion is compromised by obstructions affecting major vessels, these collateral vessels enlarge over several weeks and blood flow through them increases.[26–28] Under these conditions, perfusion via collaterals may equal or exceed perfusion via the obstructed vessel.

The functional significance of collateral vessels varies widely.[29] At best, collaterals may maintain the viability of myocardium in the presence of total occlusion. However, myocardial perfusion through collaterals cannot increase sufficiently to meet the augmented requirements of the myocardium during the stress of exercise. Therefore, when cardiac muscle is supplied entirely or largely by collateral

vessels, it often becomes ischemic if its oxygen demands increase above basal levels.

PERFUSION PRESSURE. As in any vascular bed, blood flow in the coronary bed depends on the driving pressure and the resistance offered by this bed. However, the coronary circulation differs from other circulations in that the resistance offered by the bed is influenced considerably by phasic systolic extravascular compression of the myocardium. The effective driving or perfusion pressure is the pressure gradient between the coronary arteries and the coronary sinus. However, effective perfusion pressure is not constant throughout the cardiac cycle. When the aortic valve is open and ejected blood flows rapidly past the coronary ostia, perfusion pressure is reduced slightly below aortic pressure because of the Venturi effect. In addition, phasic changes in right atrial pressure occurring during the cardiac cycle modify the effective perfusion pressure gradient, albeit only slightly, except in the presence of a tall *v* wave, as in tricuspid regurgitation.

FACTORS EXTRINSIC TO THE VASCULAR BED. Coronary vascular resistance is influenced both by factors *extrinsic* to the bed, particularly compressive forces within the myocardium (intramyocardial pressure acting on the intramyocardial vessels), and by metabolic, neural, and humoral factors *intrinsic* to the bed causing changes in the cross-sectional area of coronary resistance vessels. Intramyocardial pressure is determined primarily by the ventricular pressure throughout the cardiac cycle.[30–32] Because ventricular pressure is so much higher in systole than it is in diastole, myocardial compressive forces acting on intramyocardial vessels are much greater during this phase of the cardiac cycle. Accordingly, a large proportion of coronary blood flow to the left ventricle occurs during diastole. Since an increase in heart rate diminishes the total amount of diastolic time per minute (and increases myocardial oxygen demands), tachycardia may compromise coronary perfusion. This "throttling" effect of systole on myocardial perfusion[19] is particularly important when systolic intraventricular pressure is elevated but coronary perfusion pressure is not, as in the case of obstruction to left ventricular outflow by valvular or subvalvular aortic stenosis, or in severe aortic regurgitation.

The dramatic impact of left ventricular compression on coronary blood flow can be demonstrated experimentally with a beating heart perfused at constant pressure and ventricular asystole induced transiently by vagal stimulation. During asystole, coronary blood flow suddenly increases by approximately 50 per cent because of relief of the compressive effect.[20] Since compressive forces exerted by the right ventricle are ordinarily far less than those of the left ventricle, perfusion of the right ventricle is not interrupted during systole (Fig. 36–6).

The systolic compressive effect just discussed is much greater in subendocardial compared with subepicardial zones of the heart.[31] Under physiological conditions, marked transitory disparities exist between endocardial and epicardial wall stresses and, correspondingly, between endocardial and epicardial flow throughout the cardiac cycle. Nevertheless, under physiological conditions, the ratio of endo- to epicardial flow averaged throughout the cardiac cycle is approximately 1:1 as a consequence of preferential dilatation of the subendocardial vessels.[32,33] Inter-

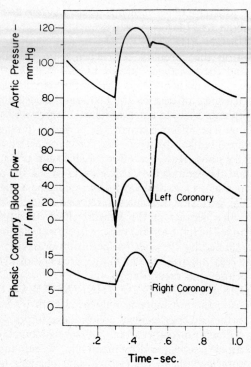

FIGURE 36–6   Phasic right and left coronary artery blood flow in relation to aortic blood pressure. (From Berne, R. M., and Levy, M. D.: Cardiovascular Physiology, 2nd ed. St. Louis, The C. V. Mosby Co., 1972.)

cardial zone include its greater potential for glycolytic metabolism[38] due to higher glycolytic enzyme activity and, consequently, higher lactate production rates[39] when coronary flow is restricted. However, even though the glycogen content of subendocardium is higher than that of the subepicardium under aerobic conditions,[40] concentrations of high-energy phosphate compounds are generally lower than those in the mid- and subepicardium when coronary flow is restricted,[41] because of the inability of anaerobic metabolism to fulfill energy requirements completely.

Hoffman, Buckberg, Griggs, and their collaborators have developed indices for the evaluation of subendocardial ischemia in the absence of coronary artery obstruction.[35,42–44] They reasoned that the driving force for subendocardial blood flow depends on the integrated pressure difference between the aorta and left ventricle, termed the *diastole pressure–time index* (DPTI), while the demand for blood flow, i.e., myocardial O_2 consumption, is closely related to the area beneath the systolic portion of the ventricular pressure curve, i.e., the *systolic pressure–time index* (SPTI). The ratio DPTI/SPTI has been used as an index of the relation between subendocardial oxygen supply and demand. This ratio can be reduced by (1) opening an arteriovenous fistula or patent ductus arteriosus or inducing aortic regurgitation to diminish aortic diastolic pressure; (2) increasing preload or afterload, causing left ventricular dysfunction, or reducing left ventricular compliance; these maneuvers all raise left ventricular diastolic pressure; and (3) inducing tachycardia to shorten diastole.[45,46] These investigators found that with reduction of the DPTI/SPTI below a critical value of approximately 0.7, the endocardial/epicardial blood flow ratio also decreased.

These observations can explain a number of clinical findings, such as the development of angina and the electrocardiographic and biochemical evidence of ischemia caused by tachycardia in patients with aortic stenosis. Indeed, myocardial lactate production has been observed to occur during beta-adrenergic receptor stimulation with isoproterenol in patients with aortic stenosis,[47] when left ventricular systolic pressure, contractility, heart rate, and, therefore, myocardial oxygen demand rise. When adrenergic stimulation was carried out in dogs with experimentally produced aortic stenosis, the myocardial lactate concentration and the lactate-pyruvate ratio rose while the reduction of ATP stores was more prominent in the inner than the outer half of the ventricle,[35] again indicating that the subendocardium is more vulnerable to ischemia and therefore becomes dependent on anaerobic metabolism more readily than does the subepicardium.

In experimentally produced aortic regurgitation, diastolic coronary blood flow falls but systolic flow rises, so the total coronary flow does not change;[48] however, with severe reductions in aortic diastolic pressure the subendocardial region exhibits biochemical evidence of anaerobic metabolism. Although metabolically stimulated coronary dilatation in the subendocardial region can maintain blood flow despite considerable reduction in aortic diastolic pressure, this compensation is often incomplete with very severe aortic regurgitation. As the DPTI/SPTI declines, the subendocardial lactate-pyruvate ratio rises, providing evidence of anaerobic metabolism by the myocardium. These experiments are clinically relevant when it is considered

ventions that reduce the perfusion pressure gradient during diastole (as occurs with coronary obstruction, elevation of ventricular diastolic pressure, and tachycardia) lower the ratio of subendocardial to subepicardial flow and may cause the subendocardium to become ischemic.

The combination of a greater wall stress, and hence greater resistance to flow, and higher metabolic demands results in lower coronary vascular tone in the subendocardium than in the subepicardium. As a consequence, the reserve for vasodilatation is also less in the subendocardium than in the subepicardium, and as perfusion is reduced the deeper layers of myocardium become ischemic before the more superficial ones. This phenomenon is manifested by reduced intracellular oxygen tension and contractility and increased production of lactate initially in the inner layers of the ventricular wall.[31,34,35]

The susceptibility of the subendocardium to ischemia by the combination of limited reserve for vasodilation, extrinsic compression from the higher wall stress to which it is subjected,[36] and the resultant high metabolic demands accounts for ST segment depression on the electrocardiogram characteristically associated with transient episodes of angina pectoris (Fig. 7–29, p. 222). Injury currents from the subendocardium, resulting in ST segment depression, accompany the maldistribution of transmural flow and metabolic impairment of subendocardial tissue under these circumstances, even though net transmural flow may remain near normal.[37] These considerations provide the basis for the recognition of myocardial ischemia by ST-segment depression during exercise stress testing (Chap. 8). When perfusion is limited, the adaptive changes of the subendo-

that angina pectoris occurs in more than one third of patients with severe aortic regurgitation in the absence of coronary artery disease[49] (p. 1110). Other conditions in which subendocardial ischemia occurs include marked systemic hypotension, regardless of etiology (Chap. 18), and pulmonary embolism; in these conditions the ischemia results from a combination of lowered coronary perfusion pressure, tachycardia, and increased subendocardial tension secondary to sympathetic stimulation of myocardial contractility.

In the presence of coronary obstruction the *effective* pressure perfusing the subendocardial region is reduced to the gradient between the diastolic coronary pressure *distal* to the obstruction and the left ventricular end-diastolic pressure; the DPTI no longer reflects the driving force for subendocardial blood flow. Since maldistribution of transmural blood flow compromises the subendocardial tissue, antianginal drugs may be effective if they improve the ratio of subendocardial to subepicardial flow even if they do not augment net transmural perfusion.[31] Analysis of the washout of ^{86}Rb and fractional uptake of radioactive labeled microspheres has shown that both nitroglycerin and propranolol redistribute blood flow to the subendocardium.[50,51] Whether or not this phenomenon reflects the direct effects of the drugs on the coronary vascular bed or, as is more likely, the reduction of extravascular compressive forces induced by a lowering of ventricular diastolic pressure resulting from a reduction of preload (nitroglycerin) or a reduction of ischemia consequent to diminishing myocardial oxygen needs (propranolol), the net result is a decline in extrinsic resistance with an augmentation of subendocardial perfusion.

INTRINSIC FACTORS. Coronary resistance is influenced markedly by changes in the tone of the vascular bed, changes that are mediated by neural, metabolic, pharmacological, and myogenic factors.[52]

The coronary arteries are richly innervated by sympathetic and parasympathetic nerves.[20] Both alpha- and beta-2 receptor activity has been demonstrated in the coronary vascular bed of the intact unanesthetized dog.[53,54] Intravenous administration of norepinephrine induces a brief fall, followed by a sustained rise, in coronary vascular resistance, accompanied by a decline in coronary sinus pO₂ (Fig. 36–7).[55] The early vasodilatation can be eliminated by beta-adrenergic blockade and presumably results from the augmented myocardial oxygen needs consequent to stimulation of myocardial beta receptors; the later increase in coronary vascular resistance can be prevented by alpha-adrenergic receptor blockade and presumably results from stimulation of alpha receptors in the coronary vascular bed.

Baroreceptor activity affects coronary vascular resistance reflexly. In the dog with sectioned vagal nerves, occlusion of the carotid arteries to produce baroreceptor hypotension induces an increase in heart rate and blood pressure, accompanied by a reduction in coronary vascular resistance.[56] When the reflex tachycardia and myocardial contractility (which would be expected to increase MV̇O₂ and lower coronary vascular resistance) are blocked with propranolol, an increase in coronary vascular resistance is observed,

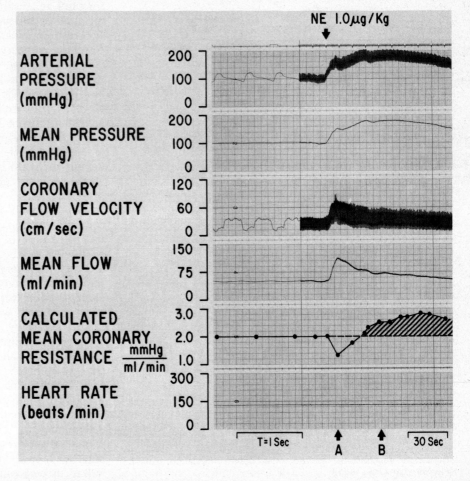

FIGURE 36–7 Effects of intravenously administered norepinephrine (NE) in the intact unanesthetized dog with heart rate held constant. Coronary vascular resistance fell initially (A) and then showed a sustained increase (B). (From Vatner, S. F., Higgins, C. B., and Braunwald, E.: Effects of norepinephrine on coronary circulation and left ventricular dynamics in the conscious dog. Circ. Res. *34*: 812, 1974, by permission of the American Heart Association, Inc.)

which can be prevented by cardiac sympathectomy. It may be concluded that with intact sympathetic nerves and beta receptors, the coronary dilatation consequent to carotid occlusion is due to heightened cardiac metabolic activity induced reflexly by baroreceptor hypotension. When this augmentation of myocardial beta-receptor–mediated activity is prevented with beta blockade, reflex coronary *vasoconstriction* secondary to carotid hypotension is unmasked.[57] Stimulation of the distal ends of the vagi produces coronary vasodilatation,[57,58] an effect that is mediated by the release of acetylcholine from vagal nerve endings and that can be blocked by atropine.[20]

There is also evidence for *tonic* coronary constriction mediated by the sympathetic nerves.[59] Acute surgical denervation of the heart produces a fall in coronary vascular resistance with a decrease in arteriovenous oxygen extraction.[60] Coronary vascular resistance in patients as well as in dogs[61] with innervated hearts declines by almost 25 per cent in response to alpha-adrenergic blockade, suggesting that basal coronary constrictor tone mediated by alpha receptors was released. However, resistance does not diminish when patients with cardiac transplants receive alpha-adrenergic blockade, suggesting that cardiac denervation had previously released the coronary constrictor tone. In the unanesthetized dog, stimulation of the carotid sinus nerves results in a substantial reduction in coronary vascular resistance (Fig. 36–8),[59] an effect which can be prevented by alpha-receptor blockade, suggesting that sympathetic coronary constrictor tone is present in the resting conscious dog and that coronary vasodilatation attendant

upon electrical stimulation of the carotid sinus nerves results from a reduction in this resting vasoconstrictor tone. Coronary vasodilatation resulting from stimulation of the carotid sinus nerves occurs also during exercise, suggesting that alpha-receptor–mediated constrictor tone persists in the coronary vascular bed during exercise, despite the coexisting metabolic vasodilatation. This conclusion is supported by studies using alpha-adrenergic blocking drugs which have shown that the increase in coronary blood flow and oxygen delivery to the myocardium during normal exercise is limited by alpha-adrenergic vasoconstriction.[62,63]

Efferent neural influences on the coronary vascular bed may also be activated reflexly by cardiopulmonary parasympathetic receptors. Stimulation of parasympathetic receptors leads to reflex systemic and coronary vasodilatation.[64] Chemoreceptor activation can also cause coronary dilatation, a reflex that is mediated by the vagi and can be abolished by atropine.[20] Intracoronary injection of veratrum alkaloids, as well as other metabolically active substances, induces reflex bradycardia and hypotension (the Bezold-Jarisch reflex),[65,66] the afferent limb of which involves the vagus nerves. The effects of efferent vagus nerve activity causing *coronary* vasodilatation[67] have been documented, indicating that the Bezold-Jarisch reflex involves coronary efferent as well as afferent parasympathetic components.[64]

Coronary beta-adrenergic receptors are similar to those in other vessels and conform to the beta-2 category.[68] Administration of a beta-1 agonist stimulates myocardial contractility and heart rate, with the enhanced production of metabolites eliciting coronary vasodilatation. Administration of propranolol, on the other hand, might be expected to reduce coronary blood flow and elevate coronary vascular resistance by two separate mechanisms: (1) blocking the effect of beta-1 receptors and thereby reducing $M\dot{V}O_2$ and the metabolic vasodilatation consequent thereto; and (2) blocking coronary vasodilator influences mediated by activation of beta-2 receptors. However, despite these theoretical considerations and the demonstration of the activity of beta-adrenergic agonists and antagonists in vitro,[69] under physiological conditions direct effects of beta-adrenergic antagonists on the coronary vascular bed are not prominent.

AUTOREGULATION. When sudden alterations in coronary perfusion pressure are imposed on an experimental preparation in which myocardial oxygen demands are held constant, the abrupt changes in coronary blood flow are only transitory, with flow promptly returning toward the previous steady-state level.[70] This phenomenon, termed autoregulation (Fig. 36–9), tends to maintain regional coronary perfusion within a relatively narrow range, regardless of transitory changes in perfusion pressure. Demonstration of autoregulation in intact animals is difficult because modification of coronary perfusion pressure also changes both $M\dot{V}O_2$ and extrinsic compression of the coronary vessels. However, under experimental conditions in which perfusion pressure is altered but ventricular pressure, cardiac contractility, and heart rate—the principal determinants of $M\dot{V}O_2$—are maintained constant, autoregulation is clearly evident. Several mechanisms have been implicated, including myogenic and metabolic factors as well as tissue pressure.[19,20]

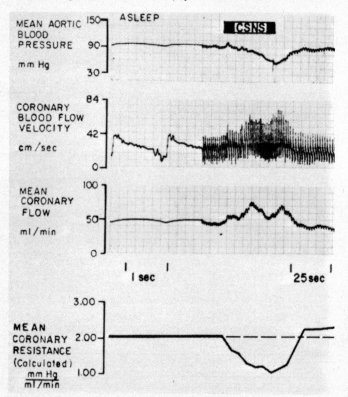

FIGURE 36–8 Responses to 30-sec periods of carotid sinus nerve stimulation (CSNS) in a conscious, sleeping dog. Responses of mean arterial pressure, phasic and mean coronary blood flow, and calculated mean coronary resistance are shown. (From Vatner, S. F., Franklin, D., and Braunwald, E.: Effects of anesthesia and sleep on circulatory response to carotid sinus nerve stimulation. Am J. Physiol. *220*:1249, 1971.)

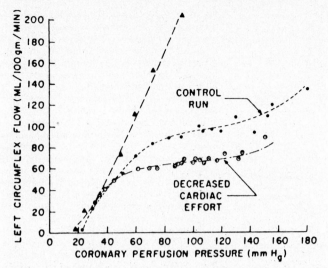

FIGURE 36–9 Relation between left circumflex coronary flow and coronary perfusion pressure. Coronary perfusion pressure has been altered independently of aortic pressure, which is maintained essentially constant. Triangles represent the immediate change in flow with various sudden increases in perfusion pressure from a pressure of 40 mm Hg. Closed circles along the middle curve represent the readjusted steady-state flow levels over a range of perfusion pressures after autoregulation has occurred. Note the relative independence of flow from coronary perfusion pressure between approximately 70 and 130 mm Hg. When cardiac effort was reduced by lowering aortic pressure (open circles), the steady-state level of left circumflex flow was also reduced but again remained relatively independent of coronary perfusion pressure over a broad range of perfusion pressure changes. (From Mosher, P., et al.: Control of coronary blood flow by an autoregulatory mechanism. Circ. Res. *14*:250, 1964, by permission of the American Heart Association, Inc.)

Myogenic Factors. Stretch of vascular smooth muscle resulting from an increase in perfusion pressure stimulates the muscle to contract.[70a] The consequent augmentation of resistance tends to return blood flow toward normal despite the higher perfusion pressure. Although the myogenic mechanism, sometimes called the Bayliss effect, appears to be a general characteristic of vascular smooth muscle,[71] its role in the regulation of coronary blood flow is probably a modest one.[20]

Metabolic Factors. It is likely that changes in regional myocardial metabolism are important determinants of autoregulation (and therefore coronary blood flow). Several mediators have been implicated, including oxygen, carbon dioxide, and vasodilator metabolites, such as adenosine, that accumulate in hypoperfused regions of myocardium. For example, a reduction in coronary arterial perfusion pressure, causing an immediate decrease in flow, might be expected to cause an increased myocardial oxygen extraction and a reduction in myocardial oxygen tension; the resultant hypoxia then causes coronary vasodilation,[72,73] presumably because oxygen acts on vascular smooth muscle directly, possibly by altering the electrochemical potential of the muscle cells. Direct vasodilating effects of diminished oxygen tension have been demonstrated in the coronary, femoral, and other vessels.[74–76] Molecular oxygen diffusing across the walls of the vessels appears to be a primary determinant of constrictor tone of precapillary sphincters under physiological conditions.[77,78] Thus, diminution of oxygen tension increases the number of capillaries perfused within a

predefined region of myocardium, presumably by relaxation of these sphincters.[79] In this manner coronary blood flow would be expected to remain constant despite a reduction of perfusion pressure. Transitory augmentation of the concentration of potassium in extracellular fluid, an early consequence of myocardial ischemia, may also modify the transmembrane potential of vascular smooth muscle cells and result in vasodilatation.

Degradation of adenine nucleotides under conditions in which ATP utilization exceeds the capacity of myocardial cells to resynthesize high-energy phosphate compounds (a process dependent on oxidative phosphorylation in mitochondria) results in the efflux of purine bases that cannot be reutilized readily by the heart. Accordingly, adenosine and its metabolites, inosine and hypoxanthine, appear in interstitial fluid and in the coronary sinus venous effluent. *Adenosine* is a powerful vasodilator[80,81] that is considered to be an important, perhaps *the critical, mediator* linking metabolically induced vasodilatation to diminish coronary perfusion (Fig. 36–10). Concentrations of adenosine in the venous effluent are much lower than those in interstitial fluid, in part because capillary endothelium rapidly converts adenosine to inosine and hypoxanthine.[82] However, when the enzyme responsible for this conversion, adenosine deaminase, is inhibited by administration of 8-azaguanine, prominent increases occur in the concentration of adenosine in the effluent.[75] If, at a constant level of myocardial metabolism, adenosine were being released at a constant rate, an elevation of coronary perfusion pressure and the resultant increase in coronary blood flow would augment the washout of adenosine, reduce its concentration, and thus increase coronary vascular resistance. Such a mechanism could provide a feedback to account for pressure-independent autoregulation of coronary blood flow and could also explain the close correlation between the metabolic activity of the heart and the level of coronary blood flow.[83] It is also possible that adenosine interacts with hypoxia in causing coronary relaxation.[84]

It appears that adenosine acts on the surface of vascular smooth muscle cells, presumably at a receptor site on the cell membrane; presumably adenosine blocks entry of Ca^{++} into these cells and thereby causes vasodilatation.[20] In addition to its potent vasodilating action, adenosine exerts a generally depressant activity on cardiac automaticity and atrioventricular conduction and attenuates the effects of adrenergic influences on myocardial contractility.[85]

Despite its importance, adenosine is almost certainly not the only metabolic factor involved. Prostaglandins, kinins,[86] potassium, and a number of metabolites alter coronary vascular resistance profoundly and may play a role in mediating vasodilatation in response to hypoxia. The infusion of at least two prostaglandins synthesized in the heart (PGI_2 and PGE_2) can cause coronary vasodilatation,[87] and the inhibition of prostaglandin synthesis with indomethacin causes an increase in coronary vascular resistance in humans.[88]

When coronary perfusion pressure falls to below 60 to 70 mm Hg, the coronary vessels become maximally dilated and flow becomes pressure-dependent[19]; i.e., coronary autoregulation is lost (Fig. 36–9). This observation explains the importance of maintaining coronary perfusion pressure in patients with acute myocardial infarction (Chap. 38). In patients with cardiogenic shock, the reduc-

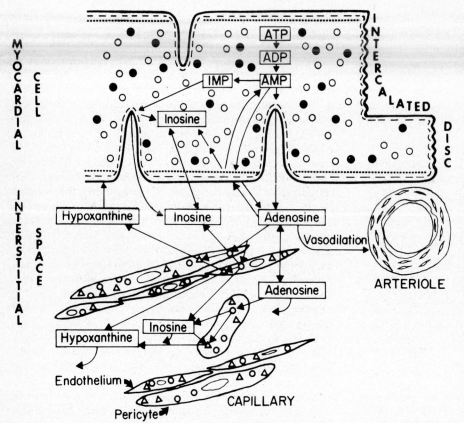

FIGURE 36–10 Schematic drawing depicting a myocardial cell, interstitial space, an arteriole, and a capillary with the localization of enzymes involved in the formation and fate of adenosine. Adenosine formed by 5'-nucleotidase from AMP (which in turn arises from ATP) can enter the interstitial space. There it can induce arteriolar dilation and reenter the myocardial cell, where it is either phosphorylated to AMP by adenosine kinase or deaminated to inosine by adenosine deaminase, or it can enter the capillaries and leave the tissue. A large fraction of adenosine that crosses the capillary wall is deaminated to inosine, which in turn is split to hypoxanthine and ribose-1-PO_4 by nucleoside phosphorylase located in the endothelial cells, pericytes, and erythrocytes. Most of the adenosine is taken up by the myocardial cells, and that escaping into the circulation is largely in the form of inosine and hypoxanthine. Since adenylic acid deaminase (which deaminates AMP to IMP) is in low concentration in heart muscle, the major degradative pathway from AMP is via dephosphorylation to adenosine.

○ = Adenosine deaminase; ● = adenylic acid deaminase; △ = nucleoside phosphorylase; (---) = 5'-nucleotidase; (·····) = adenosine kinase. (From Berne, R. M., and Rubio, R.: Coronary circulation. *In* Berne, R. M., Sperelakis, N., and Geiger, S. R. (eds.): Handbook of Physiology, Section 2. The Cardiovascular System, Bethesda, Md., American Physiological Society, 1979, p. 924.)

tion of perfusion pressure below this level lowers coronary blood flow even through nonobstructed vessels and may reduce collateral blood flow to the peri-infarction zone, thereby enlarging the infarct.[89]

As noted, with organic occlusive lesions or spasm in major coronary arteries the effective myocardial perfusion pressure is the low pressure existing *distal* to the obstruction, and autoregulation in the distal bed may be compromised because it is already maximally dilated in the basal state. As a consequence, perfusion of this distal bed becomes dependent entirely on perfusion pressure. Under these circumstances, augmentation of cardiac oxygen requirements *without* an increase in perfusion pressure results in or intensifies ischemia. Since blood flow to regions supplied by normal vessels can be increased (because regional vasodilatation in these regions is possible), while blood flow to the compromised zone cannot (because it is already maximally dilated), disparities in regional perfusion can become intensified. In addition, vasodilatation in the normal zones may reduce perfusion pressure to the ischemic zones and deprive them further of blood flow, a phenomenon sometimes termed "coronary steal."

PHARMACOLOGICAL AGENTS. Alpha-adrenergic agonists can cause constriction of both coronary conduction vessels, i.e., the large epicardial arteries, as well as coronary resistance vessels, i.e., the small intramural arteries and arterioles[90] (Fig. 36–5). This effect tends to be minimized by the passive distention of the vessels consequent to an elevation of intravascular pressure as well as by the metabolically induced coronary vasodilatation consequent to an imbalance between oxygen supply and demand resulting from the coronary constriction and from any in-

crease in $M\dot{V}O_2$ accompanying the arterial hypertension induced by these drugs. Directly acting coronary vasodilators, such as nitroglycerin and isosorbide dinitrate,[27,28] augment perfusion of ischemic zones, as reflected by increased clearance of ^{133}Xe in patients with coronary artery disease[90]; these drugs have been shown to dilate coronary conductance vessels, coronary collaterals, and even atherosclerotic stenoses,[91–93] as well as to reduce the ventricular diastolic tension which tends to limit flow to the subendocardium; they have a lesser effect on resistance vessels.[92] The effects of calcium antagonists, such as verapamil or nifedipine, on coronary perfusion appear to reflect primarily direct action on the large epicardial conductance vessels as well as on the resistance vessels.[93] These agents increase blood flow to normal as well as ischemic myocardium.[94] Dipyridamole dilates the distal (resistance) vessels; since these are also acted upon by the endogenous vasodilator (adenosine), this agent is of little if any value in the treatment of myocardial ischemia. Prostaglandin I_2, which inhibits platelet aggregation, also decreases coronary vascular resistance,[87] whereas thromboxane A_2, which aggregates platelets, is also a potent coronary vasoconstrictor.

Factors Limiting Coronary Perfusion

The normal coronary vascular bed has the capacity to reduce its resistance to approximately 25 per cent of basal levels during the stress of maximal exercise; i.e., a four- to fivefold increase in coronary blood flow can occur during maximal exercise, which is generally accompanied by an increase in arterial pressure and a marked tachycardia. It is then not surprising that, in the basal state, the cross-sectional area of a proximal coronary artery can be reduced by up to approximately 80 per cent of normal, and vasodilatation of the coronary resistance vessels distal to the obstruction can maintain blood flow without the development of ischemia at rest (p. 261). However, since coronary blood flow cannot rise with this degree of obstruction in the proximal coronary bed, any stimulus that increases $M\dot{V}O_2$, such as exercise- or pacing-induced tachycardia, will elicit ischemia. With lesser degrees of obstruction, the distal bed is not maximally dilated in the basal state and, although the capacity for further dilatation exists, this capacity is subnormal and ischemia may develop, depending on the extent to which myocardial oxygen demands are augmented. When obstruction of a proximal coronary artery reduces the lumen to less than approximately 20 per cent of normal, ischemia will be present even in the basal state, despite maximal dilatation of the resistance vessels (unless the myocardium distal to the obstructed vessel is perfused by collateral vessels). Transient severe obstruction, as may occur in coronary spasm, will result in brief periods of ischemia, chest pain, electrocardiographic changes, and myocardial dysfunction. When it persists, myocardial necrosis ensues.

Basic considerations of fluid mechanics indicate that the pressure drop across a stenosis varies directly with the length of the stenosis and inversely with the fourth power of the radius (Bernoulli's theorem). Stenosis resistance changes relatively little with mild degrees of vascular narrowing but rises progressively and precipitously with severe obstruction; indeed, resistance almost triples as stenosis severity increases from 80 to 90 per cent.[95] As a consequence, with even a slight change in the severity of stenosis—as might occur when the resistance of the distal bed and therefore the pressure distending the narrowed coronary artery declines, as during exercise or following dipyridamole—the perfusion pressure distal to the obstruction may become reduced and subendocardial perfusion impaired.[96]

Myocardial ischemia and its consequences may occur as a result of fixed, atherosclerotic lesions or may be secondary to transitory reduction of myocardial blood flow caused by coronary spasm or platelet aggregates.[97] The clinical sequelae of myocardial ischemia, whether produced by an increase in $M\dot{V}O_2$ in the face of fixed obstruction or by a reduction in myocardial oxygen supply resulting from coronary spasm or transient aggregation of platelets, may be manifest clinically as angina pectoris, electrical instability, characteristic electrocardiographic changes, and depression of myocardial function.

EFFECTS OF ISCHEMIA ON MYOCARDIAL CONTRACTILITY

EFFECTS ON VENTRICULAR CONTRACTION. In 1935 Tennant and Wiggers demonstrated that after ligation of a coronary artery the contraction of cardiac muscle supplied by this vessel ceases, and the affected area appears cyanotic, dilated, and bulging.[98] More recent studies by Vatner have shown that in the basal state there is no reserve in blood flow; any given reduction in flow, even one as small as 10 to 20 per cent, results in an approximately similar per cent reduction of myocardial segment

shortening. A reduction of blood flow of 80 per cent results in akinesis, while a 95 per cent reduction causes systolic bulging (dyskinesis).[99] Patients with coronary artery disease and a previous myocardial infarction exhibit impaired left ventricular function; in the presence of angina, transient episodes of myocardial ischemia cause left ventricular systolic and diastolic dysfunction.[100] The duration of impaired function may be quite prolonged, and postischemic depression ("stunning") of the myocardium, with impaired mechanical performance, high-energy phosphate stores, and abnormal ultrastructure may persist for a week or longer following a brief—15-minute—period of coronary occlusion, which is not enough to cause myocardial necrosis.[101] Myocardial ischemia may be associated with elimination of the normal contractile performance in a *localized area* of myocardium, resulting in an asynergic contraction.[102] Figure 36–11 shows the immediate regional myocardial functional responses to an acute coronary occlusion: paradoxical motion in the central ischemic zone, reduced contraction in the adjacent area, and compensatory hyperfunction of the uninvolved normal myocardium, the latter mediated in part by its dilation and the operation of the Frank-Starling mechanism.

Regional loss of myocardial contractile activity, whether sustained or transient, if sufficiently widespread, may depress overall left ventricular function, producing reductions of stroke volume, stroke work, cardiac output, and ejection fraction and elevation of end-diastolic volume and pressure.[103] Clinical evidence of heart failure occurs when regional asynergy is so severe and extensive that the uninvolved myocardium cannot sustain the excess load it must sustain. Hemodynamic evidence of left ventricular failure develops when contraction ceases in 20 to 25 per cent of the left ventricle; with loss of 40 per cent or more of left ventricular myocardium, severe pump failure ensues and, if this loss is acute, fatal or near-fatal cardiogenic shock usually develops (p. 591).

Since the heart has virtually no stores of oxygen, its high rate of energy expenditure results in a sudden, striking decline of myocardial oxygen tension within seconds of coronary occlusion, coincident with the loss of contractility. The marginal zone contracts weakly, whereas the nonischemic myocardium exhibits a compensatory increase in its force of contraction. The rapid decline in contractility induced by ischemia cannot be attributed to alterations in excitability.[104] Although ischemia does not produce major changes in the amplitude and upstroke velocity of the action potential, the duration of the plateau phase of the action potential is shortened, which may signify a reduction in the slow inward current, carried largely by calcium.

It is possible that the concentrations of high-energy phosphate compounds in critical locations—such as the sarcoplasmic reticulum, a locus of calcium binding and release, or the sarcolemma, where ion fluxes and cell volume may be affected—are reduced by ischemia, even when the overall intracellular concentration of these compounds is still normal or near normal.

A final possibility is that ischemia reduces the release of Ca^{++} from the sarcolemma, the sarcoplasmic reticulum, or both, and thereby interferes with the interaction of Ca^{++} with the contractile proteins.[105,106] As outlined in Chapter 13, contraction is normally initiated by the rapid release of

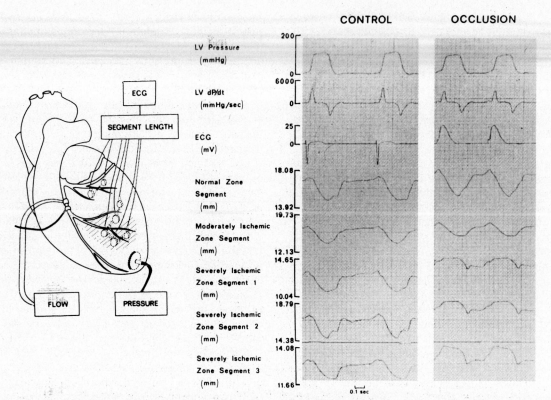

FIGURE 36–11 Effects of coronary occlusion on left ventricular (LV) pressure, LV dP/dt, and the epicardial electrogram in the severely ischemic zone, and on left ventricular dimensions in a normal segment of myocardium, a moderately ischemic segment (at the border between the normal and severely ischemic segment), and in three severely ischemic segments. The experimental preparation is illustrated on the left; an occluding cuff and flow meter are placed around the left anterior descending coronary artery, and crystals for ultrasonographic measurement of cardiac dimensions are sewn into the left ventricle. With coronary occlusion, only a slight decline in left ventricular systolic pressure and a slight elevation in left ventricular end-diastolic pressure occur, but there is a marked rise in the ST segment in the ischemic zone. The normal zone exhibits increased excursion per cardiac cycle with an increase in end-diastolic dimensions. Shortening of the segmental length per contraction decreases in the moderately ischemic zone. There is frank paradoxical pulsation in all three severely ischemic zones. (From Vatner, S. F., and Baig, H.: The effects of inotropic stimulation on ischemic myocardium in conscious dogs. Trans. Assoc. Am. Phys. *91*:283, 1978.)

Ca^{++} from the sarcoplasmic reticulum,[107] and this release is triggered by a rise in the local concentration of Ca^{++} in the vicinity of the sarcoplasmic reticulum. According to this concept, when the Ca^{++} concentration in the cytoplasm reaches a critical level, a massive release of Ca^{++} from the sarcoplasmic reticulum occurs, leading to muscle contraction.[108] Changes in intracellular pH may influence this Ca^{++} trigger mechanism—i.e., a fall in intracellular pH, as occurs in ischemia, may reduce the sensitivity of the sarcoplasmic reticulum to the local concentrations of Ca^{++}.

As discussed on p. 413, once Ca^{++} is released from the sarcoplasmic reticulum, it combines with specific receptor sites on the regulator protein, troponin, which ultimately leads to muscle tension and shortening. The high intracellular $[H^+]$ induced by ischemia may compete with Ca^{++} for the receptors on the troponin molecules. Thus, the actin-myosin interaction is impaired and it has been postulated that as a result of these two processes, i.e., reduction of the sensitivity of the sarcoplasmic reticulum to any given concentration of Ca^{++} and competition between H^+ and Ca^{++} for the troponin receptor sites, contractility is reduced.[105,109,110]

This concept of the critical importance of intracellular $[H^+]$ is supported by the observations that the functional changes induced by primary acidosis in the face of adequate myocardial oxygenation are similar to those produced by ischemia.[111] Furthermore, the reversal of acidosis by the administration of alkali improves contractile performance.[112] In addition to the role played by intracellular $[H^+]$, minor reductions of ATP may be important. Even a small reduction of intracellular ATP to levels that are still well above those required for the contractile process can be responsible for the changes in ion transport, which ultimately lead to a reduction in the delivery of Ca^{++} to the contractile sites.

In summary, it is likely that the abnormalities of contraction caused by ischemia result from the reduced release of Ca^{++} by the sarcoplasmic reticulum, ultimately making less Ca^{++} available to the contractile sites, as well as from the accumulation of intracellular H^+ and its interference with the interaction of Ca^{++} and the contractile proteins. Further exploration is needed of the roles of reduced transsarcolemmal passage of Ca^{++} during the plateau of the action potential and of lowered intracellular oxygen tension on stores of high-energy phosphate compounds in critical locations within the myocardial cell.

EFFECTS ON VENTRICULAR RELAXATION. Myocardial ischemia and infarction alter not only the contractile properties of the heart but also the diastolic pressure-volume relations of the left ventricle.[113] Myocardial ischemia impairs ventricular relaxation, as evidenced by a decreased peak negative maximal rate of pressure decline (negative dP/dt) and ventricular wall thinning and prolongs the isovolumetric relaxation period.[113-118] In turn, this impairment in ventricular relaxation increases the resistance to ventricular filling.[119,120] The combination of increased diastolic stiffness, decreased rate of wall thinning, and slow active pressure decay all contribute to the upward shift of the ventricular pressure-volume relationship observed during pacing-induced angina.[116] The mechanism responsible for the ischemia-induced impairment of myocardial relaxation has not been fully elucidated, but it has been proposed that reductions of myocardial high-energy stores impair the rate of uptake of Ca^{++} from the neighborhood of the myofilaments into the sarcoplasmic reticulum, thus prolonging contraction. Ca^{++} channel blockade will antagonize this process and by diminishing Ca^{++} influx into the cell will lower cytosolic $[Ca^{++}]$, restoring rapid relaxation. On the other hand, caffeine, an agent known to prolong Ca^{++} availability, potentiates the ischemia-induced impairment of ventricular relaxation.[121]

Ischemia thus causes impairment of cardiac contraction and incomplete ventricular emptying (systolic failure) and an elevation of ventricular end-diastolic volume. In addition, it impairs ventricular relaxation and shifts the diastolic pressure-volume curve upward (diastolic failure). The combination of systolic and diastolic failure, leads to elevated ventricular filling pressures,[115,122] ultimately causing symptoms of pulmonary congestion.

RECOGNITION OF MYOCARDIAL ISCHEMIA

ELECTROCARDIOGRAPHIC TECHNIQUES. It has been known for more than a half century that ST-segment elevation is an electrocardiographic sign of coronary artery occlusion.[123] Within 30 to 60 seconds after occlusion in dogs with open chests, epicardial leads from within the area of cyanosis show ST-segment elevation, reaching a maximum 5 to 7 minutes after occlusion. ST-segment elevation in the central area of cyanosis is usually more marked than at the periphery.[124,125] With the use of small intracavitary electrodes, simultaneous ST-segment elevation is noted on the endocardial surface, although it is less marked than that recorded on the epicardium.[124]

The electrophysiological basis of ST-segment changes in myocardial ischemia is discussed on page 223; an altered ion transport across the myocardial cell membrane apparently is the underlying cause. In the nonischemic myocardium, cell volume is regulated within narrow limits by a "sodium pump" located on the plasma membrane.[126] This active, metabolically dependent pump maintains a high extracellular $[Na^+]$ as well as high intracellular $[K^+]$ and colloids, thus stabilizing cell volume.[127] It has been postulated that with ischemia, the availability of energy necessary for this pumping is reduced. According to this concept, Na^+, accompanied by Cl^- and H_2O, accumulates intracellularly and K^+ begins to leak into the extracellular space.[128] The cells eventually lose all control of volume and have an electrolyte distribution similar to that of the extracellular fluid.[126] The reduction in intracellular $[K^+]$ or the accumulation of extracellular K^+ or both are critical in the generation of the elevated ST segment,[129] since small changes in the ratio of intracellular to extracellular $[K^+]$ have a marked effect on the polarity of cellular membranes.[130]

The magnitude of epicardial ST-segment elevation correlates, in general, with the decrease in blood flow, lactate accumulation, and depletion of high-energy phosphate compounds in the underlying myocardium.[131] In addition, ST-segment elevation is associated with a reduction in oxygen tension in the affected tissue below 65 per cent of control,[132] and the magnitude of the elevation correlates well with intramyocardial oxygen tension.[133] Measurements with a mass spectrometer have shown that intramyocardial ST-segment elevations correspond to changes in myocardial gas tensions.[134] Also, epicardial ST-segment elevations shortly after coronary artery occlusion correlate closely with subsequent depletion of myocardial creatine phosphokinase (CPK) activity and with histological evidence of necrosis in the subjacent myocardium.[135-137] It is now clear that the distribution of epicardial ST-segment elevation provides a reasonable index of the extent of myocardial ischemia and that the intramyocardial ST segment is a more sensitive index than the epicardial. However, it must be appreciated that ST-segment elevation is not specific for myocardial ischemia, since the ST segment is also affected by changes in temperature, by drugs (including the digitalis glycosides and quinidine), by sympathetic stimulation of the heart,[138] by epicardial injury due to pericarditis, and by localized intraventricular conduction defects.[139]

ALTERATIONS IN CELLULAR ELECTROPHYSIOLOGY INDUCED BY ISCHEMIA. Ischemia-induced ventricular tachyarrhythmias can be caused by increased automaticity (p. 622), triggered activity (p. 620), and reentry (p. 629). However, knowledge of the effects of acute ischemia on the electrophysiology of the human heart is limited. Although studies in animal models provide major insights, these models may differ from the clinical condition in several aspects, including the nature of the occlusive coronary artery lesion, the presence of multiple lesions, and differences in collateral blood flow. After acute coronary artery ligation *in the dog*, ventricular arrhythmias occur in three phases[140,141]:

1. An early phase begins almost immediately after coronary ligation, frequently culminates in ventricular fibrillation within 3 to 6 minutes, and usually lasts less than 30 minutes. Within minutes after coronary occlusion, marked alterations occur in the electrophysiological properties of ventricular myocardial cells, with shortening of action potential duration and decreased amplitude, upstroke velocity, and resting potential.[142] Extracellular recordings from the epicardial surface of the ischemic zone show marked loss of amplitude and delay and fractionation of recorded electrograms, suggesting that activation in myocardium is irregular and that the effects of ischemia are not uniform.[143] Available evidence suggests that reentry is responsible for ventricular tachycardia and ventricular fibrillation early during ischemia, while the cause of ventricular premature beats is less clear but may be related to the triggering of automatic activity by the current of injury.[144] This early arrhythmic phase observed in experimental animals could be related to the "prehospital" phase of arrhythmias observed in patients, which is also marked by a high incidence of ventricular fibrillation and sudden death. The arrhythmias

of the early phase are intimately rate-related.[140,143,145] Thus, vagally induced cardiac slowing can avert or abort ectopic ventricular rhythms.[143,145] Conversely, ectopic ventricular rhythm can be induced by cardiac pacing.[140]

There is evidence that regional myocardial sympathetic stimulation contributes to the early malignant phase of ventricular arrhythmia after the onset of ischemia. Sympathectomy and beta-adrenergic blockade mitigate both the regional augmentation of cyclic AMP and the frequency and severity of the early phase of ventricular arrhythmias.[146,147] On the other hand, the effectiveness of antiarrhythmic drugs such as quinidine, lidocaine, or aprindine during the early phase is controversial.[148–150]

2. After a period of quiescence, a delayed arrhythmic phase begins at about 6 to 9 hours following coronary occlusion in the dog and lasts for 24 to 72 hours. During this period spontaneous polymorphic ventricular rhythms occur, but ventricular fibrillation is uncommon. Multiple electrophysiological mechanisms are probably involved in the delayed arrhythmic phase, particularly abnormal automaticity of subendocardial Purkinje fibers.[151,152] This phase may partly correspond to ventricular tachycardia and "accelerated idioventricular rhythms" (p. 1286) commonly seen on the second and third days following infarction in humans. Antiarrhythmic drugs such as quinidine, procainamide, lidocaine, and disopyramide suppress these arrhythmias by reducing automaticity.

3. By 72 hours after coronary ligation in the dog, the spontaneous polymorphic ventricular rhythms have nearly subsided, but the heart is still prone to ventricular tachyarrhythmias and, occasionally, ventricular fibrillation. These arrhythmias may be easily induced by rapid cardiac pacing or programmed premature stimulation[153] and are the result of reentrant circuits in the subepicardial layer of the infarction, including the boundary zone between the infarction and surrounding viable myocardium. This late phase of ventricular vulnerability may correspond to the "post-coronary care unit" ventricular arrhythmias and late in-hospital ventricular fibrillation. Antiarrhythmic drugs, such as lidocaine or procainamide, seem to abolish these late reentrant arrhythmias by further depression or block of the already slowed conduction in the reentrant circuit.[154,155]

Mechanics of Arrhythmias. There has been considerable interest in the mechanism of ventricular arrhythmias that occur with release of coronary occlusion and reperfusion,[156] as opposed to occlusion arrhythmias. Ventricular fibrillation is likely to occur abruptly without warning following reperfusion, whereas it is often heralded by ventricular ectopic beats with increasing frequency following occlusion. The most likely explanation for reperfusion arrhythmias is that chemical and electrical gradients caused by washout of metabolites and electrolytes that have accumulated in the ischemic zone are responsible for the electrophysiological derangement.[157,158] Reperfusion is accompanied by changes in regional concentrations of K^+, Ca^{++}, H^+, catecholamines, and lysophosphoglycerides; the last are derived from degradation of membrane phospholipids in cells undergoing infarction.[159] There may be some relevance of reperfusion arrhythmias in experimental animals to such clinical syndromes as the abrupt onset of ventricular fibrillation in patients who are undergoing surgical, thrombolytic, or spontaneous reperfusion

after thrombotic coronary occlusion, and the malignant arrhythmias that can accompany Prinzmetal's angina; the release of coronary spasm may be a common cause of reperfusion and its attendant arrhythmias.

The biochemical correlates of ischemia-induced electrophysiological changes are not clearly identified. Ischemia depresses the energy-dependent membrane sodium-potassium pumping system, which leads to a gain in intracellular sodium and loss of intracellular potassium with consequent elevation of extracellular potassium concentration in the vicinity of the sarcolemma.[160,161] As a result of anaerobic metabolism, intracellular pH declines. Ischemia also results in release of norepinephrine from adrenergic nerve endings and an increase of tissue levels of cyclic AMP.[162] It has been postulated that in the ischemic zone, high concentrations of extracellular K^+ may depolarize the cells to the extent that the rapid Na^+ channel is inactivated, and high concentrations of catecholamines may stimulate the slow current carried principally by Ca^{++}, resulting in slow response action potentials. The latter could explain the slowed conduction and reentrant ventricular arrhythmias associated with ischemia. However, it must be acknowledged that while this hypothesis is attractive, its validity has not been established, and indeed has been questioned.[150,157,163]

The concept that slow response action potentials are responsible for ischemia-induced electrophysiological disturbances loses much of its plausibility in the later stage of myocardial infarction. The extracellular K^+ concentration is probably not as high as in the early stage of ischemia. Besides, total catecholamines in the ischemic region decline to a very low level on the day after coronary occlusion.[164] However, ischemic myocardium still shows markedly depressed action potentials, slow conduction, and a high propensity for reentrant rhythms.[165] In the later stage of ischemia, ischemic myocardial cells have been found to be exquisitely sensitive to the depressant effect of tetrodotoxin, a specific blocker of the fast Na^+ channel, and not to verapamil and D600, which are blockers of the slow Ca^{++} channel.[165] These observations suggest that poor membrane responses of ischemic myocardial cells are related to depression of the fast Na^+ channel. The clinical relevance of studies of ischemia-induced ionic conductance changes relates to the choice of ideal antiarrhythmic therapy following ischemia. Thus, the antiarrhythmic effect of lidocaine on ischemia-induced reentrant ventricular arrhythmias is due to selective depression of ischemic myocardial cells forming part of the reentrant pathway.[154,155] The finding that the effect of lidocaine on depressed ischemic cells is similar to that of tetrodotoxin suggests that lidocaine acts by further depressing the tenuous Na^+ channel in ischemic cells.[154,155]

EFFECTS OF ISCHEMIA ON MYOCARDIAL METABOLISM

HIGH-ENERGY PHOSPHATE METABOLISM. During the first minutes of severe ischemia, the production of high-energy phosphates (the sum of ATP and creatine phosphate (CP)) declines and is greatly exceeded by the utilization; hence tissue stores decline progressively, with CP stores falling more rapidly than ATP stores. CP is depleted by transferring its high-energy phosphate to ADP in an attempt to maintain ATP stores. In the presence of normal aerobic mitochondrial function, ADP is converted to ATP (through the myokinase reaction), but in the absence of normal oxidative phosphorylation it is converted to AMP (Fig. 36–12), which in turn is broken down to adenosine and ultimately to inosine, hypoxanthine, and xanthine (Fig. 36–10).[166] Reimer and Jennings have shown that when ATP was reduced below 20 per cent of control values the ability to regenerate high-energy phosphate, preserve cell volume, and maintain ionic regulation were lost. When ATP fell below 10 per cent of control, damage to the sarcolemma occurred.[167] When tissue is *reversibly* injured by ischemia (i.e., its viability can be maintained by reperfusion), ATP stores are usually greater than 60 per cent of control and electronmicroscopy may reveal only glycogen loss, nuclear chromatin clumping, intermyofibrillar edema, and mitochondrial swelling but no sarcolemma damage or amorphous dense bodies in the mitochondria. Reduction of ATP below 30 per cent is usually associated with visible sarcolemmal damage and irreversible injury (i.e., the tissue is not viable despite reperfusion).[168,169]

The technique of phosphorus-31 nuclear magnetic resonance spectroscopy (^{31}PNMR) (Chap. 11B) is providing important new information concerning high-energy phosphate stores and intracellular pH in ischemic myocardium. Multiple sequential measurements can be made on the same tissue and correlated with mechanical activity.[169] This technique has demonstrated that the magnitude of intracellular acidosis and associated increase in inorganic phosphate correlate inversely with postischemic structure and recovery of function. ATP but not CP content correlates with return of contractile function after reperfusion.[170]

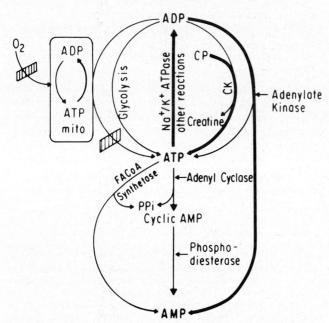

FIGURE 36–12 The major metabolic pathways of adenine nucleotide degradation during myocardial ischemia are illustrated. The quantitatively most important pathways are indicated by the solid arrows. (Reproduced with permission from Jennings, R. B., Reimer, K. A., Hill, M. L., and Mayer, S. E.: Total ischemia in dog hearts, in vitro. 1. Comparison of high energy phosphate production, utilization, and depletion, and of adenine nucleotide catabolism in total ischemia in vitro vs. severe ischemia in vivo. Circ. Res. **49**:892, 1981, by permission of the American Heart Association, Inc.)

Carbohydrate metabolism. Under normal aerobic conditions, myocardium derives its energy primarily from oxidative phosphorylation, a process localized to the mitochondria. Although many types of substrate can be utilized, oxidation of fatty acids predominates. Oxidative phosphorylation is regulated to a large extent by the phosphate potential: $(ATP)/(ADP) \times (P_i)$. When oxygen availability is limited, the rate of ATP synthesis declines and high-energy phosphate stores decline. Depletion of purine nucleotide pools is prompt. It persists for hours to days after even brief intervals of ischemia, in part because of the limited capacity of myocardium for de novo purine synthesis. The reduction in the phosphate potential and the prevailing concentrations of intermediates such as glucose-6-phosphate alter the activity of enzymes involved in intermediary metabolism. During hypoxia, glycolytic flux increases because of enhanced uptake of glucose and also phosphorylation, reflecting (1) decline of glucose-6-phosphate and release of inhibition of hexokinase; (2) release of inhibition of phosphofructokinase (PFK) by citrate and ATP; and (3) activation of PFK by inorganic phosphate. Glycogenolysis accelerates because of transformation of phosphorylase b, an inactive form of the enzyme under physiological conditions, to the active, phosphorylated form, phosphorylase a. Later, glycogenolysis is potentiated by activation of phosphorylase b itself, by accumulating metabolites such as adenosine monophosphate, and by release of inhibition by glucose-6-phosphate (Fig. 36–13).

The augmentation of glycolytic flux so characteristic of hypoxia and of the initial response to ischemia may contribute to maintenance of viability of the heart by providing ATP. The importance of glycolysis in the generation of energy is reflected in the observation that inhibition of glycolysis with iodoacetate results in cessation of beating of the anoxic heart even though the agent does not influence the apparent function of the well-oxygenated heart. Augmentation of glycolytic flux by provision of glucose or prior augmentation of glycogen stores confers some resistance to the deterioration of function induced by anoxia or ischemia. Nevertheless, even with insulin present in the perfusion medium, anaerobic metabolism can supply less than half the energy requirement for maintenance of viability of the nonworking, isolated, perfused, anoxic heart. Thus, anaerobic metabolism alone cannot maintain myocardial ATP stores indefinitely in the nonworking heart, let alone in myocardium with markedly greater energy requirements associated with contractile function.

Under aerobic conditions, carbohydrate metabolism proceeds via oxidation through the Krebs (tricarboxylic acid) cycle. However, when anoxia supervenes, the lack of oxygen inhibits Krebs cycle activity and the metabolism of glucose can proceed only via anaerobic glycolysis. When the cause of anoxia is ischemia, lactate accumulates, since oxidation of pyruvate is precluded by the inhibition of the Krebs cycle, and washout of metabolites is reduced because of the limited perfusion. The initial burst of glycolytic activity accompanying hypoxia with or without ischemia appears to depend on allosteric effects of adenine nucleotides and other regulators of enzymes such as phosphorylase b, hexokinase, and phosphofructokinase.[173] However, under conditions of limited perfusion sufficient to induce hypoxia, the rapidly increasing concentration of lactic acid within the cell, the decline of pH, and the accumulation of other metabolites inhibit glycolytic flux at the phosphofructokinase and glyceraldehyde-3-phosphate dehydrogenase[172,173] steps, among others (Fig. 36–11).

In isolated perfused hearts, lactate exerts a deleterious effect on glycolytic flux independent of pH[174] by inhibiting the glyceraldehyde-phosphate dehydrogenase reaction, which is responsible for conversion of glyceraldehyde-3-phosphate to 1,3-diphosphoglyceric acid. On the other hand, acidosis itself inhibits glycolytic flux,[174,175] left ventricular performance, and the malate-aspartate cycle.[174-176] This and other similar cycles provide a shuttle via intermediates to which the mitochondrial membranes are permeable, permitting transport of reducing equivalents formed in the cytosol across the mitochondrial membranes and thereby allowing their oxidation by the respiratory chain. Persistent or prolonged ischemia results in inhibition of the shuttle reactions because of accumulation of reducing equivalents in the mitochondria (due to the lack of oxygen as a terminal electron and hydrogen receptor), with consequent accumulation of reducing equivalents and hydrogen ions in the cytosol as well.

The acidosis and accumulation of metabolites contribute directly to inhibition of glycolytic flux.[177] Thus, because glycolytic flux in ischemic tissue becomes limited relatively soon after the initial burst of activity, it is capable of meeting only a significantly smaller proportion of energy requirements than in anoxic tissue. The decline of high-energy phosphate stores is therefore faster, perhaps contributing to the more

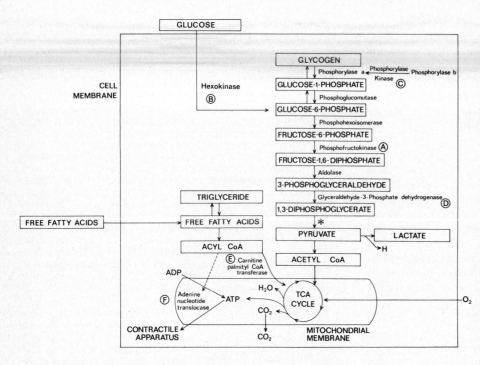

FIGURE 36–13 Effects of ischemia on glycolysis and free fatty acid metabolism. Ischemia increases intracellular lactate concentration; this accumulation inhibits several enzymes in the glycolytic pathway: Phosphofructokinase (A); hexokinase (B); and phosphorylase kinase (C), which prevents activation of phosphorylase b to phosphorylase a and therefore suppresses conversion of glycogen to glucose-1-phosphate. Glyceraldehyde-3-phosphate dehydrogenase (D) is suppressed by an elevation of intracellular lactate. (* denotes that the glycolytic pathway has been condensed at this point.) Ischemia increases the intracellular concentration of acyl CoA esters, in part because the intracellular accumulation of lactate inhibits carnitine palmityl coenzyme A transferase (E), the enzyme that catalyzes the transfer of acyl CoA from the cell cytoplasm to the mitochondria. Acyl CoA esters inhibit the effective exchange of ADP and ATP between the cytoplasm of the cell and the mitochondria by suppressing the activity of adenine nucleotide translocase (F). The antilipolytic agents are effective because they prevent a build-up of acyl CoA esters within the cytoplasm, and 1-carnitine exerts a salutary effect on ischemic myocardium by reversing the inhibition of adenine nucleotide translocase, thus allowing continued movement of ADP and ATP between the cell cytoplasm and the mitochondria. (TCA = tricarboxylic acid.) (Reproduced with permission from Hillis, L. D., and Braunwald, E.: Myocardial ischemia. N. Engl. J. Med. *296*:971, 1034, and 1093; 1977.)

rapid development of irreversible injury in ischemic compared with anoxic myocardium.

The above-described changes in carbohydrate metabolism induced by myocardial ischemia account for the relationship between lactate production and the severity of impaired perfusion; this relationship may be exploited diagnostically. Under normal aerobic conditions, myocardium extracts lactate from the arterial blood with extraction fractions in the range of 20 per cent. Extraction persists despite acceleration of ventricular rate by pacing.[178] However, when myocardial ischemia is present at rest or develops in response to stress induced by pacing or other physiological stimuli, lactate extraction declines or is replaced by net lactate production[179] (p. 1344). In general, both decreased lactate extraction and an increase in lactate production are accompanied by an increase in coronary venous lactate/pyruvate ratios, compared with values in arterial blood. Unfortunately, relationships between the concentrations of lactate in coronary sinus blood and in extracellular fluid, cytosol, and mitochondrial compartments are complex and are influenced by nonspecific factors such as acid-base balance, adrenergic stimulation of the heart, substrate availability, permeability of cell membranes to lactate and pyruvate, concomitant disorders such as diabetes mellitus, and prevailing levels of plasma free fatty acids. Furthermore, net lactate extraction is a relatively insensitive index of changes occurring in localized regions of the heart. Accordingly, the diagnostic sensitivity and specificity of altered lactate extraction for the detection or assessment of severity of ischemia are somewhat limited.

Differences Between Ischemia and Anoxia.

Although differences between anoxia and ischemia have been alluded to above, it is useful to summarize them at this point. Not only is oxidative metabolism reduced during ischemia, as it is in anoxia, but the anaerobic production of ATP also proceeds at less than maximal capacity. In the ischemic working heart the concentration of lactic acid rises and the intracellular pH falls rapidly as the acid products of glycolysis accumulate. In contrast, in the anoxic heart perfusion results in the washout of the acid products of glycolysis, thereby retarding the rate of development of intracellular acidosis. The increased lactate production is not sustained by the ischemic heart, which has a glycolytic rate about one fourth that of the anoxic heart in a steady state. This is unrelated to a reduction of substrate availability, because the addition of insulin and glucose to the perfusion medium fails to stimulate glycolysis to the extent observed in anoxia or under normal aerobic conditions. While insulin and elevated glucose in the perfusate are able to increase glucose transport and augment the intracellular glucose concentration, they do not prevent ischemia from inhibiting glucose utilization.

The lower glycolytic flux in the ischemic as compared to the anoxic heart probably results in part from the inhibition by intracellular acidosis of PFK (Fig. 36–11), a key enzyme in the glycolytic chain. The reduction of glycolytic flux through the inhibition of PFK results in the accumulation of glucose-6-phosphate, and this inhibits hexokinase, further decreasing the phosphorylation of glucose. As a consequence, glycolysis provides less energy to the ischemic than to the anoxic heart. The importance of intracellular pH is further supported by the observation that pretreatment of rat myocardium to an alkaline pH of 7.9 maintains tension during a subsequent period of hypoxia.[180]

Fatty Acid Metabolism. Under normal aerobic conditions, 60 to 90 per cent of myocardial energy requirements is met by oxidation of free fatty acids (FFA),[181] which are trapped in cells in the form of fatty (acyl) esters containing coenzyme A (acyl-CoA). The preferential utilization of FFA by myocardium appears to depend on the high activity of several enzyme systems, including the acyl-CoA–carnitine transferase systems that facilitate continuing transport of acyl-CoA from the cytosol to the mitochondria in a series of steps in which acyl-CoA and acyl-carnitine are interconverted.

After fatty acids are taken up by myocardial cells and undergo esterification with CoA, the acyl-CoA intermediates generally remain trapped in the cell. Acyl-CoA may be incorporated into triglycerides in the cytosol or oxidized after transport through the mitochondrial membrane. Under aerobic conditions, oxidation predominates since the products formed (two carbon moieties called acetyl groups) are readily incorporated as intermediates into the citric acid cycle and oxidized to CO_2 and water. Oxidation of fatty acids inhibits glucose uptake, glycolytic flux, and glycogenolysis. The increased production of acetyl-CoA accompanying fatty acid oxidation inhibits pyruvate dehydrogenase,[182] thereby limiting the flow of carbohydrate metabolism through the citric acid cycle. Accumulation of glucose-6-phosphate inhibits hexokinase, decreasing phosphorylation of glucose. The decreased phosphorylation, coupled with direct inhibition of membrane transport of glucose mediated by fatty acids, contributes to the overall reduction of carbohydrate metabolism when fatty acid availability is high and oxygenation adequate.[183]

Striking changes in fatty acid metabolism result from myocardial ischemia. The limited supply of oxygen inhibits beta-oxidation—as does the increased ratio of NADH/NAD and the reduced concentration of flavoproteins.[173] With more prolonged ischemia, oxidation of fatty acids is inhibited by another mechanism: inhibition or loss of long-chain acyl-carnitine transferase enzyme activity, necessary for transport of cytosolic acyl-CoA to the mitchondria prior to oxidation.[184] Accordingly, intracellular concentrations of acyl-CoA increase and acetyl-CoA content declines.[185,186] The increased acyl-CoA accompanied by increased production of glycerol, a byproduct of the enhanced glycolytic flux induced by ischemia, leads to increased synthesis of triglycerides,[187] which accumulate in the ischemic myocardium.

Accumulation of acyl-CoA may be deleterious because it inhibits further formation of CoA esters of fatty acids. Thus, fatty acids entering the cell cannot be esterified and trapped and are therefore prone to egress promptly. Furthermore, oxidation of fatty acids entering the cell cannot proceed without initial esterification with CoA. Accordingly, accumulation of fatty acid labeled with carbon-11, which can be monitored externally in vivo by positron tomography, is diminished in ischemic or hypoxic zones.[188,189] Restored metabolism accompanying reperfusion implemented promptly enough to maintain cell viability is reflected by a return of myocardial accumulation of fatty acid toward normal[190,191] (Fig. 36–14).

Accumulation of acyl-CoA esters also inhibits activity of an enzyme in the inner mitochondrial membrane, adenine nucleotide translocase—important in myocardial energy metabolism[192] and required for

transport of ATP synthesized in the mitchrondria to the cytosol. Although definitive information is not yet available, inhibition of the translocase and consequent failure of repletion of cytosolic ATP may be one factor accounting for the prompt decline of creatine phosphate in ischemic myocardium. Creatine kinase facilitates phosphorylation of ADP to form ATP, with concomitant conversion of creatine phosphate to creatine when cytosolic ATP concentrations decline. Thus, cytosolic creatine phosphate content declines as the cell compensates for diminished transport of ATP from mitchrondria to cytosol. Accordingly, the effects of limited oxygen availability in ischemic myocardium on fatty acid metabolism may result in impaired energy production not only by direct limitation of oxidation of fatty acids, but also because of deleterious effects of the accumulating acyl-CoA intermediates on cellular function.

Detection of altered fatty acid metabolism is the basis for recognition of ischemic myocardium in experimental animals and patients after intravenous administration of cyclotron-produced, positron-emitting, ^{11}C-labeled fatty acids. In isolated perfused hearts, transitory diminution of perfusion leads to a reversible reduction of ^{11}C-palmitate accumulation, reflecting decreased uptake and oxidation of fatty acids in the perfusate.[193,194,194a,194b,194c] The uptake of tracer is independent of flow per se, as long as metabolic activity of the myocardium remains constant. In dogs subjected to coronary occlusion, diminished accumulation of ^{11}C-palmitate is evident in computer-reconstructed images obtained by positron-emission, transaxial tomography. Because this technique permits quantitative delineation of the distribution of the tracer in a cross-section of the heart after intravenous administration, the diminution of ^{11}C-palmitate uptake detectable tomographically corresponds quantitatively to biochemical and morphometric criteria of infarction.[195] Reduced flow alone does not diminish uptake of a substrate if intermediary metabolism is not altered, since the extraction fraction increases. Thus, transitory ischemia without reduction of either myocardial oxygen consumption or fatty acid utilization would not be manifested tomographically by decreased ^{11}C-palmitate uptake.[196] However, prolonged ischemia, with impairment of oxidative metabolism but without necrosis, would give rise to a zone

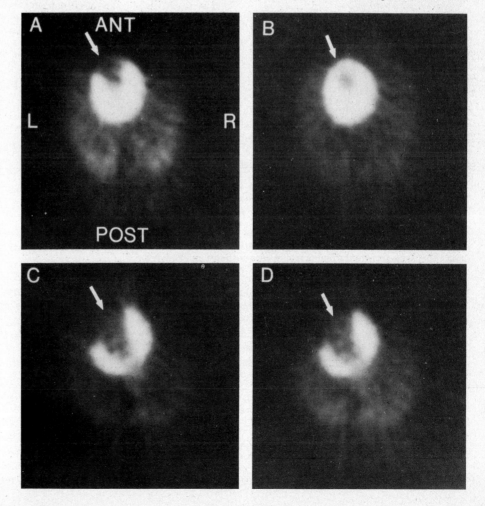

FIGURE 36–14 Transverse cardiac positron emission tomographic reconstructions obtained after intravenous administration of ^{11}C-palmitate in dogs. Reconstructions depicted are those obtained one hour after experimentally induced left anterior descending coronary artery thrombosis (*A*) and again after thrombolysis in the same dog (*B*). Normal myocardium extracts palmitate uniformly, whereas the ischemic zone exhibits diminished accumulation of tracer (arrow). The tomogram in panel *B* demonstrates substantial restoration of metabolism in the previously compromised anterior myocardium. In the lower panel, a tomogram six hours after onset of thrombosis and prior to the administration of streptokinase is shown (*C*) with a repeat tomogram (*D*) from the same dog one hour after intracoronary thrombolysis with streptokinase (confirmed angiographically). In contrast to the restoration of metabolism observed in dogs in which reperfusion was induced early after thrombosis, animals subjected to thrombolysis later than six hours after occlusion exhibited no significant restoration of metabolism despite angiographically documented lysis of coronary thrombi. (From Sobel, B. E., and Bergmann, S. R.: Coronary thrombolysis: Some unresolved issues. Am. J. Med. *72*:1, 1982. Reprinted with permission of Yorke Publishing Corporation.)

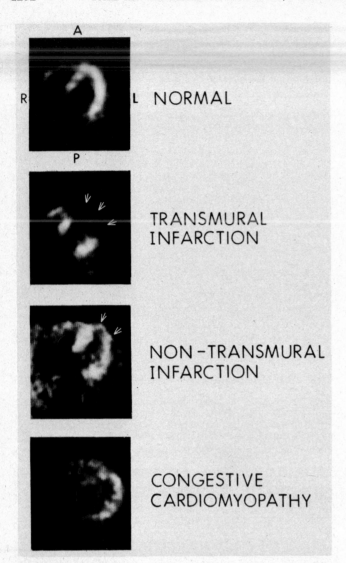

A

R   L   NORMAL

P

TRANSMURAL
INFARCTION

NON-TRANSMURAL
INFARCTION

CONGESTIVE
CARDIOMYOPATHY

FIGURE 36–15   Cardiac positron emission tomographic reconstructions obtained at the midventricular level after the intravenous injection of ^{11}C-palmitate, in a normal subject, patients with transmural and nontransmural infarction, and a patient with congestive cardiomyopathy. The horseshoe-shaped region depicts a 1.5 cm thick cross-section of the left ventricular myocardium. Accumulation of palmitate is homogeneous throughout each cross-section in the left ventricle in the normal subject. A homogeneous, intense depression of the accumulation of palmitate indicated by the arrow is found in the subject with anterior transmural infarction. The region of nontransmural infarction indicated by the arrow involves only a portion of the thickness of the anterolateral left ventricular wall. The subject with cardiomyopathy demonstrates marked left ventricular enlargement with marked spatial heterogeneity of the accumulation of palmitate within the left ventricular myocardium. A = anterior, P = posterior, L = left, R = right. (From Geltman, E. M., and Sobel, B. E.: Cardiac positron tomography. Chest, in press. Reprinted with permission of the American College of Chest Physicians.)

of decreased accumulation of the tracer evident by tomography. The two conditions (prolonged ischemia without necrosis and infarction per se) can be readily differentiated with the use of serial studies. Prolonged and persistent diminution of oxidative metabolism and hence persistently impaired regional uptake of ^{11}C-palmitate detectable tomographically are tantamount to necrosis in view of the well-established irreversibility of injury sustained by myocardium rendered ischemic for 2 hours or more[197] (Fig. 36–15).

Protein Metabolism. Characteristic changes in synthesis and degradation of myocardial proteins accompany ischemia. Synthesis decreases because of inhibition of peptide chain initiation and elongation.[198] Efflux of alanine reflects not only its diminished utilization in protein synthesis but also augmented synthesis by transamination of pyruvate, a precursor accumulating because of impaired carbohydrate exudation.[199] Thus, alanine release from the ischemic heart is analogous to lactate production.

Release of another amino acid, phenylalanine, has been employed in experimental preparations in which reincorporation into protein is prevented by pretreatment with cycloheximide (an inhibitor of protein synthesis) to provide an index of protein degradation under a variety of conditions, including normal oxygenation, anoxia, and simulated ischemia. The process of protein degradation requires energy derived from oxidative metabolism under physiological conditions based on observations with such preparations, since the rate of protein degradation declines by as much as 80 per cent in isolated hearts subjected to severe ischemia.[200] Although proteolysis mediated by lysosomal hydrolases has been implicated as a factor leading to irreversible injury in myocardium undergoing ischemic injury, increases in free and total lysosomal hydrolase activity do not occur until several hours after the onset of ischemia.[201] Accordingly, it appears likely that the early loss of functional sarcolemmal integrity accompanied by electrophysiological manifestations, subsequent impairment of cell volume regulation, and leakage of cytoplasmic constituents reflects primary damage to the cell membrane itself. Only later during the evolution of ischemic injury, when tissue pH is markedly diminished and reparative processes have already begun, do activation and liberation of lysosomal enzymes appear to be prominent. These and related observations suggest that the irreversible nature of injury sustained by ischemic myocardium is not due to proteolysis or activation of lysosomal enzymes, even though activation of these enzymes may account for the release of relatively late markers of cell death and result in protein degradation late in the evolution of necrosis.

Under physiological conditions, the myocardium extracts glutamic acid from arterial blood and produces ammonia and glutamine which appear in the coronary venous effluent. When ischemia supervenes, ammonia derived from amino acids that cannot be incorporated into protein under these conditions is incorporated into alanine and glutamine with a consequent increase in their concentrations in the coronary sinus effluent. The increased production of alanine has been viewed as analogous to the increased production of lactate. Both are markers of ischemia. In the case of alanine, transamination of pyruvate serves as a sink for ammonia that would otherwise accumulate. In the case of lactate, the pyruvate serves as a sink for hydrogen ions.

OXIDATIVE PHOSPHORYLATION. The importance of oxidative phosphorylation, i.e., the coupling of ATP synthesis to aerobic respiration, for the metabolic integrity of myocardium is underscored by some simple quantitative considerations. Complete oxidation of one mole of glucose gives rise to the net production of 36 moles of ATP. In contrast, only 2 moles of ATP are produced from complete anaerobic metabolism of 1 mole of glucose. Thus, even if the profound derangements in intermediary metabolism associated with increased production of reducing equivalents accompanying anaerobic glycolysis could be corrected, an 18-fold increase in glycolytic flux would be required for myocardium to synthesize comparable quantities of ATP via anaerobic compared to aerobic metabolism. The failure of energy production to keep pace with demand in ischemic cells is manifest by a prompt decline in the concentration of creatine phosphate, a major constituent of myocardial high-energy phosphate stores.[202]

The dependence of myocardial viability on the availability of oxygen has stimulated careful assessment of the gradients of oxygen present within ischemic zones of the heart, based on analysis of the oxidation-reduction state of specific components of the electron transport chain and different spectra reflecting changes in the oxygenation of myoglobin.[203] Results obtained with optical techniques applied to the infarcted heart in vitro suggest that individual cells, and possibly individual mitochondria, are either fully aerobic or fully anaerobic in regions of myocardium subjected to ischemia. Thus, at any given instant, borders between anoxic and oxygenated tissue are very sharp. This phenomenon is in part a reflection of the very high affinity of mitochondria for oxygen. In response to ischemia, the mitochondria remain oxidized, despite very low levels of tissue oxygen tension, and become reduced only when virtually the last remaining oxygen has been utilized within a region. However, it should be recognized that the sharp, anatomically definable, border zones detectable at a given instant with these optical techniques do not imply the absence of a time-dependent, potentially large mass of jeopardized but not yet irreversibly injured ischemic myocardium, susceptible to favorable influence by selected interventions. In fact, as ischemia persists, the locations of the discrete borders shift, judging from morphological observations in canine hearts subjected to coronary occlusion.

The percentage of transmural necrosis ultimately developing within a zone of myocardium rendered ischemic by coronary occlusion maintained for 40 minutes, 3 hours, 6 hours, and 24 hours, followed by reperfusion for 2 to 4 days, varies from 38 to 85 per cent with a "wavefront" of necrosis progressing from subendocardial to epicardial tissue.[204] Obviously, a cell may be able to tolerate severe ischemia for a brief interval although it will become necrotic after a prolonged insult. A cell with similar energy requirements will be able to tolerate a milder degree of ischemia for a longer period before becoming necrotic.[205] The extent to which ischemic myocardium may be protected by metabolic, pharmacological, or physiological interventions designed to improve the balance between myocardial oxygen supply and demand (Chap. 38) cannot be inferred from the sharpness of the border of oxygenation at a specific instant during the evolution of injury. In fact, the location of the transmural wavefront of irreversible injury is a function of the duration as well as the severity of limitation of oxygen supply and of the rate of accumulation of noxious metabolites in specific regions.

ACTIVATION OF LYSOSOMAL ENZYMES. Most tissues contain latent lysosomal hydrolases capable of mediating proteolysis under certain conditions. Lysosomal hydrolases are activated by an acid pH, although mammalian cells contain neutral proteases as well. Relatively late reparative processes in myocardium undergoing infarction are accompanied by consistent increases in lysosomal hydrolase activity in tissue extracts as well as in the circulation, suggesting that activation of proteases with dissolution of cellular debris is a component of the response to irreversible injury. However, the extent to which activation of lysosomal hydrolases contributes to early manifestations of ischemia or irreversibility remains controversial. What is clear is that much of the lysosomal activity in the heart undergoing infarction comes from cells participating in the response to inflammation, such as polymorphonuclear leukocytes rather than myocardial cells per se.

Calcium Metabolism in Ischemia

Myocardial injury induced by ischemia is associated with complexes of calcium in the tissue detectable by electron microscopy.[205-207] The interaction between myocardial ischemia and myoplasmic [Ca^{++}] is complex, as illustrated in Figure 36–16. Ischemia, however produced, is characterized by a reduction of myocardial ATP stores, which interferes with the transsarcolemmal Na$^+$-K$^+$ exchange, which in turn elevates intracellular [Na$^+$], raising intracellular [Ca^{++}] through an enhanced Na$^+$-Ca^{++} exchange. Lowered ATP stores also reduce Ca^{++} uptake by the sarcoplasmic reticulum and reduce extrusion of Ca^{++} from cells. The resultant augmented intracellular [Ca^{++}] causes mitochondrial Ca^{++} overload, which depresses ATP production further. Activation of intracellular Ca^{++} ATPases augments ATP usage and activates sarcolemmal phospholipases, which release membrane phospholipid degradation products whose detergent properties impair the integrity of the cell membrane.[208,209] Calcium-channel blockers interfere with Ca^{++} influx through voltage-dependent channels.

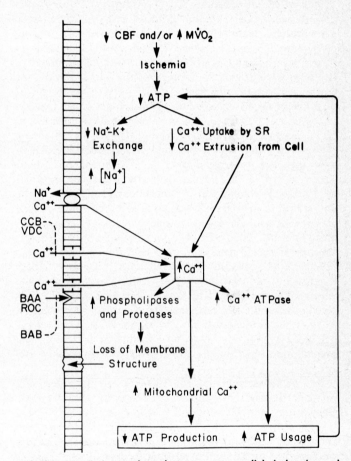

FIGURE 36–16 Interactions between myocardial ischemia and [Ca^{++}]. A reduction of coronary blood flow (CBF), sometimes accompanied by an increase in myocardial oxygen requirements (MVO$_2$), causes myocardial ischemia, which in turn reduces cellular ATP stores. This reduction interferes with the transsarcolemmal Na$^+$-K$^+$ exchange, which elevates intracellular [NA$^+$], raising intracellular [Ca^{++}] through an enhanced Na$^+$-Ca^{++} exchange. Lowered ATP stores also reduce Ca^{++} uptake by the sarcoplasmic reticulum (SR) and reduce extrusion of Ca^{++} from cells. The resultant augmented intracellular [Ca^{++}] causes mitochondrial Ca^{++} overload, which depresses ATP production further; activation of intracellular Ca^{++} ATPases, which augment ATP usage; and activation of sarcolemmal phospholipases and proteases, which impair the integrity of the cell membrane. Calcium-channel blockers (CCB) interfere with Ca^{++} influx through voltage-dependent channels (VDA). Beta-adrenergic agonists (BAA) recruit additional receptor-operated channels (ROC). Beta-adrenergic blockers (BAB) reduce Ca^{++} influx by interfering with the recruitment of ROC. (Reproduced with permission from Braunwald, E.: Mechanism of action of calcium channel blocking agents. N. Engl. J. Med. *307*:1618, 1982.)

Beta-adrenergic agonists recruit additional receptor-operated channels, and beta-adrenergic blockers reduce Ca^{++} influx by interfering with the recruitment of receptor-operated channels. Thus, one would expect beta blockers and Ca^{++}-channel blockers to have similar effects in the treatment of ischemia. Indeed, both groups of compounds delay ischemia-induced necrosis and, particularly when combined with reperfusion, reduce the extent of myocardial necrosis.[210,211]

The hypothesis that the entry of Ca^{++} into ischemic cells may be harmful is based on the observation that after a period of myocardial ischemia and subsequent reperfusion the accumulation of excess Ca^{++} in the mitochondria may interfere with their capacity to generate ATP. The destructive chain of metabolic events provoked by increased intracellular $[Ca^{++}]$ appears to be responsible, at least in part, for the death of cells in the ischemic myocardium. Henry and associates[212] found that during one hour of severe ischemia, the left ventricle undergoes progressive ischemic contracture, with the development of an elevated ventricular diastolic pressure and a fourfold increase in mitochondrial Ca^{++}. With subsequent reperfusion, both myocardial systolic function and relaxation remain abnormal, and a further marked increase in Ca^{++} accumulation occurs. Administration of nifedipine prevents ischemic contracture and permits recovery of systolic contractile function and of myocardial relaxation. These favorable hemodynamic changes are accompanied by a marked reduction in the accumulation of Ca^{++} in the mitochondria. Verapamil has also been shown to reduce myocardial damage during coronary occlusion, and particularly during reperfusion,[213] and nifedipine preserved left ventricular function in dogs with cardiopulmonary bypass that were subjected to prolonged total ischemia.[214] These experiments demonstrate that in a setting analogous to the clinical practice of cardiac surgery, Ca^{++}-channel blockers give considerable hemodynamic and histological protection to the ischemic-reperfused myocardium. Thus, Ca^{++}-channel blockers may prove to be valuable in protecting the myocardium from the Ca^{++}-associated ischemic injury occurring during open heart surgery.

The accumulation of Ca^{++} in myocardium undergoing ischemic injury has important diagnostic implications. Myocardial infarct scintigraphy with agents such as ^{99m}Tc-stannous pyrophosphate permits detection and localization of infarction after intravenous injection of tracer. The tissue's avidity for the tracer appears to depend on the accumulation of Ca^{++} (p. 380).

RELEASE OF ENZYMES IN DETECTION OF ACUTE MYOCARDIAL INFARCTION

Acute myocardial infarction is detected on the basis of clinical, electrocardiographic, biochemical, and radiographic phenomena, considered in detail in Chapter 37. Since biochemical markers of ischemic injury have become important clinical tools, some considerations required for their proper interpretation merit particular attention. Loss of functional integrity of the sarcolemma is a primary common denominator underlying liberation of cytoplasmic constituents into the circulation, such as transaminase (SGOT, AST), lactic dehydrogenase (LDH), and creatine kinase (CK).[215,216] Species of lower molecular weight, such as myoglobin, are liberated, but elevated concentrations

persist in the circulation only briefly because of rapid renal clearance. Furthermore, myoglobin released from hypoperfused skeletal muscle may cloud interpretation of elevated values in plasma.[217]

Accurate assessment of myocardial infarction based on analysis of plasma enzyme time-activity curves has been facilitated by the demonstration that one isoenzyme of creatine kinase, MB CK, is localized virtually exclusively in myocardium as opposed to other tissues in humans.[216-218] Under carefully defined conditions in experimental animals, depletion of myocardial CK activity correlates with infarct size estimated independently by morphometric techniques or with the use of radioactively labeled microspheres.[219] The corollary of these observations, namely, that increases in plasma enzyme activity reflect infarct size, has been recognized for many years.[220]

Based on review of many clinical studies[221] and observations in conscious experimental animals,[222] it has become clear that release of myocardial cytosolic enzymes into the circulation is tantamount to cell death when the cause of enzyme release is myocardial ischemia. Accordingly, infarct size has been estimated from analysis of plasma enzyme CK time-activity curves,[223-225] and recently from curves obtained by quantitative assay of plasma samples for MB CK activity.[226] Despite obvious imperfections, enzymatic estimates of infarct size have correlated with biochemical and morphological analyses of infarction in hearts of experimental animals, morbidity and mortality in patients, histochemical assessment of necrosis among patients who succumb to acute myocardial infarction,[227] early and late ventricular arrhythmia, and impairment of ventricular function.[228-230] Time-activity curves are influenced by regional myocardial perfusion, local degradation of enzyme in the heart, the ratio of enzyme released compared to that destroyed,[231] inactivation of enzyme in lymph,[232] exchange of enzyme between vascular and extravascular compartments,[224] and potential variation in the rate of inactivation and removal of enzyme once it has reached the circulation.[232] Thus, the pattern of enzyme release and its overall magnitude may be influenced by interventions resulting in early reperfusion and accelerated washout. Nevertheless, analysis of plasma time-activity curves of MB CK and other biochemical markers of ischemic injury has proved useful in quantitative assessment of the progress and extent of myocardial infarction in the clinical setting and should prove useful in dating the onset of effective reperfusion.[225]

MODIFICATION OF ISCHEMIC INJURY

A variety of interventions have been shown in animal experiments to modify the severity of ischemic injury, and in some instances parallel changes in infarct size have been observed. The theoretical basis for these interventions and the experimental results are discussed below. The clinical application of these observations is discussed on p. 1318.

The potency of any intervention designed to limit infarct size is inversely related to the interval between the onset of the ischemic stimulus and the time the intervention is applied.[234] In the normothermic working dog heart no intervention can be expected to exert a significant beneficial effect if it is begun more than six hours after the onset of severe ischemia, because by this time all tissue in the distribution of the occluded vessel has become irreversibly injured.

INTERVENTIONS THAT INCREASE MYOCARDIAL INJURY AFTER CORONARY ARTERY OCCLUSION (TABLE 36–2)

The extent and severity of myocardial ischemic injury, and ultimately of myocardial infarction after coronary occlusion, depend on the balance between oxygen supply and demand in the jeopardized myocardium. Certain interventions known to increase myocardial oxygen consumption also increase the severity and extent of myocardial injury in the presence of residual coronary blood flow. In the dog without heart failure, isoproterenol, digitalis (in the absence of heart failure), and amrinone[235,236] have a deleterious effect on ischemic myocardium. Also, pacing-induced tachycardia increases ischemic damage,[236,237] and a similar observation in patients has been reported.[238] Hypoxemia,[239] anemia,[240] and hypotension, regardless of how produced,[241] increase myocardial ischemic injury after coronary occlusion, since in all of these conditions the delivery of oxygen to the ischemic tissue is reduced; similarly, hypoglycemia augments ischemic injury.[242] Hyperthermia impairs mechanical performance of the ischemic myocardium;[243] through its direct stimulation of myocardial oxygen consumption and heart rate, it exerts an adverse effect on myocardial oxygen balance.

The positive inotropic and chronotropic effects of isoproterenol improve the function of normal myocardium and elevate $M\dot{V}O_2$. When isoproterenol is administered in the presence of global myocardial ischemia, however, myocardial function deteriorates rapidly.[244-246] The effects of isoproterenol on myocardial function in the presence of regional ischemia, a situation in which the myocardium is perfused heterogeneously, are more complex. In the conscious dog with regional myocardial ischemia, isoproterenol elicits a spectrum of reactions in areas with different degrees of ischemia.[247] Specifically, myocardial function deteriorates in severely ischemic zones but improves in normal and moderately ischemic zones. These changes in myocardial function in response to isoproterenol correlate with changes in myocardial blood flow; severely ischemic sites exhibit no increase in blood flow and a deterioration of function occurs during infusion of isoproterenol, as a result of an increase in $M\dot{V}O_2$, whereas normal or moderate-

ly ischemic areas show an improvement of both myocardial function and regional blood flow. The positive chronotropic and inotropic actions of isoproterenol cause an increase in infarct size in anesthetized dogs with open chests,[219] and myocardial lactate production increases when isoproterenol is given to patients with acute myocardial infarction.[248]

An increase in the concentration of circulating fatty acids also aggravates ischemia following coronary occlusion[249]; the augmentation of myocardial oxygen requirements[250] in the presence of limited oxygen supply, intensifies ischemia, depresses myocardial contractility, and, in all likelihood, precipitates arrhythmias.[251]

INTERVENTIONS THAT REDUCE MYOCARDIAL INJURY AFTER CORONARY ARTERY OCCLUSION (TABLE 36–3)

The balance between myocardial oxygen supply and demand in the ischemic myocardium can be improved by augmenting oxygen supply and/or reducing demand. Several studies in animals have shown that early reperfusion results in smaller infarction than if the occlusion is sustained. As might be expected, the extent of salvage depends on the duration of occlusion.[204,252,253] Reperfusion after less than 15 to 20 minutes of coronary occlusion salvages essentially all of the ischemic tissue. With longer periods of ischemia, a wavefront of necrosis beginning in the subendocardium and moving progressively outward, i.e., to the epicardium and laterally, occurs. When reperfusion is carried out after six hours of coronary occlusion, most of the jeopardized myocardium becomes necrotic and no tissue is salvaged. In some experiments histological evidence of hemorrhagic necrosis has been noted with coronary artery reperfusion.[254,255] This does not appear to be associated with extension of infarction but rather with acceleration of necrosis of tissue that had already been irreversibly injured. The inhalation of an oxy-

TABLE 36–2 SOME INTERVENTIONS THAT INCREASE MYOCARDIAL INJURY AFTER CORONARY ARTERY OCCLUSION

Increase Myocardial Oxygen Requirements
  Isoproterenol
  Digitalis and amrinone (in the absence of heart failure)
  Tachycardia
  Hyperthermia
Decrease Myocardial Oxygen Supply
  Directly
    Hypoxemia
    Anemia
  Through collateral vessels, reducing coronary perfusion pressure
    Hemorrhage
    Sodium nitroprusside
    Minoxidil
    Other vasodilators (including isoproterenol)
    Coronary vasoconstriction (indomethacin)
Decrease substrate availability
  Hypoglycemia

TABLE 36–3 SOME INTERVENTIONS THAT REDUCE EXPERIMENTAL MYOCARDIAL INJURY FOLLOWING CORONARY OCCLUSION

Increasing myocardial oxygen supply
  Directly
    Coronary artery reperfusion (surgery, thrombolysis)
    Elevating arterial pO_2
    Fluorocarbons
  Through collateral vessels
    Elevation of coronary perfusion pressure by methoxamine, neosynephrine, or norepinephrine
    Intra-aortic balloon counterpulsation
    Coronary vasodilatation (calcium blockers, nitroglycerin, prostacyclin)
Decreasing myocardial oxygen demand
  Beta-adrenergic blockers
  Cardiac glycoside in the failing heart
  Intra-aortic balloon counterpulsation
  Decreasing afterload in hypertensive individuals
  Inhibiting calcium influx
  Hypothermia
Increasing plasma osmolality
  Mannitol
  Hypertonic glucose
Augmenting anaerobic metabolism (presumed)
  Glucose-insulin-potassium
  Hypertonic glucose
Enhancing transport to the ischemic zone of substrate utilized in energy production (presumed)
Protecting against autolytic and heterolytic processes (presumed)
  Glucocorticoids
  Cobra venom factor
  Aprotinin
  Nonsteroidal anti-inflammatory agents—ibuprofen

gen-rich gas mixture exerts a slight beneficial effect on the ischemic myocardium, also presumably by enhancing delivery of O_2 to ischemic tissue through collaterals.[256] This may be greatly enhanced by combining inhalation of 100 per cent oxygen with fluorocarbon mixtures, i.e., so-called artificial blood, which greatly augments O_2 delivery.[257]

Intra-aortic balloon counterpulsation (p. 593) reduces the severity of ischemic injury, presumably by reducing $M\dot{V}O_2$, as a consequence of lowering systolic wall tension, while simultaneously augmenting oxygen delivery by increasing aortic diastolic (coronary perfusion) pressure. In experimental animals, *beta-adrenergic blockers* appear to prolong the survival of severely ischemic tissue, judging from changes in ST segments, QRS complexes, myocardial creatine kinase activity, and electronmicroscopic, histochemical, and histological criteria.[258] In addition, it appears to improve the ratio of subendocardial to subepicardial blood flow in both ischemic and normal areas of myocardium in dogs with coronary occlusion, despite failing to alter net transmural blood flow to ischemic zones. Beta blockade appears to be more useful in delaying than preventing cell death and is especially effective in limiting infarct size in animals subjected to coronary occlusion and reperfusion.[259,260] As discussed above (p. 1253), an influx of Ca^{++} into the myocardial cell is associated with and may play a role in cell necrosis. It has been observed that the Ca^{++} channel blockers verapamil,[207,210,213] nifedipine,[261] and diltiazem[261a] reduce the severity of ischemic injury as well as infarct size.

A number of *metabolic interventions* may also improve the energy balance of ischemic myocardium. As fatty acid oxidation is impaired by ischemia, glucose becomes the principal source of energy.[262] In the ischemic dog heart, oxidative phosphorylation and cardiac function are enhanced by the infusion of glucose-insulin-potassium (GIK),[263] whereas, in the anoxic, isolated heart, both electrical and mechanical function improve and recovery occurs more rapidly when glucose is added to the perfusate.[169,264] Other beneficial effects that have been attributed either to glucose alone or to glucose-insulin-potassium include an increase in contractility due to the hyperosmolar action of glucose,[265] a reduction in the concentration and myocardial uptake of circulating free fatty acids (which reduces $M\dot{V}O_2$, p. 1250), a restoration of the intracellular potassium concentration, thus stabilizing the membrane potential[266,267] and reducing the frequency of serious ventricular dysrhythmias. In the open-chest dog, administration of GIK begun 30 minutes after coronary occlusion and maintained for 24 hours reduces the extent of myocardial necrosis that eventually develops.[268] Hypertonic glucose without insulin and potassium also reduces myocardial necrosis, but its salutary effect is not as great as that of GIK. In the baboon, GIK infusion after acute coronary occlusion preserves myocardial energy stores, with greater amounts of ATP, creatine phosphate, and glycogen in the ischemic zones of treated than in those of untreated animals.[269]

In the dog with experimentally produced coronary occlusion, myocardial ischemic injury is reduced by other agents that inhibit myocardial extraction of free fatty acids (i.e., antilipolytic agents, such as beta-pyridyl carbinol, and lipid-free albumin infusion), thus indirectly favoring glucose metabolism.[270] Injury is also reduced by sodium dichloroacetate,[271] which enhances the utilization of glucose relative to that of free fatty acids and by L-carnitine,

which, by reversing the inhibition of adenine nucleotide translocase in vitro, prevents the depletion of cytoplasmic high-energy phosphate stores (Fig. 36–11).[272]

A number of agents that limit the inflammatory or immune response reduce myocardial ischemic injury in the laboratory animal, and some have been used in limited numbers of patients (Chap. 38). The activation of the complement system via its alternate pathway, a shift that characterizes ischemic tissue, releases leukotactic factors and increases capillary permeability, leading to interstitial edema. As a result, the microvasculature is compressed, further diminishing blood flow to the ischemic area.[273] *Cobra venom factor*, a protein that enzymatically cleaves C3 and prevents the effects of the complement system, reduces myocardial injury.[274] Similarly, the kallikrein system enhances leukotactic activity, capillary permeability, interstitial edema, and proteolytic activity, and *aprotinin*, an inhibitor of this system, diminishes ischemic injury.[275] A single large dose of a *glucocorticosteroid* also reduces myocardial infarct size in the dog with coronary occlusion.[276-278] These compounds limit myocardial necrosis, presumably by stabilizing lysosomal and other cellular membranes,[279] but they may also increase blood flow to the ischemic myocardium. Regardless of the effect of corticosteroids on the extent of myocardial ischemic injury, there is also evidence that when multiple doses are employed they may inhibit healing of the infarct, increasing the risk of ventricular rupture or aneurysm formation.[278-282] *Ibuprofen*, a nonsteroidal anti-inflammatory compound, has also been shown to reduce infarct size in experimental animals,[283] but, like corticosteroids, interferes with infarct healing and scar formation.[284]

Mannitol reduces the extent of ischemic injury and improves the function of the ischemic myocardium. This hyperosmotic agent reduces cell swelling and also presumably improves collateral blood flow to the ischemic myocardium.[285]

Hyaluronidase also reduces myocardial necrosis[286] in the dog and rabbit.[287] The depolymerization of mucopolysaccharides caused by hyaluronidase may increase the supply of nutrients to the myocardium or increase the washout of damaging metabolites.[288] This agent decreases ST-segment elevations in dogs with coronary occlusion and decreases the ultimate extent of damage, estimated electrocardiographically, biochemically, and morphologically.

For decades *nitroglycerin* was avoided in patients with acute myocardial infarction because nitroglycerin-induced reductions in systemic arterial pressure and concomitant reflex increases in heart rate were believed to intensify ischemic injury.[289] However, use of this drug has recently been reassessed, and it has been shown in the dog that intravenous nitroglycerin, administered at a rate sufficient to cause a mild diminution in systemic arterial pressure, reduces the magnitude and extent of ischemic injury,[290,291] and that this injury can be further lessened if the blood pressure decrease and reflex tachycardia induced by nitroglycerin are abolished by the simultaneous infusion of methoxamine and phenylephrine. In addition, the administration of nitroglycerin shortly after coronary artery occlusion partially reverses the ventricular fibrillation threshold, whereas nitroglycerin and phenylephrine in combination restore this threshold to normal.[292,293] Nitroglycerin is presumed to act by augmenting perfusion of the border of the ischemic zone[293] by dilating collaterals and by reducing myocardial oxygen demands by lowering preload and afterload.

References

1. McKeever, W. P., Gregg, D. E., and Canney, P. C.: Oxygen uptake of the nonworking left ventricle. Circ. Res. 6:612, 1958.
2. Rooke, G. A., and Feigl, E. O.: Work as a correlate of canine left ventricular oxygen consumption, and the problem of catecholamine oxygen wasting. Circ. Res. 50:273, 1982.
3. Klocke, F. J., Braunwald, E., and Ross, J., Jr.: Oxygen cost of electrical activation of the heart. Circ. Res. 18:357, 1966.
4. Evans, C. L., and Matsuoka, Y.: The effect of various mechanical conditions on the gaseous metabolism and efficiency of the mammalian heart. J. Physiol. 49:378, 1915.
5. Sarnoff, S. J., Braunwald, E., Welch, G. H., Jr., Case, R. B., Stainsby, W. N., and Macruz, R.: Hemodynamic determinants of oxygen consumption of the heart with special reference to the tension-time index. Am. J. Physiol. 192:148, 1958.
6. Braunwald, E., Sarnoff, S. J., Case, R. B., Stainsby, W. N., and Welch, G. H., Jr.: Hemodynamic determinants of coronary flow: Effect of changes in aortic pressure and cardiac output on the relationship between myocardial oxygen consumption and coronary flow. Am. J. Physiol. 192:157, 1958.
7. Rodbard, S., Williams, C. B., and Rodbard, D.: Myocardial tension and oxygen uptake. Circ. Res. 14:139, 1964.
8. Sonnenblick, E. H., Ross, J., Jr., Covell, J. W., and Braunwald, E.: Velocity of contraction as a determinant of myocardial oxygen consumption. Am. J. Physiol. 209:919, 1965.
9. Suga, H., Hayashi, T., Suehiro, S., Hisano, R., Shirahata, M., and Ninomiya, I.: Equal oxygen consumption rates of isovolumic and ejecting contractions with equal systolic pressure-volume areas in canine left ventricle. Circ. Res. 49:1082, 1981.
10. Suga, H., Hisano, R., Hirata, S., Hayashi, T., and Ninomiya, I.: Mechanism of higher oxygen consumption rate: Pressure-loaded vs. volume-loaded heart. Am. J. Physiol. 242(Heart Circ. Physiol. 11):H942, 1982.
11. Fenn, W. O.: A quantitative comparison between the energy liberated and the work performed by the isolated sartorius muscle of the frog. J. Physiol. (Lond.) 58:175, 1923.
12. Rall, J. A.: Sense and nonsense about the Fenn effect. Am. J. Physiol. 242 (Heart Circ. Physiol. 11):H1, 1982.
13. Covell, J. W., Braunwald, E., Ross, J., Jr., and Sonnenblick, E. H.: Studies on digitalis. XVI. Effects on myocardial oxygen consumption. J. Clin. Invest. 45:1535, 1966.
14. Graham, T. P., Jr., Ross, J., Jr., Covell, J. W., Sonnenblick, E. H., and Clancy, R. L.: Myocardial oxygen consumption in acute experimental cardiac depression. Circ. Res. 21:123, 1967.
15. Graham, T. P., Jr., Covell, J. W., Sonnenblick, E. H., Ross, J., Jr., and Braunwald, E.: Control of myocardial oxygen consumption: Relative influence of contractile state and tension development. J. Clin. Invest. 47:375, 1968.
16. Boerth, R. C., Covell, J. W., Pool, P. E., and Ross, J., Jr.: Increased myocardial oxygen consumption and contractile state associated with increased heart rate in dogs. Circ. Res. 24:725, 1969.
17. Urschel, C. W., Covell, J. W., Graham, T. P., Clancy, R. L., Ross, J., Jr., Sonnenblick, E. H., and Braunwald, E.: Effects of acute valvular regurgitation on the oxygen consumption of the canine heart. Circ. Res. 23:33, 1968.
18. Vik-Mo, H., and Mjos, O. E.: Influence of free fatty acids on myocardial oxygen consumption and ischemic injury. Am. J. Cardiol. 48:361, 1981.
19. Braunwald, E., Ross, J., Jr., and Sonnenblick, E. H.: Regulation of coronary blood flow. In Mechanisms of Contraction of the Normal and Failing Heart, 2nd Ed. Boston, Little, Brown, 1976, p. 200.
20. Berne, R. M., and Rubio, R.: Coronary circulation. In Berne, R. M., Sperelakis, N., and Geiger, S. R. (eds.): Handbook of Physiology; Section 2, The Cardiovascular System. Bethesda, American Physiological Society, 1979, p. 897.
20a. Feigl, E. O.: Coronary physiology. Physiol. Rev. 63:1, 1983.
21. Gorlin, R.: Coronary anatomy. In Coronary Artery Disease. Philadelphia, W. B. Saunders Co., 1976, p. 40.
22. Bell, J. R., and Fox, A. C.: Pathogenesis of subendocardial ischemia. Am. J. Med. Sci. 268:2, 1974.
23. Wearn, J. T.: Morphological and functional alterations of the coronary circulation. Harvey Lect. 35:243, 1940.
24. Provenza, D. V., and Scherlis, S.: Coronary circulation in dog's heart: Demonstration of muscle sphincters in capillaries. Circ. Res. 7:318, 1959.
25. Fulton, W. F. M.: The Coronary Arteries. Springfield, Ill., Charles C Thomas, 1965.
26. Schaper, W.: The physiology of the collateral circulation in the normal and hypoxic myocardium. Rev. Physiol. Biochem. Pharmacol. 63:102, 1971.
27. Fam, W. M., and McGregor, M.: Effect of coronary vasodilator drugs on retrograde flow in areas of chronic myocardial ischemia. Circ. Res. 15:355, 1964.
28. Cohen, M. V., Downey, J. M., Sonnenblick, E. H., and Kirk, E. S.: The effects of nitroglycerin on coronary collaterals and myocardial contractility. J. Clin. Invest. 52:2836, 1973.
29. Kolibash, A. J., Bush, C. A., Wepsic, R. A., Schroeder, D. P., Tetalman, M. R., and Lewis, R. P.: Coronary collateral vessels: Spectrum of physiologic capabilities with respect to providing rest and stress myocardial perfusion, main-

tenance of left ventricular function and protection against infarction. Am. J. Cardiol. 50:230, 1982.
30. Downey, J. M., and Kirk, E. S.: Inhibition of coronary blood flow by a vascular waterfall mechanism. Circ. Res. 36:753, 1975.
31. Moir, T. W.: Subendocardial distribution of coronary blood flow and the effect of antianginal drugs. Circ. Res. 30:621, 1972.
32. Gregg, D. E., Khouri, E. M., and Rayford, C. R.: Systemic and coronary energetics in the resting unanesthetized dog. Circ. Res. 16:102, 1965.
33. Klocke, F. J.: Coronary blood flow in man. Prog. Cardiovasc. Dis. 19:117, 1976.
34. Sonnenblick, E. H., and Kirk, E. S.: Effects of hypoxia and ischemia on myocardial contraction: Alterations in the time course of force and ischemia-dependent inhomogeneity of contractility. Cardiology 56:302, 1971/72.
35. Griggs, D. M., Jr., Chen, C. C., and Tchokoev, V. V.: Subendocardial metabolism in experimental aortic stenosis. Am. J. Physiol. 224:607, 1973.
36. Sabbah, H. N., and Stein, P. D.: Effect of acute regional ischemia on pressure in the subepicardium and subendocardium. Am. J. Physiol. 242(Heart Circ. Physiol. 11):H240, 1982.
37. Brazier, J., Cooper, N., and Buckberg, G.: The adequacy of subendocardial oxygen delivery: The interaction of determinants of flow, arterial oxygen content and myocardial oxygen need. Circulation 49:968, 1974.
38. Lundsgaard-Hansen, P., Meyer, C., and Riedwyl, H.: Transmural gradients of glycolytic enzyme activities in left ventricular myocardium. I. The normal state. Pfluegers Arch. 297:89, 1967.
39. Rovetto, M. J., Whitmer, J. T., and Neely, J. R.: Comparison of the effects of anoxia and whole heart ischemia on carbohydrate utilization in isolated working rat hearts. Circ. Res. 32:699, 1973.
40. Jedeikin, L. A.: Regional distribution of glycogen and phosphorylase in the ventricles of the heart. Circ. Res. 14:202, 1964.
41. Allison, T. B., Ramey, C. A., and Holsinger, J. W., Jr.: Transmural gradients of left ventricular tissue metabolites after circumflex artery ligation in dogs. J. Mol. Cell. Cardiol. 9:837, 1977.
42. Buckberg, G. D., Fixler, D. E., Archie, J. P., and Hoffman, J. I. E.: Experimental subendocardial ischemia in dogs with normal coronary arteries. Circ. Res. 30:67, 1972.
43. Hoffman, J. I. E.: Determinants and prediction of transmural myocardial perfusion. Circulation 58:381, 1978.
44. Oliveros, R. A., Boucher, C. A., Haycraft, G. L., and Beckmann, C. H.: Myocardial oxygen supply-demand ratio. A validation of peripherally vs. centrally determined values. Chest 75:693, 1979.
45. Becker, L. C.: Effect of tachycardia on regional left ventricular blood flow after coronary artery occlusion. Am. J. Cardiol. 35:122, 1975.
46. Neill, W. A., Oxendine, J., Phelps, N., and Anderson, R. P.: Subendocardial ischemia provoked by tachycardia in conscious dogs with coronary stenosis. Am. J. Cardiol. 35:30, 1975.
47. Fallen, E. L., Elliott, W. C., and Gorlin, R.: Mechanisms of angina in aortic stenosis. Circulation 36:480, 1967.
48. Griggs, D. M., Jr., and Chen, C. C.: Coronary hemodynamics and regional myocardial metabolism in experimental aortic insufficiency. J. Clin. Invest. 53:1599, 1974.
49. Segal, J., Harvey, W. P., and Hufnagel, C.: A clinical study of one hundred cases of severe aortic insufficiency. Am. J. Med. 21:200, 1956.
50. Becker, L. C., Fortuin, N. J., and Pitt, B.: Effect of ischemia and antianginal drugs on the distribution of radioactive microspheres in the canine left ventricle. Circ. Res. 28:263, 1971.
51. Mathes, P., and Rival, J.: Effect of nitroglycerin on total and regional coronary blood flow in the normal and ischaemic canine myocardium. Cardiovasc. Res. 5:54, 1971.
52. Belloni, F. L.: The local control of coronary blood flow. Cardiovasc. Res. 13:63, 1979.
53. Pitt, B., Elliot, E. C., and Gregg, D. E.: Adrenergic receptor activity in the coronary arteries of the unanesthetized dog. Circ. Res. 21:75, 1967.
54. Vatner, S. F., Hintze, T. H., and Macho, P.: Regulation of large coronary arteries by beta-adrenergic mechanisms in the conscious dog. Circ. Res. 51:56, 1982.
55. Vatner, S. F., Higgins, C. B., and Braunwald, E.: Effects of norepinephrine on coronary circulation and left ventricular dynamics in the conscious dog. Circ. Res. 34:812, 1974.
56. Szentivanyi, M., and Juhasz-Nagy, N.: Physiological role of the coronary constrictor fibers. Q. J. Exp. Physiol. 48:93, 1963.
57. Hackett, J. G., Abboud, F. M., Mark, A. L., Schmid, P. G., and Heistad, D. D.: Coronary vascular responses to stimulation of chemoreceptors and baroreceptors. Circ. Res. 21:8, 1972.
58. Higgins, C. B., Vatner, S. F., and Braunwald, E.: Parasympathetic control of the heart. Pharmacol. Rev. 25:119, 1973.
59. Vatner, S. F., Franklin, D., VanCitters, R. L., and Braunwald, E.: Effects of carotid sinus nerve stimulation on the coronary circulation of the conscious dog. Circ. Res. 27:11, 1970.
60. Brachfeld, N., Monroe, R. G., and Gorlin, R.: Effects of pericoronary denervation on coronary hemodynamics. Am. J. Physiol. 199:174, 1960.
61. Macho, P., and Vatner, S. F.: Effects of prazosin on coronary and left ventricular dynamics in conscious dogs. Circulation 65:1186, 1982.
62. Heyndrickx, G. R., Muylaert, P., and Pannier, J. L.: Alpha-adrenergic control of oxygen delivery to myocardium during exercise in conscious dogs. Am. J. Physiol. 242(Heart Circ. Physiol. 11):H805, 1982.
63. Murray, P. A., and Vatner, S. F.: Alpha adrenoceptor attenuation of the coro-

nary vascular response to severe exercise in the conscious dog. Circ. Res. 45: 654, 1979.

64. Feigl, E. O.: Reflex parasympathetic coronary vasodilation elicited from cardiac receptors in the dog. Circ. Res. 37:175, 1975.

65. Bezold, A., and Hirt, L.: Über die physiologischen Wirkungen des essigsauren Veratrins. Unters. Physiol. Lab. Würzburg 1:75, 1867.

66. Jarisch, A., and Zotterman, Y.: Depressor reflexes from the heart. Acta Physiol. Scand. 16:31, 1948.

67. Feigl, E. O.: Parasympathetic control of coronary blood flow in dogs. Circ. Res. 25:509, 1969.

68. Hamilton, F. N., and Feigl, E. O.: Coronary vascular sympathetic beta-receptor innervation. Am. J. Physiol. 230:1569, 1976.

69. Ross, G.: Adrenergic responses of the coronary vessels. Circ. Res. 39:461, 1976.

70. Driscol, T. E., Moir, T. W., and Eckstein, R. W.: Vascular effects of changes in perfusion pressure in the nonischemic and ischemic heart. Circ. Res. 15 (Suppl. I):I-94, 1964.

70a. Øien, A. H., and Aukland, K.: A mathematical analysis of the myogenic hypothesis with special reference to autoregulation of renal blood flow. Circ. Res. 52:241, 1983.

71. Bayliss, W. M.: On the local reaction of the arterial wall to changes in arterial pressure. J. Physiol. (Lond.) 28:220, 1902.

72. Coffman, J. D., and Gregg, D. E.: Oxygen metabolism and oxygen debt repayment after myocardial ischemia. Am. J. Physiol. 201:881, 1961.

73. Berne, R. M., Blackmon, J. R., and Gardner, T. H.: Hypoxemia and coronary flow. J. Clin. Invest. 36:1101, 1957.

74. Weglicki, W. B., Rubenstein, C. J., Entman, M. L., Thompson, H. K., Jr., and McIntosh, H. D.: Effects of hyperbaric oxygenation on myocardial blood flow and myocardial metabolism in the dog. Am. J. Physiol. 216:1219, 1969.

75. Rubio, R., Berne, R. M., and Katori, M.: Release of adenosine in reactive hyperemia of the dog heart. Am. J. Physiol. 216:56, 1969.

76. Detar, R., and Bohr, D. F.: Oxygen and vascular smooth muscle contraction. Am. J. Physiol. 214:241, 1968.

77. Duling, B. R.: Microvascular responses to alterations in oxygen tension. Circ. Res. 31:481, 1972.

78. Duling, B. R.: Changes in microvascular diameter and oxygen tension induced by carbon dioxide. Circ. Res. 32:370, 1973.

79. Martini, J., and Honig, C. R.: Direct measurement of intercapillary distance in beating rat heart in situ under various conditions of O_2 supply. Microvasc. Res. 1:244, 1969.

80. Rubio, R., and Berne, R. M.: Release of adenosine by the normal myocardium and its relationship to the regulation of coronary resistance. Circ. Res. 25:407, 1969.

81. Bardenheuer, H., and Schrader, J.: Relationship between myocardial oxygen consumption, coronary flow and adenosine release in an improved isolated working heart preparation of guinea pigs. Circ. Res. 52:263, 1983.

82. Rubio, R., Berne, R. M., and Dobson, J. G., Jr.: Sites of adenosine production in cardiac and skeletal muscle. Am. J. Physiol. 225:938, 1973.

83. McKenzie, J. E., Steffen, R. P., and Haddy, F. J.: Relations between adenosine and coronary resistance in conscious exercising dogs. Am. J. Physiol. 242:H24, 1982.

84. Gellai, M., Norton, J. M., and Detar, R.: Evidence for direct control of coronary vascular tone by oxygen. Circ. Res. 32:279, 1973.

85. Belardinelli, L., Vogel, S., Linden, J., and Berne, R. M.: Anti-adrenergic action of adenosine on ventricular myocardium in embryonic chick hearts. J. Molec. Cell. Cardiol. 14:291, 1982.

86. Needleman, P., Marshall, G. R., and Sobel, B. E.: Hormone interactions in the isolated rabbit heart: Synthesis and coronary vasomotor effects of prostaglandins, angiotensin, and bradykinin. Circ. Res. 37:802, 1975.

87. Bergman, G., Atkinson, L., Richardson, P. J., Daly, K., Rothman, M., Jackson, G., and Jewitt, D. E.: Prostacyclin: Haemodynamic and metabolic effects in patients with coronary artery disease. Lancet 1:569, 1981.

88. Friedman, P. L., Brugada, P., Kuck, K. H., Bar, F. W. H. M., and Wellens, H. J. J.: Coronary vasoconstrictor effect of indomethacin in patients with coronary artery disease. N. Engl. J. Med. 305:1171, 1981.

89. DeBoer, L. W. V., Rude, R. E., Davis, R. F., Maroko, P. R., and Braunwald, E.: Extension of myocardial necrosis into normal epicardium following hypotension during prolonged coronary occlusion. Cardiovasc. Res. 16:423, 1982.

90. Vatner, S. F., Pagani, M., Manders, T., and Pasipoularides, A. D.: Alpha adrenergic vasoconstriction and nitroglycerin vasodilation of large coronary arteries in the conscious dog. J. Clin. Invest. 65:5, 1980.

91. Feldman, R. L., Marx, J. D., Pepine, C. J., and Conti, C. R.: Analysis of coronary responses to various doses of intracoronary nitroglycerin. Circulation 66:321, 1982.

92. Macho, P., and Vatner, S. F.: Effects of nitroglycerin and nitroprusside on large and small coronary vessels in conscious dogs. Circulation 64:1101, 1981.

93. Hintz, T. H., and Vatner, S. F.: Comparison of effects of nifedipine and nitroglycerin on large and small coronary arteries and cardiac function in conscious dogs. Circulation Res. 52:I-139, 1983.

94. Engle, H.-J., and Lichten, P. R.: Beneficial enhancement of coronary blood flow by nifedipine: Comparison with nitroglycerin and beta blocking agents. Am. J. Med. 71:658, 1981.

95. Klocke, F. J.: Measurements of coronary blood flow and degree of stenosis: Current clinical implications and continuing uncertainties. J. Am. Coll. Cardiol. 1:31, 1983.

96. Gould, K. L.: Dynamic coronary stenosis. Am. J. Cardiol. 45:286, 1980.

97. Hillis, L. D., and Braunwald, E.: Coronary artery spasm. N. Engl. J. Med. 299: 695, 1978.

98. Tennant, R., and Wiggers, C. J.: The effect of coronary occlusion on myocardial contractions. Am. J. Physiol. 112:351, 1935.

99. Vatner, S. F.: Correlation between acute reductions in myocardial blood flow and function in conscious dogs. Circ. Res. 47:201, 1980.

100. Herman, M. V., Heinle, R. A., Klein, M. D., and Gorlin, R.: Localized disorders in myocardial contraction: Asynergy and its role in congestive heart failure. N. Engl. J. Med. 277:222, 1967.

101. Braunwald, E., and Kloner, R. A.: The stunned myocardium: Prolonged, postischemic ventricular dysfunction. Circulation 66:1146, 1982.

102. Osakada, G., Hess, O. M., Gallather, K. P., Kemper, W. S., and Ross, J., Jr.: End-systolic dimension-wall thickness relations during myocardial ischemia in conscious dogs. Am. J. Cardiol. 51:1750, 1983.

103. Parker, J. O., Ledwich, J. R., West, R. O., and Case, R. B.: Reversible cardiac failure during angina pectoris: Hemodynamic effects of atrial pacing in coronary artery disease. Circulation 39:745, 1969.

104. Kardesch, M., Hogancamp, C. E., and Bing, R. J.: The effect of complete ischemia on the intracellular electrical activity of the whole mammalian heart. Circ. Res. 6:715, 1958.

105. Katz, A. M.: Effects of ischemia on the contractile processes of heart muscle. Am. J. Cardiol. 32:456, 1973.

106. Chesnais, J. M., Coraboeuf, E., Sauviat, M. P., and Vassas, J. M.: Sensitivity to H, Li and Mg ions of the slow inward sodium current in frog atrial fibres. J. Mol. Cell. Cardiol. 7:627, 1975.

107. Sandow, A.: Excitation-contraction coupling in skeletal muscle. Pharmacol. Rev. 17:265, 1965.

108. Fabiato, A., and Fabiato, F.: Contractions induced by a calcium-triggered release of calcium from the sarcoplasmic reticulum of single skinned cardiac cells. J. Physiol. 249:469, 1975.

109. Katz, A. M., and Hecht, H. H.: The early "pump" failure of the ischemic heart. Am. J. Med. 47:497, 1969.

110. Braunwald, E., Ross, J., Jr., and Sonnenblick, E. H.: Mechanisms of Contractions in the Normal and Failing Heart, 2nd Ed. Boston, Little, Brown, 1976, p. 357.

111. Williamson, J. R., Schaffer, S. W., Ford, C., and Safer, B.: Contribution of tissue acidosis to ischemic injury in the perfused rat heart. Circulation 53(Suppl. 1):3, 1976.

112. Regan, T. J., Effros, R. M., Haider, B., Oldewurtel, H. A., Ettinger, P. O., and Ahmed, S. S.: Myocardial ischemia and cell acidosis: Modification by alkali and the effects on ventricular function and cation composition. Am. J. Cardiol. 37:501, 1976.

113. Barry, W. H., Brooker, J. Z., Alderman, E. L., and Harrison, D. C.: Changes in diastolic stiffness and tone of the left ventricle during angina pectoris. Circulation 49:255, 1974.

114. Hess, O. M., Osakada, G., Lavelle, J. F., Gallagher, K. P., Kemper, W. S., and Ross, J., Jr.: Diastolic myocardial wall stiffness and ventricular relaxation during partial and complete coronary occlusions in the conscious dog. Circulation Res. 52:387, 1983.

115. Grossman, W., and McLaurin, L. P.: Diastolic properties of the left ventricle. Ann. Intern. Med. 84:316, 1976.

116. Bourdillon, P. D., Lorell, B. H., Mirsky, I., Paulus, W. J., Wynne, J., and Grossman, W.: Increased regional myocardial stiffness of the left ventricle during pacing-induced angina in man. Circulation 67:316, 1983.

117. Carroll, J. D., Hess, O. M., Hirzel, H. O., and Krayenbuehl, H. P.: Exercise-induced ischemia: The influence of altered relaxation on early diastolic pressures. Circulation 67:521, 1983.

118. Kay, H. R., Levine, F. H., Grotte, G. J., Rosenthal, S., Austen, W. G., and Buckley, M. J.: Isovolumic relaxation as a critical determinant of postischemic ventricular function. J. Surg. Res. 26:659, 1979.

119. McLaurin, L. P., Rolett, E. L., and Grossman, W.: Impaired left ventricular relaxation during pacing-induced ischemia. Am. J. Cardiol. 32:751, 1973.

120. Linhart, J. W., Hildner, F. J., Barold, S. S., Lister, J. W., and Samet, P.: Left heart hemodynamics during angina pectoris induced by atrial pacing. Circulation 40:483, 1969.

121. Paulus, W. J., Serizawa, T., and Grossman, W.: Altered left ventricular diastolic properties during pacing-induced ischemia in dogs with coronary stenoses. Potentiation by caffeine. Circ. Res. 50:218, 1982.

122. McCans, J. L., and Parker, J. O.: Left ventricular pressure-volume relationships during myocardial ischemia in man. Circulation 48:775, 1973.

123. Pardee, H. E. B.: An electrocardiographic sign of coronary artery obstruction. Arch. Intern. Med. 26:244, 1920.

124. Rakita, L., Borduas, J. L., Rothman, S., and Prinzmetal, M.: Studies on the mechanism of ventricular activity. XII. Early changes in the RS-T segment and QRS complex following acute coronary artery occlusion: Experimental study and clinical applications. Am. Heart J. 48:351, 1954.

125. Ekmekci, A., Toyoshima, H., Dowczynski, J. K., Nagaya, T., and Prinzmetal, M.: Angina pectoris. IV. Clinical and experimental difference between ischemia with S-T elevation and ischemia with S-T depression. Am. J. Cardiol. 7:412, 1961.

126. Leaf, A.: Cell swelling: A factor in ischemic tissue injury. Circulation 48:455, 1973.

127. Flores, J., DiBona, D. R., Beck, C. H., and Leaf, A.: The role of cell swelling in ischemic renal damage and the protective effect of hypertonic solute. J. Clin. Invest. 51:118, 1972.

128. Opie, L. H., Owen, P., Thomas, M., and Samson, R.: Coronary sinus lactate measurements in assessment of myocardial ischemia: Comparison with changes in lactate/pyruvate and beta-hydroxybutyrate/acetoacetate ratios and with release of hydrogen, phosphate and potassium ions from the heart. Am. J. Cardiol. 32:295, 1973.

129. Johnson, E. A.: First electrocardiographic sign of myocardial ischemia: An electrophysiological conjecture. Circulation 53(Suppl. 1):82, 1976.

130. Holland, R. P., and Brooks, H.: The QRS complex during myocardial ischemia: An experimental analysis in the porcine heart. J. Clin. Invest. 57: 541, 1976.

131. Karlsson, J., Templeton, G. H., and Willerson, J. T.: Relationship between epicardial S-T segment changes and myocardial metabolism during acute coronary insufficiency. Circ. Res. 32:725, 1973.

132. Sayen, J. J., Peirce, G., Katcher, A. H., and Sheldon, W. F.: Correlation of intramyocardial electrocardiograms with polarographic oxygen and contractility in the nonischemic and regionally ischemic left ventricle. Circ. Res. 9:1268, 1961.

133. Angell, C. S., Lakatta, E. G., Weisfeldt, M. L., and Shock, N. W.: Relationship of intramyocardial oxygen tension and epicardial ST segment changes following acute coronary artery ligation: Effects of coronary perfusion pressure. Cardiovasc. Res. 9:12, 1975.

134. Khuri, S. F., Flaherty, J. T., O'Riordan, J. B., Pitt, B., Brawley, R. K., Donahoo, J. S., and Gott, V. L.: Changes in intramyocardial ST segment voltage and gas tensions with regional myocardial ischemia in the dog. Circ. Res. 37:455, 1975.

135. Braunwald, E., and Maroko, P. R.: ST-segment mapping: Realistic and unrealistic expectations. Circulation 54:529, 1976.

136. Maroko, P. R., Kjekshus, J. K., Sobel, B. E., Covell, J. W., Ross, J., Jr., and Braunwald, E.: Factors influencing infarct size following experimental coronary artery occlusions. Circulation 43:67, 1971.

137. Hillis, L. D., Askenazi, J., Braunwald, E., Radvany, P., Muller, J. E., Fishbein, M. C., and Maroko, P. R.: Use of changes in epicardial QRS complex to assess interventions which modify the extent of myocardial necrosis following coronary artery occlusion. Circulation 54:591, 1976.

138. Kralios, F. A., Martin, L., Burgess, M. J., and Millar, K.: Local ventricular repolarization changes due to sympathetic nerve-branch stimulation. Am. J. Physiol. 228:1621, 1975.

139. Muller, J. E., Maroko, P. R., and Braunwald, E.: Evaluation of precordial electrocardiographic mapping as a means of assessing changes in myocardial ischemic injury. Circulation 52:16, 1975.

140. Elharrar, V., and Zipes, D. P.: Cardiac electrophysiological alterations during myocardial ischemia. In Levy, M. N., and Vassalle, M. (Eds.): Excitation and Neural Control of the Heart. Baltimore, Williams and Wilkins, 1982, pp. 149–180.

141. Mehra, R., Zeiler, R. H., Gough, W. B., and El-Sherif, N.: Reentrant ventricular arrhythmias in the late myocardial infarction period. 9. Electrophysiologic-anatomic correlation of reentrant circuits. Circulation 67:11, 1983.

142. Downar, E., Janse, M. J., and Durrer, D.: The effect of acute coronary artery occlusion on subepicardial transmembrane potentials in the intact porcine heart. Circulation 56:217, 1977.

143. El-Sherif, N., Scherlag, B. J., and Lazzara, R.: Electrode catheter recording during malignant ventricular arrhythmias following experimental acute myocardial ischemia. Evidence for reentry, due to conduction delay and block in ischemic myocardium. Circulation 51:1003, 1975.

144. Janse, M. J., and Kleber, A. G.: Electrophysiological changes and ventricular arrhythmias in the early phase of regional myocardial ischemia. Circ. Res. 49: 1069, 1981.

145. Kent, F. K., Smith, E. R., Redwood, D. R., and Epstein, S. E.: Electrical stability of acutely ischemic myocardium. Influence of heart rate and vagal stimulation. Circulation 47:291, 1973.

146. Schaal, S. F., Wallace, A. G., and Sealy, W. C.: Protective influence of cardiac denervation against arrhythmias of myocardial infarction. Cardiovasc. Res. 3: 241, 1969.

147. Corr, P. B., Witkowski, F. X., and Sobel, B. E.: Mechanisms contributing to malignant dysrhythmias induced by ischemia in the cat. J. Clin. Invest. 61: 109, 1978.

148. Hope, R. R., Williams, D. O., El-Sherif, N., Lazzara, R., and Scherlag, B. J.: The efficacy of antiarrhythmic agents during acute myocardial ischemia and the role of heart rate. Circulation 50:507, 1974.

149. Kupersmith, J., Ontman, E. M., and Hoffman, B. F.: In vivo electrophysiological effects of lidocaine in canine acute myocardial infarction. Circ. Res. 36:84, 1975.

150. Elharrar, J., Gaum, W. E., and Zipes, D. P.: Effect of drugs on conduction delay and incidence of ventricular arrhythmias induced by acute coronary occlusion in dogs. Am. J. Cardiol. 39:544, 1977.

151. Friedman, P. L., Stewart, J. R., and Wit, A. L.: Spontaneous and induced cardiac arrhythmias in subendocardial Purkinje fibers after extensive myocardial infarction in dogs. Circ. Res. 33:612, 1973.

152. Horowitz, L. N., Spear, J. F., and Moore, E. N.: Subendocardial origin of ventricular arrhythmias in 24-hour-old experimental myocardial infarction. Circulation 53:56, 1976.

153. El-Sherif, N., Hope, R. R., Scherlag, B. J., and Lazzara, R.: Re-entrant ventricular arrhythmias in the late myocardial infarction period. 2. Patterns of initiation and termination of reentry. Circulation 55:702, 1977.

154. El-Sherif, N., Scherlag, B. J., Lazzara, R., and Hope, R. R.: Reentrant ventricular arrhythmias in the late myocardial infarction period. 4. Mechanism of action of lidocaine. Circulation 56:395, 1977.

155. Lazzara, R., Hope, R. R., El-Sherif, N., and Scherlag, B. J.: Effects of lidocaine on hypoxic and ischemic cardiac cells. Am. J. Cardiol. 41:872, 1978.

156. Murdock, D. K., Loeb, J. M., Euler, D. E., and Randall, W. C.: Electrophysiology of coronary reperfusion. A mechanism for reperfusion arrhythmias. Circulation 61:175, 1980.

157. Downar, E., Janse, M. S., and Durrer, D.: The effect of "ischemic" blood on transmembrane potentials of normal porcine ventricular myocardium. Circulation 55:455, 1977.

158. Sobel, B. E., Corr, P. B., Robinson, A. K., Goldstein, R. A., Witkowski, F. X., and Klein, M. S.: Accumulation of lysophosphoglycerides with arrhythmogenic properties in ischemic myocardium. J. Clin. Invest. 61:109, 1978.

159. Corr, P. B., Cain, M. E., Witkowski, F. X., Price, D. A., and Sobel, B. E.: Potential arrhythmogenic electrophysiological derangements in canine Purkinje fibers induced by lysophosphoglycerides. Circ. Res. 44:822, 1979.

160. Schwartz, A., Wood, J. M., Allen, J. C., Barret, E., Entman, M. L., Goldstein, M. A., Sordahl, L. Z., Suzuki, M., and Lewis, R. M.: Biochemical and morphologic correlates of cardiac ischemia. 1. Membrane systems. Am. J. Cardiol. 32:46, 1973.

161. Cherry, G., and Myers, M. B.: The relationship to ventricular fibrillation of early tissue sodium and potassium shifts and coronary vein potassium levels in experimental myocardial infarction. J. Thorac. Cardiovasc. Surg. 61:587, 1971.

162. Podzuweit, T., Dalby, A. J., Cherry, G. W., and Opie, L. H.: Tissue levels of cyclic AMP in ischemic and non-ischemic myocardium following coronary artery ligation. J. Mol. Cell. Cardiol. 10:81, 1978.

163. Kuppersmith, J., Shaing, H., Litwak, R. S., and Harman, M. V.: Electrophysiologic effects of verapamil in canine myocardial ischemia. Am. J. Cardiol. 37:149, 1976.

164. Griffith, J., and Leung, F.: The sequential estimation of plasma catecholamines and whole blood histamine in myocardial infarction. Am. Heart J. 82:171, 1971.

165. El-Sherif, N., and Lazzara, K.: Reentrant ventricular arrhythmias in the late myocardial infarction period. 7. Effect of verapamil and D-600 and role of the "slow channel." Circulation 60:3, 1979.

166. Jennings, R. B., Reimer, K. A., Hill, M. L., and Mayer, S. E.: Total ischemia in dog hearts in vitro. I. Comparison of high energy phosphate production, utilization and depletion, and of adenine nucleotide catabolism in total ischemia in vitro vs. severe ischemia in vivo. Circ. Res. 49:892, 1981.

167. Reimer, K. A., Jennings, R. B., and Hill, M. L.: Total ischemia in dog hearts, in vitro. 2. High energy phosphate depletion and associated defects in energy metabolism, cell volume regulation, and sarcolemmal integrity. Circ. Res. 49: 901, 1981.

168. Rude, R. E., DeBoer, L. W. V., Ingwall, J. S., Kloner, R. A., Hale, S. L., Davis, M., Maroko, P. R., and Braunwald, E.: Prediction of biochemical derangement in ischemic myocardium following experimental coronary artery occlusion. Am. J. Cardiol. 45:415, 1980.

169. Ingwall, J. S.: Phosphorus nuclear magnetic resonance spectroscopy of cardiac and skeletal muscles. Am. J. Physiol. 242 (Heart Circ. Physiol. 11):H729, 1982.

170. Flaherty, J. T., Weisfeldt, M. L., Bulkley, B. H., Gardner, T. J., Gott, V. L., and Jacobus, W. E.: Mechanisms of ischemic myocardial cell damage assessed by phosphorus-31 nuclear magnetic resonance. Circulation 65:561, 1982.

171. Pernot, A-C., Ingwall, J. S., Menasche, P., Grousset, C., Bercot, M., Pinwnica, A., and Fossel, E. T.: Evaluation of high-energy phosphate metabolism during cardioplegic arrest and reperfusion: A phosphorus-31 nuclear magnetic resonance study. Circulation 67:1296, 1983.

172. Sobel, B. E., and Mayer, S. E.: Cyclic adenosine monophosphate and cardiac contractility. Circ. Res. 32:407, 1973.

173. Rovetto, M. J., Lamberton, W. F., and Neely, J. R.: Mechanisms of glycolytic inhibition in ischemic rat hearts. Circ. Res. 37:742, 1975.

174. Williamson, J. R., Schaffer, S. W., Ford, C., and Safer, B.: Contribution of tissue acidosis to ischemic injury in the perfused rat heart. Circulation 53(Suppl. I):I-3, 1976.

175. Ng, M. L., Levy, M. N., and Zieske, H. A.: Effects of changes of pH and of carbon dioxide tension on left ventricular performance. Am. J. Physiol. 213: 115, 1967.

176. Williamson, J. R., Safer, B., LaNoue, K. F., Smith, C. M., and Walajtys, E.: Mitochondrial-cytosolic interactions in cardiac tissue: Role of the malate aspartate cycle in the removal of glycolytic NADH from the cytosol. Symp. Soc. Exp. Biol. 27:241, 1973.

177. LaNoue, K. F., and Williamson, J. R.: Interrelationships between malate-aspartate shuttle and critic acid cycle in rat heart mitochondria. Metabolism 20: 119, 1971.

178. Most, A. S., Gorlin, R., and Soeldner, J. S.: Glucose extraction by the human myocardium during pacing stress. Circulation 45:92, 1972.

179. Opie, L. H., Owen, P., Thomas, M., and Samson, R.: Coronary sinus lactate measurements in assessment of myocardial ischemia: Comparison with changes in lactate/pyruvate and beta-hydroxybutyrate/acetoacetate ratios and with release of hydrogen, phosphate and potassium ions from the heart. Am. J. Cardiol. 32:295, 1973.

180. Regan, T. J., Effros, R. M., Haider, R., Oldewurtel, H. A., Ettinger, P. O., and Ahmed, S. S.: Myocardial ischemia and cell acidosis: Modification by alkali and the effects on ventricular function and cation composition. Am. J. Cardiol. 27:501, 1976.

181. Neely, J. R., and Morgan, H. E.: Relationship between carbohydrate and lipid metabolism and the energy balance of heart muscle. Annu. Rev. Physiol. 36: 413, 1974.

182. Crass, M. F., III, McCaskill, E. S., and Shipp, J. C.: Glucose-free fatty acid interactions in the working heart. J. Appl. Physiol. 29:87, 1970.

183. Neely, J. R., Bowman, R. H., and Morgan, H. E.: Effects of ventricular pressure development and palmitate on glucose transport. Am. J. Physiol. 216: 804, 1969.

184. Wood, J. M., Sordahl, L. A., Lewis, R. M., and Schwartz, A.: Effect of chronic myocardial ischemia on the activity of carnitine palmityl-coenzyme A transferase of isolate canine heart mitochondria. Circ. Res. 32:340, 1973.

185. Bremer, J., and Wojtczak, A. B.: Factors controlling the rate of fatty acid β-oxidation in rat liver mitochondria. Biochim. Biophys. Acta 280:515, 1972.

186. Neely, J. R., Rovetto, M. J., Whitmer, J. T., and Morgan, H. E.: Effects of ischemia on ventricular function and metabolism in the isolated working rat heart. Am. J. Physiol. 225:651, 1973.

187. Brachfeld, N., Ohtaka, Y., Klein, I., and Kawade, M.: Substrate preference and metabolic activity of the aerobic and the hypoxic turtle heart. Circ. Res. 31:453, 1972.

188. Lerch, R. A., Bergmann, S. R., Ambos, H. D., Welch, M. J., Ter-Pogossian, M. M., and Sobel, B. E.: Effect of flow-independent reduction of metabolism on regional myocardial clearance of ¹¹C-palmitate. Circulation 65:731, 1982.

189. Sobel, B. E.: The diagnostic promise of positron tomography. Am. Heart J. 103:673, 1982.

190. Bergmann, S. R., Lerch, R. A., Fox, K. A. A., Ludbrook, P. A., Welch, M. J., Ter-Pogossian, M. M., and Sobel, B. E.: Temporal dependence of beneficial effects of coronary thrombolysis characterized by positron tomography. Am. J. Med. 73:573, 1982.

191. Sobel, B. E., and Bergmann, S. R.: Coronary thrombolysis: Some unresolved issues. Am. J. Med. 72:1, 1982.

192. Shrago, E., Shug, A., and Elson, C.: Regulation of cell metabolism by mitochondrial transport systems. In Hanson, R. W., and Mehlman, M. A. (eds.): Gluconeogenesis: Its Regulation in Mammalian Species. New York, John Wiley & Sons, 1976, p. 221.

193. Weiss, E. S., Hoffman, E. J., Phelps, M. E., Welch, M. J., Henry, P. D., Ter-Pogossian, M. M., and Sobel, B. E.: External detection and visualization of myocardial ischemia with ¹¹C-substrates in vitro and in vivo. Circ. Res. 39:24, 1976.

194. Ter-Pogossian, M. M., Klein, M. S., Markham, J., Roberts, R., and Sobel, B. E.: Regional assessment of myocardial metabolic integrity in vivo by positron-emission tomography with ¹¹C-labeled palmitate. Circulation 61:242, 1980.

194a. Geltman, E. M., and Sobel, B. E.: Cardiac positron tomography. Chest 83:553, 1983.

194b. Schelbert, H. R., Phelps, M. E., and Shine, K. I.: Imaging metabolism and biochemistry—a new look at the heart. Am. Heart J. 105:522, 1983.

194c. Schelbert, H. R., Henze, E., Schon, H. R., Keen, R., Hansen, H., Selin, C., Huang, S-C., Barrio, J. R., and Phelps, M. E.: C-11 palmitate for the noninvasive evaluation of regional myocardial fatty acid metabolism with positron computed tomography. III. In vivo demonstration of the effects of substrate availability on myocardial metabolism. Am. Heart J. 105:492, 1983.

195. Weiss, E. S., Ahmed, S. A., Welch, M. J., Williamson, J. R., Ter-Pogossian, M. M., and Sobel, B. E.: Quantification of infarction in cross sections of canine myocardium in vivo with positron emission transaxial tomography and ¹¹C-palmitate. Circulation 55:66, 1977.

196. Fox, K. A. A., Nomura, H., Sobel, B. E., and Bergmann, S. R.: Consistent substrate utilization despite reduced flow in hearts with maintained work. Am. J. Physiol. (in press).

197. Rude, R. E., Kloner, R. A., DeBoer, L. W. V., Hale, S. L., Davis, M. A., Maroko, P. R., and Braunwald, E.: A predictive index of subendocardial ischemic damage following coronary artery occlusion. Circulation 60(Suppl. 2):96, 1979.

198. Kao, R., Rannels, E., and Morgan, H. E.: Effects of anoxia and ischemia on protein synthesis in perfused rat hearts. Circ. Res. 38(Suppl. I):I-124, 1976.

199. Taegtmeyer, H., Peterson, M. B., Ragavan, V. V., Ferguson, A. G., and Lesch, M.: De novo alanine synthesis in isolated oxygen-deprived rabbit myocardium. J. Biol. Chem. 252:5010, 1977.

200. Rannels, D. E., McKee, E. E., and Morgan, H. E.: Regulation of protein synthesis and degradation in heart and skeletal muscle. In Litwack, G. (ed.): Biochemical Actions of Hormones. New York, Academic Press, 1976.

201. Weissman, G., Hoffstein, S., Gennaro, D., and Fox, A. C.: Lysosomes in ischemic myocardium, with observations on the effects of methyl-prednisolone. In Lefer, A. M., Kelliher, G. J., and Rovetto, M. J. (eds.): Pathophysiology and Therapeutics of Myocardial Ischemia. New York, Spectrum Publications, Inc., 1977, p. 367.

202. Williamson, J. R., Steenbergern, C., Rich, T., Deleeuw, G., Barlow, C., and Chance, B.: The nature of ischemic injury in cardiac tissue. In Lefer, A. M., Kelliher, G. J., and Rovetto, M. J. (eds.): Pathophysiology and Therapeutics of Myocardial Ischemia. New York, Spectrum Publications, Inc., 1977, p. 193.

203. Chance, B.: Discussion. Circ. Res. 38(Suppl. I):I-69, 1976.

204. Reimer, K. A., Lowe, J. E., Rasmussen, M. M., and Jennings, R. B.: The wavefront phenomenon of ischemic cell death. I. Myocardial infarct size vs duration of coronary occlusion in dogs. Circulation 56:786, 1977.

205. Fleckenstein, A.: Calcium Antagonism in Heart and Smooth Muscle. New York, John Wiley and Sons, 1983.

206. Shen, A. C., and Jennings, R. B.: Kinetics of calcium accumulation in acute myocardial ischemic injury. Am. J. Pathol. 67:441, 1972.

207. Braunwald, E.: Mechanism of action of calcium channel blocking agents. N. Engl. J. Med. 307:1618, 1982.

208. Corr, P. B., Gross, R. W., and Sobel, B. E.: Arrhythmogenic amphiphilic lipids and the myocardial cell membrane. J. Molec. Cell. Cardiol. 14:619, 1982.

209. Sedlis, S. P., Corr, P. B., Sobel, B. E., and Ahumada, G. G.: Lysophosphatidyl choline potentiates Ca⁺⁺ accumulation in rat cardiac myocytes. Am. J. Physiol. 13:H32, 1983.

210. Kloner, R. A., DeBoer, L. W. V., Carlson, N., and Braunwald, E.: The effect of verapamil on myocardial ultrastructure during and following release of coronary artery occlusion. Exp. Molec. Pathol. 36:277, 1982.

211. Braunwald, E., Muller, J. E., Kloner, R. A., and Maroko, P. R.: Role of beta-adrenergic blockade in the therapy of patients with myocardial infarction. Am. J. Med. 784:113, 1983.

212. Henry, P. D., Shuchleib, R., Davis, J., Weiss, E. S., and Sobel, B. E.: Myocardial contracture and accumulation of mitochondrial calcium in ischemic rabbit heart. Am. J. Physiol. (Heart Circ. Physiol.) 2:H677, 1977.

213. DeBoer, L. W. V., Strauss, H. W., Kloner, R. A., Rude, R. E., David, R. F., Maroko, P. R., and Braunwald, E.: Autoradiographic method for measuring the ischemic myocardium at risk: Effects of verapamil on infarct size after experimental coronary artery occlusion. Proc. Natl. Acad. Sci. 77:6119, 1980.

214. Clark, R. E., Christlieb, I. Y., and Ferguson, T. B.: Laboratory and initial clinical studies of nifedipine, a calcium antagonist for improved myocardial preservation. Ann. Surg. 193:719, 1981.

215. Sobel, B. E., Roberts, R., and Larson, K. B.: Considerations in the use of biochemical markers of ischemic injury. Circ. Res. 38(Suppl. I):I-99, 1976.

216. Ahumada, G., Roberts, R., and Sobel, B. E.: Evaluation of myocardial infarction with enzymatic indices. Prog. Cardiovasc. Dis. 18:405, 1976.

217. Stone, M. J., Willerson, J. T., Gomez-Sanchez, C. E., and Waterman, M. R.: Radioimmunoassay of myoglobin in human serum: Results in patients with acute myocardial infarction. J. Clin. Invest. 56:1334, 1975.

218. Wagner, G. S., Roe, C. R., Limbird, L. E., Rosati, R. A., and Wallace, A. G.: The importance of identification of the myocardial specific isoenzyme of creatine phosphokinase (MB form) in the diagnosis of acute myocardial infarction. Circulation 47:263, 1973.

219. Braunwald, E., and Maroko, P. R.: Limitation of infarct size. Curr. Probl. Cardiol. 3:51, 1978.

220. Nachlas, M. M., Friedman, M. M., and Cohen, S. P.: A method for the quantitation of myocardial infarcts and the relation of serum enzyme levels to infarct size. Surgery 55:700, 1964.

221. Sobel, B. E., and Shell, W. E.: Diagnostic and prognostic value of serum enzyme changes in patients with acute myocardial infarction. In Yu, P. N., and Goodwin, J. F. (eds.): Progress in Cardiology 4. Philadelphia, Lea and Febiger, 1975, p. 165.

222. Ahmed, S. A., Williamson, J. R., Roberts, R., Clark, R. E., and Sobel, B. E.: The association of increased plasma MB CPK activity and irreversible ischemic myocardial injury in the dog. Circulation 54:187, 1976.

223. Shell, W. E., Kjekshus, J. K., and Sobel, B. E.: Quantitative assessment of the extent of myocardial infarction in the conscious dog by means of analysis of serial changes in serum creatine phosphokinase activity. J. Clin. Invest. 50:2614, 1971.

224. Sobel, B. E., Markam, J., Karlsberg, R. P., and Roberts, R.: The nature of disappearance of creatine kinase from the circulation and its influence on enzymatic estimation of infarct size. Circ. Res. 41:836, 1977.

225. Geltman, E. M., Ehsani, A. A., Campbell, M. K., Schechtman, K., Roberts, R., and Sobel, B. E.: The influence of location and extent of myocardial infarction on long-term ventricular dysrhythmia and mortality. Circulation 60:805, 1979.

226. Roberts, R., Gowda, K. S., Ludbrook, P. A., and Sobel, B. E.: Specificity of elevated serum MB creatine phosphokinase activity in the diagnosis of acute myocardial infarction. Am. J. Cardiol. 36:433, 1975.

227. Bleifeld, W., Mathey, D., Hanrath, P., Buss, H., and Effert, S.: Infarct size estimated from serial serum creatine phosphokinase in relation to left ventricular hemodynamics. Circulation 55:303, 1977.

228. Mathey, D., Bleifeld, W., Hanrath, P., and Effert, S.: Attempt to quantitate relation between cardiac function and infarct size in acute myocardial infarction. Br. Heart J. 36:271, 1974.

229. Norris, R. M., Whitlock, R. M. L., Barratt-Boyes, C., and Small, C. W.: Clinical measurement of myocardial infarct size. Modification of a method for the estimation of total creatine phosphokinase release after myocardial infarction. Circulation 51:614, 1975.

230. Yasmineh, W. G., Pyle, R. B., Cohn, J. N., Nicoloff, D. M., Hanson, N. Q., and Steele, B. W.: Serial serum creatine phosphokinase MB isoenzyme activity after myocardial infarction. Studies in the baboon and man. Circulation 55:733, 1977.

231. Vatner, S. F., Baig, H., Manders, W. T., and Maroko, P. R.: Effects of coronary artery reperfusion on myocardial infarct size calculated from creatine kinase. J. Clin. Invest. 61:1048, 1978.

232. Clark, G. L., Robison, A. K., Gnepp, D. R., Roberts, R., and Sobel, B. E.: Effects of lymphatic transport of enzyme on plasma CK time-activity curves after myocardial infarction. Circ. Res. 43:162, 1978.

233. Sobel, B. E., Markam, J., and Roberts, R.: Factors influencing enzymatic estimates of infarct size. Am. J. Cardiol. 39:130, 1977.

234. Rude, R. E., Muller, J. E., and Braunwald, E.: Efforts to limit the size of myocardial infarcts. Ann. Intern. Med. 95:736, 1981.

235. Maroko, P. R., Kjekshus, J. K., Sobel, B. E., Watanabe, T., Covell, J. W., Ross, J., Jr., and Braunwald, E.: Factors influencing infarct size following experimental coronary artery occlusion. Circulation 43:67, 1971.

236. Kloner, R. A., and Braunwald, E.: Review—Observations on experimental myocardial ischemia. Cardiovasc. Res. 14:371, 1980.

237. Shell, W. E., and Sobel, B. E.: Deleterious effects of increased heart rate on infarct size in the conscious dog. Am. J. Cardiol. 31:474, 1973.

238. Richman, S.: Adverse effect of atropine during myocardial infarction: Enhancement of ischemia following intravenously administered atropine. J.A.M.A. 228:1414, 1974.

239. Radvany, P., Maroko, P. R., and Braunwald, E.: Effect of hypoxemia on the extent of myocardial necrosis after experimental coronary artery occlusion. Am. J. Cardiol. 35:795, 1975.

240. Yoshikawa, H., Powell, W. J., Jr., Bland, J. H. L., and Lowenstein, E.: Effect of acute anemia on experimental myocardial ischemia. Am. J. Cardiol. 32:670, 1973.

241. DeBoer, L. W. V., Rude, R. E., Davis, R. F., Maroko, P. R., and Braunwald, E.: Extension of myocardial necrosis into normal epicardium following hypotension during experimental coronary occlusion. Cardiovasc. Res. 16:423, 1982.

242. Libby, P., Maroko, P. R., and Braunwald, E.: The effect of hypoglycemia on myocardial ischemic injury during acute experimental coronary artery occlusion. Circulation 51:621, 1975.

243. Liedtke, A. J., and Hughes, H. C.: Hyperthermic insult to ischemic myocardium: Implications of fever as an energy draining process in myocardial infarct. Clin. Res. 24:227A, 1976.

244. Vatner, S. F., McRitchie, R. J., Maroko, P. R., Patrick, T. A., and Braunwald, E.: Effects of catecholamines, exercise, and nitroglycerin on the normal and ischemic myocardium in conscious dogs. J. Clin. Invest. 54:563, 1974.

245. Maroko, P. R., Libby, P., and Braunwald, E.: Effect of pharmacologic agents on the function of the ischemic heart. Am. J. Cardiol. 32:930, 1973.

246. Davidson, S., Maroko, P. R., and Braunwald, E.: Effects of isoproterenol on contractile function of the ischemic and anoxic heart. Am. J. Physiol. 227:439, 1974.

247. Vatner, S. F., Millard, R. W., Patrick, T. A., and Heyndrickx, G. R.: Effects of isoproterenol on regional myocardial function, electrogram, and blood flow in conscious dogs with myocardial ischemia. J. Clin. Invest. 57:1261, 1976.

248. Mueller, H., Ayres, S. M., Gregory, J. J., Giannelli, S., Jr., and Grace, W. J.: Hemodynamics, coronary blood flow, and myocardial metabolism in coronary shock: Response to 1-norepinephrine and isoproterenol. J. Clin. Invest. 49:1885, 1970.

249. Shug, A., and Shrago, E.: A proposed mechanism for fatty acid effects on energy metabolism of the heart. J. Lab. Clin. Med. 81:214, 1973.

250. Mjós, O. D., Kjekshus, J. K., and Lekven, J.: Importance of free fatty acids as a determinant of myocardial oxygen consumption and myocardial ischemic injury during norepinephrine infusion in dogs. J. Clin. Invest. 53:1290, 1974.

251. Kjekshus, J. K., and Mjós, O. D.: Effect of free fatty acids on myocardial function and metabolism in the ischemic dog heart. J. Clin. Invest. 51:1767, 1972.

252. Schaper, J., and Schaper, W.: Reperfusion of ischemic myocardium: Ultrastructural and histochemical aspects. J. Am. Coll. Cardiol. 1:1037, 1983.

253. Ellis, S. G., Henschke, C. I., Sandor, T., Wynne, J., Braunwald, E., and Kloner, R. A.: Time course of functional and biochemical recovery of myocardium salvaged by reperfusion. J. Am. Coll. Cardiol. 1:1047, 1983.

254. Higginson, L. A. J., Beanlands, D. S., Nair, R. C., Temple, V., and Sheldrick, K.: The time course and characterization of myocardial hemorrhage after coronary reperfusion in the anesthetized dog. Circulation 67:1024, 1983.

255. Lang, T. W., Corday, E., Gold, H., Meerbaum, S., Rubins, S., Constantini, C., Hirose, S., Osher, J., and Rosen, V.: Consequences of reperfusion after coronary occlusion: Effects on hemodynamic and regional myocardial metabolic function. Am. J. Cardiol. 33:69, 1974.

256. Maroko, P. R., Radvany, P., Braunwald, E., and Hale, S. L.: Reduction of infarct size by oxygen inhalation following acute coronary occlusion. Circulation 52:360, 1975.

257. Glogar, D. H., Kloner, R. A., Muller, J., DeBoer, L. W. V., and Braunwald, E.: Fluorocarbons reduce myocardial ischemic damage after coronary occlusion. Science 211:1439, 1981.

258. Braunwald, E., Muller, J. E., Kloner, R. A., and Maroko, P. R.: Role of beta-adrenergic blockade in the therapy of patients with myocardial infarction. Am. J. Med. 74:113, 1983.

259. Lange, R., Kloner, R. A., and Braunwald, E.: First ultra-short-acting-beta-adrenergic blocking agent: Its effect on size and segmental wall dynamics of reperfused myocardial infarcts in dogs. Am. J. Cardiol. 51:1759, 1983.

260. Hammerman, H., Kloner, R. A., Briggs, L. L., and Braunwald, E.: Combination therapy for early treatment of myocardial infarction: Beta blockade plus reperfusion. Clin. Res. 31:524a, 1983.

261. Henry, P. R., Shuchleib, R., Borda, L. J., Roberts, R., Williamson, J. R., and Sobel, B. E.: Effects of nifedipine on myocardial perfusion and ischemic injury in dogs. Circ. Res. 43:372, 1978.

261a. Drury, J. K., Haendchen, R. V., Meerbaum, S., Fishbein, M. C., Y-Rit, J., and Corday, E.: Diltiazem improves function and reduces infarct size after acute coronary occlusion. J. Am. Coll. Cardiol. 1:692, 1983.

262. Opie, L. H.: Metabolism of free fatty acids, glucose and catecholamines in acute myocardial infarction: Relation to myocardial ischemia and infarct size. Am. J. Cardiol. 36:938, 1975.

263. Calva, E., Mujica, A., Bisteni, A., and Sodi-Pallares, D.: Oxidative phosphorylation in cardiac infarct: Effect of glucose-KCl-insulin solution. Am. J. Physiol. 209:371, 1965.

264. Henry, P. D., Sobel, B. E., and Braunwald, E.: Protection of hypoxic guinea pig hearts with glucose and insulin. Am. J. Physiol. 226:390, 1974.

265. Wildenthal, K., Mierzwiak, D. S., and Mitchell, J. H.: Acute effects of increased serum osmolality on left ventricular performance. Am. J. Physiol. 216:898, 1969.

266. Regan, T. J., Harman, M. A., Lehan, P. H., Burke, W. M., and Oldewurtel, H. A.: Ventricular arrhythmias and K+ transfer during myocardial ischemia and intervention with procaine amide, insulin, or glucose solution. J. Clin. Invest. 46:1657, 1967.

267. Sodi-Pallares, D., Bisteni, A., Medrano, G. A., Testelli, M. R., and DeMicheli, A.: The polarizing treatment of acute myocardial infarction: Possibility of its use in other cardiovascular conditions. Dis. Chest. 43:424, 1963.

268. Maroko, P. R., Libby, P., Sobel, B. E., Bloor, C. M., Sybers, H. D., Shell, W. E., Covell, J. W., and Braunwald, E.: Effect of glucose-insulin-potassium infusion on myocardial infarction following experimental coronary artery occlusion. Circulation 45:1160, 1972.

269. Opie, L. H., Bruyneel, K., and Owen, P.: Effects of glucose, insulin, and potassium infusion on tissue metabolic changes within the first hour of myocardial infarction in the baboon. Circulation 52:49, 1975.

270. Kjekshus, J. K.: Effect of lipolytic and inotropic stimulation on myocardial ischemic injury. In Hjalmarson, A., and Werko, L. (eds.): Experimental and Clinical Aspects on Preservation of the Ischemic Myocardium. Sweden, Molndal, 1976, p. 35.

271. Mjós, O. D.: Effect of reduction of myocardial free fatty acid metabolism relative to that of glucose on the ischemic injury during experimental coronary artery occlusion in dogs. In Hjalmarson, A., and Werko, L. (eds.): Experimental and Clinical Aspects on Preservation of the Ischemic Myocardium. Sweden, Molndal, 1976, p. 29.

272. Folts, J. D., Shug, A. S., Koke, J. R., and Bittar, N.: Protection of the ischemic dog myocardium with L-carnitine. Clin. Res. 24:217A, 1976.

273. Flores, J., DiBona, D. R., Beck, C. H., and Leaf, A.: The role of cell swelling in ischemic renal damage and the protective effect of hypertonic solute. J. Clin. Invest. 51:118, 1972.

274. Maroko, P. R., Carpenter, C. B., Chiariello, M., Fishbein, M. C., Radvany, P., Knostman, J. B., and Hale, S. L.: Reduction by cobra venom factor of myocardial necrosis following coronary artery occlusion. J. Clin. Invest. 61:661, 1978.

275. Diaz, P. E., Fishbein, M. C., Davis, M. A., Askenazi, J., and Maroko, P. R.: Effect of kallikrein inhibitor aprotinin on myocardial ischemic injury following coronary artery occlusion in the dog. Am. J. Cardiol. 40:541, 1977.

276. Libby, P., Maroko, P. R., Bloor, C. M., Sobel, B. E., and Braunwald, E.: Reduction of experimental myocardial infarct size by corticosteroid administration. J. Clin. Invest. 52:599, 1973.

277. Masters, T. N., Harbold, N. B., Jr., Hall, D. G., Jackson, R. D., Mullen, D. C., Daugherty, H. K., and Robicsek, F.: Beneficial metabolic effects of methylprednisolone sodium succinate in acute myocardial ischemia. Am. J. Cardiol. 37:557, 1976.

278. Hammerman, H., Kloner, R. A., Hale, S. L., Schoen, F. J., and Braunwald, E.: Is scar thinning and LV topographic alterations induced by antiinflammatory agent of functional significance? Clin. Res. (abst.), in press.

279. Weissman, G.: Corticosteroids and membrane stabilization. Circulation 53 (Suppl. 1):171, 1976.

280. Kloner, R. A., Fishbein, M. C., Lew, H., Maroko, P. R., and Braunwald, E.: Mummification of the infarcted myocardium by high dose corticosteroids. Circulation 57:56, 1978.

281. Roberts, R. deMello, V., and Sobel, B. E.: Deleterious effects of methylprednisolone in patients with myocardial infarction. Circulation 53(Suppl. 1):1, 1976.

282. Maclean, D., Maroko, P. R., Fishbein, M. C., and Braunwald, E.: Effects of corticosteroids on myocardial infarct size and healing following experimental coronary occlusion. Am. J. Cardiol. 39:280, 1977.

283. Jugdutt, B. I., Hutchins, G. M., Bulkley, B. H., and Becker, L. C.: Salvage of ischemic myocardium by ibuprofen during infarction in the conscious dog. Am. J. Cardiol. 46:74, 1980.

284. Brown, E. J., Kloner, R. A., Schoen, F. J., Hammerman, H., Hale, S., and Braunwald, E.: Scar thinning due to ibuprofen administration following experimental myocardial infarction. Am. J. Cardiol. 51:877, 1983.

285. Willerson, J. T., Watson, J. T., and Platt, M. R.: Effect of hypertonic mannitol and intraaortic counterpulsation on regional myocardial blood flow and ventricular performance in dogs during myocardial ischemia. Am. J. Cardiol. 37:514, 1976.

286. Maroko, P. R., Libby, P., Bloor, C. M., Sobel, B. E., and Braunwald, E.: Reduction by hyaluronidase of myocardial necrosis following coronary artery occlusion. Circulation 46:430, 1972.

287. Wetstein, L., Simson, M. B., Haselgrove, J., Barlow, C. H., and Harken, A. H.: Mechanism of action of hyaluronidase in decreasing myocardial ischemia post coronary occlusion in the isolated perfused rabbit heart. Am. Heart J. 104:529, 1982.

288. Askenazi, J., Hillis, L. D., Diaz, P. E., Davis, M. A., Braunwald, E., and Maroko, P. R.: The effects of hyaluronidase on coronary blood flow following coronary artery occlusion in the dog. Cir. Res. 40:566, 1977.

289. Epstein, S. E., Borer, J. S., Kent, K. M., Redwood, D. R., Goldstein, R. E., and Levitt, B.: Protection of ischemic myocardium by nitroglycerin: Experimental and clinical results. Circulation 53(Suppl. 1): 191, 1976.

290. Smith, E. R., Redwood, D. R., McCarron, W. E., and Epstein, S. E.: Coronary artery occlusion in the conscious dog: Effects of alterations in arterial pressure produced by nitroglycerin, hemorrhage, and alpha-adrenergic agonists on the degree of myocardial ischemia. Circulation 47:51, 1973.

291. Myers, R. W., Scherer, J. L., Goldstein, R. A., Goldstein, R. E., Kent, K. M., and Epstein, S. E.: Effects of nitroglycerin and nitroglycerin-methoxamine during acute myocardial ischemia in dogs with preexisting multivessel coronary occlusive disease. Circulation 51:632, 1975.

292. Kent, K. M., Smith, E. R., Redwood, D. R., and Epstein, S. E.: Beneficial electrophysiologic effects of nitroglycerin during acute myocardial infarction. Am. J. Cardiol. 33:513, 1974.

293. Forman, R., Eng, C., and Kirk, E. S.: Comparative effect of verapamil and nitroglycerin on collateral blood flow. Circulation 67:1200, 1983.

37 ACUTE MYOCARDIAL INFARCTION: PATHOLOGICAL, PATHOPHYSIOLOGICAL, AND CLINICAL MANIFESTATIONS

by Joseph S. Alpert, M.D., and Eugene Braunwald, M.D.

Approximately one-third of all deaths in the United States are due to ischemic heart disease, and, of these, one-half are attributable to acute myocardial infarction (AMI). Approximately one-half of patients with AMI die suddenly, i.e., within 1 hour of onset (Chap. 23). Most of the remainder, annually approximately one-half million patients, are admitted to hospitals with AMI.[1] The mortality rates during hospitalization and during the year following infarction are approximately 15 and 10 per cent, respectively, with at least half of the post-hospitalization deaths occurring suddenly before the victim can be returned to the hospital. In addition to this high probability of death within the first year after myocardial infarction (MI), excessive mortality risk continues for a prolonged period. Indeed, a three- to fourfold excess in the risk of death persists even 10 years after infarction.[2] Recently, a modest though significant reduction in the death rate from coronary artery disease has been noted (p. 1208).[3] The cause of this decreased mortality is unknown, but it may be the result, in part, of a decreased incidence of AMI, improved treatment, or both.

PATHOLOGY OF MYOCARDIAL INFARCTION

Almost all myocardial infarctions result from atherosclerosis of the coronary arteries. The genesis of the coronary atherosclerotic lesion is a complex and controversial issue (see Chap. 34), and a number of risk factors have been associated with the development of atherosclerosis (see Chap. 35). However, regardless of the etiology and pathogenesis of the atherosclerotic process, the end result is plaques that cause luminal narrowing of the coronary arterial tree and thus reduce the blood supply to the myocardium. Below a certain critical level of blood flow, myocardial cells develop ischemic injury, a process described in detail in Chapter 36. When severe ischemia is prolonged, irreversible damage, i.e., myocardial infarction, occurs.

Since the coronary luminal narrowing affects the major coronary arteries and their various branches to a different extent, MI usually occurs focally in specific regions of the heart. The location and size of a particular infarction depend on a number of different factors: (1) the location and severity of the atherosclerotic narrowings in the coronary arterial tree; (2) the presence, site, and severity of coronary arterial spasm; (3) the size of the vascular bed perfused by the narrowed vessels; (4) the extent of development of collateral blood vessels; and (5) the oxygen needs of the poorly perfused myocardium.

GROSS PATHOLOGICAL CHANGES OF MYOCARDIAL INFARCTION

Myocardial infarction may be divided into two major types: *transmural infarcts*, in which myocardial necrosis involves the full thickness of the ventricular wall, and *subendocardial (nontransmural) infarcts*, in which the necrosis involves the subendocardium, the intramural myocardium, or both without extending all the way through the ventricular wall to the epicardium.

Gross changes do not appear in the myocardium until 6 hours after the onset of myocardial infarction.[4] Initially, the myocardium in the affected region appears pale, bluish, and slightly swollen. Eighteen to 36 hours after the onset of the infarct, the myocardium appears tan or reddish-purple, with a serofibrinous exudate evident on the epicardium in transmural infarcts. These changes persist for approximately 48 hours; the infarct then turns gray, and fine yellow lines, secondary to neutrophilic infiltration, appear at its periphery. This zone gradually widens and during the next few days extends throughout the infarct.

Eight to 10 days following infarction, the thickness of the cardiac wall in the area of the infarct is reduced as necrotic muscle is removed by mononuclear cells. The cut surface of an infarct of this age is yellow, surrounded by a reddish-purple band of granulation tissue (Fig. 37–1) that extends through the necrotic tissue by 3 to 4 weeks. Com-

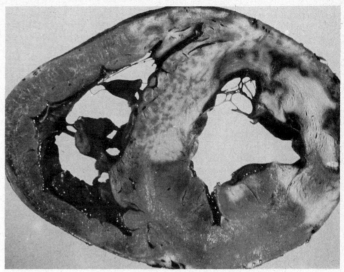

FIGURE 37–1 Acute myocardial infarct. Cross section of the heart shows myocardial infarct about 1 week old, involving the posterior half of the interventricular septum and the posterior lateral left ventricular walls. This infarct is secondary to occlusion of the left circumflex coronary artery. The myocardium has a mottled appearance, and the margins of the infarct are well demarcated. In the central portion of the infarct involving the posterior papillary muscle, there is evidence of hemorrhage. (From Bloor, C. M.: Cardiac Pathology. Philadelphia, J. B. Lippincott Co., 1978.)

mencing at this time and extending over the next 2 to 3 months, the infarcted area gradually acquires a gelatinous, ground-glass, gray appearance, eventually converting into a shrunken, thin, firm scar, which whitens and firms progressively with time;[5–7] this process begins at the periphery of the infarct and gradually moves centrally. The endocardium below the infarct increases in thickness and becomes gray and opaque.

HISTOLOGICAL AND ULTRASTRUCTURAL CHANGES

On light microscopy, severe ischemia, which is potentially reversible, causes cloudy swelling, as well as hydropic, vascular, and fatty degeneration.[8] For many years it was believed that no light microscopic changes could be seen in infarcted myocardium until 8 hours

FIGURE 37–2 Wavy and stretched appearance of necrotic muscle cells in an acute myocardial infarct. The wavy myocardial fibers have pyknotic nuclei and hypereosinophilic cytoplasm. (Hematoxylin and eosin, × 128). (Reproduced with permission from Willerson, J. T., Hillis, L. D., and Buja, L. M. [eds.]: Pathogenesis and pathology of ischemic heart disease. *In* Ischemic Heart Disease. Clinical and Pathophysiological Aspects. New York, Raven Press, 1982, p. 46.)

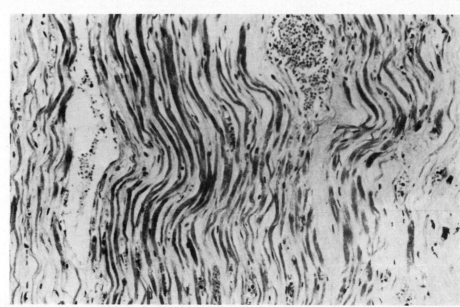

after interruption of blood flow. Bouchardy and Majno, however, have called attention to a wavy pattern of myocardial cells that occurs shortly after the onset of infarction (Fig. 37-2), a pattern that is probably the result of agonal contraction of myocardial cells.[9,10] With careful light microscopy, contraction bands and small spaces between myocardial cells are also revealed.[11] After 8 hours, edema of the interstitium becomes evident, as do increased fatty deposits in the muscle fibers, along with infiltration of neutrophilic polymorphonuclear leukocytes and red blood cells. Muscle cell nuclei become pyknotic and then undergo karyolysis, and small blood vessels undergo necrosis.

By 24 hours there is clumping of the cytoplasm and loss of cross striations, with appearance of focal hyalinization and irregular cross bands in the involved myocardial fibers. The nuclei become pyknotic and sometimes even disappear. The myocardial capillaries in the involved region dilate, and polymorphonuclear leukocytes accumulate, first at the periphery and then in the center of the infarct. During the first 3 days, the interstitial tissue becomes edematous and red blood cells may extravasate. Generally, on about the fourth day after infarction, removal of necrotic fibers begins, again commencing at the periphery. Later, lymphocytes, macrophages, and fibroblasts infiltrate between myocytes, which become fragmented. At 8 days the necrotic muscle fibers have become dissolved; by about 10 days the number of polymorphonuclear leukocytes is reduced, and granulation tissue first appears at the periphery. Ingrowth of blood vessels and fibroblasts continues, along with removal of necrotic muscle cells, until the fourth to sixth week following infarction, by which time much of the necrotic myocardium has been removed. This process continues along with increasing collagenization of the infarcted area. By the sixth week, the infarcted area has usually been converted into a firm connective tissue scar with interspersed intact muscle fibers.[6]

A variety of *histochemical* approaches have been used to detect myocardial changes compatible with infarction before routine microscopic changes become evident at 6 hours. These include estimation of glycogen, using a periodic acid–Schiff stain (PAS) and succinic dehydrogenase activity. Glycogen stores may become depleted within 3 to 4 hours after the onset of severe myocardial ischemia. However, the reliability of these procedures diminishes with lengthening of the interval between death and the examination of the myocardium.[4]

One of the most useful histochemical methods is the nitro–blue tetrazolium staining technique; the heart is sliced transversely into several sections. These sections are washed and incubated in buffered tetrazolium solution, which is reduced to a dark blue compound, formazan, in viable zones of myocardium. Reduction of tetrazolium is accomplished by endogenous substrates, coenzymes, and dehydrogenases; these are absent or deficient in necrotic areas of myocardium, which therefore remain uncolored and hence identifiable. This reaction can distinguish infarcted myocardium 6 to 8 hours after the start of infarction.[11]

Although the *alterations in cardiac ultrastructure* to be described are based on animal experiments and are not directly applicable to clinical diagnosis, they provide important information concerning the process of myocardial infarction. The earliest ultrastructural changes in cardiac muscle following ligation of a coronary artery, noted within 20 minutes, consist of reduction in the size and number of glycogen granules, development of intracellular edema, and swelling and distortion of the transverse tubular system, the sarcoplasmic reticulum, and the mitochondria (Fig. 37-3).[12-17] When these changes are relatively mild, they are compatible with reversible ischemic injury. Changes after 60 minutes of occlusion include myocardial cell swelling, mitochondrial abnormalities such as swelling and internal disruption, aggregation and margination of nuclear chromatin, and relaxation of myofibrils.[11] After 20 minutes to 2 hours of ischemia, changes in some cells become irreversible, and there is progression of these alterations; additional changes include indistinct, tight junctions at the intercalated disks, swollen sacs of the sarcoplasmic reticulum at the level of the A band, greatly enlarged mitochondria with few cristae, thinning and fractionation of myofilaments, disappearance of the heterochromatin, rarefaction of the euchromatin and peripheral aggregation of chromatin in the nucleus, disorientation of myofibrils, and clumping of mitochondria. Cells irreversibly damaged by ischemia are usually swollen, with an enlarged sarcoplasmic space; the sarcolemma may peel off the cells, defects in the plasma membrane may appear, and the mitochondria are fragmented.

The swollen mitochondria obtained from ischemic myocardium contain deposits of calcium phosphate and amorphous matrix densities;[18] many of these changes become more intense when blood flow is restored.[14,19] However, it appears unlikely that the structural and functional deterioration of mitochondria—the hallmark of ischemic injury—is the primary mediator of myocardial cell death. In experimental infarction, reflow into an area rendered ischemic for 40 to 60 minutes results in violent cell swelling with vacuolization of myocardial cell cytoplasm and marked swelling of mitochondria. Cell membranes are lifted off the myofibrils, and subsarcolemmal blebs appear. The speed with which these morphological changes occur during early postischemic reflow suggests that ischemia produces a defect of volume regulation in myocardial cells.

Three patterns of myocardial necrosis are recognized. *Coagulation necrosis*[20] results from severe, persistent ischemia and is usually present in the central region of infarcts, which results in the arrest of muscle cells in the relaxed state and the passive stretching of ischemic muscle cells. On light microscopy the myofibrils are stretched, many with unclear pyknosis, with vascular congestion and healing by phagocytosis of necrotic muscle cells. There is evidence of mitochondrial damage with prominent amorphous (flocculent) densities but no calcification.

Coagulative myocytolysis[9,21,22] (also termed contraction band necrosis)[23] results primarily from severe ischemia followed by reflow.[12] It is

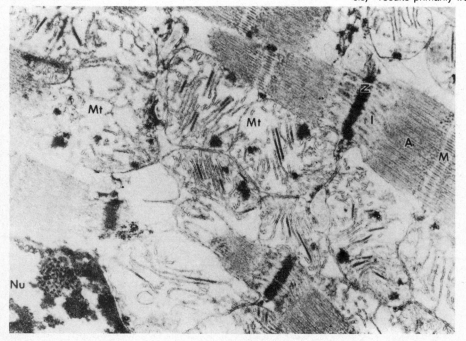

FIGURE 37–3 Electron micrograph of a muscle cell from the center of an infarct produced by permanent coronary occlusion in the dog. The myofibrils are fixed in a relaxed state and exhibit I, A, M, and Z bands. There is slight edema and no glycogen. (The clusters of granules resembling glycogen probably are ribosomes.) The mitochondria (Mt) are swollen and have linear densities and amorphous matrix (flocculent) densities. The nucleus (Nu) has clumped chromatin along the nuclear membrane and large lucent areas. (Tissue fixed with glutaraldehyde and osmium. Epoxy section stained with uranyl acetate and lead citrate, × 19,500). (Reproduced with permission from Willerson, J. T., Hillis, L. D., and Buja, L. M. [eds.]: Pathogenesis and pathology of ischemic heart disease. *In* Ischemic Heart Disease. Clinical and Pathophysiological Aspects. New York, Raven Press, 1982, p. 47.)

caused by increased Ca^{++} influx into dying cells, resulting in the arrest of cells in the contracted state. It is seen in the periphery of large infarcts or constitutes the entire infarct in patients subjected to iatrogenic reperfusion (by surgery or thrombolysis). Its presence in a large segment of some infarcts suggests that reperfusion through spontaneous thrombolysis or the release of spasm or both have occurred. It is characterized by hypercontracted myofibrils with contraction bands and mitochondrial damage, frequently with calcification, marked vascular congestion, and healing by lysis of muscle cells.

Myocytolysis results from prolonged moderate ischemia and, like coagulative myocytolysis, is also frequently seen at the borders of an infarct as well as in patchy areas of infarction in patients with chronic ischemic heart disease. It is characterized by edema and cell swelling, early lysis of myofibrils, late lysis of nuclei, no neutrophilic response, and healing by lysis and phagocytosis of necrotic myocytes.[7,21]

Relation of Myocardial Infarction to Coronary Arterial Obstruction

Myocardial infarction usually occurs in hearts with more than one severely narrowed coronary artery.[24,25] One-third to two-thirds of patients with AMI have critical obstruction (less than 25 per cent of luminal area), whereas the remainder is equally divided between patients having one-vessel disease and those having two-vessel disease.[26,27] Most transmural infarcts occur distal to a totally occluded coronary artery. However, the converse is not the case, in that total occlusion of a coronary artery is not always associated with myocardial infarction. Collateral blood flow and other factors—such as the level of myocardial metabolism, the presence and location of stenoses in other coronary arteries, the rate of development of the obstruction, and the quantity of myocardium supplied by the obstructed vessel—all influence the viability of myocardial cells distal to the occlusion. In many series of patients studied at necropsy or by coronary arteriography, a small number (< 5 per cent) of patients with MI are found to have normal coronary vessels. In these patients, an embolus that has lysed or a prolonged episode of severe coronary spasm may have been responsible for the reduction in coronary flow.

Obstruction of the left anterior descending coronary artery usually causes infarction or threatens the viability of the anterior and apical regions of the left ventricle; portions of the septum, anterolateral wall, papillary muscles, and inferoapical wall of the left ventricle may also be involved. Obstruction of the left circumflex artery can cause infarction of the lateral or inferoposterior wall of the left ventricle, whereas occlusion of the right coronary artery usually results in infarction of the inferoposterior wall of the left ventricle, the inferior portions of the septum, and the posteromedial papillary muscle. The size of the infarction and its location depend on the distribution of the obstructed coronary vessels. Thus, with occlusion of a dominant right coronary artery, which supplies the posterior descending artery and posterior left ventricular wall, the inferoposterior wall of the left ventricle becomes infarcted, whereas the same region of the myocardium becomes involved with occlusion of the left circumflex coronary artery in the presence of a dominant left coronary artery. Rather frequently, when an area of the ventricle is perfused by collateral vessels, an infarct occurs at a distance from a coronary occlusion. For example, following the gradual obliteration of the lumen of the right coronary artery, the inferior wall of the left ventricle may be maintained viable by collateral vessels arising from the left anterior descending coronary artery. In this circumstance, an occlusion of the left anterior descending artery may cause an infarct of the diaphragmatic wall.

Transmural infarctions are found at postmortem examination to be associated with fresh or organizing thrombosis of the coronary artery supplying the infarcted region in slightly more than half of the cases;[27] as discussed below, a much larger percentage of these patients are thought to have thrombi at the onset of infarct. Transmural infarcts are more frequently localized to the zone of distribution of a single coronary artery. Nontransmural infarctions (either subendocardial or multifocal), however, frequently occur in the setting of severely narrowed but still patent coronary arteries, often in patients with pulmonary embolism, hypertension, hypotension, anemia, aortic stenosis, operative procedures, or cerebrovascular accidents.[28,29] In the presence of severe atherosclerotic narrowing of the coronary arteries, these and other conditions associated with increased myocardial metabolic demands or decreased myocardial oxygen delivery or both are capable of producing patchy, nontransmural myocardial necrosis.

CORONARY ARTERIAL THROMBI. Coronary arterial thrombi, which are approximately 1 cm in length in most cases,[25] adhere to the luminal surface of an artery and are composed of platelets, fibrin, erythrocytes, and leukocytes. The composition of the thrombus may vary at different levels: A white thrombus is composed of platelets, fibrin, or both distally, and a red thrombus is composed of erythrocytes, fibrin, platelets, and leukocytes proximally. Early thrombi are usually small and nonocclusive and are composed almost exclusively of platelets.

In patients with MI, coronary thrombi are usually superimposed on or adjacent to atherosclerotic plaques; the mechanism by which thrombosis occurs in these stenotic areas remains controversial. It has been suggested that degenerative changes in the atherosclerotic intima damage supportive perivascular tissue with resultant rupture of a plaque, sometimes accompanied by intramural hemorrhage.[12,30,31] This process may enlarge the volume of the plaque so that it occludes the arterial lumen without the occurrence of thrombosis, or the hemorrhage may disrupt the intima covering the plaque, thereby exposing collagen to flowing blood, a strong stimulus for thrombus formation.[25] Another possible mechanism for coronary thrombosis is ulceration or erosion of an atherosclerotic plaque with resultant exposure of collagen and other thrombogenic materials to the bloodstream.[26] Coronary spasm in the vicinity of an atherosclerotic plaque may be responsible for the development of a platelet fibrin thrombus.[31a] Platelet aggregates, in turn, may release thromboxane A_2, a potent vasoconstrictor, which may be responsible for the development or enhancement of coronary spasm.

THE CORONARY ARTERIAL BED IN MYOCARDIAL INFARCTION. Roberts has pointed out that (1) in patients with *fatal* ischemic heart disease, the lumina of at least two of the three major coronary arteries are usually narrowed by more than 75 per cent by atherosclerotic plaques; (2) the atherosclerotic process is limited to the epicardial arteries and spares the intramural vessels; and (3) the degree of luminal narrowing by atherosclerotic plaques is similar irrespective of the type of fatal coronary event.[32,33] There has been little dispute about these points. On the other hand, there has been some controversy about the relationship between coronary occlusion and myocardial infarction. In the three decades following Herrick's description of the condition,[34] the clinical manifestations of myocardial infarction were felt to stem from sudden coronary arterial occlusion, usually due to thrombosis; hence the terms *coronary thrombosis* and *acute myocardial infarction* became almost synonymous. One weakness of this concept was shown by Blumgart, Schlesinger, and their colleagues, who demonstrated that *coronary occlusion could occur in the absence of infarction*, when the collateral circulation was adequate to maintain myocardial nutrition.[24,35] Equally important, Friedberg and Horn observed that *infarction could occur in the absence of coronary occlusion.*[28] The patients whom they described had severe coronary arterial narrowing, and the areas of patchy, subendocardial infarction which occurred were felt to have developed secondary to relative insufficiency of coronary blood flow. Miller, Burchell, and Edwards then expanded on these observations, demonstrating that predominantly subendocardial infarcts were rarely associated with coronary occlusion, whereas transmural infarctions were frequently so.[36]

In order to define the precise relationship between coronary thrombosis and MI, it is important to know the time course of thrombus formation in relation to the onset of infarction. Unfortunately, estimates of the age of coronary thrombi and myocardial infarction by histological criteria may be quite imprecise.[32,37,38] Recent studies in which coronary arteriography was performed on patients within the first few hours after the onset of myocardial infarction have demonstrated that the coronary artery supplying the area of evolving infarction is totally occluded in the majority of these individuals.[39–44] If fibrinolytic agents are infused into the occluded artery, patency is achieved in a high percentage of cases. Angiography performed after fibrinolytic therapy usually demonstrates residual high-grade stenotic lesions at the site where coronary arterial occlusion had existed. Fresh thrombi have been recovered from the majority of patients with acute myocardial infarction undergoing emergency coronary bypass surgery.[43]

It is now clear that a transmural MI is usually (in more than 90 per cent of cases) caused by coronary thrombosis, as postulated by early investigators.[34] It is still not clear whether and how often coronary spasm plays an important role in the pathophysiological sequence leading from coronary atherosclerosis to MI.[31a] Less frequently, perhaps in one-third to one-half of cases, coronary thrombosis is responsible for regional subendocardial infarction, i.e., in the distribution of a single coronary artery. Rarely, coronary thrombosis causes multifocal or circumferential infarction. The converse, however, is not often the case. It is well established that coronary thrombosis or acute coronary occlusion of any cause may not be associated with MI. The extent of coronary collaterals will determine whether acute coronary occlusion causes a transmural infarct (sparse collaterals), a subendocardial infarct (moderate collaterals), or no infarct (extensive collaterals).[12] However, coronary thrombosis is one—perhaps the most important, but not the only—cause of acute coronary occlusion; other causes include coronary spasm, as well as rupture of, or hemorrhage into, an atherosclerotic plaque. Alterations in platelet function and an imbalance of the

thromboxane A_2—prostacyclin system can play a role both in the development of coronary thrombosis and in coronary vasospasm.[12,26,45]

Nonatherosclerotic Causes of Acute Myocardial Infarction

Numerous pathological processes other than atherosclerosis can, on occasion, involve the coronary arteries and result in myocardial infarction (Table 37–1).[46] For example, coronary arterial occlusions can be the result of embolization of a coronary artery. Emboli most frequently lodge in the distribution of the left anterior descending coronary artery, commonly in the distal epicardial and intramural branches.[25] The causes of coronary embolism are numerous: infective and marantic endocarditis (Chap. 33), mural thrombi, prosthetic valves, and calcium deposits from manipulation of calcified valves at operation. In situ thrombosis of coronary arteries can occur secondary to chest-wall trauma (Chap. 44). Syphilitic aortitis may produce marked narrowing or occlusion of one or both coronary ostia,[47] whereas Takayasu's arteritis may result in obstruction of the coronary arteries (Chap. 48).[48] Necrotizing arteritis, polyarteritis nodosa, mucocutaneous lymph node syndrome (Kawasaki's disease) (p. 1053),[49,50] systemic lupus erythematosus,[51] and syphilis can cause coronary artery obstruction. Therapeutic levels of mediastinal radiation can cause thickening and hyalinization of the walls of coronary arteries, with subsequent infarction (p. 1690).[52] MI may also be the result of coronary arterial involvement in amyloidosis (Fig. 41–19, p. 1424), Hurler syndrome, pseudoxanthoma elasticum, and homocystinuria (Chap. 48).[53–55]

Involvement of the small coronary arteries (0.1 to 1.0 mm in diameter) by a number of disease processes may produce intimal and medial hyperplasia, necrosis, dissection, and thrombosis,[56] resulting in occlusions that produce *focal* areas of infarction and ultimately of fibrosis. Depending on the location and extent of the fibrotic reaction, arrhythmias, conduction defects, heart block, and heart failure can occur.

Myocardial Infarction with Angiographically Normal Coronary Vessels

Approximately 4 per cent of all patients with AMI and perhaps four times that percentage of patients with this diagnosis under the age of 35 years do not have coronary atherosclerosis demonstrated by coronary arteriography or at autopsy. Perhaps half the patients of this group, in turn, have a variety of other lesions involving the coronary vessels or myocardium (Table 37–1), whereas the others have no detectable coronary obstructive lesions.[57–60] Patients with AMI and normal coronary arteries tend to be young and to have relatively few coronary risk factors; usually they have no history of angina pectoris prior to the infarction.[58] The infarction in these patients is usually not preceded by any prodrome, but the clinical, laboratory, and electrocardiographic features of AMI are otherwise indistinguishable from those present in the overwhelming majority of patients with AMI who have classic obstructive atherosclerotic coronary artery disease.[61] In patients without coronary obstruction, the prognosis for survival of the

TABLE 37–1 SOME CAUSES OF MYOCARDIAL INFARCTION
WITHOUT CORONARY ATHEROSCLEROSIS

Coronary Artery Disease Other Than Atherosclerosis

Arteritis
  Luetic
  Granulomatous (Takayasu's disease)
  Polyarteritis nodosa
  Mucocutaneous lymph node (Kawasaki's) syndrome
  Disseminated lupus erythematosus
  Rheumatoid arthritis
  Ankylosing spondylitis
Trauma to coronary arteries
  Laceration
  Thrombosis
  Iatrogenic
Coronary mural thickening with metabolic diseases or intimal
    proliferative disease
  Mucopolysaccharidoses (Hurler's disease)
  Homocystinuria
  Fabry's disease
  Amyloidosis
  Juvenile intimal sclerosis
    (idiopathic arterial calcification of infancy)
  Intimal hyperplasia associated with contraceptive
    steroids or with the postpartum period
  Pseudoxanthoma elasticum
  Coronary fibrosis caused by radiation therapy
Luminal narrowing by other mechanisms
  Spasm of coronary arteries
    (Prinzmetal's angina with normal coronary arteries)
  Spasm after nitroglycerin withdrawal
  Dissection of the aorta
  Dissection of the coronary artery

Emboli to Coronary Arteries

Infective endocarditis
Prolapse of mitral valve
Mural thrombus from left atrium, left ventricle
Prosthetic valve emboli
Cardiac myxoma
Associated with cardiopulmonary bypass surgery and coronary
    arteriography
Paradoxical emboli
Papillary fibroelastoma of the aortic valve ("fixed embolus")

Congenital Coronary Artery Anomalies

Anomalous origin of left coronary from pulmonary artery
Left coronary artery from anterior sinus of Valsalva
Coronary arteriovenous and arteriocameral fistulae
Coronary artery aneurysms

Myocardial Oxygen Demand-Supply Disproportion

Aortic stenosis, all forms
Incomplete differentiation of the aortic valve
Aortic insufficiency
Carbon monoxide poisoning
Thyrotoxicosis
Prolonged hypotension

Hematological (in situ Thrombosis)

Polycythemia vera
Thrombocytosis
Disseminated intravascular coagulation
Hypercoagulability
Hypercoagulability, thrombosis, thrombocytopenic purpura

Miscellaneous

Myocardial contusion
Myocardial infarction with normal coronary arteries

Modified from Cheitlin, M., et al.: Myocardial infarction without atherosclerosis. J.A.M.A. *231*:951, 1975. Copyright 1975, American Medical Association.

acute event is usually excellent, but a few fatalities have occurred, and it has therefore been possible to document the presence of this syndrome at autopsy.[60,62] In 10 such patients, infarcts ranged from 5 to 33 per cent (mean of 18 per cent) of the left ventricle.[62] In patients who recover, areas of localized dyskinesis and hypokinesis can often be demonstrated by left ventricular angiography.

The long-term prognosis for patients who have survived an AMI with normal coronary vessels on arteriography appears to be substantially better than for patients with MI and obstructive coronary artery disease.[57-63] Following recovery from the initial infarct, recurrent infarction, heart failure, and death are unusual in patients with normal coronary arteries. Indeed, most of these individuals have normal exercise electrocardiograms,[64] and only a minority develop angina pectoris.

Numerous theories have been proposed to explain the occurrence of AMI in patients with normal coronary arteriograms. Suggested causes include coronary emboli, perhaps from a small mural thrombus, a prolapsed mitral valve[64a] (p. 1091), or a myxoma; coronary artery spasm;[65] coronary artery disease in vessels too small to be visualized by coronary arteriography or coronary arterial thrombosis with subsequent recanalization (Table 37–1); a variety of hematological disorders causing in situ thrombosis in the presence of normal coronary arteries,[60] such as polycythemia vera, sickle cell anemia, disseminated intravascular coagulation, thrombocytosis, and thrombotic thrombocytopenic purpura; augmented oxygen needs; hypotension secondary to sepsis, blood loss, or pharmacological agents; and anatomical changes, such as anomalous origin of a coronary artery and coronary arteriovenous fistula.[46,58,64-70] Eliot and coworkers examined the hearts of 10 patients who had died of a recent MI and in whom minimal or no coronary disease was present.[62] No thromboembolic material was seen in the coronary arterial tree despite the fact that the infarcts were only 2 days old in five patients and 3 or 4 days old in three others.

Collateral Circulation

Normal hearts contain an extensive network of interarterial anastomotic blood vessels, greater than 60 μm in diameter, involving epicardial, intramyocardial, and subendocardial connections. This collateral circulation exists at birth and apparently grows in size along with the rest of the coronary circulation but is beyond the limit of resolution of coronary arteriographic techniques and is not seen in living subjects without disease. In patients with coronary artery disease, these preexisting channels progressively enlarge, presumably as a consequence of the release of local vasodilators; flow through the collaterals will occur when pressure differences exist across these channels.[35,71-73] The coronary collateral circulation is particularly well developed in patients with (1) coronary occlusive disease, especially when it is severe, with the reduction of the luminal cross-sectional area by more than 75 per cent in one or more major vessels; (2) chronic hypoxia, as occurs in severe anemia, chronic obstructive pulmonary disease, and cyanotic congenital heart disease; and (3) left ventricular hypertrophy, which intensifies coronary collaterals.

There is considerable variability in the development of collateral channels that exists among patients with comparable degrees of coronary artery disease. Although the increases in the collateral circulation in patients with ischemic heart disease are due primarily to enlargement of already existing anastomoses, the possibility exists that new anastomotic channels are formed during the reparative phase following AMI. In animals, collateral development occurs rapidly after experimental coronary artery obstruction; Blumgart et al. noted maximum increases in collateral circulation in pigs 12 to 21 days after the production of severe coronary arterial stenoses,[73] whereas Gregg observed that a spontaneous and progressive increase in collateral blood flow was present 12 hours after coronary occlusion in dogs.[74] Eckstein noted marked increases in collateral circulation in dogs rendered anemic for 4 weeks.[72] The time course for development of collateral vessels in humans is not known. However, in an interesting case report of a 14-year-old boy who had suffered a traumatic right coronary arteriovenous fistula, collateral vessels were visible on a coronary angiogram 9 days later. Two weeks after repair of the fistula, angiographic evidence of collateral vessels was no longer evident.[75]

Collateral blood vessels are frequently noted on coronary arteriograms of patients with severe obstructive coronary vascular disease (p. 332). However, considerable debate has centered on the issue of whether collateral vessels are truly functional.[76] A number of angiographic studies have attempted to examine the functional state of these collateral vessels by quantifying left ventricular function in patients with and without evidence of collateral circulation. In several investigations, no differences in overall left ventricular performance were noted in patients with obstructive coronary artery disease, regardless of whether or not collateral vessels were present.[71,77,78] On the other hand, significantly better left ventricular function has been noted in regions of the left ventricle in the distribution of obstructed coronary vessels, supplied by collateral vessels, than in regions without collateral vessels,[79] and congestive heart failure and cardiomegaly have been reported to occur with greater frequency in patients with coronary artery disease who lack collateral vessels than in those patients who have them.[80] Also supporting the argument in favor of a functional role for coronary collateral vessels is the finding that in patients with coronary occlusion the area of myocardial necrosis is frequently smaller than the area supplied by the occluded coronary artery when collaterals are present. Indeed, it is rather common for patients with abundant collaterals to have totally occluded coronary arteries without evidence of infarction in the distribution of that coronary vessel; thus, the survival of the myocardium distal to such occlusions must be dependent on collateral blood flow.

Of interest also are reports on patients who suffered traumatic lacerations of the heart requiring ligation of the left anterior descending coronary artery but who did not develop clinical or, in one instance, postmortem evidence of myocardial necrosis.[81] Again, collateral circulation must have supplied sufficient blood flow to the myocardium distal to the ligation to have prevented MI. In addition, among patients with total coronary occlusion and AMI, the response of precordial ST-segment elevation to beta-adrenergic blockade is distinctly superior when collaterals enter the myocardium perfused by the occluded vessel.[82]

In conclusion, collateral coronary vessels, present from birth, frequently enlarge and may become functional in the presence of severe myocardial hypoxia or ischemia and following acute coronary occlusion and MI. Although blood flow through collaterals may be capable of contributing importantly to the maintenance of the resting energy requirements of the heart, and although the collaterals may limit infarct size in the face of total coronary occlusion and thereby contribute to patient survival, blood flow through collaterals is not sufficient to meet the needs of the myocardium when the latter are augmented by stress or to prevent myocardial necrosis in the majority of instances.[71]

Right Ventricular and Atrial Infarction

MI most commonly involves the left ventricle and interventricular septum; however, approximately one-third of patients with inferior infarction have some involvement of the right ventricle.[83–85,85a] Among these patients, right ventricular infarction occurs exclusively in those with transmural infarction of the inferoposterior wall and the posterior portion of the septum. The incidence of clinically significant right ventricular infarction is considerably lower than the incidence rate found at autopsy. Although right ventricular infarction almost invariably develops in association with infarction of the adjacent septum and left ventricular myocardium, *isolated* infarction of the right ventricle occurs in 3 to 5 per cent of autopsy-proved cases of myocardial infarction.

Right ventricular infarction, regardless of whether or not it is combined with involvement of the left ventricle, is generally associated with obstructive lesions of the right coronary artery. However, right ventricular infarction occurs less commonly than would be anticipated from the frequency of atherosclerotic lesions involving the right coronary artery.[86] This discrepancy can probably be explained by the lower oxygen demands of the right ventricle, since right ventricular infarcts occur more commonly in conditions associated with increased right ventricular oxygen needs.[87] Moreover, the intercoronary collateral system of the right ventricle is richer than that of the left, and the thinness of the right ventricular wall allows the chamber to derive some nutrition from blood within the right ventricular cavity. Rarely, a mural thrombus overlying a right ventricular infarct produces pulmonary embolism. Abnormal right ventricular wall motion, cavity dilatation, tricuspid regurgitation,[88] and cardiogenic shock with normal left but elevated right ventricular filling pressures have been documented in patients with infarction of the right ventricle.[83,84,86,89,89a]

Atrial infarction occurs in 7 to 17 per cent of autopsy-proved cases of myocardial infarction,[49,87,90–92] is often seen in conjunction with left ventricular infarction, can result in rupture of the atrial wall, and is more common on the right than the left side.[92] Infarcts occur more frequently in the atrial appendages than in the lateral or posterior walls of the atria. These differences in incidence might be explained by the considerably higher oxygen content of left atrial blood, which may nourish the thin atrial wall despite obstructive disease involving the coronary arterial system perfusing it. Since right atrial infarction is usually associated with obstructive disease of the sinus node artery, it is frequently accompanied by atrial arrhythmias.

Myocardial Rupture

RUPTURE OF THE FREE WALL (Table 37–2). Rupture of the free wall of the infarcted ventricle occurs in

TABLE 37–2   CLINICAL FEATURES OF CARDIAC RUPTURE

Factors Indicating Increased Risk of Cardiac Rupture

1. Recurrent chest pain without electrocardiographic changes suggestive of another infarct or extension
2. Sustained hypertension after myocardial infarction
3. First myocardial infarction; no or only recent history of angina
4. Less than 5 days since myocardial infarction
5. Patient 80 years or older

Signs and Symptoms Suggesting Cardiac Rupture

Terminal Signs

1. Pericardial blood and tamponade
2. Electromechanical dissociation
3. Failure of closed chest resuscitation to produce peripheral pulses

Preterminal Signs and Symptoms

1. Pericardial blood
2. Recurrent severe chest pain without evidence of new infarct
3. M-complex in electrocardiogram
4. Pericardial fluid on echocardiography

From Bates, R. J., et al.: Cardiac rupture—Challenge in diagnosis and management. Am. J. Cardiol. *40*:429, 1977.

up to 10 per cent of patients dying in the hospital of AMI. Thinness of the apical wall, marked intensity of necrosis at the terminal end of the blood supply, poor collateral flow, the shearing effect of muscular contraction against an inert and stiffened necrotic area, and aging of the myocardium with laceration in the myocardial microstructure have all been proposed as the local factors that lead to rupture.[93–95]

This serious complication of AMI

1. Occurs more frequently in women than in men with infarction and more frequently in the elderly;

2. Is more common in hypertensive than normotensive patients;[96]

3. Occurs approximately seven times more frequently in the left than the right ventricle and seldom occurs in the atria;

4. Usually involves the anterior or lateral walls of the ventricle in the area of the terminal distribution of the left anterior descending coronary artery;

5. Is usually associated with transmural infarction involving at least 20 per cent of the left ventricle;

6. Occurs between 1 day and 3 weeks, but most commonly 3 to 5 days, following the infarct;

7. Is usually preceded by infarct expansion, i.e., thinning and a disproportionate dilatation within the softened necrotic zone;[97]

8. Most commonly results from a distinct tear in the myocardial wall or a dissecting hematoma that perforates a necrotic area of myocardium (Fig. 37–4);

9. Usually occurs near the junction of the infarct and the normal muscle;

10. Occurs less frequently in the center of the infarct, but when rupture occurs here, it is usually during the second rather than the first week following the infarct;

11. Rarely occurs in a hypertrophied ventricle or in an area of excellent collateral vessels.[93]

Rupture of the free wall of the left ventricle usually leads to hemopericardium and immediate death from cardiac tamponade. Occasionally, rupture of the free wall of the ventricle occurs as the first clinical manifestation in patients with undetected or silent myocardial infarction, and then it may be considered a form of "sudden cardiac death" (Chap. 23).

RUPTURE OF HEART FOLLOWING
MYOCARDIAL INFARCTION

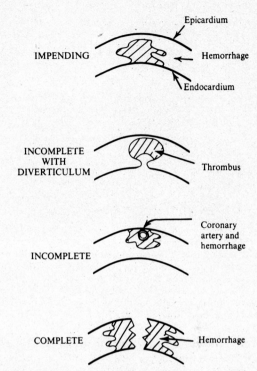

FIGURE 37–4   Range of complications that may follow an intramural hemorrhage in a patient with myocardial infarction. (From Datta, B. N., et al.: Incomplete rupture of the heart with diverticulum formation. Pathology *7*:179, 1975.)

Incomplete rupture of the heart may occur when organizing thrombus and hematoma, together with pericardium, seal a rupture of the left ventricle and thus prevent the development of hemopericardium (Figs. 37–5 and 37–6). With time, this area of organized thrombus and pericardium can become a small, left ventricular diverticulum or a large, false (pseudo) aneurysm which maintains communication with the cavity of the left ventricle.[98] In con-

LEFT VENTRICULAR ANEURYSM

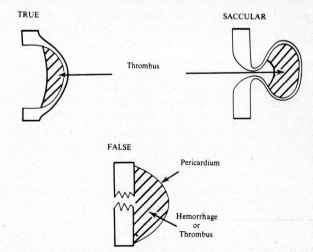

FIGURE 37–5   Appearance of aneurysms that may develop following myocardial infarction. (From Datta, B. N., et al.: Incomplete rupture of the heart with diverticulum formation. Pathology *7*:179, 1975.)

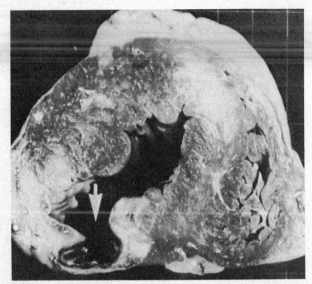

FIGURE 37–6 Heart slice showing incomplete rupture with diverticulum formation in the posterior wall of the left ventricle (arrow). Its lumen contains thrombus. Note scarring of the walls of the left ventricle. Coronary arteries have barium in their lumens. (From Datta, B. N., et al.: Incomplete rupture of the heart with diverticulum formation. Pathology 7:179, 1975.)

trast to true aneurysms, which always contain some myocardial elements in their walls, the walls of false aneurysms are composed of pericardium and organized hematoma and lack any elements of the original myocardial wall. False aneurysms can become quite large, even equaling the true ventricular cavity in size, and they communicate with the left ventricular cavity through a narrow neck. Frequently, false aneurysms contain significant amounts of old and recent thrombus, superficial portions of which can result in arterial emboli. False aneurysms can drain off a portion of each ventricular stroke volume just like true aneurysms. However, in contrast to true aneurysms, false aneurysms do have a tendency to rupture, even in late stages.[98]

RUPTURE OF THE INTERVENTRICULAR SEPTUM. Although rupture of the interventricular septum is said to be less common than rupture of the free wall,[93,96,99–101] our experience has been otherwise, perhaps because death usually is not immediate, and patients can reach a referral center where treatment of this complication is common. The perforation is usually single and ranges in length from one to several centimeters. The size of the defect determines the magnitude of the left-to-right shunt and the extent of hemodynamic deterioration, which in turn affects the likelihood of survival. As in rupture of the free wall of the ventricle, transmural infarction underlies rupture of the ventricular septum. Anterior and anterolateral myocardial infarctions are somewhat more common than inferior or inferolateral infarcts in patients with ventricular septal rupture.[99] Rupture of the septum with an anterior infarction tends to be apical in location, whereas inferior infarctions are associated with perforation of the basal septum.

RUPTURE OF PAPILLARY MUSCLES. Partial or total rupture of a papillary muscle is a rare but often fatal complication of transmural MI.[101a] Inferior wall infarction can lead to rupture of the posteromedial papillary muscle. This occurs more commonly than rupture of the anterolat-

eral muscle, a consequence of anterolateral MI; rupture of a right ventricular papillary muscle is rare but can cause massive tricuspid regurgitation and right ventricular failure. Complete transection of a left ventricular papillary muscle is incompatible with life because the sudden massive mitral regurgitation which develops cannot be tolerated.[102–104] Rupture of a portion of a papillary muscle which results in severe, though not necessarily overwhelming, mitral regurgitation is much more frequent (Fig. 32–9 and 32–10, p. 1077).

In a small number of patients, rupture of more than one cardiac structure is noted at postmortem examination; all possible combinations of rupture of the free left ventricular wall, the interventricular septum, and a papillary muscle have been described.[99]

ANEURYSM. A ventricular aneurysm, which is a circumscribed, noncontractile outpouching of the left ventricle, develops in 12 to 15 per cent of patients who survive a myocardial infarction.[105] The wall of the aneurysm is thin in comparison with the rest of the left ventricle (Fig. 37–5), and it is usually composed of fibrous tissue as well as necrotic muscle, occasionally mixed with viable myocardium.[106] Aneurysm formation presumably occurs when intraventricular tension stretches the noncontracting infarcted heart muscle, thus producing infarct expansion,[97,107] a relatively weak, thin layer of necrotic muscle, and fibrous tissue that bulges with each systole. With the passage of time, the wall of the aneurysm becomes more densely fibrotic, but it continues to bulge with systole, thus "stealing" some of the left ventricular stroke volume during each systole.[108]

Aneurysms range from 1 to 8 cm in diameter and usually involve the left ventricle.[105] They occur approximately four times more often at the apex and in the anterior wall than in the inferoposterior wall.[105] The overlying pericardium is usually densely adherent to the wall of the aneurysm, which may even become partially calcified after several years. Rarely, a true left ventricular aneurysm ruptures soon after its development. Late rupture, when the aneurysm has become stabilized by the formation of dense fibrous tissue in its wall, almost never occurs.[98,105]

Mural thrombosis is found at autopsy or operation in 15 to 77 per cent of left ventricular aneurysms. Approximately half the patients with mural thrombi at autopsy also have evidence of systemic emboli.[105,109,110]

CARDIOGENIC SHOCK (p. 591). This is the most severe and most commonly fatal complication of AMI. Page et al., who studied 20 such patients at autopsy, found that all exhibited necrosis of at least 40 per cent of the left ventricle. In contrast, 35 per cent or less of the left ventricle had been destroyed in all but 1 of 14 patients who succumbed without having been in cardiogenic shock.[111] Similar findings were reported by Alonso et al.: Patients with cardiogenic shock had lost an average of 51 per cent of the left ventricular myocardium (range: 35 to 68 per cent), whereas in a group of infarcted patients who died suddenly from arrhythmias and who had never been in cardiogenic shock, necrosis averaged 23 per cent (range: 14 to 31 per cent) of the left ventricle.[86] Patients with rupture of the ventricular septum or of a papillary muscle can also present with cardiogenic shock. These patients often have smaller infarcts than do those with cardiogenic shock sec-

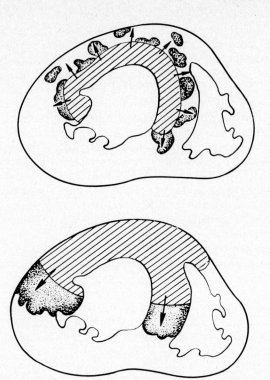

FIGURE 37–7 Two types of extension of myocardial infarction. Type A (top) was observed at the edges of an infarct, usually subepicardially. Type B (bottom) occurred at the lateral margins. (From Alonso, D. R., et al.: Pathophysiology of cardiogenic shock: Quantification of myocardial necrosis, clinical, pathologic and electrocardiographic correlation. Circulation *48*:588, 1973, by permission of the American Heart Association, Inc.)

ondary to ventricular failure without a mechanical lesion. The prognosis is better in such patients, since the smaller infarct allows their left ventricle to support the circulation once the mechanical defect has been corrected surgically.

At autopsy, patients with cardiogenic shock consistently demonstrate marginal extension of recent areas of infarction (Fig. 37–7).[111-114] Moreover, focal areas of necrosis are also frequently found in regions of the left and right ventricles that are not adjacent to the major area of recent infarction.[111] Such extensions and focal lesions are probably the result of the shock state itself, since they can also be found in the hearts of patients dying of noncardiogenic shock.

The shock state in patients with AMI would therefore appear to be the result of a vicious cycle, demonstrated in Figure 37–8. According to this formulation, coronary obstruction leads to myocardial ischemia which impairs myocardial contractility and ventricular performance; this, in turn, reduces arterial pressure and therefore coronary perfusion pressure, leading to further ischemia and extension of necrosis until the left ventricle has insufficient contracting myocardium to sustain life. Stasis in the smaller arteries and arterioles distal to a major proximal occlusion may result in secondary microvascular obstruction, further impairing myocardial perfusion. The progressive nature of the myocardial insult in this syndrome is reflected in the stuttering and progressive evolution of elevations in the plasma enzyme–time activity curves of markers specific for myocardial injury.[114]

At autopsy, more than two-thirds of patients with cardi-

ogenic shock demonstrate stenosis of 75 per cent or more of the luminal diameter of all three major coronary vessels, usually including the left anterior descending coronary artery.[115] Almost all patients with cardiogenic shock are found to have thrombosis of the artery supplying the major region of recent infarction.[111,112]

LEFT VENTRICULAR THROMBUS AND ARTERIAL EMBOLISM. Mural thrombi are common in patients succumbing to AMI.[115a] In one report, 44 per cent of 924 patients dying of AMI were found to have mural thrombi attached to the endocardium overlying the infarct;[116] thrombi are more common in patients with large than small infarcts and therefore are probably more frequently found in nonsurvivors than in survivors. They are almost universally located in the left ventricle, particularly at its apex; with extensive transmural infarction of the septum, however, mural thrombi may overlie infarcted myocardium in both ventricles. As noted earlier, mural thrombus in a ventricular aneurysm or pseudoaneurysm is rather common. Mural thrombi can be recognized pre mortem by two-dimensional echocardiography in approximately one-third of all patients with acute transmural anterior or apical infarctions (Figure 5–68, p. 127); they are extremely rare in patients with inferior-posterior infarcts.[110]

Although a mural thrombus adheres to the endocardium overlying the infarcted myocardium, superficial portions of it can become detached and produce systemic arterial emboli. In one study, systemic emboli were noted at autopsy in 10 per cent of 500 patients who died of acute myocardial infarction; half of the emboli were cerebral.[117] The other half usually lodged in the kidney or spleen or at the bifurcation of the aorta or iliac or femoral arteries; rarely, intestinal infarction results from embolization of the superior mesenteric artery. Occasionally, embolism from a mural

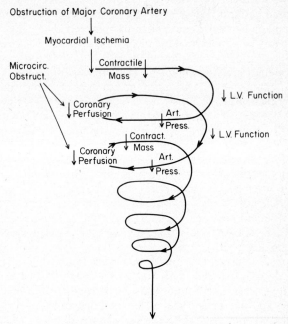

FIGURE 37–8 The sequence of events in the vicious cycle in which coronary artery obstruction leads to cardiogenic shock and progressive circulatory deterioration. (Reproduced with permission from Braunwald, E., and Alpert, J. S. *In* Petersdorf, R., et al. [eds.]: Harrison's Principles of Internal Medicine, New York, McGraw-Hill Book Co., 1983.)

thrombus is the presenting symptom, with the underlying myocardial infarction either silent or overlooked.

VENOUS THROMBOSIS AND EMBOLISM. Almost all pulmonary emboli originate from thrombi in the veins of the lower extremities (Chap. 46); much less commonly, they originate from mural thrombi overlying an area of infarction in the right atrium or ventricle. Bed rest and heart failure predispose to venous thrombosis and subsequent pulmonary embolism, and both of these factors occur commonly in patients with AMI, particularly those with large infarctions. In one autopsy study, major pulmonary emboli were present (though not always responsible for a fatal outcome) in 11 per cent of patients dying of AMI.[11]

Several decades ago, at a time when patients with AMI were subjected to prolonged periods of bed rest, significant pulmonary embolism was found in more than 20 per cent of patients with autopsy-proved myocardial infarction,[118] and massive pulmonary embolism accounted for 10 per cent of deaths from MI.[116] In recent years, with early mobilization and the widespread use of low-dose anticoagulant prophylaxis (Chap. 38), pulmonary embolism has become a rare cause of death in this condition.

PERICARDITIS (see also p. 1503).   Transmural myo-

cardial infarction, by definition, extends to the epicardial surface and is responsible for producing a local pericarditis in approximately 50 per cent of patients and diffuse, fibrinous, or serofibrinous pericarditis in about 15 per cent. This complication generally occurs between the second and fourth days following the infarction. In some patients with diffuse pericarditis, pericardial effusion may be large, but tamponade is rare. Occasionally, hemorrhagic effusion with cardiac tamponade develops in patients with post–myocardial infarction pericarditis who are treated with anticoagulants.[119]

Dressler's syndrome (p. 1513), or the *post–myocardial infarction syndrome*,[120,121] usually occurs 2 to 10 weeks after infarction. The incidence of this syndrome is difficult to define because it often blends imperceptibly with the more common early post–myocardial infarction pericarditis. At autopsy, patients with this syndrome usually demonstrate localized fibrinous pericarditis[122] containing polymorphonuclear leukocytes.[123] The post–myocardial infarction syndrome is probably the result of an autoimmune antibody response against certain pericardial and myocardial antigens exposed to the immune system at the time of infarction.[124]

PATHOPHYSIOLOGY OF
ACUTE MYOCARDIAL INFARCTION

SYSTOLIC VENTRICULAR FUNCTION. The fundamental pathological alteration underlying left ventricular dysfunction in AMI is loss of functioning segments of myocardium.[124a] Depression of cardiac function in myocardial infarction is directly related to the extent of left ventricular damage.[125,125a] Cessation of blood flow to a region of myocardium produces four sequential abnormal contraction patterns[126] (Figure 10–48, p. 339): (1) *dyssynchrony*, dissociation in the time course of contraction of adjacent segments of myocardial segments; (2) *hypokinesis*, reduction in the extent of shortening; (3) *akinesis*, cessation of shortening; and (4) *dyskinesis*, paradoxical expansion, systolic bulging.[108,127] If a sufficient amount of myocardium undergoes ischemic injury, left ventricular pump function becomes depressed, and cardiac output, stroke volume, blood pressure, and peak dp/dt are reduced.[125,127] The paradoxical systolic expansion of an area of ventricular myocardium decreases the stroke output of the left ventricle. With the passage of time, edema and cellular infiltration and ultimately fibrosis increase the stiffness of the infarcted myocardium back to and beyond control values.[128] Increasing stiffness in the infarcted zone of myocardium improves left ventricular function, since it prevents systolic paradoxical wall motion.

Areas with reduced and absent wall motion are universally seen in patients with transmural AMI. Rackley and collaborators have demonstrated a linear relationship between specific parameters of left ventricular function and clinical symptoms.[129] The earliest abnormality is a reduction in diastolic distensibility, which can be observed with infarcts that involve only 8 per cent of the total left ventricle on angiographic examination. When the abnormally contracting segment exceeds 10 per cent, the ejection fraction is reduced; with 15 per cent involvement, elevations of

left ventricular end-diastolic pressure and volume occur. Clinical heart failure accompanies areas of abnormal contraction exceeding 25 per cent, and cardiogenic shock, often fatal, accompanies loss of more than 40 per cent of the left ventricular myocardium.[129]

Unless extension of the infarct occurs, some improvement in abnormal wall motion takes place during the healing phase, as recovery of function occurs in initially reversibly injured myocardium. Regardless of the age of the infarct, patients who continue to demonstrate abnormal wall motion of 20 to 25 per cent of the left ventricle manifest hemodynamic signs of left ventricular failure.[130] Physical signs and symptoms of left ventricular failure also increase proportional to increasing areas of abnormal left ventricular wall motion.[127] These findings are of interest in view of the experimental work of Pfeffer et al., who produced infarcts of varying sizes and studied their left ventricular performance 3 weeks later.[125] Rats with relatively small infarcts (< 30 per cent of the left ventricle) had no detectable impairment of function; those with moderate-sized infarcts (31 to 46 per cent) exhibited normal baseline measurements but inadequate responses to hemodynamic stresses; rats with large infarcts (> 46 per cent) uniformly exhibited left ventricular failure. Patients with AMI often also show reduced myocardial contractile function in noninfarcted zones of myocardium.[131] This may result from obstruction of the coronary artery supplying this region of the ventricle, which is perfused by collaterals from the vessel that becomes occluded, a condition that has been termed *ischemia at a distance*.[132]

DIASTOLIC VENTRICULAR FUNCTION. As pointed out on page 1246, myocardial ischemia alters not only the systolic performance but also the diastolic characteristics of the left ventricle, ultimately raising its diastolic pressure at any given volume.[128,133-135] As outlined on page 1247, left ventricular diastolic properties are altered in infarcted and ischemic myocardium, leading initially to an increase but later to a reduction in left ventricular compliance. Patients who have recovered from an AMI frequently continue to manifest decreased left ventricular compliance secondary to the fibrous scar that remains in the left ventricle.

Pathophysiology of Left Ventricular Failure

In patients with AMI, heart failure is characterized by left ventricular diastolic and therefore pulmonary venous hypertension, leading to pulmonary congestion. The two mechanisms responsible for the pulmonary venous hypertension are (1) reduced ventricular diastolic compliance with resultant augmented resistance to left ventricular filling; and (2) reduced ventricular systolic function with resultant increases in end-diastolic volume and pressure. Both of these mechanisms are responsible for elevation of the left ventricular diastolic pressure, which is often associated with a depression of cardiac output. Clinical manifestations of both expressions of left ventricular failure become more common as the extent of the injury to the left ventricle increases.[129]

Cardiogenic Shock. The severest clinical expression of left ventricular failure, cardiogenic shock, is associated with extensive damage to the left ventricular myocardium.[111,112,112a] Patients who die as a consequence of cardiogenic shock often develop this complication of MI while in the hospital. These individuals often have a stepwise increase or progression of myocardial necrosis from marginal extension of their infarct in an ischemic zone bordering on the infarction.[136] Deterioration in left ventricular function secondary to apparent extension of infarction may, in some cases, result from *expansion* of the necrotic zone of myocardium without actual extension of the necrotic process.[137] Shearing forces that develop during ventricular systole can disrupt necrotic myocardial muscle bundles, with resultant expansion and thinning of the akinetic zone of myocardium, which in turn results in deterioration of overall left ventricular function.[138]

Alonso et al. described pathological evidence of marginal extensions of infarction in 18 of 22 patients dying of cardiogenic shock (Fig. 37-7).[112] Infarction of this ischemic periinfarction zone can be precipitated by a number of factors that adversely affect the supply of oxygen or the metabolic demand in the zone of myocardium, including a reduction of coronary perfusion pressure and an augmentation of myocardial oxygen demand resulting from the local release of catecholamines from ischemic adrenergic nerve endings in the heart as well as from circulating endogenous or infused catecholamines. Much recent work focuses on the development of strategies for limiting infarct size and prevention of infarct extension, thereby preventing the vicious downward spiral into irreversible cardiogenic shock (Fig. 37-8).[139] The experimental basis for these efforts is described on page 1255, and their clinical application is discussed on page 1318.

Swan, Forrester, and their associates have examined the cardiac output and wedge pressure together and have identified four major subsets of patients with AMI (Table 37-3): patients with normal perfusion and without pulmonary congestion (normal cardiac output and normal wedge pressure), patients with normal perfusion and pulmonary congestion (normal cardiac output and elevated wedge pressure), patients with decreased perfusion but without pulmonary congestion (reduced cardiac output and normal wedge pressure), and patients with decreased perfusion and pulmonary congestion (reduced cardiac output and elevated wedge pressure).[140] Although this classification is useful, it must be appreciated that patients frequently pass from one category to another with therapy and, sometimes, even apparently spontaneously.

The hemodynamic subsets of AMI usually reflect the clinical status of the patients.[141] Hypoperfusion usually becomes evident clinically when the cardiac index falls below approximately 2.2 liters/min/sq meter, whereas pulmonary congestion is noted when the wedge pressure exceeds approximately 20 mm Hg. However, approximately 25 per cent of patients with cardiac indices less than 2.2 liter/min/sq meter and 15 per cent of patients with elevated pulmonary capillary wedge pressures are not recognized clinically. Discrepancies in hemodynamic and clinical classification of patients with AMI arise for a variety of reasons. Patients may exhibit "phase lags" as clinical pulmonary congestion develops or resolves, symptoms secondary to chronic obstructive pulmonary disease may be confused with those resulting from pulmonary congestion, or longstanding left ventricular dysfunction may mask signs of hypoperfusion secondary to compensatory vasoconstriction.[140]

If the cardiac index is plotted as a function of the pulmonary capillary wedge pressure (a modified Starling relationship) in patients with AMI, a wide range of left ventricular performances is apparent (Fig. 37-9). It is clear from this figure that mortality in AMI increases in association with the severity of the hemodynamic deficit. In addition, one-third of patients with AMI have normal resting left ventricular hemodynamics.[140]

Certain patients present a hemodynamic pattern that is

TABLE 37-3 HEMODYNAMIC SUBSETS IN ACUTE MYOCARDIAL INFARCTION

CLINICAL SUBSET	CARDIAC INDEX (liter/min/sq meter)	PULMONARY CAPILLARY WEDGE PRESSURE (mm Hg)	MORTALITY (%)
I. No pulmonary congestion or peripheral hypoperfusion	2.7 ± 0.5	12 ± 7	2.2
II. Isolated pulmonary congestion	2.3 ± 0.4	23 ± 5	10.1
III. Isolated peripheral hypoperfusion	1.9 ± 0.4	12 ± 5	22.4
IV. Both pulmonary congestion and hypoperfusion	1.6 ± 0.6	27 ± 8	55.5

From Forrester, J. S., et al.: Medical therapy of acute myocardial infarction by application of hemodynamic subsets. N. Engl. J. Med. *295*:1404, 1976. Reprinted by permission.

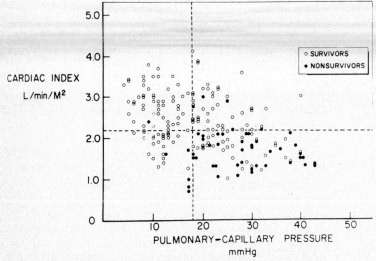

CARDIAC INDEX
L/min/M²

○ SURVIVORS
● NONSURVIVORS

PULMONARY-CAPILLARY PRESSURE
mmHg

FIGURE 37–9 Relation between pulmonary-capillary pressure and cardiac index in 200 patients with acute myocardial infarction. The dotted lines are placed at the levels of 18 mm Hg for pulmonary-capillary pressure and 2.1 liters per minute per square meter for cardiac index. There is a wide degree of variability in left ventricular performance in patients with acute myocardial infarction, and mortality rate increases as cardiac performance deteriorates. (Reproduced with permission from Forrester, J. S., et al.: Medical therapy of acute myocardial infarction by application of hemodynamic subsets. N. Engl. J. Med. *295*:1356, 1976.)

a variant of group 1 (normal or nearly normal pulmonary artery occlusive pressure and cardiac output).[141a] These patients exhibit a hyperkinetic state characterized by sinus tachycardia and hypertension in addition to normal wedge pressure and cardiac output. Presumably, the increased heart rate and blood pressure are the result of inappropriate activation of the sympathetic nervous system, possibly secondary to augmented release of catecholamines or anxiety or both. It is important to recognize this variant of group 1, since such individuals may benefit from therapy with beta-adrenergic blocking agents (p. 1321).

Physiological assessment of left ventricular function refines the information obtained by clinical means.[141] Among patients with AMI who are clinically uncomplicated (Killip Class I, p. 1280), approximately 50 per cent have a reduced cardiac output and 75 per cent have an elevated ventricular filling pressure. Patients with one or both of these hemodynamic abnormalities have a worse prognosis than those without any hemodynamic disturbance, even though they may be clinically uncomplicated.[141] Similarly, the prognosis of patients in Killip Class IV (cardiogenic shock) is a function of the hemodynamic status. Rackley et al. reported that in such patients a filling pressure greater than 29 mm Hg was associated with a mortality of 100 per cent; a filling pressure greater than 15 mm Hg and a cardiac index less than 2.0 liter/min/sq meter with a mortality of 93 per cent; and a filling pressure less than 15 mm Hg and a cardiac index less than 2.0 liters/min/sq meter with a mortality of 63 per cent.[141] Thus, it is clear that hemodynamics vary widely among patients with AMI having similar clinical presentations, and for this reason measurement of pertinent hemodynamic variables may be of great value in patients with complications.[142]

Classifications of patients with AMI by hemodynamic subsets has therapeutic relevance, as discussed in Chapter 38. For example, patients with normal wedge pressures and hypoperfusion often benefit from infusion of fluids, since the peak value of stroke volume is usually not attained until left ventricular filling pressure reaches 20 to 24 mm Hg.[141] However, a low level of left ventricular filling pressure does not imply that left ventricular damage is necessarily slight. Such patients may be relatively hypovolemic and/or may have suffered a right ventricular infarct with or without severe left ventricular damage.[143]

The relation between ventricular filling pressure and cardiac index with an increase in preload produced by an infusion of saline or dextran can provide valuable hemodynamic information, in addition to that obtained from baseline measurements. For example, the ventricular function curve rises steeply (marked increase in cardiac index, small increase in filling pressure) in patients with normal left ventricular function and hypovolemia, whereas the curve rises gradually or remains flat in those patients with a combination of hypovolemia and depressed cardiac function. The slope of the ventricular function curve, obtained 2 or 3 days following the infarction, correlates well with the ejection fraction determined 4 to 6 weeks later.[141]

HEMODYNAMIC FINDINGS IN RIGHT VENTRICULAR INFARCTION (Table 37–4). A characteristic hemodynamic pattern has been observed in patients

---

TABLE 37–4   FEATURES OF RIGHT VENTRICULAR INFARCTION

1. Inferior-posterior myocardial infarction
2. Clinical findings may include:
   A. Normal or depressed right ventricular function
   B. Shock
   C. Tricuspid regurgitation
   D. Ruptured ventricular septum
3. Hemodynamic measurements
   A. Abnormally elevated right atrial pressure
   B. Normal right ventricular and pulmonary artery systolic pressures
   C. Increased ratio of right ventricular to left ventricular filling pressure
   D. Depressed right ventricular function curve
4. Scintigraphy
   A. Uptake in right ventricular free wall
   B. Increased right ventricular dimensions and decreased wall motion
5. Echocardiography
   A. Increased right ventricular dimension
   B. Absence of pericardial effusion
6. Cardiac enzymes
   A. Increased magnitude of enzyme values to left ventricular dysfunction
7. Cardiac catheterization
   A. Involvement of right or left circumflex coronary arteries
   B. Right ventricular akinesis
8. Differential diagnosis
   A. Hypotension with acute myocardial infarction
   B. Pericardial tamponade
   C. Constrictive pericarditis
   D. Pulmonary embolus

Reproduced with permission from Rackley, C. E., Russell, R. O., Jr., Mantle, J. A., Rogers, W. J., Papapietro, S. E., and Schwartz, K. M.: Right ventricular infarction and function. Am. Heart J. *101*:215, 1981.

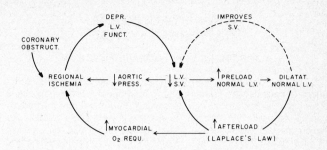

FIGURE 37–10 Changes in circulatory regulation in ischemic heart disease. DEPR. L.V. FUNCT., depressed left ventricular function; S.V., stroke volume; DILATAT., dilatation; O₂ REQU., oxygen requirements. Solid lines indicate that the effect is produced or intensified; broken lines indicate that it is diminished. (Reproduced with permission from Braunwald, E.: Regulation of the circulation. N. Engl. J. Med. *290*:1420, 1974.)

with right ventricular infarction[141b,141c] (which, as stated above, frequently accompanies inferior left ventricular infarction or less commonly occurs in isolated form): elevated right-heart filling pressures (central venous, right atrial, and right ventricular end-diastolic pressures) with normal or modestly elevated left ventricular filling pressures.[143] Right ventricular systolic and pulse pressures are decreased, and cardiac output is depressed. Many patients with the combination of normal left ventricular filling pressure and depressed cardiac index in fact have right ventricular infarcts (with accompanying inferior left ventricular infarcts). The hemodynamic picture may superficially resemble that seen in patients with pericardial disease (Chap. 42):[143] i.e., elevated right ventricular filling pressure; well-preserved, steep, right atrial *y* descent; and an early diastolic dip and plateau (square root sign) in the right ventricular pressure tracing. Moreover, Kussmaul's sign (inspiratory rise in mean right atrial pressure) and pulsus paradoxus (inspiratory fall > 10 mm Hg in systolic arterial blood pressure) may be present in patients with right ventricular infarction (Chap. 42). Echocardiography is helpful in the differential diagnosis,[89a] since in right ventricular infarction, in contrast to pericardial tamponade, no significant amounts of pericardial fluid are seen. Loss of atrial transport in patients with right ventricular infarction can result in marked decreases in stroke volume and arterial blood pressure.[144] The hemodynamic importance of right ventricular infarction in patients with inferior infarction is reflected in the observations of Marmor et al., who noted that although infarct size (reflected in CK release curves) was similar in patients with anterior and inferior infarcts, the former had more severe depression of the left ventricular ejection fraction and the latter had more severe depression of the right ventricular ejection fraction.[145]

CIRCULATORY REGULATION IN MYOCARDIAL INFARCTION

The abnormality in circulatory regulation that is present in AMI is diagrammed in Figure 37–10.[146] The process begins with an anatomical or functional obstruction in the coronary vascular bed, which results in regional myocardial ischemia and, if the ischemia persists, in infarction. If the infarct is of sufficient size, it depresses overall left ventricular function so that left ventricular stroke volume falls and filling pressures rise. The hemodynamic deterioration is more severe if an atrioventricular conduction disturbance develops or if mitral regurgitation or ventricular septal rupture occurs. A marked depression of left ventricular stroke volume ultimately lowers aortic pressure and reduces coronary perfusion pressure; this condition may intensify myocardial ischemia and thereby initiate the afore-

mentioned vicious cycle (see Fig. 37–9). The inability of the left ventricle to empty also leads to an increased preload—that is, it dilates the well-perfused, normally functioning portion of the left ventricle. This compensatory mechanism tends to restore stroke volume to normal levels. However, the dilatation of the left ventricle also elevates ventricular afterload, because Laplace's law dictates that at any given arterial pressure the dilated ventricle must develop a higher wall tension (p. 431). The increased afterload not only depresses left ventricular stroke volume but also elevates myocardial oxygen consumption, which in turn intensifies regional myocardial ischemia. When regional myocardial dysfunction is limited and the function of the remainder of the left ventricle is normal, compensatory mechanisms will sustain overall left ventricular function. If a large portion of the left ventricle becomes necrotic, pump failure occurs, i.e., overall left ventricular function becomes so depressed that the circulation cannot be sustained despite the dilatation of the remaining viable portion of the ventricle.

Some of the consequences of treating pump failure, discussed in Chapter 38, should be considered. The favorable effect of raising a depressed arterial pressure results from the increased coronary perfusion pressure and the subsequent augmented blood flow across the stenotic areas and through the collateral vessels. This improvement of coronary blood flow may limit the size of the infarction by improving oxygen delivery to the periinfarction zone. In this manner, myocardial fiber shortening may be augmented, thereby increasing stroke volume and cardiac output and elevating arterial pressure.

However, there are also some unfavorable effects of increasing arterial pressure because this intervention usually necessitates an elevation of left ventricular intracavitary pressure (unless it is achieved by a circulatory assist device, such as an intraaortic balloon). The increased afterload causes cardiac dilatation; intramyocardial tension rises, not only because of the higher intraventricular pressure but also because of the cardiac dilatation (p. 431). The increased wall tension augments myocardial oxygen needs and reduces myocardial fiber shortening (p. 1237). These changes can cause further ischemia of the marginally viable myocardium adjacent to that supplied exclusively by the occluded vessel. Thus, cardiac function may deteriorate further.

It is obvious that the circulation is delicately balanced in patients with AMI. Unless the loss of viable myocardium is so extensive that it precludes survival, or is so small that the patient's survival is not threatened, the outcome may well depend on the physician's appreciation of the interaction of the many factors that influence circulatory performance and their judicious manipulation.

PATHOPHYSIOLOGY OF OTHER ORGAN SYSTEMS

ALTERATIONS IN PULMONARY FUNCTION

Significant changes in the pulmonary function and arterial blood gases of patients with AMI are described in Chapter 54. Hypoxemia is a frequent consequence, with its severity, in general, proportional to that of left ventricular failure. Thus, there is an inverse relation between arterial oxygen tension and pulmonary artery diastolic pressure in patients with AMI (Figs. 37-11 and 54-7, p. 1788), suggesting that increased pulmonary capillary hydrostatic pressure leads to interstitial edema, which results in arteriolar and bronchiolar compression that ultimately causes perfusion of poorly ventilated alveoli with resultant hypoxemia.[147,148] In addition to hypoxemia, hyperventilation often occurs in patients with AMI and may cause hypocapnia and respiratory alkalosis, particularly in restless, anxious patients with pain. Intrapulmonary shunting of blood has been noted in patients in whom left ventricular failure complicates AMI. With improvement in heart failure, hypoxemia and intrapulmonary shunting diminish.

In patients with MI, particularly when complicated by left ventricular failure or cardiogenic shock, the affinity of hemoglobin for oxygen is reduced, i.e., the P_{50} is increased.[149,150] The increase in P_{50} results from increased levels of erythrocyte 2,3-diphosphoglycerate (2,3-DPG), is maximal after 24 hours, and constitutes an important compensatory mechanism, responsible for an estimated 18 per cent increase in oxygen release from oxyhemoglobin in patients with cardiogenic shock.[149]

With a double radioisotope indicator dilution technique, a positive correlation has been demonstrated between pulmonary extravascular (interstitial) water content, left ventricular filling pressure, and the clinical signs and symptoms of left ventricular failure.[147] Over a period of 2 to 4 days following AMI, both the pulmonary extravascular water content and the wedge pressure decline. Presumably the increased pulmonary extravascular water represents a transudate secondary to increased pulmonary capillary pressure.

The increase in pulmonary extravascular water may also be responsible for the alterations in pulmonary mechanics observed in patients with AMI, i.e., reductions of airway conductance, pulmonary compliance, forced expiratory volume and midexpiratory flow rate, and an increase in closing volume—the last presumably related to the widespread closure of small, dependent airways during the first 3 days following AMI.[151] Recovery of left ventricular function or diuresis reduces abnormally elevated values for closing volumes to normal. Presumably, competition for space between arteries and small airways in the bronchovascular sheath accounts for some of the eleva-

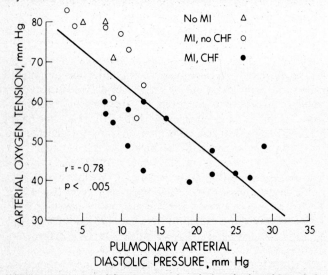

FIGURE 37-11 Arterial oxygen tension during the breathing of air, plotted in relation to pulmonary arterial diastolic pressure in patients with and without myocardial infarction (MI) and congestive heart failure (CHF). (From Fillmore, S. J., et al.: Blood-gas changes and pulmonary hemodynamics following acute myocardial infarction. Circulation 45:583, 1972, by permission of the American Heart Association, Inc.)

tion in airway resistance, particularly at left atrial pressures under 15 mm Hg. Higher left atrial pressures produce increases in airway resistance secondary to interstitial, alveolar, and peribronchial edema.

Increased pulmonary venous pressure also results in redistribution of pulmonary blood flow from the bases to the apices of the lung in patients with AMI,[152] altering the relationship between ventilation and perfusion (p. 1786). However, at follow-up examination 3 to 25 weeks after MI, the ventilation/perfusion relationship has usually returned to normal or almost so.

ALTERATIONS IN ENDOCRINE FUNCTION (Fig. 37-12)

Pancreas. Hyperglycemia and impaired glucose tolerance are common in patients with AMI. Although the absolute levels of blood insulin are often in the normal range in patients with uncomplicated AMI, they are usually inappropriately low for the level of blood sugar elevation, and there may be relative insulin resistance as well.[153] Patients with cardiogenic shock often demonstrate marked hyperglycemia and depressed levels of circulating insulin, often with complete suppression of insulin secretion in response to tolbutamide.[154] These abnormalities in insulin secretion and the resultant impaired glucose tolerance appear to be secondary to a reduction in pancreatic blood flow as a consequence of splanchnic vasoconstriction, which accompanies severe left ventricular failure. In addition, increased activity of the sympathetic nervous system with augmented circulating catecholamines[155] inhibits insulin secretion[156,157] and augments glycogenolysis, also contributing to the elevation of blood sugar.[158]

Since hypoxic heart muscle derives a considerable portion of its energy from the metabolism of glucose (Chap. 36), and since insulin is essential for the uptake of glucose by the myocardium as well as for myocardial protein synthesis and inhibition of lysosomal activity, the deleterious effects of insulin deficiency are clear.[159]

Adrenal Gland. Excessive secretion of catecholamines produces many of the characteristic signs and symptoms of AMI. The plasma and urinary catecholamine levels are highest during the first 24 hours after the onset of chest pain,[158] with the greatest rise in plasma catecholamine secretion occurring during the first hour after the onset of MI,[160] when it may be in the range observed in racing car drivers immediately upon completion of a race.[161] These high levels of circulating catecholamines in patients with AMI correlate with the occurrence of serious arrhythmias[157,162-164] and result in the stimulation of myocardial oxygen consumption, both directly and indirectly, as a consequence of catecholamine-induced elevation of circulating free fatty acids.[160] As might be anticipated, the concentration of circulating catecholamines correlates with both the incidence of cardiogenic shock and the mortality rate.[157] Circulating catecholamines enhance platelet aggregation; when this occurs in the coronary microcirculation, the release of the potent vasoconstrictor thromboxane A_2 may further impair cardiac perfusion.[158]

Plasma and urinary 17-hydroxycorticosteroids and ketosteroids, as well as aldosterone, are also markedly elevated in patients with AMI.[158,165,166] Their concentrations correlate directly with the peak level of serum glutamic oxaloacetic transaminase, implying that the stress imposed by larger infarcts is associated with greater secretion of adrenal steroids. Glucocorticosteroids also contribute to the impairment of glucose tolerance; although it has been suggested that the secretion of glucocorticoids is increased, it is inadequate to meet the demands for the stress imposed by a massive AMI, particularly if it is accompanied by cardiogenic shock.[158]

Hematological Function (see also p. 1699). AMI generally occurs in the presence of extensive coronary and systemic atherosclerotic plaques, which may serve as the site for the formation of platelet aggregates, a sequence which has been suggested as the initial step in the process of coronary thrombosis, coronary occlusion, and subsequent MI. Approximately one-third of patients with AMI demonstrate shortened platelet survival times.[167] Types III and IV hyperlipoproteinemia, frequently present in patients with AMI, can also be responsible for shortening platelet survival. Findings suggestive of a hypercoagulable state as a risk factor for AMI are discussed on page 1695.

Elevated levels of serum fibrinogen degradation products, an end product of thrombosis[168]—as well as release of distinctive proteins when platelets are activated, i.e., platelet factor 4[169]—have been reported in some patients with AMI. The interpretation of the coagulation tests in patients with AMI may be complicated by elevated blood levels of catecholamines, concomitant shock, and/or pulmonary em-

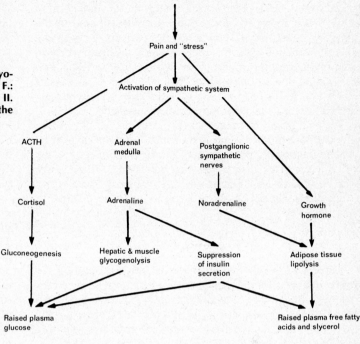

FIGURE 37–12 Principal hormonal and metabolic effects of myocardial infarction. (Reproduced with permission from Oliver, M. F.: Metabolic response during impending myocardial infarction. II. Clinical implications. Circulation *45*:491, 1972 by permission of the American Heart Association, Inc.)

bolism, conditions which are all capable of altering various tests of platelet and coagulation function.[170] Thus, it is not yet clear whether the above-mentioned changes are the causes or consequences of AMI.

An elevation of *blood viscosity* also occurs in patients with AMI.[171] During the first few days after infarction, this is mainly attributable to hemoconcentration, but later the increases in plasma viscosity and red cell aggregation correlate with elevated serum concentrations of alpha$_2$ globulin and fibrinogen, which are nonspecific reactions to tis-

sue necrosis and which are also responsible for the elevated sedimentation rate characteristic of AMI.[172] The high values of blood viscosity are observed most frequently in patients with complications, such as left ventricular failure, cardiogenic shock, and thromboembolism.

Alterations in Renal Function. Both prerenal azotemia and acute renal failure can complicate the marked reduction of cardiac output that occurs in cardiogenic shock. These conditions are discussed on pages 587 and 1752.

CLINICAL FEATURES OF ACUTE MYOCARDIAL INFARCTION

PRECIPITATING FACTORS

In most patients with AMI, no precipitating factor can be identified. An early study noted the following patient activities at the onset of AMI: heavy physical exertion, 13 per cent; modest or usual exertion, 18 per cent; surgical procedure, 6 per cent; rest, 51 per cent; and sleep, 8 per cent.[173] Another study showed similar results except that only 2 per cent of patients experienced MI during heavy physical exertion.[174] Others, however, have reported that a significant number of AMI's occur within a few hours of severe physical exertion.[175,176] It has been pointed out that the *severe exertion* which preceded an infarction was often performed at times when the patient was unduly fatigued or emotionally stressed.[177] Thus, although adequate control studies have not been carried out, there is suggestive evidence that heavy exercise may play a precipitating role in some patients. Such infarctions are presumably the result of marked increases in myocardial oxygen consumption in the presence of severe coronary arterial narrowing. Supporting this hypothesis is the finding that fatal MI occur-

ring during heavy exertion is often associated with severe coronary arterial narrowing but no occlusion.[176]

Surgical procedures associated with acute blood loss have also been noted as frequent precursors of MI (p. 1818). Reduced myocardial perfusion secondary to hypotension and increased myocardial oxygen demands secondary to fever, tachycardia, and agitation are presumably responsible for the myocardial necrosis. Other factors reported as predisposing to MI include respiratory infections, hypoxemia of any cause, pulmonary embolism, hypoglycemia, administration of ergot preparations, serum sickness, allergy, and wasp stings.[178–181] In patients with Prinzmetal's angina (p. 1360), MI may develop in the territory of the coronary artery, which repeatedly undergoes spasm. Rarely, munition workers exposed to high concentrations of nitroglycerin may develop myocardial infarction when they are withdrawn from this exposure, suggesting that it is caused by vasospasm.[182] Unstable angina (accelerating angina) and rest angina (p. 1355) may culminate as infarction of the myocardium, again in the distribution of the affected vessel.[183]

Considerable evidence has accumulated that *emotional stresses* may be a precipitating factor in the initiation of AMI.[184] A number of reports have documented that upsetting life events occur commonly in patients who subsequently suffer an MI (p. 1827).[185] Such events have been quantified and scored as *Life Change Units*. Rahe and coworkers noted, on retrospective analysis, a significant buildup in Life Change Units in patients who subsequently suffered myocardial infarction or died suddenly.

Trauma may precipitate an AMI in one of two ways. Myocardial contusion and hemorrhage into the myocardium may actually cause cell necrosis, or the injury may involve a coronary artery, causing occlusion of that vessel with resultant MI (Chap. 44). *Neurological disturbances* (transient ischemic attacks or strokes) may also precipitate AMI.[186]

HISTORY

Despite recent advances in the laboratory detection of AMI, the history remains of substantial value in establishing a diagnosis. A *prodromal history* can be elicited in 20 to 60 per cent of patients with AMI.[186,187] The prodrome is usually characterized by chest discomfort, resembling classic angina pectoris (described on pp. 5 and 1355), but it occurs at rest or with less activity than usual and can therefore be classified as unstable angina (p. 1355). However, the latter is often not disturbing enough to induce the patient to seek medical attention, and if he does, he is not usually hospitalized. Among patients who are hospitalized for unstable angina, fewer than 15 per cent develop AMI (p. 1359).

The pain of AMI is variable in intensity; in most patients it is severe and, in some instances, intolerable. The pain is prolonged, usually lasting for more than 30 minutes and frequently for a number of hours. The discomfort is described as constricting, crushing, oppressing, or compressing; often the patient complains of something sitting on or squeezing the chest. Although usually described as a squeezing, choking, viselike, or heavy pain, it may also be characterized as a stabbing, knifelike, boring, or burning discomfort. The pain is usually retrosternal in location, spreading frequently to both sides of the anterior chest, with predilection for the left side. Often the pain radiates down the ulnar aspect of the left arm, producing a tingling sensation in the left wrist, hand, and even fingers. Some patients note only a dull ache or numbness of the wrists in association with severe substernal or precordial discomfort. In some instances, the pain of AMI may begin in the epigastrium and simulate a variety of abdominal disorders, a fact which often causes MI to be misdiagnosed as "indigestion." In other patients the discomfort of AMI radiates to the shoulders, upper extremities, neck, jaw, and interscapular region, again usually favoring the left side. In patients with preexisting angina pectoris, the pain of infarction usually resembles that of angina with respect to quality and location. However, it is generally much more severe, lasts longer, and is not relieved by rest and nitroglycerin.

In some patients, particularly the elderly, AMI is manifest clinically not by chest pain but rather by symptoms of acute left ventricular failure and chest tightness or by overwhelming weakness, accompanied by diaphoresis, nausea, vomiting, and diarrhea.[186] The pain of AMI may have disappeared by the time the physician first encounters the patient (or the patient reaches the hospital), or it may persist for many hours. Opiates—in particular, morphine—usually relieve the pain, although a persistent soreness, pressure, or dull ache may remain for several hours or more despite intensive treatment with analgesics. Both angina pectoris and the pain of AMI are thought to arise from nerve endings in ischemic or injured, but not necrotic, myocardium.[188] Thus, in MI, stimulation of nerve fibers in an ischemic zone of myocardium surrounding the necrotic central area of infarction probably gives rise to the pain.

The pain of AMI may simulate the pain of *acute pericarditis*, which is usually associated with some pleuritic features, i.e., it is aggravated by respiratory movements and coughing and often involves the shoulder, ridge of the trapezius, and neck. *Pleural pain* is usually sharp, knifelike, and aggravated by each breath, which distinguishes it from the deep, dull, steady pain of AMI. *Pulmonary embolism* (Chap. 46) generally produces pain laterally in the chest, is often pleuritic in nature, and may be associated with hemoptysis. The pain due to *acute dissection of the aorta* (Chap. 45) is usually localized in the center of the chest, is extremely severe, persists for many hours, and often radiates to the lower back and sometimes into the legs. Often one or more major arterial pulses are absent. Pain arising from the *costochondral and chondrosternal articulations* may be associated with localized swelling and redness; it is usually sharp and "darting" and is characterized by marked localized tenderness.

Nausea and vomiting occur frequently in patients with AMI and severe chest pain, presumably owing to activation of a vagal reflex. These occur more commonly in patients with inferior MI than in those with anterior MI. Occasionally a patient complains of diarrhea or a violent urge to evacuate the bowels during the acute phase of MI. Moreover, nausea and vomiting are common side effects of opiates. When the pain of AMI is epigastric in location and is associated with nausea and vomiting, the clinical picture may easily be confused with that of acute cholecystitis, gastritis, or peptic ulcer. Other symptoms include feelings of profound weakness, dizziness, palpitations, cold perspiration, and a sense of impending doom. On occasion, symptoms arising from an episode of cerebral embolism or other systemic arterial embolism are the first signs of an AMI. Rarely, patients with inferior infarction report intractable hiccupping, a finding which has been attributed to diaphragmatic irritation by the infarct.[189] The aforementioned symptoms may or may not be accompanied by chest pain.[190]

Approximately one-quarter of nonfatal MI are unrecognized by the patient and are discovered only on subsequent routine electrocardiographic[191,192] or postmortem examinations. Of these unrecognized infarctions, approximately half are truly silent, with the patients unable to recall any symptoms whatsoever referable to the infarction. The other half of patients with so-called silent infarction can recall an event characterized by symptoms compatible with acute infarction when leading questions are posed after the abnormal electrocardiogram is discovered. Unrecognized or silent infarction rarely occurs in patients with antecedent angina pectoris, and it is more common in patients with diabetes and hypertension.

In an analysis of atypical presentations of AMI, Bean[193] lists the following: (1) congestive heart failure—beginning de novo or worsening of established failure; (2) classic angina pectoris without a particularly severe or prolonged attack; (3) atypical location of the pain; (4) central nervous system manifestations, resembling those of stroke, secondary to a sharp reduction in cardiac output in a patient with cerebral arteriosclerosis; (5) apprehension and nervousness; (6) sudden mania or psychosis; (7) syncope; (8) overwhelming weakness; (9) acute indigestion; and (10) peripheral embolism.

Pericarditis secondary to transmural AMI (p. 1503) may produce pain as early as the first day and as late as 6 weeks after MI and may be confused with pain resulting from persistent ischemia or extension of the infarct or both. Although transitory pericardial friction rubs are very common among patients with transmural infarction within the first 48 hours, the pain or electrocardiographic changes occur much less often. The discomfort of pericarditis usually becomes worse during a deep inspiration, but it may be somewhat relieved when the patient sits up and leans forward (Chap. 43).

Angina developing within the first 10 days following AMI is disconcerting to patients and physicians alike. In most patients, it responds to rest, nitroglycerin, beta-adrenergic blockade, and calcium channel antagonists,[194] just as does classic angina. In a minority of patients, postinfarction angina may be refractory to treatment and is provoked by minimal activity, meals, or emotional upset. When accompanied by ST-T–wave changes in the same area where Q waves have appeared, it is probably due to coronary spasm.[195,196]

It is frequently difficult to distinguish postinfarction angina from infarct extension. The latter is usually associated with more severe and prolonged discomfort, *persistent* electrocardiographic changes (ST-T changes or QRS changes or both), and reelevation of serum enzymes.

PHYSICAL EXAMINATION

GENERAL APPEARANCE. Patients suffering an AMI usually appear anxious and in considerable distress. An anguished facial expression is common, and—in contrast to patients with angina pectoris, who often lie, sit, or stand quite still, realizing that all forms of activity increase the discomfort—patients suffering an AMI are often restless and move about in an effort to find a comfortable position. They may massage or clutch their chests and frequently describe their pain with a clenched fist held against the sternum (a sign of ischemic pain popularized by Dr. Samuel A. Levine). In patients with left ventricular failure and sympathetic stimulation, cold perspiration and skin pallor may be evident; they usually sit or are propped up in bed, gasping for breath. Between breaths, they may complain of chest discomfort or a feeling of suffocation. Cough productive of frothy, pink, or blood-streaked sputum is common.

Patients in cardiogenic shock often lie listlessly, making few, if any, spontaneous movements. The skin is cool and clammy, with a bluish or mottled color over the extremities, and there is marked facial pallor with severe cyanosis of the lips and nailbeds. Depending on the degree of cerebral perfusion, the patient in shock may converse normally or may evidence confusion and disorientation.

VITAL SIGNS. The heart rate may vary from a marked bradycardia to rapid regular or irregular tachycardia, depending on the underlying rhythm and the degree of left ventricular failure. Most commonly, the pulse is rapid and regular initially (sinus tachycardia at 100 to 110 beats/min), slowing as the patient's pain and anxiety are relieved; premature ventricular beats are common, occurring in more than 95 per cent of patients evaluated early after the onset of symptoms.

The majority of patients with uncomplicated AMI are normotensive, although the reduced stroke volume accompanying the tachycardia may cause a small decline in systolic pressure and an elevation of diastolic pressure. In a minority of previously normotensive patients, a hypertensive response occurs, with the arterial pressure exceeding 160/90 mm Hg, presumably as a consequence of adrenergic discharge secondary to pain and agitation. The arterial pressure rarely exceeds 200/110 mm Hg. It is rather common for previously hypertensive patients to become normotensive without treatment following AMI, although approximately two-thirds of these previously hypertensive patients eventually regain their elevated levels of blood pressure, generally 3 to 6 months after infarction. In patients with massive infarcts, arterial pressure falls acutely, owing to left ventricular dysfunction and venous pooling secondary to administration of morphine or nitrates or both; as recovery occurs, the arterial pressure tends to return to preinfarction levels. Patients in cardiogenic shock (p. 591), by definition, have systolic pressures below 90 mm Hg. However, hypotension does not necessarily signify cardiogenic shock, since some patients with inferior infarction, in whom the Bezold-Jarisch reflex is activated, may also have systolic blood pressure below 90 mm Hg.[197,198] These patients do not demonstrate peripheral manifestations of hypoperfusion; their prognosis is generally good and their hypotension eventually resolves spontaneously, although this resolution can be accelerated by atropine and assumption of the Trendelenburg position. Other patients who are initially only slightly hypotensive may demonstrate gradually falling blood pressures with progressive reduction in cardiac output over several days as they gradually develop cardiogenic shock as a consequence of increasing ischemia and extension of infarction (Fig. 37–8).

Most patients with AMI develop *fever*, a nonspecific response to tissue necrosis, within 24 to 48 hours of the onset of infarction. Body temperature often begins to rise within 4 to 8 hours after the onset of infarction, and rectal temperature often reaches 101 to 102° F. Fever usually resolves by the seventh or eighth day following infarction.

The *respiratory rate* may be slightly elevated soon after the development of an AMI; in patients without heart failure, it results from anxiety and pain, since it returns to normal with treatment of physical and psychological discomfort. In patients with left ventricular failure, the respiratory rate correlates with the severity of failure; patients with pulmonary edema may have respiratory rates exceeding 40 per minute. However, the respiratory rate is not necessarily elevated in patients with cardiogenic shock.

Cheyne-Stokes (periodic) respiration (p. 449) may occur in elderly individuals with cardiogenic shock and heart failure, particularly after opiate therapy and in the presence of cerebrovascular disease.

THE FUNDI.   Hypertension, diabetes, and generalized atherosclerosis commonly accompany AMI, and since these conditions may produce characteristic changes in the fundus, a careful funduscopic examination may provide information concerning the underlying vascular status; this is particularly useful in patients unable to provide a detailed history.

JUGULAR VENOUS PULSE.   The height and contour of the jugular venous pulse reflect right atrial and right ventricular diastolic pressures (p. 20). Since these pressures are usually normal or only slightly elevated in patients with AMI (even in the presence of mild to moderate left ventricular failure), it is not surprising that the jugular venous pulse does not appear to be abnormal. The *a* wave may be prominent in patients with pulmonary hypertension secondary to left ventricular failure or reduced compliance.[199] In contrast, right ventricular infarction (whether or not it accompanies left ventricular infarction) often results in marked jugular venous distention and, when it is complicated by necrosis of right ventricular papillary muscles, tall *v* waves of tricuspid regurgitation are evident. In patients with AMI and cardiogenic shock, the jugular venous pressure is usually elevated. In patients with AMI, hypotension, and hypoperfusion, who may specifically resemble those with cardiogenic shock but who have flat neck veins, it is likely that the depression of left ventricular performance may be related, at least in part, to hypovolemia, but the differentiation can be made only by assessing left ventricular performance.

CAROTID PULSE.   Palpation of the carotid arterial pulse provides a clue to the left ventricular stroke volume; a small pulse suggests a reduced stroke volume, whereas a sharp, brief upstroke is often observed in patients with mitral regurgitation or ruptured ventricular septum with a left-to-right shunt. Pulsus alternans reflects severe left ventricular dysfunction.

THE CHEST.   Moist rales are audible in patients who develop left ventricular failure and/or a reduction of left ventricular compliance after AMI. As noted, the prognosis is related to the fraction of the lung field over which rales are heard (Table 37–5). Diffuse wheezing may be present in patients with severe left ventricular failure. Cough with hemoptysis, suggesting pulmonary embolism with infarction, may also occur.

THE HEART.   Despite severe symptoms and extensive myocardial damage, the findings on examination of the heart may be surprisingly unremarkable in patients with AMI. Palpation of the precordium may yield normal findings but more commonly reveals a presystolic pulsation, synchronous with an audible fourth heart sound, reflecting a vigorous left atrial contraction filling a ventricle with reduced compliance. In the presence of left ventricular systolic dysfunction, an outward movement of the left ventricle may be palpated in early diastole, coincident with a third heart sound. When the anterior or lateral portion of the ventricle is dyskinetic, an abnormal systolic pulsation is present in the third, fourth, or fifth interspaces to the left of the sternum. In some patients, this abnormal paradoxical precordial impulse is clearly separable from the point of maximal impulse, which is more lateral and to the left. In other patients, the abnormal impulse is a diffuse, rippling, precordial movement, approximately 5 to 10 cm in diameter, not clearly separable from the point of maximal impulse. Patients with longstanding hypertension or previous infarction with left ventricular hypertrophy often demonstrate a laterally displaced, sustained point of maximum impulse.

Auscultation.   The heart sounds, particularly the first sound, are frequently muffled[200] and occasionally inaudible immediately after the infarct, and their intensity increases as healing occurs.[201] A soft first sound may also reflect prolongation of the P-R interval. Patients with marked ventricular dysfunction or left bundle branch block may have paradoxical splitting of the second heart sound (p. 47). Individuals with postinfarction angina also may develop transient, paradoxically split second heart sounds during anginal episodes because of prolongation of the left ventricular preejection period.

A *fourth heart sound* is almost universally present in patients with AMI and is usually best heard between the left sternal border and the apex. This sound reflects a reduction in left ventricular compliance (p. 51) and is associated with an elevation of left ventricular end-diastolic pressure, even in the absence of left ventricular systolic dysfunction. It is of little diagnostic value, since it is commonly audible in most patients with chronic ischemic heart disease as well as in many normal subjects older than 45 years.

A *third heart sound* reflects extensive left ventricular

TABLE 37–5   KILLIP CLASSIFICATION OF PATIENTS WITH ACUTE MYOCARDIAL INFARCTION

	DEFINITION	PATIENTS WITH ACUTE MYOCARDIAL INFARCTION ADMITTED TO CCU IN THIS CATEGORY (%)	APPROXIMATE MORTALITY (%)
Class I	Absence of rales over the lung fields and absence of S3	30–40	8
Class II	Rales over 50 per cent or less of the lung fields or the presence of an S3	30–50	30
Class III	Rales over more than 50 per cent of the lung fields (frequently pulmonary edema)	5–10	44
Class IV	Shock	10	80–100

Adapted from Killip, T., and Kimball, J. T.: Treatment of myocardial infarction in a coronary care unit. A two year experience with 250 patients. Am. J. Cardiol. *20*:457, 1967.

dysfunction. It is usually heard in patients with large infarctions. This sound is heard best at the apex, with the patient in the left lateral recumbent position, and is more common in patients with transmural anterior infarctions than in those with inferior or nontransmural infarctions[202]; patients with a third heart sound often have elevated left ventricular filling pressure. The mortality of patients who manifest a third heart sound during the acute phase of MI is 40 per cent, contrasted with 15 per cent for patients without such a sound.[202] A third sound may be caused not only by left ventricular failure but also by increased inflow into the left ventricle, as occurs in mitral regurgitation or ventricular septal defect. Third and fourth heart sounds emanating from the left ventricle are heard best at the apex; in patients with right ventricular infarcts that originate from this chamber, these sounds may be heard along the left sternal border and are intensified by inspiration.

Systolic murmurs, transient or persistent, are commonly audible in patients with AMI and generally result from mitral regurgitation secondary to papillary muscle dysfunction. A new, prominent holosystolic murmur at the apex, accompanied by a thrill, may represent rupture of a head of a papillary muscle (p. 1076); the findings in rupture of the interventricular septum are similar, although the murmur and thrill are usually most prominent along the left sternal border. The systolic murmur of tricuspid regurgitation (caused by right ventricular failure due to pulmonary hypertension or right ventricular infarction or by infarction of a right ventricular papillary muscle) is also heard along the left sternal border but is characteristically intensified by inspiration and is accompanied by a prominent *v* wave in the jugular venous pulse. In evaluating systolic murmurs in patients with chest pain, it is important to note that aortic stenosis is a common cause of ischemic pain (p. 1099) and that, like coronary artery disease, it occurs most commonly in middle-aged and elderly men. Therefore, the diagnosis of aortic stenosis should be considered in patients suspected of having suffered an MI who have a systolic murmur at the base of the heart. Rarely, *diastolic murmurs* are produced by blood flowing through a severe coronary arterial stenosis.

Pericardial friction rubs are audible in up to 20 per cent of patients with AMI and in a high percentage of patients with transmural infarcts.[203] Rubs are notorious for their evanescence and, hence, are probably even more common than reported; frequent auscultation in patients with transmural infarction often results in the discovery of a rub which might otherwise have gone unnoticed. Although friction rubs may be heard by 24 hours or as late as 2 weeks after the onset of infarction, most commonly they are noted on the second or third day. Occasionally, in patients with extensive infarction, a loud rub may be heard for many days. Delayed onset of the rub and the associated discomfort of pericarditis (as late as three months postinfarction) are characteristic of the postmyocardial infarction syndrome (p. 1514).[120-124]

Pericardial rubs are most readily audible along the left sternal border or just inside the point of maximal impulse and occur after either anterior or inferoposterior transmural infarction. Loud rubs may be audible over the entire precordium and even over the back. Occasionally, only the systolic portion of a rub is heard; it may be confused with

a systolic murmur, and the diagnosis of rupture of the ventricular septum or mitral regurgitation may be considered. The presence of a pericardial friction rub does not exclude the presence of a significant pericardial effusion.

THE ABDOMEN. As noted above, in patients with AMI (particularly inferior infarcts) with diaphragmatic irritation, the pain may localize in the epigastrium or the right upper quadrant. Pain in the abdomen associated with nausea, vomiting, restlessness, and even abdominal distention is often interpreted by patients as a sign of "indigestion,"[193] resulting in self-medication with antacids, and it may suggest an acute abdominal process to the physician. A normal abdominal examination aids in ruling this out and in pointing to the correct diagnosis. Right heart failure, characterized by hepatomegaly and a positive abdominojugular reflux, is unusual in patients with acute left ventricular infarction but does occur in patients with severe and usually prolonged left ventricular failure or right ventricular infarction.

THE EXTREMITIES. Coronary atherosclerosis is often associated with systemic atherosclerosis, and it is therefore common for patients with AMI to have a history of intermittent claudication and to demonstrate physical findings of peripheral vascular disease. Thus, diminished peripheral arterial pulses, loss of hair, and atrophic skin in the lower extremities are frequently noted in patients with coronary artery disease. Peripheral edema is a manifestation of right ventricular failure and, like congestive hepatomegaly, is unusual in patients with acute left ventricular infarction. Cyanosis of the nailbeds is common in patients with severe left ventricular failure and is particularly striking in patients with cardiogenic shock.

NEUROPSYCHIATRIC EXAMINATION. Except for the altered mental status which occurs in patients with AMI who have a markedly reduced cardiac output and cerebral hypoperfusion, the neurological examination is normal unless the patient has suffered cerebral embolism secondary to a mural thrombus. Indeed, an underlying MI is common in patients with cerebral embolic stroke. There is an increased coincidence of cerebrovascular accidents and AMI. In a prospective study of patients with cerebrovascular accidents admitted to the hospital within 72 hours of the onset, 12.7 per cent has an associated AMI; in contrast, in a series of patients with AMI, only 1.7 per cent suffered a stroke. The coincidence was confined to patients with large myocardial infarcts as reflected in markedly elevated serum creatine kinase concentrations.[204] The coincidence between these two conditions may be explained by systemic hypotension due to MI precipitating a cerebral infarction and the converse, as well as by mural emboli from the heart causing cerebral emboli.

As discussed in Chapter 57, patients with AMI often exhibit alterations of the emotional state, including intense anxiety, denial, and depression.

LABORATORY EXAMINATIONS

ENZYMES. Irreversibly injured myocardial cells release a number of enzymes into the circulation, where they can be measured by specific chemical reactions (p. 1254).[205] Increased activities of many enzymes have been found in

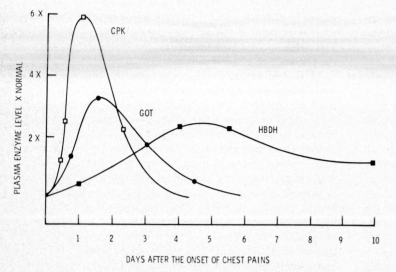

FIGURE 37–13   Typical plasma profiles for creatine kinase (CPK), glutamate oxalocetate transaminase (GOT), and hydroxybutyrate dehydrogenase (HBDH, LDH) activities following the onset of acute myocardial infarction. (From Hearse, D. J.: Myocardial enzyme leakage. J. Mol. Med. *2*: 185, 1977.)

the serum or plasma of patients with AMI.[206] Following experimental MI, a small, but significant, myocardial veno-arterial difference of enzyme activity can be measured,[207] and elevated plasma levels of enzymes correlate with corresponding depletion of these same enzymes from infarcted tissue.[208] Determinations of serum activity of creatine kinase (CK), glutamic oxaloacetic transferase (GOT), and lactic dehydrogenase (LDH) have become standard in the laboratory diagnosis of AMI. Although only one of these enzymes need be elevated to establish the diagnosis of AMI, most hospitals continue to measure all three because of the different time patterns of release.

Serum glutamic oxaloacetic transferase (SGOT) activity usually exceeds the normal range within 8 to 12 hours following the onset of chest pain; peak SGOT levels occur 18 to 36 hours after infarction and fall to normal within 3 to 4 days (Fig. 37–13). Elevated SGOT activity has been found in 97 per cent of 119 autopsy-proved cases of myocardial infarction.[209] False-positive elevations of this enzyme occur in patients with primary liver disease, hepatic congestion, and skeletal muscle disease and following intramuscular injections, pulmonary embolism, and various forms of shock.[205] Elevated levels of SGOT have also been noted in patients with pericarditis and epicardial involvement.

LDH activity rises and falls more slowly than SGOT and exceeds the normal range by 24 to 48 hours after the onset of AMI, reaches a peak 3 to 6 days after the onset of pain, and returns to normal levels 8 to 14 days after the infarction. In one study, elevations in serum LDH activity occurred in 86 per cent of 282 patients with the clinical diagnosis of AMI and in all 39 patients with autopsy-proved infarction.[209] Like SGOT, the total LDH, while sensitive, is not specific; false-positive elevations occur in patients with hemolysis, megaloblastic anemia, leukemia, liver disease, hepatic congestion, renal disease, a variety of neoplasms, pulmonary embolism, myocarditis, skeletal muscle disease, and shock.[205]

LDH has five isoenzymes, which are numbered in the order of the rapidity of their migration toward the anode of an electrophoretic field. LDH_1 moves most rapidly, whereas LDH_5 is the slowest. Fractionation of serum LDH into its five isoenzymes increases diagnostic accuracy, since the heart contains principally LDH_1, whereas liver and

skeletal muscle contain primarily LDH_4 and LDH_5. Thus, LDH_5 is commonly elevated in patients with congestive hepatomegaly. Most conditions causing elevated serum total LDH activity, such as liver or skeletal muscle disease or injury, are readily distinguished from AMI by analysis of LDH isoenzymes. Increased serum LDH_1 activity precedes elevation of serum total LDH and usually occurs within 8 to 24 hours after infarction.[210] Elevations of LDH and in the ratio of LDH_1 to total LDH occur in more than 95 per cent of patients with AMI.[205,211] Since hemolysis also raises serum LDH_1 activity, particular care must be taken in the withdrawal and handling of the blood specimens. LDH_1 reduces alpha-ketobutyric acid more readily than the more slowly moving isoenzymes of LDH; therefore, this property of the enzyme is termed hydroxybutyric dehydrogenase (HBD) activity,[205] and serum activity of alpha-HDB is often measured in patients with AMI. However, HBD should not be called a specific enzyme because its measurement actually reflects LDH_1 activity.

Serum CK activity exceeds the normal range within 6 to 8 hours following the onset of AMI, peaks at about 24 hours, and declines to normal within 3 to 4 days after the onset of chest pain (Fig. 37–13).[205] CK values in women are normally about two-thirds of those in men. Although elevation of the serum CK is the most sensitive enzymatic detector of AMI that can be used routinely,[205,210–213] 15 per cent false-positive results will occur in patients with muscle disease, alcohol intoxication, diabetes mellitus, skeletal muscle trauma, vigorous exercise, convulsions, intramuscular injections, and pulmonary embolism.[205] However, serum CK activity is normal in patients with heart failure and hepatic disease.

Three isoenzymes of CK (MM, BB, and MB) have been identified by electrophoresis. Extracts of brain and kidney contain predominantly the BB isoenzyme, skeletal muscle contains principally MM, and both MM and MB isoenzymes are present in cardiac muscle. The MB isoenzymes of CK may also be present in minor quantities in the small intestine, tongue, diaphragm, uterus, and prostate.[213,214] Despite these small amounts of CK-MB isoenzyme in tissues other than heart, elevated serum activity of CK-MB may be considered for practical purposes to be the result of AMI (except in the case of trauma or surgery on the above-mentioned organs, which contain small quantities of the enzyme). Thus, measurement of serum CK-MB isoenzyme appears to be a most useful test for myocardial necrosis.[214-216] The development of radioimmunoassay for the measurement of serum CK-MB has been helpful in increasing the accuracy, sensitivity, and specificity of this test.[217] In addition to AMI secondary to coronary obstruction, other forms of injury to cardiac muscle—such as those resulting from myocarditis, trauma, cardiac catheterization, and cardiac surgery—may also produce elevated serum CK-MB activity.[218-220] These latter causes of elevations of serum CK-MB values can usually be readily distinguished from AMI by the clinical setting. In approximately 15 per cent of patients with AMI, the CK-MB may be elevated despite a normal total CK.[221,221a] Therefore, total CK is not a sensitive adequate screening test. Serial measurement of CK-MB and application of the methods devised by Sobel and Shell (p. 1254)[205,208] allow prediction of infarct size determined at necropsy;[222] infarct size estimated by this method varies inversely with ejection fraction[223] and with survival[224] (Fig. 38–8, p. 1319).

Other Chemical Measurements. Numerous nonspecific manifestations may be recognized in patients with AMI. Although they are not generally employed in establishing the diagnosis, awareness of their coexistence with infarction is important in order to avoid misinterpretation or erroneous diagnosis of other disorders.

Hyperglycemia occurs frequently following AMI, not only in diabetic patients, in whom ketoacidosis may be precipitated, but also (with a lower frequency) in nondiabetics, in whom several weeks may elapse before carbohydrate tolerance returns to normal.[225] The plasma urea and creatinine concentrations are normal, except in patients with severe left ventricular failure, in whom reduced renal perfusion and glomerular filtration may result in azotemia (p. 1750). Hypokalemic alkalosis may be present in patients who develop an AMI while receiving thiazide or loop diuretics for antecedent hypertension or heart failure.

Serum lipids are often determined shortly after admission in patients with AMI. However, the results may be misleading, since numerous factors that can alter the values are operating at the time of the patient's admission to the hospital; for example, stress increases serum cholesterol, whereas recumbency decreases it.[226,227] Serum triglycerides are affected by caloric intake, intravenous glucose, and recumbency.[227] Therefore, it is best to defer determinations of serum lipid levels until 4 to 8 weeks after the infarction has occurred.

Release of *myoglobin* into the circulation from injured myocardial cells can be demonstrated within a few hours after the onset of infarction, and myoglobinemia is common in patients with AMI. Peak levels of serum myoglobin are reached considerably earlier (3 to 20 hours, mean = 11.4 hours after onset of infarction) than peak values of serum CK.[228] However, the time of earlier appearance of myoglobin in the serum, its peak level, and the duration of detectable myoglobin release do *not* correlate well with these same parameters for serum CK and with clinical estimates of the severity of infarction. Myoglobin appears in the serum in multiple short bursts which last for only an hour or two; in contrast to CK, myoglobin (which has a molecular weight of only 17,000) is readily excreted into the urine. This pattern of myoglobin release suggests that MI may be occurring in a series of short bursts rather than as a single episode.[228] The clinical value of serial determinations of myoglobin in AMI is limited because of the brief duration of its elevation and the lack of specificity resulting from the fact that myoglobin is a constituent of skeletal muscle and is readily detected in the serum following damage to skeletal muscle.

Alterations in serum concentrations of various *trace metals* have been noted during AMI. Elevations in serum concentration of copper and nickel have been observed which seem to parallel elevations in the sedimentation rate.[229,230] Significant decreases in serum zinc,[231] iron,[232] and magnesium[233] concentration occur within a day after infarction. The significance of alterations in serum concentrations of trace metals after infarction is currently unknown.

Hematological Manifestations. An increase in the *white blood count* occurs frequently following AMI; it may be a response to tissue necrosis or increased secretion of adrenal glucocorticoids or both. The elevation of the white count usually develops within 2 hours after the onset of chest pain, reaches a peak 2 to 4 days following infarction, and returns to normal in 1 week; the peak white blood cell count usually ranges between 12 and 15×10^3 per cubic millimeter but occasionally rises to as high as 20×10^3 per cubic millimeter. Often there is an increase in the percentage of polymorphonuclear leukocytes and a shift of the differential count to band forms. The *erythrocyte sedimentation rate* (ESR) is usually normal during the first day or two after infarction, even though fever and leukocytosis may be present. It then rises to a peak on the fourth or fifth day and may remain elevated for several weeks. The increase in the ESR is secondary to elevated plasma alpha$_2$ globulin and fibrinogen,[234] but the peak does not correlate well with the size of the infarction or with the prognosis. The *hematocrit* often increases during the first few days following infarction as a consequence of hemoconcentration.[171]

ELECTROCARDIOGRAPHIC FINDINGS
(See also p. 222)

In the majority of patients with AMI, some change can be documented when serial electrocardiographic tracings are compared. However, many factors limit the ability of the electrocardiogram to diagnose and localize myocardial infarcts: the extent of myocardial injury, the age of the infarct, its location, the presence of conduction defects, the presence of previous infarcts or acute pericarditis, changes in electrolyte concentrations, and the administration of cardioactive drugs. Nonetheless, the standard 12-lead electrocardiogram remains a clinically useful method for the detection and localization of transmural infarction.[235]

Although there is general agreement on electrocardiographic and vectorcardiographic criteria for the recognition of infarction of the anterior and inferior myocardial walls (Table 7–5, p. 230), there is less agreement on criteria for lateral and posterior infarcts.[236] Although most patients continue to demonstrate the electrocardiographic changes from an infarction for the rest of their lives, in a substantial minority the typical changes disappear and the electrocardiogram returns to normal after a number of months or, more commonly, years.[237]

The electrocardiographic diagnosis of subendocardial (nontransmural) MI is often difficult and is usually characterized by persistent ST-segment depression or T-wave inversion or both. However, ST-segment and T-wave changes are quite nonspecific and may occur in a variety of conditions, including stable and unstable angina pectoris, ventricular hypertrophy, acute and chronic pericarditis, myocarditis, early repolarization, electrolyte imbalance, shock, metabolic disorders, and following the administration of digitalis (Chap. 7).[236] Serial electrocardiograms may be of considerable aid in differentiating these conditions from subendocardial infarction: Transient changes favor angina or electrolyte disturbances, whereas persistent changes argue for infarction if other causes such as shock, administration of a glycoside, and metabolic disorders can be eliminated. In the final analysis, the diagnosis of subendocardial infarction rests more on the combination of clinical findings and the elevation of serum enzymes than on the electrocardiogram.

Right ventricular infarction is difficult to diagnose by the electrocardiogram, presumably because the right ventricular myocardial mass is small in comparison with the left.

However, ST-segment elevation in right precordial leads (V_1, V_{4R}) has been noted to be a relatively sensitive and specific sign of right ventricular infarction.[238,239] The presence of *atrial infarction* can occasionally be suspected from the electrocardiogram;[240,241] the most common electrocardiographic patterns are depression or elevation of the PQ segment, alterations in the contour of the P wave and abnormal atrial rhythms, including atrial flutter, atrial fibrillation, wandering atrial pacemaker, and AV nodal rhythm.[236]

The relative values of vectorcardiography and conventional scalar electrocardiography in the recognition of MI continue to be debated.[242–244] Table 7–5 (p. 230) lists a number of currently accepted vectorcardiographic criteria for the diagnosis and localization of MI.

ARRHYTHMIAS IN ACUTE MYOCARDIAL INFARCTION

The genesis and diagnosis of arrhythmias are presented in Chapters 19 and 21 and their treatment in Chapters 20 and 38. Discussed in this section is the role of arrhythmias in complicating the course of patients with AMI.

Some abnormality of cardiac rhythm has been noted in 72 to 96 per cent of patients with acute myocardial infarction treated in coronary care units (Table 37–6).[186,245,246] Moreover, many arrhythmias occur prior to hospitalization, before the patient is monitored.[247,247a] Thus, the overall incidence of rhythm disturbance in AMI may actually be as high as 100 per cent. However, these data are difficult to interpret, since ambulatory electrocardiographic monitoring has also disclosed arrhythmias in a high percentage of asymptomatic, middle-aged, actively employed men.[248]

Sinus Bradycardia (also see p. 690). Sinus bradycardia is the most common arrhythmia occurring during the early phases of AMI, and it is particularly frequent in patients with inferior infarction.[247–251] Observations in mobile coronary care units indicate that 40 per cent of patients with AMI have electrocardiographic evidence of sinus bradycardia within the first hour after the onset of symptoms; however, 4 hours after infarction commences, the incidence of sinus bradycardia has declined to 20 per cent. This arrhythmia occurs more frequently in patients with infarcts involving the inferior and posterior walls than in those with infarcts affecting the anterior and lateral walls. It is a manifestation of the Bezold-Jarisch reflex,[251a] is mediated by the vagi, and occurs during thrombolytic reperfusion, particularly of the right coronary artery.[252]

The clinical significance of this arrhythmia is under debate. There is evidence, on the one hand, that sinus bradycardia is an important risk factor during the very early phase of AMI and predisposes the patient to the development of repetitive ventricular arrhythmias and hypotension.[251] On the other hand, it has been suggested on the basis of data obtained in experimental infarction and from some clinical observations that the increased vagal tone that produces sinus bradycardia during the early phase of AMI may actually be protective, perhaps because it reduces myocardial oxygen demands.[250] Thus the acute mortality rate appears to be lower in patients with sinus bradycardia than in patients without this arrhythmia (Table 37–5).

Sinus Tachycardia (p. 689). Almost one-third of patients with an AMI will develop sinus tachycardia at some time during the first few days after the infarction.[246,253] The most common causes of sinus tachycardia are anxiety, persistent pain, and left ventricular failure. Other causes include fever, pericarditis, hypovolemia, atrial infarction, pulmonary embolism, and the administration of cardioaccelerator drugs such as atropine, epinephrine, or isoproterenol. Sinus tachycardia is particularly common in patients with anterior infarction. It is an undesirable rhythm in patients with AMI, since it results in an augmentation of myocardial oxygen consumption, as well as a reduction in the time available for coronary perfusion. Persistent sinus tachycardia may signify persistent heart failure and under these circumstances is a poor prognostic sign associated with an excess mortality.

Atrial Premature Contractions (p. 694). Atrial premature contractions are relatively common after MI, occurring in up to half of all patients.[246,253,254] Atrial premature contractions, and the atrial tachyarrhythmias (paroxysmal supraventricular tachycardia, atrial flutter, and atrial fibrillation) which they often herald, may be caused

TABLE 37–6   ARRHYTHMIAS DETECTED BY ECG MONITORING IN A CORONARY CARE UNIT IN 1000 CONSECUTIVE PATIENTS WITH INFARCTION 1967–71

ARRHYTHMIA	INCIDENCE (%)	MORTALITY (%)	ASSOCIATION WITH VENTRICULAR FIBRILLATION (%)
All ventricular ectopics	57	19	14
i. Salvos (runs)	17	35	26
ii. Bigemini	7	36	22
iii. R on T	6	41	40
iv. VPBs not i, ii or iii	36	15	8
Ventricular tachycardia	10	55	52
Ventricular fibrillation	8	61	
Accelerated idioventricular rhythm	9	19	12
Atrial fibrillation	11	28	
Atrial flutter	3	24	
Paroxysmal supraventricular tachycardia	3	37	
Sinus tachycardia	41	26	11
Sinus bradycardia	25	9	8
All cases		18	8

Reproduced with permission from Norris, R. M., and Singh, B. N.: Arrhythmias in acute myocardial infarction. *In* Norris, R. M. (ed.): Myocardial Infarction. Its Presentation, Pathogenesis and Treatment. Edinburgh, Churchill Livingstone, 1982, p. 55.

by atrial distention secondary to increases in left ventricular diastolic pressure, by pericarditis with its associated atrial epicarditis, or, less commonly, by ischemic injury to the atria and sinus node. Atrial premature beats per se are not associated with an increase in mortality, and cardiac output is unaffected.[255] The importance of atrial premature beats is that they often reflect an elevation of atrial (usually left atrial) pressure and that they may presage sustained supraventricular tachyarrhythmias which may impair cardiac performance. However, occasionally an atrial premature beat may initiate ventricular tachycardia[256] or even ventricular fibrillation[257] in the presence of AMI.

Paroxysmal Supraventricular Tachycardia (also see p. 702). This arrhythmia occurs in 2 to 5 per cent of patients with AMI.[258] Its deleterious effects result from the elevation of myocardial oxygen consumption and the impairment of ventricular performance consequent to the rapid ventricular rate; it is associated with an increase in mortality.

Atrial Flutter (also see p. 697). Atrial flutter is the least common atrial arrhythmia associated with AMI, occurring in only 1 to 3 per cent of all patients.[246,247,253,255] As in patients who develop this arrhythmia in the absence of infarction, atrial flutter is usually associated with 2:1 atrioventricular block. Since the atrial rate ranges from 250 to 350 beats/min, the ventricular rate is usually 125 to 175 beats/min. Atrial flutter is usually transient and is a consequence of augmented sympathetic stimulation of the atria, often occurring in patients with left ventricular failure[246] or pulmonary emboli. Atrial flutter often intensifies hemodynamic deterioration.

Atrial Fibrillation. Atrial fibrillation is far more common than flutter, occurring in 10 to 15 per cent of patients with AMI.[247,253-255,258] As with atrial premature contractions and atrial flutter, fibrillation is usually transient and tends to occur in patients with left ventricular failure but is also observed in patients with pericarditis and ischemic injury to the atria; it occurs more frequently following anterior than inferior infarction. The increased ventricular rate and the loss of the atrial contribution to left ventricular filling—i.e., the atrial kick—result in a significant reduction in cardiac output. As might be anticipated, both atrial fibrillation and flutter are associated with an increased mortality.

Junctional Rhythms (also see p. 702). Sustained junctional rhythms fall into three categories:

1. *AV junctional rhythm* at a rate of 35 to 60 beats/min in which the AV junctional tissue simply assumes the role of the dominant pacemaker when the sinus node is depressed.

2. *Accelerated junctional rhythm* in which increased rhythmicity of the junctional tissue usurps the role of pacemaker, usually at a rate of 70 to 130 beats/min.

These two arrhythmias usually develop and terminate gradually and are characterized by QRS complexes which resemble those of normally conducted beats. Retrograde P waves may be evident, or atrioventricular dissociation may occur, with the junctional rate slightly in excess of the underlying sinus rate. Disagreement exists concerning the prognostic implications of these arrhythmias; some observers attach a poor prognosis to these arrhythmias, whereas others feel that they are benign.[246,254,259] However, in patients with relatively slow junctional rhythm, the process is generally a benign protective escape rhythm and is commonly seen among patients with a slow sinus rate in the presence of inferior myocardial infarction.

3. *Paroxysmal junctional tachycardia* usually manifests rates between 160 and 220 beats/min.[246,254] This arrhythmia is uncommon in AMI, occurring in only 1 to 2 per cent of patients. In contrast to accelerated junctional rhythms, episodes of paroxysmal junctional tachycardia commence and terminate abruptly, thereby resembling other forms of paroxysmal supraventricular tachycardia, and they often occur in the presence of left ventricular failure, ischemia of the conduction system, or digitalis excess.[254] When intraventricular conduction defects are present, it may be difficult to distinguish paroxysmal atrial or junctional tachycardia from ventricular tachycardia. The hemodynamic and prognostic significance of paroxysmal junctional tachycardia is similar to that for paroxysmal atrial tachycardia except that the atrial kick is lost with the junctional rhythm.

Ventricular Premature Beats (VPB's) (see also p. 719). Although VPB's are very frequent, indeed, almost universal[260,261] in the presence of AMI, the value of the so-called warning arrhythmias in the prediction of ventricular fibrillation is not clear. It was believed that warning arrhythmias—defined as frequent VPB's (more than five per minute), VPB's with multiform configuration, early coupling (the "R-on-T" phenomenon), and repetitive patterns in the form of couplets or salvos—presage ventricular fibrillation. However, it is now clear that they are present in as many patients who develop fibrillation as who do not.[186] Several reports have shown that primary ventricular fibrillation (see below) occurs without antecedent warning arrhythmias in 40 to 83 per cent of cases.[262-265] On the other hand, frequent and complex VPB's are commonly observed in patients with AMI who never develop ventricular fibrillation.[262,263]

The prognostic significance of early coupling ("R-on-T" phenomenon) has been reassessed in several experimental[265,266] and clinical[263] studies which have shown that ventricular tachyarrhythmias in patients with AMI are often initiated by a VPB that does *not* fall on an antecedent T wave. As a matter of fact, a majority of ventricular tachycardias in patients with AMI appear to be initiated by a *late*-coupled VPB.[267,268] In two clinical reports on electrocardiographic antecedents of primary ventricular fibrillation, 45 per cent[262] and 41 per cent[263] of episodes of ventricular fibrillation, respectively, were initiated by a late-coupled VPB. However, in one study[269] frequent VPB's showing the R-on-T phenomenon did appear to herald the development of ventricular fibrillation but not of ventricular tachycardia. Thus, the prognostic value, if any, of various forms of VPB's in AMI still requires clarification.

In the post–myocardial infarction period, the prognostic significance of VPB's, particularly frequent ones, appears to be less controversial. Although there is little correlation between ventricular arrhythmias occurring in the early hours or days of AMI and those observed in the late post-infarction period,[270,271] frequent VPB's or ventricular tachycardia *following* hospital discharge do appear to be associated with increased risk of sudden death (p. 783).[272,273]

Ventricular Tachycardia (also see p. 721). Ventricular

tachycardia is generally defined as three or more consecutive ventricular ectopic beats occurring at a frequency exceeding 120 beats/min. The reported incidence of ventricular tachycardia in AMI is in the range of 10 to 40 per cent.[186,246] When this arrhythmia occurs within the first 24 hours, it is usually precipitated by a late VPB and is transient and benign. Ventricular tachycardia occurring late in the course of AMI is more common in patients with transmural infarction and left ventricular dysfunction, is sustained, usually induces marked hemodynamic deterioration, and is associated with a relatively high hospital mortality rate—40 to 50 per cent[246] (Table 37–6). However, the relative contribution to the high mortality rate of this arrhythmia per se, compared with that of the underlying impairment of left ventricular performance due to large infarction, is not clear.[274] In addition, the long-term mortality in patients who exhibit ventricular tachycardia in the late hospital phase of AMI is greatly increased.[275]

Accelerated Idioventricular Rhythm (Fig. 21–37, p. 725). Commonly defined as a ventricular rhythm with a rate of 60 to 110 (or 125) beats/min,[276,277] this arrhythmia is seen in 8 to 20 per cent of patients with AMI, usually in the first 2 days, and seems to be equally common in anterior and inferior infarctions. About half of all episodes of accelerated idioventricular rhythm manifest as an escape rhythm occurring during slowing of the sinus rhythm or gradual speeding of the ventricular pacemaker; the other half of accelerated idioventricular rhythms is initiated by a premature beat.[278] Most episodes are of short duration, and the arrhythmia may terminate abruptly, slow gradually before termination, or be overdriven by acceleration of the basic cardiac rhythm. Variation of the rate is common and may take the form of gradual acceleration, gradual slowing, or a grossly irregular rate. In a few instances, the rate may suddenly double, resulting in rapid ventricular tachycardia and suggesting the presence of a fast ectopic focus with exit block.[278] Accelerated idioventricular rhythms in patients with AMI probably results from enhanced automaticity of Purkinje fibers. In contrast to rapid ventricular tachycardia, accelerated idioventricular rhythms are thought not to affect prognosis.[186,277,278] However, accelerated idioventricular rhythms are frequently associated with episodes of rapid ventricular tachycardia, and in many patients increased automaticity is manifest at times as accelerated idioventricular rhythms and at other times as ventricular tachycardia.

Ventricular Fibrillation (also see p. 728). Ventricular fibrillation occurs in 4 to 18 per cent of patients with AMI treated in coronary care units.[262–264] It occurs with equal incidence in patients with anterior and with inferior transmural infarctions[253] and is rare in patients with nontransmural infarction. This arrhythmia may occur in three settings in hospitalized patients with AMI. Its occurrence as a mechanism of sudden death is discussed in Chapter 23. *Primary* ventricular fibrillation, responsible for more than 80 per cent of all instances of this arrhythmia,[264] occurs suddenly and unexpectedly in patients with no or few signs or symptoms of left ventricular failure. Approximately 60 per cent of episodes occur within 4 hours and 80 per cent within 12 hours of the onset of symptoms.[264] *Secondary* ventricular fibrillation, on the other hand, is the final phase of a progressive downhill course

with left ventricular failure and cardiogenic shock.[253] So-called *late* ventricular fibrillation usually occurs 1 to 6 weeks following AMI. Coronary care unit survivors with anteroseptal infarction complicated by right or left bundle branch block are particularly vulnerable to this complication.[279] The prognosis, both immediate and late, is best in the primary form, worst in the secondary form, and intermediate in the late ventricular fibrillation group.

Asystole. This arrhythmia has been reported to occur in 1 to 14 per cent of patients with AMI admitted to coronary care units.[246,253] This wide variation in incidence reflects differences in the definition of this event. The lower incidence rates include only patients who develop asystole either as a primary event or following abnormalities of atrioventricular or intraventricular conduction, whereas the higher rates include patients who develop asystole as a terminal complication. In either event, the mortality is very high, ranging upward from 90 per cent.[246]

HEMODYNAMIC CONSEQUENCES OF CARDIAC ARRHYTHMIAS. Patients with significant left ventricular dysfunction have a relatively fixed stroke volume and depend on changes in heart rate to alter cardiac output. However, there is a narrow range over which the cardiac output is maximal, with significant reductions occurring at faster and lower rates.[280] Thus, all forms of bradycardia and tachycardia may depress the cardiac output in patients with AMI. Although the optimal rate insofar as cardiac output is concerned may exceed 100 per minute, it is important to consider that heart rate is one of the major determinants of myocardial oxygen consumption (p. 1238) and that at more rapid heart rates myocardial energy needs can be elevated to levels that adversely affect ischemic myocardium. Therefore, in patients with AMI, the optimal rate is usually somewhat lower, in the range of 80 to 90 beats/min.

A second factor to consider in assessing the hemodynamic consequences of a particular arrhythmia is the loss

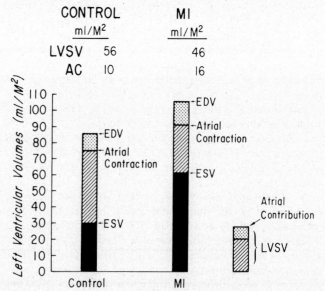

FIGURE 37–14 Average end-diastolic volumes (EDV), end-systolic volumes (ESV), left ventricular stroke volumes (LVSV), and atrial contribution (AC) in a control group of patients and in patients after myocardial infarction (MI). (From Rahimtoola, S. H., et al.: Left atrial transport function in myocardial infarction. Am. J. Med. *59*:686, 1975.)

of atrial transport function, i.e., the atrial "kick."[281] Studies in patients without AMI have demonstrated that loss of atrial transport decreases left ventricular output by 15 to 20 per cent.[282] However, in patients with reduced diastolic left ventricular compliance of any etiology (including AMI), atrial systole is of greater importance for left ventricular filling. In patients with AMI, atrial systole boosts end-diastolic volume by 15 per cent, end-diastolic pressure by 29 per cent, and stroke volume by 35 per cent (Fig. 37–14).[283]

Conduction Disturbances

Ischemic injury can produce blocks at any level of the atrioventricular or intraventricular conduction system. Such blocks may occur in the atrioventricular node, producing various grades of AV block; in either main bundle branch, producing right or left bundle branch block; and in the anterior and posterior divisions of the left bundle, producing left anterior or left posterior (fascicular) divisional blocks (Table 37–7). Disturbances of conduction can, of course, occur in various combinations. The mechanisms and recognition of intraventricular conduction disturbances are discussed in Chapter 7 and of atrioventricular conduction disturbances in Chapter 21.

First-degree AV Block (Fig. 21–42, p. 730). First-degree AV block occurs in 4 to 14 per cent of patients with AMI admitted to coronary care units. His bundle electrocardiographic studies have shown that almost all patients with first-degree AV block have disturbances in conduction *above* the bundle of His, i.e., intranodal. The localization of the site of block is of considerable importance, since the development of complete heart block and ventricular asystole is restricted almost exclusively to those patients with first-degree block in whom the conduction disturbance is *below* the bundle of His,[284] and this occurs more commonly in patients with anterior infarction and in those with associated bifascicular block.[285,286]

Second-degree AV Block

Mobitz Type I, or Wenckebach (Fig. 21–43, p. 731). Mobitz type I block occurs in 4 to 10 per cent of patients with AMI admitted to coronary care units[246,285] and accounts for about 90 per cent of all patients with second-degree AV block. This type of block (1) generally occurs within the AV node; (2) is usually associated with narrow QRS complexes; (3) is presumably secondary to ischemic injury; (4) commonly occurs in patients with inferior myocardial infarction; (5) is usually transient and does not persist for more than 72 hours after infarction; (6) may be intermittent; and (7) rarely progresses to complete AV block. First-degree and type I second-degree AV block do not appear to affect survival, are most commonly associated with inferior wall infarction, and are caused by ischemia of the AV node.

Mobitz Type II (Fig. 21–44, p. 732). This is a rare conduction defect following AMI, occurring in only 10 per cent of all cases of second-degree block;[246] thus, the overall incidence of Mobitz type II block after infarction is less than 1 per cent. In contrast to Mobitz type I block, type II second-degree block (1) usually originates from a lesion in the conduction system below the bundle of His;[285] (2) is associated with a wide QRS complex; (3) often, but not invariably, reflects trifascicular block with impaired conduction distal to the bundle of His; (4) often progresses suddenly to complete atrioventricular block; and (5) is almost always associated with anterior rather than inferior infarction.

Complete (Third-degree) AV Block. The atrioventricular conduction system has a dual blood supply, the AV branch of the right coronary artery and the septal perforating branch from the left anterior descending coronary artery. Therefore, complete AV block can occur in patients with either anterior or inferior infarction. Complete AV block develops in 5 to 8 per cent of patients with AMI. As with other forms of AV block, the prognosis depends on the anatomical location of the block in the conduction system and the size of the infarction.

In general, complete heart block in patients with inferior infarction results from an intranodal lesion and develops gradually, often progressing from first-degree and type I second-degree block. The escape rhythm is often junctional with a narrow QRS complex in 60 per cent of cases and a wide QRS in the remaining 40 per cent. This form of complete AV block is usually transient and resolves in 1 week. The mortality is approximately 20 to 25 per cent.[286,287]

In patients with anterior infarction, third-degree AV block often occurs with dramatic suddenness, 12 to 24 hours after the onset of the infarct. It is usually preceded by intraventricular block, not lower degrees of AV block. Such patients have escape rhythms with wide QRS complexes and rates less than 40 beats/min; ventricular asystole may occur quite suddenly in these patients. The mortality in this group of patients is extremely high, approximately 70 to 80 per cent.[288–291]

The prognosis for patients with AV block complicating AMI depends on the extent and secondarily on the anatomical site of the myocardial injury. Thus, patients with inferior infarction often have concomitant ischemia or infarction of the AV node secondary to hypoperfusion of the AV nodal artery. However, the His-Purkinje system usually escapes injury in such individuals. As noted above, junctional escape rhythms with narrow QRS complexes occur commonly in this setting. Hemodynamic derangements are often mild in these patients, and mortality is only slightly increased.[292] In patients with anterior infarction, AV block usually develops as a result of extensive

TABLE 37–7 INCIDENCE AND PROGNOSES OF CONDUCTION BLOCKS IN ACUTE MYOCARDIAL INFARCTION

TYPE OF CONDUCTION BLOCK	INCIDENCE OF CONDUCTION BLOCK (%)	PATIENTS WITH CONDUCTION BLOCK WHO DEVELOP COMPLETE AV BLOCK (%)	MORTALITY (%)
None		6	15
LAH	5	3	27
LPH	1	0	42
RBBB + LAH	5	46	45
RBBB + LPH	1	43	57
RBBB	2	43	46
LBBB	5	20	44

Adapted from Mullins, C. B., and Atkins, J. M.: Prognoses and management of ventricular conduction blocks in acute myocardial infarction. Mod. Concepts Cardiovasc. Dis. 45:129, 1976, by permission of the American Heart Association, Inc.

septal necrosis that involves the bundle branches; the high mortality in this group of patients with slow idioventricular rhythms and wide QRS complexes is the consequence of extensive myocardial necrosis resulting in severe left ventricular failure and often shock.[292]

Intraventricular Block (Table 37–7).   Intraventricular conduction disturbances, i.e., block within one or more of the three subdivisions (fascicles) of the His-Purkinje system (the anterior and posterior divisions of the left bundle and the right bundle, p. 217) occur in 10 to 20 per cent of patients with AMI. The right bundle branch and the left posterior division have a dual blood supply from the left anterior descending and right coronary artery, whereas the left anterior division is supplied by septal perforators originating from the left anterior descending coronary artery. Not all conduction blocks observed in patients with AMI can be considered to be complications of infarcts, since almost half are already present at the time the first electrocardiogram is recorded, and they may represent antecedent disease of the conduction system.

Preexisting bundle branch block or divisional block is less often associated with the development of complete heart block in patients with AMI than are newly acquired conduction defects. First-degree AV block adds to the risk of intraventricular conduction defects progressing to complete AV block.[293,294]

Left anterior divisional block (Fig. 7–24, p. 218) occurs in 3 to 5 per cent of patients with AMI,[295,296] and, as noted in Table 37–7, mortality is increased in these patients, though not as much as in patients with other forms of conduction block. Since left anterior divisional block may be difficult to diagnose in the presence of inferior wall infarction, it may be helpful to employ the vectorcardiogram to establish this diagnosis.

Left posterior divisional block occurs in only 1 per cent of patients with AMI admitted to coronary care units. The posterior fascicle is larger than the anterior fascicle, and, in general, a larger infarct is required to block it. As a consequence, mortality is markedly increased (Table 37–7).[295] Complete AV block is not a frequent complication of *either* form of isolated divisional block.

Right bundle branch block occurs in approximately 2 per cent of patients with AMI and frequently leads to AV block because it is often a new lesion, associated with anteroseptal infarction. The mortality is high even if complete AV block does not occur (Table 37–7).[246,293,295–297]

Bidivisional (Bifascicular) Block.   The combination of right bundle branch block with either left anterior or posterior divisional block or the combination of left anterior and posterior divisional blocks (i.e., left bundle branch block) is known as bidivisional block (p. 219). If new block occurs in two of the three divisions of the conduction system, the risk of developing complete AV block is quite high.[246,295] Mortality is also high because of the occurrence of severe pump failure secondary to the extensive myocardial necrosis required to produce such an extensive intraventricular block.[298] Left bundle branch block occurs in approximately 5 per cent of patients with AMI (Table 37–7). Although the latter defect progresses to complete AV block only half as frequently as does right bundle branch block, it is associated with as high a mortality as right bundle branch block and the other two forms of

bifascicular block,[246,293,295] and with a high late mortality.[186] Patients with intraventricular conduction defects, particularly right bundle branch block, account for the majority of patients who develop ventricular fibrillation late in their hospital stay. However, the high mortality in these patients occurs even in the absence of AV block and appears to be related to cardiac failure and massive infarction rather than to the conduction disturbance.

Roentgenographic and Radionuclide Studies

Roentgenography (see also p. 160).   The initial chest roentgenogram in patients with AMI is almost invariably a film portably obtained in the emergency room or the coronary care unit. Two findings are common: signs of left ventricular failure and cardiomegaly. Although the pulmonary vascular markings on the roentgenogram generally reflect the left ventricular end-diastolic pressure, significant discrepancies may occur because of what have been termed *diagnostic lags* and *post-therapeutic phase lags*. In the former, patients may have elevated left ventricular filling pressures and normal chest roentgenograms, and, because of the time required for pulmonary edema to accumulate after left ventricular filling pressure has become elevated, 12 hours may elapse before the radiographic findings reflect the hemodynamic status. The post-therapeutic phase lag represents the longer time interval, generally 1 or 2 days, required for pulmonary edema to resorb and the radiographic signs of pulmonary congestion to clear after left ventricular filling pressure has returned toward normal.[299–301]

Cardiomegaly in a patient with AMI usually signifies prior infarction or another form of antecedent heart disease with subsequent left ventricular dilatation, and it is usually associated with significantly impaired left ventricular function.[302] The converse is not true, however, in that patients may have increased end-diastolic volumes and still demonstrate a normal-sized heart on roentgenographic examination. The degree of congestion and the size of the left side of the heart on the initial chest film are highly useful independent predictors for defining groups of patients with AMI who are at increased risk of dying within the first year after the acute event.[303]

Radioisotopic Studies.   All major forms of cardiac imaging—radionuclide angiography, perfusion scintigraphy, infarct avid scintigraphy, and positive emission tomography—are useful in detecting AMI, in assessing infarct size, in determining the effects of the infarct on ventricular function, and in establishing prognosis. The application of these techniques is discussed in Chapter 11A.[304–306]

Echocardiography (See also p. 127)

Although *M-mode echocardiography* is a sensitive technique for examining regional left ventricular wall motion,[306a] it is limited to the imaging of small segments of the interventricular septum and posterior left ventricular wall; rarely, small segments of the anterior wall can be imaged as well. Therefore, abnormalities of regional wall motion and even left ventricular aneurysms, particularly those involving the anterior wall, may be missed completely.[307] Despite this obvious shortcoming, some useful information

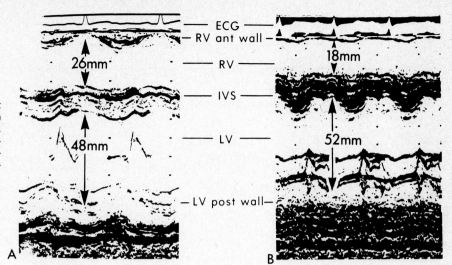

FIGURE 37–15 Echocardiograms. *A*, Patient with RV infarction and dilatation. *B*, Patient with LV inferior infarction and normal RV dimensions. (From Sharpe, D. N., et al.: The noninvasive diagnosis of right ventricular infarction. Circulation *57*:483, 1978, by permission of the American Heart Association, Inc.)

can be obtained from patients with acute or old MI, particularly in the diagnosis of complications of MI (Table 37–8). Abnormalities of left ventricular wall motion, usually corresponding to the electrocardiographic site of infarction, may be recognized in the majority of patients with transmural infarction, and exaggerated normal motion can be found in noninfarcted areas in approximately one-third of patients.[308] An increased internal diameter of the left ventricle, determined by echocardiography, correlates closely with clinical, hemodynamic, and angiographic signs of heart failure.[309] The echocardiographic distance between the E-point of the anterior mitral valve and the septum has been shown to correlate well with the global left ventricular ejection fraction in patients with AMI.[310]

M-mode echocardiography is also useful in detecting small pericardial effusions in patients with postinfarction pericarditis.[311] A number of changes—including increased amplitude of upper septal wall motion; dilatation of the right ventricle; and abnormal mitral valve motion in diastole, suggesting increased mitral valve flow—have been noted in the echocardiograms of patients with rupture of the ventricular septum after MI. Although not specific, this combination of echocardiographic findings provides a useful clue to the diagnosis of septal rupture.[312,313] M-mode echocardiography can also be employed in the noninvasive diagnosis of right ventricular infarction. Findings include an increased right ventricular end-diastolic diameter and an increased ratio of right ventricular to left ventricular end-diastolic diameter (Fig. 37–15).[314]

Two-dimensional echocardiography can provide both longitudinal and transverse views of the left ventricle, and a much larger fraction of the ventricular wall—including significant portions of the left ventricular apical, anterior, septal, inferior, and posterior walls—can be imaged[315] by this method than by the M-mode technique. Areas of abnormal regional wall motion are observed almost universally in patients with AMI (Fig. 37–16).[316,317] Left ventricular function, estimated from two-dimensional echocardiograms, correlates well and sometimes predicts the clinical course. The detection of wall-motion disorders outside the infarct zone predicts the development of heart failure or cardiogenic shock. In many patients, regional abnormalities of left ventricular wall motion detected during

AMI improve during the recovery phase. In addition, in patients with AMI who develop a loud systolic murmur, two-dimensional echocardiography can detect and localize a ventricular septal defect, as well as detect mitral regurgitation and elucidate its cause.[318–321]

Systolic Time Intervals and Apexcardiograms
(See also Chap. 4)

Systolic time intervals (preejection period [PEP] and left ventricular ejection time [LVET]) have been employed to

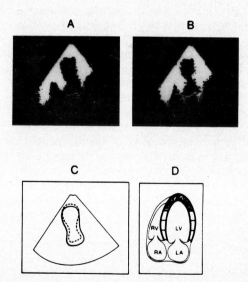

FIGURE 37–16 Panels A and B show end-diastolic and end-systolic frames of each of the three long-axis apical four-chamber views in a two-dimensional echocardiogram in a patient with an acute anterior infarction, 8 hours after onset of symptoms. Panel C shows the diastolic (solid line) and systolic (dotted line) outlines of the left ventricle. There is extensive asynergy. In Panel D the dotted segments represent the visually estimated asynergic area of the left ventricular wall, calculated at 37 per cent. Ao = aorta; LA = left atrium; LV = left ventricle; RV = right ventricle; RA = right atrium. (Reproduced with permission from Visser, C. A., Kan, G., Lie, K. I., Becker, A. E., and Durrer, D.: Apex two dimensional echocardiography. Alternative approach to quantification of acute myocardial infarction. Br. Heart J. *47*:461, 1982.)

TABLE 37–8   COMPLICATIONS OF ACUTE MYOCARDIAL INFARCTION
DETECTED BY ECHOCARDIOGRAPHY

COMPLICATION	ECHOCARDIOGRAPHIC MANIFESTATIONS
Early	
Arrhythmias	Not applicable
Heart block and/or marked bradycardia	Not applicable
Shock	Large areas of noncontractile LV myocardium
	Right ventricular infarction: impaired RV wall motion; increased RV size with or without abnormal septal motion; absence of pericardial fluid
Pulmonary edema (congestive heart failure)	Large areas of noncontractile LV myocardium and/or anatomical complications (e.g., ventricular septal defect)
Subacute	
Infarct extension/expansion	Expansion demonstrated by disproportionate transmural diastolic thinning and associated regional ventricular dilation on two-dimensional echocardiography (2DE)
Severe mitral regurgitation secondary to papillary muscle dysfunction or rupture	Rupture demonstrated by visualization of untethered mitral valve leaflet on 2DE
Acute ventricular septal defect	2DE visualization of septal rent; negative contrast effect after IV fluid injection
Subacute to late	
Ventricular aneurysm	Localized interruption in the diastolic configuration of LV wall; orifice to aneurysm is wide
Ventricular pseudoaneurysm	Demonstration of narrow neck leading into the false aneurysm cavity
Thromboembolism	Visualization of LV thrombus

Reproduced with permission from Strauss, W. E., and Parisi, A. F.: Echocardiography. *In* Morganroth, J., Parisi, A., and Pohost, G. M. (eds.): Noninvasive Cardiac Imaging. Copyright © 1983 by Year Book Medical Publishers, Inc., Chicago.

estimate the state of left ventricular function in patients with AMI, but considerable disagreement exists concerning the value of these measurements in this condition.[322-325] Because of the adrenergic hyperactivity commonly present in patients with AMI, comparison of systolic time intervals in patients with AMI with those obtained from patients with chronic, stable, left ventricular dysfunction is not valid. In general, patients with AMI demonstrate an abnormally short LVET, reflecting a reduction of stroke volume and a normal or only slightly prolonged PEP. The normal or nearly normal PEP should, in reality, be considered to be abnormally prolonged, since a markedly shortened PEP is normally obtained in the presence of excess adrenergic activity. Patients with AMI and normal PEP/LVET ratios demonstrate fewer clinical signs of left ventricular failure than do patients with abnormally elevated ratios. The PEP/LVET ratio becomes progressively increased with greater degrees of left ventricular failure, and patients who succumb to pump failure usually have the most abnormally elevated ratios.

Serial measurements of systolic time intervals usually reflect the changes in left ventricular function that frequently occur during the course of an acute myocardial infarction. Thus, the PEP/LVET ratio rises in patients with infarct extension.

Apexcardiography can be employed to gain information about left ventricular systolic and diastolic function (p. 58). Abnormalities of the *a* wave and systolic wave of the apexcardiogram correlate with measurements of left ventricular function obtained at the time of cardiac catheterization (Fig. 37–17).[326] Moreover, paradoxical motion of the left ventricle secondary to an aneurysm can be identified by apexcardiography. Thus, Khan and Haywood recorded serial apexcardiograms in 40 patients with AMI and in 21 patients with angiographically proved left ventricular aneurysms. Increased amplitude of the *a* wave and an abnormal morphology of the systolic wave (presence of an abnormally shaped systolic wave or a secondary systolic bulge) of the apexcardiogram correlated well with akinesia or dyskinesia or both identified angiographically.[326]

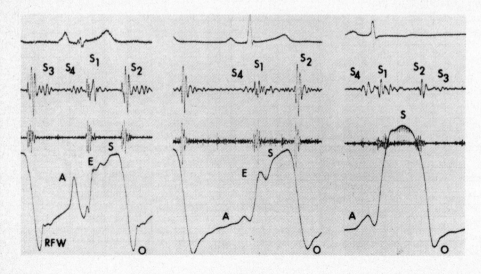

FIGURE 37–17 Examples of abnormal apexcardiograms frequently seen in acute myocardial infarction. Note tall *a* wave and prominent secondary systolic wave (S) (systolic bulge) in left panel, normal *a* wave and bifid systolic wave corresponding to E point and secondary systolic wave in middle panel, and *a* wave normal in height and monophasic secondary systolic wave in panel on right. S₂, second heart sound; and RFW, rapid filling wave. (From Khan, A. H., et al.: Value of serial apex cardiograms during and after myocardial infarction. Chest *70*:367, 1976.)

Hemodynamics and Angiography

Hemodynamic monitoring in the coronary care unit has become widespread in recent years.[140,141,327-330] A balloon-tipped catheter is advanced, usually with fluoroscopic guidance, from a peripheral vein through the right heart and into the pulmonary artery (Chap. 9). Judicious positioning of the catheter allows recording of the pulmonary arterial pressure when the balloon is deflated and of the pulmonary capillary wedge pressure when the balloon is inflated.[327] Blood may be sampled from the tip of the catheter in the pulmonary artery and, in certain models, from a second lumen opening into the right atrium. In addition, some models of pulmonary artery balloon catheters have a thermistor near the tip for recording thermodilution cardiac output.[331] Thus, a single catheter in the right heart can yield the following information: saturation of blood in the pulmonary artery and right atrium, pressures in the pulmonary artery, pulmonary wedge position, and right atrium and cardiac output. A good correlation has been found between pulmonary artery occlusive pressure (which is equal to pulmonary capillary pressure) and left ventricular diastolic pressure in patients with AMI.[332]

Pulmonary arterial systolic pressure is distinctly elevated in patients with AMI and in individuals with chronic obstructive pulmonary disease or pulmonary embolism. Patients with significant mitral regurgitation complicating MI may demonstrate tall *v* waves in the pulmonary capillary wedge positions (p. 1080) (Fig. 37-18). Patients with rupture of the interventricular septum have increased right ventricular and pulmonary arterial blood oxygen saturation, as well as wide pulmonary arterial pulse pressures.[140] These patients may also demonstrate tall *v* waves in the pulmonary wedge pressure tracing.[333]

In the past, central venous or right atrial pressure was used to gauge the degree of left ventricular failure in patients with MI. This estimate is fraught with error, since central venous pressure actually reflects *right* rather than left ventricular function (Figure 38-3, p. 1312). Right ventricular function, and therefore systemic venous pressure, may be normal or nearly so in patients with significant left ventricular failure.[140] Conversely, patients with right ven-

tricular failure due to right ventricular infarction or pulmonary embolism may exhibit elevated right atrial and central venous pressures despite normal left ventricular function.[334] Low values for right atrial and central venous pressures imply hypovolemia, whereas elevated right atrial pressures usually result from right ventricular failure secondary to left ventricular failure, pulmonary hypertension, or right ventricular infarction, or, less commonly, from tricuspid regurgitation or pericardial tamponade.

Both the prognosis and the clinical status are related to the cardiac output. Patients with normal cardiac output after MI have an expected mortality as low as 1 per cent;[141] prognosis worsens as cardiac output declines. Patients with cardiac indices in the range of 2.7 to 4.3 liters/min/sq meter usually have no clinical signs of impaired perfusion, whereas patients with cardiac indices ranging from 1.8 to 2.2 liters/min/sq meter demonstrate early signs of hypoperfusion (cool skin and decreasing urine output and mental acuity). Patients whose cardiac index is less than 1.8 liters/min/sq meter are usually in shock. The pulmonary artery occlusive pressure reflects the state of left ventricular filling, its compliance, and its ability to empty. As pulmonary pressure rises, progressive increases in pulmonary congestion occur. Increasing degrees of pulmonary congestion can also be monitored through changes in the physical examination (development of tachypnea, rales, wheezing, or pleural effusion) or on the chest roentgenogram.

Patients with intraventricular conduction defects or heart block or both after anterior infarction have lower cardiac indices and higher pulmonary capillary wedge pressures than do patients without these conduction disturbances. On the other hand, patients with these conduction defects and inferior myocardial infarction usually do not demonstrate such hemodynamic abnormalities. The difference in hemodynamic measurements between these two groups is the result of the more extensive myocardial necrosis in patients with anterior infarction.[292]

HEMODYNAMIC FINDINGS IN VENTRICULAR SEPTAL RUPTURE AND MITRAL REGURGITATION. It may be difficult, on clinical grounds, to distinguish between acute mitral regurgitation and rupture of the ventricular septum in patients with AMI who suddenly

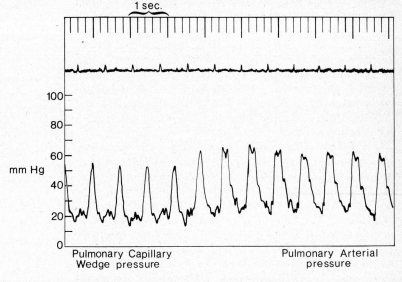

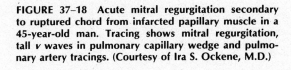

FIGURE 37-18 Acute mitral regurgitation secondary to ruptured chord from infarcted papillary muscle in a 45-year-old man. Tracing shows mitral regurgitation, tall *v* waves in pulmonary capillary wedge and pulmonary artery tracings. (Courtesy of Ira S. Ockene, M.D.)

develop a loud systolic murmur.[335] One approach to the differentiation is first-pass radionuclide ventriculography (p. 356). In addition, a right-heart catheterization with a balloon-tipped catheter can readily distinguish between these two complications. Patients with ventricular septal rupture demonstrate a "step-up" in oxygen saturation in blood samples from the right ventricle and pulmonary artery compared with those from the right atrium; patients with acute mitral regurgitation lack this step-up; they may demonstrate tall v waves in both the pulmonary capillary and the pulmonary arterial pressure tracings (Fig. 37–18). Cardiac output is usually significantly decreased in both conditions.

Left Ventricular Function after Myocardial Infarction. As noted, angiographic or echocardiographic evidence of abnormal regional left ventricular wall motion is very commonly present after AMI;[336] some improvement in function occurs during uncomplicated convalescence, whereas extension (or possibly expansion) of the infarction increases the segment of the left ventricle that is hypokinetic or akinetic.[337] Patients who have suffered a transmural MI often demonstrate increased left ventricular end-diastolic volume and pressure and reduced ejection fraction, velocity of circumferential fiber shortening, and cardiac index.[338,339] Some degree of mitral regurgitation is present in almost half of all patients following transmural infarction. Discrete aneurysmal bulges are seen on the left ventriculogram in about one-fifth of such patients.[336,340] Patients in cardiogenic shock invariably demonstrate markedly abnormal hemodynamics, with elevated pulmonary capillary wedge pressure (> 15 mm Hg), reduced cardiac index (< 2.3 liters/min/sq meter), and severely reduced ejection fractions.[341]

PROGNOSIS (Table 37–9)

Both short-term and long-term survival following an AMI depends on a number of factors;[341a,341b,341c] the most important are the state of left ventricular function and the severity of the obstructive lesions in the coronary vascular bed perfusing residual viable myocardium. At one extreme, the prognosis is best for the patient with normal intrinsic coronary vessels who has completed an infarct constituting less than 5 per cent of the left ventricle as a consequence of a coronary embolus and who has no jeopardized myocardium. At the other extreme is the patient with a massive infarct who is in cardiogenic shock and whose residual myocardium is perfused by markedly obstructed vessels; obviously, progression of atherosclerosis or lowering perfusion pressure in these vessels will impair the function and viability of the residual myocardium on which left ventricular function depends.

CLINICAL FACTORS. Soon after coronary care units were instituted, it became apparent that left ventricular function is an important early determinant of survival. Thus, Killip studied patients divided into four groups based on findings of left ventricular failure by physical examination at the time of admission to the coronary care unit; as noted in Tables 37–3 and 37–5, hospital mortality from MI depends directly on the severity of left ventricular dysfunction present at the time of admission.[342] Similarly, Peel[343] and Norris[344] and their collaborators developed

prognostic indices for patients with AMI. Although they used historical, electrocardiographic, and radiological data to predict hospital mortality, evidence of left ventricular failure heavily weights these indices in the direction of poor prognosis.

Certain demographic and historical factors are associated with a poor prognosis after infarction, including male sex, age greater than 60 years and a history of diabetes mellitus, hypertension, prior angina pectoris, and previous myocardial infarction. The last factor may contribute to a poor prognosis, since it indicates loss of viable myocardium preceding the reference infarct.

INFARCT EXTENSION. Extension occurs in 10 to 30 per cent of patients with AMI during the first 10 days.[344a] It is generally defined as reelevation or reappearance of CK-MB in the serum after the initial peak. Neither chest pain nor the electrocardiogram provides accurate markers for recognizing infarct extension. The majority of patients with cardiogenic shock have developed infarct extension.[112] In the prospective study of patients, it was found that mortality in those experiencing extension is more than double that noted in patients in whom extension did not occur.[345-348] Marmor reported that infarct extension occurred most frequently in obese females and was most common in patients with nontransmural infarction.[348] Presumably, the higher mortality associated with infarct extension is related to the larger mass of myocardium whose function becomes compromised.

HEMODYNAMICS. Physiological evidence of compromised left ventricular function also correlates with hospital mortality in AMI,[349] as already discussed (Table 37–

TABLE 37–9 FACTORS ASSOCIATED WITH POOR PROGNOSIS AFTER MYOCARDIAL INFARCTION

Left Ventricular Function

Clinical evidence of heart failure
Hemodynamic evidence of heart failure
Invasive and/or noninvasive demonstration of poor left ventricular systolic function

Electrocardiogram

Persistent, repetitive, ventricular ectopic activity
Atrioventricular and intraventricular conduction defects
Persistent ST-segment depression or elevation (the latter without pericarditis)
Persistent T-wave inversions
Abnormal Q waves in multiple leads
Atrial fibrillation
Left ventricular hypertrophy

Chest Roentgenogram

Cardiomegaly

Age > 60 Years
Male Sex
Presence of Additional Diseases

Previous myocardial infarction or angina
Post–myocardial infarction angina
Diabetes mellitus
Hypertension

Laboratory Data

Markedly elevated cardiac enzymes (e.g., GOT > 250 Karmen units; CK > 2000 IU)
Elevated blood urea nitrogen
Absence of collateral blood vessels to region of reduced perfusion by angiography

Psychological Aspects

Psychosis

3). Thus, patients with hemodynamic (elevated pulmonary capillary wedge pressure or depressed cardiac index or both) or ventriculographic (depressed ejection fraction and elevated end-systolic volume by radionuclide angiography) evidence of left ventricular failure have a worse prognosis than patients without these findings.[350,351,351a] The *chest roentgenogram* is also prognostic, since patients with cardiomegaly or increased heart volume after infarction do not fare as well as individuals without these features.[303] Since impaired ventricular function is generally a manifestation of the cumulative extent of myocardial damage sustained, one important determinant of prognosis is, therefore, *infarct size*. Thus, patients with markedly elevated plasma enzyme levels (CK > 2000 IU) often manifest left ventricular failure with concomitant poor prognosis. Furthermore, prognosis for as long as 4 years after an initial infarction is related to infarct size estimated from plasma CK time-activity curves at the time of the acute episode (Figure 38–8, p. 1319).[224] A large defect or multiple defects on a thallium-201 perfusion scintigram, obtained very early in the course of AMI, also presumably related to infarct size, is associated with a high incidence of mortality or subsequent cardiac events.[351,351a] Similarly, patients with largest infarcts on technetium-99m scintigrams have the poorest prognosis.[305,352]

ELECTROCARDIOGRAM. Patients whose electrocardiogram demonstrates persistent advanced (e.g., Mobitz type II, second-degree, or third-degree atrioventricular block) or new intraventricular conduction abnormalities (bifascicular or trifascicular) in the course of an AMI have a worse prognosis than do patients without these abnormalities (Table 37–7). Other electrocardiographic findings that augur poorly for the postinfarction patient are repetitive ventricular ectopic activity (Table 37–6) (couplets, runs), persistent horizontal or downsloping ST-segment depression and Q waves in multiple leads, atrial arrhythmias (especially atrial fibrillation), and voltage criteria for left ventricular hypertrophy.

ST-segment depressions in leads other than those with acute Q waves are also a poor prognostic sign; for example, patients with acute inferior wall infarcts who demonstrate ST-segment depressions in precordial leads have a worse prognosis than do patients without this finding. There is controversy concerning whether these ST-segment depressions reflect reciprocal electrical changes, associated disease of the left anterior descending coronary artery, or, most likely, a larger inferior infarct.[353–355,355a] Similarly, patients who develop angina during the first 10 days following infarction, with new electrocardiographic changes distant from the acute infarct, i.e., angina "at a distance," have a distinctly worse prognosis than do patients having postinfarct angina with ischemia in the infarct zone.[356]

TRANSMURAL VERSUS SUBENDOCARDIAL INFARCTION. Patients with myocardial infarction are usually classified into two groups on the basis of electrocardiographic criteria: *transmural and subendocardial (nontransmural) infarction*. Transmural infarctions demonstrate definite Q waves, loss of R-wave voltage, or both, whereas subendocardial infarctions are characterized by only ST- or T-wave changes on their electrocardiograms. Of course, subendocardial and even transmural infarction can occur in the absence of electrocardiographic changes.

Earlier workers noted a more favorable clinical course in patients with nontransmural infarctions compared with individuals having transmural infarcts,[357–359] and it is agreed that the acute mortality in patients with subendocardial infarcts is approximately half that in patients with transmural infarcts.[347,360] However, it is now clear that nontransmural infarctions are not benign conditions.[361–363] Thus, 60 per cent of patients with subendocardial infarction have critical obstruction in two or three of the major coronary arteries, and approximately 20 per cent go on to develop an acute transmural infarction within 3 months of the subendocardial infarct.[361] In one series almost half of the patients with subendocardial infarction developed unstable angina during a follow-up period averaging 11 months.[364] In another, the incidence of infarct extension or early recurrent infarction was high.[361] Hutter et al. have reported high early and late reinfarction rates in patients with subendocardial infarctions and comparable late mortalities in patients with subendocardial and transmural infarctions.[360]

The correlation between the electrocardiographic findings of transmural and subendocardial myocardial infarction and their pathological counterparts is not good.[361a] Indeed, many patients with pathological transmural infarctions have no Q waves or have loss of R waves on the electrocardiogram and vice versa. Consequently, it has been suggested that the electrocardiographic terms transmural and subendocardial be changed to "Q-wave" and "non–Q-wave infarctions."

Notwithstanding the terminology, non–Q-wave infarctions (whether they represent subendocardial infarcts or not) may be considered relatively unstable conditions associated with a low initial mortality rate, a high risk of later infarction, and a high late mortality rate. The recognition in differences between the natural histories of these two forms of infarction suggests a more aggressive diagnostic approach, perhaps followed by early surgical treatment in suitable patients who have sustained an acute non–Q-wave infarction.

LATE POSTINFARCT ASSESSMENT. Following recovery from AMI—i.e., by 2 to 4 weeks after the event—long-term prognosis can be evaluated by ambulatory electrocardiographic monitoring and exercise testing.[364a] The development of ST-segment abnormalities, typical angina or exercise limitation by dyspnea at low levels of exercise (heart rate < 120 beats/min or exercise duration < 6 minutes on the Bruce protocol [p. 266]), and a major (> 2 mm) ST-segment depression and a stress-induced fall in blood pressure at any level of exercise signify a poor prognosis (p. 274 and 1389).[351,365,365a,365b,366] Radionuclide angiography,[366a] as well as coronary arteriography and left ventriculography, can provide additional important prognostic information, but the invasive tests are ordinarily carried out only if the patient is symptomatic or if the noninvasive tests suggest a poor prognosis and if the results of these examinations would alter the management (p. 1327) (Chap. 39).[361,368] Recent evidence indicates that electrical instability, as reflected in frequent, multiple, or complex ventricular extrasystoles, and left ventricular dysfunction, as reflected in a depressed left ventricular ejection fraction (< 40 per cent) 10 days after the occurrence of an AMI, are independent risk factors; the presence of both risk factors was associated with an increased 15-month mortality.[369,370]

References

1. May, G. S., Furberg, C. D., Eberlein, K. A., and Gerard, B. J.: Secondary prevention after myocardial infarction: a review of short term acute phase trials. Prog. Cardiovasc. Dis. 25:335, 1983.
2. Blackburn, H.: Progress in the epidemiology and prevention of coronary heart disease. In Yu, P. N., and Goodwin, J. F. (eds.): Progress in Cardiology. Philadelphia, Lea and Febiger, 1974, p. 1.
3. Feinleib, M., Havlik, R. J., and Thom, T. J.: The changing pattern of ischemic heart disease. J. Cardiovasc. Med. 7:139, 1982.

PATHOLOGY

4. Bloor, C. M.: Cardiac Pathology. Philadelphia, J. B. Lippincott Co., 1978, p. 176.
5. Mallory, G. K., White, P. D., and Salcedo-Salger, J.: The speed of healing of myocardial infarction: A study of the pathological anatomy in seventy-two cases. Am. Heart J. 18:647, 1939.
6. Fishbein, M. C., Maclean, D., and Maroko, P. R.: The histopathological evolution of myocardial infarction. Chest 73:843, 1978.
7. Buja, L. M., and Willerson, J. T.: Clinicopathologic correlates of acute ischemic heart disease syndromes. Am. J. Cardiol. 47:343, 1981.
8. Schlesinger, M. J., and Reiner, L.: Focal myocytolysis of the heart. Am. J. Pathol. 31:443, 1955.
9. Bouchardy, B., and Majno, G.: Histopathology of early myocardial infarcts. Am. J. Pathol. 74:301, 1974.
10. Derias, N. W., and Adams, C. W. M.: The non-specific nature of the myocardial wave fiber. Histopathology 3:241, 1979.
11. Kloner, R. A., Ganote, C. E., Whalen, D. A., Jr., and Jennings, R. B.: Effect of a transient period of ischemia on myocardial cells: Fine structure during the first few minutes of reflow. Am. J. Pathol. 74:399, 1974.
12. Willerson, J. T., Hillis, L. D., and Buja, L. M.: Ischemic Heart Disease. New York, Raven Press, 1982, 374 pp.
13. Sybers, H. D., Maroko, P. R., Ashraf, M., Libby, P., and Braunwald, E.: The effect of glucose-insulin-potassium on cardiac ultrastructure following acute experimental coronary occlusion. Am. J. Pathol. 70:401, 1973.
14. Jennings, R. B., and Ganote, C. E.: Structural change in myocardium during acute ischemia. Circ. Res. 35(Suppl. 3):156, 1974.
15. Kloner, R. A., Rude, R. E., Carlson, N., Maroko, P. R., Karaffa, S., DeBoer, L. W. V., and Braunwald, E.: Ultrastructural evidence of microvascular damage and myocardial cell injury after coronary artery occlusion: Which comes first? Circulation 62:945, 1980.
16. Kloner, R. A., and Braunwald, E.: Review—Observations on experimental myocardial ischemia. Cardiovasc. Res. 14:371, 1980.
17. Kloner, R. A., DeBoer, L. W. V., Carlson, N., and Braunwald, E.: The effect of verapamil on myocardial ultrastructure during and following release of coronary artery occlusion. Exp. Mol. Pathol. 36:277, 1982.
18. Caulfield, J., and Klionsky, B.: Myocardial ischemia and early infarction: An electron microscopic study. Am. J. Pathol. 35:489, 1959.
19. Shen, A. C., and Jennings, R. B.: Kinetics of calcium accumulation in acute myocardial ischemic injury. Am. J. Pathol. 67:441, 1972.
20. Kloner, R. A., Fishbein, M. C., Hare, C. M., and Maroko, P. R.: Early ischemic ultrastructural and histochemical alterations in the myocardium of the rat following coronary artery occlusion. Exp. Mol. Pathol. 30:129, 1979.
21. Baroldi, G.: Different types of myocardial necrosis in coronary heart disease: A pathophysiologic review of their functional significance. Am. Heart J. 89:742, 1975.
22. Hagler, H. K., Sherwin, L., and Buja, L. M.: Effect of different methods of tissue preparation on mitochondrial inclusions of ischemic and infarcted canine myocardium: Transmission and analytical electron microscopic study. Lab. Invest. 40:529, 1979.
23. Hutchins, G. M., and Bulkley, B. H.: Correlation of myocardial contraction band necrosis and vascular patency: A study of coronary artery bypass graft anastomoses at branch points. Lab Invest. 36:642, 1977.
24. Blumgart, H. L., Schlesinger, M. J., and Davis, D.: Studies on the relation of the clinical manifestations of angina pectoris, coronary thrombosis, and myocardial infarction to the pathologic findings with particular reference to the significance of the collateral circulation. Am. Heart J. 19:1, 1940.
25. Roberts, W. C.: Coronary arteries in fatal acute myocardial infarction. Circulation 45:215, 1972.
26. Betriu, A., Castaner, A., Sanz, G. A., Pare, J. C., Roig, E., Coll, S., Magrina, J., and Navarro-Lopez, F.: Angiographic findings 1 month after myocardial infarction: A prospective study of 259 survivors. Circulation 65:1099, 1982.
27. Silver, M. D., Baroldi, G., and Mariani, F.: The relationship between acute occlusive coronary thrombi and myocardial infarction studied in 100 consecutive patients. Circulation 61:219, 1980.
28. Friedberg, C. K., and Horn, H.: Acute myocardial infarction not due to coronary artery occlusion. J.A.M.A. 112:1675, 1939.
29. Allison, R. B., Rodriguez, F. L., Higgins, E. A., Jr., Leddy, J. P., Abelmann, W. H., Ellis, L. B., and Robbins, S. L.: Clinicopathologic correlations in coronary atherosclerosis. Four hundred thirty patients studied with post-mortem coronary angiography. Circulation 27:170, 1963.
30. Paterson, J. C.: Capillary rupture with intimal hemorrhage as a causative factor in coronary thrombosis. Arch. Pathol. 25:474, 1938.
31. Paterson, J. C.: Relation of physical exertion and emotion to precipitation of coronary thrombi. J.A.M.A. 112:895, 1939.

31a. Dalen, J. E., Ockene, I. S., and Alpert, J. S.: Coronary spasm, coronary thrombosis and myocardial infarction. Am. Heart J. 104:1119, 1982.
32. Roberts, W. C.: The coronary arteries in fatal coronary events. In Chung, E. K. (ed.): Controversies in Cardiology. New York, Springer-Verlag, 1976, p. 1.
33. Chandler, A. B., Chapman, I., Erhardt, L. R., Roberts, W. C., Schwartz, C. J., Sinapius, D., Spain, D. M., Sherry, S., Ness, P. M., and Simon, T. L.: Coronary thrombosis in myocardial infarction. Report of a workshop on the role of coronary thrombosis in the pathogenesis of acute myocardial infarction. Am. J. Cardiol. 34:823, 1974.
34. Herrick, J. B.: Clinical features of sudden obstruction of the coronary arteries. J.A.M.A. 59:2015, 1912.
35. Blumgart, H. L., Schlesinger, M. J., and Zoll, P. M.: Angina pectoris, coronary failure, and acute myocardial infarction; Role of coronary occlusions and collateral circulation. J.A.M.A. 116:91, 1941.
36. Miller, R. D., Burchell, H. B., and Edwards, J. E.: Myocardial infarction with and without acute coronary occlusion; A pathologic study. Arch. Intern. Med. 88:597, 1951.
37. Chandler, A. B.: Relationship of coronary thrombosis to myocardial infarction. Mod. Concepts Cardiovasc. Dis. 44:1, 1975.
38. Barold, G.: Pathological anatomy of myocardial infarction. In Wilhelmsen, L., and Hjalmarson, A. (eds.): Acute and Long-Term Medical Management of Myocardial Ischemia. Sweden, Mölndal, 1978, p. 41.
39. Ganz, W., Buchbinder, N., Marcus, H., Mondkar, A., Maddahi, J., Charuzi, Y., O'Connor, L., Shell, W., Fishbein, M. C., Kass, R., Miyamoto, A., and Swan, H. J. C.: Intracoronary thrombolysis in evolving myocardial infarction. Am. Heart J. 101:4, 1981.
40. Mathey, D. G., Kuck, K. H., Tilsner, V., Krebber, H. J., and Bleifeld, W.: Nonsurgical coronary artery recanalization in acute myocardial infarction. Circulation 63:489, 1981.
41. Rentrop, P., Blanke, H., Karsch, K. R., Kaiser, H., Kostering, H., and Leitz, K.: Selective intracoronary thrombolysis in acute myocardial infarction and unstable angina pectoris. Circulation 63:307, 1981.
42. Markis, J. E., Malagold, M., Parker, J. A., Silverman, K. J., Barry, W. H., Als, A. V., Paulin, S., Grossman, W., and Braunwald, E.: Myocardial salvage after intracoronary thrombolysis with streptokinase in acute myocardial infarction. N. Engl. J. Med. 305:777, 1981.
43. DeWood, M. A., Spores, J., and Notske, R.: Prevalence of total coronary occlusion during the early hours of transmural myocardial infarction. N. Engl. J. Med. 303:897, 1980.
44. Gagnon, R. M., Morissette, M., Bensimon, H., Beaudet, R., Poirier, N., Noel, C., Presant, S., and Lemire, J.: The role of coronary thrombosis in myocardial infarction: Further evidence shown by intracoronary thrombolysis with streptokinase. Cathet. Cardiovasc. Diagn. 8:393, 1982.
45. Oliva, P. B.: Pathophysiology of acute myocardial infarction, 1981. Ann. Intern. Med. 94:236, 1981.
46. Cheitlin, M. D., McAllister, H. A., and deCastro, C. M.: Myocardial infarction without atherosclerosis. J.A.M.A. 231:951, 1975.
47. Connolley, J. E., Eldridge, F. L., Calvin, J. W., and Stemmer, E. A.: Proximal coronary artery obstruction. N. Eng. J. Med. 271:213, 1964.
48. Roberts, W. C., MacGregor, R. R., DeBlanc, H. J., Beiser, G. D., and Wolff, S. M.: The prepulseless phase of pulseless disease, or pulseless disease with pulses. Am. J. Med. 46:313, 1969.
49. Laurie, W., and Woods, J. D.: Infarction (ischemic fibrosis) in the right ventricle of the heart. Acta Cardiol. 18:399, 1963.
50. Kegel, S. M., Dorsey, T. J., Rowen, M., and Taylor, W. F.: Cardiac death in mucocutaneous lymph node syndrome. Am. J. Cardiol. 40:282, 1977.
51. Liberthson, R. R., Homcy, C., Fallon, J. T., Gross, S., Leppo, J., and Miller, L.: Systemic lupus erythematosis and heart disease. Primary Cardiol. 9:77, 1983.
52. Cohn, K. E., Stewart, J. R., Fajardo, L. F., and Hancock, E. W.: Heart disease following radiation. Medicine 46:281, 1967.
53. Perloff, J. K.: Coronary artery disease—Antidote to a stereotype. Am. J. Cardiol. 30:437, 1972.
54. Bonfiglio, T. A., Botti, R. E., and Hagstrom, J. W. C.: Coronary arteritis, occlusion, and myocardial infarction due to lupus erythematosus. Am. Heart J. 83:153, 1972.
55. Huang, S., Kumar, G., Steele, H. D., and Parker, J. O.: Cardiac involvement in pseudoxanthoma elasticum. Am. Heart J. 74:680, 1967.
56. James, T. N.: Small arteries of the heart. Circulation 56:2, 1977.
57. Thompson, S. I., Vieweg, W. V. R., Alpert, J. S., and Hagan, A. D.: Incidence and age distribution of patients with myocardial infarction and normal coronary arteriograms. Cathet. Cardiovasc. Diagn. 3:1, 1977.
58. Rosenblatt, A., and Selzer, A.: The nature and clinical features of myocardial infarction with normal coronary arteriograms. Circulation 55:578, 1977.
59. Glover, M. V., Kuber, M. T., Warren, S. E., and Vieweg, W. V. R.: Myocardial infarction before age 36: Risk factor and arteriographic analysis. Am. J. Cardiol. 49:1600, 1982.
59a. Ciraulo, D. A., Bresnahan, G. F., Frankel, P. S., Isely, P. E., Zimmerman, W. R., and Chesne, R. B.: Transmural myocardial infarction with normal coronary angiograms and with single vessel coronary obstruction. Clinical-angiographic features and five-year follow-up. Chest 83:196, 1983.
60. Achuff, S. C., Bell, W. R., and Bulkley, B. H.: Thromboses in previously normal coronary arteries. Primary Cardiol. 8:137, 1982.
61. Khan, A. H., and Haywood, L. J.: Myocardial infarction in nine patients with radiologically patent coronary arteries. N. Engl. J. Med. 291:428, 1974.

62. Eliot, R. S., Baroldi, G., and Leone, A.: Necropsy studies in myocardial infarction with minimal or no coronary luminal reduction due to atherosclerosis. Circulation 49:1127, 1974.

63. Eslami, B., Russell, R. O., Jr., Bailey, M. T., Oberman, A., Tieszen, R. L., and Rackley, C. E.: Acute myocardial infarction in the absence of coronary arterial insufficiency. Ala. J. Med. Sci. 12:322, 1975.

64. Arnett, E. N., and Roberts, W. C.: Acute myocardial infarction and angiographically normal coronary arteries: An unproven combination. Circulation 53:395, 1976.

64a. Makino, H., and Al-Sadir, J.: Myocardial infarction in patients with mitral valve prolapse and normal coronary arteries. J. Am. Coll. Cardiol. 1:661, 1983.

65. Braunwald, E.: Editorial. Coronary spasm and acute myocardial infarction — New possibility for treatment and prevention. N. Engl. J. Med. 299:1301, 1978.

66. Sasse, L., Wagner, R., and Murray, F. E.: Transmural myocardial infarction during pregnancy. Am. J. Cardiol. 35:448, 1975.

67. Chesler, E., Matisonn, R. E., Lakier, J. B., Pocock, W. A., Obel, I. W. P., and Barlow, J. B.: Acute myocardial infarction with normal coronary arteries. A possible manifestation of the billowing mitral leaflet syndrome. Circulation 54:203, 1976.

68. Regan, T. J., Wu, C. F., Weisse, A. B., Moschos, C. B., Ahmed, S. S., and Lyons, M. D.: Acute myocardial infarction in toxic cardiomyopathy without coronary obstruction. Circulation 51:453, 1975.

69. Hallman, G. L., Cooley, D. A., and Singer, D. B.: Congenital anomalies of the coronary arteries. Surgery 59:133, 1966.

70. James, T. N.: Angina without coronary disease. Circulation 42:189, 1970.

71. Gorlin, R.: Coronary collaterals. In Coronary Artery Disease. Philadelphia, W. B. Saunders Co., 1976, p. 59.

72. Eckstein, R. W.: Development of interarterial coronary anastomoses by chronic anemia: Disappearance following correction of anemia. Circ. Res. 3:306, 1955.

73. Blumgart, H. L., Zoll, P. M., Paul, M. H., and Norman, L. R.: The effect of experimental acute coronary occlusion on stimulation of intercoronary collateral anastomoses. Trans. Assoc. Am. Phys. 68:155, 1955.

74. Gregg, D. E.: Coronary Circulation in Health and Disease. Philadelphia, Lea and Febiger, 1950.

75. Siepser, S. L., Kaltman, A. J., Mills, N., Pughkem, T., and Fox, A. C.: Coronary collateral flow after traumatic fistula between right coronary artery and right atrium. N. Engl. J. Med. 287:754, 1972.

76. Wiggers, C. J.: The functional importance of coronary collaterals. Circulation 5:609, 1952.

77. Helfant, R. H., Vokonas, P. S., and Gorlin, R.: Functional importance of human coronary collateral circulation. N. Engl. J. Med. 284:1277, 1971.

78. Carroll, R. J., Verani, M. S., and Falsetti, H. L.: The effect of collateral circulation on segmental left ventricular contraction. Circulation 50:709, 1974.

79. Levin, D. C.: Pathways and functional significance of the coronary collateral circulation. Circulation 50:831, 1974.

80. Hamby, R. I., Aintablian, A., and Schwartz, A.: Reappraisal of the functional significance of the coronary collateral circulation. Am. J. Cardiol. 38:304, 1976.

81. Carlton, R. A., and Boyd, T.: Traumatic laceration of the anterior descending coronary artery treated by ligation without myocardial infarction: Report of a case with review of the literature. Am. Heart J. 56:136, 1958.

82. Gold, H. K., Leinbach, R. C., and Maroko, P. R.: Propranolol-induced reduction of signs of ischemic injury during acute myocardial infarction. Am. J. Cardiol. 38:689, 1976.

83. Wackers, F. J. T., Lie, K. I., Sokole, E. B., Res, J., Schoot, J. B. V. D., and Durrer, D.: Prevalence of right ventricular involvement in inferior wall infarction assessed with myocardial imaging with thallium-201 and technetium-99m pyrophosphate. Am. J. Cardiol. 42:358, 1978.

84. Isner, J. M., and Roberts, W. C.: Right ventricular infarction complicating left ventricular infarction secondary to coronary heart disease. Frequency, location, associated findings and significance from analysis of 236 necropsy patients with acute or healed myocardial infarction. Am. J. Cardiol. 42:885, 1978.

85. Nixon, J. V.: Right ventricular myocardial infarction. Arch. Intern. Med. 142:945, 1982.

85a. Haupt, H. M., Hutchins, G. M., and Moore, G. W.: Right ventricular infarction: Role of the moderator band artery in determining infarct size. Circulation 67:1268, 1983.

86. Rackley, C. E., Russell, R. O., Jr., Mantle, J. A., Rogers, W. J., Papapietro, S. E., and Schwartz, K. M.: Right ventricular infarction and function. Am. Heart J. 101:215, 1981.

87. Wade, W. G.: The pathogenesis of infarction of the right ventricle. Br. Heart J. 21:545, 1957.

88. Silverman, B. D., Carabajal, N. R., Chorches, M. A., and Taranto, A. I.: Tricuspid regurgitation and acute myocardial infarction. Arch. Intern. Med. 142:1394, 1982.

89. Lloyd, E. A., Gersh, B. J., and Kennelly, B. M.: Hemodynamic spectrum of dominant right ventricular infarction. Am. J. Cardiol. 48:1016, 1981.

89a. Lopez-Sendon, J., Garcia-Fernandez, M. A., Coma-Canella, I., Yanguela, M. M., and Banuelos, F.: Segmental right ventricular function after acute myocardial infarction: Two-dimensional echocardiographic study in 63 patients. Am. J. Cardiol. 51:390, 1983.

90. Cushing, E. H., Feil, H. S., Stanton, E. J., and Wartman, W. B.: Infarction of the cardiac auricles (atria): Clinical, pathological and experimental studies. Br. Heart J. 4:17, 1942.

91. Wartman, W. B., and Hellerstein, H. K.: The incidence of heart disease in 2000 consecutive autopsies. Ann. Intern. Med. 28:41, 1948.

92. Lowe, T. E., and Wartman, W. B.: Myocardial infarction. Br. Heart J. 6:115, 183, 1944.

93. London, R. E., and London, S. B.: Rupture of the heart. A critical analysis of 47 consecutive autopsy cases. Circulation 31:202, 1965.

94. Björck, G., Mogensen, L., Nyquist, O., Orinius, E., and Sjögren, A.: Studies of myocardial rupture with cardiac tamponade in acute myocardial infarction. Chest 61:4, 1972.

95. Kassis, E., Vogelsang, M., and Lyngborg, K.: Cardiac rupture complicating myocardial infarction. A study concerning early diagnosis and possible management. Dan. Med. Bull. 48:164, 1981.

96. Edmondson, H. A., and Hoxie, H. J.: Hypertension and cardiac rupture: Clinical and pathological study of 72 cases, in 13 of which rupture of the interventricular septum occurred. Am. Heart J. 24:719, 1942.

97. Schuster, E. H., and Bulkley, B. H.: Expansion of transmural myocardial infarction: A pathophysiologic factor in cardiac rupture. Circulation 60:1532, 1979.

98. Vlodaver, Z., Coe, J. L., and Edwards, J. E.: True and false left ventricular aneurysms. Circulation 51:567, 1975.

99. Vlodaver, Z., and Edwards, J. E.: Rupture of ventricular septum or papillary muscle complicating myocardial infarction. Circulation 55:815, 1977.

100. Radford, M. J., Johnson, R. A., Daggett, W. M., Fallon, J. T., Buckley, M. J., Gold, H. K., and Leinbach, R. C.: Ventricular septal rupture: A review of clinical and physiologic features and an analysis of survival. Circulation 64:545, 1981.

101. Matsui, K., Kay, J. H., Mendez, M., Zubiate, P., Vanstrom, N., and Yokoyama, T.: Ventricular septal rupture secondary to myocardial infarction. Clinical approach and surgical results. J.A.M.A. 245:1537, 1981.

101a. Nishimura, R. A., Schaff, H. V., Shub, C., Gersh, B. J., Edwards, W. D., and Tajik, A.: Papillary muscle rupture complicating acute myocardial infarction: Analysis of 17 patients. Am. J. Cardiol. 51:373, 1983.

102. Roberts, W. C., and Cohen, L. D.: Left ventricular papillary muscles. Description of the normal and a survey of conditions causing them to be abnormal. Circulation 46:138, 1972.

103. Roberts, W. C., and Perloff, J. K.: Mitral valvular disease — A clinicopathologic survey of the conditions causing the mitral valve to function abnormally. Ann. Intern. Med. 77:939, 1972.

104. Wei, J. Y., Hutchins, G. M., and Bulkley, B. H.: Papillary muscle rupture in fatal acute myocardial infarction. Ann. Intern. Med. 90:149, 1979.

105. Abrams, D. L., Edelist, A., Luria, M. H., and Miller, A. J.: Ventricular aneurysm: A reappraisal based on a study of 65 consecutive autopsied cases. Circulation 27:164, 1963.

106. Schlicter, J., Hellerstein, H. K., and Katz, L. N.: Aneurysm of the heart: A correlative study of one hundred and two proved cases. Medicine 33:43, 1954.

107. Eaton, L. W., and Bulkley, B. H.: Expansion of acute myocardial infarction: Its relationship to infarct morphology in a canine model. Circ. Res. 49:80, 1981.

108. Swan, H. J. C., Forrester, J. S., Diamond, G., Chatterjee, K., and Parmley, W. W.: Hemodynamic spectrum of myocardial infarction and cardiogenic shock. Circulation 45:1097, 1972.

109. Graber, J. D., Oakley, C. M., Pickering, J. F., Goodwin, J. F., Raphael, M. J., and Steiner, R. E.: Ventricular aneurysm, an appraisal of diagnosis and surgical therapy. Br. Heart J. 34:830, 1972.

110. Asinger, R. W., Mikell, F. L., Elsperger, J., and Hodges, M.: Incidence of left ventricular thrombosis after acute transmural myocardial infarction. Serial evaluation of two-dimensional echocardiography. N. Engl. J. Med. 305:297, 1981.

111. Page, D. L., Caulfield, J. B., Kastor, J. A., DeSanctis, R. W., and Sanders, C. A.: Myocardial changes associated with cardiogenic shock. N. Engl. J. Med. 285:133, 1971.

112. Alonso, D. R., Scheidt, S., Post, M., and Killip, T.: Pathophysiology of cardiogenic shock; quantification of myocardial necrosis, clinical, pathologic and electrocardiographic correlation. Circulation 48:588, 1973.

112a. Resnekov, L.: Cardiogenic shock. Chest 83:893, 1983.

113. Fraker, T. D., Jr., Wagner, G. S., and Rosati, R. A.: Extension of myocardial infarction: Incidence and prognosis. Circulation 60:1126, 1979.

114. Gutovitz, A. L., Sobel, B. E., and Roberts, R.: Progressive nature of myocardial injury in selected patients with cardiogenic shock. Am. J. Cardiol. 41:469, 1978.

115. Wackers, F. J., Lie, K. I., Becker, A. E., Durrer, D., and Wellens, H. J. J.: Coronary artery disease in patients dying from cardiogenic shock or congestive heart failure in the setting of acute myocardial infarction. Br. Heart J. 38:906, 1976.

115a. Visser, C. A., Kan, G., Lie, K. I., and Durrer, D.: Incidence and one-year follow-up of left ventricular thrombus following acute myocardial infarction: An echocardiographic study of 96 patients. J. Am. coll. Cardiol. 1:648, 1983.

116. Hellerstein, H. K., and Martin, J. W.: Incidence of thrombo-embolic lesions accompanying myocardial infarction. Am. Heart J. 33:443, 1947.

117. Davies, M. J., Woolf, N., and Robertson, W. B.: Pathology of acute myocardial infarction with particular reference to occlusive coronary thrombi. Br. Heart J. 38:659, 1976.

118. Eppinger, E. C., and Kennedy, J. A.: The cause of death in coronary thrombo-

sis, with special reference to pulmonary embolism. Am. J. Med. Sci. *195*:104, 1938.

119. Blau, N., Shen, B. A., Pittman, D. E., and Joyner, C. E.: Massive hemopericardium in a patient with post-myocardial infarction syndrome. Chest *71*:549, 1977.

120. Dressler, W.: The post-myocardial infarction syndrome: A report of forty-four cases. Arch. Intern. Med. *103*:28, 1959.

121. Lichstein, E., Arsura, E., Hollander, G., Greengart, A., and Sanders, M.: Current incidence of postmyocardial infarction (Dressler's) syndrome. Am. J. Cardiol. *50*:1269, 1982.

122. Lichstein, E., Lin, H. M., and Gupta, P.: Pericarditis complicating acute myocardial infarction: Incidence of complications and significance of electrocardiogram on admission. Am. Heart J. *87*:246, 1974.

123. Soloff, L. A.: Pericardial cellular response during the post-myocardial infarction syndrome. Am. Heart J. *82*:812, 1971.

124. McCabe, J. C., Ebert, P. A., Engle, M. A., and Zabriskie, J. B.: Circulating heart-reactive antibodies in the postpericardiotomy syndrome. J. Surg. Res. *14*:158, 1973.

124a.Spann, J. F.: Changing concepts of pathophysiology, prognosis and therapy in acute myocardial infarction. Am. J. Med. *74*:877, 1983.

PATHOPHYSIOLOGY

125. Pfeffer, M. A., Pfeffer, J. M., Fishbein, M. C., Fletcher, P. J., Spadaro, J., Kloner, R. A., and Braunwald, E.: Myocardial infarct size and ventricular function in rats. Circ. Res. *44*:503, 1979.

125a.Slutsky, R. A., Mattrey, R. F., Long, S. A., and Higgins, C. B.: In vivo estimation of myocardial infarct size and left ventricular function by prospectively gated computerized transmission tomography. Circulation *67*:759, 1983.

126. Herman, M. V., Heinle, R. A., Klein, M. D., and Gorlin, R.: Localized disorders in myocardial contraction. N. Engl. J. Med. *277*:222, 1967.

127. Forrester, J. S., Wyatt, H. L., DaLuz, P. L., Tyberg, J. V., Diamond, G. A., and Swan, H. J. C.: Functional significance of regional ischemic contraction abnormalities. Circulation *54*:64, 1976.

128. Diamond, G., and Forrester, J. S.: Effect of coronary artery disease and acute myocardial infarction on left ventricular compliance in man. Circulation *45*:11, 1972.

129. Rackley, C. E., Russell, R. O., Jr., Mantle, J. A., and Rogers, W. J.: Modern approach to the patient with acute myocardial infarction. Curr. Prob. Cardiol. *1*:49, 1977.

130. Klein, M. D., Herman, M. V., and Gorlin, R. G.: A hemodynamic study of left ventricular aneurysm. Circulation *35*:614, 1967.

131. Wynne, J., Sayres, M., Maddox, D. E., Idoine, J., Alpert, J. S., Neill, J., and Holman, B. L.: Regional left ventricular function in acute myocardial infarction: Evaluation with quantitative radionuclide ventriculography. Am. J. Cardiol. *45*:203, 1980.

132. Weiss, J. L., Bulkley, B. H., Hutchins, G. M., and Mason, S. J.: Two-dimensional echocardiographic recognition of myocardial injury in man: Comparison with postmortem studies. Circulation *63*:401, 1981.

133. Forrester, J. S., Diamond, G., Parmley, W., and Swan, H. J. C.: Early increase in left ventricular compliance after myocardial infarction. J. Clin. Invest. *51*:598, 1972.

134. Pirzada, F. A., Ekong, E. A., Vokonas, P. S., Apstein, C. S., and Hood, W. B., Jr.: Experimental myocardial infarction. XIII. Sequential changes in left ventricular pressure-length relationships in the acute phase. Circulation *53*:970, 1976.

135. Smith, M., Ratshin, R. A., Harrel, F. E., Jr., Russell, R. O., Jr., and Rackley, C. E.: Early sequential changes in left ventricular dimensions and filling pressure in patients after myocardial infarction. Am. J. Cardiol. *33*:363, 1974.

136. Ratshin, R. A., Rackley, C. E., and Russell, R. O., Jr.: Hemodynamic evaluation of left ventricular function in shock complicating myocardial infarction. Circulation *45*:127, 1972.

137. Eaton, L. W., and Bulkley, B. H.: Expansion of acute myocardial infarction. Its relationship to infarct morphology in a canine model. Circ. Res. *49*:80, 1981.

138. Erlebacher, J. A., Weiss, J. L., Eaton, L. W., Kallman, C., Weisfeldt, M. L., and Bulkley, B. H.: Late effects of acute infarct dilation on heart size: A two-dimensional echocardiographic study. Am. J. Cardiol. *49*:1120, 1982.

139. Rude, R. E., Muller, J. E., and Braunwald, E.: Efforts to limit the size of myocardial infarcts. Ann. Intern. Med. *95*:736, 1981.

140. Forrester, J. S., Diamond, G., Chatterjee, K., and Swan, H. J. C.: Medical therapy of acute myocardial infarction by application of hemodynamic subsets. N. Engl. J. Med. *295*:1356, 1404, 1976.

141. Russell, R. O., Jr., Mantle, J. A., Rogers, W. J., and Rackley, C. E.: Current status of hemodynamic monitoring: Indications, diagnosis and complications. *In* Rackley, C. E. (ed.): Critical Care Medicine. Cardiovascular Clinics. Philadelphia, F. A. Davis, 1981, pp. 1–14.

141a.Rabinowitz, B., Elazar, E., and Neufeld, H. N.: A hemodynamic and autonomic profile of patients belonging to the hyperkinetic subset of acute myocardial infarction. J. Am. Coll. Cardiol. *1*:649, 1983.

141b.Chou, T-C., Fowler, N. O., Gabel, M., van der Bel-Kahn, J., and Feltner, E. J.: Electrocardiographic and hemodynamic changes in experimental right ventricular infarction. Circulation *67*:1258, 1983.

141c.Baigrie, R. S., Haq, A., Morgan, C. D., Rakowski, H., Drobac, M., and

McLaughlin, P.: The spectrum of right ventricular involvement in inferior wall myocardial infarction: A clinical, hemodynamic and noninvasive study. J. Am. Coll. Cardiol. *1*:1396, 1983.

142. Carabello, B., Cohn, P. F., and Alpert, J. S.: Hemodynamic monitoring in patients with hypotension after myocardial infarction. Chest *74*:5, 1978.

143. Coma-Canella, I., Lopez-Sendon, J., and Gamallo, C.: Low output syndrome in right ventricular infarction. Am. Heart J. *98*:613, 1979.

144. Haffajee, C. I., Love, J., Gore, J. M., and Alpert, J. S.: Reversibility of shock by atrial or atrioventricular sequential pacing in right ventricular infarction. Am. J. Cardiol. *49*:1025, 1982.

145. Marmor, A., Geltman, E. M., Biello, D. R., Sobel, B. E., Siegel, B. S., and Roberts, R.: Functional response to the right ventricle to myocardial infarction: Dependence on the site of left ventricular infarction. Circulation *64*:1005, 1981.

146. Braunwald, E.: Regulation of the circulation. N. Engl. J. Med. *290*:1124, 1420, 1974.

147. Biddle, T. L., Yu, P. N., Hodges, M., Chance, J. R., Ehrlich, D. A., Kronenberg, M. W., and Roberts, D. L.: Hypoxemia and lung water in acute myocardial infarction. Am. Heart J. *92*:692, 1976.

148. Biddle, T. L., Khanna, P. K., Yu, P. N., Hodges, M., and Shah, P. M.: Lung water in patients with acute myocardial infarction. Circulation *49*:115, 1974.

149. Lichtman, M. A., Cohen, J., Young, J. A., Whitbeck, A. A., and Murphy, M.: The relationships between arterial oxygen flow rate, oxygen binding by hemoglobin, and oxygen utilization after myocardial infarction. J. Clin. Invest. *54*:501, 1974.

150. DaLuz, P. L., Cavanilles, J. M., Michaels, S., Weill, M. H., and Shubin, H.: Oxygen delivery, anoxic metabolism and hemoglobin-oxygen affinity (P_{50}) in patients with acute myocardial infarction and shock. Am. J. Cardiol. *36*:148, 1975.

151. Hales, C. A., and Kazemi, H.: Small-airways function in myocardial infarction. N. Engl. J. Med. *290*:761, 1974.

152. Kazemi, H., Parsons, E. F., Valenca, L. M., and Strieder, D. J.: Distribution of pulmonary blood flow after myocardial ischemia and infarction. Circulation *41*:1025, 1970.

153. Datey, K. K., and Nanda, N. C.: Hyperglycemia after acute myocardial infarction. N. Engl. J. Med. *276*:262, 1976.

154. Vetter, N. J., Adams, W., Strange, R. C., and Oliver, M. F.: Initial metabolic and hormonal response to acute myocardial infarction. Lancet *1*:284, 1974.

155. Bertel, O., Buhler, F. R., Baitsch, G., Ritz, R., and Burkart, F.: Plasma adrenaline and noradrenaline in patients with acute myocardial infarction. Relationship to ventricular arrhythmias in varying severity. Chest *82*:64, 1982.

156. Taylor, S. H., Majid, P. A., Saxton, C., and Sharma, B.: Insulin secretion in heart failure. Am. Heart J. *83*:281, 1972.

157. Taylor, S. H., Saxton, C., Majid, P. A., Dykes, J. R. W., Ghosh, P., and Stoker, J. B.: Insulin secretion following myocardial infarction with particular respect to pathogenesis of cardiogenic shock. Lancet *2*:1373, 1969.

158. Ceremuzynski, L.: Hormonal and metabolic reactions evoked by acute myocardial infarction. Circ. Res. *48*:767, 1981.

159. Jefferson, L. S., Rannels, D. E., Munger, B. L., and Morgan, H. E.: Insulin in the regulation of protein turnover in heart and skeletal muscle. Fed. Proc. *33*:1098, 1974.

160. Opie, L. H.: Metabolism of free fatty acids, glucose, and catecholamines in acute myocardial infarction: Relation to myocardial ischemia and infarct size. Am. J. Cardiol. *36*:938, 1975.

161. Taggart, P., and Carruthers, M.: Endogenous hyperlipidemia induced by emotional stress of racing driving. Lancet *1*:363, 1971.

162. Valori, C., Thomas, M., and Shillingford, J.: Free noradrenaline and adrenaline excretion in relation to clinical syndromes following myocardial infarction. Am. J. Cardiol. *20*:605, 1969.

163. Gupta, D. K., Young, R., Jewitt, D. E., Hartog, M., and Opie, L. H.: Increased plasma free fatty acids and their significance in patients with acute myocardial infarction. Lancet *2*:1209, 1969.

164. Jequier, E., and Perret, C.: Urinary excretion of catecholamines and their main metabolites after myocardial infarction: Relationship to the clinical syndrome. Eur. J. Clin. Invest. *1*:77, 1970.

165. Logan, R. W., and Murdoch, W. R.: Blood levels of hydrocortisone, transaminases and cholesterol after myocardial infarction. Lancet *2*:521, 1966.

166. Baily, R. R., Abernethy, M. H., and Beaven, D. W.: Adrenocortical response to the stress of an acute myocardial infarction. Lancet *1*:970, 1976.

167. Steele, P., Rainwater, J., and Vogel, R.: Abnormal platelet survival time in men with myocardial infarction and normal coronary arteriogram. Am. J. Cardiol. *41*:60, 1978.

168. Laursen, B., and Gormsen, J.: Spontaneous fibrinolysis demonstrated by immunological technique. Thromb. Diath. Haemorrh. *17*:42, 1967.

169. Handin, R. I., McDonough, M., and Lesch, M.: Elevation of platelet factor 4 in acute myocardial infarction: Measurement by radioimmunoassay. J. Lab. Clin. Med. *91*:340, 1978.

170. Rickman, F. D., Handin, R., Howe, J. P., Alpert, J. S., Dexter, L., and Dalen, J. E.: Fibrin split products in acute pulmonary embolism. Ann. Intern. Med. *79*:664, 1973.

171. Jan, K. M., Chien, S., and Bigger, J. T., Jr.: Observation on blood viscosity changes after acute myocardial infarction. Circulation *51*:1079, 1972.

172. Hershberg, P. I., Wells, R. E., and McGandy, R. B.: Hematocrit and prognosis in patients with acute myocardial infarction. J.A.M.A. *219*:855, 1972.

CLINICAL FEATURES

173. Phipps, C.: Contributory causes of coronary thrombosis. J.A.M.A. *106*:761, 1936.
174. Master, A. M., Dack, S., and Jaffe, H. L.: Factors and events associated with onset of coronary artery thrombosis. J.A.M.A. *109*:546, 1937.
175. Smith, C., Sauls, H. C., and Ballew, J.: Coronary occlusion: A clinical study of 100 patients. Ann. Intern. Med. *17*:681, 1942.
176. French, A. J., and Dock, W.: Fatal coronary arteriosclerosis in young soldiers. J.A.M.A. *124*:1233, 1944.
177. Fitzhugh, G., and Hamilton, B. E.: Coronary occlusion and fatal angina pectoris: Study of the immediate causes and their prevention. J.A.M.A. *100*:475, 1933.
178. Knapp, R. B., Topkins, M. J., and Artusio, J. F., Jr.: The cerebrovascular accident and coronary occlusion in anesthesia. J.A.M.A. *182*:332, 1962.
179. Goldfischer, J. D.: Acute myocardial infarction secondary to ergot therapy. N. Engl. J. Med. *262*:860, 1960.
180. Roussak, N. J.: Myocardial infarction during serum sickness. Br. Heart J. *16*:218, 1954.
181. Levine, H. D.: Acute myocardial infarction following wasp sting. Report of two cases and critical survey of the literature. Am. Heart J. *91*:365, 1976.
182. Lange, R. L., Reid, M. S., Tresch, D. D., Keelan, M. H., Bernhard, V. M., and Coolidge, G.: Nonatheromatous ischemic heart disease following withdrawal from chronic industrial nitroglycerin exposure. Circulation *46*:666, 1972.
183. Maseri, A., L'Abbate, A., Baroldi, G., Chierchia, S., Marzilli, M., Ballestra, A. M., Severi, S., Parodi, O., Biagini, A., Distante, A., and Pesola, A.: Coronary vasospasm as a possible cause of myocardial infarction. A conclusion derived from the study of "preinfarction" angina. N. Engl. J. Med. *299*:1271, 1978.
184. Jenkins, C. D.: Recent evidence supporting psychologic and social risk factors for coronary disease. N. Engl. J. Med. *294*:987, 1033, 1976.
185. Rahe, R. H., Romo, M., Bennett, L., and Siltanen, P.: Recent life changes, myocardial infarction, and abrupt coronary death. Arch. Intern. Med. *133*:221, 1974.
186. Norris, N. M.: Myocardial Infarction. Edinburgh, Churchill Livingstone, 1982, 322 pp.
187. Alonzo, A. M., Simon, A. B., and Feinleib, M.: Prodromata of myocardial infarction and sudden death. Circulation *52*:1056, 1975.
188. Malliani, A., and Lombardi, F.: Consideration of the fundamental mechanisms eliciting cardiac pain. Am. Heart J. *103*:575, 1982.
189. Ikram, H., Orchard, R. T., and Read, S. E. C.: Intractable hiccupping in acute myocardial infarction. Br. Med. J. *2*:504, 1971.
190. Uretsky, B. F., Farquhar, D. S., Borezin, A., and Hood, W. B.: Symptomatic myocardial infarction without chest pain: Prevalence and clinical course. Am. J. Cardiol. *40*:498, 1977.
191. Margolis, J. R., Kannel, W. B., Feinleib, M., Dawber, T. R., and McNamara, P. M.: Clinical features of unrecognized myocardial infarction — Silent and symptomatic. Eighteen year follow-up: The Framingham Study. Am. J. Cardiol. *32*:1, 1973.
192. Sullivan, W., Vlodaver, Z., Tuna, N., Long, L., and Edward, J. E.: Correlation of electrocardiographic and pathologic findings in healed myocardial infarction. Am. J. Cardiol. *42*:724, 1978.
193. Bean, W. B.: Masquerade of myocardial infarction. Lancet *1*:1044, 1977.
194. Stone, P., and Muller, J. E.: Nifedipine therapy for recurrent ischemic pain following myocardial infarction. Clin. Cardiol. *5*:223, 1982.
195. Moran, T. J., French, W. J., Abrams, H. F., and Criley, J. M.: Post–myocardial infarction angina and coronary spasm. Am. J. Cardiol. *50*:197, 1982.
196. Koiwaya, Y., Torii, S., Takeshita, A., Nakagaki, O., and Nakamura, M.: Postinfarction angina caused by coronary arterial spasm. Circulation *65*:275, 1982.
197. Thoren, P. N.: Activation of left ventricular receptors with nonmedullated vagal afferent fibers during occlusion of a coronary artery in the cat. Am. J. Cardiol. *37*:1046, 1976.
198. Chadda, K. D., Lichstein, E., Gupta, P. K., and Choy, R.: Bradycardia-hypotension syndrome in acute myocardial infarction. Reappraisal of the overdrive effects of atropine. Am. J. Med. *59*:158, 1975.
199. Chizner, M. A.: Bedside diagnosis of the acute myocardial infarction and its complications. Curr. Probl. Cardiol. *7*:1, 1982.
200. Renner, W. F., and Renner, G. W.: The quality of resonance of the first heart sound after myocardial infarction: Clinical significance. Circulation *59*:1144, 1979.
201. Stein, P. D., Sabbah, H. N., and Barr, I.: Intensity of heart sounds in the evaluation of patients following myocardial infarction. Chest *75*:679, 1979.
202. Riley, C. P., Russell, R. O., Jr., and Rackley, C. E.: Left ventricular gallop sound and acute myocardial infarction. Am. Heart J. *86*:598, 1973.
203. Sawaya, J. I., Mujais, S. K., and Armenian, H. K.: Early diagnosis of pericarditis in acute myocardial infarction. Am. Heart J. *100*:144, 1980.
204. Thompson, P. L., and Robinson, J. S.: Stroke after acute myocardial infarction: Relation to infarct size. Br. Med. J. *2*:457, 1978.
205. Sobel, B. E., and Shell, W. E.: Serum enzyme determinations in the diagnosis and assessment of myocardial infarction. Circulation *45*:471, 1972.
206. Hearse, D. J.: Myocardial enzyme leakage. J. Mol. Med. *2*:185, 1977.
207. Pasyk, S., Bloor, C. M., Khouri, E. M., and Gregg, D. E.: Systemic and coronary effects of coronary artery occlusion in the unanesthetized dog. Am. J. Physiol. *220*:646, 1971.
208. Shell, W. E., Kjekshus, J. K., and Sobel, B. E.: Quantitative assessment of the extent of myocardial infarction in the conscious dog by means of analysis of serial changes in serum creatine phosphokinase activity. J. Clin. Invest. *50*:2614, 1971.
209. Agress, C. M., and Kin, J. H. C.: Evaluation of enzyme tests in the diagnosis of heart disease. Am. J. Cardiol. *6*:641, 1960.
210. Vasudevan, G., Mercer, D. W., and Varat, M. A.: Lactic dehydrogenase isoenzyme determination in the diagnosis of acute myocardial infarction. Circulation *57*:1055, 1978.
211. Weidner, N.: Laboratory diagnosis of acute myocardial infarct. Usefulness of determination of lactate dehydrogenase (LDH)–1 level and the ratio of LDH–1 to total LDH. Arch. Pathol. Lab. Med. *106*:375, 1982.
212. Goldberg, D. M., and Windfield, D. A.: Diagnostic accuracy of serum enzyme assays for myocardial infarction in a general hospital population. Br. Heart J. *34*:597, 1972.
213. Roberts, R., and Sobel, B. E.: Isoenzymes of creatine phosphokinase and diagnosis of myocardial infarction. Ann. Intern. Med. *79*:741, 1973.
214. Tsung, S. H.: Several conditions causing elevation of serum CK-MB and CK-BB. Am. J. Clin. Pathol. *75*:711, 1981.
215. Roberts, R., Gowda, K. S., Ludbrook, P. A., and Sobel, B. E.: Specificity of elevated serum MB creatine phosphokinase activity in the diagnosis of acute myocardial infarction. Am. J. Cardiol. *36*:433, 1975.
216. Roberts, R., and Sobel, B. E.: Creatine kinase isoenzymes in the assessment of heart disease. Am. Heart J. *95*:521, 1978.
217. Roberts, R., Sobel, B. E., and Parker, C. W.: Radioimmunoassay for creatine kinase isoenzymes. Science *194*:855, 1976.
218. Alderman, E. L., Matlof, H. J., Shumway, N. E., and Harrison, D. C.: Evaluation of enzyme testing for the detection of myocardial infarction following direct coronary surgery. Circulation *48*:135, 1973.
219. Klein, M. S., Colemen, R. E., Weldon, C. S., Sobel, B. E., and Robert, R.: Concordance of electrocardiographic and scintigraphic criteria of myocardial injury after cardiac surgery. J. Thorac. Cardiovasc. Surg. *71*:934, 1976.
220. Roberts, R., Sobel, B. E., and Ludbrook, P. A.: Determination of the origin of elevated plasma CPK after cardiac catheterization. Cathet. Cardiovasc. Diagn. *2*:239, 1976.
221. Heller, G. V., Blaustein, A. S., and Wei, J. Y.: Implications of increased myocardial isoenzyme level in the presence of normal serum creatine kinase activity. Am. J. Cardiol. *51*:24, 1983.
221a. Smith, J. L., Ambos, D., Gold, H. K., Muller, J. E., Poole, W. K., Raabe, D. S., Jr., Rude, R. E., Passamani, E., Braunwald, E., Sobel, B. E., Roberts, R., and the MILIS Study Group. Am. J. Cardiol. *51*:1294, 1983.
222. Grande, P., Hansen, B. F., Christiansen, C., and Naestoft, J.: Estimation of acute myocardial infarct size in man by serum CK-MB measurements. Circulation *65*:756, 1982.
223. Hori, M., Inoue, M., Fukui, S., Shimazu, T., Mishima, M., Ohgitani, N., Minamino, T., and Abe, H.: Correlation of ejection fraction and infarct size estimated from the total CK released in patients with acute myocardial infarction. Br. Heart J. *41*:433, 1979.
224. Geltman, E. M., Ehsani, A. A., Campbell, M. K., Schechtman, K., Roberts, R., and Sobel, B. E.: The influence of location and extent of myocardial infarction on long-term ventricular dysrhythmia and mortality. Circulation *60*:805, 1979.
225. Goldberger, E., Alesio, J., and Woll, F.: The significance of hyperglycemia in myocardial infarction. N.Y. State Med. J. *45*:391, 1945.
226. Rahe, R. H., Rubin, R. T., Arthur, R. J., and Clark, B. R.: Serum uric acid and cholesterol variability. J.A.M.A. *206*:2875, 1973.
227. Tan, M. H., and Wilmshurst, E. G., Gleason, R. E., and Soeldner, J. S.: Effect of posture on serum lipids. N. Engl. J. Med. *289*:416, 1973.
228. Kagen, L., Scheidt, S., and Butt, A.: Serum myoglobin in myocardial infarction: The "staccato phenomenon." Is acute myocardial infarction in man an intermittent event? Am. J. Med. *62*:86, 1977.
229. Vallee, B. L.: The time course of serum copper concentrations of patients with myocardial infarction. Metabolism *1*:420, 1952.
230. Sunderman, F. W., Jr., Nomoto, S., Pradhan, A. M., Levine, H., Bernstein, S. H., and Hirsch, R.: Increased concentration of serum nickel after acute myocardial infarction. N. Engl. J. Med. *283*:896, 1970.
231. Wacker, W. E. C., Ulmer, D. D., and Vallee, B. L.: Metalloenzymes and myocardial infarction. II. Malic and lactic dehydrogenase activities and zinc concentrations in serum. N. Engl. J. Med. *255*:449, 1956.
232. Fitzsimons, E. J., and Kaplan, K.: Rapid drop in serum iron concentration in myocardial infarction. Am. J. Clin. Pathol. *73*:552, 1980.
233. Rector, W. G., Jr., DeWood, M. A., Williams, R. V., and Sullivan, J. F.: Serum magnesium and copper levels in myocardial infarction. Am. J. Med. Sci. *281*:25, 1981.
234. Eastham, R. D., and Morgan, E. H.: Plasma-fibrinogen levels in coronary-artery disease. Lancet *2*:1196, 1963.
235. Savage, R. M., Wagner, G. S., Ideker, R. E., Podolsky, S. A., and Hackel, D. B.: Correlation of postmortem anatomic findings with electrocardiographic changes in patients with myocardial infarction. Circulation *55*:279, 1977.
236. Cooksey, J. D., Dunn, M., and Massie, E.: Clinical Vectorcardiography and Electrocardiography. 2nd Ed. Chicago, Year Book Medical Publishers, 1977, p. 361.

237. Haiat, R., Worthington, F. X., Castellanos, A., and Lemberg, L.: Unusual normalization of the electrocardiogram on the 6th day of myocardial infarction. J. Electrocardiol. *4*:363, 1971.

238. Candell-Riera, J., Figueras, J., Valle, V., Alvarez, A., Gutierrez, L., Cortadellas, J., Cinca, J., Salas, A., and Rius, J.: Right ventricular infarction: Relationships between ST segment elevation in V$_{4R}$ and hemodynamic, scintigraphic, and echocardiographic findings in patients with acute inferior myocardial infarction. Am. Heart J. *101*:281, 1981.

239. Chou, T., Van Der Bel-Kahn, J., Allen, J., Brockmeier, L., and Fowler, N.O.: Electrocardiographic diagnosis of right ventricular infarction. Am. J. Med. *70*: 1175, 1981.

240. Lieu, C. K., Greenspan, G., and Piccirillo, R. T.: Atrial infarction of the heart. Circulation *23*:331, 1961.

241. Silvertssen, E., Hoel, B., Bay, G., and Jorgensen, L.: Electrocardiographic atrial complex and acute atrial myocardial infarction. Am. J. Cardiol. *31*:450, 1973.

242. Stein, P. D., and Simon, A. P.: Vectorcardiographic diagnosis of diaphragmatic myocardial infarction. Am. J. Cardiol. *38*:568, 1976.

243. Howard, P. F., Benchimol, A., Desser, K. B., Reich, F. D., and Graves, C.: Correlation of electrocardiogram and vectorcardiogram with coronary occlusion and myocardial contraction abnormality. Am. J. Cardiol. *38*:582, 1976.

244. Levine, H. D., Young, E., and Williams, R. A.: Electrocardiogram and vectorcardiogram in myocardial infarction. Circulation *45*:457, 1972.

245. Yu, P. N., Fox, S. M., Imboden, C. A., Jr., and Killip, T.: Coronary care unit. I. A specialized intensive care unit for acute myocardial infarction. Mod. Concepts Cardiovasc. Dis. *34*:23, 1965.

246. Meltzer, L. E., and Cohen, H. E.: The incidence of arrhythmias associated with acute myocardial infarction. *In* Meltzer, L. E., and Dunning, A. J. (eds.): Textbook of Coronary Care. Philadelphia, Charles Press, 1972.

247. Pantridge, J. F., and Adgey, A. A. J.: Pre-hospital coronary care. The mobile coronary care unit. Am. J. Cardiol. *24*:666, 1969.

247a.Julian, D. G., Valentine, P. A., and Miller, G. G.: Disturbances of rate, rhythm and conduction in acute myocardial infarction. Am. J. Med. *37*:915, 1964.

248. Hinkel, L. E., Jr., Carver, S. T., and Stevens, M.: The frequency of asymptomatic disturbances of cardiac rhythm and conduction in middle-aged men. Am. J. Cardiol. *24*:629, 1969.

249. Adgey, A. A. J., Alley, J. D., Geddes, J. S., James, R. G. G., Webb, S. W., and Zaidi, S. A.: Acute phase of myocardial infarction. Lancet *2*:501, 1971.

250. Graner, L. E., Gershen, B. J., Orlando, M. M., and Epstein, S. E.: Bradycardia and its complications in the pre-hospital phase of acute myocardial infarction. Am. J. Cardiol. *32*:607, 1973.

251. Zipes, D. P.: The clinical significance of bradycardic rhythms in acute myocardial infarction. Am. J. Cardiol. *24*:814, 1969.

251a.Mark, A. L.: The Bezold-Jarisch reflex revisited: Clinical implications of inhibitory reflezes originating in the heart. J. Am. Coll. Cardiol. *1*:90, 1983.

252. Wei, J. Y., Markis, J. E., Malagold, M., and Braunwald, E.: Cardiovascular reflexes stimulated by reperfusion of ischemic myocardium in acute myocardial infarction. Circulation *67*:796, 1983.

253. Meltzer, L. E., and Kitchell, J. B.: The incidence of arrhythmias associated with acute myocardial infarction. Prog. Cardiovasc. Dis. *9*:50, 1966.

254. DeSanctis, R. W., Block, P., and Hutter, A. M.: Tachyarrhythmias in myocardial infarction. Circulation *45*:681, 1972.

255. Jewitt, D. E., Balcon, R., Raftery, E. B., and Oram, S.: Incidence and management of supraventricular arrhythmias after acute myocardial infarction. Lancet *2*:734, 1967.

256. Rothfeld, E. L., Parsonnet, J., McGorman, W., and Linden, S.: Harbingers of paroxysmal ventricular tachycardia in acute myocardial infarction. Chest *71*: 142, 1977.

257. El-Sherif, N., Gann, D., and Sung, R. J.: Initiation of ventricular fibrillation by supraventricular beats in patients with acute myocardial infarction. (Abstr.). Circulation *58*(Suppl. II):195, 1978.

258. James, T. N.: Myocardial infarction and atrial arrhythmias. Circulation *24*: 761, 1961.

259. Konecke, L. L., and Knoebel, S. B.: Nonparoxysmal junctional tachycardia complicating acute myocardial infarction. Circulation *45*:367, 1972.

260. Lown, B., Fakhro, A., Hood, W. B., and Thorn, G. W.: The coronary care unit—New perspectives and directions. J.A.M.A. *199*:188, 1967.

261. Julian, D. T., Valentine, P. Z., and Miller, G. G.: Disturbances of rate, rhythm and conduction in acute myocardial infarction. A prospective study of 100 consecutive unselected patients with the aid of electrocardiographic monitoring. Am. J. Med. *37*:915, 1964.

262. Lie, K. J., Wellens, H. J. J., Dorsnar, E., and Durrer, D.: Observations on patients with primary ventricular fibrillation complicating acute myocardial infarction. Circulation *52*:755, 1975.

263. El-Sherif, N., Myerburg, R. J., Scherlag, B. J., Befeler, B., Aranda, J. M., Castellanos, A., and Lazzara, R.: Electrocardiographic antecedents of primary ventricular fibrillation. Value of the R-on-T phenomenon in myocardial infarction. Br. Heart J. *38*:415, 1976.

264. Lawrie, D. M., Higgins, M. R., Godman, M. J., Julian, D. G., and Donald, K. W.: Ventricular fibrillation complicating acute myocardial infarction. Lancet *2*:523, 1968.

265. Williams, D. O., Scherlag, B. J., Hope, R. R., El-Sherif, N., and Lazzara, R.: The pathophysiology of malignant ventricular arrhythmias during acute myocardial ischemia. Circulation *50*:1163, 1974.

266. El-Sherif, N., Scherlag, B. J., and Lazzara, R.: Electrode catheter recordings during malignant ventricular arrhythmias following experimental acute myocardial ischemia. Evidence for reentry due to conduction delay and block in ischemic myocardium. Circulation *51*:1003, 1975.

267. DeSoyza, N., Meacham, D., Murphy, M. L., Kane, J. J., Doherty, J. E., and Bissett, J. K.: Evaluation of warning arrhythmias before paroxysmal ventricular tachycardia during acute myocardial infarction in man. Circulation *60*:814, 1979.

268. Roberts, R., Ambos, H. D., Loh, C. W., and Sobel, B. E.: Initiation of repetitive ventricular depolarizations by relatively late premature complexes in patients with acute myocardial infarction. Am. J. Cardiol. *41*:678, 1978.

269. Campbell, R. W. F., Murray, A., and Julian, D. G.: Relation of ventricular arrhythmias to ventricular fibrillation. Br. Heart J. *43*:109, 1980.

270. Wenger, T. L., Bigger, J. T., Jr., and Merrill, G. S.: Ventricular arrhythmias in the late hospital phase of acute myocardial infarction. Circulation *52*:110, 1975.

271. Schulze, R. A., Rouleau, J., Rigo, P., Bowers, S., Strauss, H. W., and Pitt, B.: Ventricular arrhythmias in the late phase of acute myocardial infarction: Relation to left ventricular function detected by gated cardiac blood pool scanning. Circulation *52*:1006, 1975.

272. Oliver, G. C., Nolle, F. M., and Tiefenbrunn, J.: Ventricular arrhythmias associated with sudden death in survivors of acute myocardial infarction. Am. J. Cardiol. *33*:160, 1974.

273. Moss, A. J., De Camilla, J. J., Davis, H. P., and Bayer, L.: Clinical significance of ventricular ectopic beats in the early post-hospital phase of myocardial infarction. Am. J. Cardiol. *39*:635, 1977.

274. Anderson, K. P., De Camilla, J., and Moss, A. J.: Clinical significance of ventricular tachycardia (three beats or longer) detected during ambulatory monitoring after myocardial infarction. Circulation *57*:890, 1978.

275. Bigger, J. T., Jr., Weld, F. M., and Rolnitzky, L. M.: Prevalence, characteristics and significance of ventricular tachycardia (three or more complexes) detected with ambulatory electrocardiographic recording in the late hospital phase of acute myocardial infarction. Am. J. Cardiol. *48*:815, 1981.

276. DeSoyza, N., Bissett, J. K., Kane, J. J., Murphy, M. L., and Doherty, J. E.: Association of accelerated idioventricular rhythm and paroxysmal ventricular tachycardia in acute myocardial infarction. Am. J. Cardiol. *34*:667, 1974.

277. Sclarovsky, S., Strasberg, B., Martonovich, G., and Agmon, J.: Ventricular rhythms with intermediate rates in acute myocardial infarction. Chest *74*:180, 1978.

278. Lichstein, E., Ribas-Meneclier, C., Gupta, P. K., and Chadda, K. D.: Incidence and description of accelerated idioventricular rhythm complicating acute myocardial infarction. Am. J. Med. *58*:192, 1975.

279. Lie, K. I., Liem, K. L., Schuilenburg, R. M., David, G. K., and Durrer, D.: Early identification of patients developing late in-hospital ventricular fibrillation after discharge from the coronary care unit. Am. J. Cardiol. *41*:674, 1978.

280. Shillingford, J., and Thomas, M.: Hemodynamic effects of acute myocardial infarction in man. Prog. Cardiovasc. Dis. *9*:571, 1967.

281. Lassers, B. E., Anderton, J. L., George, M., Muir, A. L., and Julian, D. G.: Hemodynamic effects of artificial pacing in complete heart block complicating acute myocardial infarction. Circulation *38*:308, 1968.

282. Ruskin, J., McHale, P. A., Harley, A., and Greenfield, J. C., Jr.: Pressure-flow studies in man; effects of atrial systole on left ventricular function. J. Clin. Invest. *49*:472, 1970.

283. Rahimtoola, S. H., Ehsani, A., Sinno, M. Z., Loeb, H. S., Rosen, K. M., and Gunnar, R. M.: Left atrial transport function in myocardial infarction; Importance of its booster function. Am. J. Med. *59*:686, 1975.

284. Damato, A. N., and Lau, S. H.: Clinical value of the electrogram of the conduction system. Prog. Cardiovasc. Dis. *13*:119, 1970.

285. Johansson, B. W.: Atrioventricular and bundle branch block in acute myocardial infarction. Natural history and prognosis. *In* Meltzer, L. E., and Dunning. A. J. (eds.): Textbook of Coronary Care. Philadelphia, Charles Press, 1972, p. 328.

286. Rotman, M., Wagner, G. S., and Wallace, A. G. P.: Bradyarrhythmias in acute myocardial infarction. Circulation *45*:703, 1972.

287. Friedberg, C. K., Cohen, H., and Donoso, E.: Advanced heart block as a complication of acute myocardial infarction. Role of pacemaker therapy. Prog. Cardiovasc. Dis. *10*:466, 1968.

288. Beregovich, J., Fenig, S., and Lassers, J.: Management of acute myocardial infarction complicated by advanced atrioventricular block: Role of artificial pacing. Am. J. Cardiol. *23*:54, 1969.

289. Lassers, B. W., and Julian, D. G.: Artificial pacing in management of complete heart block complicating myocardial infarction. Br. Med. J. *2*:142, 1968.

290. Chatterjee, K., Harris, A., and Leatham, A.: The risk of pacing after infarction, and current recommendation. Lancet *2*:1061, 1969.

291. Kostuk, W. J., and Beanland, D. S.: Complete heart block associated with acute myocardial infarction. Am. J. Cardiol. *26*:380, 1970.

292. Biddle, T. L., Ehrich, D. A., Hu, P. N., and Hodges, M.: Relation of heart block and left ventricular dysfunction in acute myocardial infarction. Am. J. Cardiol. *39*:961, 1977.

293. Hindman, M. C., Wagner, G. S., Jaro, M., Atkins, J. M., Scheinman, M. M., DeSanctis, R. W., Hutter, A. H., Yeatman, L., Rubenfire, M., Pujure, C., Rubvin, M., and Morris, J. J.: The clinical significance of bundle branch block complicating acute myocardial infarction. I. Clinical characteristics, hospital mortality and one-year follow-up. Circulation *58*:679, 1978.

294. Lie, K. I., Wellens, H. J., and Schuilenburg, R. M.: Bundle branch block and

acute myocardial infarction. *In* Wellens, H. J. J., Lie, K. I., and Janse, M. J. (eds.): The Conduction System of the Heart: Structure, Function and Clinical Implications. Philadelphia, Lea and Febiger, 1976, pp. 662–672.

295. Mullins, C. B., and Atkins, J. M.: Prognoses and management of ventricular conduction blocks in acute myocardial infarction. Mod. Concepts Cardiovasc. Dis. *45*:129, 1976.

296. Scheinman, M. M., and Gonzalez, R. P.: Fascicular block and acute myocardial infarction. J.A.M.A. *244*:2646, 1980.

297. Atkins, J. M., Leshin, S. J., Blomquist, G., and Mullins, C. B.: Ventricular conduction blocks and sudden death in acute myocardial infarction. N. Engl. J. Med. *288*:281, 1973.

298. Godman, M. J., Lassers, B. W., and Julian, D. G.: Complete bundle branch block complicating acute myocardial infarction. N. Engl. J. Med. *282*:237, 1970.

299. Kostuk, W., Barr, J. W., Simon, A. L., and Ross, J., Jr.: Correlations between the chest film and hemodynamics in acute myocardial infarction. Circulation *48*:624, 1973.

300. McHugh, T. J., Forrester, J. S., Adler, L., Zion, D., and Swan, H. J. C.: Pulmonary vascular congestion in acute myocardial infarction: Hemodynamic and radiologic correlations. Ann. Intern. Med. *79*:29, 1972.

301. Timmis, A. D., Fowler, M. B., Burwood, R. J., Gishen, P., Vincent, R., and Chamberlain, D. A.: Pulmonary oedema without critical increase in left atrial pressure in acute myocardial infarction. Br. Med. J. *283*:636, 1981.

302. Field, B. J., Russell, R. O., Jr., Moraski, R. E., Soto, B., Hood, W. P., Jr., Burdenshaw, J. A., Smith, M., Maurer, B. J., and Rackley, C. E.: Left ventricular size and function and heart size in the year following myocardial infarction. Circulation *50*:331, 1974.

303. Brattler, A., Karliner, J. S., Higgins, C. B., Slutsky, R., Gilpin, E. A., Froelicher, V. F., and Ross, J., Jr.: The initial chest x-ray in acute myocardial infarction. Prediction of early and late mortality and survival. Circulation *61*:1004, 1980.

304. Gibson, R. S., Taylor, G. J., Watson, D. D., Stebbins, P. T., Martin, R. P., Crampton, R. S., and Beller, G. A.: Predicting the extent and location of coronary artery disease during the early postinfarction period by quantitative thallium-201 scintigraphy. Am. J. Cardiol. *47*:1010, 1981.

305. Willerson, J. T., Parkey, R. W., Lewis, S. E., Bonte, F. J., and Buja, L. M.: Hot-spot imaging for patients with acute myocardial infarction. J. Cardiovasc. Med. *7*:291, 1982.

306. Geltman, E. M., Biello, D., Welch, M. J., Ter-Pogossian, M. M., Roberts, R., and Sobel, B. E.: Characterization of nontransmural myocardial infarction by positron-emission tomography. Circulation *65*:747, 1982.

306a. Lindvall, K., Erhardt, L., and Sjogren, A.: Serial M-mode echocardiographic mapping in myocardial infarction: A quantitative evaluation of left ventricular wall motion abnormalities. Clin. Cardiol. *6*:220, 1983.

307. Teichholz, L. E., Kreulen, T., Herman, M. V., and Gorlin, R.: Problems in echocardiographic volume determinations; echocardiographic-angiographic correlations in the presence or absence of asynergy. Am. J. Cardiol. *37*:7, 1976.

308. Corya, B. C., Rasmussen, S., Knoebel, S. B., and Feigenbaum, H.: Echocardiography in acute myocardial infarction. Am. J. Cardiol. *36*:1, 1975.

309. Nieminen, M., and Heikkilä, J.: Echoventriculography in acute myocardial infarction. II. Monitoring of left ventricular performance. Br. Heart J. *38*:271, 1976.

310. Fletcher, P. J., Berning, J., Wynne, J., Ostriker, G., Sayres, M., Holman, B. L., and Alpert, J. S.: Prospective evaluation of M-mode echocardiography in acute myocardial infarction: Comparison of gated radionuclide ventriculography. Br. Heart J.

311. Feigenbaum, H., Corya, B. C., Dillon, J. C., Weyman, A. E., Rasmussen, S., Black, M. J., and Chang, S.: Role of echocardiography in patients with coronary artery disease. Am. J. Cardiol. *37*:775, 1976.

312. Chandraratna, P. A. N., Balachandran, P. K., Shah, P. M., and Hodges, M.: Echocardiographic observation on ventricular septal rupture complicating acute myocardial infarction. Circulation *51*:506, 1975.

313. DeJoseph, R. L., Seides, S. F., Lindner, A., and Damato, A. N.: Echocardiographic findings of ventricular septal rupture in acute myocardial infarction. Am. J. Cardiol. *36*:346, 1975.

314. Sharpe, D. N., Botvinick, E. H., Shames, D. M., Schiller, N. B., Massie, B. M., Chatterjee, D., and Parmley, W. W.: The noninvasive diagnosis of right ventricular infarction. Circulation *57*:483, 1978.

315. Heger, J. J., Weyman, A. E., Wann, L. S., Dillon, J. C., and Feigenbaum, H.: Cross-sectional echocardiography in acute myocardial infarction: Detection and localization of regional left ventricular asynergy. Circulation *60*:531, 1979.

316. Visser, C. A., Lie, K. I., Becker, A. E., and Durrer, D.: Apex two-dimensional echocardiography. Alternative approach to quantification of acute myocardial infarction. Br. Heart J. *47*:461, 1982.

317. Gibson, R. S., Bishop, H. L., Stamm, R. B., Crampton, R. S., Beller, G. A., and Martin, R. P.: Value of early two dimensional echocardiography in patients with acute myocardial infarction. Am. J. Cardiol. *49*:1110, 1982.

318. Richards, K. L., Hoekenga, D. E., Leach, J. K., and Blaustein, J. C.: Dopplercardiographic diagnosis of interventricular septal rupture. Chest *76*:101, 1979.

319. Bishop, H. L., Gibson, R. S., Stamm, R. B., Beller, G. A., and Martin, R. P.: Role of two-dimensional echocardiography in the evaluation of patients with ventricular septal rupture postmyocardial infarction. Am. Heart J. *102*:965, 1981.

320. Donaldson, R. M., and Ballester, M.: Echocardiographic visualization of the anatomic causes of mitral regurgitation resulting from myocardial infarction. Postgrad. Med. J. *58*:257, 1982.

321. Morganroth, J., Parisi, A., and Pohost, G. M. (eds.): Noninvasive Cardiac Imaging. Chicago, Year Book Medical Publishers, 1983, p. 203.

322. Hamosh, P., Cohn, J. N., Engleman, K., Broder, M. I., and Freis, E. D.: Systolic time intervals and left ventricular function in acute myocardial infarction. Circulation *45*:375, 1972.

323. Inoue, K., Young, G. M., Brievson, A. L., Smulyan, H., and Eich, R. H.: Isometric contraction period of the left ventricle in acute myocardial infarction. Circulation *42*:79, 1970.

324. Parker, M. E., and Just, H. G.: Systolic time intervals in coronary artery disease as indices of left ventricular function: Fact or fancy? Br. Heart J. *36*:368, 1974.

325. Brubakk, O., and Overskeid, K.: Systolic time intervals in acute myocardial infarction. Acta Med. Scand. *199*:33, 1976.

326. Khan, A. H., and Haywood, L. J.: Value of serial apexcardiograms during and after myocardial infarction. Chest *70*:367, 1976.

327. Swan, H. J. C., Ganz, W., Forrester, J. S., Marcus, H., Diamond, G., and Chonette, D.: Catheterization of the heart in man with use of a flow-directed balloon-tipped catheter. N. Engl. J. Med. *283*:447, 1970.

328. Russell, R. O., Jr., Rackley, C. E., Pombo, J., Hunt, D., Potanin, C., and Dodge, H. T.: Effects of increasing left ventricular filling pressure in patients with acute myocardial infarction. J. Clin. Invest. *49*:1539, 1970.

329. Crexells, C., Chatterjee, K., Forrester, J. S., Dikshit, K., and Swan, H. J. C.: Optimal level of filling pressure in the left side of the heart in acute myocardial infarction. N. Engl. J. Med. *289*:1263, 1973.

330. Raphael, L. D., Mantle, J. A., Moraski, R. E., Rogers, W. J., Russell, R. O., Jr., and Rackley, C. E.: Quantitative assessment of ventricular performance in unstable ischemic heart disease by dextran function curves. Circulation *55*:858, 1977.

331. Weisel, R. D., Berger, R. L., and Hechtman, H. B.: Measurement of cardiac output by thermodilution. N. Engl. J. Med. *292*:682, 1975.

332. Rahimtoola, S. H., Loeb, H. S., Ehsani, A., Sinno, Z., Chuquimia, R., Lal, R., Rosen, K. M., and Gunnar, R. M.: Relationship of pulmonary artery to left ventricular diastolic pressures in acute myocardial infarction. Circulation *46*:283, 1972.

333. Fuchs, R. M., Heuser, R.R., Yin, F. C. P., Brinker, J. A.: Limitations of pulmonary wedge V waves in diagnosing mitral regurgitation. Am. J. Cardio. *49*:849, 1982.

334. Gewirtz, H., Gold, H. K., Fallon, J. T., Pasternak, R. C., and Leinbach, R. C.: Role of right ventricular infarction in cardiogenic shock associated with inferior myocardial infarction. Br. Heart J. *42*:719, 1979.

335. Meister, S. G., and Helfant, R. H.: Rapid bedside differentiation of ruptured interventricular septum from acute mitral insufficiency. N. Engl. J. Med. *287*:1024, 1972.

336. Rigaud, M., Rocha, P., Boschat, J., Favcot, J. C., Bardet, J., and Bourdarias, J. P.: Regional left ventricular function assessed by contrast angiography in acute myocardial infarction. Circulation *60*:130, 1979.

337. Stewart, D. K., Hamilton, G. W., Murray, J. A., and Kennedy, J. W.: Left ventricular function and coronary artery anatomy before and after myocardial infarction: A study of six cases. Circulation *49*:47, 1974.

338. Baxley, W. A., Jones, W. B., and Dodge, H. T.: Left ventricular anatomical and functional abnormalities in chronic postinfarction heart failure. Ann. Intern. Med. *74*:499, 1971.

339. Moraski, R. E., Russell, R. O., Jr., Smith, M., and Rackley, C. E.: Left ventricular function in patients with and without myocardial infarction and one, two, or three vessel coronary artery disease. Am. J. Cardiol. *35*:1, 1975.

340. Bertrand, M. E., Rousseau, M. F., Lablanche, J. M., Carre, A. G., and Lekieffre, J. P.: Cineangiographic assessment of left ventricular function in the acute phase of transmural myocardial infarction. Am. J. Cardiol. *43*:472, 1979.

341. Ratshin, R. A., Rackley, C. E., and Russell, R. O., Jr.: Hemodynamic evaluation of left ventricular function in shock complicating myocardial infarction. Circulation *45*:127, 1972.

341a. Rapaport, E., and Remedios, P.: The high risk patient after recovery from myocardial infarction: Recognition and management. J. Am. Coll. Cardiol. *1*:391, 1983.

341b. Coll, S., Castaner, A., Sanz, G., Roig, E., Magrina, J., Navarro-Lopez, F., and Betriu, A.: Prevalence and prognosis after a first nontransmural myocardial infarction. Am. J. Cardiol. *51*:1584, 1983.

341c. Madsen, E. B., Hougaard, P., and Gilpin, E.: Dynamic evaluation of prognosis from time-dependent variables in acute myocardial infarction. Am. J. Cardiol. *51*:1579, 1983.

342. Killip, T., and Kimball, J. I.: Treatment of myocardial infarction in a coronary care unit. A two year experience with 250 patients. Am. J. Cardiol. *20*:457, 1967.

343. Peel, A. A. F., Semple, T., Wang, I., Lancaster, W. M., and Dall, J. L. G.: A coronary prognostic index for grading the severity of infarction. Br. Heart J. *24*:745, 1962.

344. Norris, R. M., Brandt, P. W. T., Caughey, D. E., Lee, A. J., and Scott, P. J.: A new coronary prognostic index. Lancet *1*:274, 1969.

344a. Buda, A. J., Macdonald, I. L., Dubbin, J. D., Orr, S. A., and Strauss, H. D.: Myocardial infarct extension: Prevalence, clinical significance, and problems in diagnosis. Am. Heart J. *105*:744, 1983.

345. Strauss, H. D.: Myocardial infarction extension: Clinical significance. Primary Cardiol. *8*:14, 1982.

346. Baker, J. T., Bramlet, D. A., Lester, R. M., Harrison, D. G., Roe, C. R., and Cobb, F. R.: Myocardial infarct extension: Incidence and relationship to survival. Circulation 65:918, 1982.

347. Marmor, A., Geltman, E. M., Schechtman, K., Sobel, B. E., and Roberts, R.: Recurrent myocardial infarction: Clinical predictors and prognostic implications. Circulation 66:415, 1982.

348. Marmor, A., Sobel, B. E., and Roberts, E.: Factors presaging early recurrent myocardial infarction ("extension"). Am. J. Cardiol. 48:603, 1981.

349. Verdouw, P. D., Hagemeijer, F., van Dorp, W. G., van der Vorm, A., and Hugenholtz, P. G.: Short-term survival after acute myocardial infarction predicted by hemodynamic parameters. Circulation 52:413, 1975.

350. Sanford, C. F., Corbett, J., Nicod, P., Curry, G. L., Lewis, S. E., Dehmer, G. J., Anderson, A., Moses, B., and Willerson, J. T.: Value of radionuclide ventriculography in the immediate characterization of patients with acute myocardial infarction. Am. J. Cardiol. 49:637, 1982.

351. Miller, D. H., and Borer, J. S.: Exercise testing early after myocardial infarction. Risks and benefits. Am. J. Med. 72:427, 1982.

351a. Becker, L. C., Silverman, K. J., Bulkley, B. H., Kallman, C. H., Mellits, E. D., and Weisfeldt, M.: Comparison of early thallium-201 scintigraphy and gated blood pool imaging for predicting mortality in patients with acute myocardial infarction. Circulation 67:1272, 1983.

352. Holman, B. L., Chisholm, R. J., and Braunwald, E.: The prognostic implications of acute myocardial infarct scintigraphy with 99mTc-pyrophosphate. Circulation 57:320, 1978.

353. Nasmith, J., Marpole, D., Rahal, D., Homan, J., Stewart, S., and Sniderman, A.: Clinical outcomes after inferior myocardial infarction. Ann. Intern. Med. 96:22, 1982.

354. Gibson, R. S., Crampton, R. S., Watson, D. D., Taylor, G. J., Carabello, B. A., Holt, N. D., and Beller, G. A.: Precordial ST segment depression during acute inferior myocardial infarction: Clinical, scintigraphic and angiographic correlations. Circulation 66:732, 1982.

355. Salcedo, J. R., Baird, M. G., Chambers, R. J., and Beanlands, D. S.: Significance of reciprocal S-T segment depression in anterior precordial leads in acute inferior myocardial infarction: Concomitant left anterior descending coronary artery disease? Am. J. Cardiol. 48:1003, 1981.

355a. Ong, L., Valdellon, B., Coromilas, J., Brody, R., Reiser, P., and Morrison, J.: Precordial S-T segment depression in inferior myocardial infarction. Evaluation by quantitative thallium-201 scintigraphy and technetium-99m ventriculography. Am. J. Cardiol. 51:734, 1983.

356. Schuster, E. H., and Bulkley, B. H.: Early post-infarction angina. Ischemia at a distance and ischemia in the infarct zone. N. Engl. J. Med. 305:1101, 1981.

357. Edson, J. N.: Subendocardial myocardial infarction. Am. Heart J. 60:323, 1960.

358. Erikssen, J., Muller, C., and Anderssen, J. N.: Atypical case histories and electrocardiograms in myocardial infarction. Acta Med. Scand. 188:95, 1970.

359. Friedberg, C. K.: Symposium: Myocardial infarction 1972. Part 1. Introduction. Circulation 45:179, 1972.

360. Hutter, A. M., Jr., DeSanctis, R. W., Flynn, T., and Yeatman, L. A.: Nontransmural myocardial infarction: A comparison of hospital and late clinical course of patients with that of matched patients with transmural anterior and transmural inferior myocardial infarction. Am. J. Cardiol. 48:595, 1981.

361. Madias, J. E., Chahine, R. A., Gorlin, R., and Blacklow, D. J.: A comparison of transmural and nontransmural acute myocardial infarction. Circulation 49:498, 1974.

361a. Phibbs, B.: "Transmural" versus "Subendocardial" myocardial infarction: An electrocardiographic myth. J. Am. Coll. Cardiol. 1:561, 1983.

362. Rigo, R., Murray, M., Taylor, D. R., Weisfeldt, M. L., Strauss, H. W., and Pitt, B.: Hemodynamic and prognostic findings in patients with transmural and nontransmural infarction. Circulation 51:1064, 1975.

363. Madias, J. E., and Gorlin, R.: They myth of "mild" myocardial infarction. Ann. Intern. Med. 86:347, 1977.

364. Madigan, N. P., Rutherford, B. D., and Frye, R. L.: The clinical course, early prognosis and coronary anatomy of subendocardial infarction. Am. J. Med. 60:634, 1976.

364a. DeFeyter, P. J., van Eenige, M. J., Dighton, D. H., and Roos, J. P.: Exercise testing early after myocardial infarction. Chest 83:853, 1983.

365. Fuller, C. M., Raizner, A. E., Verani, M., Nahormek, P. A., Chahine, R. A., McEntee, C. W., and Miller, R. R.: Early post–myocardial infarction treadmill stress testing. Ann. Intern. Med. 94:734, 1981.

365a. Nair, R., Allan, K., Reg, N., Baird, M. G., Beanlands, D. S., and Higginson, L. A.: A comparison of clinical and treadmill predictors of prognosis following acute myocardial infarction. J. Am. Coll. Cardiol. 1:717, 1983.

365b. Gibson, R. S., Watson, D. D., Crampton, R. S., Beller, G. A.: Prospective comparison of submaximal exercise TL-201 scintigraphy 2 weeks after and symptom-limited maximal testing 3 months after myocardial infarction. J. Am. Coll. Cardiol. 1:654, 1983.

366. Corbett, J. R., Dehmer, G. J., Lewis, S. E., Woodward, W., Henderson, E., Parkey, R. W., Blomqvist, C. G., and Willerson, J. T.: The prognostic value of submaximal exercise testing with radionuclide ventriculography before hospital discharge in patients with recent myocardial infarction. Circulation 64:535, 1981.

366a. Hung, J., Goris, M. L., Nash, E., Kraemer, H. C., and DeBusk, R. F.: The comparative prognostic value of standard treadmill testing, rest and exercise thallium myocardial perfusion scintigraphy and radionuclide ventriculography 3 weeks after myocardial infarction. J. Am. Coll. Cardiol. 1:654, 1983.

367. Sanz, G., Castaner, A., Betriu, A., Magrina, J., Roig, E., Coll, S., Pare, J. C., and Navarro-Lopez, F.: Determinants of prognosis in survivors of myocardial infarction. A prospective clinical angiographic study. N. Engl. J. Med. 306:1065, 1982.

368. Borer, J. S., Rosing, D. R., Miller, R. H., Stark, R. M., Kent, K. M., Bacharach, S. L., Green, M. V., Lake, C. R., Cohen, H., Holmes, D., Donohue, D., Baker, W., and Epstein, S. E.: Natural history of left ventricular function during 1 year after acute myocardial infarction: Comparison with clinical, electrocardiographic and biochemical determinations. Am. J. Cardiol. 46:1, 1980.

369. Mukharji, J., Rude, R., Gustafson, N., Poole, K., Passamani, E., Thomas, L. J., Jr., Strauss, H. W., Muller, J. E., Roberts, R., Raabe, D. S., Jr., Braunwald, E., Willerson, J. T., and cooperating investigators, MILIS: Late sudden death following myocardial infarction: Interdependence of risk factors. J. Am. Coll. Cardiol. 1:585, 1983.

370. Moss, A. J., Bigger, J. T., Case, R. B., Gillespie, J., Goldstein, R., Greenberg, H., Krone, R., Marcus, F. I., Odoroff, C. L., and Oliver, G. C.: Risk stratification and prognostication after myocardial infarction. J. Am. Coll. Cardiol. 1:716, 1983.

38 THE MANAGEMENT OF ACUTE MYOCARDIAL INFARCTION

by Burton E. Sobel, M.D., and Eugene Braunwald, M.D.

More than 60 per cent of the deaths associated with acute myocardial infarction (AMI) occur within one hour of the event and are attributable to malignant arrhythmias, usually ventricular fibrillation. This manifestation of ischemic heart disease is discussed in Chapter 23. Despite the importance of sudden death, more than 500,000 patients are hospitalized annually in the United States for AMI.[1] The pathological, physiological, and clinical features of this condition are presented in Chapter 37, while its management is considered here.

Careful monitoring of cardiac rhythm and the prompt treatment of arrhythmias have reduced sharply the incidence of in-hospital deaths from AMI.[2] Accordingly, most deaths among patients with this condition who reach the hospital are now attributable to left ventricular failure and shock and occur within the three or four days after the onset of infarction.[3] Only a minority of in-hospital deaths now result from intractable arrhythmias, and most of these occur in settings where monitoring and/or treatment is inadequate or are secondary to extensive infarction and left ventricular failure.[2,4–6]

Prior to the advent of coronary care units, treatment of AMI was directed almost exclusively toward allowing healing of the infarct, preventing cardiac rupture and other complications such as pulmonary and systemic embolism, and sustaining arterial pressure and urine output. Subsequently, the major emphasis of therapeutic strategy was on the prevention and aggressive treatment of arrhythmias. The concept that infarct size is an important determinant of prognosis (Fig. 37–8, p. 1271) and that its ultimate extent might be modified favorably by early implementation of selected physiological and pharmacological interventions has directed attention to protection of jeopardized myocardium by restoring perfusion to ischemic tissue or by a variety of pharmacological interventions.[7,8] However, as discussed later, the ultimate clinical benefits of this approach have yet to be realized. The treatment of AMI is discussed under five headings:

1. General measures
2. Treatment and prophylaxis of arrhythmias
3. Treatment of hemodynamic disturbances
4. Minimization of infarct size
5. Convalescence

GENERAL MEASURES

MOBILE CORONARY CARE UNITS. It is now well established that most deaths associated with AMI occur within the first hour after its onset and that death is usually due to ventricular fibrillation (Chap. 23).[9,10] Accordingly, the importance of the immediate implementation of definitive resuscitative efforts and of rapidly transporting the patient to a hospital cannot be overemphasized. Well-equipped ambulances, staffed by personnel trained in the care of the infarct victim, allow definitive therapy to commence while the patient is being transported to the hospital.[11,12] These specially equipped and staffed ambulances have been termed mobile coronary care units; to be used effectively, they must be placed strategically within a community and excellent radio-communication systems must be available. They should be equipped with a battery-operated monitoring oscilloscope and direct writing electrocardiograph; a battery-operated DC defibrillator; oxygen, endotracheal tubes, and suction apparatus; and commonly used cardiovascular drugs. A radiotelemetry system that allows transmission of the electrocardiogram to the hospital is desirable but not essential.

The effectiveness of these systems in Belfast, Ireland,[11] Seattle, Washington,[13] and Columbus, Ohio[14] has been amply documented. The rapid initiation of prehospital cardiopulmonary resuscitation facilitated by mobile coronary care units and trained paramedical personnel results in initially successful resuscitation in approximately two thirds of patients. It has been demonstrated that the frequency of death during transportation can be diminished from 22 to 9 per cent when defibrillation equipment and trained paramedical personnel are available.[15] In addition to prompt defibrillation, the efficacy of prehospital care appears to depend on several factors, including early relief of pain with its deleterious physiological sequelae, the reduction of excessive activity of the autonomic nervous system, and abolition of prelethal arrhythmias, such as ventricular tachycardia.

CORONARY CARE UNITS.   During the past two decades the mortality of patients with AMI treated in coronary care units has declined significantly from what it had been before the introduction of these units.[4] Reduction in mortality has resulted almost entirely from the elimination of primary arrhythmias as a cause of death.[2] Most instances of this arrhythmia occur *before* the patient reaches the hospital, and only about 5 per cent of patients develop a primary ventricular arrhythmia *after* they reach the hospital, an average of five to six hours after the onset of the attack in most series. Deaths from primary ventricular fibrillation have been prevented because the coronary care unit allows continuous monitoring of cardiac rhythm by highly trained nurses with the authority to administer immediate treatment and prophylaxis of arrhythmias in the absence of physicians, and because of the specialized equipment (defibrillators, pacemakers) and drugs available for instantaneous use.[16] Although all these benefits can certainly be achieved for patients scattered throughout the hospital, the clustering of patients with AMI has greatly improved the efficient use of the trained personnel, facilities, and equipment. In recent years, with increasing emphasis on hemodynamic monitoring and treatment of the serious complications of AMI with such modalities as afterload reduction and intra-aortic balloon counterpulsation, the coronary care unit has assumed even greater importance.

At the same time, the value of coronary care units for patients with *uncomplicated AMI* has been questioned and restudied.[17] In one widely publicized randomized trial, patients with suspected infarction were evaluated initially at home; after a two-hour observation interval they were divided at random into home-management and hospital-management groups.[18] Although the six-week mortality rate among patients with infarction in the two groups was similar (13 per cent and 11 per cent, respectively), such low overall mortality rates make detection of small although real differences difficult. Furthermore, approximately one fourth of the patients with significant electrophysiological or hemodynamic complications were excluded. Thus, hospital care was provided for all high-risk patients. Furthermore, under the general conditions of medical practice in the United States, it is difficult to provide the same immediate intensive care at home for all patients with suspected infarction that was made available in this study. Since prediction of the occurrence of early complications is imperfect, we believe that the observation and prompt treatment possible in a well-staffed coronary care unit continue to justify the reliance placed upon this setting as the primary one for early management of patients with suspected or confirmed AMI. Patient delay in seeking medical attention and the medical system's delay in responding reduce the potential impact of the coronary care unit because the patients do not reach the unit until the maximum danger has passed. Therefore, education of the public, of patients at high risk of AMI, and those members of the medical profession involved in responding to the initial complaints of these patients is likely to be rewarded by further reductions of mortality.[17,19]

INTERMEDIATE CORONARY CARE UNITS. Since the hazard of *primary* ventricular fibrillation is essentially over in 24 to 36 hours, there is little need for patients with entirely *uncomplicated* infarcts to remain in a coronary care unit for more than two days. Obviously, patients with complicated infarcts, particularly those with arrhythmias and pump failure, require continued care in such a unit. There is an increased risk of ventricular tachycardia and ventricular fibrillation in the late MI period, and an increased vulnerability to ventricular fibrillation is responsible for these arrhythmias four to ten days after AMI, accounting for between 10 and 30 per cent of total hospital deaths.[20,21] In view of this significant in-hospital mortality after discharge from the coronary care unit, continued surveillance in intermediate coronary care units (also called "step-down units") is justifiable.

Risk factors for sudden death in the hospital *after* discharge from the coronary care unit include intraventricular conduction defects,[22] sinus tachycardia persisting for more than two days, and extensive anterior infarction, as well as episodes of ventricular fibrillation and of atrial flutter or fibrillation occurring while the patient is in the coronary care unit, and, possibly, marked electrocardiographic ST-segment abnormalities induced by low levels of activity.[23] Although not established with certainty, it is suspected that substantial reduction in the late hospital death rate can be achieved with the use of intermediate coronary care units, which permit prolonged continuous monitoring of the electrocardiogram and prompt, effective treatment of ventricular fibrillation and other serious arrhythmias.[2,4,10,22] The availability of these units may be useful also in helping to identify those patients who remain free from complications for a minimum of one week, since early discharge from the hospital appears to be feasible for this subset.[24,25] An additional potential advantage is facilitation of patient education in a group setting with formal lectures and videotape programs.

ANALGESIA. The alleviation or reduction of pain is a critical factor in the care of patients with AMI. Although a wide variety of agents has been used to treat the pain associated with MI, including meperidine, pentazocine, and morphine, the latter agent remains the drug of choice except in patients with well-documented morphine hypersensitivity. Four to 8 mg should be administered intravenously and doses of 2 to 8 mg repeated at intervals of 5 to 15 minutes until the pain is relieved or evident toxicity—i.e., hypotension, depression of respiration, or severe vomiting—precludes further administration of the drug. In some patients, remarkably large cumulative doses of morphine (2 to 3 mg/kg) may be required and are usually tolerated.

The reduction of anxiety resulting from morphine diminishes the patient's restlessness and the activity of the autonomic nervous system, with a consequent reduction of the heart's metabolic demands. The beneficial effect of morphine in patients with pulmonary edema is unequivocal (p. 571) and may relate to several factors, including peripheral arterial and venous dilatation (particularly among patients with excessive sympathoadrenal activity), reduction of the work of breathing, and slowing of heart rate secondary to combined withdrawal of sympathetic tone and augmentation of vagal tone.[26]

Hypotension following the administration of morphine can be minimized by maintaining the patient in a supine position and elevating the lower extremities if systolic arterial pressure declines below 100 mm Hg. Obviously, such positioning is undesirable in the presence of pulmonary edema, but morphine rarely produces hypotension under these circumstances. The concomitant administration of atropine in doses of 0.5 to 1.5 mg intravenously may be helpful in reducing the excessive vagomimetic effects of morphine, particularly when hypotension and bradycardia are present before it is administered. Respiratory depression is an unusual complication of morphine in the presence of severe pain or pulmonary edema, but as the patient's cardiovascular status improves, impairment of ventilation may supervene and should be watched for. It can be treated with Narcan, in doses of 0.4 mg intravenously at 5-minute intervals to a maximum of 1.2 mg. Nausea and vomiting may be troublesome side effects following large doses of morphine and may be treated with a phenothiazine in order to avoid the marked stress on the circulation resulting from emesis.

Other analgesics such as meperidine are less effective than is morphine but equally likely to produce side effects and prone to augment ventricular rate. Inhalation of *nitrous oxide*, in concentrations of from 20 to 50 per cent, combined with oxygen, has been utilized widely in Europe and with increasing frequency in the United States. It frequently provides effective analgesia, particularly in patients with relatively mild pain[27,28] and in those having recurrent prolonged episodes of pain. Nitrous oxide appears to influence myocardial oxygen demands favorably, since its sedative action diminishes the patient's total metabolic needs. It does not depress left ventricular function or produce significant hemodynamic changes or adverse reactions.

OXYGENATION. Hypoxemia is common in patients with AMI and is usually secondary to ventilation-perfusion abnormalities[29] (pp. 1276 and 1787), which are sequelae of left ventricular failure; patchy pneumonia and intrinsic pulmonary disease are additional causes of hypoxemia. It is common practice to treat all patients hospitalized with AMI with oxygen for 24 to 48 hours, based on the very common occurrence of arterial hypoxemia and both experimental[30] and clinical[31] evidence that increased oxygen in the inspired air protects ischemic myocardium. However, augmentation of the fraction of oxygen in the inspired air does not elevate oxygen delivery significantly in patients who are not hypoxemic. Furthermore, it may increase systemic vascular resistance and arterial pressure and thereby lower cardiac output slightly.

In view of these considerations, arterial oxygen tension should be measured at the time of the patient's admission to the coronary care unit; oxygen therapy may be omitted if it is normal. On the other hand, oxygen should be administered to patients with AMI when arterial hypoxemia is clinically evident or can be documented.[32] In these patients, serial arterial blood gas measurements may be employed to follow the efficacy of oxygen therapy. Although patients with AMI may exhibit a reduction in precordial ST-segment elevation during 100 per cent oxygen breathing, no long-term effect on survival or on the development of complications has been documented.[31]

In general, the delivery of 2 to 4 L/min of 100 per cent oxygen by mask or nasal prongs for two to three days is satisfactory for most patients with mild hypoxemia. If arterial oxygenation is still depressed on this regimen, the flow rate may have to be increased. In patients with pulmonary edema, endotracheal intubation and controlled ventilation at a positive pressure may be necessary. Although hyperbaric oxygen has been evaluated in experimental animals[33] and in patients[34] with AMI, routine implementation of this intervention in the conventional clinical setting is impractical, and no long-term benefit has been established. Alternative approaches designed to facilitate delivery of oxygen to ischemic myocardium, such as intravenous administration of fluorocarbon preparations, capable of enhancing oxygen-carrying capacity and reducing viscosity of the circulating blood, although promising in animal experiments, have not yet been evaluated clinically.

PHYSICAL ACTIVITY. In the absence of all complications, patients with AMI need not be confined to bed for more than 24 to 36 hours and may use a bedside commode from the time of admission. They may sit in a chair for two half-hour periods on the second and for two one-hour periods on the third day. If arrhythmia, heart failure, and other significant complications have not occurred or if they are controlled, the patient may be transferred out of the coronary care unit after three days. Monitoring for an additional two days in an intermediate care unit is desirable. A nurse should help wash the patient during the first five days. If the convalescence continues uneventfully, limited ambulation within the room can be begun on the fourth or fifth day. Activity can then increase progressively, and a shower may be allowed on the ninth or tenth day.

Hospitalization and enforced bed rest for any illness may lead to complications, particularly in elderly patients, such as constipation, decubitus ulcers, excessive resorption of bone with formation of renal calculi, atelectasis, thrombophlebitis, pulmonary emboli, urinary retention, mild anemia due to repetitive blood sampling for diagnostic tests, impaired oral intake of fluids, bleeding from the gastrointestinal tract due to stress ulcers, and deconditioning of cardiovascular reflex responses to postural changes. Because of the precarious status of the heart recovering from AMI, avoidance of such complications is of primary importance. For example, constipation may lead to straining, transitory reduction of venous return and diminution of cardiac output, impaired coronary perfusion, and ventricular arrhythmias, occasionally culminating in ventricular fibrillation. Early implementation of a bed-chair regimen appears to be useful in avoiding many of the difficulties encountered previously among patients confined to bed for several weeks.

Other general measures include (1) A liquid diet for 24 hours, because of the risk of nausea and vomiting or cardiac arrest early after infarction and the need to reduce the risk of aspiration. This should be followed by a 1500 calorie soft diet, with no added salt, divided into multiple small feedings for several days. Then, in the absence of heart failure, a regular diet, low in cholesterol and saturated fats, is appropriate. Caffeine-rich beverages should be avoided because of their possible arrhythmogenic effects. (2) Dioctyl sodium sulfosuccinate, 100 mg daily, or another stool softener should be used to prevent constipation and straining. (3) The emotional impact of an AMI and of hospitalization in a coronary care unit (p. 1829) should be offset by thoughtful explanations of the nature of the illness, the function of the equipment, and the purpose of the procedures. A deliberate effort should be made to maintain the atmosphere in the coronary care unit as quiet and restful as possible. Diazepam, 2 to 5 mg orally four times a day, is useful to allay the anxiety that is so common in this setting. Flurazepam, 15 to 30 mg, or an equivalent narcotic may be given for sleep. (4) Derangements potentially contributing to arrhythmias, such as hypoxemia, hypovolemia, disturbances of acid-base balance or of electrolytes, and digitalis toxicity should be identified and corrected. (5) The treatment of post–myocardial infarction pericarditis and Dressler's syndrome are discussed on pp. 1505 and 1514.

ANTICOAGULANTS. There are at least three theoretical reasons for anticipating that anticoagulants might be beneficial in the management of AMI: (1) Since the coronary occlusion responsible for the AMI is often a thrombus (p. 1265), anticoagulants might be expected to halt or slow progression and to prevent the development of new thrombi elsewhere in the coronary arterial tree (2) Anticoagulants might be expected to diminish the formation of mural thrombi (p. 1271) and resultant systemic embolization (3) Anticoagulants might be expected to reduce the incidence of venous thrombosis and pulmonary embolization.

Despite several decades of evaluation, the results of the treatment of AMI with anticoagulants are inconclusive. However, sporadic reports continue to appear of the favorable effects of anticoagulants on mortality among patients hospitalized with AMI.[36–39] Salutary effects on the underlying coronary disease, progression, or recurrence of infarction have not been clearly demonstrated with conventional anticoagulant drugs, yet it is clear that they decrease the incidence of cerebral emboli resulting from mural thrombi from approximately 10 to 4 per cent.[40] In addition, the administration of heparin in doses sufficient to influence activation of Factor X without affecting conventional laboratory tests of the coagulation system substantially diminish the incidence of deep vein thrombosis[41] and thereby reduce the incidence of pulmonary emboli. It appears advisable, therefore, to administer minidose heparin (5000 units subcutaneously) every 8 to 12 hours in the absence of specific contraindications.[42–44] The drug should be continued until two to three days prior to hospital discharge, although it is recognized that in patients with uncomplicated AMI's, there is no evidence that it reduces mortality.

In patients with high risk of embolism (e.g., those with ventricular aneurysm, marked obesity, cardiogenic shock, low output state, present or past thrombophlebitis, arterial or pulmonary embolism), there is evidence that in the absence of contraindications, anticoagulant treatment does exert a favorable effect on survival, and full-dose anticoagulation with heparin is indicated (e.g., intravenous administration of 15,000 units, followed by continuous infusion of 1000 units per hour) to maintain the clotting time and partial thromboplastin time at 1.5 to 2.5 times normal. After five to seven days of therapy, prothrombinopenic drugs or continued administration of subcutaneous, adjusted doses of heparin may be employed if conditions exist which suggest that venous thrombosis and embolism are likely to recur. These include continued or worsening heart failure, persistent thrombophlebitis, or the need for prolonged bed rest.

The long-term benefit of anticoagulants *following hospital discharge* is especially controversial. In one well-designed clinical trial on survivors of AMI exceeding 60 years of age, intensive and stable anticoagulant therapy reduced the risk of recurrent infarction and of cardiac death.[45] If these findings are confirmed, it will be essential to reconsider our present policy which limits the use of chronic anticoagulants to patients in the post-hospital phase to those with specific indications, including thrombophlebitis, a history of pulmonary or systemic embolism, evidence of a mural thrombus in the left ventricle on two-dimensional echocardiography (Fig. 5–68, p. 127), and severe heart failure. The role, if any, of sulfinpyrazone, aspirin, dipyridamole, and other antiplatelet agents in both the acute and the chronic convalescent phases of MI is unsettled and controversial at this time.

TREATMENT AND PROPHYLAXIS OF ARRHYTHMIAS

The electrophysiological mechanisms responsible for arrhythmias in patients with AMI are discussed on pp. 619 to 629. The incidence and consequences of arrhythmias and atrioventricular and intraventricular conduction defects in these patients are presented on p. 1284, the action of antiarrhythmic drugs on p. 653, and the role of cardiac pacing and of electric cardioversion on p. 669.

Arrhythmias occurring in patients with AMI require vigorous treatment when they impair hemodynamics, compromise myocardial viability by augmenting myocardial oxygen requirements, or predispose to malignant ventricular arrhythmias, i.e., ventricular tachycardia, ventricular fibrillation, or asystole.[46] There is evidence that both the diminished threshold to ventricular fibrillation[5] and the incidence of malignant ventricular arrhythmias associated with infarction[47-49] are affected by the extent of the underlying infarction.

When patients are seen early during the course of MI they almost invariably exhibit evidence of increased activity of the autonomic nervous system. Sinus bradycardia, sometimes associated with AV block, often reflecting augmented vagal activity, is particularly common in patients with inferoposterior infarction and is often accompanied by hypotension. Hypotension, regardless of cause, is hazardous in patients with AMI, since it impairs perfusion of marginally ischemic zones, intensifies ischemia, and may initiate or perpetuate the vicious circle illustrated in Figure 37–8, p. 1271.

Bradyarrhythmias and Conduction Defects

SINUS BRADYCARDIA (see also p. 1284). The cause of the vagotonia and resultant bradycardia and hypotension that often accompany AMI, particularly in patients with inferior and posterior infarcts, is not entirely clear. One factor appears to be stimulation of cardiac vagal afferent receptors[50] (which are more common in the inferoposterior than the anterior or lateral portions of the left ventricle), with resulting efferent cholinergic stimulation of the heart. In the first four to six hours following infarction, if the sinus rate is slow (under 60/min), administration of intravenous atropine in aliquots of 0.3 to 0.6 mg every 3 to 10 minutes (with a total dose not exceeding 2 mg) to bring heart rate up to approximately 60/min often abolishes premature ventricular beats commonly associated with sinus bradycardia.[51-54] Atropine often contributes to restoration of arterial pressure[9] and hence coronary perfusion. These favorable effects are frequently accompanied by regression of ST-segment elevation (Fig. 38–1). Elevation of the lower extremities will also often elevate arterial pressure by redistributing blood from the systemic venous bed to the thorax, thereby augmenting ventricular preload, cardiac output, and arterial pressure.

Sinus bradycardia occurring more than six hours after the onset of the AMI is often transitory, is caused by sinus node dysfunction or atrial ischemia rather than vagal hyperactivity, is usually not accompanied by hypotension, and does not usually predispose to ventricular arrhythmias. Treatment is not required unless ventricular performance is compromised or administration of propranolol or high doses of antiarrhythmic drugs, which may slow the sinus rate further, is planned. When atropine is ineffective and the patient is symptomatic and/or hypotensive, electrical pacing is indicated. In patients with depressed ventricular performance, who require the "atrial kick," atrial pacing or atrioventricular sequential pacing is superior to simple ventricular pacing.[55]

ATRIOVENTRICULAR BLOCK (see also pp. 730 and 1287). *First degree AV block* generally does not require specific treatment. However, if digitalis intoxication is sus-

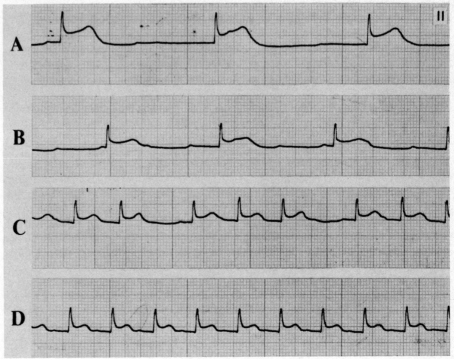

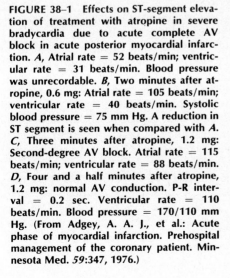

FIGURE 38–1 Effects on ST-segment elevation of treatment with atropine in severe bradycardia due to acute complete AV block in acute posterior myocardial infarction. *A*, Atrial rate = 52 beats/min; ventricular rate = 31 beats/min. Blood pressure was unrecordable. *B*, Two minutes after atropine, 0.6 mg: Atrial rate = 105 beats/min; ventricular rate = 40 beats/min. Systolic blood pressure = 75 mm Hg. A reduction in ST segment is seen when compared with *A*. *C*, Three minutes after atropine, 1.2 mg: Second-degree AV block. Atrial rate = 115 beats/min; ventricular rate = 88 beats/min. *D*, Four and a half minutes after atropine, 1.2 mg: normal AV conduction. P-R interval = 0.2 sec. Ventricular rate = 110 beats/min. Blood pressure = 170/110 mm Hg. (From Adgey, A. A. J., et al.: Acute phase of myocardial infarction. Prehospital management of the coronary patient. Minnesota Med. *59*:347, 1976.)

pected as the etiology, this drug should be discontinued. If the block is a manifestation of excessive vagotonia and is associated with sinus bradycardia and hypotension, administration of atropine, as outlined above, may be helpful. In all circumstances, careful surveillance is important in view of the possibility of progression to higher degrees of block.[56]

Specific therapy also is not required in patients with *second-degree AV block of the Mobitz type I* variety (Wenckebach), when the average ventricular rate is adequate and ventricular irritability, heart failure, or bundle branch block are absent. However, if these complications develop of if the ventricular rate falls below 60/min, immediate treatment with a temporary transvenous pacemaker is indicated. *Mobitz type II second-degree AV block* (p. 731) is relatively rare in AMI, but because of its potential for progression to complete heart block, it should be treated with a demand transvenous pacemaker with the rate set at approximately 60/min.[57]

Definitive data are not available concerning the importance of *complete AV block* as an *independent* risk factor for mortality and whether temporary transvenous pacing per se improves survival of patients with AMI. Some contend that ventricular pacing is useless when employed to correct complete AV block in patients with *anterior* infarction in view of the poor prognosis in this group regardless of therapy and therefore that ventricular pacing should be initiated only for complete AV block in association with inferior infarction and only when hemodynamic impairment is present. We believe, however, that ventricular or atrioventricular sequential pacing is indicated in essentially *all* patients with AMI with complete AV block. Pacing is likely to protect against transient hypotension with its attendant risks of extending infarction and precipitating malignant ventricular arrhythmias. Also, pacing protects against asystole, a particular hazard in patients with anterior infarction and infranodal block. Improved survival with pacing probably occurs in only a small fraction of patients with complete AV block and anterior wall infarcts, since the extensive destruction of the myocardium that almost invariably accompanies this condition results in a very high mortality rate, even in paced patients. Therefore, a large series of patients would be required to demonstrate the small reduction of mortality that might be achieved by pacing. The absence of data supporting such an effect, however, by no means excludes the possibility that it may be present. While it is generally agreed that pacing is indicated in patients with *inferior* wall infarction and complete AV block, it is of particular importance if the ventricular rate is very slow (<45 beats/min), if ventricular irritability is present, or if pump failure develops; atropine is of little value in these patients.

INTRAVENTRICULAR BLOCK. Complete bundle branch block (either left or right), the combination of right bundle branch block and left anterior divisional (fascicular) block, or any of the various forms of trifascicular block are more often associated with anterior than inferoposterior infarction. The poor prognosis associated with these intraventricular conduction defects is probably related more to the extent of infarction than to the direct consequences of the block itself.[57,58] Although, just as is the case for complete AV block, transvenous ventricular pacing has not resulted in statistically demonstrable improve-

ment in prognosis among patients with AMI who develop intraventricular conduction defects, we believe that pacing is advisable in patients at high risk of developing complete AV block. This includes patients with *new* bilateral bundle branch block, i.e., right bundle branch block with left anterior or posterior divisional block and alternating right and left bundle branch block; first degree AV block adds to this risk. Isolated new block in only one of the three fascicles poses somewhat less risk; these patients can have a prophylactic pacemaker inserted or may be monitored closely and insertion of a pacemaker deferred unless conduction in a second fascicle becomes impaired or the P-R interval becomes prolonged. In our opinion, failure to demonstrate improved prognosis statistically does not belie the potential value of pacemaker therapy; it probably reflects the overriding impact on mortality of the extensive infarction responsible for the development of the conduction abnormality and the large number of patients required to permit statistical documentation of reduction of mortality. The presence of an intraventricular conduction defect *antedating* the AMI does not appear to predispose the patient to the development of complete AV block, and prophylactic pacing is not ordinarily indicated.

The question of permanent pacing in survivors of AMI associated with conduction defects is still controversial.[58–62] Patients with inferior infarction with *transient* Type II second-degree block or complete AV block without an associated intraventricular conduction defect do not appear to require permanent pacing. Some contend that prophylactic pacing makes little difference in the long-term survival of patients with AMI and bundle branch block complicated by transient high-degree block.[59] On the other hand, in a retrospective multicenter study, survivors of AMI and bundle branch block who experienced transient high-degree (Mobitz Type II second-degree, or third-degree) block had a high incidence of recurrent high-degree AV block and sudden death, and this incidence was reduced by insertion of a permanent demand pacemaker.[61–63] Thus, these findings suggest a role for prophylactic permanent pacing in patients with AMI and bundle branch block with transient high-degree atrioventricular block.

The question of the advisability of permanent pacemaker insertions is complicated by the fact that not all sudden deaths in this population are due to recurrent high-degree block. A high incidence of late in-hospital ventricular fibrillation occurs in coronary care unit survivors with anteroseptal myocardial infarction complicated by either right or left bundle branch block,[21] and if the propensity for this arrhythmia continued, ventricular fibrillation rather than asystole due to failure of atrioventricular conduction and of the infranodal pacemaker could be responsible for late sudden death.

VENTRICULAR ASYSTOLE. Sudden death associated with AMI is almost always due to ventricular fibrillation. Appearance of apparent ventricular asystole on oscilloscopic displays of continuously recorded electrocardiograms may be misleading, since the mechanism may in fact be fine ventricular fibrillation. Because of the predominance of ventricular fibrillation as the cause of cardiac arrest in this setting, initial therapy should include electrical countershock, even if definitive electrocardiographic documentation of this arrhythmia is not available. In the rare instance in which asystole can be documented to be the responsible electrophysiological disturbance, immediate transthoracic pacing (or stimulation with a transvenous pacemaker if one is already in place) is indicated.

Supraventricular Tachyarrhythmias and Premature Beats

Activation of receptors within atrial and ventricular myocardium by necrotic tissue may cause enhanced efferent sympathetic activity, increased concentrations of circulating catecholamines, and local release of catecholamines from nerve endings within the heart.[64] The latter may also result from direct ischemic damage of adrenergic neurons. In addition, ischemic myocardium may be hyperreactive to the arrhythmogenic effects of norepinephrine,[65,66] which may vary strikingly in concentration in different portions of the ischemic heart.[67] Sympathetic stimulation of the heart may also enhance the automaticity of ischemic Purkinje fibers. Furthermore, catecholamines facilitate propagation of slow current responses mediated by calcium (p. 624), and stimulation of ischemic myocardium by catecholamines may exacerbate arrhythmias dependent on such currents.[65,68,69] Cardiac catecholamine depletion induced by mediastinal ablation[70] or reduction of adrenergic stimulation by pharmacological means[6] protects against ventricular arrhythmias in experimental animals. Thus, although ventricular premature beats in patients with MI can usually be suppressed by administration of antiarrhythmic agents such as lidocaine, beta-adrenergic blocking agents may also be helpful in the treatment of ventricular arrhythmias, particularly when the latter are associated with other signs of heightened adrenergic activity such as sinus tachycardia.

Tachyarrhythmias of any origin may be deleterious, since they increase myocardial oxygen requirements, limit the time available for coronary perfusion and ventricular filling during diastole, and compromise cardiac output. Even electrophysiologically mild disturbances may have grave import in patients with AMI. For example, while atrial transport plays only a modest role in sustaining stroke volume in patients with normal hearts, cardiac output may be remarkably dependent upon maintenance of a properly timed atrial contraction in patients with AMI (Fig. 37–14, p. 1286). Therefore, aggressive management is indicated when hemodynamics are compromised by arrhythmias that disturb the sequence of atrial and ventricular contractions, such as wandering atrial pacemaker, AV junctional escape rhythms, frequent premature atrial contractions, accelerated idioventricular rhythm, and atrial fibrillation or flutter, even when the ventricular response is not excessively rapid, as well as when more serious derangements such as paroxysmal supraventricular tachycardia, AV dissociation with nodal tachycardia, and high degrees of AV block are present. The treatment of tachyarrhythmias involves not only the use of antiarrhythmic drugs but also correction of abnormalities of plasma electrolyte concentrations, acid-base balance disturbances, hypoxemia, and anemia. In addition, it is essential to treat pericarditis, pulmonary emboli, and pneumonia or other infections, which may give rise to sinus tachycardia or other supraventricular tachyarrhythmias.

SINUS TACHYCARDIA. This arrhythmia occurs in approximately one third of patients with AMI and may be associated with transient hypertension or hypotension and augmented sympathetic activity.[64,71] Sinus tachycardia may result from pain and fright or may be the only overt evidence of pump failure; it may result from associated infection or pulmonary embolism, pericarditis, hypovolemia, or fever. The etiology should be sought and appropriate treatment instituted, e.g., analgesics for pain, diuretics for heart failure, oxygen, beta blockers and nitroglycerin for ischemia, and aspirin for pericarditis.[72]

Administration of beta-adrenergic blocking agents, in the dosage and manner described on p. 1320, may be helpful in the treatment of sinus tachycardia, particularly when this arrhythmia is a manifestation of a hyperdynamic circulation, which is seen particularly in young patients with an initial MI without extensive cardiac damage (p. 1274). However, beta blockade is contraindicated in patients in whom the sinus tachycardia is a manifestation of pump failure, as reflected in a systolic arterial pressure below 100 mm Hg, rales involving more than one third of the lung fields, a pulmonary capillary wedge pressure exceeding 20 to 25 mm Hg, or a cardiac index below approximately 2.5 L/min/m².

ATRIAL FLUTTER AND FIBRILLATION (see pp. 626 and 1285). Both of these arrhythmias are more common during the first 24 hours after infarction than subsequently and are associated with increased mortality, particularly in patients with anterior wall infarction. However, because they are more common in patients with clinical and hemodynamic manifestations of extensive infarction and a poor prognosis, their *independent* contributions to increased mortality are not clear. Unfortunately, their management is complicated by frequent recurrence, particularly when they result from left atrial dilatation secondary to left ventricular failure.

Management of atrial flutter and fibrillation in patients with AMI is usually similar to their management in other settings (pp. 698 and 700). However, because of the possibility that a rapid ventricular rate can increase infarct size and because of the important role played by atrial contraction in the support of cardiac output in patients with AMI (Fig. 37–14, p. 1286), treatment must be prompt, especially when the ventricular rate exceeds 100/min. *Digitalis glycosides* are the principal agents used to slow the ventricular response. Digitalis may be supplemented by small intravenous doses of a beta blocker which also prolongs the AV nodal refractory period: 1 to 4 mg of propranolol in divided doses is often quite effective in reducing the ventricular rate and is well tolerated even in patients with mild heart failure and a rapid ventricular rate. Reduction of the rate of ventricular response to atrial fibrillation may be achieved also with verapamil administered intravenously[73] via bolus injections of 60 to 120 µg/kg, followed by a continuous infusion of 2.5 to 5.0 µg/kg/min, although caution must be exercised to avoid systemic arterial hypotension. On the other hand, when hemodynamic decompensation is prominent, electrical cardioversion with anterior and laterally placed paddles[74] employing low-energy, 5 to 20 watt-second discharges is indicated. An additional important option for the treatment of atrial flutter is the use of rapid atrial stimulation via a transvenous intraatrial electrode (p. 672); in contrast to DC cardioversion, this technique can be employed in the presence of possible digitalis intoxication, is less prone than DC countershock to elicit bradycardia after conversion to sinus rhythm, provides control of ventricular rate via atrial or ventricular pacing should this be necessary, and can be reapplied with less difficulty than cardioversion, should the patient experience recurrent atrial flutter. Following restoration of sinus rhythm, attention should be directed to the management of the underlying cause, usually heart failure, and to the prevention of recurrences, with antiarrhythmic agents such as quinidine.[75] Patients with recurrent episodes should be treated with oral anticoagulants.

OTHER ATRIAL ARRHYTHMIAS. *Premature atrial contractions* require no specific therapy. However, since they often herald more serious forms of atrial tachyarrhythmias, they merit attention. As is the case for patients with atrial flutter and fibrillation, premature atrial contractions may indicate atrial dilatation or excessive autonomic stimulation and they often reflect the presence of overt or occult heart failure; therefore they may respond to treatment of this condition. *Wandering atrial pacemaker* and *AV junctional rhythm* are important in patients with AMI because, as indicated above, the loss of atrial transport function may be tolerated poorly. Transvenous sequential atrioventricular pacing may be required to facilitate ventricular performance and maintain adequate peripheral perfusion.

Aggressive management is indicated for *paroxysmal supraventricular tachycardia* due to reentry involving the AV node (p. 626 and 707) because of the very rapid ventricular rate and its potentially adverse effects in patients with AMI. Augmentation of vagal tone by manual carotid sinus stimulation or intravenous administration of 10 mg of edrophonium (Tensilon) may restore sinus rhythm. Alpha-adrenergic agonists to increase arterial pressure and activate carotid sinus baroreceptors, an acceptable form of therapy for paroxysmal supraventricular tachycardia under other circumstances, are hazardous in patients with AMI, and intravenous verapamil is preferable.[73,76] Although digitalis glycosides may be useful in augmenting vagal tone, thereby terminating the arrhythmia, their effect is often delayed. Accordingly, low-energy DC countershock or rapid atrial stimulation via a transvenous intra-atrial electrode should be utilized just as for atrial flutter, particularly if hemodynamic decompensation occurs or if the rhythm is refractory to conventional measures. *Paroxysmal atrial tachycardia with AV block* (p. 701) may be a manifestation of digitalis intoxication and should be treated by withholding this drug and instituting potassium therapy, when it is accompanied by hypokalemia.

Ventricular Arrhythmias

VENTRICULAR PREMATURE CONTRACTIONS (see also pp. 719 and 1285). The suppression of ventricular premature contractions is based on the concept that in the face of myocardial ischemia the threshold for ventricular fibrillation is reduced and otherwise innocuous ventricular premature contractions may trigger ventricular fibrillation. While frequent ventricular premature contrac-

tions in the setting of ischemia are often used as a marker of the heart's propensity to fibrillate, successful suppression of ventricular premature contractions provides no assurance that ventricular fibrillation will not occur. Indeed, in more than half of the patients with AMI developing ventricular fibrillation, there are no premonitory ventricular premature contractions (p. 1286).[78] Furthermore, a large number of randomized trials have compared the routine administration of several potent antiarrhythmic drugs —lidocaine, quinidine, procainamide, and disopyramide, as well as beta-adrenergic blocking agents—against placebo. All of these agents reduced the frequency of ventricular premature contractions, and in the case of lidocaine, routine administration lowered the incidence of ventricular fibrillation.[79-81] None of the agents administered in this fashion, however, reduced mortality.[82]

Despite the results of these large trials and despite the complexity of the relationship between ventricular premature contractions and ventricular fibrillation, we favor the prophylactic administration of antiarrhythmic drugs in selected patients. This position is based partly on the concept that the abolition or reduction of ventricular premature contractions serves as a useful end-point that reflects an adequate overall pharmacological effect. Thus, when an appropriately selected agent is administered in sufficiently high doses, it can reduce the incidence of ventricular fibrillation even though its antifibrillatory activity can be monitored only indirectly, i.e., by reducing the incidence of ventricular premature contractions. It seems eminently desirable to reduce the incidence of ventricular fibrillation; although this potentially lethal arrhythmia may be treated effectively in centers where clinical trials on patients with AMI are being carried out, which usually have well-staffed and equipped coronary care units, this does not guarantee similar results in different settings.

Frequent ventricular premature contractions occurring very soon after the onset of MI, particularly during the first hour, may depend primarily on reentry rather than on increased automaticity.[81a] At this time, lidocaine, which impairs conduction in ventricular myocardium and diminishes automaticity, may be somewhat less effective than it is later.[82] When, at the very inception of an infarction, ventricular premature contractions are encountered in the presence of sinus tachycardia, augmented sympathoadrenal stimulation is often a contributing factor, and beta-adrenergic blockade is usually effective. Indeed, the effectiveness of beta-adrenergic blocking drugs under these circumstances may, in fact, play a role in the reduction in sudden deaths reported in patients who have recovered from AMI and are at high risk of recurrence.[83,84] The dose and mode of administration as well as the contraindications to beta-blockade are discussed on p. 1320.

In the absence of specific, correctable factors, such as sympathoadrenal hyperactivity with tachycardia, lidocaine should be administered to patients with AMI and frequent ventricular premature contractions (>6/min), multiform premature contractions and extrasystoles occurring in pairs or salvos, and early premature contractions (R on T), even though it is acknowledged that it may not be appropriate to consider these to be "warning arrhythmias." We favor the prophylactic administration of lidocaine, as described below, particularly in patients with AMI at high risk of developing ventricular fibrillation. This includes younger patients (< 50 years) without a prior history of heart failure or AMI and who present within the first six hours of infarction. Older patients (> 70 years) who are seen more than six hours after the onset of the MI are less likely to develop ventricular fibrillation and are at higher risk of developing lidocaine toxicity and should probably not receive prophylaxis routinely. The management of other patients must be individualized. The setting in which the patient is treated must also be considered. Obviously, the risk to life of ventricular fibrillation is greater at home or on a general hospital floor than in an expertly and fully staffed and equipped coronary care unit.

The pharmacology and pharmacokinetics of lidocaine are discussed on p. 653. With regimens depending on continuous infusion alone, therapeutic blood levels (1.5 to 5 μg/ml) are reached only after several hours because of the short half-life of the drug. Therefore, a loading dose of 100 mg or 1 mg/kg should be given intravenously as a bolus injection at the time of admission or during the patient's transportation to the hospital, followed in 5 to 10 minutes by an injection of 0.5 mg/kg. An intravenous infusion should be started concomitantly; a dose of 50 μg/kg/min in patients without heart failure and of 20 μg/kg/min in patients with heart failure is advised.[85] Intramuscular injections into the deltoid or gluteal muscles with conventional syringes and needles do not achieve therapeutic concentrations as promptly as those following intravenous injection.

The maintenance dose of lidocaine should be adjusted within the range of 1 to 4 mg/min to reduce sharply or abolish premature ventricular contractions. It should be recognized that the metabolism of lidocaine is slowed not only in patients with heart failure but also in those with diminution of hepatic blood flow due to effects of pharmacological agents such as propranolol.[86] Therefore, careful titration is needed to avoid toxicity, manifested primarily by central nervous system hyperactivity, as well as by depression of intraventricular and atrioventricular conduction and cardiac contractility (p. 656). Saturation of an extravascular pool normally occurs after a continuous infusion of approximately three hours, at which time blood levels will increase despite maintenance of a constant infusion rate.[87] At this time, it may be desirable to reduce the rate of administration by about 25 per cent.

This regimen is effective in suppressing ventricular premature contractions in approximately 75 per cent of patients seen within the first hour after the onset of ischemia;[9] it is effective in an even higher percentage—80 to 90 per cent—of patients seen later after the onset of ischemia, perhaps because enhanced automaticity becomes a progressively more important factor in the etiology of ventricular premature contractions with the passage of time from the onset of infarction and because of the particular effectiveness of the drug for arrhythmias on this basis.[88-91] Lidocaine has been shown to abolish reentrant ventricular arrhythmias in the late myocardial infarction phase by further depression and block of conduction in the reentrant pathway.[92]

When ventricular premature contractions compromise hemodynamics and persist despite administration of lidocaine, administration of *procainamide* intravenously in bolus doses of approximately 1 to 2 mg/kg intravenously over intervals of 5 minutes to a cumulative dose of approximately 1000 mg, followed by maintenance therapy with an intravenous infusion (20 to 80 μg/kg/min), may be effective.

Ventricular premature contractions that are unresponsive to lidocaine and procainamide in approximately the first six hours following AMI, particularly in the presence of sinus tachycardia, may be responsive to beta-adrenergic blocking agents. Newer investigational antiarrhythmic agents with actions resembling those of procainamide, such as acetyl procainamide,[93] aprindine,[76] and encainide[77] (p. 667), may be given to patients unresponsive to lidocaine and/or procainamide. Efficacy of these agents is noted in some patients with AMI and frequent ventricular premature contractions refractory to therapy with conventionally available agents.

Although *phenytoin* (Dilantin) (p. 661) (50 to 100 mg intravenously at 5 to 10 minute intervals to a total of 1000 mg) may diminish ventricular arrhythmia by decreasing the rate of phase IV depolarization, suppressing efferent cardiac sympathetic stimulation,[94] and further depressing and blocking conduction in ischemia-induced reentrant pathways,[95] it does not confer protection against ventricular fibrillation either in the first few hours[96] or later in the course of AMI. On the other hand, this drug may be effective when ventricular arrhythmias are initiated or potentiated by digitalis intoxication.

If ventricular premature contractions recur following initial intravenous treatment, oral administration of conventional antiarrhythmic agents is justified, including quinidine, procainamide, disopyramide, phenytoin, and propranolol, selected on the basis of the criteria outlined above and described in Chapter 20.

ACCELERATED IDIOVENTRICULAR RHYTHM (see also pp. 724 and 1286). The need for treatment of this arrhythmia with rates in the range of 60 to 100 beats/min remains controversial. Since these rhythms may deteriorate into ventricular tachycardia and since they may compromise cardiac function because of impairment of the physiological sequential relationship between atrial and ventricular contraction, it may be prudent to treat them by accelerating the sinus rate with atropine or atrial pacing or by suppressing the ventricular pacemaker with the administration of lidocaine intravenously. However, there is no definitive evidence that this arrhythmia, when left untreated, increases the incidence of either ventricular fibrillation or mortality.[10]

VENTRICULAR TACHYCARDIA (see also pp. 721 and 1286). Rapid abolition of this arrhythmia in patients with AMI is mandatory because of its deleterious effect on pump function and because it frequently deteriorates into ventricular fibrillation. When the ventricular rate is rapid (> 150/min) and/or there is a decline in arterial pressure, a single attempt at "thump version," i.e., striking a sharp blow to the precordium, is indicated (Fig. 38–2). If this maneuver is unsuccessful, it should be followed immediately by synchronized DC countershock, with the use of relatively low energies, i.e., 10 to 25 watts. When the ventricular rate is very rapid and synchronization is not possible, a defibrillatory impulse of 100 to 200 watt-seconds should be delivered. When the ventricular rate is slower than approximately 150/min and the arrhythmia is

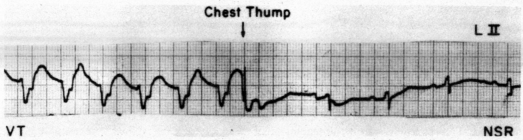

FIGURE 38–2   An example of reversion of ventricular tachycardia by a precordial thump. (Reproduced with permission from Pennington, J. E. Taylor, J., and Lown, B.: Chest thump for reverting ventricular tachycardia. N. Engl. J. Med. *283*:1192, 1970.)

well tolerated hemodynamically, a brief (15 to 20 min) trial of treatment with lidocaine or procainamide, using the loading doses described above, is in order. After reversion to sinus rhythm, every effort should be made to correct underlying abnormalities such as hypoxia, hypotension, acid-base or electrolyte disturbances, and digitalis excess. If these measures are unsuccessful, an infusion of bretylium tosylate (1–2 mg/min) may be tried. Recurrent or refractory ventricular tachycardia may respond to aneurysm resection, encircling endocardial ventriculotomy, or endocardial resection with or without coronary artery bypass grafting; these surgical procedures are generally reserved for use until after the acute phase.[97–99]

VENTRICULAR FIBRILLATION (see also pp. 728 and 1286).   Several forms of ventricular fibrillation associated with acute ischemic episodes can be distinguished. Two forms are associated with the syndrome of sudden cardiac death among ambulatory patients (Chap. 23): (1) In the first, the majority of survivors do not evolve AMI, although they usually have serious coronary artery disease. Therefore this form, although a manifestation of acute myocardial ischemia, should not be classified as one associated with AMI. (2) The second form is seen among survivors of resuscitation from sudden out-of-hospital ventricular fibrillation and occurs within minutes or a very few hours after the onset of other symptoms of ischemia such as pain. Patients evolve an MI, and in them the arrhythmia may well be identical to another form, generally called (3) *primary ventricular fibrillation*. This form occurs usually during the first 24 hours (most commonly during the first six to eight hours) in the course of AMI in the absence of cardiac failure or shock, and accounts for approximately 80 per cent of in-hospital episodes of ventricular fibrillation. (4) The fourth form, *secondary ventricular fibrillation*, occurs most commonly between 12 hours and four days after infarction, and is accompanied by and is probably a consequence of heart failure, hypotension, cardiogenic shock, or all three. (5) The fifth form, termed *late in-hospital ventricular fibrillation*, usually occurs after the third or fourth day—often after discharge from the coronary care unit but prior to hospital discharge. It is the risk of developing this form of ventricular fibrillation that has served as a stimulus to the development of intermediate coronary care (step-down) units (p. 1302). Patients may have heart failure but are rarely in cardiogenic shock. Patients with intraventricular conduction defects, extensive anterior wall infarction, persistent sinus tachycardia, as well as atrial flutter or fibrillation early in their course, are at higher risk of suffering late in-hospital ventricular fibril-

lation than patients without these features. Thus, this form of ventricular fibrillation merges with the first form, i.e., that responsible for sudden death after hospital discharge in patients with healed infarcts.

Procainamide,[100] lidocaine,[101] and the beta-adrenergic blocker, metoprolal,[101a] administered prophylactically have all been reported to reduce the incidence of ventricular fibrillation in hospitalized patients.[88,102,103] However, they may not reduce overall mortality substantially because treatment of this arrhythmia is so successful in an effectively staffed coronary care unit. Despite the potentially lethal nature of primary ventricular fibrillation, the bulk of evidence (with one exception[104]) suggests that when it is treated promptly with electrical countershock, ventricular fibrillation does not affect prognosis adversely, either in the hospital or following discharge. On the other hand, secondary ventricular fibrillation occurring in association with marked left ventricular failure or hypotension entails a dire prognosis, with only 20 to 25 per cent of patients surviving hospitalization;[10] the prognosis is intermediate in so-called late in-hospital ventricular fibrillation.[2] In the latter two forms it is the impairment of cardiac function consequent to the loss of contracting myocardium rather than the arrhythmia *per se* which is responsible for the poor prognosis.

The treatment of ventricular fibrillation, described in detail on p. 729, is *electrical countershock*, implemented as rapidly as possible. The likelihood of successful restoration of an effective cardiac rhythm declines rapidly with time after the onset of uncorrected ventricular fibrillation. Irreversible brain damage may occur within 1 to 2 minutes, particularly in elderly patients. Despite the superficial appeal of "thump version," which may sometimes terminate ventricular tachycardia (as opposed to fibrillation), no time should be lost before treating patients with ventricular fibrillation with electrical countershock.

Prompt electrical countershock generally interrupts fibrillation and restores an effective cardiac rhythm in patients under direct medical observation in the coronary care unit. When ventricular fibrillation occurs outside of an intensive care unit, resuscitative efforts are much less likely to be successful, primarily because the time interval between the onset of the episode and institution of definitive therapy tends to be prolonged. Since closed-chest cardiopulmonary resuscitation with external cardiac compression provides only a marginal cardiac output even under optimal circumstances, countershock should be implemented as soon as possible after the detection of ventricular fibrillation rather than deferred under the mistaken impression that adequate circulatory and respiratory support can be maintained in the interim. Failure of electrical countershock to restore an effective cardiac rhythm is due almost always to rapidly recurrent ventricular tachycardia or ventricular fibrillation, to electromechanical dissociation, or, very rarely, to electrical asystole.

Ventricular fibrillation often recurs rapidly and repeatedly when the metabolic milieu of the heart has been compromised by severe or prolonged hypoxemia, acidosis, or electrolyte abnormalities. Under these conditions, continued cardiopulmonary resuscitation, prompt implementation of pharmacological and ventilatory maneuvers designed to correct these abnormalities, treatment with antiarrhythmic agents such as lidocaine, and rapidly repeated attempts with electrical countershock may be effective. Even though repeated shocks with excessive energy may damage the myocardium[105-107] and elicit arrhythmias,[108] speed is essential and prompt efforts with high-intensity shocks (generally 300-400 watts initially) are justified. When ventricular fibrillation persists without documented interruption by electrical countershock, the intracardiac administration of epinephrine (up to 10 ml of a 1:10,000 concentration) or calcium gluconate (up to 15 ml of 10 per cent calcium gluconate) may facilitate success in a subsequent attempt. Conversion of fine to coarse ventricular fibrillation by either or both of these drugs may augur well for subsequent successful defibrillation.

Successful interruption of ventricular fibrillation or prevention of refractory recurrent episodes may be facilitated by administration of bretylium tosylate, 5 mg/kg I.V., repeated 20 minutes later if necessary (p. 663).[109] When synchronous cardiac electrical activity is restored by countershock, but contraction is ineffective, i.e., during electromechanical dissociation—the usual underlying cause is very extensive myocardial ischemia, or necrosis, or rupture of the ventricular free wall or septum. If rupture has not occurred, intracardiac administration of calcium gluconate or epinephrine may facilitate restoration of an effective heart beat. Another antifibrillatory agent is amiodarone (p. 666) (investigational in the United States). It has a slow onset of action, and therefore its principal role may prove to be in the prevention rather than treatment of ventricular fibrillation. Despite the unequivocal antiarrhythmic efficacy of this agent[110] and its potential value in limiting infarct size,[111] ocular, cutaneous, endocrine, and pulmonary toxicities may preclude its widespread clinical use.

TREATMENT OF HEMODYNAMIC DISTURBANCES

As indicated on p. 1274, hemodynamic assessment of patients with AMI has delineated several subsets with characteristic hemodynamic profiles. A convenient classification is (1) normal hemodynamics, (2) hyperdynamic circulatory state, (3) hypovolemic hypotension, (4) left ventricular failure, and (5) cardiogenic shock.[112-114] As indicated in Table 38-1, therapy designed to maintain ventricular performance, support hemodynamics, and protect jeopardized myocardium should be selected with consideration of the class of each patient. This classification can be achieved most readily by means of hemodynamic monitoring.

HYPOTENSION IN THE PREHOSPITAL PHASE. During the prehospital phase of AMI, invasive hemodynamic monitoring is usually not practical, and during this period, therapy should be guided by frequent clinical assessment and measurement of arterial pressure by the cuff method, with the recognition that intense vasoconstriction can provide a falsely low pressure measured by this method. Hypotension associated with bradycardia often reflects excessive vagotonia, which may be responsive to atropine and elevation of the lower extremities. Relative or absolute hypovolemia is often present when hypotension occurs with a normal or rapid heart rate, particularly among patients receiving diuretics just prior to the occurrence of infarction. Marked diaphoresis, reduction of fluid intake, or vomiting during the period preceding and accompanying the onset of AMI may all contribute to the development of hypovolemia. Even if the effective vascular volume is normal, relative hypovolemia may be present, since ventricular compliance is reduced in AMI (p. 1247) and a left

TABLE 38-1 POTENTIALLY USEFUL THERAPEUTIC INTERVENTIONS IN HEMODYNAMIC CATEGORIES OF PATIENTS WITH ACUTE MYOCARDIAL INFARCTION*

HEMODYNAMIC CATEGORY	P_a†	$\overline{PA}_o$‡	CI§	SUGGESTED INTERVENTION	REMARKS
Normal	≤ 15	≤ 12	2.7–3.5	None	β-blockade may be beneficial
Hyperdynamic state	≤ 15	≤ 12	≥ 3.0	β-adrenergic blockage	Tachycardia is a hallmark of subset
Hypotension or shock secondary to hypovolemia	≤ 15	≤ 9	≤ 2.7	Repletion of vascular volume	Reclassification may be necessary after PA_o is increased to range of 14 to 18 mm Hg
LV failure					
Mild	≥ 22	≥ 18– ≤ 22	≤ 2.5	Diuretics	Dyspnea, hypoxemia, or mild pulmonary vascular congestion
Severe	≥ 25	≥ 22	≤ 1.8	Vasodilators + diuretics	Pulmonary vascular congestion and pulmonary edema; cardiac glycosides; positive pressure ventilation and/or circulatory assist may be useful
Cardiogenic hypotension or shock	≥ 22	≥ 18	≤ 1.8	Circulatory assist	Sympathomimetic agents with positive inotropic effects such as dopamine or dobutamine may be useful

*Modified from references 3, 112, and 113.
†P_a, mean pulmonary artery pressure in mm Hg.
‡$\overline{PA}_o$, mean pulmonary artery occlusive pressure in mm Hg.
§CI, cardiac index in liters/minute/m².

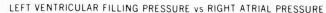

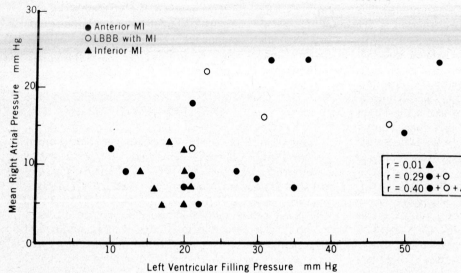

FIGURE 38–3 Comparison between left ventricular filling pressure and right atrial pressure in patients with acute myocardial infarction did not reveal a significant relationship. (From Rackley, C. E., et al.: Recognition of acute myocardial infarction. *In* Rackley, C. E., and Russell, R. O., Jr. (eds.): Coronary Artery Disease: Recognition and Management. Mt. Kisco, N.Y., Futura Publishing Co., 1979, p. 315.)

ventricular filling pressure as high as 20 to 24 mm Hg may be needed to provide an optimal preload.

In the absence of rales involving more than one third of the lung fields, the reverse Trendelenburg position should be assumed and in patients with sinus bradycardia, atropine should be administered (p. 690). If these measures do not correct the hypotension, crystalloid solutions should be administered intravenously, beginning with a bolus of 100 ml followed by 50-ml increments every five minutes. The patient should be carefully observed and the infusion stopped when the systolic pressure returns to approximately 100 mm Hg, if the patient becomes dyspneic or if pulmonary rales develop or increase. Because of the poor correlation between left ventricular filling pressure and mean right atrial pressure (Fig. 38–3), assessment of systemic venous pressure is of limited value as a guide to fluid therapy. Administration of cardiotonic agents (see below) is indicated during the prehospital phase if systemic arterial hypotension persists and is refractory to correction of hypovolemia and excessive vagotonia.

In the absence of invasive hemodynamic monitoring, assessment of peripheral vascular resistance must be based on clinical observations. If cutaneous vasoconstriction is present, therapy with dobutamine, which stimulates cardiac contractility without unduly accelerating heart rate and which does not increase the impedance to ventricular outflow, may be helpful (p. 543). In hypotensive patients with AMI, when there is clinical evidence of vasodilatation, an uncommon circumstance, norepinephrine is preferable.

INDICATIONS FOR INVASIVE HEMODYNAMIC MONITORING. Hemodynamic assessment becomes possible once the patient reaches the hospital. An estimation of the presence or absence of gross abnormalities in cardiac index and left ventricular filling pressure can be made on the basis of clinical examination in approximately 80 per cent of patients. Additional insights can sometimes be obtained with the use of noninvasive methods such as echocardiography to estimate the left atrial pressure, based on the timing of mitral valve closure and the interval from aortic valve closure to mitral valve opening.[115] Echocardiography can also demonstrate the presence of right

ventricular dilatation in patients with right ventricular infarcts (Fig. 37–15, p. 1289). However, severe depression of cardiac index and/or elevation of left ventricular filling pressure may be unsuspected in as many as 15 per cent of patients when estimates are based exclusively on clinical criteria.[116]

In patients with *clinically uncomplicated AMI*, invasive hemodynamic monitoring is generally not necessary, since the status of the circulation can be assessed by careful clinical evaluation. This ordinarily consists of monitoring of heart rate and rhythm, measurement of systemic arterial pressure by cuff, obtaining chest roentgenograms to detect heart failure, careful and repeated auscultation of the lung fields for pulmonary congestion, measurement of urine flow, examination of the skin and mucous membranes for evidence of the adequacy of perfusion, and arterial sampling for pO_2, pCO_2, and pH when hypoxemia or metabolic acidosis is suspected.

Invasive monitoring ordinarily consists of inserting an arterial line for the continuous measurement of arterial pressure, and a balloon flotation catheter for measurement of pulmonary artery, pulmonary artery occlusive (equivalent to pulmonary wedge) and right atrial pressures, and cardiac output by thermodilution (p. 290); in patients with hypotension, a Foley catheter provides accurate and continuous measurement of urine output.

The importance of invasive hemodynamic monitoring[116] is based on the following principal factors:

1. The difficulty of interpreting clinical and radiographic findings of pulmonary congestion because of phase lags, such as those occurring after diuretic therapy.

2. The need for identifying noncardiac causes of arterial hypotension, particularly hypovolemia.

3. Possible contributions of reduced ventricular compliance to impaired hemodynamics, requiring judicious adjustment of intravascular volume to optimize left ventricular filling pressure.

4. Difficulty in assessing the severity and sometimes even the presence of lesions such as mitral regurgitation

and ventricular septal defect when the cardiac output or the systemic pressures are depressed.

5. Establishing a baseline of hemodynamic measurements and guiding therapy in patients with clinically apparent pulmonary edema or cardiogenic shock.

6. The underestimation of systemic arterial pressure by the cuff method in patients with intense vasoconstriction (p. 22).

Therefore, we believe the following to be indications for invasive hemodynamic monitoring in patients with AMI: (1) hypotension unresponsive to simple measures, such as elevation of the lower extremities and the administration of atropine in patients with accompanying bradycardia; (2) moderate or severe left ventricular failure, manifested by persistent or excessive dyspnea, rales, or radiographic evidence of pulmonary vascular congestion, pulmonary edema, or cardiomegaly; (3) unexplained or refractory sinus tachycardia or other tachyarrhythmias; (4) unexplained or severe cyanosis, hypoxemia, tachypnea, diaphoresis, or acidosis; and (5) clinical signs suggestive of mitral regurgitation, ventricular septal defect, or pericardial effusion.

HYPERDYNAMIC STATE. When infarction is not complicated by hemodynamic impairment, no therapy other than general supportive measures and treatment of arrhythmias is necessary. However, if the hemodynamic profile is of the hyperdynamic state, i.e., elevation of sinus rate, arterial pressure, and cardiac index, occurring singly or together in the presence of a normal or low left ventricular filling pressure, and if other causes of tachycardia such as fever, infection, and pericarditis can be excluded, treatment with beta-adrenergic blocking agents is indicated. The rationale, dose, and mode of administration are discussed on p. 1320.

HYPOVOLEMIC HYPOTENSION. Recognition of hypovolemia is of particular importance in hypotensive patients with AMI, because improvement in circulatory dynamics is so readily and safely achieved by augmentation of vascular volume. Since hypovolemia is often occult, it is frequently overlooked in the absence of invasive hemodynamic monitoring. It may be absolute, with low left ventricular filling pressure (< 8 mm Hg), or relative, with normal (8 to 12 mm Hg) or even modestly increased (13 to 18 mm Hg) left ventricular filling pressures. Because of the reduction of left ventricular compliance that occurs

with acute ischemia and infarction (p. 1246), left ventricular filling pressures between 13 and 18 mm Hg, while above the upper limits of normal, may be suboptimal.

Exclusion of hypovolemia as the cause of hypotension requires documentation of a reduced cardiac output despite left ventricular filling pressure of more than approximately 17 mm Hg. If, in a hypotensive patient, the pulmonary capillary wedge pressure (ordinarily measured as the pulmonary artery occlusive pressure) is below this level, fluid challenge should be carried out with sequential 50-ml intravenous bolus infusions[117] and serial assessments should be made of pulmonary capillary wedge pressure and cardiac output. Elevation of pulmonary capillary wedge pressure to between 18 and 24 mm Hg reflects the achievement of a left ventricular filling pressure associated with an optimal cardiac output (Fig. 38–4). If hypovolemia is documented, the fluid replaced should resemble the fluid lost. Thus, when a low hematocrit complicates AMI, infusion of whole blood is the treatment of choice. On the other hand, crystalloid or colloid solutions should be administered when the hematocrit is normal or elevated.

Hypotension Due to Right Ventricular Infarction. Hypotension caused by right ventricular infarction may be confused with that caused by hypovolemia, because both are associated with a low, normal, or minimally elevated left ventricular filling pressure. However, hypotension secondary to right ventricular infarction (which is frequently associated with inferior left ventricular infarction) is generally recognizable from discordant elevation of right compared to left ventricular filling pressure, diminution of right ventricular ejection fraction by radionuclide ventriculography,[118,119] and right ventricular dilatation on echocardiography (Fig. 37–15, p. 1289). The hypotension associated with right ventricular infarction often responds to the vigorous administration of fluid, and positive inotropic agents such as dobutamine;[118–120] the treatment of cardiogenic shock associated with right ventricular infarction is discussed on p. 1317).

Treatment of Left Ventricular Failure

The treatment of left ventricular failure with AMI requires meticulous attention to ventilation, since hypoxemia can impair the function of ischemic tissue at the margin of

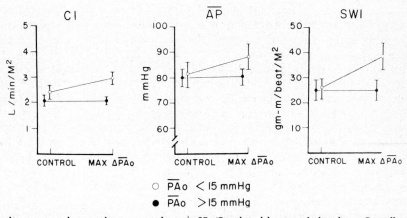

FIGURE 38–4 Effects of augmentation of vascular volume on ventricular function in patients with AMI who were categorized according to levels of pulmonary artery occlusive ($\overline{PAo}$) pressure (pulmonary capillary wedge pressure) as soon as possible after hospitalization. Vascular volume was augmented by infusion with dextran or hypertonic glucose solutions. As can be seen, among patients with high initial $\overline{PAo}$ pressure, cardiac index (CI) and mean aortic pressure ($\overline{AP}$) did not increase as a result of volume expansion, nor did the stroke work index (SWI) rise. On the other hand, in patients in whom initial values of $\overline{PAo}$ were not elevated substantially above the normal range, expansion of plasma volume led to an increase in cardiac index, elevation of mean aortic pressure, and an increased stroke work index—all compatible with improved ventricular performance achieved by the induction of more favorable loading conditions. Results expressed comprise mean values ± SE. (Reprinted by permission from Crexells, C., et al.: Optimal level of filling pressure in the left side of the heart in acute myocardial infarction. N. Engl. J. Med. *289*:1264, 1973.)

the infarct and thereby initiate the vicious circle, ultimately leading to the patient's demise (Fig. 37–8, p. 1271). The combination of pulmonary vascular congestion (or when it is severe, pulmonary edema), reduced pulmonary compliance, and the respiratory depression that may be associated with excessive doses of analgesics conspires to impair ventilatory function and arterial oxygenation (pp. 1276 and 1786). When arterial oxygen tension cannot be maintained above 60 to 70 mm Hg despite inhalation of 100 per cent oxygen delivered at 8 L/min by mask and the adequate use of bronchodilators, endotracheal intubation, assisted ventilation, and positive pressure should be considered. The improvement of arterial oxygenation and hence myocardial oxygen supply may help to restore ventricular performance. Invasive hemodynamic monitoring is necessary to guide therapy under these circumstances, since positive end-expiratory pressure may diminish systemic venous return and reduce effective left ventricular filling pressure.

When wheezing complicates pulmonary congestion, bronchodilators that act primarily on beta-2 adrenergic receptors, such as isoetharine or metaproterenol, given as aerosols, or terbutaline, which can be administered subcutaneously or orally, are more desirable than conventional bronchodilators, such as isoproterenol or epinephrine, whose primary effects are on beta-1 receptors.

Although positive inotropic agents may be useful, they do *not* represent the *initial* therapy of choice in patients with AMI. Instead, heart failure in this setting is managed most effectively first by reduction of blood volume and ventricular preload, and, if possible, by lowering afterload.

DIURETICS (also see p. 527).   Mild heart failure in patients with AMI frequently responds well to diuretics such as furosemide, administered intravenously in doses of 40 mg, repeated at 3- to 4-hour intervals if necessary. The resultant reduction of pulmonary capillary pressure reduces dyspnea, and the lowering of left ventricular wall tension that accompanies the reduction of left ventricular diastolic volume diminishes myocardial oxygen requirements and may lead to improvement of contractility and augmentation of the ejection fraction, stroke volume, and cardiac output. The reduction of elevated left ventricular filling pressure may also enhance myocardial oxygen delivery by diminishing the impedance to coronary perfusion attributable to elevated ventricular wall tension (p. 1239). It may also improve arterial oxygenation by reducing pulmonary vascular congestion.

The intravenous administration of furosemide reduces pulmonary vascular congestion and pulmonary venous pressure within 15 minutes, before renal excretion of sodium and water have occurred; presumably this action results from a direct dilating effect of this drug on the systemic arterial bed (p. 527). It is important not to "overshoot" the mark by reducing left ventricular filling pressure much below 18 mm Hg, the lower range associated with optimal left ventricular performance, since this may reduce cardiac output further and cause arterial hypotension. Excessive diuresis may also result in hypokalemia, with its attendant risk of digitalis intoxication.

VASODILATORS (see p. 534).   Myocardial oxygen requirements depend on left ventricular wall stress, which in turn is proportional to the product of peak developed left ventricular pressure, volume, and wall thickness (p.

1535). Vasodilator therapy is not recommended in patients with uncomplicated AMI, but is useful in patients whose MI is complicated by heart failure unresponsive to treatment with diuretics, hypertension, mitral regurgitation, or ventricular septal defect. In these patients, treatment with vasodilator agents increases stroke volume and reduces myocardial oxygen consumption. The necessity for hemodynamic monitoring of systemic arterial and pulmonary capillary wedge (or at least pulmonary artery) pressure of cardiac output in patients treated with these agents must be emphasized, since improvement of cardiac performance and energetics requires three simultaneous effects: (1) reduction of impedance to ventricular ejection; (2) avoidance of excessive systemic arterial hypotension in order to maintain effective coronary perfusion pressure; and (3) avoidance of excessive reduction of ventricular filling pressure with consequent diminution of cardiac output. In general, pulmonary capillary wedge pressure should be maintained at approximately 20 mm Hg and arterial diastolic blood pressure above 60 mm Hg in patients who were normotensive prior to the development of the AMI.

Appropriate doses of vasodilators generally enhance stroke volume and cardiac output, reduce left ventricular filling pressure and volume and calculated systemic vascular resistance, without causing serious reflex tachycardia. While available data are not conclusive and do not apply to all subsets of patients with AMI, at least one vasodilator, nitroglycerin, when given early in the course of AMI, has been reported also to protect ischemic myocardium and limit infarct size (p. 1322). Excessive doses of vasodilators may decrease cardiac output by reducing preload and left ventricular filling pressure below optimal levels or may decrease coronary perfusion by excessive depression of systemic arterial pressure. Compromise of coronary perfusion, in turn, may impair ventricular performance further, extend infarction, and give rise to lethal arrhythmias.

Vasodilator therapy is particularly useful when AMI is complicated by mitral regurgitation or rupture of the ventricular septum. In such patients, vasodilators alone or in combination with intra-aortic balloon counterpulsation can sometimes serve as a "holding maneuver" and provide hemodynamic stabilization to permit definitive catheterization and angiographic studies to be carried out and to prepare the patient for early surgical intervention. Because of the precarious state of patients with complicated infarcts and the need for meticulous adjustment of dosage, therapy is best initiated with agents that can be administered intravenously and that have a short duration of action, such as nitroprusside,[121–124] trimethaphan,[125] nitroglycerin,[126–133] isosorbide dinitrate,[134] or phentolamine.[135,136] After initial stabilization, oral medication with hydralazine;[137,138] long-acting nitrates given by mouth, sublingually, by ointment or transdermally;[139,140] prazosin;[141] calcium antagonists such as nifedipine;[142] and angiotensin-converting enzyme inhibitors such as captopril[143] may be useful.

There has been more experience with the intravenous infusion of *nitroprusside* in patients with AMI than with other vasodilators. It is generally given initially in doses of 0.5 μg/kg/min[145,146] and may be gradually and progressively increased up to 50 μg/kg/min. While increasing cardiac output in patients with AMI and left ventricular failure (Fig. 38–5),[147] nitroprusside diminishes arteriolar resistance

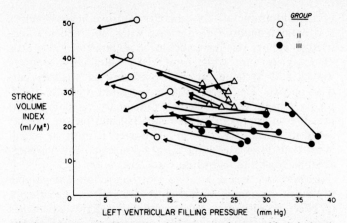

FIGURE 38–5 Hemodynamic responses to nitroprusside infusion in patients with acute myocardial infarction. Patients in Groups II and III with elevated left ventricular filling pressures (20 mm Hg or more) tend to respond to the vasodilator with an increase in the stroke volume and a marked drop in the filling pressure, whereas patients with left ventricular filling pressures below 15 mm Hg (Group I) show a reduction in the stroke volume and tend to have less marked decreases in filling pressures during nitroprusside infusion. Group III patients had stroke work indices below 20 g-m/m². (Reproduced with permission from Chatterjee, K., and Parmley, W. W.: The role of vasodilator therapy in heart failure. Prog. Cardiovasc. Dis. *19*:301, 1977.)

and impedance to left ventricular ejection, pulmonary capillary wedge pressure, myocardial oxygen requirements, and sometimes the frequency of ventricular premature contractions. With optimization of dose, improved segmental ventricular function of zones of apparent infarction has been observed.[124] Nitroprusside may augment cardiac output even in patients with cardiogenic shock, if arterial diastolic and coronary perfusion pressure are maintained by concomitant intra-aortic balloon counterpulsation.

Nitroglycerin has been shown in animal experiments to be less likely than nitroprusside to produce a "coronary steal," i.e., to divert blood flow from the ischemic to the nonischemic zone,[127] and therefore when it (or isosorbide dinitrate, which has a similar action[134]) is used intravenously it may be a particularly useful vasodilator in patients with AMI.[128] Ten to 15 μg/min is infused and the dose is increased by 5 μg/min every five minutes until the desired effect (improvement of hemodynamics or relief of ischemic chest pain) or a decline in systolic arterial pressure to 90 mm Hg, or by more than 15 mm Hg, has occurred. Since nitroglycerin adheres to polyvinyl chloride, this drug should be administered through specially available kits. Although both nitroglycerin and nitroprusside lower systemic arterial pressure, systemic vascular resistance, and the heart rate–systolic blood pressure product, the reduction of left ventricular filling pressure is more prominent with nitroglycerin because of its relatively greater effect than nitroprusside on venous capacitance vessels. Nevertheless, in patients with severe left ventricular failure, cardiac output often increases despite the reduction in left ventricular filling pressure produced by nitroglycerin.

Favorable effects on ventricular performance and jeopardized ischemic myocardium in patients with AMI have been obtained with *phentolamine* (at doses of 0.1 to 2.0 mg/min), an alpha-adrenergic blocking agent whose predominant effects are on arteriolar resistance vessels;[135,136]

unfortunately, this agent is extremely expensive and causes tachycardia. Reduction of ventricular afterload with intravenous infusions of a ganglionic blocking agent, *trimethaphan*, in doses of 100 to 1000 μg/min in patients with AMI, associated with acute or chronic hypertension has been shown to protect ischemic myocardium and to reduce infarct size and early mortality in hypertensive patients with AMI.[125] This agent is less likely to produce reflex tachycardia than are directly acting vasodilators because of its inhibitory effects on sympathetic ganglia and therefore on baroreceptor-mediated reflexes.

The use of oral vasodilators in the treatment of chronic congestive heart failure is discussed on pp. 534 to 541. Here we focus on their use in the patients with AMI, which is generally begun after their condition has been stabilized with an intravenous agent.

Hydralazine (p. 538) (10 to 100 mg four times a day) is an orally effective vasodilator acting directly on arterioles. Although useful as an afterload-reducing agent in patients with chronic heart failure, it may be hazardous in patients in the first few days following AMI because of the tachycardia it sometimes induces owing to reflex stimulation. Furthermore, some[148,149] but not all[150,151] investigators have reported the development of pharmacological or physiological tolerance with prolonged use.

Prazosin (p. 539) (0.5 mg. with gradual increments to a maximum of 10 mg, three times daily), an orally active adrenergic-blocking agent, improves cardiac function in patients with chronic congestive heart failure.[141] Although it has not been evaluated extensively in the treatment of AMI, its unique pharmacological properties, compared with those of other alpha-adrenergic receptor antagonists, appear promising. In contrast to other alpha-receptor blocking agents, prazosin does not inhibit presynaptic sites, i.e., so-called alpha-2 receptors (Fig. 27–9, p. 914). Accordingly, negative feedback on presynaptic receptors by norepinephrine released from the nerve endings remains intact. This may account for the absence of tachycardia after administration of the drug, which should make it particularly useful in patients with AMI. Prazosin, like nitroprusside, affects both arteriolar and venous tone; effects persist for up to six hours after an oral dose.

Captopril (p. 539) (25 to 100 mg three times daily)[151] elicits sustained increases in cardiac index and diminution of left ventricular filling pressure, even among patients with congestive heart failure complicated by impaired renal function. Its inhibition of formation of angiotensin II results in retention of potassium due to decreased aldosterone levels, and hence it should be used with caution with potassium-sparing diuretics such as spironolactone, triamterene, or amiloride. It may potentiate the hypotensive effects of other agents such as thiazide or "loop" diuretics, which should therefore be used judiciously and sometimes at reduced dosage if employed concomitantly. Rare toxic effects on the hematopoietic system or on glomerular functional integrity and proteinuria are generally seen only with high doses. Captopril has not been evaluated extensively in patients with AMI, but it is of interest that it has been shown, in experimental studies, to reduce infarct size in dogs with coronary occlusion.[152]

Digitalis (see p. 508). Although digitalis increases contractility and the oxygen consumption of normal hearts, when heart failure is present the diminution of heart size and wall tension frequently results in a net reduction of myocardial oxygen requirements.[153] In animal experiments acetylstrophanthidin fails to improve ventricular performance immediately following experimental coronary occlusion, but salutary effects are elicited when it is administered several days later.[154] The absence of early beneficial effects may be due to the inability of ischemic tissue to respond to digitalis, the already maximal stimulation of contractility of the normal heart by circulating and neuronally released catecholamines, or the dissipation of the force of contraction of normal myocardium into dyskinetic areas. In experimental animals without congestive heart failure who are subjected to coronary occlusion, digitalis increases the distribution and severity of ischemia, presumably by stimulating oxygen requirements,[155] although it augments blood flow to ischemic zones in conscious dogs.[156] Digitalis reduces the severity of ischemia occurring in the presence of experimentally induced congestive heart failure,[157] presumably because of the reduction in myocardial oxygen requirements.

Although the issue is still controversial, arrhythmias may be increased by digitalis glycosides when they are given to patients in the first few hours after the onset of MI, particularly in the presence of hypokalemia. Also, undesirable peripheral systemic and coronary vasoconstriction may result from the rapid intravenous administration of these agents.[158]

Administration of digitalis to patients hospitalized with AMI should generally be reserved for the management of supraventricular tachyarrhythmias such as atrial flutter and fibrillation and of heart failure that persists despite treatment with diuretics. Digitalis causes modest improvement of cardiac performance in patients with mild heart failure (Killip Class II).[159,160] There is no indication for its use as an inotropic agent in patients without clinical evidence of left ventricular dysfunction (Killip Class I), and it is too weak an inotropic agent to be relied upon as the principal cardiac stimulant in patients in overt pulmonary edema or cardiogenic shock (Classes III or IV). It may, however, be useful as a supplement to vasodilator agents and in the treatment of persistent or recurrent left ventricular failure. Cardiac glycosides appear to become progressively more effective in the treatment of heart failure as the interval from the acute events lengthens; i.e., they are more effective in the treatment of chronic than of acute heart failure secondary to ischemic heart disease. However, the possibility that continued administration of digitalis might contribute to late mortality in the two years following AMI has been raised[161] and debated.[162] The possible long-term hazards of digitalis administration must be clarified before a definitive recommendation about its use in the convalescent phase can be made. At this time, it would appear to be indicated only if there is overt heart failure and/or supraventricular tachyarrhythmias, but it is of interest that it has been shown, in experimental studies, to reduce the area of infarct size in dogs with coronary occlusion and heart failure.[166]

BETA-ADRENERGIC AGONISTS (see also p. 542). When left ventricular failure is severe, as manifested by marked reduction of cardiac index (<2 L/min/m^2), and pulmonary capillary wedge pressure is at optimal (18 to 24 mm Hg) or excessive (>24 mm Hg) levels despite therapy with diuretics, beta-adrenergic agonists are indicated. Although isoproterenol is a potent cardiac stimulant and improves ventricular performance, it also causes tachycardia and augments myocardial oxygen consumption and lactate production;[163] in addition, it reduces coronary perfusion pressure by causing systemic vasodilation and increases the extent of experimentally induced infarction in animals.[155,164] Norepinephrine and metaraminol also increase myocardial oxygen consumption because of their peripheral vasoconstrictor as well as positive inotropic actions.

Dopamine and dobutamine, which are relatively cardioselective and stimulate beta-1 receptors, exert predominantly positive inotropic effects (p. 418) and may be particularly useful in patients with AMI and reduced cardiac output, increased left ventricular filling pressure, pulmonary vascular congestion, and hypotension.[164a] Fortunately, the potentially deleterious alpha-adrenergic vasoconstrictor effects exerted by *dopamine* occur only at higher doses than those required to increase contractility. Its vasodilating actions on renal and splanchnic vessels and its positive inotropic effects generally improve hemodynamics and renal function.[165] In patients with AMI and left ventricular failure, this drug should be administered at a dose of 3 μg/kg/min, while monitoring pulmonary capillary wedge and systemic arterial pressures as well as cardiac output. The dose may be increased stepwise to 20 μg/kg/min, in order to reduce pulmonary capillary wedge pressure to approximately 20 mm Hg and elevate cardiac index to exceed 2 L/min/m^2. However, it must be recognized that doses exceeding 5 μg/kg/min activate peripheral alpha receptors and cause vasoconstriction.

Dobutamine has a positive inotropic effect comparable to that of dopamine but a slightly less positive chronotropic effect,[166] with less vasoconstrictor activity at higher doses. In patients with AMI dobutamine improves left ventricular performance without augmenting enzymatically estimated infarct size.[167-169,169a] It may be administered in a starting dose of 2.5 μg/kg/min and increased stepwise to a maximum of 30 μg/kg/min. Both dopamine and dobutamine must be given carefully and with constant monitoring of the electrocardiogram, systemic arterial pressure, pulmonary artery or pulmonary artery occlusive pressure, and, if possible, frequent measurements of cardiac output. The dose must be reduced if systolic pressure exceeds 130 to 140 mm Hg, heart rate exceeds 100 to 110 beats/min, or supraventricular or ventricular tachyarrhythmias are precipitated.

TREATMENT OF CARDIOGENIC SHOCK
(see also p. 593)

Massive AMI may produce global impairment of left ventricular function which is so profound that cardiogenic shock supervenes. The etiology, pathophysiology, and clinical picture of this syndrome are considered in detail on pp. 591 and 1270. Cardiogenic shock is characterized by marked hypotension with systolic arterial pressure less than 80 mm Hg and a marked reduction of cardiac index (generally <1.8 L/min/m^2) in the face of elevated left ventricular filling pressure (pulmonary capillary wedge pressure >18 mm Hg).[169b] Spurious estimates of left ventricular filling pressure based on measurements of the pulmonary artery occlusive pressure can occur in the presence of marked mitral regurgitation, in which the tall v wave in the left atrial (and pulmonary artery occlusive) pressure tracing elevates the mean pressure above left ventricular end-diastolic pressure. Accordingly, mitral regurgitation and other mechanical lesions such as ventricular septal defect, ventricular aneurysm, and pseudoaneurysm must be excluded before the diagnosis of cardiogenic shock due to global impairment of left ventricular function can be established. These potentially catastrophic mechanical complications should be suspected in any patient with AMI in whom circulatory collapse occurs. Immediate hemodynamic and angiographic evaluations are necessary if these complications are likely to be responsible for the impairment of left ventricular performance, since primary therapy of such lesions usually requires immediate operative treatment with intervening support of the circulation by intra-aortic balloon counterpulsation.

Cardiotonic agents, particularly dopamine and dobutamine, are employed extensively in the treatment of cardiogenic shock owing to global impairment of left ventricular function.[170] While these drugs can improve hemodynamics in the absence of the above-mentioned mechanical complications, unfortunately they do not appear to affect mortality significantly. Similarly, vasodilators have been utilized in an effort to elevate cardiac output and to reduce left ventricular filling pressure. However, by lowering the already markedly reduced coronary perfusion pressure, myocardial perfusion can be compromised further, accelerating the vicious circle illustrated in Figure 37–8 p. 1271. Vasodilators may nonetheless be employed in conjunction with intra-aortic balloon counterpulsation and/or inotropic agents in an effort to increase cardiac output while sustaining or elevating coronary perfusion pressure.

The systemic vascular resistance is usually elevated in patients with cardiogenic shock, but occasionally resistance is normal, and in some instances vasodilation actually predominates. When systemic vascular resistance is *not* elevated in patients with cardiogenic shock, norepinephrine (in doses ranging from 2 to 10 μg/min), which has both alpha- and beta-adrenergic agonist properties, is often employed to increase diastolic arterial pressure, maintain coronary perfusion, and improve contractility, but, again, there is no definitive evidence that ultimate outcome is affected by this drug.[163,171] Norepinephrine should be used only when other means, including balloon counterpulsation, fail to maintain systemic arterial diastolic pressure above 50 to 60 mm Hg in a previously normotensive patient. The use of alpha-adrenergic agents such as phenylephrine or methoxamine is contraindicated in patients with cardiogenic shock.

INTRAAORTIC BALLOON COUNTERPULSATION.

The implementation, underlying principles, and physiological consequences of this procedure in patients with cardiogenic shock are discussed on p. 593 and illustrated in Figure 18–10. This form of circulatory assistance augments diastolic aortic pressure and thereby facilitates coronary perfusion; it reduces left ventricular afterload and thereby reduces myocardial oxygen consumption;[172,173] as a consequence anaerobic metabolism[174] and myocardial ischemia are diminished. Favorable effects are sometimes reflected in prompt resolution of electrocardiographic signs of ischemia (Fig. 38–6).

Intraaortic balloon counterpulsation is utilized in the treatment of AMI in three groups of patients: (1) those who are hemodynamically unstable and in whom support of the circulation is required for the performance of diagnostic studies which are carried out to assess lesions that are potentially correctable surgically; (2) in cardiogenic shock that is unresponsive to medical management; and (3) in the presence of persistent ischemic pain that is unresponsive to treatment with inhalation of 100 per cent oxygen, beta-adrenergic blockade, nitrates, and calcium channel blocking agents during the postinfarction state. Unfortunately, among patients with cardiogenic shock, improvement is often only temporary, and "balloon dependence" is common.[175,176] Patients with cardiogenic shock treated with this modality can be successfully weaned from the supporting system only occasionally, and counterpulsation alone does not improve overall mortality, either in patients with or those without a surgically remediable mechanical lesion.[177,178] However, it may be life-saving

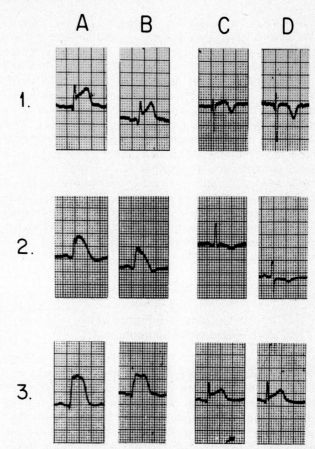

FIGURE 38–6 Precordial lead showing maximal ST-segment elevation in patients with acute myocardial infarction 1 hour before intraaortic balloon pumping (IABP) (column A), immediately before IABP (column B), 30 minutes after commencing IABP (column C), and 1 hour after IABP had begun (column D). The fall in ST-segment elevation in these leads during the hour before IABP was 26 per cent, compared with 84 per cent during the post-IABP hour. In all cases the ST response was greatest during the first 30 minutes of treatment. (Modified from Leinbach, R. C., et al.: Early intraaortic balloon pumping for anterior myocardial infarction without shock. *Circulation 58*:204, 1978, by permission of the American Heart Association, Inc.)

in allowing the patient to tolerate catheterization and coronary arteriography and to be brought to the operating room for definitive treatment without irreversible organ damage. It is possible that left ventricular bypass, a technique that reduces left ventricular oxygen demands more drastically (p. 548), may ultimately prove to be more effective in improving survival in patients with cardiogenic shock than intraaortic balloon counterpulsation;[179] however, at the present time it is still experimental.

Noninvasive approaches to circulatory assistance have been developed, such as external devices that apply pressure to the lower extremities during diastole, thereby promoting increased runoff during systole. However, this form of therapy likewise does not alter outcome decisively; its hemodynamic effects are, in fact, less than those of intraaortic counterpulsation.[180]

RIGHT VENTRICULAR INFARCTION (see also p. 1274). Unlike cardiogenic shock due solely or predominantly to left ventricular involvement, hemodynamics may be improved in patients with right ventricular infarction by a combination of expanding plasma volume to augment right ventricular preload and cardiac output, and the administration of arterial vasodilators. These drugs reduce the impedance to left ventricular outflow and in turn left ventricular diastolic, left atrial, and pulmonary (arterial) pressures, thereby lowering the impedance to right ventricular outflow and enhancing right ventricular output. A remarkably high survival rate of 60 per cent, albeit in a small series, makes recognition and vigorous medical therapy of this syndrome particularly important.[120] Since right ventricular infarction is so common among patients with inferior left ventricular infarction, otherwise unexplained systemic arterial hypotension or diminished cardiac output in such patients should lead to the prompt consideration of this diagnosis. Replacement of the tricuspid valve has been carried out in the treatment of severe tricuspid regurgitation secondary to right ventricular infarction.[181]

Surgical Treatment of Hemodynamic Impairment

Operative intervention is most successful in patients with AMI and circulatory collapse when a surgically correctable mechanical lesion can be identified and repaired, such as ventricular septal defect,[182,183] acute mitral regurgitation resulting from rupture of the head of a papillary muscle or of chordae tendineae, aneurysm, or pseudoaneurysm (p. 1270).[184] In such patients the circulation should at first be supported by intraaortic balloon pulsation and a positive inotropic agent such as dopamine or dobutamine in combination with a vasodilator unless the patient is hypotensive. Operation should not be delayed in patients with a correctable lesion who require pharmacologic and/or mechanical (counterpulsation) support (Fig. 38–7).[182,185,186] Such patients frequently develop a serious complication—infection, adult respiratory distress syndrome, extension of the infarct, renal failure, etc.—if operation is delayed. On the other hand, when the hemodynamic status of a patient with one of these mechanical lesions complicating an AMI remains stable after the patient has been weaned off pharmacologic and/or mechanical support, it may be desirable to postpone operation for two to four weeks to allow some healing of the infarct to occur.

Some favorable results have been reported from early revascularization and infarctectomy in patients who have cardiogenic shock due to ventricular failure without mechanical complications and who are unresponsive to all other measures.[187,188] However, this approach has not received widespread acceptance because of the high mortality rate, and the difficulties involved in selecting the proper time for operation—after it has become clear that the patient is in cardiogenic shock despite optimal medical management, yet before a critical quantity of myocardium has become irreversibly damaged.

Although cardiac rupture (p. 1268) is generally immediately fatal pericardiocentesis to abort cardiac tamponade, followed immediately by resection of the necrotic and ruptured myocardium with primary reconstruction, has on rare occasion been lifesaving.[188,189]

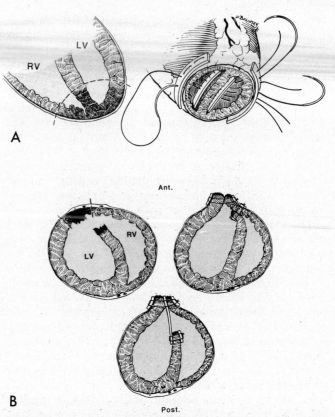

FIGURE 38–7 *A,* Closure of apical ventricular septal rupture. The infarcted apex is resected, and the remaining viable myocardium of the septum and the left and right ventricular free walls are buttressed together using Teflon felt inside and outside the ventricle. LV = left ventricle; RV = right ventricle. *B,* Closure of a ventricular septal rupture with an extensive anterior infarct. The septum is reconstructed with a heavy Dacron patch that is sewn to the base of remaining septum using Teflon bolsters on both sides. The free edge of the patch is then brought out and the left and right ventricular free walls are attached to it, as shown in *C.* Ant. = anterior; LV = left ventricle; Post = posterior; RV = right ventricle. (Reproduced with permission from Kopf, G. S., Meshkov, A., Laks, H., Hammond, G. L., and Geha, A. S.: Changing patterns in the surgical management of ventricular septal rupture after myocardial infarction. Am. J. Surg. **143:**465, 1982.)

LIMITATION OF INFARCT SIZE

As already noted, infarct size is an important determinant of prognosis in patients with AMI. Patients who succumb from cardiogenic shock exhibit massive infarcts,[191,192] and early impairment of ventricular function, presaging a poor prognosis, is correlated with extensive infarcts.[192–196] Survivors with large infarcts frequently exhibit late impairment of ventricular function, and the long-term mortality rate is higher than that for survivors with small infarcts (Fig. 38–8), who tend not to develop cardiac decompensation.[49,193,194,197–201] The influence of infarct size on mortality is most apparent during the patient's hospital course and in the first few months after infarction. The hospital mortality of patients with large infarcts, as estimated by technetium pyrophosphate scanning, is several-fold greater than it is in patients with small infarcts (Fig. 11–24, p. 387).[201] However, the importance of infarct size declines

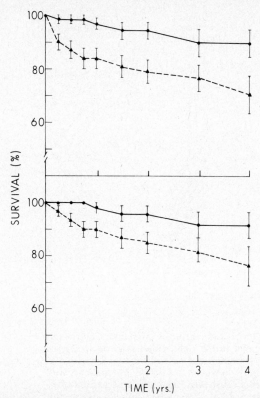

FIGURE 38–8 The influence of the extent of initial myocardial infarction on survival. Survival is shown after initial myocardial infarction in a total of 173 patients with infarct size index (expressed in terms of CK-gram-equivalents/m²) of <15 (solid line) vs. ≥15 (interrupted line). Brackets indicate standard errors. The upper panel depicts survival curves for all patients who survived for at least 24 hours after the onset of an initial myocardial infarction. The lower panel depicts curves for those patients who survived at least 21 days after infarction. In both groups, survival was significantly greater for patients with small compared to large infarcts (p <0.05). (From Geltman, E. M., et al.: The influence of location and extent of myocardial infarction on long-term ventricular dysrhythmia and mortality. Circulation *60*:805, 1979, by permission of the American Heart Association, Inc.)

somewhat with time after the initial episode;[49] after recovery from an AMI it is the quantity of remaining myocardium whose viability is threatened because it is perfused by obstructed coronary vessels (p. 340) that becomes critical to the prognosis.

THE DYNAMIC NATURE OF INFARCTION. AMI is a dynamic process that often does not occur instantaneously but sometimes evolves relatively slowly (Fig. 37–7, p. 1271). As has been pointed out (p. 1256), in experimental animals the fate of jeopardized, ischemic tissue may be affected favorably by interventions that restore perfusion, reduce myocardial oxygen requirements, inhibit accumulation or facilitate washout of noxious metabolites, augment the availability of substrate for anaerobic metabolism,[7,8,155,202–204] or blunt the effects of mediators of injury such as calcium (Fig. 36–16, p. 1253),[205,206] metabolites, and constituents of cell membranes.[207,208]

The perfusion of the myocardium associated with AMI appears to be reduced maximally immediately following coronary occlusion. In experimental animals, increases in blood flow to the peripheral portions of the ischemic zones become evident within 24 hours of acute coronary occlusion,[209,210] suggesting that dynamic factors contribute to the early limitation of perfusion; these may include release of catecholamines as a consequence of ischemia of adrenergic neurons, as well as the efflux of potassium from injured myocardial cells.[211] Spasm of coronary vessels has been implicated not only in Prinzmetal's variant angina (p. 1360) but also in association with MI induced by atherosclerosis,[212–215] as well as in patients experiencing postinfarction angina at rest.[216,217]

Relatively prompt, *partial* restoration of reduced blood flow to the ischemic zone may result from spontaneous thrombolysis, from relief of coronary spasm, or from improved systemic hemodynamics; the latter includes augmented coronary perfusion pressure and reduced left ventricular end-diastolic pressure. Subsequently, perfusion may be enhanced by the development of collateral circulation.[218] The prompt implementation of measures designed to protect ischemic myocardium and support myocardial perfusion may provide sufficient time for the development of anatomical and physiological compensatory mechanisms that limit the ultimate extent of infarction.

AMI in hospitalized patients may be complicated by extension of infarction or early reinfarction (p. 1292). Depending on the criteria utilized for detection, the incidence of these complications ranges from 8 to 30 per cent.[219–221] It is possible that interventions designed to protect ischemic myocardium during the initial event may also reduce the incidence of extension of infarction or early reinfarction. On the other hand, it has been suggested that preservation of ischemic myocardium could lead to persistent survival of cells in regions subjected to repetitive episodes of severe ischemia, leading to the development of arrhythmias. The relatively poor late prognosis of patients with subendocardial infarction[222,223] and the very high risk of sudden death among patients with serious coronary artery disease but without MI who are successfully resuscitated from ventricular fibrillation[13] (Chap. 23) are consistent with this possibility. However, despite these hazards, there is no evidence that the implementation of interventions designed to protect ischemic myocardium results in any late deleterious effects. Furthermore, it has been reported that preservation of ischemic myocardium by trimethaphan in hypertensive patients with evolving infarction,[125] by intravenous nitroglycerin in normotensive patients,[132] and by the early administration of beta-adrenergic blocking agents[224–226] is actually associated with a reduced rather than an increased mortality.

Proof of the clinical efficacy of specific interventions has been difficult to acquire, in part because of the wide variations in the size of infarcts and their rate of evolution, in part because of the difficulties involved in measuring infarct size, and in part because it is difficult to predict what the size of any given infarction would have been had the intervention under study not been administered. In addition, since many patients usually reach the hospital five hours or even later after the onset of ischemia, it may be too late in these patients to salvage substantial quantities of ischemic myocardium in the first place. In addition, from a statistical point of view, detection of a 15 per cent difference in an estimate of infarct size would require anal-

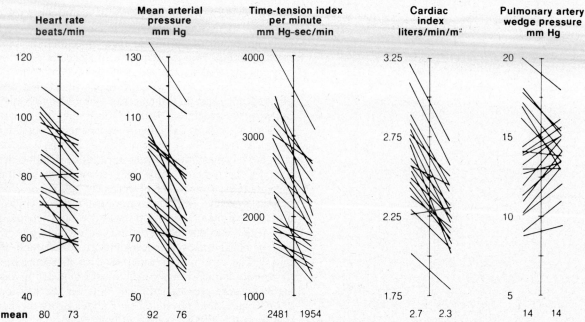

FIGURE 38–9   Hemodynamic effects of propranolol in patients with acute myocardial infarction. Control values are shown to the left of each scale and results after propranolol to the right. Heart rate, mean arterial pressure, and time-tension index are uniformly decreased after propranolol, and cardiac index is decreased in all but one patient. The response of pulmonary artery wedge pressure, however, is variable; in 6 patients with pressures above 15 mm Hg before treatment, propranolol produced a substantial reduction, whereas in the remaining patients, pressure was slightly increased. (From Mueller, H. S., et al.: How, when and why to use propranolol in acute MI. Cardiovasc. Med. *2*:321, 1977.)

ysis of the results in as many as 3000 patients initially entering a prospective study of the effects of treatment according to a rigorous protocol. With mortality as an endpoint, detection of a significant difference attributable to an intervention would require study of an even larger number of patients. Despite the difficulties in the unequivocal demonstration of efficacy of interventions designed to limit infarct size, we believe that therapeutic nihilism is not justified. By analogy, the well-documented high mortality in essential hypertension and the potential benefits of antihypertensive drugs led to their extensive and effective utilization long before improved survival with treatment was demonstrated unequivocally.

BETA-ADRENERGIC BLOCKADE. Beta blockers decrease cardiac index, stroke index, heart rate, blood pressure, and tension-time index (Fig. 38–9). The net effect of these drugs is a reduction in myocardial oxygen consumption per minute and per beat, in the setting of increased concentrations of circulating catecholamines and sympathetic nerve stimulation associated with AMI.[226] Favorable effects of beta-adrenergic blockade on the balance of myocardial oxygen supply and demand are reflected in the reduction of myocardial lactate production[227–229] and the diminution of ventricular arrhythmias.[230] Since beta-adrenergic blockade diminishes circulating levels of free fatty acids by antagonizing the lipolytic effects of catecholamines, and since elevated levels of fatty acids augment myocardial oxygen consumption and probably increase the incidence of arrhythmias, these metabolic actions of beta-blocking agents may be beneficial to the ischemic heart.[228,229]

Objective evidence of beneficial effects of beta-blockers in acute myocardial ischemia in patients has been reported by several investi-

gators using various modifications of the precordial ST-segment mapping technique (Fig. 38–10).[231–234] Gold et al.[231] found that the likelihood of a beneficial clinical and electrocardiographic response increased in the presence of residual antegrade or collateral blood flow to the infarct zone, as determined by coronary arteriography. Waagstein and Hjalmarson[235] demonstrated, in a double-blind controlled study, that each of three cardioselective beta blockers decreased ST-segment elevations in transmural infarction and reduced ischemic chest pain in patients with transmural and nontransmural infarction; no diminution of ST-segment elevation occurred with the administration of saline or an analgesic. In addition, intravenous pindolol, a beta blocker with some intrinsic sympathomimetic activity, has been shown to reduce ST-segment elevation, relieve ischemic pain, and improve regional wall motion in patients with transmural AMI.[236]

However, just as is the case in the experimental situations (p. 1256), not all clinical trials of beta blockers in AMI have reported salutary effects. Thus, practolol (oral or intravenous followed by oral) begun early during the course of AMI did not result in major differences in the clinical course, although there was a lower mortality in the subgroup of practolol-treated patients who had tachycardia at the time of entry into the study.[237]

Studies of the effect of beta blockade on indexes of infarct size in patients are limited. Peter et al.[238] reported the results of a randomized trial of propranolol (0.1 mg/kg intravenously, followed by 320 mg orally over the next 27 hours). The patients treated *within four hours of onset of symptoms* of uncomplicated MI had significantly lower peak serum creatine kinase levels and less cumulative creatine kinase release into plasma than did patients without specific therapy (Figure 38–11). The same group[239] also found that patients with suspected MI, treated with propranolol within four hours of the onset of symptoms, had a significantly lower incidence of infarction, as indicated by electrocardiographic changes and serum creatine kinase elevation, suggesting that threatened infarction might actually be prevented by early beta blockade. Similarly, Yusuf et al. have reported that intravenous atenolol, given a median of four hours following symptoms of AMI, decreased the incidence of AMI, MB creatine kinase release, electrocardiographic evolution of infarction,[240] and the severity of ischemic pain.[241] Two randomized double-blind controlled studies with beta blockade carried out in the acute phase of infarction have indicat-

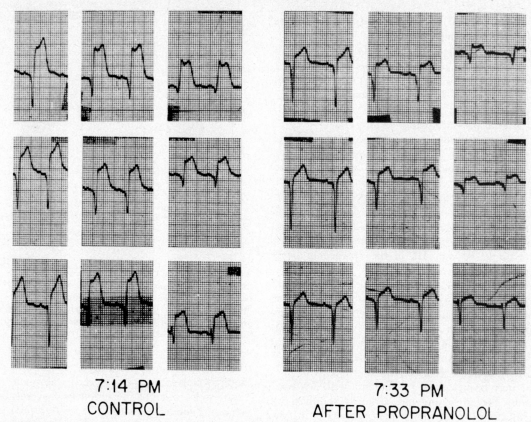

7:14 PM
CONTROL

7:33 PM
AFTER PROPRANOLOL

FIGURE 38–10 The effect of propranolol in the reduction of ST-segment elevation in a patient with acute myocardial infarction. The nine leads, depicted from the V_1, V_3, and V_5 positions, and the corresponding sites are one intercostal space above and below the standard positions. Note the marked reduction in ST-segment elevations after propranolol administration. (From Gold, H. K., et al.: Propranolol-induced reduction of signs of ischemic injury during acute myocardial infarction. Am. J. Cardiol. *38*:689, 1976.)

cated that such therapy can limit enzymatically estimated infarct size. One involved alprenolol[242] and the other the cardioselective beta-blocker metoprolol.[242a] In both of these investigations, beta-blocker therapy was initiated early in the course of infarction and was then maintained.

Although the precise indications for beta blockade in AMI are controversial, on the basis of available information, patients with the hyperdynamic state (sinus tachycardia, hypertension, no evidence of heart failure) as well as patients seen in the first four hours who will not be subjected to thrombolytic therapy would appear to be the best candidates; in addition, unless there are contraindications, beta blockade should probably be continued in patients who develop an AMI while receiving one of these agents. In addition, propranolol is indicated in patients in whom infarction is complicated by persistent or recurrent ischemic pain, progressive or repetitive serum enzyme elevations suggestive of infarct extension, or tachyarrhythmias refractory to lidocaine and procainamide early after the onset of infarction. On the other hand, it is unlikely that beta blockade (or any intervention) can reduce infarct size significantly if it is applied much later than six hours after the onset of the event, because by this time, the ultimate size of the infarct has been established in many patients.

In patients who have not received beta blockers in the preceding 24 hours, propranolol may be administered in initial amounts of 0.1 mg/kg intravenously, divided into three equal doses given at 5-minute intervals. During this

period, heart rate and arterial pressure should be determined, either through an indwelling arterial catheter or by the cuff method, and an electrocardiographic strip should be recorded after each injection. Intravenous propranolol

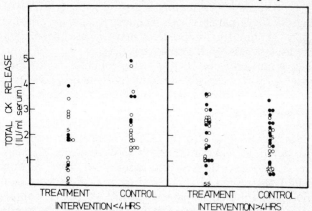

FIGURE 38–11 Effect of propranolol on total CK release after infarction as a function of the time of onset of myocardial infarction. Total calculated CK appearance in treated and control patients entering the trial, less than 4 hours (*left*) or more than 4 hours (*right*) after the onset of infarction. Solid circles indicate patients with anterior infarction and open circles indicate those with inferior infarction. Total CK appearance was 30 per cent less ($p < 0.025$) in patients treated within 4 hours of the onset than in control patients. No significant improvement occurred in patients treated more than 4 hours after the onset. (From Peter, T., et al.: Reduction of enzyme levels by propranolol after acute myocardial infarction. Circulation *57*:1091, 1978, by permission of the American Heart Association, Inc.)

should *not* be administered or its administration should be halted if any of the following events occur:

1. Second- or third-degree AV block or lengthening of the P-R interval beyond 0.24 sec.

2. Rales extending more than one third of the way up the lung fields, or wheezes detected on auscultation.

3. Ventricular rate below 50 per minute.

4. Systolic arterial pressure below 95 mm Hg.

5. Pulmonary artery wedge pressure above 24 mm Hg. (While it is useful, it is by no means necessary to monitor this pressure in patients in whom a beta blocker will be administered.)

The intravenous administration of propranolol is followed one hour later by oral propranolol given in a dose, generally 20 to 80 mg every six hours, adjusted to keep the heart rate between 50 and 65 beats/min and the systolic pressure above 95 mm Hg in the absence of heart failure, wheezing, or advanced AV block.

With the availability of cardioselective beta-adrenergic blocking agents such as alprenolol and metoprolol, and the favorable effects of alprenolol,[243] timolol,[83] metoprolol,[225] and propranolol[84] in double-blind, prospective, *secondary prevention* trials, it appears likely that the beneficial effects of all of these agents are attributable to their beta-1 receptor blocking actions. Some of the alternatives to propranolol that may be beneficial for patients with AMI include alprenolol (40 to 50 mg intravenously followed by 100 to 200 mg orally twice daily), metoprolol (15 mg intravenously followed by 100 mg orally twice daily), and timolol (10 mg orally twice daily). As experience with other available beta-blocking agents such atenolol, nadolol, and pindolol increases, their use in the setting of AMI will undoubtedly be evaluated and clarified as well.

Although antagonism of sympathetic stimulation to the heart might be expected to exacerbate pulmonary edema in patients with occult heart failure, only directionally inconsistent and small changes in pulmonary capillary wedge pressure occur when the drug is used in patients with AMI (Fig. 38–9); in patients with pulmonary capillary pressures below 25 mm Hg, propranolol may elevate the pressure but usually not to excess of this level.[227,228] In an equal number of patients, the elevated pulmonary capillary wedge pressure actually declines, presumably because of the lessening of ischemia and the resultant increase in ventricular compliance and improvement of ventricular performance.

NITRATES (see also p. 1256). Intravenous nitroglycerin has been reported to affect measurements of infarct size in patients. Derrida and associates[243] have reported preliminary results of a randomized trial of prolonged nitroglycerin infusion in patients with AMI. ECG mapping showed a greater reduction in ST-segment elevations after the start of nitroglycerin therapy and less R-wave fall at initially ischemic sites in the nitroglycerin-treated group. Furthermore, in patients with heart failure, mortality and serious ventricular arrhythmias appeared to be reduced in the nitroglycerin-treated group. Bussmann and associates[244] have also reported on a prospective, randomized trial of intravenous nitroglycerin in patients with AMI. Findings included significantly lower values of peak serum CK, lower rates of CK release, and smaller calculated infarct sizes in nitroglycerin-treated patients (Fig. 38–12). Becker and colleagues[245,246] have shown in a prospective, randomized

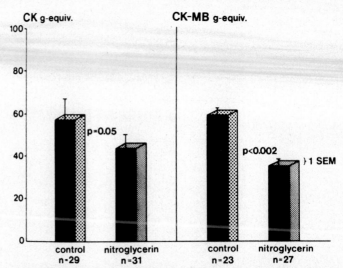

FIGURE 38–12 CK and CK-MB infarct size were significantly reduced in nitroglycerin-treated patients (n = 31) compared with untreated controls (n = 29). (Reproduced with permission from Bussmann, W. D., Passek, D., Seidel, W., and Kaltenbach, M.: Reduction of CK and CK-MB indexes of infarct size by intravenous nitroglycerin. Circulation *63*:615, 1981.)

trial that treatment with intravenous nitroglycerin for 48 hours followed by nitroglycerin ointment therapy for 72 hours enhanced postinfarction improvement of myocardial perfusion measured with ^{201}Tl scintigraphy; there is preliminary evidence from the same trial that nitroglycerin reduces the frequency of infarct extension and late ventricular arrhythmias.[247] Kim and Williams have reported that large and frequent doses of nitroglycerin used in the first four hours after the onset of the infarct limited the electrocardiographic signs of myocardial necrosis,[248] a finding consistent with that of other workers using intravenous nitroglycerin.[245,249,250]

In experimental animals, nitrates elicit small reductions in total coronary vascular resistance with improvement in the ratio of endocardial to epicardial flow in ischemic myocardium. Myocardial lactate production declines, reflecting diminished myocardial dependence on anaerobic metabolism. However, beneficial effects on coronary blood flow are blunted by the systemic hypotension and reflex tachycardia that are sometimes induced. In contrast to agents such as nitroprusside, nitroglycerin does not appear to produce a "coronary steal."[127] In dogs subjected to coronary occlusion, nitroglycerin reduces the incidence of spontaneous ventricular fibrillation, increases the threshold to induced fibrillation, and diminishes ST-segment elevation.[250] When systemic arterial hypotension and reflex tachycardia are prevented by the concomitant administration of methoxamine or phenylephrine, there is a marked reduction of ST-segment elevation accompanied by a reduction in experimental infarct size.[130]

In patients with AMI, the administration of nitroglycerin and other nitrates such as isosorbide dinitrate diminishes pulmonary capillary wedge pressure and systemic arterial pressure as well as left ventricular end-systolic and end-diastolic volumes. It also reduces ventricular asynergy, to the extent that the local impairment of the left ventricular function is due to reversibly injured, depressed myocardium rather than to zones of completed infarction or scar.[252]

As is true in experimental animals, the administration of nitroglycerin to patients with AMI depends on the existing hemodynamics. When systemic arterial and pulmonary capillary wedge pressures are normal or low prior to the administration of nitroglycerin, reflex tachycardia may result from the further reduction of ventricular filling and arterial pressures; nitroglycerin is probably contraindicated under these circumstances, although the administration of an alpha-adrenergic agonist such as methoxamine (5 mg intravenously or 10 to 15 mg intramuscularly) to augment systemic arterial resistance may be helpful.[130]

Intravenous nitroglycerin can be administered safely to patients with evolving MI as long as the dose is titrated carefully to avoid induction of reflex tachycardia or systemic arterial hypotension (systolic blood pressure $\leq$ 95 mm Hg).[254,255] One useful regimen employs an initial infusion rate of 10 μg/min with stepwise increases of 10 μg/min. Alternatively, it may be administered sublingually at doses of 0.3 to 0.6 mg. This route may be more hazardous, since the rate of absorption is difficult to control and arterial pressure may decline precipitously. Nitroglycerin is often useful for the relief of persistent pain and as a vasodilator in patients with infarction associated with left ventricular failure.

OTHER POTENTIALLY USEFUL APPROACHES TO PROTECTION OF ISCHEMIC MYOCARDIUM

The experimental observations indicating the potential usefulness of the agents described below are summarized on pp. 1255 to 1257.

Hyaluronidase. In several small prospective randomized trials, hyaluronidase diminished development of Q waves or loss of R waves in electrocardiographic sites initially exhibiting ST-segment elevation,[256-258] suggesting that ischemic myocardium was protected and that the evolution of infarction in jeopardized zones was limited. In other studies, it was associated with a small reduction in mortality.[259] It is ordinarily administered intravenously in doses of 500 NF units per kg every 6 hours for 48 hours. An advantage of this agent is the absence of any detectable hemodynamic action and the lack of adverse effects except for rare allergic reactions. It is undergoing further clinical trials.

Glucose-Insulin-Potassium. Administration of a solution of glucose-insulin-potassium (300 gm of glucose, 50 units of insulin, and 80 mEq of KCl in 1000 ml of H_2O administered at a rate of 1.5 ml/kg/hr) lowers the concentration of plasma free fatty acids and improves ventricular performance, as reflected in systolic arterial pressure, cardiac output, and stroke work at any level of left ventricular filling pressure (Fig. 14-3, p. 470)[260,261]; also the frequency of ventricular premature beats decreases.[262,263] In a nonrandomized study, mortality appeared to be reduced,[264,265] hemodynamics improved, global ejection fraction increased, and asynergy in the ischemic zone and pulmonary artery diastolic pressure reduced.[266,266a] However, no definitive effect on enzymatically estimated infarct size or long-term mortality has been described in a prospective, controlled, randomized trial.

Corticosteroids. Administration of a single large dose of methylprednisolone has been reported to decrease infarct size, estimated enzymatically.[267] However, the control and treated groups were not strictly comparable with respect to the apparent extent of infarction prior to the administration of the drug. In contrast to these favorable effects, in another study infarct size estimated enzymatically appeared to be *increased* by multiple doses of methylprednisolone.[268] Administration of the drug has led to persistent elevation of plasma MB-CK and the suspicion of an excessively high incidence of ventricular rupture, as well as an increase in mortality, perhaps because administration of corticosteroids inhibits healing of the infarct.[269-271] Accordingly, administration of multiple high doses of corticosteroids beginning several hours after the onset of ischemic injury appears to be deleterious rather than beneficial. However, on the basis of recent experimental work, it is possible that a single large dose of a glucocorticosteroid may reduce infarct size without interfering with myocardial healing.[272]

Intraaortic Balloon Counterpulsation. From a theoretical standpoint, intra aortic or external[273] balloon counterpulsation might be expected to limit infarct size for several reasons. In experimental animals, intra aortic balloon counterpulsation decreases afterload and myocardial oxygen consumption,[274] decreases preload, increases coronary blood flow, and improves cardiac performance.[173] When intra-aortic balloon counterpulsation is carried out in experimental animals immediately after coronary occlusion, ischemic myocardium appears to be protected, based on analysis of ST-segment elevations, myocardial CK depletion, and histological and histochemical criteria of necrosis.[275-277] No definitive information is available indicating that intra-aortic balloon counterpulsation alters the prognosis in patients with relatively uncomplicated infarction. Leinbach et al., however, have reported an immediate, persistent fall in ST-segment elevation. This occurred in patients with anterior MI who had preservation of precordial R waves and good ventricular function,[278] in whom the left anterior descending coronary artery was not totally occluded and who underwent intra-aortic balloon pumping within six hours.

REPERFUSION

When carried out within the first several hours after coronary occlusion, reperfusion improves hemodynamics and decreases infarct size, as assessed by epicardial ST-segment recordings, precordial QRS maps, myocardial CK depletion, positron emission tomography and morphology, in several species of experimental animals;[279-287] the extent of protection appears to be directly related to the rapidity with which reperfusion is implemented after the onset of coronary occlusion.[288] Potentially deleterious effects that may accompany reperfusion in experimental animals include myocardial hemorrhage[280,289] and ventricular fibrillation,[280-282] complications that may be particularly prominent when sufficient time (i.e., more than four or five hours) has elapsed after coronary occlusion such that microvascular integrity has become compromised.[282,284] Fortunately, it appears that hemorrhage occurs into tissue that is either already necrotic or destined to become so; therefore, reperfusion does not appear to *extend* infarction.[286]

SURGICAL REPERFUSION. Recent modifications of surgical technique and extensive improvements in intraoperative myocardial preservation with cardioplegia and hypothermia have allowed surgical reperfusion to be carried out at a very low mortality—approximately 2 per cent, in selected centers. This has kindled enthusiasm for emergency coronary revascularization as a possible therapy to protect jeopardized myocardium in patients undergoing AMI.[290-294] As appears to be the case for all methods designed to limit infarct size, this therapy can be successful only if it is applied within the first four or five hours of the onset of the acute event. It is logistically very difficult in the usual patient who develops an AMI outside of the hospital, to bring the patient to the hospital, carry out a clinical evaluation, outline the coronary anatomy by arteriography, assemble the surgical team, commence operation, and place the patient on cardiopulmonary bypass in less than four hours after the onset of the event. It is therefore unlikely that surgical reperfusion can or will be widely applied on a regular basis in the treatment of AMI. Indeed, operation is *contraindicated* in patients with uncomplicated transmural infarcts more than six hours after the onset of the event.

However, in some patients with AMI, including some with cardiogenic shock, infarction appears to occur in a stuttering fashion over an interval of several days.[295] Theoretically, revascularization carried out more than six hours after the onset of the event might be of benefit in this group, but this has yet to be established. Also, coronary bypass surgery can be carried out promptly in patients who appear to develop infarction in the course of cardiac catheterization, coronary arteriography, and transluminal coronary angioplasty,[296-298] as well as in patients whose coronary anatomy has been recently assessed by coronary arteriography and who develop an infarction in the hospital while awaiting operation. In these selected groups of patients, coronary artery bypass surgery is likely to be effective in limiting myocardial infarct size, since it can be carried out before irreversible myocardial damage has occurred. At the same time, bypass of non–infarct-related coronary obstructions can be expected to exert additional benefit. It must be appreciated, however, that definitive diagnostic criteria, such as elevations of plasma enzyme activity indicative of infarction, do not evolve instantaneously, and the decision to intervene surgically must often be implemented on the basis of clinical suspicion and at a time when the diagnosis of infarction cannot be established with certainty. These circumstances make objective evaluation of this form of therapy difficult.

INTRACORONARY THROMBOLYSIS.   The appreciation that coronary thrombosis is often responsible for the initiation and/or the perpetuation of infarction (p. 1265) and the discovery that intracoronary administration of thrombolytic agents restores angiographic patency to coronary vessels in a majority of cases[300,301] have sparked interest in the potential value of clot lysis in salvaging jeopardized tissue and limiting the extent of injury sustained in patients evolving MI.

On the basis of experience gathered in several laboratories,[302–306] it now appears that:

1. Coronary arteriography can be carried out safely by a skilled and experienced team in patients presenting within the first four hours of what appears, on clinical grounds, to be an AMI with electrocardiographic evidence of early infarction, i.e., ST-segment elevation and early changes in the QRS complex.

2. A total occlusion that appears on coronary arteriography to be produced by a thrombus will be found in the infarct-related artery in approximately 95 per cent of such patients.

3. The direct intracoronary injection of nitroglycerin will relieve the obstruction in only a very small minority of such patients, i.e., less than 5 per cent.

4. Intracoronary infusion of streptokinase, according to the technique outlined on p. 336, will lyse the clot in 70 to 80 per cent of patients; large bolus doses of streptokinase (approximately 1.0 million units) administered intravenously will be successful in lysing clots in approximately 50 per cent (Fig. 38–13).

5. At least a portion of the successfully reperfused myocardium will show evidence of viability, as reflected in the uptake and concentration of Thallium-201 in previously unperfused areas (Fig. 38–14), or restoration of wall motion in previously akinetic segments, in approximately two thirds of patients treated within four hours.[306a,306b]

6. When carried out by experienced groups, the procedure is associated with a small risk of serious bleeding; reperfusion ventricular tachyarrhythmias are common[307] but can usually be controlled by lidocaine or DC cardioversion; therefore coronary thrombolysis is associated with a low mortality.

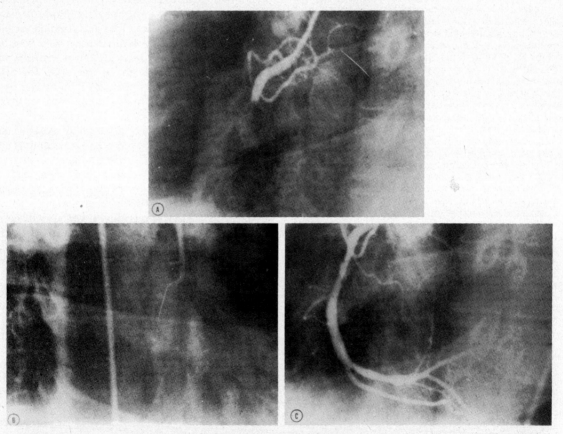

FIGURE 38–13   *A*, Complete occlusion of the right coronary artery in a 38-year-old male patient with evolving inferoposterolateral myocardial infarction. *B*, Infusion catheter advanced to site of occlusion. *C*, The artery was patent after 20 minutes of Thrombolysin infusion at a rate of 4,000 IU/min. The arteriogram was taken after an additional infusion of Thrombolysin, 120,000 IU in 60 minutes, which further improved patency. (Reproduced with permission from Ganz, W., Buchbinder, N., Marcus, H., Mondkar, A., Maddahi, J., Charuzi, Y., O'Connor, L., Shell, W., Fishbein, M. C., Kass, R., Miyamoto, A., and Swan, H. J. C.: Intracoronary thrombolysis in evolving myocardial infarction. Am. Heart J. *101*:4, 1981.)

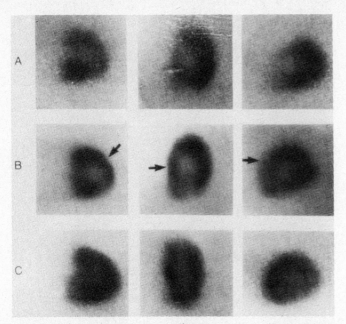

FIGURE 38–14   Intracoronary thallium-201 scintiscans performed in a patient before thrombolysis (*A*), immediately after thrombolysis (*B*), and three months after thrombolysis (*C*). There was a recanalization of the totally obstructed left anterior descending coronary artery. Views, from left to right, are the anterior, modified left anterior oblique, and 70-degree left anterior oblique. Panel *B* shows an increase in perfusion to the anteroseptal region (arrows). In Panel B in the modified left anterior oblique view at seven o'clock, there is an area of improved perfusion, which enhances a persistent filling defect present in the same view in Panel *A* at six o'clock. There is persistence of perfusion of the anteroseptal region at three months after thrombolysis (Panel *C*). (Reproduced with permission from Markis, J. E., Malagold, M., Parker, J. A., Silverman, K. J., Barry, W. H., Als, A. V., Paulin, S., Grossman, W., and Braunwald, E.: Myocardial salvage after intracoronary thrombolysis with streptokinase in acute myocardial infarction. N. Engl. J. Med. *305*:777, 1981.)

Despite the promise of this approach, its ultimate utility remains to be proven because of several unresolved issues.[308,308a] These include (1) difficulty in interpreting the significance of accelerated electrocardiographic changes and the appearance of enzymes in plasma; (2) problems in determining the presence of infarction definitively when thrombolysis is initiated early; (3) problems in interpreting an enhanced ejection fraction or wall motion following thrombolysis, which does not always portend myocardial salvage (the role of augmented sympathetic stimulation and of arterial pressure reduction due to the hypotensive effect of streptokinase infusion in improving myocardial wall remain to be established); (4) the potentially deleterious effects of reperfusion injury when lysis is induced late; (5) lack of proof, at this time, that survival is enhanced; and (6) lack of knowing the optimal manner of treatment following successful reperfusion (i.e., coronary artery bypass grafting,[309,309a] percutaneous transluminal angioplasty,[310,310a] or medical therapy with streptokinase or with clot-selective activators of the fibrinolytic system that do not induce a systemic lytic state. Thus, despite its distinct promise as a technique to limit infarct size, coronary thrombolysis remains an investigational modality at the time of this writing. The possibility that large doses of intravenous streptokinase may also lyse intracoronary thrombi is also under intense investigation.[310b]

IMPLICATIONS OF THE CONCEPT OF INFARCT SIZE LIMITATION FOR ROUTINE MANAGEMENT OF AMI

The recognition that the ultimate size of an MI does not depend solely on the pathological anatomy of the coronary vascular bed, but also on a variety of physiological variables, suggests emphasis on a number of principles in the management of AMI. These principles can and should be applied in routine care despite the fact that the clinical efficacy of the specific interventions described above has not yet been definitively established. First, and of greatest importance, it is mandatory to maintain an optimal balance between myocardial oxygen supply and demand so that as much of the jeopardized zone of the myocardium surrounding the most profoundly ischemic zones of the infarct can be salvaged. Myocardial oxygen consumption is minimized by maintaining the patient at rest, physically and emotionally, and by utilizing mild sedation and a quiet atmosphere that may lower heart rate, a major determinant of myocardial oxygen consumption. If the patient was receiving a beta-adrenergic blocking agent at the time the clinical manifestations of the infarct commenced, the drug should not be discontinued unless a specific contraindication develops, such as left ventricular failure or a bradyarrhythmia. Marked sinus bradycardia (heart rate less than approximately 50 beats/min) and the frequently coexisting hypotension should be treated with postural maneuvers (the reverse Trendelenburg position) to increase central blood volume and atropine or electrical pacing, but not with isoproterenol. On the other hand, the *routine* administration of atropine, with the resultant increase in heart rate, to patients without serious bradycardia is contraindicated. All forms of tachyarrhythmias require prompt and direct treatment, since they increase myocardial oxygen needs.

Diuretics are the first line of drugs indicated in the treatment of heart failure. If insufficient, vasodilators should be added,[255] unless the patient is already hypotensive. Inotropic agents such as the digitalis glycosides and cardioactive sympathomimetics should be added only if there is evidence of persistent ventricular failure despite diuretics and vasodilators; these agents should not be given prophylactically. Of the various sympathomimetic amines available, isoproterenol with its chronotropic and vasodilator effects is the most hazardous. Dobutamine, or small doses of dopamine, which has less effect on heart rate and systemic vascular resistance than do norepinephrine, epinephrine or isoproterenol is the drug of choice when cardiac contractility *must* be augmented.

Particular attention must be paid to preserving arterial oxygenation in patients with hypoxemia, such as occurs in patients with chronic pulmonary disease, pneumonia, or left ventricular failure. Oxygen-enriched air should be administered to patients with hypoxemia, and bronchodilators and expectorants should be used when indicated. Severe anemia, which can also extend the area of ischemic injury, should be corrected by the cautious administration of packed red cells, accompanied by a diuretic if there is any evidence of left ventricular failure. Associated conditions, particularly infections and the accompanying tachycardia, fever, and elevated myocardial oxygen needs, require immediate attention.

Systolic arterial pressure should not be allowed to deviate by more than approximately 25 to 30 mm Hg from the patient's usual level. In regard to the effect of changes in arterial pressure on myocardial injury, it is likely that each patient has an optimum level of arterial pressure. As coronary perfusion pressure deviates from this level, the unfavorable balance between oxygen supply (which is related to coronary perfusion pressure) and myocardial oxygen demand (which is related to ventricular wall tension) that ensues will increase the extent of ischemic injury.

Rather than simply maintaining the patient's vital signs, the physician's attention should be directed toward preserving the myocardium as well as maintaining perfusion of peripheral organs. However, these two objectives may sometimes conflict. In the first four to six hours following the onset of the clinical event, when the ultimate size of the infarct has not yet been established, myocardial preservation should ordinarily be given the highest priority. This may mean foregoing the stimulation of cardiac contractility by inotropic agents. Later, once the size of the infarct is fixed and if heart failure supervenes, it may be appropriate to stimulate the heart with positive inotropic agents, i.e., to employ an intervention that might have increased infarct size if given at an earlier time.

In some patients, particularly those with cardiogenic shock, tissue damage occurs in a "stuttering" manner with persistent release of CK into the blood stream (Fig. 38–15) rather than abruptly, a condition that might more properly be termed *subacute infarction*.[49,192] This concept of the dynamic nature of the infarct process as well as the observa-

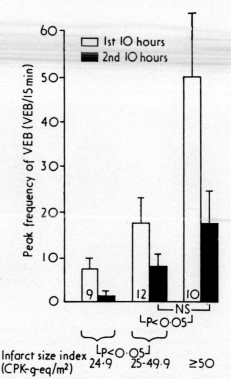

FIGURE 38–16 Dependence of ventricular ectopic activity, expressed as ventricular ectopic beats (VEB's), during the first 20 hours after admission in patients with acute myocardial infarction. Patients were divided into three groups according to infarct size index, expressed in terms of CPK-gram-equivalents/m². VEB frequency was greater in patients with larger infarcts during the first 10 hours after admission, as shown by the clear bars. A similar trend was evident during the second 10 hours after admission, as shown by the solid bars, although the overall frequency of VEB's was less during this interval compared with the first 10 hours after admission. Results expressed are means ±SE. (From Roberts, R., et al.: Relation between infarct size and ventricular arrhythmia. Br. Heart J. *37*:1169, 1975.)

tion that the incidence of ventricular ectopic activity in both the early (Fig. 38–16) and late (Table 38–2) post-infarct periods greatly expands the horizon for what can *potentially* be accomplished by techniques to limit myocardial necrosis.

However, it must be acknowledged that *definitive* proof that substantial quantities of tissue can be salvaged and that prognosis can thereby be improved is not yet available, despite (1) the inherent logic in attempting to reduce infarct size; (2) the availability of a wide variety of interventions that are effective in experimental animals; (3) the ability to apply these techniques with reasonable safety in patients; and (4) the results of an increasing number of trials in patients with encouraging results.

CONVALESCENCE

The time of discharge from the hospital is variable. It may be as early as one week after admission for patients who experience no complications, who can be followed readily at home, and for whom the family setting is conducive to convalescence.[311,312] Most complications that would preclude early discharge occur within the first day or two of admission and therefore, patients suitable for early dis-

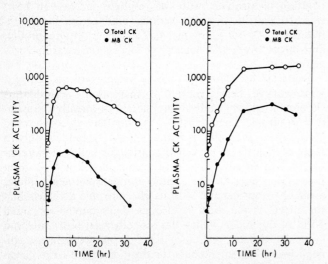

FIGURE 38–15 Plasma CK time-activity curves in a patient with uncomplicated acute myocardial infarction (*left*) and one with acute myocardial infarction associated with cardiogenic shock (*right*). As shown on the left, hemodynamically uncomplicated acute myocardial infarction is characterized by a relatively early occurrence of peak total and MB-CK activity, with a gradual subsequent smooth decline. On the other hand, as shown on the right, myocardial infarction associated with cardiogenic shock is characterized by a more prolonged interval prior to occurrence of peak enzyme activity in blood, indicative of persistent release of enzyme reflecting progressive damage of myocardium. Total CK activity may remain elevated in patients with myocardial infarction because of extracardiac release of enzyme, but the sustained elevation of MB-CK activity accompanying cardiogenic shock, as evident in the example shown on the right, is attributable to continuing cardiac damage. (From Gutovitz, A. L., et al.: The progressive nature of myocardial injury in selected patients with cardiogenic shock. Am. J. Cardiol. *41*:469, 1978.)

TABLE 38–2   RELATION BETWEEN VENTRICULAR ECTOPIC ACTIVITY AND INFARCT SIZE LATE AFTER INFARCTION

LOCATION OF INFARCTION	IN PVC's/24 HR	
Transmural		
All patients	4.17(66)	
ISI < 15	2.93(20)	
ISI ≥ 15	4.71(46)	(P < 0.005)
Inferior (Transmural)		
All patients	4.52(40)	
ISI < 15	3.81(14)	
ISI ≥ 15	4.90(26)	(P = N.S.)
Anterior (Transmural)		
All patients	3.64(26)	
ISI < 15	0.88(6)	
ISI ≥ 15	4.47(20)	(P < 0.001)
Subendocardial		
All patients	3.64(15)	
ISI < 15	2.48(11)	
ISI ≥ 15	6.81(4)	(P < 0.02)

The significance of relationships between infarct location, infarct size index (ISI) expressed as CK-gram-equivalents, and the frequency of premature ventricular complexes (PVC's). Numbers in parentheses indicate the number of patients sustaining an initial infarction occurring at the locus specified, with follow-up obtained from 3 to 38 months after infarction. Results are expressed as the natural logarithm (ln) of PVC frequency because the statistical distribution of PVC's is not normal but the distribution of ln PVC's is. (Reproduced with permission from Geltman, E. M., et al.: The influence of location and extent of myocardial infarction on long-term ventricular dysrhythmia and mortality. Circulation 60:805, 1979, by permission of the American Heart Association, Inc.)

charge can be identified very early during the hospitalization.[312] Ordinarily, discharge of patients without complications is deferred until 10 to 12 days following infarction, at a time when the patient has become fully ambulatory. For patients who have experienced a complication, discharge is deferred until their condition has been stable for several days and it is clear that they are responding appropriately to necessary medications such as antiarrhythmic agents, vasodilators, or positive inotropic agents.

Before discharge from the hospital, the patient should receive detailed instruction concerning physical activity. Initially, this should consist of being ambulatory at home but avoiding isometric activity such as lifting; several rest periods should be taken daily. In addition, the patient should be given fresh nitroglycerin tablets and instructed in their use. As convalescence progresses, graded resumption of activity should be encouraged. Many approaches have been utilized, ranging from formal rigid guidelines to general advice advocating moderation and avoidance of any activity that evokes symptoms. There is some evidence that behavior alteration is possible after recovery from MI and that this may improve prognosis.[313,313a] The physical and psychological rehabilitation of patients convalescing from AMI are discussed in Chapters 40 and 57.

The concept of *secondary prevention* of reinfarction and death after recovery from an AMI has been actively investigated during the past two decades. Until quite recently, however, nearly all efforts at demonstrating secondary prevention had failed. Thus, studies of antiplatelet agents (aspirin, sulfinpyrazone[314]), lipid-lowering drugs, antiarrhythmic agents, anticoagulants, and even beta blockers had not provided undisputed proof of improvement of long-term survival following myocardial infarction. However, large trials with three beta blockers—timolol,[83] propranolol,[84] and metoprolol[225]—have demonstrated that these drugs do improve survival in a wide spectrum of

postinfarction patients and also reduce the incidence of sudden death and reinfarction.

While the exact mechanism of this beneficial effect is unknown, it appears to be due to a "class" effect, i.e., it is secondary to beta blockade, since neither cardioselectivity, intrinsic sympathomimetic activity, or membrane stabilizing activity appear to be requisite. The reduction in mortality is seen in all age groups, for all types of infarction, and in all risk groups. Therefore, based on currently available evidence, patients without contraindication to beta blockade (asthma, congestive heart failure, bradyarrhythmias) should have prophylactic treatment with beta blockers initiated between one and four weeks after AMI. The dosage should be sufficient to blunt the heart rate response to exercise, and therapy should be continued for at least two years. The effectiveness of secondary prevention with other agents, including calcium-channel blockers, antiplatelet agents, anticoagulants, lipid lowering drugs, antiarrhythmics, prostacyclin analogs, and thromboxane synthetase inhibitors, requires further investigation.

In addition to exercise testing in the early convalescent phase (p. 1386), in many centers cardiac catheterization and angiography are being carried out more or less routinely in most survivors of AMI, regardless of whether or not they are symptomatic. Similar anatomical findings have been observed independent of the patient's postinfarction course; approximately one third of patients each have serious obstruction in one, two, and three vessels, while 10 per cent have left main coronary artery disease.[315] Two thirds of the patients have residual viable myocardium that is seriously jeopardized because it is perfused by critically narrowed vessels.[316] These provocative findings have raised the question of whether or not it is advisable to carry out coronary arteriography routinely in survivors of AMI in order to detect patients who might benefit from coronary artery bypass grafting. Insufficient information is available to take a firm position on this question,[317] but since it is possible to identify high-risk patients from their clinical course, combined with noninvasive exercise testing, including myocardial perfusion scintigraphy[318–320] (p. 374) as well as ambulatory electrocardiography,[320a,320b] it seems reasonable at this time to limit these invasive studies to such high-risk patients, as well as to those who have significant postinfarct angina, despite a good medical regimen, including a calcium-channel blocker.[321]

References

1. Hillis, L. D., and Braunwald, E.: Myocardial ischemia. N. Engl. J. Med. *296*: 971, 1034, 1093, 1977.
2. Norris, R. M.: Myocardial Infarction. Edinburgh, Churchill Livingstone, 1982.
3. Gillespie, T. A., and Sobel, B. E.: A rationale for therapy of acute myocardial infarction: Limitation of infarct size. Adv. Intern. Med. *22*:319, 1976.
4. Karliner, J. S., and Gregoratos, G.: Coronary Care. Edinburgh, Churchill Livingstone, 1981.
5. Bloor, C. M., Ehsani, A., White, F. C., and Sobel, B. E.: Ventricular fibrillation threshold in acute myocardial infarction and its relation to myocardial infarct size. Cardiovasc. Res. *9*:468, 1975.
6. Spann, J. F.: Changing concepts of pathophysiology, prognosis, and therapy in acute myocardial infarction. Am. J. Med. *74*:877, 1983.
7. Rude, R. E., Muller, J. E., and Braunwald, E.: Efforts to limit the size of myocardial infarcts. Ann. Intern. Med. *95*:736, 1981.
8. Lange, L. G., and Sobel, B. E.: Pharmacological salvage of myocardium. Ann. Rev. Pharmacol. Toxicol. *22*:115, 1982.
9. Pantridge, J. F., Webb, S. W., Adgey, A. A. J., and Geddes, J. S.: The first hour after the onset of acute myocardial infarction. *In* Yu, P. N., and

Goodwin, J. F. (eds.): Progress in Cardiology.Philadelphia, Lea and Febiger, 1974, p. 173.

10. Bigger, J. T., Jr., Dresdale, R. J., and Heissenbuttel, R. H., Weld, F. M., and Wit, A. L.: Ventricular arrhythmias in ischemic heart disease: Mechanism, prevalence, significance, and management. Prog. Cardiovasc. Dis. *19*:255, 1977.

11. Pantridge, J. R., and Geddes, J. S.: Diseases of the cardiovascular system. Management of acute myocardial infarction. Br. Med. J. *2*:168, 1976.

12. Adgey, A. A. J., Clements, I. P., Mulholland, H. C., Wilson, C., and Webb, S. W.: Acute phase of myocardial infarction. Prehospital management of the coronary patient. Minnesota Med. *59*:347, 1976.

13. Cobb, L. A., Baum, R. S., Alvarez, H., III, and Schaffer, W. A.: Resuscitation from out-of-hospital ventricular fibrillation: 4 years' follow-up. Circulation *51-52* (Suppl. III):223, 1975.

14. Lewis, R. P., Lanese, R. R., Stang, J. M., Chirikos, T. N., Keller, M. D., and Warren, J. V.: Reduction of mortality from prehospital myocardial infarction by prudent patient activation of mobile coronary care system. Am. Heart J. *103*:123, 1982.

15. Crampton, R. S., Aldrich, F. R., Gascho, J. A., Miles, J. R., Jr., and Stillerman, R.: Reduction of prehospital, ambulance and community coronary death rates by the community-wide emergency cardiac care system. Am. J. Med. *58*:151, 1975.

16. Goldman, L.: Coronary care units: A perspective on their epidemiologic impact. Int. J. Cardiol., *2*:284, 1982.

17. Morris, A. L., Nernberg, V., Roos, N. P., Henteleff, P., and Ross, L., Jr.: Acute myocardial infarction: Survey of urban and rural hospital mortality. Am. Heart J. *105*:44, 1983.

18. Hill, J. D., Hampton, J. R., and Mitchell, J. R. A.: A randomized trial of home-versus-hospital management for patients with suspected myocardial infarction. Lancet *1*:837, 1978.

19. Rowley, J. M., Hill, J. D., Hampton, J. R., and Mitchell, J. R. A.: Early reporting of myocardial infarction: Impact of an experiment in patient education. Br. Med. J. *284*:1741, 1982.

20. Graboys, T. B.: In-hospital sudden death after coronary care unit discharge: A high-risk profile. Arch. Intern. Med. *135*:512, 1975.

21. Wilson, C., and Adgey, A. A. J.: Survival of patients with late ventricular fibrillation after acute myocardial infarction. Lancet *2*:214, 1974.

22. Lie, K. I., Liem, K. L., Schuilenburg, R. M., David, G. K., and Durrer, B.: Early identification of patients developing late in-hospital ventricular fibrillation after discharge from the Coronary Care Unit. Am. J. Cardiol. *41*:674, 1978.

23. Starling, M. R., Crawford, M. H., Kennedy, G. T., and O'Rourke, R. A.: Treadmill exercise tests predischarge and six week post-myocardial infarction to detect abnormalities of known prognostic value. Ann. Intern. Med. *94*:721,1981.

24. McNeer, J. F., Wagner, G. S., Ginsburg, P. B., Wallace, A. G., McCants, C. B., Conley, M. J., and Rosati, R. A.: Hospital discharge one week after acute myocardial infarction. N. Engl. J. Med. *298*:229, 1978.

25. Severance, H. W., Jr., Morris, K. G., and Wagner, G. S.: Criteria for early discharge after acute myocardial infarction. Validation in a community hospital. Arch. Intern. Med. *142*:39, 1982.

26. Zelis, R., Mansour, E. J., Capone, R. J., and Mason, D. T.: The cardiovascular effects of morphine: The peripheral capacitance and resistance vessels in human subjects. J. Clin. Invest. *54*:1247, 1974.

27. Wynne, J., Mann, T., Alpert, J. S., and Grossman, W.: Beneficial effects of nitrous oxide in patients with ischemic heart disease. Circulation *55-56* (Suppl. III):18, 1977 (Abstr.).

28. Thompson, P. L., and Lown, B.: Nitrous oxide as an analgesic in acute myocardial infarction. J.A.M.A. *235*:924, 1976.

29. Fillmore, S. J., Shapiro, M., and Killip, T.: Arterial oxygen tension in acute myocardial infarction. Serial analysis of clinical state and blood gas changes. Am. Heart J. *79*:620, 1970.

30. Maroko, P. R., Radvany, P., Braunwald, E., and Hale, S. L.: Reduction of infarct size by oxygen inhalation following acute coronary occlusion. Circulation *52*:360, 1975.

31. Madias, J. E., and Hood, W. B., Jr.: Reduction of precordial ST-segment elevation in patients with anterior myocardial infarction by oxygen breathing. Circulation *53*(Suppl. I):198, 1976.

32. Singer, M. M., Wright, F., Stanley, L. K., Roe, B. B., and Hamilton, W. K.: Oxygen toxicity in man: A prospective study in patients after open-heart surgery. N. Engl. J. Med. *283*:1473, 1970.

33. Mogelson, S., Davidson, J., Sobel, B. E., and Roberts, R.: The effect of hyperbaric oxygen on infarct size in the conscious animal. Eur. J. Cardiol. *12*:135, 1980.

34. Meijne, N. G.: Hyperbaric Oxygen and Its Clinical Value: With Special Emphasis on Biochemical and Cardiovascular Aspects. Springfield, Ill., Charles C Thomas, 1970.

35. Glogar, D. H., Kloner, R. A., Muller, J., DeBoer, L. W. V., Braunwald, E., and Clark, L. C., Jr.: Fluorocarbons reduce myocardial ischemic damage after coronary occlusion. Science *211*:1439, 1981.

36. Modan, B., Shani, M., Schor, S., and Modan, M.: Reduction of hospital mortality from acute myocardial infarction by anticoagulant therapy. N. Engl. J. Med. *292*:1359, 1975.

37. Wessler, S.: Antithrombotic agents are indicated in the therapy of acute myocardial infarction. Cardiovasc. Clin. *8*:131, 1977.

38. Tonaschia, J., Gordis, L., and Schmerler, H.: Retrospective evidence favoring use of anticoagulants for myocardial infarctions. N. Engl. J. Med. *292*:1362, 1975.

39. Horwitz, R. I., and Feinstein, A. R.: The application of therapeutic trial principles to improve the design of epidemiologic research: A case-control study suggesting that anticoagulants reduce mortality in patients with myocardial infarction. J. Chron. Dis. *34*:575, 1981.

40. Anticoagulants in acute myocardial infarction: Results of a cooperative clinical trial. J.A.M.A. *225*:724, 1973.

41. Wray, R., Maurer, B., and Shillingford, J.: Prophylactic anticoagulant therapy in the prevention of calf-vein thrombosis after myocardial infarction. N. Engl. J. Med. *288*:815, 1973.

42. Rosenberg, R. D.: Actions and interactions of antithrombin and heparin. N. Engl. J. Med. *292*:146, 1975.

43. Hull, R., Delmore, T., Carter, C., Hirsh, J., Genton, E., Gent, M., Turpie, G., and McLaughlin, D.: Adjusted subcutaneous heparin versus warfarin sodium in the long-term treatment of venous thrombosis. N. Engl. J. Med. *306*:189, 1982.

44. Pitt, A., Anderson, S. T., Habersberger, P. G., and Rosengarten, D. S.: Low dose heparin in the prevention of deep vein thromboses in patients with acute myocardial infarction. Am. Heart J. *99*:574, 1980.

45. A double-blind trial to assess long-term oral anticoagulant therapy in elderly patients with myocardial infarction. Report of the sixty-plus reinfarction study research group. Lancet *2*:989, 1980.

46. Corday, E., and Corday, S. R.: Advances in clinical management of acute myocardial infarction in the past 25 years. J. Am. Coll. Cardiol. *1*:126, 1983.

47. Cox, J. R., Jr., Roberts, R., Ambos, H. D., Oliver, G. C., and Sobel, B. E.: Relations between enzymatically estimated myocardial infarct size and early ventricular dysrhythmia. Circulation *53*(Suppl. I):150, 1976.

48. Roberts, R., Husain, A., Ambos, H. D., Oliver, G. C., Cox, J., Jr., and Sobel, B. E.: Relation between infarct size and ventricular arrhythmia. Br. Heart J. *37*:1169, 1975.

49. Geltman, E. M., Ehsani, A. A., Campbell, M. K., Schechtman, K., Roberts, R., and Sobel, B. E.: The influence of location and extent of myocardial infarction on long-term ventricular dysrhythmia and mortality. Circulation *60*:805, 1979.

50. Thorén, P. N.: Activation of left ventricular receptors with nonmedullated vagal afferent fibers during occlusion of a coronary artery in the cat. Am. J. Cardiol. *37*:1046, 1976.

51. Adgey, A. A. J., Geddes, J. S., Mulholland, H. C., Keegan, D. A. J., and Pantridge, J. F.: Incidence, significance, and management of early brady-arrhythmia complicating acute myocardial infarction. Lancet *2*:1097, 1968.

52. Han, J.: Mechanisms of ventricular arrhythmias associated with myocardial infarction. Am. J. Cardiol. *24*:800, 1969.

53. Chadda, K. D., Lichstein, E., Gupta, P. K., and Choy, R.: Bradycardia-hypotension syndrome in acute myocardial infarction: Reappraisal of the overdrive effects of atropin. Am. J. Med. *59*:158, 1975.

54. Warren, J. V., and Lewis, R. P.: Beneficial effects of atropine in the pre-hospital phase of coronary care. Am. J. Cardiol. *37*:68, 1976.

55. Topol, E. J., Goldschlager, N., Ports, T. A., DiCarlo, L. A., Jr., Schiller, N. B., Botvinick, E. H., and Chatterjee, K.: Hemodynamic benefit of atrial pacing in right ventricular myocardial infarction. Ann. Intern. Med. *96*:594, 1982.

56. Norris, R. M., and Mercer, C. J.: Significance of idioventricular rhythms in acute myocardial infarction. Prog. Cardiovasc. Dis. *16*:455, 1974.

57. Haft, J. I.: Clinical implications of atrioventricular and intraventricular conduction abnormalities. II. Acute myocardial infarction. *In* Rios, J. C. (ed.): Clinical-Electrocardiographic Correlations. Philadelphia, F. A. Davis Co., 1977, p. 65.

58. Ritter, W. S., Atkins, J. M., Blomqvist, C. G., and Mullins, C. B.: Permanent pacing in patients with transient trifascicular block during acute myocardial infarction. Am. J. Cardiol. *38*:205, 1976.

59. Ginks, W. R., Sutton, R., Oh, W., and Leatham, A.: Long-term prognosis after acute inferior infarction with atrioventricular block. Br. Heart J. *39*:186, 1977.

60. Waters, D. D., and Mizgala, H. F.: Long-term prognoses of patients with incomplete bundle branch block complicating acute myocardial infarction. Am. J. Cardiol. *34*:1, 1974.

61. Hindman, M. C., Wagner, G. S., JaRo, M., Atkins, J. M., Scheinman, M. M., DeSanctis, R. W., Hutter, A. H., Jr., Yeatman, L., Rubenfire, M., Pujura, C., Rubin, M., and Morris, J. J.: The clinical significance of bundle branch block complicating acute myocardial infarction. I. Clinical characteristics, hospital mortality, and one-year followup. Circulation *58*:679, 1978.

62. Hindman, M. C., Wagner, G. S., JaRo, M., Atkins, J. M., Scheinman, M. M., DeSanctis, R. W., Hutter, A. H., Jr., Yeatman, L., Rubenfire, M., Pujura, C., Rubin, M., and Morris, J. J.: The clinical significance of bundle branch block complicating acute myocardial infarction. 2. Indications for temporary and permanent pacemaker insertion. Circulation *58*:689, 1978.

63. Hindman, M. C., and Wagner, G. S.: Bundle branch block during acute myocardial infarction. Primary Cardiol. *6*:73, 1980.

64. Malliani, A., Schwartz, P. J., and Zanchetti, A.: A sympathetic reflex elicited by experimental coronary occlusion. Am. J. Physiol. *217*:703, 1969.

65. Corr, P. B., and Gillis, R. A.: Autonomic neural influences on the dysrhythmias resulting from myocardial infarction. Circ. Res. *43*:1, 1978.

66. Harris, A. S., Otero, H., and Bocage, A. J.: The induction of arrhythmias by sympathetic activity before and after occlusion of a coronary artery in the canine heart. J. Electrocardiol. *4*:34, 1971.

67. Han, J., and Moe, G. K.: Nonuniform recovery of excitability in ventricular muscle. Circ. Res. *14*:44, 1964.

68. Cranefield, P. F.: The Conduction of the Cardiac Impulse: The Slow Response and Cardiac Arrhythmias. Mount Kisco, N.Y., Futura Publishing Company, 1975.

69. Wit, A. L., Hoffman, B. F., and Rosen, M. R.: Electrophysiology and pharmacology of cardiac arrhythmias. IX. Cardiac electrophysiologic effects of beta adrenergic receptor stimulation and blockade. Part A. Am. Heart J. *90*: 521, 1975.

70. Ebert, P. A., Venderbeek, R. B., Allgood, R. J., and Sabiston, D. C., Jr.: Effect of chronic cardiac denervation on arrhythmias after coronary artery ligation. Cardiovasc. Res. *4*:141, 1970.

71. Peterson, D. F., and Brown, A. M.: Pressor reflexes produced by stimulation of afferent fibers in the cardiac sympathetic nerves of the cat. Circ. Res. *28*: 605, 1971.

72. Berman, J., Haffajee, C. I., and Alpert, J. S.: Therapy of symptomatic pericarditis after myocardial infarction: Retrospective and prospective studies of aspirin, indomethacin, prednisone, and spontaneous resolution. Am. Heart J. *101*: 750, 1981.

73. Krikler, D. M., and Rowland, E.: The role of calcium-ion antagonists in cardiac arrhythmias. *In* Fleckenstein, A., and Roskamm, G. (eds.): Calcium Antagonismus. Berlin, Springer-Verlag, 1980, p. 55.

74. Kerber, R. E., Jensen, S. R., Grayzel, J., Kennedy, J., and Hoyt, R.: Elective cardioversion: Influence of paddle-electrode location and size on success rates and energy requirements. N. Engl. J. Med. *305*:658, 1981.

75. Pantridge, J. F.: Emergency treatment of cardiac arrhythmias in myocardial infarction. *In* Scott, D. B., and Julian, D. G. (eds.): Lidocaine in the Treatment of Ventricular Arrhythmias. Edinburgh, E. & S. Livingstone, 1971, p. 77.

76. Zipes, D. P., and Troup, P. J.: New antiarrhythmic agents: Amiodarone, aprindine, disopyramide, ethmozin, mexiletine, tocainide, verapamil. Am. J. Cardiol. *41*:1005, 1978.

77. Abitbol, H., Califano, J. E., Abate, C., Beilis, P., and Castanellos, H.: Use of flecainide acetate in the treatment of premature ventricular contractions. Am. Heart J. *105*:227, 1983.

78. Dhurandher, R. W., MacMillan, R. L., and Brown, K. W. G.: Primary ventricular fibrillation complicating acute myocardial infarction. Am. J. Cardiol. *27*:347, 1971.

79. Lie, K. I., Wellens, H. J., and Van Capelli, F. J.: Lidocaine in the prevention of primary ventricular fibrillation. A double blind randomized study of 212 consecutive patients. N. Engl. J. Med. *291*:1324, 1974.

80. Routledge, P. A., Stargel, W. W., Barchowsky, A., Wagner, G. S., and Shand, D. G.: Control of lidocaine therapy: New perspectives. Therap. Drug Monitoring *4*:265, 1982.

81. DeSilva, R. E., Hennekens, C. H., Lown, B., and Casscells, S. W.: Lidocaine prophylaxis in acute myocardial infarction: An evaluation of methodology. Lancet *1*:855, 1981.

81a. Mehra, R., Zeiler, R. H., Gough, W. B. and El-Sherif, N.: Reentrant ventricular arrhythmias in the later myocardial infarction period. 9. Electrophysiologic-anatomic correlation of reentrant circuits. Circulation *67*:11, 1983.

82. May, G. S., Furberg, C. D., Eberlein, K. A., and Geraci, B. J.: Secondary prevention after myocardial infarction. A review of short-term acute phase trials. Prog. Cardiovasc. Dis. *25*:335, 1983.

83. The Norwegian Multicenter Study Group: Timolol-induced reduction in mortality and reinfarction in patients surviving acute myocardial infarction. N. Engl. J. Med. *304*:801, 1981.

84. The Beta-Blocker Heart Attack Trial. Beta Blocker Heart Attack Study Group. J.A.M.A. *246*:2073, 1981.

85. Lopez, L. M., Mehta, J. L., Robinson, J. D., and Roberts, R. J.: Optimal lidocaine dosing in patients with myocardial infarction. Therap. Drug. Monitoring *4*:271, 1982.

86. Prescott, L. F., Adjepon-Yamoah, K. K., and Talbot, R. G.: Impaired lignocaine metabolism in patients with myocardial infarction and cardiac failure. Br. Med. J. *1*:939, 1976.

87. LeLorier, J., Grenon, D., Latour, Y., Caille, G., Dumont, G., Brosseau, A., and Solignac, A.: Pharmacokinetics of lidocaine after prolonged intravenous infusions in uncomplicated myocardial infarction. Ann. Intern. Med. *87*:700, 1977.

88. Corr, P. B., and Sobel, B. E.: Mechanisms contributing to dysrhythmias induced by ischemia and their therapeutic implications. Adv. Cardiol. *22*:110, 1978.

89. Chopra, M. P., Portal, R. W., and Aber, C. P.: Lignocaine therapy after acute myocardial infarction. Br. Med. J. *1*:213, 1969.

90. Lown, B., and Vassaux, C.: Lidocaine in acute myocardial infarction. Am. Heart J. *76*:586, 1968.

91. Fehmers, M. C. O., and Dunning, A. J.: Intramuscularly and orally administered lidocaine in the treatment of ventricular arrhythmias in acute myocardial infarction. Am. J. Cardiol. *29*:514, 1972.

92. El-Sherif, N., Scherlag, B. J., Lazzara, R., and Hope, R. R.: Reentrant ventricular arrhythmias in the late myocardial infarction period. 4. Mechanism of action of lidocaine. Circulation *56*:395, 1977.

93. Kluger, J., Drayer, D. E., Reidenberg, M. M., and Lahita, R.: Acetylprocainamide therapy in patients with previous procainamide-induced lupus syndrome. Ann. Intern. Med. *95*:18, 1981.

94. Gillis, R. A., McClellan, J. R., Sauer, T. S., and Standaert, F. G.: Depression of cardiac sympathetic nerve activity by diphenylhydantoin. J. Pharmacol. Exp. Ther. *179*:599, 1971.

95. El-Sherif, N., and Lazzara, R.: Reentrant ventricular arrhythmias in the late myocardial infarction period. 5. Mechanism of action of diphenylhydantoin. Circulation *57*:405, 1978.

96. Lown, B., and Wolf, M.: Approaches to sudden death from coronary heart disease. Circulation *44*:130, 1971.

97. Wald, R. W., Waxman, M. B., Corey, P. N., Gunstensen, J., and Goldman, B. S.: Management of intractable ventricular tachyarrhythmias after myocardial infarction. Am. J. Cardiol. *44*:329, 1979.

98. Guiraudon, G., Fontaine, G., Frank, R., Escande, G., Etievent, P., and Cabrol, C.: Encircling endocardial ventriculotomy: A new surgical treatment for life-threatening ventricular tachycardias resistant to medical treatment following myocardial infarction. Ann. Thorac. Surg. *26*:438, 1978.

99. Josephson, M. E., Harken, A. H., and Horowitz, L. N.: Endocardial excision: A new surgical technique for the treatment of recurrent ventricular tachycardia. Circulation *60*:1430, 1979.

100. Wyman, M. G., and Hammersmith, L.: Comprehensive treatment plan for the prevention of primary ventricular fibrillation in acute myocardial infarction. Am. J. Cardiol. *33*:661, 1974.

101. Lie, K. I., Wellens, H. J., van Capelle, F. J., and Durrer, D.: Lidocaine in the prevention of primary ventricular fibrillation: A double-blind, randomized study of 212 consecutive patients. N. Engl. J. Med. *291*:1324, 1974.

101a. Ryden, L., Ariniego, R., Arnman, K., Herlitz, J., Hjalmarson, A., Holmberg, S., Reyes, C., Smedgard, P., Svedberg, K., Vedin, A., Waagstein, F., Waldenstrom, A., Wilhelmsson, C., Wedel, H., and Yamamoto, M.: A double-blind trial of metoprolol in acute myocardial infarction. Effects on ventricular tachyarrhythmias. N. Engl. J. Med. *308*:614, 1983.

102. Engler, R. L., and LeWinter, M. M.: Ventricular arrhythmias: Diagnosis, treatment and prognosis. *In* Karliner, J. (ed.): Coronary Care. Edinburgh, Churchill Livingstone, 1981, pp. 367–390.

103. Jewitt, D. E., Kishon, Y., and Thomas, M.: Lignocaine in the management of arrhythmias after acute myocardial infarction. Lancet *1*:266, 1968.

104. Conley, M. J., McNeer, J. F., Lee, K. L., Wagner, G. S., and Rosati, R. A.: Cardiac arrest complicating acute myocardial infarction. Predictability and prognosis. Am. J. Cardiol. *39*:7, 1977.

105. Davis, J. S., Lie, J. T., Bentinck, D. C., Titus, J. L., Tacker, W. A., and Geddes, L. A.: Cardiac damage due to electric current and energy: Light microscopic and ultrastructural observations of acute and delayed myocardial cellular injuries. *In* Proceedings, Cardiac Defibrillation Conference, Purdue University, W. Lafayette, Ind., 1975.

106. Van Vleet, J. F., Tacker, W. A., Jr., Geddes, L. A., and Ferrans, V. J.: Acute cardiac damage in dogs given multiple transthoracic shocks with a trapezoidal wave-form defibrillator. Am. J. Vet. Res. *38*:617, 1977.

107. Ehsani, A., Ewy, G. A., and Sobel, B. E.: Effects of electrical countershock on serum creatine phosphokinase (CPK) isoenzyme activity. Am. J. Cardiol. *37*: 12, 1976.

108. Abboud, F. M., Pansegrau, D. G., and Mark, A. L.: Autonomic responses to ventricular defibrillation. *In* Proceedings, Cardiac Defibrillation Conference, Purdue University, W. Lafayette, Ind., 1975.

109. Heissenbuttel, R. H., and Bigger, J. T., Jr.: Bretylium tosylate, a newly available antiarrhythmic drug for ventricular arrhythmias. Ann. Intern. Med. *91*: 229, 1979.

110. Kaski, J. C., Girotti, L. A., Messuti, H., Rutitzky, B., and Rosenbaum, M. B.: Long-term management of sustained, recurrent symptomatic ventricular tachycardia with amiodarone. Circulation *64*:273, 1981.

111. DeBoer, L. W. V., Nosta, J. J., Kloner, R. A., and Braunwald, E.: Studies of amiodarone during experimental myocardial infarction: Beneficial effects on hemodynamics and infarct size. Circulation *65*:508, 1982.

112. Forrester, J. S., Diamond, G., Chatterjee, K., and Swan, H. J. C.: Medical therapy of acute myocardial infarction by application of hemodynamic subsets (First of Two Parts). N. Engl. J. Med. *295*:1356, 1976.

113. Forrester, J. S., Diamond, G., Chatterjee, K., and Swan, H. J. C.: Medical therapy of acute myocardial infarction by application of hemodynamic subsets (Second of Two Parts). N. Engl. J. Med. *295*:1404, 1976.

114. Klein, M. S., and Sobel, B. E.: Medical management of myocardial infarction. Ann. Rev. Med. *27*:89, 1976.

115. Askenazi, J., Koenigsberg, D. I., Ziegler, J. H., and Lesch, M.: Echocardiographic estimates of pulmonary artery wedge pressure. N. Engl. J. Med. *305*:1566, 1981.

116. Russell, R. O., Jr., Mantle, J. A., Rogers, W. J., and Rackley, C. E.: Current status of hemodynamic monitoring: Indications, diagnosis and complications. *In* Rackley, C. E. (ed.): Critical Care Medicine, Cardiovascular Clinics. Philadelphia, F. A. Davis, 1981, pp. 1–14.

117. Russell, R. O., Jr., Rackley, C. E., Pambo, J., Hunt, D., Potanin, C., and Dodge, H. T.: Effects of increasing left ventricular filling pressure in patients with acute myocardial infarction. J. Clin. Invest. *49*:1539, 1970.

118. Strauss, H. D., Sobel, B. E., and Roberts, R.: The influence of occult right ventricular infarction on enzymatically estimated infarct size, hemodynamics and prognosis. Circulation *62*:503, 1980.

119. Marmor, A., Geltman, E. M., Biello, D. R., Sobel, B. E., Siegel, B. A., and Roberts, R.: Functional response of the right ventricle to myocardial infarction: Dependence on the site of left ventricular infarction. Circulation *64*: 1005, 1981.

120. Lorell, B., Leinbach, R. C., Pohost, G. M., Gold, H. K., Dinsmore, R. E.,

Hutter, A. M., Jr., Pastore, J. O., and DeSanctis, R. W.: Right ventricular infarction. Clinical diagnosis and differentiation from cardiac tamponade and pericardial constriction. Am. J. Cardiol. 43:465, 1979.

121. Durrer, J. D., Lie, K. I., VanCapelle, F. J. L., and Durrer, D.: Effect of sodium nitroprusside on mortality in acute myocardial infarction. N. Engl. J. Med. 306:1121, 1982.

122. Cohn, J. N., Franciosa, J. A., Francis, G. S., Archibald, D., Tristani, F., Fletcher, R., Montero, A., Cintron, G., Clarke, J., Hager, D., Saunders, R., Cobb, F., Smith, R., Hoeb, H., and Settle, H.: Effect of short-term infusion on sodium nitroprusside in mortality rate in acute myocardial infarction complicated by left ventricular failure. Results of a Veterans Administration Cooperative study. N. Engl. J. Med. 306:1129, 1982.

123. Passamani, E. R.: Nitroprusside in myocardial infarction. N. Engl. J. Med. 306:1168, 1982.

124. Bodenheimer, M. M., Ramanathan, K., Banka, V. S., and Helfant, R. H.: Effect of progressive pressure reduction with nitroprusside on acute myocardial infarction in humans: Determination of optimal afterload. Ann. Intern. Med. 94:435, 1981.

125. Shell, W. E., and Sobel, B. E.: Protection of jeopardized ischemic myocardium by reduction of ventricular afterload. N. Engl. J. Med. 291:481, 1974.

126. Flaherty, J. T., Reid, P. R., Kelly, D. T., Taylor, D. R., Weisfeldt, M. L., and Pitt, B.: Intravenous nitroglycerin in acute myocardial infarction. Circulation 51:132, 1975.

127. Chiariello, M., Gold, H. K., Leinbach, R. C., Davis, M. A., and Maroko, P. R.: Comparison between the effects of nitroprusside and nitroglycerin on ischemic injury during acute myocardial infarction. Circulation 54:766, 1976.

128. Flaherty, J. T.: Intravenous nitroglycerin. Johns Hopkins Med. J. 151:36, 1982.

129. Bussmann, W. D., Barthe, G., Klepzig, H., Jr., and Kaltenbach, M.: Controlled study of intravenous nitroglycerin treatment for two days in patients with recent myocardial infarction. Clin. Cardiol. 3:399, 1980.

130. Borer, J. S., Redwood, D. R., Levitt, B., Cagin, N., Bianchi, C., Vallin, H., and Epstein, S. E.: Reduction in myocardial ischemia with nitroglycerin or nitroglycerin plus phenylephrine administered during acute myocardial infarction. N. Engl. J. Med. 293:1008, 1975.

131. Come, P. C., Flaherty, J. T., Baird, M. G., Rouleau, J. R., Weisfeldt, M. L., Greene, H. L., Becker, L., and Pitt, B.: Reversal by phenylephrine of the beneficial effects of intravenous nitroglycerin in patients with acute myocardial infarction. N. Engl. J. Med. 293:1004, 1975.

132. Derrida, J. P., Sal, R., and Chiche, P.: Nitroglycerin infusion in acute myocardial infarction. N. Engl. J. Med. 297:336, 1977.

133. Awan, N. A., Amsterdam, E. A., Zakuddin, V., DeMaria, A. N., Miller, R. R., and Mason, D. T.: Reduction of ischemic injury by sublingual nitroglycerin in patients with acute myocardial infarction. Circulation 54:761, 1976.

134. Rabinowitz, B., Tamari, I., Elazar, E., and Neufeld, H. N.: Intravenous isosorbide dinitrate in patients with refractory pump failure and acute myocardial infarction. Circulation 65:771, 1982.

135. Kelly, D. T., Delgado, C. E., Taylor, D. R., Pitt, B., and Ross, R. S.: Use of phentolamine in acute myocardial infarction associated with hypertension and left ventricular failure. Circulation 47:729, 1973.

136. Chatterjee, K., Parmley, W. W., Ganz, W., Forrester, J., Walinsky, P., Crexells, C., and Swan, H. J. C.: Hemodynamic and metabolic responses to vasodilator therapy in acute myocardial infarction. Circulation 48:1183, 1973.

137. Franciosa, J. A., Pierpont, G., and Cohn, J. N.: Hemodynamic improvement after oral hydralazine in left ventricular failure. Ann. Intern. Med. 86:388, 1977.

138. Chatterjee, K., Parmley, W. W., Massie, B., Greenberg, B., Werner, J., Klausner, S., and Norman, A.: Oral hydralazine therapy for chronic refractory heart failure. Circulation 54:879, 1976.

139. Franciosa, J. A., Mikulic, E., Cohn, J. N., Jose, E., and Fabie, A.: Hemodynamic effects of orally administered isosorbide dinitrate in patients with congestive heart failure. Circulation 50:1020, 1974.

140. Gold, H. K., Leinbach, R. C., and Sanders, C. A.: Use of sublingual nitroglycerin in congestive failure following acute myocardial infarction. Circulation 46:839, 1972.

141. Magorien, R. D., Triffon, D. W., Desch, C. E., Bay, W. H., Unverferth, D. V., and Leier, C. V.: Prazosin and hydralazine in congestive heart failure. Ann. Intern. Med. 95:5, 1981.

142. Cohen, R. A., Shepherd, J. T., and Vanhoutte, P. M.: Prejunctional and postjunctional actions of endogenous norepinephrine at the sympathetic neuroeffector junction in canine coronary arteries. Circ. Res. 52:16, 1983.

143. Jaffe, A. S., Henry, P. D., Vacek, J. L., Sobel, B. E., and Roberts, R.: Administration of nifedipine to patients with acute myocardial infarction. In Vogel, J. H. K. (ed.): Cardiovascular Medicine 1982. New York, Raven Press, 1982, p. 91.

144. Cohn, J. N.: Editorial—Progress in vasodilator therapy for heart failure. N. Engl. J. Med. 302:1414, 1980.

145. Kötter, V., Von Leitner, E. R., Wunderlich, J., and Schröder, R.: Comparison of haemodynamic effects of phentolamine, sodium nitroprusside, and glyceryl trinitrate in acute myocardial infarction. Br. Heart J. 39:1196, 1977.

146. Franciosa, J. A., Guiha, N. H., Limas, C. J., Rodriguera, E., and Cohn, J. N.: Improved left ventricular function during nitroprusside infusion in acute myocardial infarction. Lancet 1:650, 1972.

147. Hockings, B. E. F., Cope, G. D., Clarke, G. M., and Taylor, R. R.: Randomized controlled trial of vasodilator therapy after myocardial infarction. Am. J. Cardiol. 48:345, 1981.

148. Packer, M., Meller, J., Medina, N., Yushak, M., and Gorlin, R.: Hemodynamic characterization of tolerance to long-term hydralazine therapy in severe chronic heart failure. N. Engl. J. Med. 306:57, 1982.

149. Colucci, W. S., Williams, G. H., Alexander, R. W., and Braunwald, E.: Mechanisms and implications of vasodilator tolerance in the treatment of congestive heart failure. Am. J. Med. 71:89, 1981.

150. Chatterjee, K., Ports, T. A., Brundage, B. H., Massie, B., Holly, A. N., and Parmley, W. W.: Oral hydralazine in chronic heart failure: Sustained beneficial hemodynamic effects. Ann. Intern. Med. 92:600, 1980.

151. Dzau, V. J., Colucci, W. S., Williams, G. H., Curfman, G., Meggs, L., and Hollenberg, N. K.: Sustained effectiveness of converting-enzyme inhibition in patients with severe congestive heart failure. N. Engl. J. Med. 302:1373, 1980.

152. Ertl, G., Kloner, R. A., Alexander, R. W., and Braunwald, E.: Limitation of experimental infarct size by angiotensin-converting enzyme inhibitor. Circulation 65:40, 1982.

153. Covell, J. W., Braunwald, E., Ross, J., Jr., and Sonnenblick, E. H.: Studies on digitalis XVI. Effects on myocardial oxygen consumption. J. Clin. Invest. 45:1535, 1966.

154. Kumar, R., Hood, W. B., Jr., Joison, J., Gilmour, D. P., Norman, J. C., and Abelmann, W. H.: Experimental myocardial infarction. VI. Efficacy and toxicity of digitalis in acute and healing phase in intact conscious dog. J. Clin. Invest. 49:358, 1970.

155. Maroko, P.R., Kjekshus, J. K., Sobel, B. E., Watanabe, T., Covell, J. W., Ross, J., Jr., and Braunwald, E.: Factors influencing infarct size following experimental coronary artery occlusions. Circulation 43:67, 1971.

156. Vatner, S. F., Baig, H., Manders, W. T., and Murray, P. A.: Effects of a cardiac glycoside on regional function, blood flow, and electrograms in conscious dogs with myocardial ischemia. Circ. Res. 43:413, 1978.

157. Watanabe, T., Covell, J. W., Maroko, P. R., Braunwald, E., and Ross, J., Jr.: The effects of increased arterial pressure and positive inotropic agents on the severity of myocardial ischemia in the acutely depressed heart. Am. J. Cardiol. 30:371, 1972.

158. Ross, J., Jr., Waldhausen, J. S., and Braunwald, E.: Studies on digitalis. I. Direct effects on peripheral vascular resistance. J. Clin. Invest. 39:930, 1960.

159. Morrison, J., Coromilas, J., Robbins, M., Ong, L., Eisenberg, S., Stechel, R., Zema, M., Reiser, P., and Scherr, L.: Digitalis and myocardial infarction in man. Circulation 62:8, 1980.

160. Marcus, F. I.: Editorial—Use of digitalis in acute myocardial infarction. Circulation 62:17, 1980.

161. Moss, A. J., Davis, H. T., Conard, D. L., DeCamilla, J. J., and Odoroff, C. L.: Digitalis-associated cardiac mortality after myocardial infarction. Circulation 64:1150, 1981.

162. Ryan, T. J., McCabe, C. H., Bailey, D., Papapietro, S. E., Fisher, L. D., Mock, M., and Killip, T.: The effect of digitalis on survival in high risk patients (CASS). Circulation 64 (Suppl. 4): 43, 1981.

163. Mueller, H., Ayres, S. M., Giannelli, S., Jr., Conklin, E. F., Mazzara, J. T., and Grace, W. J.: Effect of isoproterenol, 1-norepinephrine, and intra-aortic counterpulsation on hemodynamics and myocardial metabolism in shock following acute myocardial infarction. Circulation 45:335, 1972.

164. Shell, W. E., and Sobel, B. E.: Deleterious effects of increased heart rate on infarct size in the conscious dog. Am. J. Cardiol. 31:474, 1973.

164a. Ichard, C., Ricome, J. L., Rimailho, A., Bottineau, G., and Auzepy, P.: Combined hemodynamic effects of dopamine and dobutamine in cardiogenic shock. Circulation 67:620, 1983.

165. Holzer, J., Karliner, J. S., O'Rourke, R. A., Pitt, W., and Ross, J., Jr.: Effectiveness of dopamine in patients with cardiogenic shock. Am. J. Cardiol. 32:79, 1973.

166. Tuttle, R. R., and Mills, J.: Development of a new catecholamine to selectively increase cardiac contractility. Circ. Res. 36:185, 1975.

167. Gillespie, T. A., Ambos, H. D., Sobel, B. E., and Roberts, R.: Effects of dobutamine in patients with acute myocardial infarction. Am. J. Cardiol. 39:588, 1977.

168. Keung, E. C. H., Siskind, S. J., Sonnenblick, E. H., Ribner, H. S., Schwartz, W. J., and LeJemtel, T. H.: Dobutamine therapy in acute myocardial infarction. J.A.M.A. 245:144, 1981.

169. Goldstein, R. A., Passamani, E. R., and Roberts, E.: Comparison of digoxin and dobutamine in patients with acute infarction and cardiac failure. N. Engl. J. Med. 303:846, 1980.

169a. Maekawa, K., Liang, C-S., and Hood, W. B., Jr.: Comparison of dobutamine and dopamine in acute myocardial infarction. Effects of systemic hemodynamics, plasma catecholamines, blood flows and infarct size. Circulation 67:750,1983.

169b. Resnevkov, L.: Cardiogenic shock. Chest 83:893, 1983.

170. Gunnar, R. M., and Loeb, H. S.: Shock in acute myocardial infarction: Evolution of physiologic therapy. J. Am. Coll. Cardiol. 1:154, 1983.

171. Mueller, H., Ayres, S. M., Gregory, J. J., Gianelli, S., Jr., and Grace, W. J.: Hemodynamics, coronary blood flow, and myocardial metabolism in coronary shock; Response to L-norepinephrine and isoproterenol. J. Clin. Invest. 49:1885, 1970.

172. Mueller, H., Ayres, S. M., Conklin, E. F., Giannelli, S., Jr., Mazzara, J. T., Grace, W. T., and Nealon, T. F., Jr.: The effects of intra-aortic counterpulsation on cardiac performance and metabolism in shock associated with acute myocardial infarction. J. Clin. Invest. 50:1885, 1971.

173. Saini, V. K., Hood, W. B., Jr., Hechtman, H. B., and Berger, R. L.: Nutrient myocardial blood flow in experimental myocardial ischemia. Circulation 52:1086, 1975.

174. Gold, H. K., Leinbach, R. C., Mundth, E. D., Sanders, C. A., and Buckley,

M. J.: Reversal of myocardial ischemia complicating acute infarction by intra-aorta balloon pumping (IABP). Circulation *45–46*(Suppl. II):22, 1972.

175. DeLaria, G. A., Johansen, K. H., Sobel, B. E., Sybers, H. D., and Bernstein, E. F.: Delayed evolution of myocardial ischemic injury after intra-aortic balloon counterpulsation. Circulation *50*(Suppl. II):242, 1974.

176. Johnson, S. A., Scanlon, P. J., Loeb, H. S., Moran, J. M., Pifarre, R., and Gunnar, R. M.: Treatment of cardiogenic shock in myocardial infarction by intraaortic balloon counterpulsation and surgery. Am. J. Med. *62*:687, 1977.

177. O'Rourke, M. F., Norris, R. M., Campbell, T. J., Chang, V. P., and Sammel, N. L.: Randomized controlled trial of intra-aortic balloon counterpulsation in early myocardial infarction with acute heart failure. Am. J. Cardiol. *47*:815, 1981.

178. Bitran, D., Hasin, Y., Weiss, A., Shefer, A., Freiman, I., Shimon, D., and Gotsman, M. S.: Intra-aortic balloon counterpulsation in acute myocardial infarction. Israel J. Med. Sci. *18*:215, 1982.

179. Pae, W. E., Jr., and Pierce, W. S.: Temporary left ventricular assistance in acute myocardial infarction and cardiogenic shock. Rationale and criteria for utilization. Chest *79*:692, 1981.

180. Gowda, S. K., Gillespie, T. A., Byrne, J. D., Ambos, H. D., Sobel, B. E., and Roberts, R.: Effects of external counterpulsation on enzymatically estimated infarct size and ventricular arrhythmia. Br. Heart J. *40*:308, 1978.

181. Korr, K. S., Lewvinson, H., Bough, E. W., Gheorghiade, M., Stone, J., McEnany, T., and Shulman, R. S.: Tricuspid valve replacement for cardiogenic shock after acute right ventricular infarction. J.A.M.A. *244*:1958, 1980.

182. Kopf, G. S., Meshkov, A., Laks, H., Hammond, G. L., and Beha, A. S.: Changing patterns in the surgical management of ventricular septal rupture after myocardial infarction. Am. J. Surg. *143*:465, 1982.

183. Montoya, A., McKeever, L., Scanlon, P., Sullivan, H. J., Gunnar, R. M., and Pifarre, R.: Early repair of ventricular septal rupture after infarction. Am. J. Cardiol. *45*:345, 1980.

184. Catherwood, E., Mintz, G. S., Kotler, M. N., Parry, W. R., and Segal, B. L.: Two-dimensional echocardiographic recognition of left ventricular pseudoaneurysm. Circulation *62*:294, 1980.

185. Miller, D. C., and Stinson, E. B.: Surgical management of acute mechanical defects secondary to myocardial infarction. Am. J. Surg. *141*:677, 1981.

186. Thomas, C. S., Jr., Alford, W. C., Jr., Burrus, G. R., Glassford, D. M., Jr., and Stoney, W. S.: Urgent operation for acquired ventricular septal defect. Ann. Surg. *195*:706, 1982.

187. Mundth, E. D.: Surgical treatment of cardiogenic shock and of acute mechanical complications following myocardial infarction. Cardiovasc. Clin. *8*:241, 1977.

188. Johnson, S. A., Scanlon, P. J., and Loeb, H. S.: Treatment of cardiogenic shock in myocardial infarction by intraaortic balloon counterpulsation and surgery. Am. J. Med. *62*:687, 1977.

189. Eisenmann, B., Bareiss, P., Pacifico, A. D., Jeanblanc, B., Kretz, J. G., Baehret, B., Warter, J., and Kieny, R.: Anatomic, clinical and therapeutic features of acute cardiac rupture. J. Thorac. Cardiovasc. Surg. *76*:78, 1978.

190. Russell, R. O., Jr., Turner, J. D., Rogers, W. J., Mantle, J. A., and Rackley, C. E.: Mortality reduction after acute myocardial infarction in a myocardial infarction research unit. Clin. Res. *26*:752A, 1978.

191. Page, D. L., Caulfield, J. B., Kastor, J. A., DeSanctis, R. W., and Sanders, C. A.: Myocardial changes associated with cardiogenic shock. N. Engl. J. Med. *285*:133, 1971.

192. Gutovitz, A. L., Sobel, B. E., and Roberts, R.: Progressive nature of myocardial injury in selected patients with cardiogenic shock. Am. J. Cardiol. *41*:469, 1978.

193. Kostuk, W. J., Ehsani, A. A., Karliner, J. S., Ashburn, W. L., Peterson, K. L., Ross, J., Jr., and Sobel, B. E.: Left ventricular performance, after myocardial infarction assessed by radioisotope angiocardiography. Circulation *47*:242, 1973.

194. Rogers, W. J., McDaniel, H. G., Smith, L. R., Mantle, J. A., Russell, R. O., Jr., and Rackley, C. E.: Correlation of angiographic estimates of myocardial infarct size and accumulated release of creatine kinase MB isoenzyme in man. Circulation *56*:199, 1977.

195. Peel, A. A. F., Semple, T., Wang, I., Lancaster, W. M., and Dall, J. L. G.: A coronary prognostic index for grading the severity of infarction. Br. Heart J. *24*:745, 1962.

196. Norris, R. M., Brandt, P. W. T., and Lee, A. J.: Mortality in a coronary-care unit analysed by a new coronary prognostic index. Lancet *1*:278, 1969.

197. Sobel, B. E., Bresnahan, G. F., Shell, W. E., and Yoder, R. D.: Estimation of infarct size in man and its relation to prognosis. Circulation *46*:640, 1972.

198. Shell, W. E., and Sobel, B. E.: Biochemical markers of ischemic injury. Circulation *53*(Suppl. I):98, 1976.

199. Bleifield, W., Mathey, D., Hanrath, P., Buss, H., and Effert, S.: Infarct size estimated from serial serum creatine phosphokinase in relation to left ventricular hemodynamics. Circulation *55*:303, 1977.

200. Mathey, D., Bleifield, W., Hanrath, P., and Effert, S.: Attempt to quantitate relation between cardiac function and infarct size in acute myocardial infarction. Br. Heart J. *36*:271, 1974.

201. Holman, B. L., Chisholm, R. J., and Braunwald, E.: The prognostic implications of acute myocardial infarct scintigraphy with [99]m Tc-pyrophosphate. Circulation *57*:320, 1978.

202. Sobel, B. E., and Shell, W. E.: Jeopardized, blighted and necrotic myocardium. Circulation *47*:215, 1973.

203. Braunwald, E., and Maroko, P. R.: The reduction of infarct size—an idea whose time (for testing) has come. Circulation *50*:206, 1974.

204. Braunwald, E., and Maroko, P. R.: Limitation of infarct size. Curr. Probl. Cardiol. *3*:1, 1978.

205. Christlieb, I. Y., Clark, R. E., and Sobel, B. E.: Three-hour preservation of the hypothermic globally ischemic heart with nifedipine. Surgery *90*:947, 1981.

206. Snyder, D. W., and Sobel, B. E.: Treatment of ischemic heart disease: Clinical therapy of ischemic heart disease. *In* Rosen, M., and Hoffman, B. (eds.): Medical Management of Ischemic Heart Disease. The Hague, The Netherlands, Martinus Nijhoff Publishers, in press.

207. Corr, P. B., Snyder, D. W., Lee, B. I., Gross, R. W., Keim, C. R., and Sobel, B. E.: Pathophysiological concentrations of lysophosphatides and the slow response. Am. J. Physiol., *12:187, 1982.*

208. Gross, R. W., Corr, P. B., Lee, B. I., Saffitz, J. E., Crafford, W. A., Jr., and Sobel, B. E.: Incorporation of radiolabeled lysophosphatidyl choline into canine Purkinje fibers and ventricular muscle: Electrophysiological, biochemical and autoradiographic correlations. Circ. Res., *51*:27, 1982.

209. Schaper, W., and Pasyk, S.: Influence of collateral flow on the ischemic tolerance of the heart following acute and subacute coronary occlusion. Circulation *53*(Suppl. I):57, 1976.

210. Bishop, S. P., White, F. C., and Bloor, C. M.: Regional myocardial blood flow during acute myocardial infarction in the conscious dog. Circ. Res. *38*:429, 1976.

211. Borda, L., Shuchleib, R., and Henry, P. D.: Effects of potassium on isolated canine coronary arteries. Circ. Res. *41*:778, 1977.

212. Oliva, P. B., and Breckinridge, J. C.: Arteriographic evidence of coronary arterial spasm in acute myocardial infarction. Circulation *56*:366, 1977.

213. Braunwald, E.: Coronary artery spasm as a cause of myocardial ischemia. J. Lab Clin. Med. *97*:299, 1981.

214. Maseri, A., L'Abbate, A., Baroldi, G., Chierchia, S., Marzilli, M., Ballestra, A. M., Severi, S., Parodi, O., Biagini, A., Distante, A., and Pesola, A.: Coronary vasospasm as a possible cause of myocardial infarction. N. Engl. J. Med. *299*:1271, 1978.

215. Henry, P. D., and Yokoyama, M.: Supersensitivity of atherosclerotic rabbit aorta to ergonovine: Mediation by aserotonergic mechanism. J. Clin. Invest. *66*:306, 1980.

216. Moran, T. J., French, W. J., Abrams, H. F., and Criley, J. M.: Post-myocardial infarction angina and coronary spasm. Am. J. Cardiol. *50*:192, 1982.

217. Koiwaya, Y., Torii, S., Takeshita, A., Nakagaki, O., and Nakamura, M.: Postinfarction angina caused by coronary arterial spasm. Circulation *65*:275, 1982.

218. Williams, D. O., Amsterdam, E. A., Miller, R. R., and Mason, D. T.: Functional significance of coronary collateral vessels in patients with acute myocardial infarction: Relation to pump performance, cardiogenic shock and survival. Am. J. Cardiol. *37*:345, 1976.

219. Strauss, H. D.: Myocardial infarction extension: Clinical significance. Primary Cardiol. *8*:14, 1982.

220. Baker, J. T., Bramlet, D. A., Lester, R. M., Harrison, D. C., Roe, C. R., and Cobb, F. R.: Myocardial infarct extension: Incidence and relationship to survival. Circulation *65*:918, 1982.

221. Marmor, A., Sobel, B. E., and Roberts, R.: Factors presaging early recurrent myocardial infarction ("extension"). Am. J. Cardiol. *48*:603, 1981.

222. Cannom, D. S., Levy, W., and Cohen, L. S.: The short- and long-term prognosis of patients with transmural and nontransmural myocardial infarction. Am. J. Med. *61*:452, 1976.

223. Hutter, A. M., Jr., DeSanctis, R. W., Flynn, T., and Yeatman, L. A.: Nontransmural myocardial infarction. A comparison of hospital and late clinical course of patients with that of matched patients with transmural anterior and transmural inferior myocardial infarction. Am. J. Cardiol. *48*:595, 1981.

224. Yusuf, S., Ramsdale, E., Peto, R., Furse, L., Bennet, D., Bray, C., and Sleight, P.: Early intravenous atenolol treatment in suspected acute myocardial infarction. Preliminary report of a randomized trial. Lancet *2*:73, 1980.

225. Lange, R., Kloner, R. A., and Braunwald, E.: First ultra-short-acting beta-adrenergic blocking agent: Its effect on size and segmental wall dynamics of reperfused myocardial infarcts in dogs. Am. J. Cardiol. *51*:1759, 1983.

226. Braunwald, E., Muller, J. E., Kloner, R. A., and Maroko, P. R.: Role of beta-adrenergic blockade in the therapy of patients with myocardial infarction. Am. J. Med. *74*:113, 1983.

227. Mueller, H. S., Ayres, S. M., Religa, A., and Evans, R. G.: Propranolol in the treatment of acute myocardial infarction: Effect on myocardial oxygenation and hemodynamics. Circulation *49*:1078, 1974.

228. Mueller, H. S., and Ayres, S. M.: The role of propranolol in the treatment of acute myocardial infarction. Prog. Cardiovasc. Dis. *19*:405, 1977.

229. Opie, L. H.: Metabolism of free fatty acids, glucose and catecholamines in acute myocardial infarction: Relation to myocardial ischemia and infarct size. Am. J. Cardiol. *36*:938, 1975.

230. Ahumada, G. G., Karlsberg, R. P., Jaffe, A. S., Ambos, H. D., Sobel, B. E., and Roberts, R.: Reduction of early ventricular arrhythmia by acebutolol in patients with acute myocardial infarction. Br. Heart J. *41*:654, 1979.

231. Gold, H. K., Leinbach, C., and Maroko, P. R.: Propranolol-induced reduction of signs of ischemic injury during acute myocardial infarction. Am. J. Cardiol. *38*:689, 1976.

232. Libby, P., Maroko, P. R., Covell, J. W., Malloch, C. I., Ross, J., Jr., and Braunwald, E.: Effect of practolol on the extent of myocardial ischemic injury after experimental coronary occlusion and its effect on ventricular function in the normal and ischemic heart. Cardiovasc. Res. *7*:167, 1973.

233. Muller, J. E., Maroko, P. R., and Braunwald, E.: Precordial electrocardio-

graphic mapping: A technique to assess the efficacy of interventions designed to limit infarct size. Circulation 57:1, 1978.

234. Pelides, L. J., Reid, D. S., Thomas, M., and Shillingford, J. P.: Inhibition by beta-blockade of the ST segment elevation after acute myocardial infarction in man. Cardiovasc. Res. 2:295, 1972.

235. Waagstein, F., and Hjalmarson, A. C.: Effect of cardioselective beta blockade on heart function and chest pain in acute myocardial infarction. Acta Med. Scand. 587(Suppl.):201, 1975.

236. Heikkila, J., and Nieminen, M. S.: Failure of methylprednisolone to protect acutely ischemic myocardium: A contrast with subsequent beta-adrenergic blockade in man. Chest 73:577, 1978.

237. Barber, J. M., Boyle, D. M., Chaturvedi, N. C., Singh, N., and Walsh, M. J.: Practolol in acute myocardial infarction. Acta Med. Scand. 587(Suppl.):213, 1976.

238. Peter, T., Norris, R. M., and Clarke, E. D.: Reduction of enzyme levels by propranolol after acute myocardial infarction. Circulation 57:1091, 1978.

239. Norris, R. M., Clarke, E. D., Sammel, N. L., Smith, W. M., and Williams, B.: Protective effect of propranolol in threatened myocardial infarction. Lancet 2: 907, 1978.

240. Yusuf, S., Sleight, P., Rossi, P., Ramsdale, D., Peto, R., Furze, L., Sterry, H., Pearson, M., Motwani, R., Parish, S., Gray, R., Bennett, D., and Bray, C.: Reduction in infarct size, arrhythmias and chest pain by early intravenous beta blockade in suspected acute myocardial infarction. Circulation 67:12, 1983.

240a. Yusuf, S., Ramsdale, D., Rossi, P., Peto, R., Pearson, M., Sterry, H., Furse, L., Motwani, R., Parish, S., Gray, R., Bennett, D., Bray, C., and Sleight, P.: Reduction in infarct size, morbidity and short term mortality by early intravenous beta blockade. J. Am. Coll. Cardiol. 1:676, 1983.

241. Ramsdale, D. R., Faragher, E. B., Bennett, D. H., Bray, C. L., Ward, C., Cruickshank, J. M., Yusuf, S., and Sleight, P.: Ischemic pain relief in patients with acute myocardial infarction by intravenous atenolol. Am. Heart J. 103: 459, 1982.

242. Jurgensen, H. J., Frederiksen, J., Hansen, D. A., and Pedersen-Bjorgaard, D.: Limitation of myocardial infarct size in patients less than 66 years treated with alprenolol. Br. Heart J. 45:583, 1981.

242a. Hjalmarson, A., Herlitz, J., Holmberg, S., Ryden, L., Swedberg, K., Vedin, A., Waagstein, F., Waldenstrom, A., Waldenstrom, J., Wedel, H., Wilhelmsen, L., and Wilhelmsson, C.: The Goteborg metoprolol trial. Effects on mortality and morbidity in acute myocardial infarction. Circulation 67:26, 1983.

243. Andersen, M. P., Fredriksen, J., and Jurgensen, H. J.: Effect of alprenolol on mortality among patients with definite or suspected acute myocardial infarction: Preliminary results. Lancet 2:865, 1979.

244. Bussman, W. D., Passek, D., Seidel, W., and Kaltenbach, M.: Reduction of CK and CK-MB indexes of infarct size by intravenous nitroglycerin. Circulation 63:615, 1981.

245. Becker, L. C., Bulkley, B. J., and Pitt, B.: Enhanced reduction of thallium-201 defects in acute myocardial infarction by nitroglycerin treatment: Initial results of a prospective randomized trial. Clin. Res. 26:219A, 1978 (abst.).

246. Becker, L. C., Fortuin, N. J., and Pitt, B.: Effect of ischemia and antianginal drugs on the distribution of radioactive microspheres in the canine left ventricle. Circ. Res. 28:263, 1971.

247. Flaherty, J. T., Becker, L. C., and Weisfeldt, M. L.: Results of a prospective randomized clinical trial of intravenous nitroglycerin in acute myocardial infarction. Circulation 62(Suppl. 3):82, 1980 (abst.).

248. Kim, Y. I., and Williams, J. F., Jr.: Large dose sublingual nitroglycerin in myocardial infarction: Relief of chest pain and reduction of Q wave randomized prospective study. Circulation 64(Suppl. 4):195, 1981.

249. Gold, H. K., Chiariello, M., Leinbach, R. C., Davis, M. A., and Maroko, P. R.: Deleterious effects of nitroprusside on myocardial injury during acute myocardial infarction. Herz 1:161, 1976.

250. Jaffe, A. S., Geltman, E. M., Tiefenbrunn, A. J., Ambos, H. D., Snyder, D., Dukuyama, O., Bauwens, D., Sobel, B. E., and Roberts, R.: Reduction of the extent of inferior myocardial infarction with intravenous nitroglycerin: A randomized prospective study. Circulation 64(Suppl. 4):195, 1981.

251. Borer, J. S., Kent, K. M., Goldstein, R. E., and Epstein, S. E.: Nitroglycerin-induced reduction in the incidence of spontaneous ventricular fibrillation during coronary occlusion in dogs. Am. J. Cardiol. 33:517, 1974.

252. Shah, R., Bodenheimer, M. M., Banka, V. S., and Helfant, R. H.: Nitroglycerin and ventricular performance: Differential effect in the presence of reversible and irreversible asynergy. Chest 70:473, 1976.

253. Myers, R. W., Scherer, J. L., Goldstein, R. A., Goldstein, R. E., Kent, K. M., and Epstein, S. E.: Effects of nitroglycerin and nitroglycerin-methoxamine during acute myocardial ischemia in dogs with pre-existing multivessel coronary occlusive disease. Circulation 51:632, 1975.

254. Hill, N. S., Antman, E. M., Green, L. H., and Alpert, J. S.: Intravenous nitroglycerin. A review of pharmacology, indications, therapeutic effects and complications. Chest 79:69, 1981.

255. Chatterjee, K., and Parmley, W. W.: Vasodilator therapy for acute myocardial infarction and chronic congestive heart failure. J. Am. Coll. Cardiol. 1:133, 1983.

256. Maroko, P. R., Hillis, L. D., Muller, J. E., Tavazzi, L., Heyndrickx, G. R., Ray, M., Chiariello, M., Distante, A., Askenazi, J., Salerno, J., Carpentier, J., Reshetnaya, N. I., Radvany, P., Libby, P., Raabe, D. S., Chazov, E. I., Bobba, P., and Braunwald, E.: Favorable effects of hyaluronidase on electrocardiographic evidence of necrosis in patients with acute myocardial infarction. N. Engl. J. Med. 296:898, 1977.

257. Saltissi, S., Coltart, D. J., Robinson, P. S., Webb-Peploe, M. M., and Croft, D. N: Effects of early administration of a highly purified hyaluronidase preparation (GL enzyme) on myocardial infarct size. Lancet 1:867, 1982.

258. Henderson, A., Campbell, R. W. F., and Julian, D. G.: Effect of a highly purified hyaluronidase preparation (GL enzyme) on electrocardiographic changes in acute myocardial infarction. Lancet 1:874, 1982.

259. Flint, E. J., Cadigan, P. J., DeGiovanni, J., Lamb, P., and Pentecost, B. L.: Effect of GL enzyme (a highly purified form of hyaluronidase) on mortality after myocardial infarction. Lancet 1:871, 1982.

260. Rackley, C. E., Russell, R. O., Jr., Rogers, W. J., and Mantle, J. A.: Glucose-insulin-potassium infusion in acute myocardial infarction: Review of clinical experience. Postgrad. Med. 65:93, 1979.

261. Mantle, J. A., Rogers, W. J., McDaniel, H. G., Holmes, R. A., Russell, R. O., Jr., and Rackley, C. E.: Metabolic support of mechanical performance in myocardial infarction in man—a randomized clinical trial of glucose-insulin-potassium. Am. J. Cardiol. 43:395, 1979.

262. Rogers, W. J., Russel, R. O., Jr., McDaniel, H. G., and Rackley, C. E.: Acute effects of glucose-insulin-potassium infusion on myocardial substrates, coronary blood flow and oxygen consumption in man. Am. J. Cardiol. 40:421, 1977.

263. Rogers, W. J., Segall, P. H., McDaniel, H. G., Mantle, J. A., Russell, R. O., Jr., and Rackley, C. E.: Prospective randomized trial of glucose-insulin-potassium in acute myocardial infarction. Am. J. Cardiol. 43:801, 1979.

264. Russell, R. O., Jr., Rogers, W. J., Mantle, J. A., McDaniel, H. G., and Rackley, C. E.: Glucose-insulin-potassium, free fatty acids and acute myocardial infarction in man. Circulation 53 (Suppl. I):I–207, 1975.

265. Heng, M. K., Norris, R. M., Singh, B. N., and Barratt-Boyes, C.: Effects of glucose and glucose-insulin-potassium on haemodynamics and enzyme release after acute myocardial infarction. Br. Heart J. 39:748, 1977.

266. Whitlow, P. L., Rogers, W. J., Smith, L. R., McDaniel, H. G., Papapietro, S. E., Mantle, J. A., Logic, J. R., Russell, R. O., Jr., and Rackley, C. E.: Enhancement of left ventricular function by glucose-insulin-potassium infusion in acute myocardial infarction. Am. J. Cardiol. 49:811, 1982.

266a. Rogers, W. J., McDaniel, H. G., Mantle, J. A., and Rackley, C. E.: Prospective randomized trial of glucose-insulin-potassium in acute myocardial infarction: Effects on hemodynamics, short- and long-term survival. J. Am. Coll. Cardiol. 1:628, 1983.

267. Morrison, J., Reduto, L., Pizzarello, R., Geller, K., Maley, T., and Gulotta, S.: Modification of myocardial injury in man by corticosteroid administration. Circulation 53 (Suppl. I):200, 1976.

268. Roberts, R., DeMello, V., and Sobel, B. E.: Deleterious effects of methylprednisolone in patients with myocardial infarction. Circulation 53 (Suppl. I):204, 1976.

269. Bulkley, B. H., and Roberts, W. C.: Steroid therapy during acute myocardial infarction: A cause of delayed healing and of ventricular aneurysm. Am. J. Med. 56:244, 1974.

270. Kloner, R. A., Fishbein, M. C., Lew, H., Maroko, P. R., and Braunwald, E.: Mummification of the infarcted myocardium by high dose corticosteroids. Circulation 57:56, 1978.

271. Maclean, D., Maroko, P. R., Fishbein, M. C., and Braunwald, E.: Effects of corticosteroids on myocardial infarct size and healing following experimental coronary occlusion. Am. J. Cardiol. 39:280, 1977.

272. Hammerman, H., Kloner, R. A., Hale, S. L., Schoen, F. J., and Braunwald, E.: Is scar thinning and LV topographic alterations induced by anti-inflammatory agent of functional significance? Clin. Res., in press.

273. Amsterdam, E. A., et al.: Clinical assessment of external pressure circulatory assist in acute myocardial infarction. Report of a cooperative clinical trial. Am. J. Cardiol. 45:349, 1980.

274. Powell, W. J., Jr., Daggett, W. M., Magro, A. E., Bianco, J. A., Buckley, M. J., Sanders, C. A., Kantrowitz, A. R., and Austen, W. G.: Effects of intra-aortic balloon counterpulsation on cardiac performance, oxygen consumption, and coronary blood flow in dogs. Circ. Res. 26:753, 1970.

275. Maroko, P. R., Bernstein, E. F., Libby, P., DeLaria, G. A., Covell, J. W., Ross, J., Jr., and Braunwald, E.: Effects of intraaortic balloon counterpulsation on the severity of myocardial ischemic injury following acute coronary occlusion: Counterpulsation and myocardial injury. Circulation 45: 1150, 1972.

276. Nachlas, M. M., and Siedband, M. P.: The influence of diastolic augmentation on infarct size following coronary artery ligation. J. Thorac. Cardiovasc. Surg. 53:698, 1967.

277. Sugg, W. L., Webb, W. R., and Ecker, R. R.: Reduction of extent of myocardial infarction by counterpulsation. Ann. Thorac. Surg. 7:310, 1969.

278. Leinbach, R. C., Gold, H. K., Harper, R. W., Buckley, M. J., and Austen, W. G.: Early intraaortic balloon pumping for anterior myocardial infarction without shock. Circulation 58:204, 1978.

279. Ginks, W. R., Sybers, H. D., Maroko, P. R., Covell, J. W., Sobel, B. E., and Ross, J., Jr.: Coronary artery reperfusion: II. Reduction of myocardial infarct size at 1 week after the coronary occlusion. J. Clin. Invest. 51:2717, 1972.

280. Lang, T., Corday, E., Gold, H., Meerbaum, S., Rubins, S., Costantini, C., Hirose, S., Osher, J., and Rosen, J.: Consequences of reperfusion after coronary occlusion: Effects on hemodynamic and regional myocardial metabolic function. Am. J. Cardiol. 33:69, 1974.

281. Smith, G. T., Soeter, J. R., Haston, H. H., and McNamara, J. J.: Coronary reperfusion in primates: Serial electrocardiographic and histologic assessment. J. Clin. Invest. 54:1420, 1974.

282. Symes, J. F., Arnold, I. M. F., and Blundell, P. E.: Early revascularization of the acute myocardial pulfarction: The critical time factor. Can. Med. Assoc. J. 107:636, 1972.

283. Kloner, R. A., Fishbein, M. C., Cotran, R. S., Braunwald, E., and Maroko, P. R.: The effect of propranolol on microvascular injury in acute myocardial ischemia. Circulation 55:872, 1977.

284. Deloche, A., Fabiani, J. N., Camilleri, J. P., Relland, J., Joseph, D., Carpentier, A., and Dubost, C.: The effect of coronary artery reperfusion on the extent of myocardial infarction. Am. Heart J. *93*:358, 1977.
285. Kloner, R. A., Rude, R. E., Carlson, N., Maroko, P. R., DeBoer, L. W. V., and Braunwald, E.: Ultrastructural evidence of microvascular damage and myocardial cell injury after coronary artery occlusion: Which comes first? Circulation *62*:945, 1980.
286. Kloner, R. A., Ellis, S. G., Lange, R., and Braunwald, E.: Studies of experimental coronary artery reperfusion: Effects on infarct size, myocardial function, biochemistry, ultrastructure and microvascular damage. Circulation, in press.
287. Bergmann, S. R., Lerch, R. A., Fox, K. A. A., Ludbrook, P. A., Welch, M. J., Ter-Pogossian, M. M., and Sobel, B. E.: The temporal dependence of beneficial effects of coronary thrombolysis characterized by positron tomography. Am. J. Med., *73*:573, 1982.
288. Reimer, K. A., and Jennings, R. B.: The wavefront phenomenon of myocardial ischemic cell death. II. Transmural progression of necrosis within the framework of ischemic bed size (myocardium at risk) and collateral flow. Lab. Invest. *40*:633, 1979.
289. Bresnahan, G. F., Roberts, R., Shell, W. E., Ross, J., Jr., and Sobel, B. E.: Deleterious effects due to hemorrhage after myocardial reperfusion. Am. J. Cardiol. *33*:82, 1974.
290. Hammermeister, K. E.: The effect of coronary bypass surgery on survival. Prog. Cardiovasc. Dis. *25*:297, 1983.
291. Phillips, S. J., Kongtahworn, C., Zeff, R. H., Benson, M., Iannone, L., Brown, T., and Gordon, D. F.: Emergency coronary artery revascularization: A possible therapy for acute myocardial infarction. Circulation *60*:241, 1979.
292. McIntosh, H. D., and Buccino, R. A.: Editorial—Emergency coronary artery revascularization of patients with acute myocardial infarction. You can . . . but should you? Circulation *60*:247, 1979.
293. Bery, R., Jr., Selinger, S. L., and Leonard, J. J.: Immediate coronary artery bypass for acute evolving myocardial infarction. J. Thorac. Cardiovasc. Surg. *81*:493, 1981.
294. DeWood, M. A., Spores, J., Notske, R. N., Lang, H. T., Shields, J. P., Simpson, C. S., Rudy, L. W., and Grunwald, R.: Medical and surgical management of myocardial infarction. Am. J. Cardiol. *44*:1356, 1979.
294a. DeWood, M. A., Heit, J., Spores, J., Berg, R., Jr., Selinger, S. L., Rudy, L. W., Hensley, G. R., and Shields, J. P.: Anterior transmural myocardial infarction: Effects of surgical coronary reperfusion on global and regional left ventricular function. J. Am. Coll. Cardiol. *1*:1223, 1983.
295. Kagen, L., Scheidt, S., and Butt, A.: Serum myoglobin in myocardial infarction: The "staccato phenomenon": Is acute myocardial infarction in man an intermittent event? Am. J. Med. *62*:86, 1977.
296. Loop, F. D., Cheanvechai, C., Sheldon, W. C., Taylor, P. C., and Effler, D. B.: Early myocardial revascularization during acute myocardial infarction. Chest *66*:478, 1974.
297. Gruntzig, A. R., Senning, A., and Siegenthaler, W. E.: Nonoperative dilatation of coronary artery stenosis. N. Engl. J. Med. *301*:61, 1979.
298. Kent, K. M., Bonow, R. O., Rosing, D. R., Ewels, C. J., Lipson, L. C., McIntosh, C. L., Bacharach, S., Green, M., and Epstein, S. E.: Improved myocardial function during exercise after successful percutaneous transluminal coronary angioplasty. N. Engl. J. Med. *306*:441, 1982.
299. DeWood, M. A., Spores, J., Notske, R., Mouser, L. T., Burroughs, R., Golden, M. S., and Lang, H. T.: Prevalence of total coronary occlusion during the early hours of transmural myocardial infarction. N. Engl. J. Med. *303*:897, 1980.
300. Rentrop, P., Blanke, H., Marsch, K. R., Kaiser, H., Kostering, H., and Leitz, K.: Selective intracoronary thrombolysis in acute myocardial infarction and unstable angina pectoris. Circulation *63*:307, 1981.
301. Ganz, W., Buchbinder, N., Marcus, H., Mondkar, A., Maddahi, J., Charuzi, Y., O'Conner, L., Shell, W., Fishbein, M. C., Cass, R., Miyamoto, A., and Swan, H. J. C.: Intracoronary thrombolysis in evolving myocardial infarction. Am. Heart J. *101*:4, 1981.
301a. Schroder, R., Biamino, G., Leitner, E-R. V., Linderer, T., Bruggemann, T., Heitz, J., Vohringer, H-F., and Wegscheider, K.: Intravenous short-term infusion of streptokinase in acute myocardial infarction. Circulation *67*:536, 1983.
301b. Feit, F., and Rentrop, K. P.: Thrombolytic therapy in acute myocardial infarction. Cardiovasc. Rev. Rep. *4*:426, 1983.
302. Markis, J. E., Malagold, M., Parker, J. A., Silverman, K. J., Barry, W. H., Als, A. V., Paulin, S., Grossman, W., and Braunwald, E.: Myocardial salvage after intracoronary thrombolysis with streptokinase in acute myocardial infarction: Assessment of intracoronary thallium-201. N. Engl. J. Med. *305*:777, 1981.
303. Mathey, D. G., Kuck, K-H., Tilsner, V., Krebber, H-J., and Bleifeld, W.: Nonsurgical coronary artery recanalization in acute transmural myocardial infarction. Circulation *63*:489, 1981.
304. Ganz, W., Geft, I., Maddahi, J., Berman, D., Charuzi, Y., Shah, P. K., and Swan, H. J. C.: Nonsurgical reperfusion in evolving myocardiol infarction. J. Am. Coll. Cardiol. *1*:1247, 1983.
305. Anderson, J. L., Marshall, H. W., Bray, B. E., Lutz, J. R., Frederick, P. R., Yanowitz, F. G., Datz, F. L., Klausner, S. C., and Hagan, A. D.: A randomized trial of intracoronary streptokinase in the treatment of acute myocardial infarction. N. Engl. J. Med. *308*:1312, 1983.
306. Maddahi, J., Ganz, W., Ninomiya, K., Hashida, J., Fishbein, M. C., Mondkar, A., Buchbinder, N., Marcus, H., Geft, I., Shah, P. K., Rozanski, A., Swan, H. J. C., and Berman, D. S.: Myocardial salvage by intracoronary thrombolysis in evolving acute myocardial infarction. Evaluation using intracoronary injection of thallium-201. Am. Heart J. *102*:664, 1981.
306a. Blanke, H., Schicha, H., Kaiser, H., Karsch, K. R., and Rentrop, K. P.: Long-term left ventricular function after intracoronary streptokinase therapy. J. Am Coll. Cardiol. *1*:579, 1983.
306b. Schwarz, F., Faure, A., Katus, H., VonOlshausen, K., Hofmann, M., Schuler, G., Manthey, J., and Kubler, W.: Intracoronary thrombolysis in acute myocardial infarction: An attempt to quantitate its effects by comparison of enzymatic estimate of myocardial necrosis with left ventricular ejection fraction. Am. J. Cardiol. *51*:1573, 1983.
307. Fujimoto, T., Peter, T., Hamamoto, H., and Mandel, W. J.: Electrophysiologic observations on ventricular tachyarrhythmias following reperfusion. Am. Heart J. *105*:201, 1983.
308. Sobel, B. E., and Bergmann, S. R.: Coronary thrombolysis: Some unresolved issues. Am. J. Med. *72*:1, 1982.
308a. Khaja, F., Walton, J. A., Jr., Brymer, J. F., Lo, E., Osterberger, L., O'Neill, W. W., Colfer, H. T., Weiss, R., Lee, T., Kurian, T., Goldberg, A. D., Pitt, B., and Goldstein, S.: Intracoronary fibrinolytic therapy in acute myocardial infarction. Report of a prospective randomized trial. N. Engl. J. Med. *308*:1305, 1983.
309. Krebber, H. J., Mathey, D., Kuck, K. J., Kalmar, P., and Rodewald, G.: Management of evolving myocardial infarction by intracoronary thrombolysis and subsequent aorta-coronary bypass. J. Thorac. Cardiovasc. Surg. *83*:186, 1982.
309a. Lolley, D. M., Fulton, R., Hamman, J., Reader, G. S., Johnson, J. L., Clarke, J. A., Sheth, M. K., and Hearne, M. J.: Early coronary artery surgery after intracoronary streptokinase thrombolytic therapy. J. Am. Coll. Cardiol. *1*:632, 1983.
310. Meyer, J., Merx, W., Dorr, R., Lambertz, H., Bethge, C., and Effert, S.: Successful treatment of acute myocardial infarction shock by combined percutaneous transluminal coronary recanalization (PTCR) and percutaneous transluminal coronary angioplasty (PTCA) Am. Heart J. *103*:132, 1982.
310a. Papapietro, S. E., MacLean, W. A. H., Stanley, A. W. H., Jr., Cooper, T. B., Hess, R. G., Siler, W., and Geer, D. A.: Percutaneous transluminal coronary angioplasty in acute myocardial infarction. J. Am. Coll. Cardiol. *1*:580, 1983.
310b. Schroder, R.: Systemic versus intracoronary streptokinase infusion in the treatment of acute myocardial infarction. J. Am. Coll. Cardiol. *1*:1254, 1983.
311. Ahlmark, G., Ahlberg, G., Saetre, H., Haglund, I., and Korsgren, M.: A controlled study of early discharge after uncomplicated myocardial infarction. Acta Med. Scand. *206*:87, 1979.
312. Lau, Y. K., Smith, J., Morrison, S. L., and Chamberlain, D. A.: Policy for early discharge after acute myocardial infarction. Br. Med. J. *281*:1489, 1980.
313. Friedman, M., Thoresen, C. E., Gill, J. J., Ulmer, D., Thompson, L., Powell, L., Price, V., Elek, S. R., Rabin, D. D., Breall, W. S., Piaget, G., Dixon, T., Bourg, E., Levy, R. A., and Tasto, D. L.: Feasibility of altering type A behavior pattern after myocardial infarction. Recurrent coronary prevention project study: Methods, baseline results and preliminary findings. Circulation *66*:83, 1982.
313a. Ewart, C. K., Taylor, C. B., Reese, L., and Debusk, R. F.: Effects of early postinfarction exercise testing on self perception and subsequent physical activity. J. Am. Coll. Cardiol. *1*:662, 1983.
314. Hood, W. B., Jr.: More on sulfinpyrazone after myocardial infarction. N. Engl. J. Med. *306*:988, 1982.
315. Rackley, C. E., Russell, R. O., Mantle, J. A., Rogers, W. J., and Papapietro, S. E.: Modern approach to myocardial infarction: Determination of prognosis and therapy. Am. Heart J. *101*:75, 1981.
316. Turner, J. D., Schwartz, K. M., Logic, J. R., Sheffield, L. T., Rensal, S., Roitman, D. I., Mantle, J. A., Russell, R. O., Rackley, C. E., and Rogers, W. J.: Detection of residual jeopardized myocardium three weeks after myocardial infarction by exercise testing with thallium 201 myocardial scintigraphy. Circulation *61*:729, 1980.
317. Forrester, J. S.: Do you routinely recommend coronary angiography after uncomplicated MI? J. Cardiovasc. Med. *6*:393, 1981.
318. Willerson, J. T., and Buja, L. M.: Cause and course of acute myocardial infarction. Am. J. Med. *69*:903, 1980.
319. Miller, D. H., and Borer, J. S.: Exercise testing early after myocardial infarction. Risks and benefits. Am. J. Med. *72*:427, 1982.
320. Fuller, C. M., Raizner, A. E., Verani, M. S., Nahormek, P. A., Chahine, R. A., McEntee, C. W., and Miller, R. R.: Early post-myocardial infarction treadmill stress testing. Ann. Intern. Med. *94*:734, 1981.
320a. Rapaport, E., and Remedios, P.: The high risk patient after recovery from myocardial infarction: Recognition and management. J. Am. Coll. Cardiol. *1*: 391, 1983.
320b. Mukharji, J., Rude, R., Gustafson, N., Poole, K., Passamani, E., Thomas, L. J., Jr., Strauss, H. W., Muller, J. E., Roberts, R., Raabe, D. S., Jr., Braunwald, E., Willerson, J. T., and cooperating investigators, MILIS: Late sudden death following myocardial infarction: Interdependence of risk factors. J. Am. Coll. Cardiol. *1*:585, 1983
321. Stone, P. H., and Muller, J. E.: Nifedipine therapy for recurrent ischemic pain following myocardial infarction. Clin. Cardiol. *5*:223, 1982.

39 CHRONIC ISCHEMIC HEART DISEASE

by Peter F. Cohn, M.D., and Eugene Braunwald, M.D.

Chronic ischemic heart disease is most commonly due to obstruction of the coronary arteries, which in turn usually results from atherosclerosis, a condition described in Chapter 34. The importance of ischemic heart disease in contemporary society is attested to by the almost epidemic number of persons afflicted—especially when this number is compared with the anecdotal reports of its occurrence in the medical literature prior to this century. Coronary artery disease causes more deaths, disability, and economic loss in industrialized nations than any other group of diseases. In the United States arteriosclerosis is responsible for nearly half of all deaths: almost one million annually. Each year, 200,000 Americans under the age of 65 years die with what has been called *premature* ischemic heart disease and another two million people are afflicted with it. In addition to enormous personal and family suffering, it has been estimated that these diseases cost the United States more than $50 billion in health expenditures and lost productivity.

HISTORICAL PERSPECTIVES

To appreciate this disease entity, some historical perspective is useful. Angina pectoris serves as a useful example, since it is the most common clinical presentation of chronic ischemic heart disease. The term was first used by Dr. William Heberden in a report published in 1772.[1] Unlike the word "dolor," which means pain, the word "angina" was intended to indicate a sense of *strangling*. Heberden noted that fear of death ("angor animi") often accompanies this sensation in the chest (or rather, observed with this symptom complex, episodes of discomfort in the "breast"). Heberden's description of angina is as accurate today as it was more than two centuries ago: "There is a disorder of the breast, marked with strong and peculiar symptoms considerable for the kind of danger belonging to it, and not extremely rare, of which I do not recollect any mention among medical authors. The seat of it, and sense of strangling and anxiety, with which it is attended, may make it not improperly be called angina pectoris. Those, who are afflicted with it, are seized while they are walking and most particularly when they walk soon after eating, with a painful and most disagreeable sensation in the breast, which seems as if it would take their life away, if it were to increase or to continue; the moment they stand still, all this uneasiness vanishes."

The pathophysiological mechanism of angina pectoris as being related to an imbalance between myocardial oxygen supply and demand was first appreciated in 1799 by C.H. Parry: "The rigidity of the coronary arteries may act, proportionately to the extent of the ossification, as a mechanical impediment to the free motion of the heart; and though a quantity of blood may circulate through these arteries, sufficient to nourish the heart, yet there may probably be less than what is requisite for ready and vigorous action. Hence, though a heart so diseased may be fit for the purposes of common circulation, during a state of bodily and mental tranquility, and of health otherwise good, yet when any unusual exertion is required, its powers may fail, under the new and extraordinary demand."[2]

An indirect commentary on the incidence of coronary atherosclerosis is provided by the medical literature dealing with angina. Following Heberden's original account of angina pectoris, few reports dealt with this syndrome before the beginning of the 20th century. For example, in a textbook of medicine by Austin Flint published in 1866,[3] only two pages were devoted to angina pectoris. There appears to have been far less coronary artery disease 100 years ago than now, for it seems hard to believe that it could have escaped attention if acute myocardial infarction and sudden death occurred with any frequency in young and middle-aged men. In the mid-19th century, renewed interest in angina pectoris was stimulated by Brunton's report on the use of amyl nitrate for the treatment of angina pectoris,[4] yet when William Osler published his textbook of medicine in 1892,[5] he still referred to angina as a rare condition. Osler believed that complete obliteration of a coronary artery, if produced suddenly, was usually fatal. Although he recognized different gradations of anginal pain,[6] nonfatal acute myocardial infarction as a separate entity was appreciated for the first time with the reports of Obraztov and Strazhesko in Russia in 1910[7] and of Herrick in the United States in 1912.[8]

The work of these clinical pioneers did not receive much attention initially, possibly because the condition was not yet common enough for physicians to appreciate its importance. This may be due to the fact that even in the early 20th century, the large hospitals of the country were "reserved" for the indigent, who were often malnourished; the more affluent private patients in whom the incidence of ischemic heart disease was greater, were seen at home. P. D. White became interested in coronary artery disease early in the 20th century; however, while in medical school and as an intern and resident in Boston, he stated that he received no instruction or experience that helped him recognize this condition. In 1968, he reviewed the hospital records of 800 patients who had been under his care as an intern at the Massachusetts General Hospital in 1912–1913.[9] Of 700 men, mainly between the ages of 20 and 60 years, only eight were diagnosed as having angina pectoris; three had syphilitic aortitis as the cause of their pain, and one had rheumatic aortic regurgitation. Thus, it appears that symptomatic ischemic heart disease was quite uncommon at the Massachusetts General Hospital at the beginning of the 20th century. In the early 1920's, ischemic heart disease aroused more interest, and there were increasing reports of its occurrence. Wearn, at the Peter Bent Brigham Hospital, described a premonitory chest pain syndrome before the actual myocardial infarction occurred —a forerunner of the syndrome currently named unstable angina.[10]

With the development of cardiology as a specialty, interest in coronary artery disease grew rapidly. The diagnostic value of the electrocardiogram became appreciated, as did the importance of electrocardiographic abnormalities occasioned by exercise. Perhaps the most important next step in understanding the pathophysiology of chronic ischemic heart disease was the clinical-pathological correlation described by Blumgart, Schlesinger, and Zoll at Boston's Beth Israel Hospital.[11] Their studies were particularly important because they demonstrated the different histopathological findings in patients with angina pectoris and myocardial infarction, and they stressed the importance of the collateral circulation. Two decades after the work of Blumgart and associates the modern era of study of coronary artery disease began with the introduction of coronary arteriography by Sones in 1959,[12] allowing the evaluation of coronary anatomy in vivo.

There is no uniform presenting syndrome for chronic ischemic heart disease. Although chest discomfort is usually the predominant symptom in chronic (stable), unstable, or variant angina and acute myocardial infarction, syndromes of ischemic heart disease also occur in which ischemic chest discomfort is absent or not prominent. These include asymptomatic myocardial ischemia, cardiac arrhythmias, and congestive heart failure. Myocardial ischemia may also occur in the absence of coronary atherosclerosis (as in aortic valve disease, hypertrophic cardiomyopathy, and syphilitic aortitis), and coronary artery disease may occur together with these other forms of heart disease. Finally, the various syndromes characteristic of ischemic heart disease may complicate noncardiac disease, e.g., coronary artery disease may occur in patients with chronic renal failure requiring dialysis.

CHRONIC (STABLE) ANGINA PECTORIS

CLINICAL MANIFESTATIONS

CHARACTERISTICS OF ANGINA (see also p. 5). Heberden's initial description of the chest discomfort as conveying a sense of "strangling and anxiety" is still remarkably pertinent today, although adjectives used to describe this distress now include "viselike," "constricting," "suffocating," "crushing," "heavy," and "squeezing." In other patients, the quality of the sensation is even more vague and may be described as a mild pressure-like discomfort or an uncomfortable numb sensation. The site of the discomfort is usually retrosternal, but radiation is common and usually occurs down the ulnar surface of the left arm; commonly, the right arm and the outer surfaces of both arms are also involved.[13] Sampson and Cheitlin have documented the large number of regions that can be sites of radiation, with neck, jaw, and throat pain observed most commonly.[14] Headache is uncommon,[15] and discomfort below the epigastrium due to angina is rare. Anginal "equivalents" (i.e., symptoms of myocardial ischemia other than angina) such as breathlessness, faintness, fatigue, and belching have also been reported.

The etiology of the discomfort is complex and not fully understood.[16] For example, the specific substance that actually stimulates sympathetic afferents and begins the series of interactions that culminate in chest discomfort has not been identified.[17] Some evidence favors agents that are released from cells as a result of transient ischemia, such as bradykinin, histamine, or serotonin.[18] Acidosis or elevated potassium concentration in the involved tissues may trigger release of these substances to which the sensory end-plates of the intracardiac sympathetic nerves appear to be particularly sensitive. The end-plates are the receptors of a network of unmyelinated nerves that lie between cardiac muscle fibers and that are also found around coronary vessels, travel to the cardiac plexus, and then ascend to the sympathetic ganglia (C7-T4). Impulses are transmitted to corresponding spinal ganglia, then via the spinal cord to the thalamus, and finally to the cerebral cortex.

The discomfort of myocardial ischemia is perceived in various regions of the chest because it is "referred" to the corresponding peripheral dermatomes that supply afferent nerves to the same segment of the spinal cord as the heart. A plausible explanation is that a common pool of secondary neurons can be stimulated by somatic and visceral afferent impulses.[19] If visceral stimuli are excessive, the nearby intermediate neurons that are receptors for somatic impulses may be excited, and the discomfort will then be perceived as being cutaneous in origin. Thus, pain impulses can be referred to the medial aspects of the arm via common connections to the brachial plexus and can be referred to the neck via connections with the cervical roots.

It is not clear why some patients with clear-cut evidence of ischemic heart disease experience no chest discomfort; diabetics, in particular, appear to have a higher frequency of "silent" ischemia, presumably because of autonomic denervation. In some patients chest pain disappears after a myocardial infarction, even though other evidence of paroxysmal ischemia, such as ST-segment depression, may persist. It is postulated that in these patients the nerve endings may have been damaged as a result of the infarction. Finally, patients with reproducible evidence of myocardial ischemia may or may not experience chest pain with each of the various episodes. Ambulatory electrocardiography has revealed that the majority of patients with angina also experience numerous episodes of silent ischemia, i.e., ST-segment and T-wave changes, identical to those occurring during typical angina but unaccompanied by chest discomfort; the frequency of these episodes is reduced by treatment with beta blockers and calcium-channel blockers, supporting the contention that they represent instances of myocardial ischemia.

The fact that the discomfort of angina is not uniform and that other entities can mimic it often makes the differential diagnosis of chest pain difficult[13,17,20] (Table 1–1, p. 5). Differentiating the discomfort resulting from these noncardiac disorders from angina pectoris is usually possible when the *quality* of the pain and its *duration, precipitating factors*, and *associated symptoms* are taken into consideration (Table 39–1).[14] Thus, the *typical* anginal episode usually begins gradually and reaches maximum intensity over a period of minutes before dissipating—usually as a result of cessation of the activity that precipitated it. One should consider *noncoronary* causes in patients with sharp, stabbing, or burning chest pain that comes and goes in a matter of seconds or with a dull, continuous ache in the chest. Similarly, changes in posture do not usually affect the discomfort of myocardial ischemia, and this maneuver helps to distinguish angina from pericardial disease or hiatus hernia. In typical angina, the pain is related to

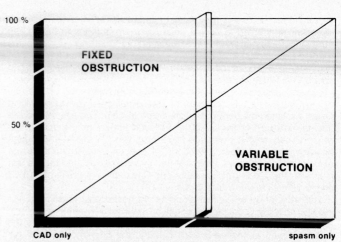

FIGURE 39–1   Different mixtures of fixed and variable obstruction may produce myocardial ischemia. The vertical bar represents a patient in whom both spasm (variable obstruction) and fixed obstruction play significant roles in occluding a coronary artery. This variable mixture of spasm and fixed obstruction may be present not only in Prinzmetal's angina but in classic angina and acute myocardial infarction as well. (From Muller, J. E.: Prinzmetal's angina: A model for the role of spasm in ischemic heart disease. J. Cardiovasc. Med. *5*:19, 1980.)

an increase in myocardial oxygen demands, most commonly brought about by physical activity; the *rate* at which a task is carried out is important. Hurrying is particularly likely to precipitate angina, as are efforts involving motion of the hands over the head. Emotion or eating, particularly when combined with physical activity, commonly causes angina, as do a variety of other factors, including the excessive metabolic demands imposed by chills and fever, thyrotoxicosis, tachycardia from any cause, severe anemia, and hypoglycemia. In all these conditions, underlying fixed coronary artery obstruction in the form of atheromatous disease is usually present, and the other factors (e.g., exercise, fever) increase the activity of the heart, stimulate myocardial oxygen needs in the presence of a fixed and limited oxygen-supply, and thus precipitate ischemia and chest discomfort.

There is increasing evidence, however, that angina may also be caused by transient reductions of oxygen supply as a consequence of *coronary vasoconstriction*.[21–24,24a,24b] As pointed out on page 1241, the coronary arterial bed is well innervated and a variety of stimuli alter coronary tone. There is a reciprocal relation between the severity of dynamic and organic obstruction required to cause myocardial ischemia. Thus, in persons with no organic lesions, only severe dynamic obstruction—as occurs in the coronary spasm of Prinzmetal's angina—can cause myocardial ischemia and resultant angina. On the other hand, in patients with severe, although subcritical, fixed obstruction to coronary flow, only a minor increase in dynamic obstruction is necessary to cause blood flow to fall below a critical level and cause myocardial ischemia (Fig. 39–1).

FIXED- VS. VARIABLE-THRESHOLD ANGINA. The variability of the threshold for angina differs among patients. In patients with *fixed-threshold angina*, with few if any dynamic (vasoconstrictive) components, the level of physical activity, a reflection of myocardial oxygen consumption, required to precipitate angina is relatively constant. Characteristically, these patients can predict with

---

TABLE 39–1   CHARACTERISTICS OF ANGINA PECTORIS

Quality
　Sensation of pressure or heavy weight on the chest
　Burning sensation
　Feeling of tightness
　Shortness of breath with feeling of constriction about the larynx or
　　upper trachea
　Visceral quality (deep, heavy, squeezing, aching)
　Gradual increase in intensity followed by gradual fading away
Location
　Over the sternum or very near to it
　Anywhere between epigastrium and pharynx
　Occasionally limited to left shoulder and left arm
　Rarely limited to right arm
　Limited to lower jaw
　　Lower cervical or upper thoracic spine
　Left interscapular or suprascapular area
Duration
　0.5 to 30 minutes
Precipitating Factors
　Relationship to exercise
　Effort which involves use of arms above the head
　Cold environment
　Walking against the wind
　Walking after a large meal
　Emotional factors involved with physical exercise
　Fright, anger
　Coitus
Nitroglycerin Relief
　Relief of pain occurring within 45 seconds to 5 minutes of taking ni-
　　troglycerin
Radiation
　Medial aspect of left arm
　Left shoulder
　Jaw
　Occasionally right arm

From Helfant, R. H., and Banka, V. S.: A Clinical and Angiographic Approach to Coronary Heart Disease. Philadelphia, F. A. Davis Co., 1978, p. 47.

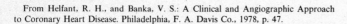

precision the amount of physical activity that causes angina, e.g., walking up exactly two and a half flights of stairs. When these patients are tested on a treadmill or bicycle, the pressure-rate product that elicits angina and/or electrocardiographic evidence of ischemia is fixed or almost so. Patients with *variable-threshold angina*, who may or may not have a fixed obstructive lesion but in whom dynamic obstruction caused by vasoconstriction plays an important role in causing myocardial ischemia, typically have "good days," when they are capable of substantial physical activity, and "bad days," when even minimal activity can cause clinical and/or electrocardiographic evidence of myocardial ischemia or when angina occurs at rest. Often, even in the course of a single day, they may be capable of substantial physical activity at one time, while at another time minimal activity will result in angina. Patients with variable-threshold angina typically complain occasionally of angina at rest, nocturnal angina, and angina precipitated by the cold, emotion, and meals. It is presumed that coronary vasoconstriction is responsible for or contributes to the development of angina under all these circumstances. The anginal threshold tends to be lower in the morning than in the afternoon, correlating with the angiographic finding of smaller coronary arterial lumina at that time of day.[25] Many patients fall between these two extremes (Fig. 39–1), i.e., their anginal threshold is moderately variable; the term *mixed angina* is suggested to describe this large group.

Changes in the blood pressure–heart rate product (the double product) provide a rough approximation of myocardial oxygen requirements (p. 1238). In patients with effort-induced fixed-threshold angina, the threshold at which ischemia develops (as reflected in angina and ST-segment depression) is a function of myocardial oxygen requirement. In patients with (relatively) fixed-threshold angina, the time and effort required for the development of angina during treadmill exercise is relatively predictable and reproducible; it is probable that as the performance of the ventricle (and therefore its oxygen consumption) increases, a point is reached at which myocardial perfusion distal to a major coronary arterial obstruction can no longer increase, and ischemia ensues.

Observations in patients experiencing angina under circumstances other than exercise help to explain the pathophysiological bases of angina. For example, some patients with ischemic heart disease characteristically experience angina on exposure to *cold weather* or *during or after meals*. A cold environment has been shown to increase peripheral resistance at rest and during exercise.[26] The rise in arterial pressure, by augmenting myocardial oxygen requirements, lowers the threshold for the development of angina. An alternative, or additional, explanation is the development of coronary spasm.[27,28] The reduction in exercise capacity during or after meals has been explained by a more rapid rise in heart rate and blood pressure compared to preprandial values,[29] but the postprandial increase in myocardial oxygen needs may not be sufficient to explain the development of ischemia, and a dynamic component, i.e., coronary vasoconstriction, may also be involved.[30] Similarly, during angina induced by *emotional stress*, heart rate and blood pressure and therefore myocardial oxygen needs rise but usually not to the level required to produce

angina during exercise. Therefore, a dynamic component probably plays a role as well.[31]

Relief of anginal discomfort is usually afforded by rest (not by "walking through") and by sublingual nitroglycerin; indeed, the response to the drug is often a useful diagnostic tool.[32] A longer delay before relief is obtained, i.e., more than 5 to 10 minutes, suggests that the pain is not ischemic in origin. As described by Levine, carotid sinus pressure can also often bring about rapid alleviation of discomfort.[33]

In *atypical angina* the precipitating factors may be similar, but the quality of the discomfort is different (sharp and stabbing, for example); or, if the quality of the discomfort is angina-like, the precipitating causes are unusual, such as varying body positions; or the discomfort may be typical in quality and occur only at rest but may not be accompanied by characteristic ST-segment changes. *Nonanginal chest pain* has neither the quality of typical angina nor its usual precipitating causes.

CLINICAL-PATHOLOGICAL CORRELATIONS OF ANGINA. The prevalence of coronary artery disease in subsets of patients with typical angina, atypical angina, and nonanginal chest pain has been estimated by Diamond and Forrester to be about 90 per cent, 50 per cent, and 16 per cent, respectively, while the prevalence of coronary artery disease in asymptomatic adults of comparable age is estimated to be 3 to 4 per cent.[34] Pasternak et al. reported that among 3242 patients in whom coronary angiograms were obtained for chest pain, 175 (5.4%) had essentially normal coronary vessels. Of the latter, about one-third had chest pain typical of angina and in two-thirds it was atypical.[35] There is a suggestion from a number of reports[36–39] that on the whole the clinical manifestations of ischemia may be more severe in patients with multivessel than single-vessel disease, but in any individual patient the nature of the underlying disease cannot be predicted from the severity, nature, duration, or quality of the discomfort. Perhaps the best examples of this lack of clinical-pathological correlation are two groups of patients who are relatively common: those with advanced obstructive disease and so-called "silent ischemia"[40–42] (p. 1362) and those with Prinzmetal's angina (p. 1360). For comparable degrees of obstructive coronary artery disease, as defined arteriographically, asymptomatic or minimally symptomatic patients have a better prognosis than do those with severe angina.[42] When infarction (without angina) is the first manifestation of ischemic heart disease, it is usually associated with single-vessel disease; when angina occurs before and/or after infarction, two- or three-vessel disease is usually present.[43]

Differential Diagnosis of Chest Pain
(Table 1–1, p. 5)

The differentiation of various disorders from coronary artery disease is challenging because the severity of the chest pain and the seriousness of the underlying disorder are not necessarily related. Compounding the difficulty in differential diagnosis is the common myth that pain in the left arm or left side of the chest is an ominous sign signifying the presence of coronary artery disease. A host of disorders can cause these types of discomfort.[20] *Esophagitis* can produce discomfort that can mimic that of myocardial ischemia because it is usually substernal in location and may have a "burning" component. Because there is usually an element of esophageal spasm, discomfort is often relieved by nitroglycerin or, unlike angina, by milk or antacids as well. Acid infusion studies, radiological studies, and esophagoscopy are helpful in confirming the diagnosis of this disorder.[44] Gastric reflux is often associated with *hiatus hernia*, which can also be diagnosed radiographically; postprandial distress is most marked in the recumbent position, and this feature helps to differentiate it from angina pectoris.[45] Distention of the splenic flexure of the colon can mimic anginal pain, but, unlike angina, relief of symptoms often follows a bowel movement. The major *musculoskeletal disorders* that can mimic angina include subacromial bursitis and costochondritis.[46] Cervical radiculitis may occur as a constant ache, often resulting in a sensory deficit. The pain may be related to motion of the neck, just as motion of the shoulder triggers attacks of pain that are due to *bursitis*. The full-blown *Tietze syndrome*, i.e., painful swelling of the costochondral junctions, is uncommon, whereas costochondritis causing tenderness of the costochondral joints is relatively common[47]; pain on palpation of these joints is a useful clinical sign. Physical examination may also detect pain brought about by movement of an arthritic shoulder, a calcified shoulder tendon, and the like. Occasionally, pain mimicking angina can be due to compression of the brachial plexus by a cervical rib.

Other cardiovascular diseases may also mimic angina pectoris. In addition to *aortic dissection*, which usually is characterized by sharp, intense, retrosternal pain with radiation to the back (p. 1550), *pulmonary hypertension* may also be a problem in differential diagnosis (p. 840). The discomfort produced by the latter is generally precordial and, although often precipitated by exertion, is usually more persistent than angina. Pulmonary hypertension must be severe to cause chest pain and may be readily recognized by the findings of right ventricular hypertrophy on physical examination and electrocardiography. The discomfort that is perhaps most difficult to differentiate from angina is that produced by *acute pericarditis* (p. 1474), which is usually relieved by sitting up and leaning forward and is intensified by the supine posture. A friction rub often helps to confirm the diagnosis.

In many of the disorders just mentioned, angina pectoris can usually be excluded by a careful history and physical examination. Brief episodes of sharp, stabbing pain or continual dull aches of a burning or boring quality commonly observed with gastrointestinal disorders are not characteristic of angina, nor is the response to antacids or eating. On the other hand, the major point in differentiating between angina and musculoskeletal disorders usually relates to an abnormality found on physical examination, with tenderness either on palpation or on movement of the affected part. It must be stressed, however, that ischemic heart disease can and frequently does *coexist* with any of these other disorders and that occasionally noncardiac disease can trigger a true anginal attack in a patient with coronary artery disease. For example, the sympathoadrenal discharge that accompanies biliary colic may increase heart rate and blood pressure and thereby increase myocardial oxygen requirements, so that myocardial ischemia may develop in a patient with obstructive coronary artery disease.

Chest Pain with Normal Coronary Arteriogram

The syndrome of angina or angina-like chest pain with a normal coronary arteriogram is an important clinical entity to be differentiated from classic ischemic heart disease caused by coronary atherosclerosis.[35,48–55] In this condition, the prognosis is usually excellent—contrasted with that in patients with coronary atherosclerosis—and hence its recognition is of critical importance. Patients with chest pain who have normal coronary arteries may constitute as many as 20 per cent of individuals undergoing coronary arteriography because of the strong suspicion of angina. The etiology of the syndrome is unknown. True myocardial ischemia, reflected in the production of lactate by the myocardium during exercise or pacing, is present in only a small fraction of these patients. However, in one study, the increase in coronary blood flow following dipyridamole, a potent coronary vasodilator, was found to be reduced, and this inability to augment coronary blood flow was associated with a decline of left ventricular function during exercise; presumably an abnormality of the small arteries was responsible for the angina and ischemia.[54] Some patients with angina and normal coronary arteries are found on extensive investigation to have a cardiomyopathy—either hypertrophic or congestive—and in these cases reduced perfusion, especially of the subendocardium, may be responsible for myocardial ischemia and resultant angina.[55] Herman et al. discussed some of the theories proffered for this syndrome; an abnormal oxyhemoglobin dissociation curve, misinterpretation of arteriography, occult cardiomyopathy, and psychomotor factors.[51] Patients with psychogenic chest pain, neurocirculatory asthenia, and Da Costa's syndrome (p. 6) also fall into this category. These patients are not considered to have coronary spasm because of the absence of a typical response to ergonovine (p. 1361); they rarely develop acute myocardial infarction, but if they do, their long-term prognosis tends to be favorable because they do not have diffuse coronary artery disease. The syndrome of angina or angina-like chest pain occurs more frequently in women, while obstructive coronary artery disease is far more common in men. Fewer than half the patients with chest pain with normal coronary arteriograms have typical angina; the majority have a variety of forms of atypical chest pain.

Abnormal physical findings such as precordial bulges, gallop sounds, and murmurs of mitral regurgitation are uncommon. The resting electrocardiogram may be normal, but nonspecific ST-T abnormalities are often observed. A minority, approximately 20 per cent of the patients with chest pain and normal coronary arteriograms, have positive exercise tests. Left ventricular function is usually normal at rest and after pacing,[56–58] unlike the situation in obstructive coronary artery disease in which function is or becomes impaired during stress. However, a small number of these patients exhibit lactate production and electrocardiographic changes (ST-segment depression) during stress, signifying ischemia, for as yet unexplained reasons. Myocardial perfusion studies have not shown any consistent pattern of abnormal myocardial blood flow,[59,60] although coronary vasodilator reserve may be impaired.[52,54] *Management* of patients with this syndrome is focused on the explanation of the relatively benign nature of the condition to the patient, psychological counseling, and analgesics to provide pain relief. However, many of these patients continue to remain disabled with chest discomfort despite these measures.[51]

Physical Examination of the Patient with Chronic Stable Angina

General physical examination of the patient with chronic ischemic heart disease and angina pectoris may be entirely normal or may reveal the presence of risk factors for the development of coronary atherosclerosis. Thus, the blood pressure either may be chronically elevated or may rise acutely (along with the heart rate) during an anginal attack.[61,62] The general examination may also reveal xanthomas suggestive of hypercholesterolemia (p. 17); arcus senilis in patients under 50 years of age also suggests this metabolic abnormality, but this sign is less significant in older persons. Precordial tenderness is uncommon in angina, and the presence of costosternal tenderness suggests that angina is not responsible for the chest discomfort. An interesting finding is the diagonal earlobe crease, reportedly more prevalent in patients with coronary artery disease[63]; however, the interpretation of this sign is controversial.[64] Retinal arteriolar changes are common in patients with coronary artery disease, even in those without diabetes mellitus or hypertension; an abnormal light reflex is the most sensitive sign, while abnormal vessel tortuosity and decreased caliber are less sensitive but more specific signs.[65]

The *cardiac examination*, long considered of little help in the diagnosis of chronic coronary artery disease, especially in patients with only a history of angina pectoris, actually may supply useful clues to both the diagnosis of ischemic heart disease and the functional state of the myocardium. First, the presence of murmurs of hypertrophic obstructive cardiomyopathy or aortic valve disease suggests that the ischemic chest pain may be due to conditions other than, or in addition to, coronary artery disease. Second, certain findings suggest ischemia as the basis for the chest pain if other obvious cardiac diseases are absent. A prime example is the presence of a third or a loud fourth heart sound,[66,67] and the presence of prominent early diastolic or presystolic filling waves on the apexcardiogram. Although these are common findings in patients with angina at rest,[66] their frequency is increased during handgrip exercise,[68] even if the latter does not precipitate angina pectoris. These sounds and pulsations are related to the functional state of the left ventricle, particularly its pressure and compliance during diastole (p. 50)[66–69]; their absence does not exclude significant coronary atherosclerosis but instead suggests the absence of left ventricular dysfunction. Although the specificity of the fourth heart sound as a finding diagnostic of cardiac disease has been questioned, since it is heard in many apparently normal subjects over 45 years of age,[70,71] we agree with Tavel[72] that a clear, loud fourth heart sound accompanied by a palpable presystolic wave is an abnormal finding. It is not specific for ischemic heart disease but may also be elicited in other conditions associated with left ventricular hypertrophy, like aortic stenosis and hypertension, in which left ventricular compliance is reduced. Paradoxical splitting of the second heart sound may occur transiently during an anginal attack. It appears to be related to asynergy and

prolongation of left ventricular contraction. Abnormal left ventricular function may also be documented by abnormalities in systolic time intervals, i.e., prolongation of the preejection period (PEP), shortening of the systolic ejection period (SEP), and an increase in PEP/SEP (p. 55).

When patients with ischemic heart disease lie in the left lateral recumbent position, dyskinetic bulges at the apex may be palpated or recorded by means of apexcardiography (p. 62); the bulges correspond to dyskinetic areas and often complement the auscultatory findings of diastolic filling sounds. Transient or persistent apical systolic murmurs are quite common and have been attributed to papillary muscle dysfunction secondary to myocardial ischemia.[67] They are more prevalent in patients with extensive coronary artery disease, especially those with prior myocardial infarction and left ventricular dysfunction. The systolic murmur may assume a variety of configurations (early, late, or holosystolic) and may be accentuated by exertion or during angina. A midsystolic click, often followed by a late systolic murmur characteristic of mitral valve prolapse produced by papillary muscle dysfunction (p. 1076), also occurs in patients with coronary artery disease.[73] A diastolic murmur or a continuous murmur is a rare finding and has been attributed to turbulent flow across a proximal coronary artery stenosis.[74]

ELECTROCARDIOGRAM. The resting electrocardiogram is normal in one-fourth to one-half of patients with chronic stable angina pectoris, depending on the incidence of previous myocardial infarction in the particular series of patients.[75] Patients with normal tracings may have severe angina, but they usually have not previously suffered large infarctions. When the electrocardiogram is abnormal, the most common findings are nonspecific ST-T changes with or without evidence of prior transmural infarction; however, a variety of conduction disturbances, most frequently left bundle branch block and left anterior divisional block, have also been reported. However, these are nonspecific signs and occur in many conditions other than ischemic heart disease. A variety of arrhythmias, especially ventricular premature beats, may be present, but they too are nonspecific. P-wave abnormalities indicative of left atrial enlargement are frequently associated with impairment of left ventricular contractility. Q waves are specific although insensitive indicators of abnormal wall motion. Correlation between the electrocardiographic pattern of myocardial infarction and total obstruction of the coronary artery perfusing that segment of the ventricle is excellent.[76]

NONINVASIVE STRESS TESTING

The contemporary approach to the use of noninvasive stress testing in the diagnosis and evaluation of patients with known or suspected ischemic heart disease has been well summarized by Gibson and Beller.[77] For appropriate application of noninvasive tests, it is important to consider Bayes theorem (p. 273), which states that while the reliability of any test is defined by its sensitivity and specificity,* its predictability depends on the prevalence of the disease in the population under study (Fig. 39–2). In interpreting the results of stress tests for the diagnosis of

---

*For definition of these terms; see page 273.

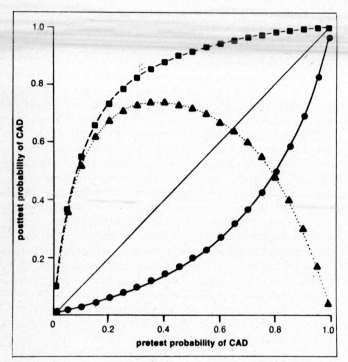

FIGURE 39–2 Pre- and posttest probability of CAD for abnormal and normal results of exercise-redistribution thallium-201 scintigraphy. The curve describing the difference between posttest probability of a normal and abnormal test result indicates the range of disease prevalence for which ²⁰¹Tl at exercise and redistribution discriminates most effectively between the presence and absence of disease. ²⁰¹Tl stress scintigraphy is most useful when the pretest prevalence of CAD is 20 to 60 per cent. *Example*: In a patient with a pretest probability of CAD of 60 per cent, a positive ²⁰¹Tl stress test increases the probability of CAD to about 95 per cent, but a negative test decreases it to about 25 per cent. On the other hand, at a very high or very low pretest probability of disease, not much will be gained by either a positive or a negative test result. ■ = abnormal; ▲ = posttest probability difference; ● = normal. (From Hamilton, G. W., et al.: Semin. Nucl. Med. *8*:358, 1978.)

ischemic heart disease, it is vital to consider the patient population being studied, i.e., the estimated prevalence of the disease *prior* to testing. Thus, if the pretest likelihood of the patient having coronary artery disease is low (less than 15 per cent), as occurs in asymptomatic persons or patients with so-called nonanginal chest pain, a normal result on any of the three commonly employed noninvasive tests (exercise electrocardiography, stress myocardial perfusion scintigraphy, and stress radionuclide angiography) may be used to exclude coronary disease. However, when a positive test in these individuals is a false-positive response, as often occurs, a second noninvasive test is indicated; if it too is positive, coronary artery disease is likely. On the other hand, when the pretest likelihood of disease is high, approximately 85 per cent, as in patients with typical angina pectoris, a positive test is helpful in that it confirms the disease and often provides an indication of its severity.[77] An unexpected negative result does not exclude the diagnosis of coronary disease; under these circumstances, a second or third noninvasive test would be of value, since it might identify the first test as being falsely negative. On the other hand, if the second test is also negative, reevaluation of the patient is clearly in order. Maximal benefit from noninvasive diagnostic testing is obtained when the pretest likelihood for disease is approximately 50

per cent, as in patients with atypical angina pectoris. In them, a positive test raises the likelihood of significant coronary artery disease to approximately 85 per cent and a negative test reduces it to 15 per cent.

EXERCISE ELECTROCARDIOGRAPHY (p. 267).

The recording of an electrocardiogram during and after exercise, especially if angina is precipitated, can be a valuable adjunct in the evaluation of patients suspected of having ischemic heart disease[78,79]; this important technique is the subject of Chapter 8. The degree of ST-segment depression has been combined with the configuration, time of onset, and persistence of depression during treadmill testing to increase the sensitivity and specificity of the test.[80] Early onset of ST-segment depression, its long persistence following exercise, and most importantly its shape, i.e., the slope of the segment (Fig. 39–3), are all strongly associated with extensive coronary artery disease (Table 39–2). Increases in R-wave height with exercise in one or more leads, possibly reflecting an increase in left ventricular volume, are often associated with coronary artery disease and left ventricular dysfunction.[81]

There is increasing interest in *nonelectrocardiographic findings* during exercise testing as indicators of severe coronary artery disease. In particular, attention has been called to the development of hypotension as important in predicting the presence of coronary artery disease.[82,83] Multifactorial approaches are being utilized[84–86] that include both electrocardiographic and nonelectrocardiographic measurements, such as the duration of the test and the heart rate response, to improve the accuracy of the exercise test. The occurrence of chest pain early during the test has been correlated with increased risk of future myocardial infarction and coronary death[87] and appears to be an-

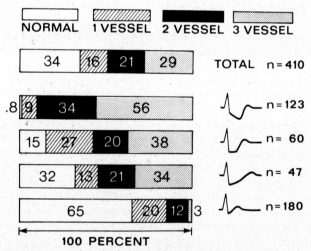

FIGURE 39–3 Relation between the type of ST-segment response in an exercise test and the extent of coronary artery disease. All numbers represent percentages. The total study population is represented at the top. Downsloping ST segments are highly specific for coronary disease, with only one false-positive response (0.8 per cent) encountered; most patients with this response (90 per cent) have double- and triple-vessel involvement. Neither the horizontal nor the slowly upsloping ST segments aid in identifying severe disease. A small percentage (15 per cent) of patients with entirely normal treadmill tests have double- and triple-vessel disease. (From Goldschlager, N., et al.: Treadmill stress tests as indicators of presence and severity of coronary artery disease. Ann. Intern. Med. *85*: 277, 1976.)

TABLE 39–2 CAUSES OF FALSE-POSITIVE EXERCISE ST-SEGMENT
RESPONSE

1. Abnormality in baseline ECG at rest due to digitalis, left ventricular hypertrophy, Wolff-Parkinson-White syndrome and other preexcitation variants, hypokalemia, bundle branch block, or vasoregulatory asthenia.
2. Failure before exercise to exclude hyperventilation-induced ST abnormality, recent food intake, or anemia.
3. ECG baseline instability during test simulating ST-segment displacement.
4. Sudden excessive exercise with excessive double product.
5. Various cardiac disorders, such as valvular or congenital heart disease, cardiomyopathy, mitral valve prolapse syndrome, hypertension, hypertrophic obstructive cardiomyopathy, and pericardial disorders.

Exercise Test Variables Associated with Multivessel Coronary Artery Disease and Increased Risk for Subsequent Myocardial Infarction or Sudden Death

ST-segment response:
    1. 2 mm or more horizontal or downsloping ST-segment depression at heart rate ≤ 130 beats/min.
    2. Postexercise ST-segment depression persisting ≥ 5 min.
Systolic blood pressure response to progressive exercise:
    1. Flat response (< 10 mm Hg rise for 2 stages).
    2. Sustained decrease of ≥ 10 mm Hg.
Exercise capacity:
    1. Inability to complete stage II of Bruce protocol or equivalent.
    2. Maximal heart rate < 70 per cent of age-predicted maximum.
Frequent or complex ventricular arrhythmias at low heart rate.

From Gibson, R. S., and Beller, G. A.: Should exercise electrocardiographic testing be replaced by radioisotope methods? *In* Rahimtoola, S. H. (ed.): Controversies in Coronary Artery Disease. Philadelphia, F. A. Davis Co., 1983, p. 1–31.

other useful diagnostic feature. In patients with coronary arteriographically proven ischemic heart disease, survival correlated directly with the duration of exercise that the patient could tolerate[79] and with the time during the test at which ST-segment depression occurred (Figs. 8–11, p. 274, and 8–12, p. 275).

The exercise test is also useful for exposing ventricular ectopic activity[88] but is less sensitive in this regard than is *ambulatory electrocardiographic monitoring* for 24 hours.[89] Patients with the more severe forms of coronary artery disease and abnormal left ventricular function have been shown to have a greater prevalence of exercise-induced arrhythmias.[90,91] Ambulatory electrocardiographic monitoring can also document the presence of ischemia in patients with coronary artery disease, with a good correlation between ST-segment depression occurring during normal activity and severe arteriographic abnormalities having been reported[92]; pain often does not accompany the ST-segment depression.[93] However, false-positive responses in patients free of coronary artery disease limit the usefulness of ambulatory 24-hour monitoring.[94]

In 16 studies summarized by Gibson and Beller in which results of exercise electrocardiography and coronary arteriography were compared, the overall sensitivity of the former test averaged 64 per cent and the specificity 89 per cent.[77] The extent of coronary artery disease affects the sensitivity of the test, i.e., the test is substantially more sensitive as the number of involved coronary vessels increases, rising from 44 per cent in patients with one-vessel disease to 85 per cent in patients with three-vessel and left main coronary artery disease. Thus, in view of the relatively low sensitivity of the test, a negative result does not rule out ischemic heart disease; however, it does make three-

vessel or left main disease much less likely. Conversely, an adequate maximum exercise test, one achieving more than 85 per cent of the predicted maximal heart rate, is unlikely to miss significant three-vessel or left main coronary artery disease. In normal asymptomatic persons, the incidence of false-positive exercise electrocardiograms is relatively high, approximately 40 per cent. Although the test is not very helpful for evaluating individual asymptomatic individuals, it is of great value in epidemiological studies, since *groups* of asymptomatic and apparently normal persons with a positive test are at much higher risk of developing overt coronary disease in the future than are those with negative tests.

A major limitation of the sensitivity of the exercise electrocardiogram is that it cannot be interpreted in many patients, including patients who are incapable of reaching the level of exercise required for near-maximal effort (85 per cent or more of maximal predicted heart rate), particularly those on propranolol or those who develop fatigue, leg cramps, or dyspnea, and patients with abnormalities in the baseline electrocardiogram, including those on digitalis (Table 39–2). The findings on exercise electrocardiograms in patients with multivessel coronary artery disease and those at high risk for subsequent myocardial infarctions and sudden death are shown in Table 39–2.

STRESS THALLIUM-201 MYOCARDIAL PERFUSION IMAGING (p. 369). In this technique, the radionuclide is injected at peak exercise and the image is obtained several minutes later when the patient is at rest; it demonstrates the regional perfusion pattern that existed during the stress of exercise. Defects represent either areas of stress-induced impairment of blood flow or infarction. If a delayed image is obtained 2 to 3 hours later and the initial defect persists, it is probably due to an infarction. On the other hand, if it exhibits delayed uptake, it represents an area of ischemic, transiently hypoperfused but viable myocardium.

In a summary of 22 published studies involving more than 2000 patients, the stress thallium-201 scintigram was usually superior to the exercise electrocardiogram, with a sensitivity of 83 per cent (compared with 73 per cent for the electrocardiogram) and a specificity of 90 per cent (compared with 82 per cent).[77,95] In patients with single-vessel coronary artery disease, the sensitivity of the electrocardiographic exercise test is particularly low, but this is not the case for thallium scintigraphy. Thallium defects in two or three vascular segments correctly predict multivessel disease in approximately 75 per cent of patients. Failure of normal redistribution into a defect is usually associated with wall motion abnormalities and with irreversible asynergy after a premature ventricular contraction on ventriculography, while asynergic segments at rest with redistribution on postexercise scintigrams usually show transient reversibility of the wall motion defect as well.[96] Patients with multiple defects of the redistribution type, with abnormal lung uptake during exercise-induced ischemia, reflecting a sudden rise in left ventricular diastolic pressure,[97,97a] are at particularly high risk for subsequent ischemic events. The thallium-perfusion defect can also be used to predict the ejection fraction[98] and the potential reversibility of perfusion abnormalities following surgical treatment.[99]

EXERCISE RADIONUCLIDE ANGIOGRAPHY (p. 365). In this test, measurements of ejection fraction and of regional wall motion are obtained both at rest and at increasing workloads.[100,100a,100b,100c] In a summary of 12 published studies comprising 771 patients, Gibson and Beller reported that the radionuclide angiogram had both sensitivity and specificity of approximately 90 per cent when both failure of a rise in ejection fraction and presence of a new regional wall motion abnormality were required for the test to be deemed positive.[77] (It is important to include exercise-induced regional wall motion abnormalities in order to define a positive exercise radionuclide angiogram, since the ejection fraction may fail to rise in patients with conditions other than ischemic heart disease, including cardiomyopathies, valvular heart disease, or hypertension, and in normal individuals receiving propranolol.)

The greater sensitivity of the two radionuclide techniques, i.e., exercise radionuclide angiography and stress thallium perfusion scintigraphy, compared to exercise electrocardiography, is probably related to the fact that abnormalities of perfusion and left ventricular contraction occur at a lower ischemic threshold than does exercise-induced ST-segment depression. Both radionuclide techniques are superior to exercise electrocardiography primarily because they allow evaluation of patients with electrocardiographic abnormalities at rest and of those who are unable to achieve adequate levels of exercise (Table 39–2).[100]

The sensitivity and specificity of both radionuclide techniques have been found to be similar in seven studies, comprising a total of 391 patients.[77] There is no consensus as to which of the two tests should be carried out first. We prefer to obtain the stress thallium-201 scintigram initially, since exercise radionuclide angiography can usually be performed on the same day after myocardial perfusion scintigraphy if the need arises, whereas the converse is not possible.

CLINICAL APPLICATION OF NONINVASIVE TESTS. In asymptomatic persons or in those with nonanginal chest pain who are being screened or evaluated for coronary artery disease, i.e., patients in whom the pretest likelihood of coronary disease is low (less than 15 per cent), a negative exercise electrocardiogram generally provides sufficient information to confirm the absence of ischemic heart disease; a positive test result should be followed by a thallium perfusion scan. When both of these tests are abnormal, the likelihood of significant coronary artery disease exceeds 80 per cent; however, if there is a discrepancy in the results of the two tests, either coronary arteriography or radionuclide angiography (and arteriography if the result is positive) is in order.

In patients with *atypical angina*, if two noninvasive tests are abnormal, the likelihood of coronary artery disease exceeds 95 per cent; if both tests are normal, this likelihood falls below 5 per cent. Results of noninvasive stress tests are independent of each other, and whenever they are discordant, a third noninvasive test will often be helpful. Also, when test results are discordant, they should be evaluated in the light of the level of exercise achieved as well as the degree of positivity (e.g., the presence of accompanying symptoms, the depth of the ST-segment response, the heart rate at which it occurred, and the persistence of the ST-segment response on the stress electrocardiogram;

the size and number of perfusion defects on the stress perfusion scintigram; and the magnitude of the exercise-induced change in ejection fraction and regional wall motion disorder on the exercise radionuclide angiogram). Thus, a patient with a normal exercise electrocardiogram who develops multiple large perfusion defects on a thallium-201 scintigram (accompanied by chest pain at a heart rate of 160 beats/min) is more likely to have ischemic heart disease than one who has a normal exercise electrocardiogram and develops a single small perfusion defect without chest pain at a heart rate of 195 beats/min.

In patients with *typical angina* (i.e., those with a high pretest likelihood of disease) noninvasive testing is most valuable for establishing the extent and severity of underlying coronary artery disease. The development of exertional hypotension, marked or prolonged ST-segment depression at low work levels and/or heart rate, striking decreases in ejection fraction and wall motion, and large or multiple defects on the exercise thallium scintigram all point to severe multivessel disease in patients at high risk of subsequent coronary events, including sudden death.[101]

OTHER LABORATORY TESTS

In patients with angina pectoris, the *echocardiogram* may show abnormalities of motion of the septum and posterior wall, corresponding to obstruction of the left anterior descending and right or left circumflex coronary arteries, respectively (Fig. 5–64, p. 125).[102,103] These abnormalities are particularly marked in patients who have had a myocardial infarction in those regions. However, the areas of the ventricle that can be imaged by the conventional M-mode echocardiogram are limited; the apex and inferior and lateral walls of the left ventricle are usually missed. Larger sections of the ventricle can be visualized by two-dimensional echocardiography (p. 93),[104] and this technique is of substantial value for defining noninvasively those areas of the left ventricle which show abnormal wall motion and for assessing left ventricular function (Fig. 5–65, p. 126). Serial tracings often reveal disorders of wall motion as ischemia waxes or wanes. Two-dimensional echocardiography is also useful for defining obstructive lesions of the left main coronary artery.[105]

Serum levels of cardiac enzymes are normal in angina pectoris and serve to differentiate these patients from those with acute myocardial infarction. One of the striking features of chronic ischemic heart disease in relatively young persons is the frequency with which certain metabolic abnormalities are detected. Since *hyperlipidemia* and *carbohydrate intolerance* are recognized as risk factors for the development of ischemic heart disease, this finding is not unexpected, and the prevalence of these abnormalities, particularly in patients under the age of 50 years, is impressive (Chap. 35). Two studies found that over 90 per cent of patients under the age of 50 years with angiographically proven ischemic heart disease had either carbohydrate intolerance or Type II or IV hyperlipoproteinemia.[106,107]

The *chest roentgenogram* is usually within normal limits in patients with chronic ischemic heart disease. However, coronary artery calcification detected fluoroscopically may be more diagnostic of coronary artery disease than was once thought, especially in young people.[108,109] More than 90 per cent of patients with coronary artery calcification were found to have critical coronary artery obstruction;

however, coronary calcification on fluoroscopy is not a very sensitive test, since it is found in only 40 per cent of patients with angiographically documented coronary artery disease.[108] When fluoroscopic evidence of coronary calcification is present in combination with a positive exercise test, the probability of finding coronary artery disease on subsequent coronary angiography is very high.[34]

CATHETERIZATION, ANGIOGRAPHY, AND CORONARY ARTERIOGRAPHY

Although the clinical examination and noninvasive techniques described above are valuable, the definitive diagnosis of coronary artery disease and a precise assessment of its anatomical severity and its effects on cardiac performance and myocardial metabolism require cardiac catheterization (Chap. 9), left ventricular angiography (Chap. 6), and coronary arteriography (Chap. 10). Among patients with chronic stable angina pectoris, coronary arteriography usually reveals relatively equal distribution (approximately 25 per cent each) of one-, two-, and three-vessel disease; about 5 to 10 per cent of patients have obstruction of the left main coronary artery, and in approximately 15 per cent no critical obstruction is detectable (p. 1338). Total occlusion of at least one major coronary artery is more common in patients with chronic angina who have had prior infarctions than in those without infarction.[43]

Coronary artery ectasia, i.e., aneurysmal dilatation, is present in approximately 5 per cent of patients with ischemic heart disease. This angiographic lesion does not appear to affect either survival or the incidence of myocardial infarction; it is considered to be a variant of coronary atherosclerosis rather than a distinct clinical entity.[110] Coronary collaterals are observed only when there is 50 to 75 per cent stenosis* of a coronary artery, but in 15 to 20 per cent of patients with this degree of stenosis, no collaterals are visible.[111] The functional significance of collateral vessels is unclear (p. 1267).[112,113] When they are well developed, coronary collaterals may be adequate to protect against resting ischemia but may fail to meet the increased needs of exercise and therefore may not reduce the frequency or severity of angina. Also, patients with abundant collaterals appear to suffer smaller myocardial infarctions.[114,115] On the basis of canine experiments, it is not clear whether or not exercise alters the development of collaterals.[116,117]

Diastolic ventricular performance, as reflected in the early diastolic ventricular filling rate, is abnormally reduced at rest in many patients with chronic stable angina, even when systolic performance, as reflected in the ejection fraction, is normal. Diastolic filling becomes even more abnormal during exercise.[118]

The frequency of abnormal elevations of left ventricular end-diastolic pressure and of reduced cardiac output increases with the number of vessels exhibiting critical narrowing and with the number of prior infarctions,[119] but there is a great deal of overlap among individual patients[120] so that the severity of coronary arterial or left ventricular disease cannot be predicted from this measurement. The left ventricular end-diastolic pressure may be elevated be-

cause of reduced ventricular compliance, left ventricular failure, or a combination of these two processes[121-123]; both reduced compliance and left ventricular failure may occur as a consequence of acute ischemia and chronic scar formation. The elevation of left ventricular diastolic pressure has its clinical correlate in the presence of diastolic (third and fourth) heart sounds.

In the resting state, i.e., in the absence of active or recent ischemia, hemodynamic abnormalities in patients with chronic stable angina usually reflect the presence of prior myocardial infarction, but in many patients with normal hemodynamics in the basal state, abnormalities of left ventricular function can be elicited by dynamic or static exercise.[124,125] Elevations of left ventricular end-diastolic pressure usually occur *before* the patient complains of chest discomfort and before there is electrocardiographic ST-segment depression.

Pacing-induced and post-pacing angina can also be observed in the catheterization laboratory (Fig. 39–4, p. 1344). This form of stress testing is especially useful for combined hemodynamic-metabolic-ventriculographic studies[126] because quantitative left ventricular angiography and myocardial lactate metabolism can be studied during or immediately after pacing, uncomplicated by an elevation of systemic arterial lactate levels, as occurs in dynamic exercise. When atrial pacing to induce ischemia is carried out in patients with chronic angina secondary to chronic obstructive coronary artery disease, elevations in ventricular end-diastolic pressure occur frequently and usually in association with the development of typical anginal discomfort at a reproducible heart rate–blood pressure product.[126,127] Impaired ventricular relaxation and increased regional myocardial stiffness have also been demonstrated during pacing-induced ischemia[128] and may be one component of the altered diastolic properties of the ischemic ventricle (p. 1246).

Abnormalities of left ventricular wall motion on biplane left ventriculography (asynergy) occur in approximately two-thirds of patients with ischemic heart disease and chronic stable angina pectoris, often in conjunction with abnormal hemodynamic findings (Fig. 10–48, p. 339).[129] Asynergy in the basal state is usually due to necrotic tissue, reflecting prior infarction, and there is a good correlation between electrocardiographic evidence of infarction (Q waves) and corresponding regional asynergy.[130,131] In many other patients with chronic ischemic heart disease, areas of abnormal wall motion are apparent only after ischemia is induced acutely—as with atrial pacing[132] or with exercise[133] —and the asynergy is "reversible," that is, it reverts to normal when the ischemic episode ceases.

The potential reversibility of localized asynergy evident on the basal ventriculogram has become the center of intensive investigation using several approaches. The purpose of these studies has been to devise techniques to distinguish between areas that are irreversibly damaged as a result of infarction and those that are "stunned,"[134] i.e., reversibly ischemic, even in the absence of angina or acute electrocardiographic changes. Techniques to identify the latter areas, i.e., to study the "contractile reserve" of the left ventricle, make use of inotropic stimulation (epinephrine and postextrasystolic potentiation[135] as well as preload reduction with nitroglycerin[135,136]). A reversibly damaged portion of the left ventricle begins to contract normally

---

*Unless otherwise noted, "per cent stenosis" refers to reduction of luminal diameter.

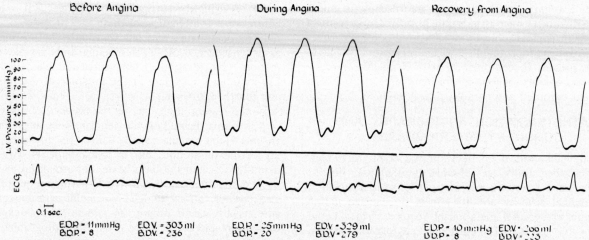

FIGURE 39–4   Records demonstrating changes in left ventricular pressure and an electrocardiographic tracing of a patient before angina, during angina, and after recovery from angina. Angina was produced by a brief period of atrial pacing at 140 beats/min, and the heart rate was maintained at approximately 95 beats/min during pressure recording. The beginning- and end-diastolic pressure (BDP and EDP, respectively) and corresponding ventricular volumes (BDV and EDV, respectively) are noted below each condition. (From Barry, W. H., et al.: Changes in diastolic stiffness and tone of the left ventricle during angina pectoris. Circulation *49*:255, 1974, by permission of the American Heart Association, Inc.)

when these interventions are applied, while irreversibly damaged myocardium does not. Histopathological studies performed on myocardial biopsy specimens obtained at the time of coronary artery bypass operations have demonstrated that those segments which exhibit reversible asynergy at angiography are made up predominantly of histologically normal myocardium, while the nonresponsive segments exhibit marked muscle loss and replacement by fibrous tissue.[137] The more responsive areas are usually better perfused, either by the native coronary artery or by collateral vessels, and are associated with a lower frequency of Q waves on the electrocardiogram.[138] The most severe aspect of left ventricular asynergy is the well-demarcated aneurysm, which not only exhibits contractile failure but also is unable to resist expansion during ventricular systole; in other words, it exhibits dyskinesis (paradoxical pulsation).

In addition to demonstrating areas of asynergy, left ventriculography may also show mitral valve prolapse (p. 1093), which occurs in 20 to 25 per cent of patients with obstructive coronary artery disease[139,140] and probably results from impaired contractility of the ventricular myocardium and papillary muscles.

Abnormal myocardial metabolism has also been documented by means of cardiac catheterization in patients with chronic stable angina. With a catheter in place in the coronary sinus, coronary arteriovenous lactate measurements are obtained at rest and after suitable stresses, such as the infusion of isoproterenol[141] or pacing.[142] Since lactate is a byproduct of anaerobic glycolysis, its production by the heart and subsequent appearance in coronary sinus blood is a sign of myocardial ischemia. When combined with coronary arteriography, this technique may be helpful in localizing significant coronary obstructive lesions and myocardial ischemia.[141]

MYOCARDIAL PERFUSION STUDIES.   Several techniques based on washout of radioactive inert gases from the myocardium following injection into the coronary

arteries can be used to measure regional myocardial blood flow, as described on page 377. Using these techniques, Cannon et al. have shown reductions in the perfusion of areas of myocardium subserved by totally obstructed coronary arteries compared with areas that are normally perfused. Less striking differences were observed with lesions compromising the lumen by 50 to 90 per cent.[143,144] Coronary blood flow measured by the regional xenon-133 technique has also been shown to be diminished in areas of abnormal ventricular wall motion, both at sites of previous infarction[145] and in noninfarcted regions.[146] This reduction in blood flow can be caused by coronary arterial stenosis or the reduced myocardial oxygen requirements of a noncontracting region or both. Whether any given area with low flow measured by this technique is contracting poorly because of reversible ischemia or is irreversibly damaged by scar formation is unclear, but there is evidence, obtained by means of postextrasystolic potentiation, that in regions with blood flow $\leq$ 50 ml/min/100 g in the basal state, the myocardium usually lacks contractile reserve and is probably irreversibly injured.[147] Atrial pacing has also been used with the xenon-133 technique to accentuate the differences between regions that are normally and poorly perfused in the basal state.[148] Regional myocardial blood flow can also be assessed noninvasively by myocardial perfusion scintigraphy, described in detail on page 369.[149]

MEDICAL MANAGEMENT

The medical management of ischemic heart disease involves four aspects: (1) correction of specific coronary risk factors, discussed in Chapter 35; (2) general and nonpharmacological methods, with particular attention toward adjustment of the patient's lifestyle;[150] (3) various specific medications used to treat angina; and (4) percutaneous transluminal angioplasty.

General Treatment

Fever, anemia, thyrotoxicosis, infection, tachycardia, hypoxemia, and certain drugs used to treat noncardiac diseases (such as amphetamines and isoproterenol mists) all increase myocardial oxygen needs and may precipitate or intensify angina. It is generally appreciated that cigarette smoking, the inhalation of smog, and ascent to high altitudes all lower the threshold for angina. It is less well known that breathing smoke-filled air from *other* people's cigarettes, i.e., passive smoking, may also aggravate angina.[151] These drugs and conditions should be eliminated. Congestive heart failure, by causing cardiac dilatation and cardiac tachyarrhythmias, can increase myocardial oxygen needs, and their treatment, as outlined in Chapters 16 and 21, will frequently diminish the frequency and severity of angina.

Other general measures include the treatment of hypertension (Chap. 27), which not only is a risk factor for the progression of atherosclerosis but also augments myocardial oxygen requirements. Attainment of an ideal weight is particularly important in the obese patient, since weight reduction raises the threshold for the development of angina pectoris.

Effective communication with both the patient and the family is essential. The psychosocial issues faced by the patient who develops chronic stable angina are similar to, though usually less intense than, those experienced by the patient with an acute myocardial infarction, discussed on page 1828. Many patients have an unrealistically gloomy perception of their prognosis; they should be offered a realistic appraisal, together with an understandable explanation of the pertinent clinical features of the disease. The advantages to the patient of having an effective anginal "warning system"[40] to prevent damage to the heart should be stressed. The role of personality type as an independent risk factor for coronary artery disease is discussed on pp. 1826 to 1828; some evidence indicates that counseling efforts to reduce the features of the "Type A" personality may improve prognosis in patients following myocardial infarction.[152] An important aspect of the physician's role is to counsel patients in the kind of work they can do, in their leisure activities, eating habits, vacation plans, and the like. It is desirable, if possible, to consult with the closest member(s) of the family, both to insure an accurate and full assessment of the patient's activities and to inform the family of what can be expected in the course of the patient's disease.

Certain changes in life style may be helpful, such as modifying strenuous activities if they constantly and repeatedly produce angina. These changes may be minor in many instances. For example, golfing could be modified to include use of a golfcart instead of walking. Many activities, such as shopping or climbing stairs, need not be discontinued. Often, it is merely necessary to perform them more slowly or to pause for brief periods of rest. The patient with chronic stable angina should avoid excessive fatigue and exhaustion; one or two regular rest periods during each day are often helpful. While it is desirable to minimize the number of bouts of angina, an occasional episode is not to be feared. The vast majority of patients with chronic stable angina should not be treated like invalids. Often, the propensity for angina actually declines,[153] per-

haps as a result of the development of collaterals or because of training effects, discussed later; indeed, unless patients occasionally reach their anginal thresholds, they may not appreciate the extent of their exercise capacity.

Eliminating or reducing the factors that precipitate anginal episodes is of obvious importance. Each patient learns what his usual threshold is by trial and error. Since many anginal episodes are precipitated by increases in the mechanical activity of the heart (due to increases in heart rate and blood pressure), the patient should avoid *sudden* bursts of activity, particularly after long periods of rest. Thus, morning activities such as showering, shaving, and dressing should be done at a slower pace, and at certain times, prophylactic nitroglycerin is extremely useful (discussed below). The stress of sexual intercourse is ordinarily approximately equal to that of climbing one flight of stairs at a normal pace or of any activity that induces a heart rate of approximately 120 beats/min. With proper precautions, i.e., commencing more than 2 hours postprandially and taking an additional dose of propranolol one hour before and nitroglycerin 15 minutes before, the majority of patients with chronic stable angina are able to continue a satisfactory sexual life.

Just as there is a role for exercise in the management of coronary artery disease, so is there a role for rest, especially in situations in which angina has become frequent or severe. Marked restriction of activity or even complete bed rest, in addition to drug therapy, may be necessary to control symptoms. In less critical situations, merely reducing the amount of time spent working or increasing the rest periods will have a beneficial effect. For example, a long lunch break including a short nap may be beneficial. It may be necessary for the patient to use a face mask or scarf to cover the mouth or nose in cold weather. A hot, humid environment may also precipitate angina, and air conditioning may be a necessity rather than a luxury for patients with ischemic heart disease. Large meals can have a similar effect if they are followed by exertion. An effort should be made to minimize emotional outbursts, since they too increase myocardial oxygen requirements and sometimes induce coronary vasoconstriction. Occasionally antianxiety drugs or sedation may be useful.

Exercise (see also Chapter 40). There is a growing interest in the use of *physical exercise*, either in prevention of ischemic heart disease or in the reduction of complications once clinical manifestations occur. Despite observations that physical training has a beneficial effect on cardiac performance,[154] the relationship between physical activity and the development of coronary artery disease is unclear. Whether the widespread adoption of regular dynamic exercise (jogging, swimming, walking, bicycling) influences the development or rate of progression of coronary artery disease remains to be determined. Although the question of whether or not regular exercise accelerates the development of collateral vessels is still unsettled,[116,117] exercise does have a place, not only in the rehabilitation of individuals recovering from myocardial infarction, but in the management of patients with chronic angina as well.

The *conditioning effect of exercise* on skeletal muscle allows the patient to expend a greater physical effort at any level of total body oxygen consumption, and the conditioning effect of exercise on the heart, by decreasing the

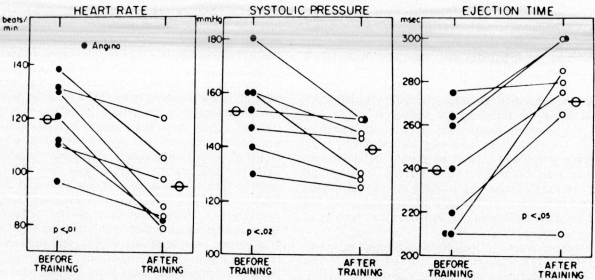

FIGURE 39–5   Effects ot training on the response of heart rate, systolic aortic pressure, and ejection time to exercise. In each panel the points at the left represent pre-training values obtained during exercise at the onset of angina, and the points at the right represent post-training values measured at the same intensity and duration of exercise as in the pre-training studies. Mean values are represented by the barred circles. (From Redwood, D. R. et al.: Circulatory and symptomatic effects of physical training in patients with coronary artery disease and angina pectoris. N. Engl. J. Med. *286*:959, 1972.)

heart rate at any level of exercise, allows a higher cardiac output to be achieved at any level of myocardial oxygen consumption. The combination of these two effects of exercise permits the patient with chronic stable angina to increase his physical performance substantially following institution of a chronic exercise program. The reduced pressure-rate product reduces myocardial oxygen requirements during exertion and enables the patient with coronary artery disease to perform at higher workloads before reaching the ischemic threshold.[154] Therefore, physical conditioning reduces the amount of oxygen needed by the heart for any given amount of total body work. An example of this effect is seen in the study of Redwood et al. who noted that a six-week training program improved exercise performance by reducing the responses of heart rate and arterial pressure to bicycle exercise (Fig. 39–5) and by prolonging the duration of exercise before angina occurred.[155] There is also some evidence that in patients with chronic ischemic heart disease after training, a greater ejection fraction was achieved at equivalent workloads.[156] For all the aforementioned reasons, patients are urged to participate in regular exercise programs—usually walking (see below)—in conjunction with their drug therapy.[157] Patients who are involved in exercise programs are also usually more apt to be health conscious, to pay attention to diet and weight, and to discontinue cigarette smoking. Thus, in addition to a conditioning effect on skeletal and cardiac muscle, regular dynamic exercise provides the individual with a feeling of well-being, an important consideration in the management of any chronic disease. The rationale and specific details for establishing an exercise program in patients with coronary artery disease are outlined in Chapter 40.

Nitrates

Mechanism of Action.   Although the clinical effectiveness of amyl nitrite was first described in 1867 by Brun-

ton,[4] organic nitrates are still the most common medications physicians employ to treat patients with angina pectoris. The basic pharmacological action of these agents is to relax vascular smooth muscle.[158] The vasodilator effects of nitrates are evident in both systemic arteries and veins in normal subjects and in patients with ischemic heart disease,[159,160] but they appear to be predominant in the venous circulation.[161] The decrease in venous tone reduces the return of blood to the heart and reduces preload and ventricular dimensions,[162–164] which in turn reduces wall tension and afterload. The actions of nitrates to reduce preload and afterload also make them useful in the treatment of heart failure (p. 538).

Posture is important in evaluating the hemodynamic effects of nitrates. In the supine position, venous return is normally greater while exercise tolerance and the anginal threshold are lower than in the upright position.[165] The hemodynamic and angina-relieving effects of nitrates are most marked when patients are sitting or standing,[166] i.e., when these drugs can reduce preload, and these effects resemble those of phlebotomy.[167] By reducing the heart's mechanical activity, volume, and oxygen consumption, nitrates increase exercise capacity in patients with ischemic heart disease,[168,169] i.e., a greater total body workload can be achieved before the anginal threshold is reached.

A vasodilating effect of the nitrates on the larger (conductance) coronary arteries can also be readily demonstrated,[170] and there is recent evidence, obtained from quantitative, computer-assisted measurements of coronary arterial diameter, that nitroglycerin causes vasodilatation of epicardial stenoses. Presumably, these are eccentric lesions, and nitroglycerin causes relaxation of smooth muscle in the wall of the coronary artery not encompassed by the plaque. Even a small increase in the narrowed arterial lumen can produce a significant reduction in resistance to blood flow across the narrowed lesion (Fig. 39–6).[171]

Studies in experimental animals with coronary obstruc-

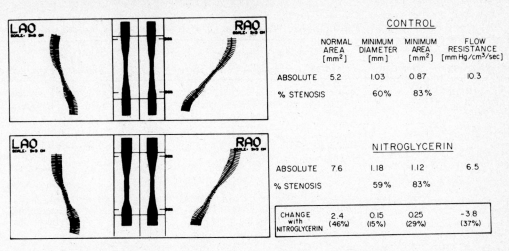

FIGURE 39–6 Representative computer printout of segmental stenosis images and dimensional data for pre- and post-nitroglycerin (0.4 mg, sublingual) angiograms of this 60 per cent midright coronary artery stenosis. Each value is averaged from eight estimates. LAO = left anterior oblique; RAO = right anterior oblique. (From Brown, B. G., et al.: The mechanisms of nitroglycerin action: Stenosis vasodilatation as a major component of the drug response. Circulation *64*:1089, 1981, by permission of the American Heart Association, Inc.)

	NORMAL AREA [mm²]	MINIMUM DIAMETER [mm]	MINIMUM AREA [mm²]	FLOW RESISTANCE [mm Hg/cm³/sec]
CONTROL				
ABSOLUTE	5.2	1.03	0.87	10.3
% STENOSIS		60%	83%	
NITROGLYCERIN				
ABSOLUTE	7.6	1.18	1.12	6.5
% STENOSIS		59%	83%	
CHANGE with NITROGLYCERIN	2.4 (46%)	0.15 (15%)	0.25 (29%)	-3.8 (37%)

tion have shown that nitroglycerin causes redistribution of blood flow to ischemic areas, particularly in the subendocardium,[172-174] perhaps mediated in part by an increase in collateral blood flow[175,176] and in part by a lowering of ventricular diastolic pressure, reducing subendocardial compression. Results of studies of nitroglycerin on coronary blood flow have been conflicting. Some studies in patients have reported increased blood flow after sublingual or intravenous nitroglycerin,[177] but most report no change or reduced flow as myocardial oxygen demands fell.[160,178-180] In studies employing intracoronary injections of xenon-133[181,182] (as well as in retrograde perfusion studies performed during coronary bypass surgery[183]), regional myocardial blood flow in areas perfused by stenotic coronary arteries rose after nitroglycerin when well-developed collaterals supplying those regions were present. Atrial pacing studies indicate that after nitroglycerin the heart can be paced to higher rates before angina occurs.[184] The nitrates have also been shown to improve ventricular wall motion in patients with ischemic heart disease, as demonstrated by contrast ventriculography,[136,185] echocardiography,[164] and radionuclide ventriculography, at rest[186] and during exercise.[187]

The mechanism of the nitrates' antianginal actions is complex. Apparently, their major action is to reduce the mechanical activity of the heart through the previously noted systemic effects, with subsequent reduction in development of the left ventricular wall tension (which results from reduction of arterial pressure and ventricular volume) and of myocardial oxygen consumption (Fig. 39–7).[164,170,188-190] Reduced left ventricular end-diastolic pressure may also decrease the resistance to coronary blood flow. It is probable that the coronary actions of the nitrates—dilating epicardial stenoses, dilating coronary collateral vessels, and reducing ventricular diastolic pressure and thereby lowering extravascular resistance to endocardial perfusion—all act to increase oxygen delivery to ischemic myocardium. In the final analysis, some combination of a reduction of myocardial oxygen requirements and increased oxygen delivery to the ischemic area relieves or prevents the development of myocardial ischemia in patients with chronic stable angina. Nitrates are not considered to exert a *direct* effect on the contractile state of the heart, although heart rate may rise reflexly as a consequence of the decline in blood pressure.

An assessment of the relative importance of these two

actions of nitroglycerin (reducing oxygen demand and increasing oxygen supply) has been complicated by the differing results of studies on the effects of intracoronary nitroglycerin.[171,191] Any effect of the drug administered by this route must derive from its direct action on the coronary vascular bed, i.e., by improving myocardial oxygen supply; some studies have demonstrated a beneficial effect of intracoronary nitroglycerin,[171] while others have not.[191] Perhaps the principal action of nitrates differs in different patients; they increase oxygen delivery to ischemic myocardium in patients with a strong vasoconstrictive component and reduce oxygen needs in patients with relatively fixed lesions and constant-threshold angina.

Types of Preparations and Routes of Administration. Nitroglycerin given *sublingually* is the drug of choice for treatment of the acute anginal attack. It is also available in oral, ointment, and transdermal forms (Table 39–3). The usual sublingual dose is 0.3 to 0.4 mg, and most patients respond within 5 minutes to one or two tablets. Intolerance is rarely a problem with intermittent usage. Sublingual nitroglycerin is also useful when it is taken prophylactically shortly before beginning activities likely

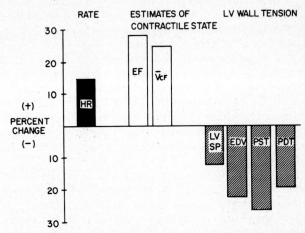

FIGURE 39–7 The effect of sublingually administered nitroglycerin on determinants of myocardial oxygen consumption. HR = heart rate; EF = ejection fraction; = VCF = mean circumferential fiber shortening velocity; LVSP = left ventricular systolic pressure; EDV = end-diastolic volume; PST = peak systolic tension; PDT = peak developed tension. (From Greenberg, H., et al.: Effects of nitroglycerin on the major determinants of myocardial oxygen consumption. An angiographic and hemodynamic assessment. Am. J. Cardiol. *36*:426, 1975.)

TABLE 39–3   DOSAGE AND ACTIONS OF NITROGLYCERIN FOR ANGINAL THERAPY

NAME		EFFECTS°		DOSAGE						SIDE EFFECTS
Nonproprietary	Proprietary	Physiologic	Therapeutic	Beginning	Average	Maximal	Formulation	Route	Supplied	
Glyceryl trinitrate (nitroglycerin)	Nitrostat	Relaxes vascular smooth muscle	Decreases venous return	0.3 mg	0.6 mg	As needed	Sublingual tablets	SL	0.3, 0.4, and 0.6 mg	Headache Flushing Tachycardia
	Nitrobid	Dilates arterioles	Decreases blood pressure	2.5 mg bid	2.5 mg tid; 6.5 mg bid	6.5 mg tid	Sustained-release capsules	PO	2.5 and 6.5 mg	Dizziness Postural hypotension
	Nitroglyn	Reduces peripheral vascular resistance	Decreases net myocardial oxygen consumption	1.3 mg bid	1.3 mg tid; 6.5 mg bid	6.5 mg tid	Sustained-action tablets	PO	1.3, 2.6, and 6.5 mg	
	Nitrospan	Reduces mean arterial pressure		2.5 mg before breakfast and at hour of sleep			Sustained-release microdialysis cells	PO	2.5 mg	
	Nitro-SA	Reflex tachycardia		2.5 mg bid	2.5 mg bid	2.5 mg tid	Sustained-release capsules	PO	2.5 mg	
	Nitrong			2.6 mg tid			Controlled release tablets	PO	2.6 mg	
	Nitrol ointment			1 to 2 inches hs	2 inches hs	6 inches hs	Lanolin, petrolatum	Topically	1- and 2-oz tubes 2% TNG	

°These effects refer to all formulations of nitroglycerin.

Reproduced with permission from Wolfson, S., and Costin, J. C.: Medical therapy in angina pectoris. *In* Donoso, E., and Gorlin, R. (eds.): Angina Pectoris. Vol. III. New York, Stratton Intercontinental Medical Book Corp., 1977, p. 121.

to cause angina.[192,193] Used for this purpose, it may prevent anginal attacks for 30 to 45 minutes. Nitroglycerin tablets tend to lose their potency, especially if exposed to light, and should therefore be kept in dark containers. Adverse reactions are common and include headache, flushing, and hypotension. The last is only rarely severe but can be potentially dangerous if the chest pain is due to a myocardial infarction rather than angina and arterial pressure had already declined because of pump failure and/or a vagal reaction or hypovolemia. In addition, the partial pressure of oxygen in arterial blood may fall after nitroglycerin administration because of an increasing ventilation-perfusion imbalance owing to impairment of the lung's ability to vasoconstrict in areas of alveolar hypoxia and thereby redirect perfusion to less hypoxic tissue.[194] Methemoglobinemia is a rare complication of very large doses of nitrates (p. 1694).

Other nitrate preparations are available in sublingual, buccal, oral, and ointment form (Table 39–4). Isosorbide dinitrate and other long-acting preparations are available in 2.5- and 5.0-mg sublingual tablets, a 10-mg buccal (chewable) form, and 5-, 10-, and 20-mg tablets for oral use as well as in 40-mg "sustained-release" capsules. Since orally administered nitrates undergo rapid hepatic metabolism,[195] large doses (5 mg nitroglycerin and 20 mg isosorbide dinitrate or pentaerythritol tetranitrate) may be required. Oral nitrates are not very potent agents but they can raise the threshold of activity required for the development of angina and reduce the incidence of anginal attacks

and the need for sublingual nitroglycerin.[196,197] They do not appear to cause tolerance to sublingual nitroglycerin.[198] Thadani et al. have reported that isosorbide dinitrate should be administered as frequently as every 2 to 3 hours for a continued beneficial effect.[199]

Topical Nitroglycerin.   Nitroglycerin ointment (15 mg/ inch) is efficacious when applied (most commonly to the chest) in strips of 0.5 to 2.0 inches. This form of the drug is particularly useful in patients with severe angina who are confined to bed and chair; since it is effective for 4 to 6 hours, it may also be used prophylactically after retiring by patients with nocturnal angina. While ordinary nitroglycerin ointment is not suitable for ambulatory patients, *sustained-release transdermal preparations* offer an alternative. A nitroglycerin-impregnated polymer is bonded to an adhesive bandage that should be applied to a site free of hair. Physically, these products resemble a "Band-Aid"; the drug is delivered at the inner surface, the outer layer is impermeable, and the entire unit is attached to the skin by an adhesive. The rate of delivery of the drug is determined by several means in different preparations, including a semipermeable membrane placed between the drug reservoir and the skin.[200] The dose depends on the size of the unit (5 to 30 cm^2) which releases 25 to 154 mg nitroglycerin over a 24-hour period. Clinical efficacy over a 24-hour period has been established.[201] Therapeutic plasma levels are achieved within 30 to 60 minutes of application and are maintained for at least 30 minutes after removal of the patch. Thus, transdermal delivery devices, suitable for

TABLE 39–4 DOSAGE AND ACTIONS OF LONG-ACTING NITRATES FOR ANGINAL THERAPY

NAME		EFFECTS°		DOSAGE						SIDE EFFECTS
Nonproprietary	Proprietary	Physiologic	Therapeutic	Beginning	Usual	Maximal	Formulation	Route	Supplied	
Isosorbide dinitrate	Isordil and Sorbitrate	Relaxes vascular smooth muscle	Decreases venous return	5 mg q 2–3 hr	5 to 10 mg q 3 hr	20 mg	Sublingual† tablets	SL	2.5, 5, 10, 20 mg	Headache Flushing Tachycardia Dizziness
				5 mg qid or 40 mg bid	5 to 30 mg qid or 40 mg bid	30 mg qid or 40 mg tid	Tablets and capsules	PO	5 and 10 mg	
Pentaerythritol tetranitrate	Peritrate	Dilates arterioles; reduces peripheral vascular resistance	Decreases blood pressure; decreases net myocardial oxygen consumption	10 mg qid	10 to 20 mg qid or 80 mg bid	60 mg q 4 hr	Oral†	PO	10 and 20 mg	Postural hypotension
Erythrityl tetranitrate	Cardilate	Reflex tachycardia		5 mg qid	5 to 15 mg qid	45 mg q 2 hr	Oral, sublingual, and chewable tablets	SL or PO	5, 10, 15 mg; 10-mg chewable	Possibly causes tachyphylaxis to nitroglycerin with prolonged use

°These effects refer to all long-acting nitrates.
†Also available as "sustained-action" tablets; efficacy not well documented.
Reproduced with permission from Wolfson, S., and Costin, J. C.: Medical therapy in angina pectoris. *In* Donoso, E., and Gorlin, R. (eds.): Angina Pectoris. Vol. III. New York, Stratton Intercontinental Medical Book Corp., 1977, p. 121.

once-a-day application in ambulatory patients, may prove to be a more convenient way to deliver the time-honored drug. Absorption through the skin by ointment or the transdermal route is advantageous, since it reaches target organs without being inactivated by the liver. Allergic contact dermatitis is occasionally associated with topical nitroglycerin.

Although chronic administration of nitrates does not usually induce clinically important tolerance or cross-tolerance to nitroglycerin, the lowest effective dosage of long-acting nitrates should be employed, since the development of tolerance to large doses does occasionally occur.[192] Because of the suggestion of nitrate dependence, nitrate therapy should be carefully withdrawn. Indeed, in individuals exposed to industrial doses of nitroglycerin, nitrate tolerance, nitrate dependence, and withdrawal symptoms may cause serious problems.[202]

The chronic combined administration of nitrates and beta-adrenergic blockers reduces the frequency of anginal episodes. Some investigators have reported an additive effect of the two drugs in increasing exercise tolerance.[203] Certainly, beta blockers have the desirable effect of blocking the reflex tachycardia that may accompany nitrate-induced hypotension.[204]

Beta-Adrenergic Blocking Agents

These drugs constitute a cornerstone of therapy for effort-induced, chronic stable angina.[205] A number of randomized, double-blind studies have shown that beta-adrenergic blockers, in doses that are generally well tolerated, reduce the frequency of anginal episodes and raise the anginal threshold.[206,207,207a] This action is dependent on their ability to cause competitive inhibition of the effects of neuronally released and circulating catecholamines on beta-adrenergic receptors (p. 418).[208] In this manner, these drugs attenuate the cardiac responses to adrenergic stimulation (chiefly increases in heart rate and contractility). Thus, beta blockers reduce myocardial oxygen demands primarily during activity or excitement when surges of increased sympathetic activity occur. Effects on heart rate and myocardial contractility at rest are less profound because of the lower adrenergic drive to the heart in the basal state. Beta-adrenergic blockers also lower myocardial oxygen needs by reducing arterial pressure and they are extremely useful antihypertensive agents (p. 916).

For optimal results, the dose of beta blocker should be carefully titrated. It is useful to start with 80 mg of propranolol daily (20 mg four times a day), or comparable doses of one of the other beta blockers, in an effort to reduce resting heart rates to 50 to 60 beats/min and to cause less than a 20-beat/min increase with modest exercise (e.g., climbing one flight of stairs). The usual dosage of propranolol ranges from 80 to 320 mg/day, but some patients require (and tolerate) doses as high as 1000 mg daily. Serum levels of 30 ng/ml are usually required to achieve a 25 per cent or greater reduction in the frequency of angina.[209,210]

Adverse Reactions. Beta blocking drugs may induce fatigue, mental depression, gastrointestinal upset, intensification of insulin-induced hypoglycemia, cutaneous reactions, bronchoconstriction, and heart block.[211,212] In patients who already have impaired left ventricular function, congestive heart failure may ensue or may be intensified, an effect that can be counteracted by the use of digitalis or diuretics. Beta blockers should *not* be used in patients with bradyarrhythmias of any kind unless a pacemaker is in place.

TABLE 39–5 PHARMACOKINETICS AND PHARMACOLOGY OF SOME BETA-ADRENERGIC BLOCKERS

	DRUG					
	Atenolol	*Metoprolol*	*Nadolol*	*Pindolol*	*Propranolol*	*Timolol*
Extent of absorption (%)	$\simeq$50	> 95	$\simeq$30	> 90	90	> 90
Extent of bioavailability (% of dose)	$\simeq$40	$\simeq$50	$\simeq$30	$\simeq$90	$\simeq$30	75
Beta-blocking plasma concentration	0.2 to 0.5 μg/ml	50 to 100 ng/ml	50 to 100 ng/ml	50 to 100 ng/ml	50 to 100 ng/ml	5 to 10 ng/ml
Protein binding (%)	< 5	12	$\simeq$30	57	93	$\simeq$10
Lipophilicity*	Low	Moderate	Low	Moderate	High	Low
Elimination half-life (hr)	6 to 9	3 to 4	14 to 25	3 to 4	3.5 to 6.0	3 to 4
Urinary recovery of unchanged drug (% of dose)	$\simeq$40	$\simeq$3	70	$\simeq$40	< 1	$\simeq$20
Total urinary recovery (% of dose)	> 95	> 95	70	> 90	> 90	65
Drug accumulation in renal disease	Yes	No	Yes	No	No	No
Predominant route of elimination†	RE (mostly unchanged)	HM	RE	RE ($\simeq$40% unchanged) and HM	HM	RE ($\simeq$20% unchanged) and HM
Active metabolites	No	No	No	No	Yes	No
β_1-blocker potency ratio (propranolol = 1)	1.0	1.0	1.0	6.0	1.0	6.0
Relative β_1 sensitivity	+	+	0	0	0	0
Intrinsic sympathetic activity	0	0	0	+	0	0
Membrane-stabilizing activity	0	0	0	+	+ +	0
Usual maintenance dose	50 to 100 mg/qd	50 to 100 mg/qid	40 to 80 mg/qd	5 to 20 mg/tid	60 mg/qid	20 mg/bid

*Determined by the distribution ratio between octanol and water.
†RE = renal excretion; HM = hepatic metabolism.

Modified from Frishman, W. H.: Beta-adrenoceptor antagonists: New drugs and new indications. N. Engl. J. Med. *305*:500, 1981.

Sudden withdrawal of the drug in ambulatory patients has been reported to result in acute ischemic episodes.[213] There are several possible mechanisms for this "rebound" phenomenon; since the drug prevents or reduces the frequency of angina, patients increase their activities to a level that previously would have resulted in chest pain. When the drug is discontinued, they maintain their higher levels of activity but without the drug's protective effects. Since the greatest clinical benefit occurs in patients who were previously most disabled, the rebound effects might be expected to be most marked in those patients readily prone to myocardial ischemia. Other possible mechanisms involve the unmasking of the underlying coronary obstruction that has progressed during the course of drug administration, the elevation of arterial pressure, and an increase in the number of adrenergic beta receptors ("up-regulation").[214] The rebound phenomenon is much less marked in hospitalized patients, suggesting that the higher "set" of activity level is the major mechanism.

Blockade of noncardiac (i.e., beta$_2$) receptors inhibits catecholamine-induced glycogenolysis and the vasodilating effects of catecholamines in peripheral blood vessels. Therefore, noncardioselective beta blockers may impair the defense of insulin-induced hypoglycemia, may precipitate episodes of Raynaud's phenomenon, and may cause uncomfortable coldness of the distal extremities. Blockade of vasodilatory (beta$_2$) receptors by noncardioselective beta blockers, such as propranolol, leaves the constrictor (alpha-adrenergic) receptors unopposed and thereby enhances vasoconstriction. Indeed, Kern et al. have shown in patients with chronic obstructive coronary artery disease that the coronary vasoconstriction that normally occurs during the cold pressor test is intensified by beta-adrenergic blockade with propranolol.[215] Propranolol prolongs episodes of myocardial ischemia in patients with Prinzmetal's angina[216] and is ordinarily contraindicated in this condition (p. 1360).

Six beta blockers are currently available in the United States (Table 39–5). They appear to be equally effective in

the treatment of angina pectoris, but their differences in membrane-stabilizing properties, lipo- or hydrophilicity, cardioselectivity, and intrinsic sympathomimetic activity affect the other actions of these compounds. The hydrophilic beta blockers, i.e., atenolol and nadolol, are not as readily absorbed from the gastrointestinal tract as are the more lipophilic agents.[217] On the other hand, they are not as extensively metabolized and have relatively long plasma half-lives. Hydrophilic beta blockers tend not to penetrate into the central nervous system and therefore appear to be associated with less mental depression and sleep disturbances. Bronchoconstriction results from blockade of beta$_2$ receptors in the tracheobronchial tree; as a consequence, asthma and chronic obstructive lung disease are contraindications to the use of these agents. Since cardioselectivity is only relative, the use of such drugs (metoprolol and atenolol) in doses sufficient to prevent angina may still cause bronchoconstriction in susceptible patients.

One group of beta blockers with so-called intrinsic stimulating activity (ISA) cause not only blockade but also stimulation of beta receptors. Pindolol, a beta blocker with partial agonist activity, causes little if any slowing of heart rate, depression of atrioventricular (AV) conduction, and depression of contractility at rest but still blocks the effects of exercise on these parameters. Its partial agonist activity also induces bronchodilatation.[218–220] Accordingly, there is at least some theoretical advantage to using this beta blocker in patients with sinus bradycardia, AV block, left ventricular dysfunction and bronchospasm. However, additional clinical evidence is required to support these theoretical advantages.[207]

Calcium-Channel Blockers

The critical role played by calcium ions in the normal contraction of cardiac and vascular smooth muscle is discussed on page 413 and in myocardial ischemia on page 1253. Calcium-channel blocking agents have been found to be effective in the treatment of chronic stable angina, either alone or in combination with beta-adrenergic blockers and nitrates.[221,222,222a,222b,222c,222d] Three calcium-channel blocking agents—nifedipine, verapamil, and diltiazem—are now available in the United States. All three agents are effective in causing relaxation of vascular smooth muscle, in both the systemic arterial and the coronary arterial beds.

Nifedipine is the most potent vasodilator of the three. Although in vitro its actions on the myocardium and specialized cardiac tissue (i.e., the sinoatrial and AV nodes) are similar to those of the other agents, the concentration required to reproduce this effect is not reached in vivo because of its powerful vasodilating effects. Therefore, nifedipine's beneficial effects in the treatment of angina result from its capacity to reduce myocardial oxygen needs consequent to afterload reduction and to increase coronary blood flow consequent to its dilating action on the coronary vascular bed. Nifedipine decreases left ventricular afterload, while ejection fraction, velocity of circumferential fiber shortening, heart rate, and cardiac index all show slight reflex increases. In patients with elevated left ventricular end-diastolic volumes and pressures, nifedipine reduces ventricular end-diastolic pressure and left ventricular end-diastolic and end-systolic volumes and enhances ejection fraction more than it does in patients with normal baseline left ventricular function (Fig. 39–8 and Table 39–6).[223]

Side effects include headache, dizziness, flushing, nausea, and leg edema not related to heart failure. In a small number of patients, a paradoxical increase in myocardial ischemia may occur, presumably resulting from excessive lowering of arterial pressure and reflex tachycardia; cardiac depression is very rarely seen. The dose is 10 mg orally every 8 (or 6) hours increased to 20 mg every 8 (or 6) hours, guided by blood pressure response; 160 mg daily is considered to be the maximum dose.

Verapamil appears to decrease myocardial oxygen demand without any change in the anginal threshold (i.e., in the rate-pressure product) at the onset of angina, suggesting that increased oxygen delivery is not a principal mechanism of action.[224,225,225a] Charlap and Frishman[226] have summarized nine trials comparing verapamil with beta blockade (usually propranolol) in the treatment of effort-related angina. The two drugs were found to be comparable, both producing dose-dependent reductions in the frequency of anginal attacks (Fig. 39–9). In a comparison of propranolol, 480 mg/day, and verapamil, 320 mg/day, Leon et al. found verapamil to be superior.[227] Left ventricular diastolic filling is enhanced by verapamil in patients

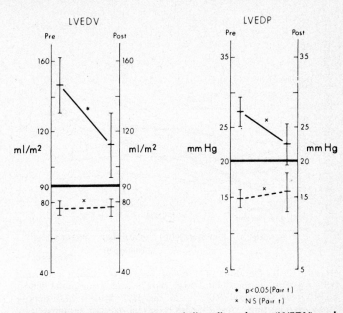

FIGURE 39–8 Left ventricular end-diastolic volume (LVEDV) and end-diastolic pressure (LVEDP) before and after nifedipine. Average EDV declined significantly in group 2 patients, in whom baseline LVEDV exceeded 90 ml/m², but was unchanged in group 1 patients, in whom initial LVEDV was normal. Average LVEDP declined in group 2 patients but did not change significantly in those in group 1. (From Ludbrook, P. A., et al.: Acute hemodynamic responses to sublingual nifedipine: Dependence on left ventricular function. Circulation *65*:489, 1982, by permission of the American Heart Association, Inc.)

with chronic stable angina both at rest and during exercise, but beta blockade does not have this effect.[227] The dose is *80 to 120* mg, *three or four times daily* (Table 39–7).

Diltiazem's actions are similar to those of verapamil—lowering arterial pressure at rest and during exertion and increasing the workload required to produce myocardial ischemia—but there is also some evidence that the drug may increase myocardial oxygen delivery.[228] Its action on the coronary vasculature is relatively selective, and this may explain the remarkably low incidence of adverse effects that have been reported. Like verapamil, diltiazem should be used only with great caution in patients with sick sinus syndrome and advanced degrees of AV block and left ventricular dysfunction. The dose is 30 to 60 mg four times daily.[229,229a]

Verapamil and diltiazem in doses used clinically not only cause systemic coronary vascular dilatation but also inhibit calcium influx into the myocardial and specialized cardiac cells, sometimes causing slowing of heart rate and AV conduction and impairing myocardial contractility.

TABLE 39–6 COMPARISON OF DRUG EFFECTS ON GLOBAL AND REGIONAL LEFT VENTRICULAR FUNCTION DURING EXERCISE (VS. CONTROL)

	GLOBAL LV FUNCTION								REGIONAL LV FUNCTION		
	HR	*SBP*	*DBP*	*PAPD*	*CI*	*TVR*	*EF*	*EDVI*	*NL*	*ISCH*	*SCAR*
Nitroglycerin	(↑)	—	(↓)	↓	—	—	(↑)	(↓)	—	↑	—
Nifedipine	↑	↓	↓	↓	↑	↓	(↑)	—	—	↑	—
Metoprolol	↓	↓	—	↑	(↓)	↑	—	—	↓	(↑)	—

Significant group differences are represented by different symbols: arrows indicate changes vs. control; arrows in parentheses indicate changes that are significant by single comparison but not by multiple group comparison.

Abbreviations: LV = left ventricular; HR = heart rate; SBP = systolic blood pressure; DBP = diastolic blood pressure; PAPD = pulmonary artery diastolic pressure; CI = cardiac index; TVR = total vascular resistance; EF = ejection fraction; EDVI = end-diastolic volume index; NL = normal segment; ISCH = ischemic segment; SCAR = scar segment; ↑ = increase; ↓ = decrease; — = no significant change vs. control.

From Pfisterer, M., et al.: Comparative effects of nitroglycerin, nifedipine and metoprolol on regional left ventricular function in patients with one-vessel coronary disease. Circulation *67*: 291, 1983.

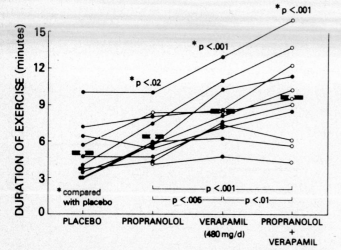

FIGURE 39–9 Duration of exercise in patients taking verapamil (480 mg/day), propranolol ("best dose"), and propranolol ("best dose") plus verapamil (407 ± 25 mg/day). Broken bars denote mean exercise time, closed circles represent exercise terminated by angina, and open circles represent exercise limited by fatigue or shortness of breath. (From Leon, M. B., et al.: Clinical efficacy of verapamil alone and combined with propranolol in treating patients with chronic stable angina pectoris. Am. J. Cardiol. 48:131, 1981.)

The principal side effects of these three calcium-channel blockers are contrasted with those of beta blockers and nitrates in Table 39–8. The major side effects of nifedipine are hypotension, flushing, and headache. The drug lowers arterial pressure and may produce a mild reflex tachycardia and augmentation of myocardial contractility. On the other hand, verapamil and diltiazem, by blocking the influx of calcium ions into cardiac tissue, cause a depression of cardiac contractility and a slowing of heart rate and of AV conduction. Therefore, nifedipine is contraindicated in patients who are already hypotensive,[230] while verapamil and diltiazem should probably not be administered to patients with left ventricular dysfunction, sinus bradycardia, sick sinus syndrome, and AV block, particularly if they are already receiving a beta-adrenergic blocker that can exert similar deleterious effects. In such patients, nifedipine is the calcium-channel blocker of choice, since it has less negative effects on myocardial contractility or on the specialized automatic or conduction system than does verapamil or diltiazem.

RELATIVE ADVANTAGES OF BETA BLOCKERS AND CALCIUM ANTAGONISTS. There is some controversy at the present time about whether a calcium-channel blocking agent or a beta blocker should be employed first in the treatment of chronic stable angina if more than an occasional sublingual nitroglycerin tablet is required. As indicated in the foregoing discussion, both classes of agents appear to be about equally effective. Chronic administration of beta-adrenergic blockers has been found to prolong life in patients after acute myocardial infarction,[231,232] but this has not yet been demonstrated for calcium-channel blockers. Since many patients with chronic stable angina either have suffered a myocardial infarction or have a similar pathophysiological process, not only might they benefit from the symptomatic relief provided by beta-adrenergic blockade, but conceivably these agents may also improve survival and diminish mortality in patients with chronic stable angina. On the other hand, a number of conditions, such as moderate to severe left ventricular failure, sinus bradycardia, sick sinus syndrome, and advanced AV block as well as obstructive lung disease, are contraindications to beta blockade, and in such patients nifedipine is preferable. Hypertensive patients do well with both beta blockers and calcium-channel blockers, since both agents have antihypertensive effects.

One logical way to make a choice between a calcium antagonist and a beta blocker is to take a detailed history and determine whether the patient's anginal threshold is fixed or variable, as discussed on page 1336. When it is relatively fixed, it may be presumed that myocardial ischemia is caused primarily by an increase in myocardial oxygen needs during exercise in the face of a fixed supply, and a beta blocker would be considered the agent of choice; conversely, in patients with variable-threshold angina, in whom a reduction of myocardial blood supply caused by coronary vasospasm plays a role in the development of ischemia and angina, a calcium-channel blocking agent may be preferable to a beta blocker.

COMBINATION THERAPY. In patients with more severe angina, a combination of a beta-adrenergic blocker, a calcium antagonist, and long-acting nitrates may be employed. The hemodynamic spectrum of action of nitroglycerin, calcium antagonists, and beta blockers is sufficiently different to suggest that combination therapy might be useful (Table 39–6).[233] Indeed, a number of studies[234-239] have shown that the combination of a beta blocker and a calcium-channel blocker is superior to either drug alone (Fig. 39–9). While combined blockade of calcium entry and beta-adrenergic receptors is usually well tolerated, this combination should be approached with caution, since it can occasionally produce severe left ventricular dysfunction.[240,241] It is often possible to use low doses of each agent, so that the adverse effects of each drug are diminished.

In patients with angina severe enough to require combination therapy but without specific contraindications to any antianginal agents, the combination of a beta blocker

TABLE 39–7   CLINICAL PHARMACOKINETICS OF MAJOR CALCIUM ANTAGONISTS

AGENT	USUAL ADULT DOSE	ABSORPTION	ONSET OF ACTION	PEAK EFFECT	PLASMA HALF-LIFE
Verapamil	IV: 0.075 to 0.15 mg/kg	—	≈2 min	3 to 5 min	<½ hr
	Oral: 80 to 120 mg tid or qid	90%	2 hr	3 to 4 hr	3 to 7 hr*
Nifedipine	SL: 10 to 30 mg tid or qid	90%	<3 min	Not available	
	Oral: 10 to 30 mg tid or qid	90%	<20 min	1 to 2 hr	4 hr
Diltiazem	IV: 0.075 to 0.15 mg/kg	—		Not available	
	Oral: 30 to 90 mg tid or qid	90%	<15 min	30 min	4 hr

IV = intravenous; SL = sublingual.
*Single dose; may be lengthened to 4.5 to 12 hours after 6 to 10 consecutive oral doses.
From Singh, B. N.: Clinical pharmacology of calcium antagonist drugs. Cornell Postgraduate Course on Calcium Antagonists. New York, Medcom, Inc., 1982, p. 5.

TABLE 39–8 SIDE EFFECTS OF ANTIANGINAL DRUGS*

	HYPOTENSION FLUSHING, HEADACHE	LEFT VENTRICULAR DYSFUNCTION	DECREASED HEART RATE ATRIO-VENTRICULAR BLOCK[†]	GASTRO-INTESTINAL SYMPTOMS	BRONCHO-CONSTRICTION[‡]
Beta blockers	0	+ +	+ + +	+	+ + +
Nitrates	+ + +	0	0	0	0
Diltiazem	+	+	+	0	0
Nifedipine	+ + +	0	0	0	0
Verapamil	+	+	+ +	+ +	0

*0 = absent; + = mild; + + = moderate; + + + sometimes severe.
[†]In patients with sick sinus node syndrome or conduction system disease.
[‡]In patients with obstructive lung disease.
From Braunwald, E.: Mechanism of action of calcium channel blocking agents. N. Engl. J. Med. *307*:1618, 1982.

and nifedipine or of verapamil or diltiazem with a long-acting nitrate is appropriate. As already stated, since beta blockers and both verapamil and diltiazem exert negative inotropic effects and depress cardiac automaticity and conduction, this combination may be hazardous in patients who already have left ventricular dysfunction and in those with impaired function of the sinoatrial or AV nodes. The combination of nifedipine and nitrates may also be less than ideal, since both agents are potent vasodilators. In practice, antianginal drugs are begun in low doses and are gradually raised to tolerance. If the patient's lifestyle is limited by persistent angina despite all the aforementioned measures, and if there are no contraindications, surgical treatment should be considered.

OTHER ANTIANGINAL THERAPIES. Anticoagulant therapy with coumarin derivatives is no longer recommended for patients with chronic stable angina without other factors predisposing to venous thrombosis. Its use in the postmyocardial infarction state is discussed on page 1304. Whether treatment with sulfinpyrazone and other drugs that impair platelet function is of value is not yet clear.[242]

Percutaneous Transluminal Angioplasty (PTCA)

This technique consists of introducing a catheter incorporating a balloon under local anesthesia across a stenotic segment in a coronary artery and relieving the stenosis by inflating the balloon (Fig. 9–12, p. 298).[243,243a,243b,243c] Morphological studies have shown that this procedure, when successful, disrupts the intima and splits the atherosclerotic plaque.[244] The most appropriate candidates for this procedure are patients with (1) stable angina refractory to medical therapy and severe enough to warrant surgical revascularization; (2) a relatively proximal stenosis in one of the three major coronary arteries; and (3) a discrete stenosis, less than 1 cm in length, that is readily accessible.[245] Patients with left main coronary artery disease are *not* good candidates, and the role of this procedure in patients with multivessel disease is not yet clear.[245a,245b] Approximately 10 per cent of patients who are candidates for coronary artery bypass grafting are candidates for angioplasty.

Depending on the skill and experience of the operator, PTCA is successful in dilating the stenosis in 60 to 80 per cent of cases.[245–247] In these patients, angina is usually relieved and left ventricular function improves, as reflected

in an elevation of the ventricular ejection fraction during exercise.[246,248] Coronary occlusion occurs in about 5 per cent of patients, and in these, myocardial infarction can sometimes be averted or limited by immediate coronary artery bypass grafting. Accordingly, a cardiac surgical team must be available on standby for treatment of this complication. Mortality rate changes from 0.5 to 1.0 per cent.[245,247] In about 20 per cent of the patients in whom the procedure is initially successful, stenosis recurs, usually during the first 6 months.[247a] In about two-thirds of these patients, a second angioplasty will be successful, with symptomatic improvement for more than one year.[247b] Exercise electrocardiography and [201]thallium perfusion imaging are helpful in following patients after angioplasty;[248a, 248b] recurrence of symptoms and abnormal findings on these noninvasive tests are useful in determining when arteriography should be repeated.[249,250]

Successful vaporization of atherosclerotic plaques and intracoronary thrombi using an argon laser passed through a fiberoptic catheter (i.e., transluminal laser coronary angioplasty) has been reported in a variety of animal and human necropsy models.[251,252,252a,252b,252c] This technique, like percutaneous transluminal coronary angioplasty, appears to be promising for the treatment of chronic stable angina in selected patients. Balloon angioplasty has also been employed successfully in the course of surgical revascularization to improve perfusion of vessels that cannot be reached by grafts.[253,254]

Guidelines for Medical Treatment of Chronic (Stable) Angina

Risk factor modification is most important in younger patients with chronic stable angina (under age 50). This is most easily accomplished by cessation of cigarette smoking and treatment of hypertension. What effect reduction of serum cholesterol levels will have on regression of atheromas is unclear, but it is unlikely to be significant unless a means is found to produce a radical reduction of markedly elevated serum cholesterol. Perhaps currently available methods of diet and drug therapy may slow the progression of the disease. Similarly, the relationship between maintenance of blood sugar within the normal range in diabetics and preventing vascular disease is far from settled.

In mild chronic stable angina, drug therapy may be limited to sublingual nitroglycerin on an "as necessary" basis if pain episodes are relatively infrequent (once or twice a week). It should also be used prophylactically in situations known to precipitate angina. If nitroglycerin is required on a daily basis, either long-acting nitrate preparations or moderate doses of a beta blocker (propranolol, 20 mg four times a day, or an equivalent dose of another beta blocker) or both may also be employed. The doses of the drugs will depend on how well they are tolerated and on the clinical response. Resting heart rate should be lowered to 50 to 60 beats/min to assure adequate beta blockade. The clinical response can often be estimated by an improvement in exercise tolerance or the degree of ST-segment depression during a standard treadmill test. If the patient is still symptomatic at high doses of propranolol (>320 to 400 mg/day) and long-acting nitrates (e.g., isosorbide dinitrate, 40 to 80 mg/day), a calcium-channel blocking agent should be added.

There is no unanimity concerning when a patient with chronic angina pectoris should undergo cardiac catheterization, coronary arteriography, and left ventriculography. Some physicians take a more aggressive posture with patients under 50 years of age, with the hope of finding a lesion that demands surgical correction or angioplasty; others prefer to wait for refractoriness to medical therapy to develop, regardless of the patient's age. We believe that the use of noninvasive tests, as outlined on page 1342, can be extremely helpful in identifying patients with chronic stable angina at high risk of coronary events or early death; if there are no contraindications to coronary artery surgery in such patients, they should be subjected to coronary arteriography. Similarly, patients for whom medical therapy fails should undergo coronary arteriography.

PROGNOSIS

The natural history of coronary artery disease is outlined in Figure 39–10.

NONANGIOGRAPHIC CRITERIA FOR PROGNOSTIC EVALUATION. Of the nonarteriographic investigations, the Framingham study, in which a sample population in one geographic area has been followed prospectively, is well known.[255] In this group, the annual mortality of patients with angina was 4 per cent. Remission may occur in one-third of patients with angina of recent onset[153] but is rare in patients whose angina has been present for several years. The annual mortality in the Framingham study of patients who had suffered a nonfatal myocardial infarction was 5 per cent after the first postinfarct year.[255] Other groups have reported similar,[256] higher,[257] and lower mortality rates.[258] In a recent report on 586 men who survived an attack of unstable angina or acute myocardial infarction and who are treated conservatively, survival at 5 years was 80 per cent; at 10 years it was 61 per cent, and at 15 years 43 per cent.[258] Although the adverse influence of hypertension on prognosis in patients with established coronary artery disease was reported by Frank et al.,[259] the effect on mortality of other risk factors, such as diabetes mellitus and hyperlipidemia in such patients, is not clear[260]; however, cigarette smoking does appear to increase the incidence of sudden death.[261] Electrocardiographic abnormalities, particularly multiple Q waves, intraventricular conduction defects, left ventricular hypertrophy, and ventricular ectopic activity, especially of the higher grades (p. 786), are also associated with a poor prognosis in patients with coronary artery disease.[262–264]

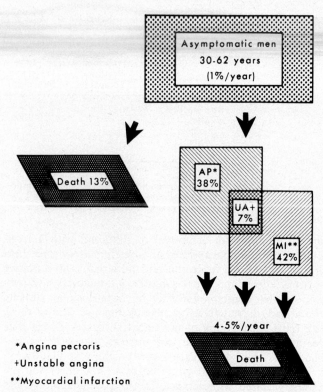

*Angina pectoris
+Unstable angina
**Myocardial infarction

FIGURE 39–10 The natural history of coronary artery disease: manifestations of coronary heart disease at onset and subsequent mortality in men ages 30 to 62. Of the 1 per cent asymptomatic men per year who develop manifestations of coronary artery disease, 13 per cent may be expected to die suddenly. The remaining 87 per cent will develop one of the three forms of clinically recognizable ischemic syndrome: angina pectoris (AP), unstable angina (UA), or acute myocardial infarction (MI). The mortality rate for the year following myocardial infarction, including the period of hospitalization, approximates 20 per cent. Thereafter, the annual mortality in all three groups approximates 4 to 5 per cent. (From Oberman, A., et al.: Long-term results of the medical treatment of coronary artery disease. Angiology *28*:160, 1977.)

ANGIOGRAPHIC CRITERIA FOR PROGNOSTIC EVALUATION. With the development of coronary arteriography and left ventriculography, it became possible to relate the natural history of ischemic heart disease both to the severity of the obstructive lesions in the coronary arterial bed and to left ventricular wall motion abnormalities. A combination of studies in symptomatic patients from several major centers indicates that if only one of the three major coronary arterial branches has more than 50 per cent stenosis, the annual mortality rate will be approximately 2 per cent.[265] In a study of unoperated patients with one-vessel disease, Califf et al. reported a 5-year survival of 95 per cent; lesions of the right coronary artery were particularly benign, while patients with proximal obstruction of the left anterior descending coronary artery were at higher risk than were those with more distal lesions; however, even in this group, 90 per cent were alive after 5 years.[266] If two of the three major arteries are stenotic, the annual mortality rate rises to about 7 per cent in symptomatic patients; if all three vessels are stenotic, this rate is approximately 11 per cent.[267–269] Annual mortality is about 20 per cent in patients with disease involving the left main coronary artery (Table 39–9). In addition to the number of vessels involved, the degree of obstruction is also impor-

TABLE 39–9 EXPECTED CARDIAC MORTALITY: NONSURGICAL TREATMENT

	MORTALITY	
	Per Year (%)	5 Years (%)
Normal arteriogram	0	0
Single-vessel obstruction		
LAD	2 to 4	10 to 20
RCA	1 to 2	2 to 8
CIRC	0 to 1	0 to 2
Two-vessel obstruction		
LAD plus RCA or CIRC	7 to 10	35 to 50
Before FSP		40
After FSP		12
RCA and CIRC	3 to 6	15 to 30
Three-vessel obstruction	10 to 12	50 to 60
Left main obstruction	15 to 25	70

LAD = left anterior descending artery; RCA = right coronary artery; CIRC = left circumflex artery; FSP = first septal perforating artery.

From Humphries, J. O.: Expected course of patients with coronary artery disease. *In* Rahimtoola, S. H. (ed.): Coronary Bypass Surgery. Philadelphia, F. A. Davis Co., 1977, p. 48.

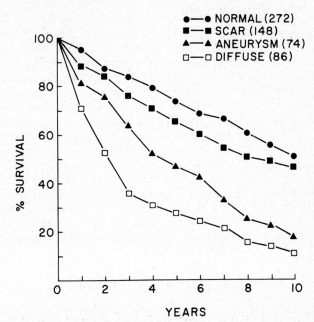

FIGURE 39–11 Ten-year survival curves from the Cleveland Clinic series based on ventriculographic findings. Numbers in parentheses indicate numbers of patients in groups (From Proudfit, W. L., et al.: Natural history of obstructive coronary artery disease: Ten year study of 601 nonsurgical cases. Progr. Cardiovasc. Dis. *41:*53, 1978.)

tant. Thus, the prognosis for patients with 50 to 75 per cent narrowing is clearly better than for those with more than 75 per cent narrowing.[270]

The severity of symptoms also influences prognosis. In asymptomatic or mildly symptomatic patients with one- or two-vessel disease, the prognosis is excellent, i.e., an annual mortality of 1.5 per cent. In patients with three-vessel disease with good exercise capacity, the annual mortality was 4 per cent, but in those with poor exercise capacity, it was 9 per cent.[271] An important feature of studies done at the Cleveland Clinic was the inclusion of left ventricular wall motion abnormalities, which significantly affect prognosis (Fig. 39–11).[272,273] In patients whose natural history could be followed because surgical revascularization was not carried out, the ejection fraction was again confirmed as an important prognostic determinant.[274] Among patients with three-vessel disease, a higher mortality rate has been reported in patients with depressed ejection fractions (36 per cent after 2 years) compared with that in patients with normal ejection fractions (12 per cent after 2 years).[275] Survival can also be estimated from more easily available measurements reflecting left ventricular function: both cardiomegaly on a routine chest radiograph and the presence of a third heart sound on physical examination have adverse effects on prognosis.[276]

High-grade lesions of the *left main coronary artery* are particularly life-threatening, with the Cleveland Clinic reporting a 5-year mortality of 57 per cent.[277] Other groups have also studied this subset of patients and have confirmed these results.[278,278a] Survival appears to be better for patients with 50 to 70 per cent stenosis compared with those having over 70 per cent stenosis; in addition, prog-

nosis is worse in those with a left rather than a right dominant system.

One of the benefits of the arteriographic approach to the estimation of prognosis has been the ability to characterize progression of atherosclerosis in patients with the clinical manifestations of ischemic heart disease. Coronary atherosclerosis is a dynamic rather than static disorder, and the development of new lesions or progression of old ones directly influences prognosis. Progression of coronary obstructive lesions is associated with the development of myocardial infarction but not necessarily with worsening angina pectoris.[279] The time interval between arteriograms is a significant determinant of the extent of progression, but risk factors are probably of less importance.[280,281]

EFFECT OF MEDICAL THERAPY ON PROGNOSIS

Medical therapy differed in the natural history just cited. Since 1975, most patients not subjected to surgical treatment have received beta blockers, which improve survival in those in whom the drug is begun within a month of myocardial infarction (p. 1352).[231,232,281a] The ability of these drugs to exert a similar effect in patients with chronic stable angina without prior infarction is not illogical but entirely conjectural.

UNSTABLE ANGINA

Unstable angina (also known as preinfarction angina, crescendo angina, [acute] coronary insufficiency, and intermediate coronary syndrome) is clinically important because of its frightening and disabling nature and the possibility that it heralds acute myocardial infarction.[282]

The existence of the syndrome was appreciated early in this century, when Osler[6] and later Herrick[8] described cardiac pain that was more severe than angina and often preceded a myocardial infarction. The term "unstable angina" was first proposed in 1971 by Fowler.[283] Pathological studies of patients with this syndrome who do *not* develop an acute fatal myocardial infarction are rare, but those that are available usually reveal multivessel disease but a low incidence of recent occlusive thrombi; these findings suggest that coronary vasospasm and/or transient platelet aggregation may play a role in the development of the acute ischemic episodes occurring in the presence of severe organic obstructive disease.[284] Microinfarcts may occur in many patients suffering from angina (stable as well as unstable) as suggested by pathological studies showing patchy fibrosis in patients without a history or electrocardiographic evidence of frank infarction.[285] Thus, ischemic heart disease may really represent a spectrum of severity of myocardial necrosis, with transmural infarction at one end of the spectrum, ranging through acute subendocardial infarction, to unstable angina, to chronic stable angina at the other end of the spectrum.

CLINICAL MANIFESTATIONS

DEFINITION. In addition to the absence of clear-cut electrocardiographic and cardiac enzyme changes diagnostic of a myocardial infarction, the currently used definition of unstable angina pectoris depends on the presence of *one* or more of the following three historical features, accompanied by electrocardiographic changes: (1) crescendo angina (more severe, prolonged, or frequent) superimposed on a preexisting pattern of relatively stable, exertion-related angina pectoris; (2) angina pectoris at rest as well as with minimal exertion; or (3) angina pectoris of new onset (usually within one month), which is brought on by minimal exertion. The ischemic episodes of unstable angina pectoris are *not* related to obvious precipitating factors, such as anemia, infection, thyrotoxicosis, or cardiac arrhythmias. Prinzmetal's ("variant") angina is a different entity and is discussed on page 1360.

The chest discomfort in this syndrome is similar in quality to that of classic effort-induced angina, although it is usually more intense, is usually described as pain, may persist for as long as 30 minutes, and occasionally awakens the patient from sleep. Longer episodes of ischemic pain are usually associated with acute myocardial infarction. The usual therapeutic regimen of nitroglycerin administration and physical rest often provides only incomplete relief. Several clues should alert the physician to a changing anginal pattern and the development of unstable angina; these include an abrupt and persistent reduction in the threshold of physical activity that provokes angina; an increase in the frequency, severity, and duration of angina; radiation of the discomfort to a new site; and onset of new features associated with the pain, such as diaphoresis, nausea, or palpitation.

The proportion of patients with unstable angina who have angina of new onset, a crescendo pattern superimposed on stable angina, or rest angina varies among different series and depends on how the observers defined the syndrome. In the few studies in which a breakdown of the data is possible (more than one type of pain pattern and large numbers of patients), one group reported 88 patients with new onset of angina versus 79 with either crescendo or rest angina.[286] The National Cooperative Study reported 69 patients with new onset of angina versus 81 with a crescendo pattern and/or rest angina.[287] In a third series, 27 had angina of new onset versus 109 with the crescendo type.[288] Patients in whom unstable angina is superimposed on longstanding, stable angina almost always have significant multivessel obstructive disease, while patients with new onset of severe angina may have a strong dynamic (vasoconstrictive) component superimposed on fixed obstructive disease, involving only a single coronary artery.[289]

PHYSICAL EXAMINATION. This may reveal transient diastolic (third and fourth) heart sounds and dyskinetic apical impulses, suggesting left ventricular dysfunction, or a transient murmur of mitral regurgitation during or immediately after an ischemic episode.[290] These findings are nonspecific, since they may also be present in patients with chronic angina pectoris or acute myocardial infarction.

ELECTROCARDIOGRAM. After the history, the most important feature in the diagnosis of unstable angina is the electrocardiogram; indeed, transient deviations of the ST segment (depression or elevation) often associated with T-wave inversions is the rule. These ST-segment/T-wave changes clear completely or partially with relief of the pain. Persistence of electrocardiographic changes for more than 6 to 12 hours suggests that a subendocardial infarction has occurred. In the National Cooperative Study (which required electrocardiographic changes to establish the diagnosis of unstable angina), only 19 of 150 patients did not have ST-segment changes during angina, and all 19 had T-wave inversions.[287] In one study in which 18 patients with ST-segment elevation during pain were compared with 64 patients with ST-segment depression, no differences in age, sex, history of previous myocardial infarctions, or angiographic features were found.[291] While the presence of the electrocardiographic changes greatly increases the certainty of diagnosis, their absence does not exclude unstable angina. In particular, in patients with a typical history (as outlined above) and established coronary artery disease (previous myocardial infarction, abnormal coronary arteriograms, or a history of a positive noninvasive stress test), the diagnosis can be made with reasonable reliability.

It is in the subgroup of patients without evidence of previous coronary artery disease and no electrocardiographic changes associated with the pain that the chance of finding no underlying coronary artery disease at coronary arteriography is greatest. Patients with unstable angina do not have new Q waves on the surface leads or when intraoperative epicardial electrograms are recorded nor are histopathological abnormalities apparent in biopsy specimens taken from the ischemic area,[292] indicating that the transient ST-T abnormalities are not indicative of infarction.

Standard Laboratory Tests. Findings on chest roentgenogram, serum cholesterol level, and carbohydrate tolerance are similar to those observed in patients with stable angina (p. 1342). Unlike acute myocardial infarction, nonspecific indicators of gross tissue necrosis, such as leukocytosis and fever, are usually absent. Cardiac enzymes are not abnormally elevated; when cardiac-specific enzymes are elevated, by definition the diagnosis is acute myocardial infarction and not unstable angina.

CARDIAC CATHETERIZATION AND CORONARY ARTERIOGRAPHY. Coronary arteriographic findings in patients with unstable angina have generally shown the same distribution of no disease and one-, two-, and three-vessel disease found in patients with chronic angina pectoris and in patients who have suffered a myocardial infarction[293]; the incidence of left main coronary artery disease may be somewhat higher.[294] The left anterior descending coronary artery is the most commonly affected vessel in patients with unstable (as well as stable) angina.[295] The collateral circulation appears less well developed in patients with unstable angina than in those with stable angina pectoris,[290] an arteriographic impression that is supported by findings at operation in which retrograde flow, measured directly by cannulation of the opened artery, was less in patients with unstable angina than in those with chronic stable angina.[296] The incidence of normal coronary arteriograms among patients with unstable angina varies among different series and averages 5 per cent. No obvious explanation other than coronary spasm exists for this finding.

Findings on left ventriculography are similar to those in patients with chronic stable angina and generally show good wall motion *between* episodes of acute ischemia, except of course in patients who have had prior myocardial infarctions. During episodes of acute ischemia, localized areas of asynergy are present and stroke volume and ejection fraction decline, while left ventricular end-systolic and end-diastolic volumes rise, as does left ventricular filling pressure[297]; nitroglycerin restores both global and regional left ventricular function (Fig. 39–12).

PATHOPHYSIOLOGY. Since most patients with unstable angina have severe obstructive coronary artery disease, the episodes of ischemia could be precipitated by an increase in myocardial oxygen demand and/or a reduction in myocardial oxygen supply. In 1966, Roughgarden reported that arterial hypertension *preceded* episodes of spontaneous (rest) angina.[298] Thus, as is the case for exertion-related fixed-threshold angina pectoris, increases in myocardial oxygen requirements appeared to precipitate angina; these observations have been confirmed.[299] However, Maseri and his colleagues have demonstrated that a reduction of myocardial oxygen supply, i.e., coronary vasospasm, may be responsible for many cases of angina at rest and not merely those associated with Prinzmetal's type.[300] In carefully monitored patients, it was observed that a reduction of coronary sinus oxygen saturation, sig-

nifying a reduction of coronary blood flow in the presence of constant oxygen needs, is followed in turn by the characteristic electrocardiographic changes and chest discomfort, and only then does blood pressure and/or heart rate rise.[301] Thus, it now appears that the pathogenesis of unstable angina is more complex than was previously thought. In some patients, oxygen demands rise, even at rest, and outstrip the limited oxygen availability. In others, oxygen requirements remain constant, but the oxygen supply is reduced as a consequence of vasospasm, platelet aggregates, or thrombus formation.[302,303] Both mechanisms (increased demand and reduced supply) probably operate simultaneously in some patients. Indeed, the elevation of arterial pressure and heart rate and coronary vasoconstriction may result from a generalized increase in sympathetic discharge and might well occur simultaneously. The observation that coronary vasoconstriction can occur during exercise in patients with chronic stable angina[304] is an example of the simultaneous augmentation of myocardial oxygen needs with reduced oxygen availability, and a similar mechanism may be operative in patients with unstable angina. Myocardial ischemia probably occurs more commonly than does anginal discomfort in unstable angina, with many patients exhibiting multiple asymptomatic episodes of ST-T changes during continuous electrocardiographic monitoring.[305] Patients with frequent transient ST-segment alterations accompanied by bursts of ventricular tachycardia are a high-risk group, with a high incidence of left main or three-vessel disease and a poor prognosis.[306]

NONINVASIVE TESTS. Approximately one-third of patients with unstable angina have positive technetium-99m stannous pyrophosphate myocardial scintigrams, suggesting diffuse subendocardial necrosis, without electrocardiographic or enzyme changes diagnostic of acute myocardial infarction.[307] These patients either sustained minor degrees of otherwise unrecognized subendocardial necrosis, or their persistently positive scintigrams resulted from infarction that had occurred at some time in the past. Thallium scintigraphy often reveals a transient defect of myocardial perfusion in patients developing angina at rest, accompanied by ST-segment alterations, supporting the concept that a reduction of blood flow is responsible.[308] Two-dimensional echocardiography reveals transient abnormalities of wall motion; patients with unstable angina (without old myocardial infarction) and persistent wall motion abnormalities have a poor prognosis.[309]

INDICATIONS FOR CATHETERIZATION AND ANGIOGRAPHY. As is the case in patients with chronic stable angina, several questions need to be resolved: How will these tests aid in further management of the syndrome? In what patients should they be performed? What are the risks involved? Are any special precautions necessary? Although there is no unanimity of opinion regarding the answers to these questions, we believe that in most instances coronary arteriography is very helpful in the management of patients with unstable angina. For patients in whom medical therapy fails and who require balloon counterpulsation, coronary arteriography should be carried out immediately, i.e., as soon as their condition has been stabilized, unless there are obvious contraindications to coronary bypass surgery. On the other hand, in patients who respond to medical therapy, we recommend catheterization and arteriography several days after symptoms

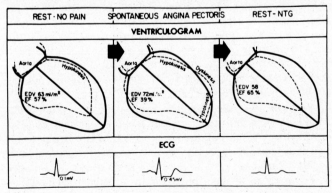

FIGURE 39–12 Diagrammatic representation of left ventricular end-systolic and end-diastolic frames. Note that during spontaneous angina pectoris, when ST-segment depression of 0.45 mV develops, there is an increase in end-diastolic volume (EDV) with a decrease in ejection fraction (EF); regional wall motion abnormality also develops. These values revert to normal after nitroglycerin (NTG) therapy. (From Sharma, B., et al.: Left ventricular function during spontaneous angina pectoris: Effect of sublingual nitroglycerin. Am. J. Cardiol. *46*:34, 1980.)

have stabilized. These procedures are helpful in that they identify several subgroups of patients with unstable angina pectoris and can thus be used to dictate therapy: (1) Patients with left main coronary artery disease—the most life-threatening form of the disease—in whom there is now general agreement that urgent surgery is indicated. (2) Patients in whom a large segment of remaining viable myocardium is perfused by a critically narrowed vessel, which, if occluded, would be likely to result in a fatal or life-threatening infarction; these patients should also be operated upon on an urgent basis. (3) Patients with three-vessel obstructive disease; unless there are contraindications, we recommend that operation be planned on a semiurgent basis (within 10 days) after the patient's condition has stabilized. (4) A small number of patients (about 5 per cent of all patients with unstable angina) with no demonstrable coronary artery disease, in whom the prognosis appears excellent and no further surgical consideration is necessary. In many of these patients coronary spasm is responsible for the angina, and this can be established by an ergonovine test at the time of coronary arteriography (p. 1361); intensification of therapy with nitrates and calcium-channel blockers would then be indicated. (5) Patients with single-vessel disease with a discrete narrow proximal lesion amenable to percutaneous transluminal angioplasty (p. 1353). (6) Patients with diffuse distal coronary artery disease unsuitable for bypass grafting.

Which patients are unsuitable for study? Obviously, patients who are suffering from another serious life-threatening illness with a poor prognosis do not require study. Age is not considered to be a contraindication; arteriography may be of value if unstable angina is present in patients who are in their 70's but who are otherwise fit. The risks of coronary arteriography may be somewhat greater in patients with unstable angina than in those with chronic stable angina. For example, 5 of 136 patients with unstable angina suffered myocardial infarctions with two deaths[310,311] as a consequence of invasive studies, but these were performed before intraaortic balloon counterpulsation was used. The addition of the latter modality to assist in coronary arteriography has reduced mortality to near zero.[312,313] Maximal medical therapy, as described below, should be maintained up to and continued through the time of cardiac catheterization and arteriography.

Other measures must be considered in treatment failures, i.e., in patients with recurrent episodes of myocardial ischemia at low levels of activity or at rest (10 to 15 per cent of all patients). Anticoagulants are not generally employed unless the patient has a history of thromboembolic disease. Intraaortic balloon counterpulsation is often effective in arresting episodes of ischemia in these patients, but improvement is usually only transient, persisting only for as long as counterpulsation is continued. Therefore, this technique is used primarily as an aid in supporting patients while they undergo cardiac catheterization, angiography, and coronary arteriography.[311-313]

MANAGEMENT

Unstable angina pectoris is a serious, potentially dangerous condition, and its management must be approached with this in mind. The patient should be admitted to the hospital and immediately placed at bed rest. Removal from an emotionally taxing situation, a quiet atmosphere, physical and emotional rest, the physician's reassurance, mild sedation, and antianxiety drugs are all helpful and will diminish or relieve episodes of rest pain in perhaps half of all patients. A vigorous effort must be immediately undertaken to diagnose and treat conditions that may be responsible for transient increases in myocardial oxygen demands, such as infection, fever, thyrotoxicosis, anemia, exacerbation of preexisting heart failure, concurrent illnesses (particularly of the pulmonary tract, leading to coughing and hypoxemia, and acute gastrointestinal disturbances, causing vomiting, wretching, or severe diarrhea), tachyarrhythmias that increase myocardial oxygen demand, and severe bradyarrhythmias that reduce myocardial perfusion. Control of these aggravating factors will be helpful in 10 to 15 per cent of patients.[314,315] Placing the bed into the reverse Trendelenburg position (feet down) is a simple measure that may be helpful[316] as may the inhalation of 100 per cent oxygen during periods of pain.

The electrocardiogram should be monitored continuously; diagnostic tests to rule out a myocardial infarction should include serial CK-MB enzymes. Invasive monitoring is usually not necessary unless a serious hemodynamic disturbance is suspected. Frequent radionuclide angiograms, thallium perfusion scans, and two-dimensional echocardiograms, although useful in elucidating the mechanism and consequences of unstable angina, are not very helpful in acute patient management and may actually be harmful in that they disturb the patient's rest.

Nitrates are a mainstay of therapy. In addition to frequently relieving and preventing the pain of unstable angina, they have been shown to improve global and regional left ventricular function, as indicated above (Fig. 39–12). Nitrates may be given sublingually, orally, topically, or intravenously, and they may be of the short- or long-acting variety. The route of administration is probably not very important, except that intravenous nitroglycerin offers the advantage of more consistent control of ischemic episodes during the first 24 hours of treatment.[317] The dose of nitrates should be sufficient to lower arterial pressure by 15 mm Hg or to 100 to 110 mm Hg systolic, whichever represents a smaller reduction. *Beta-adrenergic blockers* also play a key role in the pharmacological treatment of unstable angina pectoris. In patients who are already on beta blockers at the time when unstable angina develops, the drug should be continued unless contraindications have developed. The dosage of the beta blocker should be increased so that resting heart rate drops to between 50 and 60 beats/min.[290] This usually requires 240 to 320 mg of propranolol per day (or the equivalent for other beta blockers). Beta blockade may improve pulmonary congestion if the elevated pulmonary venous pressure is due to an ischemia-induced reduction of left ventricular compliance or left ventricular systolic failure. Rarely, heart failure may be precipitated by beta blockade in patients with previous infarction, and in them the drug should be discontinued or the dose reduced and treatment with diuretics instituted.

Calcium-channel blockers are also helpful in the treatment of unstable angina, either as initial therapy or along with nitrates, and they appear to be about as effective as beta-adrenergic blockers.[318] Alternatively, calcium blockers may be added to nitrates and beta blockers[319]; they appear both to offer symptomatic relief and to lessen failure of

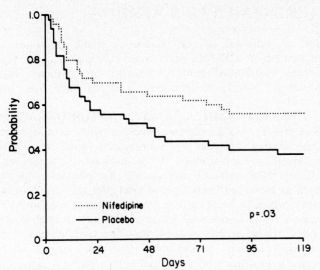

FIGURE 39–13 Effect of nifedipine on the cumulative probability of no failure of medical therapy in all patients. (From Gerstenblith, G., et al.: Nifedipine in unstable angina. A double-blind, randomized trial. N. Engl. J. Med. *306*:885, 1982.)

medical therapy, defined as sudden death, myocardial infarction, or the need for bypass surgery (Fig. 39–13).[320,320a]

Patients in whom medical management fails require *intraaortic balloon counterpulsation*, which results in the prompt relief of chest pain. In many instances the pain recurs when intraaortic balloon pulsation is discontinued; therefore this technique is useful primarily because it allows the safe performance of coronary arteriography.

There is considerable controversy concerning the role of coronary arteriography and coronary artery bypass grafting in the management of unstable angina. It is our policy to recommend urgent surgery (i.e., within 2 days) for patients (with no contraindication to operation) who are medical failures, have a suitable coronary anatomy, and require intraaortic balloon counterpulsation to control or prevent recurrent ischemic episodes as well as for patients with left main coronary artery disease. Other patients are gradually ambulated, and if rest angina or angina on mild effort recurs despite maximal medical therapy and if the coronary anatomy is suitable for bypass grafting, they are operated upon promptly, i.e., during the same period of hospitalization, if possible. Patients with unstable angina and one-vessel disease and discrete proximal lesions may undergo percutaneous transluminal angioplasty, with excellent results.[321,322] Other patients who improve on medical management may be discharged from the hospital, and the decision for operation can be made on the basis of their symptoms and anatomical findings, just as is done for patients with chronic stable angina.

Unstable angina may be associated with enhanced platelet reactivity, as reflected in increased plasma concentrations of platelet factor 4 and beta-thromboglobulin, as well as release of thromboxane B_2 into the coronary sinus.[323,324] It is possible that platelet aggregation at the site of critical obstruction in the coronary vascular bed may intensify ischemia.[325] These considerations have led to a large randomized trial, lasting 12 weeks, in which men with unstable angina regularly took aspirin, a potent antiplatelet drug. One aspirin tablet daily (324 mg) resulted in a 50 per cent reduction in mortality and nonfatal myocardial infarctions.[326]

PROGNOSIS

Early studies of unstable angina consisted of retrospective surveys relating prodromal events to subsequent myocardial infarction; therefore, unstable angina pectoris was considered to be "preinfarction angina," a term that has since outlived its usefulness. It is now appreciated that most patients with unstable angina do not, in fact, develop infarction over the short term. For example, Fulton et al. combined the experience of a large group of general practitioners in Edinburgh, Scotland,[286] with crescendo angina and/or angina at rest. Of 167 patients, only 16 per cent developed a myocardial infarction and 2 per cent died within 3 months. Krauss et al. reviewed 100 patients with angina at rest[327]; immediate hospital mortality was only 1 per cent and the myocardial infarction rate was 7 per cent. However, after one year of followup, mortality was 15 per cent, with a 22 per cent incidence of infarction. The study by Gazes et al., the first reported *long-term* followup study, included 140 patients with unstable angina diagnosed prior to 1961 and followed for 10 years.[288] At 3 months, the incidence of myocardial infarction was 21 per cent and mortality was 10 per cent; at 1 year, mortality was 18 per cent, at 5 years it had risen to 39 per cent, and at 10 years to 52 per cent. Although the overall survival rate was 82 per cent at one year, it was only 57 per cent in the subgroup of patients with persistent pain after 48 hours of bed rest compared with 96 per cent in those patients whose pain was quickly relieved. It appears that patients with unstable angina at highest risk of death and/or infarction are those whose pain does not respond rapidly and in whom the pattern of unstable angina is superimposed on previously stable coronary disease. This correlates with the finding that patients with new onset unstable angina often have one-vessel disease.[289] The prognosis over a 6-month period has been reported to be similar for patients discharged from the hospital with the diagnosis of acute myocardial infarction and for those admitted to the Coronary Care Unit suspected of having an infarction that was subsequently ruled out,[328] i.e., patients with unstable angina.

One of the threads that runs through reports on patients with unstable angina is the *prodrome* of myocardial infarction that many patients experience. This was commented on as early as 1923 by Wearn in describing cases of myocardial infarction at the Peter Bent Brigham Hospital.[10] As Solomon et al. have noted, nearly 50 years later, 65 of 100 patients with acute myocardial infarction reported more intense angina or longer periods of angina (in other words, unstable angina) shortly before infarction.[329] It should be stressed, however, that while a prodrome of unstable angina often precedes acute myocardial infarction, the opposite is not the case, i.e., only a minority of cases of unstable angina pectoris terminate in early infarction.

Clearly, the prognosis of unstable angina has improved over the past 15 years. During this period, the current therapy of unstable angina pectoris evolved in a piecemeal fashion. At the same time, the definition of unstable angina has broadened, and cardiologists have lowered their threshold for making this diagnosis. Whether either of these events (or perhaps their combination) is responsible for the improved prognosis is not clear.

VARIANT ANGINA PECTORIS (PRINZMETAL'S ANGINA)

In 1959, Prinzmetal et al. described an unusual syndrome of cardiac pain that occurs almost exclusively at rest, is not precipitated by physical exertion or emotional stress, and is associated with ST-segment elevations on the electrocardiogram.[330] This syndrome, now known as *Prinzmetal's or variant angina*, may be associated with severe cardiac arrhythmias, including ventricular tachycardia and fibrillation, and acute myocardial infarction as well as sudden death. Its incidence relative to that of the other forms of ischemic heart disease has not been established.

CLINICAL MANIFESTATIONS

The history in patients with this form of angina differs from that of typical angina: the principal finding is angina *at rest*.[331] In contrast to unstable angina, the rest pain does not usually represent an "evolution" from an earlier period in which pain occurred with decreasing levels of effort. Although exercise capacity is usually well preserved, some patients experience their typical pain and ST-segment elevations not only at rest but during or after exertion as well[304,332]; the anginal discomfort may be extremely severe and accompanied by syncope, the latter presumably caused by arrhythmias. Attacks of variant angina tend to be clustered between midnight and 8 A.M.[333] Some patients have a combination of fixed-threshold, exertion-induced angina with ST-segment depression, and variant angina (rest angina with ST-segment elevation).[334-339] Rarely, variant angina develops following coronary artery bypass grafting.[340] In approximately one-fourth of patients variant angina appears to be a manifestation of a generalized vasospastic disorder, with accompanying attacks of migraine and Raynaud's phenomenon.[341] Patients with Prinzmetal's angina are often younger than patients with classic exertion-induced angina, and the great preponderance among males that is characteristic of stable angina is not seen.[342] Many patients are heavy cigarette smokers.

On *physical examination*, patients with Prinzmetal's angina do not usually exhibit the risk factors for coronary atherosclerosis. Cardiac examination is usually normal in the absence of ischemia (unless the patient has previously suffered a myocardial infarction) but often reveals signs of impaired left ventricular function during episodes of myocardial ischemia.

ELECTROCARDIOGRAM. The electrocardiogram is the key to the diagnosis of variant angina. ST segments, usually normal at rest, develop characteristic elevations with pain (Fig. 39–14). In some patients episodes of ST-segment elevation alternate with episodes of ST-segment depression accompanied by pseudonormalization of the T waves. Many patients exhibit multiple attacks of asymptomatic ST-segment deviation. The ST-segment deviations may be present in any leads but are particularly frequent in inferior leads and disappear as pain subsides. Arrhythmias and conduction disturbances are rather common during episodes of ischemia[343]; experimental work and clinical observations suggest that the incidence of arrhythmias depends on the severity of the ischemia and that the risk of ventricular fibrillation during release of coronary spasm may be greater in patients *without* collateral blood flow induced by fixed coronary lesions.[344,345] Myocardial cell damage, as reflected in the release of small quantities of myoglobin or CK-MB, may occur in the absence of persistent electrocardiographic changes in patients with prolonged attacks.[346] Transient Q waves have been observed.[347]

HEMODYNAMIC AND ARTERIOGRAPHIC STUDIES. Unlike chronic stable angina, hemodynamic data during episodes of spontaneous pain have been obtained only fortuitously.[348,349] In contrast to patients with classic (effort-related) angina, no hemodynamic factors such as increased heart rate, arterial pressure and contractility, which increase cardiac work or oxygen consumption, appear to be responsible for precipitating the anginal episodes. These studies suggest that the pathophysiological mechanisms that precipitate Prinzmetal's angina differ from those causing effort-related angina pectoris. Spasm of a proximal coronary artery with resultant transmural ischemia, first postulated as the cause of variant angina, has now been convincingly documented (Fig. 10–41, p. 335).

The *coronary anatomy* in Prinzmetal's angina has been

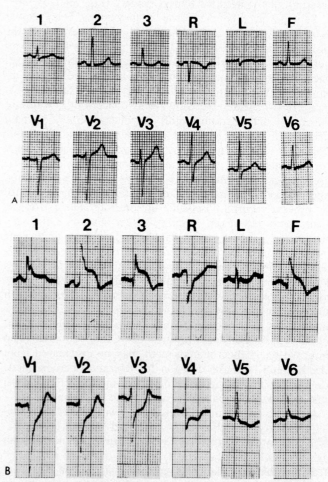

FIGURE 39–14 Electrocardiogram (*A*) prior to an episode of Prinzmetal's angina and (*B*) during an episode of Prinzmetal's angina. ST segments are now markedly elevated in the inferior leads, with reciprocal depression in the anterior leads. After nitroglycerin was given, the ECG returned to baseline. (From Berman, N. D., et al.: Prinzmetal's angina with coronary artery spasm. Angiographic, pharmacologic, metabolic and radionuclide perfusion studies. Am. J. Med. 60:727, 1976.)

defined both at autopsy and during coronary arteriography; severe proximal coronary atherosclerosis of at least one major vessel is a common finding, but many patients apparently have normal coronary arteries in the absence of ischemia.[350,351] Selzer et al. noted that patients with variant angina who had normal coronary arteriograms, i.e., no evidence of fixed obstruction, were more likely to have purely nonexertional angina and ST-segment elevations involving inferior leads, while patients with variant angina who had organic obstructive lesions with superimposed coronary spasm often had associated effort angina and ischemia in anterolateral leads.[351] During followup, patients with no or mild fixed coronary obstruction exhibit a more benign course than do patients with associated severe obstructive lesions.[352]

THE ERGONOVINE TEST. A number of provocative tests for coronary spasm have been developed. Of these, the ergonovine test is the most sensitive and useful. Ergonovine maleate, an ergot alkaloid that stimulates both alpha-adrenergic and serotonergic receptors and therefore exerts a direct constrictive effect on vascular smooth muscle, has been used to induce coronary artery spasm in patients with Prinzmetal's angina. Coronary arteries that constrict spontaneously appear to be supersensitive to this agent. When administered intravenously in doses ranging from 0.05 to 0.40 mg, ergonovine provides a sensitive and specific test for provoking coronary artery spasm.[353,354,354a] There is a rough correlation between the dose of ergonovine required to induce a positive test and the frequency of spontaneous attacks[355]. In low doses and in carefully controlled clinical situations, ergonovine is a relatively safe drug, but prolonged coronary artery spasm precipitated by ergonovine may cause myocardial infarction. Because of this hazard, it is recommended that ergonovine be administered only to patients in whom coronary arteriography has demonstrated normal or nearly normal coronary arteries and in gradually increasing doses, beginning with a very low dose. The test should be carried out only in a setting where appropriate resuscitation equipment, drugs, and personnel are readily available, usually in the cardiac catheterization laboratory, so that the angiographic diagnosis of spasm can be made and intracoronary nitroglycerin can be administered to abolish the spasm. Some investigators have also found that the ergonovine test can be carried out safely in the coronary care unit, with a positive test being reflected in the development of chest pain and ST-segment depression[355–357]; however, the safety of the test in this setting has not been firmly established.[358,359]

Methacholine,[360] a parasympathomimetic drug, and *histamine*[361] can also induce coronary artery spasm. Like ergonovine, these agents are capable of producing marked coronary artery spasm both in patients with variant angina who have severe underlying arteriosclerotic coronary artery narrowing and in those without such fixed stenoses. Exercise, the cold pressor test, and induced alkalosis can all cause coronary spasm in patients with variant angina, but none of these tests is as sensitive as ergonovine.[362] Catheter-induced coronary ostial spasm is nonspecific and not helpful in the diagnosis of Prinzmetal's angina.

Myocardial Perfusion Studies. Localization of the myocardial perfusion defect to an area perfused by a coronary artery in which spasm can be demonstrated by arteriography has been reported using intravenous thallium-

201,[363,364] and a reduction in coronary sinus flow during episodes of spasm has also been noted.[365] These studies support the relationship between coronary spasm causing impaired myocardial perfusion and ischemia.

MANAGEMENT

Although the management of Prinzmetal's variant angina is similar in some respects to that of chronic stable angina pectoris, there are important differences:

1. Patients with both forms of angina respond promptly to nitrates; sublingual or intravenous nitroglycerin can abolish attacks promptly, and long-acting nitrates are useful in preventing attacks.[366] However, the mechanism of action of the drugs may differ in the two types of angina. As already discussed (p. 1347), in chronic (effort-induced) stable angina, an important action of the nitrates appears to involve reducing myocardial oxygen needs, with augmentation of the oxygen supply a secondary effect. In Prinzmetal's angina, the nitrates abolish or prevent myocardial ischemia by exerting a direct vasodilating effect on the coronary arteries.

2. In patients with chronic stable angina pectoris, beta-adrenergic blockade is usually beneficial, but the response of patients with Prinzmetal's angina is variable. Some of the latter, particularly those with associated fixed lesions, exhibit a reduction in the frequency of exertion-induced anginal episodes produced primarily by an augmentation of myocardial oxygen requirements. In others, however, propranolol or any nonselective beta-adrenergic blocker may actually be detrimental, since blockade of the beta$_2$ receptors, which subserve coronary dilation, allows unopposed alpha-receptor–mediated coronary artery vasoconstriction to occur. The duration of episodes of vasotonic angina have been reported to be prolonged by propranolol.[216]

3. The calcium-channel blockers have been found to be extremely effective in preventing the coronary artery spasm of variant angina.[342,367–369] In a multicenter trial with nifedipine, there were dramatic reductions in the frequency of episodes and in the need for nitroglycerin (Fig. 39–15). Since calcium-channel blockers act through different mechanisms, the vasodilatory actions of these drugs may add to those of nitroglycerin. Prazosin, a selective alpha-adrenergic blocker[370] (p. 916), has also been found to be of value in patients with Prinzmetal's angina,[371] while aspirin, helpful in unstable angina (p. 1359), may actually be harmful in patients with Prinzmetal's angina, since in large doses aspirin inhibits the biosynthesis of the naturally occurring coronary vasodilator prostaglandin I$_2$.[372]

Coronary artery bypass surgery is not indicated for patients with isolated coronary spasm but may be helpful in patients who also have severe fixed lesions. In these patients, surgical treatment can abolish the exertion-induced angina,[373] and subsequently, a combination of calcium-channel blockers and nitrates may be used to treat the spastic component.

PROGNOSIS

Patients with variant angina with normal coronary arteriograms have a more benign course than do patients with associated coronary atherosclerosis.[351] Sudden death has

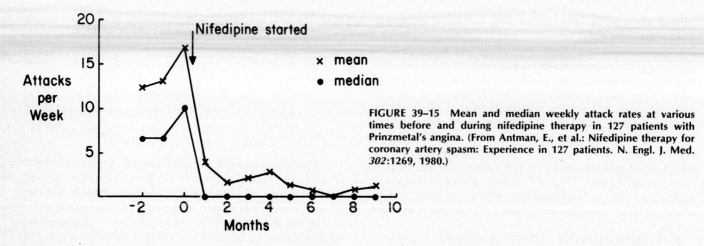

FIGURE 39–15   Mean and median weekly attack rates at various times before and during nifedipine therapy in 127 patients with Prinzmetal's angina. (From Antman, E., et al.: Nifedipine therapy for coronary artery spasm: Experience in 127 patients. N. Engl. J. Med. *302*:1269, 1980.)

been reported in about 15 per cent of patients with variant angina, with half occurring in the first 3 months after the onset of symptoms. Of 132 consecutive patients studied by Waters et al.,[374] 18 died or experienced a myocardial infarction within one month of the development of this condition. Severe ischemia, pain, and ST-segment elevation unrelieved by calcium-channel blockers or nitroglycerin may cause cardiogenic shock prior to elevation of enzyme levels, and myocardial infarction may occur in the absence of fixed lesions and in spite of clinical improvement with a calcium-channel blocking drug.[374] In most patients who survive an infarction, the condition stabilizes, presumably because the myocardium perfused by the vessel that undergoes spasm is no longer viable; in others, there is also a tendency for symptoms to stabilize and to diminish with time. Thus, variant angina may go into remission, and the results of the ergonovine test may become negative.[355]

Patients with Prinzmetal's angina who have no associated fixed organic obstruction represent one end of a spectrum of coronary artery disease; the other end of this spectrum is represented by patients with fixed lesions without associated vasospasm (see Fig. 39–1, p. 1336). The former patients present with angina at rest—these cases are the extreme forms of variable-threshold angina due to vasospasm causing reduction of oxygen supply—while the latter cases are the extreme forms of fixed-threshold angina due to increased oxygen need in the face of a restricted but constant oxygen supply. As noted earlier (p. 1336), Maseri has indicated that a vasospastic element is common in many patients with rest angina, whether of the Prinzmetal type with ST-segment elevation or associated with ST-seg-

ment depression.[300] Careful and prolonged monitoring has revealed that in many patients angina at rest may be associated with ST-segment elevation and at other times with ST-segment depression, blurring the distinction between variant angina and unstable angina. These observations reinforce the pathophysiological importance of coronary spasm in *both* Prinzmetal's angina and in some instances of typical angina.

It is now clear that in many—perhaps most—patients with symptomatic coronary artery disease, there is some combination of these two causes of myocardial ischemia. As pointed out above, many patients with Prinzmetal's variant angina have one or more discrete obstructive lesions, while many patients with chronic stable angina can exhibit dynamic obstruction,[375] i.e., they may evidence coronary vasoconstriction during the cold pressor test,[376,377] during emotion,[31] and on exercise; frequently this can be abolished by calcium-channel blockade. Also, the ergonovine test may be positive in 20 per cent of patients with recent transmural infarction.[378] It is important to determine the position of a given patient with coronary artery disease within this spectrum and to adjust therapy appropriately. Patients in whom myocardial ischemia is caused largely by spasm respond best to nitroglycerin and calcium-channel blockers; beta-adrenergic blockers and coronary artery bypass grafting are of little, if any, value. On the other hand, for patients in whom ischemia is caused primarily by fixed obstructive lesions, beta-adrenergic blockers and surgical therapy are the mainstays of therapy; however, in these patients, nitrates and calcium-channel blockers are also useful.[379,380]

ISCHEMIC HEART DISEASE IN WHICH DISCOMFORT IS NOT THE DOMINANT SYMPTOM

"SILENT" MYOCARDIAL ISCHEMIA

Epidemiological studies of sudden death[381] (Chap. 23) as well as clinical and postmortem studies of patients with "silent" myocardial infarction[382] suggest that many individuals with extensive coronary artery obstruction do not

have angina pectoris in any of its recognized forms (stable, unstable, or variant). These individuals have no anginal "warning system,"[40] and both patient and physician may be unaware of the presence of ischemic heart disease until a fatal event ensues or an old infarction is detected on a routine electrocardiogram. In many other patients, a myocardial infarction is the first clinical manifestation of ischemic heart disease, although necropsy or angiographic studies indicate that the coronary atherosclerosis must have been of many years' duration. Not enough is known about the clinical state of these patients without angina *prior* to the morbid event to permit a description of findings at physical examination or on laboratory studies, except to note that some of them can be identified prior to such an event because of the presence of cardiac arrhythmias or abnormal electrocardiograms (occasionally at rest, more commonly during exercise) or by means of coronary arteriography performed in response to a positive exercise test.[383]

Several factors may explain the difference in symptoms among patients with extensive coronary obstructive disease. These include differences in the amount of myocardium in jeopardy, different thresholds of pain sensitivity, the presence of autonomic neuropathies (sensory denervation) as occurs in diabetics, psychological denial, and the influence of cultural norms concerning the "acceptability" of symptoms in otherwise healthy persons.

Thus, the detection of patients with extensive coronary artery disease without angina is fortuitous at the present time. The cost-benefit ratio of carrying out screening exercise electrocardiograms or radionuclide studies on large numbers of asymptomatic individuals is not clear, and many false-positive tests occur in this patient group (p. 274).[384,385] An extensive effort to detect such patients was carried out in Norway, where a combination of screening techniques (questionnaires, resting and exercise electrocardiograms) was utilized in over 2000 asymptomatic and presumably healthy men 40 to 50 years of age[386]; patients known to have heart disease, hypertension, or diabetes were excluded. As a result of the screening, more than 105 men were referred for coronary angiography: only 20 on the basis of a suspicious history, and the rest because of electrocardiographic abnormalities. Two-thirds were found to have coronary artery disease. Overall, less than 4 per cent of this population had silent myocardial ischemia, i.e., more than 75 per cent luminal stenosis of one or more coronary arteries. This figure is close to the 4 to 5 per cent of the population estimated by others to be the size of this subgroup.[34,41]

Silent myocardial ischemia can also be demonstrated in asymptomatic post-infarction patients, as well as in patients who *do* complain of angina. In these persons, the pain pattern is variable and cannot always be correlated with objective evidence of myocardial ischemia, especially ST-segment deviations detected on ambulatory electrocardiography or myocardial perfusion abnormalities.[387,388] In the absence of angina, signs and symptoms aside from an electrocardiographic abnormality may suggest ischemic heart disease. These include cardiac arrhythmias and, in patients who have suffered previous myocardial infarctions, congestive heart failure. Even when angina pectoris is present, these features may dominate the clinical picture.

Management of patients with silent coronary artery disease is unresolved. Modification of risk factors is recommended, as it is for all patients with ischemic heart disease. The role, if any, of prophylactic nitrates and beta blockers is unclear. The prognosis is uncertain because of the lack of any large-scale studies; however, available data[389] suggest that the prognosis for patients with this syndrome may be better than that for patients with similar coronary obstructive disease and typical angina.

CONGESTIVE HEART FAILURE

Manifestations of congestive heart failure are common in patients with coronary artery disease but may be predominant in some, especially those who have sustained prior myocardial infarctions and in whom the ischemic focus may have become replaced by fibrous scar, with disappearance or reduction of the angina. The three most common causes of congestive heart failure are (1) left ventricular aneurysm, (2) mitral regurgitation due to papillary muscle dysfunction, and (3) an inadequate quantity of normally contracting myocardium.

LEFT VENTRICULAR ANEURYSM. This is usually defined as paradoxical (dyskinetic) systolic expansion of a portion of the ventricular wall, most commonly the anterior or apical segment.[390] In vitro length-tension studies of tissue taken from human ventricular aneurysms have demonstrated that chronic fibrous aneurysms interfere with ventricular performance principally through loss of contractile tissue but that the extent of expansion and "lost work" by the normal left ventricle is minor.[391] These might be considered to be anatomical but not functional aneurysms (Fig. 39–16). In contrast, aneurysms made up largely of a mixture of scar tissue and viable myocardium or of thin scar tissue produce a mechanical disadvantage by a combination of paradoxical expansion and loss of effective contraction[392]; these might be considered to be functional aneurysms. *False aneurysms* (pseudoaneurysms), which represent localized myocardial rupture, in which the hemorrhage is limited by pericardial adhesions (Fig. 37–5, p. 1269, and Fig. 39–16) have a mouth that is considerably smaller than the maximal diameter.

The frequency of the development of true and false ventricular aneurysms after myocardial infarction depends on the incidence of transmural myocardial infarction and congestive heart failure in the population studied. Left ventricular aneurysm in the absence of coronary artery disease but with prior infarction has been reported,[393] but it is a rare occurrence.

The usual clinical manifestation of large aneurysms is heart failure due to decreased viable myocardium and the "lost work" referred to above, although many patients with large aneurysms do *not* manifest heart failure. Others may have angina or systemic embolization[394] from thrombi that can be detected by angiography, two-dimensional echocardiography,[395–397] or indium-111–labeled autologous platelets[398] (Fig. 39–17), with or without congestive heart failure. In addition, patients with ventricular aneurysms have a high incidence of arrhythmias. Diagnostic clues to the presence of an aneurysm include persistent ST-segment elevations on the electrocardiogram and a characteristic contour (bulge) of the cardiac silhouette of the left ventricle on a chest roentgenogram (Fig. 6–3B, p. 149). Although the last two findings, when clear-cut, are relatively specific, they have limited sensitivity. Furthermore, while phonocardiography, apexcardiography, and M-mode echocardiography display only nonspecific abnormalities and

LEFT VENTRICULAR ANEURYSM IN CORONARY HEART DISEASE

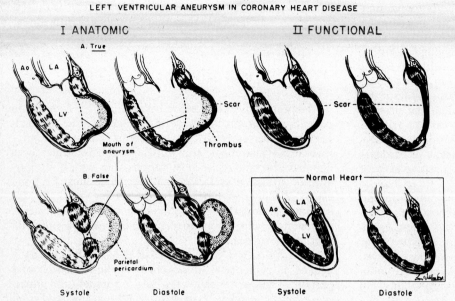

FIGURE 39–16 Diagrams of hearts in systole and diastole with true and false anatomical and functional left ventricular aneurysms and healed myocardial infarction. A diagram of a normal heart in systole and diastole is shown for comparison. The *true anatomical left ventricular aneurysm* protrudes during both systole and diastole, has a mouth that is as wide as or wider than the maximal diamete has a wall that was formerly the wall of the left ventricle, and is composed of fibrous tissue with or without residual myocardial fibers. A true aneurysm may or may not contain thrombus and almost never ruptures once the wall is healed. The *false anatomical left ventricular aneurysm* protrudes during both systole and diastole, has a mouth that is considerably smaller than the maximal diameter of the aneurysm and represents a myocardial rupture site, has a wall made up of parietal pericardium, virtually always contains thrombus, and often ruptures. The *functional left ventricular aneurysm* protrudes during ventricular systole but not during diastole and consists of fibrous tissue with or without myocardial fibers. (From Cabin, H. S., and Roberts, W. C.: Left ventricular aneurysm, intraaneurysmal thrombus and systemic embolus in coronary heart disease. Chest *77*:586, 1980.)

cannot confirm the diagnosis, radionuclide ventriculography[399] (Fig. 11–12, p. 368) and two-dimensional echocardiography[400] (Fig. 5–67, p. 127) can demonstrate aneurysms. Left ventricular angiography is the most precise method available for outlining a left ventricular aneurysm.

True ventricular aneurysms do not rupture, and operative excision is carried out in order to improve left ventricular function in patients with severe heart failure or intractable arrhythmias (p. 1374). Pseudoaneurysms do rupture, on the other hand, and they should be resected on an urgent basis as soon as the diagnosis is established.

MITRAL REGURGITATION.[401,402] Rupture of a papillary muscle, or of the head of a papillary muscle, usually causes severe acute mitral regurgitation in the course of an acute myocardial infarction (p. 1076). Chronic mitral regurgitation in patients with ischemic heart disease is caused, most commonly, by papillary muscle dysfunction due to ischemia or fibrosis and/or by dilatation of the mitral annulus; many of the latter patients have ventricular aneurysms (p. 1074). Most patients with chronic coronary artery disease and mitral regurgitation suffered prior myocardial infarction, but the frequency of this syndrome (as with aneurysm) varies depending on the population studied. In one series, a 31 per cent incidence of mitral regurgitation on left ventricular angiograms of patients with

documented coronary artery disease was reported.[403] Clinical features that help to identify mitral regurgitation due to papillary muscle dysfunction as the cause of acute pulmonary edema or of milder symptoms of left-sided failure include a heart murmur and demonstration of a prolapsing mitral valve leaflet on echocardiography. The latter is the preferred diagnostic technique, since the timing and duration of the murmur are variable. Instead of being only mid- to late systolic, as was originally thought, murmurs may be holosystolic or early systolic. The left atrium is usually not greatly enlarged unless severe mitral regurgitation has been present for almost a year. The electrocardiogram is nonspecific, and most patients have angiographic evidence of multivessel coronary artery disease.[404] Mitral valve replacement alone is rarely indicated but may be undertaken in the course of coronary artery bypass grafting.

ISCHEMIC CARDIOMYOPATHY. The term *ischemic cardiomyopathy*, first used by Burch and colleagues, refers to the condition in which ischemic heart disease results in severe myocardial dysfunction, often indistinguishable from the manifestations of primary cardiomyopathy.[405] Angina may or may not be present, but congestive heart failure, caused by diffuse fibrosis or multiple infarctions but not by a single discrete ventricular aneurysm, dominates the clinical picture. In some patients angina had

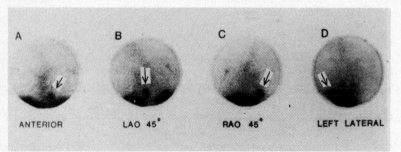

FIGURE 39–17 This scintiphoto was obtained 96 hours after injection of the platelet suspension. Images are oriented with the top of the figure cephalad. Activity in the left lower quadrant in panels *A* and *B* is from the liver. The cardiac blood pool and blood pool from the great vessels are clearly delineated. LAO = left anterior oblique; RAO = right anterior oblique. In panel *C* the liver is superimposed on the spleen and occupies the lower zone of the frame. In all four views, the round homogeneous areas of increased and abnormal indium-III activity (arrows) represent active thrombus in a large anteroapical left ventricular aneurysm. (From Ezekowitz, M. D., et al.: Identification of left ventricular thrombi in man using indium-III–labeled autologous platelets. A preliminary report. Circulation *63*:803, 1981, by permission of the American Heart Association, Inc.)

been the principal clinical manifestation at one time but then diminished or even disappeared as heart failure became more prominent. Generalized abnormalities of left ventricular wall motion dominate the angiographic picture; in some patients, mitral regurgitation due to annular dilatation is also present.[406,407] A history of multiple prior infarctions is very common and is usually associated with severe, multivessel coronary artery disease. A small number of patients have no history of angina, and in them, ischemic cardiomyopathy may be confused with dilated cardiomyopathy (p. 1400); the diagnosis is made clinically by the history of a prior infarction, often with a typical electrocardiogram; some patients do not even have a history of infarction, but the electrocardiogram usually suggests this diagnosis, which can be confirmed by coronary arteriography.

Medical therapy is similar to that for other patients with congestive heart failure (Chap. 16), but the prognosis is poor. In one study, a 31 per cent one-year mortality was reported.[406] At the Cleveland Clinic, 27 of 32 (84 per cent) patients with congestive heart failure and coronary artery disease had died 5 years after presentation.[277] The prognosis may depend on the diffuseness of left ventricular dysfunction. Thus, patients with relatively well-demarcated wall motion disorders and heart failure may have a somewhat more favorable clinical course than do patients with diffuse disease.[277] The prognosis also depends on the degree of electrical instability of the heart as well as the extent of atherosclerosis in vessels perfusing residual viable myocardium and the likelihood of additional infarction with further compromise of left ventricular performance.

CARDIAC ARRHYTHMIAS. Many patients with ischemic heart disease with serious cardiac arrhythmias have other manifestations of myocardial ischemia, such as acute myocardial infarction. Various degrees of ventricular ectopic activity are the most common arrhythmias. The frequency and severity of ventricular arrhythmias induced during exercise tests[84,85] and ambulatory monitoring correlate with the degree of arteriographically documented coronary artery disease. Patients with severe left ventricular dysfunction associated with multivessel disease have more high-grade ectopic activity than do those with normal ventricular function and single-vessel disease.[408] The fraction of patients with ischemic heart disease in whom cardiac arrhythmias are the *predominant* manifestation of chronic coronary artery disease is not known. That there is a substantial subgroup of patients with coronary artery disease and occult arrhythmias is suggested by the frequency with which sudden death is the first manifestation of ischemic heart disease (Chap. 23). When arrhythmias are the predominant clinical manifestation, they are also the main focus of therapeutic interventions.

CORONARY ARTERY DISEASE COMPLICATING VALVULAR AND NONCARDIAC DISORDERS

Atherosclerotic coronary disease may occur in the presence of any other form of cardiac disease. It may occur concomitantly with pericardial disease or cardiomyopathy (including hypertrophic obstructive cardiomyopathy, where it can pose a diagnostic problem that may ne-

cessitate coronary arteriography [p. 1409]), and it is a common associated finding in patients with valvular heart disease (Chap. 32). For many years, ischemic heart disease was considered to be an uncommon occurrence in patients with rheumatic mitral valve disease. In the era preceding coronary arteriography, *clinical* evidence of atherosclerotic coronary artery disease was rare among several large groups of patients with mitral stenosis or regurgitation.[409,410] More recent coronary arteriographic and autopsy studies continue to show that ischemic heart disease occurs relatively infrequently in patients with rheumatic mitral valve disease, perhaps because of the relative youth of these patients and the preponderance of women with symptomatic mitral stenosis, but the concurrence of these two conditions is not as rare as was once believed. For example, in one series, 5 of 26 male patients with mitral stenosis had significant coronary obstruction on coronary arteriography[411]; 8 had discrete but nonobstructive atherosclerotic luminal irregularities, and the remaining 13 had normal coronary arteries.

The frequency of angina pectoris in patients with significant *aortic valve disease* has been reported to range from 40 to 80 per cent in those with predominant aortic stenosis[412] and 3 to 60 per cent in those with predominant aortic regurgitation.[412,413] In a more recent series, typical angina pectoris occurred in 52 per cent of patients with aortic stenosis, in 35 per cent of patients with aortic regurgitation, and in 45 per cent of patients with combined aortic stenosis and regurgitation.[414] Angina may occur in patients with aortic valve disease with or without concomitant coronary artery obstruction, and the frequency of associated coronary disease has varied widely, from 10 to 56 per cent.[412-416] The reported frequency of coronary artery obstruction in patients with severe aortic valve disease and at least one critically narrowed coronary artery without angina has been reported to vary in incidence from 0 to 25 per cent. Although many adults with aortic valve disease and angina do not have associated coronary artery disease, the incidence of coronary artery disease is sufficiently high that we believe that coronary arteriography is indicated *prior* to aortic valve replacement in patients with typical or even atypical anginal pain, so that, if necessary, coronary revascularization can be carried out during the course of this procedure.

The treatment of coronary artery disease occurring in patients with aortic valve disease should be modified; beta-adrenergic blockade is generally contraindicated in patients with critical aortic stenosis and in patients with aortic regurgitation and left ventricular dilatation because of the hazard of any reduction in left ventricular contractility in the face of fixed stenosis. Also, the hypotensive effects of nitrates and nifedipine can be hazardous in patients with critical aortic stenosis. However, these vasodilators are usually well tolerated in patients with aortic regurgitation.

Coronary artery disease can complicate any systemic disorder, but it is now recognized that patients undergoing chronic hemodialysis for renal failure and those who have received kidney transplants may exhibit accelerated atherogenesis involving all arteries, including the coronary vessels (p. 1753).[417,418] Therefore, the frequency of cardiovascular morbidity and mortality consequent to coronary atherosclerosis is strikingly increased in these patients.[419-420]

NONATHEROMATOUS CORONARY ARTERY DISEASE

Nonatheromatous ischemic heart disease may result from congenital abnormalities in the origin or distribution of the coronary arteries (p. 971). The most important of these are anomalous origin of a coronary artery (usually the left) from the pulmonary artery, origin of both coronary arteries from either the right or left sinus of Valsalva, and coronary arteriovenous fistula. This last lesion may also develop as a result of trauma (p. 1536).

A number of inherited connective tissue disorders are frequently associated with myocardial ischemia.[421] These include the Marfan syndrome (aortic dissection) (p. 1665), Hurler's syndrome (coronary obstruction) (p. 1670), homocystinuria (coronary artery thrombosis) (Chap. 34), Ehlers-Danlos syndrome (coronary arterial dissection) (p. 1668), and pseudoxanthoma elasticum (accelerated coronary artery disease) (p. 1669). The mucocutaneous lymph node syndrome may cause coronary artery aneurysms and ischemic heart disease in children (p. 1053).

Perhaps the most common cause of nonatheromatous coronary disease resulting in myocardial ischemia is the syndrome of angina-like pain despite normal coronary arteriograms, discussed on page 1338. Myocardial ischemia not caused by coronary atherosclerosis can also result from embolism, as in infective endocarditis (Chap. 33); mitral valve prolapse (p. 1089); prosthetic valve thrombosis; primary tumors of the heart (Chap. 42); calcific emboli from calcified aortic valves; especially during operation; mural thrombi in patients with cardiomyopathy and myocardial infarction; and aortitis (lues, arteritis) (Chap. 45).

An interesting nonatherosclerotic ischemic syndrome has been described in workers in the nitrate industry who apparently experience nitrate withdrawal symptoms on weekends, presumed to be secondary to coronary spasm when there is no counterstimulation to the vasoconstriction that they undergo as an adaptation to the vasodilating actions of the high concentrations of nitrates to which they are exposed.[422]

SURGICAL MANAGEMENT OF ISCHEMIC HEART DISEASE

HISTORICAL PERSPECTIVE

Numerous operations have been proposed for the treatment of coronary artery disease. The earliest was cardiac denervation, consisting of excision of cardiac fibers. Although many patients reported relief of angina, this procedure did not gain wide acceptance. Procedures to revascularize the myocardium have included suturing the omentum directly to the epicardium,[423] obstruction of coronary venous outflow,[424] application of irritants to the epicardium in the hope that new blood vessels would form, and ligation of the distal internal mammary artery in order to increase blood flow through the pericardial branches.[425] These approaches were of little value because they did not take into account the magnitude of the blood flow deficit nor the fact that the major site of diminished perfusion was in the deep rather than superficial layers of the myocardium.[426]

In 1964, Vineberg and Walter reported on the generally favorable clinical course of 140 patients in whom the more physiologic operation (carried out over the preceding 13 years) of implantation of a systemic (internal mammary) artery deep into the myocardium, beyond the area of obstruction, resulted in the formation of new blood vessels that communicated with the distal branches of the obstructed coronary artery.[427] A beneficial effect on myocardial lactate metabolism as well as on myocardial blood flow was demonstrated in some patients.[428] Patency of the implants to the preexisting coronary circulation was demonstrated on selective arteriography in about half the cases. Although sustained relief of angina and reductions in mortality or in the rate of recurrent myocardial infarction, compared with medically treated patients, were never clearly demonstrated,[426,429] there is little doubt that in individual patients an internal mammary artery implant can act as the crucial source of blood to an otherwise severely underperfused region. In most patients, however, blood flow through the grafts is simply too low for adequate revascularization.[430]

Cardiovascular surgeons at the Cleveland Clinic then introduced or popularized several surgical procedures that directly involved the coronary arteries, including "roofing over" an atheromatous plaque with a pericardial patch graft, resecting the obstructed portion of the coronary artery and interposing a venous graft, and/or endarterectomy,[431,432] but none of these operations was shown to provide sustained benefit and all were often associated with a high operative mortality rate. A major advance took place in 1964, when DeBakey and colleagues anastomosed portions of an autologous saphenous vein proximally to the aorta and distally to the diseased coronary artery beyond the obstruction.[433] The internal mammary artery was then used for the same purpose.[434] These procedures were soon found to be qualitatively superior to the earlier operations because they were capable of delivering substantial quantities of blood to previously ischemic myocardium, providing marked and sustained relief of angina pectoris in most patients. These direct revascularization procedures are now being used widely on more than 100,000 patients per year in the United States. Thus, aortocoronary bypass grafting not only has become the most widely applied cardiac operation but is now one of the most frequently practiced of all major surgical procedures.

OPERATIVE PROCEDURE
(See also Chapter 55)

Beta-adrenergic blockers, nitrates, and calcium-channel blockers are continued until surgery, and anesthesia is

employed to maintain a normal rate-pressure product during induction. Most surgeons employ coronary revascularization, carried out with the aid of cardiopulmonary bypass at moderate hypothermia (24° to 32° C) and hemodilution. A motionless heart is achieved by continuous aortic cross-clamping with profound cardiac hypothermia and cardioplegia with cold potassium solution.[435] The vein grafts are inverted so that the distal end of the vein is placed proximally as an end-to-side anastomosis on the aorta (Fig. 39–18). The distal end of the vein is then placed as an end-to-side anastomosis on the coronary artery (Fig. 39–19); side-to-side anastomoses permit revascularization of several coronary artery branches with a single saphenous vein graft. In order to avoid obstruction of the graft by thrombotic occlusion or kinking, care must be exercised in the physical handling of the veins used as bypass grafts as well as in the positioning and arching of the vessels as they exit from the aorta and at-

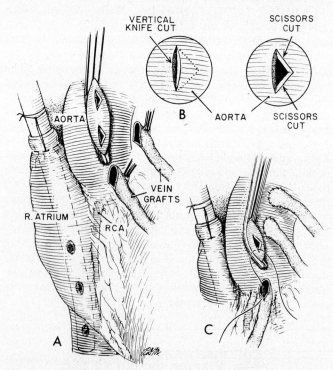

FIGURE 39–18   The aorticovenous anastomosis. *A* shows the direction of the anastomotic site for left-sided grafts; *B* shows details of aortic orifices; *C* shows the direction of right coronary artery (RCA) grafts. (From Cohn, L. H.: Surgical techniques of emergency coronary revascularization. *In* Cohn, L. H. (ed.): The Treatment of Acute Myocardial Ischemia: An Integrated Medical-Surgical Approach. Mt. Kisco, N.Y., Futura Publishing Co., 1979, p. 87.)

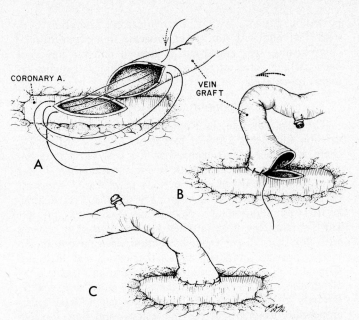

FIGURE 39–19 The venocoronary anastomosis to the proximal portion of the arteriotomy. (From Cohn, L. H.: Surgical techniques of emergency coronary revascularization. *In* Cohn, L. H. (ed.): The Treatment of Acute Myocardial Ischemia: An Integrated Medical-Surgical Approach. Mt. Kisco, N.Y., Futura Publishing Co., 1979, p. 87.)

tach to a coronary artery. Revascularization should include bypass of all major arterial segments with greater than 50 per cent stenosis of the luminal diameter.[436,437,437a]

Internal mammary artery bypass grafts may have certain advantages over vein grafts. The size of the internal mammary artery is similar to that of the native coronary vessel, and there is apparently little tendency for this graft to develop fibrous intimal hyperplasia, which may account for its reported higher patency rate.[434] However, because of its smaller internal diameter, it delivers less blood than do saphenous vein bypass grafts[438] and is also of limited value for revascularization of the posterior surface of the heart, because it is often too short to be used for more distal anastomoses. In general, internal mammary artery grafting also requires a longer time to perform and is therefore less desirable than saphenous vein grafting for emergency procedures. It is best suited for those patients in whom saphenous veins are not available because of prior bypass surgery or venous stripping of the leg for varicosities. Comparison of the efficacy of artery versus vein techniques must await followup results.

PATIENT SELECTION FOR CORONARY ARTERY SURGERY

To undergo coronary artery bypass grafting, patients must usually meet certain clinical, coronary arteriographic, and hemodynamic criteria.[439]

CLINICAL FACTORS

Chronic Stable Angina. We still agree with the Report of the Inter-Society Commission for Heart Disease Resources, presented in 1972, that the most widely accept-ed indication for coronary artery bypass surgery in stable angina is significant disability from moderate to severe angina pectoris, despite optimal medical care.[440] The threshold for "significant" disability varies widely among patients. Obviously, it differs for a relatively young man (under age 45) who is dependent on heavy physical work for his livelihood and an older woman (over age 75) who is sedentary and retired. In general, however, we would define "significant" disability as one that clearly interferes with the patient's desired lifestyle. Although this disability usually results from the coronary artery disease itself, it may be related to the side effects of the medications required to control the discomfort of myocardial ischemia. Angina pectoris can be controlled in most patients but sometimes only with excessive doses of antianginal agents. Optimal medical care, as described earlier (p. 1345), involves achievement of optimal weight; treatment of associated illnesses that can intensify myocardial ischemia, such as thyrotoxicosis or anemia; control of blood pressure, arrhythmias, and metabolic abnormalities such as carbohydrate intolerance and hyperlipidemias; abstinence from smoking; and most importantly, medication with beta blockers as well as short- and long-acting nitrates and calcium-channel blockers.

In published reports in the early 1970's, the majority of patients selected for operation were, in fact, in functional Classes III and IV.[441,442] However, with the reduction in perioperative mortality, a trend toward operating on less symptomatic or intensively treated patients has been noted. Other clinical factors considered in the selection of patients with arteriographically proven coronary obstructive disease include an increased concern for younger patients with coronary disease and evidence of previous myocardial infarction, even in patients with few symptoms. In many centers, the average age at operation is approximately 50 years, and more than half these patients have suffered previous myocardial infarction.[442]

Unstable Angina. The indications for operation in patients with unstable angina are more clear-cut than are those for stable angina and are discussed on page 1358. Initial medical management with bed rest, sedation, nitrates, beta blockade, and, if necessary, intraaortic balloon counterpulsation is the treatment of choice; *emergency* surgery is recommended only when this therapy fails to stabilize the patient. Patients with left main coronary artery disease should be operated upon on an urgent basis. In patients with coronary artery anatomy suitable for bypass who have been successfully treated medically, we recommend that operation be carried out 1 to 2 weeks after symptoms subside, generally during the same hospital stay. These patients could also return home, gradually increase activity, and maintain therapy with beta-adrenergic blockade, calcium-channel blocking agents, and nitrates; operation would be deferred until the patient developed either a second episode of unstable angina or sufficiently disabling chronic stable angina to satisfy the surgical requirements for the condition, as described above. It has been our experience that many patients with unstable angina will present one of these two indications within 6 months of discharge from the hospital, and the relatively high incidence of surgical treatment in the patients selected at random for medical therapy in the National Cooperative

Study confirms this.[287,443] It is for this reason and because of the relatively low risk of operation in the hands of a skilled surgical team and the excellent symptomatic results that we recommend early operation, i.e., prior to hospital discharge for the majority of patients with unstable angina. However, a number of randomized studies in addition to the National Cooperative Study have shown no advantage to urgent operation in this condition, and it must be acknowledged that firm data are lacking on the comparative advisability of early operation as opposed to the conservative course of postponing the procedure until required by the development of symptoms despite optimal medical management.

It is generally agreed that (1) patients with unstable angina treated surgically within the first 24 hours of presenting to the hospital have higher mortality and periinfarction rates than those operated upon later[444]; (2) the survival of patients operated upon early (1 to 2 weeks) after hospital admission is similar to that of medically treated patients; (3) surgically treated patients do better symptomatically than those treated medically; and (4) many medically treated patients ultimately require operation because of the recurrence of unstable angina or the development of severe chronic stable angina.

Prinzmetal's Angina. Although coronary artery bypass grafting is generally successful in relieving the pain of chronic stable angina pectoris, it is of little if any value in patients with *Prinzmetal's variant angina* without organic obstructive coronary artery disease. Since episodes of coronary artery spasm continue after operation, blood flow may be reduced sufficiently to cause thrombosis if spasm occurs in the area of insertion of the anastomosis of the graft into the native coronary artery. Patients with coronary artery spasm superimposed on obstructive arteriosclerotic coronary artery disease may fare better with coronary artery bypass than those in whom spasm occurs in unobstructed coronary arteries. Although some patients with variant angina clearly derive benefit from the bypass operation,[373] their response generally is inferior to that of patients with typical angina pectoris.

Heart Failure and Myocardial Infarction. In the absence of severe angina, patients with *heart failure* secondary to diffuse coronary artery disease (i.e., patients with ischemic cardiomyopathy) are not good candidates for coronary revascularization, since the mortality rate is higher than in patients with well-preserved left ventricular function.[445,446] However, there is some evidence that in patients in whom left ventricular dysfunction is due to chronically ischemic but not irreversibly damaged fibrotic tissue, surgical revascularization can improve left ventricular function[447,448] and perhaps survival as well.[449,450] Patients with heart failure should be studied carefully to exclude a mechanical lesion, such as mitral regurgitation or a ventricular aneurysm, which is usually amenable to surgical treatment.

Indications for coronary revascularization in patients with *acute myocardial infarction* or *cardiogenic shock* and *intractable ventricular arrhythmias* are discussed elsewhere (p. 1318). The number of patients with these manifestations of coronary artery disease subjected to these procedures has been relatively small, and suitable control series are not available. Although favorable results have been reported in patients with acute myocardial infarction both with [451–453] and without[454–456] cardiogenic shock, appropriate comparisons with nonsurgically treated patients have not been carried out, and the question of clinical benefits remains unresolved.

ARTERIOGRAPHIC FACTORS

The view stated in the Report of the Inter-Society Commission for Heart Disease Resources in 1972 still holds: there is "general agreement that the best candidates for bypass surgery are those with severe (greater than 75 per cent) luminal diameter obstructions in proximal segments of major branches of the coronary arteries," as demonstrated by high-quality angiograms taken in multiple views.[440] Intraoperative studies have shown that arteries with less than 50 per cent obstruction often have minimal, if any, pressure gradients across the lesions and little difference in blood flow through the artery, as measured by clearance of xenon-133, when the bypass graft is opened.[457] Patients with higher-grade obstructions usually have greater pressure gradients across the lesions, and flow through the artery could be shown to increase significantly when the bypass graft is opened.

The state of the distal vasculature is equally important. This can be evaluated directly by an angiographic assessment and indirectly by flow measurements. In one series of 154 venous grafts studied 2 months and 1 year after operation, it was concluded that late patency of the grafts was related to coronary arterial runoff, as determined by the diameter of the coronary artery into which the graft was inserted, the size of the distal vascular bed, and, to a lesser degree, the severity of coronary atherosclerosis distal to the site of insertion of the graft.[458] The highest graft patency rates were found when the lumina of the vessels distal to the graft insertion were greater than 1.5 mm in diameter, perfused a large peripheral vascular bed, and were free of atheromas occluding more than 25 per cent of the vessel lumen. Vessel diameters measured at coronary arteriography correlated satisfactorily with those obtained at operation.[459] The most accurate appraisal of the vascular bed distal to the principal obstruction can be made when the vessels fill in an antegrade manner. Assessment is less accurate when there is total proximal occlusion and distal filling occurs through adequate collaterals. In many such instances, the vessels are actually larger than the arteriogram suggests. Whenever there is any question about the ability of a vessel to accept a graft, the surgeon should attempt the anastomosis (consistent with patient safety, of course), since subjective improvement clearly depends on the completeness of revascularization.[460,461]

Flow rates through saphenous vein grafts measured at the time of operation average nearly 70 ml/min; those in which the flow is less than 45 ml/min—and especially less than 25 ml/min—are frequently associated with graft closure, whereas closure is less common at flow rates exceeding 45 ml/min.[462,463] The possible causes for reduced flow include subcritical obstruction of a proximal coronary artery; a technically poor anastomosis, with narrowing of the lumen due to kinking of the vessel or pinching at the site of the anastomosis; and a small myocardial mass perfused by the graft, which may in turn be due to diseased distal vasculature.

Ventricular Function. The relation between the presence of clinical evidence of congestive heart failure, hemodynamic evidence of left ventricular dysfunction, extensive wall motion disorders on left ventricular angiography, and poor surgical outcome is now well appreciated.[463–466] Clinical descriptors such as a history of heart failure, pulmonary rales, previous need of a diuretic or digitalis, and a cardiothoracic ratio of 0.50 or more are all associated with a significantly higher operative risk. In the Collaborative Study in Coronary Artery Surgery (CASS), the operative mortality was 1.9 per cent in patients with ejection fractions of 50 per cent or more and 6.7 per cent in those with ejection fractions below 19 per cent; these rates were 1.7 per cent in those with normal or minimally impaired wall motion and 9.1 per cent in those with greatly impaired wall motion.[467]

In estimating ejection fraction and wall motion in patients with coronary artery disease, it is important to analyze ventricular wall motion in the basal state as well as after inotropic stimulation or afterload reduction, in order to show enhancement of otherwise depressed wall motion.[135–137] As noted earlier, "contractile reserve" is the term used to describe the ability of ventricular wall segments that contract abnormally in the basal state to exhibit augmented contractility, often with an increase in overall ejection fraction, in response to a suitable stimulus.[468]

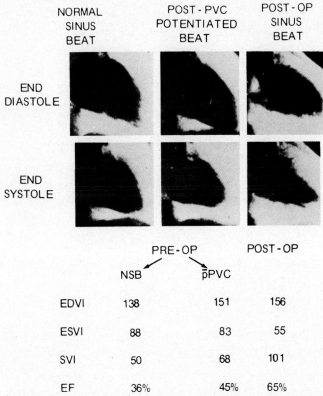

	PRE-OP		POST-OP
	NSB	pPVC	
EDVI	138	151	156
ESVI	88	83	55
SVI	50	68	101
EF	36%	45%	65%

FIGURE 39–20 Examples of the ventriculographic analysis performed to evaluate the effects of an inotropic stimulus, including some of the calculations made. PVC = premature ventricular contraction; PRE-OP = preoperative; POST-OP = postoperative; NSB = normal sinus beat; pPVC = after premature ventricular contraction; EDVI = end-diastolic volume index (ml/m²); ESVI = end-systolic volume index (ml/m²); SVI = stroke volume index (ml/m²); EF = ejection fraction. (From Popio, K. A., et al.: Post extrasystolic potentiation as a predictor of potential myocardial viability. Am. J. Cardiol. *39*:944, 1977.)

Zones of the myocardium responding to inotropic stimulation or to a decrease in afterload may improve functionally after revascularization (Fig. 39–20).[469] The demonstration of augmentation of contractility acutely and similar improvement after revascularization are related to the finding that many hypokinetic (and even akinetic) areas of the ventricular wall are composed either of ischemic, though viable, muscle or of a mixture of the latter and fibrous scar; the viable muscle is capable of responding to stimulation and, after operation, to improved perfusion.[137] In contrast, necrotic tissue obviously cannot be stimulated to contract by any pharmacological or hemodynamic intervention nor by improved perfusion. In patients with poor left ventricular function and poor contractile reserve (less than 0.10 increase in ejection fraction with inotropic stimulation), perioperative mortality is higher and long-term survival is poorer than in patients with equally depressed left ventricular function but with normal contractile reserve.[468–470]

Although, as stated above, the risk of operation is higher in patients with depressed left ventricular function, many such patients will nonetheless experience striking relief of anginal discomfort, and symptoms of heart failure may diminish somewhat after coronary bypass grafting. Therefore, we generally recommend surgical treatment for patients with heart failure and disabling angina, recognizing the higher risks involved.

RESULTS

OPERATIVE MORTALITY. Operative mortality for the treatment of stable and unstable angina pectoris has been declining steadily. In the CASS, the overall mortality for 6630 patients operated upon between 1975 and 1978 was 2.3 per cent. In addition to being affected by left ventricular function, as described above, mortality increased with age (0 in patients under 30 years to 7.9 per cent in those over 70 years). It was higher in women than in men, varied with the number of vessels involved, and was highest in patients with left main coronary artery stenosis. Operative mortality was 1.7 per cent for elective surgery, 3.5 per cent for urgent surgery, and 10.8 per cent for emergency surgery.[467] Additional cardiac surgical procedures raised the risk to 8 per cent in patients undergoing resection or plication of aneurysm and to 24 per cent in patients undergoing mitral valve replacement.

As with other operations, the risks depend on the patient's general medical status and the presence of associated conditions, such as pulmonary or renal disease. It must be recognized that the surgical results reported in the literature are usually the best in the field and may be substantially superior to those in the institution where the patient under consideration is going to receive surgical care. Thus, operative mortality among the 15 participating centers ranged from 0.3 to 6.4 per cent, emphasizing that the experience and skill of the team (surgeons, anesthesiologists, and cardiologists) play decisive roles in determining the outcome. The presence of risk factors for coronary artery disease and a previous myocardial infarction did not appear to affect operative mortality. Kuchoukos et al. have emphasized that improved perioperative management, including anesthetic techniques, intraoperative protection of the myocardium, and preoperative stabilization of patients, have all played important roles in the steady decline of operative mortality.[436] In patients with active ischemia or extremely poor left ventricular function, operative mortality may be reduced when the intraaortic balloon is used to support the circulation during the perioperative period. Finally, the physician considering referral of a particular patient for surgical treatment must fully appreciate the recent results obtained by the surgical group selected.

LATE SURVIVAL. Lack of controlled studies in most series makes evaluation of the effect of surgical treatment of survival difficult. In large series, 4-year mortality rates range from 9 to 18 per cent.[471,472] Although operative mortality is also considered in these analyses, survival figures must be evaluated with the realization that, in general, operated patients have been preselected for good left ventricular function. Left ventricular function, reflected in the ejection fraction[473] and the qualitative assessment of left ventricular contraction,[474] influences late postoperative survival. The presence of associated peripheral vascular disease signifying diffuse atherosclerosis, cigarette smoking, hypertension, and hypercholesterolemia all correlate with an increased likelihood of late death.[475]

SYMPTOMATIC RESULTS.   Between 70 and 95 per cent of patients with chronic stable angina operated upon report relief of anginal symptoms and reduction of nitroglycerin and propranolol use[429,475a]; 33 to 55 per cent of patients become totally asymptomatic, while symptoms increase in approximately 5 per cent.[474] In many reports, this improvement in symptoms is a subjective impression and open to criticism in view of the profound placebo effect of a thoracotomy. However, unlike a placebo effect, which is usually transient, the improvement persists, and the results of exercise testing carried out pre- and postoperatively often substantiate the belief that true clinical benefit has been achieved. Techniques that combine pre- and postoperative myocardial imaging with thallium-201 often indicate that the improved symptomatic state results from improved regional myocardial perfusion via patent grafts.[476] In general, the clinical benefits of the operation can be related to graft patency and completeness of revascularization.[441,472] Return of angina with graft closure implies that a placebo effect is not of major importance with this kind of surgery. However, recurrence of symptoms, which occurs at an annual rate of 3.5 per cent is related to obstruction of vein grafts in one-fourth of patients, to progression of atherosclerosis in native ungrafted vessels in half the patients, and to both in the remaining one-fourth.[474,447] However, despite the salutary clinical results, the employment rate among these patients shows little tendency to rise postoperatively.[478,479]

VENTRICULAR FUNCTION. Determining whether or not coronary revascularization improves left ventricular function is complicated by the occasional occurrence of perioperative myocardial infarction, progression of disease in the native coronary arteries, and closure of bypass grafts. Improvement in function, no change, and worsening have been reported to varying degrees.[480,481] Improvement in symptoms of cardiac failure is also variable. In most patients in whom pre- and postoperative comparisons were made at rest, the cardiac output, stroke volume, left ventricular end-diastolic pressure and volume, and ejection fraction show no significant change for the group as a whole, although in individual patients there may be sub-

stantial changes in either direction. On the other hand, an improvement in left ventricular function during exercise can often be demonstrated by means of radionuclide cine ventriculography (Fig. 39–21).[475] In addition, if motion of left ventricular wall segments improved with nitroglycerin, they will usually improve with coronary bypass grafting, as will some persistent deficits on thallium perfusion scans.[472] Coronary artery bypass grafting has also been shown to reverse exertional hypotension, a manifestation of acute left ventricular dysfunction caused by widespread ischemia. Thus, in most cases, failure to demonstrate that surgery leads to improvement in the resting state suggests that the reperfused myocardium is not ischemic at rest; rather, it is the stress-induced depression of left ventricular function that can be improved by revascularization.

PERIOPERATIVE COMPLICATIONS.   The rate of perioperative *myocardial infarction* that has been reported to be associated with elective coronary revascularization is approximately 5 per cent.[436,481,482] The most accurate method for diagnosing this complication relies on electrocardiographic evidence of new and persistant Q waves combined with marked elevation of cardiac enzymes, especially the

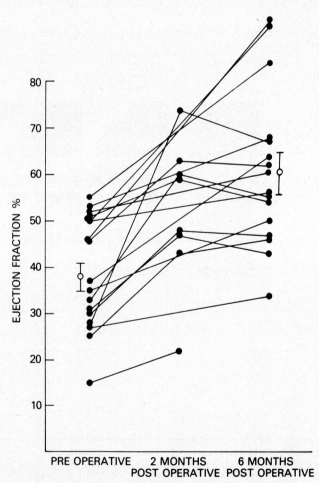

FIGURE 39–21 Radionuclide ejection fraction during exercise in 17 of 23 patients who showed improvement after operation. All 17 patients improved symptomatically (12 were entirely asymptomatic). By contrast, in the six patients with unchanged or decreased ejection fraction (not shown in figure), four had unchanged symptoms. (From Kent, K. M., et al.: Effects of coronary-artery bypass on global and regional left ventricular function during exercise. N. Engl. J. Med. *298*:1434, 1978.)

CK-MB fraction, and positive postoperative pyrophosphate scans.[483] The incidence of perioperative infarction is usually related to obstruction of a graft and correlates with the number of bypass grafts. Therefore, meticulous attention to anastomosis of the graft to the coronary artery is vital.[482] Although the loss of viable myocardium is obviously undesirable, in most patients the perioperative infarcts are small.

The development of *hypertension*[484] represents another postoperative problem peculiar to direct coronary revascularization. This complication, which may occur in up to one-third of all patients, can lead to fatal hemorrhage, cardiac failure, and arrhythmias. The mechanism responsible for the hypertension is unclear, but it may be related to increased levels of circulating catecholamines and renin. Intravenous sodium nitroprusside is effective for short-term management until appropriate oral antihypertensive agents, such as alpha-methyldopa, can be started.

GRAFT PATENCY RATE AND CHANGES IN THE NATIVE CIRCULATION. Overall, vein graft patency rates 6 to 12 months after operation range from 75 to 87 per cent[472]; since most patients receive multiple grafts, a larger percentage of patients, 84 to 95 per cent, have at least one patent graft.[429] Perhaps the most important single factor influencing graft patency is the flow rate through the graft, which in turn is a function of the severity of the obstruction in the native vessel proximal to the graft, the capacity of the distal arterial bed to accept the flow, and the technical adequacy of the operation; kinking or angulation of the graft, which diminishes flow rate, is particularly hazardous.[472a] Graft occlusion occurring within 6 to 12 months of operation is usually due to thrombosis; approximately half the occlusions occur within the first month after surgery.[472] Vein grafts may also undergo fibrous intimal, medial, and adventitial proliferation (Fig. 39–22) as well as atherosclerosis-like changes (Fig. 39–23),[485,486] and these morphological changes may represent a major cause of late graft closure,[487] which is approximately 2 per cent per year after the first year.[477,488] In a larger number of patients, particularly those with hyperlipidemia, progressive narrowing of the graft without total occlusion occurs.[485]

Contrast-enhanced computed tomography[489,490] represents a useful, relatively noninvasive way to assess patency of saphenous vein grafts (p. 191). In one prospective, randomized, double-blind trial, the effects of two platelet in-

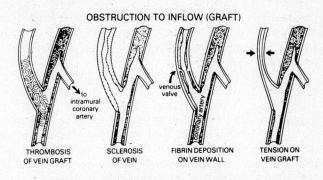

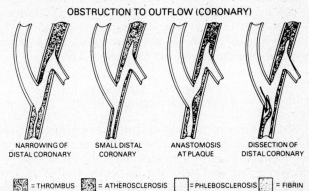

OBSTRUCTION TO INFLOW (GRAFT)

THROMBOSIS OF VEIN GRAFT   SCLEROSIS OF VEIN   FIBRIN DEPOSITION ON VEIN WALL   TENSION ON VEIN GRAFT

OBSTRUCTION TO OUTFLOW (CORONARY)

NARROWING OF DISTAL CORONARY   SMALL DISTAL CORONARY   ANASTOMOSIS AT PLAQUE   DISSECTION OF DISTAL CORONARY

= THROMBUS   = ATHEROSCLEROSIS   = PHLEBOSCLEROSIS   = FIBRIN

FIGURE 39–22 Anatomical and technical factors that can produce obstruction of a vein graft (top) and of arterial outflow (bottom). (From Spray, T. L., and Roberts, W. C.: Morphologic observations in biologic conduits between aorta and coronary artery. *In* Rahimtoola, S. (ed.): Coronary Bypass Surgery. Philadelphia, F. A. Davis, 1977, p. 11.)

hibitors on early postoperative vein graft patency were studied. Dipyridamole, begun 2 days before operation, and aspirin, begun 7 hours after operation, markedly reduced graft occlusion during a 4-month period.[491] Sulfinpyrazone has also been reported to reduce the incidence of early closure in grafts with flow rates exceeding 30 ml/min.[492]

Progression of atherosclerosis in the native coronary circulation may also contribute to poor clinical results. The tendency for proximal lesions to progress to complete stenosis is greater in operated than nonoperated vessels, but this is of little importance if the graft is patent; progression of disease distal to the graft can be expected to have more serious side effects. At an average followup of one

FIGURE 39–23 Postmortem histological sections through coronary artery (CA) anastomosis sites of saphenous vein bypass grafts (SVBG) show extensive fibrous tissue proliferation in the grafts' intimal layers. In the graft at left, the circumferential intimal fibrous plaque (IFP) developed in 5 months. In the graft at right, the process resulted in greater than 90 per cent stenosis 8 months after implantation. With time, such fibrous plaques may become infiltrated with lipids and calcium and increasingly resemble atherosclerotic plaques. (From Bulkley, B. H.: Why coronary bypass grafts fail: Early and late pathologic changes. J. Cardiovasc. Med. *5*:1025, 1980.)

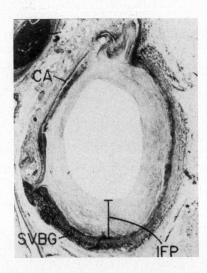

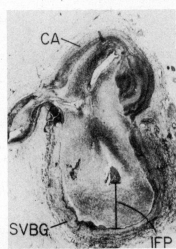

year, the frequency of distal progression ranged from 27 to 35 per cent in two studies.[493,494] However, based on 5- to 7-year followup, grafting does not appear to accelerate distal progression.[495]

REOPERATION.   Reoperation is indicated in patients with minimal relief of angina after the initial procedure or with recurrence of this symptom due to graft closure or progression of disease in unoperated arteries and in whom the distal vasculature and state of left ventricular function are still adequate for surgery. The procedure can be carried out with a relatively low mortality, only slightly higher than that for the initial procedure; relief of angina occurs in about two-thirds of the patients.[496,497] Reoperation tends to be more successful in relieving angina when it is performed in patients with new lesions in unoperated vessels than when carried out for graft occlusion.

EFFECT OF SURGICAL
TREATMENT ON SURVIVAL

The question of whether or not coronary artery bypass grafting affects long-term survival is one of the most pressing questions in cardiology and can be answered only by a comparison of medically and surgically treated patients. This can be accomplished by the use of randomized trials as well as by comparing the outcome in suitably matched patients treated medically and surgically. There is general agreement that surgical treatment improves survival in patients with *left main coronary artery obstruction*[498-501] (Fig. 39-24). The greatest difference occurred in patients with associated disease of the right coronary artery and some degree of left ventricular dysfunction.

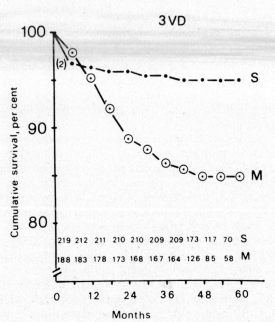

FIGURE 39-25   Cumulative survival curves for patients with three-vessel disease from the European Coronary Surgery Study. M = medical group; S = surgical group. Numbers along the bottom represent patients at risk at the beginning of each 6-month period. Numbers within parentheses indicate preoperative deaths in the surgical group. (From Varnauskas, E.: Prospective randomized study of coronary artery bypass surgery in stable angina pectoris. Lancet 2: 491, 1980.)

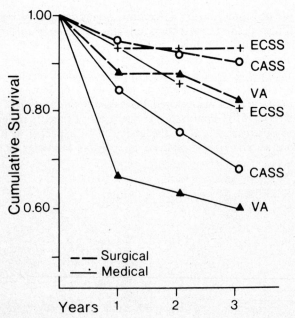

FIGURE 39-24   Cumulative 3-year survival rates of medically treated patients with left main coronary artery disease in three studies: Collaborative Study in Coronary Artery Surgery (CASS), the European Study (ECSS), and the Veterans Administration (VA) Study. (From Chaitman, B. R., et al.: Effect of coronary bypass surgery on survival patterns in subsets of patients with left main coronary artery disease. Am. J. Cardiol. 48:765, 1981.)

Randomized trials in patients with chronic stable angina have shown that surgical treatment also prolongs life in patients with three-vessel disease (Fig. 39-25).[498,502] Among patients with two-vessel disease, those with proximal left anterior descending obstruction appeared to do better after surgery while other patients with two-vessel disease showed no change.[445] In one trial, surgical treatment has also been shown to improve longevity in patients at high risk, defined by four noninvasively determined characteristics: New York Heart Association Class III or IV, a history of hypertension, a history of prior myocardial infarction, and ST-segment depression on the resting electrocardiogram[503]; however, surgery did not have this effect in "low risk" patients. There is no evidence that surgical treatment improves survival in patients with any form of single-vessel disease, including isolated proximal left anterior descending coronary artery obstruction.[445] Asymptomatic or mildly symptomatic patients appear to have better prognoses than do seriously symptomatic patients,[389] and surgery appears to improve prognosis only in that subgroup of asymptomatic or mildly symptomatic patients who have three-vessel disease with some impairment of left ventricular function.[445] On the other hand, there is no evidence that surgery improves survival in asymptomatic survivors of two or three myocardial infarctions with multivessel disease.[450] Whether coronary surgery improves the prognosis of survivors of out-of-hospital ventricular fibrillation is unsettled, but based on some theoretical reasons and a few observations it may do so.[504]

INDICATIONS FOR SURGICAL TREATMENT (Table 39-10).   Surgical treatment for chronic stable angina must be individualized. All patients in whom medical treatment has failed and who have persistent angina are

TABLE 39–10 CORONARY BYPASS SURGERY FOR ANGINA

Prolongs life
1. In LMCAD, particularly if LV function is moderately impaired
2. In three-vessel disease
3. In angina and ST depression on resting ECG + at least two of the following:
   NYHA Class III or IV
   History of myocardial infarction
   History of systemic hypertension *or* all three of the above with ECG changes

Symptomatic improvement
1. 50 to 70% asymptomatic — (0 to 9% with medical therapy)
2. 85 to 90% improved — (50% with medical therapy)
3. 81% no angina at rest — (65% with medical therapy)
4. 82% no unstable angina — (55% with medical therapy)
5. 75% no nitroglycerin — (36% with medical therapy)
6. 87% no propranolol — (33% with medical therapy)
7. 50% event-free course up to 7 years — (12% with medical therapy)

Risks
1. Operative mortality*
   a. 1.3%; varies from 0 to 3.5% in various subgroups:

Extent of CAD	All patients	Normal LV function	Abnormal LV function
One-vessel disease	0.5%	0.0%	1.7%
Two-vessel disease	0.8%	1.5%	0.0%
Three-vessel disease	1.5%	0.7%	2.1%
LMCAD	2.5%	0.0%	3.5%

   b. LV function: Normal 0.7%
      Abnormal 1.8%
   c. Age
      <45 years 0.0%
      45 to 65 years 1.3%
      >65 years 2.0%
2. Perioperative myocardial infarction ≤ 10% (may be as low as 2.5%)
3. Vein graft occlusion rate 10 to 15% (depends on state and location of grafted coronary artery; vein graft patency is 92% for LAD, 80% for RCA, and 70% for OM).
4. No patent grafts — 0 to 10% (depending on the number of grafts inserted)
5. No relief of pain — 5 to 10% (50% with medical therapy)
6. Angina worse — 6% (12% with medical therapy)
7. Recurrence of angina — 2 to 4% per year

Late survival
1. At 4 years 92.5% (91 to 94% is the 95% confidence interval)
2. Four-year survival in various subgroups:

a.

Extent of CAD	All patients	Normal LV function	Abnormal LV function
One-vessel disease	97%	98%	94%
Two-vessel disease	95%	92%	97%
Three-vessel disease	90%	94%	87%
LMCAD	95%	97%	94%

   b. LV function: Normal 95%
      Abnormal 90%
   c. Age
      <45 years 98%
      45 to 65 years 93%
      ≥ 66 years 84%

*A 0% operative mortality means the operative mortality is very low but will not necessarily be 0% as more patients are operated.
  Abbreviations: LMCAD = left main coronary artery disease; NYHA = New York Heart Association; LV = left ventricular; CAD = coronary artery disease; LAD = left anterior descending coronary artery; RCA = right coronary artery; OM = obtuse marginal coronary artery.
  From Rahimtoola, S. H.: Coronary bypass surgery for chronic angina — A Perspective. Circulation 65:225, 1982.

usually candidates for operation (or angioplasty). Patients with single-vessel disease are operated upon only to improve symptoms, not to prolong survival. Patients with left main coronary artery disease, with three-vessel coronary artery disease, and with two-vessel disease involving the proximal left anterior descending coronary artery who are moderately or severely symptomatic (but not necessarily medical failures) are ordinarily referred for surgery, unless there are specific contraindications.

The multicenter National Cooperative Study to Compare Medical and Surgical Therapy of Unstable Angina Pectoris evaluated 288 patients between 1972 and 1976.[286,443]

One randomly selected group received intensive pharmacological treatment with nitrates and propranolol and another underwent emergency coronary revascularization. The surgical group had a higher early myocardial infarction rate and significantly improved long-term quality of life, compared with the medically treated group; almost half the latter eventually required surgical treatment. The finding of greater symptomatic relief with operation but without increased longevity has also been reported from smaller randomized series.[445] A major conclusion from these studies is that immediate bypass surgery can be reserved for patients with unstable angina who have significant disease of the left main coronary artery or who have undergone an unsuccessful trial of optimal medical management.

At the time of this writing, we do *not* ordinarily recommend *surgical treatment* for asymptomatic patients with normal left ventricular function, unless they have left main coronary artery disease. Surgical treatment is also often recommended to asymptomatic and symptomatic patients after a myocardial infarction with three-vessel coronary disease or two-vessel disease involving the proximal left anterior descending coronary artery, although it is acknowledged that the evidence that such treatment will prolong survival is still incomplete. A symptomatic survivors of out-of-hospital ventricular fibrillation with silent myocardial ischemia may also be considered for surgery if they have similar anatomical findings. It is not our policy, at this time, to recommend surgery to patients with heart failure who do not have angina (unless a substantial quantity of myocardium is reversibly damaged and function can be improved by nitroglycerin or an inotropic intervention) nor to patients with acute myocardial infarction with or without cardiogenic shock.

Since totally asymptomatic patients are usually not candidates for surgery, and since the false-positive rate of noninvasive tests is high, we do not recommend that totally asymptomatic persons or populations be subjected to screening with noninvasive tests unless there are compelling reasons to do so. These reasons include multiple risk factors, family history of premature coronary disease, or as part of the evaluation for entry into strenuous conditioning programs. Patients with mild or atypical angina should undergo noninvasive stress testing with exercise electrocardiography and perhaps one of the radionuclide tests, as described on page 1342. Coronary arteriography may be carried out if results of these tests indicate that the patient is at high risk and/or has impaired left ventricular function. This procedure, of course, is also carried out for patients who are symptomatic despite therapy and who have no obvious contraindication to operation. The results obtained are critical for reaching a decision as to whether or not to advise surgical treatment.

There is no simple formula for recommending operation, and the decision must be made on an individual basis. Among the factors to be considered are the patient's lifestyle, age, and general health; the presence of disease of other organs and of atherosclerosis involving other vascular beds; and the capability and experience of the surgical team.

OTHER SURGICAL PROCEDURES FOR ISCHEMIC HEART DISEASE. Replacement of the aortic or mitral valve or both and left ventricular aneurysmectomy may be performed with or without associated bypass grafting in patients with ischemic heart disease. When valve replacement or aneurysmectomy is carried out as the sole procedure, it is usually because of the presence of heart failure refractory to medical management. In most instances, these procedures are performed along with coronary revascularization; the fact that these procedures may add to the operative risk of simple bypass grafting[467] may be related to the fact that they are carried out on patients with left ventricular failure who are poor operative risks.

Resection (or plication) of a left ventricular aneurysm for treatment of congestive heart failure has been associated

with a surgical mortality of 5 to 15 per cent; clinical results depend on the quantity of residual contractile tissue[505,506,506a] and the extent of obstructive coronary artery disease.[507] Experiments in the normal canine heart have demonstrated that up to 42 per cent of left ventricular cavity volume can be functionally eliminated with retention of adequate mechanical performance.[508] In followups exceeding 5 years, clinical improvement of left ventricular function is usually impressive in most patients,[509–511] although hemodynamic results are variable. However, a host of postoperative problems (including systemic embolism, arrhythmias, and progression of coronary artery disease) can cause disability after a successful operation. The effects of aneurysmectomy on survival are encouraging but not definitive. As an isolated procedure (without coronary artery bypass grafting), aneurysmectomy should be reserved for patients with intractable congestive heart failure.

ASSOCIATED CORONARY AND CAROTID ARTERY DISEASE. Since both carotid and coronary artery disease are manifestations of the same underlying disease process, it is not surprising that there is a relatively high incidence of carotid arterial disease in patients who are candidates for coronary bypass surgery; in one series, 12 per cent of such patients had serious carotid obstruction.[512] Although there is no agreement about the ideal manner in which these patients should be managed,[513] many surgeons now prefer to perform combined carotid endarterectomy and coronary artery bypass surgery in patients who require both procedures. A similar approach is taken with patients who are to undergo coronary revascularization and are found to have critical obstruction of a carotid artery on noninvasive testing but remain asymptomatic. Patients who require coronary bypass grafting but who have only a carotid bruit or less than 50 per cent reduction of the carotid artery lumen do not require carotid surgery.

References

1. Heberden, W.: Some account of a disorder of the breast. Med. Trans. Coll. Physicians (Lond.) *2*:59, 1772.
2. Parry, C. H.: An inquiry into the symptoms and causes of the syncope anginosa, commonly called angina pectoris. Vols. 3 and 4. Bath, England, R. Cuttwell, 1799, p. 113.
3. Flint, A.: Diseases affecting the circulatory system. *In* A Treatise on the Principles and Practice of Medicine. Philadelphia, Henry C. Lea, 1866.
4. Brunton, T. L.: On the use of nitrite of amyl in angina pectoris. Lancet *2*:97, 1867.
5. Osler, W.: The Principles and Practice of Medicine. New York, Appleton, 1892.
6. Osler, W.: Angina pectoris. Lancet *1*:839, 1910.
7. Muller, J. E.: Diagnosis of myocardial infarction: Historical notes from the Soviet Union and the United States. Am. J. Cardiol. *40*:269, 1977.
8. Herrick, J. B.: Clinical features of sudden obstruction of the coronary arteries. J.A.M.A. *59*:2015, 1912.
9. White, P. D.: The prevalence of coronary heart disease. *In* Blumgart, H. L. (ed.): Symposium on Coronary Heart Disease. New York, American Heart Association, 1968.
10. Wearn, J. T.: Thrombosis of the coronary arteries, with infarction of the heart. Am. J. Med. Sci. *165*:250, 1923.
11. Blumgart, H. L., Schlesinger, M. J., and Zoll, P. M.: Angina pectoris, coronary failure and acute myocardial infarction: The role of coronary occlusions and collateral circulation. J.A.M.A. *116*:91, 1941.
12. Sones, F. M., Jr.: Acquired heart disease: Symposium on present and future of cineangiography. Am. J. Cardiol. *3*:710, 1959.

CHRONIC (STABLE) ANGINA PECTORIS

13. Christie, L. G., Jr., and Conti, C. R.: Systematic approach to evaluation of angina-like chest pain: Pathophysiology and clinical testing with emphasis on objective documentation of myocardial ischemia. Am. Heart J. *102*:897, 1981.

14. Sampson, J. J., and Cheitlin, M. D.: Pathophysiology and differential diagnosis of cardiac pain. Progr. Cardiovasc. Dis. *13*:507, 1971.
15. Lefkowitz, D., and Biller, J.: Bregmatic headache as a manifestation of myocardial ischemia. Arch. Neurol. *39*:130, 1982.
16. Malliani, A., and Lombardi, F.: Consideration of the fundamental mechanisms eliciting cardiac pain. Am. Heart J. *103*:575, 1982.
17. Levine, H. J.: Difficult problems in the diagnosis of chest pain. Am. Heart J. *100*:108, 1980.
18. Del Banco, P. L., Del Bene, E., and Sicuteri, F.: Heart pain. *In* Bonica, J. J. (ed.): Advances in Neurology. Vol. 4. New York, Raven Press, 1974, p. 375.
19. Mountcastle, V. B.: Pain and temperature sensibilities. *In* Mountcastle, V. B. (ed.): Medical Physiology. 13th ed. St. Louis, The C. V. Mosby Co., 1974.
20. Branch, W. T., Jr.: Severe chest pain: Noncardiac emergencies. J. Cardiovasc. Med. *8*:159, 1983.
21. Hillis, L. D., and Braunwald, E.: Coronary artery spasm. N. Engl. J. Med. *299*:695, 1978.
22. Epstein, S. E., and Talbot, T. L.: Dynamic coronary tone in precipitation, exacerbation and relief of angina pectoris. Am. J. Cardiol. *48*:797, 1981.
23. Maseri, A., and Chierchia, S.: Angina pectoris—A new dimension, a new approach. Primary Cardiol. *6*:10 and 123, 1980.
24. DeServi, S., Specchia, G., Falcone, C., Gavazzi, A., Mussini, A., Angoli, L., Bramucci, E., Ardissino, D., Vaccari, L., Salerno, J., and Bobba, P.: Variable threshold exertional angina in patients with transient vasospastic myocardial ischemia. Am. J. Cardiol. *51*:397, 1983.
24a. Gorlin, R.: Dynamic vascular factors in the genesis of myocardial ischemia. J. Am. Coll. Cardiol. *1*:897, 1983.
24b. Pepine, C. J., and Feldman, R. L.: Dynamic coronary blood flow reduction: Supply side considerations. Int. J. Cardiol. *3*:3, 1983.
25. Yasue, H.: Pathophysiology and treatment of coronary arterial spasm. Chest *78*:216, 1980.
26. Epstein, S. E., Stampfer, M., Beiser, G. D., Goldstein, R. E., and Braunwald, E.: Effect of a reduction in environmental temperature on the circulatory response to exercise in man. Implications concerning angina pectoris. N. Engl. J. Med. *280*:7, 1969.
27. Mudge, G. H., Jr., Grossman, W., Mills, R. M., Jr., Lesch, M., and Braunwald, E.: Reflex increase in coronary vascular resistance in patients with ischemic heart disease. N. Engl. J. Med. *295*:1333, 1976.
28. Mudge, G. H., Jr., Goldberg, S., Gunther, S., Mann, T., and Grossman, W.: Comparison of metabolic and vasoconstrictor stimuli on coronary vascular resistance in man. Circulation *59*:544, 1979.
29. Goldstein, R. E., Redwood, D. R., Rosing, D. R., Beiser, G. D., and Epstein, S. E.: Alterations in the circulatory response to exercise following a meal and their relationship in postprandial angina pectoris. Circulation *44*:90, 1971.
30. Figueras, J., Singh, B. N., Ganz, W., and Swan, H. J. C.: Hemodynamic and electrocardiographic accompaniments of resting postprandial angina. Br. Heart J. *42*:402, 1979.
31. Schiffer, F., Hartley, L. W., Schulman, C. L., and Abelmann, W. H.: Evidence for emotionally-induced coronary arterial spasm in patients with angina pectoris. Br. Heart J. *44*:62, 1980.
32. Horwitz, L. D., Herman, M. V., and Gorlin, R.: Clinical response to nitroglycerin as a diagnostic test for coronary artery disease. Am. J. Cardiol. *29*:149, 1972.
33. Levine, S. A.: Carotid sinus massage: A new diagnostic test for angina pectoris. J.A.M.A. *182*:1332, 1962.
34. Diamond, G. A., and Forrester, J. S.: Analysis of probability as an aid in the clinical diagnosis of coronary artery disease. N. Engl. J. Med. *300*:1350, 1979.
35. Pasternak, R. C., Thibault, G. E., Savoia, M., DeSanctis, R. W., and Hutter, A. M., Jr.: Chest pain with angiographically insignificant coronary arterial obstruction. Clinical presentation and long-term follow-up. Am. J. Med. *68*:813, 1980.
36. Proudfit, W. L., Shirey, E. K., Sheldon, W. C., and Sones, F. M., Jr.: Certain clinical characteristics correlated with extent of obstructive lesions demonstrated by selective cine-coronary arteriography. Circulation *38*:947, 1968.
37. Cohen, L. S., Elliott, W. C., Klein, M. D., and Gorlin, R.: Coronary heart disease: Clinical, cinearteriographic, and metabolic correlations. Am. J. Cardiol. *17*:153, 1966.
38. Hamby, R. I., Gupta, M. P., and Young, M. W.: Clinical and hemodynamic aspects of single vessel coronary artery disease. Am. Heart J. *85*:458, 1973.
39. Welch, C. C., Proudfit, W. L., and Sheldon, W. C.: Coronary arteriographic findings in 1000 women under age 50. Am. J. Cardiol. *35*:211, 1975.
40. Cohn, P. F.: Silent myocardial ischemia in patients with a defective anginal warning system. Am. J. Cardiol. *45*:697, 1980.
41. Cohn, P. F.: Asymptomatic coronary artery disease: Pathophysiology, diagnosis, management. Mod Conc. Cardiovasc. Dis. *50*:55, 1981.
42. Cohn, P. F., Harris, P., Barry, W. H., Rosati, R. A., Rosenbaum, P., and Waternaux, C.: Prognostic importance of anginal symptoms in angiographically defined coronary artery disease. Am. J. Cardiol. *47*:233, 1981.
43. Midwall, J., Ambrose, J., Pichard, A., Abedin, Z., and Herman, M. V.: Angina pectoris before and after myocardial infarction. Angiographic correlations. Chest *81*:681, 1982.
44. Winnan, G. R., Meyer, C. T., and McCallum, R. W.: Interpretation of the Bernstein Test: A reappraisal of criteria. Ann. Intern. Med. *96*:320, 1982.
45. Long, W. B., and Cohen, S.: The digestive tract as a cause of chest pain. Am. Heart J. *100*:567, 1980.
46. Levine, H. J.: Difficult problems in the diagnosis of chest pain. Am. Heart J. *100*:108, 1980.
47. Wolf, E., and Stern, S.: Costosternal syndrome. Its frequency and importance in differential diagnosis of coronary heart disease. Arch. Intern. Med. *136*:189, 1976.
48. Likoff, W., Segal, B. L., and Kasparian, H.: Paradox of normal selective coronary arteriograms in patients considered to have unmistakable coronary heart disease. N. Engl. J. Med. *276*:1063, 1967.
49. Kemp, H. G., Vokonas, P. S., Cohn, P. F., and Gorlin, R.: The anginal syndrome associated with normal coronary arteriograms. Report of a six year experience. Am. J. Med. *54*:735, 1973.
50. Bemiller, C. R., Pepine, C. J., and Rogers, A. K.: Long-term observations in patients with angina and normal coronary arteriograms. Circulation *47*:36, 1973.
51. Cannon, R. O., III, Watson, R. M., Rosing, D. R., and Epstein, S. E.: Angina caused by reduced vasodilator reserve of the small coronary arteries. J. Am. Coll. Cardiol. *1*:1359, 1983.
52. Gorlin, R.: A quantitative clinical index for the diagnosis of symptomatic coronary artery disease. N. Engl. J. Med. *286*:501, 1972.
53. Ockene, I. S., Shay, M. J., Alpert, J. S., Weiner, B. H., and Dalen, J. E.: Unexplained chest pain in patients with normal coronary arteriograms. N. Engl. J. Med. *303*:1249, 1980.
54. Opherk, D., Zebe, H., Weihe, E., Mall, G., Durr, C., Gravert, B., Mehmel, H. C., Schwarz, F., and Kubler, W.: Reduced coronary dilatory capacity and ultrastructural changes of the myocardium in patients with angina pectoris but normal coronary arteriograms. Circulation *63*:817, 1981.
55. Pasternac, A., Noble, J., Streulens, Y., Elie, R., Henschke, C., and Bourassa, M. G.: Pathophysiology of chest pain in patients with cardiomyopathies and normal coronary arteries. Circulation *65*:778, 1982.
56. Arbogast, R., and Bourassa, M. G.: Myocardial function during atrial pacing in patients with angina pectoris and normal coronary arteriograms. Am. J. Cardiol. *32*:257, 1973.
57. Boudoulas, H., Cobb, T. C., Leighton, R. F., and Wilt, S. M.: Myocardial lactate production in patients with angina-like chest pain and angiographically normal coronary arteries and left ventricle. Am. J. Cardiol. *34*:501, 1974.
58. Mammohansingh, P., and Parker, J. O.: Angina pectoris with normal coronary arteriograms: Hemodynamic and metabolic response to pacing. Am. Heart J. *90*:555, 1975.
59. Meller, J., Goldsmith, S. J., Rudin, A., Pichard, A. D., Gorlin, R., Teichholz, L. E., and Herman, M. V.: Spectrum of exercise thallium-201 myocardial perfusion imaging in patients with chest pain and normal coronary angiograms. Am. J. Cardiol. *43*:717, 1979.
60. Green, L. H., Cohn, P. F., Holman, B. L., Adams, D. F., and Markis, J. E.: Regional myocardial blood flow in patients with chest pain syndromes and normal coronary arteriograms. Br. Heart J. *40*:242, 1978.
61. Robinson, B. F.: Relation of heart rate and systolic blood pressure to the onset of pain in angina pectoris. Circulation *35*:1073, 1967.
62. Proudfit, W. L., and Hodgman, J. R.: Physical signs during angina pectoris. Progr. Cardiovasc. Dis. *10*:283, 1968.
63. Lichstein, E., Chapman, I., and Gupta, P. K., et al.: Diagonal ear-lobe crease and coronary artery sclerosis. Ann. Intern. Med. *85*:337, 1976.
64. Fisher, J. R., and Sievers, M. L.: Ear-lobe crease in American Indians. Ann. Intern. Med. *93*:512, 1980.
65. Michelson, E. L., Morganroth, J., Nichols, C. W., and MacVaugh, H., III: Retinal arteriolar changes as an indicator of coronary artery disease. Arch. Intern. Med. *139*:1139, 1979.
66. Cohn, P. F., Vokonas, P. S., Williams, R. A., Herman, M. V., and Gorlin, R.: Diastolic heart sounds and filling waves in coronary artery disease. Circulation *44*:196, 1971.
67. Martin, C. E., Shaver, J. A., and Leonard, J. J.: Physical signs, apexcardiography, photocardiography and systolic time intervals in angina pectoris. Circulation *46*:1098, 1972.
68. Cohn, P. F., Thompson, P., Strauss, W., Todd, J., and Gorlin, R.: Diastolic heart sounds during static (handgrip) exercise in patients with chest pain. Circulation *47*:1217, 1973.
69. Voigt, G. C., and Friesinger, G. C.: The use of apexcardiography in the assessment of left ventricular diastolic pressure. Circulation *41*:1015, 1970.
70. Spodick, D. H., and Quarry, V. M.: Prevalence of the fourth heart sound by phonocardiography in the absence of cardiac disease. Am. Heart J. *87*:11, 1974.
71. Benchimol, A., and Desser, K. B.: The fourth heart sound in patients without demonstrable heart disease. Am. Heart J. *93*:298, 1977.
72. Tavel, M. E.: The fourth heart sound—a premature requiem? Circulation *49*:4, 1974.
73. Steelman, R. B., White, R. S., Hill, J. C., Nagle, J. P., and Cheitlin, M. D.: Midsystolic clicks in arteriosclerotic heart disease. A new facet in the clinical syndrome of papillary muscle dysfunction. Circulation *44*:503, 1971.
74. Sangster, J. F., and Oakley, C. M.: Diastolic murmur of coronary artery stenosis. Br. Heart J. *35*:840, 1973.
75. Gorlin, R.: Evaluation of the patient with coronary heart disease. *In* Gorlin, R.: Coronary Artery Disease. Philadelphia, W. B. Saunders Co., 1976, p. 178.
76. McQueen, M. J., Holder, D., and El-Maraghi, N. R. H.: Assessment of the accuracy of serial electrocardiograms in the diagnosis of myocardial infarction. Am. Heart J. *105*:258, 1983.
77. Gibson, R. S., and Beller, G. A.: Should exercise electrocardiographic testing be replaced by radioisotope methods? *In* Rahimtoola, S. H. (ed.): Controversies in Coronary Artery Disease. Philadelphia, F. A. Davis Co., 1983, pp. 1–31.

78. Faris, J. V., McHenry, P. L., and Morris, S. N.: Concepts and applications of treadmill exercise testing and the exercise electrocardiogram. Am. Heart J. *95*: 102, 1978.

79. Dagenais, G. R., Rouleau, J. R., Christen, A., and Fabia, J.: Survival of patients with a strongly positive exercise electrocardiogram. Circulation *65*:452, 1982.

80. Goldschlager, N., Selzer, A., and Cohn, K.: Treadmill stress tests as indicators of presence and severity of coronary artery disease. Ann. Intern. Med. *85*:277, 1976.

81. Bonoris, P. E., Greenberg, P. S., Castellanet, M. D., and Ellestad, M. H.: Significance of changes in R-wave amplitude during treadmill stress testing: Angiographic correlation. Circulation *57*:904, 1978.

82. Irving, J. B., Bruce, R. A., and DeRouen, T. A.: Variations in and significance of systolic pressure during maximal exercise (treadmill) testing. Relation to severity of coronary artery disease and cardiac mortality. Am. J. Cardiol. *39*: 841, 1977.

83. Thompson, P. D., and Kelemer, M. H.: Hypotension accompanying the onset of exertional angina. A sign of severe compromise of left ventricular blood supply. Circulation *52*:28, 1975.

84. Berman, J. L., Wynne, J., and Cohn, P. F.: Value of multivariate approach for interpreting treadmill exercise tests in coronary artery disease. Circulation *58*: 515, 1978.

85. McNeer, J. F., Margolis, J. R., Lee, K. L., Kisslo, J. A., Peter, R. H., Kong, Y., Behar, V. S., Wallace, A. G., McCantis, C. B., and Rosati, R. A.: The role of the exercise test in the evaluation of patients for ischemic heart disease. Circulation *57*:64, 1978.

86. Chaitman, B. R., Bourassa, M. G., Wagniart, P., Corbara, F., and Ferguson, R. J.: Improved efficiency of treadmill exercise testing using a multiple lead ECG system and basic hemodynamic exercise response. Circulation *57*:71, 1978.

87. Cale, J. R., and Ellestad, M. H.: Significance of chest pain during treadmill exercise: Correlation with coronary events. Am. J. Cardiol. *41*:227, 1978.

88. Jelinek, M. V., and Lown, B. L.: Exercise stress testing for exposure of cardiac arrhythmias. Progr. Cardiovasc. Dis. *16*:497, 1974.

89. Ryan, M., Lown, B., and Horn, H.: Comparison of ventricular ectopic activity during 24-hour monitoring and exercise testing in patients with coronary heart disease. N. Engl. J. Med. *292*:224, 1975.

90. Helfant, R. H., Pine, R., Kabde, V., and Banka, V. S.: Exercise-related ventricular premature complexes in coronary heart disease. Correlations with ischemia and angiographic severity. Ann. Intern. Med. *80*:589, 1974.

91. McHenry, P. L., Morris, S. N., Kavalier, M., and Jordan, J. W.: Comparative study of exercise-induced ventricular arrhythmias in normal subjects and patients with documented coronary artery disease. Am. J. Cardiol. *37*:609, 1976.

92. Stein, S., Tzivoni, D., and Stern, Z.: Diagnostic accuracy of ambulatory ECG monitoring in ischemic heart disease. Circulation *52*:1045, 1975.

93. Schang, S. J., and Pepine, C. J.: Transient asymptomatic ST-segment depression during daily activity. Am. J. Cardiol. *39*:396, 1971.

94. Crawford, M. H., Mendoza, C. A., O'Rourke, R. A., White, P. H., Boucher, C. A., and Gorwit, J.: Limitations of continuous ambulatory electrocardiogram monitoring for detecting coronary artery disease. Ann. Intern. Med. *89*: 1, 1978.

95. Iskandrian, A. S., Wasserman, L. A., Anderson, G. S., Hakki, H., Segal, B. L., and Kane, S.: Merits of stress thallium-201 myocardial perfusion imaging in patients with inconclusive exercise electrocardiograms: Correlation with coronary arteriograms. Am. J. Cardiol. *46*:553, 1980.

96. Gibson, R. S., Taylor, G. J., Watson, D. D., Stebbins, P. T., Martin, R. P., Crampton, R. S., and Beller, G. A.: Predicting the extent and location of coronary artery disease during the early postinfarction period by quantitative thallium-201 scintigraphy. Am. J. Cardiol. *47*:1010, 1981.

97. Gibson, R. S., Watson, D. D., Carabello, B. A., Holt, N. D., and Beller, G. A.: Clinical implications of increased lung uptake of thallium-201 during exercise scintigraphy 2 weeks after myocardial infarction. Am. J. Cardiol. *49*:1586, 1982.

97a. Wilson, R. A., Okada, R. D., Boucher, C. A., Strauss, H. W., and Pohost, G. M.: Radionuclide-determined changes in pulmonary blood volume and thallium lung uptake in patients with coronary artery disease. Am. J. Cardiol. *51*: 741, 1983.

98. DePace, N. L., Iskandrian, A. S., Hakki, A., Kane, S. A., and Segal, B. L.: Use of QRS scoring and thallium-201 scintigraphy to assess left ventricular function after myocardial infarction. Am. J. Cardiol. *50*:1262, 1982.

99. Bungo, M. W., and Leland, O. S., Jr.: Discordance of exercise thallium testing with coronary arteriography in patients with atypical presentations. Chest *83*: 112, 1983.

100. Pitt, B., Kalff, V., Rabinovitch, M. A., Buda, A. J., Colfer, H. T., Vogel, R. A., and Thrall, J. H.: Impact of radionuclide techniques on evaluation of patients with ischemic heart disease. J. Am. Coll. Cardiol. *1*:63, 1983.

100a. Manyari, D. E., and Kostuk, W. J.: Left and right ventricular function at rest and during bicycle exercise in the supine and sitting positions in normal subjects and patients with coronary artery disease. Assessment by radionuclide ventriculography. Am. J. Cardiol. *51*:36, 1983.

100b. Osbakken, M. D., Boucher, C. A., Okada, R. D., Bingham, J. B., Strauss, H. W., and Pohost, G. M.: Spectrum of global left ventricular responses to supine exercise. Limitation in the use of ejection fraction in identifying patients with coronary artery disease. Am. J. Cardiol. *51*:28, 1983.

100c. Campos, C. T., Chu, H. W., D'Agostino, H. J., Jr., and Jones, R. H.: Comparison of rest and exercise radionuclide angiocardiography and exercise treadmill testing for diagnosis of anatomically extensive coronary artery disease. Circulation *67*:1204, 1983.

101. Patterson, R. E., Horowitz, S. F., Eng, C., Meller, J., Goldsmith, S. J., Pichard, A. D., Halgash, D. A., Herman, M. V., and Gorlin, R.: Can noninvasive exercise test criteria identify patients with left main or 3-vessel coronary disease after a first myocardial infarction? Am. J. Cardiol. *51*:361, 1983.

102. Feigenbaum, H., Corya, B. C., Dillon, J. C., Weyman, A. E., Rasmussen, S., Black, M. J., and Chang, S.: Role of echocardiography in patients with coronary artery disease. Am. J. Cardiol. *37*:775, 1976.

103. Corya, B. C.: Echocardiography in ischemic heart disease. Am. J. Med. *63*:10, 1977.

104. Limacher, M. C., Quinones, M. A., Poliner, L. R., Nelson, J. G., Winters, W. L., Jr., and Waggoner, A. D.: Detection of corconary artery disease with excercise two-dimensional echocardiography. Description of a clinically applicable method and comparison with radionuclide ventriculography. Circulation *67*:1211, 1983.

105. Rink, L. D., Feigenbaum, H., Godley, R. W., Weyman, A. E., Dillon, J. C., Phillips, J. F., and Marshall, J. E.: Echocardiographic detection of left main coronary artery obstruction. Circulation *65*:719, 1982.

106. Neinle, R. A., Levy, R. I., Frederickson, D. S., and Gorlin, R.: Lipid and carbohydrate abnormalities in patients with angiographically documented coronary artery disease. Am. J. Cardiol. *24*:178, 1969.

107. Falsetti, H. L., Schnatz, J. D., Greene, D. G., and Bunnell, I. L.: Lipid and carbohydrate studies in coronary artery disease. Circulation *37*:184, 1968.

108. Margolis, J. R., Chen, J. T. T., Kong, Y., Peter, R. H., Behar, V. S., and Kisslo, J. A.: The diagnostic and prognostic significance of coronary artery calcification. A report of 800 Cases. Radiology *137*:609, 1980.

109. Rifkin, R. D.: Coronary calcification: A neglected clue to coronary artery disease. J. Cardiovasc. Med. *5*:343, 1980.

110. Swaye, P. S., Fisher, L. D., Litwin, P., Vignola, P. A., Judkins, M. P., Kemp, H. G., Mudd, J. G., and Gosselin, A. J.: Aneurysmal coronary artery disease. Circulation *67*:134, 1983.

111. Gorlin, R.: Coronary collaterals. *In* Gorlin, R.: Coronary Artery Disease. Philadelphia, W. B. Saunders Co., 1976, p. 65.

112. Newman, P. E.: The coronary collateral circulation: Determinants and functional significance in ischemic heart disease. Am. Heart J. *102*:431, 1981.

113. Schwarz, F., Flameng, W., and Ensslen, R.: Effect of coronary collaterals on left ventricular function at rest and during stress. Am. Heart J. *95*:570, 1978.

114. Newman, P. E.: The coronary collateral circulation: Determinants and functional significance in ischemic heart disease. Am. Heart J. *102*:431, 1981.

115. Gregg, D. E., and Patterson, R. E.: Functional importance of the coronary collaterals. N. Engl. J. Med. *303*:1404, 1980.

116. Schaper, W.: Influence of physical exercise on coronary collateral blood flow in chronic experimental two-vessel occlusion. Circulation *65*:905, 1982.

117. Cohen, M. V., Yipintsol, T., and Scheuer, J.: Coronary collateral stimulation by exercise in dogs with stenotic coronary arteries. J. Appl. Physiol. Resp. Environ. Exercise Physiol. *52*:664, 1982.

118. Reduto, L. A., Wickemeyer, W. J., Young, J. B., DelVentura, L. A., Reid, J. W., Glaeser, D. H., Quinones, M. A., and Miller, R. R.: Left ventricular diastolic performance at rest and during exercise in patients with coronary artery disease. Circulation *63*1228, 1981.

119. Moraski, R. E., Russel, R. O., Jr., Smith, M., and Rackley, C. E.: Left ventricular function in patients with and without myocardial infarction and one, two or three vessel coronary artery disease. Am. J. Cardiol. *35*:1, 1975.

120. Cohn, P. F., and Gorlin, R.: Ventricular dysfunction in coronary artery disease. Am. J. Cardiol. *33*:307, 1974.

121. McCans, J. L., and Parker, J. O.: Left ventricular pressure-volume relationships during myocardial ischemia in man. Circulation *48*:775, 1973.

122. Barry, W. H., Brooker, J. Z., Alderman, E. L., and Harrison, D. C.: Changes in diastolic stiffness and tone of the left ventricle during angina pectoris. Circulation *49*:255, 1974.

123. Mann, T., Brodie, B. R., Grossman, W., and McLaurin, L. P.: Effect of angina on the left ventricular diastolic pressure-volume relationship. Circulation *55*: 761, 1977.

124. Wiener, L., Dwyer, E. M., Jr., and Cox, J. W.: Left ventricular hemodynamics in exercise-induced angina pectoris. Circulation *38*:240, 1968.

125. Parker, J. O., DiGiorgi, S., and West, R. O.: A hemodynamic study of acute coronary insufficiency precipitated by exercise: With observations on the effect of nitroglycerin. Am. J. Cardiol. *17*:470, 1966.

126. Helfant, R. H., Forrester, J. S., Hampton, J. R., Haft, J. I., Kemp, H. G., and Gorlin, R.: Coronary heart disease. Differential hemodynamic, metabolic, and electrocardiographic effects in subjects with and without angina pectoris during atrial pacing. Circulation *42*:601, 1970.

127. Linhart, J. W.: Myocardial function in coronary artery disease determined by atrial pacing. Circulation *44*:203, 1971.

128. Bourdillon, P. D., Lorell, B. H., Mirsky, I., Paulus, W. J., Wynne, J., and Grossman, W.: Increased regional myocardial stiffness of the left ventricle during pacing-induced angina in man. Circulation *67*:316, 1983.

129. Helfant, R. H., Bodenheimer, M. M., and Banka, V. S.: Asynergy in coronary heart disease. Evolving clinical and pathophysiologic concepts. Ann. Intern. Med. *87*:475, 1977.

130. Williams, J. F., Cohn, P. F., Vokonas, P. S., Young, E., Herman, M. V., and Gorlin, R.: Electrocardiographic, arteriographic and ventriculographic correlations in transmural myocardial infarction. Am. J. Cardiol. *31*:595, 1973.

131. Bodenheimer, M. M., Banka, V. S., and Helfant, R. H.: Q waves and ventricular asynergy: Predictive value and hemodynamic significance of anatomical localization. Am. J. Cardiol. *35*:615, 1975.

132. Pasternac, A., Gorlin, R., Sonnenblick, E. H., Haft, J. I., and Kemp, H. G.:

Abnormalities of ventricular motion induced by atrial pacing in coronary artery disease. Circulation 45:1195, 1972.

133. Sharma, B., and Taylor, S. H.: Localization of left ventricular ischemia in angina pectoris by cineangiography during exercise. Br. Heart J. 37:963, 1975.

134. Braunwald, E., and Kloner, R. A.: The stunned myocardium: Prolonged, postischemic ventricular dysfunction. Circulation 66:1146, 1982.

135. Cohn, P. F.: Contractile reserve in coronary heart disease: Detection and clinical importance. Primary Cardiol. 7:48, 1981.

136. McAnulty, J. H., Hattenhauer, M. T., Rosche, J., Kloster, F. E., and Rahimtoola, S. H.: Improvement in left ventricular wall motion following nitroglycerin. Circulation 51:140, 1975.

137. Bodenheimer, M. M., Banka, V. S., Hermann, G. A., Trout, R. G., Pasdar, H., and Helfant, R. H.: Reversible asynergy: Histopathologic and electrographic correlations in patients with coronary artery disease. Circulation 53:792, 1976.

138. Banka, V. S., Bodenheimer, M. M., and Helfant, R. H.: Determinants of reversible asynergy: The native coronary circulation. Circulation 52:810, 1975.

139. Verani, M. S., Carroll, R. J., and Falsetti, H. L.: Mitral valve prolapse in coronary artery disease. Am. J. Cardiol. 37:1, 1976.

140. Aranda, L. M., Befeler, B., Lazzaro, R., Embi, A., and Machado, H.: Mitral valve prolapse and coronary artery disease. Clinical, hemodynamic and angiographic correlations. Circulation 52:245, 1975.

141. Herman, M. V., Elliott, W. C., and Gorlin, R.: An electrocardiographic, anatomic, and metabolic study of zonal myocardial ischemia in coronary heart disease. Circulation 35:834, 1967.

142. Gertz, E. W., Wisneski, J. A., Neese, R., Bristow, J. D., Searle, G. L., and Hanlon, J. T.: Myocardial lactate metabolism: Evidence of lactate release during net chemical extraction in man. Circulation 63:1273, 1981.

143. Cannon, P. J., Sciacca, R. R., Fowler, D. L., Weiss, M. B., Schmidt, D. H., and Casarella, W. J.: Measurement of regional myocardial blood flow in man: Description and critique of the method using xenon-133 and a scintillation camera. Am. J. Cardiol. 36:783, 1975.

144. Cannon, P. J., Weiss, M. B., and Sciacca, R. R.: Myocardial blood flow in coronary artery disease: Studies at rest and during stress with inert gas washout techniques. Progr. Cardiovasc. Dis. 20:95, 1977.

145. Dwyer, E. M., Jr., Dell, R. B., and Cannon, P. J.: Regional myocardial flow in transmural myocardial infarction. Circulation 48:924, 1973.

146. See, J. R., Cohn, P. F., Holman, B. L., Roberts, B. H., and Adams, D. F.: Angiographic abnormalities associated with alterations in regional myocardial blood flow in coronary artery disease. Br. Heart J. 38:1278, 1976.

147. See, J. R., Cohn, P. F., Holman, B. L., Maddox, D. E., and Adams, D. F.: Significance of reduced regional myocardial blood flow in asynergic areas evaluated with two-state (intervention) ventriculography. Results of studies combining washout of xenon-133 and postextrasystolic potentiation. Am. J. Cardiol. 43:179, 1979.

148. Maseri, A., L'Abbate, A., Pesola, A., Michelassi, C., Marzilli, M., and DeNes, M.: Regional myocardial perfusion in patients with atherosclerotic coronary artery disease at rest and during angina pectoris induced by tachycardia. Circulation 55:423, 1977.

149. Okada, R. D., Pohost, G. M., Kirshenbaum, H. D., Kushner, F. G., Boucher, C. A., Block, P. C., and Strauss, H. W.: Radionuclide-determined change in pulmonary blood volume with exercise. N. Engl. J. Med. 301:569, 1979.

150. Sostman, H. D., and Langou, R. A.: Contemporary medical management of stable angina pectoris. Am. Heart J. 95:775, 1978.

151. Aronow, W. S.: Effect of passive smoking on angina pectoris. N. Engl. J. Med. 299:21, 1978.

152. Friedman, M., Thoresen, C. E., Gill, J. J., Ulmer, D., Thomas, L., Powell, L., Price, V., Elek, S. R., Rabin, D. D., Breall, W. S., Piaget, G., Dixon, T., Bourg, E., Levy, R. A., and Tasto, D. L.: Feasibility of altering Type A behavior pattern after myocardial infarction. Recurrent coronary prevention project study: Methods, baseline results and preliminary findings. Circulation 66:83, 1982.

153. Kannel, W. B., and Sorlie, P. D.: Remission of clinical angina pectoris: The Framingham Study. Am. J. Cardiol. 42:119, 1978.

154. Clausen, J. P., and Trap-Jensen, J.: Heart rate and arterial blood pressure during exercise in patients with angina pectoris: Effect of training and of nitroglycerin. Circulation 53:436, 1976.

155. Redwood, D. R., Rosing, D. R., and Epstein, S. E.: Circulatory and symptomatic effects of physical training in patients with coronary artery disease and angina pectoris. N. Engl. J. Med. 286:959, 1972.

156. Jensen, D., Atwood, J. E., Froelicher, V., McKirnan, M. D., Battler, A., Ashburn, W., and Ross, J., Jr.: Improvement in ventricular function during exercise studied with radionuclide ventriculography after cardiac rehabilitation. Am. J. Cardiol. 46:770, 1980.

157. Fox, S. M., Naughton, J. P., and Gorman, P. A.: Physical activity and cardiovascular health: The exercise prescription. Mod. Conc. Cardiovasc. Dis. 41:21, 1972.

158. Cohn, P. F., and Gorlin, R.: Physiologic and clinical actions of nitroglycerin. Med. Clin. North Am. 58:407, 1974.

159. Brachfeld, N., Bozer, J., and Gorlin, R.: Action of nitroglycerin on the coronary circulation in normal and mild cardiac subjects. Circulation 19:697, 1959.

160. Gorlin, R., Brachfeld, N., MacLeod, C., and Bopp, P.: Effect of nitroglycerin on the coronary circulation in patients with coronary artery disease or increased left ventricular work. Circulation 19:705, 1959.

161. Mason, D. T., and Braunwald, E.: The effects of nitroglycerin and amyl nitrite on arteriolar and venous tone in the human forearm. Circulation 32:755, 1965.

162. Williams, J. F., Jr., Glick, G., and Braunwald, E.: Studies on cardiac dimen-

sions in intact unanesthetized man. V. Effects of nitroglycerin. Circulation 32:76, 1965.

163. Burggraf, G. W., and Parker, J. O.: Left ventricular volume changes after amyl nitrite and nitroglycerin in man as measured by ultrasound. Circulation 49:136, 1974.

164. DeMaria, A. N., Vismara, L. A., Auditore, K., Amsterdam, E. A., Zelis, R., and Mason, D. T.: Effects of nitroglycerin on left ventricular cavity size and cardiac performance determined by ultrasound in man. Am. J. Med. 57:754, 1974.

165. Lecerof, H.: Influences of body position on exercise tolerance, heart rate, blood pressure and respiration rate in coronary insufficiency. Brit. Heart J.33:78, 1971.

166. Christensson, B., Nordenfelt, I., Westling, H., and White, T.: Hemodynamic effects of nitroglycerin in normal subjects during supine and sitting exercise. Br. Heart J. 31:80, 1969.

167. Parker, J. O., Case, R. B., Khaja, F., Ledwich, J. R., and Armstrong, P. W.: The influence of changes in blood volume on angina pectoris: A study of the effect of phlebotomy. Circulation 41:593, 1976.

168. Parker, J. O., DiGiorgi, S., and West, R. O.: A hemodynamic study of acute coronary insufficiency precipitated by exercise: With observations on the effect of nitroglycerin. Am. J. Cardiol. 17:470, 1966.

169. Robinson, B. F.: Mode of action of nitroglycerin in angina pectoris. Correlation between hemodynamic effects during exercise and prevention of pain. Br. Heart J. 30:295, 1968.

170. Likoff, W., Kasparian, H., Lehman, J. S., and Segal, B. L.: Evaluation of "coronary vasodilators" by coronary arteriography. Am. J. Cardiol. 13:7, 1964.

171. Brown, B. G., Bolson, E., Petersen, R. B., Pierce, C. D., and Dodge, H. T.: The mechanisms of nitroglycerin action: Stenosis vasodilation as a major component of the drug response. Circulation 64:1089, 1981.

172. Becker, L. C., Fortuin, N. J., and Pitt, B.: Effect of ischemia and antianginal drugs on radioactive microspheres in the canine left ventricle. Circ. Res. 28:263, 1971.

173. Winbury, M. W., Howe, B. B., and Weiss, H. R.: Effect of nitroglycerin and dipyridamole on epicardial and endocardial oxygen tension—further evidence for redistribution of myocardial blood flow. J. Pharmacol. Exp. Ther. 176:184, 1971.

174. Bache, R. J., Ball, R. M., Cobb, F. R., Rembert, J. C., and Greenfield, J. C., Jr.: Effects of nitroglycerin on transmural myocardial blood flow in the unanesthetized dog. J. Clin. Invest. 55:1219, 1975.

175. Fam, W. M., and McGregor, M.: Effect of coronary vasodilator drugs on retrograde flow in areas of chronic myocardial ischemia. Circ. Res. 15:355, 1964.

176. Cohen, M. V., Downey, J. M., Sonnenblick, E. H., and Kirk, E. S.: The effects of nitroglycerin on coronary collaterals and myocardial contractility. J. Clin. Invest. 52:2836, 1973.

177. Cowan, C., Duran, P. V. M., Corsini, G., Goldschlager, N., and Bing, R. J.: The effects of nitroglycerin on myocardial blood flow in man. Measured by coincidence counting and bolus injections of [84]rubidium. Am. J. Cardiol. 24:154, 1969.

178. Parker, J. O., West, R. O., and DiGiorgi, S.: The effect of nitroglycerin on coronary blood flow and the hemodynamic response to exercise in coronary artery disease. Am. J. Cardiol. 27:59, 1971.

179. Ganz, W., and Marcus, H. S.: Failure of intracoronary nitroglycerin to alleviate pacing-induced angina. Circulation 46:880, 1972.

180. Bernstein, L., Friesinger, G. C., Lichtlen, P. R., and Ross, R. S.: The effect of nitroglycerin on the systemic circulation in man and dog. Circulation 33:107, 1966.

181. Maseri, A.: Regional myocardial blood flow in man—evaluation of drugs. In Strauss, H. W., Pitt, B., and James, A. E., Jr. (eds.): Cardiovascular Nuclear Medicine. St. Louis, The C. V. Mosby Co., 1974, p. 171.

182. Cohn, P. F., Maddox, D. E., Holman, B. L., Markis, J. E., Adams, D. F., and See, J. R.: Effect of sublingually administered nitroglycerin on regional myocardial blood flow in patients with coronary artery disease. Am. J. Cardiol. 39:672, 1977.

183. Goldstein, R. E., Stinson, E. B., Scherer, J. L., Seningen, R. P., Grehl, T. M., and Epstein, S. E.: Intraoperative coronary collateral function in patients with coronary occlusive disease. Nitroglycerin responsiveness and angiographic correlations. Circulation 49:298, 1974.

184. Chiong, M. A., West, R. O., and Parker, J. O.: Influence of nitroglycerin on myocardial metabolism and hemodynamics during angina induced by atrial pacing. Circulation 45:1044, 1972.

185. Dove, J. T., Shah, P. M., and Schreiner, B. F.: Effects of nitroglycerin on left ventricular wall motion in coronary artery disease. Circulation 49:682, 1974.

186. Salel, A. F., Berman, D. S., DeNardo, G. L., and Mason, D. T.: Radionuclide assessment of nitroglycerin influence on abnormal left ventricular segmental contraction in patients with coronary artery disease. Circulation 53:975, 1976.

187. Borer, J. S., Bacharach, S. L., Green, M. V., Kent, K. M., Johnston, G. S., and Epstein, S. E.: Effect of nitroglycerin on exercise-induced abnormalities of left ventricular regional function and ejection fraction in coronary artery disease. Assessment by radionuclide cineangiography in symptomatic and asymptomatic patients. Circulation 57:314, 1978.

188. Dimond, E. G., and Benchimol, A.: Correlation of intracardiac pressure and precordial movement in ischemic heart disease. Br. Heart J. 25:389, 1963.

189. Lee, S. J. K., Sung, Y. K., and Zaragoza, A. J.: Effects of nitroglycerin on left ventricular volumes and wall tension in patients with ischemic heart disease. Br. Heart J. 32:790, 1970.

190. Muller, O., and Rorvik, R.: Hemodynamic consequences of coronary heart disease: With observations during anginal pain and on the effect of nitroglycerin. Br. Heart J. 20:302, 1958.

191. Hood, W. P., Jr., Amende, I., Simon, R., and Lichtlen, P. R.: The effects of intracoronary nitroglycerin on left ventricular and diastolic function in man. Circulation *61*:1098, 1980.
192. Abrams, J.: Nitroglycerin and long-acting nitrates. N. Engl. J. Med. *302*:1234, 1980.
193. Alpert, J. S.: Toward the more effective use of nitroglycerin. J. Cardiovasc. Med. *7*:598, 1982.
194. Hales, C. A., and Westphal, D.: Hypoxemia following the administration of sublingual nitroglycerin. Am. J. Med. *65*:911, 1978.
195. Needleman, P., Lang, S., and Johnson, E. M., Jr.: Organic nitrates: Relationship between biotransformation and rational angina pectoris therapy. J. Pharmacol. Exp. Ther. *181*:489, 1972.
196. Glancy, D. L., Richter, M. A., Ellis, E. V., and Johnson, W.: Effect of swallowed isosorbide dinitrate on blood pressure, heart rate and exercise capacity in patients with coronary artery disease. Am. J. Med. *62*:39, 1977.
197. Markis, J. E., Gorlin, R., Mills, R. M., Williams, R. A., Schweitzer, P., and Ransil, B. J.: Sustained effect of orally administered isosorbide dinitrate on exercise performance of patients with angina pectoris. Am. J. Cardiol. *43*:265, 1979.
198. Lee, G., Mason, O. T., and DeMaria, A. N.: Effects of long-term oral administration of isosorbide dinitrate on the antianginal response to nitroglycerin. Am. J. Cardiol. *41*:82, 1978.
199. Thadani, U., Fung, H. L., Darke, A. C., and Parker, J. O.: Oral isosorbide dinitrate in angina pectoris: Comparison of duration of action and dose-response relation during acute and sustained therapy. Am. J. Cardiol. *49*:411, 1982.
200. Transdermal delivery systems for nitroglycerin. Med. Lett. *24*:35, 1982.
201. Thompson, R. H.: The clinical use of transdermal delivery devices with nitroglycerin. Cardiovasc. Rev. Rep. *4*:91, 1983.
202. Abrams, J.: Nitrate tolerance and dependence. Am. Heart J. *99*:113, 1980.
203. Bassan, M. M., and Weiler-Ravell, D.: The additive antianginal action of oral isosorbide dinitrate in patients receiving propranolol. Magnitude and duration of effect. Chest *83*:233, 1983.
204. Epstein, S. E., and Braunwald, E.: Inhibition of the adrenergic nervous system in the treatment of angina pectoris. Med. Clin. North Am. *52*:1031, 1968.
205. Braunwald, E. (ed.): Beta-Adrenergic Blockade—A New Era in Cardiovascular Medicine. New York, Excerpta Medica, 1978, 309 pp.
206. Miller, R. R., Olson, H. G., and Pratt, C. M.: Efficacy of beta-adrenergic blockade in coronary heart disease: Propranolol in angina pectoris. Clin. Pharmacol. Ther. *18*:598, 1975.
207. Manyari, D. E., Kostuk, W. J., Carruthers, G., Johnston, D. J., and Purves, P.: Pindolol and propranolol inpatients with angina pectoris and normal or near-normal ventricular function. Lack of influence of intrinsic sympathomimetic activity on global and segmental left ventricular function assessed by radionuclide ventriculography. Am. J. Cardiol. *51*:427, 1983.
207a. Harris, F. J., Low, R. I., Palmer, L., Amsterdam, E. A., and Mason, D. T.: Antianginal efficacy and improved exercise performance with timolol. Twice-daily beta blockade in ischemic heart disease. Am. J. Cardiol. *51*:13, 1983.
208. Watanabe, A. G.: Recent advances in knowledge about beta-adrenergic receptors: Application to clinical cardiology. J. Am. Coll. Cardiol. *1*:82, 1983.
209. Alderman, E. L., Davies, R. O., Crowley, J. J., Lopes, M. G., Brooker, J. Z., Friedman, J. P., Graham, A. F., Matlof, H. J., and Harrison, D. C.: Dose response effectiveness of propranolol for the treatment of angina pectoris. Circulation *51*:964, 1975.
210. Pine, M., Favrot, L., Smith, S., McDonald, K., and Chidsey, C. A.: Correlation of plasma propranolol concentration with therapeutic response in patients with angina pectoris. Circulation *52*:886, 1975.
211. Parmley, W. W.: Beta blockers in coronary artery disease. Cardiovasc. Rev. Rep. *2*:655, 1981.
212. Koch-Weser, J.: Beta-adrenoceptor antagonists: New drugs and new indications. N. Engl. J. Med. *305*:500, 1981.
213. Miller, R. R., Olson, H. G., Amsterdam, E. A., and Mason, D. T.: Propranolol withdrawal rebound phenomenon. Exacerbation of coronary events after abrupt cessation of antianginal therapy. N. Engl. J. Med. *293*:416, 1975.
214. Aarons, R. D., and Molinoff, P. B.: Changes in the density of beta adrenergic receptors in rat lymphocytes, heart and lung after chronic treatment with propranolol. J. Pharmacol. Exp. Ther. *221*:439, 1982.
215. Kern, M. J., Ganz, P., Horowitz, J. D., Gaspar, J., Barry, W. H., Lorell, B. H., Grossman, W., and Mudge, G. H., Jr.: Potentiation of coronary vasoconstriction by beta-adrenergic blockade. Circulation *67*:1178, 1983.
216. Robertson, R. M., Wood, A. J. J., Vaughn, W. K., and Robertson, D.: Exacerbation of vasotonic angina pectoris by propranolol. Circulation *65*:281, 1982.
217. Cruickshank, J. M.: The clinical importance of cardioselectivity and lipophilicity in beta blockers. Am. Heart J. *100*:160, 1980.
218. Frishman, W. H., and Kostis, J.: The significance of intrinsic sympathomimetic activity in beta-adrenoceptor blocking drugs. Cardiovasc. Rev. Rep. *3*:503, 1982.
219. Kostis, J. B., Frishman, W., Hosler, M. H., Thorsen, N. L., Gonasun, L., and Weinstein, J.: Treatment of angina pectoris with pindolol: The significance of intrinsic sympathomimetic activity of beta blockers. Am. Heart J. *104*:496, 1982.
220. Cannon, R. E., Slavin, R. G., and Gonasun, L. M.: The effect on asthma of a new beta blocker, pindolol. Am. Heart J. *104*:438, 1982.
221. Krikler, D. M., and Rowland, E.: Clinical value of calcium antagonists in treatment of cardiovascular disorders. J. Am. Coll. Cardiol. *1*:355, 1983.
222. Fleckenstein, A.: Calcium Antagonist in Heart and Smooth Muscle. New York, John Wiley and Sons, 1983.
222a. Sherman, G., and Liang, C-S.: Nifedipine in chronic stable angina: A double-blind placebo-controlled crossover trial. Am. J. Cardiol. *51*:706, 1983.
222b. Stone, P. H., Turi, Z., Muller, J. E., Geltman, E., Jaffe, A., and Braunwald, E.: Experience with nifedipine in 845 patients with refractory angina pectoris. J. Am. Coll. Cardiol. *1*:596, 1983.
222c. Subramanian, B.: Long-term therapy of angina with calcium antagonists. Cardiovasc. Rev. Rep. *4*:493, 1983.
222d. Subramanian, V. B., Khurmi, N. S., Bowles, M. J., O'Hara, M., and Raftery, E. B.: Objective evaluation of three dose levels of diltiazem in patients with chronic stable angina. J. Am. Coll. Cardiol. *1*:1144, 1983.
223. Ludbrook, P. A., Tiefenbrunn, A. J., Reed, F. R., and Sobel, B. E.: Acute hemodynamic responses to sublingual nifedipine: Dependence on left ventricular function. Circulation *65*:489, 1982.
224. Klein, H. O., Ninio, R., Oren, V., Lang, R., Sareli, P., DiSegni, E., David, D., Guerrero, J., and Kaplinsky, E.: The acute hemodynamic effects of intravenous verapamil in coronary artery disease. Assessment by equilibrium-gated radionuclide ventriculography. Circulation *67*:101, 1983.
225. Rouleau, J., Chatterjee, K., Ports, T. A., Doyle, M. B., Hiramatsu, B., and Parmley, W. W.: Mechanism of relief of pacing-induced angina with oral verapamil: Reduced oxygen demand. Circulation *67*:94, 1983.
225a. Chew, C. Y. C., Brown, B. G., Singh, B. N., Wong, M. M., Pierce, C., and Petersen, R.: Effects of verapamil on coronary hemodynamic function and vasomobility relative to its mechanism of antianginal action. Am. J. Cardiol. *51*:699, 1983.
226. Charlap, S., and Frishman, W. H.: Comparative effects of verapamil and beta blockers in the therapy for patients with stable angina pectoris. Cardiovasc. Rev. Rep. *4*:66, 1983.
227. Leon, M. B., Rosing, D. R., Bonow, R. O., Lipson, L. C., and Epstein, S. E.: Clincial efficacy of verapamil alone and combined with propranolol in treating patients with chronic stable angina pectoris. Am. J. Cardiol. *48*:131, 1981.
228. Wagniart, P., Ferguson, R. J., Chaitman, B. R., Achard F., Benacerraf, A., Delanguenhagen, B., Morin, B., Pasternac, A., and Bourassa, M. G.: Increased exercise tolerance and reduced electrocardiographic ischemia with diltiazem in patients with stable angina pectoris. Circulation *66*:23, 1982.
229. Schroeder, J. S., McAuley, B., and Ginsburg, R.: Diltiazem: A clinical and pharmacologic profile. J. Cardiovasc. Med. *8*:41, 1983.
229a. Smith, M. S., Verghese, C. P., Shand, D. G., and Pritchett, E. L. C.: Pharmacokinetic and pharmacodynamic effects of diltiazem. Am. J. Cardiol. *51*:1369, 1983.
230. Marra, S., Paolillo, V., Baduini, G., Spadaccini, F., and Angelino, P. F.: Acute effects of chewable nifedipine on hemodynamic responses to upright exercise in patients with prior myocardial infarction and effort angina. Chest *83*:50, 1983.
231. Furberg, C. D., Friedewald, W. T., and Eberlein, K. A. (eds.): Proceedings of the workshop on implications of recent beta-blocker trials for post-myocardial infarction patients. Circulation *67*:1–111, 1983.
232. Turi, Z. G., and Braunwald, E.: The use of beta blockers after myocardial infarction. JAMA *249*:2512, 1983.
233. Pfisterer, M., Glaus, L., and Burkart, F.: Comparative effects of nitroglycerin, nifedipine and metoprolol on regional left ventricular function in patients with one-vessel coronary disease. Circulation *67*:291, 1983.
234. Johnson, S. M., Mauritson, D. R., Corbett, J. R., Woodward, W., Willerson, J. T., and Hillis, L. D.: Double-blind, randomized, placebo-controlled comparison of propranolol and verapamil in the treatment of patients with stable angina pectoris. Am. J. Med. *71*:443, 1981.
235. Braunwald, E.: Mechanism of action of calcium-channel-blocking agents. N. Engl. J. Med. *307*:1618, 1983.
236. Dargie, H. J., Lynch, P. G., Krikler, D. M., Harris, L., and Krikler, S.: Nifedipine and propranolol: A beneficial drug interaction. Am. J. Med. *71*:676, 1981.
237. Pfisterer, M., Muller-Brand, J., and Burkart, F.: Combined acebutolol/nifedipine therapy in patients with chronic coronary artery disease: Additional improvement of ischemia-induced left ventricular dysfunction. Am. J. Cardiol. *49*:1259, 1982.
238. Bassan, M., Weiler-Ravell, D., and Shalev, O.: The additive antianginal action of oral nifedipine in patients receiving propranolol. Magnitude and duration of effect. Circulation *66*:710, 1982
239. Winniford, M. D., Huxley, R. L., and Hillis, L. D.: Randomized, double-blind comparison of propranolol alone and a propranolol-verpamil combination in patients with severe angina of effort. J. Am. Coll. Cardiol. *1*:492, 1983.
239a. Johnston, D. L., Gebhart, V., Lesoway, R., and Kostuk, W. J.: Hemodynamic evaluation of verapamil and propranolol alone and in combination: Assessment of radionuclide ventriculography. J. Am. Coll. Cardiol. *1*:679, 1983.
239b. Lessem, J.: Combined therapy with verapamil and atenolol in chronic stable angina. J. Am. Coll. Cardiol. *1*:596, 1983.
240. Packer, M., Meller, J., Medina, N., Yushak, M., Smith, H., Holt, J., Guererro, J., Todd, G. D., McAllister, R. G., Jr., and Gorlin, R.: Hemodynamic consequences of combined beta-adrenergic and slow calcium channel blockade in man. Circulation *65*:660, 1982.
241. Kieval, J., Kirsten, E. B., Kessler, K. M., Mallon, S. M., and Myerburg, R. J.: The effects of intravenous verapamil on hemodynamic status of patients with coronary artery disease receiving propranolol. Circulation *65*:653, 1982.
242. Hood, W. B., Jr.: More on sulfinpyrazone after myocardial infarction (Editorial). N. Engl. J. Med. *306*:988, 1982.
243. Grüntzig, A. R., and Meier, B.: Percutaneous transluminal coronary angioplasty. The first five years and the future. Intern. J. Cardiol. *2*:319, 1983.
243a. Dorros, G., Cowley, M. J., Simpson, J., Bentivoglio, L. G., Block, P. C., Bourassa, M., Detre, K., Goselin, A. J., Gruntzig, A. R., Kelsey, S. F., Kent, K. M., Mock, M. B., Mulin, S. M., Myuler, R. K., Passamani, E. R., Stertzer, S. H., and Williams, D. O.: Percutaneous transluminal coronary angioplasty: Report of complications from the National Heart, Lung and Blood Institute PTCA registry. Circulation *67*:723, 1983.
243b. Holmes, D. R., Jr., Vlietstra, R. E., Mock, M. B., Reeder, G. S., Smith, H. C., Bove, A. A., Bresnahan, J. F., Piehler, J. M., Schaff, H. V., and Orszulak,

T. A.: Angiographic changes produced by percutaneous transluminal coronary angioplasty. Am. J. Cardiol. 51:676, 1983.

243c. Meier, B., Hollman, J., and Gruentzig, A. R.: Percutaneous transluminal coronary angioplasty. Circulation 67:1155, 1983.

244. Block, P. C., Myler, R. K., Stertzer, S., and Fallon, J. T.: Morphology after transluminal angioplasty in human beings. N. Engl. J. Med. 305:382, 1981.

245. Meier, B., Grüntzig, A. R., Hollman, J., Ischinger, T., and Bradford, J. M.: Does length or eccentricity of coronary stenoses influence the outcome of transluminal dilatation? Circulation 67:497, 1983.

245a. Vlietstra, R. E., Holmes, D. R., Jr., Mock, M. B., Smith, H. C., Reeder, G. S., Bresnahan, J. F., Bove, A. A., and Piehler, J. M.: Balloon angioplasty in multivessel coronary disease: Mayo Clinic experience. J. Am. Coll. Cardiol. 1: 656, 1983.

245b. Williams, D. O., Kurzrok, S., Riley, R., Singh, A., and Most, A.: Partial revascularization by single vessel coronary angioplasty: Efficacious therapy of multivessel coronary artery disease. J. Am. Coll. Cardiol. 1:655, 1983.

246. Kent, K. M., Bonow, R. O., Rosing, D. R., Ewels, C. J., Lipson, L. C., McIntosh, C. L., Bacharach, S., Green, M., and Epstein, S. E.: Improved myocardial function during exercise after successful percutaneous transluminal coronary angioplasty. N. Engl. J. Med. 306:441, 1982.

247. Kent, K. M., Bentivoglio, L. G., Block, P. C., Cowley, M. J., Dorros, G., Gosselin, A. J., Grüntzig, A., Myler, R. K., Simpson, J., Stertzer, S. H., Williams, D. O., Fisher, L., Gillespie, M. J., Detre, K., Kelsey, S., Mullin, S. M., and Mock, M. B.: Percutaneous transluminal coronary angioplasty: Report from the registry of the National Heart, Lung, and Blood Institute. Am. J. Cardiol. 49:2011, 1982.

247a. Hollman, J., Gruentzig, A., Meier, B., Bradford, J., and Galan, K.: Factors affecting recurrence after successful coronary angioplasty. J. Am. Coll. Cardiol. 1:644, 1983.

247b. Williams, D. O., Gruntzig, A., Kent, K., Detre, K., Kelsey, C., Shalloner, K., and members of the Executive Committee, NHLBI: Role of repeated percutaneous transluminal coronary angioplasty (PTCA) for coronary restenosis: A report of the NHLBI PTCA registry. J. Am. Coll. Cardiol. 1:644, 1983.

248. Sigwart, U., Grbic, M., Essinger, A., Bischof-Delaloye, A., Sadeghi, H., and Rivier, J.-L.: Improvement of left ventricular function after percutaneous transluminal coronary angioplasty. Am. J. Cardiol. 49:651, 1982.

248a. Williams, D., Singh, A., and Most, A.: Sustained efficacy of coronary angioplasty documented by stress testing at one year. J. Am. Coll. Cardiol. 1:724, 1983.

249. Hirzel, H. O., Nuesch, K., Grüntzig, A. R., and Leutolf, U. M.: Short- and long-term changes in myocardial perfusion after percutaneous transluminal coronary angioplasty assessed by thallium-201 exercise scintigraphy. Circulation 63:1001, 1981.

250. Scholl, J. M., Chaitman, B. R., David, P. R., Dupras, G., Bevers, G., Val, P. G., Crepeau, J., Lesperance, J., and Bourassa, M. G.: Exercise electrocardiography and myocardial scintigraphy in the serial evaluation of the results of percutaneous transluminal coronary angioplasty. Circulation 66:380, 1982.

251. Choy, D. S. J., Stertzer, S., Rotterdam, H. Z., Sharrock, N., and Kaminow, I. P.: Transluminal laser catheter angioplasty. Am. J. Cardiol. 50:1206, 1982.

252. Choy, D. S. J., Stertzer, S. H., Rotterdam, H. Z., and Bruno M. S.: Laser coronary angioplasty: Experience with 9 cadaver hearts. Am. J. Cardiol. 50:1209, 1982.

252a. Lee, G., Ikeda, R., Herman, I., Dwyer, R. M., Bass, M., Hussein, H., Kozina, J., and Mason, D. T.: The qualitative effects of laser irradiation on human arteriosclerotic disease. Am. Heart J. 105:885, 1983.

252b. Choy, D. S., Stertzer, S. H., Quilici, P., Wallsh, E., Bruno, M. S., Loubeau, J-M., Kaminow, I., and Rotterdam, H.: Argon laser angioplasty in cadaver and animal models. J. Am. Coll. Cardiol. 1:690, 1983.

252c. Gessman, L. J., Reno, C. W., and Hastie, R.: Model for testing coronary angioplasty by laser catheter. J. Am. Coll. Cardiol. 1:690, 1983.

253. Mills, N. L., and Doyle, D. P.: Does operative transluminal angioplasty extend the limits of coronary artery bypass surgery? A preliminary report. Circulation 66(Suppl. 1):26, 1982.

254. Jones, E. L., and King, S. B.: Intraoperative angioplasty in the treatment of coronary artery disease. J. Am. Coll. Cardiol. 1:970, 1983.

255. Kannel, W. B., and Feinleib, M.: Natural history of angina pectoris in the Framingham study: Progress and survival. Am. J. Cardiol. 29:154, 1972.

256. Frank, C. W., Weinblatt, W., and Shapiro, S.: Angina pectoris in men: Prognostic significance of related medical factors. Circulation 47:509, 1973.

257. Vedin, A., Wilhelmsson, C., Elmfeldt, D., Save-Soderbergh, J., Tibblin, G., and Wilhelmsen, L.: Death and non-fatal reinfarctions during two years' follow-up after myocardial infarction. Acta Med. Scand. 198:353, 1975.

258. Graham, I., Mulcahy, R., Hickey, N., O'Neill, W., and Daly, L.: Natural history of coronary heart disease: A study of 586 men surviving an initial acute attack. Am. Heart J. 105:249, 1983.

259. Frank, C. W., Weinblatt, E., Shapiro, S., and Sager, R. V.: Prognosis of men with coronary heart disease as related to blood pressure. Circulation 38:432, 1968.

260. Gorlin, R.: Natural history of coronary heart disease. In Gorlin, R.: Coronary Artery Disease. Philadelphia, W. B. Saunders Co., 1976, p. 195.

261. Spain, D. M., and Bradess, V. A.: Sudden death from coronary heart disease: Survival time, frequency of thrombi and cigarette smoking. Chest 58:107, 1970.

262. Blackburn, H.: The prognostic importance of the electrocardiogram after myocardial infarction: Experience in the coronary drug project. Ann. Intern. Med. 77:677, 1972.

263. Kotler, M. N., Tabatznik, B., Mower, M. M., and Tominaga, S.: Prognostic significance of ventricular ectopic beats with respect to sudden death in the late postinfarction period. Circulation 47:959, 1973.

264. Kannel, W. B., Boyle, J. T., McNamara, P., Quickenton, P., and Gordon, T.: Precursors of sudden coronary death: Factors related to the incidence of sudden death. Circulation 51:606, 1975.

265. Reeves, T. J., Oberman, A., Jones, W. B., and Sheffield, L. T.: Natural history of angina pectoris. Am. J. Cardiol. 33:423, 1974.

266. Califf, R. M., Tomabechi, Y., Lee, K. L., Phillips, H., Pryor, D. B., Harrell, F. E., Jr., Harris, P. J., Peter, R. H., Behar, V. S., Kong, Y., and Rosati, R. A.: Outcome in one-vessel coronary artery disease. Circulation 67:283, 1983.

267. Burggraf, G. W., and Parker, J. O.: Prognosis in coronary artery disease—angiographic, hemodynamic and clinical factors. Circulation 51:146, 1975.

268. Humphries, J. O., Kuller, L., Ross, R. S., Friesinger, G. C., and Page, E. E.: Natural history of ischemic heart disease in relation to arteriographic findings. Circulation 49:489, 1974.

269. Oberman, A., Jones, W. B., and Riley, C. P.: Natural history of coronary artery disease. Bull. N.Y. Acad. Med. 48:1109, 1972.

270. Harris, P. J., Behar, V. S., Conley, M. J., Harrell, F. E., Jr., Lee, K. L., Peter, R. H., Kong, Y., and Rosati, R. A.: The prognostic significance of 50 per cent coronary stenosis in medically treated patients with coronary artery disease. Circulation 62:240, 1980.

271. Kent, K. M., Rosing, D. R., Ewels, C. J., Lipson, L., Bonow, R., and Epstein, S. E.: Prognosis of asymptomatic or mildly symptomatic patients with coronary artery disease. Am. J. Cardiol. 49:1823, 1982.

272. Proudfit, W. L., Bruschke, A. V., and Sones, F. M., Jr.: Natural history of obstructive coronary artery disease: Ten-year study of 601 nonsurgical cases. Progr. Cardiovasc. Dis. 22:53, 1978.

273. Bruschke, A. V., Proudfit, W. L., and Sones, F. M., Jr.: Progress study of 490 consecutive nonsurgical cases of coronary disease followed 5–9 years. II. Ventriculographic and other correlations. Circulation 47:1154, 1973.

274. Gross, H., Vaid, A. K., and Cohen, M. K.: Prognosis in patients rejected for coronary revascularization surgery. Am. J. Med. 64:9, 1978.

275. Nelson, G. R., Cohn, P. F., and Gorlin, R.: Prognosis in medically treated coronary artery disease. The value of the ejection fraction compared with other measurements. Circulation 52:408, 1975.

276. Harlan, W. R., Oberman, A., Grimm, R., and Rosati, R. A.: Chronic congestive heart failure in coronary artery disease: Clinical criteria. Ann. Intern. Med. 86:133, 1977.

277. Bruschke, A. V., Proudfit, W. L., and Sones, F. M., Jr.: Progress study of 490 consecutive nonsurgical cases of coronary disease followed 5–9 years. I. Arteriographic correlations. Circulation 47:1147, 1973.

278. Conti, C. R., Selby, J. H., and Christie, L. G.: Left main coronary artery stenosis: Clinical spectrum, pathophysiology and management. Progr. Cardiovasc. Dis. 22:73, 1979.

278a. Takaro, T., Peduzzi, P., Detre, K. M., Hultgren, H. N., Murphy, M. L., Bel-Kahn, J., Thomsen, J., and Meadows, W. R.: Survival in subgroups of patients with left main coronary artery disease. Veterans Administration Cooperative Study of Surgery for Coronary Arterial Occlusive Disease. Circulation 66:14, 1982.

279. Bemis, C. E., Gorlin, R., Kemp, H. G., and Herman, M. V.: The progression of coronary obstructive disease. A clinical arteriographic study. Circulation 47: 455, 1973.

280. Kramer, J. R., Matsuda, Y., Mulligan, J. C., Aronow, M., and Proudfit, W. L.: Progression of coronary atherosclerosis. Circulation 63:519, 1981.

281. Bruschke, A. V. G., Wijers, T. S., Kolsters, W., and Landmann, J.: The anatomic evolution of coronary artery disease demonstrated by coronary arteriography in 256 nonoperated patients. Circulation 63:527, 1981.

281a. Hansteen, V., Moinichen, E., Lorenstsen, E., Andersen, A., Strom, O., Soiland, K., Dyrbekk, D., Refsum, A.-M., Tromsdal, A., Knudsen, K., Eika, C., Bakken, J., Jr., Smith, P., and Hoff, P. I.: One year's treatment with propranolol after myocardial infarction: Preliminary report of Norwegian multicentre trial. Br. Med. J. 284:155, 1982.

UNSTABLE ANGINA

282. Adelman, A. G., and Goldman, B. S. (Eds.): Unstable Angina. Recognition and Management. Littleton, Col., 1981, PSG Publishing Co., Inc.

283. Fowler, N. O.: Preinfarction angina. Circulation 44:775, 1971.

284. Willerson, J. T., Hillis, L. D., and Buja, L. M.: Ischemic Heart Disease. New York, Raven Press, 1982.

285. Robbins, S. L.: Clinicopathologic correlations in coronary atherosclerosis. Four hundred and thirty patients studied with postmortem coronary angiography. Circulation 27:170, 1963.

286. Fulton, M., Lutz, W., Donald, K. W., Kirby, B. J., Duncan, B., Morrison, S. L., Kerr, F., Julian, D. G., and Oliver, M. F.: Natural history of unstable angina. Lancet 1:860, 1972.

287. Report of the Unstable Angina Pectoris Study Group: Unstable angina pectoris: National Cooperative Group to Compare Medical and Surgical Therapy. II. In-hospital experience and initial follow-up results in patients with one, two, and three vessel disease. Am. J. Cardiol. 42:839, 1978.

288. Gazes, P. C., Mobley, E. M., Jr., Faris, H. M., Jr., Duncan, R. C., and Humphries, G. B.: Preinfarctional (stable) angina—a prospective study; Ten year follow-up. Prognostic significance of electrocardiographic changes. Circulation 48:331, 1973.

289. Victor, M. F., Likoff, M. J., Mintz, G. S., and Likoff, W.: Unstable angina pectoris of new onset: A prospective clinical and arteriographic study of 75 patients. Am. J. Cardiol. 47:228, 1981.

290. Fischl, S., Gorlin, R., and Herman, M. V.: The intermediate coronary syndrome: Clinical, angiographic and therapeutic aspects. N. Engl. J. Med. 288: 1193, 1973.

291. Plotnick, G. D., and Conti, C. R.: Transient ST-segment elevation in unstable angina. Clinical and hemodynamic significance. Circulation 51:1015, 1975.

292. Bodenheimer, M. M., Banka, V. S., Trout, R. G., Hermann, G. A., Pasdar, H., and Helfant, R. H.: Pathophysiologic significance of ST and T wave abnormalities in patients with the intermediate coronary syndrome. Am. J. Cardiol. 39:153, 1977.

293. Rackley, C. E., Russell, R. O., Jr., Rogers, W. J., Mantle, J. A., and Papapietro, S. E.: Unstable angina pectoris: Is it time to change our approach? Am. Heart J. 103:154, 1982.

294. Alison, H. W., Russel, R. O., Jr., Mantle, J. A., Kouchoukos, N. T., and Rackley, C. E.: Coronary anatomy and arteriography in patients with unstable angina pectoris. Am. J. Cardiol. 41:204, 1978.

295. Roberts, W. C., and Virmani, Z.: Quantitation of coronary arterial narrowing in clinically isolated unstable angina pectoris: An analysis of 22 necropsy patients. Am. J. Med. 67:792, 1979.

296. Parker, F. B., Jr., Neville, J. F., Jr., Hanson, E. C., and Webb, W. R.: Retrograde and antegrade pressures and flows in preinfarction syndrome. Circulation 50(Suppl. 11):122, 1974.

297. Sharma, B., Hodges, M., Asinger, R. W., Goodwin, J. F., and Francis, G. S.: Left ventricular function during spontaneous angina pectoris: Effect of sublingual nitroglycerin. Am. J. Cardiol. 46:34, 1980.

298. Roughgarden, J. W.: Circulatory changes associated with spontaneous angina pectoris. Am. J. Med. 41:947, 1966.

299. Cannom, D. S., Harrison, D. C., and Schroeder, J. S.: Hemodynamic observations in patients with unstable angina pectoris. Am. J. Cardiol. 33:17, 1974.

300. Maseri, A.: Variant angina and coronary vasospasm: Clues to a broader understanding of angina pectoris. Cardiovasc. Med. 4:647, 1979.

301. Chierchia, S., Brunelli, C., Simonetti, I., Lazzari, M., and Maseri, A.: Sequence of events in angina at rest: Primary reduction in coronary flow. Circulation 61:759, 1980.

302. Holmes, D. R., Jr., Hartzler, G. O., Smith, H. C., and Fuster, V.: Coronary artery thrombosis in patients with unstable angina. Br. Heart J. 45:411, 1981.

303. Neill, W. A., Wharton, T. P., Jr., Fluri-Lundeen, J., and Cohen, I. S.: Acute coronary insufficiency—Coronary occlusion after intermittent ischemic attacks. N. Engl. J. Med. 302:1157, 1980.

304. Specchia, G., de Servi, S., Falcone, C., Bramucci, E., Angoli, L., Mussini, A., Marioni, G. P., Montemartini, C., and Bobba, P.: Coronary arterial spasm as a cause of exercise-induced ST-segment elevation in patients with variant angina. Circulation 59:948, 1979.

305. Biagini, A., Mazzei, M. G., Carpeggiani, C., Testa, R., Antonelli, R., Michelassi, C., L'Abbate, A., and Maseri, A.: Vasospastic ischemic mechanism of frequent asymptomatic transient ST-T changes during continuous electrocardiographic monitoring in selected unstable angina patients. Am. Heart J. 103:13, 1982.

306. Johnson, S. M., Mauritson, D. R., Winniford, M. D., Willerson, J. T., Firth, B. G., Cary, J. R., and Hillis, L. D.: Continuous electrocardiographic monitoring in patients with unstable angina pectoris: Identification of high-risk subgroup with severe coronary disease, variant angina, and/or impaired early prognosis. Am. Heart J. 103:4, 1982.

307. Donsky, M. S., Curry, G. C., Parkey, R. W., Meyer, S. L., Bonte, F. J., Platt, M. R., and Willerson, J. T.: Unstable angina pectoris. Clinical, angiographic, and myocardial scintigraphic observations. Br. Heart J. 38:257, 1976.

308. Uthurralt, N., Davies, G. J., Parodi, O., Bencivelli, W., and Maseri, A.: Comparative study of myocardial ischemia during angina at rest and on exertion using thallium-201 scintigraphy. Am. J. Cardiol. 48:410, 1981.

309. Nixon, J. V., Brown, C. N., and Smitherman, T. C.: Identification of transient and persistent segmental wall motion abnormalities in patients with unstable angina by two-dimensional echocardiography. Circulation 65:1497, 1982.

310. Conti, R., Brawley, R., Pitt, B., and Ross, J.: Unstable angina: Morbidity and mortality in 57 consecutive patients evaluated angiographically. Am. J. Cardiol. 32:745, 1973.

311. Scanlon, P. J., Nemickas, R., Moran, J. F., Talano, J. V., Amirparviz, F., and Pifane, R.: Accelerated angina pectoris. Clinical, hemodynamic, arteriographic and therapeutic experience in 85 patients. Circulation 47:19, 1973.

312. Weintraub, R. M., Aroesty, J. M., Paulin, S., Levine, F. H., Markis, J. E., LaRaia, P. J., Cohen, S. I., and Kurland, G. S.: Medically refractory unstable angina pectoris. I. Long-term follow-up of patients undergoing intraaortic balloon counterpulsation and operation. Am. J. Cardiol. 43:877, 1979.

313. Levine, F. H., Gold, H. K., Leinbach, R. C., Daggett, W. M., Austen, W. G., and Buckley, M. J.: Management of acute myocardial ischemia with intraaortic balloon pumping and coronary bypass surgery. Circulation 58(Suppl. 1):69, 1978.

314. Conti, C. R.: Treatment of unstable angina: A model for step therapy. Cardiovasc. Rev. Rep. 3:1306, 1982.

315. Cohn, P. F., and Cohn, L. H.: Medical/surgical treatment of unstable angina. In Cohn, L. H. (ed.): The Treatment of Acute Myocardial Ischemia: An Integrated Medical-Surgical Approach, Mt. Kisco, N.Y., Futura Publishing Co., 1979, p. 105.

316. Mohr, R., Smolinsky, A., and Goor, D. A.: Treatment of nocturnal angina with 10° reverse Trendelenburg bed position. Lancet 1:1325, 1982.

317. Curfman, G. D., Heinsimer, J. A., Lozner, E. C., and Fung, H.: Intravenous nitroglycerin in the treatment of spontaneous angina pectoris: A prospective, randomized trial. Circulation 67:276, 1983.

317a. Kaplan, K., Davison, R., Parker, M., Przybylek, J., Teagarden, J. R., and Lesch, M.: Intravenous nitroglycerin for the treatment of angina at rest unresponsive to standard nitrate therapy. Am. J. Cardiol. 51:694, 1983.

318. Mehta, J., Pepine, C. J., Day, M., Guerrero, J. R., and Conti, C. R.: Short-

term efficacy of oral verapamil in rest angina. A double-blind placebo controlled trial in CCU patients. Am. J. Med. 71:977, 1981.

319. Moses, J. W., Wertheimer, J. H., Bodenheimer, M. M., Banka, V. S., Feldman, M., and Helfant, R. H.: Efficacy of nifedipine in rest angina refractory to propranolol and nitrates in patients with obstructive coronary artery disease. Ann. Intern. Med. 94:425, 1981.

320. Gerstenblith, G., Ouyang, P., Achuff, S. C., Bulkley, B. H., Becker, L. C., Mellits, E. D., Baughman, K. L., Weiss, J. L., Flaherty, J. T., Kallman, C. H., Llewellyn, M., and Weisfeldt, M. L.: Nifedipine in unstable angina: A double-blind, randomized trial. N. Engl. J. Med. 306:885, 1982.

320a. Robertson, R. M., Robertson, D., Davison, R., Kaplan, K., Haywood, L. J., Goldstein, S., Lee, T. G., Mehta, J., Conti, C. R., Simpson, R. J., and Singh, B.: Angina at rest: A double-blind, placebo-controlled, multicenter study of oral verapamil. J. Am. Coll. Cardiol. 1:595, 1983.

321. Williams, D. O., Riley, R. S., Singh, A. K., Gewirtz, H., and Most, A. S.: Evaluation of the role of coronary angioplasty in patients with unstable angina pectoris. Am. Heart J. 102:1, 1981.

322. Meyer, J., Schmidtz, H., Erbel, R., Kiesslich, T., Bocker-Josephs, B., Krebs, W., Braun, P. C., Bardos, P., Minale, C., Messmer, B. J., and Effert, S.: Treatment of unstable angina pectoris with percutaneous transluminal coronary angioplasty (PTCA). Cath. Cardiovasc. Diagn. 7:361, 1981.

323. Hirsh, P. D., Hillis, L. D., Campbell, W. B., Firth, B. G., and Willerson, J. T.: Release of prostaglandins and thromboxane into the coronary circulation in patients with ischemic heart disease. N. Engl. J. Med. 304:685, 1981.

324. Smitherman, T. C., Milam, M., Woo, J., Willerson, J. T., and Frenkel, L. P.: Elevated beta thromboglobulin in peripheral venous blood of patients with acute myocardial ischemia: Direct evidence for enhanced platelet reactivity in vivo. Am. J. Cardiol. 48:395, 1981.

325. Tolts, J. D., Crowell, E. B., and Rowe, G. G.: Platelet aggregation in partially obstructed vessels and its elimination with aspirin. Circulation 54:365, 1976.

326. Lewis, H. D., Davis, J. W., Archibald, D. G., Steinke, W. E., Smitherman, T. C., Doherty, J. E., LeWinter, M. M., Linares, E. Pouget, J. M., Sabharwal, S. C., Chesler, E., and DeMots, H.: Protective effects of 324 mg. aspirin daily in men with unstable angina: Results of a VA Cooperative Study. Circulation 66 (Part II):17, 1982 (Abstr.).

327. Krauss, K. R., Hutter, A. M., and DeSanctis, R. W.: Acute coronary insufficiency: Course and follow-up. Circulation 45(Suppl. 1):66, 1972.

328. Schroeder, J. S., Lamb, I. H., and Hu, M.: Do patients in whom myocardial infarction has been ruled out have a better prognosis after hospitalization than those surviving infarction? N. Engl. J. Med. 303:1, 1980.

329. Solomon, H. A., Edwards, A. L., and Killip, T.: Prodromata in acute myocardial infarction. Circulation 40:463, 1969.

VARIANT ANGINA

330. Prinzmetal, M., Kennamer, R., Merliss, R., Wada, T., and Bor, N.: A variant form of angina pectoris. Am. J. Med. 27:375, 1959.

331. Stein, J. H., Ambrose, J. A., King, B. D., and Herman, M. V.: An integrated approach to the recognition and treatment of variant angina. Cardiovasc. Rev. Rep. 3:1297, 1982.

332. Weiner, L., Kasparian, H., Duca, P. R., Walinsky, P., Gottlieb, R.S., Hanckel, F., and Brest, A. N.: Spectrum of coronary arterial spasm. Clinical angiographic and myocardial metabolic experience in 29 cases. Am. J. Cardiol. 38:945, 1976.

333. Yasue, H., Omote, S., Takizawa, A., Nagao, M., Miwa, K., and Tanaka, S.: Cardiac variations of exercise capacity in patients with Prinzmetal's variant angina: Role of exercise-induced coronary arterial spasm. Circulation 59:938, 1979.

334. Weiner, D. A., Schick, E. C., Jr., Hood, W. B., Jr., and Ryan, T. J.: ST-segment elevation during recovery from exercise. Chest 74:133, 1978.

335. Oliva, P. B., Potts, D. E., and Pluss, R. G.: Coronary arterial spasm in Prinzmetal angina. Documentation by coronary arteriography. N. Engl. J. Med. 288:745, 1973.

336. Dhurandhar, R. W., Watt, D. L., Silber, M. D., Trimble, A. S., and Adelman, A. G.: Prinzmetal's variant form of angina with arteriographic evidence of coronary arterial spasm. Am. J. Cardiol. 30:902, 1972.

337. Higgins, C. B., Wexler, L., Silverman, J. F., and Schroeder, J. S.: Clinical and arteriographic features of Prinzmetal's variant angina: Documentation of etiology factors. Am. J. Cardiol. 37:831, 1976.

338. Berman, N. D., McLaughlin, P. R., Huckell, V. F., Mahon, W. A., Morch, J. E., and Adelman, A. G.: Prinzmetal's angina with coronary artery spasm. Angiographic, pharmacologic, metabolic and radionuclide perfusion studies. Am. J. Med. 60:727, 1976.

339. Freedman, B., Dunn, R. F., Richmond, D. R., and Kelly, D. T.: Coronary artery spasm during exercise: Treatment with verapamil. Circulation 64:68, 1981.

340. Waters, D D., Theroux, P., Crittin, J., Dauwe, F., and Mizgala, H. F.: Previously undiagnosed variant angina as a cause of chest pain after coronary artery bypass surgery. Circulation 61:1159, 1980.

341. Miller, D., Waters, D. D., Warnica, W., Szlachcic, J., Kreeft, J., and Theroux, P.: Is variant angina the coronary manifestation of a generalized vasospastic disorder? N. Engl. J. Med. 304:763, 1981.

342. Antman, E., Muller, J., Goldberg, S., MacAlpin, R., Rubenfire, M., Tabatznik, B., Liang, C., Heupler, F., Achuff, S., Reichek, N., Geltman, E., Kerin, N. Z., Neff, R. K., and Braunwald, E.: Nifedipine therapy for coronary-artery spasm. Experience in 127 patients. N. Engl. J. Med. 302:1269 1980.

343. Kerin, N. Z., Rubenfire, M., Naini, M., Wajszczuk, W. J., Pamatmat, A., and

Cascade, P. N.: Arrhythmias in variant angina pectoris: Relationship of arrhythmias to ST-segment elevation and R-wave changes. Circulation 60:1343, 1979.

344. Sheehan, F. H., and Epstein, S. E.: Determinants of arrhythmic death due to coronary spasm: Effect of preexisting coronary artery stenosis on the incidence of reperfusion arrhythmia. Circulation 65:259, 1982.

345. Kerin, N. Z., Rubenfire, M., Naini, M., Wajszezuk, W. J., Pamatmat, A., and Cascade, P. N.: Arrhythmias in variant angina pectoris. Relationship or arrhythmias to ST-segment elevation and R-wave changes. Circulation 60:1343, 1979.

346. Biagini, A., Mazzei, M. G., Carpeggiani, C., Buzzigoli, G., Zucchelli, G., Parodi, O., L'Abbate, A., and Maseri, A.: Myocardial cell damage during attacks of vasospastic angina in the absence of persistent electrocardiographic changes. Clin. Cardiol. 4:315, 1981.

347. Meller, J., Conde, C. A., Donoso, E., and Dack, S.: Transient Q waves in Prinzmetal's angina. Am. J. Cardiol. 35:691, 1975.

348. Guazzi, M., Polese, A., Fiorentini, C., Magrini, F., and Bartorelli, C.: Left ventricular performance and related hemodynamic changes in Prinzmetal's variant angina pectoris. Br. Heart J. 33:84, 1971.

349. Gaasch, W. H., Adyantha, A. V., Wang, V. H., Pickering, E., Quinons, M. A., and Alexander, J. K.: Prinzmetal's variant angina: Hemodynamic and angiographic observations during pain. Am. J. Cardiol. 35:683, 1977.

350. Muller, J. E.: Prinzmetal's angina—A model for the role of spasm in ischemic heart disease. J. Cardiovasc. Med. 5:19, 1980.

351. Selzer, A., Langston, M., Ruggeroli, C., and Cohn, K.: Clinical syndrome of variant angina with normal coronary arteriogram. N. Engl. J. Med. 295:1343, 1976.

352. Cipriano, P. R., Koch, F. H., Rosenthal, S. J., and Schroeder, J. S.: Clinical course of patients following the demonstration of coronary artery spasm by angiography. Am. Heart J. 101:127, 1981.

353. Waters, D. D., Theroux, P., Szlachcic, J., and Dauwe, F.: Provocative testing with ergonovine to assess the efficacy of treatment with nifedipine, diltiazem and verapamil in variant angina. Am. J. Cardiol. 48:123, 1981.

354. Curry, R. C., Jr., Pepine, C. J., Sabom, M. B., Feldman, R. L., Christie, L. G., and Conti, C. R.: Effects of ergonovine in patients with and without coronary artery disease. Circulation 56:803, 1977.

354a.Winniford, M. D., Johnson, S. M., Mauritson, D. R., and Hillis, L. D.: Ergonovine provocation to assess efficacy of long-term therapy with calcium antagonists in Prinzmetal's variant angina. Am. J. Cardiol. 51:684, 1983.

355. Waters, D. D., Szlachcic, J., Theroux, P., Dauwe, F., and Mizgala, H. F.: Ergonovine testing to detect spontaneous remissions of variant angina during long-term treatment with calcium antagonist drugs. Am. J. Cardiol. 47:179, 1981.

356. Ginsburg, R., Lamb, I. H., Bristow, M. R., Schroeder, J. S., and Harrison, D. C.: Application and safety of outpatient ergonovine testing in accurately detecting coronary spasm in patients with possible variant angina. Am. Heart J. 102:698, 1981.

357. Waters, D. D., Theroux, P., Szlachcic, J., Dauwe, F., Crittin, J., Bonan, R., and Mizgala, H. F.: Ergonovine testing in a coronary care unit. Am. J. Cardiol. 46:922, 1980.

358. Buxton, A., Goldberg, S., Hirshfeld, J. W., Wilson, J., Mann, T., Williams, O., Overlie, P., and Oliva, P.: Refractory ergonovine-induced coronary vasospasm: Importance of intracoronary nitroglycerin. Am. J. Cardiol. 46:329, 1980.

359. Heupler, F. A., Jr.: Provocative testing for coronary arterial spasm: Risk, method and rationale. Am. J. Cardiol. 46:335, 1980.

360. Yasue, H., Touyama, M., Shimamoto, M., Kato, H., Tanaka, S., and Akiyama, F.: Role of autonomic nervous system in the pathogenesis of Prinzmetal's variant form of angina. Circulation 50:534, 1974.

361. Ginsburg, R., Bristow, M. R., Kantrowitz, N., Baim, D. S., and Harrison, D. C.: Histamine provocation of clinical coronary artery spasm: Implications concerning pathogenesis of variant angina pectoris. Am. Heart J. 102:819, 1981.

362. Waters, D. D., Szlachcic, J., Bonan, R., Miller, D. D., Dauwe, F., and Theroux, P.: Comparative sensitivity of exercise, cold pressor and ergonovine testing in provoking attacks of variant angina in patients with active disease. Circulation 67:310, 1983.

363. Maseri, A., Parodi, O., Severi, S., and Pesola, A.: Transient transmural reduction of myocardial blood flow, demonstrated by thallium-201 scintigraphy, as a cause of variant angina. Circulation 54:280, 1976.

364. McLaughlin, P. R., Doherty, P. W., Martin, P. R., Goris, M. L., and Harrison, D. L.: Myocardial imaging in a patient with reproducible variant angina. Am. J. Cardiol. 39:129, 1977.

365. Ricci, D. R., Orlick, A. E., Doherty, P. W., Cipriano, P. R., and Harrison, D. R.: Reduction of coronary blood flow during coronary artery spasm occurring spontaneously and after provocation by ergonovine maleate. Circulation 57:392, 1978.

366. Ginsburg, R., Lamb, I. H., Schroeder, J. S., Hu, M., and Harrison, D. C.: Randomized double-blind comparison of nifedipine and isosorbide dinitrate therapy in variant angina pectoris due to coronary artery spasm. Am. Heart J. 103:44, 1982.

367. Schroeder, J. S., Lamb, I. H., Bristow, M. R., Ginsburg, R., Hung, J., and McAuley, B. J: Prevention of cardiovascular events in variant angina by long-term diltiazem therapy. J. Am. Coll. Cardiol. 1:1507, 1983.

368. Braunwald, E.: Coronary artery spasm as a cause of myocardial ischemia. J. Lab. Clin. Med. 97:299, 1981.

369. Gunther, S., Muller, J. E., Mudge, G. H., Jr., and Grossman, W.: Therapy of coronary vasoconstriction in patients with coronary artery disease. Am. J. Cardiol. 47:157, 1981.

370. Colucci, W. S.: Alpha-adrenergic receptor blockade with prazosin. Consideration of hypertension, heart failure and potential new applications. Ann. Intern. Med. 97:67, 1982.

371. Tzivoni, D., Keren, A., Benhorin, J., Gottlieb, S., Atlas, D., and Stern, S.: Prazosin therapy for refractory variant angina. Am. Heart J. 105:262, 1983.

372. Miwa, K., Kambara, H., and Kawai, C.: Effect of aspirin in large doses on attacks of variant angina. Am. Heart J. 105:351, 1983.

373. Schick, E. C., Jr., Davis, Z., Lavery, R. M., McCormick, J. R., Fay, M., and Berger, R. L.: Surgical therapy for Prinzmetal's variant angina. Ann. Thorac. Surg. 33:359, 1982.

374. Waters, D. D., Szlachcic, J., Miller, D., and Theroux, P.: Clinical characteristics of patients with variant angina complicated by myocardial infarction or death within 1 month. Am. J. Cardiol. 49:658, 1982.

375. Brunelli, C., Lazzari, M., Simonetti, I., L'Abbate, A., and Maseri, A.: Variable threshold of exertional angina: A clue to a vasopastic component. Eur. Heart J. 2:155, 1981.

376. Ahmad, M., Dubiel, J. P., and Haibach, H.: Cold pressor thallium-201 myocardial scintigraphy in the diagnosis of coronary artery disease. Am. J. Cardiol. 50:1253, 1982.

377. Mueller, H. S., Rao, P. S., Rao, P. B., Gory, D. J., Mudd, J. G., and Ayres, S. M.: Enhanced transcardiac l-norepinephrine response during cold pressor test in obstructive coronary artery disease. Am. J. Cardiol. 50:1223, 1982.

378. Bertrand, M. E., LaBlanche, J. M., Tilmant, R. Y., Thieuleux, F. A., Delforge, M. R., Carre, A. G., Asseman, P., Berzin, B., Libersa, C., and Laurent, J. M.: Frequency of provoked coronary arterial spasm in 1089 consecutive patients undergoing coronary arteriography. Circulation 65:1299, 1982.

379. Koiwaya, Y., Nakamura, M., Mitsutake, A., Tanaka, S., and Takeshita, A.: Increased exercise tolerance after oral diltiazem, a calcium antagonist, in angina pectoris. Am. Heart J. 101:143, 1981.

380. Pine, M. B., Citron, P. D., Bailly D. J., Butman, S., Plasencia, G. O., Landa, D. W., and Wong, R. K.: Verapamil versus placebo in relieving stable angina pectoris. Circulation 65:17, 1982.

ISCHEMIC HEART DISEASE IN WHICH DISCOMFORT IS NOT THE DOMINANT SYMPTOM

381. Kannel, W. B., Doyle, J. T., McNamara, P. M., Quickenton, P., and Gordon, T.: Precursors of sudden coronary death. Factors related to the incidence of sudden death. Circulation 51:606, 1975.

382. Master, A. M., and Geller, A. M.: The extent of completely asymptomatic coronary artery disease. Am. J. Cardiol. 23:173, 1969.

383. Cohn, P. F.: Severe asymptomatic coronary artery disease. A diagnostic, prognostic and therapeutic puzzle. Am. J. Med. 62:565, 1977.

384. Froelicher, V. F., Yanowitz, F. G., Thompson, A. J., and Lancaster, M. C.: The correlation of coronary angiography and the electrocardiographic response to maximal threadmill testing in 76 asymptomatic men. Circulation 48:597,1973.

385. Borer, J. S., Brensike, J. D., Redwood, D. R., Itscoitz, S. B., Passamanin, E. R., Stone, N. J., Richardson, J. M., Levy, R. I., and Epstein, S. E.: Limitations of electrocardiographic response to exercise in predicting coronary artery disease. N. Engl. J. Med. 293:367, 1975.

386. Erikssen, J., Enge, I., Forfang, K., and Storstein, O.: False positive diagnostic tests and coronary angiographic findings in 105 presumably healthy males. Circulation 54:371, 1976.

387. O'Rourke, R. A., and Ross, J. R., Jr.: Ambulatory electrocardiographic monitoring to detect ischemic heart disease. Ann. Intern. Med. 81:696, 1974.

388. Stern, S., and Tzivoni, D.: Early detection of silent ischemic heart disease by 24-hour electrocardiographic monitoring of active subjects. Br. Heart J. 36:481, 1976.

389. Cohn, P. F., Prognosis and treatment of asymptomatic coronary artery disease. J. Am. Coll. Cardiol. 1:959, 1983.

390. Gorlin, R., Klein, M. D., and Sullivan, J. M.: Prospective correlative study of ventricular aneurysm. Mechanistic concept and clinical recognition. Am. J. Med. 42:512, 1967.

391. Parmley, W. W., Chuck, L., Kivowitz, C., Matloff, J. M., and Swan, H. J. C.: In vitro length-tension relations of human ventricular aneurysms. Relation of stiffness to mechanical disadvantage. Am. J. Cardiol. 32:889, 1973.

392. Erikson, U., Hallen, A., Helmius, G., and Sawada, S.: On the pathophysiology of left ventricular aneurysm. An analysis by cineangiography and videodensitometry. Fortschr. Röntgenstr. 137:85, 1982.

393. Esente, P., Gensini, G. G.: Huntington, P. P., Kelly, A. E., and Black, A.: Left ventricular aneurysm without coronary arterial obstruction or occlusion. Am. J. Cardiol. 34:658, 1974.

394. Cabin, H. S., and Roberts, W. C.: Left ventricular aneurysm, intraaneurysmal thrombus and systemic embolus in coronary heart disease. Chest 77:586, 1980.

395. Stratton, J. R., Lighty, G. W., Jr., Pearlman, A. S., and Ritchie, J. L.: Detection of left ventricular thrombus by two-dimensional echocardiography: Sensitivity, specificity, and causes of uncertainty. Circulation 66:156, 1982.

396. Froehlich, R. T., Falsetti, H. L., Doty, D. B., and Marcus, M.: Recognizing and treating left ventricular aneurysm. J. Cardiovasc. Med. 6:465, 1981.

397. van Meurs-van Woezik, H., Meltzer, R. S., van den Brand, M., Essed, C. E., Michels, R. H. M., and Roelandt, J.: Superiority of echocardiography over angiocardiography in diagnosing a left ventricular thrombus. Chest 80:321, 1981.

398. Ezekowitz, M. D., Leonard, J. C., Smith, E. O., Allen, E. W., and Taylor, F. B.: Identification of left ventricular thrombi in man using indium-111–labeled autologous platelets. A preliminary report. Circulation 63:803, 1981.

399. Rigo, P., Murray, M., Strauss, H. W., and Pitt, B.: Scintiphotographic evalua-

tion of patients with suspected left ventricular aneurysm. Circulation 50:985, 1974.

400. Parisi, A. F., Moynihan, P. F., Ray, B. J., and Pietro, D. A.: Two-dimensional echocardiography. J. Cardiovasc. Med. 5:39, 1980.

401. Burch, G. E., DePasquale, N. P., and Phillips, J. H.: The syndrome of papillary muscle dysfunction. Am. Heart J. 75:399, 1968.

402. Balu, V., Hershowitz, S., Zaki Masud, A. R., Bhayana, J. N., and Dean, D. C.: Mitral regurgitation in coronary artery disease. Chest 81:550, 1982.

403. Gahl, K., Sutton, R., Pearson, M., Caspari, P., Lairet, A., and McDonald, L.: Mitral regurgitation in coronary heart disease. Br. Heart J. 39:13, 1977.

404. Shelburne, J. C., Rubinstein, D., and Gorlin, R.: A reappraisal of papillary muscle dysfunction. Correlative, clinical and angiographic study. Am. J. Med. 46:862, 1969.

405. Burch, G. E., Giles, T. D., and Colcolough, H. L.: Ischemic cardiomyopathy. Am. Heart J. 79:291, 1970.

406. Yatteau, R. F., Peter, R. H., Behar, V. S., Bartel, A. G., Rosati, R. A., and Kong, Y.: Ischemic cardiomyopathy: The myopathy of coronary artery disease. Natural history and results of medical versus surgical treatment. Am. J. Cardiol. 34:520, 1974.

407. Dash, H., Johnson, R. A., Dinsmore, R. E., and Harthorne, J. W.: Cardiomyopathic syndrome due to coronary artery disease. I. Relation to angiographic extent of coronary disease and to remote myocardial infarction. Br. Heart J. 39:733, 1977.

408. Calvert, A., Lown, B., and Gorlin, R.: Ventricular premature beats and anatomically defined coronary heart disease. Am. J. Cardiol. 39:4, 1977.

409. Levine, S. A., and Kauvar, A. J.: Association of angina pectoris or thrombosis with mitral stenosis. J. Mt. Sinai Hosp. 8:754, 1942.

410. Gardner, F. E., and White, P. D.: Coronary occlusion and myocardial infarction associated with chronic rheumatic heart disease. Ann. Intern. Med. 31:1003, 1949.

411. Befeler, B., Kamen, A. R., and MacLeod, M. B.: Coronary artery disease and left ventricular function in mitral stenosis. Chest 57:435, 1970.

412. Basta, L. L., Raines, D., Najjar, S., and Kioschos, J. M.: Clinical, haemodynamic, and coronary angiographic correlates of angina pectoris in patients with severe aortic valve disease. Br. Heart J. 37:150, 1975.

413. Graboys, T. B., and Cohn, P. F.: The prevalence of angina pectoris and abnormal coronary arteriograms in severe aortic valvular disease. Am. Heart J. 93:683, 1977.

414. Hakki, A., Kimbiris, D., Iskanadrian, A. S., Segal, B. L., Mintz, G. S., and Bemis, C. E.: Angina pectoris and coronary artery disease in patients with severe aortic valvular disease. Am. Heart J. 100:441, 1980.

415. Hancock, E. W.: Clinical assessment of coronary artery disease in patients with aortic stenosis. Am. J. Cardiol. 35:142, 1975.

416. Harris, C. N., Kaplan, M. A., Parker, D. P., Dunne, E. F., Cowell, H. S., and Ellestad, M. H.: Aortic stenosis, angina, and coronary artery disease-interrelations. Br. Heart J. 37:656, 1975.

417. Bagdade, J. D.: Atherosclerosis in patients undergoing maintenance hemodialysis. Kidney Int. (Suppl.)(3):370, 1975.

418. Gurland, H. J., Brunner, F. P., Dehn, H., Harlen, H., Parsons, F. M., and Scharer, K.: Combined report on regular dialysis and transplantation in Europe. Proc. Eur. Dial. Transpl. Assoc. 10:17, 1973.

419. Lowrie, E. G., Lazarus, J. M., Mocelin, A. J., Bailey, G. L., Hampers, C. L., Wilson, R. E., and Merrill, J. P.: Survival of patients undergoing chronic hemodialysis and renal transplantation. N. Engl. J. Med. 288:863, 1973.

420. Lindner, A., Charra, B., Sherrard, D. J., and Scribner, B. H.: Accelerated atherosclerosis in prolonged maintenance dialysis. N. Engl. J. Med. 290:697, 1974.

421. Oakley, C. M.: Non-atheromatous ischemic heart disease. Postgrad. Med. J. 52:438, 1976.

422. Lange, R. L., Reid, M. S., Tresch, D. D., Keelan, M. H., Bernhard, J. M., and Coolidge, G.: Nonatheromatous ischemic heart disease following withdrawal from chronic industrial nitroglycerin exposure. Circulation 46:666, 1972.

SURGICAL TREATMENT

423. O'Shaughnessy, L.: Surgical treatment of cardiac ischemia. Lancet 1:185, 1937.

424. McAllister, F. F., Leighninger, D., and Beck, C. S.: Revascularization of the heart by graft of systemic artery into coronary sinus. J.A.M.A. 137:436, 1948.

425. Glover, R. P., Davila, J. C., Kyle, R. H., Beard, J. C., Jr., Trout, R. G., and Kitchell, J. R.: Ligation of the internal mammary arteries as a means of increasing blood supply to the myocardium. J. Thorac. Surg. 34:661, 1957.

426. Gorlin, R.: Revascularization of the myocardium. In Gorlin, R.: Coronary Artery Disease. Philadelphia, W. B. Saunders Co., 1976, p. 263.

427. Vineberg, A., and Walker, J.: The surgical treatment of coronary artery heart disease by internal mammary artery implantation: Report of 140 cases followed up to thirteen years. Dis. Chest. 45:190, 1964.

428. Gorlin, R., and Taylor, W. J.: Myocardial revascularization with internal mammary artery implantation: Current status. J.A.M.A. 207:907, 1969.

429. Mundth, E. D., and Austen, W. G.: Surgical measures for coronary heart disease. N. Engl. J. Med. 293:13, 1975.

430. Participants of the Veterans Administration Coronary Bypass Surgery Cooperative Study Group: Long-term results of internal mammary artery implantation for coronary artery disease: A controlled trial. Ann. Thorac. Surg. 29:234, 1980.

431. Favalora, R.: Direct and indirect coronary surgery. Circulation 46:1197, 1972.

432. Effler, D. B.: Myocardial revascularization surgery since 1945. Its evolution and impact. J. Thorac. Cardiovasc. Surg. 72:823, 1976.

433. DeBakey, M. Garrett, H. E., and Dennis, E. W.: Aorto-coronary bypass with saphenous vein graft. Seven-year follow-up. J.A.M.A. 223:792, 1973.

434. Green, G. E.: Internal mammary artery to coronary artery anastomosis: Three year experience with 165 patients. Ann. Thorac. Surg. 14:260, 1972.

435. Loop, F. D., Sheldon, W. C., Lytle, B. W., Cosgrove, D. M., III, and Proudfit, W. L.: The efficacy of coronary artery surgery. Am. Heart J. 101:86, 1981.

436. Kouchoukos, N. T., Oberman, A., Kirklin, J. W., Russell, R. O., Jr., Karp, R. B., Pacifico, A. D., and Zorn, G. L.: Coronary bypass surgery: Analysis of factors affecting hospital mortality. Circulation 62(Suppl. I):84, 1980.

437. Frye, R. L., and Frommer, P. L. (eds.): Consensus Development Conference on Coronary Bypass Surgery. Medical and scientific aspects. Circulation 65 (Suppl. II):1–129, 1982.

437a.Jones, E. L., Carver, J. M., Guyton, R. P., Bone, D. K., Hatcher, C. R., Jr., and Riechwalt, N.: Importance of complete revascularization in performance of the coronary bypass operation. Am. J. Cardiol. 51:7, 1983.

438. Dobrin, P., Canfield, T., Moran, J., Sullivan, H., and Pifarre, R.: Coronary artery bypass. The physiological basis for differences in flow with internal mammary artery and saphenous vein grafts. J. Thorac. Cardiovasc. Surg. 74:445, 1977.

439. Cohn, P. F.: Clinical angiographic, and hemodynamic factors influencing selection of patients for coronary artery bypass surgery. Progr. Cardiovasc. Dis. 18:223, 1975.

440. Report of Inter-Society Commission for Heart Disease Resources: Optimal resources for coronary artery surgery. Circulation 46:A-325, 1972.

441. Alderman, E. L., Matlof, H. J., Wexler, L., Shumway, N. E., and Harrison, D. C.: Results of direct coronary artery surgery for the treatment of angina pectoris. N. Engl. J. Med. 388:535, 1973.

442. McNeer, J. F., Starmer, C. F., Bartel, A. G., Behar, V. S., Kong, Y., Peter, R. H., and Rosati, R. A.: The nature of treatment selection in coronary artery disease. Experience with medical and surgical treatment of a chronic disease. Circulation 49:606, 1974.

443. Report of the Unstable Angina Pectoris Study Group: Unstable angina pectoris: National Cooperative Group to Compare Medical and Surgical Therapy. I. Report of protocol and patient population. Am. J. Cardiol. 37:896, 1976.

444. Scanlon, P. J.: The intermediate coronary syndrome. Progr. Cardiovasc. Dis. 23:351, 1981.

445. Hammermeister, K. E.: The effect of coronary bypass surgery on survival. Progr. Cardiovasc. Dis. 15:297, 1983.

446. Tyers, G. F. O., Williams, D. R., and Babb, J. D.: The changing status of ejection fraction as a predictor of early mortality following surgery for acquired heart disease. Chest 71:371, 1977.

447. Rozanski, A., Berman, D. S., Gray, R., Levy, R., Raymond, M., Maddahi, J., Pantaleo, N., Waxman, A. D., Swan, H. J. C., and Matloff, J.: Use of thallium-201 redistribution scintigraphy in the preoperative differentiation of reversible and nonreversible myocardial asynergy. Circulation 64:936, 1981.

448. Rozanski, A., Berman, D., Gray, R., Diamond, G., Raymond, J., Prause, J., Maddahi, J., Swan, H. J. C., and Matloff, J.: Preoperative prediction of reversible myocardial asynergy by postexercise radionuclide ventriculography. N. Engl. J. Med. 307:212, 1982.

449. Manley, J. C., King, J. F., and Zeft, H. J.: The "bad" left ventricle. Results of coronary surgery and effect on late survival. J. Thorac. Cardiovasc. Surg. 72:841, 1976.

450. Norris, R. M., Agnew, T. M., and Brandt, P. W. T.: Coronary surgery after recurrent myocardial infarction: Progress of a trial comparing surgical with nonsurgical management for asymptomatic patients with advanced coronary disease. Circulation 63:785, 1981.

451. Faulkner, S. L., Stoney, W. S., and Alford, W. C.: Ischemic cardiomyopathy: Medical versus surgical treatment. J. Thorac. Cardiovasc. Surg. 74:77, 1977.

452. Leinbach, R. C., Gold, H. K., and Dinsmore, R. E.: The role of angiography in cardiogenic shock. Circulation 48(Suppl. III):95, 1976.

453. Johnson, S. A., Scanlon, P. J., and Loeb, H. S.: Treatment of cardiogenic shock in myocardial infarction by intraaortic balloon counterpulsation and surgery. Am. J. Med. 62:687, 1977.

454. Berg, R., Jr., Selinger, S. L., and Leonard, J. J.: Immediate coronary artery bypass for acute evolving myocardial infarction. J. Thorac. Cardiovasc. Surg. 81:493, 1981.

455. Phillips, S. J., Kongtahworn, C., and Zeff, R. H.: Emergency coronary artery revascularization: A possible therapy for acute myocardial infarction. Circulation 60:241, 1979.

456. Selinger, S. L., Berg, R., Jr., and Leonard, J. J.: Surgical treatment of acute evolving anterior myocardial infarction. Circulation 64(Suppl. II):28, 1981.

457. Smith, S. C., Jr., Gorlin, R., Herman, M. V., Taylor, W. J., and Collins, J. J., Jr.: Myocardial blood flow in man. Effect of coronary collateral circulation and coronary artery bypass surgery. J. Clin. Invest. 51:2556, 1972.

458. Lesperance, J., Bourassa, M. G., Biron, P., Campeau, L., and Saltiel, J.: Aorta to coronary artery saphenous vein grafts. Preoperative angiographic criteria for successful surgery. Am. J. Cardiol. 30:459, 1972.

459. Rosch, J., Dotter, C. T., Antonovic, R., Bonchek, L., and Starr, A.: Angiographic appraisal of distal vessel suitability for aortocoronary bypass graft surgery. Circulation 48:202, 1973.

460. Cukingnan, R. A., Carey, J. S., Wittig, J. H., and Brown, B. G.: Influence of complete coronary revascularization on relief of angina. J. Thorac. Cardiovasc. Surg. 79:188, 1980.

461. Murphy, E. S., and Kloster, F. E.: Coronary bypass surgery: What are the indications? J. Cardiovasc. Med. 8:57, 1983.

462. Walker, J. A., Friedberg, H. D., Flemma, R. J., and Johnson, W. D.: Determinants of angiographic patency of aortocoronary vein bypass grafts. Circulation 45, 46(Suppl. 1):86, 1972.

463. Grondin, C. M., Lapage, G., Castoguay, Y. R., Meere, C., and Grondin, P.:

Aorto-coronary bypass graft. Initial blood flow through the graft, and early postoperative patency. Circulation *44*:815, 1971.

464. Spencer, F. C., Green, G. E., Tice, D. A., Wallsh, E., Mills, N. L., and Glassman, E.: Coronary artery bypass grafts for congestive heart failure. A report of experiences with 40 patients. J. Thorac. Cardiovasc. Surg. *62*:529, 1971.

465. Kouchoukos, N. T., Doty, D. B., Buettner, L. E., and Kirklin, J. W.: Treatment of postinfarction cardiac failure by myocardial excision and revascularization. Circulation *45*(Suppl. 1):72, 1972.

466. Loop, F. D., Brettoni, J. N., Pichard, A., Siegel, W., Razani, M., and Effler, D. B.: Selection of the candidate for myocardial revascularization. A profile of high risk based on multivariate analysis. J. Thorac. Cardiovasc. Surg. *69*:40, 1975.

467. Kennedy, J. W., Kaiser, G. C., Fisher, L. D., Fritz, J. K., Myers, W., Mudd, J. G., and Ryan, T. J.: Clinical and angiographic predictors of operative mortality from the collaborative study in coronary artery surgery (CASS). Circulation *63*:793, 1981.

468. Cohn, P. F., Gorlin, R., Herman, M. V., Sonnenblick, E. H., Horn, H. R., Cohn, L. H., and Collins, J. J., Jr.: Relation between contractile reserve and prognosis in patients with coronary artery disease and a depressed ejection fraction. Circulation *51*:414, 1975.

469. Popio, K. A., Gorlin, R., Bechtel, D. L., and Levine, J. A.: Post extrasystolic potentiation as a predictor of potential myocardial viability. Am. J. Cardiol. *39*: 944, 1977.

470. Nesto, R. W., Cohn, L. H., Collins, J. J., Jr., Wynne, J., Holman, L., and Cohn, P. F.: Inotropic contractile reserve: A useful predictor of increased 5-year survival and improved postoperative left ventricular function in patients with coronary artery disease and reduced ejection fraction. Am. J. Cardiol. *50*: 39, 1982.

471. Starek, P. J. K.: Effects of coronary artery surgery and early and late survival. Cardiovasc. Rev. Rep. *4*:551, 1983.

472. Rahimtoola, S. H.: Coronary bypass surgery for chronic angina — 1981: A perspective. Circulation *65*:225, 1982.

472a. Waller, B. F., and Roberts, W. C.: Severe coronary narrowing at the site of or distal to the bypass graft anastomosis — the most important cause of early and late graft closure: analysis of 102 necropsy patients (108 arteries and 185 grafts) having an isolated aorto-coronary bypass operation. J. Am. Coll. Cardiol. *1*:719, 1983.

473. Solignac, A., Gueret, P., and Bourassa, M. G.: Influence of left ventricular function on survival 3 to 4 years after aortocoronary bypass. Eur. J. Cardiol. *2*: 421, 1975.

474. Hacker, R. W., Torka, M., and von der Emde, J.: Influence of preoperative variables upon the results of coronary artery bypass surgery. Cardiovascular Diseases, Bull Texas Heart Institute *7*:20, 1980.

475. Barboriak, J. J., Rimm, A. A., and Anderson, A. J.: Risk factors and mortality in patients with aortocoronary vein bypass operations. Cardiology *63*:237, 1978.

475a. Frick, M. H., Harjola, P-T., and Valle, M.: Persistent improvement after coronary bypass surgery: Ergometric and angiographic correlations at 5 years. Circulation *67*:491, 1983.

476. Greenberg, B. H., Hart, R., Botvinick, E. H., Werner, J. A., Brundage, B. H., Shames, P. M., Chatterjee, K., and Parmley, W. W.: Thallium-201 myocardial perfusion scintigraphy to evaluate patients after coronary bypass surgery. Am. J. Cardiol. *42*:167, 1978.

477. Seides, S. F., Borer, J. S., Kent, K. M., Rosing, D. R., McIntosh, C. L., and Epstein, S. E.: Long-term anatomic fate of coronary-artery bypass grafts and functional status of patients five years after operation. N. Engl. J. Med. *298*: 1213, 1978.

478. Johnson, W. D., Kayser, K. L. Pedraza, P. M., and Shore, R. T.: Employment patterns in males before and after myocardial revascularization surgery. A study of 2229 consecutive male patients followed for as long as 10 years. Circulation *65*:1086, 1982.

479. Danchin, N., David, P., Bourassa, M. G., Robert, P., and Chaitman, B. R.: Factors predicting working status after aortocoronary bypass surgery. Canad. Med. Assoc. J. *126*:255, 1982.

480. Freeman, M. R., Gray, R. J., Berman, D. S., Maddahi, J., Raymond, M. J., Forrester, J. S., and Matloff, J. M.: Improvement in global and segmental left ventricular function after coronary bypass surgery. Circulation *64*:II-34, 1981.

481. Hammermeister, K. E., Kennedy, J. W., Hamilton, G. W., Stewart, D. K., Gould, K. L., Lipscomb, K., and Murray, J. A.: Aortocoronary saphenous vein bypass. Failure of successful grafting to improve resting left ventricular function in chronic angina. N. Engl. J. Med. *290*:186, 1974.

482. Burton, J. R., FitzGibbon, G. M., Keon, W. J., and Leach, A. J.: Perioperative myocardial infarction complicating coronary bypass. Clinical and angiographic correlations and prognosis. J. Thorac. Cardiovasc. Surg. *82*:758, 1981.

483. Righetti, A., Crawford, M. H., O'Rourke, R. A., Hardason, T., Schelbert, H., Daily, P. O., De Luca, M., Ashburn, W., and Ross, J., Jr.: Detection of perioperative myocardial change after coronary artery bypass surgery. Circulation *55*:173, 1977.

484. Roberts, A. J., Subramanian, V. A., Herman, S. D., Case, D. B., Johnson, G. A., Jr., and Gay, W. A., Jr.: Systemic hypertension associated with coronary artery bypass surgery. J. Thorac. Cardiovasc. Surg. *74*:846, 1977.

485. Palac, R. T., Meadows, W. R., Hwang, M. H., Loeb, H. S., Pifarre, R., and Gunnar, R. M.: Risk factors related to progressive narrowing of aortocoronary vein grafts studied 1 and 5 years after surgery. Circulation *66*(Suppl. 1):40, 1982.

486. Bulkley, B. H.: Why coronary bypass grafts fail: Early and late pathologic changes. J. Cardiovasc. Med. *5*:1025, 1980.

487. Spray, T. L., and Roberts, W. C.: Changes in saphenous veins used as aortocoronary bypass grafts. Am. Heart J. *94*:500, 1977.

488. Campeau, L., Lesperance, J., Corbara, F., Hermann, J., Grondin, C. M., and Bourassa, M. G.: Aortocoronary saphenous vein bypass graft changes 5 to 7 years after surgery. Circulation *58*(Suppl.):170, 1978.

489. Albrechtsson, U. J., Stahl, E., and Tylen, U.: Evaluation of coronary artery bypass graft patency with computed tomography. J. Computer Asst. Tomog. *5*: 822, 1981.

490. Ullyot, D. J., Turley, K., McKay, C. R., Brundage, B. H., Lipton, M. J., and Ebert, P. A.: Assessment of saphenous vein graft patency by contrast-enhanced computed tomography. J. Thorac. Cardiovasc. Surg. *83*:512, 1982.

491. Chesebro, J. H., Clements, I. P., Fuster, V., Elveback, L. R., Smith, H. C., Bardsley, W. T., Frye, R. L., Holmes, D. R., Jr., Vlietstra, R. E., Pluth, J. R., Wallace, R. B., Puga, F. J., Orszulak, T. A., Piehler, J. M., Schaff, H. V., and Danielson, G. K.: A platelet-inhibitor drug trial in coronary artery bypass operations. Benefit of perioperative dipyridamole and aspirin therapy on early postoperative vein graft patency. N. Engl. J. Med. *307*:73, 1982.

492. Baur, H. R., VanTassel, R. A., Pierach, C. A., and Gobel, F. L.: Effects of sulfinpyrazone on early graft closure after myocardial revascularization. Am. J. Cardiol. *49*:420, 1982.

493. Griffith, L. S. C., Achuff, S. C., Conti, C. R., Humphries, J. O., Brawley, R. K., Gott, V. L., and Ross, R. S.: Changes in intrinsic coronary circulation and segmental ventricular motion after saphenous-vein coronary bypass graft surgery. N. Engl. J. Med. *288*:589, 1973.

494. Levine, J. A., Bechtel, D. J., Gorlin, R., Cohn, P. F., Herman, M. V., Cohn, L. H., and Collins, J. J., Jr.: Coronary artery anatomy before and after direct revascularization surgery: Clinical and cinearteriographic studies in 67 selected patients. Am. Heart J. *89*:561, 1975.

495. Palac, R. T., Hwang, M. H., Meadows, W. R., Croke, R. P., Pifarre, R., Loeb, H. S., and Gunnar, R. M.: Progression of coronary artery disease in medically and surgically treated patients 5 years after randomization. Circulation *64*:II-17, 1981.

496. Shark, W. M., and Kass, R. M.: Repeat myocardial revascularization in coronary disease therapy: Consideration of primary bypass failure and success of second graft surgery. Am. Heart J. *102*:303, 1981.

497. Loop, F. D.: Is there a role for repeat coronary bypass surgery? J. Cardiovasc. Med. *6*:233, 1981.

498. European Coronary Surgery Study Group: Prospective randomized study of coronary artery bypass surgery in stable angina pectoris. Lancet *2*:491, 1980.

499. Chaitman, B. P., Fisher, L. D., and Bourassa, M. G.: Effect of coronary bypass surgery on survival patterns in subsets of patients with left main coronary artery disease. Report of the Collaborative Study in Coronary Artery Surgery (CASS). Am. J. Cardiol. *48*:765, 1981.

500. Takaro, T., Hultgren, H. N., and Lipton, M. J.: The VA Cooperative Randomized Study of surgery for coronary arterial occlusive disease. II. Subgroup with significant left main lesions. Circulation *54*(Suppl. III):107, 1976.

501. Oberman, A., Harrell, R. R., and Russel, R. O.: Surgical versus medical treatment in disease of the left main coronary artery. Lancet *2*:591, 1976.

502. Takaro, T., Hultgren, H. N., Detre, K. M., and Peduzzi, P.: The Veterans Administration Cooperative Study of Stable Angina: Current status. Circulation *65*(Part II):60, 1982.

503. Detre, K., Peduzzi, P., Murphy, M., Hultgren, H., Thomsen, J., Oberman, A., and Takaro, T.: Effect of bypass surgery on survival in patients in low- and high-risk subgroups delineated by the use of simple clinical variables. Circulation *63*:1329, 1981.

504. Myerburg, R. J., Ghahramani, A., and Mallon, S. M.: Coronary revascularization in patients surviving unexpected ventricular fibrillation. Circulation *52*(Suppl. III):219, 1975.

505. Cooperman, M., Stinson, E. B., Griepp, R. B., and Shumway, N. E.: Survival and function after left ventricular aneurysmectomy. J. Thorac. Cardiovasc. Surg. *69*:321, 1975.

506. Watson, L. E., Dickhaus, D. W., and Martin, R. H.: Left ventricular aneurysm. Preoperative hemodynamics, chamber volume, and results of aneurysmectomy. Circulation *52*:868, 1975.

506a. Cohen, M., Packer, M., and Gorlin, R.: Indication for left ventricular aneurysmectomy. Circulation *67*:717, 1983.

507. Lee, D. C., Johnson, R. A., Boucher, C. A., Wexler, L. F., and McEnany, M. T.: Angiographic predictors of survival following left ventricular aneurysmectomy. Circulation *56*(Suppl. II):12, 1977.

508. Liedtke, A. J., Hughes, H. C., and Zelis, R.: Functional reductions in left ventricular volume. Minimum chamber size consonant with effective hemodynamic performance. J. Thorac. Cardiovasc. Surg. *71*:195, 1976.

509. Stephens, J. D., Dymond, D. S., Stone, D. L., Rees, G. M., and Spurrell, R. A. J.: Left ventricular aneurysm and congestive heart failure: Value of exercise stress and isosorbide dinitrate in predicting hemodynamic results of aneurysmectomy. Am. J. Cardiol. *45*:932, 1980.

510. Froehlich, R. T., Falsetti, H. L., Doty, D. B., and Marcus, M. L.: Prospective study of surgery for left ventricular aneurysm. Am. J. Cardiol. *45*:923, 1980.

511. Aranda, J. M., Befeler, B., Thurer, R., Vargas, A., El-Sherif, W., and Lazana, R.: Long-term clinical and hemodynamic studies after ventricular aneurysmectomy and aorto-coronary bypass. J. Thorac. Cardiovasc. Surg. *73*:772, 1977.

512. Barnes, R. W., Liebman, P. R., Marszalek, P. B., Kirk, C. L., and Goldman, M. H.: The natural history of asymptomatic carotid disease in patients undergoing cardiovascular surgery. Surgery *90*:1075, 1981.

513. Mannick, J. A.: Editorial — Combined carotid and coronary surgery. J. Cardiovasc. Med. (*in press*).

40

REHABILITATION OF PATIENTS WITH CORONARY ARTERY DISEASE

by Albert Oberman, M.D., M.P.H.

Cardiovascular rehabilitation aims to improve and extend the quality of life for the cardiac patient by allowing him to function at the highest level compatible with the extent of his disease. A comprehensive program emphasizes physical fitness, intervention measures to retard the underlying disease process, and psychosocial adaptations. The ultimate goal of these activities is to enable the cardiac patient, largely by his own efforts, to regain his pre-illness capabilities or make the adjustments necessary for an active, productive life. Historically, cardiac rehabilitation has evolved from the techniques and principles developed from the long-term care of survivors of myocardial infarction.[1,2] Nevertheless, these same techniques can be applied to patients with other cardiac problems, including those who have had bypass grafting,[3] heart valve surgery,[4] and even cardiac transplantation.[5]

Cardiac rehabilitation is justified by the profound influence of cardiovascular disease on health and its overall costs, currently estimated for the U.S. at over $50 billion per annum.[6] The primary focus for cardiac rehabilitation has been coronary artery disease because of its high prevalence and adverse influence on disability and mortality. Coronary artery disease, the most prominent cause of premature disability in the American labor force, continues to be the leading cause of death among adults at all ages. In addition, the indirect health care costs for coronary artery disease are more than three times the direct costs, with lost income, lower productivity, disability, insurance expenses, and workman's compensation exceeding $20 billion, in comparison to the $5.5 billion spent directly for medical care.

Many patients remain incapacitated unnecessarily. They fail to return to ordinary activities owing to an overly restrictive approach in their management, even though coronary registries indicate the maximal physical capacity for patients after infarction is only 10 per cent less than healthy men of the same age.[7] Despite therapeutic advances, physicians have estimated declines in return to work since 1970 for patients with uncomplicated myocardial infarction;[8] in 1970, 85 to 89 per cent of previously employed patients less than 55 years of age returned to work, whereas only 79 to 84 per cent did so in 1979. Many do not work because of problems related to physical deconditioning, inappropriate medical advice, and psychological maladaptations rather than actual physical limitations.[9,10] Debusk and Davidson[11] determined on the basis of myocardial infarction alone that as many as 150,000 patients aged 35 to 65 and employed outside the home have special needs because of physical, psychosocial, and related vocational disabilities. Those patients afflicted with angina or valvular heart disease or those undergoing cardiac surgery add to this burden.

The magnitude of the problem plus the anticipated tendency toward an older work force in the next decade strongly point out the need for rehabilitation services.[12] The vast majority of cardiac patients, even those with complex medical, psychological, and vocational problems, referred to special work evaluation units can return to nearly normal levels of work and leisure activities.[11] However, it should be emphasized that return to work is but one of several potential benefits arising from successful rehabilitation efforts. Other outcome measures useful in assessing the value of a cardiac rehabilitation program include improvement in functional capacity, favorable physiological adaptations, symptomatic relief, lessened anxiety and depression, and the preservation of the patient's role in family and societal activities. Less certain is whether a comprehensive rehabilitation program with an exercise component can retard atherosclerosis, protect against further cardiac complications, and prolong life.

EXERCISE PROGRAM

RATIONALE. Exercise, a key element in the rehabilitative process, leads to various training adaptations, alleviating both the physiological and the psychological disorders brought about by cardiac disease.

Musculoskeletal Disability. Prolonged immobilization causes negative nitrogen and protein balance and decreases skeletal muscle mass, contractile strength, and efficiency.[13] After hospitalization, the cardiac patient experiences degeneration of the skeletal muscles and general deconditioning as a result of the prolonged bed rest. Perhaps the ideal candidate for an exercise program to relieve musculoskeletal disabilities is the patient who has had cardiac surgery, which has involved (1) restriction of activities prior to the operation as well as afterward, (2) manipulation of the sternum and chest wall, (3) immobilization in awkward positions during the operation, and (4) edema and paresthesias at the site of saphenous vein extraction after bypass grafting. Musculoskeletal problems also affect the morale of the patient and, if not managed properly, become sources of chronic disability. An appropriate conditioning routine allows a return to daily activities by restoring strength, flexibility, muscle coordination, and joint mobility.

Functional Capacity. Exercise involving large muscle groups at sufficient intensity and duration improves oxygen transport within the circulatory system and oxidative metabolic capacity of skeletal muscles, thus enhancing physical capacity for work and leisure time activities. The circulatory demands depend primarily on the relative workload, the proportion of maximal oxygen uptake required. Multiple studies have demonstrated that properly designed physical training programs increase maximal oxygen uptake and lower the relative aerobic requirements at submaximal workloads, lessening the metabolic and circulatory demands for most coronary patients, even those with impaired left ventricular function.[14-17] The percentage increase in maximal oxygen uptake depends on several factors; however, those patients initially with low capacity but *without* left ventricular dysfunction tend to show the greatest improvement. Those previously symptomatic with ordinary activities now may exert themselves at the same level without distress because the effort required represents a lesser percentage of maximal capacity. Ordinarily, the threshold for symptoms becomes manifest at about 75 per cent of functional capacity so that any exertion less than this threshold should not trouble patients.[18] Thus, even a *modest* increment in physical capacity may permit a *marked* improvement in the quality of life by allowing stair climbing, shopping, and other common activities. A patient unable to walk at 4 mph who increases his oxygen capacity from 20 ml/kg-min to 30 ml/kg-min after training should be able to walk comfortably at this same rate

and conduct activities previously causing symptoms (Fig. 40–1). Not infrequently, patients are limited by leg fatigue or intermittent claudication. Though data are sparse, training appears to increase walking distance over a period of 3 or more months when conducted to the point of leg intolerance.[19,20]

Psychological Changes. Low-level exercise appears sufficient to stimulate positive psychosocial changes among men who have had myocardial infarctions.[21] Physical conditioning provides the means for allaying anxiety and preventing the onset and progression of depression, two major disorders encountered in cardiac patients. In contrast to the many restrictions imposed, exercise offers a positive and constructive approach by encouraging new activities and dispelling those fears associated with tasks requiring physical exertion. Such improvement in physical capacity encourages the patient to see himself in the context of previous health rather than as a cardiac cripple, strengthening feelings of well-being, self-esteem and self-confidence.[9,10,18] Psychological studies demonstrate that patients who exercise and become physically fit reduce their level of anxiety and suffer less depression and consequently are better able to tolerate life's stresses.[18,22]

Assessment for Exercise

Appropriate clinical evaluation and exercise testing allow selection of patients most likely to benefit from training programs and maximize compliance. The physician must determine whether the patient has any medical conditions that might preclude vigorous activity or influence the response to exercise. Quantification and prescription of exercise patterns for such a program can best be made by multistage exercise testing. However, a number of factors outside the exercise testing laboratory can also influence the patient's response to training: adverse environmental conditions (temperature, altitude, and air pollutants), prolonged exercise, competitive activities, noncompliance to the exercise regimen, and changes in health status. Careful observation of the patient in training through monitored exercise sessions for a period of at least 2 to 6

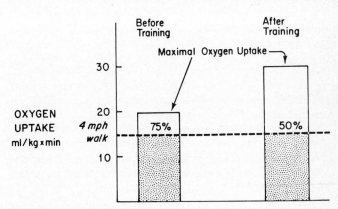

FIGURE 40–1 Effect of training on maximal oxygen uptake and relative oxygen cost (per cent VO_2max = VO_2/VO_2max) of walking at 4 mph on a level grade. (From Dehn, M. M., Pansegrau, D. G., and Mitchell, J. H.: Exercise training after acute myocardial infarction. *In* Wenger, N. K. (ed.): Exercise and the Heart. Philadelphia, F. A. Davis Co., 1978, pp. 117–132.)

weeks prior to more intense activities necessary for training adaptation allows more precise recommendations for long-term exercise.

CLINICAL EVALUATION. There are few absolute contraindications to exercise, but any acute illness, poorly controlled systemic disease, or unstable condition carries an unacceptable risk with exertion beyond that required for sedentary activities or more than several times, basal metabolic needs. Cardiovascular contraindications to exercise requiring special consideration include (1) acute myocardial infarction, (2) unstable angina pectoris, (3) arrhythmias (ventricular tachycardia or any rhythm significantly compromising cardiac function), (4) congestive heart failure, (5) severe aortic stenosis or left ventricular outflow tract obstruction, (6) aortic dissection, (7) cardiomyopathy or myocarditis within the past year, (8) thrombophlebitis, and (9) recent embolism. Complete lists of possible contraindications and precautions for exercise are reviewed in recent publications.[23–27] Patients with diabetes, obstructive lung disease, renal disease, hernia, anemia, orthopedic disabilities, or other chronic illnesses deserve special attention but such disorders rarely constitute absolute contraindications. Drugs frequently alter the exercise response and cannot be ignored in establishing training guidelines but do not necessarily preclude training effects.[26,28,29] Agents such as beta blockers or antisympathetic drugs limit the heart rate response, whereas "cold" remedies and "mood elevators" exaggerate the sympathetic response to exercise and may predispose to dysrhythmias. Individuals on anticoagulants must be carefully watched to avoid local trauma and possible bleeding; insulin requirements for diabetics may decrease considerably with exercise. Digitalis, diuretics, tranquilizers, and antihypertensives augment ST-segment depression, whereas drug-induced hypokalemia can alter exercise tolerance.[24,26,30]

EXERCISE TESTING (see Chap. 8). Although a variety of protocols can be used for exercise testing, the procedures should be conducted in a standard fashion in order to compare data at different points in time between patients and longitudinally in the same patient. Submaximal exercise tests can be used, but it must be realized that age-predicted heart rates do not always apply to patients with symptomatic coronary disease. Maximal heart rate can be highly variable among individuals of the same sex and age; moreover, cardiac diseases and drugs commonly used for treatment attenuate the heart rate response to exercise by influencing the sinus node or atrioventricular (AV) node. Maximal capacity cannot be reliably estimated or accurately measured in this fashion. An exercise test is considered maximal when a peak exertional effort is reached or the test is terminated because of electrocardiographic or clinical endpoints. Generally, ischemic symptoms and signs occur at the same heart rate or at the same double product (product of heart rate and systolic pressure), regardless of environmental conditions and the mix of dynamic-static exercise, permitting extrapolation of the standard exercise test to a variety of vocational and leisure tasks.[11,31]

The multistage exercise test defines the patient's functional capacity; provokes heart rate, blood pressure, and electrocardiographic abnormalities not apparent at rest; furnishes prognostic information; and provides baseline data for evaluating progress. Opinions vary regarding the importance of exercise-induced premature ventricular contractions (PVC's) compared with those occurring at rest but decreasing with exercise.[32,33] Neither exercise testing nor prolonged ambulatory monitoring for PVC's has clarified the significance of such dysrhythmias for patients entering an exercise program.[32–34] However, recent data indicate a characteristic and reproducible relationship between PVC frequency and heart rate over the range of heart rates encountered during routine activities.[35]

The test situation can be used to great advantage in observing the patient during exercise for symptoms, signs, and general appearances and for teaching him how to judge his own performance. The Borg Scale is a technique for quantifying perceived exertion by having the patient rate the workload on a scale from 6 to 20.[36] Each odd number of 15 grade categories is characterized by appropriate descriptors, ranging from very, very light (7 rating) to very, very hard (19 rating). Such ratings can be used for assessing the patient's work tolerance and as an educational tool by which the patient can estimate whether he is achieving his training level independent of heart rate measurement.

Exercise Training

To be worthwhile, exercise must tax the cardiorespiratory system; yet the musculoskeletal and cardiovascular hazards to unfit middle-aged adults with coronary disease who undertake strenuous exercise cannot be overemphasized. The likelihood of such problems depends in large part on age, athletic abilities, prior inactivity, extent of coronary atherosclerosis, left ventricular dysfunction, and general health. Although these immutable variables can increase the risk of complications, an exercise program can be conducted in a fashion that will minimize any potential hazards. Regular exercise, even of high intensity, is safe for cardiac patients if they follow an individualized but well-structured program. The primary determinants of the magnitude of the adaptive response to such a program involve the intensity, frequency, and duration of the exercise session and the type of exercise.

INTENSITY. This appears to be the single most important determinant in achieving the desired training effects. The cardiac patient should train at 50 to 75 per cent of his maximal oxygen uptake, although a relative load of 40 per cent has sufficed in some instances.[14,23–27,37–39] As with normal subjects, the degree of improvement tends to be inversely proportional to the pretraining capacity for patients with coronary disease.[14] Because of the high linear correlation between oxygen uptake and heart rate at submaximal workloads, the heart rate may be substituted for the more difficult measurement of oxygen consumption. Available tables for predicting maximal heart rate by age cannot be used for this purpose. These predicted heart rates represent the average values for "normal" persons not on medication and therefore can be misleading and can negate the purpose of the individual prescription. Cardiac patients should have a target that takes into consideration symptoms and signs, so that the training intensity never exceeds the point at which ischemia becomes manifest. By actually testing the patient, the monitoring physician can take into account aberrant heart rate responses due to intrinsic cardiac disease or medications such as beta blockers. The usual effects of training are observed in patients on beta blockers, and the exercise heart rate, although lower than that in patients not receiving these drugs, remains a useful guide to their evaluation throughout a physicial training program.[28,29]

Ample data indicate that a training heart rate at 70 to 85 per cent of maximal capacity corresponds to the levels of maximal oxygen uptake (57 to 78 per cent) required for training (Fig. 40–2).[14–16,26,27,37–39] Another approach for estimating the target heart rate is to add 60 to 70 per cent of the difference between resting heart rate and maximal heart rate attained to the resting heart rate.[36–39] This technique takes the variability of the resting heart rate into account and generally gives a slightly higher target heart rate. The relationship of per cent maximal heart rate and per cent maximal oxygen uptake remains consistent for persons of all ages in the presence or absence of coronary disease and at all levels of training.[37] In practice, the target heart rate determined by either procedure applies to all training activities for the patient under usual environmental conditions.

Besides oxygen consumption and heart rate, the dosage intensity may be prescribed in METS. A MET is a unit of energy that approximates the amount of oxygen required under basal conditions at rest and is 3.5 ml/kg-min. Published tables[39,40] transform METS into energy requirements for common activities at work and home (Table 40–1). METS can be used only as a crude index because differences in individual energy expenditure vary according to environmental factors, physical condition, skills, and moti-

vation. Yet the MET is recommended for translation into exercise programs, since it is easily understood by both the patient and the physician, can be applied to various tasks, and can be monitored by heart rate response. The average 40-year-old male in the U.S. can function at 10 METS at his maximum capacity; therefore, the concept of 1 MET as the energy cost of sitting provides a scale of 1 to 10 for applying physical activity components to the functional capacity of the average adult man.[24]

DURATION. Although training adaptations can occur with brief sessions at high intensity, this is not advisable from the standpoint of safety. In addition, the logistics of getting to and from supervised sessions make a 30- to 45-minute exercise session more practical. However, frequent brief sessions may be necessary for those individuals unable to tolerate 30 minutes of moderate intensity (70 to 80 per cent or lower of maximal capacity). Training effects may be noted as soon as 2 weeks or as late as 6 weeks after starting but can be highly variable among individuals, depending upon initial functional capacity, health status, and response to specific activities.[37]

FREQUENCY OF TRAINING. To improve cardiovascular fitness, the exercise program should be performed at least 3 days a week, preferably nonconsecutively to avoid musculoskeletal stress. Maintenance programs of 2 to 3 days per week suffice to retain exercise adaptations. Frequency of training appears to be less important than either intensity or duration.

TYPE OF EXERCISE. The mode of exercise should be dynamic (isotonic) activities involving large muscle groups, designed to overload the oxygen transport system of the body, such as walking, jogging, swimming, and bicycling. Swimming, an ideal exercise from the standpoint of involving large muscle groups in the arms and legs, also provides relief for weight-bearing joints but has a high relative energy cost and can mask ischemic symptoms.[41,42] Recent studies suggest no difference between combined dynamic-static exercise compared with dynamic exercise alone at peak loads in causing induced ischemia, left ventricular dysfunction, or ventricular arrhythmias.[31,43] Adaptive training responses are peculiar to the muscle group exercised so that the patient's occupational and leisure time activities should be considered in order to establish appropriate exercises.[14–16] Most rehabilitation programs incorporate interval training techniques, a series of repeated bouts of exercise alternated with periods of relief during the exercise session. For most situations, such intermittent exercise offers several advantages over continuous training techniques: (1) The patient will be able to achieve higher intensity levels with less probability of leg fatigue by virtue of the rest periods; (2) it allows more diverse activities; (3) changing modes of exercise permit different muscle groups to be stressed; and (4) ischemic signs can be monitored more carefully during the recovery intervals.

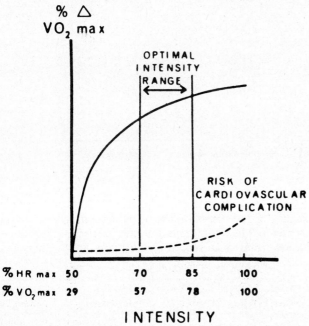

FIGURE 40–2 Relationship between per cent gain in aerobic capacity ($\triangle VO_2$max) and intensity of exercise expressed as per cent of maximal heart rate (HR max) or per cent of VO_2max. The optimal intensity range is 70 to 85 per cent of HR max equivalent to 57 to 78 per cent VO_2max. As the intensity of exercise exceeds 85 per cent of HR max, the relative risks of arrhythmias, angina pectoris, and other ischemic manifestations increase abruptly, whereas the improvement in aerobic capacity levels off. (Adapted from Hellerstein, H. K., and Franklin, B. A.: Exercise testing and prescription. *In* Wenger, N. K., and Hellerstein, H. K. (eds.): Rehabilitation of the Coronary Patient. New York, John Wiley and Sons, 1978, pp. 149–202.)

Phases of Rehabilitation

The exercise program is divided into three phases: (1) early convalescence during hospitalization; (2) intermediate convalescence, the transition period between hospital and resumption of ordinary activities; and (3) the long-term program for maintenance of health (Table 40–2). Although guidelines for exercise remain the same throughout these

TABLE 40–1 APPROXIMATE ENERGY REQUIREMENTS FOR SELECTED ACTIVITIES

ENERGY CATEGORY	SELF-CARE OR HOME	OCCUPATIONAL	RECREATIONAL	PHYSICAL CONDITIONING
Very Light < 3 METS < 10 ml/kg-min < 4 kcal	Washing, shaving, dressing Desk work, writing Washing dishes Driving auto	Sitting (clerical, assembling) Standing (store clerk, bartender) Driving truck Janitorial work	Playing cards Horseshoes Bait casting Billiards Sewing, knitting Golf (cart)	Walking (level at 2 mph) Stationary bicycle (very low resistance) Very light calisthenics
Light 3–5 METS 11–18 ml/kg-min 4–6 kcal	Cleaning windows Raking leaves Weeding Power lawn mowing Waxing floors (slowly) Painting Carrying objects (15–30 lb)	Stocking shelves (light objects) Light welding Light carpentry Machine assembly Auto repair Paperhanging	Dancing (social and square) Golf (walking) Sailing Horseback riding Volleyball (6 man) Tennis (doubles)	Walking (3–4 mph) Level bicycling (6–8 mph) Light calisthenics
Moderate 5–7 METS 18–25 ml/kg-min 6–8 kcal	Easy digging in garden Level hand lawn mowing Climbing stairs (slowly) Carrying objects (30–60 lb) Splitting wood	Carpentry (exterior home building) Shoveling dirt Pneumatic tools	Light backpacking Tennis (singles) Water skiing Skating (ice and roller) Horseback riding (gallop)	Walking (4.5–5 mph) Bicycling (9–10 mph) Swimming (breast stroke)
Heavy 7–9 METS 25–32 ml/kg-min 8–10 kcal	Sawing wood Heavy shoveling Climbing stairs (moderate speed) Carrying objects (60–90 lb)	Tending furnace Digging ditches Pick and shovel	Canoeing Mountain climbing Touch football Paddleball	Jog (5 mph) Swim (crawl stroke) Rowing machine Bicycling (12 mph) Heavy calisthenics
Very Heavy > 9 METS > 32 ml/kg-min > 10 kcal	Carrying loads upstairs Carrying objects (> 90 lb) Climbing stairs (quickly) Shoveling heavy snow	Lumber jack Heavy laborer	Handball Squash Ski touring over hills	Running (≥ 6 mph) Bicycle (≥ 13 mph or up steep hill) Rope jumping

Adapted from Haskell, W. L.: Design and implementation of cardiac conditioning programs. *In* Wenger, N. K., and Hellerstein, H. (eds.): Rehabilitation of the Coronary Patient. New York, John Wiley and Sons, 1978, pp. 203–241.

program phases, the objectives and methods differ somewhat in each.

PHASE ONE—IN HOSPITAL. Traditionally, 6 to 8 weeks of absolute bed rest was the rule for patients sustaining a myocardial infarction, although as early as the 1940's, Dr. Tinsley Harrison questioned the wisdom of undue restriction.[44] Deleterious effects of such mobilization include a decrement of 20 per cent or more in physical work capacity, hypovolemia, depression of pulmonary ventilation, and muscle degeneration.[13] Controversy surrounded early mobilization after infarction until a series of investigations, progressing from a "chair regimen"[45] to rapid mobilization, demonstrated the safety and efficacy of such activities for selected patients.[13,46-53] Coronary artery bypass grafting creates a situation not unlike that after myocardial infarction, in which carefully supervised activity programs during hospitalization result in shortened hospital stays, with no greater immediate risk than prolonged bed rest.[54]

Mobilization early in convalescence has become an integral part of the rehabilitation of patients free of continued ischemia, cardiac failure, and electrical instability. Patients with recurrent pain requiring morphine and with a CK-

TABLE 40–2 EXERCISE PROGRAM SCHEDULE

PHASE OF CONVALESCENCE*	TIME	ACTIVITIES	AVERAGE WORKLOAD
Early	1–3 weeks	Self care activities, low-level calisthenics, walking	2–4 METS
Intermediate	4–12 weeks	Moderate-level calisthenics, walking, structured endurance training	5–7 METS
Long-term	12 + weeks	High-level calisthenics, high-level endurance training	7 + METS

*Following myocardial infarction or coronary artery bypass surgery.

MB persisting for 72 hours or longer representing possible extension of the infarction[55] must be approached more cautiously. Most data reveal no immediate adverse effects of early mobilization and discharge,[56] but one randomized controlled trial noted an unexplained lower mortality during the second and third years of follow-up in the late mobilization group.[52] Although in-hospital exercise improved functional status at the time of discharge and led to an earlier and more complete return to work in some studies,[56] Sivarajan and colleagues[57] were unable to detect any significant beneficial or deleterious efforts of an early in-hospital exercise program combined with early evaluation and discharge. Another study showed significant functional improvement from early low-intensity exercises but only in a small subgroup able to exercise without evidence of ischemia.[58]

Early exercise testing (see also pp. 1293 and 1327) is useful for rehabilitation assessment in patients without congestive heart failure, severe arrhythmias, orthopedic complications, or other severe disabilities.[59-61,61a] Testing may merely involve monitoring the patient as he walks in a hospital corridor, with observation for angina, dyspnea, new murmurs, gallops, abnormalities of heart rate or blood pressure, and electrocardiographic changes. Of more value is a low-level testing protocol[11,60,62] to detect the threshold for adverse symptoms or signs, to judge whether a patient can tolerate self-care activities at home, and to provide prognostic information.[62a] The safety of early testing appears to be more related to the severity of disease than to the length of the interval following infarction or to details of the test protocol.

As early as the first few days after infarction, patients without complications can be started on self-care activities limited to several METS (Fig. 40–3). This modest exertional level rarely increases the heart rate more than 10 beats/min and permits the patient to feed himself, wash his hands and face, shave, and use the bedside commode with assistance. Activities as minimal as getting up and sitting in a chair several times daily, suggested by Levine and Lown years ago,[45] prevent orthostatic intolerance from protracted bed rest.[63] Programmed and progressive self-care activities allow patients to maintain the expectation of an independent life style. Calisthenics, valuable for flexibility, strength, and even endurance, may be started in conjunction with a walking program. Specific exercises to increase the strength of the pectoral muscles have been developed for the postoperative patient.[3] Isometric exercises are avoided because of the presumed excessive myocardial oxygen consumption and dysrhythmias imposed by the predominantly "pressure" workload, though recent studies question this concept.[31,43] Physical activities should be carried out under the supervision of the nursing staff with frequent reassessment of symptoms and signs during the early exercise sessions; just prior to discharge, physical activity should be monitored for abnormal responses to exercise. If problems occur, the level of activities should be either reduced or discontinued temporarily until the patient can resume progressive exercise safely.

PHASE TWO—INTERMEDIATE CONVALESCENCE. At the time of discharge from the hospital, the patient should be able to perform activities at peak levels of 3.5 to 4.0 METS for short durations corresponding to usual activities at home.[64] During initial days at home, patients continue the activities started at the hospital—dynamic warm-up exercises followed by walking at a graduated distance and pace. After the initial post-hospitalization examination, further advice about exercise can be given to those ready. During this period, the patient is asked first to walk at least a half mile in 10 minutes, then a mile in 20 minutes, subsequently decreasing the time to 15 minutes by increasing the speed. Provided there are no contraindications, the walking program is accelerated, first in distance and then in pace. Generally, if the duration can be doubled at a given intensity without producing symptoms or excessive heart rate response, the next higher level of intensity may be undertaken.[25] Next the walk is lengthened to 2 miles daily, with the speed maintained at 4 mph or the distance covered in 30 minutes. If a patient can maintain the pace, the distance can be increased to 3 or 4 miles per day at his physician's discretion. Not all patients can achieve this goal, but almost all can obtain great satisfaction in the attempt.

At 6 to 8 weeks after hospitalization, the emphasis shifts toward *dynamic exercises* to improve cardiopulmonary function. At this point, patients must be carefully reevaluated to determine possible adverse reactions to exercise or conditions requiring special precautions with more vigorous exertion. Some examples include prolonged fatigue, worsening angina or congestive failure, dysrhythmias, signs of cerebral dysfunction, development of orthopedic problems, electrocardiographic changes, or altered drug regimens. Recommendations for exercise should be made with the same care as for any other prescription. An inappropriately high intensity of exercise can lead to clinical events, orthopedic problems, and generally poor compliance, whereas homeopathic doses nullify any likely improvement and discourage patients from resuming ordinary activities. An appropriate prescription requires a maximal or symptom-sign–limited exercise test. In addition to the objective measurements of work capacity during the test, the patient's subjective estimate of exertion (Borg Scale) can be helpful in formulating the exercise prescription and in monitoring training effects.[36] At this stage of convalescence, the exercise prescription recommended for endurance training is based on the lower boundary of the target range, or about 60 per cent of the patient's maximal oxygen uptake, corresponding to 70 to 75 per cent of the maximal heart rate, achieved on the exercise test. For example, if the maximal heart rate achieved before termination of the exercise test is 160 beats/min, the target heart rate will be 75 per cent of 160 (160×0.75) = 120 beats per minutes. With interval (intermittent) exercise, the changing energy demands may result in heart rates varying by about 10 per cent from the prescribed target heart rate. However, the heart rate should average out to the prescribed level over the total duration of the training session. Patients able to perform at levels of 5 METS or more should exercise at least three times per week, preferably on alternate days to avoid excessive bone-joint stress. The duration of the exercise may range from 20 to 30 minutes during the first few weeks of conditioning, after which the duration can be increased to as much as 45 minutes. Duration can be set empirically for those patients with functional capacities below 5 METS and can be adjusted thereafter, depending on the individual response to exercise. The frequency of exercise should be prescribed for

POST MYOCARDIAL INFARCTION			POST CARDIAC SURGERY	
STEP/DAY/WHERE	ACTIVITY/EXERCISE		STEP/DAY/WHERE	ACTIVITY/EXERCISE
Step 1/Day 1/ Cardiac Care Unit	Bedside commode; self feeding and grooming; chair 10-15 min. twice per day/active assisted ROM exercises to all extremities performed supine (5x per day) ①		Step 1/Day 1/ Surgical Intensive Care Unit	Sit on side of bed in a.m.; chair 15 min. in p.m.; diaphragmatic breathing; feed self/active assisted ROM (5x) ① Ankle dorsiflexion (10x)
Step 2/Day 3-4/ Cardiac Care Unit	Chair 20 min. 3x per day; bed bath (staff to assist with back and lower legs)/active ROM (5x per day) ①		Step 2/Day 2/ General Nursing Area	Bedside commode or bathroom with assistance; self grooming; chair 20 min. 3x per day; walk back and forth in room (1x)/active ROM (5x) ①
Step 3/Day 5-7/ Cardiac Care Unit or General Nursing Area	Bathe self (tub or bed bath); bathroom privileges if in room; chair 30 min. 4x per day; walk back and forth in room 1x on Day 6; 2x on Day 7/active ROM 7x per day) ①		Step 3/Day 3/ General Nursing Area	Bathe self at bedside or basin; chair 30 min. 4x per day; walk 30-60 feet/ active ROM (5x) ①
Step 4/Day 8-9/ General Nursing Area	Stand at sink to shave; walk 60 feet on Day 8; 100 feet on Day 9 (3x per day)/active ROM (8x per day) ① Leg exercises while supine; arm exercises while sitting.		Step 4/Day 4/ General Nursing Area	Chair as desired; walk 100 feet with assistance 2x per day and as desired/ active ROM (5x) ① Leg exercises while supine; arm exercises while sitting.
Step 5/Day 10-11 General Nursing Area	Up as desired in chair; walk 200 feet 3x per day/same as Step 4 (10x per day) ①		Step 5/Day 5/ General Nursing Area	Up as desired in room; walk 200 feet 2x per day and as desired/do all exercises in sitting position (5x) ①
Step 6/Day 12/ General Nursing Area	May shower; low level exercise test; climb one flight of stairs; walk 300 feet 3x per day/same as Step 5. ADD: standing: arm exercises (5x)①; lateral bends (5x)②; sitting: knee bends (5x)③; knee raises (5x) ④		Step 6/Day 6/ General Nursing Area	Walk 300 feet 3x per day and as desired/same as Step 5. ADD: standing: arm exercises (5x)①; sitting: knee bends (5x)③; knee raises (5x) ④ Add home instructions.
Step 7/Day 13/ General Nursing Area	Walk 400 feet 2x per day and as desired/same as Step 6. ADD: sitting: toe touch (5x)⑤; trunk twist (5x) ⑥ Add home instructions.		Step 7/Day 7/ General Nursing Area	Walk 400 feet 3x per day and as desired; up as desired/same as Step 6. ADD: standing: lateral bends (5x)②
Step 8/Day 14-21 General Nursing Area	Up as desired.		Step 8/Day 8/ General Nursing Area	May bathe in tub or shower after removal of stitches; up as desired; low level exercise/ same as Step 7.

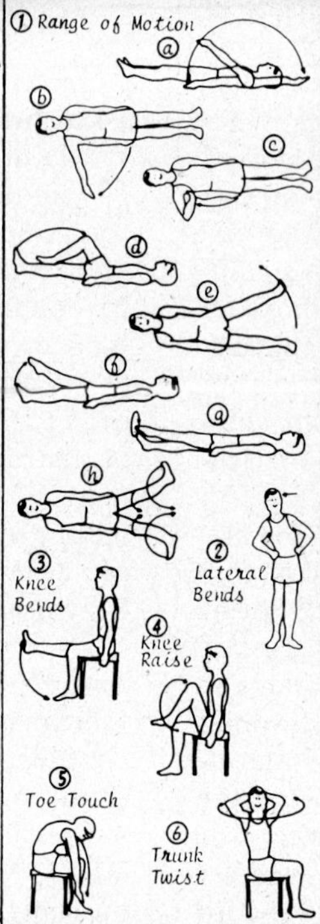

FIGURE 40–3 Inpatient activity schedule. Exercise instructions:
1. Range of motion (ROM):
   a. With elbow straight, lift arm straight over head and return to side. Relax and repeat with opposite arm.
   b. With elbow straight, lift arm away from body and over head, and then return to side. Relax and repeat with opposite arm.
   c. With arm straight down by side, bend elbow and touch shoulder with fingertips. Relax and repeat with opposite arm.
   d. Raise knee toward chest and return to starting position. Relax and repeat with opposite leg.
   e. With leg straight, move leg out to side of body and return to starting position. Relax and repeat with opposite leg.
   f. Straight leg raise.
   g. Make circular patterns with both feet. Relax and repeat.
   h. Roll legs in and out simultaneously. Relax and repeat.
2. Lateral bends: standing erect, bend trunk laterally to left then to right. Relax and repeat.
3. Knee bends: sitting erect, straighten and bend knees alternately. Relax and repeat.
4. Knee raise: sitting erect, raise knees toward the chest alternately. Relax and repeat.
5. Toe touch: sitting erect, bend trunk forward trying to touch toes with fingertips. Relax and repeat.
6. Trunk twist: sitting erect, twist trunk to left and then to right. Relax and repeat.
(Adapted from Georgia Baptist Medical Center, Cardiac Rehabilitation Unit, Atlanta, Georgia.)

three to five periods per week. Daily sessions for persons with capacities between 3 and 5 METS may be advisable, and for patients with functional capacities less than 3 METS, sessions of 5 minutes several times daily.[26] Within these guidelines, the exercise prescription for most patients will result in training adaptations without undue fatigue or hazard.

Group activities at an exercise facility offer certain advantages—trained personnel, established emergency routines, and motivation by other participants.[65] A model training session might proceed as follows: After 5 minutes of warm-up calisthenics, the patient exercises at the target rate set at about 75 per cent of the maximal heart rate achieved on the prior exercise test. Useful training devices include the treadmill, stationary bicycle, steps, rowing machine, arm ergometer, and arm wheel. On each device, the patient reaches his target rate within a minute or two and maintains this heart rate within 10 beats/min for the remainder of the 4-minute exercise period. After the fourth

minute, there is a 2-minute recovery period before the patient moves to the next exercise station, with the patient alternating between arm and leg device stations. In this way the patient achieves a larger overall workload before the onset of fatigue or symptoms. After six exercise periods, or a total of 24 minutes of exercise, the patient walks around the room for a 5-minute cool-down period. Most patients are ready to begin their own long-term program after 6 to 12 of these supervised exercise sessions.

PHASE THREE—LONG-TERM PROGRAM. The long-term program is designed to retain training adaptations and stimulate further progress. The need for supervision is critical during the transition to more vigorous exertion with less structured routines, yet economic and other concerns necessitate the judicious use of unsupervised exercise programs for coronary patients.[66–69] Except for those patients benefiting from low-level activities such as walking, it is best to delay an unsupervised program. Patients may proceed to an unsupervised maintenance program after thorough evaluation on the basis of (1) a stable health status, (2) relatively low risk for subsequent cardiac events, (3) functional performance of at least 8 METS or more, and (4) a full understanding of the principles of exercise training and the disease process.[23,26]

Recreational activities equivalent to the peak energy requirements of the previous exercise test can be introduced in the absence of possible hazards, such as adverse environmental conditions, intensive competition, or marked emotional involvement. Sports and games vary in promoting the components of fitness—endurance, strength, and flexibility—and should be selected accordingly. A typical long-term exercise session for a patient attaining a maximal heart rate of 140 beats/min and 6 METS on the exercise test before developing angina would consist of the following components: (1) warm-up exercises for 5 minutes; (2) endurance training consisting of 20 to 30 minutes of walking, jogging, or cycling, at the target exertional level (85 per cent of maximal capacity, which is about 120 beats/min, or 5 METS); (3) a 5-minute cool-down period; (4) a 5-minute warm-up period; (5) a 20- to 30-minute recreational period; and (6) a final cool-down 5-minute walk (Fig. 40–4). The allotted time for structured endurance and recreational activities depends on individual preference, capabilities, and facilities. Heart rate estimates are more difficult to make with recreational activities, and the patient's subjective feelings of exertion (Borg Scale) become more important.[36] As the patient adapts to the training routine, the heart rate for a given exertional task will decrease, allowing progressive increments in the workload. Periodic evaluation will aid in adjusting the exercise prescription and in assessing progress. Recent publications review in detail exercise prescriptions, appropriate physical activities, and topics pertinent to cardiac rehabilitation programs.[70]

SECONDARY PREVENTION

Once manifest, coronary heart disease increases susceptibility to infarction, congestive failure, stroke, and premature death.[71] New rehabilitation studies document the importance of intervention programs in reducing the sequellae of coronary dise se, prolonging life, and having a positive effect on life styl .[72–76,76a] In addition to physical training, a rehabilitation program should incorporate risk factor intervention as well as clinical measures likely to alter the progression of disease and improve the long-term prognosis. Several clinical trials (p. 1352)[77,77a,77b,77c,77d,78] have now demonstrated that beta-blocking drugs can substantially reduce the rate of death during the first 2 years after myocardial infarction. Whether other kinds of coronary artery disease patients can benefit from these agents, the best time to initiate treatment, and the duration of therapy required for optimal benefits remain unknown. Recent reviews[79–81] corroborate the value of coronary artery bypass grafting in affecting the quality of life by relieving symptoms in 80 to 90 per cent of patients with angina, by increasing functional capacity, by reducing the number of cardiac related events, and by prolonging survival in patients with substantial stenosis of the left main coronary artery or "three-vessel" disease (p. 1372). These findings emphasize the importance of optimal clinical management in the rehabilitation process for selected categories of patients.

Risk Factor Modification (See Chap. 35)

The prognosis after myocardial infarction as well as the development of coronary artery disease is associated with major risk factors.[71,82–84] Patients should be advised to discontinue all forms of smoking, even filtered cigarettes,[85] as

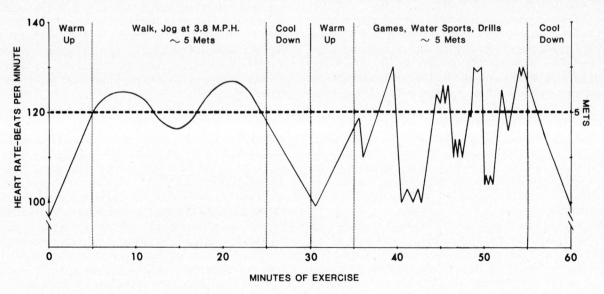

- - - - Prescribed Level of Exertion

FIGURE 40–4 Long-term exercise program. The example is for the hypothetical patient who completed Stage 6 of the prior exercise test, attaining a maximum heart rate of 140 beats/min before developing angina. The program contains variable amounts of recreational activities in addition to the basic endurance exercises to maintain the patient's interest. The actual heart rate tends to fluctuate about the desired target level and is more difficult to approximate with recreational activities. With adequate supervision, the heart rate can be maintained within 10 beats of the prescribed target rate for most of the session. (From Oberman, A., and Kouchoukos, N. T.: Role of exercise after coronary artery surgery. *In* Wenger, N. K. (ed.): Exercise and the Heart. Philadelphia, F. A. Davis Co., 1978, pp. 155–172.)

early in the course of the disease as possible. Among coronary patients, ex-smokers have only one-half the subsequent mortality of those who continue to smoke;[71] in the Coronary Artery Surgery Study registry, 5-year survival was significantly less for those who continued to smoke.[86] Weight reduction favorably modifies cholesterol levels, blood pressure, glucose tolerance, and other metabolic factors associated with atherosclerotic disease.[71,87] Persuasive evidence exists that an elevated serum cholesterol level, especially with a low proportion of high-density lipoprotein cholesterol,[88] accelerates the progression of atherosclerosis and its complications,[84,89,90] yet data from the controlled trials justifying reduction of plasma lipids by means of drugs are not encouraging.[72,91]

One must extrapolate from the studies on the efficacy of antihypertensive treatment for the general population[92] and the anticipated greater myocardial oxygen costs in hypertension to justify treating hypertension in patients with coronary artery disease. Lowering elevated blood pressure in patients with coronary artery disease should diminish symptoms, enhance left ventricular function, and retard progression of disease, but no documentation from controlled trials among such populations is available. The situation is complicated by hemodynamic changes resulting from the myocardial infarction itself. In the Framingham experience, a decrease in blood pressure at 1 year after infarction adversely affected mortality;[71] however, by excluding those patients who had sustained a fall in blood pressure post infarction, the usual direct relationship between blood pressure and mortality was found. For the long-term management of coronary patients, optimal blood pressure levels have yet to be determined.

Exercise

In the past 10 years, multiple controlled randomized trials of exercise for survivors of myocardial infarction have supported the value of physical activity in reducing long-term mortality.[72] Possible mechanisms for secondary prevention involve retardation of the atherosclerotic process or protection against the occurrence of clinical manifestations.

Retardation of Atherosclerosis. Modification of atherogenic traits that are influenced by physical activity may improve the subsequent clinical course by retarding the atherosclerotic process. For those patients undergoing coronary artery bypass grafting, the prevention of atherosclerosis in the vein grafts themselves is an important long-term concern.[93]

Some atherogenic factors influenced by a training program include the following: (1) reduction in weight with a constant caloric intake and increased lean body mass;[94-96] (2) changes in the lipoprotein profile, including reduced levels of serum triglycerides and an increased amount of cholesterol carried by high-density lipoproteins,[94-98] but no clear concensus exists regarding the relationship of total cholesterol concentration to habitual exercise;[99] (3) increased cellular sensitivity to insulin, resulting in improved glucose tolerance;[95,100] (4) minimal blood pressure changes but generally a lowered resting diastolic blood pressure with a decrease in mean blood pressure during submaximal exercise;[15,16,96,101] (5) stimulation of desirable

health habits, including modification of Type A behavior (p. 1826);[102,103] (6) decreased platelet adhesiveness and enhanced fibrinolysis;[104,105] (7) and a lessened adrenergic response to stress.[96,101,106]

Yet it is unlikely that coronary patients in a supervised exercise program not using additional intervention modalities will exhibit marked improvement in major risk factors.[107,108] Insufficient training adaptations due to poor compliance and the inability to attain the levels of exertion or the duration necessary for major changes in risk factors have been offered as explanations.[98,102,107-109] Alternatively, it is possible that exercise might act indirectly by blocking the effect of major risk factors. For example, training adaptations lower heart rate and blood pressure at submaximal work levels, accelerate carbon monoxide metabolism, and diminish platelet aggregation; any or all of these metabolic changes might counter the adverse effects of smoking.[107]

Protection Against Clinical Manifestations of Coronary Artery Disease. Properly executed physical training programs generally increase exercise tolerance by at least 20 per cent in most patients with coronary artery disease[15,25,110] and in some instances allow coronary patients to reach a degree of fitness seldom attained even by healthy individuals—that required for marathon races.[111-113] Training adaptations result in relative bradycardia at submaximal levels of exercise but induce little change in stroke volume. The increased maximum oxygen uptake depends primarily upon enhanced peripheral extraction of oxygen by redistribution of blood to working skeletal muscles and local adaptive changes in the skeletal muscle's capacity for aerobic metabolism.[15,16] Such training effects reduce cardiac work in proportion to total body work and enable an individual to respond to exertion without taxing the circulation and compromising myocardial oxygen needs.[14] Myocardial oxygen consumption, as estimated indirectly, is less for a given task owing to a systematic decrease in exercise heart rate and blood pressure.[101] More recent data suggest that training actually improves myocardial oxygen delivery or utilization, leading to an increased exercise tolerance and higher values for heart rate and systolic blood pressure before myocardial ischemia develops.[110,115-117]

Ehsani and colleagues[115] found that patients able to exercise at 65 to 85 per cent of maximum $\dot{V}O_2$ for 1 hour per day, 4 or 5 days per week, achieved a 38 per cent increase in maximum $\dot{V}O_2$ and increased the double product threshold. The extent of ST-segment displacement at the same double product and at the maximum workload was less after training, implying a reduction in myocardial ischemia. Presumably, skeletal muscle and autonomic nervous system adaptations occur rapidly, bringing about increased exercise capabilities, but cardiac adaptations occur later, only with more intense exertion over a period of months.[118,119] In addition, improvement in exercise performance[120-122] has been attributed to enhanced left ventricular function and increased stroke volume with prolonged, intensive exercise training. Failure to improve ventricular function during rest and exercise may be due to insufficient training levels.[118,119] Indirect evidence for favorable cardiovascular changes includes reversion of aberrant ballistocardiographic waveforms,[123] fewer electrocardiographic abnormalities,[124,125] and less ventricular ectopic activity[83,101] in men participating in vigorous exercise. Still uncertain is the degree to which the consequences of a myocardial infarct can be corrected or compensated for by an exercise program.

Experimental data from animals with surgically induced coronary artery lesions subjected to physical training suggest cardiovascular adaptations that might diminish myocardial ischemia: (1) improved myocardial function and metabolism and (2) augumented myocardial perfusion, possibly resulting from increased coronary vasculature, capillary to myocardial fiber ratio, and collateral circulation.[124,126] Monkeys fed an atherogenic diet and then exercised demonstrated larger coronary arteries and less surface area involved with atherosclerotic plaques than did sedentary controls, suggesting that exercise may prevent coronary artery disease in primates by augmenting the coronary vascular bed.[127] Nevertheless, studies of physical activity in patients with coronary artery disease have not demonstrated expanded collateral circulation,[116,126,128-130] but evaluation during exercise or more sensitive methods for determining myocardial perfusion might be needed.

Over the last decade a growing series of randomized trials[131-135] have demonstrated a differential mortality among survivors of myocardial infarction randomized to a physical training program compared with those in a "control" group (Table 40–3). These studies were based on supervised training programs consisting of two to four sessions per week lasting 20 to 60 minutes each. Despite major problems in adherence to the exercise regimen, all the trials but one showed reductions in mortality ranging from 20.6 to 37.0 per cent for the exercise group. Little effect on the incidence of reinfarction was noted. However, such trials were inadequate to test the hypothesis that exercise reduces overall mortality, as they were not designed with this as the primary outcome. The National Exercise and Heart Disease Project showed a substantial, but nonsignificant, 37 per cent reduction in total mortality, primarily due to fewer deaths from recurrent myocardial infarction.[135] The benefits of exercise were greatest in those patients whose physical capacity exceeded 7 METS, in cigarette smokers, and in those whose systolic blood pressure response to exercise testing exceeded 140 mm Hg. These data support an assumption of substantial benefit from supervised exercise among survivors of a myocardial infarction. Pooling of the results from these five comparable studies is consistent with a 19 per cent reduction ($p < 0.05$) in total mortality in the exercise intervention group.[72] In any event, these trials conclusively demonstrated that there was no additional hazard from supervised exercise among postinfarction patients. Haskell surveyed 30 rehabilitation programs in the U.S. and Canada treating 13,570 patients during the period evaluated and found the rate for all complications was 1 per 25,715 patient-hours and the fatal complication rate was 1 fatality per 116,402 patient-hours of participation.[136]

Comprehensive Rehabilitation Programs

There is now long-term information on several comprehensive Scandinavian rehabilitation intervention programs. In these studies a multidisciplinary rehabilitation team emphasized exercise, health education (advice on smoking cessation, diet, and stress reduction), and pharmacological management. Intervention included individual and group counseling with involvement of the spouses and specific informational material supplemented by audiovisual techniques. In the North Karelia Study,[73,74] 1300 patients with an acute myocardial infarction under the age of 65 participated in a special program for rehabilitation and secondary prevention from 1973 to 1977; these participants experienced a reduction in the incidence of recurrent infarction and new vocational invalidity pensions. A collaborative study from two Finnish centers assessed the effects of comprehensive rehabilitation on morbidity and mortality as well as on return to work and various other outcomes.[75] In this program, beginning 2 weeks after hospital discharge, the cumulative coronary mortality was 18.6 per cent in the intervention group and 29.4 per cent in the control group at the 3-year follow-up with differences due mainly to reduced numbers of sudden deaths following infarction. In a special clinic in Göteborg, there was a significant reduction in nonfatal reinfarction and new coronary events after 2 years of attendance.[76] New coronary rates were reduced by 50 per cent despite comparable values for initial risk factors between the intervention and reference group; total mortality was not changed significantly by intervention.

Substantial opportunities exist for secondary prevention

TABLE 40–3 SECONDARY PREVENTION WITH PHYSICAL TRAINING
(PREVIOUS RANDOMIZED CONTROLLED TRIALS)

| TRIAL | N | INTERVENTION | FOLLOW-UP (MONTHS) | MORTALITY (%) | | EFFECTIVENESS (%)* |
				Control	Intervention	
Sweden (1968–72)	315	Supervised exercise, 3×/week	48	22.3	17.7	20.6
Finland (1969–72)	298	Supervised exercise, 2–3×/week	12	21.9	17.1	21.9
Finland (1969–72)	380	Daily home exercise	29	14.0	10.0	28.6
Canada (1972–78)	733	Partially supervised exercise, 2–4×/week	48	7.3	9.5	−30.0
United States (1974–79)	651	Supervised exercise, 3×/week	36	7.3	4.6	37.0

*Effectiveness = $\dfrac{\text{control mortality} - \text{intervention mortality}}{\text{control mortality}} \times 100$

among patients with coronary artery disease based on recent pharmacological and surgical trials.[77-80] Other promising interventions, especially exercise, require further testing in selected subgroups most likely to derive benefits from the regimen and in adequate numbers to test definitively the hypothesis that the intervention will reduce mortality.

PSYCHOSOCIAL CONCERNS
(See also Chap. 57)

During recovery, the patient and his family are forced to make a number of social and psychological adjustments. The emotional problems of the patient, from the onset of pain, through the period of hospitalization, and until he resumes ordinary activities, have been well described.[9,10,137-139] Post–myocardial infarction depression and anxiety are almost universal and can lead to permanent psychological problems unless they are anticipated and counteracted by appropriate counseling.[7] Fear of death, reinfarction, or inability to resume former living patterns is common[140] and should be amenable to rehabilitation. The patient's perception of his physical handicap is greatly influenced by his emotional state; not surprisingly, disability varies markedly at comparable levels of disease.

Impairment of personality and psychological functioning has been observed in a number of studies after open-heart surgery and specifically after coronary artery bypass procedures. Heller and coworkers[141] have reported that despite physical improvement after surgery, psychological problems remain a major barrier to rehabilitation in approximately one-third of patients. Even 1 year after operation, these patients were more passive, anxious, and depressed, and experienced increased somatic preoccupation, loss of self-esteem, and impaired sexual and marital functioning. Asymptomatic patients after operation are uncertain about their limitations and are fearful of precipitating pain, whereas those with continued symptoms or problems become discouraged and depressed. The patient's perception of his health status is probably as important as his actual functional capacity in determining the extent of disability after operation.[142]

Although the hospital setting provides an appropriate environment for motivating the patient to adapt to a healthier life style, the anxiety, fatigue, and acuteness of the situation limit educational opportunities. After the patient has left the hospital and resumed home activities, a more detailed educational program is possible. At this time explanation of the illness, the natural history of the disease, and the possibilities for long-term management should be addressed. An assortment of recent instructional materials and books can be used advantageously.[70,143-150] Involving the patient in planning for recovery, by teaching self-monitoring responses to physical activities and identifying areas in which he can make decisions for his own care, helps to encourage adherence to the medical regimen. Group discussions are especially helpful for both the patients and their families at various stages in the rehabilitation program. At all stages of convalescence, the spouse must be involved. Typically, the spouse has guilt feelings and is unable to express his or her own inadequacies in dealing with the situation; the spouse's anxiety and uncertainty may be as great as the patient's.[10,139] The spouse finds it difficult to help the patient while allowing him or her to be independent and resume activities. As a result of these conflicts and the major changes in life-long roles, marital tensions increase.

Resumption of sexual activity may be important in the marital relationship during these stressful readjustment periods. A common misconception is that sexual intercourse may be too strenuous for patients with coronary artery disease, yet the average rate of peak sexual activity is less than 120 beats/min and exertional requirements are no more than those of walking up one or two flights of stairs or taking a brisk walk for several blocks (p. 1832).[151-153] Family counseling should include discussion of life style adjustments to be anticipated during convalescence and the harm of unnecessary restriction. Although some patients profit from formal support and intervention, it is best that patients and their families assume responsibility for their rehabilitation and deal with the emotional aspects of their illness. Medical practitioners must recognize the importance of informal counseling and social support mechanisms for effecting optimal long-term recovery from cardiac disease.[154]

Early identification of those patients likely to have special psychological problems can speed recovery because few patients will express their fears or difficulties to the physician. In one controlled study, psychotherapy initiated during the hospitalization period resulted in fewer days in the intensive care unit with fewer medical and psychological problems.[155] Cay[137] has summarized the methods of treatment as informing the patient of the natural history of the disease, explaining the rationale of treatment, reassuring and encouraging him, giving practical help with concrete problems, nondirective guidance, drug therapy, and gradually increasing physical exercise. Patients and their families should be informed about community resources, including counseling services, home care agencies and services, vocational rehabilitation facilities, and coronary clubs. Group sessions allow patients to exchange information, gain social group support, express their feelings, and share common problems and solutions. Controlled studies of group psychotherapy in a variety of settings indicate its value.[156-158] Friedman and coworkers[159] found the infarction rate and cardiovascular mortality to be significantly lower in postinfarction patients who received both behavioral counseling to diminish Type A behavior and cardiological advice compared to the control subjects. Other management techniques involve medication, relaxation techniques, and follow-up counseling.[160] The marked psychological improvements may be the most striking aspect of a comprehensive rehabilitation program and may do much to restore overall performance and to enable the patient to return to as normal an active life as possible.

EMPLOYABILITY

Many consider the return to work to be *the* goal of cardiac rehabilitation. Actually, work outcomes can be viewed from several perspectives: the time required for resumption of usual work activities, current occupational activities compared with the patient's usual profession, the number of hours worked per week, or work capabilities. Currently, about 80 to 85 per cent of patients with an uncomplicated post-hospitalization course can return to their former jobs within 3 months of infarction;[8,64,161] about 65 per cent return to gainful employment post–coronary artery bypass grafting,[142] compared with an anticipated loss of 4 per cent per year in the general population in this age group.[162] Physiological improvements suffice in many instances to bring patients back to work, but other patients require additional motivation and reassurance from their physician and their families. Nonmedical factors appear paramount; the presence or absence of angina pectoris has limited impact on the percentage of patients returning to work after infarction,[163,164] although alleviation of postoperative symptoms plays a role in some studies.[142,162,164] Patients with more extensive coronary artery disease may delay their return to work, but the proportion returning to work is not substantially different from those with less disease; little correlation exists between employability and the severity or distribution of coronary artery disease.[142,165]

What does seem to be important in determining whether individuals will return to work is their ability to work *prior* to an infarction or cardiac operation. Individuals previously unemployed or retired rarely seek employment after medical treatment.[163] In fact, "doctor's advice" has been cited as another major reason for not working after myocardial infarction and coronary artery bypass grafting.[162,166] A number of factors have proved useful in determining whether a patient will return to work: employment and occupational type at admission to hospital, work history, nonwork income, availability to the previous job, perception of health, educational level, family and social stability, and psychological factors.[142,167] Cardiac rehabilitation has significantly helped in returning to employment men otherwise at high risk of remaining unemployed.[167]

In certain occupations—airplane pilots, truck drivers, and other positions where health is critical to the public welfare—resumption of previous activities is precluded. Other barriers to work rehabilitation include noncardiac disabilities, unsatisfactory work records, low occupational skills, unavailability of jobs, workmen's compensation and related legal decisions, and a variety of societal factors.[168] The misconception that myocardial infarction patients are not capable of hard physical work has led firms to reject cardiac patients from industrial positions, even though fewer than 10 per cent of occupational tasks are considered "heavy."[11] A useful publication for disability evaluation for cardiac disease is the American Medical Association's *Guide to the Evaluation of Permanent Impairment.*[169] Historically, determination of fitness to work has been established by work evaluation units. Although nonmedical factors greatly influence individual decisions on return to work, valuable information about prognosis and physical work capacity can be clarified by special evaluation techniques, especially exercise testing. If a patient exhibits no cardiovascular abnormalities under the physical stress of symptom-limited treadmill exercise testing, the probability is high that he will not encounter these abnormalities during ordinary working conditions.

DeBusk and Davidson[11] believe that short-term observation of the cardiovascular response during treadmill exercise testing is adequate to assess work potential, thus eliminating the need for simulation of the patient's occupational tasks. The job can be tailored to achievement on the exercise test using the maximal workload, heart rate, blood pressure response, and ischemic changes as guidelines for work activities. Ambulatory electrocardiograms or monitoring may be of value in special circumstances, but generally these more cumbersome methods are not necessary. The mean oxygen transport capacity for patients after a myocardial infarction ranges from 7 to 9 METS.[65,161] Such patients should be able to work easily at usual sedentary job requirements throughout the 8-hour day at an *average* level of 30 percent capacity,[24,170] or roughly 3 METS (Table 40–1). For those jobs involving strenuous activity, exertion tends to be of short duration, so that myocardial work is less than that during longer steady-state efforts. If the peak exertion required is brief, with the usual rest periods interspersed, even individuals with low physical work capacity can reach surprisingly high work levels before developing symptoms or signs of ischemia. However, both peak loads and average work requirements must be considered in evaluating work opportunities. The physician must understand the occupational requirements of patients and help them return to gainful employment.[12,162,171,172] Medical practitioners can work with employers to establish a satisfactory work environment perceived by the patients as nonthreatening to their health by recommending temporary limited-duty jobs, alternative job assignments, and job transfers that do not involve severe physiological or psychological stress.

Much remains to be done to identify and remove potential impediments to work for individuals with a standard of living or work ethic incompatible with early retirement. Delay in return to work or threatened loss of jobs poses major problems for them and society. Competition for jobs by younger individuals should be eliminated by the forthcoming shortage of younger workers during the next decade as the population ages. Such developments are likely to exaggerate the cost of failing to return to work cardiac patients capable of productive employment, as the rising cost of social services may well extend our working lifetimes past the current customary retirement age of 65.[12]

References

1. Hellerstein, H. K.: Cardiac rehabilitation: A retrospective view. *In* Pollock, M. L., and Schmidt, D. H. (eds.): Heart Disease Rehabilitation. Boston, Houghton Mifflin, 1979, pp. 509–520.
2. Kellerman, J.: Rehabilitation of patients with coronary heart disease. Prog. Cardiovasc. Dis. *17*:303, 1975.
3. Oberman, A., and Kouchoukos, N. T.: Role of exercise after coronary artery surgery. *In* Wenger, N. K. (Ed.): Exercise and the Heart. Philadelphia, F. A. Davis Co., 1978, pp. 155–172.
4. Newell, J. P., Kappagoda, C. T., Stoker, J. B., Deverall, P. B., Watson, D. A., and Linden, R. J.: Physical training after heart valve replacement. Br. Heart J. *44*:638, 1980.
5. Hassell, L. A., Fowles, R. E., and Stinson, E. B.: Patients with congestive cardiomyopathy as cardiac transplant recipients. Am. J. Cardiol. *47*:1205, 1981.
6. Arteriosclerosis 1981: Report of the Working Group on Arteriosclerosis for the National Heart, Lung, and Blood Institute, Vol. 2, June, 1981.
7. Sanne, H.: Selection of patients for cardiac rehabilitation. *In* James, W. E., and Amsterdam, E. A. (eds.): Coronary Heart Disease, Exercise Testing and Cardiac Rehabilitation. New York, Symposia Specialists, 1977, pp. 247–257.
8. Wenger, N. K., Hellerstein, H. K., and Blackburn, H.: Physician practice in the management of patients with uncomplicated myocardial infarction: Changes in the past decade. Circulation *65*:421, 1982.
9. Eliot, R. S.: Stress and the Major Cardiovascular Disorders. New York, Futura Publishing Co., 1979.
10. Croog, S. H., and Levine, S.: The Heart Patient Recovers. New York, Human Sciences Press, 1977.
11. DeBusk, R. F., and Davidson, D. M.: The work evaluation of the cardiac patient. J. Occup. Med. *22*:715, 1980.

12. Oberman, A., and Finklea, J. F.: Return to work after coronary artery bypass grafting. Ann. Thorac. Surg. 34:353, 1982.

13. Wenger, N.: Research related to rehabilitation. Circulation 60:1636, 1979.

14. Blomqvist, C. G., and Lewis, S. F.: Physiological effects of training: General circulatory adjustments. In Cohen, L. S., Mock, M. B., and Ringqvist, I. (eds.): Physical Conditioning and Cardiovascular Rehabilitation. New York, John Wiley and Sons, 1981, pp. 57–76.

15. Clausen, J. P.: Circulatory adjustments to dynamic exercise and effect of physical training in normal subjects and in patients with coronary artery disease. Prog. Cardiovasc. Dis. 18:459, 1976.

16. Scheuer, J., and Tipton, C. M.: Cardiovascular adaptations to physical training. Ann. Rev. Physiol. 39:221, 1977.

17. Conn, E. H., Williams, R. S., and Wallace, A. G.: Exercise responses before and after physical conditioning in patients with severely depressed left ventricular function. Am. J. Cardiol. 49:296, 1982.

18. Report of the Task Force on Cardiovascular Rehabilitation of the National Heart and Lung Institute: Needs and Opportunities for Rehabilitating the Coronary Heart Disease Patient. Washington, D.C., DHEW Publication No. (NIH) 75–750, 1974.

19. Jonason, A., Jonzon, B., Ringqvist, I., and Omar-Rydbert, A.: Effect of physical training on different categories of patients with intermittent claudication. Acta Med. Scand. 206:253, 1979.

20. Saltin, B.: Physical training in patients with intermittent claudication. In Cohen, L. S., Mock, M. B., and Ringqvist, I. (eds.): Physical Conditioning and Cardiovascular Rehabilitation. New York, John Wiley and Sons, 1981, pp. 181–196.

21. Stern, M. J., and Cleary, P.: National Exercise and Heart Disease Project: Psychosocial changes observed during a low-level exercise program. Arch. Intern. Med. 141:1463, 1981.

22. Hackett, T. P., and Cassem, N. H.: Psychological aspects of rehabilitation after myocardial infarction factors related to exercise. In Wenger, N. K., and Hellerstein, H. K. (eds.): Rehabilitation of the Coronary Patient. New York, John Wiley and Sons, 1978, pp. 243–253.

23. Council on Scientific Affairs: Physician-supervised exercise programs in rehabilitation of patients with coronary heart disease. J.A.M.A. 245:1463, 1981.

24. American Heart Association: The Exercise Standards Book. Circulation 59:421A, 1979.

25. The Committee on Exercise: Exercise Testing and Training of Individuals with Heart Disease or at High Risk for its Development: A Handbook for Physicians. Dallas, American Heart Association, 1975.

26. American College of Sports Medicine: Guidelines for Graded Exercise Testing and Exercise Prescription. Philadelphia, Lea and Febiger, 1980.

27. Pollock, M. L., Ward, A., and Foster, C.: Exercise prescription for rehabilitation of the cardiac patient. In Pollock, M. L., and Schmidt, D. H. (eds.): Heart Disease Rehabilitation. Boston, Houghton Mifflin, 1979, pp. 413–445.

28. Pratt, C. M., Welton, D. E., Squires, W. G., Kirgy, T. E., Hartung, G. H., and Miller, R. R.: Demonstration of training effect during chronic beta-adrenergic blockade in patients with coronary artery disease. Circulation 64:1125, 1981.

29. Vanhees, L., Fagard, R., and Amery, A.: Influence of beta adrenergic blockage on effects of physical training in patients with ischaemic heart disease. Br. Heart J. 48:33, 1982.

30. Myocardial infarction, exercise and prognosis. Lancet 1:78, 1980.

31. Hung, J., McKillip, J., Savin, W., Magder, S., Kraus, R., Houston, N., Goris, M., Haskell, W., and DeBusk, R.: Comparison of cardiovascular response to combined static-dynamic effort, postprandial dynamic effort and dynamic effort alone in patients with chronic ischemic heart disease. Circulation 65:1411, 1982.

32. Viitasalo, M. T., Kala, R., Eisalo, A., and Halonen, A.: Ventricular arrhythmias during exercise testing, jogging, and sedentary life. Chest 76:21, 1979.

33. McKinnis, R. A., Burks, H., Lee, K. L., Harrell, F. E., Behar, V. S., Pryor, V. S., Pryor, D. B., Wagner, G. S., and Rosati, R. A.: Prognostic implications of ventricular arrhythmias during 24 hour ambulatory monitoring in patients undergoing cardiac catheterization for coronary artery disease. Am. J. Cardiol. 50:23, 1982.

34. Simoons, M., Lap, C., and Pool, J.: Heart rate levels and ventricular ectopic activity during cardiac rehabilitation. Am. Heart J. 100:9, 1980.

35. Winkle, R. A.: The relationship between ventricular ectopic beat frequency and heart rate. Circulation 66:439, 1982.

36. Borg, G. A.: Psychophysical bases of perceived exertion. Med. Sci. Sports Exercise 14:377, 1982.

37. Wilson, P. K., Fardy, P. S., and Froelicher, V. F.: Cardiac Rehabilitation, Adult Fitness, and Exercise Testing. Philadelphia, Lea and Febiger, 1981, pp. 333–351.

38. Hellerstein, H. K., and Franklin, B. A.: Exercise testing and prescription. In Wenger, N. K., and Hellerstein, H. K. (eds.): Rehabilitation of the Coronary Patient. New York, John Wiley and Sons, 1978, pp. 149–202.

39. Haskell, W. L.: Design and implementation of cardiac conditioning programs. In Wenger, N. K., and Hellerstein, H. K. (eds.): Rehabilitation of the Coronary Patient. New York, John Wiley and Sons, 1978, pp. 203–241.

40. Fox, S. M., Naughton, J. P., and Gorman, P. A.: Physical activity and cardiovascular health: III. The exercise prescription: frequency and type of activity. Mod. Concepts Cardiovasc. Dis. 41:25, 1972.

41. Magder, S., Linnarsson, D., and Gullstrand, L.: The effect of swimming on patients with ischemic heart disease. Circulation 63:979, 1981.

42. Fletcher, G. F., Cantwell, J. D., and Watt, E. W.: Oxygen consumption and hemodynamic response of exercises used in training of patients with recent myocardial infarction. Circulation 60:140, 1979.

43. Ferguson, R. J., Cote, P., Bourassa, M. G., and Corbara, F.: Coronary blood flow during isometric and dynamic exercise in angina pectoris patients. J. Cardiac Rehabil. 1:21, 1981.

44. Harrison, T. R.: Abuse of rest as a therapeutic measure for patients with cardiovascular disease. J.A.M.A. 125:1075, 1944.

45. Levine, S. A., and Lown, B.: "Armchair" treatment of acute coronary thrombosis. J.A.M.A. 148:1365, 1952.

46. Harpur, J., Kellett, R. J., Conner, W. T., Galbraith, H. J. B., Hamilton, M., Murray, J. J., Swallow, J. H., and Rose, G. A.: Controlled trial of early mobilization and discharge from hospital in uncomplicated myocardial infarction. Lancet 2:1331, 1971.

47. Lamers, H. J., Drost, W. S. J., Kroon, B. J. M., van Es, L. A., Meilink-Holdemaker, L. J., and Birkenhager, L. H.: Early mobilization after myocardial infarction.: A controlled study. Br. Med. J. 1:277, 1973.

48. Boyle, J. A., and Lorimer, A. R.: Early mobilisation after uncomplicated myocardial infarction. Prospective study of 538 patients. Lancet 2:346, 1973.

49. Hayes, M. J., Morris, G. K., and Hampton, J. R.: Comparison of mobilization after two and nine days in uncomplicated myocardial infarction. Br. Med. J. 3:10, 1974.

50. Thornley, P. E., and Turner, R. W. D.: Rapid mobilisation after acute myocardial infarction; first step in rehabilitation and secondary prevention. Br. Heart J. 39:471, 1977.

51. Lindvall, K., Erhardt, L. R., Lundman, T., Rehnqvist, N., and Sjögren, A.: Early mobilization and discharge of patients with acute myocardial infarction. A prospective study using risk indicators and early exercise tests. Acta Med. Scand. 206:169, 1979.

52. West, R. R., and Henderson, A. H.: Randomized multicentre trial of early mobilisation after uncomplicated myocardial infarction. Br. Heart J. 42:381, 1979.

53. Block, A., Maeder, J. P., Haissly, J. C., Felix, J., and Blackburn, H.: Early mobilization after myocardial infarction: A controlled study. Am. J. Cardiol. 34:152, 1974.

54. Silvidi, G. E., Squires, R. W., Pollock, M. L., and Foster, C.: Hemodynamic responses and medical problems associated with early exercise and ambulation in coronary artery bypass graft surgery patients. J. Cardiac Rehab. 2:355–362, 1982.

55. Baker, J. T., Bramlet, D. A., Lester, R. M., Harrison, D. G., Roe, C. R., and Cobb, F. R.: Myocardial infarct extension: Incidence and relationship to survival. Circulation 65:918, 1982.

56. Wenger, N. K.: Rehabilitation of the coronary patient: Scope of the problem and responsibility of the primary care physician. Cardiovasc. Rev. Rep. 12:1249, 1981.

57. Sivarajan, E. S., Bruce, R. A., Almes, M. J., Green, B., Belanger, L., Lindskog, B. D., Newton, K. M., and Mansfield, L. W.: In-hospital exercise after myocardial infarction does not improve treadmill performance. N. Engl. J. Med. 305:358, 1981.

58. DeBusk, R. F., Houston, N., Haskell, W., Fry, G., and Parker, M.: Exercise training soon after myocardial infarction. Am. J. Cardiol. 44:1225, 1979.

59. Vaisrub, S.: Editorial: Exercise tests after myocardial infarction. J.A.M.A. 243:261, 1980.

60. Jelinek, M. V., Ziffer, R. W., McDonald, D. G., Wasir, H., and Hale, S. G.: Early exercise testing and mobilization after myocardial infarction. Med. J. Aust. 29:589, 1977.

61. Theroux, P., Waters, D. D., Halphen, C., Debaisieux, J. C., and Mizgala, H. F.: Prognostic value of exercise testing soon after myocardial infarction. N. Engl. J. Med. 301:341, 1979.

61a. Ewart, C. K., Taylor, B., Reese, L., and DeBusk, R. F.: Effects of early postinfarction exercise testing on self perception and subsequent physical activity. J. Am. Coll. Cardiol. 1:662, 1983.

62. Bruce, R. A.: Exercise tests. In Cohen, L. S., Mock, M. B., and Ringqvist, I., (eds.): Physician Conditioning and Cardiovascular Rehabilitation. New York, John Wiley and Sons, 1981, pp. 3–22.

62a. Ewart, C. K., Taylor, C. B., Reese, L. B., and DeBusk, R. F.: Effects of early postmyocardial infarction exercise testing on self-perception and subsequent physical activity. Am. J. Cardiol. 51:1076, 1983.

63. Hung, J., Criley, J. M., and Corne, R. A.: Effects of bedrest and deconditioning on exercise ventricular function in middle-aged men. American College of Cardiology Extended Learning Tape, Vol. 13, No. 11, November, 1981.

64. Acker, J. E., Jr.: Medical benefits and concerns in cardiac rehabilitation. In Pollock, M. L., and Schmidt, D. H. (eds.): Heart Disease and Rehabilitation. Boston, Houghton Mifflin Professional Publishers, 1979, pp. 654–662.

65. Naughton, J.: The National Exercise and Heart Disease Project: Development, Recruitment, and Implementation. In Wenger, N. K. (ed.): Exercise and the Heart. Philadelphia, F. A. Davis Co., 1978.

66. Williams, R. S., Miller, H., Koisch, F. P., Ribisl, P. and Graden, H.: Guidelines for unsupervised exercise in patients with ischemic heart disease. J. Cardiac Rehabil. 1:213, 1981.

67. Pyfer, H. R.: Guidelines for unsupervised exercise in patients with ischemic heart disease, Commentary 1. J. Cardiac Rehabil. 1:217, 1981.

68. Oberman, A.: Guidelines for unsupervised exercise in patients with ischemic heart disease, Commentary 2. J. Cardiac Rehabil. 1:218, 1981.

69. Kavanagh, T., and Shephard, R. J.: Exercise for postcoronary patients: An assessment of infrequent supervision. Arch. Phys. Med. Rehabil. 61:114, 1980.
70. Oberman, A.: Cardiac rehabilitation, key references. Circulation 62:909, 1980.
71. Kannel, W. B.: Prospects for risk factor modification to reduce risk of reinfarction and premature death. J. Cardiac Rehabil. 1:63, 1982.
72. May, G. S., Eberlein, K. A., Furberg, C. D., Passamani, E. R., and DeMets, D. L.: Secondary prevention after myocardial infarction: A review of long-term trials. Prog. Cardiovasc. Dis. 24:331, 1982.
73. Salonen, J. T., and Puska, P.: A community programme for rehabilitation and secondary prevention for patients with acute myocardial infarction as part of a comprehensive community programme for control of cardiovascular disease (North Karelia Project). Scand. J. Rehabil. Med. 12:33, 1980.
74. Puska, P., Tuomilehto, J., Salonen, J. T., et al.: Community control of cardiovascular disease: Evaluation of a comprehensive community programme for control of cardiovascular diseases in 1972–77 in North Karelia, Finland. Geneva, WHO Monograph Series, 1981.
75. Kallio, V., Hamalainen, H., Hakkila, J., and Luurila, O. J.: Reduction in sudden deaths by a multifactorial intervention programme after acute myocardial infarction. Lancet 2:1091, 1979.
76. Vedin, A., Wilhemsson, C., Tibblin, G., and Wilhelmsen, L.: The post-infarction clinic in Göteborg, Sweden. A controlled trial of a therapeutic organization. Acta Med. Scand. 200:453, 1976.
76a. Vermeulen, A., Lie, K. I., and Durrer, D.: Effects of cardiac rehabilitation after myocardial infarction: Changes in coronary risk factors and long-term prognosis. Am. Heart J. 105:798, 1983.
77. The Norwegian Multicenter Study Group: Timolol-induced reduction in mortality and reinfarction in patients surviving acute myocardial infarction. N. Engl. J. Med. 304:801, 1981.
77a. Hansteen, V.: Beta blockade after myocardial infarction: The Norwegian propranolol study in high-risk patients. Circulation 67 (Suppl. 1):57, 1983.
77b. Goldstein, S.: Propranolol therapy in patients with acute myocardial infarction: The beta-blocker heart attack trial. Circulation 67 (Suppl. 1):53, 1983.
77c. Turi, Z. G., and Braunwald, E.: The use of beta blockers after myocardial infarction. JAMA 249:2512, 1983.
77d. Furberg, C. D., Friedewald, W. T., and Eberlein, K. A. (eds.): Proceedings of the workshop on implications of recent beta-blocker trials for post-myocardial infarction patients. Circulation 67:1–111, 1983.
78. β-Blocker Heart Attack Trial Research Group: A randomized trial of propranolol in patients with acute myocardial infarction. I. Mortality Results. J.A.M.A. 247:1707, 1982.
79. National Institutes Of Health Consensus Development Conference Statement on Coronary Bypass Surgery. Scientific and Clinical Aspects. Circulation 65 (Suppl. II):126, 1982.
80. Rahimtoola, S. H.: Coronary bypass surgery for chronic angina — 1981: a perspective. Circulation 65:225, 1982.
81. Ross, J. K., Monro, J. L., Diwell, A. E., Mackean, J. M., Marsh, J., and Barjer, D. H. P.: The quality of life after cardiac surgery. Br. Med. J. 282:451, 1981.
82. Kannel, W. B., Doyle, J. T., and Ostfeld, A. M.: American Heart Association Committee Report: Risk factors and coronary disease. Circulation 62:449A, 1980.
83. Oberman, A.: Natural history of coronary artery disease. In Racklay, C. E., and Russell, R. O. (eds.): Coronary Artery Disease: Recognition and Management. New York, Futura Publishing Co., 1979, pp. 1–30.
84. Schlant, R. C., Forman, S., Stamler, J., and Canner, P. L.: The natural history of coronary heart disease: Prognostic factors after recovery from myocardial infarction in 2789 men. The five-year findings of the Coronary Drug Project. Circulation 66:401, 1982.
85. Castelli, W. P., Dawber, T. R., Feinleib, M., Garrison, R. J., McNamara, P. M., and Kannel, W. B.: The filter cigarette and coronary heart disease: The Framingham Study. Lancet 2:109, 1981.
86. Vliestra, R. E., Kronmal, R. A., and Oberman, A.: Stopping smoking improves survival in patients with angiographically proven coronary artery disease (Abstr.). Am. J. Cardiol. 49:984, 1982.
87. Ashley, F. W., Jr., and Kannel, W. B.: Relation of weight change to changes in atherogenic traits: The Framingham Study. J. Chron. Dis. 27:103, 1974.
88. Castelli, W. P., Doyle, J. T., Gordon, T., Hames, C. G., Hjortland, M. C., Hulley, S. B., Kagan, A., and Zukel, W. J.: HDL-cholesterol and other lipids in coronary heart disease. The cooperative lipoprotein phenotyping study. Circulation 55:767, 1977.
89. Joint Recommendations by the International Society and Federation of Cardiology Scientific Councils on Arteriosclerosis, Epidemiology and Prevention, and Rehabilitation. Br. Med. J. 282:894, 1981.
90. Rationale of the diet-heart statement of the American Heart Association: Report of the AHA Nutrition Committee. Arteriosclerosis 4:177, 1982.
91. Oliver, M. F.: Serum cholesterol — the knave of hearts and the joker. Lancet 2:1090, 1981.
92. Hypertension Detection and Follow-Up Cooperative Group: Five-year findings of the Hypertension Detection and Follow-Up Program: I. Reduction in mortality of persons with high blood pressure, including mild hypertension. J.A.M.A. 242:2562, 1979.
93. Bukley, B. H., and Hutchins, G. M.: Accelerated "atherosclerosis": A morphologic study of 97 saphenous vein coronary artery bypass grafts. Circulation 55:163, 1977.
94. Hartung, G. H., Squires, W. G., and Gotto, A. M.: Effect of exercise training on plasma high-density lipoprotein cholesterol in coronary disease patients. Am. Heart J. 101:181, 1981.
95. Bjorntorp, P., Berchtold, P., Grimby, G., Lindholm, B., Sanne, H., Tibblin, G., and Wilhelmsen, L.: Effects of physical training on glucose tolerance, plasma insulin after lipids and on body composition in men after myocardial infarction. Acta Med. Scand. 192:439, 1972.
96. Fletcher, G. F., and Cantwell, J. D.: Exercise and Coronary Heart Disease. Springfield, Ill., Charles C Thomas, 1974, pp. 31–45.
97. Ballantyne, F. C., Clark, R. S., Simpson, H. S., and Ballantyne, D.: The effect of modern physical exercise on the plasma lipoprotein subfractions of male survivors of myocardial infarction. Circulation 65:913, 1982.
98. Berg, A., Keul, J., Ringwald, G., Stippig, J., and Deus, B.: Serum lipoprotein cholesterol in sedentary and trained male patients with coronary heart disease. Clin. Cardiol. 4:233, 1981.
99. Haskell, W. L.: Influence of habitual physical activity on blood lipids and lipoproteins. In Cohen, L. S., Mock, M. B., and Ringqvist, I. (eds.): Physical Conditioning and Cardiovascular Rehabilitation. New York, John Wiley and Sons, 1981, pp. 87–102.
100. Pedersen, O., Beck-Nielsen, H., and Heding, L.: Increased insulin receptors after exercise in patients with insulin-dependent diabetes mellitus. N. Engl. J. Med. 302:886, 1980.
101. Haskell, W. L.: Mechanisms by which physical activity may enhance the clinical status of cardiac patients. In Pollock, M. L., and Schmidt, D. (eds.): Heart Disease and Rehabilitation. Boston, Mass., Houghton Mifflin Professional Publishers, 1979, pp. 276–296.
102. Stern, M. J., and Cleary, P.: Long-term psychosocial outcome. Arch. Intern. Med. 152:1093, 1982.
103. Blumenthal, J. A., Williams, S., Williams, R. B., and Wallace, A. G.: Effects of exercise on the type A (coronary prone) behavior pattern. Psychosom. Med. 42:289, 1980.
104. Epstein, S. E., Rosing, D. R., and Brakman, P.: Impaired fibrinolytic response to exercise in patients with type IV hyperlipoproteinemia. Lancet 2:631, 1970.
105. Williams, R. S., Logue, E. E., and Lewis, J. L.: Physical conditioning augments the fibrinolytic response to venous occlusion in healthy adults. N. Engl. J. Med. 302:987, 1980.
106. Fox, S. M., Naughton, J. P., and Gorman, P. A.: Physical activity and cardiovascular health (Part I). Mod. Concepts Cardiovasc. Dis. 41:17, 1972.
107. Oberman, A., Cleary, P., LaRosa, J. C., Hellerstein, H. K., and Naughton, J.: Changes in risk factors among long-term exercise rehabilitation program participants. Adv. Cardiol. 31, 1983.
108. Shephard, R. J.: Cardiac rehabilitation in prospect. In Pollock, M. L., and Schmidt, D. H. (eds.): Heart Disease and Rehabilitation. Boston, Houghton Mifflin Professional Publishers, 1979, pp. 521–547.
109. Williams, P. T., Wood, P. D., Haskell, W. L., and Vranizan, K.: The effect of running mileage and duration on plasma lipoprotein levels. J.A.M.A. 247:2674, 1982.
110. Redwood, D. R., Rosing, D. R., and Epstein, S. E.: Circulatory and symptomatic effects of physical training in patients with coronary-artery disease and angina pectoris. N. Engl. J. Med. 286:959, 1972.
111. Dressendorfer, R. H., and Scaff, J. H.: Cardiorespiratory responses to marathon running in cardiac patients. Med. Sci. Sports 7:71, 1975.
112. Kavanagh, T., Shephard, R. H., and Pandit, V.: Marathon running after myocardial infarction. J.A.M.A. 229:1602, 1974.
113. Kavanagh, T., Shephard, R. J., and Kennedy, J.: Characteristics of postcoronary marathon runners. In Milvy, P. (ed.): The Marathon: Physiological, Medical, Epidemiological, and Psychological Studies. New York, New York Academy of Sciences, 1977, pp. 455–515.
114. Gobel, F. L., Nordstrom, L. A., Nelson, R. R., Jorgensen, C. R., and Wang, Y.: The rate-pressure product as an index of myocardial oxygen consumption during exercise in patients with angina pectoris. Circulation 57:549, 1978.
115. Ehsani, A. A., Heath, G. W., Hagberg, J. M., Sobel, B. E., and Holloszy, J. O.: Effects of 12 months of intense exercise training on ischemic ST-segment depression in patients with coronary artery disease. Circulation 64:1116, 1981.
116. Sim, D. N., and Neill, W. A.: Investigation of the physiological basis for increased exercise threshold for angina pectoris after physical conditioning. J. Clin. Invest. 54:763, 1974.
117. Detry, J. M., and Bruce, R. A.: Effects of physical training on exertional ST segment depression in coronary heart disease. Circulation 44:390, 1971.
118. Ehsani, A. A., Martin, W. H., Heath, G., and Coyle, E. F.: Cardiac effects of prolonged and intense exercise training in patients with coronary artery disease. Am. J. Cardiol. 50:246, 1982.
119. Paterson, D. H., Shephard, R. J., Cunningham, D., Jones, N. L., and Andrew, G.: Effects of physical training on cardiovascular function following myocardial infarction. J. Appl. Physiol. 47:482, 1979.
120. Cobb, F. R., Williams, R. S., McEwan, P., Jones, R. H., Coleman, R. E., and Wallace, A. G.: Effects of exercise training on ventricular function in patients with recent myocardial infarction. Circulation 66:100, 1982.
121. DeMaria, A. N., Neumann, A., Lee, G., Fowler, W., and Mason, D. T.: Alterations in ventricular mass and performance induced by exercise training in man evaluated by echocardiography. Circulation 57:237, 1978.
122. Jensen, D., Atwood, J. E., Froelicher, V., McKirnam, M. D., Battler, A., Ashburn, W., and Ross, J.: Improvement in ventricular function during exercise studied with radionuclide ventriculography after cardiac rehabilitation. Am. J. Cardiol. 46:770, 1980.
123. Holloszy, J. O., Skinner, J. S., Barry, A. J., et al.: Effect of physical condition-

ing on cardiovascular function—a ballistocardiographic study. Am. J. Cardiol. *14:*761, 1964.

124. Froelicher, V. F., and Brown, P.: Exercise and coronary heart disease. J. Cardiac Rehabil. *1:*277, 1981.

125. Epstein, L., Miller, G. J., Stitt, F. W., and Morris, J. N.: Vigorous exercise in leisure time, coronary risk factors, and resting electrocardiogram in middle-aged male civil servants. Br. Heart J. *38:*403, 1976.

126. Scheuer, J.: Effects of physical training on myocardial vascularity and perfusion. Circulation *66:*491, 1982.

127. Kramsch, D. M., Aspen, A. J., Abramowitz, B. M., Kreimendahl, T., and Hood, W. B.: Reduction of coronary atherosclerosis by moderate conditioning exercise in monkeys on an atherogenic diet. N. Engl. J. Med. *305:*1483, 1981.

128. Kennedy, C. C., Spiekerman, R. E., Lindsay, M. I., et al.: One-year graduated exercise program for men with angina pectoris. Mayo Clin. Proc. *51:*231, 1976.

129. Ferguson, R. J., Petitclerc, R., Choquette, G., et al.: Effect of physical training on treadmill exercise capacity, collateral circulation and progression of coronary disease. Am. J. Cardiol. *134:*764, 1974.

130. Nolewajka, A. J., Kostuk, W. J., Rechnitzer, P. A., and Cunningham, D. A.: Exercise and human collateralization: An angiographic scintigraphic assessment. Circulation *60:*114, 1979.

131. Wilhelmsen, L., Sanne, H., Elmfeldt, D., Grimby, G., Tibblin, G., and Wedel, H.: A controlled trial of physical training after myocardial infarction. Prev. Med. *4:*491, 1975.

132. Kentala, E.: Physical fitness and feasibility of physical rehabilitation after myocardial infarction in men of working age. Ann. Clin. Res. *4*(Suppl. 9):1, 1972.

133. Palatsi, I.: Feasibility of physical training after myocardial infarction and its effect on return to work, morbidity and mortality. Acta Med. Scand. (Suppl.):599, 1976.

134. Shephard, R. J.: Evaluation of earlier studies: Canada. *In* Cohen, L. S., Mock, M. B., and Ringqvist, I. (eds.): Physical Conditioning and Cardiovascular Rehabilitation. New York, John Wiley and Sons, 1981, pp. 271–288.

135. Shaw, L. W.: Effects of a prescribed supervised exercise program on mortality and cardiovascular morbidity in patients after a myocardial infarction. Am. J. Cardiol. *48:*39, 1981.

136. Haskell, W. L.: Cardiovascular complications during exercise training of cardiac patients. Circulation *57:*920, 1974.

137. Cay, E. L.: Psychological approach in patient after a myocardial infarction. Adv. Cardiol. *24:*120, 1978.

138. Stern, M. J., and Pascale, L.: Psychosocial adaptation post myocardial infarction: The spouse's dilemma. J. Psychosom. Res. *23:*83, 1979.

139. Davidson, D. M.: The family and cardiac rehabilitation. J. Fam. Pract. *8:*253, 1979.

140. International Society of Cardiology, Scientific Council on Rehabilitation of Cardiac Patients: Myocardial Infarction: How to Prevent, How to Rehabilitate, Mannheim, West Germany, Boehringer, 1973.

141. Heller, S. S., Frank, K. A., Kornfeld, D. S., et al.: Psychological outcome following open-heart surgery. Arch. Intern. Med. *5:*67, 1974.

142. Oberman, A., Wayne, J. B., Kouchoukos, N. T., Charles, E. D., Russell, R. O., and Rogers, W. J.: Employment status after coronary artery bypass surgery. Circulation *65*(Suppl. II):115, 1982.

143. Alpert, J. S.: The Heart Attack Handbook: A Common Sense Guide to Treatment, Recovery and Prevention. Boston, Little Brown and Co., 1978.

144. Farquhar, J. W.: The American Way of Life Need Not be Hazardous to Your Health. New York, W. W. Norton, 1978.

145. Halhuber, M. J.: Health education in cardiac rehabilitation. Adv. Cardiol. *24:*146, 1978.

146. Brammell, H. L., McDaniel, J. W., Niccoli, S. A., Darnell, R., and Roberson, D. R.: Cardiac Rehabilitation: A Handbook for Vocational Rehabilitation Counselors. Denver, University of Colorado Medical Center, Webb-Waring Lung Institute, 1979.

147. Cohn, K., Duke, D., and Madrid, J. A.: Coming Back: A guide to recovering from heart attack and living confidently with coronary disease. Reading, Mass., Addison-Wesley Publishing Co., 1979.

148. Zohman, L. R., Kattus, A. A., and Softness, D. G.: The Cardiologists' Guide to Fitness and Health Through Exercise. New York, Simon and Schuster, 1979.

149. American Medical Association: Book of Heart Care. New York, Random House, 1982.

150. An Active Partnership for the Health of Your Heart. Audiovisual modules. Santa Clara, Cal., American Heart Association, 1976.

151. Kavanagh, T., and Shephard, R. J.: Sexual activity after myocardial infarction. Can. Med. Assoc. J. *116:*1250, 1977.

152. Hellerstein, H. K., and Friedman, E. H.: Sexual activity and the postcoronary patient. Med. Aspects Hum. Sex. *3:*70, 1973.

153. McLane, M., Krop, H., and Mehta, J.: Psychosexual adjustment and counseling after myocardial infarction. Ann. Intern. Med. *92:*514, 1980.

154. Smith, R. T.: The role of social resources in cardiac rehabilitation. *In* Cohen, L. S., Mock, M. B., Ringqvist, I. (eds.): Physical Conditioning and Cardiovascular Rehabilitation. New York, John Wiley and Sons, 1981, pp. 221–232.

155. Gruen, W.: Effects of brief psychotherapy during the hospitalization period on the recovery process in heart attacks. J. Consult. Clin. Psychol. *43:*223, 1975.

156. Hackett, T. P.: The use of groups in the rehabilitation of the postcoronary patient. Adv. Cardiol. *24:*127, 1978.

157. Munford, E., Schlesinger, H. J., and Glass, G. V.: The effects of psychological intervention on recovery from surgery and heart attacks: An analysis of the literature. Am. J. Pub. Health *72:*141, 1982.

158. Rahe, R. H., Ward, H. W., and Hayes, V.: Brief group therapy in myocardial infarction rehabilitation; three- to four-year follow-up of a controlled trial. Psychosom. Med. *41:*229, 1979.

159. Friedman, M., Thoresen, C. E., Gill, J. J., Ulmer, D., Thompson, L., Powell, L., Price, V., Elek, S. R., Rabin, D. D., Breall, W. S., Piaget, G., Dixon, T., Bourg, E., Levy, R. A., and Tasto, D. L.: Feasibility of altering type A behavior pattern after myocardial infarction. Circulation *66:*83, 1982.

160. Hackett, T. P., and Rosenbaum, J. F.: Emotion, psychiatric disorders, and the heart. *In* Braunwald, E. (ed.): Heart Disease: A Textbook of Cardiovascular Medicine. Philadelphia, W. B. Saunders Co., 1984, pp. 1826–1844.

161. Muir, J. R.: The rehabilitation of cardiac patients. Proc. R. Soc. Med. *70:*655, 1977.

162. Johnson, W. D., Kayser, K. L., Pedraza, P. M., and Shore, R. T.: Employment patterns in males before and after myocardial revascularization surgery. A study of 229 consecutive male patients followed for as long as 10 years. Circulation *65:*1086, 1982.

163. Davidson, D. M., Taylor, C. B., and DeBusk, R. F.: Factors influencing return to work after myocardial infarction or coronary artery bypass surgery. J. Cardiac Rehabil. *10:*1, 1979.

164. Guvendik, L., Rahan, M., and Yacoub, M.: Symptomatic status and pattern of employment during a five year period following myocardial revascularization for angina. Ann. Thorac. Surg. *34:*383, 1982.

165. Nitter-Hauge, S., Noreik, K., Simonsen, S., Storstein, O., Bjorbaek, T., and Steen, A.: Studies of correlation between progression of coronary artery disease, as assessed by coronary arteriography, left ventricular end-diastolic pressure, ejection fraction, and employability. Br. Heart J. *39:*884, 1977.

166. Oberman, A., and Kouchoukos, N.: Working status of patients following coronary bypass surgery. Am. Heart J. *98:*132, 1979.

167. Schiller, E., and Baker, J.: Return to work after a myocardial infarction; evaluation of planned rehabilitation and of a predictive rating scale. Med. J. Austr. *1* :859, 1976.

168. American Heart Association: Report of the Committee on Stress, Strain and Heart Disease. Dallas, Texas, News from the AHA, 825A–835A, 1976.

169. American Medical Association, Committee on Rating of Mental and Physical Impairment: Guides to the evaluation of permanent impairment. Monroe, Wisconsin, 1977.

170. Astrand, P. O., and Rodahl, K.: Textbook of Work Physiology: Physiological Bases of Exercise. 2nd ed. New York, McGraw-Hill Book Co., 1977.

171. Liddle, H. V., Jenson, R., and Clayton, P. D.: The rehabilitation of coronary surgical patients. Ann. Thorac. Surg. *34:*374, 1982.

172. Horgan, J. H., Teo, K. K., Murren, K. M., and O'Riodan, J. M.: The response to exercise training and vocational counseling in post myocardial infarction and coronary artery bypass surgery patients. Ir. Med. J. *73:*444, 1980.

41

THE CARDIOMYOPATHIES AND MYOCARDITIDES

by Joshua Wynne, M.D., and Eugene Braunwald, M.D.

CLASSIFICATION

The cardiomyopathies are diseases involving the heart muscle itself.[1-3] They are unique in that they are not the result of ischemic,* hypertensive, congenital, valvular, or pericardial diseases (Table 41-1). While exclusion of these etiological factors is necessary for the diagnosis of cardiomyopathy, this form of heart disease is often sufficiently distinctive—both clinically and hemodynamically—to allow a positive diagnosis to be made.[4] With increasing awareness of this condition by clinicians, along with improvements in diagnostic techniques, cardiomyopathy is being recognized as a major cause of morbidity and mortality. In some areas of the world, it accounts for 30 per cent or more of all deaths due to heart disease.[5]

A variety of schemes have been proposed for classifying the cardiomyopathies.[2,3,5-8] Most useful from a clinical standpoint is a *functional* classification that emphasizes common pathophysiological abnormalities. Three basic categories of functional impairment have been described (Table 41-2): (1) *dilated* (formerly called congestive), characterized by ventricular dilatation, contractile dysfunction, and often symptoms of congestive heart failure; (2) *hypertrophic*, recognized by inappropriate left ventricular hypertrophy, often with asymmetrical involvement of the septum, with preserved or enhanced contractile function; and (3) *restrictive*, marked by endocardial scarring of the ventricle, with impairment of diastolic filling. The distinctions between these three functional categories are not absolute, and there is often overlap; in particular, patients with hypertrophic cardiomyopathy also have increased wall stiffness (as a consequence of the myocardial hypertrophy) and thus present some of the features of a restrictive cardiomyopathy.[9] Table 41-3 shows the echo-cardiographic characteristics of the three types of cardiomyopathies. We believe it is useful to divide the cardiomyopathies into primary and secondary forms. *Primary cardiomyopathies* are conditions in which: (1) the basic pathological process involves the myocardium rather than the valves or other cardiac structures, and (2) the cause of the heart disease is unknown and not part of a disorder affecting other organs. *Secondary cardiomyopathies* are conditions in which the cause of the myocardial abnormality is known or in which the cardiomyopathy is one manifestation of a systemic disease process, such as sarcoid.

ENDOMYOCARDIAL BIOPSY. Evaluation of the patient suspected of suffering from a cardiomyopathy has been facilitated by the use of endomyocardial biopsy (p. 297). Using a flexible bioptome, the clinician may obtain a tissue sample from the right or left ventricle via a transvenous or transarterial approach. Endomyocardial biopsy results in a small tissue sample (average size < 1 mm^3),[10] and five or more biopsies are often required to be certain of a given histological finding, since pronounced topographic variations may be found within the myocardium.[11] It remains controversial as to which patients with cardiomyopathy should be subjected to biopsy, but there is general agreement that biopsy may be of benefit in certain specific situations (Table 41-4). Although on occasion endomyocardial biopsy may identify a specific etiological agent in an individual patient with cardiac disease of uncertain cause (Table 41-5 and Fig. 41-1), the clinical utility of routine biopsy in cardiomyopathy remains uncertain.[10,11] While diagnostic abnormalities may be detected in the hypertrophic and restrictive cardiomyopathies, no definitive pattern has been found in dilated cardiomyopathy.[10]

DILATED CARDIOMYOPATHY

IDIOPATHIC DILATED CARDIOMYOPATHY

Dilated cardiomyopathy is a syndrome characterized by cardiac enlargement and often by the development of congestive heart failure. Formerly called congestive cardiomyopathy, the term *dilated cardiomyopathy* is now preferred, since the earliest abnormality is ventricular enlargement and systolic contractile dysfunction, with congestive heart failure often (but not invariably) developing later. It is characterized principally by impaired systolic pump function,[9,12] and both the end-diastolic and end-systolic volumes are increased. Ventricular wall thickness may be normal, increased, or decreased, and left ventricular filling pressure is usually elevated as a consequence of the poorly contractile left ventricle,[13] although decreased left ventricular compliance may contribute to the elevated filling pressures.[14]

Although the etiology is not definable in many cases, the dilated cardiomyopathies probably represent a final common pathway that is the end result of myocardial damage produced by a variety of toxic, metabolic, or infectious agents.[12,13] Alcohol, for example, may lead to severe

---

*The term *ischemic cardiomyopathy* refers to the condition in which ischemic heart disease causes diffuse fibrosis or multiple infarctions and leads to heart failure with left ventricular dilatation; it may or may not be associated with angina pectoris (p. 1363).

TABLE 41–1   IMPORTANT CAUSES OF CARDIOMYOPATHY AND MYOCARDITIS

1. Inflammatory
   a. Infective
      Viral
      Rickettsial
      Bacterial
      Mycobacterial
      Spirochetal
      Fungal
      Parasitic
   b. Noninfective
      Collagen diseases
2. Metabolic
   a. Nutritional
      Thiamine
      Kwashiorkor
      Pellagra
      Scurvy
      Hypervitaminosis D
      Obesity
   b. Endocrine
      Acromegaly
      Thyrotoxicosis
      Myxedema
      Uremia
      Cushing's disease
      Pheochromocytoma
      Diabetes mellitus
   c. Altered metabolism
      Gout
      Oxalosis
      Porphyria
   d. Electrolyte imbalance
3. Toxic
   a. Cobalt
   b. Alcohol
   c. Bleomycin
   d. Adriamycin
   e. Phenothiazines
   f. Antimony compounds
   g. Carbon monoxide
   h. Lead
   i. Emetine and dehydroemetine
   j. Chloroquine
   k. Lithium
   l. Cyclophosphamide
   m. Hydrocarbons
   n. Catecholamines
   o. Phosphorus
   p. Mercury
   q. Insect stings
   r. Snake bites
   s. Paracetamol
   t. Reserpine
   u. Corticosteroids

4. Infiltrative
   a. Amyloidosis
   b. Hemochromatosis
   c. Neoplastic
   d. Glycogen storage disorders
   e. Sarcoidosis
   f. Mucopolysaccharidosis
   g. Fabry's disease
   h. Whipple's disease
   i. Gaucher's disease
5. Fibroplastic
   a. Endomyocardial fibrosis
   b. Endocardial fibroelastosis
   c. Löffler's fibroplastic endocarditis
   d. Becker's disease
   e. Carcinoid
6. Hematological
   a. Sickle cell anemia
   b. Polycythemia vera
   c. Thrombotic thrombocytopenic purpura
   d. Leukemia
7. Hypersensitivity
   a. Methyldopa
   b. Penicillin
   c. Sulfonamides
   d. Tetracycline
   e. Phenindione
   f. Phenylbutazone
   g. Antituberculous drugs
   h. Giant cell myocarditis
   i. Cardiac transplant rejection
8. Genetic
   a. Hypertrophic cardiomyopathy
      With gradient
      Without gradient
   b. Neuromuscular
      Duchenne's muscular dystrophy
      Facioscapulohumeral muscular dystrophy
      Limb-girdle dystrophy of Erb
      Myotonia dystrophica
      Friedreich's ataxia
9. Miscellaneous acquired
   a. Postpartum cardiomyopathy
   b. Obesity
10. Idiopathic
    a. Idiopathic dilated cardiomyopathy
    b. Idiopathic restrictive cardiomyopathy
    c. Idiopathic hypertrophic cardiomyopathy
11. Physical agents
    a. Heat stroke
    b. Hypothermia
    c. Radiation

cardiac dysfunction and congestive heart failure and present clinical, hemodynamic, and pathological findings identical to those present in idiopathic dilated cardiomyopathy, which, in the final analysis, is a diagnosis of exclusion. The course of idiopathic dilated cardiomyopathy is usually one of progressive deterioration[8a]; the majority of patients succumb within four years after the onset of symptoms,[9] although a minority improve, with a reduction in cardiac size and longer survival.[15] Age greater than 55 years, a cardiothoracic ratio greater than 0.55, and a cardiac index less than 3.0 liters/min/m² each identifies patients with a greater than 85 per cent mortality (Fig. 41–2).[15]

PATHOLOGY. *Postmortem examination* discloses enlargement and dilatation of all four chambers; the ventricles are more dilated than the atria. While the thickness of the ventricular wall is increased in some cases, the degree of hypertrophy is often inadequate for the severe dilatation present.[16] The development of left ventricular hypertrophy may have a protective or beneficial role in dilated cardio-

myopathy, since it may serve to reduce systolic wall stress and protect against further cavity dilatation.[17] In patients with equivalent degrees of chamber enlargement, survival is longer in those with a greater degree of left ventricular hypertrophy.[17] The cardiac valves are intrinsically normal, and intracavitary thrombi, particularly in the ventricular apex, are common.[9,16] A nonspecific form of endocardial thickening that underlies the ventricular thrombi is often observed.[16,18] The coronary arteries are usually normal.[18]

Histological examination reveals extensive areas of interstitial and perivascular fibrosis, occasionally associated with calcification, within the walls of the ventricles.[16,19] Small areas of necrosis and cellular infiltrate are seen on occasion, but these are not prominent features.[18] Quantitative analysis of myocardial samples has shown a reduction in the number of neurons in dilated cardiomyopathy, but the significance of this finding is unclear at present.[20] Cardiac biopsy specimens obtained during life by a transvenous or transthoracic approach demonstrate a variety of

TABLE 41–2   FUNCTIONAL CLASSIFICATION OF THE CARDIOMYOPATHIES

	DILATED	RESTRICTIVE	HYPERTROPHIC
Symptoms	Congestive heart failure, particularly left-sided	Dyspnea, fatigue	Dyspnea, angina pectoris
	Fatigue and weakness	Right-sided congestive heart failure	Fatigue, syncope, palpitations
	Systemic or pulmonary emboli	Signs and symptoms of systemic disease: amyloidosis, iron storage disease, etc.	
Physical Examination	Moderate to severe cardiomegaly; S_3 and S_4	Mild to moderate cardiomegaly; S_3 or S_4	Mild cardiomegaly
			Apical systolic thrill and heave; brisk carotid upstroke
	Atrioventricular valve regurgitation, especially mitral	Atrioventricular valve regurgitation; inspiratory increase in venous pressure (Kussmaul's sign)	S_4 common
			Systolic murmur that increases with Valsalva maneuver
Chest Roentgenogram	Moderate to marked cardiac enlargement, especially left ventricular	Mild cardiac enlargement	Mild to moderate cardiac enlargement
	Pulmonary venous hypertension	Pulmonary venous hypertension	Left atrial enlargement
Electrocardiogram	Sinus tachycardia	Low voltage	Left ventricular hypertrophy
	Atrial and ventricular arrhythmias	Intraventricular conduction defects	ST-segment and T-wave abnormalities
	ST-segment and T-wave abnormalities	AV conduction defects	Abnormal Q waves
	Intraventricular conduction defects		Atrial and ventricular arrhythmias
Echocardiogram	Left ventricular dilatation and dysfunction	Increased left ventricular wall thickness and mass	Asymmetrical septal hypertrophy (ASH)
	Abnormal diastolic mitral valve motion secondary to abnormal compliance and filling pressures	Small or normal-sized left ventricular cavity	Narrow left ventricular outflow tract
		Normal systolic function	Systolic anterior motion (SAM) of the mitral valve
		Pericardial effusion	Small or normal-sized left ventricle
Radionuclide Studies	Left ventricular dilatation and dysfunction (RVG)	Infiltration of myocardium (^{201}Tl)	Small or normal-sized left ventricle (RVG)
		Small or normal-sized left ventricle (RVG)	Vigorous systolic function (RVG)
		Normal systolic function (RVG)	Asymmetrical septal hypertrophy (RVG or ^{201}Tl)
Cardiac Catheterization	Left ventricular enlargement and dysfunction	Diminished left ventricular compliance	Diminished left ventricular compliance
	Mitral and/or tricuspid regurgitation	"Square root sign" in ventricular pressure recordings	Mitral regurgitation
	Elevated left- and often right-sided filling pressures	Preserved systolic function	Vigorous systolic function
	Diminished cardiac output	Elevated left- and right-sided filling pressures	Dynamic left ventricular outflow gradient

RVG = Radionuclide ventriculogram; ^{201}Tl = thallium-201

abnormalities, including interstitial fibrosis, cellular hypertrophy, and myocardial cell degeneration.[19,20a] The mitochondria of myocytes are frequently abnormal, with swelling and loss of cristae, but specific and diagnostic electron microscopic findings are lacking.[19] Both left and right ventricular tissues possess reduced activities of mitochondrial enzymes, with elevated levels of lactate dehydrogenase.[21] These abnormalities of mitochondrial function are not unexpected in view of the known ultrastructural abnormalities of the mitochondria, and it is thought that the elevated levels of lactate dehydrogenase result from enhanced anaerobic glycolysis due to mitochondrial dysfunction.[21] No viruses or other etiological agents have been identified with any regularity in tissue from patients with dilated cardiomyopathy. Particularly disappointing has been the failure to identify any immunological, histochemical, morphological, ultrastructural, or microbiological

TABLE 41–3   ECHOCARDIOGRAPHIC FINDINGS IN THREE TYPES OF CARDIOMYOPATHY

	DILATED	HYPERTROPHIC	RESTRICTIVE
LV cavity	+ +	− or N	N
LV wall thickness	N	+	+
LV contractility	−	+ or N	N or −

LV = left ventricular; − = decreased; N = normal; + = increased.
From DeMaria, A. N., Bommer, W., Lee, G., and Mason, D. T.: Value and limitations of two dimensional echocardiography in assessment of cardiomyopathy. Am. J. Cardiol. 46:1225, 1980.

TABLE 41–4   COMMON INDICATIONS FOR ENDOMYOCARDIAL BIOPSY

1. To differentiate restrictive from constrictive disease.
2. To evaluate cardiac involvement in systemic disease.
3. To evaluate myocarditis.
4. To detect cardiotoxicity due to cardiotoxic agents.
5. To evaluate cardiac transplant rejection.
6. To evaluate cardiac tumors.

markers that might be used to establish the diagnosis of idiopathic dilated cardiomyopathy or to clarify its cause. Because there are no specific morphological features that characterize the dilated cardiomyopathies, it is not surprising that endomyocardial biopsy is not widely used for diagnosis of this condition. However, biopsy may be useful in *excluding* other conditions, such as endomyocardial fi-

TABLE 41–5   SPECIFIC PATHOLOGICAL ENTITIES DETECTED BY ENDOMYOCARDIAL BIOPSY

1. Cardiac transplant rejection
2. Myocarditis
3. Adriamycin cardiotoxicity
4. Amyloidosis
5. Sarcoidosis
6. Hemochromatosis
7. Endocardial fibroelastosis
8. Endomyocardial fibrosis
9. Carcinoid
10. Glycogen storage disease
11. Cardiac tumor
12. Fabry's disease

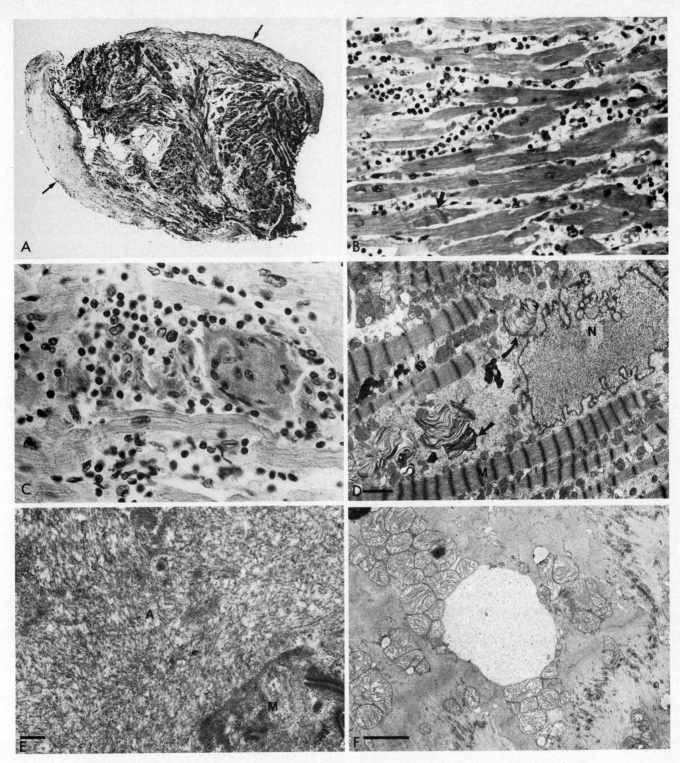

FIGURE 41–1 Representative examples of findings by endomyocardial biopsy. *A*, Low-power view of an entire transvenous right ventricular endomyocardial biopsy specimen. The endocardial surface is indicated by arrows. (Hematoxylin and eosin stain; original magnification × 90.) *B*, Inflammatory myocarditis with moderate, predominantly lymphocytic interstitial infiltrate throughout the myocardium. Focal myocardial cell necrosis is indicated by the arrow. (Hematoxylin and eosin stain; original magnification × 550.) *C*, Typical myocardial lesion in giant cell myocarditis with foci of mixed inflammatory infiltrate and multinucleated giant cells. (Hematoxylin and eosin stain; original magnification × 550.) *D*, Endomyocardial biopsy in patient with Fabry's disease. Transmission electron micrograph of cardiac muscle cell showing nucleus (N), myofibrils (M), and cytoplasmic inclusions (arrows) characteristic of Fabry's disease. (Original magnification × 3000. Bar at lower left-hand corner = 2 μm.) *E*, Cardiac amyloidosis revealed by endomyocardial biopsy. A very high magnification transmission electron photomicrograph (× 50,000) shows finely fibrillar amyloid material (A) in the interstitium surrounding individual myocytes. A portion of one myocyte is seen (M). (Bar at lower left = 0.1 μm.) *F*, Electron micrograph of endomyocardial biopsy specimen from a patient with adriamycin cardiotoxicity. The myocyte shown demonstrates swelling of the sarcoplasmic reticulum and diffuse myofibrillar loss. (Original magnification × 4500. Bar at lower left = 2 μm.) (Courtesy of Dr. Frederick J. Schoen, Department of Pathology, Brigham and Women's Hospital.)

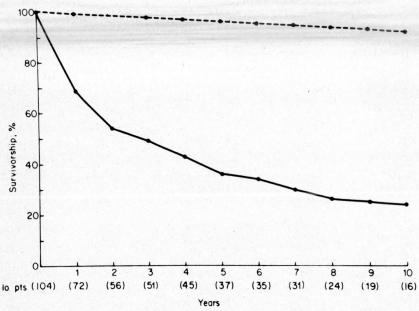

FIGURE 41–2 Observed survival plotted against time in years in 104 patients (pts.) with the diagnosis of idiopathic dilated cardiomyopathy (solid line). The dashed line represents the control expected survival, on the basis of age and sex distribution, according to the death rates of the Minnesota 1970 White Population Life Table. The number of living patients under observation at each followup interval is indicated in parentheses. (From Fuster, V., et al.: The natural history of idiopathic dilated cardiomyopathy. Am. J. Cardiol. *47*:525, 1981.)

brosis, myocarditis, and infiltrative diseases of the myocardium.[22] Also, by using a semiquantitative grading scale of the severity of histological changes in biopsy specimens, it may be possible to separate patients into groups with a poor prognosis (0 per cent survival at 4 years) and a better prognosis (better than 50 per cent 4-year survival), although there is disagreement on this point.[11,23]

ETIOLOGY. It is likely that primary dilated cardiomyopathy is a common expression of myocardial damage that has been produced by a variety of myocardial insults.[24] While the cause or causes remain unclear, at least four conditions, if not etiologically linked, appear to lower the threshold for the development of cardiomyopathy, and it is possible that in some cases a combination of factors results in severe myocardial damage.[24] Alcohol, pregnancy (see Chap. 53), systemic hypertension (see Chap. 26), and a variety of infections (pp. 1432 to 1442) may each be associated with myocardial dysfunction and congestive failure and are important causes of secondary dilated cardiomyopathy. Other causes include selenium deficiency and a variety of toxic agents, including cyclophosphamide (p. 1692) and adriamycin (p. 1690).

The possible progression of infective, particularly viral, myocarditis to cardiomyopathy has engendered the greatest speculation as a possible cause of "idiopathic" dilated cardiomyopathy.[24,25] While this hypothesis is inviting, it remains largely unsupported; there have been few observations of a transition from myocarditis to dilated cardiomyopathy and almost no evidence to suggest prior viral infections in patients with unequivocal cardiomyopathy.[26] However, there are patients who present with the clinical features of a dilated cardiomyopathy in which the apparent cause of the left ventricular enlargement and contractile dysfunction is an inflammatory myocarditis, possibly postviral (see p. 1433). Unlike the histological features of dilated cardiomyopathy, this form of myocarditis is characterized by a prominent round cell infiltrate. Identification of such patients requires endomyocardial biopsy, although myocardial uptake of the radionuclide gallium-67 may provide a noninvasive means of selecting patients for biopsy.[28,28a]

A variety of other possible causes has been proposed, again with little supportive evidence. Thus, endocrine and immunological abnormalities[27] as well as the effects of chemical or physical toxins have been suggested as possible etiological factors. Heart muscle from patients with dilated cardiomyopathy has been shown to bind immunoglobulins preferentially, and circulating antimyocardial antibodies may be demonstrated in many patients, although the significance and reproducibility of these findings remain unclear.[29,30] The observation that circulating lymphocytes of patients with idiopathic dilated cardiomyopathy demonstrate defective suppressor cell function in vitro is intriguing, but its significance, too, is not clear nor have the findings been completely reproducible.[31,32] It has been suggested that microvascular hyperreactivity (spasm) may lead to myocellular necrosis and scarring, with resultant heart failure, although this hypothesis remains speculative.[33]

In contrast to hypertrophic cardiomyopathy, in which familial transmission is quite common, in dilated cardiomyopathy it is rare. Occasional instances have been reported, and a genetic abnormality may be implicated in a small fraction of patients with dilated cardiomyopathy.[34–36]

Clinical Manifestations

Symptoms usually develop gradually in patients with dilated cardiomyopathy. Some patients may be asymptomatic yet have left ventricular dilatation for months or even years.[37,38] An unrecognized illness may result in left ventricular dilatation, which is clinically recognized only years later when symptoms develop or when routine chest roentgenography demonstrates cardiomegaly.[37] Although patients of any age may be affected, the disease is most common in middle age[37,39] and is more frequent in men than in women.[40]

The most striking symptoms are those of left ventricular failure. Dyspnea on exertion and, in more severe cases, orthopnea, paroxysmal nocturnal dyspnea, and dyspnea at rest are prominent.[38] Fatigue and weakness due to diminished cardiac output are common. Peripheral edema, hepatomegaly, and ascites are late and ominous signs. Vague chest pain is not uncommon, although angina pectoris is unusual and suggests the presence of coronary artery disease rather than dilated cardiomyopathy. In some patients there appears to be a reduction in myocardial perfusion despite normal coronary arteries, suggesting that subendocardial ischemia may play a role in the genesis of chest pain.[41] Chest pain secondary to pulmonary embolism and abdominal pain secondary to congestive hepatomegaly are frequent in the late stages of the illness.

Physical examination reveals variable degrees of cardiac enlargement and findings of congestive heart failure. The systolic blood pressure is usually normal or low, and the pulse pressure is narrow, reflecting a diminished stroke volume. The arterial pulse is of low amplitude and volume. Pulsus alternans (p. 25) is common when severe left ventricular failure is present. The jugular veins are frequently distended. Prominent *a* and *v* waves are visible—the latter a late manifestation of the presence of tricuspid valvular regurgitation. The liver may be engorged and pulsatile. Peripheral edema and ascites may be present.

The precordium usually reveals left and, occasionally, right ventricular impulses, but the heaves are not sustained, as they are in patients with considerable ventricular hypertrophy (p. 27). The apical impulse is usually displaced laterally, reflecting left ventricular dilatation. A presystolic *a* wave may be palpable. The second heart sound is usually normally split, although paradoxical splitting (p. 47) may be detected in the presence of left bundle branch block, an electrocardiographic finding which is not unusual in dilated cardiomyopathy. The pulmonary component of the second heart sound may be accentuated, and the splitting may be narrow if pulmonary hypertension is present.[42] Presystolic gallop sounds (S_4) often precede the development of overt congestive heart failure. Ventricular gallops (S_3) are the rule once cardiac decompensation occurs, and a summation gallop is often heard when there is tachycardia. Systolic murmurs are common and are usually due to mitral or, less commonly, tricuspid valvular regurgitation. Atrioventricular valvular regurgitation results from ventricular dilatation and resultant distortion of the geometry of the subvalvar apparatus.[43] Gallop sounds and regurgitant murmurs can often be elicited or intensified by isometric handgrip exercise[42] with its attendant enhancement of systemic vascular resistance and impedance to left ventricular outflow. Systemic emboli resulting from dislodgment of intracardiac thrombi from the left atrium and ventricle[38,42] and pulmonary emboli that originate in the venous system of the legs are common late complications.

NONINVASIVE EXAMINATION. The *chest roentgenogram* usually reveals left ventricular enlargement, although generalized cardiomegaly is often seen. Left ventricular failure may result in signs of pulmonary venous hypertension (i.e., pulmonary vascular redistribution) as well as interstitial and even alveolar edema (p. 173). Pleural effusions may be present, and the azygos vein and superior vena cava may be dilated when right heart failure supervenes. The *electrocardiogram* often shows sinus tachycardia when heart failure is present. The entire spectrum of atrial and ventricular tachyarrhythmias and atrioventricular conduction disturbances may be seen. Indeed, arrhyth-

mias are second in frequency only to heart failure as clinical manifestations of congestive cardiomyopathy.[38,38a] A variety of intraventricular conduction defects is common, and Q waves may be present when there is extensive left ventricular fibrosis without discrete myocardial infarction;[37] ST-segment and T-wave abnormalities are common.

Systolic time intervals (p. 54) are usually abnormal in dilated cardiomyopathy and are useful in estimating and following the severity of left ventricular dysfunction in patients with this condition. The left ventricular ejection time (LVET) is reduced, the preejection period (PEP) is prolonged, and the ratio of the PEP/LVET exceeds the upper limits of normal, i.e., 0.43.[44]

Both M-mode and two-dimensional *echocardiography* are useful in assessing the degree of impairment of left ventricular function and for excluding concomitant valvular or pericardial disease (Chap 5). In addition to examination of all four cardiac valves for evidence of structural or functional abnormalities, the size of the ventricular cavity may be assessed, the thickness of the left and right ventricular walls evaluated, and an estimate made of ventricular function.[45] Left ventricular enlargement, with increased end-diastolic and end-systolic volumes, and reduced ejection fraction and fractional shortening are characteristically found. Mitral valve motion may be abnormal and may reflect the effects of diminished left ventricular compliance and elevated end-diastolic pressure. Right ventricular enlargement occurs late in the stage of the illness. A pericardial effusion may sometimes by demonstrated. *Thallium-201 imaging* at rest and with exercise is of limited value in distinguishing left ventricular enlargement due to dilated cardiomyopathy from that due to coronary artery disease unless a large defect indicative of a myocardial infarction is seen.[46]

Radionuclide ventriculography, like echocardiography, reveals elevated end-diastolic and end-systolic left ventricular volumes, reduced ejection fractions in both ventricles and wall-motion abnormalities.[46a] This technique is helpful both in the assessment of ventricular function and in evaluating the response to therapy.[47] In many cases, however, it is not necessary to carry out serial batteries of noninvasive tests in order to follow patients with dilated cardiomyopathy and evaluate their response to treatment. This is true particularly when the studies are performed only with the patient at rest, since clinical symptoms correlate best with exercise capacity, which in turn bears only a general relationship to resting ventricular performance.[48]

To identify potentially reversible secondary causes of dilated cardiomyopathy, several basic screening tests are often indicated, including determinations of serum phosphorus (hypophosphatemia), serum calcium (hypocalcemia), serum creatinine and urea nitrogen (uremia), and serum iron (hemochromatosis).[49]

CARDIAC CATHETERIZATION AND ANGIOCARDIOGRAPHY. The left ventricular end-diastolic, left atrial, and pulmonary artery wedge pressures are usually elevated. Modest degrees of pulmonary arterial hypertension are common.[42] Advanced cases may demonstrate right ventricular dilatation and failure as well, with resultant elevation of the right ventricular end-diastolic, right atrial, and central venous pressures. However, the end-diastolic pressure in the left ventricle usually exceeds that in the right by at least 5 mm Hg. Cardiac output is reduced,[50] often markedly.

Left ventriculography demonstrates enlargement of this chamber with diffuse reduction in wall motion.[9,42] The ejection fraction is decreased and the end-systolic volume is increased as a result of the impairment of left ventricular contractility. Sometimes left ventricular thrombi may be visualized within the left ventricle as intracavitary filling defects. Mild mitral regurgitation is often present.[42] On occasion, it may be difficult to distinguish left ventricular dilatation secondary to severe mitral regurgitation from a dilated cardiomyopathy with secondary mitral regurgitation. The left ventricular wall may be thickened, but this is usually not a prominent finding.[9]

Coronary arteriography usually reveals normal vessels.[50] This technique may be of particular value in patients with abnormal Q waves on the electrocardiogram, since such a pattern may be due to myocardial infarction as a result of obstructive coronary artery disease or, alternatively, extensive myocardial fibrosis secondary to severe dilated cardiomyopathy in the absence of coronary artery obstruction.

Treatment

Since the cause of idiopathic dilated cardiomyopathy is unknown, specific therapy is not possible. Treatment, therefore, is on the same basis as that for heart failure, discussed in detail in Chapter 16. Physical, dietary, pharmacological, mechanical, and surgical interventions may help to control symptoms,[51] although their role in prolonging life has not been established.

Patients with moderately severe left ventricular failure may be comfortable at rest but may develop severe symptoms with exercise, when they are unable to increase their cardiac output commensurately. It is reasonable to restrict activity for these patients to avoid precipitation of unwanted and poorly tolerated symptoms (Fig. 16–1, p. 504). Marked curtailment of exercise in the form of prolonged bed rest may result not only in improvement of symptoms but also in a reduction in heart size and an improvement in prognosis.[16] However, many patients are unable psychologically to tolerate strict bed rest, and the efficacy of immobilization per se has not been documented.[12,52] Perhaps prolonged bed rest in the hospital is helpful by ensuring a nutritious diet and removal of a toxin (e.g., alcohol). A reasonable compromise can usually be achieved in reducing activity without totally incapacitating the patient.[52] It has been suggested that in patients with heart failure due to dilated cardiomyopathy a beneficial effect may be seen with beta-adrenergic blockade[53,53a] along with deterioration on withdrawal of therapy.[54] The mechanism of improvement is said to be protection against the increased sympathetic nervous activity that may accompany heart failure. The results have not been confirmed in adequately controlled trials, and at this final the use of beta-adrenergic blockade in dilated cardiomyopathy should be considered speculative, experimental, and potentially dangerous.[55,55a] Prolonged improvement in clinical status and left ventricular function has been noted following a 3-day infusion of the synthetic catecholamine dobutamine.[56] Further trials should clarify the role of these experimental approaches in patients with dilated cardiomyopathy.

Antiarrhythmic agents should be used to treat symptomatic or serious arrhythmias. Because of the adverse effects of most available agents, many of which depress myocardial contractility (Chap. 20), treatment should be individualized, with both efficacy and toxicity carefully monitored. Because of the frequency and hazards of embolization,[56a] patients with dilated cardiomyopathy and heart failure should be treated with anticoagulants, even without direct evidence of thrombus formation if there are no specific contraindications to these agents.[14,38,52] Corticosteroids appear to have no place in the treatment of chronic idiopathic dilated cardiomyopathy.

Surgical replacement of regurgitant valves has been attempted rarely in patients with progressive atrioventricular valvular regurgitation (almost always mitral) which appeared to result in progressive cardiac enlargement and failure. The results of operation are often less than satisfactory because of the degree of preexisting cardiac dysfunction and damage. In appropriate patients, cardiac transplantation may be an alternative (p. 547),[57] with a 3-year survival rate of nearly 70 per cent compared with less than 5 per cent in nontransplanted patients.[58] The enormous emotional and economic investments required for carrying out this procedure must be appreciated, however.

ALCOHOLIC CARDIOMYOPATHY

Excessive consumption of alcohol is the major cause of secondary, non-ischemic dilated cardiomyopathy in the Western world,[59] resulting in cardiomegaly and low cardiac output. It is estimated that two-thirds of the adult population use alcohol to some extent, and greater than 10 per cent are heavy users. Therefore, it is not surprising that alcoholic cardiomyopathy is a major problem. Ceasing alcohol consumption may halt the progression or even reverse alcoholic cardiomyopathy,[60] which, unlike idiopathic or primary dilated cardiomyopathy, is usually marked by progressive deterioration.

The consumption of alcohol may result in myocardial damage by three basic mechanisms: (1) direct toxic effects; (2) nutritional effects, most commonly in association with thiamine deficiency, which leads to beriberi heart disease (p. 814); and (3) rarely, toxic effects due to additives in the alcoholic beverage (cobalt)[61] (p. 1408). There had been considerable speculation that alcohol caused myocardial damage only through dietary deficiencies, but it is now clear that alcoholic cardiomyopathy occurs in the absence of nutritional deficiencies.[59]

Typical Oriental beriberi is distinguished from alcoholic cardiomyopathy by the presence of high output failure in the former (p. 817); peripheral vasodilatation is prominent, with increased venous return and resultant high cardiac output.[62] This condition responds to thiamine administration, often in a dramatic fashion.[63] The existence of a variant of beriberi heart disease, termed Occidental beriberi, has been proposed; in contrast to the high output state in Oriental beriberi, Occidental beriberi heart disease is marked by cardiac dilatation, congestive failure, and diminished cardiac output without peripheral vasodilatation, increased venous return, or elevated cardiac output.[64] Because it occurs almost exclusively in alcoholic patients, is not usually observed in individuals with solely a dietary thiamine deficiency, does not respond well to thiamine administration, and is otherwise identical clinically to alcoholic cardiomyopathy, Occidental beriberi heart disease in fact is probably the same as alcoholic cardiomyopathy.[39]

Alcohol results in acute as well as chronic depression of myocardial contractility[65] and may produce demonstrable cardiac dysfunction even when ingested by normal individuals in quantities consumed in social drinking.[66] When conscious, chronically instrumented, but otherwise healthy dogs are given intravenous infusions of ethanol to produce blood levels well below the usual legal human limit for the operation of motor vehicles (150 mg/dl), cardiac dilatation and systolic dysfunction occur, with a fall in cardiac output and the maximum dP/dt.[67] The acute hemodynamic effects of alcohol appear to depend on its blood levels, since ventricular dysfunction following acute ethanol ingestion may be reversed within 15 to 30 minutes of hemodialysis.[68] Prior exposure to alcohol appears to modulate the hemodynamic response to acute challenge with alcohol. Larger doses of alcohol are required to produce cardiac dysfunction in chronic alcoholic patients without obvious heart disease than in normal subjects. On the other hand, the alcoholic person with clinically evident cardiac dysfunction appears to be more susceptible to the deleterious effects of alcohol than normal.[68]

The mechanism of the cardiac depression produced by alcohol remains unclear, and a direct causal relationship between alcohol and the development of cardiomyopathy has not been proved.[66] In acute studies, alcohol and its metabolite acetaldehyde have been shown to interfere with a number of cellular functions that involve the transport and binding of calcium, mitochondrial respiration, myocardial lipid metabolism, myocardial protein synthesis, and myofibrillar ATPase.[59,69,70,70a] Alcohol results in loss of potassium ions from myocardial cells, along with diminished uptake of free fatty acids but enhanced myocardial extraction of triglyceride.[71] The major unanswered question is how these metabolic effects result in persistent myocardial injury. It is possible that factors such as magnesium deficiency or the presence of a separate toxic compound associated with the alcohol may be involved in the production of alcoholic cardiomyopathy.[66]

Several studies in experimental animals and in chronic alcoholic patients admitted to the hospital have demonstrated cardiac dysfunction even when adequate nutrition was ensured.[60] Chronic experimental studies in a well-nourished alcoholic person given 12 to 16 ounces of whiskey per day for several months demonstrated the gradual development of heart failure. Without specific therapy, the features of congestive failure resolved within several weeks following the cessation of alcohol intake[71] (Fig. 41–3).

PATHOLOGY. The gross and microscopic pathological findings are nonspecific and similar to those observed in idiopathic dilated cardiomyopathy.[19,39] Edema of the vascular wall and perivascular fibrosis of the intramyocardial coronary arteries has been observed,[72,73] and it has been suggested that the myocardial damage in alcoholic cardiomyopathy may be the result of ischemia produced by disease of the small intramural coronary arteries.[73] Alcohol, even in small amounts, may result in alterations of mitochondrial structure.[74,75]

CLINICAL MANIFESTATIONS

Alcoholic cardiomyopathy is most commonly seen in males 30 to 55 years of age who have been heavy consumers of whiskey, wine, or beer, usually for more than 10 years.[60,68,76,77] The male predominance appears to be largely the result of the higher frequency of alcoholism in this sex, although noninvasive testing of cardiac function in male and female alcoholic patients suggests that cardiac dysfunction is more likely in men than in women.[78] While alcoholic cardiomyopathy may be observed in the homeless, malnourished, "skid row" alcoholic man who is a candidate for and may often suffer from alcoholic cirrhosis, many patients are well-nourished individuals in the middle and even upper socioeconomic brackets without liver disease or peripheral neuropathy.[39,60,68,79] Therefore, unless a high index of suspicion is maintained, it may be easy to miss a history of alcohol abuse. Persistent questioning of the patient and particularly the relatives of patients with unexplained cardiomegaly or cardiomyopathy is often required to elicit a history of alcoholism.

It is frequently possible to demonstrate mild depression of cardiac function in chronic alcoholics even before cardiac dysfunction becomes clinically manifest.[68,80,81] Abnormalities of both systolic function (reduced ejection fraction) and diastolic function (increased myocardial wall stiffness) have been demonstrated in alcoholic patients without cardiac symptoms by a variety of invasive and noninvasive techniques.[68,80,81] Two basic patterns have been observed: (1) left ventricular dilatation with impaired systolic function and (2) left ventricular hypertrophy with diminished compliance and normal or increased contractile performance; left ventricular size is most substantially increased.[82–84] The development of symptoms may be insidious, although

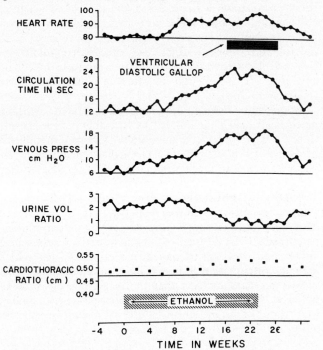

FIGURE 41–3 Development of cardiac decompensation and congestive heart failure in a well-nourished patient receiving alcohol daily. The congestive failure resolved without specific treatment within several weeks of the cessation of alcohol consumption. (From Regan, T. J., et al.: Ventricular function in noncardiacs with alcoholic fatty liver: Role of ethanol in the production of cardiomyopathy. J. Clin. Invest. 48:397, 1969.)

some patients present acute and florid left-sided congestive heart failure.[76] A paroxysm of atrial fibrillation is a relatively frequent initial presenting finding.[79] More advanced cases present findings of biventricular failure, with left ventricular dysfunction usually dominating.[39,76,79] Dyspnea, orthopnea, and paroxysmal nocturnal dyspnea are frequently observed.[79] Palpitations and syncope due to cardiac arrhythmias, usually supraventricular, are occasionally present.[76] Angina pectoris does not occur unless there is concomitant coronary artery disease or aortic stenosis.

Physical examination usually reveals a narrow pulse pressure, often with an elevated diastolic pressure secondary to excessive peripheral vasoconstriction.[39,76,79] There is cardiomegaly, and protodiastolic (S_3) and presystolic (S_4) gallop sounds are common. An apical systolic murmur of mitral regurgitation due to papillary muscle dysfunction is often found.[79] The severity of right heart failure varies, but jugular venous distention and peripheral edema are common.

LABORATORY EXAMINATION. The *chest roentgenogram* demonstrates cardiac enlargement, pulmonary congestion, and pulmonary venous hypertension. Pleural effusions are often seen. *Electrocardiographic abnormalities* are common and are frequently the only indication of alcoholic heart disease during the preclinical phase. Alcoholic patients without other evidence of heart disease often are seen after developing palpitations, chest discomfort, or syncope typically following a binge of alcohol consumption on a weekend, particularly during the year-end holiday season.[85] This is dubbed the "holiday heart syndrome." The most common arrhythmia observed is atrial fibrillation, followed by atrial flutter and frequent ventricular premature contractions.[85,86] Hypokalemia may play a role in the genesis of some of these arrhythmias. Supraventricular arrhythmias are also frequently observed in patients with overt alcoholic cardiomyopathy. Sudden, unexpected death is not uncommon in young adult alcoholics, and it is likely that ventricular fibrillation is responsible.[68] On the other hand, arrhythmias often cease in patients who abstain from alcohol.[85]

Atrioventricular conduction disturbances (most commonly first-degree heart block), bundle branch block, and left ventricular hypertrophy[79,87] are common electrocardiographic findings. Prolongation of the Q-T interval is noted frequently.[84] ST-segment and T-wave changes are often restored to normal within several days after cessation of alcohol consumption.[88] Q waves, presumably reflecting myocardial fibrosis, are usually not prominent.[76]

The hemodynamic findings observed at cardiac catheterization and the assessment of left ventricular function by noninvasive methods (echocardiography, isotope angiography, and systolic time intervals) resemble those found in idiopathic dilated cardiomyopathy.

The *natural history* of alcoholic cardiomyopathy depends on the drinking habits of the patient. Total abstinence in the earlier stages of the disease frequently leads to resolution of the manifestation of congestive heart failure and a return of heart size to normal.[77,79,89,90] Continued alcohol consumption leads to further myocardial damage and fibrosis, and the congestive heart failure becomes increasingly refractory to treatment, resulting eventually in the demise of the patient.[79] Death may also be due to arrhythmia, heart block, and systemic or pulmonary embolism.[39,79]

TREATMENT.   The key to the long-term treatment of alcoholic cardiomyopathy is *complete abstinence,* as early in the course of the disease as possible. The prognosis in patients who continue to drink, particularly if they have been symptomatic for a long period, is poor. In one study, 80 per cent of such patients died within a 3-year period.[77] In the overall population of patients with alcoholic cardiomyopathy, between 40 and 50 per cent succumb within a 3- to 6-year period.[77,89] Prolonged bed rest is also thought to result in functional improvement,[89] although its major benefit may simply be the decreased alcohol consumption.

The management of acute episodes of congestive heart failure is similar to that of idiopathic dilated cardiomyopathy. For patients with severe congestive heart failure, it is probably prudent to administer thiamine on the remote chance that beriberi may be contributing to the heart failure.

COBALT CARDIOMYOPATHY

A previously unrecognized syndrome of fulminating congestive heart failure appeared in 1966, first in Quebec City, Canada, and subsequently in Omaha, Nebraska; Minneapolis, Minnesota; and Belgium.[61] The disease was found in people who drank a particular brand of beer to which cobalt sulfate had been added as a foam stabilizer. After cobalt was removed from the process, no more cases of the disease were reported. Rare cases of cobalt cardiomyopathy have been found after industrial exposure to cobalt[91] and after the therapeutic ingestion of cobalt salts in the treatment of anemia.[92]

Pathological findings are those of a dilated, hypertrophied heart, often surrounded by a sizable pericardial effusion.[39] Microscopic examination reveals myofibrillar hyaline necrosis as well as myocardial vacuolization and degeneration. The mechanism responsible for the development of cobalt cardiotoxicity remains unclear.

Clinical Manifestations.   The typical patient who developed cobalt-beer cardiomyopathy was a middle-aged man who had consumed large quantities of the contaminated beer.[61] The disease was characterized by severe heart failure, with death occurring in more than 40 per cent of patients, often within 3 days of hospital admission.[39,61] The typical presentation was that of the abrupt onset of left followed by right heart failure. Hemodynamic findings were those of biventricular failure with depressed cardiac output.[61]

HYPERTROPHIC CARDIOMYOPATHY

DEFINITIONS. The gross pathological features of hypertrophic obstructive cardiomyopathy (HOCM) were first systematically described in 1958.[93] The characteristic finding is pronounced myocardial hypertrophy, particularly involving the interventricular septum of a nondilated left ventricle. A distinctive clinical feature was soon recognized in many patients with hypertrophic cardiomyopathy: a dynamic pressure gradient in the subaortic area, evanescent in some patients, which divides the left ventricle into a high-pressure apical region and a lower-pressure subaortic region.[94] Hence the term *idiopathic hypertrophic subaortic stenosis* (*IHSS*) was suggested, although subsequent findings have indicated that many patients do not, in fact, ever have obstruction to left ventricular outflow, and thus *hypertrophic cardiomyopathy* is a more appropriate and inclusive way to describe the disease.

Much of the initial investigation in this disease was stimulated by the unique dynamic pressure gradient.[94] Unlike the constant gradient produced by fixed orifice obstruction (as in patients with valvular aortic stenosis or a discrete subaortic membrane), the gradient in HOCM often demonstrates wide fluctuations and in some patients varies between absent and severe. Other patients do not have gradients at rest, but these can be provoked by a variety of physiological or pharmacological interventions (Table 41–6).

Because of the unique obstructive features in hypertrophic cardiomyopathy, the names used to designate this disorder emphasized this characteristic. In the United States, the disease was called idiopathic hypertrophic subaortic stenosis (IHSS) and in Canada *muscular subaortic stenosis*. Investigations over the last 20 years have helped clarify the etiological, clinical, and pathological features of hypertrophic cardiomyopathy, but as a result of the rapid growth in the field, the disorder has been referred to by a bewildering array of more than 50 names![95–97] As we now understand the disease, many of the terms used to designate it are in reality merely *features* of the disease that may be seen in a greater or lesser percentage of afflicted patients.

The older terms, such as IHSS, which emphasized the obstructive features of the disease, have fallen into disfavor, since it is now clear that many and perhaps most patients do not in fact demonstrate an intraventricular pressure gradient. The most characteristic pathophysiological abnormality is not systolic but rather *diastolic* dysfunction.[24] Thus, hypertrophic cardiomyopathy is characterized by abnormal stiffness of the left ventricle during diastole, with resultant impaired ventricular filling. This abnormality in diastolic relaxation results in elevation of the left ventricular end-diastolic pressure. The elevated left ventricular filling pressure is associated with elevated left atrial, pulmonary venous, and pulmonary capillary pressures, causing dyspnea—the most common symptom in hypertrophic cardiomyopathy, despite typically *hypercontractile* left ventricular function. The disease appears to be genetically transmitted as an autosomal dominant trait with a high degree of penetrance in most patients, although sporadic cases occur, some of which may represent new mutations.[98] As might be expected with such a mode of inheritance, evidence of the disease is found in almost half the first-degree relatives of a patient with hypertrophic cardiomyopathy; in many of the relatives the disease is milder than in the propositus, the degree of hypertrophy is less, and outflow gradients are usually lacking. Symptoms are often absent, and the disease may be detected only by echocardiography.[98]

PATHOLOGY

Gross examination of the heart discloses a marked increase in myocardial mass, and the ventricular cavities are small (Fig. 41–4). The atria are dilated and often hypertrophied,[99] reflecting the high resistance to filling of the ventricles and the effects of atrioventricular valve regurgitation (Table 41–7). The pattern of hypertrophy of the left ventricle, at least in certain population groups, is distinctive and differs from that seen with secondary hypertrophy (as in systemic hypertension or discrete obstruction to left ventricular outflow, i.e., subaortic, valvular, or supravalvular aortic stenosis) in that it is commonly associated with disproportionate involvement of the interventricular septum compared with the free wall of the left ventricle (Fig. 41–4). In both normal subjects as well as patients with left ventricular hypertrophy without HOCM, the ratio of the thickness of the interventricular septum to that of the left ventricular free wall has been shown at autopsy and by echocardiography to be around 1.0 and nearly always less than 1.3. However, this ratio usually exceeds 1.3 in HOCM. Asymmetrical septal hypertrophy (ASH) was at one time felt to be pathognomonic of HOCM, but modifications of this concept have been required.[100–111] Thus, it is now recognized that concentric left ventricular hypertrophy, with symmetrical thickening of the left ventricle, involving the septum and free wall equally, may oc-

TABLE 41–6 EFFECTS OF INTERVENTIONS ON OUTFLOW GRADIENT AND SYSTOLIC MURMUR IN HOCM

	CONTRACTILITY	PRELOAD	AFTERLOAD
Increase in Gradient and Murmur			
Valsalva maneuver (during strain)	—	↓	↓
Standing	—	↓	—
Postextrasystole	↑	↑	—
Isoproterenol	↑	↓	↓
Digitalis	↑	↓	—
Amyl nitrite	— then ↑	↓ then ↑	↓
Nitroglycerin	—	↓	↓
Exercise	↑	↑	↑
Tachycardia	↑	↓	—
Hypovolemia	↑	↓	↓
Decrease in Gradient and Murmur			
Mueller maneuver	—	↑	↑
Valsalva overshoot	—	↑	↑
Squatting	—	↑	↑
Alpha-adrenergic stimulation (phenylephrine)	—	—	↑
Beta-adrenergic blockade	↓	↑	—
General anesthesia	↓	—	↑
Isometric handgrip	—	—	↑

↑ = increase; ↓ = decrease; — = no major change.

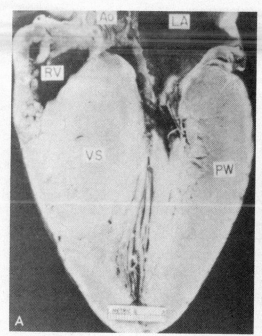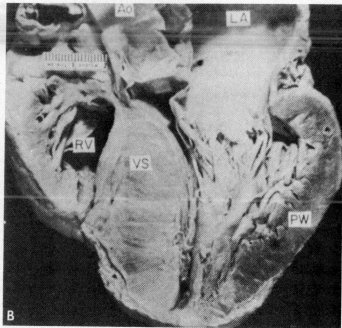

FIGURE 41-4 Two hearts showing hypertrophic cardiomyopathy, one with obstruction (*A*) and one without (*B*). The ventricular septum is markedly thickened in both, but the posterior wall is thickened only in the patient in *A*. Ao = aorta, LA = left atrium, RV = right ventricle, VS = ventricular septum, PW = posterior left ventricular wall. (From Henry, W. L., et al.: Differences in the distribution of myocardial abnormalities in patients with obstructive and nonobstructive asymmetric septal hypertrophy (ASH). Echocardiographic and gross anatomic findings. Circulation *50*:447, 1974, by permission of the American Heart Association, Inc.)

casionally be seen in patients with the genetically transmitted as well as the sporadic forms of hypertrophic cardiomyopathy.[101,102] Even in the majority of patients who manifest ASH the hypertrophy often extends beyond the septum to involve portions of the anterolateral left ventricular wall.[112] In some patients with hypertrophic cardiomyopathy there is substantial hypertrophy in unusual locations, such as the posterior portion of the septum; this may result in diagnostic confusion, since the hypertrophy may not be detectable by M-mode echocardiography but only by two-dimensional echocardiography.[113,113a]

Two types of an unusual form of hypertrophic cardiomyopathy localized to the *apical* portion of the left ventricle have been noted. One form, described in Japanese patients, imparts a characteristic spadelike configuration to the left ventricular chamber on two-dimensional echocardiographic or contrast ventriculographic study. Patients with apical hypertrophy of this type may demonstrate giant negative T waves in the precordial electrocardiographic leads, but they typically do not demonstrate pressure gra-

dients.[114] The other form demonstrates a small, poorly contractile apical segment that communicates with the subaortic area through a markedly narrowed midventricular channel. In this form of apical hypertrophic cardiomyopathy the T waves are not deeply inverted, and an intraventricular pressure gradient may be found.[115] Disproportionate septal hypertrophy may be found in patients with a variety of acquired or congenital lesions in the absence of hypertrophic cardiomyopathy.[103–110] Thus, ASH is a normal finding during fetal life, in neonates, and in infants but normally disappears by the age of 1 or 2 years.[109,116] Conditions resulting in right ventricular pressure overload and thus right ventricular hypertrophy, such as pulmonic stenosis or primary pulmonary hypertension, often result in thickening of the interventricular septum, without affecting the free wall of the left ventricle.[108,109] Abnormal thickness of the septum relative to that of the free wall may also occur in coronary artery disease, presumably when infarction leads to fibrosis and thinning of the free wall of the left ventricle, while the noninfarcted septum exhibits compensatory hypertrophy.[117,118] Other conditions that may present similar patterns of disproportionate septal hypertrophy include lentiginosis, Turner's syndrome, acromegaly, hyperthyroidism, and Friedreich's ataxia, and HOCM may develop after aortic valve replacement.[119,119a] Athletes, weight lifters, and infants of diabetic mothers may demonstrate similar patterns. Rarely, apparent left ventricular hypertrophy is due to infiltration of the septum by tumor,[120,121] Pompe's disease,[122] or Fabry's disease.[123] To differentiate the various causes of septal–free wall disproportion, the term *disproportionate septal thickening* (DST) has been used to indicate the secondary form, while ASH is often reserved for the primary form found in HOCM. The degree of thickening of the interventricular septum ap-

TABLE 41-7   PATHOLOGICAL FINDINGS IN HYPERTROPHIC CARDIOMYOPATHY

FINDING	FREQUENCY (%)
Asymmetrical septal hypertrophy	95
Small or normal-sized ventricular cavities	95
Mural plaque in left ventricular outflow tract	75
Thickened mitral valve	75
Dilated atria	100
Abnormal intramural coronary arteries	50
Disarray of ventricular septal myocardial fibers	95

Data from Roberts, W. C., and Ferrans, V. J.: Pathologic anatomy of the cardiomyopathies. Idiopathic dilated and hypertrophic types, infiltrative types and endomyocardial disease with and without eosinophilia. Hum. Pathol. *6*:287, 1975.

pears to be unrelated to the presence or absence of a pressure gradient.[99] However, patients who have had a left ventricular outflow gradient during life demonstrate secondary hypertrophy of the posterobasal wall, including the area immediately behind the posterior leaflet of the mitral valve and below the mitral annulus.[124] While hypertrophied, bizarrely shaped, and abnormally arranged myocardial cells are commonly present in the septum (Fig. 41–4), such abnormalities may be less common in the free wall,[125] although these findings are controversial.[119] The gross and histological appearance in the free wall resembles that seen in valvular aortic stenosis, suggesting that these changes are secondary to the high ventricular pressure caused by the pressure gradient. In patients *without* a gradient, por-

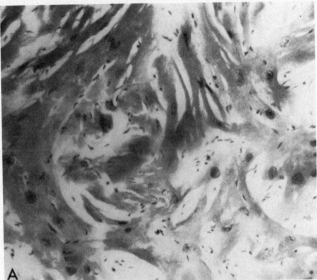

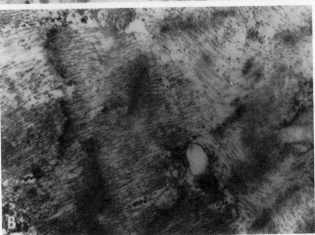

FIGURE 41–5 *A,* Photomicrograph of myocardium from the septal region in a patient firmly diagnosed clinically as suffering from hypertrophic cardiomyopathy. Extensive disarray of myocardial fibers and attempts at whorl formation are present. In addition, severe hypertrophy and an increase in collagen tissue, interrupting muscle bundles, can be seen. Nuclear changes are not prominent, and perinuclear halos are absent. Although not all diagnostic criteria are seen here, the combination of changes present characterizes this condition. (Hematoxylin and eosin stain; original magnification × 650.) *B,* Electron micrograph showing disarray of myocardial fibrils and widening of Z bands. (Lead citrate and uranyl acetate; original magnification × 38,400.) (From Olsen, E. G. J.: The pathology of idiopathic hypertrophic subaortic stenosis (hypertrophic cardiomyopathy): A critical review. Am. Heart J. *100*:553, 1980.)

tions of the free wall are hypertrophied and extensively involved by bizarre and disorganized myocardial fibers identical to those found in the septum, suggesting a diffuse myopathic process.[124,126]

A "contact lesion" in the form of a mural plaque on the endocardium of the left ventricular outflow tract is frequently found in patients with marked gradients at rest[99] (Table 41–7). This fibrous thickening appears to result from the trauma of the anterior mitral valve leaflet apposing the septum during systole. The thickening of the mitral valve that is often seen[99] is probably explained on a similar basis.

The bizarre form of myocardial fiber hypertrophy that results in myocardial fiber disarray is a prominent feature of HOCM[118] (Fig. 41–5). The disorganization and disarray seen in the septum is not confined to the muscle cell bundles but involves the myofibrils and myofilaments within individual cells as well[127,128] (Fig. 41–5). The myocardial cells are wider and shorter than in other conditions, but they often have bizarre shapes.[124,128] Foci of disorganized cells are often interspersed between areas of hypertrophied but otherwise normal-appearing muscle cells.[124] Similar cellular disorganization is found in a spontaneously occurring primary myocardial disease of dogs and cats.[129] While initially considered specific for HOCM, it is now recognized that abnormally arranged cardiac muscle cells in the septum may be found not only in a variety of disease states, including concentric left ventricular hypertrophy secondary to pressure overload, coronary artery disease, congenital heart disease, and cor pulmonale, but in normal hearts as well.[129a] However, there appears to be a quantitative relationship between the extent of cellular disarray and the underlying disease process, since the disorganization of myocardial fibers is far greater in HOCM than in other disorders.[127] There is a suggestion that the greater the extent of cellular disorganization, the worse the clinical outcome.[126] However, a somewhat surprising finding is that there is little correlation between the extent of cellular disorganization in surgically excised septectomy samples in patients with HOCM and the amount observed at subsequent necropsy.[130]

ETIOLOGY

The cause of the myocardial hypertrophy in HOCM remains unclear. While there are persuasive data that in most patients the disease is inherited,[113a] and in some instances linked to the HLA system,[130a] the basic defect is unknown. The disorganized myocardial fibers may be the result of mechanical stresses within the septum, since myocardial disarray is also seen frequently in other conditions characterized by excessive systolic pressure.[131,132] It has been suggested that the genetic defect in HOCM results in a catenoid shape and configuration of the septum that is concave to the left in the transverse plane but concave to the right in the apex-to-base plane. This abnormal configuration of the septum leads to prominent isometric contraction which might result in fiber disarray.[133] The reverse argument has also been made that the isometric contraction inherent in malaligned cells itself stimulates hypertrophy.[134]

Other suggested etiologies of HOCM include (1) abnormal sympathetic stimulation because of excessive production of or heightened responsiveness of the heart to circulating catecholamines[24,134]; (2) abnormal intramural coronary arteries that lead to myocardial ischemia, with resultant fibrosis and abnormal compensatory hypertrophy[135]; (3) abnormal rapid atrioventricular conduction that leads to asynchronous ventricular contraction resulting in abnormal myocardial hypertrophy[135]; (4) a primary abnormality of collagen that may lead to an abnormal and disorganized fibrous skeleton which, with the development of hypertrophy, leads to myocardial cellular disorganization and disarray[135]; and (5) subendocardial ischemia that depletes the energy stores essential for the sequestration of calcium during diastole, resulting in persistent interaction of the contractile elements during diastole and attendant increased diastolic stiffness.[136]

PATHOPHYSIOLOGY

Since the initial descriptions of hypertrophic cardiomyopathy, the feature that has attracted the greatest attention and has been the source of considerable controversy is the dynamic pressure gradient (Fig. 41–6). While this pressure gradient was initially felt to be due to a muscular sphincter action in the subaortic region, it appears to be related to further narrowing of an already smalltract (narrowed by the prominent septal hypertrophy and possibly abnormal location of the mitral valve) by systolic anterior motion (SAM) of the mitral valve against the septum. Even the view that the pressure gradient in HOCM is the result of mechanical obstruction as a consequence of SAM may require modification. The generation of a pressure gradient due to subaortic obstruction would imply that left ventricular ejection is slowed or impeded at some point during systole. Yet characteristic features of HOCM are rapid ventricular emptying and high ejection fractions. Hemodynamic studies have shown that the majority of flow (at least 80 per cent) is unusually rapid in hypertrophic cardiomyopathy and is completed earlier in systole than normal, regardless of whether gradients are absent, provocable, or present.[137] Since the total duration of systole is prolonged only in patients with gradients,[137] it is likely that a small residual amount of blood is in fact impeded in its ejection from the left ventricle as a consequence of dynamic obstruction.

CLINICAL MANIFESTATIONS

Symptoms. Although symptomatic HOCM is most commonly a disease of young adulthood (the average age of presentation is 26 years[138]), one-third of symptomatic

patients coming to cardiac catheterization are over the age of 60 years.[139] The condition has been observed at necropsy in stillborns and both clinically and pathologically in octogenarians.[139–144] The importance of recognizing this disorder in children at the earliest possible time is highlighted by the high mortality rate; death is often sudden and unexpected. Since syncope and sudden death have been associated with competitive sports and severe exertion in patients with hypertrophic cardiomyopathy, these activities should be proscribed. A particularly high index of suspicion of this condition must be maintained to make the clinical diagnosis in the elderly, since their symptoms may easily be confused with those of coronary artery or aortic valve disease.[139,144] No sex predilection is apparent[145] although females are more likely to be severely disabled and may initially present at a younger age than males.[146]

The clinical picture varies considerably, ranging from the asymptomatic relative of a patient with recognized HOCM who has ASH on echocardiogram but no other manifestation of the illness to the patient with incapacitating symptoms.[138] Most patients with HOCM are asymptomatic and consist of the relatives of patients with known disease. Unfortunately, the first clinical manifestation of the disease in asymptomatic individuals may be sudden death (Fig. 41–7).[147]

The most common symptom is *dyspnea*,[138] which is largely a consequence of the elevated left ventricular diastolic (and therefore left atrial and pulmonary venous) pressure, which results largely from impaired ventricular filling and increased wall stiffness secondary to ventricular hypertrophy.[148] Angina pectoris, fatigue, and syncope are also common.[138,148] Palpitations, paroxysmal nocturnal dyspnea, overt congestive heart failure, and dizziness are found less frequently,[138] although marked congestive heart failure culminating in death may be seen in infants with hypertrophic cardiomyopathy.[149] Exertion tends to exacerbate many of the symptoms. A variety of mechanisms may contribute to the production of angina pectoris. It is at least in part the result of an imbalance between oxygen supply and demand as a consequence of the greatly increased myocardial mass.[150] Transmural infarction may occur in the absence of narrowing in the extramural coronary arteries.[151] Narrowing of the small coronary arteries may contribute to myocardial ischemia,[135] and a few patients with hypertrophic cardiomyopathy may also have atheromatous obstructive coronary artery disease. Impaired diastolic relaxation may produce subendocardial

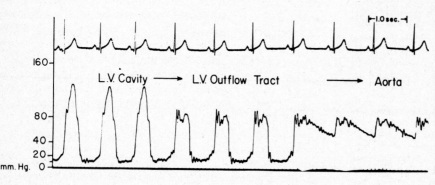

L.V. Cavity ⟶ L.V. Outflow Tract ⟶ Aorta

FIGURE 41–6 Pressure tracing recorded as retrograde aortic catheter was withdrawn from the left ventricular (LV) cavity through the left ventricular outflow tract and into the ascending aorta. Note that the pressure gradient occurs within the left ventricle. There is a notch on the left ventricular pressure pulse at approximately 100 mm Hg, the value of the peak systolic pressure distal to the obstruction. In the left ventricular outflow tract the pressure pulse exhibits a midsystolic dip and a secondary elevation late in systole. A similar contour is present during systole in the aortic pressure pulse. (From Braunwald, E., et al.: Idiopathic hypertrophic subaortic stenosis. Circulation *30*(Suppl. IV):67, 1964, by permission of the American Heart Association, Inc.)

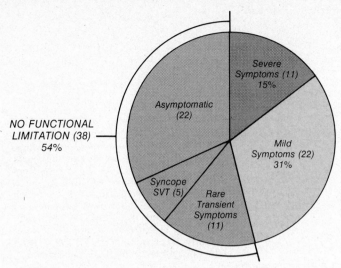

FIGURE 41-7 Functional state before sudden death or cardiac arrest in 71 patients with hypertrophic cardiomyopathy. SVT = supraventricular tachycardia. (From Maron, B. J., et al.: Sudden death in hypertrophic cardiomyopathy: A profile of 78 patients. Circulation 65:1388, 1982, by permission of the American Heart Association, Inc.)

ischemia as a result of prolonged maintenance of wall tension with a concomitant slower-than-normal decrease in the impedance to coronary blood flow. As in patients with valvular aortic stenosis, syncope may result from an inability to increase cardiac output with exertion or from cardiac arrhythmias (p. 1099).[152] Near-syncopal ("graying out") spells that occur in the erect posture and that can be relieved by immediately lying down are common. However, in contrast to valvular aortic stenosis, syncope or near-syncope may not be an ominous finding in hypertrophic cardiomyopathy; some patients have a history of such episodes dating back many years without deterioration in the condition.[138]

Physical Examination. This may be normal in asymptomatic patients without gradients, save for a left ventricular lift and a loud fourth heart sound, but there are usually prominent findings in patients with a pressure gradient in the left ventricular outflow tract. The apical precordial impulse is often displaced laterally and is usually abnormally forceful and enlarged.[138,145] Because of decreased left ventricular compliance, a prominent presystolic apical impulse which results from forceful atrial systole is often present.[148] This may result in a double apical impulse as a result of the prominent *a* wave. A more characteristic but less frequently recognized abnormality is a triple apical beat, the third impulse being a late systolic bulge that occurs when the heart is nearly empty and is performing near-isometric contraction. These findings may be readily recorded by apexcardiography (Fig. 41-8).

A systolic thrill is commonly present, is most frequently palpable at the apex or along the lower left sternal border,[146] and bears only a rough relationship to the severity of the pressure gradient.[138,146] The jugular venous pulse usually demonstrates a prominent *a* wave, reflecting diminished right ventricular compliance secondary to the massive hypertrophy of the ventricular septum. The carotid pulse typically rises briskly and then declines in midsystole as the gradient develops, followed by a secondary rise. This may be well appreciated on physical examination and can be

demonstrated more clearly by means of indirect pulse tracings (Figs. 41-8 and 41-9).

The first heart sound is normal and is often preceded by a fourth heart sound[138,146] that corresponds to the apical presystolic impulse.[145] The second heart sound is usually normally split. In some patients, however, it is narrowly split and in others, particularly those with severe outflow gradients, paradoxical splitting may be noted.[138,146] A third heart sound is common but does not have the same ominous significance as in patients with valvular aortic stenosis. Systolic ejection sounds are rare.[138] The auscultatory hallmark of HOCM is a systolic murmur (Fig. 41-8), which is typically harsh and crescendo-decrescendo in configuration; it often begins well after the first heart sound and is best heard between the apex and the left sternal border. It often radiates well to the lower sternal border, the axillae, and base of the heart but not into the neck vessels.[138,148] The murmur is often more holosystolic and blowing at the apex and in the axillae (probably due to mitral regurgitation) and midsystolic and harsher along the lower sternal border (due to flow across the outflow tract).[146,148]

The murmur is labile in intensity and duration, and a variety of maneuvers may be utilized to augment or suppress it (Table 41-6, p. 1409). The systolic murmur is due both to turbulence as the blood passes through the narrowed left ventricular outflow tract and to mitral regurgitation, which is invariably found when obstruction is present.[148] A diastolic rumbling murmur,[139] reflecting increased transmitral flow, may occur in patients with marked mitral regurgitation. The murmur of aortic regur-

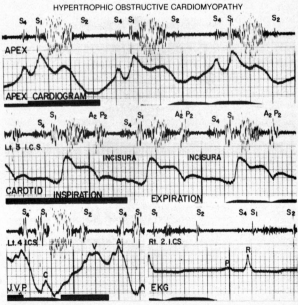

FIGURE 41-8 Phonocardiogram recorded at the apex, the third left intercostal space (Lt. 3 I.C.S.), the fourth left intercostal space (Lt. 4 I.C.S.), and the second right intercostal space (Rt. 2 I.C.S.). S₁ = first heart sound, S₂ = second heart sound, S₄ = fourth heart sound, J.V.P. = jugular venous pulse. Note the prominent S₄ and the presystolic expansion of the apexcardiogram, the prominent *a* wave of the J.V.P., and the rapid upstroke of the indirect carotid arterial pulse. The apexcardiogram exhibits early systolic collapse followed by late systolic expansion. The diamond-shaped midsystolic murmur is recorded best at the apex and is less prominent along the second right intercostal space. (From Braunwald, E., et al.: Idiopathic hypertrophic subaortic stenosis. Circulation 30(Suppl. IV):14, 1964, by permission of the American Heart Association, Inc.)

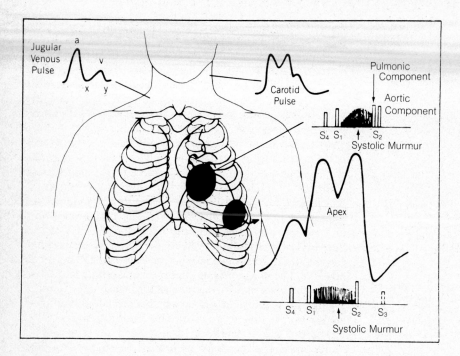

gitation is observed only rarely in patients with HOCM, although it may develop after surgery to correct the outflow gradient[138,146] or following bacterial endocarditis.[153]

It is important to know the features of physical examination that permit differentiation of HOCM from fixed orifice obstruction, most commonly due to valvular aortic stenosis (Table 32–10, p. 1100). The character of the carotid pulse is the most useful feature in this regard. Because there is obstruction to left ventricular emptying from the beginning of systole with fixed valvular stenosis, the carotid upstroke is slowed and of low amplitude (pulsus parvus et tardus) (Fig. 3–22, p. 56, and Fig. 4–4, p. 70). With HOCM, initial ejection of blood from the left ventricle is unimpeded, and therefore the arterial upstroke is brisk. Other features that may be helpful but are of considerably less significance are the location of the murmur (it radiates along the carotid arteries in valvular aortic stenosis but not in HOCM), an ejection sound (present in patients with valvular aortic stenosis in the absence of calcification of the aortic valve and absent in HOCM), and the location of the systolic thrill (most prominent in the second right intercostal space in valvular aortic stenosis and in the fourth interspace along the left sternal border in HOCM).

ELECTROCARDIOGRAM. This is usually abnormal in hypertrophic cardiomyopathy and invariably so in symptomatic patients with left ventricular outflow gradients[153a] (Fig. 41–10). Normal electrocardiograms are seen in only one-fourth of asymptomatic patients without gradients.[138,154] The most common abnormalities are ST-segment and T-wave abnormalities, followed by evidence of left ventricular hypertrophy, with QRS complexes that are tallest in the midprecordial leads.[154,155,155a] There may be progressive electrocardiographic evidence of hypertrophy over time.[155b] Prominent, abnormal Q waves are relatively common, occurring in 20 to 50 percent of patients.[146,148] The Q-wave abnormalities often involve the inferior (II, III, aV_f) and/or lateral (V_4–V_6) leads (Fig. 41–10). They appear to be due to depolarization of myopathic cells in the septum that have abnormal electrophysiological prop-

erties.[156] A variety of other electrocardiographic abnormalities may occur, including abnormal electrical axis (usually left-axis deviation) and P-wave abnormalities (usually left atrial enlargement). Accessory atrioventricular pathways have been found in hypertrophic cardiomyopathy, although they appear to be rare. A short P-R interval followed by slurring of a tall R wave with normal QRS duration is a relatively frequent finding;[138] in many cases this appears to be unassociated with evidence of preexcitation.[157] Clinically significant abnormalities of AV conduction are unusual, but disturbances of AV nodal electrophysiology are surprisingly common in the small number of patients who have undergone electrophysiological study.[158,159] The electrophysiological abnormalities may be subtle manifestations of the fibrotic and cystic changes that have been found at necropsy in the conducting system of patients with HOCM.[160]

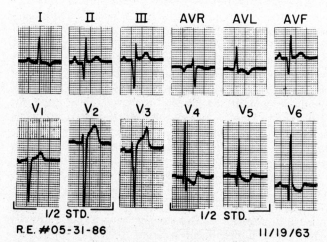

R.E. #05-31-86   11/19/63

FIGURE 41–10 Electrocardiogram showing abnormal Q waves in leads II, III, aV_F, V_5, and V_6 in a patient with HOCM. Precordial leads exhibit the voltage criteria for left ventricular hypertrophy. (From Braunwald, E., et al.: Idiopathic hypertrophic subaortic stenosis. Circulation *30*(Suppl. IV):26, 1964, by permission of the American Heart Association, Inc.)

Although a hemodynamic mechanism may play a role in the demise of patients with hypertrophic cardiomyopathy, many and perhaps most deaths, particularly those that are known to have been sudden, are probably due to an arrhythmia. Because of the systolic and diastolic abnormalities in this disorder, rhythm disturbances are less well tolerated.

Ventricular arrhythmias are common in patients with hypertrophic cardiomyopathy, occurring in over three-fourths of patients undergoing continuous ambulatory electrocardiographic monitoring.[161,162] Ventricular tachycardia is found in about one-fourth of the patients studied, and in some it is a harbinger of subsequent sudden death.[161,162a] A similar spectrum of arrhythmias may be detected in those asymptomatic relatives of patients with hypertrophic cardiomyopathy who themselves have the disease (often undiagnosed).[163] Treadmill testing may expose arrhythmias that are not present at rest, although continuous ambulatory monitoring is superior in detecting repetitive ventricular tachyarrhythmias.[162,164] Supraventricular tachycardia may be found in one-fourth of patients.[165] Atrial fibrillation occurs in 5 to 10 per cent of patients, and the resultant loss of the atrial contribution to the filling of a hypertrophied, stiff ventricle may result in marked clinical deterioration—as a consequence of a reduction in cardiac output or elevation of the left atrial pressure or both.[146,148]

CHEST ROENTGENOGRAM. The findings on radiographic examination are variable; heart size, principally the left ventricle, may range from normal to markedly enlarged, but there is little correlation between heart size and the severity of the outflow tract gradient. Left atrial enlargement is frequently observed, especially when significant mitral regurgitation is present.[138,145,148] Aortic root enlargement and valvular calcification are not seen unless associated diseases are present, although calcification of the mitral annulus is common in HOCM.[166]

ECHOCARDIOGRAPHY (see also p. 128). Because echocardiography combines the attributes of high resolution and no known risk, it has been widely utilized in the evaluation of hypertrophic cardiomyopathy,[100,167–169] (Fig. 41–11, Fig. 5–36, p. 108, and Figs. 5–69 to 5–71, pp. 128 and 129). It is useful in the study of patients with suspected hypertrophic cardiomyopathy and also in the screening of relatives of patients with documented HOCM. The echocardiogram is of value in identifying and quantifying morphological (e.g., asymmetrical septal hypertrophy) as well as functional features (e.g., hypercontractile left ventricle).

The cardinal echocardiographic feature of hypertrophic cardiomyopathy is left ventricular hypertrophy. Maximal hypertrophy of the septum often occurs midway between the base and apex of the left ventricle. The finding of a thickened septum that is 1.3 or more times the thickness of the posterior wall when measured in diastole just prior to atrial systole has been the time-honored criterion for the diagnosis of asymmetrical septal hypertrophy (ASH).[100,170] The septum not only is relatively thicker than the posterior wall but is typically at least 15 mm in thickness (normal $\leq$ 11 mm). Approximately half the first-degree relatives of patients with hypertrophic cardiomyopathy will have such an abnormal septal/free wall ratio, despite the fact that they are often asymptomatic, have normal physical examinations, and are often unaware of any cardiac disease.[94] In patients with concentric left ventricular hypertrophy (due to systemic hypertension or aortic valve disease, for example), the septal/free wall ratio will often be close to 1:1,[171] although it has been reported on the basis of M-mode echocardiograms that many such patients will have ASH.[172,173] The use of a septal/free wall ratio of 1.5:1 may be more specific for hypertrophic cardiomyopathy, although some patients with HOCM will not be identified.[174]

M-mode echocardiography will not always provide accurate measurements of true septal thickness, however. In many cases in which the M-mode echocardiogram falsely suggests ASH, the finding is due to oblique imaging of an acutely anteriorly angled interventricular septum.[175] Two-dimensional echocardiography should be used to clarify septal orientation and thickness in such questionable or equivocal cases, although optimally it should be part of the routine examination of all patients with hypertrophic cardiomyopathy. Two-dimensional echocardiography is also useful for identifying patients with localized hypertrophy in unusual locations not accessible to the M-mode beam such as the posterior or apical septum, the anterior or lateral left ventricular free wall,[113] and the apex.[114,115] An unusual echocardiographic pattern consisting of a ground-glass appearance has been noted in portions of the hypertrophied myocardium in HOCM. It has been speculated

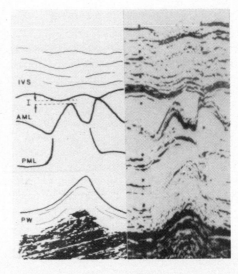
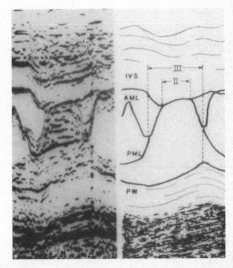

FIGURE 41–11 Determination of degree of systolic anterior motion of mitral valve. *Left,* Echocardiogram and line diagram from a patient with moderate systolic anterior motion. *Right* , A patient with severe systolic anterior motion. PML = posterior mitral leaflet; AML = anterior mitral leaflet; IVS = interventricular septum; PW = posterior left ventricular wall. (From Gilbert, B. W., et al.: Hypertrophic cardiomyopathy: Subclassification by M mode echocardiography. Am. J. Cardiol. *45*:861, 1980.)

that this pattern may be related to the abnormal cellular architecture and myocardial fibrosis that has been noted in pathological studies.[95] Two-dimensional echocardiograms in HOCM have suggested, in concordance with autopsy specimens, that the interventricular septum is configured in the shape of a catenoid, i.e., a curved surface with net zero curvature at all points.[176]

A second echocardiographic feature often found in hypertrophic cardiomyopathy in addition to ASH is narrowing of the left ventricular outflow tract, which is formed by the interventricular septum anteriorly and the anterior leaflet of the mitral valve posteriorly. The mitral valve apparatus is positioned abnormally close to the septum,[167] possibly the result of the posterior bulging of the septum. When hypertrophic cardiomyopathy is associated with a pressure gradient, there is abnormal systolic anterior motion (SAM) of the anterior leaflet of the mitral valve (Fig. 41–11).[167] Although the role of SAM in *producing* the gradient is controversial, there is a close relationship between the degree of SAM and the size of the outflow gradient.[177,178] Prolonged interventricular septal contact of the mitral apparatus is limited to hypertrophic cardiomyopathy with resting pressure gradients,[179] and there is a close temporal relationship between the onset of the pressure gradient and the onset of septal apposition of the mitral apparatus.[180]

Three explanations have been offered for SAM: (1) the mitral valve is *pulled* against the septum by contraction of the papillary muscles, because of the abnormal location and orientation of these muscles resulting from septal hypertrophy; (2) the mitral valve is *pushed* against the septum because of its abnormal position in the outflow tract;[181] (3) the mitral valve is drawn toward the septum because of the lower pressure that occurs as blood is ejected at a high velocity through a narrowed outflow tract (Venturi effect).[148] However, contrary to initial reports, SAM of the mitral valve and dynamic left ventricular gradients are not pathognomonic of HOCM but may be found in a variety of other conditions,[101,102] including hypercontractile states, left ventricular hypertrophy, transposition of the great arteries, and infiltration of the septum.[101,102,182–185] In many cases in conditions other than HOCM, SAM is due to buckling of the chordae tendineae rather than to movement of the anterior mitral valve leaflet as occurs in HOCM (although the chordae tendineae and papillary muscles may contribute to SAM in HOCM).[186]

Several other echocardiographic findings may be present: (1) a small left ventricular cavity;[187] (2) reduced septal motion and thickening during systole (presumably because of the disarray of the myofibrillar architecture and abnormal contractile function);[167] (3) normal or increased motion of the posterior wall; (4) a reduced rate of closure of the mitral valve in mid-diastole secondary to a decrease in left ventricular compliance[187] or abnormal transmitral flow during diastole;[188] (5) mitral valve prolapse;[189] and (6) partial systolic closure or, more commonly, coarse systolic fluttering of the aortic valve related to turbulent blood flow in the outflow tract.[190] The echocardiographic findings that accompany a left ventricular outflow tract gradient (SAM and aortic valve partial closure) may be quite labile, and provocative measures such as the Valsalva maneuver or pharmacologically induced vasodilatation with amyl nitrite (Fig. 3–23, p. 56), stimulation of contractility with

isoproterenol, or an induced premature ventricular contraction may be required to precipitate the findings.[178]

Abnormalities of diastolic function may be shown by echocardiography in many patients with hypertrophic cardiomyopathy, independent of the presence or absence of a systolic pressure gradient. The isovolumetric relaxation time, measured from aortic valve closure to mitral valve opening, is frequently prolonged and the peak velocity of left ventricular filling is reduced.[191,192] Because the septum is typically hypokinetic, the rate of left ventricular filling is determined primarily by the rate of free wall thinning.[191]

RADIONUCLIDE SCANNING TECHNIQUES. These techniques are gaining popularity in the detection of hypertrophic cardiomyopathy. Thallium-201 myocardial imaging permits direct determination of the relative thicknesses of the septum and free wall and may be of particular value when technical constraints limit the reliability of echocardiographic evaluation in a given patient with presumed HOCM.[193] The utility of rest and exercise thallium-201 scintigraphy in identifying patients with hypertrophic cardiomyopathy whose angina pectoris is due to obstructive epicardial coronary artery disease is controversial;[194,195] at least in some patients, thallium-201 defects suggestive of regional myocardial ischemia are found despite angiographically normal coronary arteries.[194] Gated radionuclide ventriculography with blood pool labeling permits the evaluation of not only the size but also the motion of the septum and left ventricle.[196] Disproportionate upper septal thickening is a distinctive scintigraphic feature that may be seen in the steep left anterior oblique view.[196] As with the echocardiogram, abnormal diastolic filling of the ventricle has been observed in patients with hypertrophic cardiomyopathy (both with and without gradients) by computer analysis of the blood pool scan.[197]

Hemodynamics

Cardiac catheterization discloses diminished diastolic left ventricular compliance and a pressure gradient within the body of the left ventricle, which is separated from a subaortic chamber by the thickened septum and the anterior leaflet of the mitral valve that abuts the septum (Figs. 41–6 and 41–12). The pressure gradient may be quite labile and may vary between 0 and 175 mm Hg. There is often a notch on the ascending limb of the left ventricular pressure curve, occurring at the onset of left ventricular ejection.[138] The arterial pressure tracing may demonstrate a "spike and dome" configuration similar to the carotid pulse recording. As a consequence of diminished left ventricular compliance, the mean and particularly the *a* wave in the left atrial pressure pulse and the left ventricular end-diastolic pressures are usually elevated.[138] Artifact stimulation of an outflow gradient may occur if the left ventricular catheter becomes entrapped in the trabeculae of a markedly hypertrophied left ventricle.[148] Proper technique and choice of catheters with side holes should clarify the mechanism of such gradients. Cardiac output may be depressed in patients with longstanding severe gradients. In the majority of patients it is normal; occasionally it is elevated.

Hemodynamic abnormalities in hypertrophic cardiomy-

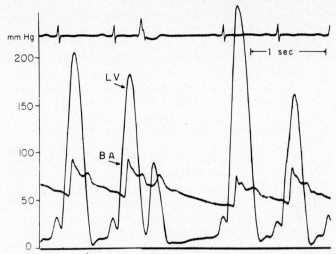

opathy are not limited to the left heart. Approximately one-fourth of patients demonstrate pulmonary hypertension, which is usually mild but occasionally may be moderate to severe. This may be due to elevated mean left atrial pressures. A pressure gradient in the right ventricular outflow tract is seen in approximately 15 per cent of patients who have obstruction to left ventricular outflow[138,146] and appears to result from muscular contraction of the infundibulum. Right atrial and right ventricular end-diastolic pressures may be slightly elevated.

Angiocardiography. Left ventriculography shows a hypertrophied ventricle in which the anterior leaflet of the mitral valve moves anteriorly during systole and encroaches upon the outflow tract (Fig. 41–13). Associated with this motion of the leaflet is mitral regurgitation, which appears to be a constant finding in patients with gradients.[148] The left ventricular cavity is often small, and systolic ejection is typically vigorous, resulting in virtual obliteration of the cavity at end systole, although reduced afterload (end-systolic wall stress) may be related to the apparent hypercontractile state.[198,199] The papillary muscles are often prominent and may fill the left ventricular cavity in late systole. In some cases, the hypertrophy of the papillary muscles and midventricular myocardium may result in true muscular stenosis owing to a sphincter mechanism.[200]

It is often helpful to supplement angiographic evaluation of the left ventricle with simultaneous right ventriculography in a cranially angulated LAO projection in order to obtain optimal visualization of the size, shape, and configuration of the interventricular septum[201] (Fig. 41–14). The hypertrophy appears maximal in the lower portion of the

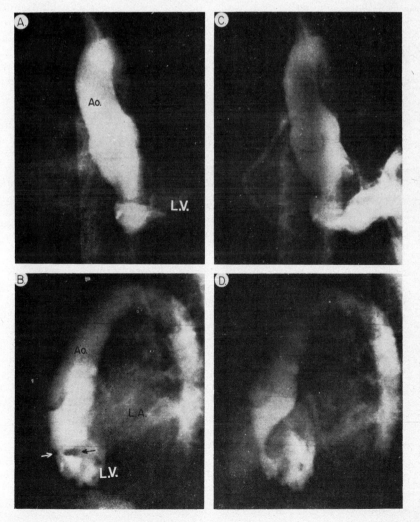

FIGURE 41–13 Angiograms showing obstruction in a patient with familial HOCM. Films were obtained during selective left ventricular angiography, in the frontal (*A* and *C*) and lateral (*B* and *D*) projections. During systole (*A* and *B*), a linear area of narrowing is apparent (arrows), which lies at the point where the hypertrophied septum impinges on the closed anterior leaflet of the mitral valve. Films exposed in diastole (*C* and *D*) also reveal the site of the mitral valve leaflet. Ao. = aorta, L.A. = left atrium, L.V. = left ventricle. (From Ross, J., Jr., Braunwald, E., Gault, J. H., Mason, D. T., and Morrow, A. G.: The mechanism of the intraventricular pressure gradient in idiopathic hypertrophic subaortic stenosis. Circulation *34*:558, 1966, by permission of the American Heart Association, Inc.)

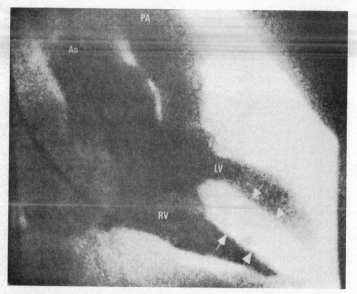

FIGURE 41–14 Right anterior oblique angiocardiogram showing HOCM. Selected systolic cine frame with simultaneous injection of contrast media into both right (RV) and left (LV) ventricles demonstrates the massive hypertrophy of the interventricular septum (arrows). The aorta (Ao) and pulmonary artery (PA) are simultaneously opacified. (From Van Houten, F. X., et al.: Radiology of valvular heart disease. *In* Sonnenblick, E. H., and Lesch, M. (eds.): Valvular Heart Disease. New York, 1974, p. 42, by permission of Grune and Stratton.)

septum, giving it a characteristic triangular appearance.[202] The left septal surface either is flat or bulges into the left ventricular cavity at its mid or lower portion, in contrast to the normal findings of the septum curving toward the right ventricle.[201]

In patients over 45 years of age, coronary artery obstructive disease is rather common, although the symptoms of ischemic pain are indistinguishable from those of patients with normal coronary angiograms and hypertrophic cardiomyopathy.[203] The left anterior descending[204] and septal perforator coronary arteries may demonstrate phasic narrowing during systole in the absence of fixed obstructive lesions.[205]

LABILITY OF GRADIENT

A feature characteristic of HOCM already referred to is the variability and lability of the left ventricular outflow gradient. A given patient may demonstrate a large outflow gradient on one occasion but have none at another time. In some patients without a resting gradient, it may be temporarily provoked.[178,206] Three basic mechanisms are involved in the production of dynamic gradients, all of which act by reducing ventricular volume and presumably accentuate the apposition of the anterior mitral leaflet against the septum: (1) increased contractility, (2) decreased preload, and (3) decreased afterload.[138,206] In a minority of patients with HOCM, the gradient is midventricular[200] and may be intensified by increased contractility, which exerts a direct muscular sphincteric action. The stimuli that provoke or intensify left ventricular outflow tract gradients in HOCM generally improve myocardial performance in normal subjects and in patients with most forms of heart disease[145] (Fig. 41–15). Conversely, reductions in contractility or increases in preload or

afterload, which increase left ventricular dimensions, reduce or abolish the left ventricular outflow gradient.

Alterations in the magnitude of the gradient are reflected by changes in the findings on physical examination, noninvasive tests, and catheterization findings (Fig. 41–16). An increase in the gradient results in a louder murmur, a longer ejection period with a more characteristic spike and dome configuration in the carotid pulse, and more flagrant echocardiographic evidence of SAM of the anterior mitral leaflet. *It is this dynamic characteristic of HOCM that distinguishes it from the discrete forms of obstruction to ventricular outflow.*

A number of bedside procedures may be useful in the evaluation of suspected hypertrophic cardiomyopathy.[207] Perhaps the most helpful is sudden standing from a squatting position. Squatting results in an increase in venous return and an increase in aortic pressure, which increases the ventricular volume, diminishing the gradient and decreasing the intensity of the murmur. Sudden standing has the opposite effects and results in accentuation of the gradient and the murmur. The Valsalva maneuver is another useful bedside technique for eliciting or exacerbating the gradient, (Table 41–6 and Fig. 41–16). Following a transient increase in arterial pressure that usually lasts for four or five cardiac cycles after the onset of the strain coincident with an increase in heart rate, the arterial systolic and pulse pressures and ventricular volume decline, and the gradient (and murmur) increase. Following release of the strain, there is a compensatory overshoot of arterial pressure and venous return and cardiac slowing, all of which increase ventricular volume and reduce the magnitude of the gradient and the murmur.[207] In occasional patients, there may be paradoxical attenuation of the systolic murmur despite an increase in the pressure gradient.[208] The Mueller maneuver, i.e., deep inspiration against a closed glottis (the opposite of the Valsalva maneuver), results in the *lessening* of dynamic obstruction to left ventricular outflow.[209] Inhalation of amyl nitrite also intensifies the murmur and the abnormality of the arterial pulse (Fig. 3–23, p. 56).

One of the most potent stimuli for enhancing the gradient is *postextrasystolic potentiation* (p. 437), which may occur following a spontaneous premature contraction or be induced by mechanical stimulation with a catheter or an external precordial mechanical stimulator.[145,178] The resultant increase in contractility in the beat following the extrasystole is so marked that it outweighs the otherwise salutary effect of increased ventricular filling caused by the compensatory pause and produces an increase in the gradient and murmur. A characteristic change often occurs in the directly recorded arterial pressure tracing, which, in addition to displaying a more marked spike and dome configuration, exhibits a pulse pressure that fails to increase as expected or actually decreases (Fig. 41–12). This is one of the most reliable signs of dynamic obstruction of the left ventricular outflow tract.[210]

Digitalis glycosides and the beta-adrenergic agonist isoproterenol result in an increase in the gradient, since they increase myocardial contractility, while nitroglycerin and amyl nitrite exaggerate the gradient by decreasing arterial pressure and ventricular volume.[138,145] Hypovolemia (as a result of hemorrhage or overly aggressive diuresis) may also provoke overt obstruction to left ventricular outflow.

FIGURE 41–15 *Top,* Simultaneous pressures recorded in the left ventricle (L.V.) and brachial artery (B.A.) before and immediately after the injection of 2 μg of isoproterenol. The broken lines indicate the fall in the brachial artery pressure and the simultaneous elevation of the left ventricular systolic pressure. (From Braunwald, E., et al.: Idiopathic hypertrophic subaortic stenosis. Circulation *30*(Suppl. IV):87, 1964, by permission of the American Heart Association, Inc.) *Bottom,* Effects of 2 mg of methoxamine in a patient with HOCM. *A,* Simultaneous left ventricular (LV) and brachial artery (BA) pressure pulses prior to the injection, showing a large pressure gradient. *B,* Continuous recording at a slow paper speed immediately after the injection, as the gradient gradually disappeared. *C,* Absence of a pressure gradient during the full effect of methoxamine. Note also that as the gradient disappeared, the brachial arterial pressure pulse became more normal and less characteristic of HOCM than it was prior to methoxamine administration (*A*). (From Braunwald, E., et al.: Idiopathic hypertrophic subaortic stenosis. Circulation *30*(Suppl. IV):91, 1964, by permission of the American Heart Association, Inc.)

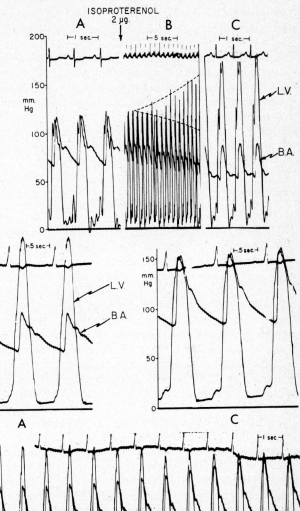

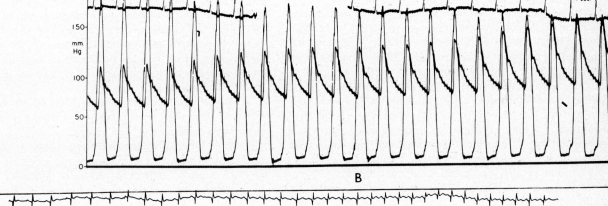

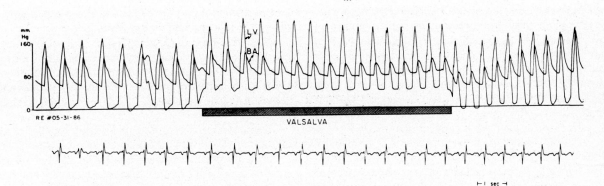

FIGURE 41–16 Effect of the Valsalva maneuver on simultaneous pressures recorded in the left ventricle (LV) and brachial artery (BA) of a patient with HOCM. Note that during the Valsalva maneuver a striking increase in the pressure gradient occurs, which diminishes following release of the Valsalva maneuver. (From Braunwald, E., et al.: Idiopathic hypertrophic subaortic stenosis. Circulation *30*(Suppl. IV):100, 1964, by permission of the American Heart Association, Inc.)

The intensity of the murmur and the left ventricular outflow gradient may be decreased by beta-adrenergic blockade, although the effect is often not dramatic and is of most hemodynamic benefit in protecting against the *increase* in the gradient that may be provoked by exercise. It has also been suggested that propranolol may exert a beneficial effect on diastolic compliance and result in an improvement in myocardial distensibility.[211] In most patients the severity of mitral regurgitation and the intensity of the apical blowing regurgitant murmur vary with the degree of obstruction of left ventricular outflow.[148,207]

TREATMENT

Interventions that decrease ventricular contractility or increase ventricular volume, systemic arterial pressure, the dimensions of the outflow tract, or ventricular distensibility in general exert a salutary effect on the symptoms and vice versa. Since digitalis glycosides increase contractility and thus the gradient, these drugs are generally proscribed unless atrial fibrillation with a very rapid ventricular rate and/or left ventricular dilatation and dysfunction without a gradient are present. Similarly, nitrates and beta-adrenergic stimulants are best avoided. Dyspnea is a prominent symptom in patients with hypertrophic cardiomyopathy but is not usually due to systolic dysfunction, and diuretics should be used sparingly, if at all, since reduction of intravascular volume may reduce ventricular size and increase the systolic pressure gradient.

The mainstay of medical therapy is beta-adrenergic blockade; most of the experience to date has been with propranolol. In addition to possible salutary effects on left ventricular compliance, beta blockade may prevent the increase in outflow obstruction that accompanies exercise, although resting gradients are largely unchanged.[9,212] It decreases the determinants of myocardial oxygen consumption and thus angina pectoris, and perhaps exerts an antiarrhythmic action.[9] Angina pectoris generally responds more favorably to treatment with a beta blocker than does dyspnea.[9] It has also been suggested that beta blockade may prevent sudden death, but its efficacy for this purpose has not been established.[9] Propranolol also blunts the chronotropic response, thus limiting the demand for increased myocardial oxygen delivery.[144a] Beta-adrenergic blockade may also have a beneficial effect on diastolic ventricular filling possibly by improving the distensibility of the left ventricle.[214] The overall clinical response to beta blockade is disappointing, however, since less than one-third of patients experience sustained symptomatic improvement.[131,215] It is reasonable to try large doses of propranolol (greater than 320 mg per day) in patients without contraindications who have not experienced adequate symptomatic improvement with conventional doses.[216]

The calcium-channel blocking agents, principally verapamil and nifedipine, are an increasingly popular alternative to beta-adrenergic blockade in the management of hypertrophic cardiomyopathy. Both the hypercontractile systolic function and the abnormalities of diastolic filling may be related to abnormal calcium kinetics, and drugs that block the inward transport of calcium across the myocardial cell membrane may be able to rectify both abnormalities.

Verapamil has been the most widely studied calcium-channel blocking agent in this condition. Its use was suggested, at least in part, by the observation that it produces a protective and beneficial effect in the hereditary cardiomyopathy of the Syrian hamster, a condition marked by intracellular calcium overload, in which propranolol is ineffective.[217] Although the vasodilator effects of verapamil should not be helpful in HOCM, it appears that by depressing myocardial contractility, verapamil can decrease the left ventricular outflow gradient when given intravenously or orally.[218–220,220a] Perhaps more important from a symptomatic point of view, verapamil improves diastolic filling in hypertrophic cardiomyopathy.[197,221,221a] While variable clinical responses have been reported with verapamil, some patients show increased exercise capacity and an improved symptomatic status.[220] Sustained symptomatic improvement has been noted with the long-term administration of verapamil in ambulatory patients,[222] although important adverse effects, including sudden death, may be seen in a small fraction of patients so treated.[223] Complications with verapamil include suppression of sinus node automaticity and inhibition of atrioventricular conduction, vasodilatation, and negative inotropic effects. These side effects may culminate in hypotension, pulmonary edema, and death; there is a suggestion that antiarrhythmic agents, especially quinidine, may exacerbate the deleterious hemodynamic effects of verapamil.[223] Because of these adverse effects, it has been suggested that verapamil should not be used, or be used only with extreme caution, in patients with high left ventricular filling pressure or symptoms of paroxysmal nocturnal dyspnea or orthopnea.[223] Unfortunately, these are usually precisely the patients who are in greatest need of therapy. In addition, patients with abnormalities of electrical impulse generation or conduction should not receive verapamil unless a pacemaker is in place.

Nifedipine is another calcium-channel blocking agent that has been used in hypertrophic cardiomyopathy, and it may have advantages over verapamil, since it causes less depression of atrioventricular conduction, although it is a more potent vasodilator.[136] It improves diastolic function in HOCM without depressing systolic function, apparently by increasing left ventricular compliance.[136] Nifedipine may also improve the chest pain associated with hypertrophic cardiomyopathy.[224] Combined administration of nifedipine and propranolol may be of benefit in some patients, particularly those with outflow gradients.[225]

Disopyramide, an antiarrhythmic drug that alters calcium kinetics, has produced symptomatic improvement and abolition of the pressure gradient in a small number of patients with hypertrophic cardiomyopathy, presumably as a consequence of depression of left ventricular systolic performance.[226]

Strenuous exercise should be avoided because of the risk of sudden death; it is the major cause of a fatal outcome in hypertrophic cardiomyopathy.[215] Atrial fibrillation should usually be electrically converted to sinus rhythm without delay because of the often catastrophic hemodynamic consequences of the loss of the atrial contribution to ventricular filling in this disorder. Infective endocarditis may occur in as many as 9 per cent of patients,[146,227,228] and antibiotic prophylaxis is indicated.[229] The infection usually occurs on the aortic valve or mitral apparatus, on the endocardium, or at the site of the contact lesion on the septum; thus, chronic endocardial trauma may provide a nidus for subsequent infection.[228] Anticoagulants should be given to patients with chronic atrial fibrillation when no contraindication exists.

Surgical Treatment

A variety of surgical procedures aimed at reducing the outflow gradient have been developed and are most commonly utilized in the markedly symptomatic patient who has not responded well to medical management. The most popular operation for HOCM consists of excising a portion of the hypertrophied septum (Fig. 41–17). A transaortic approach with septal myotomy-myectomy[230,231] is probably the most widely utilized procedure, although left transventricular[232] as well as combined transaortic and left ventricular approaches[233] have also been employed successfully. Operation often relieves the obstruction as well as the mitral regurgitation, although even when performed by surgeons experienced with this procedure, operative mortality is in the range of 5 to 10 per cent.[9,131,234–236] Even patients over the age of 65 years have undergone successful surgery, with benefits and risks comparable to those of younger adults.[237] Since symptoms are not closely correlated with the presence or magnitude of the pressure gradient, it is possible that the operation produces beneficial effects aside from the reduction in outflow gradient. Although replacement of the mitral valve has been advocated,[238] myotomy-myectomy alone is usually adequate and remains the surgical procedure of choice.[207,234,238a] Surgery results in improved exercise capacity with an increase in the peak exercise cardiac output.[239] Furthermore, septal myotomy-myectomy does not produce important impairment of global left ventricular function at rest or during exercise.[240]

Natural History

The clinical course in hypertrophic cardiomyopathy is varied, although in most patients symptoms remain stable or even improve over a period of 5 to 10 years.[146,215] The annual attrition is about 4 per cent a year, and clinical deterioration (aside from sudden death) is usually slow. Although symptoms are unrelated to the severity or even the presence of a gradient, the percentage of severely symptomatic patients does increase with age.[24,146,215] The onset of atrial fibrillation usually leads to a striking increase in symptoms, and prompt cardioversion is usually indicated.[24] Pregnancy appears to be well tolerated.[241,242]

Progression of HOCM to left ventricular dilatation and dysfunction without a gradient, i.e., dilated cardiomyopathy, is an interesting, serious, but unusual occurrence.[215,243] It usually takes place either after prior surgical resection of the septum[243,244] or as a consequence of myocardial infarction.[150,245] In patients with infarction, the extramural coronary arteries may be normal. Extensive areas of the myocardium may be scarred, resulting in left ventricular dilatation.[150]

Death is usually sudden in HOCM and may occur in previously asymptomatic patients, in individuals who were unaware they had the disease, or in patients with an otherwise stable course.[24,146,215,246,247] Paradoxically, younger patients, those without functional limitation, and those with mild or no gradients appear to be at particular risk of sudden death.[147,248] There is a subgroup of patients with hypertrophic cardiomyopathy in whose families premature death is unusually frequent.[247] Even individuals without such "malignant" family histories are at risk of sudden death. No specific clinical feature (other than a family history of sudden death due to hypertrophic cardiomyopathy and young age) appears to identify patients at risk of sudden death,[248] although it has been suggested that a history of syncope and severe dyspnea may be more common in patients at risk of sudden death.[249] Sudden death often occurs during exercise, and strenuous exertion should probably be proscribed in all patients with HOCM whether or not symptoms are prominent, although the risk of sudden death appears to decrease above the age of 40 years.[147,248] Unsuspected hypertrophic cardiomyopathy is the most common abnormality found at autopsy in young competitive athletes who die suddenly.[250]

It is presumed, but not established, that sudden death is due to a ventricular arrhythmia, although atrial arrhythmias may play a role in sensitizing the heart so that ventricular arrhythmias appear subsequently.[147] The protective effect of beta-adrenergic blockade, calcium-channel blockade, or antiarrhythmic agents in preventing sudden death has still not been established. Amiodarone is effective in suppressing repetitive ventricular tachyarrhythmias in hypertrophic cardiomyopathy, although whether this will translate into improved survival remains to be seen.[251]

The risk of sudden death appears to be reduced in patients surviving left ventricular myotomy-myectomy. A small number of patients with outflow gradients, minimal or absent symptoms, and prior cardiac arrest have undergone prophylactic surgery with encouraging short-term results, although whether surgery itself prevents repeat cardiac arrest is unclear, since these patients ordinarily receive antiarrhythmic agents after surgery.[252] Because an effective therapeutic strategy—either medical or surgical—has yet to demonstrate efficacy in preventing sudden death in hypertrophic cardiomyopathy, the results of ongoing investigative efforts are eagerly awaited, particularly those employing a variety of antiarrhythmic agents.[251]

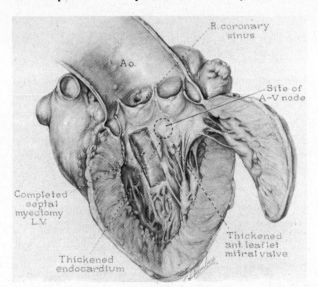

FIGURE 41–17 Appearance of the left ventricle after septal myotomy-myectomy. Ao = aorta. (From Morrow, A. G.: Hypertrophic subaortic stenosis. Operative methods utilized to relieve left ventricular outflow obstruction. J. Thorac. Cardiovasc. Surg. *76*:423, 1978.)

RESTRICTIVE AND INFILTRATIVE CARDIOMYOPATHIES

Of the three major functional categories of the cardiomyopathies (dilated, hypertrophic, and restrictive), the restrictive are the least common in Western countries.[37] The hallmark of the restrictive cardiomyopathies is abnormal diastolic function; the ventricular walls are excessively rigid and impede ventricular filling. Contractile function, on the other hand, is relatively unimpaired, with normal systolic emptying of the ventricles. Thus, restrictive cardiomyopathy bears some functional resemblance to constrictive pericarditis, which is also characterized by normal or near-normal systolic function but abnormal ventricular filling[253] (p. 1490).

A variety of specific pathological processes may result in restrictive cardiomyopathy, although the cause often remains unknown. Myocardial fibrosis, hypertrophy, or infiltration is usually responsible for the abnormal diastolic behavior. Myocardial involvement with amyloid is a common cause of secondary restrictive cardiomyopathy, although restriction is also seen in hemochromatosis, glycogen deposition, endomyocardial fibrosis, and, less commonly, fibroelastosis, the eosinophilias, neoplastic infiltration, pseudoxanthoma elasticum, and myocardial fibrosis of diverse etiologies.[4,37,42,254,255]

In a minority of cases, no specific etiology is apparent. Some patients may manifest all the features of a restrictive cardiomyopathy and exhibit the pathological findings of left ventricular hypertrophy and fibrosis;[12] certainly ventricular hypertrophy can cause diminished ventricular compliance (Fig. 12–23, p. 428 and p. 454). It has been suggested that myocardial fibrosis of any cause may result in restrictive physiology when it is sufficiently severe.[254] Rare patients may present with findings of restrictive physiology but without fibrosis, infiltration, or other pathological findings demonstrable in the heart. It has been suggested that a defect in myocardial relaxation is present in these patients.[254]

To be useful as a clinical descriptor, the term "restrictive cardiomyopathy" must be limited to those patients who are characterized *primarily* by abnormal cardiac stiffness, rather than used to describe patients who have abnormal ventricular filling dynamics associated with impaired ventricular systolic function.[256] Thus, while the hearts of patients with grossly dilated, hypocontractile left ventricles (dilated cardiomyopathy) may well have abnormal diastolic properties, their *primary* abnormality is impairment of systolic function, leading to left ventricular enlargement and, often, asynergic contraction. Similarly, it is clear that while the diastolic properties of the heart are frequently, perhaps universally, abnormal in hypertrophic cardiomyopathy, the hallmark of this condition, by definition, is ventricular hypertrophy.

HEMODYNAMICS. The clinical and hemodynamic features of restrictive heart disease simulate those of chronic constrictive pericarditis,[4,253,256] and endomyocardial biopsy may be particularly useful in this setting. Exploratory thoracotomy may be required on rare occasions.[256] The characteristic hemodynamic feature in both conditions occurs in the ventricular pressure recording, which shows a deep and rapid early decline in ventricular pressure at the onset of diastole, with a rapid rise to a plateau in early diastole. This dip and plateau has been termed the "square root" sign[257] (Fig. 43–16, p. 1490) and is manifested in the atrial pressure tracing as a prominent y descent followed by a rapid rise and plateau. The x descent may also be rapid, and the combination results in the characteristic M or W waveform in the atrial pressure tracing. The a wave is prominent and often is of the same amplitude as the v wave.[4,258] Both systemic and pulmonary venous pressures are elevated, although patients with restrictive heart disease typically have higher left than right ventricular filling pressures, and this difference is accentuated by exercise.[256] In this respect they differ from patients with constrictive pericarditis, in whom diastolic pressures are similar in both ventricles. The pulmonary artery systolic pressure is usually greater than 50 mm Hg in patients with restrictive cardiomyopathy but is lower in constrictive pericarditis.[253,258] Furthermore, the plateau of the right ventricular diastolic pressure is usually at least one-third of the peak right ventricular systolic pressure in patients with constrictive pericarditis, while it is frequently less in restrictive cardiomyopathy.[253]

CLINICAL MANIFESTATIONS. Exercise intolerance is frequent because of the inability of patients with restrictive cardiomyopathy to increase their cardiac output by tachycardia without further compromising ventricular filling.[37] Weakness and dyspnea are often prominent.[256] Chest pain may be prominent in a small fraction of patients but is usually absent. Particularly in advanced cases, an elevated central venous pressure, with peripheral edema, enlarged liver, ascites, and anasarca may be present.[4,256] *Physical examination* may reveal jugular venous distention; an S_3, S_4, or both; and, occasionally, systolic murmurs reflecting atrioventricular valvular regurgitation.[4,256] An inspiratory increase in venous pressure (Kussmaul sign) may be seen.[4] However, in contrast to constrictive pericarditis, the apex impulse is usually palpable, and the apexcardiogram demonstrates a prominent rapid filling wave in restrictive cardiomyopathy.

Various ancillary laboratory findings in addition to endomyocardial biopsy may be useful in distinguishing between constrictive and restrictive disease. While pericardial calcification is neither absolutely sensitive nor specific for constrictive pericarditis[256] (p. 1492), its presence in a patient in whom the differential diagnosis rests between restrictive cardiomyopathy and constrictive pericarditis lends strong support to the latter diagnosis. The echocardiogram may demonstrate thickening of the left ventricular wall and an increase of left ventricular mass in patients with infiltrative disease causing restrictive cardiomyopathy.[259]

AMYLOIDOSIS

ETIOLOGY AND TYPES. Amyloidosis is a disease complex that results from deposition of unique twisted β-pleated sheet fibrils formed from various proteins by several different pathogenic mechanisms.[260] Amyloid may be found in almost any organ, but clinically evident disease does not appear unless there is extensive infiltration. Several different types of amyloid fibrils have been described; the two most common are those composed of immunoglobulin light chains (designated AL) and those composed of a nonimmunoglobulin protein (designated AA).[260-262]

Amyloidosis presents in one of three clinicopathological forms: (1) acquired systemic amyloidosis, (2) organ-limited amyloidosis, and (3) localized deposition. Three forms of acquired systemic amyloidosis are seen: (a) associated with an immunocyte dyscrasia (e.g., multiple myeloma), (b) reactive (e.g., due to chronic infectious or inflammatory conditions), and (c) heredofamilial. Three different forms of familial involvement are recognized, depending upon the principal organ system involved: nephropathic, neuropathic, and cardiopathic.[263] Organ-limited amyloidosis may involve several organ systems, including the heart, and is more common with aging, thus the designation *senile* amyloidosis.

Senile amyloidosis is becoming increasingly common as the average age of the population increases. Indeed, involvement of the heart by senile amyloidosis may be found in more than 10 per cent of routinely autopsied individuals over the age of 75 years, and the prevalence and severity of involvement increases with advancing age. The fibrillar protein is unlike that found in other forms of amyloidosis. Small deposits of amyloid may often be found in the pulmonary vessels or the vessels of other organs as well.[264]

Cardiac Amyloidosis

Involvement of the heart is a common finding and is the most frequent cause of death in amyloidosis associated with an immunocyte dyscrasia.[265] In reactive amyloidosis, on the other hand, clinically significant cardiac involvement is uncommon;[260,261] the myocardial deposits are typically small and perivascular and usually do not result in significant myocardial dysfunction.[266] Familial amyloidosis is only occasionally associated with overt cardiac involvement; the clinical course is usually dominated by neurological or renal dysfunction, particularly in familial Mediterranean fever, in which death at an early age from renal failure is common.[263] Cardiac involvement in senile amyloidosis varies from small atrial deposits that do not result in functional impairment to extensive ventricular involvement with resultant cardiac failure.[267]

Cardiac amyloidosis occurs more commonly in men than in women (except for the senile form), and it is rare before the age of 40 years.[261,267-269] Even in the familial form, the onset of clinical cardiac disease usually does not occur before the age of 35 years and generally occurs much later in life.[263]

PATHOLOGY. The pathological findings often include mild cardiac enlargement, usually without significant ventricular dilatation. The walls of both ventricles are typically firm, rubbery, noncompliant, and thickened.[268] Amyloid is present between the myocardial fibers, with extensive deposition in the papillary muscles occurring commonly.[269a] Serial sections of the sinoatrial and atrioventricular nodes and the bundle branches may disclose amyloid deposits,[268] but fibrosis of these structures is perhaps more common.[270] In addition, endocardial involvement of the atria and ventricles is frequent, often associated with overlying thrombi. The pericardium may contain focal deposits of amyloid as

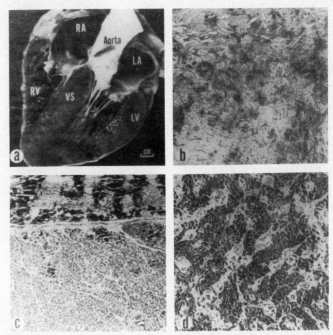

FIGURE 41–18 *a,* Gross appearance of unfixed heart in generalized cardiac amyloidosis. Note hypertrophied left ventricle (LV), right ventricle (RV), and ventricular septum (VS); rigid left atrium (LA) and right atrium (RA); and nodular thickening of mitral valve (*). *b,* Photomicrograph of mitral valve with extensive amyloid deposits (dark-staining patches) (× 64). *c,* Photomicrograph of left atrial wall. Note concentration of amyloid deposits in endocardium (dark-staining patches in upper part) (× 64). *d,* Photomicrograph of ventricular myocardium with diffuse amyloid deposits in interstitium and small blood vessels (pale-staining areas) surrounding irregular islands of muscle fibers (dark-staining areas) (× 64). (From Lie, J. T.: Amyloidosis and amyloid heart disease. Primary Cardiol. *8:*75, 1982.)

well. Amyloidosis often results in focal thickening or deposits on the cardiac valves, but these abnormalities do not appear to interfere with valvular function. The intramural coronary arteries and veins frequently contain amyloid deposits in the media and adventitia, occasionally compromising the lumina of the vessels,[270a] with attendant localized areas of ischemic necrosis that may produce intractable congestive heart failure (Fig. 41–19).[268,271]

CLINICAL MANIFESTATIONS. Involvement of the cardiovascular system by amyloidosis occurs in one of four general patterns:

1. The most common is congestive heart failure due to systolic dysfunction, which occurs in half or more patients.[265,268] Hemodynamic evidence of restriction of ventricular filling may not be prominent in these patients. The course of this form of the disease is often one of gradual progression, usually poorly responsive to treatment. The progress is usually rapid, with death due to cardiac failure generally occurring between 4 months and 2 years after the onset of symptoms.[261,265,268] Cardiomegaly is often demonstrated on chest roentgenography, although massive cardiac enlargement is uncommon. Angina pectoris occurs in one-third of the patients, often reflecting amyloid involvement of the coronary arteries.[268]

2. A second presentation of cardiac amyloidosis is that of a restrictive cardiomyopathy.[272] Right-sided findings dominate the clinical presentation, with peripheral edema a prominent finding while paroxysmal nocturnal dyspnea and orthopnea are absent. The amyloid infiltration of the

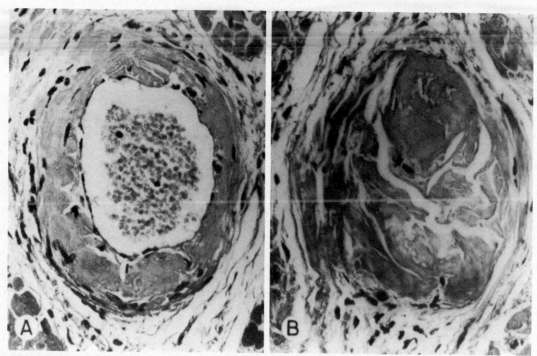

FIGURE 41–19 Amyloidosis of intramyocardial arteries. *A,* Extensive medial deposition of amyloid with preservation of the vascular lumen. *B,* Complete loss of luminal patency as a result of the amyloid. (Hematoxylin and eosin stain; × 400, reduced by 28 per cent.) (From Smith, R. R. L., and Hutchins, G. M.: Ischemic heart disease secondary to amyloidosis of intramyocardial arteries. Am. J. Cardiol. *44*:413, 1979.)

myocardium results in increased stiffness of the myocardium, producing the characteristic diastolic dip and plateau (square root sign) in the ventricular pressure pulse.[256] In contrast to the accelerated early left ventricular diastolic filling found in constrictive pericarditis, cardiac amyloidosis is marked by an impaired rate of early diastolic filling, as a consequence of the stiffness of the ventricle[273] (Fig. 43–21, p. 1494).

3. An abnormality of cardiac impulse formation and conduction is a third mode of presentation and may result in arrhythmias and conduction disturbances, which are common in cardiac amyloidosis. One-third or more of patients with primary amyloidosis may experience lightheadedness or syncope.[261,265] Sudden death, presumably arrhythmic in origin, is relatively common.[272]

4. Orthostatic hypotension is the fourth mode of presentation. Although most likely due to amyloid infiltration of the autonomic nervous system or of blood vessels (p. 930), amyloid deposition in the heart and adrenals may contribute to this manifestation.[274] Hypovolemia as a result of the nephrotic syndrome secondary to renal amyloidosis may aggravate the postural hypotension.

Physical examination often reveals findings of congestive heart failure,[268] with systolic murmurs due to atrioventricular valvular regurgitation. Particularly in patients with restrictive cardiomyopathy, jugular venous distention, a protodiastolic gallop, hepatomegaly, peripheral edema, and a narrow pulse pressure are present.[274]

The *chest roentgenogram* usually shows cardiomegaly in patients with the clinical and hemodynamic picture of congestive cardiomyopathy, although heart size may be normal in patients with the restrictive form. Pulmonary congestion may be prominent in patients with congestive

heart failure. Pleural effusions are common. *The electrocardiogram* is frequently abnormal;[268] the most characteristic feature is diffusely diminished voltage, occurring in approximately half the patients. Myocardial infarction is often simulated because of small or absent R waves in right precordial leads or, less frequently, by Q waves in the inferior leads. Left-axis deviation is seen in more than half the patients. Arrhythmias are common, particularly atrial fibrillation, which has been reported in 20 per cent of the patients. Various forms of AV conduction defects are often seen and have been found in one-third of patients with cardiac amyloidosis. Abnormalities of AV conduction appear to be particularly common in familial amyloidosis with polyneuropathy.[275] Sinus node involvement is common, and the clinical and electrocardiographic features of the sick sinus syndrome may be present (p. 693).[276] Patients with cardiac amyloidosis appear to be particularly sensitive to digitalis preparations, and the use of ordinary doses of digitalis glycosides may lead to serious arrhythmias.

Echocardiography (Fig. 5–73, p. 130) most commonly reveals increased thickness of the walls of the ventricles and an increased left ventricular mass.[259,272,277,278] The left ventricular cavity is usually normal or small in size, and wall excursions are often reduced.[259,272,277] A pericardial effusion is common, but rarely results in tamponade.[279] The appearance of the thickened cardiac walls is often distinctive on two-dimensional echocardiography, demonstrating a granular sparkling texture, presumably due to the amyloid deposit.[280] Echocardiographic demonstration of thick left ventricular walls with concomitant low voltage on the electrocardiogram appears to distinguish cardiac amyloidosis from pericardial disease or left ventricular hypertrophy, and this distinctive voltage/mass ratio is characteristic of myocardial infiltration by the amyloid fibrils.[281] Computer-assisted analysis of echocardiograms in amyloidosis has shown reduced ventricular distensibility and impaired diastolic filling.[282]

DIAGNOSIS. Whereas two or three decades ago the clinical diagnosis of systemic amyloidosis was made correctly antemortem only 25 per cent of the time, with more recent clinical awareness of the disease and the utilization of *biopsy techniques* the diagnosis is now made antemortem in almost 80 per cent of cases.[265,274] Rectal biopsy has been the single most useful diagnostic procedure, combining the attributes of relative ease of performance, sensitivity, and safety.[265] Biopsy of gingiva, bone marrow, liver, kidney, and various other tissues has also been employed. Endomyocardial biopsy of the right[283,284] or left ventricles[285] may be helpful in establishing the diagnosis of cardiac amyloidosis.

TREATMENT. The treatment of cardiac amyloidosis is generally ineffective, since there is no way to halt the progression of the underlying disease,[261] although several experimental trials are under way. Digitalis glycosides should be used with caution because patients with cardiac amyloidosis appear to be particularly sensitive to digitalis preparations, and the use of ordinary doses may lead to serious arrhythmias; this may relate to selective binding of digoxin to amyloid fibrils in the myocardium.[286] Insertion of a permanent pacemaker may be beneficial in patients with symptomatic conducting system disease.

INHERITED INFILTRATIVE DISORDERS CAUSING CARDIOMYOPATHY

The inherited disorders of Fabry's disease and Gaucher's disease are associated with the abnormal intramyocardial accumulation of a metabolic product. Such myocardial involvement results primarily in abnormal systolic contractile performance. However, the accumulation of the metabolic product in the myocardium may also impair the filling of the ventricles, thereby adding a restrictive component.

FABRY'S DISEASE. Fabry's disease (angiokeratoma corporis diffusum universale) is an X-linked disorder of glycosphingolipid metabolism due to a deficiency of the enzyme ceramide trihexosidase. It is characterized by an intracellular accumulation of a neutral glycolipid, with prominent involvement of the skin and kidneys as well as the myocardium. *Histological examination* often reveals widespread involvement of the myocardium, vascular endothelium, conducting tissues, and valves—particularly the mitral valve.[287,288] The major clinical manifestations of the disease result from the accumulation of the glycolipid substrate in endothelial cells, with eventual occlusion of small arterioles.[289] The accumulation of the glycolipid occurs in the lysosomes of the cardiac tissues and is responsible for the multiple cardiovascular manifestations of Fabry's disease.[287] Symptomatic cardiovascular involvement occurs eventually in most affected males, while female carriers are usually asymptomatic or only minimally symptomatic.[287] Systemic hypertension, myocardial ischemia or infarction, and congestive heart failure are common clinical manifestations.[287] Electrocardiographic abnormalities include left ventricular hypertrophy, P-wave abnormalities,

conduction defects, and arrhythmias.[290] The echocardiogram usually reveals increased left ventricular wall thickness, presumably the result of glycolipid deposition.[289]

GAUCHER'S DISEASE. Gaucher's disease is an uncommon, inherited disorder of glycosyl ceramide metabolism. It is secondary to a deficiency of the enzyme beta-glucosidase and results in accumulation of cerebrosides in the spleen, liver, bone marrow, lymph nodes, brain, and myocardium. Diffuse interstitial infiltration of the left ventricle by cells laden with cerebroside occurs in Gaucher's disease, associated with reduced left ventricular compliance and cardiac output. Clinical evidence of cardiac involvement is uncommon, but when present it is characterized by left ventricular dysfunction.[291]

Hemochromatosis and Hemosiderosis
(See also p. 1682)

Hemochromatosis is characterized by excessive deposition of iron in a variety of parenchymal tissues (heart, liver, gonads, and pancreas). It may occur (1) as a familial or idiopathic disorder, (2) in association with a defect in hemoglobin synthesis resulting in ineffective erythropoiesis, (3) in chronic liver disease, and (4) with excessive oral intake of iron over many years. While patients who have iron deposits in the myocardium virtually always have deposits in other organs (e.g., liver, spleen, pancreas, bone marrow), the severity of myocardial involvement varies widely and parallels only roughly that in other organs.[292]

The *pathological findings* (Fig. 49–7, p. 1683) are a dilated heart with thickened ventricular walls. Myocardial iron deposits, often grossly visible, are most common in the subepicardial region, followed by the subendocardial region and papillary muscles, and are least common in the midmyocardial wall. They are more extensive in ventricular than atrial myocardium.[292] Iron deposits in myocardial cells are typically perinuclear in location initially but eventually occupy much of the fiber. Involvement of the cardiac conducting system is limited, compared with the relatively heavy infiltration of contracting cells.[293] Myocardial degeneration and fibrosis may also occur.

The severity of myocardial dysfunction is proportional to the amount of iron present in the myocardium.[293] Extensive deposits of cardiac iron (particularly those grossly visible at postmortem examination) are invariably associated with cardiac dysfunction—usually chronic congestive heart failure, which is often the cause of death. Extensive cardiac deposits usually occur in patients who receive more than 100 blood transfusions (unless there is associated iron loss due to bleeding).[292]

The *clinical manifestations* vary widely, depending on the extent of myocardial involvement. Some patients remain asymptomatic despite echocardiographic evidence of myocardial infiltration, which is expressed as an increase in left ventricular wall thickness.[259,293] Symptomatic cardiac involvement is usually associated with electrocardiographic abnormalities, including ST-segment and T-wave changes, as well as supraventricular arrhythmias; these electrocardiographic changes correlate with the degree of iron deposits in the heart.[292] Atrioventricular conduction disturbances and ventricular arrhythmias are uncommon.

Severe iron storage disease involving the heart usually produces a dilated and rarely a restrictive cardiomyopathy, characterized by exertional dyspnea, orthopnea, peripheral edema, and protodiastolic gallop sounds. The diagnosis is aided by finding elevated plasma iron levels (180 to 300 μg/dl; normal = 50 to 150), a normal or low total iron-binding capacity (200 to 300 μg/dl; normal = 250 to 370), and markedly elevated values for saturation of transferrin (80 to 100 per cent; normal = 22 to 46 per cent), serum ferritin (900 to 6000 ng/ml; normal = 3 to 180), urinary iron (9 to 23 mg/24 hr; normal = 0 to 2), and liver iron (600 to 1800 μg/100 mg dry wt; normal = 30 to 140).[294] Cardiac failure is usually progressive and largely refractory to therapy,[292] although repeated phlebotomies or the use of the chelating agent desferrioxamine may be beneficial.[295,296] (See further discussion of the treatment of iron storage disease on p. 1684.)

SARCOIDOSIS

Sarcoidosis is a granulomatous disorder of unknown etiology, characterized by multisystem involvement. Infiltration of the lungs, reticuloendothelial system, and skin usually dominates the clinical picture, but virtually any tissue may be affected. The most important manifestation results from pulmonary involvement. This often leads to diffuse fibrosis which may result in fatal right heart failure[297] (p. 1595). Primary cardiac involvement is not often recognized clinically, although it may be demonstrated at autopsy in 20 to 30 per cent of cases of sarcoid, most of which demonstrate generalized sarcoidosis.[298,299] Clinical manifestations of sarcoid heart disease are present in less than 5 per cent of patients, although myocardial involvement may result in heart block, congestive heart failure, and sudden death.[300,301] Myocardial sarcoidosis may have restrictive as well as congestive features, since cardiac infiltration by sarcoid granulomas results not only in increased stiffness of the ventricular wall but diminished systolic contractile function as well. Myocardial sarcoidosis typically affects young or middle-aged adults (mean age, 40 years) of either sex; there is usually evidence of generalized sarcoidosis.[297,302]

PATHOLOGY. The typical pathological feature of sarcoidosis is the presence of noncaseating granulomas,[303,304] which occur in many organs.[305] They infiltrate the myocardium and may eventually become fibrotic scars[306] (Fig. 41–20). The granulomas may involve any region of the heart, although the left ventricular free wall and the interventricular septum are the most common sites, and extensive granulomas and scar tissue in the cephalad portion of the interventricular septum is a constant finding in patients with abnormalities of the conduction system.[300,302] Occasional patients may have preferential and extensive involvement of the septum with minimal disease elsewhere in the heart.[307] Transmural involvement is common,[302] and large portions of the ventricular wall may be replaced by sarcoid tissue, which may lead to aneurysm formation. Even apparently uninvolved myocardium may demonstrate extensive mitochondrial damage upon examination by electron microscopy.[308] While involvement of small coronary artery branches may be found in sarcoidosis, the pathophysiological importance of this observation remains unclear.[309]

CLINICAL MANIFESTATIONS. Death was sudden in two-thirds of the patients in a large autopsy study of sarcoidosis of the heart; indeed, sudden death is the most common manifestation of cardiac sarcoidosis.[302] Many of the patients experienced antecedent arrhythmias or complete AV block.[302,309–312] Conduction disturbance is the most frequent clinical indication of myocardial sarcoid in nonfatal cases.[298] Syncope is common and may reflect paroxysmal arrhythmias or conduction disturbances.[307,313] Atrial and ventricular arrhythmias, especially ventricular tachycardia, are observed frequently.[301,302,314,315] Congestive heart failure is the other major manifestation of myocardial involvement. While cor pulmonale accounts for some of the symptoms of heart failure, many symptoms are caused by direct myocardial involvement by granulomas and scar tissue, and the patients show the clinical features of restrictive or dilated cardiomyopathy.[302,311,312,316] Symptoms of myocardial sarcoid may be present for variable lengths of time, with survival for up to 15 years reported.[300] However, the disease often progresses rapidly to death, and in the majority of patients the interval from the onset of the cardiac symptoms to death is less than 2 years.[302]

Cardiac dysfunction is often severe and progressive and

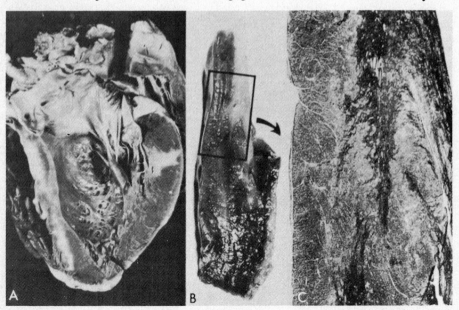

FIGURE 41–20 A, Cardiac sarcoidosis, with hypertrophied and dilated left ventricle, diffuse fibrosis of the interventricular septum, and a focal discrete scar in the free left ventricular wall. B, Fibrosis in the region of interventricular septum. C, Histological section from the area delineated in B, demonstrating the darker staining fibrosed areas. (Original magnification × 5.) (From Lie, J. T., et al.: Sudden death from cardiac sarcoidosis with involvement of conduction system. Am. J. Med. Sci. 267:123, 1974.)

usually refractory to therapy.[298] Occasionally, patients with extensive involvement develop overt left ventricular aneurysms.[301,302,317] Pericardial effusions and valvular involvement sometimes occur.[304,310] Calcification of the mitral valve annulus, probably reflecting the effects of the hypercalcemia that may accompany sarcoidosis, is sometimes found.[302]

The *physical examination* may reveal findings of extracardiac sarcoid or may be totally normal. Cardiac murmurs are common, usually reflecting mitral regurgitation.[298,302] This appears to be more the result of left ventricular dilatation or infiltration than of direct sarcoid involvement of the papillary muscles.[302]

The *electrocardiogram* is frequently abnormal in patients with known sarcoid and most commonly demonstrates T-wave abnormalities.[318] Sarcoidosis appears to have an affinity for involvement of the AV junction and bundle of His, and thus varying degrees of AV block are common.[298,302,309,311,319] With extensive myocardial involvement, pathological Q waves may appear and simulate myocardial infarction.[301,307]

DIAGNOSIS. In many cases the diagnosis may be suspected in patients with bilateral hilar lymphadenopathy on chest roentgenogram in whom there is clinical or electrocardiographic evidence of myocardial disease. Some patients may have myocardial involvement without other overt systemic indications of disease. In this situation, percutaneous endomyocardial biopsy may be particularly useful.[320] Myocardial imaging with thallium-201 may also be helpful in demonstrating segmental filling defects representing areas of infiltration of the myocardium[321] and may indicate myocardial involvement in more than one-third of patients with sarcoid but without clinical evidence of cardiac involvement.[322] Imaging may also indicate the presence of right ventricular hypertrophy in patients with right ventricular overload due to pulmonary fibrosis and pulmonary hypertension. Myocardial uptake of technetium pyrophosphate and gallium in myocardial sarcoidosis has also been reported.[322a]

TREATMENT. The treatment of myocardial sarcoidosis is difficult. Arrhythmias are often refractory to antiarrhythmic drugs, although quinidine with or without propranolol is sometimes efficacious.[300,323,324] Permanent pacing may be helpful,[300,309,324] and since sudden death is so common in sarcoid, it should be applied in all patients with advanced heart block.[324]

The evaluation of the response of sarcoidosis to therapy is made even more difficult by the occasional spontaneous improvement in conduction that may occur.[300] While the matter is not settled, it appears that corticosteroids may be of some benefit in treating the conduction disturbances, arrhythmias, and myocardial dysfunction of sarcoidosis.[300,325,326] Since the risk of the sudden death appears to be greatest in patients with extensive myocardial involvement, it is reasonable to attempt to halt the progression of the disease with steroids before irreversible fibrosis occurs.[299,319] Some evidence suggests that steroids may result in the healing of granulomas, although formation of a ventricular aneurysm may be a possible side effect.[302]

Whipple's Disease

Intestinal lipodystrophy, or Whipple's disease, may be associated with myocardial involvement, and PAS-positive macrophages may be found in the myocardium, pericardium, and heart valves of patients with this disorder.[327] Electron microscopy has demonstrated rod-shaped structures in the myocardium similar to those found in the small intestine, and it has been suggested that they are the causative agent of the myocardial abnormalities. There is often an associated inflammatory infiltrate and foci of fibrosis. The valvular fibrosis may be severe enough to result in malfunction. While asymptomatic, nonspecific electrocardiographic changes are most common, systolic murmurs, pericarditis, and even overt congestive heart failure may occur.[327]

BECKER'S DISEASE

Becker's disease (also called African cardiomyopathy) is an uncommon condition of obscure etiology that occurs most commonly in South Africa. It is characterized by cardiac dilatation without hypertrophy and by fibrosis of the papillary muscles, subendocardium, and endocardium; it is associated with pericardial effusion, myocardial necrosis, and mural thrombosis.[328,329] The disease appears to progress from an acute edematous serous myocarditis marked by fibrinoid necrosis to a chronic stage with endocardial necrosis and fibrosis, mural thrombosis, and organization leading to endocardial sclerosis.

At necropsy, the heart is dilated but not hypertrophied; a pericardial effusion is often present. White patches of endocardial thickening, composed of fibroelastic tissue, typically involve the apex, the papillary muscles, atria, and the outflow portion of the interventricular septum.[329] A thin fibrin layer usually covers the endocardium, but the cardiac valves are uninvolved. Mural thrombi are a ubiquitous finding, occurring most commonly in the left ventricle, followed in frequency by the left atrium, right atrium, and, rarely, the right ventricle.[328] There is marked interstitial edema of the myocardium, with a serous myocarditis and degenerated and necrotic muscle fibers. Perivascular fibrosis may be prominent. The aorta and its vasa vasorum may show focal nodular swellings and fibrinoid necrosis, and giant cells may be found within the intima of the pulmonary artery.[328,329]

ETIOLOGY. Although nutritional, toxic, hypersensitivity, and infectious causes of the disease have been suggested, the actual mechanism remains obscure. It is intriguing that patients at risk of developing Becker's disease appear to ingest a diet deficient in tryptophan[330] and that rats fed a similar diet for long periods of time develop cardiac lesions similar to those found in humans.[331] Jamaican cardiomyopathy[332] may represent the same or a closely related pathological process.

CLINICAL MANIFESTATIONS. The disease occurs in all ages and in all races in South Africa. It may present as congestive heart failure, which may be acute and rapidly progressive, with death occurring within 6 months, or may be chronic, with survival for up to three years.[329] Patients may show an acute illness marked by fever; leukocytosis (without eosinophilia); multiple emboli with infarction of the lungs, spleen, kidneys, or brain; and progressive congestive heart failure.[328,329] Dyspnea is an almost ubiquitous symptom, often associated with cough, peripheral edema, chest pain, and hemoptysis.[328] *Physical examination* reveals jugular venous distention, tachycardia, pulmonary congestion, edema, cardiomegaly, gallop rhythm, and a systolic murmur of atrioventricular valvular regurgitation.[329]

Chest roentgenography reveals an enlarged cardiac silhouette due to both cardiomegaly and pericardial effusion.[328] Findings typical of pulmonary congestion are common. The *electrocardiogram* is virtually always abnormal, principally with ST-segment and T-wave abnormalities.

ENDOMYOCARDIAL FIBROSIS

Endomyocardial fibrosis is a disease of unknown etiology that occurs most commonly in the residents of tropical and subtropical Africa, particularly Uganda and Nigeria. It is typified by fibrous endocardial lesions of the inflow portion of the right or left ventricle or both and often involves the atrioventricular valves, resulting in regurgitation. It is a relatively frequent cause of heart failure and death in equatorial Africa, accounting for 15 to 25 per cent of deaths due to heart disease.[329,333,334]

While most prominent in Africa, it is also found in tropical and subtropical regions in the rest of the world, including India, Brazil, Colombia, and Ceylon.[335–338] It is most common in specific ethnic groups, notably the Rwanda tribe in Uganda[339] and in people of low socioeconomic status.[334] The disease is equally frequent in both sexes, and, although most common in children and young adults, its reported age range is from 4 to 70 years of age.[329] It is most common in blacks, but cases have been reported occasionally in Caucasians in temperate climates who previously resided in tropical areas.[338]

PATHOLOGY. A pericardial effusion, which may be quite large, may be present. The heart is normal in size or slightly enlarged, but massive cardiomegaly does not occur.[337] Hypertrophy is typically absent. The right atrium is often dilated, and in patients with severe right ventricular involvement there may be massive enlargement of this chamber. Indentation of the right border of the heart above the apex as a result of apical scarring may occur. The right ventricular outflow tract is often dilated above this indentation.[339]

Combined right and left ventricular disease occurs in about half the cases, with pure left ventricular involvement occurring in 40 per cent and pure right ventricular involvement in the remaining 10 per cent of patients who are examined post mortem.[337] When affected, the right ventricle exhibits extensive, dense, fibrous thickening of the inflow tract and apex, with involvement of the papillary muscles and chordae tendineae. Involvement of the right ventricle may lead to obliteration of the apex, with a mass of thrombus and fibrous tissue filling the cavity.[329,337] The tricuspid valve is often pulled down and distorted by the fibrous process involving the supporting structures.[329] Right atrial thrombi occur commonly.[337,339] Left ventricular involvement is similar, with fibrosis extending from the apex up the inflow portion of the left ventricle to the posterior mitral valve leaflet. The anterior leaflet of the mitral valve and the outflow portion of the left ventricle are usually spared.[337] Thrombi may overlie the endocardial lesions, but obliteration of the left ventricular cavity does not occur.

Microscopically, the involved endocardium demonstrates

a thick layer of hyalinized fibrous tissue on top of a layer of collagen fibers;[329] foci of calcification may be present,[340] and thrombus may cover the outer layer of fibrous tissue. Septa composed of fibrous and granulation tissue extend for variable distances into the myocardium.[329,340] The myocardial fibers may show degeneration, particularly in areas adjacent to the fibrous plaques.[339] Interstitial edema is often present, but there is no cellular infiltration.[329] Small patches of fibroelastosis may occur in both ventricular outflow tracts beneath the semilunar valves but are felt to be a secondary phenomenon due to local trauma rather than a result of the basic pathological process.[329] The coronary arteries and great vessels are uninvolved, as is the remainder of the body.

ETIOLOGY. A variety of causes of endomyocardial fibrosis have been suggested, but the true etiology remains unclear. Perhaps the most intriguing hypothesis involves the role of diet. Patients in whom the disease occurs often consume large quantities of bananas, which have a high serotonin content, and an analogy has been drawn between the fibrotic cardiac lesions seen in carcinoid heart disease (p. 1431) and those in endomyocardial fibrosis.[337] However, it is now generally accepted that neither malnutrition nor massive consumption of plantains is the critical variable that causes this disease.[341] Other hypotheses incriminate infection with viruses, streptococci, filaria, or infestation with *Loa loa*.[337,341] It has also been suggested that endomyocardial fibrosis may represent an immunological response to streptococcal infection in individuals who are particularly susceptible to malaria, although the nature of the relationship remains unclear. Whatever the nature of the inciting agent, it appears that endomyocardial fibrosis is one part of a spectrum of a disease process that includes Löffler's endocarditis[342] (p. 1430).

CLINICAL MANIFESTATIONS. Endomyocardial fibrosis may involve both ventricles or either ventricle selectively; left-sided involvement results in symptoms of pulmonary congestion, while predominant right-sided disease may present features of a restrictive cardiomyopathy and therefore simulate constrictive pericarditis. Frequently, the disease is discovered as an incidental finding at necropsy.[337] There is often regurgitation of one or both atrioventricular valves. The onset of the disease is usually insidious, but it is sometimes ushered in by an acute febrile illness.[329,336,337,339] Patients present symptoms of cardiac decompensation, including dyspnea, cough, tender hepatomegaly, ascites, edema, and palpitations.[343] Rarely, the disease appears to stabilize, and survival for up to 12 years has been observed, but it is usually relentlessly progressive, with poor response to treatment.[329,339] Progressive heart failure is the rule. In contrast to Becker's disease, pulmonary or systemic embolization is uncommon.[329] Death is due to progressive myocardial failure, often associated with pulmonary congestion, infection, or infarction.[343] The most important immediate cause of death is sudden, unexpected cardiovascular collapse, presumably arrhythmic in origin.[343] Patients with prominent involvement of the right side of the heart appear to survive longer than those with principally left-sided involvement.[343]

Right Ventricular Endomyocardial Fibrosis. Pure or predominant right ventricular involvement is characterized by fibrous obliteration of the right ventricular apex that diminishes the capacity of this chamber.[337] The fibrosis often extends to the supporting apparatus of the tricuspid valve, resulting in tricuspid regurgitation. Therefore, clinical manifestations in patients with right-sided involvement include an elevated jugular venous pressure, a prominent *v* wave, and a rapid *y* descent. A rapid subsequent ascent is often observed.[337,339] A protodiastolic gallop sound may be heard along the lower sternal border, reflecting right ventricular dysfunction. The liver is usually large and pulsatile, and ascites, splenomegaly, and peripheral edema are common.[339] Although cyanosis and clubbing of the digits may be seen, the cause is unclear.[336] Pulmonary congestion is not present in the absence of left-sided involvement, and the pulmonary artery and pulmonary capillary wedge pressures are normal. A pericardial effusion, which is sometimes quite large, may be present.[337] The right atrium is often enlarged, sometimes massively so.[335,336,339]

The *electrocardiogram* is usually abnormal, with diminished QRS voltage (probably resulting from the presence of a pericardial effusion), ST-segment and T-wave abnormalities, and findings of right atrial enlargement.[336,337,339] Occasionally, atrial fibrillation occurs.[337,339] The *chest roentgenogram* demonstrates cardiac enlargement, usually with gross prominence of the right atrium and a pericardial effusion. Calcification in the region of the right ventricular apex may be found.[337,339] The pulmonary vasculature is typically normal.[336] At *angiography* the right ventricular apex is characteristically not visualized because of obliteration by the fibrous endocardium,[336,337] but tricuspid regurgitation, right atrial enlargement, and filling defects in the right atrium due to intraatrial thrombi are sometimes seen.[336]

Left Ventricular Endomyocardial Fibrosis. Predominant *left-sided* involvement results in a different clinical picture. The endomyocardial fibrosis involves the apex of the ventricle and usually the chordae tendineae of the posterior mitral valve leaflet as well,[337] leading to mitral regurgitation.[339] The murmur may be confined to late systole, as is characteristic of the papillary muscle dysfunction type of murmurs, or it may be pansystolic.[337,339] Findings of pulmonary hypertension may be prominent, with a closely split second heart sound and an accentuated pulmonary component, right ventricular hypertrophy with a parasternal lift, a palpable pulmonary artery impulse, and, occasionally, the murmur of functional pulmonary regurgitation. A protodiastolic gallop is commonly heard.[337,339]

The *electrocardiogram* usually shows T-wave abnormalities and diminished QRS voltage. There may be findings of left atrial and right ventricular enlargement. Occasionally, atrial fibrillation is present.[337,339] *Cardiac catheterization* usually reveals pulmonary hypertension, with elevated left ventricular filling pressures and a reduced cardiac index. The left ventriculogram usually shows extensive left ventricular asynergy and mitral regurgitation.[335] A filling defect due to an intracavitary thrombus within the ventricle may be seen on occasion.

Biventricular Endomyocardial Fibrosis. This form of endomyocardial fibrosis occurs more frequently than either isolated right- or left-sided disease. If there is more than minimal right ventricular involvement, severe pulmonary hypertension does not occur, and the right-sided findings dominate the clinical presentation.[337] The typical patient with biventricular involvement may have the features of right ventricular endomyocardial fibrosis, as described above, with only a mitral regurgitant murmur to suggest left ventricular involvement.[337] Rarely, in patients with biventricular involvement, the left-sided features dominate the clinical picture.[339] Systemic embolization may occur in up to 15 per cent of patients; infective endocarditis is even less frequent and is found in less than 2 per cent.[337]

DIAGNOSIS. This is based on the presence of the typical clinical features in an individual from the appropriate geographical area. Eosinophilia is usually not a prominent feature and, when present, may reflect associated parasitic infestation.[339] The *chest roentgenogram* usually shows mild cardiomegaly and sometimes intracardiac calcification. Right ventricular involvement often results in characteristic findings on *echocardiography*, including right ventricular dilatation, abnormal septal motion, and thickening of the ventricular wall.[344,344a] *Endomyocardial biopsy* may occasionally be helpful in establishing the diagnosis.[338] However, this risks dislodging a mural thrombus, with resultant embolization. In addition, because the disease is often focal, the biopsy may miss the pathological process, particularly if a right ventricular biopsy is performed in a patient with isolated left-sided disease.[338] The typical findings at *cardiac catheterization*[334,335,337,337a] (impairment of ventricular filling, diminished ventricular stroke volume due to partial obliteration of the ventricular apex as well as atrioventricular valve regurgitation, and systolic dysfunction) are helpful but not specific for this condition.

TREATMENT. The treatment of endomyocardial fibrosis is often difficult. Digitalis glycosides may be helpful in controlling the ventricular rate in patients with atrial fibrillation, but the response of congestive symptoms is disappointing. Diuretics are not particularly helpful in the treatment of ascites.[337] Insertion of a subcutaneous pericardioperitoneal shunt may be of some benefit in patients with massive recurrent pericardial effusion.[345] Operative excision of the fibrotic endocardium and replacement of the mitral

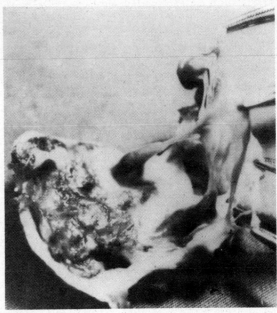

FIGURE 41–21 Appearance of the excised left ventricular endocardium and mitral valve. (From Moraes, C. R., et al.: Endomyocardial fibrosis: Report of 6 patients and review of the surgical literature. Ann. Thorac. Surg. *29*:243, 1980.)

or tricuspid valves has led to substantial symptomatic improvement (Fig. 41–21).[334,337a,346–348,348a,348b] Postoperative catheterization has also provided objective evidence of hemodynamic improvement with a reduction in ventricular filling pressures and an increase in cardiac output.[334,346] Although only a limited number of patients have undergone operation, this approach appears to be a promising alternative to medical treatment, which is often disappointing,[349] although operative mortality may be as high as 20 per cent.[350]

Löffler's Endocarditis
(Hypereosinophilic Syndrome)

A variety of disease states are marked by prolonged and profound eosinophilia associated with localized or widespread eosinophilic infiltrates.[351,352] Cardiac involvement is the rule, occurring in more than 95 per cent of such patients.[352] The characteristic cardiac lesion is dense endocardial fibrosis with superimposed thrombus. Three general causes of the so-called hypereosinophilic syndrome (i.e., profound eosinophilia with tissue involvement) have been suggested: (1) leukemia; (2) reactive—that is, secondary to polyarteritis nodosa, Hodgkin's disease, tumors, parasitic infestation, asthma, or drug reaction; and (3) idiopathic. The last is the most common.[353,354]

One of the major unanswered questions in Löffler's endocarditis is the relation between the eosinophilia and the mechanism of the cardiac damage. It has been suggested that marked eosinophilia occurs in response to profound antigenic stimulation of unknown cause.[337] It appears that the cardiac damage itself may be the result of prolonged release of products from circulating eosinophils.[355] It has been proposed that, unlike normal eosinophils, those from patients with the hypereosinophilic syndrome possess receptors that result in their degranulation in response to soluble bloodborne substances, and this degranulation may in turn release unknown cardiotoxic substances.[355]

PATHOLOGY. The pathological findings in Löffler's endocarditis may be divided into three sequential stages.[340,353] The *first stage* is an acute inflammatory infiltrate, characterized by an eosinophilic myocarditis particularly prominent in the inner layers of the myocardium.[340,353] Myocardial necrosis and arteritis of the small intramural arterioles are common. Mural thrombi may be superimposed over the thickened but intact endocardium. The duration of illness from onset of symptoms to death in patients who demonstrate these acute findings averages less than 2 months.[340]

The *second stage* is characterized by thrombus formation over a thickened myocardium which is infiltrated by eosinophils,[340] while the *third stage* is one of fibrosis, with a prominent layer of hyaline fibrous tissue in the thickened endocardium. Mural thrombi are almost always present[353] in this stage of the disease. Arteritis and the eosinophilic infiltrate present in the earlier stages are now scanty or absent. The fibrotic lesions are located primarily in the inflow tract and apex of the ventricles, with frequent involvement of the papillary muscles and chordae tendineae.[353] The pathological findings in the third stage of Löffler's endocarditis are identical to those in endomyocardial fibrosis[340] (p. 1428), and there are no reliable gross or histological features to distinguish the two diseases.

The *hypereosinophilic syndrome* is characterized by the combination of a persistent eosinophilia, i.e., ≥ 1500 eosinophils/mm^3 for at least 6 months or until death, and evidence of organ involvement. A variety of organs are frequently involved besides the heart, including the lungs, bone marrow, and brain. Renal, gastrointestinal, dermatological, and hepatic involvement is observed less frequently.[337] The majority of patients are Caucasian men living in temperate climates.[353] The disease is primarily one of middle age, and, although any age group may be involved, children are least often affected.

CLINICAL MANIFESTATIONS. The principal clinical features include weight loss, fever, cough, skin rash, and congestive heart failure. Overt cardiac dysfunction occurs in more than half the patients with cardiac involvement and may be either right- or left-sided.[352] Cardiomegaly, often without overt symptoms of congestive heart failure, may be present, and the murmur of mitral regurgitation is common. Systemic embolism is frequent and may lead to neurological and renal dysfunction.[353,356] Once the disease becomes clinically evident, survival is usually brief, averaging nine months, although a minority of patients survive for four years or more. More recent reports have suggested a more benign course, with average survivals exceeding five years;[352] the reason for this apparent improvement in prognosis is unclear but may be related to improvement in therapy.[357] Death is usually due to congestive heart failure, often with associated renal, hepatic, or respiratory dysfunction.

LABORATORY EXAMINATION. A variety of abnormalities of the blood may be seen in addition to the eosinophilia. The erythrocyte sedimentation rate is frequently elevated, and occasionally patients have abnormal or depressed leukocyte alkaline phosphatase levels and chromosomal abnormalities (including the Philadelphia [Ph^1] chromosome).[352]

The *chest roentgenogram* may reveal cardiomegaly and pulmonary congestion or, less commonly, pulmonary infiltrates. The *electrocardiogram* most commonly shows nonspecific ST-segment and T-wave abnormalities. Left ventricular hypertrophy, arrhythmias, and conduction defects, particularly right bundle branch block, may also be present.[352,358]

The *echocardiogram* commonly demonstrates thickening of the right and left ventricular walls with an increase of the left ventricular mass.[359] Localized thickening of the posterobasal left ventricular wall may lead to mitral regurgitation.[359a] Enlargement of the left atrium and right and/or left ventricles may be seen; abnormal mitral valve motion reflecting diminished left ventricular compliance and pericardial effusions are found in one-fourth to one-third of patients.[357]

The *hemodynamic consequences* of the dense endocardial scarring seen in Löffler's endocarditis are those of a restrictive cardiomyopathy as described above (p. 1422) with abnormal diastolic filling due to increased stiffness of the ventricles and a reduction in the size of the ventricular cavity by organized thrombus. Systolic performance is also impaired and atrioventricular valvular regurgitation may occur because of involvement of the supporting apparatus of the mitral or tricuspid valves.[360] In rare cases the mitral and tricuspid valves themselves may become fibrotic, and stenosis may result.[360] *Cardiac catheterization* reveals markedly elevated ventricular filling pressures, and there may be evidence of tricuspid or mitral regurgitation. On angiography, contraction of the ventricles, particularly the right ventricle, is often asynergic.[351,356] Occasionally, verrucous deposits and friable vegetations on the valves are noted on angiography.[353]

TREATMENT. Therapy is generally unsatisfactory.[351] Digitalis is usually ineffective, and the congestive failure is inexorable.[361] Short-lived improvement after steroid therapy has been reported, but sustained efficacy has not been demonstrated.[351,352,361] Eosinophilia may be diminished by treatment with hydroxyurea and vincristine, a wide range of other myelo- and immunosuppressive agents, antihistamines, radiation, splenectomy, and antiparasitic drugs, but whether this results in any change in the natural history of the disease is not clear. A rare patient has undergone surgical removal of the fibrotic endocardial tissue and has shown clinical improvement.[362,363]

RELATION BETWEEN ENDOMYOCARDIAL FIBROSIS AND LÖFFLER'S ENDOCARDITIS. There are both important similarities and differences between endomyocardial fibrosis and Löffler's endocarditis. The similarities in the histological and the gross anatomical findings as well as the clinical and hemodynamic manifestations of advanced Löffler's endocarditis and endomyocardial fibrosis have led to the suggestion that they are related entities.[353,364]

In fact, a continuum has been suggested from tropical eosinophilia to Löffler's endocarditis to, finally, endomyocardial fibrosis.[364] According to this formulation, endocardial fibrosis may be the final expression of damage initially mediated through eosinophils, and endomyocardial fibrosis may be a late form of Löffler's endocarditis.[353] It may be that eosinophilia occurs early in the course of endomyocardial fibrosis, perhaps resulting from parasitic infection, only to disappear later.[365] A number of important differences between the two diseases should be borne in mind. They occur in different geographical areas and age groups. Endomyocardial fibrosis is associated with less thrombus formation than is Löffler's endocarditis, while Löffler's endocarditis may be associated with a generalized arteritis not found in endomyocardial fibrosis.[364] Despite these differences, we favor the view that endomyocardial fibrosis may, at least in some instances, be a later, "burned-out" phase of Löffler's endocarditis that is no longer associated with eosinophilia.[364]

Endocardial Fibroelastosis (See page 1049)

Carcinoid Heart Disease

Etiology and Pathology. The carcinoid syndrome is caused by a metastasizing carcinoid tumor and is characterized by cutaneous flushing, diarrhea, bronchoconstriction, and endocardial plaques composed of a unique type of fibrous tissue.[366] The vasomotor, bronchoconstrictor, and cardiac manifestations are undoubtedly related to circulating humoral substances secreted by the tumor.[367] The diarrhea is probably caused by serotonin, which is secreted in large amounts by carcinoid tumors, while the dermal flushes and bronchospasm appear to be related to the release of kinin peptides. Virtually all patients develop diarrhea and flushing, while cardiac abnormalities occur in over half the patients and bronchospasm in one third.[366,368]

Sixty to 90 per cent of tumors arise in the appendix, while the rest originate in the ileum, stomach, duodenum, or other areas of the gastrointestinal tract.[369] Only the carcinoid tumors of the ileum tend to metastasize, with involvement of the regional lymph nodes and liver. Also, only carcinoid tumors that invade the liver result in carcinoid heart disease.[370] The cardiac lesions may be related to large circulating quantities of serotonin (5-hydroxytryptamine) or other substances secreted by the tumor, which are usually inactivated by the liver, lungs, and brain.[369] Hepatic metastases apparently allow large quantities of tumor products to reach the heart without being inactivated by the liver.[369,371] Left-sided cardiac involvement is rare in the carcinoid syndrome, probably because of the inactivation of the offending humoral substance(s) by the lungs, although left-sided lesions may occur in the presence of an intracardiac communication that allows right-to-left shunting, thus avoiding the pulmonary circulation.[370]

The characteristic lesions are fibrous plaques that involve the tricuspid and pulmonic valves, the endocardium of the cardiac chambers, and the intima of the venae cavae, pulmonary artery, and coronary sinus (Fig. 41–22).[366,367,370] The fibrous tissue in the plaques results in distortion of the valves, leading to pulmonic stenosis and tricuspid regurgitation (p. 1117).[367] Histologically, the plaques consist of deposits of fibrous tissue located superficially on the endocardium with little or no extension into the underlying layers.[367] Ultrastructural studies have demonstrated that the plaques are composed of smooth muscle cells embedded in a stroma rich in acid mucopolysaccharides and collagen.[366] The plaques may form as a result of healing of a superficial endocardial injury, which is produced by a compound secreted by or derived from the tumor.[366]

Clinical Manifestations. *Physical examination* usually reveals a systolic murmur along the left upper sternal border, produced by valvular pulmonic stenosis, tricuspid regurgitation, or both. A right ventricular heave and systolic thrill are often present.[370]

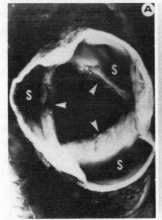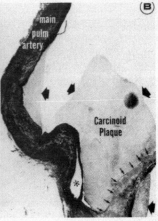

FIGURE 41–22 *A,* Gross photograph of deformed pulmonic valve with fixed, stenotic, triangular-shaped orifice (arrowheads) and sinuses (S) accentuated by thickened, retracted valve cusps. *B,* Photomicrograph of pulmonic valve cusp with a large carcinoid plaque (broad arrows) on the arterial surface (outlined by small arrows) and a smaller plaque on the ventricular surface of the valve cusp. A small plaque is also present on the intima of the buckled pulmonary artery. Empty space in pulmonary artery wall (*) is a section-preparation artifact. (Elastic Van Gieson's stain; × 16.) (From Lie, J. T.: Carcinoid tumors, carcinoid syndrome, and carcinoid heart disease. Primary Cardiol. *8:*163, 1982.)

The *chest roentgenogram* may reveal enlargement of the heart, although the pulmonary artery trunk is typically of normal size, without evidence of poststenotic dilatation. No specific *electrocardiographic pattern* is diagnostic of carcinoid heart disease, although low voltage is often present. Evidence of right atrial enlargement may be seen on occasion, but electrocardiographic evidence of right ventricular hypertrophy is usually lacking. Nonspecific ST-segment and T-wave abnormalities and right bundle branch block have also been reported.[370] *Echocardiography* may reveal evidence of tricuspid or pulmonary valve thickening.[371a]

The *hemodynamic findings* most commonly encountered are those of tricuspid regurgitation and pulmonic stenosis. Some patients with the carcinoid syndrome appear to be in a profound hyperkinetic state, which may lead to high-output heart failure[372] (p. 820). Cardiac catheterization appears to be hazardous in patients with the malignant carcinoid syndrome, and several deaths have been reported.[370,373]

Treatment.   Treatment of patients with mild congestive heart failure consists of digitalis and diuretics.[367] Some of the vasomotor symptoms may be controlled with alpha-adrenergic blockers and serotonin antagonists.[367] Surgical replacement of the tricuspid valve and pulmonic valvotomy may be beneficial in severely symptomatic patients with serious valvular dysfunction and may permit prolonged survival.[369]

Obesity Heart Disease (See page 1741)

Diabetic Cardiomyopathy (See page 1738)

MYOCARDITIS

When the heart is involved in an inflammatory process, often caused by an infectious agent, myocarditis is said to be present. The inflammation may involve the myocytes, interstitium, vascular elements, and/or pericardium; involvement of the latter structure is discussed in Chapter 43.

Myocarditis is a common cause of acute congestive cardiomyopathy and has been described during and following a wide variety of viral, rickettsial, bacterial, protozoal, and metazoal diseases; indeed, virtually any infectious agent may produce cardiac inflammation. Infectious agents cause myocardial damage by three basic mechanisms: (1) invasion of the myocardium, e.g., by echovirus[374]; (2) production of a myocardial toxin, e.g., diphtheria[375]; and (3) autoimmunity, as occurs in acute rheumatic fever[376] and systemic lupus erythematosus (p. 1660). Myocarditis may also be caused by radiation and other physical agents, chemicals (e.g., lead), pharmacological agents (e.g., adriamycin, p. 1690), and metabolic disorders (e.g., uremia, p. 1760), as is discussed later in this chapter. In an unknown number of patients, acute myocarditis becomes chronic dilated cardiomyopathy. Conversely, an unknown number of cases of chronic dilated cardiomyopathy commence as acute myocarditis.

Myocarditis may be an acute or a chronic process. In North America, viruses are the most common agents producing myocarditis, while in South America, Chagas' disease (produced by *Trypanosoma cruzi*) is far more common. The identification of the specific etiological agent responsible for infectious myocarditis usually rests on the associated extracardiac findings, since the cardiovascular signs and symptoms are often nonspecific. The histological findings vary, depending on the stage of the disease, the mechanism of myocardial damage, and the specific etiological agent. Myocardial involvement may be focal or diffuse, but the myocardial lesions are generally randomly distributed in the heart, and thus the clinical consequences depend to a large extent on the size and number of the lesions. However, a single small lesion may have profound consequences if it is located within the cardiac conducting system.[377] The histological findings are usually nonspecific (except for some parasitic and granulomatous forms of myocarditis), and, with the exception of adriamycin cardiotoxicity,[378] myocardial biopsy is usually not rewarding in elucidating the etiology.

INFECTIOUS MYOCARDITIS

Clinical Manifestations

The clinical expression of myocarditis ranges from the asymptomatic state secondary to focal inflammation to fulminant fatal congestive heart failure due to diffuse myocarditis. An initial episode of viral myocarditis, perhaps unrecognized and forgotten, may be the initial event that eventually culminates in an "idiopathic" dilated cardiomyopathy (Fig. 41–23).[379] In support of this view is the observation in experimental animals that structural and functional myocardial alterations following viral myocarditis may persist well beyond the stage of viral replication and myocardial inflammatory response.[380]

While transient electrocardiographic abnormalities suggesting myocardial involvement are noted in many patients with infectious diseases,[381,382] most patients do not have other clinical manifestations of myocarditis. It is postulated that these electrocardiographic changes reflect subclinical myocardial involvement. That frequent but unrecognized myocardial involvement occurs with systemic infections is supported by histological evidence of myocarditis in 4 to 10 per cent of routine postmortem examinations.[383–387] Some degree of myocardial involvement, often subepicardial in location, also frequently occurs in patients with acute pericarditis.[388,389]

Since myocardial involvement is subclinical in most acute infectious diseases, the majority of patients have no specific complaints referable to the cardiovascular system;

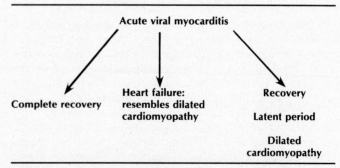

FIGURE 41–23 Viral myocarditis and cardiomyopathy. (From Goodwin, J. F.: The frontiers of cardiomyopathy. Br. Heart J. *48*:1, 1982.)

the presence of myocarditis is often inferred from the ST-segment and T-wave changes on the electrocardiogram.[383] From a clinical viewpoint, myocardial involvement is associated with nonspecific symptoms, including fatigue, dyspnea, palpitations, and precordial discomfort. Chest pain usually reflects associated pericarditis,[389] but precordial discomfort suggestive of myocardial ischemia is occasionally observed.[390]

On *physical examination*, tachycardia is usual and may be out of proportion to the temperature elevation.[385,391] The first heart sound is often muffled, and a protodiastolic gallop may be present. A transient apical systolic murmur may appear, but diastolic murmurs are rare.[381,384] Clinical evidence of congestive heart failure occurs only in the more severe cases.[381,383,385,390] Pulsus alternans is rare and is limited to patients with fulminant disease.[384] The heart is usually normal in size in the clinically silent cases, but it may be dilated in patients with congestive heart failure.[384] Pulmonary and systemic emboli may occur.[389,391]

As already indicated, *electrocardiographic* abnormalities are usually transient and occur far more frequently than does clinical myocardial involvement.[392] The most common changes are abnormalities of the ST segment and T wave, but atrial and in particular ventricular arrhythmias, atrioventricular (AV) and intraventricular conduction defects, and, rarely, Q waves may be seen.[379,393,394] Complete AV block is usually transient and resolves without sequelae, but it is occasionally a cause of sudden death in patients with myocarditis. On *radiological examination*, heart size may range from normal to markedly enlarged, and pulmonary congestion may be present in patients with fulminant disease. *Radionuclide scanning* after the administration of gallium-67 or technetium-99m pyrophosphate may identify inflammatory and necrotic changes characteristic of myocarditis.[396,397]

The *diagnosis* is often predicated on the identification of the associated systemic illness and its characteristic features. The diagnosis of viral myocarditis is supported by the identification of the virus in stool, throat washings, blood, myocardium, feces, or pericardial fluid, or by a distinct (usually fourfold) increase in virus neutralizing antibody, complement-fixation, or hemagglutination inhibition titers.[379] Even in fatal cases, isolation of virus from the myocardium at necropsy is difficult and is accomplished with regularity only with the Coxsackie, echo-, and poliomyelitis viruses.[380]

Most patients recover completely. The myocarditis frequently is clinically silent, and suspected only because of electrocardiographic changes.[394,398] However, some asymptomatic patients with prior myocarditis have left ventricular dysfunction that is not apparent clinically but may be demonstrated by exercise radionuclide ventriculography.[399] Some patients, most commonly infants and children, may succumb to the acute process. An unknown number of patients, probably a minority, develop chronic myocarditis, which may eventually culminate in "idiopathic" dilated cardiomyopathy.[392,400]

Pathology. Patients dying of or with myocarditis demonstrate a wide spectrum of gross and histological pathological changes, reflecting the range of disease seen clinically. Grossly, the hearts may be normal, dilated, hypertrophied, or flabby. An interstitial inflammatory reaction is usually observed and myocytolysis and necrosis

may be seen.[401] Routine histological examination of the heart rarely provides a specific diagnosis, although in some instances electron microscopic and immunofluorescent techniques may allow elucidation of a specific etiology.

Treatment. Therapy is often supportive and is usually directed at the more prominent systemic manifestations of the disease. The demonstration of a particular predilection for involvement of the AV conducting system in some forms of myocarditis[402] suggests that patients with suspected myocarditis should be observed closely for any evidence of conduction abnormality. Since hypoxia and exercise intensify the damage from myocarditis in experimental animals, adequate oxygenation and rest are indicated.[403,404] Congestive heart failure responds to routine management, including digitalization and diuresis, although patients with myocarditis appear to be particularly sensitive to digitalis, and toxicity should be watched for.[389] Significant arrhythmias should be treated with antiarrhythmic agents, although beta-adrenergic blockers are probably best avoided in view of their negative inotropic action. The use of corticosteroids is controversial, but they are proscribed in acute viral myocarditis, since increased tissue necrosis and viral replication have been demonstrated following their use.[404] In some patients with rapidly progressive congestive heart failure of no identifiable cause, an inflammatory myocarditis may be demonstrable by right ventricular endomyocardial biopsy. A small number of patients have responded favorably to treatment with immunosuppressive agents, usually prednisone and azathioprine.[404a] Serial endomyocardial biopsies have confirmed the resolution of the inflammatory infiltrate with treatment.[405] Prolonged bed rest has been advocated, but its utility in preventing long-term sequelae has not been established.[401]

It is hoped that effective antiviral agents for treating viral myocarditis will be developed. It may also be possible, in the future, to treat patients with myocarditis with agents that stimulate production of interferon, since this substance affords protection against the effects of viral myocarditis, at least in experimental animals.[406] Antibiotics may also be employed with benefit in infections caused by atypical pneumonia and psittacosis.

Viral Myocarditis*

Systemic infection with numerous viruses may be associated with clinical evidence of myocarditis[407] (Table 41–8). The myocarditis characteristically presents after a lag period of several weeks following the initial systemic infection, suggesting involvement of an immunological mechanism.[392] In animals, a variety of factors appears to enhance susceptibility to myocardial damage, including radiation, malnutrition, steroids, exercise, and previous myocardial injury.[400] Viral myocarditis may be particularly virulent in infants and in pregnant women.[404]

Coxsackie Virus. Both Coxsackie A and B viruses may produce myocarditis, although infection with Coxsackie B is more common,[400] and this agent is the most frequent cause of viral myocarditis.[393] The myocardium appears to be particularly susceptible to the effects of this virus because of the apparent affinity of myocardial membrane receptors for the viral particles.[404] Necropsy often demonstrates a

---

*Myocarditis secondary to psittacosis and *Mycoplasma pneumoniae* is described later in this chapter.

TABLE 41–8   PRINCIPAL
VIRAL CAUSES OF MYOCARDITIS

Coxsackie (Groups A and B)
Echovirus
Adenovirus
Influenza
Varicella
Poliomyelitis
Mumps
Rabies
Viral hepatitis
Infectious mononucleosis
Cytomegalovirus
Arbovirus (Groups A and B)
Variola and vaccinia
Viral encephalitis
Yellow fever
Herpes simplex

pericardial effusion, pericarditis, cardiac enlargement, and a predominantly mononuclear inflammatory infiltrate, with necrosis of the atrial and ventricular myocardium.[39,408] In some cases, focal myocardial necrosis simulating myocardial infarction is seen, despite normal coronary arteries.[409]

Although most infections are probably subclinical,[410,411] Coxsackie myocarditis appears to be particularly virulent in the neonate. In most infections in adults, the other clinical manifestations of viral involvement, such as pleurodynia, myalgia, upper respiratory tract symptoms, and arthralgias, predominate. Severe cases in the adult are characterized by myopericardial involvement with pleuritic or pericarditic chest pain, palpitations, and fever. Many patients with overt myocardial involvement develop congestive heart failure with cardiomegaly and pulmonary edema.

The *electrocardiogram* is virtually always abnormal, with ST-segment and T-wave changes and arrhythmias, often ventricular in origin; AV conduction disturbances are common.[412] Blood levels of myocardial enzymes (serum glutamic oxaloacetic transaminase, creatine kinase) may be normal or elevated, reflecting the absence or presence of variable degrees of myocardial necrosis.[413]

Most patients recover completely within weeks, although it may require months for the electrocardiogram to return to normal.[414] Rarely, Coxsackie myocarditis is fatal in adults. Some patients become symptomatic following resolution of the infection, and they may present years later with dilated cardiomyopathy.[412] Occasionally, patients appear to recover completely only to develop symptoms subsequently.[415,416]

Treatment is symptomatic, and despite occasional postmortem evidence of intracardiac thrombi, anticoagulation should probably be avoided because of the risk of a hemorrhagic pericardial effusion.[412] Bed rest is indicated during the acute course of myocarditis, but there is no convincing evidence that a period of prolonged rest after apparent resolution of the acute process is useful.[417] Heart failure and cardiac arrhythmias are treated in the usual fashion.

Echovirus.   Closely akin to the Coxsackie virus, the echoviruses may also be associated with myopericarditis, often during the course of an acute, pleurodynia-like illness,[418,419] although clinically apparent myocardial involvement during the course of an echovirus infection is rare.[401] Ventricular arrhythmias, complete AV block, and transient, nonspecific electrocardiographic changes have been reported.[420]

Adenovirus.   Myocarditis is rare in adenovirus infection. Postmortem findings include dilated right and left ventricles, with a mononuclear infiltrate with fragmentation of the myocardial fibers.[421]

Influenza.   Cardiovascular involvement may play an important role in patients with influenza, since one-third of fatal cases have evidence of active myocarditis.[422] Postmortem findings in fatal cases include biventricular dilatation, with evidence of subendocardial and subepicardial petechiae and hemorrhage. A mononuclear inflammation is prominent, especially in perivascular areas. Occasional fibrinoid necroses of the myocardial arterioles may be seen.[423] The earliest histological abnormalities include petechial hemorrhages and loss of myofibrillar striations. Then, fragmentation of the myocardial fibers becomes marked, and there is interstitial edema and hemorrhage.[422]

Cardiac involvement typically occurs within 1 to 2 weeks of the onset of the illness and may be severe, sometimes contributing to mortality.[423,424] The *clinical manifestations* include dyspnea, palpitations,

anginal chest pain, arrhythmia, and heart failure[425]; there is often concomitant involvement of the pericardium. Sinus tachycardia or, less commonly, sinus bradycardia may be seen. The *electrocardiogram* may show transient ST-segment and T-wave abnormalities, conduction defects, and even complete AV block.[422] Sudden death is common and may be associated with massive hemorrhagic pulmonary edema due to viral involvement of the lungs.[422]

Varicella.   Clinical myocarditis is a rare finding in varicella. Occasionally a patient may develop overt evidence of myocarditis with congestive heart failure.[426] Histological findings include rare but characteristic intranuclear inclusion bodies within the myocardial cells, along with interstitial edema, cellular infiltrates, and myonecrosis.[427] The electrocardiogram may show conduction abnormalities, and sudden death occurs rarely.[428]

Poliomyelitis.   Myocarditis is a frequent finding in fatal cases of poliomyelitis, particularly during epidemics,[429] occurring in half or more of all patients dying with this disease. While myocardial involvement is usually focal and minimal in extent, some patients with bulbar disease succumb early in the course of the illness, often with cardiovascular collapse.[429,430] These patients all have viral infection of the medulla and severe systemic vasoconstriction that leads to pulmonary edema. Myocarditis appears to contribute to the heart failure.[429] The *electrocardiogram* is frequently abnormal, with ST-segment and T-wave abnormalities, prolongation of the P-R and Q-T intervals,[431] extrasystoles, tachycardia, and atrial fibrillation.[382] *Treatment* is symptomatic, with aggressive support of pulmonary function; tracheostomy and prolonged mechanical ventilatory support may be required. Fortunately, this disease has been largely eliminated by immunization.

Mumps.   Myocardial involvement during the course of mumps is a rare phenomenon, occurring in less than 10 per cent of adults infected with this virus, and even less frequently in children.[432] The hearts of only a few patients with mumps have come to postmortem examination and they have been found to be both dilated and hypertrophied. Histologically, there is diffuse interstitial fibrosis, with infiltration of mononuclear cells and areas of focal necrosis.[433]

Cardiac involvement is usually unrecognized clinically, and the diagnosis of myocarditis is based on nonspecific electrocardiographic changes.[434] Transient ST-segment and T-wave abnormalities are most common, but extrasystoles and AV conduction block may occur; in a rare case, persistent complete heart block requires insertion of a permanent pacemaker.[435] Myocarditis generally occurs in the first week of illness and is transient, in most cases resolving within several weeks.[382,434] A few patients develop precordial chest pain, dyspnea, palpitations, and fatigue; cardiomegaly and congestive heart failure occur on occasion.[433] Tachycardia, a transient apical systolic murmur, and protodiastolic gallop may be present.[434]

Viral Hepatitis.   The characteristic *pathological changes* in the myocardium associated with viral hepatitis are minute foci of necrosis of isolated muscle bundles, often surrounded by lymphocytes, and a diffuse serous inflammation.[436] The ventricles may be dilated, with petechial hemorrhages.[437] Hemorrhage into the interventricular septum involving the area of the conduction system is a conspicuous finding,[436,437] and electrocardiographic surveillance for evidence of conduction defects may be warranted in patients with clinical evidence of myocarditis during the course of viral hepatitis.

Electrocardiographic changes, including bradycardia, ventricular premature beats, and ST-segment and T-wave changes, may be seen during the course of hepatitis.[401,436,438] These abnormalities are usually transient and asymptomatic, although congestive heart failure, cardiomegaly, and sudden death have been reported.[437] Patients may present dyspnea, palpitations, and an anginal type of chest pain. Symptomatic myocarditis is generally observed during the first to third week of the disease.[438]

Infectious Mononucleosis.   Examination of the hearts of patients with the myocarditis associated with infectious mononucleosis may reveal atypical lymphocytes within the myocardium, along with focal myocardial infiltrates and necrosis.[439] *Electrocardiographic changes* associated with infectious mononucleosis are common, although symptomatic cardiac involvement is only rarely observed.[439-441] ST-segment and T-wave changes may be observed, along with varying degrees of AV block. Ventricular arrhythmias occur rarely but may be fatal. Symptomatic patients may demonstrate a pericardial friction rub, an apical systolic murmur, and evidence of congestive heart failure.[439] Most patients follow an uncomplicated and nonfatal clinical course.[442]

Rubella and Rubeola. Congenital cardiovascular lesions may develop in the offspring when *rubella* is contracted by the mother during the first trimester of pregnancy, with persistent ductus arteriosus and pulmonary artery maldevelopment as prominent anomalies (p. 942). Abnormalities of the conduction system have been reported in postnatal rubella, but myocarditis does not appear to occur.[443]

In *rubeola,* transient electrocardiographic abnormalities,[444,445] including prolongation of the P-R interval, ST-segment and T-wave changes, AV conduction abnormalities, and ventricular tachycardia, have been reported.[381,444,445] The electrocardiographic changes are usually transient. Congestive heart failure occurs on rare occasions, and its appearance is a poor prognostic sign, often indicating a fatal outcome.[382] Histological examination of the heart in fatal cases has revealed evidence of myocarditis characterized predominantly by a perivascular lymphocytic infiltrate.[445]

Cytomegalovirus. Unrecognized infection with cytomegalovirus (CMV) is extremely common in childhood, and the majority of the adult population have antibodies to CMV.[446,447] Primary infection after the age of 35 years is uncommon, and generalized infection usually occurs only in immunosuppressed patients with neoplastic disease. The cardiovascular manifestations in adults are generally limited to asymptomatic and transient electrocardiographic changes. Symptomatic cardiac involvement is rare, although a hemorrhagic pericardial effusion may occur.[448] While fatalities are unusual, when they do occur histological examination of the heart may reveal focal lymphocytic infiltration and fibrosis.[448]

Arbovirus. Infections due to group A arbovirus (e.g., chikungunya) and group B arbovirus (e.g., dengue) often result in symptomatic cardiac involvement. In addition to symptoms due to systemic involvement (fever, headache, sweating), chest pain, dyspnea, palpitations, fatigue, dizziness, and paroxysmal nocturnal dyspnea are often prominent features. A protodiastolic gallop, apical systolic murmur,

and cardiomegaly are common.[449-451] The latter often persists after the acute illness has resolved. The *electrocardiogram* is virtually always abnormal in patients with myocardial involvement, and ST segment and T wave abnormalities, sinus tachycardia, sinus bradycardia, conduction disturbances, and arrhythmias are found.[451] Atrial fibrillation, atrial premature depolarizations, and ventricular premature depolarizations are also seen. Sudden death may occur, most often due to ventricular arrhythmias or embolization.[449] Complete recovery is unusual, and most patients have persistent cardiomegaly and abnormalities of the electrocardiogram.[449,451]

Variola and Vaccinia. Cardiac involvement following smallpox is rare, although several cases of myocarditis associated with acute cardiac failure and death have been reported.[452] Myocarditis with pericardial effusion and congestive heart failure has also been observed as a complication of smallpox vaccination;[453] an immunological mechanism has been suggested and dramatic responses to steroids have been reported. The histological changes include a mixed mononuclear infiltrate, with interstitial edema and occasional degenerating or necrotic muscle bundles.[454]

Yellow Fever. Myocardial changes are occasionally seen in fatal cases of yellow fever, with petechial hemorrhages of the endocardial and epicardial surfaces, foci of myocardial necrosis, and cellular infiltration.[455]

Respiratory Syncytial Virus. Although respiratory syncytial virus is an important cause of respiratory disease, particularly in children, it rarely results in cardiac involvement.[456] Several patients have developed clinical congestive heart failure after an infection with this virus, with symptoms appearing several days after the initial respiratory manifestations[456,457] (Fig. 41–24). Complete heart block is a prominent feature, although cardiomegaly, ventricular arrhythmias, and cardiac decompensation may also be noted.

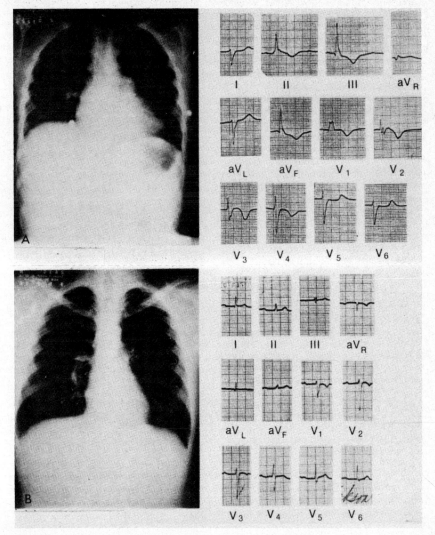

FIGURE 41–24 Recovery from myocardial involvement with respiratory syncytial virus. *A,* On admission, there is generalized cardiomegaly, prominence of the hilar vessels, and a pacing catheter within the right ventricle. The electrocardiogram demonstrates complete heart block with an idioventricular rhythm. *B,* One month later, following clinical recovery, the chest roentgenogram is normal, and the electrocardiogram is normal except for first-degree heart block. (From Giles, T. D., and Gond, R. S.: Respiratory syncytial virus and heart disease. A report of two cases. J.A.M.A. *236*:1128, 1976. Copyright 1976, American Medical Association.)

Mycoplasma pneumoniae.   Electrocardiographic abnormalities are common during the course of atypical pneumonia, occurring in up to one-third of patients.[458] Nonspecific ST-segment and T-wave abnormalities are most common, particularly involving the right-sided precordial leads, but first-degree AV block is occasionally seen.[382,458] The electrocardiographic findings usually resolve within 1 to 2 weeks. Pericarditis may be a prominent finding, and congestive heart failure is occasionally seen.[459,460] A protodiastolic gallop and pericardial friction rub may be noted in occasional cases.[382] No specific treatment for the cardiovascular involvement is usually indicated. Complete recovery is the rule in most patients.[459]

Psittacosis.   Myocarditis complicating psittacosis is a relatively common occurrence and is characterized by congestive heart failure and acute pericarditis.[461,462] *Pathological changes* include a fibrinous pericarditis, subendocardial hemorrhages, and interstitial edema, with lymphocytic and plasma cell infiltrates. Fatty degeneration or cloudy swelling of the muscle fibers may be seen. Fever, chest pain, electrocardiographic changes, cardiomegaly, systemic emboli, tachycardia, and hypotension may occur. While most patients recover completely, fatalities have been reported in a small fraction.[461] The systemic infection may be treated effectively with tetracycline, but the effect of the antibiotic on the myocardium is unknown.

Rickettsial Myocarditis

The rickettsial diseases are frequently associated with evidence of myocardial involvement. Transient ST-segment and T-wave alterations in particular are observed commonly.[463] The circulatory collapse that may accompany these diseases is largely a manifestation of abnormalities of the peripheral vascular bed, but a myocardial component may also be present. The basic histopathological process is a vasculitis, with a periarterial interstitial infiltrate.[464]

Scrub Typhus.   Myocarditis is common during the course of scrub typhus (tsutsugamushi disease, caused by *R. tsutsugamushi*). The histological findings are those of a focal panvasculitis involving the small blood vessels. Myocardial necrosis is unusual, but hemorrhage into the heart and subepicardial petechiae may occur. Clinical evidence of myocardial involvement typically is not severe and is usually not associated with residual cardiac damage.[465,466] The electrocardiogram may show nonspecific ST-segment and T-wave abnormalities, as well as first-degree AV block. A protodiastolic gallop and apical systolic murmur suggestive of mitral regurgitation are occasionally found.

Rocky Mountain Spotted Fever.   Clinical evidence of myocarditis is *not* usually a prominent feature of Rocky Mountain spotted fever (caused by *R. rickettsii*), although the heart is involved in the multisystem damage that occurs as the result of a widespread vasculitis.[467,468]

Q Fever.   Endocarditis is the most common cardiac manifestation of infection with *R. burnettii* (Q fever). Myocarditis is not a prominent feature, although dyspnea and chest pain, perhaps reflecting associated pericarditis, occur frequently.[469] The electrocardiogram may demonstrate transient ST-segment and T-wave changes as well as paroxysmal ventricular arrhythmias.[469,470]

Bacterial Myocarditis

Diphtheria.   Myocardial involvement is one of the most serious complications of diphtheria[471] and occurs in at least one fourth of cases. Indeed, myocardial involvement is the most common cause of death in this infection.[472] Cardiac damage is due to the liberation by the diphtheria bacillus of a toxin that inhibits protein synthesis by interfering with the transfer of amino acids from soluble RNA to polypeptide chains under construction.[473]

Pathological findings include a flabby and dilated heart with a myocardium that has a "streaky" appearance. Microscopic examination reveals characteristic fatty infiltration of the myocytes, often with an interstitial inflammatory infiltrate, myocytolysis, and hyaline necrosis of muscle fibers.[382] With time, fibrosis and hypertrophy of the remaining myocardial cells develop. The conduction system is often involved.

Typically, *clinical signs* of cardiac dysfunction appear at the end of the first week of the illness.[471] Cardiomegaly and severe congestive heart failure are often present.[382] A protodiastolic gallop and pulmonary congestion may be prominent features. Elevation of the serum transaminase levels may be seen; a high level is associated with a

poor prognosis.[471] Sudden circulatory failure and death may occur.[382] Many patients develop ST-segment and T-wave abnormalities, but atrial and ventricular arrhythmias, bundle branch block, and various grades of AV conduction defects may also occur.[474] Persistently abnormal electrocardiograms are common following diphtheritic myocarditis, as are cardiomegaly and symptoms of reduced cardiac reserve.[382] Some patients recover fully.[471]

Because of the serious effects of the toxin on the myocardium, antitoxin should be administered as rapidly as possible. Antibiotic therapy is of less urgency. General supportive measures are indicated. Overt congestive heart failure may be resistant to therapy with cardiac glycosides. The development of complete AV block is a serious complication, but it may be amenable to treatment with a transvenous pacemaker.[475]

Salmonella.   Symptomatic myocardial involvement during salmonella infections is rare, although electrocardiographic abnormalities are often seen, suggesting subclinical myocarditis. *Postmortem findings* in salmonella myocarditis may reveal a shaggy, fibrinous pericarditis and, in some cases, evidence of endocarditis.[476,477] Myocardial petechiae and hemorrhagic necrosis may occur, with evidence of biventricular dilatation. A polymorphonuclear leukocytic infiltrate with evidence of coronary arteritis may be found.[478] The arteritis may lead to thrombosis, infarction, and death. Other cardiovascular complications include infected mural thrombi, occasionally resulting in pulmonary and systemic emboli, and mycotic aneurysms.[476] Myocardial abscesses often develop and may rupture, producing fatal cardiac tamponade.[476] Myocarditis with congestive heart failure occurs most commonly in children who are severely ill with salmonellosis, and it is associated with a high mortality.[479] When myocarditis occurs, it often develops rapidly, with evidence of biventricular failure, tachycardia, a protodiastolic gallop, an apical systolic murmur of mitral regurgitation, and peripheral edema.[480]

Electrocardiographic abnormalities include ST-segment and T-wave changes, and prolonged P-R or Q-T intervals. These electrocardiographic changes typically appear in the second week of illness and usually resolve completely within a week.[480,481]

Tuberculosis.   Tuberculous involvement of the myocardium is rare, particularly since the introduction of drugs effective against tuberculosis.[482] Children are more susceptible than adults to myocardial involvement.[483] Cardiac involvement may occur by direct extension from tuberculous hilar lymph nodes (probably the most common); lymphatic spread; and hematogenous spread.[484,485]

Miliary involvement of the heart is most common in children and occurs in 15 to 50 per cent of cases of miliary tuberculosis. The nodular and diffuse varieties are more common in adults.[483] The pericardium is typically free of tuberculous involvement in miliary tuberculosis, while the right side of the heart and interventricular septum are most commonly involved. *Nodular* myocardial involvement is the most common type of myocarditis in adults. Tuberculomas are isolated or multiple, rounded, circumscribed, firm nodules 2 to 70 mm in diameter.[486] The cardiac involvement may lead to compression of cardiac chambers with resulting functional abnormalities.[483] *Diffuse* infiltrating myocardial tuberculosis is the least common form of myocardial tuberculosis.[483] The myocardial involvement may lead to formation of a tuberculous aneurysm, and rupture with cardiac tamponade and death has been reported.[487] Infiltrative involvement of the heart appears to be predominantly right-sided, particularly the right atrium.[485,488] Most cases of myocardial tuberculosis are clinically silent and are diagnosed only at postmortem examination.[482,488] On rare occasions, tuberculous involvement of the myocardium may lead to arrhythmias, including atrial fibrillation and ventricular tachycardia, complete AV block, and congestive heart failure.

Streptococcus.   The most common detected cardiac finding following beta-hemolytic streptococcal infection is acute rheumatic fever, which is discussed in detail in Chapter 48.

Direct infection of the heart by the streptococcus produces a myocarditis that is distinct from acute rheumatic carditis. It is characterized by an interstitial infiltrate composed of mononuclear cells with occasional polymorphonuclear leukocytes; the infiltrate may be focal or diffuse and may be localized to the subendocardial or perivascular region. There may be small areas of myocardial necrosis,[489] and direct bacterial invasion of the myocardium can sometimes be detected. *Electrocardiographic abnormalities*, including prolongation of the P-R and Q-T intervals, occur frequently;[382] while these abnormalities are rarely associated with other clinical manifestations of myocardial involvement, sudden death, conduction disturbances, and arrhythmias may occur.[490]

Meningococcus. Myocardial involvement is common during the course of meningococcal infections, particularly in men with fatal meningococcal infections.[491] *Pathological findings* include hemorrhagic myocardial lesions, occasionally associated with intracellular organisms. An interstitial myocarditis composed of lymphocytes, plasma cells, and polymorphonuclear leukocytes is often observed, occasionally with muscle necrosis.[393, 491] Fulminating meningococcemia associated with the Waterhouse-Friderichsen syndrome may exhibit focal muscle necrosis, severe fatty change, and cloudy swelling of the myocytes.[492]

Meningococcal myocarditis may result in congestive heart failure, which may be fatal, as well as in pericardial effusion.[493] Death may also occur suddenly and be associated with involvement of the AV node.[393] It is advisable to monitor the rhythm of patients with meningococcemia. In milder cases, transient electrocardiographic abnormalities, principally ST-segment and T-wave changes, are often seen and may resolve completely with time.[493]

Clostridia. Cardiac involvement is common in patients with clostridial infections with multiple organ involvement[494]; the myocardial damage results from the toxin elaborated by the bacteria. The *pathological findings* are distinctive, with gas bubbles usually present in the myocardium. Areas of degenerated muscle fibers are apparent, but an inflammatory infiltrate is usually absent.[494] *C. perfringens* may cause myocardial abscess formation with myocardial perforation and resultant purulent pericarditis.[495]

Bacterial Endocarditis. Myocardial infection is frequently observed as a consequence of infective endocarditis (Chap. 33).

Legionnaire's Disease. Although pneumonia, rhabdomyolysis, renal failure, and hepatic as well as central nervous system involvement are common with *Legionella pneumophila*, overt cardiac involvement is not. Occasional electrocardiograpic changes may be noted, consisting primarily of ST-segment and T-wave abnormalities. Rarely, myocarditis with evidence of myocardial necrosis and congestive heart failure may be seen.[496]

Spirochetal Infections

Syphilis. Aortitis is the most common manifestation of luetic involvement of the cardiovascular system. Aortic regurgitation and coronary ostial narrowing are associated findings (p. 1562). Syphilitic involvement of the myocardium itself in the form of gumma formation is rare and is usually unsuspected clinically. Involvement of the interventricular septum may result in damage to the conducting system and AV block.[497] Gummae may also impinge on the heart valves and interfere with their function.[498] While congenital syphilis may lead to a diffuse myocarditis,[499] the existence of this in adults is disputed.[500]

Leptospirosis [Weil's Disease]. Cardiac involvement is common in leptospirosis. The *pathological findings* include petechiae or larger foci of hemorrhage, often located in the epicardium.[501] An interstitial myocardial infiltration, often subendocardial in location, may occur, with involvement of the papillary muscles.[501] Involvement of the AV conduction system may be a prominent feature. The most common manifestations of cardiac involvement are ST-segment and T-wave changes; atrial and ventricular arrhythmias, sinus bradycardia, and conduction defects may occur.[502,503] Cardiomegaly, pulmonary congestion, a protodiastolic gallop, pericarditis, and symptoms of congestive heart failure occur rarely.[502]

Relapsing Fever. Many infections are currently observed in Ethiopia. During pandemics, mortality may be particularly high, reaching 70 per cent. Cardiac involvement is a common complication and is often implicated as a cause of death. AV conduction defects occur frequently and may be responsible for sudden death, although tachyarrhythmias have also been implicated.[504] Numerous petechiae are observed with a diffuse histiocytic interstitial infiltrate, particularly around small arterioles in the left ventricle.

Fungal Infections

Systemic fungal infections often occur in individuals with reduced resistance to infection, who are frequently patients with malignant disease and/or those receiving chemotherapy, steroids, radiation, or immunosuppressive therapy.

Aspergillosis. Myocardial involvement is not uncommon in generalized aspergillosis. On *pathological examination*, myocardial necro-

sis and infarction caused by thrombosis of vessels that contain fungal mycelia are commonly seen. The fungus often extends beyond the vessel walls and invades the surrounding necrotic myocardium.[505] The electrocardiogram may be normal in the face of significant myocardial damage but T-wave changes may be present.[506] The *diagnosis* of aspergillus infection is often difficult. Identification of aspergillus through open lung biopsy, aspiration lung biopsy, transtracheal aspiration, or bronchial brush technique is usually successful. Early institution of prolonged therapy with amphotericin B may result in significant improvement.[505]

Actinomycosis. Myocarditis is a rare complication of actinomycotic infection, occurring in less than 2 per cent of patients.[507] However, cardiac involvement is quite serious when it does occur. Involvement of the heart most commonly is the result of direct extension of disease within the thorax.[507] Initially the pericardium is invaded, with eventual obliteration of the pericardial space.[508] The myocardium is commonly involved by extension of the pericardial process. Myocardial seeding is less common. The myocardial lesion is a suppurative, necrotizing abscess containing the organism, surrounded by granulation tissue.[508] Both right- and left-sided failure are common manifestations.[508] A pericardial rub may be heard, sometimes associated with clinical evidence of a pericardial effusion. Arrhythmias occur infrequently.[507]

Blastomycosis. Blastomycosis involves the myocardium by spread from mediastinal lymph nodes, by hematogenous miliary seeding,[509,510] and most frequently by direct extension from the pericardium. *Pathological findings* include cardiac dilatation without hypertrophy but with caseation and tubercle formation. Thrombi may form above the endocardial lesions. Dyspnea, cyanosis, and peripheral edema may be prominent. Tachycardia and a systolic murmur are often present.[510]

Cryptococcosis. Cryptococcal infection of the myocardium occurs most commonly in patients with disseminated malignancy.[511] *Pathological examination* may show cardiac dilatation, with epithelial granulomas and giant cells and variable degrees of fibrosis.[512] Congestive heart failure occurs[512]; pulmonary congestion and muffled heart sounds may be found on physical examination, and cardiomegaly on the chest roentgenogram. The *electrocardiogram* may show first-degree AV block and T-wave inversions; ventricular arrhythmias have been observed.

Candidiasis. Disseminated monilial infections are common opportunistic infections, particularly in the compromised host.[513] Endocardi-

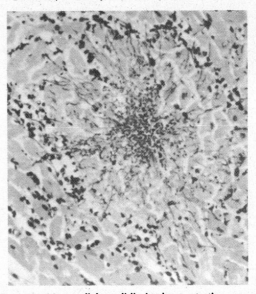

FIGURE 41–25 Myocardial candidiasis, demonstrating a necrotizing myocarditis with a surrounding inflammatory infiltrate. Fungal growth is apparent in the center of the figure. (Original magnification × 360.) (From Brooks, S. E. H., and Young, E. G.: Clinicopathologic observations on systemic moniliasis: A case report and review of the literature. Arch. Pathol. *73*:383, 1962. Copyright 1962, American Medical Association.)

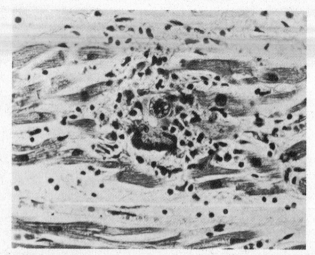

FIGURE 41-26 Disseminated coccidioidomycosis with myocardial involvement. There is a coccidioidal granuloma with evidence of necrosis, multinucleated giant cells, mononuclear cells, lymphocytes, and a coccidioidal spherule. (From Reingold, I. M.: Myocardial lesions in disseminated coccidioidomycosis. Am. J. Clin. Pathol. *20*: 1044, 1950.)

tis is the most frequent manifestation of cardiac involvement (p. 1170), although abscesses of the myocardium may occur as associated or independent findings. Complete heart block may be caused by microabscesses of the conduction system. Pseudohyphae and yeast forms are often found, and multiple foci in the myocardium are usually present.[514] The abscesses are composed of tubercles, with pseudohyphae in the center of the lesions and surrounding yeast forms; there may be polymorphonuclear leukocytes in the periphery of the lesion[514] (Fig. 41-25).

Coccidioidomycosis. Involvement of the heart is seen on occasion in patients with generalized coccidioidomycosis. The hearts may be grossly normal, although epicardial lesions with resultant pericarditis are frequent,[515] and progression to constrictive pericarditis may occur[516] (p. 1502). A nonspecific, focal, interstitial, and perivascular cellular infiltrate with associated muscle fiber degeneration and interstitial edema is commonly found, although granulomas containing fungi are also seen sometimes[515] (Fig. 41-26).

Histoplasmosis. Cardiac involvement in histoplasmosis is rare and usually is in the form of endocarditis (Chap. 33).[517] Pericarditis with effusion may also occur (p. 1502) and superior vena caval obstruction has been observed.[518] Myocardial involvement occurs less frequently, although atrial arrhythmias and T-wave abnormalities have been reported.[518]

Protozoal Myocarditis

TRYPANOSOMIASIS (CHAGAS' DISEASE)

Chagas' disease is caused by the protozoan *Trypanosoma cruzi.* The major cardiovascular manifestation is an extensive myocarditis that typically becomes evident years after the initial infection. The disease is prevalent in Central and South America, particularly in Brazil, Argentina, and Chile, where it is a major public health problem. More than 10 million people in South America may be afflicted.[519]

The natural history of Chagas' disease is characterized by three phases: acute, latent, and chronic. During the *acute phase,* the disease is transmitted to humans through the bite of a reduviid bug (subfamily *Triatominae*), which harbors the parasite in its gastrointestinal tract. This insect acquires the disease from feeding on infected animals, including the armadillo, raccoon, opossum, and skunk as well as domestic dogs and cats. The reduviid bug, popularly known in Argentina as "vinchuca," meaning "to let oneself drop," lives in the walls and roofs of houses and,

during nocturnal feeding, drops from the ceiling onto the sleeping person below.[520] The bug then often bites the person around the eyes, and infection of the human host occurs when the trypanosomes in the animal's feces gain entry through abraded skin or through the conjunctivae. Occasionally, this results in unilateral periorbital edema and swelling of the eyelid, termed *Romaña's sign,* while entry through the skin may result in a lesion called a *chagoma.* Transmission may also occur through blood transfusions as well as congenitally.

ACUTE TRYPANOSOMIASIS. Following inoculation, the protozoa multiply and then migrate widely throughout the body. In a minority of cases an acute illness occurs, although inapparent acute infections are more common.[520,521] There appears to be a depression of T-cell function in those with inapparent acute infections, while those with evident acute disease have normal T-cell function.[521]

Pathological examination during the acute phase often reveals parasites in the cardiac fibers with a marked cellular infiltrate, particularly around cardiac cells that have ruptured and released the parasites. The cellular infiltrate is typically milder around intact muscle fibers harboring parasites. Degeneration of the myocardial fibers may occur. Involvement may extend into the endocardium, resulting in thrombus formation, and into the epicardium, resulting in pericardial effusion.[522] The pathogenesis of the myocardial lesions of acute Chagas' disease appears to relate in large part to immune lysis by antibody and cell-mediated immunity directed against antigens released from *T. cruzi*–infected cells, which become adsorbed onto the surface of infected and noninfected host cells.[523–525]

Clinical Manifestations. These include fever, muscle pains, sweating, hepatosplenomegaly, myocarditis, and, occasionally, meningoencephalitis.[520] The congestive heart failure is characterized by tachycardia, a protodiastolic gallop, arrhythmias, pulmonary congestion, and peripheral edema. Most patients recover, and their symptoms resolve over several months. Occasionally, patients develop fulminant necrotizing panmyocarditis, often with electrocardiographic evidence of right bundle branch block and findings suggesting extensive myocardial necrosis.[520] Young children most commonly develop clinical acute disease and generally are the most seriously ill.

CHRONIC TRYPANOSOMIASIS. The disease then enters a *latent phase,* not to reappear for 10 to 30 years. At an average of 20 years after the initial (and usually unrecognized) infestation, approximately 30 per cent of infected individuals develop findings of *chronic Chagas' disease,* characterized by cardiomegaly, congestive heart failure, arrhythmias, and right bundle branch block (Fig. 41-27). In this stage, cardiac dilatation typically involves all the cardiac chambers, although right-sided enlargement may predominate.[526] The right ventricle may exhibit increased compliance, dilatation and inflammation, with areas of necrosis.

The pathogenesis of chronic chagasic cardiomyopathy is becoming clearer. The central paradox in this disorder is the negative correlation between the severity of disease and the level of parasitemia.[524] It is not unusual to be unable to detect parasites in patients dying of Chagas' disease.[527] An autoimmune mechanism is thus suggested. It appears (at least in an animal model) that self-reactive cytotoxic T

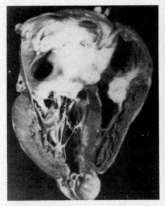
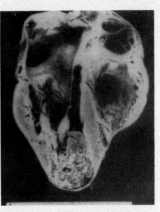

FIGURE 41–27 *Left*, Chagas' heart disease with apical aneurysm. *Right*, Thrombosis of the apical aneurysm. (From Oliveira, J. S. M., et al.: Apical aneurysm of Chagas' heart disease. Br. Heart J. *46*: 432, 1981.)

lymphocytes develop following the initial infection, and these lymphocytes are able to lyse normal host cells in the absence of parasite antigens.[523] It is thought that the acute phase results in the release from parasite-modified host cells of self components that are immunogenic.

Pathology. Nerves and autonomic ganglia are frequently abnormal; megaesophagus and megacolon may occur; less commonly, there is dilatation of the stomach, duodenum, ureter, and bronchi.[528] Different strains of *T. cruzi* may account for the geographic differences in the expression of Chagas' disease; in Brazil, megaesophagus and megacolon are uncommon, but these conditions are usual in Venezuela.[529] Lesions of the cardiac nerves are routinely found in patients with chronic Chagas' disease.[526] Pathological cardiac findings include cardiac enlargement with dilatation and hypertrophy of all cardiac chambers.[520,526,528] The left ventricular apex is often thin and bulging, resembling an aneurysm[530] (Fig. 41–27). Thrombus formation is frequent and may fill much of the apex; the right atrium also frequently contains thrombus.[528]

The microscopic findings are principally those of extensive fibrosis, particularly of the left ventricle.[531] A chronic cellular infiltrate composed of lymphocytes, plasma cells, and macrophages is often present[528,531] (Fig. 41–28). In rare cases, granulomatous lesions or an arteritis is apparent.[528] Preferential involvement of the right bundle branch and the anterior fascicle of the left bundle branch by inflammatory and fibrotic changes explains the frequent occurrence of right bundle branch and left anterior fascicular block.[532] Parasites may be identified in one-fourth of patients[526]; the frequency with which they are found depends upon the diligence of the search for them.

Clinical Manifestations. Chronic progressive heart failure, often predominantly right-sided, is the rule. Thus, while pulmonary congestion is occasionally noted, the usual findings generally include fatigue due to diminished cardiac output, peripheral edema, ascites, and hepatic congestion.[520] Tricuspid regurgitation is often present, particularly in patients with severe right-sided heart failure, although mitral regurgitation is frequently present as well.[528] The second heart sound is widely split, often with an accentuated pulmonic component,[520] reflecting the combined effects of right bundle branch block and pulmonary hypertension.

The *chest roentgenogram* often demonstrates severe car-

diomegaly, with or without pulmonary venous hypertension.[528] *Electrocardiographic abnormalities* are the rule, with right bundle branch block and left anterior hemiblock being the most common changes in patients with chronic Chagas' disease[520,528,528a] (Fig. 41–29). Left bundle branch block is uncommon. ST-segment and T-wave abnormalities are common,[520] while Q waves involving the inferior leads,[528] P-wave abnormalities, and AV block are occasionally seen.[522] Early in the disease, the electrocardiogram may be normal or nearly so. Administration of the antiarrhythmic agent ajmaline may precipitate the appearance of electrocardiographic abnormalities and thus identify patients with as yet clinically silent cardiac involvement.[533,534a]

Ventricular arrhythmias are a prominent feature of chronic Chagas' disease. Frequent ventricular premature depolarizations, often with multiple morphologies, are seen often, and bouts of ventricular tachycardia may occur. Ventricular arrhythmias are particularly common during and following exercise, occurring in the majority of patients subjected to stress electrocardiographic testing.[528] Syncope and sudden death due to ventricular fibrillation are a constant threat and may develop even before cardiomegaly or heart failure.[520] Sinus bradycardia may also be seen, even in patients with severe heart failure when a tachycardia would be expected.[520,526] Atrial arrhythmias, including atrial fibrillation, may also occur. Thromboembolic phenomena are a frequent complication.[528]

The *echocardiographic findings* in some are those of a dilated cardiomyopathy (Fig. 5–72, p. 130), with dilatation, increased end-diastolic and end-systolic volumes, reduced fractional systolic shortening of the left ventricle, and ejection fraction, often with enlargement of the left atrium and right ventricle.[528] In the majority of patients, the echocardiographic appearance is distinctive, with left ventricular posterior wall hypokinesis and relatively preserved interventricular septal motion; an apical aneurysm is often seen on two-dimensional echocardiography.[519]

Left ventricular cineangiography in advanced cases shows a dilated, hypokinetic left ventricle with a large apical aneurysm containing intracavitary thrombus, often with evidence of mitral regurgitation (Fig. 41–27). Mild

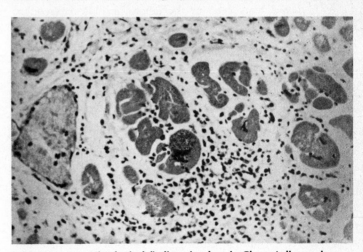

FIGURE 41–28 Histological findings in chronic Chagas' disease include myocardial cell hypertrophy with numerous small *T. cruzi* organisms and a surrounding chronic inflammatory infiltrate. (Original magnification × 400.) (From Puigbo, J. J., et al.: Diagnosis of Chagas' cardiomyopathy. Noninvasive techniques. Postgrad. Med. J. *53*: 527, 1977.)

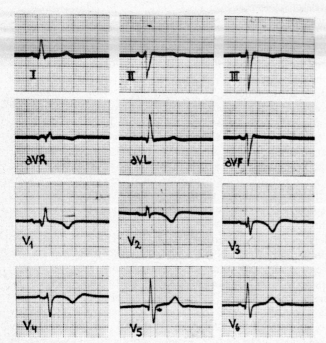

FIGURE 41–29 Electrocardiogram typical of chronic Chagas' disease, demonstrating left anterior hemiblock, right bundle branch block, and T-wave changes. (From Rosenbaum, M. B.: Chagasic myocardiopathy. Progr. Cardiovasc. Dis. 7:199, 1964, by permission of Grune and Stratton.)

asynergy in the anteroapical region may be seen in some patients despite the absence of clinical, radiological or electrocardiographic evidence of cardiac involvement.[534,534a]

The *complement-fixation* test (Machado-Guerreiro test) is useful in diagnosis; it has a sensitivity of greater than 90 per cent, with a specificity of 99 per cent[520] for the identification of chronic Chagas' disease. Also used in diagnosis are the indirect immunofluorescent antibody, the enzyme-linked immunosorbent assay (ELISA), and the hemagglutination tests.[535,536] Another test that is occasionally useful is the detection of parasites in the blood of patients with chronic Chagas' disease (which occurs in 30 to 40 per cent of cases) by means of *xenodiagnosis.* The patient is bitten by reduviid bugs bred in the laboratory; the subsequent identification of parasites in the intestine of the insect is proof of infection in the human host.[520]

Diagnosis. Three forms of evidence should be available to establish a diagnosis of chronic Chagas' cardiomyopathy: (1) *epidemiological evidence*—the patient should be from a geographical area where the vectors are available and the disease occurs; (2) *clinical evidence*—the patient should have findings of a dilated cardiomyopathy with arrhythmias or conduction abnormalities, without evidence of intrinsic valvular, pericardial, coronary, or congenital disease; (3) *laboratory evidence*—the serological or xenodiagnostic test should be positive.[520]

Treatment. The management of Chagas' disease remains difficult; once cardiac decompensation develops, there is usually a rapid and inexorable progression to death. While antiparasitic agents such as nifurtimox and benzimidazole are effective in reducing parasitemia, there is no evidence that they are efficacious in curing the disease.[537] A more promising avenue of approach appears to be immunoprophylaxis, although a clinically useful vaccine is not yet available.[524]

African Trypanosomiasis. African sleeping sickness, due to *Trypanosoma gambiense* or *T. rhodesiense,* may be associated with myocardial abnormalities, although they are usually of less functional significance than in so-called American trypanosomiasis (Chagas' disease).[538] *T. rhodesiense,* in particular, may lead to cardiac failure, although the central nervous system findings (excessive somnolence) usually dominate the clinical picture.

Pathological examination uniformly reveals pericardial fluid. The heart is not as greatly dilated and hypertrophied as it is in Chagas' disease and may appear grossly to be normal. There is often epicardial thickening with a cellular exudate composed of lymphocytes, plasma cells, and histiocytes.[539] The myocardium typically displays a diffuse interstitial infiltrate, often with zones of patchy fibrosis and interstitial edema.[539,540]

Nonspecific *electrocardiographic changes,* usually T-wave abnormalities and prolongation of the Q-T interval,[538] are often observed. Unlike Chagas' disease, arrhythmias and conduction disturbances are usually not prominent features and the arterial pressure is usually normal. Some of the patients have asymptomatic cardiomegaly, although both pulmonary congestion and peripheral edema have been reported.

Toxoplasmosis. *Toxoplasma* infections are caused by an obligate intracellular parasite (*T. gondii*); both congenital and acquired forms may occur. Symptomatic, acquired, toxoplasmic infections occur most commonly in patients with malignant diseases who are being treated with corticosteroids, chemotherapy, radiation, or immunosuppressive drugs.[541] *Pathological findings* include cardiac enlargement and hypertrophy, with occasional endocardial thrombi.[542] Petechial hemorrhages, an inflammatory infiltrate with variable degrees of edema and degeneration of the muscle bundles, and pericardial effusion are often present.

Most adult cases are asymptomatic, but *Toxoplasma* infections may produce a severe, fatal disease with multisystem involvement.[541] Toxoplasmic myocarditis, often with pericarditis, may occur as an isolated disease process or as part of a multisystem disseminated disease. Manifestations may include arrhythmia (atrial and ventricular), AV block, pericarditis, and heart failure.[543] Large pericardial effusions may be seen on occasion.[544] Palpitations, tachycardia, chest discomfort, fatigue, pulmonary congestion, and peripheral edema may be prominent symptoms. *Physical examination* usually reveals cardiomegaly, congestive heart failure, gallop rhythm, systolic murmurs, and hypotension. The *electrocardiogram* may show a variety of abnormalities, including atrial and ventricular arrhythmias, bundle branch block or hypertrophy patterns, or AV conduction defects.[541,542,545] When the myocardial involvement is one manifestation of disseminated disease, the antibody titers are typically quite high or rise rapidly. On the other hand, isolated myocarditis may be associated with low and nondiagnostic titers.

Treatment is with a combination of pyrimethamine and triple sulfonamides, but the response to therapy is variable.[541,545] Corticosteroids may be helpful in treating arrhythmias or conduction defects.

Malaria. While myocardial changes may be demonstrated during the course of malaria, particularly with *Plasmodium falciparum,* clinical findings to indicate cardiac involvement are rare. The heart generally demonstrates few gross abnormalities. The principal findings are histological. The capillaries are often filled and even distended with an accumulation of parasites, sometimes totally occluding the lumen of the vessels. Thrombosis of the capillaries and ischemic myocardial changes may be seen.[546,547] Focal myocardial damage may be present, along with an interstitial infiltrate composed of lymphocytes, plasma cells, and macrophages. In rare cases, cardiac failure may contribute to or even cause death,[548] although it has not been demonstrated that chronic heart disease results from malaria. Slight ST-segment and T-wave changes on the electrocardiogram may be the only clinical indications of myocarditis.[549]

Metazoal Myocardial Disease

Schistosomiasis. Schistosomiasis is a major public health problem, with an infection rate as high as 85 per cent in heavily endemic areas, such as the Nile River basin in Africa and the Yangtze River basin in the Orient. Its principal cardiac effect is right heart overload secondary to pulmonary hypertension. Embolization of the schistosomal ova to the pulmonary vasculature results in an allergic pulmonary arteritis and a paravascular granulomatous reaction, which results in pulmonary hypertension. Right ventricular hypertrophy and right heart failure with chronic cor pulmonale occur typically in young adults.[550,551]

Direct myocardial involvement, on the other hand, is quite infrequent.[552] Myocardial invasion by the ova may result in an inflammatory myocarditis, with a perivasculitis composed principally of mononuclear cells and eosinophils.[552] It has also been proposed that a myocarditis may occur in the absence of direct invasion by the parasite, and a toxic or allergic etiology has been postulated.[553]

Heterophyiasis. This condition results from infestation by several intestinal flukes and is common, particularly in the Far East. The heart may become involved, presumably by hematogenous spread. The heart may be slightly dilated, particularly the right side, with prominent subepicardial hemorrhages. Chronic congestive heart failure is present for some time and may eventually culminate in the patient's demise.[553,554]

Cysticercosis. Cardiac involvement with *Cysticercus cellulosae*, the larval form of *Taenia solium*, is occasionally seen following a disseminated systemic infection. While electrocardiographic changes, including P- and T-wave abnormalities, as well as congestive heart failure have been reported, most cases of cardiac involvement are not apparent clinically.[555-557]

Echinococcus (Hydatid Cyst). *Echinococcus* is endemic in many sheep-raising areas of the world, particularly Argentina, Uruguay, New Zealand, Greece, North Africa, and Iceland, but cardiac involvement in hydatid disease is uncommon, occurring in less than 2 per cent of cases.[558] The usual host of *Echinococcus granulosus* is the dog, but human beings may serve as intermediate hosts (rather than the sheep, the usual intermediate host) if they accidentally ingest ova from contaminated dog feces. The parasites leave the intestine and enter the portal circulation, where the majority are trapped by the liver. Some of the parasites may escape the hepatic and pulmonary bed and become trapped in the myocardium.[559] Once in the myocardium, the parasite grows and a cyst is formed, which may range from a few millimeters to many centimeters in diameter; most exceed 5 centimeters.[560]

The left ventricle is the most common site of cardiac involvement, presumably because of its richer coronary circulation.[560-563] Involvement of the interventricular septum and right ventricle may also occur.[39,564-566] A myocardial cyst may degenerate and calcify, develop daughter cysts, or rupture. Rupture of the cyst is the most dreaded complication; rupture into the pericardium may result in acute pericarditis, which may progress to chronic constrictive pericarditis. Rupture into the cardiac chambers may result in systemic or pulmonary emboli. The liberation of hydatid fluid into the circulation may produce profound, fatal circulatory collapse due to an anaphylactic reaction to the protein constituents of the fluid.

Most patients with cardiac involvement are in the second to fourth decades, and men predominate.[560-562] The diagnosis may be made from the *chest roentgenogram*, which typically shows an abnormal cardiac silhouette with a distinct bulge of the cardiac border.[558,559,561] Expansion of the cyst may result in myocardial compression and damage, sometimes resulting in angina pectoris and electrocardiographic abnormalities.[565] The *electrocardiogram* often reflects the location of the cyst; T-wave changes and loss of QRS voltage may occur with left ventricular involvement, while AV conduction defects or right bundle branch block may be seen with involvement of the interventricular septum. P-wave abnormalities occur in the rare cases of atrial involvement. Arrhythmias are occasionally seen as well.[559] Chest pain is usually due to rupture of the cyst into the pericardial space wth resultant pericarditis.[558] Protrusion of a cyst from the interventricular septum into the right ventricular outflow tract may result in partial obstruction.[558,562,566]

Diagnosis of an echinococcal cyst of the heart is a relatively simple matter if there is evidence of cysts in other organs, particularly the liver and lung.[553,558] Unfortunately, the cardiac cyst is often an isolated, solitary finding. The *chest roentgenogram* frequently shows a calcified lobular mass adjacent to the left ventricle,[562] and fluoroscopy and tomography may furnish additional details regarding location, size, shape, and degree of cyst calcification. Two-dimensional echocardiography may prove useful in the early detection of cardiac involvement.[567] Definitive diagnosis is provided by cardiac catheterization and angiography.[558,559,562] Left ventricular angiography may be particularly helpful in differentiating a cyst from a ventricular aneurysm.[563] Coronary arteriography may be useful in defining the extent

of the cyst by its displacement of the coronary vasculature.[559] Hemodynamic measurements may demonstrate a gradient between the right ventricle and pulmonary artery in patients with obstruction to right ventricular outflow.

Eosinophilia, present in some patients, is a useful adjunctive finding. The Casoni skin test is not very helpful because both false-positive and false-negative results occur. Serological tests, including hemagglutination and complement-fixation, are more useful.[559]

Until recently, *treatment* for hydatid disease was limited to surgical excision.[558,559] Recent experience suggests that the benzimidazole derivative mebendazole may be an effective agent in the medical management of this disease.[568] Because of the significant risk of rupture of the cyst and its attendant serious and sometimes fatal consequences, surgical excision is generally recommended for asymptomatic patients.[562] The surgical results have been favorable, with complete recovery in many cases.[562]

Visceral Larva Migrans. People are occasional accidental hosts of the roundworm infestations of dogs due to *Toxocara canis*. Most cases occur in children one to three years of age.[569] Myocarditis may occur in association with invasion of the myocardium by larvae. The myocardial lesions include granulomas or extensive inflammatory infiltrates with foci of muscle necrosis.[570] Congestive failure and death may occur, although complete recovery following the use of corticosteroids has been reported.[569,570]

TRICHINOSIS. Infestation with *Trichinella spiralis* is the most common human helminthic disease, and evidence of involvement may be found in almost 1 per cent of routine autopsies.[571] Unlike some parasitic diseases with cardiac involvement, myocarditis plays a prominent role in trichinosis and is in fact responsible for the majority of fatalities.[572] The mortality of acute trichinosis is reported to be approximately 5 per cent. Less frequently, death is due to pulmonary embolism secondary to venous thrombosis as well as encephalitis.[572]

Although the parasite frequently invades the heart, it does not usually encyst there, and it is rare to find larvae or larval fragments in the myocardium.[573] Nonetheless, *pathological findings* at postmortem examination may be impressive. The heart may be dilated and flabby and a pericardial effusion may be present. A prominent focal infiltrate composed of lymphocytes and eosinophils, with interstitial edema, hyperemia, and scattered hemorrhages, is commonly found.[553,571-573] Areas of muscle degeneration and necrosis are present. The lesions may be due to toxic effects of the products produced in the course of the host reaction.

The *clinical manifestations*, congestive heart failure and chest pain, usually appear around the third week of the disease, when the general constitutional symptoms are abating.[571,574] Often, the cardiac symptoms are mild or absent or are overshadowed by other symptoms. Physical examination may be normal, or there may be gross cardiomegaly with severe congestive heart failure.[573,575,576] Sudden death may occur, usually in the fourth to eighth week of the illness.[553,574]

Electrocardiographic abnormalities may be detected in one-fourth of patients with trichinosis[573] and parallel the time course of clinical cardiac involvement, initially appearing in the second or third week and usually resolving by the seventh week of the illness.[571,576] The most common electrocardiographic abnormalities are T-wave changes, followed by prolongation of the QRS complex, diminished QRS voltage, first-degree AV block,[576] and ventricular arrhythmias.[575] The electrocardiographic changes usually resolve completely.

The definitive *diagnosis* is based on the demonstration of

larval forms in tissue biopsy samples, usually of the gastrocnemius muscle. Eosinophilia, when present, is a supportive finding.[553] The skin test is usually but not invariably positive. Treatment is with corticosteroids; dramatic improvement in cardiac function has been reported following their use.[571,575] Recovery from myocarditis may occur without residual cardiac damage.

NONINFECTIOUS MYOCARDIAL DAMAGE

A wide variety of stimuli other than those produced by infection may act on the heart and damage the myocardium.[577,578] In some cases, the damage is acute, transient, and associated with evidence of myocardial inflammation (myocarditis). Other agents that damage the myocardium may lead to chronic changes with resulting histological evidence of fibrosis and a clinical picture of a dilated cardiomyopathy. Furthermore, many offending stimuli may be associated with both acute and chronic phases (e.g., alcohol, adriamycin). The response often is related to the dose and rate of exposure.

Numerous chemicals and drugs (both industrial and therapeutic) may lead to cardiac damage and dysfunction. Several physical agents (e.g., radiation and excessive heat) may also result in myocardial damage. Furthermore, myocardial involvement may be evident in a variety of systemic diseases, which are described in Part IV of this book.

Toxic, Chemical, and Drug Effects

Tricyclic Antidepressants (see also p. 1839). Although sudden death, disturbances in rhythm, and abnormalities of AV conduction may be seen with the tricyclic antidepressants, important depression of left ventricular function is usually not seen, even in patients with preexisting heart disease.[579] Postural hypotension may be exacerbated, however.

Phenothiazines (see also p. 1840). The phenothiazines may be associated with a variety of cardiac disturbances, including electrocardiographic changes, atrial and ventricular arrhythmias, and sudden death.[580–582] Of the most commonly used agents, evidence of cardiac involvement is most common with thioridazine (Mellaril), less common with chlorpromazine (Thorazine), and least common with trifluoperazine (Stelazine). The cardiac effects are largely dose-dependent. Electrocardiographic abnormalities may be seen with as little as 200 milligrams of thioridazine per day and consist of lengthening of the Q-T interval and T-wave changes.[583] Higher doses may lead to frank T-wave inversion and increase in the amplitude of the U wave.[580] Changes in the P wave, QRS complex, and ST segment are usually absent.

The phenothiazines appear to have a quinidine-like effect, except that they do not prolong the duration of the QRS complex.[583] Although the phenothiazines may lead to ventricular arrhythmias, they also apparently suppress atrial and ventricular ectopic beats, at least in experimental animals.[584] The electrocardiographic abnormalities and arrhythmias resolve with discontinuation of the drug, usually within 48 hours.[585] Ventricular irritability apparently is caused by the facilitation of reentry by the phenothiazines.

Pathological changes in the hearts of patients who have received psychotropic drugs and who have died suddenly include the deposition of acid mucopolysaccharide between muscle bundles in periarteriolar regions as well as the conduction system, with myofibrillar degeneration, and endothelial proliferation in the smaller blood vessels. A variety of explanations have been invoked for the cardiac damage, including direct toxic effects of the phenothiazines on the myocardium, stimulation of higher autonomic centers, and changes in circulating or myocardial levels of catecholamines.[586]

Emetine. Cardiovascular changes are common with the use of emetine, a drug often employed in the treatment of amebiasis and schistosomiasis.[587] Myocardial lesions may be observed in some but not all patients at autopsy, and similar cardiac damage is noted in experimental animals given emetine.[580,587,588] The myocardial lesions consist of myofibrillar degeneration and necrosis, with an interstitial infiltrate of mononuclear cells and histiocytes. Emetine appears to inhibit oxidative phosphorylation and results in reversible damage to the mitochondria.[587,589] However, the observation that potassium administration often results in normalization of the T waves suggests that the electrocardiographic changes are due to transient intracellular ionic shifts.[588,590]

The *electrocardiogram* most commonly shows reduced T-wave amplitude or inversion. Prolongation of the Q-T interval and ST-segment shifts may also be seen, although abnormalities of the P wave, P-R segment, and QRS complex are infrequent. The electrocardiographic changes usually resolve within weeks or months after cessation of treatment. Sinus tachycardia and hypotension may also be seen, although clinical evidence of myocardial toxicity is usually lacking.[588] Only rare fatalities have been reported. *Dehydroemetine* results in electrocardiographic abnormalities similar to those of emetine, but they are less prominent and of shorter duration.[588]

Emetine and dehydroemetine therapy should be discontinued upon appearance of clinical evidence of cardiac toxicity, but treatment may be continued cautiously if electrocardiographic changes are the only manifestation. Potassium supplementation may be employed so long as the serum potassium level is closely monitored.

Chloroquine. This drug has been widely used in the prophylaxis and treatment of a variety of parasitic diseases and has potent toxic cardiac effects, which appear to be related to its ability to inhibit cellular respiration by blocking the Krebs cycle.[591] It is a myocardial depressant in large doses, although routine doses are not usually associated with clinical evidence of cardiac dysfunction.[590,591] Electrocardiographic changes occur routinely and are similar to those seen with emetine, although they are less pronounced and of shorter duration. In toxic doses, chloroquine may result in depressed cardiac output, bradycardia, arrhythmias, heart block, and death.[591]

Antimony Compounds. Various antimony compounds, such as stibophen and tartar emetic, have been widely used in the treatment of schistosomiasis; less toxic agents are now becoming available. The antimony compounds are associated with electrocardiographic changes in almost all patients. Typical *electrocardiographic changes* include prolongation of the Q-T interval with flattening or inversion of T waves. ST-segment shifts and P-wave changes may be seen, although the QRS complex usually demonstrates no abnormality.[580] Most patients do not demonstrate cardiac findings, although chest pain, bradycardia, hypotension, ventricular arrhythmias (including paroxysmal ventricular tachycardia), and sudden death may occur.[592]

Lithium (see also p. 1841). Lithium carbonate, used in the treatment of manic-depressive disorders, is associated with T-wave changes in one-fourth or more of patients who receive the drug. Clinical evidence of myocardial involvement is usually lacking, although intoxication with lithium may be associated with ventricular arrhythmias, symptomatic sinus node abnormalities, atrioventricular conduction disturbances, and death.[593–595] In fatal lithium toxicity, the heart is dilated and there is evidence of myofibrillar degeneration associated with a lymphocytic interstitial infiltrate and fibrosis.[595]

Hydrocarbons. Ingestion of hydrocarbons may result in fragmentation and vacuolization of the muscle fibers with loss of cross-striations.[596] Electrocardiographic changes, arrhythmias, and cardiomegaly may occur. Involvement of the central nervous, renal, hepatic, and pulmonary systems may dominate the clinical presentation and obscure the myocardial damage, which may well contribute to the mortality of hydrocarbon ingestion.[596] The electrocardiographic changes include ST-segment and T-wave abnormalities, although patterns suggesting acute myocardial injury have been noted.[597]

The *fluorinated hydrocarbons*, commonly used as aerosol propellants, appear to be cardiac toxins, contrary to their reputation of being inert. In animal preparations, at least, the aerosol propellants cause ventricular tachyarrhythmias, depress myocardial contractility, and lower systemic vascular resistance and arterial pressure.[598] These cardiovascular effects may be involved in the sudden deaths seen in individuals who abuse aerosols for their psychotropic effect.

Catecholamines. Myocarditis is frequently observed in conjunction with pheochromocytoma, and the myocardial damage has been attributed to high levels of circulating catecholamines[599,600] (p. 1734). Similar changes have been demonstrated in experimental animals treated with prolonged infusions of L-norepinephrine. Catecholamines may produce an acute myocarditis, with focal myocardial necrosis, inflammation, epicardial hemorrhages, tachycardia, and arrhythmias.[601] Phenylpropanolamine, a sympathomimetic amine used in decongestants and appetite suppressants, may result in similar findings.[602]

A variety of mechanisms have been suggested. A direct toxic effect may be involved, or the damage may be secondary to relative tissue hypoxia because of heightened metabolic demands. Alternatively, the damage may result from changes in autonomic tone or enhanced lipid mobility induced by epinephrine.[603] Aspirin and dipyridamole appear to offer some protection against experimental myocardial necrosis by catecholamines, suggesting that platelet aggregation plays a major role. It has been suggested that the rare development of a myocardial infarction after prolonged stress may result from intravascular platelet thrombosis induced by catecholamines, which may lead to occlusion of a coronary artery previously narrowed by an atheroma.[603]

Lead. The prominent features in lead poisoning generally center on the gastrointestinal and central nervous systems. However, myocardial involvement may contribute to or be the principal cause of death in some cases.[577,604] Reported pathological changes include cloudy swelling of the myofibers, with interstitial fibrosis and edema but without much of a cellular infiltrate. Electrocardiographic changes, chest pain, atrioventricular conduction defects, and overt congestive heart failure may occur.[605] The electrocardiographic and myocardial changes appear to be reversible.

Carbon Monoxide. Both acute and chronic carbon monoxide toxicity are common. While central nervous system findings usually dominate the clinical presentation, significant and occasionally fatal cardiac abnormalities are often present. Because carbon monoxide has a higher affinity for hemoglobin than does oxygen, insufficient oxygen is transported to the tissues.[606] Thus, the cardiac toxicity is the result of myocardial hypoxia, but a direct toxic effect of the gas on myocardial mitochondria may also play a role.[607] The *histological features* include focal areas of necrosis, most marked in the subendocardium. Focal perivascular infiltrates and punctate hemorrhages are also seen.[606] The *electrocardiographic changes* in survivors are transient.[606] Administration of 100 per cent oxygen, bed rest, and surveillance for serious rhythm or conduction abnormalities will usually permit rapid recovery.[606]

Cardiac involvement may appear promptly after exposure or it may be delayed for up to several days. Palpitations, sinus tachycardia, and various arrhythmias, including ventricular extrasystoles and atrial fibrillation, are common.[606,608] Bradycardia and AV block may occur in more severe cases. In patients with ischemic heart disease, angina pectoris and myocardial infarction may be precipitated. Electrocardiographic ST-segment and T-wave abnormalities are quite common. Transient left ventricular wall motion abnormalities may be present.[609]

Mercury. Electrocardiographic abnormalities, principally ST-segment depression, T-wave changes, and prolongation of the Q-T interval, are common findings in mercury poisoning. However, no specific cardiac symptoms occur.[610]

Phosphorus. Ingestion of phosphorus leads to death in 30 to 50 per cent of individuals, with most deaths occurring within 36 hours.[611] The heart is dilated, with diffuse interstitial edema but without a cellular infiltrate. Electrocardiographic abnormalities occur in the majority of patients and consist of ST-segment and T-wave abnormalities, prolongation of the QRS complex and Q-T interval, and atrial arrhythmias.[611,612] Prominent clinical features include severe biventricular depression of contractile function, peripheral vasodilatation, and marked hypotension.

Hypocalcemia. In rare patients with chronic hypocalcemia (often due to hypoparathyroidism), congestive heart failure may occur and resolve only when the serum calcium level is raised.[613,614]

Selenium Deficiency. Dietary deficiency of the trace element selenium appears to be one of the principal factors responsible for a form of dilated cardiomyopathy endemic to certain rural areas in China that are deficient in selenium.[615] Termed *Keshan disease*, it affects mainly children and young women and can be prevented by the prophylactic administration of sodium selenite tablets.[616] A similar cardiomyopathy may be found in Occidentals subjected to prolonged parenteral hyperalimentation.[617]

Scorpion Sting. The venom of the scorpion is mainly neurotoxic, but cardiac findings may be prominent and even fatal, particularly in children.[577,618] Hearts are normal on gross examination with prominent microscopic changes usually but not invariably present, particularly in the subendocardial regions and papillary muscles.[618,619] Degeneration and necrosis of muscle fibers are noted, with interstitial edema and a mononuclear infiltrate. The histological features of scorpion sting suggest high levels of circulating catecholamines[618-620] and are similar to those seen with experimental catecholamine infusion and in pheochromocytoma (p. 1734). The parasympathetic system appears to be stimulated as well.[621]

The *electrocardiogram* often initially shows tall peaked T waves that progress to inversions and ST-segment shifts. Q waves may appear, and the Q-T interval is usually prolonged. Atrial, junctional, and ventricular arrhythmias may occur. Tachycardia, hypertension, anxiety, diaphoresis, and pulmonary edema—findings resembling those of a massive catecholamine effect—are striking in many patients.[618-620] A smaller number of patients are seen in shock with peripheral vascular collapse. Most deaths are due to pulmonary edema, presumably the result of left ventricular dysfunction. Occasionally, sudden and unexpected deaths occur in a smaller percentage of patients, presumably as a consequence of arrhythmias. Adrenergic blocking agents may be useful in the management of the cardiovascular manifestation of scorpion stings.[618]

Wasp and Spider Stings. Stings by the vespine wasps may lead to hypotension, circulatory collapse, and cyanosis,[622] manifestations of anaphylaxis. Occasional patients may have chest pain and clinical findings compatible with acute myocardial infarction. The mechanism of myocardial damage is unclear; perhaps it merely reflects necrosis from profound hypotension, although a direct toxic effect on the myocardium or an indirect effect on the coronary arteries may be involved.

Cardiovascular collapse may also appear after stings due to the "black widow" spider (*Latrodectus mactans*). Atrial arrhythmias, labile blood pressure, and increased urinary levels of vanillylmandelic acid suggest that the stings may result in increased catecholamine levels.[623]

Snake Bite. Cardiac complications are usually not prominent features of snake bites, and the clinical picture is usually dominated by the neurological, hematological, and vascular damage produced by the snakebite toxin.[624] Myocardial involvement is seen on occasion and may rarely contribute to morbidity and mortality.[577] T-wave abnormalities are the most common manifestation of myocardial involvement, although ST-segment depression and QRS prolongation may also be seen. The electrocardiographic changes are usually transient, but when persistent they are attributed to direct myocardial damage due to the toxin.[625] Death may occur from circulatory collapse in adder bites, and myocardial infarction due to hypotension and coronary artery thrombosis has been reported.[626]

Arsenic. Arsenicals are currently utilized in pesticides. Myocardial involvement may be seen in both acute and chronic poisoning; the heart may be dilated, with accumulation of pericardial fluid.[627] Multiple focal and confluent areas of subepicardial and subendocardial hemorrhage are characteristic findings.[627,628] The myocardium is usually abnormal, with evidence of a perivascular mononuclear infiltrate.

Clinically unrecognized, toxic, interstitial myocarditis[629] is reflected in T-wave inversions and ST-segment depressions, along with prolongation of the Q-T interval. The electrocardiographic changes usually revert to normal within two to four weeks. The electrocardiographic abnormalities appear to resolve more rapidly when BAL (British antilewisite, dimercaprol) is utilized in therapy.[630] Death is often due to acute renal failure, although circulatory collapse may occur.[627,628]

Industrial exposure to *arsine gas* is often rapidly fatal, with deaths due to myocardial failure and uremia.[631] The principal toxic effect of arsine is on the red blood cells, with the production of massive hemolysis. Cardiac dilatation is typically present at postmortem examination. Myocardial edema with subepicardial hemorrhage, fibrosis, cloudy swelling, and fragmentation of muscle fibers with a minimal cellular infiltrate constitute the principal histological findings. T-wave changes are common. Death from pulmonary edema usually occurs within two days of exposure.

Cyclophosphamide (see also p. 1692). High doses of cyclophosphamide (greater than 45 mg/kg/24 hr) have been associated with electrocardiographic changes, congestive heart failure, and death from a hemorrhagic myocarditis.[632,633] In the majority of patients treated a reversible decrease in QRS voltage and systolic function is seen, often asymptomatic, although more than 20 per cent may succumb owing to myopericarditis.[634] The hearts are dilated, with subepicardial and subendocardial ecchymoses, and the left ventricle is thickened.[634] The myocardial damage appears to result from direct endothelial damage and resultant fibrin microthrombi in the capillaries. Myopericarditis may occur within the first two weeks of the initiation of therapy, with development of dyspnea, tachycardia, orthopnea, hypotension, fluid retention, and decreased QRS voltage.[632]

Paracetamol. Paracetamol, a phenacetin metabolite, may result in massive liver necrosis. On occasion it also results in fatty degeneration and focal necrosis of the myocardium, typically on the second to fourth day after an overdose.[635]

Thyroid Hormone. Rare cases of sudden death have been seen with thyroid hormone abuse, and pathological examination has revealed evidence of myocarditis with focal leukocytic infiltration and fibrosis.[636]

Miconazole. Anaphylaxis and cardiac arrest may be seen in patients with hematological malignancies treated with the antifungal agent miconazole.[637] The mechanism of apparent cardiotoxicity is unclear.

Disopyramide (see also p. 659). The antiarrhythmic agent disopyramide may lead to depression of left ventricular function when given either intravenously or orally, although this effect usually is seen only in patients with preexisting left ventricular dysfunction.[638] In addition to an exacerbation of congestive failure, disopyramide may also precipitate profound cardiovascular collapse and death.[639]

5-Fluoro-uracil. This antineoplastic agent has rarely been associated with cardiotoxicity manifested by chest pain, electrocardiographic changes, and arrhythmia. Swelling of myocardial fibers has been demonstrated in an animal preparation.[640]

Daunorubicin and Adriamycin (see page 1690 to 1692).

Hypersensitivity

Hypersensitivity to a variety of agents may result in allergic reactions that involve the myocardium.[641] In addition to anaphylaxis and serum sickness, allergies to a variety of drugs or other sensitizers may lead to an allergic myocarditis, characterized by eosinophilia, and a perivascular infiltration of the myocardium by eosinophils, multinucleated giant cells, and leukocytes.

Methyldopa. This drug is widely used in the treatment of hypertension (p. 915). Although hepatitis is the most frequently encountered serious adverse reaction, sudden and unexpected death has been reported in a number of patients found at necropsy to have had an unsuspected myocarditis.[578] The *histological findings* have the characteristics of an allergic myocarditis, showing an interstitial inflammatory infiltrate with abundant eosinophils, a vasculitis, and focal myocardial necrosis.[642]

Penicillin. Allergic reactions to penicillin are fairly common, but myocardial involvement is rare.[577,578] *Histological findings* consist of a perivascular and interstitial infiltrate composed of eosinophils, plasma cells, lymphocytes, and histiocytes.[643] Both myocardial infarction and pericarditis may occur and account for some of the electrocardiographic changes.[644] Transient electrocardiographic changes may be the only manifestation of cardiac involvement, with bradycardia, ST-segment elevation, and T-wave inversion.

Sulfonamides. Sulfonamides may result in myocardial damage owing to a hypersensitivity vasculitis as well as a myocarditis.[645] Fatal cases usually demonstrate an eosinophilic myocarditis, sometimes with granulomas.[646] While usually clinically silent, severe and even fatal congestive heart failure may occur.[647] Electrocardiographic changes are usually absent, but nonspecific ST-segment and T-wave abnormalities may be seen.[580,647]

Tetracycline. Allergic reactions to antibiotics of the tetracycline class include fever, tachycardia, and first-degree AV block. Postmor-

tem findings include cardiac dilatation, fibrinoid muscle cell degeneration, and a diffuse interstitial and perivascular infiltrate.[577,578,648]

Phenindione. Marked congestive heart failure with cardiomegaly and pulmonary edema has been reported following the use of phenindione. The electrocardiogram may show sinus tachycardia, low QRS voltage, and T-wave inversion.[578,649]

Phenylbutazone. Myocarditis is an uncommon complication[578] but is characterized by dyspnea, chest pain, hypotension, and extensive ST-segment elevations.[650] Pericardial effusions with a prominent perivascular infiltrate may be seen in the myocardium.[651]

Antituberculous Drugs. Most reactions to antituberculous drugs consist of a fever, rash, or both, but serious and fatal cardiac reactions may occur. *Paraaminosalicylic acid* may lead to the development of interstitial edema, acute inflammatory infiltrate, refractory congestive heart failure, hypotension, and ventricular irritability.[652] It is commonly associated with transient arrhythmias or cardiac dilatation.[653]

Streptomycin has been implicated as a rare cause of myocarditis. Pathological findings may include cardiac dilatation, myocarditis with necrosis, hemorrhage, and a fibrinous pericardial effusion.[654] Clinically, it may be associated with chest pain, dyspnea, fever, and rash, followed by collapse and death.

Lyme Carditis. Lyme disease is a process of uncertain etiology that appears to be transmitted by the tick *Ixodes dammini*. The disease is found only in areas of tick distribution, the majority of cases emanating from the northeastern coast of the United States.[655] Lyme disease usually begins during the summer months with a characteristic skin rash (erythema chronicum migrans), followed in days to months by neurological, joint, or cardiac involvement.[656] It is thought that the tick bite transmits an infectious agent that produces the initial skin eruption. The later manifestations, including carditis, appear to be immune-mediated, perhaps related to circulating immune complexes.[657]

About 10 per cent of patients with Lyme disease develop evidence of cardiac involvement, the most common manifestation being variable degrees of AV block. Syncope due to complete heart block is frequent with cardiac involvement, as are diffuse ST-segment and T-wave abnormalities.[657] Transient asymptomatic left ventricular dysfunction may be detected by radionuclide ventriculography in as many as one-third of patients, although cardiomegaly or symptoms of congestive heart failure are rare.[657]

The value of specific therapy in Lyme carditis remains uncertain. Although the skin eruption responds to penicillin or tetracycline, a beneficial effect of antibiotics on the carditis is unestablished.[657] Advanced AV block is usually treated with salicylates or prednisone, although patients with the most severe involvement (meningoencephalitis, complete AV block for longer than one week, or cardiomegaly) are treated routinely with corticosteroids. Temporary transvenous pacing may be required for up to a week in patients with complete heart block.[657]

Giant Cell Myocarditis. Giant cell myocarditis is a rare disease of unknown etiology characterized by the presence of multinucleated giant cells in the myocardium. Variously called acute isolated myocarditis and granulomatous myocarditis, this condition is typically a rapidly fatal disease of young to middle-aged adults.[658,659] *Pathological findings* are usually impressive. The ventricles are dilated, and when death is not sudden, mural thrombi may be present. A serpiginous area of myocardial necrosis may be seen involving the right as well as the left ventricle.[659] Multinucleated giant cells are found, particularly at the margins of the areas of myocardial necrosis. An extensive inflammatory infiltrate is present within the necrotic areas, composed of eosinophils, histiocytes, and other cells[658,659]; fibrosis is absent.[658]

Although giant cell myocarditis appears to be associated with thymoma, systemic lupus erythematosus, and thyrotoxicosis,[659,660] the cause of the disease remains obscure. In many ways the clinical features suggest a viral myocarditis except for the rapid and virulent course. However, despite careful investigation there has been no serological or bacteriological evidence of an infectious etiology.[658,661] Sarcoid, syphilis, and tuberculosis have all been proposed as possible causes, although these usually present distinctive histological

rysm—A comparison with idiopathic dilated cardiomyopathy. J. Am. Coll. Cardiol. *1*:704, 1983.

57. Schroeder, J. S.: Current status of cardiac transplantation, 1978. J.A.M.A. *241*: 2069, 1979.

58. Hassell, L. A., Fowles, R. E., and Stinson, E. B.: Patients with congestive cardiomyopathy as cardiac transplant recipients: Indications for and results of cardiac transplantation and comparison with patients with coronary artery disease. Am. J. Cardiol. *47*:1205, 1981.

59. Rubin, E.: Alcoholic myopathy in heart and skeletal muscle. N. Engl. J. Med. *301*:28, 1979.

60. Regan, T. J., Haider, B., Ahmed, S. S., Lyons, M. M., Oldewurtel, H. A., and Ettinger, P. O.: Whiskey and the heart. Cardiovasc. Med. *2*:165, 1977.

61. Alexander, C. S.: Cobalt-beer cardiomyopathy. A clinical and pathological study of twenty-eight cases. Am. J. Med. *53*:395, 1972.

62. Albarian, M., Yankopoulos, N. A., and Abelmann, W. H.: Hemodynamic studies in beriberi heart disease. Am. J. Med. *41*:197, 1966.

63. Jeffrey, F. E., and Abelmann, W. H.: Recovery from proved Shoshin beriberi. Am. J. Med. *50*:123, 1971.

64. Weiss, S.: Occidental beriberi with cardiovascular manifestations. Its relation to thiamine deficiency. J.A.M.A. *115*:832, 1940.

65. Segel, L. D., Rendig, S. V., and Mason, D. T.: Left ventricular dysfunction of isolated working rat hearts after chronic alcohol consumption. Cardiovasc. Res. *13*:136, 1979.

66. Friedman, H. S., and Lieber, C. S.: Cardiotoxicity of alcohol. Cardiovasc. Med. *2*:111, 1977.

67. Horwitz, L. D., and Atkins, J. M.: Acute effects of ethanol on left ventricular performance. Circulation *49*:124, 1974.

68. Regan, T. J., Ettinger, P. O., Lyons, M. M., Moschos, C. B., and Weisse, A. B.: Ethyl alcohol as a cardiac risk factor. Cur. Probl. Cardiol. *2*:1, 1977.

69. Bing, R. J.: Cardiac metabolism: Its contribution to alcoholic heart disease and myocardial failure. Circulation *58*:965, 1978.

70. Rubin, E.: Alcoholic myopathy in heart and skeletal muscle. N. Engl. J. Med. *301*:28, 1979.

70a. Lange, L. G., and Sobel, B. E.: Impaired cardiac mitochondrial function induced by specific metabolites of ethanol: Fatty acid ethyl esters. J. Am. Coll. Cardiol. *667*:1983.

71. Regan, T. J., Levinson, G. E., Oldewurtel, H. A., Frank, M. J., Weisse, A. B., and Moschos, C. B.: Ventricular function in noncardiacs with alcoholic fatty liver: Role of ethanol in the production of cardiomyopathy, J. Clin. Invest. *48*: 397, 1969.

72. Burch, G. E., and Giles, T. D.: The small coronary arteries in alcoholic cardiomyopathy. Am. Heart J. *94*:471, 1977.

73. Factor, S. M.: Intramyocardial small-vessel disease in chronic alcoholism. Am. Heart J. *92*:561, 1976.

74. Klein, H., and Harmjanz, D.: Effect of ethanol infusion on the ultrastructure of human myocardium. Postgrad. Med. J. *51*:325, 1975.

75. Weisharr, R., Sarma, J. S. M., Maruyama, Y., Fischer, R., Bertuglia, S., and Bing, R. J.: Reversibility of mitochondrial and contractile changes in the myocardium after cessation of prolonged ethanol intake. Am. J. Cardiol. *40*:556, 1977.

76. Bridgen, W.: Alcoholic cardiomyopathy. *In* Burch, G. E. (ed.): Cardiomyopathy. (Cardiovascular Clinics Series.) Philadelphia, F. A. Davis Co., 1972, p. 188.

77. Demakis, J. G., Proskey, A., Rahimtoola, S. H., Jamil, M., Sutton, G. C., Rosen, K. M., Gunnar, R. M., and Tobin, J. R., Jr.: The natural course of alcholic cardiomyopathy. Ann. Intern. Med. *80*:293, 1974.

78. Wu, C. F., Sudhaker, M., Jaferi, G., Ahmed, S. S., and Regan, T. J.: Preclinical cardiomyopathy in chronic alcoholics: A sex difference. Am. Heart J. *91*: 291, 1976.

79. Burch, G. E., and DePasquale, N. P.: Alcoholic cardiomyopathy. Am. J. Cardiol. *23*:723, 1969.

80. Spodick, D. H., Pigott, V. M., and Chirife, R.: Preclinical cardiac malfunction in chronic alcoholism. N. Engl. J. Med. *287*:677, 1972.

81. Levi, G. F., Quadri, A., Ratti, S., and Basagni, M.: Preclinical abnormality of left ventricular function in chronic alcoholics. Br. Heart J. *39*:35, 1977.

82. Mathews, E. C., Gardin, J. M., Henry, W. L., Del Negro, A. A., Fletcher, R. D., Snow, J. A., and Epstein, S. E.: Echocardiographic abnormalities in chronic alcoholics with and without overt congestive heart failure. Am. J. Cardiol. *47*:570, 1981.

83. Askanas, A., Udoshi, M., and Sadjadi, S. A.: The heart in chronic alcoholism. A noninvasive study. Am. Heart J. *99*:9, 1980.

84. Kino, M., Imamitchi, H., Morigutchi, M., Kawamura, K., and Takatsu, T.: Cardiovascular status in asymptomatic alcoholics, with reference to the level of ethanol consumption. Br. Heart J. *46*:545, 1981.

85. Ettinger, P. O., Wu, C. F., De La Cruze, C., Jr., Weisse, A. B., Ahmed, S. S., and Regan, T. J.: Arrhythmias and the "holiday heart": Alcohol-associated cardiac rhythm disorders. Am. Heart J. *95*:555, 1978.

86. Greenspan, A. J., and Schaal, S. F.: The "holiday heart": Electrophysiologic studies of alcohol effects in alcoholics. Ann. Intern. Med. *98*:135, 1983.

87. Bashour, T. T., Fahdul, H., and Cheng, T. O.: Electrocardiographic abnormalities in alcoholic cardiomyopathy. A study of 65 patients. Chest *68*:24, 1975.

88. Lacour, F., Sr., and Suire, E. M.: The diagnosis of alcohol cardiomyopathies. J. La. State Med. Soc. *130*:159, 1978.

89. McDonald, C. D., Burch, G. E., and Walsh, J. J.: Alcoholic cardiomyopathy managed with prolonged bed rest. Ann. Intern. Med. *74*:681, 1971.

90. Schwartz, L., Sample, K. A., and Wigle, E. D.: Severe alcoholic cardiomyopathy reversed with abstention from alcohol. Am. J. Cardiol. *36*:963, 1975.

91. Barborik, M., and Dusek, J.: Cardiomyopathy accompanying industrial cobalt exposure. Br. Heart J. *34*:113, 1972.

92. Manifold, I. H., Platts, M. M., and Kennedy, A.: Cobalt cardiomyopathy in a patient on maintenance haemodialysis. Br. Med. J. *2*:1609, 1978.

HYPERTROPHIC CARDIOMYOPATHY

93. Teare, R. D.: Asymmetrical hypertrophy of the heart in young adults. Brit. Heart J. *20*:1, 1958.

94. Morrow, A. G., and Braunwald, E.: Functional aortic stenosis: A malformation characterized by resistance to left ventricular outflow without anatomic obstruction. Circulation *20*:181, 1959.

95. Martin, R. P., Rakowski, H., French, J., and Popp, R. L.: Idiopathic hypertrophic subaortic stenosis viewed by wide-angle, phased-array echocardiography. Circulation *59*:1206, 1979.

96. Maron, B. J., and Epstein, S. E.: Hypertrophic cardiomyopathy: Recent observations regarding the specificity of three hallmarks of the disease: asymmetric septal hypertrophy, septal disorganization and systolic anterior motion of the anterior mitral leaflet. Am. J. Cardiol. *45*:141, 1980.

97. Doi, Y. L., McKenna, W. J., Gehrke, J., Oakley, C. M., and Goodwin, J. F.: M-mode echocardiography in hypertrophic cardiomyopathy: Diagnostic criteria and prediction of obstruction. Am. J. Cardiol. *45*:6, 1980.

98. Clark, C. E., Henry, W. L., and Epstein, S. E.: Familial prevalence and genetic transmission of idiopathic hypertrophic subaortic stenosis. N. Engl. J. Med. *289*:709, 1973.

99. Roberts, W. C., and Ferrans, V. J.: Pathologic anatomy of the cardiomyopathies. Idiopathic dilated and hypertrophic types, infiltrative types and endomyocardial disease with and without eosinophilia. Hum. Pathol. *6*:287, 1975.

100. Epstein, S. E., Henry, W. L., Clark, C. E., Roberts, W. C., Maron, B. J., Ferrans, V. J., Redwood, D. R., and Morrow, A. G.: Asymmetric septal hypertrophy. Ann. Intern. Med. *81*:650, 1974.

101. Maron, B. J., Gottdiener, J. S., Roberts, W. C., Henry, W. L., Savage, D. D., and Epstein, S. E.: Left ventricular outflow tract obstruction due to systolic anterior motion of the anterior mitral leaflet in patients with concentric left ventricular hypertrophy. Circulation *57*:527, 1978.

102. Come, P. C., Bulkley, B. H., Goodman, Z. D., Hutchins, G. M., Pitt, B., and Fortuin, N. J.: Hypercontractile cardiac states simulating hypertrophic cardiomyopathy. Circulation *55*:901, 1977.

103. Buxton, A. E., Morganroth, J., Josephson, M. E., Perloff, J. K., and Shelborne, J. C.: Isolated dextroversion of the heart with asymmetric septal hypertrophy. Am. Heart J. *92*:785, 1976.

104. Sommerville, J., and Becu, L.: Congenital heart disease associated with hypertrophic cardiomyopathy. Johns Hopkins Med. J. *140*:151, 1977.

105. Maron, B. J., Gottdiener, J. S., Roberts, W. C., Hammer, W. J., and Epstein, S. E.: Nongenetically transmitted disproportionate ventricular septal thickening associated with left ventricular outflow obstruction. Br. Heart J. *41*:345, 1979.

106. Sommerville, J., and Becu, L.: Congenital heart disease associated with hypertrophic cardiomyopathy. Br. Heart J. *40*:1034, 1978.

107. Abbasi, A., Slaughter, J. C., and Allen, M. W.: Asymmetrical septal hypertrophy in patients with long-term hemodialysis. Chest *74*:548, 1978.

108. Maron, B. J., Clark, C. E., Henry, W. L., Fukuda, T., Edwards, J. E., Mathews, E. C., Jr., Redwood, D. R., and Epstein, S. E.: Prevalence and characteristics of disproportionate ventricular septal thickening in patients with acquired or congenital heart disease. Echocardiographic and morphologic findings. Circulation *55*:489, 1977.

109. Larter, W. E., Allen, H. D., Sahn, D. J., and Goldberg, S. J.: The asymmetrically hypertrophied septum. Further differentiation of its causes. Circulation *53*: 19, 1976.

110. Stern, A., Kessler, K. M., Hammer, W. J., Kreulen, T., and Spann, J. F.: Septal-free wall disproportion in inferior infarction: The echocardiographic differentiation from hypertrophic cardiomyopathy. Circulation *58*:700, 1978.

111. Raj, M. V. J., Srinivas, V., Graham, I. M., and Evans, D. W.: Coexistence of asymmetric septal hypertrophy and aortic valve disease in adults. Thorax *34*: 91, 1979.

112. Maron, B. J., Gottdiener, J. S., and Epstein, S. E.: Patterns and significance of distribution of left ventricular hypertrophy in hypertrophic cardiomyopathy: A wide-angle two-dimensional echocardiographic study of 125 patients. Am. J. Cardiol. *48*:418, 1981.

113. Maron, B.J., Gottdiener, J. S., Bonow, R. O., and Epstein, S. E.: Hypertrophic cardiomyopathy with unusual locations of left ventricular hypertrophy undetectable by M-mode echocardiography: Identification by wide-angle two-dimensional echocardiography. Circulation *63*:409, 1981.

113a. Ciro, E., Nichols, P. F., III, and Maron, B. J.: Heterogeneous morphologic expression of genetically transmitted hypertrophic cardiomyopathy. Circulation *67*:1227, 1983.

114. Yamaguchi, H., Ishimura, T., Nishiyama, S., Nagasaki, F., Nakanishi, S., Takatsu, F., Nishijo, T., Umeda, T., and Machii, K.: Hypertrophic nonobstructive cardiomyopathy with giant negative T waves (apical hypertrophy): Ventriculographic and echocardiographic features in 30 patients. Am. J. Cardiol. *44*:401, 1979.

115. Maron, B. J., Bonow, R. O., Seshagiri, T. N. R., Roberts, W. C., and Epstein, S. E.: Hypertrophic cardiomyopathy with ventricular septal hypertrophy localized to the apical region of the left ventricle (apical hypertrophic cardiomyopathy). Am. J. Cardiol. *49*:1838, 1982.

116. Bulkley, B. H., Weisfeldt, M. L., and Hutchins, G. M.: Asymmetric septal hypertrophy and myocardial fiber disarray. Features of normal, developing and malformed hearts. Circulation 56:292, 1977.

117. Rassmussen, S., Corya, B. C., Feigenbaum, H., and Knoebel, S. B.: Detection of myocardial scar tissue by M-mode echocardiography. Circulation 57:230, 1978.

118. Maron, B. J., Savage, D. D., Clark, C. E., Henry, W. L., Vlodaver, Z., Edwards, J. E., and Epstein, S. E.: Prevalence and characteristics of disproportionate ventricular septal thickening in patients with coronary artery disease. Circulation 57:250, 1978.

119. Olsen, E. G. J.: The pathology of idiopathic hypertrophic subaortic stenosis (hypertrophic cardiomyopathy). A critical review. Am. Heart J. 100:553, 1980.

119a. Thompson, R., Ahmed, M., Pridie, R., and Yacoub, M.: Hypertrophic cardiomyopathy after aortic valve replacement. Am. J. Cardiol. 45:33, 1980.

120. Isner, J. M., Falcone, M. W., Virmani, R., and Roberts, W. C.: Cardiac sarcoma causing "ASH" and simulating coronary heart disease. Am. J. Med. 66:1025, 1979.

121. Cabin, H. S., Costello, R. M., Vasudevan, G., Maron, B. J., and Roberts, W. C.: Cardiac lymphoma mimicking hypertrophic cardiomyopathy. Am. Heart J. 102:466, 1981.

122. Bulkley, B. H., and Hutchins, G. M.: Pompe's disease presenting as hypertrophic myocardiopathy with Wolff-Parkinson-White syndrome. Am. Heart J. 96:246, 1978.

123. Colucci, W. S., Lorell, B. H., Schoen, F. J., Warhol, M. J., and Grossman, W.: Hypertrophic obstructive cardiomyopathy due to Fabry's disease. N. Engl. J. Med. 307:926, 1982.

124. Henry, W. L., Clark, C. E., Roberts, W. C., Morrow, A. G., and Epstein, S. E.: Differences in the distribution of myocardial abnormalities in patients with obstructive and nonobstructive asymmetric septal hypertrophy (ASH). Echocardiographic and gross anatomic findings. Circulation 50:447, 1974.

125. Maron, B. J., Ferrans, V. J., Henry, W. L., Clark, C. E., Redwood, D. R., Roberts, W. C., Morrow, A. G., and Epstein, S. E.: Differences in distribution of myocardial abnormalities in patients with obstructive and nonobstructive asymmetric septal hypertrophy (ASH). Light and electron microscopic findings. Circulation 50:436, 1974.

126. Maron, B. J., Anan, T. J., and Roberts, W. C.: Quantitative analysis of the distribution of cardiac muscle cell disorganization in the left ventricular free wall of patients with hypertrophic cardiomyopathy. Circulation 63:882, 1981.

127. Maron, B. J., and Roberts, W. C.: Quantitative analysis of cardiac muscle cell disorganization in the ventricular septum of patients with hypertrophic cardiomyopathy. Circulation 59:689, 1979.

128. Ferrans, V. J., Morrow, A. G., and Roberts, W. C.: Myocardial ultrastructure in idiopathic hypertrophic subaortic stenosis. A study of operatively excised left ventricular outflow tract muscle in 14 patients. Circulation 45:769, 1972.

129. Maron, B. J., and Roberts, W. C.: Hypertrophic cardiomyopathy and cardiac muscle cell disorganization revisited: Relation between the two and significance. Am. Heart J. 102:95, 1981.

129a. Wigle, E. D., and Silver, M. D.: Editorial: Myocardial fiber disarray and ventricular septal hypertrophy in asymmetrical hypertrophy of the heart. Circulation 58:398, 1978.

130. Isner, J. M., Maron, B. J., and Roberts, W. C.: Comparison of amount of myocardial cell disorganization in operatively excised septectomy specimens with amount observed at necropsy in 18 patients with hypertrophic cardiomyopathy. Am. J. Cardiol. 46:42, 1980.

130a. Kishimoto, C., Kaburagi, T., Takayama, S., Yokoyama, S., Hanyu, I., Takatsu, Y., and Tomimoto, K.: Two forms of hypertrophic cardiomyopathy distinguished by inheritance of HLA haplotypes and left ventricular outflow tract obstruction. Am. Heart J. 105:988, 1983.

131. Shah, P. M.: Idiopathic hypertrophic subaortic stenosis (hypertrophic obstructive cardiomyopathy). Changing concepts—1975. Chest 68:814, 1975.

132. Hamby, R. I., Roberts, G. S., and Meron, J. M.: Hypertension and hypertrophic subaortic stenosis. Am. J. Med. 51:474, 1971.

133. Hutchins, G. M., and Bulkley, B. H.: Catenoid shape of the interventricular septum: Possible cause of idiopathic hypertrophic subaortic stenosis. Circulation 58:392, 1978.

134. Perloff, J. K.: Pathogenesis of hypertrophic cardiomyopathy: Hypothesis and speculation. Am. Heart J. 101:219, 1981.

135. James, T. N., and Marshall, T. K.: De Subitaneis Mortibus. XII. Asymmetrical hypertrophy of the heart. Circulation 51:1149, 1975.

136. Lorell, B. H., Paulus, W. J., Grossman, W., Wynne, J., and Cohn, P. F.: Modification of abnormal left ventricular diastolic properties by nifedipine in patients with hypertrophic cardiomyopathy. Circulation 65:499, 1982.

137. Murgo, J. P., Alter, B. R., Dorethy, J. F., Altobelli, S. A., and McGrawahan, G. M., Jr.: Dynamics of left ventricular ejection in obstructive and nonobstructive hypertrophic cardiomyopathy. J. Clin. Invest. 66:1369, 1980.

138. Braunwald, E., Lambrew, C. T., Rockoff, S. D., Ross, J., Jr., and Morrow, A. G.: Idiopathic hypertrophic subaortic stenosis. Circulation 29/30 (Suppl. IV):1, 1964.

139. Whiting, R. B., Powell, W. J., Jr., Dinsmore, R. E., and Sanders, C. A.: Idiopathic hypertrophic subaortic stenosis stenosis in the elderly. N. Engl. J. Med. 285:196, 1971.

140. Neufeld, H. N., Ongley, P. A., and Edwards, J. E.: Combined congenital subaortic stenosis and infundibular pulmonary stenosis. Br. Heart. J. 22:686, 1960.

141. Maron, B. J., Edwards, J. E., Henry, W. L., Clark, C. E., Bingle, G. J., and Epstein, S. E.: Asymmetric septal hypertrophy (ASH) in infancy. Circulation 50:809, 1974.

142. Fiddler, G. I., Tajik, A. J., Weidman, W. H., McGoon, D. C., Ritter, D. G., and Guiliani, E. R.: Idiopathic hypertrophic subaortic stenosis in the young. Am. J. Cardiol. 42:793, 1978.

143. Hamby, R. I., and Aintablian, A.: Hypertrophic subaortic stenosis is not rare in the eighth decade. Geriatrics 31:71, 1976.

144. Krasnow, N., and Stein, R. A.: Hypertrophic cardiomyopathy in the aged. Am. Heart J. 96:326, 1978.

145. Spodick, D. H.: Hypertrophic obstructive cardiomyopathy of the left ventricle (idiopathic hypertrophic subaortic stenosis). In Burch, G. E. (ed.): Cardiomyopathy. (Cardiovascular Clinics Series.) Philadelphia, F. A. Davis Co., 1972, p. 133.

146. Frank, S., and Braunwald, E.: Idiopathic hypertrophic subaortic stenosis. Clinical analysis of 126 patients with emphasis on the natural history. Circulation 37:759, 1968.

147. Maron, B. J., Roberts, W. C., Edwards, J. E., McAllister, H. U., Jr., Foley, D. D., and Epstein, S. E.: Sudden death in patients with hypertrophic cardiomyopathy: Characterization of 26 patients without functional limitation. Am. J. Cardiol. 41:803, 1978.

148. Wigle, E. D., Felderhof, C. H., Silver, M. D., and Adelman, A. G.: Hypertrophic obstructive cardiomyopathy (muscular or hypertrophic subaortic stenosis). In Fowler, N. O. (ed.): Myocardial Diseases. New York, Grune and Stratton, 1973, p. 297.

149. Maron, B. J., Tajik, A. J., Ruttenberg, H. D., Graham, T. P., Atwood, G. F., Victorica, B. E., Lie, J. T., and Roberts, W. C.: Hypertrophic cardiomyopathy in infants: Clinical features and natural history. Circulation 65:7, 1982.

150. Sutton, M. G. St. J., Tajik, A. J., Smith, H. C., and Ritman, E. L.: Angina in idiopathic hypertrophic subaortic stenosis. A clinical correlation of regional left ventricular dysfunction: A videometric and echocardiographic study. Circulation 61:561, 1980.

151. Maron, B. J., Epstein, S. E., and Roberts, W. C.: Hypertrophic cardiomyopathy and transmural myocardial infarction without significant atherosclerosis of the extramural coronary arteries. Am. J. Cardiol. 43:1086, 1979.

152. McKenna, W., Harris, L., and Deanfield, J.: Syncope in hypertrophic cardiomyopathy. Br. Heart J. 47:117, 1982.

153. Wiener, M. W., Vondoenhoff, L. J., and Cohen, J.: Aortic regurgitation first appearing 12 years after successful septal myectomy for hypertrophic obstructive cardiomyopathy. Am. J. Med. 72:157, 1982.

153a. Henderson, M. A., Ruddy, T. D., Makowski, H., and Wigle, E. D.: Left ventricular hypertrophy by ECG in hypertrophic cardiomyopathy. J. Am. Coll. Cardiol. 1:693, 1983.

154. Savage, D. D., Seides, S. F., Clark, C. E., Henry, W. L., Maron, B. J., Robinson, F. C., and Epstein, S. E.: Electrocardiographic findings in patients with obstructive and nonobstructive hypertrophic cardiomyopathy. Circulation 58:402, 1978.

155. Chen, C-H., Nobuyoshi, M., and Kawai, C.: ECG pattern of left ventricular hypertrophy in nonobstructive hypertrophic cardiomyopathy: The significance of the mid-precordial changes. Am. Heart J. 97:687, 1979.

155a. Maron, B. J., Wolfson, J. K., Ciro, E., and Spirito, P.: Relation of electrocardiographic abnormalities and patterns of left ventricular hypertrophy identified by 2-dimensional echocardiography in patients with hypertrophic cardiomyopathy. Am. J. Cardiol. 51:189, 1983.

155b. McKenna, W. J., Borggrefe, M., England, D., Deanfield, J., Oakley, C. M., and Goodwin, J. F.: The natural history of left ventricular hypertrophy in hypertrophic cardiomyopathy: An electrocardiographic study. Circulation 66:1233, 1982.

156. Cosio, F. G., Moro, C., Alonso, M., de la Calzada, C. S., and Llovet, A.: The Q waves of hypertrophic cardiomyopathy: An electrophysiologic study. N. Engl. J. Med. 302:96, 1980.

157. Krikler, D. M., Davies, M. J., Rowland, E., Goodwin, J. F., Evans, R. C., and Shaw, D. B.: Sudden death in hypertrophic cardiomyopathy: Associated accessory atrioventricular pathways. Br. Med. J. 43:245, 1980.

158. Ingham, R. E., Mason, J. W., Rossen, R. M., Goodman, D. J., and Harrison, D. C.: Electrophysiologic findings in patients with idiopathic hypertrophic subaortic stenosis. Am. J. Cardiol. 41:811, 1978.

159. Spilkin, S., Mitha, A. S., Matisonn, R. E., and Chesler, E.: Complete heart block in a case of idiopathic hypertrophic subaortic stenosis. Noninvasive correlates with the timing of atrial systole. Circulation 55:418, 1977.

160. Bharati, S., McAnulty, J. H., Lev, M., and Rahimtoola, S. H.: Idiopathic hypertrophic subaortic stenosis with split His bundle potentials: Electrophysiologic and pathologic correlations. Circulation 62:1373, 1980.

161. McKenna, W. J., Chetty, S., Oakley, C. M., and Goodwin, J. F.: Arrhythmia in hypertrophic cardiomyopathy: Exercise electrocardiographic and 48 hour ambulatory electrocardiographic assessment with and without beta adrenergic blocking therapy. Am. J. Cardiol. 45:1, 1980.

162. Savage, D. D., Seides, S. F., Maron, B. J., Myers, D. J., and Epstein, S. E.: Prevalence of arrhythmias during 24-hour electrocardiographic monitoring and exercise testing in patients with obstructive and nonobstructive hypertrophic cardiomyopathy. Circulation 59:866, 1979.

162a. Anderson, K. P., Stinson E. B., Derby, G. C., Oyer, P. E., and Mason, J. W.: Vulnerability of patients with obstructive hypertrophic cardiomyopathy to ventricular arrhythmia induction in the operating room. Analysis of 17 patients. Am. J. Cardiol. 51:811, 1983.

163. Bjarnason, I., Hardarson, T., and Jonsson, S.: Cardiac arrhythmias in hypertrophic cardiomyopathy. Br. Heart J. 48:198, 1982.

164. Ingham, R. E., Rossen, R. M., Goodman, D. T., and Harrison, D. C.: Treadmill arrhythmias in patients with idiopathic hypertrophic subaortic stenosis. Chest 68:759, 1975.

165. McKenna, W. J., England, D., Doi, Y. L., Deanfield, J. E., Oakley, C., and Goodwin, J. F.: Arrhythmia in hypertrophic cardiomyopathy. I. Influence on prognosis. Br. Heart J. 46:168, 1981.

166. Kronzon, I., and Glassman, E.: Mitral ring calcification in idiopathic hypertrophic subaortic stenosis. Am. J. Cardiol. 42:60, 1978.

167. Shah, P. M., and Sylvester, L. J.: Echocardiography in the diagnosis of hypertrophic obstructive cardiomyopathy. Am. J. Med. 62:830, 1977.

168. Schapira, J. N., Stemple, D. R., Martin, R. P., Rakowski, H., Stinson, E. B., and Popp, R. L.: Single and two-dimensional echocardiographic visualization of the effects of septal myectomy in idiopathic hypertrophic subaortic stenosis. Circulation 58:850, 1978.

169. Weyman, A. E., Feigenbaum, H., Hurwitz, R. A., Girod, D. A., Dillon, J. C., and Chang, S.: Localization of left ventricular outflow obstruction by cross-sectional echocardiography. Am. J. Med. 60:33, 1976.

170. Maron, B. J., Henry, W. L., and Epstein, S. E.: Pathophysiology of asymmetric septal hypertrophy. Ann. Radiol. 20:359, 1977.

171. Abbasi, A. S., MacAlpin, R. N., Eber, L. M., and Pearce, M. L.: Left ventricular hypertrophy diagnosed by echocardiography. N. Engl. J. Med. 289:118, 1973.

172. Wei, J. Y., Weiss, J. L., and Bulkley, B. H.: The heterogeneity of hypertrophic cardiomyopathy: An autopsy and one-dimensional echocardiographic study. Am. J. Cardiol. 45:24, 1980.

173. Doi, Y. L., Deanfield, J. E., McKenna, W. J., Dargie, H. J., Oakley, C. M., and Goodwin, J. F.: Echocardiographic differentiation of hypertensive heart disease and hypertrophic cardiomyopathy. Br. Heart J. 44:395, 1980.

174. Kansal, S., Roitman, D., and Sheffield, L. T.: Interventricular septal thickness and left ventricular hypertrophy. An echocardiographic study. Circulation 60:1058, 1979.

175. Fowles, R. E., Martin, R. P., and Popp, R. L.: Apparent asymmetric septal hypertrophy due to angled interventricular septum. Am. J. Cardiol. 46:386, 1980.

176. Silverman, K. J., Hutchins, G. M., Weiss, J. L., and Moore, G. W.: Catenoid shape of the interventricular septum in idiopathic hypertrophic subaortic stenosis: Two-dimensional echocardiographic confirmation. Am. J. Cardiol. 49:27, 1982.

177. Henry, W. L., Clark, C. E., Glancy, L., and Epstein, S. E.: Echocardiographic measurement of the left ventricular outflow gradient in idiopathic hypertrophic subaortic stenosis. N. Engl. J. Med. 288:989, 1973.

178. Angoff, G. H., Wistran, D., Sloss, L. J., Markis, J. E., Come, P. C., Zoll, P. M., and Cohn, P. F.: Value of a noninvasively induced ventricular extrasystole during echocardiographic and phonocardiographic assessment of patients with idiopathic hypertrophic subaortic stenosis. Am. J. Cardiol. 42:919, 1978.

179. Gilbert, B. W., Pollick, C., Adelman, A. G., and Wigle, E. D.: Hypertrophic cardiomyopathy: Subclassification by M mode echocardiography. Am. J. Cardiol. 45:861, 1980.

180. Pollick, C., Morgan, C. D., Gilbert, B. W., Rakowski, H., and Wigle, E. D.: Muscular subaortic stenosis: The temporal relationship between systolic anterior motion of the anterior mitral leaflet and the pressure gradient. Circulation 66:1087, 1982.

181. Henry, W. L., Clark, C. E., Griffith, J. M., and Epstein, S. E.: Mechanism of left ventricular outflow obstruction in patients with obstructive asymmetric septal hypertrophy (idiopathic hypertrophic subaortic stenosis). Am. J. Cardiol. 35:337, 1975.

182. Awdeh, N., Ervin, S., Young, J. M., and Nunn, S.: Systolic anterior motion of the mitral valve caused by sarcoid involving the septum. South Med. J. 71:969, 1978.

183. Rees, A., Elbl, F., Minhas, K., and Solinger, R.: Echocardiographic evidence of outflow tract obstruction in Pompe's disease (glycogen storage disease of the heart). Am. J. Cardiol. 37:1103, 1976.

184. Crawford, M.H., Groves, B. M., and Horwitz, L. D.: Dynamic left ventricular outflow tract obstruction and systolic anterior motion of the mitral valve in the absence of asymmetric septal hypertrophy. Am. J. Med. 65:703, 1978.

185. Maron, B. J., Gottdiener, J. S., and Perry, L. W.: Specificity of systolic anterior motion of anterior mitral leaflet for hypertrophic cardiomyopathy: Prevalence in large population of patients with other cardiac diseases. Br. Heart J. 45:206, 1981.

186. Gardin, J. M., Talano, J. V., Stephanides, L., Fizzano, J., and Lesch, M.: Systolic anterior motion in the absence of asymmetric septal hypertrophy: A buckling phenomenon of the chordae tendineae. Circulation 63:181, 1981.

187. Feizi, O., and Emmanuel, R.: Echocardiographic spectrum of hypertrophic cardiomyopathy. Br. Heart J. 37:1286, 1975.

188. Venco, A., Recusani, F., and Sgalambro, A.: Diastolic movement of mitral valve in hypertrophic cardiomyopathy: An echocardiographic study. Br. Heart J. 43:159, 1980.

189. Chandraratna, P. A. N., Tolentino, A. O., Mutricumarana, W., and Lomez, A. L.: Echocardiographic observations on the association between mitral valve prolapse and asymmetric septal hypertrophy. Circulation 55:622, 1977.

190. Sabbah, H. N., Alam, M., Anbe, D. T., and Stein, P. D.: Mid-systolic closure of the aortic valve in hypertrophic obstructive cardiomyopathy: A pressure-related phenomenon induced by turbulent blood flow. Cath. Cardiovasc. Diag. 6:397, 1980.

191. St. John Sutton, M. G., Tajik, A. J., Gibson, D. G., Brown, D. J., Seward, J. B., and Giuliani, E. R.: Echocardiographic assessment of left ventricular filling and septal and posterior wall dynamics in idiopathic hypertrophic subaortic stenosis. Circulation 57:512, 1978.

192. Hanrath, P., Mathey, D. G., Siegert, R., and Bleifeld, W.: Left ventricular relaxation and filling pattern in different forms of left ventricular hypertrophy: An echocardiographic study. Am. J. Cardiol. 45:15, 1980.

193. Bulkley, B. H., Rouleau, J., Strauss, H. W., and Pitt, B.: Idiopathic hypertrophic subaortic stenosis: Detection by thallium-201 myocardial perfusion imaging. N. Engl. J. Med. 293:1113, 1975.

194. Pitcher, D., Wainwright, R., Maisey, M., Curry, P., and Sowton, E.: Assessment of chest pain in hypertrophic cardiomyopathy using exercise thallium-201 myocardial scintigraphy. Br. Heart J. 44:650, 1980.

195. Rubin, K. A., Morrison, J., Padnick, M. B., Binder, A. J., Chiaramida, S., Margouleff, D., Padmanabhan, V. T., and Gulotta, S. J.: Idiopathic hypertrophic subaortic stenosis: Evaluation of anginal symptoms with thallium-201 myocardial imaging. Am. J. Cardiol. 44:1040, 1979.

196. Pohost, G. M., Vignola, P. A., McKusick, K. E., Block, P. C., Myers, G. S., Walker, H. J., Copen, D. L., and Dinsmore, R. E.: Hypertrophic cardiomyopathy. Evaluation by gated cardiac blood pool scanning. Circulation 55:92, 1977.

197. Bonow, R. O., Rosing, D. R., Bacharach, S. L., Green, M. V., Kent, K. M., Lipson, L. C., Maron, B. J., Leon, M. B., and Epstein, S. E.: Effects of verapamil on left ventricular systolic function and diastolic filling in patients with hypertrophic cardiomyopathy. Circulation 64:787, 1981.

198. Raizner, A. E., Chahine, R. A., Ishimon, T., and Audek, M.: Clinical correlates of left ventricular cavity obliteration. Am. J. Cardiol. 40:303, 1977.

199. Hirota, Y., Furubayashi, K., Kaku, K., Shimizu, G., Kino, M., Kawamura, K., and Takatsu, T.: Hypertrophic nonobstructive cardiomyopathy: A precise assessment of hemodynamic characteristics and clinical implications. Am. J. Cardiol. 50:990, 1982.

200. Falicov, R. E., and Resnekov, L.: Mid ventricular obstruction in hypertrophic obstructive cardiomyopathy. New diagnostic and therapeutic challenge. Br. Heart J. 39:701, 1977.

201. Redwood, D. R., Scherer, J. L., and Epstein, S. E.: Biventricular cineangiography in the evaluation of patients with asymmetric septal hypertrophy. Circulation 49:1116, 1974.

202. Delius, W., Wirtzfeld, A., Schinz, A., Mathes, P., Sebening, H., and Blomer, H.: Evaluation of the ventricular septum by biventricular cineangiography in congestive and hypertrophic cardiomyopathies. Ann. Radiol. 21:463, 1978.

203. Walston, A., II, and Behar, V. S.: Spectrum of coronary artery disease in idiopathic hypertrophic subaortic stenosis. Am. J. Cardiol. 38:12, 1976.

204. Brugada, P., Bär, F. W. H. M., de Zwaan, C., Roy, D., Green, M., and Wellens, H. J. J.: "Sawfish" systolic narrowing of the left anterior descending coronary artery: An angiographic sign of hypertrophic cardiomyopathy. Circulation 66:800, 1982.

205. Pichard, A. D., Meller, J., Teichholz, L. E., Lipnik, S., Gorlin, R., and Herman, M. V.: Septal perforator compression (narrowing) in idiopathic hypertrophic subaortic stenosis. Am. J. Cardiol. 40:310, 1977.

206. Glancy, D. L., Shephard, R. L., Beiser, G. D., and Epstein, S. E.: The dynamic nature of left ventricular outflow obstruction in idiopathic hypertrophic subaortic stenosis. Ann. Intern. Med. 75:589, 1971.

207. Delman, A. J., and Stein, E.: Dynamic Auscultation and Phonocardiography. Philadelphia, W. B. Saunders Co., 1979, p. 825.

208. Stefadouros, M. A., Mucha, E., and Frank, M. J.: Paradoxic response of the murmur of idiopathic hypertrophic subaortic stenosis to the Valsalva maneuver. Am. J. Cardiol. 37:89, 1976.

209. Bartall, H., Amber, S., Desser, K. B., and Benchimol, A.: Normalization of the external carotid pulse tracing of hypertrophic subaortic stenosis during Müller's maneuver. Chest 74:77, 1978.

210. Brockenbrough, E. C., Braunwald, E., and Morrow, A. G.: A hemodynamic technic for the detection of hypertrophic subaortic stenosis. Circulation 23:189, 1961.

211. Saenz de la Calzada, C., Ziady, G. M., Hardarson, T., Curiel, R., and Goodwin, J. F.: Effect of acute administration of propranolol on ventricular function in hypertrophic obstructive cardiomyopathy measured by noninvasive techniques. Br. Heart J. 38:798, 1976.

212. Cohen, L. S., and Braunwald, E.: Amelioration of angina pectoris in idiopathic hypertrophic subaortic stenosis with beta-adrenergic blockade. Circulation 35:847, 1967.

213. Thompson, D. S., Haqvi, N., Juul, S. M., Swanton, R. H., Coltart, D. J., Jenkins, D. S., and Webb-Peploe, M. M.: Effects of propranolol on myocardial oxygen consumption, substrate extraction and haemodynamics in hypertrophic cardiomyopathy. Br. Heart J. 44:488, 1980.

214. Alvares, R. F., and Goodwin, J. F.: Noninvasive assessment of diastolic function in hypertrophic cardiomyopathy on and off beta adrenergic blocking drugs. Br. Heart J. 48:204, 1982.

215. Shah, P. M., Adelman, A. G., Wigle, E. D., Gobel, F. L., Burchell, H. B., Hardarson, T., Curill, R., de al Calzada, C., Oakley, C. M., and Goodwin, J. F.: The natural (and unnatural) history of hypertrophic obstructive cardiomyopathy. Circ. Res. 34/35 (Suppl. II):11, 1974.

216. Canedo, M. I., Frank, M. J., and Abdulla, A. M.: Rhythm disturbances in hypertrophic cardiomyopathy: Prevalence, relation to symptoms and management. Am. J. Cardiol. 45:848, 1980.

217. Rouleau, J.-L., Chuck, L. H. S., Hollosi, G., Kidd, P., Sievers, R. E., Wikman-Coffelt, J., and Parmley, W. W.: Verapamil preserves myocardial contractility in the hereditary cardiomyopathy of the Syrian hamster. Circ. Res. 50:405, 1982.

218. Kaltenbach, M., Hopf, R., Kober, G., Bussmann, W.-D., Keller, M., and Petersen, Y.: Treatment of hypertrophic obstructive cardiomyopathy with verapamil. Br. Heart J. 42:35, 1979.

219. Rosing, D. R., Kent, K. M., Borer, J. S., Seides, S. F., Maron, B. J., and Epstein, S. E.: Verapamil therapy: A new approach to the pharmacologic treatment of hypertrophic cardiomyopathy. I. Hemodynamic effects. Circulation 60:1201, 1979.

220. Rosing, D. R., Kent, K. M., Maron, B. J., and Epstein, S. E.: Verapamil therapy: A new approach to the pharmacologic treatment of hypertrophic cardiomyopathy. II. Effects on exercise capacity and symptomatic status. Circulation 60:1208, 1979.

220a. Spicer, R. L., Rocchini, A. P., Crowley, D. C. Vasiliades, J., and Rosenthal, A.: Hemodynamic effects of verapamil in children and adolescents with hypertrophic cardiomyopathy. Circulation 67:413, 1983.

221. Hanrath, P., Mathey, D. G., Kremer, P., Sonntag, F., and Bleifeld, W.: Effect of verapamil on left ventricular isovolumic relaxation time and regional left ventricular filling in hypertrophic cardiomyopathy. Am. J. Cardiol. 45:1258, 1980.

221a. Bonow, R. O., Frederick, T. M., Bacharach, S. L., Green, M. V., Goose, P. W., and Rosing, D. R.: Atrial systole and left ventricular filling in patients with hypertrophic cardiomyopathy: Effect of verapamil. J. Am. Coll. Cardiol. 1: 738, 1983.

222. Rosing, D. R., Condit, J. R., Maron, B. J., Kent, K. M., Leon, M. B., Bonow, R. O., Lipson, L. C., and Epstein, S. E.: Verapamil therapy: A new approach to the pharmacologic treatment of hypertrophic cardiomyopathy. III. Effects of long-term administration. Am. J. Cardiol. 48:545, 1981.

223. Epstein, S. E., and Rosing, D. R.: Verapamil: Its potential for causing serious complications in patients with hypertrophic cardiomyopathy. Circulation 64: 437, 1981.

224. Koide, T., Kakihana, M., Takabatake, Y., Iizuka, M., Uchida, Y., Ozeki, K., Morooka, S., Kato, A., Tanaka, S., Oya, T., Momomura, S., and Murao, S.: Long term clinical effects of calcium inhibitors in hypertrophic cardiomyopathy compared to the effect of beta-blocking agents. Jap. Heart J. 22:87, 1981.

225. Landmark, K., Sire, S., Thaulow, E., Amlie, J. P., and Nitter-Hauge, S.: Haemodynamic effects of nifedipine and propranolol in patients with hypertrophic obstructive cardiomyopathy. Br. Heart J. 48:19, 1982.

226. Pollick, C.: Muscular subaortic stenosis. Hemodynamic and clinical improvement after disopyramide. N. Engl. J. Med. 307:997, 1982.

227. Adelman, A. G., Wigle, E. D., Ranganathan, N., Webb, G. D., Kidd, B. S. L., Bigelow, W. G., and Silver, M. D.: The clinical course in muscular subaortic stenosis. A retrospective and prospective study of 60 hemodynamically proven cases. Ann. Intern. Med. 77:515, 1972.

228. LeJemtel, T. H., Factor, S. M., Koenigsberg, M., O'Reilly, M., Frater, R., and Sonnenblick, E. H.: Mural vegetations at the site of endocardial trauma in infective endocarditis complicating idiopathic hypertrophic subaortic stenosis. Am. J. Cardiol. 44:569, 1979.

229. Chagnac, A., Rudniki, C., Loebel, H., and Zahavi, I.: Infectious endocarditis in idiopathic hypertrophic subaortic stenosis: Report of three cases and review of the literature. Chest 81:346, 1982.

230. Morrow, A. G.: Hypertrophic subaortic stenosis. Operative methods utilized to relieve left ventricular outflow obstruction. J. Thorac. Cardiovasc. Surg. 76: 423, 1978.

231. Maron, B. J., Koch, J.-P., Kent, K. M., Epstein, S. E., and Morrow, A. G.: Results of surgery for idiopathic subaortic stenosis. J. Cardiovasc. Med. 5:145, 1980.

232. Senning, A.: Transventricular relief of idiopathic hypertrophic subaortic stenosis. J. Cardiovasc. Surg. 17:371, 1976.

233. Agnew, T. M., Barratt-Boyes, B. G., Brandt, P. W. T., Roche, A. H. G., Lowe, J. B., and O'Brien, K. P.: Surgical resection in idiopathic hypertrophic subaortic stenosis with a combined approach through aorta and left ventricle. J. Thorac. Cardiovasc. Surg. 74:307, 1977.

234. Roberts, W. C.: Operative treatment of hypertrophic obstructive cardiomyopathy. The case against mitral valve replacement. Am. J. Cardiol. 32:377, 1973.

235. Maron, B. J., Merrill, W. H., Freier, P. A., Kent, K. M., Epstein, S. E., and Morrow, A. G.: Long-term clinical course and symptomatic status of patients after operation for hypertrophic subaortic stenosis. Circulation 57:1205, 1978.

236. Tajik, A. J., Giuliani, E. R., Weidman, W. H., Brandenburg, R. O., and McGoon, D. C.: Idiopathic hypertrophic subaortic stenosis. Long-term surgical followup. Am. J. Cardiol. 34:815, 1974.

237. Koch, J.-P., Maron, B. J., Epstein, S. E., and Morrow, A. G.: Results of operation for obstructive hypertrophic cardiomyopathy in the elderly: Septal myotomy and myectomy in 20 patients 65 years of age or older. Am. J. Cardiol. 46:963, 1980.

238. Cooley, D. A., Leachman, R. D., and Wukasch, D. C.: Diffuse muscular subaortic stenosis: Surgical management. Am. J. Cardiol. 31:1, 1973.

238a. Beahrs, M. M., Tajik, A. J., Seward, J. B., Giuliani, E. R., and McGoon, D. C.: Hypertrophic obstructive cardiomyopathy: Ten- to 21-year followup after partial septal myectomy. Am. J. Cardiol. 51:1160, 1983.

239. Redwood, D. R., Goldstein, R. E., Hirshfeld, J., Borer, J. S., Morganroth, J., Morrow, A. G., and Epstein, S. E.: Exercise performance after septal myotomy and myectomy in patients with obstructive cardiomyopathy. Am. J. Cardiol. 44:215, 1979.

240. Borer, J. S., Bacharach, S. L., Green, M. V., Kent, K. M., Rosing, D. R., Seides, S. F., Morrow, A. G., and Epstein, S. E.: Effect of septal myotomy and myectomy on left ventricular systolic function at rest and during exercise in patients with IHSS. Circulation 60(Suppl. I):I-82, 1979.

241. Kolibash, A. J., Ruiz, D. E., and Lewis, R. P.: Idiopathic hypertrophic subaortic stenosis in pregnancy. Ann. Intern. Med. 82:791, 1975.

242. Oakley, G. D. G., McGarry, K., Limb, D. G., and Oakley, C. M.: Management of pregnancy in patients with hypertrophic cardiomyopathy. Br. Med. J. 1:1749, 1979.

243. Beder, S. D., Gutgesell, H. P., Mullins, C. E., and McNamara, D. G.: Progression from hypertrophic obstructive cardiomyopathy to congestive cardiomyopathy in a child. Am. Heart J. 104:155, 1982.

244. ten Cate, F. J., and Roelandt, J.: Progression of left ventricular dilatation in patients with hypertrophic obstructive cardiomyopathy. Am. Heart J. 97:762, 1979.

245. Waller, B. F., Maron, B. J., Epstein, S. E., and Roberts, W. C.: Transmural myocardial infarction in hypertrophic cardiomyopathy: A cause of conversion from left ventricular asymmetry to symmetry and from normal-sized to dilated left ventricular cavity. Chest 79:461, 1981.

246. Powell, W. J., Jr., Whiting, R. B., Dinsmore, R. E., and Sanders, C. A.: Symptomatic prognosis in patients with idiopathic hypertrophic subaortic stenosis (IHSS). Am. J. Med. 55:15, 1973.

247. Maron, B. J., Lipson, L. C., Roberts, W. C., Savage, D. D., and Epstein, S. E.: "Malignant" hypertrophic cardiomyopathy: Identification of a subgroup of families with unusually frequent premature deaths. Am. J. Cardiol. 41:1133, 1978.

248. Baron, B. J., Roberts, W. C., Epstein, S. E.: Sudden death in hypertrophic cardiomyopathy: A profile of 78 patients. Circulation 65:1388, 1982.

249. McKenna, W., Deanfield, J., Faruqui, A., England, D., Oakley, C., and Goodwin, J.: Prognosis in hypertrophic cardiomyopathy: Role of age and clinical, electrocardiographic and hemodynamic features. Am. J. Cardiol. 47:532, 1981.

250. Maron, B. J., Roberts, W. C., McAllister, H. A., Rosing, D. R., and Epstein, S. E.: Sudden death in young athletes. Circulation 62:218, 1980.

251. McKenna, W. J., Harris, L., Perez, G., Krikler, D. M., Oakley, C., and Goodwin, J. F.: Arrhythmia in hypertrophic cardiomyopathy. II. Comparison of amiodarone and verapamil in treatment. Br. Heart J. 46:173, 1981.

252. Morrow, A. G., Koch, J.-P., Maron, B. J., Kent, K. M., and Epstein, S. E.: Left ventricular myotomy and myectomy in patients with obstructive hypertrophic cardiomyopathy and previous cardiac arrest. Am. J. Cardiol. 46:313, 1980.

RESTRICTIVE AND INFILTRATIVE CARDIOMYOPATHIES

253. Hirschmann, J. V.: Pericardial constriction. Am. Heart J. 96:110, 1978.

254. Benotti, J. R., Grossman, W., and Cohn, P. F.: The clinical profile of restrictive cardiomyopathy. Circulation 61:1206, 1980.

255. Navarro-Lopez, F., Llorian, A., Ferrer-Roca, O., Betriu, A., and Sanz, G.: Restrictive cardiomyopathy in pseudoxanthoma elasticum. Chest 78:113, 1980.

256. Meaney, E., Shabetai, R., Bhargana, V., Shearer, M., Weidner, C., Mangiardi, L. M., Smalling, R., and Peterson, K.: Cardiac amyloidosis, constrictive pericarditis and restrictive cardiomyopathy. Am. J. Cardiol. 38:547, 1976.

257. Hansen, A. T., Eskildsen, P., and Gotzsche, H.: Pressure curves from the right auricle and the right ventricle in chronic constrictive pericarditis. Circulation 3: 881, 1951.

258. Shabetai, R.: Profiles in constrictive pericarditis, cardiac tamponade and restrictive cardiomyopathy. In Grossman, W. (ed.): Cardiac Catheterization and Angiography. Philadelphia, Lea and Febiger, 1974, p. 304.

259. Borer, J. S., Henry, W. L., and Epstein, S. E.: Echocardiographic observations in patients with systemic infiltrative disease involving the heart. Am. J. Cardiol. 39:184, 1977.

260. Glenner, G. C.: Amyloid deposits and amyloidosis: The β-fibrilloses. N. Engl. J. Med. 302:1283 and 1333, 1980.

261. Kyle, R. A., and Baynd, E. D.: Amyloidosis: Review of 236 cases. Medicine 54:271, 1975.

262. Pear, B. L.: Big heart, tongue, and kidneys—stiff intestines: The roentgenographic diagnosis of amyloidosis. J.A.M.A. 241:58, 1979.

263. Gafni, J., Sohar, E., and Heller, H.: The inherited amyloidoses. Their clinical and theoretical significance. Lancet 1:71, 1964.

264. Westermark, P., Natvig, J. B., and Johansson, B.: Characterization of an amyloid fibril protein from senile cardiac amyloid. J. Exp. Med. 146:631, 1977.

265. Barth, W. F.: Amyloidosis: Review of cardiac and renal manifestations. Med. Ann. D.C. 36:228, 266, 1967.

266. Dahlin, D. C.: Classification and general aspects of amyloidosis. Med. Clin. North Am. 34:1107, 1950.

267. Hodkinson, H. M., and Pomerance, A.: The clinical significance of senile cardiac amyloidosis: A prospective clinicopathological study. Q. J. Med. 46:381, 1977.

268. Buja, L. M., Khoi, N. B., and Roberts, W. C.: Clinically significant cardiac amyloidosis. Am. J. Cardiol. 26:394, 1970.

269. Pomerance, A.: Senile cardiac amyloidosis. Br. Heart J. 27:711, 1965.

269a. Maule, W. F., and Martin, R. H.: Primary cardiac amyloidosis: An angiographic clue to early diagnosis. Ann. Intern. Med. 98:177, 1983.

270. Ridolfi, R. L., Bulkley, B. H., and Hutchins, G. M.: The conduction system in cardiac amyloidosis. Clinical and pathologic features of 23 patients. Am. J. Med. 62:677, 1977.

270a. Saffitz, J. E., Sazama, K., and Roberts, W. C.: Amyloidosis limited to small arteries causing angina pectoris and sudden death. Am. J. Cardiol. 51:1234, 1983.

271. Smith, R. R. L., and Hutchins, G. M.: Ischemic heart disease secondary to amyloidosis of intramyocardial arteries. Am. J. Cardiol. 44:413, 1979.

272. Chew, C., Ziady, G. M., Raphael, M. J., and Oakley, C. M.: The functional defect in amyloid heart disease: The "stiff heart" syndrome. Am. J. Cardiol. 36: 438, 1975.

273. Tyberg, T. I., Goodyer, A. V., Hurst, V. W., III, Alexander, J., and Langou, R. A.: Left ventricular filling in differentiating restrictive amyloid cardiomyopathy and constrictive pericarditis. Am. J. Cardiol. 47:791, 1981.

274. Garcia, R., and Saleh, S. M.: Amyloidosis. Cardiovascular manifestations in five illustrative cases. Arch. Intern. Med. *121*:259, 1968.

275. Olofsson, B. O., Andersson, R., and Furberg, B.: Atrioventricular and intraventricular conduction in familial amyloidosis with polyneuropathy. Acta Med. Scand. *208*:77, 1980.

276. Gray, L. W., Duca, P. R., and Chung, E. K.: Sick sinus syndrome due to cardiac amyloidosis. Cardiology *63*:212, 1978.

277. Giles, T. D., Leon-Galindo, J., and Burch, G. E.: Echocardiographic findings in amyloid cardiomyopathy. South. Med. J. *71*:1393, 1978.

278. Child, J. S., Krivokapich, J., and Abbasi, A. S.: Increased right ventricular wall thickness on echocardiography in amyloid infiltrative cardiomyopathy. Am. J. Cardiol. *44*:1391, 1979.

279. Brodarick, S., Paine, R., Higa, E., and Carmichael, K. A.: Pericardial tamponade, a new complication of amyloid heart disease. Am. J. Med. *73*:133, 1982.

280. Siqueira-Filho, A. G., Cunha, C. L. P., Tajik, A. J., Seward, J. B., Schattenberg, T. T., and Giuliani, E. R.: M-mode and two-dimensional echocardiographic features in cardiac amyloidosis. Circulation *63*:188, 1981.

281. Carroll, J. D., Gaasch, W. H., and McAdam, K. P. W. J.: Amyloid cardiomyopathy: Characterization by a distinctive voltage/mass relation. Am. J. Cardiol. *49*:9, 1982.

282. St. John Sutton, M. D., Reicheck, N., Kastor, J. A., and Giuliani, E. R.: Computerized M-mode echocardiographic analysis of left ventricular dysfunction in cardiac amyloid. Circulation *66*:790, 1982.

283. Schroeder, J. S., Billigham, M. E., and Rider, A. K.: Cardiac amyloidosis. Diagnosis by transvenous endomyocardial biopsy. Am. J. Med. *59*:269, 1975.

284. Hedner, P., Rausing, A., Steen, K., and Torp, A.: Diagnosis of cardiac amyloidosis by myocardial biopsy. Acta Med. Scand. *198*:525, 1975.

285. Chan, W., and Ikram, H.: Primary amyloidosis with cardiac involvement diagnosed by left ventricular endomyocardial biopsy. Aust. N.Z. J. Med. *7*:427, 1977.

286. Rubinow, A., Skinner, M., and Cohen, A. S.: Digoxin sensitivity in amyloid cardiomyopathy. Circulation *63*:1285, 1981.

287. Desnick, R. J., Blieden, L. C., Sharp, H. L., Hofschire, P. J., and Moller, J. H.: Cardiac valvular anomalies in Fabry disease. Clinical, morphologic and biochemical studies. Circulation *54*:818, 1976.

288. Becker, A. E., Schoorl, R., Balk, A. G., and van der Heide, R. M.: Cardiac manifestations of Fabry's disease. Report of a case with mitral insufficiency and electrocardiographic evidence of myocardial infarction. Am. J. Cardiol. *36*:829, 1975.

289. Bass, J. L., Shrivastava, S., Grabowski, G. A., Desnick, R. J., and Moller, J. H.: The M-mode echocardiogram in Fabry's disease. Am. Heart J. *100*:807, 1980.

290. Mehta, J., Tuna, N., Moller, J. H., and Desnick, R. J.: Electrocardiographic and vectorcardiographic abnormalities in Fabry's disease. Am. Heart J. *93*:699, 1977.

291. Smith, R. R. L., Hutchins, G. M., Sack, G. H., and Ridolfi, R. L.: Unusual cardiac, renal and pulmonary involvement in Gaucher's disease. Interstitial glucocerebroside accumulation, pulmonary hypertension, and fatal bone marrow embolization. Am. J. Med. *65*:352, 1978.

292. Buja, L. M., and Roberts, W. C.: Iron in the heart. Etiology and clinical significance. Am. J. Med. *51*:209, 1971.

293. Arnett, E. N., Nienhuis, A. W., Henry, W. L., Ferrans, V. J., Redwood, D. R., and Roberts, W. C.: Massive myocardial hemosiderosis: A structure-function conference at the National Heart and Lung Institute. Am. Heart J. *90*:777, 1975.

294. Cartwright, G. E.: Hemochromatosis. *In* Thorn, G. W., Adams, R. D., Braunwald, E., Isselbacher, K. J., and Petersdorf, R. G. (eds.): Harrison's Principles of Internal Medicine. New York, McGraw-Hill, 1977, p. 652.

295. Cutler, D. J., Isner, J. M., Bracey, A. W., Hufnagel, C. A., Conrad, P. W., Roberts, W. C., Kerwin, D. M., and Weintraub, A. M.: Hemochromatosis heart disease: An unemphasized cause of potentially reversible restrictive cardiomyopathy. Am. J. Med. *69*:923, 1980.

296. Short, E. M., Winkle, R. A., and Billingham, M. E.: Myocardial involvement in idiopathic hemochromatosis. Morphologic and clinical improvement following venesection. Am. J. Med. *70*:1275, 1981.

297. Editorial: Sarcoid heart disease. Br. Med. J. *4*:627, 1972.

298. Gozo, E. G., Jr., Cosnow, I., Cohen, H. C., and Okun, L.: The heart in sarcoidosis. Chest *60*:379, 1971.

299. Silverman, K. J., Hutchins, G. M., and Bulkley, B. H.: Cardiac sarcoid: A clinicopathologic study of 84 unselected patients with systemic sarcoidosis. Circulation *58*:1204, 1978.

300. Lie, J. T., Hunt, D., and Valentine, P. A.: Sudden death from cardiac sarcoidosis with involvement of conduction system. Am. J. Med. Sci. *267*:123, 1974.

301. Lull, R. J., Dunn, B. E., Gregoratos, G., Cox, W. A., and Fisher, G. W.: Ventricular aneurysm due to cardiac sarcoidosis with surgical cure of refractory ventricular tachycardia. Am. J. Cardiol. *30*:282, 1972.

302. Roberts, W. C., McAllister, H. A., and Ferrans, V. J.: Sarcoidosis of the heart. A clinicopathologic study of 35 necropsy patients (Group I) and review of 78 previously described necropsy patients (Group II). Am. J. Cardiol. *63*:86, 1977.

303. Fawcett, F. J., and Goldberg, M. J.: Heart block resulting from myocardial sarcoidosis. Br. Med. J. *36*:220, 1974.

304. Porter, G. H.: Sarcoid heart disease. N. Engl. J. Med. *263*:1350, 1960.

305. Ghosh, P., Fleming, H. A., Gresham, G. A., and Stonin, P. G. I.: Myocardial sarcoidosis. Br. Heart J. *34*:769, 1972.

306. Bulkley, B. H., and Hutchins, G. M.: Sarcoidosis, myocarditis and sudden death. Primary Cardiology July/Aug:38, 1977.

307. Phinney, A. O., Jr.: Sarcoid of the myocardial septum with complete heart block: Report of two cases. Am. Heart J. *62*:270, 1961.

308. Ferrans, V. J., Hibbs, R. G., Block, W. C., Walsh, J. J., and Burch, G. E.: Myocardial degeneration in cardiac sarcoidosis: Histochemical and electron microscopic studies. Am. Heart J. *69*:159, 1965.

309. James, T. N.: De Subitaneis Mortibus. XXV. Sarcoid heart disease. Circulation *56*:320, 1977.

310. Shiff, A. D., Blatt, C. J., and Colp, C.: Recurrent pericardial effusion secondary to sarcoidosis of the pericardium. A biopsy-proved case. N. Engl. J. Med. *281*:141, 1969.

311. McTaggart, D. R.: Sarcoidosis with cardiac involvement. Med. J. Aust. *2*:689, 1973.

312. Fleming, H. A.: Sarcoid heart disease. Br. Heart J. *36*:54, 1974.

313. Abeler, V.: Sarcoidosis of the cardiac conducting system. Am. Heart J. *97*:701, 1979.

314. Walsh, M. J.: Systemic sarcoidosis with refractory ventricular tachycardia and heart failure. Br. Heart J. *40*:931, 1978.

315. Serwer, G. A., Edwards, S. B., Benson, W., Jr., Anderson, P. A. W., and Spack, M.: Ventricular tachycardia due to cardiac sarcoidosis in a child. Pediatrics *62*:322, 1978.

316. Miller, A., Jackler, I., and Chuang, M.: Onset of sarcoidosis with left ventricular failure and multisystem involvement. Chest *70*:302, 1976.

317. Ahmed, S. S., Rozefort, R., Taclob, L. T., and Brancato, R. W.: Development of ventricular aneurysm in cardiac sarcoidosis. Angiology *28*:323, 1977.

318. Stein, E., Jackler, I., Stimmel, B., Stein, W., and Siltzbach, L. E.: Asymptomatic electrocardiographic alterations in sarcoidosis. Am. Heart J. *86*:474, 1973.

319. Strauss, G. S., Lawton, B. R., Wenzel, F. J., and Ray, J. F., III: Detection of covert myocardial sarcoidosis by scalene node biopsy. Chest *69*:790, 1976.

320. Lorell, B., Alderman, E. L., and Mason, J. W.: Cardiac sarcoidosis. Diagnosis with endomyocardial biopsy and treatment with corticosteroids. Am. J. Cardiol. *42*:143, 1978.

321. Bulkley, B. H., Rouleau, J. R., Whitaker, J. Q., Strauss, H. W., and Pitt, B.: The use of ^{201}thallium for myocardial perfusion imaging in sarcoid heart disease. Chest *72*:27, 1977.

322. Kinney, E. L., Jackson, G. L., Reeves, W. C., and Zelis, R.: Thallium-scan myocardial defects and echocardiographic abnormalities in patients with sarcoidosis without clinical cardiac dysfunction. An analysis of 44 patients. Am. J. Med. *68*:497, 1980.

323. Stein, E., Stimmel, B., and Siltzbach, L. E.: Clinical course of cardiac sarcoidosis. Ann. N.Y. Acad. Sci. *278*:470, 1976.

324. Duvernoy, W. F. C., and Garcia, R.: Sarcoidosis of the heart presenting with ventricular tachycardia and atrioventricular block. Am. J. Cardiol. *28*:348, 1971.

325. Friedman, H. S., Parikh, N. K., Chandler, N., and Calderon, J.: Sarcoidosis with incomplete bilateral bundle branch block pattern disappearing following steroid therapy. An electrophysiological study. Eur. J. Cardiol. *4*:141, 1976.

326. Bashour, F. A., McConnell, J., Skinner, W., and Hanson, M.: Myocardial sarcoidosis. Dis. Chest *53*:413, 1968.

327. McAllister, H. A., and Fenoglio, J. J.: Cardiac involvement in Whipple's disease. Circulation *52*:152, 1975.

328. Becker, B. J. P., Chatgidakis, C. B., and Van Lingen, B.: Cardiovascular collagenosis with parietal endocardial thrombosis. A clinicopathological study of forty cases. Circulation *7*:345, 1953.

329. Davies, J. N. P., and Coles, R. M.: Some considerations regarding obscure disease affecting the mural endocardium. Am. Heart J. *59*:606, 1960.

330. Reid, J. V. O., and Berjak, P.: Tryptophan and serotonin levels in patients with or susceptible to African cardiomyopathy. Am. Heart J. *74*:337, 1967.

331. Reid, J. V. O., and Berjak, P.: Dietary production of myocardial fibrosis in the rat. Am. Heart J. *71*:240, 1966.

332. Hill, K. R., Still, W. J. S., and McKinney, B.: Jamaican cardiomyopathy. Br. Heart J. *29*:594, 1967.

333. Brink, A. J., and Lewis, C. M.: Coronary blood flow, energetics, and myocardial metabolism in idiopathic mural endomyocardiopathy. Am. Heart J. *73*:339, 1967.

334. Lepley, D., Jr., Aris, A., Korns, M. E., Walker, J. A., and D'Cunha, R. M.: Endomyocardial fibrosis. A surgical approach. Ann. Thorac. Surg. *18*:626, 1974.

335. Vijayaraghavan, G., Cherian, G., Krishnaswami, S., and Sukumar, I. P.: Left ventricular endomyocardial fibrosis in India. Br. Heart J. *39*:563, 1977.

336. Guimaraes, A. C., Esteves, J. P., Filho, A. S., and Macedo, V.: Clinical aspects of endomyocardial fibrosis in Bahia, Brazil. Am. Heart J. *81*:7, 1971.

337. Shaper, A. G., Hutt, M. S. R., Edington, G. M., Somers, K., and Fowler, J. M.: Endomyocardial fibrosis. Cardiologia *52*:20, 1968.

337a. Cherian, G., Vijayaraghavan, G., Krishnaswami, S., Sukumar, I. P., John, S., Jairaj, P. S., and Bhaktaviziam, A.: Endomyocardial fibrosis: Report on the hemodynamic data in 29 patients and review of the results of surgery. Am. Heart J. *105*:659, 1983.

338. Beck, W., and Schrire, V.: Endomyocardial fibrosis in Caucasians previously resident in tropical Africa. Br. Heart J. *34*:915, 1972.

339. Connor, D. H., Somers, K., Hutt, M. S. R., Manion, W. C., and D'Arbela, P. G.: Endomyocardial fibrosis in Uganda (Davies disease): Part I. An epidemiologic, clinical and pathologic study. Am. Heart J. *74*:687; *75*:107, 1968.

340. Olsen, E. G.: Endomyocardial fibrosis and Löffler's endocarditis parietalis fibroplastica. Postgrad. Med. J. *53*:538, 1977.

341. Carlisle, R., Ogunba, E. D., McFarlane, H., Onayemi, D. A., and Oyeleye, V. O.: Immunoglobulins and antibody to *Loa loa* in Nigerians with endomyocardial fibrosis and other heart disease. Br. Heart J. *34*:678, 1972.

342. Roberts, W. C., Liegler, D. G., and Carbone, P. P.: Endomyocardial disease and eosinophilia: A clinical and pathologic spectrum. Am. J. Med. *46*:28, 1969.

343. D'Arbela, P. G., Mutazindwa, T., Patel, A. K., and Somers, K.: Survival after first presentation with endomyocardial fibrosis. Br. Heart J. *34*:403, 1972.

344. George, B. O., Talabi, A. I., Gaba, F. E., and Adeniyi, D. S.: Echocardiography in the diagnosis of right ventricular endomyocardial fibrosis. Postgrad. Med. J. *58*:467, 1982.

344a. Acquatella, H., Schiller, N. B., Puigbo, J. J., Gomez-Mancebo, J. R., Suarez, C., and Acquatella, G.: Value of two-dimensional echocardiography in endomyocardial disease with and without eosinophilia. A clinical and pathologic study. Circulation *67*:1219, 1983.

345. Adebonojo, S. A., and Jaiyesimi, F.: Pericardioperitoneal shunt for massive recurrent pericardial effusion in patients with endomyocardial fibrosis. Int. Surg. *62*:349, 1977.

346. Hess, O. M., Turina, M., Senning, A., Goebel, N. H., Scholer, Y., and Krayenbuehl, H. P.: Pre- and postoperative findings in patients with endomyocardial fibrosis. Br. Heart J. *40*:406, 1978.

347. Sheikhzadeh, A. H., Tarbiat, S., Nazarian, I., Aryanpur, I., and Sening. Å.: Constrictive endocarditis: Report of a case with successful surgery. Br. Heart J. *42*:224, 1979.

348. Goebel, N., Gander, M. P., and Hess, O. M.: Angiographic aspects of endomyocardial fibrosis. Ann. Radiol. *21*:475, 1978.

348a. Cherian, K. M., John, T. A., and Abraham, K. A.: Endomyocardial fibrosis: Clinical profile and role of surgery in management. Am. Heart J. *105*:706, 1983.

348b. Gonzalez-Lavin, L., Friedman, J. P., Hecker, S. P., and McFadden, P. M.: Endomyocardial fibrosis: Diagnosis and treatment. Am. Heart J. *105*:699, 1983.

349. Dubost, C., Prigent, C., Gerbaux, A., Maurice, P., Passelecq, J., Rulliere, R., Carpentier, A., and Deloche, A.: Surgical treatment of constrictive fibrous endocarditis. J. Thorac. Cardiovasc. Surg. *82*:585, 1981.

350. Metras, D., Coulibaly, A. O., Chauvet, J., Ekra, A., Longechaud, A., and Bertrand, E.: Endomyocardial fibrosis. J. Thorac. Cardiovasc. Surg. *83*:52, 1982.

351. Hall, S. W., Jr., Theologides, A., From, A. H. L., Gobel, F. L., Fortuny, I. E., Lawrence, C. J., and Edwards, J. E.: Hypereosinophilic syndrome with biventricular involvement. Circulation *55*:217, 1977.

352. Chusid, M. J., Dale, D. C., West, B. C., and Wolff, S. M.: The hypereosinophilic syndrome: Analysis of fourteen cases with review of the literature. Medicine *51*:1, 1975.

353. Brockington, I. F., and Olsen, E. G. J.: Löffler's endocarditis and Davies' endomyocardial fibrosis. Am. Heart J. *85*:308, 1973.

354. Brink, A. J., and Weber, W. H.: Fibroplastic parietal endocarditis with eosinophilia: Löffler's endocarditis. Am. J. Med. *34*:52, 1963.

355. Spry, C. J. F., and Tai, P. C.: Studies on blood eosinophils. II. Patients with Löffler's cardiomyopathy. Clin. Exp. Immunol. *24*:423, 1976.

356. Bell, J. A., Jenkins, B. S., and Webb-Peploe, M. M.: Clinical, haemodynamic, and angiographic findings in Löffler's eosinophilic endocarditis. Br. Heart J. *38*:541, 1976.

357. Parrillo, J. E., Borer, J. S., Henry, W. L., Wolff, S. M., and Fauci, A. S.: The cardiovascular manifestations of the hypereosinophilic syndrome. Prospective study of 26 patients, with review of the literature. Am. J. Med. *67*:573, 1979.

358. Raizner, A. E., Silverman, M. E., and Waters, W. C., III: Conduction disturbances and pacemaker failure in Löffler's endomyocarditis. Am. J. Med. *53*:343, 1972.

359. Rodger, J. C., Irvine, K. G., and Lerski, R. A.: Echocardiography in Löffler's endocarditis. Br. Heart J. *46*:110, 1981.

359a. Gottdiener, J. S., Maron, B. J., Schooley, R. T., Harley, J. B., Roberts, W. C., and Fauci, A. S.: Two dimensional echocardiographic assessment of the idiopathic hypereosinophilic syndrome. Anatomic basis of mitral regurgitation and peripheral embolization. Circulation *67*:572, 1983.

360. Weyman, A. E., Rankin, R., and King. H. Löffler's endocarditis presenting as mitral and tricuspid stenosis. Am. J. Cardiol. *40*:438, 1977.

361. Scott, M. E., and Bruce, J. H.: Löffler's endocarditis. Brit. Heart J. *37*:534, 1975.

362. Fournier, G., Schlanger, B., Berthoumieu, F., Pris, J., Marco, J., and Eschapasse, H.: Surgery for cardiac complications caused by endocardial mural fibrin deposits in a hypereosinophilic syndrome. Circulation *65*:1010, 1982.

363. Cohen, J., Davies, J., Goodwin, J. F., and Spry, C. J. F.: Arrhythmias in patients with hypereosinophilia: A comparison of patients with and without Löffler's endomyocardial disease. Postgrad. Med. J. *56*:828, 1980.

364. Oakley, C. M., and Olsen, E. G. J.: Eosinophilia and heart disease. Brit. Heart J. *39*:233, 1977.

365. Andy, J. J., Bishara, F. F., and Soyinka, O. O.: Relation of severe eosinophilia and microfilariasis to chronic African endomyocardial fibrosis. Br. Heart J. *45*:672, 1981.

366. Ferrans, V. J., and Roberts, W. C.: The carcinoid endocardial plaque. An ultrastructural study. Hum. Pathol. *7*:387, 1976.

367. Grahame-Smith, D. G.: The carcinoid syndrome. Am. J. Cardiol. *21*:376, 1968.

368. Grahame-Smith, D. G.: The carcinoid syndrome. *In* Bondy, P. K., and Rosenberg, L. E. (eds.): Metabolic Control and Disease. 9th ed. Philadelphia, W. B. Saunders Co., 1980, p. 1703.

369. Hendel, N., Leckie, B., and Richards, J.: Carcinoid heart disease: Eight-year survival following tricuspid valve replacement and pulmonary valvotomy. Ann. Thorac. Surg. *30*:391, 1980.

370. Roberts, W. C., and Sjoerdsma, A.: The cardiac disease associated with the carcinoid syndrome (carcinoid heart disease). Am. J. Med. *36*:5, 1969.

371. Stephan, E., and deWit J.: Carcinoid heart disease from primary carcinoid tumour of the ovary. Haemodynamic and cine coronary angiocardiographic study after operation. Br. Heart J. *36*:613, 1974.

371a. Howard, R. J., Drobac, M., Rider, W. D., Keane, T. T., Finlayson, J., Silver, M. D., Wigle, E. D., and Rakowski, H.: Carcinoid heart disease: Diagnosis by two-dimensional echocardiography. Circulation *66*:1059, 1982.

372. Schwaber, J. R., and Lukas, D. S.: Hyperkinemia and cardiac failure in the carcinoid syndrome. Am. J. Med. *32*:846, 1962.

373. Biörck, G., Axen, O., and Thorson, A.: Unusual cyanosis in a boy with congenital pulmonary stenosis and tricuspid insufficiency. Fatal outcome after angiocardiography. Am. Heart J. *44*:143, 1952.

MYOCARDITIS

374. Monif, G. R. G., Lee, C. W., and Hsiung, G. D.: Isolated myocarditis with recovery of ECHO type 9 virus from the myocardium. N. Engl. J. Med. *277*:1353, 1967.

375. Morales, A. R., Vichitbhandha, P., Chandruang, P., Evans, H., and Bourgeois, C. H.: Pathologic features of cardiac conduction disturbances in diphtheritic myocarditis. Arch. Pathol. *91*:1, 1971.

376. Kaplan, M. H., and Meyeserian, M.: An immunological cross-reaction between Group-A streptococcal cells and human heart tissue. Lancet *1*:706, 1962.

377. James, T. N., Schlant, R. C., and Marshall, T. K.: De Subitaneis Mortibus. XXIX. Randomly distributed focal myocardial lesions causing destruction in the His bundle or a narrow origin left bundle branch. Circulation *57*:816, 1978.

378. Friedman, M. A., Bozdeck, M. J., Billingham, M. E., and Rider, A. K.: Daunorubicin cardiotoxicity. Serial endomyocardial biopsies and systolic time intervals. J.A.M.A. *240*:1603, 1978.

379. Ablemann, W. H.: Viral myocarditis and its sequelae, Annu. Rev. Med. *24*:145, 1973.

380. Adesanya, C. O.: Heart muscle performance after experimental viral myocarditis. J. Clin. Invest. *57*:569, 1976.

381. Fine, I., Brainerd, H., and Sokolow, M.: Myocarditis in acute infectious diseases: A clinical and electrocardiographic study. Circulation *2*:859, 1950.

382. Weinstein L.: Cardiovascular manifestations in some of the common infectious diseases. Mod. Concepts Cardiovasc. Dis. *23*:229, 1954.

383. Abelmann, W. H.: Myocarditis. N. Engl. J. Med. *275*:832, 944, 1966.

384. De La Chapelle, C. E., and Kossmann, C. E.: Myocarditis. Circulation *10*:747, 1954.

385. Saphir, O., Wile, S. A., and Reingold, J. M.: Myocarditis in children. Am. J. Dis. Child. *67*:294, 1944.

386. Saphir, O.: Myocarditis: A general review with an analysis of two hundred and forty cases. Arch. Pathol. *32*:1000, 1941; *33*:88, 1942.

387. Stevens, P. J., and Underwood Ground, K. E.: Occurrence and significance of myocarditis in trauma. Aerospace Med. *41*:776, 1970.

388. Pankey, G. A.: Effect of viruses on the cardiovascular system. Am. J. Med. Sci. *250*:103, 1965.

389. Woodward, T. E., Togo, Y., Lee, Y-C., and Hornick, R. B.: Specific microbial infections of the myocardium and pericardium. A study of 82 patients. Arch. Intern. Med. *120*:270, 1967.

390. Gore, I., and Saphir, O.: Myocarditis: A classification of 1402 cases. Am. Heart J. *34*:827, 1947.

391. Editorial: Non-rheumatic myopericarditis. Br. Med. J., *2*:544, 1971.

392. Sanders, V.: Viral myocarditis. Am. Heart J. *66*:707, 1963.

393. Robboy, S. J.: Atrioventricular-node inflammation. Mechanisms of sudden death in protracted meningococcemia. N. Engl. J. Med. *286*:1091, 1972.

394. Gerzen, P., Granath, A., Holmgren, B., and Zetterquist, S.: Acute myocarditis. A followup study. Br. Heart J. *34*:575, 1972.

395. Lim, C. H., Toh, C. C. S., Chia, B-L., and Low, L-P.: Stokes-Adams attacks due to acute nonspecific myocarditis. Am. Heart J. *90*:172, 1975.

396. Reeves, W. C., Jackson, G. L., Flickinger, F. W., Divee, H. G., Schwiter, E. J., Werner, J., Whitesell, L., Bidde, M. A., Copenhover, G., Shaikh, B. S., and Zelis, R.: Radionuclide imaging of experimental myocarditis. Circulation *63*:640, 1981.

397. Matsumori, A., Kadota, K., and Kawai, C.: Technetium-99m pyrophosphate uptake in experimental viral perimyocarditis. Sequential study of myocardial uptake and pathologic correlates. Circulation *61*:802, 1980.

398. Bengtsson, E., and Lamberger, B.: Five-year followup study of cases suggestive of acute myocarditis. Am. Heart J. *72*:751, 1966.

399. Das, S. K., Brady, T. J., Thrall, J. H., and Pitt, B.: Cardiac function in patients with prior myocarditis. J. Nucl. Med. *21*:689, 1980.

400. Burch, G. E., and Giles, T. D.: The role of viruses in the production of heart disease. Am. J. Cardiol. *29*:231, 1972.

401. Abelmann, W. H.: Clinical aspects of viral cardiomyopathy. *In* Fowler, N. O. (ed.): Myocardial Diseases. New York, Grune and Stratton, 1973, p. 253.

402. Wenger, N. K.: Infectious myocarditis. *In* Burch, G. E. (ed.): Cardiomyopathy. (Cardiovascular Clinics Series.) Philadelphia, F. A. Davis Co., 1972, p. 168.

403. Pearce, J. H.: Heart disease and filtrable virus. Circulation *21*:448, 1960.

404. Lerner, A. M.: Coxsackie virus myocardiopathy. J. Infect. Dis. *120*:496, 1969.

404a. Fenoglio, J. J., Ursell, P. C., Kellogg, C. F., Drusin, R. E., and Weiss, M. B.: Diagnosis and classification of myocarditis by endomyocardial biopsy. N. Engl. J. Med. *308*:12, 1983.

405. Mason, J. W., Billingham, M. E., and Ricci, D. R.: Treatment of acute inflammatory myocarditis assisted by endomyocardial biopsy. Am. J. Cardiol. *45*: 1037, 1980.

406. Norris, D., and Loh, P. C.: Coxsackie virus myocarditis: Prophylaxis and therapy with an interferon stimulator. Proc. Soc. Exp. Biol. Med. *142*:133, 1973.

407. Levine, H. D.: Virus myocarditis: A critique of the literature from clinical, electrocardiographic, and pathologic standpoints. Am. J. Med. Sci. *277*:132, 1979.

408. Price, R. A., Garcia, J. H., and Rightsel, W. A.: Choriomeningitis and myocarditis in an adolescent with isolation of Coxsackie B-5 virus. Am. J. Clin. Pathol. *53*:825, 1970.

409. Desa'Neto, A., Bullington, D., Bullington, R. H., Desser, K. B., and Benchimol, A.: Coxsackie B5 heart disease. Demonstration of inferolateral wall myocardial necrosis. Am. J. Med. *68*:295, 1980.

410. Grist, N. R., and Bell, E. J.: Coxsackie viruses and the heart. Am. Heart J. *77*: 295, 1969.

411. Ray, C. G., Portman, J. N., Stamm, S. J., and Hickman, R. O.: Hemolytic-uremic syndrome and myocarditis. Association with coxsackievirus B infection. Am. J. Dis. Child. *122*:418, 1970.

412. Smith, W. G.: Coxsackie B myopericarditis in adults. Am. Heart J. *80*:34, 1970.

413. Hirschman, S. F., and Hammer, G. S.: Coxsackie virus myopericarditis. A microbiological and clinical review. Am. J. Cardiol. *34*:224, 1974.

414. Sainani, G. S., Dekate, M. P., and Rao, C. P.: Heart disease caused by Coxsackie virus B infection. Br. Heart J. *37*:819, 1975.

415. Rose, H. D.: Recurrent illness following acute Coxsackie B-4 myocarditis. Am. J. Med. *54*:544, 1973.

416. Burch, G. E., and Colcolough, H. L.: Progressive Coxsackie viral pericarditis and nephritis. Ann. Intern. Med. *71*:963, 1969.

417. Editorial: Acute myocarditis and its sequelae. Br. Med. J. *3*:783, 1972.

418. Bell, E. J., and Grist, N. R.: Echoviruses, carditis and acute pleurodynia. Am. Heart J. *82*:133, 1971.

419. Bell, E. J., and Grist, N. R.: Echovirus, carditis and actue pleurodynia. Lancet *1*:326, 1970.

420. Schleissner, L. A., Fiala, M., Imagawa, D. T., and Casaburi, R.: Application of systolic time intervals to acute cardiomyopathy with echovirus 2. Chest *69*: 563, 1976.

421. Henson, D., and Nufson, M. A.: Myocarditis and pneumonitis with type 21 adenovirus infection. Association with fatal myocarditis and pneumonitis. Am. J. Dis. Child *121*:334, 1971.

422. Verel, D., Warrack, A. J. N., Potter, C. W., Ward, C., and Rickards, D. F.: Observations on the A₂ England influenza epidemic: A clinicopathological study. Am. Heart J. *92*:290, 1976.

423. Oseasohn, R., Adelson, L., and Kaji, M.: Clinicopathological study of thirty-three fatal cases of Asian influenza. N. Engl. J. Med. *260*:509, 1959.

424. Coltman, C. A., Jr.: Influenza myocarditis: Report of a case with observations on serum glutamic oxaloacetic transaminase. J.A.M.A. *180*:204, 1962.

425. Adams, C. W.: Postviral myopericarditis associated with the influenza virus. Am. J. Cardiol. *4*:56, 1959.

426. Moore, C. M., Henry, J., Benzing, G., III, and Kaplan, S.: Varicella myocarditis. Am. J. Dis. Child *118*:899, 1969.

427. Hackel, D. B.: Myocarditis in association with varicella. Am. J. Pathol. *29*: 369, 1953.

428. Morales, A. R., Adelman, S., and Fine, G.: Varicella myocarditis: A case of sudden death. Arch. Pathol. *91*:29, 1971.

429. Hildes, J. A., Schaberg, A., and Alcock, A. J. W.: Cardiovascular collapse in acute poliomyelitis. Circulation *12*:986, 1955.

430. Teloth, H. A.: Myocarditis in poliomyelitis. Arch. Pathol. *55*:408, 1953.

431. Weinstein, L., and Shelokov, A.: Cardiovascular manifestations of acute poliomyelitis. N. Engl. J. Med. *244*:281, 1951.

432. Mohammed, I., and Carlisle, R.: Cardiac and renal involvement in mumps. West Afr. Med. J.: *20*:367, 1971.

433. Roberts, W. C., and Fox, S. M., III: Mumps of the heart: Clinical and pathologic features. Circulation *32*:342, 1965.

434. Bengtsson, E., and Orndahl, G.: Complications of mumps with special reference to the incidence of myocarditis. Acta Med. Scand. *149*:381, 1954.

435. Arita, M., Ueno, Y., and Masuyama, Y.: Complete heart block in mumps myocarditis. Br. Heart J. *46*:342, 1981.

436. Saphir, O., Amromin, G. D., and Yokoo, H.: Myocarditis in viral (epidemic) hepatitis. Am. J. Med. Sci. *231*:168, 1956.

437. Bell, H.: Cardiac manifestations of viral hepatitis. J.A.M.A. *218*:387, 1971.

438. Nagaratnam, N., deSilva, D. P. K. M., and Gunawardene, K. R. W.: Myocardial involvement in infectious hepatitis. Postgrad. Med. J. *47*:785, 1971.

439. Webster, B. H.: Cardiac complications of infectious mononucleosis: A review of the literature and report of five cases. Am. J. Med. Sci. *234*:62, 1957.

440. Frishman, W., Kraus, M. E., Zabkar, J., Brooks, V., Alonso, D., and Dixon, L. M.: Infectious mononucleosis and fatal myocarditis. Chest *72*:535, 1977.

441. Miller, R., Ward, C., Amsterdam, E., Mason, D. T., and Zelis, R.: Focal mononucleosis myocarditis simulating myocardial infarction. Chest *63*:102, 1973.

442. Hudgins, J. M.: Infectious mononucleosis complicated by myocarditis and pericarditis. J.A.M.A. *235*:2626, 1976.

443. Goldfinger, D., Schreiber, W., and Wosika, P. H.: Permanent heart block following German measles. Am. J. Med. *2*:320, 1947.

444. Goldfield, M., Bayer, N. H., and Weinstein, L.: Electrocardiographic changes during the course of measles. J. Pediatr. *46*:30, 1955.

445. Degen, J. A.: Visceral pathology in measles: A clinico-pathologic study of 100 cases. Am. J. Med. Sci. *194*:104, 1937.

446. Wilson, R. S., Morris, T. H., and Rossell Rees, J.: Cytomegalovirus myocarditis. Br. Heart J. *34*:865, 1972.

447. Wink, K., and Schmitz, H.: Cytomegalovirus myocarditis. Am. Heart J. *100*: 667, 1980.

448. Tuila, E., and Leinikki, P.: Fatal cytomegalovirus infection in a previously healthy boy with myocarditis and consumption coagulopathy as presenting signs. Scand. J. Infect. Dis. *4*:57, 1972.

449. Obeyesekere, I., and Herman, Y.: Arbovirus heart disease: Myocarditis and cardiomyopathy following dengue and chikungunya fever—a follow-up study. Am. Heart J. *85*:186, 1973.

450. Nagaratham, N., Siripala, K., and deSilva, N.: Arbovirus (dengue type) as a cause of acute myocarditis and pericarditis. Br. Heart J. *35*:204, 1973.

451. Obeyesekere, I., and Herman, Y.: Myocarditis and cardiomyopathy after arbovirus infections (dengue and chikungunya fever). Br. Heart J. *34*:821, 1972.

452. Anderson T., Foulis, M. A., Grist, N. R., and Landsman, J. B.: Clinical and laboratory observations in a smallpox outbreak. Lancet *1*:1248, 1951.

453. Matthews, A. W., and Griffiths, I. D.: Post-vaccinal pericarditis and myocarditis. Br. Heart J. *36*:1043, 1974.

454. Finlay-Jones, L. R.: Fatal myocarditis after vaccinations for smallpox. N. Engl. J. Med. *270*:41, 1964.

455. Connell, D. E.: Myocardial degeneration in yellow fever. Am. J. Pathol. *4*:431, 1928.

456. Gills, T. D., and Gohd, R. S.: Respiratory syncytial virus and heart disease. A report of two cases. J.A.M.A. *236*:1128, 1976.

457. Bairan, A. C., Cherry, J. D., Fagan, L. F., and Coff, J. E., Jr.: Complete heart block and respiratory syncytial virus infection. Am. J. Dis. Child. *127*:264, 1974.

458. Lewes, D., Rainsford, D. J., and Lane, W. F.: Symptomless myocarditis and myalgia in viral and *Mycoplasma pneumoniae* infections. Br. Heart J. *36*:924, 1974.

459. Sands, M. J., Jr., Satz, J. E., Turner, W. E., and Soloff, L. A.: Pericarditis and perimyocarditis associated with active *Mycoplasma pneumoniae* infection. Ann. Intern. Med. *86*:544, 1977.

460. Pickens, S., and Catterall, J. R.: Disseminated intravascular coagulation and myocarditis associated with *Mycoplasma pneumoniae* infection. Br. Med. J. *1*: 1526, 1978.

461. Dymock, I. W., Lawson, J. M., MacLennan, W. J., and Ross, C. A. C.: Myocarditis associated with psittacosis. Br. J. Clin. Pract. *25*:240, 1971.

462. Sutton, G. C., Morrissey, R. A., Tobin, J. R., Jr., and Anderson, T. V.: Pericardial and myocardial disease associated with serologic evidence of infection by agents of the psittacosis-lymphogranuloma venereum group (Chlamydiaceae). Circulation *36*:830, 1967.

463. Woodward, I. E., McCrumb, F. R., Jr., Carey, I. N., and Tago, Y.: Viral and rickettsial causes of cardiac disease including the Coxsackie virus etiology of pericarditis and myocarditis. Ann. Intern. Med. *53*:1130, 1960.

464. Allen, A. C., and Spitz, S.: A comparative study of the pathology of scrub typhus (tsutsugamushi disease) and other rickettsial diseases. Am. J. Pathol. *21*: 603, 1945.

465. Ognibane, A. J., O'Leary, D. S., Czarnocki, S. W., Flannery, E. P., and Grove, R. B.: Myocarditis and disseminated intravascular coagulation in scrub typhus. Am. J. Med. Sci. *262*:233, 1971.

466. Levine, H. D.: Pathologic study of thirty-one cases of scrub typhus fever with special reference to the cardiovascular system. Am. Heart J. *31*:314, 1946.

467. Bradford, W. D., and Hackel, D. B.: Myocardial involvement in Rocky Mountain spotted fever. Arch. Pathol. Lab. Med. *102*:357, 1978.

468. Hand, W. L., Miller, J. B., Reinary, J. A., and Sanford, J. P.: Rocky Mountain spotted fever: A vascular disease. Arch. Intern. Med. *125*:879, 1970.

469. Sheridan, P., MacCraig, J. N., and Hart, R. J. C.: Myocarditis complicating Q fever. Br. Med. J. *2*:155, 1974.

470. Barraclough, D., and Popert, A. J.: Q fever presenting with paroxysmal ventricular tachycardia. Br. Med. J. *2*:423, 1975.

471. Taheinia, A. C.: Electrocardiographic abnormalities and serum transaminase levels in diphtheritic myocarditis. J. Pediatr. *75*:1008, 1969.

472. Riley, H. D., Jr., and Weaver, T. S.: Cardiovascular and nervous system complications of diphtheria. Am. Pract. *3*:536, 1952.

473. Collier, R. J., and Pappenheimer, A. M.: Studies on the mode of action of diphtheria toxin. J. Exp. Med. *120*:1007; 1018, 1964.

474. Ledbetter, M. K., Cannon, A. B., and Costa, A. F.: The electrocardiogram in diphtheritic myocarditis. Am. Heart J. *68*:599, 1964.

475. Matisonn, R. E.: Successful electrical pacing for complete heart block complicating diphtheritic myocarditis. Br. Heart J. *38*:423, 1976.

476. Sanders, V., and Misanik, L. F.: Salmonella myocarditis: Report of a case with ventricular rupture. Am. Heart J. *68*:682, 1964.

477. Hennigar, G. R., Thabet, R., Bundy, W. C., and Sutton, L. E.: Salmonellosis complicated by pancarditis. J. Pediatr. *43*:524, 1953.

478. Shilkin, K. B.: *Salmonella typhimurium* pancarditis. Postgrad. Med. J. *45*:40,1969.

479. Le-Van-Diem, A. K.: Typhoid fever with myocarditis. Am. J. Trop. Med. Hyg. *23*:218, 1974.

480. Mainzer, F.: Electrocardiographic study of typhoid myocarditis. Br. Heart J. *9*: 145, 1947.

481. Thiruvengadam, K. V., Shetty, M. R., and Mallick, M. A.: Myocarditis in enteric fever. J. Indian Med. Assoc. *48*:115, 1967.
482. Kinare, S. G., and Deshmulh, M. M.: Complete atrioventricular block due to myocardial tuberculosis. Arch. Pathol. *88*:684, 1969.
483. Auerbach, O., and Guggenheim, A.: Tuberculosis of the myocardium: A review of the literature and a report of six new cases. Q. Bull. Sea View Hosp. *2*: 264, 1937.
484. Horn, H., and Saphir, O.: The involvement of the myocardium in tuberculosis. A review of the literature and report of 3 cases. Am. Rev. Tuberc. *32*:492, 1935.
485. Rosenbaum, H., and Linn, H. J.: Tuberculosis of myocardium. Am. J. Clin. Pathol. *18*:162, 1948.
486. Claiborne, T. S.: Caseating granuloma of the heart. Am. J. Cardiol. *33*:920, 1974.
487. Jones, K. P., and Tilden, I. L.: Tuberculous myocardial aneurysm, with rupture and sudden death from tamponade: Review of the literature and report of a case. Hawaii Med. J. *1*:295, 1942.
488. Rawls, W. J., Shuford, W. H., Kogan, W. D., Hurst, J. W., and Schlant, R. C.: Right ventricular outflow tract obstruction produced by a myocardial abscess in a patient with tuberculosis. Am. J. Cardiol. *21*:738, 1968.
489. Gore, I.: Myocarditis in infectious diseases. Am. Pract. *1*:292, 1947.
490. Brody, A., and Smith, L. W.: Visceral pathology in scarlet fever and related streptococcal infections. Am. J. Pathol. *12*:373, 1936.
491. Hardman, J. M., and Earle, K. M.: Myocarditis in 200 fatal meningococcal infections. Arch. Pathol. *87*:318, 1969.
492. d'Agati, V., and Marangoni, B. A.: The Waterhouse-Friderichsen syndrome. N. Engl. J. Med. *232*:1, 1945.
493. Denmark, I. C., and Knight, E. L.: Cardiovascular and coagulation complications of Group C meningococcal disease. Arch. Intern. Med. *127*:238, 1971.
494. Roberts, W. C., and Beard, G. W.: Gas gangrene of the heart in clostridial septicemia. Am. Heart J. *74*:482, 1967.
495. Guneratre, P.: Gas gangrene (abscess) of heart. N.Y. State J. Med. *75*:1766, 1975.
496. Gross, D., Willens, H., and Zeldis, S. M.: Myocarditis in Legionnaire's disease. Chest *79*:232, 1981.
497. Doscia, J. L., Fisco, J. M., and Brace, W. T.: Complete heart block due to a solitary gumma. Am. J. Cardiol. *13*:553, 1964.
498. Spain, D. M., and Johannsen, M. W.: Three cases of localized gummatous myocarditis. Am. Heart J. *241*:689, 1942.
499. Boss, J. H., Liftkowtiz, M., and Freud, M.: Unusual manifestations of syphilitic cardiovascular disease. Ann. Intern. Med. *55*:824, 1961.
500. Saphir, O.: Syphilitic myocarditis. Arch. Pathol. *13*:266, 1932.
501. Arean, V. M.: Leptospiral myocarditis. Lab. Invest. *6*:462, 1957.
502. Edwards, G. A., and Damm, B. M.: Human leptospirosis. Medicine *39*:117, 1960.
503. Sodeman, W. A., and Kellough, J. H.: The cardiac manifestations of Weil's disease. Am. J. Trop. Med. *31*:479, 1957.
504. Judge, D. M., Samuel, I., Perine, P. L., Vukotic, D., and Ababa, A.: Louseborne relapsing fever in man. Arch. Pathol. *97*:136, 1974.
505. Williams, A. H.: Aspergillus myocarditis. Am. J. Clin. Pathol. *61*:247, 1974.
506. Cade, J. F.: Pulmonary aspergillosis with myocarditis. Med. J. Aust. *1*:581, 1966.
507. Zoeckler, S. J.: Cardiac actinomycosis: A case report and survey of the literature. Circulation *3*:854, 1951.
508. Edwards, A. C.: Actinomycosis in children: A review of the literature and report of cases. Am. J. Dis. Child. *41*:1419, 1931.
509. Martin, D. S., and Smith, D. T.: Blastomycosis (American blastomycosis, Gilchrist's disease). I. A review of the literature. Am. Rev. Tuberc. *39*:275, 1939.
510. Baker, R. D., and Brian, E. W.: Blastomycosis of the heart: Report of two cases. Am. J. Pathol. *13*:139, 1937.
511. Hutter, R. V. P., and Collins, H. S.: The appearance of opportunistic fungus infections in a cancer hospital. Lab. Invest. *11*:1035, 1962.
512. Jones, I., Nassau, E., and Smith, P.: Cryptococcosis of the heart. Br. Heart J. *27*:462, 1965.
513. Van Kirk, J. E., Simon, A. B., and Armstrong, U. R.: Candida myocarditis causing complete atrioventricular block. J.A.M.A. *227*:931, 1974.
514. Brooks, S. E. H., and Young, E. G.: Clinicopathologic observations on systemic moniliasis: A case report and review of the literature. Arch. Pathol. *73*:383, 1962.
515. Reingold, I. M.: Myocardial lesions in disseminated coccidioidomycosis. Am. J. Clin. Pathol. *20*:1044, 1950.
516. Larson, R., and Schert, R. E.: Coccidioidal pericarditis. Circulation *7*:211, 1953.
517. Merchant, R. K., Louria, D. B., Geisler, P. H., Edgcomb, J. H., and Utz, S. P.: Fungal endocarditis. Review of the literature and report of three cases. Ann. Intern. Med. *48*:242, 1958.
518. Owen, G. E., Scherr, W. N., and Segre, E. J.: Histoplasmosis involving the heart and great vessels. Am. J. Med. *32*:552, 1962.
519. Acquatella, H., Schiller, N. B., Puigbo, J. J., Giordano, H., Suarez, J. A., Casal, H., Arreaza, N., Valecillos, R., and Hirschhaut, E.: M-mode and two-dimensional echocardiography in chronic Chagas' heart disease. A clinical and pathologic study. Circulation *62*:787, 1980.
520. Rosenbaum, M. B.: Chagasic myocardiopathy. Progr. Cardiovasc. Dis. *7*:199, 1964.
521. Teixeira, A. R. L., Teixeira, G., Macedo, V., and Prata, A.: Acquired cell-mediated immunodepression in acute Chagas' disease. J. Clin. Invest. *62*:1132, 1978.
522. Winslow, D. J., and Chaffee, E. F.: Preliminary investigations in Chagas disease. Milit. Med. *130*:826, 1965.
523. Ribeiro Dos Santos, R., and Hudson, L.: *Trypanosoma cruzi*: Immunological consequences of parasite modification of host cells. Clin. Exp. Immunol. *40*:36, 1980.
524. Editorial: Chagas' disease: Potential for immunoprophylaxis. Lancet *1*:466, 1980.
525. Ribeiro Dos Santos, R., and Hudson, L.: *Trypanosoma cruzi*: Binding of parasite antigens to mammalian cell membranes. Parasite Immunol. *2*:1, 1980.
526. Mott, K. E., and Hagstrom, J. W. C.: The pathologic lesions of the cardiac autonomic nervous system in chronic Chagas' myocarditis. Circulation *31*:273, 1965.
527. Teixeira, A. R. L.: Chagas' disease: Trends in immunological research and prospects for immunoprophylaxis. Bull. WHO *57*:697, 1979.
528. Puigbó, J. J., Valecillos, R., Hirschhault, E, Giordano, H., Boccalandro, I., Suarez, C., and Aparicio, J. M.: Diagnosis of Chagas' cardiomyopathy. Noninvasive techniques. Postgrad. Med. *53*:527, 1977.
528a. Maguire, J. H., Mott, K. E., Lehman, J. S., Hoff, R., Muniz, T. M, Guimāraes, A. C., Sherlock, I., and Morrow, R. H. : Relationship of electrocardiographic abnormalities and seropositivity to Trypanosoma cruzi within a rural community in Northeast Brazil. Am. Heart J. *105*:287, 1983.
529. Miles, M. A., Cedillos, R. A., Povoa, M. M., De Souza, A. A., Prata, A., and Macedo, V.: Do radically dissimilar *Trypanosoma cruzi* strains (zymodemes) cause Venezuelan and Brazilian forms of Chagas' disease? Lancet *1*:1338, 1981.
530. Oliveira, J. S. M., Oliveira, J. A. M., Frederigue, V., Jr., and Filho, E. C. L.: Apical aneurysm of Chagas' heart disease. Br. Heart J. *46*:432, 1981.
531. Laranja, F. S., Dias, E., Nobrega, G., and Miranda, A.: Chagas' disease: A clinical, epidemiologic, and pathologic study. Circulation *14*:1035, 1956.
532. Andrade, Z. A., Andrade, S. G., Oliveira, G. B., and Alonso, D. R.: Histopathology of the conducting tissue of the heart in Chagas' myocarditis. Am. Heart J. *95*:316, 1978.
533. Chiale, P. A., Przybylski, J., Laino, R. A., Halpern, M. S., Sanchez, R. A., Gafrieli, A., Elizari, M. V., and Rosenbaum, M. B.: Electrocardiographic changes evoked by ajmaline in chronic Chagas' disease without manifest myocarditis. Am. J. Cardiol. *49*:14, 1982.
534. Carrasco, H. A., Barboza, J. S., Inglessis, G., Fuenmayor, A., and Molina, C.: Left ventricular cineangiography in Chagas' disease: Detection of early myocardial damage. Am. Heart J. *104*:595, 1982.
535. Araujo, F., Chiari, E., and Dias, J. C. P.: Demonstration of *Trypanosoma cruzi* antigen in serum from patients with Chagas' disease. Lancet *1*:246, 1981.
536. Mott, K. E., Lehman, J. S., Jr., Hoff, R., Morrow, R. H., Muniz, T. M., Sherlock, I., Draper, C. C., Pugliese, C., and Guimaraes, A.: The epidemiology and household distribution of seroreactivity to Trypanosoma cruzi in a rural community in northeast Brazil. Am. J. Trop. Med. Hyg. *25*:552, 1976.
537. Brener, Z., and Andrade, Z. A. (eds.): *Trypanosoma cruzi* e Doenca de Chagas. Rio de Janeiro, Guanabara Koogan, 1979, p. 362.
538. Francis, T. I.: Visceral complications of Gambian trypanosomiasis in a nigerian. Trans. R. Soc. Trop. Med. Hyg. *66*:140, 1972.
539. deRaadt, P., and Koten, J. W.: Myocarditis in rhodesiense trypanosomiasis. East Afr. Med. J. *45*:128, 1968.
540. Poltera, A. A., Cox, N., and Owor, R.: Pancarditis affecting the conducting system and all valves in human African trypanosomiasis. Br. Heart J. *38*:827, 1976.
541. Theologides, A., and Kennedy, B. J.: Toxoplasmic myocarditis and pericarditis (editorial). Am. J. Med. *47*:169, 1969.
542. Van der Horst, R., Kleverman, P., Schonland, M., and Gotsman, M.: Fatal myocardial necrosis probably due to toxoplasma myocarditis. S. Afr. Med. J. *46*:949, 1972.
543. Leak, D., and Meghji, M.: Toxoplasmic infection in cardiac disease. Am. J. Cardiol. *43*:841, 1979.
544. Sagrista-Sauleda, J., Permanyer-Miralda, G., Juste-Sanchez, C., de Buen-Sanchez, M. L., Pujadas-Capmany, R., Arcalis-Arce, L., and Soler-Soler, J.: Huge chronic pericardial effusion caused by *Toxoplasma gondii*. Circulation *66*: 895, 1982.
545. Mary, A. S., and Hamilton, M.: Ventricular tachycardia in a patient with toxoplasmosis. Br. Heart J. *35*:349, 1973.
546. Rojas, R. A., and Deza, D.: Cardiac changes in malarial patients. Am. Heart J. *33*:702, 1947.
547. Merkel, W. C.: *Plasmodium falciparum* malaria: The coronary and myocardial lesions observed at autopsy in two cases of acute fulminating *Plasmodium falciparum* infection. Arch. Pathol. *41*:290, 1946.
548. Herrera, J. M.: Cardiac lesions in vivax malaria: Study of a case with coronary and myocardial damage. Arch. Inst. Cardiol. Mex. *30*:26, 1960.
549. Simonson, E., and Keys, A.: Experimental malaria in man. III. The changes in the electrocardiogram. J. Clin. Invest. *29*:68, 1950.
550. Wessel, H. U., Sommers, H. M., Cugell, D. W., and Paul, M. H.: Variants of cardiopulmonary manifestations of Manson's schistosomiasis: Report of two cases. Ann. Intern Med. *62*:757, 1965.
551. Bedford, D. E., Aidaros, S. M., and Girgis, B.: Bilharzial heart disease in Egypt: Cor pulmonale due to bilharzial pulmonary endarteritis. Br. Heart J. *8*: 87, 1946.
552. Zahawi, S., and Shukri, N.: Histopathology of fatal myocarditis due to ectopic schistosomiasis. Trans. R. Soc. Trop. Med. Hyg. *50*:166, 1956.
553. Kean, B. H., and Breslou, R. C.: Parasites of the Human Heart. New York, Grune and Stratton, 1964.

554. Africa, C. M., Garcia, E. Y., and DeLeon, W.: Intestinal heterophyiasis with cardiac involvement. A contribution to the etiology of heart failure. J. Philipp. Isl. Med. Assoc. 15:358, 1935.

555. Helimsky, A. M.: Cysticercosis of the brain, heart and skeletal muscles. Med. Parazitol. (Mosk.) 31:610, 1962.

556. Goldsmid, J. M.: Two unusual cases of cysticercosis in man in Rhodesia. J. Helminthol. 40:331, 1966.

557. Ibarra-Perez, C., Fernandez-Diez, J., and Rodriguez-Trujillo, F.: Myocardial cysticercosis: Report of two cases with coexisting heart disease. South. Med. J. 65:484, 1972.

558. Murphy, T. E., Kean, B. H., Venturine, A., and Lillekei, C. W.: Echinococcus cyst of the left ventricle: Report of a case with review of the pertinent literature. J. Thorac. Cardiovasc. Surg. 61:443, 1970.

559. Dodek, A., DeMots, H., Antonomic, J. A., and Hodam, R. P.: Echinococcus of the heart. Am. J. Cardiol. 30:293, 1972.

560. DiBello, R., Urioste, H. A., and Rubio, R.: Hydatid cysts of the ventricular septum of the heart: A study based on two personal cases and forty-one observations in the literature. Am. J. Cardiol. 14:237, 1964.

561. Dighiero, J., Canabal, E. J., Aguirre, C. V., Hazan, J., and Horjales, J. O.: Echinococcus disease of the heart. Circulation 17:127, 1958.

562. Heilbrunn, A., Kittle, C. F., and Dunn, M.: Surgical management of echinococcal cysts of the heart and pericardium. Circulation 27:219, 1963.

563. Gibson, D. S.: Cardiac hydatid cysts. Thorax 19:151, 1964.

564. Artucio, R., Roglia, J. L., DiBello, R., Dubra, J., Gorlero, A., Polero, J., and Urioste, H. A.: Hydatid cyst of the interventricular septum of the heart with rupture into the right ventricle. J. Thorac. Cardiovasc. Surg. 44:110, 1962.

565. De Los Arcos, E., Madurga, M. P., Leon, J. P., Martinez, J. L., and Urquira, M.: Hydatid cyst of the interventricular septum causing left anterior hemiblock. Br. Heart J. 33:623, 1971.

566. Naaman, Y. D., Samarrai, A. A. R., and al-Omeri, M. M.: Hydatid disease of the heart. A report of four cases. J. Cardiovasc. Surg. 14:95, 1973.

567. Oliver, J. M., Benito, L. P., Ferrufino, O., Sotillo, J. F., and Nunez, L.: Cardiac hydatid cysts diagnosed by two-dimensional echocardiography. Am. Heart J. 104:164, 1982.

568. Editorial: Medical treatment of hydatid disease. Br. Med. J. 2:563, 1979.

569. Becroft, D. M. O.: Infection by the dog roundworm Toxocara canis and fatal myocarditis. N. Engl. J. Med. 63:729, 1964.

570. Friedman, S., and Hervada, A. R.: Severe myocarditis with recovery in a child with visceral larva migrans. J. Pediatr. 56:91, 1960.

571. Barr, R.: Human trichinosis: Report of four cases, with emphasis on central nervous system involvement, and a survey of 500 consecutive autopsies at the Ottawa Civic Hospital. Can. Med. Assoc. J. 95:912, 1966.

572. Edwards, J. L., Hood, C. I., and Laite, H. B.: Studies on the pathogenesis of cardiac and cerebral lesions of experimental trichinosis in rabbits. Am. J. Pathol. 40:711, 1962.

573. Chase, G. O.: Death due to eosinophilic myocarditis related to trichinosis. J.A.M.A. 165:1826, 1957.

574. Grey, D. F., Morse, B. S., and Phillips, W. F.: Trichinosis with neurologic and cardiac involvement: Review of the literature and report of three cases. Ann. Intern. Med. 57:230, 1962.

575. Segar, L. F., Kashtan, H. A., and Miller, P. B.: Trichinosis with myocarditis. Report of a case treated with ACTH. N. Engl. J. Med. 252:397, 1955.

576. Solarz, S. D.: An electrocardiographic study of one hundred and fourteen consecutive cases of trichinosis. Am. Heart J. 34:230, 1947.

577. Van Stee, E. W. (ed.): Cardiovascular Toxicology. New York, Raven Press, 1982, 388 pp.

578. Bristow, M. R. (ed.): Drug-Induced Heart Disease. Amsterdam, Elsevier Press, 1980, 476 pp.

579. Veith, R. C., Raskind, M. A., Caldwell, J. H., Barnes, R. F., Gumbrecht, G., and Ritchie, J. L.: Cardiovascular effects of tricyclic antidepressants in depressed patients with chronic heart disease. N. Engl. J. Med. 306:954, 1982.

580. Surawicz, B., and Lasseter, K. C.: Effect of drugs on the electrocardiogram. Prog. Cardiovasc. Dis. 13:26, 1970.

581. Fletcher, G. F., Kazamias, T. M., and Wenger, N. K.: Cardiotoxic effect of mellaril: Conduction disturbances and supraventricular arrhythmias. Am. Heart J. 78:135, 1969.

582. Fowler, N. O., McCall, D., Chou, T. C., Holmes, J. C., and Hanenson, I. B.: Electrocardiographic changes and cardiac arrhythmias in patients receiving psychotropic drugs. Am. J. Cardiol. 37:223, 1976.

583. Kelley, H. G., Fay, J. E., and Laverty, S. G.: Thioridazine hydrochloride (Mellaril): Its effect on the electrocardiogram and a report of two fatalities with electrocardiographic abnormalities. Can. Med. Assoc. J. 89:546, 1963.

584. Madan, B. R., and Pendse, V. K.: Antiarrhythmic activity of thioridazine hydrochloride (Mellaril). Am. J. Cardiol. 11:78, 1963.

585. Burda, D. C.: Electrocardiographic abnormalities induced by thioridazine (Mellaril). Am. Heart J. 76:153, 1968.

586. Raisfeld, I. H.: Cardiovascular complications of antidepressant therapy. Interactions at the adrenergic neuron. Am. Heart J. 83:129, 1972.

587. Pearce, M. B., Bullock, R. T., and Murphy, M. L.: Selective damage of mitochondria due to emetine hydrochloride. Arch. Pathol. 91:8, 1971.

588. Dempsy, J. J., and Salem, H. H.: An enzymatic electrocardiographic study on toxicity of dehydroemetine. Br. Heart J. 28:505, 1966.

589. Murphy, M. L., Bullock, R. T., and Pearce, M. B.: The correlation of metabolic and ultrastructural changes in emetine myocardial toxicity. Am. Heart J. 87:105, 1974.

590. Sanghri, L. M., and Mathur, B. B.: Electrocardiogram after chloroquine and emetine. Circulation 32:281, 1965.

591. Michael, T. A. D., and Arivazzadek, S.: The effects of acute chloroquine poisoning with special reference to the heart. Am. Heart J. 79:831, 1970.

592. Honey, M.: The effects of sodium antimony tartrate on the myocardium. Br. Heart J. 22:601, 1960.

593. Wellens, H. J., Cats, V. M., and Duren, D. R.: Symptomatic sinus node abnormalities following lithium carbonate therapy. Am. J. Med. 59:285, 1975.

594. Tilkian, A., Schroeder, J. S., Kao, J., and Hultgren, H.: Effect of lithium on cardiovascular performance: Report on extended ambulatory monitoring and exercise testing before and during lithium therapy. Am. J. Cardiol. 38:701, 1976.

595. Tseng, H. C.: Interstitial myocarditis probably related to lithium carbonate intoxication. Arch. Pathol. 92:444, 1971.

596. James, F. W., Kaplan, S., and Benzing, G., III: Cardiac complications following hydrocarbon ingestion. Am. J. Dis. Child 121:431, 1971.

597. Steiner, M. H.: Syndromes of kerosene poisoning in children. Am. J. Dis. Child. 74:32, 1947.

598. Harris, W. S.: Toxic effects of aerosol propellants on the heart. Arch. Intern. Med. 131:162, 1973.

599. Bagnell, W. E., Salway, S. G., and Jackson, E. W.: Phaeochromocytoma with myocarditis managed with l-methyl-p-tyrosine. Postgrad. Med. J. 52:653, 1976.

600. Van Vliet, P. D., Burchell, H. B., and Titus, J. L.: Focal myocarditis associated with pheochromocytomas. N. Engl. J. Med. 274:1102, 1966.

601. Szakacs, J. E., and Mehlman, B.: Pathologic changes induced by l-norepinephrine: Quantitative aspects. Am. J. Cardiol. 5:619, 1960.

602. Pentel, P. R., Mikell, F. L., and Zavoral, J. H.: Myocardial injury after phenylpropanolamine ingestion. Br. Heart J. 47:51, 1982.

603. Haft, J. I., Gershengorn, K., Kranz, P. D., and Oestreicher, R.: Protection against epinephrine-induced myocardial necrosis by drugs that inhibit platelet aggregation. Am. J. Cardiol. 30:838, 1972.

604. Kline, T. S.: Myocardial changes in lead poisoning. Am. J. Dis. Child. 99:48, 1960.

605. Freeman, R.: Reversible myocarditis due to chronic lead poisoning in childhood. Arch. Dis. Child. 40:389, 1965.

606. Anderson, R. F., Allensenarth, D. C., and DeGroot, W. J.: Myocardial toxicity from carbon monoxide poisoning. Ann. Intern. Med. 67:1172, 1967.

607. Hayes, J. M., and Hall, G. V.: The myocardial toxicity of carbon monoxide. Med. J. Aust. 1:865, 1964.

608. Shafer, N., Smilay, M. G., and MacMillan, F. P.: Primary myocardial disease in man resulting from acute carbon monoxide poisoning. Am. J. Med. 38:316, 1965.

609. Corya, B. C., Black, M. J., and McHenry, P. L.: Echocardiographic findings after acute carbon monoxide poisoning. Br. Heart J. 38:712, 1976.

610. Dahhan, S. S., and Orfaly, H.: Electrocardiographic changes in mercury poisoning. Am. J. Cardiol. 14:178, 1964.

611. Talley, R. C., Tinhart, J. W., Trevino, A. J., Moore, C., and Beller, B. M.: Acute elemental phosphorus poisoning in man: Cardiovascular toxicity. Am. Heart J. 84:139, 1972.

612. Diaz-Rivera, R. S., Ramos-Morales, R., Garcia-Palmieri, M. R., and Ramirez, E. A.: The electrocardiographic changes in acute phosphorus poisoning in man. Am. J. Med. Sci. 241:758, 1961.

613. Connor, T. B., Rosen, B. L., Blaustein, M. P., Applefeld, M. M., and Doyle, L. A.: Hypocalcemia precipitating congestive heart failure. N. Engl. J. Med. 307:869, 1982.

614. Giles, T. D., Iteld, B. J., and Rives, K. L.: The cardiomyopathy of hypoparathyroidism. Chest 79:225, 1981.

615. Editorial: Selenium in the heart of China. Lancet 2:889, 1979.

616. Keshan Disease Research Group of the Chinese Academy of Medical Sciences: Observations on the effect of sodium selenite in prevention of Keshan disease. Chin. Med. J. (Engl.) 92:471, 1979.

617. Johnson, R. A., Baker, S. S., Fallon, J. T., Maynard, E. P., III, Ruskin, J. N., Wen, A., Ge, K., and Cohen, H. J.: An occidental case of cardiomyopathy and selenium deficiency. N. Engl. J. Med. 304:1210, 1981.

618. Gueron, M., and Yarom, R.: Cardiovascular complications of severe scorpion sting: Clinicopathologic correlations. Chest 57:156, 1970.

619. Gueron, M., Stern, J., and Cohen, W.: Severe myocardial damage and heart failure in scorpion sting: Report of five cases. Am. J. Cardiol. 19:719, 1967.

620. Bisarya, B. N., Vasavada, J. P., Bhatt, A., Nair, P. N. R., and Sharma, V. R.: Hemiplegia and myocarditis following scorpion bite (a case report). Indian Heart J. 29:97, 1977.

621. Gueron, M., Adolph, R. J., Grupp, I. L., Gabel, M., Grupp, G., and Fowler, N. O.: Hemodynamic and myocardial consequences of scorpion venom. Am. J. Cardial. 45:979, 1980.

622. Levine, H. D.: Acute myocardial infarction following wasp sting: Report of two cases and critical survey of the literature. Am. Heart J. 91:365, 1976.

623. Weitzman, S., Margulis, G., and Lehmann, E.: Uncommon cardiovascular manifestations and high catecholamine levels due to "black widow" bite. Am. Heart J. 93:89, 1977.

624. Reid, H. A.: Snakebite in the tropics. Br. Med. J. 3:359, 1968.

625. Reid, H. A., Thean, P. C., Chan, K. E., and Baharom, A. R.: Clinical effects of bites by Malayan viper (Ancistrodon rhodostoma). Lancet 1:617, 1963.

626. Chadha, J. S., Ashby, D. W., and Brown, J. O.: Abnormal electrocardiogram after adder bite. Br. Heart J. 30:138, 1968.

627. Weinberg, S. L.: The electrocardiogram in acute arsenic poisoning. Am. Heart J. 60:971, 1960.

628. Barry, K. G., and Herndon, E. G., Jr.: Electrocardiographic changes associated with acute arsenic poisoning. Med. Ann. D.C. 31:25, 1962.

629. Wenzel, D. G.: Drug-induced cardiomyopathies. J. Pharm. Sci. 56:1209, 1967.

630. Glazener, F. S., Ellis, J. G., and Johnson, P. K.: Electrocardiographic findings with arsenic poisoning. Calif. Med. *109*:158, 1968.

631. McKinstry, W. J., and Hicks, V. M.: Emergency-arsine poisoning. Arch. Intern. Med. *100*:34, 1957.

632. Appelbaum, F., Strauchen, J. A., and Graw, R. G., Jr.: Acute lethal carditis caused by high-dose combination chemotherapy. A unique clinical and pathological entity. Lancet *1*:58, 1976.

633. O'Connell, T. X., and Berenbaum, M. C.: Myocardial and pulmonary effects of high doses of cyclophosphamide and isophosphamide. Cancer Res. *34*:1586, 1974.

634. Gottdiener, J. S., Appelbaum, F. R., Ferrans, V. J., Deisseroth, A., and Ziegler, J.: Cardiotoxicity associated with high-dose cyclophosphamide therapy. Arch. Intern. Med. *141*:758, 1981.

635. Sanerkin, N. G.: Acute myocardial necrosis in paracetamol poisoning. Br. Med. J. *3*:478, 1971.

636. Bhasin, S., Wallace, W., Lawrence, J. B., and Lesch, M.: Sudden death associated with thyroid hormone abuse. Am. J. Med. *71*:887, 1981.

637. Fainstein, V., and Bodey, G. P.: Cardiorespiratory toxicity due to miconazole. Ann. Intern. Med. *93*:432, 1980.

638. Kowey, P. R., Friedman, P. L., Podrid, P. J., Zielonka, J., Lown, B., Wynne, J., and Holman, B. L.: Use of radionuclide ventriculography for assessment of changes in myocardial performance by disopyramide phosphate. Am. Heart J. *104*:769, 1982.

639. Morady, F., Scheinman, M. M., and Desai, J.: Disopyramide. Ann. Intern. Med. *96*:337, 1982.

640. Vorobiof, D. A.: Cardiotoxicity of 5-fluoro-uracil. A case report. South Africa Med. J. *61*:634, 1982.

641. Harkavy, J.: Cardiac manifestations due to hypersensitivity. Ann. Allergy *28*:242, 1970.

642. Mullick, F. G., and McAllister, H. A.: Myocarditis associated with methyldopa therapy. J.A.M.A. *237*:1699, 1977.

643. Plafker, J.: Penicillin-related nephritis and myocarditis: A case report. South. Med. J. *64*:852, 1971.

644. Schoenivetter, A. H., and Silber, E. N.: Penicillin hypersensitivity, acute pericarditis, and eosinophilia. J.A.M.A. *191*:672, 1965.

645. Simon, M. A.: Pathologic lesions following the administration of sulfonamide drugs. Am. J. Med. Sci. *205*:439, 1943.

646. Blanchard, A. J., and Mertens, G. A.: Hypersensitivity myocarditis occurring with sulphamethoxypyridazine therapy. Can. Med. Assoc. J. *79*:627, 1958.

647. MacSearraegh, E. T. M., and Patel, I. C. M.: Cardiomyopathy as a complication of sulphonamide therapy. Br. Med. J. *3*:33, 1968.

648. Kline, L. K., Kline, T. S., and Saphir, O.: Myocarditis in senescence. Am. Heart J. *65*:446, 1963.

649. Kerwin, A. J.: Fatal myocarditis due to sensitivity to phenindione. Can. Med. Assoc. J. *90*:1418, 1964.

650. Hodge, P. R., and Lawrence, J. R.: Two cases of myocarditis associated with phenylbutazone therapy. Med. J. Aust. *1*:640, 1957.

651. Edelstein, J. M.: Butazolidin angiitis and periangiitis simulating Aschoff nodule. Am. Heart J. *69*:573, 1965.

652. Barrett, D. A., II, Dalldorf, F. G., Barnwell, W. H., II, and Hudson, R. P.: Allergic giant cell myocarditis complicating tuberculosis chemotherapy. Arch. Pathol. *91*:201, 1971.

653. Hubaytar, R. T., and Simpson, D. G.: Atrial fibrillation due to hypersensitivity due to para-aminosalicylic acid. Am. Rev. Respir. Dis. *86*:720, 1962.

654. Chatterjee, S. S., and Thakre, M. W.: Fiedler's myocarditis; Report of a fatal case following intramuscular injection of streptomycin. Tubercle *39*:240, 1958.

655. Schrock, C. G.: Lyme disease: Additional evidence of widespread distribution. Recognition of a tick-borne dermatitis-encephalitis-arthritis syndrome in an area of known Ixodes tick distribution. Am. J. Med. *72*:700, 1982.

656. Steere, A. C., Malawista, S. E., Newman, J. H., Spiebler, P. N., and Bartenhagen, N. H.: Antibiotic therapy in Lyme disease. Ann. Intern. Med. *93*:1, 1980.

657. Steere, A. C., Batsford, W. P., Weinberg, M., Alexander, J., Berger, H. J., Wolfson, S., and Malawista, S. E.: Lyme carditis: Cardiac abnormalities of Lyme disease. Ann. Intern. Med. *93*:8, 1980.

658. Peison, B., and Lowenstein, E. C.: Giant-cell myocarditis. N.Y. State J. Med. *73*:2259, 1973.

659. Davies, M. J., Pomerance, A., and Teare, R. D.: Idiopathic giant cell myocarditis—a distinctive clinicopathological entity. Br. Heart J. *37*:192, 1975.

660. Pyun, K. S., Kim, Y. H., Katzenstein, R. E., and Kikkawn, Y.: Giant cell myocarditis. Light and electron microscopic study. Arch. Pathol. *90*:181, 1970.

661. Nakahara, K.: Giant cell myocarditis. Hawaii Med. J. *34*:56, 1975.

662. Dragatakis, L. M., Klassen, J., Hüttner, I., Fraser, D. G., Poirier, N. L., and Klassen, G. A.: Autoimmune myocarditis: A clinical entity. Canad. Med. Assoc. J. *120*:317, 1979.

663. Graham, A. F., Rider, A. K., Caves, P. K., Stinson, E. B., Harrison, D. C., and Schroeder, J. S.: Acute rejection in the long-term cardiac transplant survival. Clinical diagnosis, treatment and significance. Circulation *49*:361, 1974.

664. Gripp, R. B., Stinson, E. B., Dong, E., Jr., Clark, D. A., and Shumway, N. E.: Acute rejection of the allografted human heart. Diagnosis and treatment. Ann. Thorac. Surg. *12*:113, 1971.

665. Caves, P. K., Stinson, E. B., Billingham, M. E., Rider, A. K., and Shumway, N. E.: Diagnosis of human cardiac allograft rejection by serial cardiac biopsy. J. Thorac. Cardiovasc. Surg. *66*:461, 1973.

666. Caves, P. K., Stinson, E. B., Graham, A. F., Billingham, M. E., Grehl, T. M., and Shumway, N. E.: Percutaneous transvenous endomyocardial biopsy. J.A.M.A. *225*:288, 1973.

667. Bieber, C. P., Stinson, E. B., Shumway, N. E., Payne, R., and Kosek, J.: Cardiac transplantation in man. VII. Cardiac allograft pathology. Circulation *41*:753, 1970.

668. Thomson, J. G.: Production of severe atheroma in a transplanted human heart. Lancet *2*:1088, 1969.

669. Griepp, R. B., Stinson, E. B., Bieher, C. P., Reitz, B. A., Copeland, J. G., Oyer, P. E., and Shumway, N. E.: Control of graft arteriosclerosis in human heart transplant recipients. Surgery *81*:262, 1977.

670. Kew, M. C., Tucker, R. B. K., Bersohn, I., and Seftel, H. C.: The heart in heatstroke. Am. Heart J. *77*:324, 1969.

671. Malamud, N., Haymaker, W., and Luster, R. F.: Heatstroke: A clinicopathological study of 125 fatal cases. Milit. Surg. *99*:397, 1946.

672. Duguid, H., Simpson, R. G., and Stowers, R. G.: Accidental hypothermia. Lancet *2*:1213, 1961.

673. Read, A. E., Ainslie-Smith, D., Gough, K. R., and Holmes, R.: Pancreatitis and accidental hypothermia. Lancet *2*:1219, 1961.

674. Biran, S., Hochmann, A., and Stern, S.: Therapeutic irradiation of the chest and electrocardiographic changes. Clin. Radiol. *20*:433, 1969.

675. McReynolds, R. A., Gold, G. L., and Roberts, W. C.: Coronary heart disease after mediastinal irradiation for Hodgkin's disease. Am. J. Med. *60*:39, 1976.

675a. Applefeld, M. M., and Wiernik, P. H.: Cardiac disease after radiation therapy for Hodgkin's disease: Analysis of 48 patients. Am. J. Cardiol. *51*:1679, 1983.

675b. Totterman, K. J., Pesonen, E., and Siltanen, P.: Radiation-related chronic heart disease. Chest *83*:875, 1983.

676. Arom, K. V., Bishop, V. S., Grover, F. L., and Trinkle, J. K.: Effect of therapeutic-dose irradiation of left ventricular function in conscious dogs. Ann. Thorac. Surg. *28*:166, 1979.

677. Weinstein, P., Greenwald, E. S., and Grossman, J.: Unusual cardiac reaction to chemotherapy following mediastinal irradiation in a patient with Hodgkin's disease. Am. J. Med. *60*:152, 1976.

678. Stewart, J. R., and Fajardo, C. F.: Radiation-induced heart disease. Clinical and experimental aspects. Radiol. Clin. North Am. *9*:511, 1971.

678a. Gottdiener, J. S. Katin, M. J., Borer, J. S., Bacharach, S. L., and Green, M. V.: Late cardiac effects of therepeutic mediastinal irradiation. Assessment by echocardiography and radionuclide ventriculography. N. Engl. J. Med. *308*:569, 1983.

678b. Burns, R. J., Bar-Shlomo, B-Z., Druck, M. N., Herman, J. G., Gilbert, B. W., Perrault, D. J., and McLaughlin, P. R.: Detection of radiation cardiomyopathy by gated radionuclide angiography. Am. J. Med. *74*:297, 1983.

679. Brosius, F. C., III, Waller, B. F., and Roberts, W. C.: Radiation heart disease: Analysis of 16 young (aged 15 to 33 years) necropsy patients who received over 3,500 rads to the heart. Am. J. Med. *70*:519, 1981.

680. Reeves, W. C., Cunningham, D., Schwiter, E. J., Abt, A. Skarlatos, S., Wood, M. A., and Whitesell, L.: Myocardial hydroxyproline reduced by early administration of methylprednisolone or ibuprofen to rabbits with radiation-induced heart disease. Circulation *65*:924, 1982.

42 PRIMARY TUMORS OF THE HEART

by Wilson S. Colucci, M.D., and Eugene Braunwald, M.D.

"A diagnosis is easy as long as you think of it."
SOMA WEISS

The incidence of primary tumors of the heart* in autopsy series ranges from 0.0017 to 0.28 per cent.[1–5] Thus, these tumors are far less common than metastatic tumors to the heart.[6] The diagnosis is further complicated by an extraordinary variety of nonspecific clinical signs and symptoms that are capable of masquerading as many other more common cardiovascular and systemic diseases (Table 42–1). Prior to the advent of modern cardiopulmonary bypass surgical techniques, the correct antemortem diagnosis of an intracardiac tumor was largely academic, since effective therapy was not possible. However, now that many cardiac tumors are curable by operation, it is critically important to establish this diagnosis whenever possible. During the last decade, major advances in noninvasive cardiovascular diagnostic techniques have greatly facilitated this task, and it is now possible safely and readily to screen patients suspected of having a cardiac tumor, in many cases arriving at a definitive diagnosis preoperatively. Nevertheless, a high index of suspicion remains the most important element in diagnosing a cardiac tumor.

HISTORICAL PERSPECTIVE

Although primary tumors of the heart have been recognized since at least as early as the sixteenth century,[6a] a correct antemortem diagnosis was not recorded until 1934.[7] The modern era of diagnosis began with the development of angiography, which permitted the visualization of cardiac tumors during life, and, in 1952, Goldberg et al. reported the first angiographic diagnosis of a left atrial myxoma.[8]

Before the development of modern open heart surgical techniques, there were only rare reports of the successful removal of cardiac tumors, most on the epicardial surface.[9,10] Prior to the use of cardiopulmonary bypass, most attempts to remove intracardiac were unsuccessful.[11] In 1954, Crafoord performed the first successful excision of an intracardiac tumor, a left atrial myxoma, utilizing total cardiopulmonary bypass under direct vision.[12] The successful surgical excision of a wide variety of cardiac tumors is now possible, and in many instances a complete cure has been achieved.[11,13–17]

Advances in the field of noninvasive cardiovascular diagnosis have had a major impact on the ability of physicians to recognize correctly cardiac tumors antemortem. A cardiac tumor was first demonstrated by M-mode echocardiography in 1959,[18] and, subsequently, echocardiography has become the cornerstone of the noninvasive diagnosis of cardiac tumors. Cross-sectional echocardiography has proved to be extremely useful and, in most situations, superior to M-mode echocardiography[18–24]. Radionuclide gated blood pool scanning[25–27] and computed tomography[28–32] have also been shown to be of value in the diagnosis of cardiac tumors. Thus, during the past quarter century it has become possible to diagnose and successfully treat the majority of primary cardiac tumors. An appreciation of the clinical features, therefore, is now of far greater importance than heretofore.

CLINICAL PRESENTATION (Table 42–1)

SYSTEMIC FINDINGS. Cardiac tumors can produce a broad array of systemic (i.e., noncardiac) findings, including fever, cachexia, malaise, arthralgias, Raynaud's phenomenon, rash, clubbing, and episodic bizarre behavior,[33–37] as well as systemic and pulmonary emboli. A variety

---

*Tumors arising elsewhere in the body and metastasizing to the pericardium and heart are discussed in Chapter 43 (Diseases of the Pericardium) and Chapter 49 (Hematologic-Oncologic Disorders and Heart Disease).

TABLE 42–1   CLINICAL PRESENTATIONS OF CARDIAC TUMORS

CARDIOVASCULAR SIGNS AND SYMPTOMS

1. Chest pain
2. Syncope
3. Congestive heart failure (left and/or right heart)
4. Valvular stenosis and/or insufficiency
5. Constrictive pericarditis
6. Pericardial effusion or tamponade
7. Arrhythmias
8. Conduction blocks
9. Intracardiac shunts

SYSTEMIC SIGNS AND SYMPTOMS

1. Systemic embolization
2. Pulmonary embolization and pulmonary hypertension
3. Fever
4. Cachexia and malaise
5. Arthralgia
6. Rash
7. Clubbing
8. Raynaud's phenomenon
9. Hypergammaglobulinemia
10. Anemia or polycythemia
11. Thrombocytosis or thrombocytopenia
12. Leukocytosis

of laboratory findings have been reported, including hypergammaglobulinemia, an elevated erythrocyte sedimentation rate, thrombocytosis, thrombocytopenia, polycythemia, leukocytosis, and anemia.[33–35,38–40] The mechanism by which cardiac tumors cause these systemic manifestations is not known with certainty, but it has been attributed to secretory products of the tumor or to tumor necrosis.[33,34,41] An immunological basis for the systemic manifestations is suggested by the finding of an increased titer of antimyocardial antibodies in a patient with a myxoma and a fall in the titer following surgical removal of the tumor.[42] A case of multiple myeloma has been attributed to continuous immunological stimulation by a left atrial myxoma.[43] Because the cardiac findings are nonspecific and may be subtle or absent, it is not unusual for these systemic findings to lead to a diagnosis of collagen vascular disease, infection, or noncardiac malignancy.[44–46] Rarely, myxomas may be superinfected by bacteria or fungi.[47]

EMBOLIC PHENOMENA.   The embolization of tumor fragments or of thrombi from the surface of a tumor is a frequent and often dramatic clinical occurrence.[48–55] Although myxomas are the source of most tumor emboli because of the combination of their friable consistency and intracavitary location, other types of cardiac tumors occasionally may embolize.

The distribution of tumor emboli depends upon the location of the tumor and the presence or absence of intracardiac shunts. Left-sided tumors embolize to the systemic circulation, resulting in infarction and hemorrhage of viscera, including the heart, as well as peripheral limb ischemia and vascular aneurysms.[35,48–57] The diagnosis of an intracardiac tumor may be made after histological examination of systemic embolic material,[48,51,56] and, therefore, it is of critical importance to make every effort to recover and examine embolic material. In some cases, particularly when petechiae are present, biopsy of skin or muscle[35] may demonstrate intravascular tumor emboli.

Multiple systemic emboli may mimic systemic vasculitis[35,44,46] or infective endocarditis,[45,52] especially when associated with other manifestations of a systemic illness such as fever, weight loss, arthralgias, elevated erythrocyte sedimentation rate, and elevated serum gamma globulins. The finding at angiography of multiple vascular aneurysms secondary to tumor emboli in the cerebral, renal, femoral, and coronary arteries may lead to the diagnosis of polyarteritis nodosa.[53] The neurological consequences of embolization include transient ischemic attacks, seizures, syncope, and cerebral, cerebellar, brain stem, spinal cord or retinal infarction.[54,55,58] The neurological event may occasionally be the first or only clinical manifestation of a cardiac tumor. An embolic stroke in a young person without evidence of cerebrovascular disease, particularly in the presence of sinus rhythm, should raise the possibility of intracardiac myxoma, as well as infective endocarditis (p. 1155) and prolapse of the mitral valve (p. 1094).

Right-sided cardiac tumors, and left-sided cardiac tumors proximal to left-to-right intracardiac shunts, may result in pulmonary emboli.[59–61] Indeed, serious pulmonary hypertension and secondary cor pulmonale due to chronic recurrent pulmonary emboli from a right atrial myxoma have been noted.[60] Clinically, the findings may be indistinguishable from pulmonary emboli secondary to venous thromboembolism (p. 1582). Although the findings on chest roentgenogram are relatively nonspecific,[61] perfusion lung scanning in such patients (pp. 390 and 1586) may be atypical of pulmonary embolism in two respects: (1) The tumor-produced perfusion defects may remain static for long periods of time, as opposed to typical pulmonary embolic disease in which the defects usually resolve over the course of a few weeks; and (2) there may be complete absence of flow to one lung in the presence of completely normal perfusion of the opposite lung, a pattern unusual with typical pulmonary emboli.[61,62]

Cardiac Manifestations

The specific signs and symptoms produced by tumors are more closely related to their precise anatomical location than to their histological types.[63] Thus, it is useful to consider the constellation of findings which is typical of each location. The presentation of *pericardial tumors* is considered on pages 1507 to 1509 and will not be discussed here except to point out that primary tumors of the myocardium and endocardium may extend into the pericardial space and produce many of the clinical manifestations of pericardial tumors, including hemorrhagic pericardial effusion and compression of the heart by the effusion or the tumor itself.

MYOCARDIAL TUMORS.   When clinically apparent, myocardial tumors most commonly result in disturbances of conduction or rhythm,[63–66] the precise nature of which is determined by the location of the tumor. Thus, tumors in the area of the atrioventricular node, typically angiomas and mesotheliomas, may produce atrioventricular (AV) conduction disturbances, including complete heart block and asystole, and can lead to sudden death.[64,65] A wide variety of arrhythmias may be produced, including atrial fibrillation or flutter, paroxysmal atrial tachycardia with or without block, nodal rhythm, ventricular premature beats, ventricular tachycardia, and ventricular fibrillation.[63] Intramural tumors may also produce symptoms by virtue of their size and location. Impairment of ventricular performance may simulate congestive, restrictive, or hypertrophic cardiomyopathy (Chap. 41).[67,68] Myocardial rupture rarely may result from tumor infiltration of the myocardial wall.

LEFT ATRIAL TUMORS. Mobile, predunculated, left atrial tumors may prolapse to variable degrees into the mitral valve orifice, resulting in obstruction to atrioventricular blood flow and, frequently, mitral regurgitation. The resultant signs and symptoms often mimic those of mitral valve disease[60] (Chap. 32) and include dyspnea, orthopnea, paroxysmal nocturnal dyspnea, acute pulmonary edema, cough, hemoptysis, chest pain, peripheral edema, and fatigue. However, weight loss, pallor, syncope, and sudden death—manifestations uncommon for mitral valve disease—also occur.[63] It is not unusual for the symptoms to be sudden in onset, intermittent, and related to the patient's body position.[52,63] Although the majority of symptoms produced by left atrial tumors are nonspecific, the occurrence of paroxysmal symptoms that arise characteristically in a particular body position and are out of proportion to the clinical findings should raise the possibility of a left atrial tumor.

Physical examination may disclose signs of pulmonary congestion, an S_4, a loud S_1 which is often widely split, a holosystolic murmur which is loudest at the apex and resembles mitral regurgitation, and a diastolic murmur resulting from the obstruction to flow through the mitral orifice produced by the tumor. In many cases an early diastolic sound, termed a tumor "plop," can be identified (Fig. 42–1). It is thought to be produced as the tumor strikes the endocardial wall or as its excursion is abruptly halted[70] (Fig. 3–15, p. 50). Although in most cases the tumor "plop" occurs later than the opening snap of the mitral valve and earlier than the S_3, it is not surprising that this sound is frequently confused with the opening snap or the S_3.

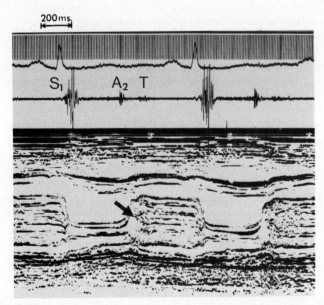

200 ms.

S_1 A_2 T

FIGURE 42–1 Simultaneous phonocardiogram and echocardiogram of a 68-year-old woman with a left atrial myxoma. S_1 is loud and prolonged as a result of tumor interference with mitral valve closure. A characteristic tumor "plop" (T) occurs approximately 100 msec after A_2 and corresponds with movement of the tumor into the mitral valve orifice (arrow) on the echocardiogram. (Courtesy of L.J. Sloss, M.D., Brigham and Women's Hospital, Boston.)

RIGHT ATRIAL TUMORS. Right atrial tumors frequently produce symptoms of right heart failure, including fatigue, peripheral edema, ascites, hepatomegaly, and prominent *a* waves in the jugular venous pulse.[52,71] The average time interval from the symptomatic presentation to the correct diagnosis of right atrial tumor is 3 years.[72] The development of right heart failure may be rapidly progressive and is often associated with new systolic or diastolic murmurs or both.[61,73] The murmurs are generally the result of tumor obstruction to tricuspid valve flow, or of tricuspid regurgitation caused by tumor interference with valve closure or valve destruction as a result of trauma by the tumor.[74] It is not surprising that right atrial tumors have been misdiagnosed as Ebstein's anomaly of the tricuspid valve, constrictive pericarditis, tricuspid stenosis, carcinoid syndrome, superior vena caval syndrome, and cardiomyopathy.[52] Pulmonary embolism and pulmonary hypertension occur and may simulate classic thromboembolic disease.[60-62] Right atrial hypertension may cause right-to-left shunting through a patent foramen ovale, with systemic hypoxia, cyanosis, clubbing, and polycythemia.[61,62,71]

Physical examination may reveal peripheral edema, superior vena caval syndrome, hepatomegaly, and ascites. An early diastolic rumbling murmur, alone or in combination with a holosystolic murmur secondary to tricuspid regurgitation, may be heard and may demonstrate respiratory or positional variation.[52] Because of the rarity of isolated rheumatic tricuspid valvular disease, the lack of other valvular findings should raise the question of a right atrial tumor.[71] A protodiastolic tumor plop has been described and is thought to be similar in etiology to that produced by the left atrial tumor.[74a] The jugular venous pressure may be elevated, and a prominent *a* wave and steep *y* descent have been described.[75]

RIGHT VENTRICULAR TUMORS. Right ventricular tumors often present with right heart failure as a result of obstruction to right ventricular filling or outflow. Clinical manifestations include peripheral edema, hepatomegaly, ascites, shortness of breath, syncope, and sudden death.[76]

A systolic ejection murmur at the left sternal border is usually found on physical examination.[77] A presystolic murmur[78] and a diastolic rumble[63] have been noted and are thought to be due to obstruction of the tricuspid valve. An S_3 may be audible, and a low-pitched diastolic sound that coincides with the maximal anterior excursion of the tumor has been ascribed either to tumor or to late closure of the pulmonary valve.[76] P_2 is often delayed, and its intensity may be normal, decreased, or increased. Tumor emboli to the pulmonary arteries may result in pulmonary hypertension, and the presence of tumor in the pulmonic valve orifice may lead to pulmonary regurgitation. The jugular veins are frequently distended with a prominent *a* wave and may demonstrate a Kussmaul's sign (p. 21).[78]

The cardiac findings often lead to a diagnosis of pulmonic stenosis, restrictive cardiomyopathy, or tricuspid regurgitation.[77,79] Whereas pulmonic stenosis is often asymptomatic and slowly progressive, the symptoms of right ventricular tumors are often rapidly progressive, and there is no poststenotic dilatation or systolic ejection click.

LEFT VENTRICULAR TUMORS. When left ventricular tumors are predominantly intramural in location, they are often asymptomatic, or they may present as conduction disturbances, arrhythmias, or interference with ventricular function. However, when the tumor also has a significant intracavitary component, there may be obstruction to left ventricular outflow, resulting in syncope and findings consistent with left ventricular failure. Atypical chest pain has also been reported on occasion and in some cases may reflect obstruction of a coronary artery either directly by tumor involvement or as a result of a tumor embolus to the coronary artery.

On physical examination a systolic murmur may be noted, and both the murmur and the blood pressure may vary with position.[80] Left ventricular tumors may simulate the findings of aortic stenosis, subaortic stenosis, hypertrophic cardiomyopathy,[67,68] endocardial fibroelastosis, and coronary artery disease.[81]

BENIGN VERSUS MALIGNANT TUMORS

The type of benign and malignant mesenchymal tumors that may develop in the heart is typical of that occurring in any mass of striated muscle and connective tissue. Although the exact incidence of each specific tumor type cannot be stated, about 75 per cent of all cardiac tumors are benign histologically and the remainder are malignant.[3,82,83] The majority of benign cardiac tumors are myxomas, followed in frequency by a wide variety (Table 42–2). Almost all malignant cardiac tumors are sarcomas, and of these the rhabdomyosarcoma and angiosarcoma are the most common forms.[4,82]

Although it is often difficult or impossible to differentiate histologically benign from malignant tumors prior to operation, certain findings may be helpful. Characteristics suggestive of malignancy include the presence of distant metastases, local mediastinal invasion, evidence of rapid growth in tumor size, hemorrhagic pericardial effusion, precordial pain, and location of the tumor on the right side of the heart. Benign tumors are more likely to occur in the left atrium and to grow slowly. Although benign tumors do not metastasize, distant tumor emboli may mimic peripheral or pulmonary metastases. The preoperative differentiation between benign and malignant tumors may occasionally be made by examination of peripheral tumor emboli recovered by arteriotomy or by biopsy of skin or muscle.[48,51,56]

Benign Tumors

MYXOMAS. As already pointed out, myxomas are the most common type of primary cardiac tumor, composing 30 to 50 per cent of the total in most pathological series.[3,4,82,84] They have been reported in patients ranging in age from 3 to 83 years, but the majority occur between the ages of 30 and 60 years. There are now several reports of the familial occurrence of myxomas,[24,49,85–87] and the observation of myxomas in a mother and her three sons suggests that this condition may be transmitted as an autosomal dominant.[85] Therefore, routine echocardiographic screening of asymptomatic first-degree relatives of patients with myxoma appears warranted. Multiple atrial and ventricular tumors appear to be more common in patients with a familial history of myxoma.[24]

The pathological features of myxoma are very similar to those of an organized thrombus, a finding which has led to the suggestion that myxomas are not true neoplasms but may represent one form of organization of an endocardial thrombus.[88] Most investigators, however, favor the view that myxomas are a true neoplastic process.[3,4,82,87,89] This view is supported by ultrastructural evidence,[90,91,92] the elaboration of factor VIII by myxoma cells,[93] and the fact that when cardiac myxomas are grown in tissue culture, a distinctive polygonal cell results that has the characteristics of a multipotential mesenchymal cell.[94] In addition, it has been argued that the ability of myxomas to recur and their occurrence in multiple sites, in the ventricles, and in families all favor a neoplastic nature. Although histologically benign, occasional reports suggest that myxomas have the ability to implant and grow at distant foci such as in brain or bone.[95,96]

Over 90 per cent of myxomas occur in the atria, with three to four times as many occurring on the left as on the right.[4] There are also several reports of biatrial tumors[97,98] and occasional reports of right ventricular, left ventricular, biventricular, and combined left atrial and left ventricular tumors.[4,99] A myxoma of the mitral valve has been reported.[100] The usual site of attachment of atrial myxomas is in the area of the fossa ovalis, although they have been found rarely on the posterior wall of the atrium.

The clinical signs and symptoms produced by cardiac myxomas include nonspecific manifestations, as discussed above, embolization, and mechanical interference with cardiac function, the precise nature of which is determined by the size and location of the tumor. The clinical presentation of cardiac myxoma in 130 patients reviewed at the Armed Forces Institute of Pathology is summarized in Table 42–3.

Pathology. Grossly, myxomas are generally pedunculated, with a fibrovascular stalk. Most sessile tumors probably represent the base

TABLE 42–2 RELATIVE INCIDENCE OF TUMORS OF THE HEART

Type	Number	Per Cent
Benign		
Myxoma	130	30.5
Lipoma	45	10.5
Papillary fibroelastoma	42	9.9
Rhabdomyoma	36	8.5
Fibroma	17	4.0
Hemangioma	15	3.5
Teratoma	14	3.3
Mesothelioma of the AV node	12	2.8
Granular cell tumor	3	–
Neurofibroma	3	–
Lymphangioma	2	–
Subtotal	319	75.1
Malignant		
Angiosarcoma	39	9.2
Rhabdomyosarcoma	26	6.1
Fibrosarcoma	14	3.3
Malignant lymphoma	7	1.6
Extraskeletal osteosarcoma	5	–
Neurogenic sarcoma	4	–
Malignant teratoma	4	–
Thymoma	4	–
Leiomyosarcoma	1	–
Liposarcoma	1	–
Synovial sarcoma	1	–
Subtotal	106	24.9
TOTAL	425	100.0

Modified from McAllister, H. A., and Fenoglio, J. J.: Tumors of the cardiovascular system. *In* Atlas of Tumor Pathology. Washington, D.C., Armed Forces Institute of Pathology, 1978. Fasc. 15, 2nd series.

TABLE 42–3 CLINICAL PRESENTATION OF CARDIAC
MYXOMA IN 130 PATIENTS°

Signs and symptoms of mitral valve disease	57
Embolic phenomena	36
No cardiac symptoms—incidental finding	16
Signs and symptoms of tricuspid valve disease	6
Sudden unexpected death	5
Pericarditis	4
Myoc ardial infarction	3
Signs and symptoms of pulmonary valve disease	2
Fever of undetermined origin	2

°One patient with multiple myxomas had signs and symptoms of mitral and
tricuspid valve disease.
Reproduced from McAllister, H. A., and Fenoglio, J. J.: Tumors of the
cardiovascular system. *In* Atlas of Tumor Pathology. Washington, D.C., Armed
Forces Institute of Pathology, 1978. Fasc. 15, 2d series.

of the pedicle, which remains after the body has embolized.[4] The tumors average 4 to 8 cm in diameter, although tumors of up to 15 cm
have been reported. Most myxomas are gelatinous and polypoid, although they may also be smooth and round with a glistening surface;
areas of hemorrhage are not unusual.

By *light microscopy*, the cells are uniform, small, and polygonal in
shape with round or oval nuclei and a moderate amount of cytoplasm. The cells are surrounded by myxomatous stroma composed
predominantly of an eosinophilic matrix which appears to be composed of an acid mucopolysaccharide similar to chondroitin-C.[3] The
cells and the stroma are frequently positive with periodic acid–Schiff
stain, whereas only stroma is stained with alcian blue stain.[82] Elastic
fibers, reticular fibers, smooth muscle cells, collagen, calcium, and
bone may be seen. Other cellular elements include lymphocytes,
plasma cells, mast cells, histiocytes, and, rarely, fibrocytes. Thin-
walled vessels simulating primitive capillaries are present. The surface of the tumor consists of the typical myxoma cells and, in some
cases, thrombus.

On electron microscopic examination, the myxoma cells demonstrate areas of intracellular junctions (zonulae adherentes), single nuclei with finely dispersed chromatin and nucleoli, rough endoplasmic
reticulum, free ribosomes, mitochondria, Golgi complexes, and cytoplasmic filaments.[4,90,101,102] On examination with scanning electron microscopy, myxomas are covered by endothelium and possess endothelium-lined crevices and clefts, features not seen in atrial
thrombus.[92]

Papillary Tumors of Heart Valves. Papillary tumors of the cardiac valves and adjacent endocardium, occasionally seen post mortem,
may result in clinically significant valvular dysfunction or, rarely, angina as a result of obstruction of a coronary ostium.[3,4,103] These lesions
have a characteristic frondlike appearance, may be up to 3 or 4 cm in
diameter, are single or multiple, and may occur on any valve; most
often the ventricular surface of semilunar valves and the atrial surface of AV valves are affected. Rarely, they may be present on papillary muscle, chordae tendineae, or endocardium.[104] The tricuspid
valve is most commonly involved in children and the aortic valve in
adults.[82] Histologically, the tumor is covered by endothelium that sur-
rounds a core of loose connective tissue consisting of an acid mucopolysaccharide matrix, smooth muscle cells, and collagen and elastic
fibers.[4] The pathogenesis of these lesions is unsettled, but it appears
that they may originate from organized mural thrombi.[3,4,88,104] Papillary
tumors are generally distinguished from *Lambl's excrescences*, which
are ubiquitous acellular deposits covered by a single layer of endothelium and found on heart valves at the site of endothelial damage
in over 70 per cent of adults[3,4,105,106]

Rhabdomyomas. These are the most common cardiac tumors of
infants and children, the large majority occurring in patients younger
than 1 year.[107] Morphological evidence suggests that rhabdomyomas
are actually myocardial hamartomas rather than true neoplasms.[107,108]
Consistent with this view is the complete lack of any mitotic activity[107]
and the observation at the ultrastructural level that the characteristic
glycogen-laden cells are typical of immature myocytes.[108] Alternatively, it has been suggested that rhabdomyomas may represent a nodular form of a diffuse cardiac glycogen storage disease.[109]

One-third to one-half of patients with cardiac rhabdomyoma have tuberous sclerosis; adenoma sebaceum and benign kidney tumors
(angiomyolipomas and hamartomas) are seen less frequently.[3,107]
Rhabdomyomas causing significant intracavitary obstruction may re-

sult in death within the first 24 hours of life, whereas less severe involvement may remain asymptomatic or become apparent during
infancy or early childhood.[107]

Rhabdomyomas invariably involve the ventricles, affecting the left
and right sides equally. Ninety per cent are multiple, and in 30 per
cent there is involvement of at least one of the atria. Approximately
50 per cent of rhabdomyomas are large enough to cause significant
obstruction of a cardiac chamber or valvular orifice.[107] Nonspecific
clinical manifestations—including cardiomegaly, right and/or left ventricular failure, and S_3, S_4, and systolic or diastolic murmurs—may
mimic mitral stenosis, mitral atresia, aortic stenosis, subaortic stenosis, and infundibular pulmonic stenosis.[110]

Rhabdomyomas are yellow-gray and range from 1 to 20 mm in diameter. The microscopic hallmark, termed the "spider cell," is a cell
containing a central cytoplasmic mass that is suspended by fine fibrillar processes radiating to the periphery, thus giving the appearance
of a spider hanging in a net.[3] The cytoplasm is rich in glycogen and
stains positively with periodic acid–Schiff reagent.[4] Electron microscopy demonstrates myofibrils, cytoplasmic and mitochondrial glycogen,
and apparent intercellular junctions similar to intercalated disks.[107]

Fibromas and Hamartomas. Fibromas are benign, connective
tissue tumors that occur predominantly in children. The majority occur
before the age of 10 years, and about 40 per cent are diagnosed in
infants less than 1 year of age.[111] Males and females appear equally
affected. Fibromas constitute the second most common type of primary cardiac tumor occurring in infants and children.[110,111,112] Whether
fibromas represent hamartomas or true neoplasms is debated.[112,113]
The histological criteria for diagnosis are not uniformly agreed upon,
and therefore several designations are employed, including fibromyxoma, fibroelastic hamartoma, embryonic mesenchymoma, fibroma,
and fibrous rhabdomyoma.[82]

Almost all fibromas occur within the ventricular myocardium—most
frequently within the anterior free wall of the left ventricle or the interventricular septum and much less often in the posterior left ventricular wall or right ventricle.[3] Typically, they are gray, firm, circumscribed,
not capsulated, and range in size from 3 to 7 cm. Grossly, they resemble fibroids and exhibit a whorled appearance on cut sections.
Microscopically, cardiac fibromas consist of elongated fibroblasts
admixed with fibrous tissue consisting of collagen and elastic fibers.
Their cellularity is variable, and mitotic figures are rarely, if ever,
seen. Fibrous tissue is intermingled with adjacent myocardial fibers at
the margins of the lesion.[112] Calcification and fossae of bone formation may be seen microscopically and occasionally radiographically.

Although fibromas may be incidental findings at postmortem examination, approximately 70 per cent at some time show signs or symptoms due to mechanical interference with intracardiac flow, ventricular
contraction, or conduction disturbances.[3] Clinical manifestations are
protean and include murmurs, atypical chest pain, congestive heart
failure and signs of subaortic stenosis, valvular or infundibular pulmonic stenosis with right ventricular hypertrophy,[114] tricuspid stenosis,[111]
conduction disturbances, and sudden death.

Lipomas and Lipomatous Hypertrophy of the Atrial Septum.
Lipomas occur at all ages and with equal frequency in both sexes.
Most range in diameter from 1 to 15 cm, although some have been
reported to weigh more than 2 kg.[10,115] Most tumors are sessile or
polypoid in configuration and occur in the subendocardium or subepicardium, although about one-fourth are completely intramuscular.[2]
Subendocardial tumors with intracavitary extension produce symptoms that are characteristic of their location, whereas subepicardial
tumors may cause compression of the heart and pericardial effusion.
The most common chambers affected are the left ventricle, right atrium, and interatrial septum.[82] Intramural tumors may be asymptomatic
or result in arrhythmias, AV or intraventricular conduction disturbances, or mechanical interference.[116] Many tumors are clinically silent and are found only at autopsy or become apparent on a routine
chest roentgenogram.

Microscopically, the lesions are usually well encapsulated, composed of typical mature fat cells, and occasionally contain fibrous
connective tissue (fibrolipoma), muscular tissue (myolipoma), or vacu-
olated brown fat resembling a hibernoma.

Whereas lipomas are true neoplasms, a condition termed *lipomatous hypertrophy of the interatrial septum* represents the occurrence
of an accumulation of mature adipose tissue within the interatrial septum.[4,117,118] These lesions range from 1 to 6.5 cm in dimension, most
often protrude into the right atrium, and are more common in obese,
elderly, or female patients.[118] A variety of atrial arrhythmias have been

attributed to these lesions, but a cause-and-effect relationship has been difficult to establish.[117-119] Rarely, the lesion may result in a clinical syndrome resembling congestive heart failure, constrictive pericarditis, or pericardial effusion.[4,120] Since this lesion may occasionally be detected by cineangiography or other diagnostic techniques, the major clinical dilemma is the differential diagnosis and treatment of an intraatrial filling defect.

Angiomas. Benign vascular tumors, including hemangiomas, lymphangiomas, and angioreticulomas, are extremely rare.[121] Anatomically, they may occur in any part of the heart but usually are intramural, often in the interventricular septum[82,83] or AV node, where they may cause complete heart block and sudden death.[122] Cardiac tamponade due to hemopericardium may be the presenting clinical syndrome. More commonly found in the right heart chambers, hemangiomas are generally sessile or polypoid subendocardial nodules ranging from 2 to 3.5 cm in diameter. Histologically, the tumors consist of endothelium-lined spaces which may contain blood, lymph, or thrombi; they are classified according to the predominant type of proliferating vascular channel.

Benign Cystic Tumors. Benign epithelium lined cystic tumors, including mesotheliomas and benign epithelium-lined cysts, occur within or immediately adjacent to the AV node.[64] The embryogenetic and histological classifications of these tumors are controversial and preclude a precise classification.

Mesotheliomas are small (generally <15 mm) cystic lesions lined with mesothelial epithelium which is devoid of mitotic activity but may have secretory function.[64,82] They typically present during the first or second decade, exhibit a marked female predominance, and are frequently noted at the time of puberty or pregnancy, thus suggesting a hormonal role in their development and expression.[66] Because of their location in the area of the AV node, they most often present as progressive heart block, syncope, or sudden death, although many are asymptomatic and consistent with a long life. Ventricular tachycardia progressing to ventricular fibrillation has been observed, perhaps explaining the poor results obtained with cardiac pacemakers in this condition.[64,66]

Epithelium-lined cysts are extremely rare lesions which are usually an incidental postmortem finding.[2,82] They are 4 to 25 mm in diameter and are lined with cuboidal or columnar ciliated epithelium.

Malignant Tumors—Sarcomas

About one-fourth of all cardiac tumors exhibit typically malignant histological characteristics and invasive behavior[2-4,82] (Table 42–2). Virtually all of these are sarcomas, thus making these tumors second in overall frequency only to myxomas. Sarcomas may occur at any age but are most common between the third and fifth decades and show no sex preference. In decreasing order of frequency, the chambers involved are the right atrium, left atrium, right ventricle, left ventricle, and interventricular septum.[82]

Sarcomas derive from mesenchyme and therefore may display a wide variety of morphological types which may be subtyped as angiosarcoma, rhabdomyosarcoma, fibrosarcoma, and lymphosarcoma.[4,82,123-125]

From a clinical viewpoint, sarcomas characteristically display a rapidly downhill course. Death most often occurs from a few weeks to 2 years after the onset of symptoms. These tumors proliferate rapidly and generally cause death through widespread infiltration of the myocardium, obstruction of flow within the heart, or distant metastases. About 75 per cent of all patients with cardiac sarcomas have pathological evidence of distant metastases at the time of death.[126] The most frequent sites are the lungs, thoracic lymph nodes, mediastinum, and vertebral column; less often, the liver, kidneys, adrenals, pancreas, bone, spleen, and bowel are involved.

The cardiac findings are determined primarily by the location of the tumor and by the extent of intracavitary obstruction. Typical presentations include progressive, unex-

plained, congestive heart failure, particularly of the right side; precordial pain; pericardial effusion; tamponade; arrhythmias; conduction disturbances; obstruction of the venae cavae; and sudden death. Tumors limited to the myocardium without intracavitary extension may produce no cardiac symptoms or may cause arrhythmias and conduction disturbances. Because of the rapid growth potential of sarcomas, they commonly extend into the cardiac chambers, the pericardial space, or both. In about 20 per cent of cases, the tumor is sessile or polypoid in configuration.[127] When there is extension into the pericardial space, hemorrhagic pericardial effusion is common, and tamponade may occur. Because the right side of the heart is most commonly affected, sarcomas frequently cause signs of right heart failure as a result of obstruction of the right atrium, right ventricle, or tricuspid or pulmonic valves. In addition, obstruction of the superior vena cava may result in swelling of the face and upper extremities, whereas obstruction of the inferior vena cava may result in visceral congestion.

Angiosarcomas. Included within this category are malignant hemangioendotheliomas, angiosarcomas, Kaposi's sarcomas, angioreticuloendotheliomas, and cavernous angiosarcomas.[82] All 40 patients in one series were adults.[128] In distinction to most other cardiac sarcomas, in which the sex distribution is equal, there appears to be a 2:1 male-to-female ratio among patients with angiosarcomas.[4] These tumors have a striking predilection for the right atrium, most often arising from the interatrial septum,[129] and may be infiltrative or polypoid in nature. Microscopically, angiosarcomas are characterized by ill-defined anastomotic vascular channels which are lined with atypical, often heaped-up, endothelial cells.[130] By electron microscopy, immature endothelial cells, primitive pericytes, and undifferentiated mesenchymal cells may be identified.[131] Associated cavernous hemangiomas of the liver have been reported.[2]

Rhabdomyosarcomas. These are tumors of striated muscle which most often diffusely infiltrate the myocardium but which may also, on occasion, form a polypoid extension into the cardiac chambers and therefore have been clinically mistaken for myxoma.[2] Rhabdomyoblasts are the histological hallmark of this tumor, and 20 to 30 per cent of the tumors have cross-striations.[82,84] "Strap cells," "tennis racquet cells," and "spider cells" with periodic acid–Schiff–positive cytoplasm may be seen.[82]

Fibrosarcomas. Fibrosarcomas of the heart resemble the soft, whitish "fish flesh" characteristic of this tumor type elsewhere in the body. They may contain areas of hemorrhage and necrosis and extensively infiltrate the heart, often involving more than one cardiac chamber. A thrombus may form in an obstructed pulmonary vein or the vena cava or over the mural surface of the tumor.[3]

Lymphosarcomas. Although cardiac involvement of systemic lymphoma has been reported in 25 to 36 per cent of cases, primary lymphosarcoma involving only the heart or pericardium appears to be much less common.[132] Myocardial infiltration by lymphoma may be nodular or diffuse, and the clinical syndrome of hypertrophic cardiomyopathy has been mimicked.[133]

DIAGNOSTIC TECHNIQUES

Although certain clinical manifestations may be suggestive of a cardiac tumor, no clinical finding or set of findings is pathognomonic. Furthermore, the majority of cardiac tumors produce signs and symptoms typical of the common forms of heart disease. The development of modern diagnostic methods has had a major impact on the diagnosis and hence the natural history of cardiac tumors. Whereas only 20 years ago the diagnosis of a cardiac tumor was rarely made ante mortem, it is now not unusual for cardiac tumors to be diagnosed and cured in patients who are totally asymptomatic or without signs of cardiovascular disease.[134-136] Although cardiac catheterization made possible the definitive preoperative diagnosis of cardiac tumor, it was not until the advent of echocardiography that it was feasible to evaluate all patients suspected of this diagnosis. Both M-mode and two-dimensional echocardiography are effective screening techniques. However, two-dimensional echocardiography is more sensitive and provides considerably more information regarding the site of tumor attachment, pattern of tumor movement, and size. In many centers, the information provided by two-dimensional echocardiography is considered sufficient to proceed directly to surgery without cardiac catheterization.[19,20,22] M-mode echocardiography alone does not provide adequate information in the majority of cases to proceed to surgery without catheterization, nor should catheterization be omitted in the absence of a technically adequate two-dimensional echocardiographic study that has visualized all four cardiac chambers. As discussed below, gated blood pool scanning and cardiac computed tomography may provide enough information in conjunction with M-mode or two-dimensional echocardiography to allow a direct move to surgery. However, more experience is required with both techniques in order to define their diagnostic sensitivity and specificity.

It is imperative that noninvasive evaluation, preferably by two-dimensional echocardiography, be performed whenever cardiac catheterization is planned and the diagnosis of cardiac tumor is considered. Thus, when left atrial myxoma is suspected, it is safest to visualize the left atrium by injecting the contrast agent into the pulmonary artery and filming during the levophase. It is particularly important to avoid the transseptal approach, since this risks dislodgement of fragments of tumor that may be attached in the region of a fossa ovalis. Furthermore, since cardiac tumors may be multiple and present in more than one chamber, all four chambers should be visualized noninvasively prior to cardiac catheterization whenever possible. Because the diagnosis of cardiac tumor may be missed at cardiac catheterization, it has been suggested that echocardiography be performed routinely before cardiac catheterization, particularly in patients with the clinical diagnosis of mitral stenosis.

RADIOLOGICAL EXAMINATION

Cardiac tumors may display several findings on plain chest roentgenograms. These include alterations in cardiac contour, changes in overall cardiac size, specific chamber enlargement, alterations in pulmonary vascularity, and intracardiac calcification.[137-139] The cardiac contour may be normal, may display generalized or specific chamber enlargement that mimics virtually any type of valvular heart disease, or may demonstrate a bizarre appearance. Pericardial effusions are rather common and generally indicate invasion of the pericardial space by a malignant tumor. Mediastinal widening, due to hilar and paramediastinal adenopathy, may indicate spread of a malignant cardiac tumor.[137] A bumpy, irregular, or fuzzy cardiac border may be seen when pericardium is involved. Cardiac enlargement may reflect rapid tumor growth, particularly in the case of sarcomas, whereas specific chamber enlargement is frequently due to intracavitary obstruction, particularly by pedunculated tumors such as myxomas. Thus, left atrial myxoma may produce the radiological pattern characteristic of mitral stenosis. Occasionally a large tumor mass displaces the heart and may simulate enlargement of a specific chamber.

Calcification visible by roentgenographic methods may occur with several types of cardiac tumor, including rhabdomyomas, fibromas, hamartomas, teratomas, myxomas, and angiomas.[138-140] Visualization of intracardiac calcium in an infant or a child is unusual and should immediately raise the question of an intracardiac tumor. Cardiac fluo-

roscopy and laminagraphy may be helpful in differentiating calcification of cardiac tumor from that of other structures, such as cardiac valves, coronary arteries, pericardium, and mural thrombus. Occasionally, calcified atrial polypoid tumors may be seen to prolapse into the ventricle during diastole.[141] Fluoroscopy is also useful in differentiating cardiac tumor from ventricular aneurysm, both of which may result in a localized protrusion on plain chest roentgenogram. However, on fluoroscopic examination, cardiac tumors do not display the paradoxical motion during ventricular contraction that is characteristic of ventricular aneurysm.

ECHOCARDIOGRAPHY
(See Figs. 5–79 and 5–80, p. 134).

M-Mode. M-mode echocardiography has been extensively used in the diagnosis and evaluation of cardiac tumors.[142-149,149a] This technique is most useful for pedunculated tumors of the left atrium, primarily left atrial myxomas, and is generally less sensitive for the detection of intramural and sessile tumors.

Left atrial tumors are often pedunculated myxomas that traverse the mitral valve during diastole.[142] Thus, during diastole when the tumor extends into the atrioventricular canal, a mass of echoes is visualized behind the anterior leaflet of the mitral valve (Figs. 42–1 and 5–79, p. 134). During systole, the mitral valve is closed, the tumor is confined to the left atrium, and therefore, the mass of echoes is no longer seen in the atrioventricular canal. Posterior descent of the anterior mitral leaflet may also be slow as a result of mechanical interference by the tumor. In some cases the tumor is less mobile and therefore may not traverse the mitral orifice; it may be detected only if the left atrium is carefully imaged from several different angles.[143] It has been suggested that in order to diagnose left atrial tumors reliably the ultrasound beam should be directed in turn (1) through both leaflets of the mitral valve, (2) through the aorta and left atrium, (3) in an intermediate direction through the anterior mitral leaflet and left atrium, and (4) caudally, with a suprasternal transducer position.[142]

Right atrial tumors generally appear as echoes behind the tricuspid valve, prolapsing into the right ventricle during diastole.[74,144] Because myxomas frequently occur biatrially, it is vital that when the diagnosis of myxoma is suspected the echocardiographic examination be thorough and include both atria.[19,98,145]

Ventricular tumors are less frequently diagnosed by M-mode echocardiography.[99] Left ventricular tumors may be visualized as a mass of echoes interposed between the interventricular septum and the anterior leaflet of the mitral valve and are present during both systole and diastole. Large left ventricular tumors may cause apparent filling of the left ventricular cavity by an echo-dense mass. *Right ventricular tumors* may be visualized as intracavitary echoes in the right ventricle and, in addition, may result in a paradoxical square wave motion of the interventricular septum.[78,147] Although reverberations produced by a right ventricular mass may be imaged in a position posterior to the tricuspid valve, the right atrial cavity is free of echoes in such cases.[147]

Two-Dimensional Echocardiography (Fig. 42–2). This technique (p. 134) provides substantial advantages over conventional M-mode echocardiography for the diagnosis and preoperative evaluation of intracardiac tumors.[20-24,148,148a] These advantages are derived primarily from the ability to evaluate tumor size, point of attachment, and

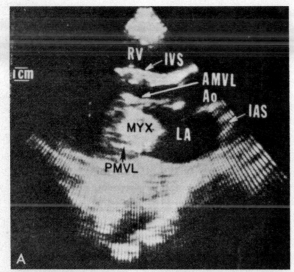

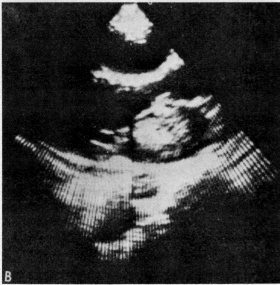

FIGURE 42–2 Two-dimensional sagittal echocardiogram, showing highly mobile tumor, 3 × 4 cm, prolapsing well into the left ventricle during diastole (*A*, top) and returning to left atrium (LA) during systole (*B*, bottom). Note normal-appearing echoes of mitral valve. RV = right ventricle; IVS = interventricular septum; AMVL = anterior mitral valvular leaflet; Ao = aorta; IAS = interatrial septum; MYX = myxoma; and PMVL = posterior mitral valvular leaflet. (From Lappe, D.L., et al.: Two-dimensional echocardiographic diagnosis of left atrial myxoma. Chest *74*:55, 1978.)

mobility.[19] In addition, the cross-sectional method is more sensitive than the M-mode for the detection of small tumors[19] and is especially useful in the detection of left ventricular tumors and tumors that do not prolapse through the mitral or tricuspid valve orifices. Phased-array techniques may facilitate the differentiation between left atrial thrombus and myxoma, because the former typically produces a layered appearance and is generally situated in the posterior portion of the atrium, whereas the latter is often mottled in appearance[150] and rarely occurs in the posterior portion of the atrium. In some atrial myxomas, areas of echolucency may be seen within the tumor mass, corresponding to areas of hemorrhage within the tumor.[151] Since these areas of echolucency are not found in thrombotic or infective lesions, this finding may be of value in the differential diagnosis of an intraatrial mass.

Radionuclide Imaging (Fig. 42–3). Gated blood pool scanning has been used to identify atrial, ventricular, and intramuscular tumors.[25–27,152,153] Radionuclide ventriculography generally has a lower rate of resolution than does echocardiography or contrast injection angiography and therefore may be less sensitive for the detection of small filling defects. However, radionuclide ventriculography may provide clear visualization of filling defects in some cases when other methods are nondiagnostic, particularly in the case of ventricular or intramural tumors.[25,26] In some cases, gated blood pool scanning may provide more detailed information regarding myocardial geometry and tumor size and location than that obtained by echocardiography.[25] Mobile left atrial tumors may be seen to prolapse into the left ventricle during diastole.[25] Thus, gated blood pool scanning may, in some cases, provide information complementary to that obtained by echocardiography.[25–27]

Computed Tomography (p. 189). Computed tomography of the heart has been used in several cases to demonstrate cardiac tumors[28–32] (Fig. 42–4). Although more experience will be necessary in order to establish its role, certain advantages and disadvantages are already apparent. The former include a high degree of tissue discrimination, which may allow definition of the degree of intramural tumor extension; evaluation of the extracardiac structures; and the ability to construct images in any plane. Disadvantages include poor resolution consequent to movement and long exposure times, and patient exposure to contrast agents and radiation.[29] At present, computed tomography appears to be most useful in the evaluation of suspected malignant tumors in order to determine the degree of myocardial invasion and the involvement of pericardial and extracardiac structures.

Other Noninvasive Methods. Cardiac tumors cannot be diagnosed by phonocardiography, apex cardiography, or jugular venous or carotid pulse analysis. However, when valvular or myocardial disease is suspected on clinical grounds, certain atypical findings may raise the question of cardiac tumor. The intensity of the systolic or diastolic murmur caused by a left atrial myxoma is often exquisitely sensitive to positional change, a finding atypical of valvular heart disease.[63] The first heart sound may be delayed as a consequence of an elevated left atrial pressure, as in mitral stenosis (p. 1068) It is often intense and widely split, and an early systolic sound may occur, representing tumor movement toward the atrium during systole.[154] In addition, a tumor "plop" may be present about 100 msec after the second heart sound, which appears to result from the sudden tensing

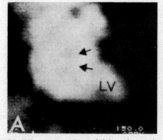
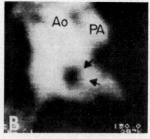

FIGURE 42–3 Gated blood pool scan of a patient with a left atrial myxoma. During systole (*A*) the tumor is faintly visualized in the left atrium (arrows). However, during diastole (*B*) the tumor is clearly seen as a filling defect in the left ventricle (arrows). Ao = aorta; PA = pulmonary artery; LV = left ventricle. (From Pohost, G.M., et al.: Detection of left atrial myxoma by gated radionuclide cardiac imaging. Circulation *55*:88, 1977, by permission of the American Heart Association, Inc.)

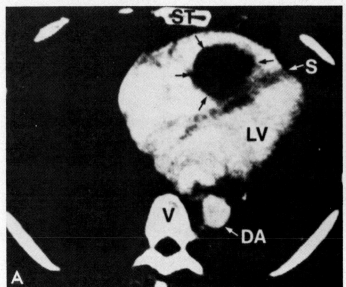

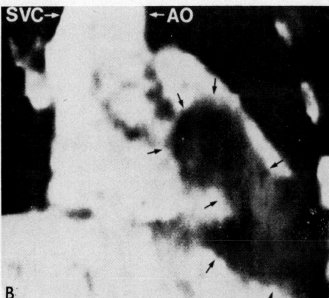

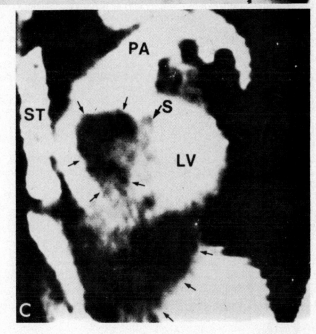

FIGURE 42–4 A, Transverse computed tomographic (CT) scan through the right and left ventricles (RV and LV) during IV infusion of 76 per cent diatrizoate of a patient with a cardiac liposarcoma. The patient's right side is projected at the left side of the illustration, as in a conventional radiograph of the chest. The sternum (ST) and vertebral body (V) are marked for orientation. Contrast fills the ventricles and descending aorta (DA). The large, low-density tumor (arrows) occupies the cavity of the right ventricle and lies alongside the interventricular septum (S). B, Reformatted CT image made from contiguous transverse CT slices taken during contrast infusion. The plane of reformatting passes through the RV, corresponding to the right anterior oblique projection of an angiocardiogram. The low-density tumor (arrows) forms a pedunculated mass in the cavity of the RV with invasion through the myocardium of the apex of the RV into the pericardial sac. The lowermost arrows indicate the intrapericardial component of the tumor. SVC = superior vena cava; AO = ascending aorta. C, Reformatted CT image made from contiguous transverse CT slices taken during contrast infusion. The plane of reformatting passes through both ventricles, corresponding to the left anterior oblique projection of an angiocardiogram, but the plane is also angled along the axis extending from the right ventricular apex to the outflow tract, roughly corresponding to a half-axial projection. The pedunculated, low-density tumor (arrows) is again visualized in the right ventricular cavity and extending through the apex into the pericardial sac (lowermost arrows). ST = sternum; PA = pulmonary artery; S = interventricular septum; LV = left ventricular cavity. (Reproduced with permission from Godwin, J.D., et al.: Computed tomography: A new method for diagnosing tumor of the heart. Circulation 63:448, 1981.)

of the tumor stalk as it prolapses into the left ventricle during diastole or from the tumor striking the myocardium[63,70] (Figs. 42–1 and 3–15, p. 50). The tumor "plop" *precedes* the end of the rapidly filling wave of the apex cardiogram and can thereby be differentiated from an S_3; as noted, it usually occurs later than an opening snap. Systolic time intervals are usually consistent with a reduced stroke volume (p. 54). The apexcardiography often shows a deep notch on the upstroke which occurs at the time of extrusion of the tumor through the mitral valve in early systole.

Right atrial tumors may also result in a widely split first heart sound and an early systolic sound. The second heart sound may be paradoxically split as a result of early pulmonic valve closure.[155] A tumor "plop" and systolic and diastolic murmurs which are increased by inspiration may also occur with right atrial tumors.[154] The jugular venous pulse tracing may reflect obstruction of the tricuspid orifice, demonstrating an accentuated *a* wave, attenuation of the *x* descent, or an early, broad *v* wave.[154]

ANGIOGRAPHY

Cardiac catheterization and selective angiocardiography are not necessary in all cases of cardiac tumors, since, as discussed above, in many cases adequate preoperative information may be obtained by echocardiography, gated blood pool scanning, and/or computed tomography. However, several circumstances exist in which the risk of cardiac catheterization is outweighed by the supplemental information it may provide. These situations include cases in which (1) noninvasive evaluation has not been fully adequate in defining tumor location or attachment; (2) all four cardiac chambers have not been adequately visualized noninvasively; (3) a malignant cardiac tumor is considered likely; or (4) other cardiac lesions may coexist with a cardiac tumor and possibly dictate a different surgical approach. For instance, when a malignant cardiac tumor is suspected, cardiac angiography may provide valuable information regarding the degree of myocardial, vascular, and/or pericardial invasion. Likewise, in certain cases, such as the presence of pulmonary hypertension or the coexistence of significant valvular or coronary artery lesions, cardiac catheterization and angiography may provide information that significantly affects the surgical approach.

The major angiographic findings in patients with cardiac tumors include (1) compression or displacement of cardiac chambers or large vessels, (2) deformity of cardiac chambers, (3) intracavitary filling defects, (4) marked variations in myocardial thickness, (5) pericardial effusion, and (6) local alterations in wall motion.[137,138] Displacement of the cardiac chambers or the great vessels without deformation of the internal contour may be observed in both benign and malignant tumors, whereas deformation of a cardiac chamber usually indicates an infiltrating malignant lesion.[138] The most frequent angiographic findings are intracavitary filling defects, which may be either fixed or mobile. Fixed defects may be lobulated or appear as a coarse nodularity of the myocardium often difficult to distinguish from a mural thrombus. Such defects may reflect endocardial tumors with broad attachments or intramural tumors with intracavitary extension. Mobile intracavitary defects are usually pedunculated tumors, typically myxomas, although the stalk may be difficult to visualize. Such tumors may prolapse into the atrioventricular valve orifice during diastole (Fig. 42–5) or, in the case of ventricular tumors, into the left ventricular outflow tract during systole. An atrial ball thrombus may mimic a pedunculated tumor but is more likely to be associated with clot in the atrial appendage.

A localized increase in myocardial wall thickness, especially when accompanied by a pericardial effusion, suggests an infiltrating malignant tumor. It is often difficult to differentiate myocardial thickening from pericardial effusion, but this may be aided by observation of the thickness of the right atrial wall. Since the right atrial wall is seldom infiltrated by tumor, the finding of right atrial thickening to greater than 5 mm suggests a pericardial effusion.[138] In myocardial infiltration, localized areas of disordered wall motion may also be noted by cineangiography. Coronary arteriography may in some cases allow visualization of the vascular supply of the tumor, thus demarcating the extent of tumor invasion, the source of its blood supply, and its relation to the coronary arteries. However, the vascular pattern of cardiac tumors has not proved to be a useful sign of malignancy.[138]

False-negative angiographic studies generally occur when the diagnosis is not suspected prior to catheterization.[23,142] False-positive studies are most often the result of thrombus, but may also be produced by many entities: such as streaming of nonopaque venous blood, a hematoma in the atrial septum, an aneurysm of the muscular or membranous ventricular septum, Bernheim syndrome, congenital septal dysplasia, and hydatid cysts of the interventricular septum.[138,156]

The major risk of angiography is peripheral embolization due to dislodgement of a fragment of tumor or of an associated throm-

bus.[138,157] Therefore, the thorough evaluation of all cardiac chambers by *noninvasive* methods prior to catheterization is to be recommended in patients suspected of having cardiac tumors so that contrast material can be injected into the chamber proximal (upstream) to the location of the tumor.[138] The transseptal approach to the left atrium (p. 283) is particularly hazardous because of the frequent occurrence of left atrial myxomas in the region of the fossa ovalis.

TREATMENT AND PROGNOSIS

BENIGN TUMORS. Operative excision is the treatment of choice for most benign cardiac tumors and in many cases results in a complete cure.[4,11,13,14,17] Although many tumors are histologically benign, all cardiac tumors are potentially lethal as a result of intracavitary or valvular obstruction, peripheral embolization, and disturbances of rhythm or conduction. Unfortunately, it is not unusual for patients to die or experience a major complication while awaiting operation, and therefore it is mandatory to carry out the operation promptly after the diagnosis has been established.

Although some epicardial tumors may be removed without the aid of extracorporeal circulation, most mural and intracavitary tumors must be excised under direct vision, with use of the heart-lung machine.[11] Closed approaches, although occasionally used in the past,[158] are not now recommended because of increased risk of dislodging tumor fragments. In addition, excision cannot be as complete, and adequate inspection of the other cardiac chambers for additional tumors is not possible.

The dislodgement of tumor fragments constitutes a major risk of operation and may result in peripheral emboli or the dispersion of micrometastases, which may seed peripherally. To reduce this risk, manipulation of the heart prior to cardiopulmonary bypass should be minimized. Some surgeons recommend that venous cannulation for cardiopulmonary bypass be performed via the femoral or azygous veins rather than through the right atrium in order to avoid dislodging an unsuspected right atrial tumor.[121] In addition, the tumor should be removed en bloc when possible, and the chamber then irrigated well with saline.

Atrial Myxomas. Numerous reports document complete cure of left and right atrial myxomas with follow-up periods of 10 to 15 years.[4,11,16,17] However, in about 1 to 5 per cent of cases, a recurrence or second cardiac myxoma has been reported following resection of the initial myxoma.[159] Possible etiologies of the second tumor include incomplete excision of the original tumor with regrowth, growth from a second "pretumorous" focus, or intracardiac implantation from the original tumor.[159] Because of the first two possibilities, some surgeons advocate excision of the entire region of the fossa ovalis and repair of the resultant atrial septal defect in order to remove presumably high concentrations of "pretumor" cells thought to be located in that region.[160,161] Other surgeons have reported equally successful long-term recurrence-free periods with simple excision of the tumor and a small rim at the base.[13,16] Regardless of the extent of tumor resection performed, such patients should receive periodic long-term follow-up by cross-sectional echocardiography.

Other Benign Tumors. Although the majority of operations for cardiac tumors have been performed for atrial myxomas owing to their high frequency, successful exci-

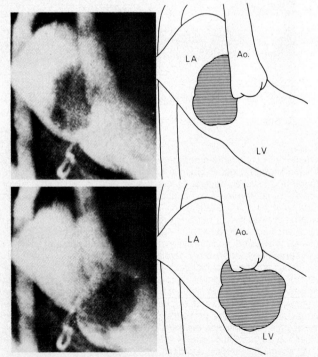

FIGURE 42–5 Cineangiogram of a patient with left atrial myxoma. The tumor appears as a filling defect in the left atrium during systole (upper panel) and prolapses into the left ventricle during diastole (lower panel). LA = left atrium; Ao. = aorta; LV = left ventricle. (From Selzer, A., et al.: Protean clinical manifestations of primary tumors of the heart. Am. J. Med. *52*:9, 1972.)

sion has also been reported for ventricular myxomas, as well as most other types of benign cardiac tumor, including rhabdomyoma, hamartoma, fibroma, lipoma, hemangioma, and papillary fibroelastoma.[17,99,102,110,112,120,162-166] The major surgical considerations in excision of ventricular tumors include preservation of adequate ventricular myocardium, maintenance of proper atrioventricular valve function, and preservation of as much of the conduction system as possible. Often, however, papillary muscles, chordae tendineae, or the AV conduction system must be sacrificed during the resection of a tumor, thereby necessitating replacement of the atrioventricular valve, implantation of a pacemaker, or both.

MALIGNANT TUMORS. Operation is not an effective treatment for the great majority of primary malignant tumors of the heart because of the large mass of cardiac tissue involved or the presence of metastases. The major role for surgery in such cases is to establish a diagnosis in order to exclude the possibility of a curable benign tumor. Nevertheless, in some cases palliation of hemodynamic and/or constitutional symptoms and extension of life may be achieved by aggressive therapy. Survivals of from 1 to 3 years have been reported following partial resection, chemotherapy, radiation therapy, or various combinations of these modalities.[123,131,167-169] In some instances, localized recurrences have been eliminated by as many as five operations.[14,15] Some success in palliation of symptoms has been reported following the combination of chemotherapy and radiation therapy[170] and radiation therapy alone.[171] Lymphosarcoma of the heart frequently responds to chemotherapy, radiation therapy, or both.[172,173] Unfortunately, many other reports indicate a failure to alter the course of cardiac sarcomas despite various combinations of surgery, chemotherapy, and radiation therapy.

References

1. Straus, R., and Merliss, R.: Primary tumors of the heart. Arch. Pathol. 39:74, 1945.
2. Fine, G.: Neoplasms of the pericardium and heart. In Gould, S. E. (ed.): Pathology of the Heart and Blood Vessels. Springfield, Ill., Charles C Thomas, 1968, p. 851.
3. Heath, D.: Pathology of cardiac tumors. Am. J. Cardiol. 21:315, 1968.
4. McAllister, H. A., and Fenoglio, J. J.: Tumors of the cardiovascular system. In Atlas of Tumor Pathology. Washington, D. C., Armed Forces Institute of Pathology, 1978. Fasc. 15, 2nd series.
5. McAllister, H. A., Jr.: Primary tumors of the heart and pericardium. Pathol. Ann. 17:325, 1979.
6. Fabian, J. T., and Rose, A. G.: Tumours of the heart. S. Afr. Med. J. 61:71, 1982.
6a.Mahaim, I.: Les Tumeurs et les Polypes de Coeur: Étude Anatomo-Clinique. Paris, Masson, 1945.
7. Barnes, A. R., Beaver, D. C., and Snell, A. M.: Primary sarcoma of the heart: Report of a case with E. C. G. and pathological studies. Am. Heart J. 9:480, 1934.
8. Goldberg, H. P., Glenn, F., Dotter, C. T., and Steinberg, I.: Myxoma of the left atrium. Diagnosis made during life with operative and postmortem findings. Circulation 6:762, 1952.
9. Beck, C. S.: An intrapericardial teratoma and a tumor of the heart: Both removed operatively. Ann. Surg. 116:161, 1942.
10. Maurer, E. R.: Successful removal of tumor of the heart. J. Thorac. Surg. 23:473, 1952.
11. Castaneda, A. R., and Varco, R. L., Tumors of the heart: Surgical considerations. Am. J. Cardiol. 21:357, 1968.
12. Crafoord, C. L.: Case report. In Lam, C. R. (ed.): Proceedings, International Symposium on Cardiovascular Surgery. Philadelphia, W. B. Saunders Co., 1955, p. 202.
13. Melo, J., Ahmad, A., Chapman, R., Wood, J., and Starr, A.: Primary tumors of the heart: A rewarding challenge. Am. Surg. 45:681, 1979.
14. Gabelman, C., Al-Sadir, J., Lamberti, J., Fozzard, H. A., Laufer, E., Replogle, R. L., and Myerowitz, P. D.: Surgical treatment of recurrent primary malignant tumor of the left atrium. J. Thorac. Cardiovasc. Surg. 77:914, 1979.

15. Yashar, J., Witoszka, M., Savage, D. D., Klie, J., Dyckman, J., Yashar, J. J., Reddick, R. L., Watson, D. C., and McIntosh, C. L.: Primary osteogenic sarcoma of the heart. Ann. Thorac. Surg. 28:594, 1979.
16. Silverman, N. A.: Primary cardiac tumors. Ann. Surg. 191:127, 1980.
17. Houser, S., Forbes, N., and Stewart, S.: Rhabdomyoma of the heart: A diagnostic and therapeutic challenge. Ann. Thorac. Surg. 29:373, 1980.
18. Effert, S., and Domanig, E.: The diagnosis of intra-atrial tumor and thrombi by the ultrasonic echo method. Ger. Med. Mon. 4:1, 1959.
19. Lappe, D. L., Bulkley, G. H., and Weiss, J. L.: Two-dimensional echocardiographic diagnosis of left atrial myxoma. Chest 74:55, 1978.
20. Lewis, B. S., Lewis, N., Popp, R. L., Weiss, A. T., Borman, J. B., and Gotsman, M. S.: Diagnostic value of cross-sectional echocardiography in left atrial myxoma. Isr. J. Med. Sci. 15:426, 1979.
21. Come, P. C., Kurland, G. S., and Vine, H. S.: Two dimensional echocardiography in differentiating right atrial and tricuspid valve mass lesions. Am. J. Cardiol. 44:1207, 1979.
22. Fye, W. B., and Molina, J. E.: Right atrial angiosarcoma: Echocardiographic diagnosis and surgical correction. Johns Hopkins Med. J. 147:111, 1980.
23. Fowles, R. E., Miller, C., Egbert, B. M., Fitzgerald, J. W., and Popp, R. L.: Systemic embolization from a mitral valve papillary endocardial fibroma detected by two-dimensional echocardiography. Am. Heart J. 102:128, 1981.
24. Tway, K. P., Shah, A. A., and Rahimtoola, S. H.: Multiple biatrial myxomas demonstrated by two-dimensional echocardiography. Am. J. Med. 71:896, 1981.
25. Pohost, G. M., Pastore, J. O., McKusick, K. A., Chiotellis, P. N., Kapeliakis, G. Z., Myers, G. S., Dinsmore, R. E., and Block, P. C.: Detection of left atrial myxoma by gated radionuclide cardiac imaging. Circulation 55:88, 1977.
26. Pitcher, D., Wainwright, R., Brennand-Roper, D., Deverall, P., Sowton, E., and Maisey, M.: Cardiac tumors: Non-invasive detection and assessment by gated blood pool radionuclide imaging. Br. Heart J. 44:143, 1980.
27. Winzelberg, G. G., Rapoport, F., Boucher, C. A., Carey, R. W., McKusick, K. A., and Strauss, H. W.: Combined gated cardiac blood pool scintigraphy and 67Ga-citrate scintigraphy for detection of cardiac lymphoproliferative disorders. Radiology 141:191, 1981.
28. Huggins, T. J., Huggins, M. J., Schnapf, D. J., Brott, W. H., Sinnott, R. C., and Shawl, F. A.: Left atrial myxoma: Computed tomography as a diagnostic modality. J. Comput. Assist. Tomogr. 4:253, 1980.
29. Godwin, J. D., Axel, L., Adams, J. R., Schiller, N. B., Simpson, P. C., Jr., and Gertz, E. W.: Computed tomography: A new method for diagnosing tumor of the heart. Circulation 63:448, 1981.
30. Köhler, E., Bocker, K., Leuner, C., Jungblut, R., Schoppe, W., Nessler, L., Minami, K., and Loogen, F.: The diagnostic value of M-mode, two-dimensional echocardiography, and computed tomography in comparison to the results of cardiac catheterization in the diagnosis of tumors of the heart. Z. Kardiol. 70:571, 1981.
31. Sutton, D., Al-Kutoubi, M. A., and Lipkin, D. P.: Left atrial myxoma diagnosed by computerized tomography. Br. J. Radiol. 55:80, 1982.
32. Lackner, K., Heuser, L., Friedman, G., and Thurn, P.: Computer-kardiotomographie bei Tumoren des linken Vorhofes. Forstchr. Roentgenstr. 129:735, 1978.
33. Goodwin, J. F.: Symposium on cardiac tumors. The spectrum of cardiac tumors. Am. J. Cardiol. 21:307, 1968.
34. MacGregor, G. A., and Cullen, R. A.: The syndrome of fever, anaemia and high sedimentation rate with an atrial myxoma. Br. Med. J. 5:158, 1959.
35. Huston, K. A., Combs, J. J., Lie, J. T., and Giuliani, E. R.: Left atrial myxoma simulating peripheral vasculitis. Mayo Clin. Proc. 53:752, 1978.
36. Caralis, D. G., Kennedy, H. L., Bailey, I., and Bulkley, B. H.: Primary right cardiac tumor. Chest 77:100, 1980.
37. Willey, R. F., Mathews, M. B., and Walbaum, P. R.: An unusual case of large right atrial myxoma. Br. Heart J. 44:108, 1980.
38. Firor, W. B., Aldridge, H. E., and Bigelow, W. G.: A follow-up study of three patients after removal of left atrial myxoma five to ten years previously. J. Thorac. Cardiovasc. Surg. 51:515, 1966.
39. Levinson, J. P., and Kincaid, O. W.: Myxoma of the right atrium associated with polycythemia. N. Engl. J. Med. 264:1187, 1961.
40. Vuopio, P., and Nikkila, E. A.: Hemolytic anemia and thrombocytopenia in a case of left atrial myxoma associated with mitral stenosis. Am. J. Cardiol. 17:585, 1966.
41. Boss, J. H., and Bechar, M.: Myxoma of the heart. Report based on four cases. Am. J. Cardiol. 3:823, 1959.
42. Curry, H. L. F., Mathews, J. A., and Robinson, J.: Right atrial myxoma mimicking a rheumatic disorder. Br. Med. J. 1:542, 1967.
43. Graham, S. L., and Sellers, A. L.: Atrial myxoma with multiple myeloma. Arch. Intern. Med. 139:116, 1979.
44. Kaminsky, M. E., Ehlers, K. H., Engle, M. A., Klein, A. A., Levin, A. R., and Subramanian, V. A.: Atrial myxoma mimicking a collagen disorder. Chest 75:93, 1979.
45. Rajpal, R. S., Leibsohn, J. A., Liekweg, W. G., Gross, C. M., Olinger, G. N., Rose, H. D., and Bamrah, V. S.: Infected left atrial myxoma with bacteremia simulating infective endocarditis. Arch. Intern. Med. 139:1176, 1979.
46. Byrd, W. E., Matthews, O. P., and Hunt, R. E.: Left atrial myxoma presenting as a systemic vasculitis. Arth. Rheum. 23:240, 1980.
47. Joseph, P., Himmelstein, D. U., Mahowald, J. M., and Stullman, W. S.: Atrial myxoma infected with Candida: First survival. Chest 78:340, 1980.
48. Silverman, J., Olwin, J. S., and Graettinger, J. S.: Cardiac myxomas with systemic embolization. Circulation 26:99, 1962.

49. Farah, M. G.: Familial atrial myxoma. Ann. Intern. Med. *83*:358, 1975.

50. Burton, C., and Johnston, J.: Multiple cerebral aneurysms and cardiac myxoma. N. Engl. J. Med. *282*:35, 1970.

51. Koikkalainen, K., Kostiainen, S., and Luosto, R.: Left atrial myxoma revealed by femoral embolectomy. Scand. J. Thorac. Cardiovasc. Surg. *11*:33, 1977.

52. Greenwood, W. F.: Profile of atrial myxoma. Am. J. Cardiol. *21*:367, 1968.

53. Leonhardt, E. T. G., and Kullenberg, K. P. G.: Bilateral atrial myxomas with multiple arterial aneurysms—A syndrome mimicking polyarteritis nodosa. Am. J. Med. *62*:792, 1977.

54. Yufe, R., Karpati, G., and Carpenter, S.: Cardiac myxoma: A disgnostic challenge for the neurologist. Neurology *26*:1060, 1976.

55. Cogan, D. G., and Wray, S. H.: Vascular occlusions in the eye from cardiac myxomas. Am. J. Ophthalmol. *80*:396, 1975.

56. Schweiger, M. J., Hafer, J. G., Jr., Brown, R., and Gianelly, R. E.: Spontaneous cure of infected left atrial myxoma following embolization. Am. Heart J. *99*:630, 1980.

57. Tanabe, J., Williams, R. L., and Diethrich, E. B.: Left atrial myxoma: Association with acute coronary embolization in an 11-year-old boy. Pediatrics *63*:778, 1979.

58. Sandok, B. A., van Estorff, I., and Giuliani, E. R.: CNS embolism due to atrial myxoma. Arch. Neurol. *37*:485, 1980.

59. Gonzalez, A., Altieri, P. I., Marquez, E., Cox, R. A., and Castillo, M.: Massive pulmonary embolism associated with a right ventricular myxoma. Am. J. Med. *69*:795, 1980.

60. Heath, D., and Mackinnon, J.: Pulmonary hypertension due to myxoma of the right atrium. With special reference to the behavior of emboli of myxoma in the lung. Am. Heart J. *68*:227, 1964.

61. Muroff, L. R., and Johnson, P. M.: Right atrial myxoma presenting as non-resolving pulmonary emboli: Case report. J. Nucl. Med. *17*:890, 1976.

62. Tai, A. R., Gross, H., and Siegelman, S. S.: Right atrial myxoma and pulmonary hypertension. N.Y. State J. Med. *70*:2996, 1970.

63. Harvey, W. P.: Clinical aspects of cardiac tumors. Am. J. Cardiol. *21*:328, 1968.

64. James, T. N., and Galakhov, I.: De subitaneis mortibus XXVI. Fatal electrical instability of the heart associated with benign congenital polycystic tumor of the atrioventricular node. Circulation *56*:667, 1977.

65. Bharati, S., Bicoff, J. P., Fridman, J. L., Lev, M., and Rosen, K. M.: Sudden death caused by benign tumor of the atrioventricular node. Arch. Intern. Med. *136*:224, 1976.

66. Hawthorne, J. W., and Fallon, J. T.: Case Records of the Massachusetts General Hospital. Case 1–1982: A 42-year-old woman with longstanding heart block. N. Engl. J. Med. *306*:32, 1982.

67. Isner, J. M., Falcone, M. W., Virmani, R., and Roberts, W. C.: Cardiac sarcoma causing "ASH" and simulating coronary heart disease. Am. J. Med. *66*:1025, 1979.

68. Cabin, H. S., Costello, R. M., Vasudevan, G., Maron, B. J., and Roberts, W. C.: Cardiac lymphoma mimicking hypertrophic cardiomyopathy. Am. Heart J. *102*:466, 1981.

69. Hamada, N., Matsuzaki, M., Kusukawa, R., Fujii, Y., Yamaki, R., Masuda, M., and Tani, S.: Malignant fibrous histiocytoma of the heart. Jpn. Circ. J. *44*:361, 1980.

70. Bass, N. M., and Sharratt, G. J. P.: Left atrial myxoma diagnosed by echocardiography, with observations on tumor movement. Br. Heart J. *35*:1332, 1973.

71. Talley, R. C., Baldwin, B. J., Symbas, P. N., and Nutter, D. O.: Right atrial myxoma. Unusual presentation with cyanosis and clubbing. Am. J. Med. *48*:256, 1970.

72. Hansen, J. F., Lyngborg, K., Andersen, M., and Wennevold, A.: Right atrial myxoma. Acta Med. Scand. *186*:165, 1969.

73. Goldschlager, A., Popper, R., Goldschlager, N., Gerbode, F., and Prozan, G.: Right atrial myxoma with right to left shunt and polycythemia presenting as congenital heart disease. Am. J. Cardiol. *30*:82, 1972.

74. Waxler, E. B., Kawai, N., and Kasparian, H.: Right atrial myxoma: Echocardiographic, phonocardiographic and hemodynamic signs. Am. Heart J. *82*:251, 1972.

74a. Massumi, R.: Bedside diagnosis of right heart myxomas through detection of palpable tumor shocks and audible plops. Am. Heart J. *105*:303, 1983.

75. Saunerstedt, R., Varnauskas, E., Paulin, S., Linder, E., Ljunggren, H., and Werko, L.: Right atrial myxoma. Report of a case and review of the literature. Am. Heart J. *64*:243, 1962.

76. Hada, Y., Wolfe, C., Murry, C. F., and Craige, E.: Right ventricular myxoma. Case report and review of phonocardiographic and auscultatory manifestations. Am. Heart J. *100*:871, 1980.

77. Goldstein, S., and Mahoney, E. B.: Right ventricular fibrosarcoma causing pulmonic stenosis. Am. J. Cardiol. *17*:570, 1966.

78. Sasse, L., Lorentzen, D., and Alvarez, H.: Paradoxical septal motion secondary to right ventricular tumor. J.A.M.A. *234*:915, 1975.

79. Mahoney, L., Schieken, R. M., and Doty, D.: Cardiac rhabdomyoma simulating pulmonic stenosis. Cathet. Cardiovasc. Diagn. *5*:385, 1979.

80. de Paiva, E. C., Maciera-Coelko, E., Amram, S. S., Duarte, C., and Coelho, E.: Intracavitary left ventricular myxoma. Am. J. Cardiol. *20*:260, 1967.

81. Hoen, A. G., and Ellis, E. J.: Intramural fibroma of the heart. Am. J. Cardiol. *17*:579, 1966.

82. Bloor, C. M.: Cardiac pathology. *In* Neoplastic Heart Disease. Philadelphia, J. B. Lippincott Co., 1978, pp. 386–418.

83. Pritchard, R. W.: Tumors of the heart. Arch. Pathol. *51*:98, 1951.

84. Bulkley, B. H., and Hutchins, G. M.: Atrial myxomas: A fifty year review. Am. Heart J. *97*:639, 1979.

85. Siltanen, P., Tuuteri, L., Norio, R., Tala, P., Ahrenberg, P., and Halonen, P. I.: Atrial myxoma in a family. Am. J. Cardiol. *38*:252, 1976.

86. Powers, J. C., Falkoff, M., Heinle, R. A., Nanda, N. C., Ong, L. S., Weiner, R. S., and Barold, S. S.: Familial cardiac myxoma. Emphasis on unusual clinical manifestations. J. Thorac. Cardiovasc. Surg. *77*:782, 1979.

87. Bashey, R. I., and Nochumson, S.: Cardiac myxoma. Biochemical analyses and evidence for its neoplastic nature. N.Y. State J. Med. *79*:29, 1979.

88. Sayler, W. R., Page, D. L., and Hutchins, G. M.: The development of cardiac myxomas and papillary endocardial lesions from mural thrombus. Am. Heart J. *89*:4, 1975.

89. Glasser, J. P., Bedynek, J. L., Hall, R. J., Hopeman, A. R., Treasure, R. L., McAllister, H. A., Jr., Esterly, J. A., Manion, W. C., and Sanford, H. S.: Left atrial myxoma. Report of a case including hemodynamic, surgical, histologic and histochemical characteristics. Am. J. Med. *50*:113, 1971.

90. Ferrans, V. J., and Roberts, W. C.: Structural features of cardiac myxomas. Hum. Pathol. *4*:111, 1973.

91. Frishman, W., Factor, S., Jordan, A., Hellman, C., Elkayam, U., LeJemtel, T., Strom, J., Unschuld, H., and Becker, R.: Right atrial myxoma: Unusual clinical presentation and atypical glandular history. Circulation *59*:1070, 1979.

92. Wold, L. E., and Lie, J. T.: Scanning electron microscopy of intracardiac myxoma. Mayo Clin. Proc. *56*:198, 1981.

93. Morales, A. R., Fine, G., Castro, A., and Nadji, M.: Cardiac myxoma. Hum. Pathol. *12*:896, 1981.

94. Powers, J. C., Falkoff, M., Heinle, R. A., Nanda, N. C., Ong, L. S., Weiner, R. S., and Barold, S. S.: Familial cardiac myxoma: Emphasis on unusual clinical manifestations. J. Thorac. Cardiovasc. Surg. *77*:782, 1979.

95. Seo, I. S., Warner, T. F. C. S., Colyer, R. A., and Winkler, R. F.: Metastasizing atrial myxoma. Am. J. Surg. Pathol. *4*:391, 1980.

96. Budzilovich, G., Aleksic, S., Greco, A., Fernandez, J., Harris, J., and Finegold, M.: Malignant cardiac myxoma with cerebral metastases. Surg. Neurol. *11*:461, 1979.

97. Dashkoff, N., Boersma, R. B., Nanda, N. C., Gramiak, R., Anderson, M. N., and Subramanian, S.: Bilateral atrial myxomas. Echocardiographic considerations. Am. J. Med. *65*:361, 1978.

98. Imperio, J., Summers, D., Krasnow, N., and Piccone, V. A., Jr.: The distribution pattern of biatrial myxomas. Ann. Thorac. Surg. *29*:469, 1980.

99. Morgan, D. L., Palazola, J., Reed, W., Bell, H. H., Kindred, L. H., and Beauchamp, G. D.: Left heart myxomas. Am. J. Cardiol. *40*:611, 1977.

100. Sandrasagra, A., Oliver, W. A., and English, T. A. H.: Myxoma of mitral valve. Br. Heart J. *42*:221, 1979.

101. Williams, W. J., Jenkins, D., and Erasmus, D.: The ultrastructure of cardiac myxomas. Thorax *25*:756, 1970.

102. Feldman, P. S., Horvath, E., and Kovacs, K.: An ultrastructural study of seven cardiac myxomas. Cancer *40*:2216, 1977.

103. Pomerance, A.: Papillary "tumours" of the heart valves. J. Pathol. Bacteriol. *81*:135, 1961.

104. Lichtenstein, H. L., Lee, J. C. K., and Stewart, S.: Papillary tumor of the heart: Incidental finding at surgery. Hum. Pathol. *10*:473, 1979.

105. Lambl, V. A.: Papillare Excrescenzen an der Semilunar-Klappe der Aorta. Wien Med. Wchnschr. *6*:244, 1856.

106. Cha, S. D., Incarvito, J., Fernandez, J., Chang, K. S., Maranho, V., and Gooch, A. S.: Giant Lambl's excrescences of papillary muscle and aortic valve: Echocardiographic, angiographic, and pathologic findings. Clin. Cardiol. *4*:51, 1981.

107. Fenoglio, J. J., McAllister, H. A., and Ferrans, V. J.: Cardiac rhabdomyoma: A clinicopathologic and electron microscopic study. Am. J. Cardiol. *38*:241, 1976.

108. Bruni, C., Prioleau, P. G., Ivey, H. H., and Nolan, S. P.: New fine structural features of cardiac rhabdomyoma: A case report. Cancer *46*:2068, 1980.

109. Shrivastava, S., Jacks, J. J., White, R. S., and Edwards, J. E.: Diffuse rhabdomyomatosis of the heart. Arch. Pathol. Lab. Med. *101*:78, 1977.

110. Mair, D. D., Titus, J. L., Davis, G. D., and Ritter, D. G.: Cardiac rhabdomyoma simulating mitral atresia. Chest *71*:102, 1977.

111. Van der Hauwaert, L. G.: Cardiac tumours in infancy and childhood. Br. Heart J. *33*:125, 1971.

112. Feldman, P. S., and Meyer, M. W.: Fibroelastic hamartoma (fibroma) of the heart. Cancer *38*:314, 1976.

113. Calhoun, T. R., Terry, E. E., Best, E. B., and Sunbury, T. R.: Myocardial fibroma or fibrous hamartoma. Ann. Thorac. Surg. *32*:406, 1981.

114. Nicks, R.: Hamartoma of the right ventricle. J. Thorac. Cardiovasc. Surg. *47*:762, 1964.

115. Moulton, A. L., Jaretzki, A., 3rd, Bowman, F. O., Jr., Silverstein, E. F., and Bregman, D.: Massive lipoma of the heart. N.Y. State J. Med. *76*:1820, 1976.

116. Reyes, L. H., Rubio, P. A., Korompai, F. L., and Guinn, G. A.: Lipoma of the heart. Int. Surg. *61*:179, 1976.

117. Reyes, C. V., and Jablokow, V. R.: Lipomatous hypertrophy of the cardiac interatrial septum. Am. J. Clin. Pathol. *72*:785, 1979.

118. Prior, J. T.: Lipomatous hypertrophy of cardiac interatrial septum. Arch. Pathol. *78*:11, 1964.

119. Hutter, A. M., Jr., and Page, D. L.: Atrial arrhythmias and lipomatous hypertrophy of the cardiac interatrial septum. Am. Heart J. *82*:16, 1971.

120. Tschirkov, A., and Stegaru, B.: Lipomatous hypertrophy of interatrial septum

presenting as recurring pericardial effusion and mistaken for constrictive pericarditis. Thorac. Cardiovasc. Surg. *27*:400, 1979.

121. Tabry, I. F., Nasser, V. H., Rizk, G., Touma, A., and Dagher, I. K.: Cavernous hemangioma of the heart: Case report and review of the literature. J. Thorac. Cardiovasc. Surg. *69*:415, 1975.

122. Grant, R. T., and Camp, P. D.: A case of complete heart block due to an arterial angioma. Heart *16*:137, 1933.

123. Gough, J. C., Connolly, C. E., and Kennedy, J. D.: Primary sarcoma of the heart: A light and electron microscopic study of two cases. J. Clin. Pathol. *32*: 601, 1979.

124. Mahar, L. J., Lie, J. T., Groover, R. V., Seward, J. B., Puga, F. J., and Feldt, R. H.: Primary cardiac myxosarcoma in a child. Mayo Clin. Proc. *54*:261, 1979.

125. Stoupel, E., Primo, G., Kahn, R. J., le Clerc, J. L., de Wilde, P., Deuvaert, F., and Toussaint, C.: Cardiac tamponade with renal failure due to hemangioma of the heart. Acta Cardiol. (Brux.) *34*:345, 1979.

126. Whorton, C. M.: Primary malignant tumor of the heart. Cancer *2*:245, 1949.

127. Goldberg, H. P., and Steinberg, I.: Primary tumors of the heart. Circulation *11*: 963, 1955.

128. Glancy, L., Morales, J. B., and Roberts, W. C.: Angiosarcoma of the heart. Am. J. Cardiol. *21*:413, 1968.

129. Rossi, N. P., Kioschos, J. M., Ascenbrener, C. A., and Ehrenhaft, J. L.: Primary angiosarcoma of the heart. Cancer *37*:891, 1976.

130. Panella, J. S., Paige, M. L., Victor, T. A., Semerdjian, R. A., and Hueter, D. C.: Angiosarcoma of the heart. Diagnosis by echocardiography. Chest *76*:221, 1979.

131. Yang, H.-Y., Wasielewski, J. F., Lee, W., Lee, E., and Paik, Y. K.: Angiosarcoma of the heart: Ultrastructural study. Cancer *47*:72, 1981.

132. Roberts, W. C., Glancy, D. L., and DeVita, V. T., Jr.: Heart in malignant lymphoma. A study of 196 autopsy cases. Am. J. Cardiol. *22*:85, 1968.

133. Fiester, R. F.: Reticulum cell sarcoma of the heart. Arch. Pathol. *99*:80, 1975.

134. Galton, B. B.: Left atrial myxoma without significant cardiac manifestations. J. Med. Soc. N.J. *76*:754, 1979.

135. Roudaut, R., Pouget, B., Videau, P., Clementy, J., Choussat, A., Baudet, E., and Dallocchio, M.: Right atrial myxoma in an asymptomatic child. Eur. Heart J. *1*:453, 1980.

136. Oldershaw, P. J., Sutton, M. St. J., and Gibson, R. V.: Long asymptomatic period of atrial myxomas. Thorax *35*:70, 1980.

137. Steiner, R. E.: Radiologic aspects of cardiac tumors. Am. J. Cardiol. *21*:344, 1968.

138. Abrams, H. L., Adams, D. F., and Grant, H. A.: The radiology of tumors of the heart. Radiol. Clin. North Am. *9*:299, 1971.

139. Sharratt, G. P., Grover, M. L., and Monro, J. L.: Calcified left atrial myxoma with floppy mitral valve. Br. Heart J. *42*:608, 1979.

140. Davis, G., Kincaid, O., and Hallermann, F.: Roentgen aspects of cardiac tumors. Semin. Roentgenol. *4*:384, 1969.

141. Buenger, R., Ogelsby, P., and Egbert, H.: Calcified polyp of the heart. Radiology *67*:531, 1956.

142. Petsas, A. A., Gottlieb, S., Kingsley, B., Segal, B. L., and Myerburg, R. J.: Echocardiographic diagnosis of left atrial myxoma. Usefulness of suprasternal approach. Br. Heart J. *38*:627, 1976.

143. Nasser, W. K., Davis, R. H., Dillon, J. C., Travel, M. E., Helmen, C. H., Feigenbaum, H., and Fisch, C.: Atrial myxoma: I. Clinical and pathologic features in nine cases: II. Phonocardiographic, echocardiographic, hemodynamic and angiographic features in nine cases. Am. Heart J. *83*:694, 810, 1972.

144. Sabot, G., Fauvel, J. M., and Bounhoure, J. P.: Echocardiographic diagnosis of mobile left ventricular tumour. Br. Heart J. *42*:113, 1979.

145. Fitterer, J. D., Spicer, M. J., and Nelson, W. P.: Illustrative echocardiogram. Echocardiographic demonstration of bilateral atrial myxomas. Chest *70*:282, 1976.

146. Levisman, J. A., MacAlpin, R. N., Abbasi, A. S., Ellis, N., and Eber, L. M.: Echocardiographic diagnosis of a mobile, pedunculated tumor in the left ventricular cavity. Am. J. Cardiol. *36*:957, 1975.

147. Nanda, N. C., Barold, S. S., Gramiak, R., Ong, L. S., and Heinle, R. A.: Echocardiographic features of right ventricular outflow tumor prolapsing into the pulmonary artery. Am. J. Cardiol. *40*:272, 1977.

148. Donahoo, J. S., Weiss, J. L., Gardner, T. J., Fortuin, N. J., and Brawley, R. K.: Current management of atrial myxoma with emphasis on a new diagnostic technique. Ann. Surg. *189*:763, 1979.

148a. Green, S. E., Joynt, L. E., Fitzgerald, P. J., Rubenson, D. S., and Popp, R. L.: In vivo ultrasonic tissue characterization of human intracardiac masses. Am. J. Cardiol. *51*:231, 1983.

149. Berning, J., Egeblad, H., Lauridsen, P., and Wennevold, A.: The diagnostic challenge of left atrial myxoma. Acta Med. Scand. *206*:115, 1979.

149a. Salcedo, E. E., Adams, K. V., Lever, H. M., Gill, C. C., and Lombardo, H.: Echocardiographic findings in 25 patients with left atrial myxoma. J. Am. Coll. Cardiol. *1*:1162, 1983.

150. Tallury, V. K., and DePasquale, N. P.: Ultrasound cardiography in the diagnosis of left atrial thrombus. Chest *59*:501, 1971.

151. Rahilly, G. T., and Nanda, N. C.: Two-dimensional echocardiographic identification of tumor hemorrhages in atrial myxomas. Am. Heart J. *101*:237, 1981.

152. Bonte, F. J., and Curry, T. S.: Technetium-99m HSA blood pool scan in diagnosis of an intracardiac myxoma. J. Nucl. Med. *8*:35, 1967.

153. Zaret, B. L., Hurley, P. J., and Pitt, B.: Noninvasive scintiphotographic diagnosis of left atrial myxoma. J. Nucl. Med. *13*:81, 1972.

154. Tavel, M. E.: Clinical Phonocardiography and External Pulse Recording. 2nd ed. Chicago, Year Book Medical Publishers, 1972, pp. 248–249.

155. Kaufmann, G., Rutishauser, W., and Hegglin, R.: Heart sounds in atrial tumors. Am. J. Cardiol. *8*:350, 1961.

156. Wollenweber, J., Giuliani, E. R., Harrison, C. E., and Kincaid, O. W.: Pseudotumors of the right heart. Arch. Intern. Med. *121*:169, 1968.

157. Pendyck, F., Pierce, E. C., Baron, M. G., and Lukban, S. B.: Embolization of left atrial myxoma after transseptal cardiac catheterization. Am. J. Cardiol. *30*: 569, 1972.

158. Differding, J. T., Gardner, R. E., and Towe, B. B.: Intracardial myxoma with report of two unusual cases and successful removal. Circulation *23*:929, 1961.

159. Dang, C. R., and Hurley, E. J.: Contralateral recurrent myxoma of the heart. Ann. Thorac. Surg. *21*:59, 1976.

160. Larmi, T. K. I., Karkola, P., Kairaluoma, M. I., and Takkunen, J.: Surgical treatment of cardiac myxoma. A case report. Ann. Chir. Gynaecol. *66*:18, 1977.

161. Kabbani, S. S., and Cooley, D. A.: Atrial myxoma — Surgical considerations. J. Thorac. Cardiovasc. Surg. *65*:731, 1973.

162. Gottsegen, G., Wessely, J., Arvay, A., and Temesvari, A.: Right ventricular myxoma simulating pulmonary stenosis. Circulation *27*:95, 1963.

163. Taber, R. E., and Lam, C. R.: Diagnosis and surgical treatment of intracardiac myxoma and rhabdomyoma. J. Thorac. Cardiovasc. Surg. *40*:337, 1960.

164. Parks, F. R., Adams, F., and Longmire, W. P.: Successful excision of a left ventricular hamartoma. Circulation *26*:1316, 1962.

165. Etches, P. C., Gribbin, B., and Gunning, A. J.: Echocardiographic diagnosis and successful removal of cardiac fibroma in 4-year old child. Br. Heart J. *43*: 360, 1980.

166. Bradford, J. H., Nomeir, A. M., and Watts, L. E.: Left ventricular lipoma: Echocardiographic and angiographic features. South. Med. J. *73*:663, 1980.

167. Hager, W., Kremer, K., and Muller, W.: Angiosarkom des Herzens. Dtsch. Med. Wchschr. *95*:680, 1970.

168. Sagerman, R., Hurley, E., and Bagshaw, M.: Successful sterilization of a primary cardiac sarcoma by supervoltage radiation therapy. Am. J. Roentgenol. *92*:942, 1964.

169. Laws, J. W., Annes, G. P., and Bogren, H. G.: Primary malignant tumors of the heart. Calif. Med. *118*:11, 1973.

170. Hollingworth, J. H., and Sturgill, B. C.: Treatment of primary angiosarcoma of the heart. Am. Heart J. *78*:254, 1969.

171. Allaire, F. J., Grimm, C. A., Taylor, L. M., and Pfaff, J. P.: Primary hemangioendothelioma of the heart. Rocky Mt. Med. J. *61*:34, 1964.

172. Terry, L. N., and Kilgerman, M. M.: Pericardial and myocardial involvement by lymphomas and leukemias. The role of radiotherapy. Cancer *25*:1003, 1970.

173. Garfein, O. B.: Lymphosarcoma of the right atrium: Angiographic and hemodynamic documentation of response to chemotherapy. Arch. Intern. Med. *135*:325, 1975.

43 PERICARDIAL DISEASE

by Beverly H. Lorell, M.D., and Eugene Braunwald, M.D.

HISTORICAL BACKGROUND[1,2]

In the ancient world knowledge of the pericardium was gained from anatomical observations of animal sacrifices and human corpses during war. Both Homer and Pliny wrote about the anatomical finding of "hairy hearts" in warriors who died on the battlefield. Hippocrates accurately described the normal pericardium as "a smooth mantle surrounding the heart and containing a small amount of fluid resembling urine." In the Dead Sea Scrolls (A.D. 1) the pericardium was referred to as "the foreskin of the heart." Galen (A.D. 131–201) named the pericardium and recognized its protective function.

In the 17th century, Riolan advocated the technique of pericardial aspiration for treating patients with large pericardial effusions, and William Harvey vividly demonstrated to King Charles that much of the visceral pericardium is pain-insensitive by palpating the beating heart of a young nobleman who had a large defect in the left chest. In the same century, the Cornish physiologist Richard Lower made remarkable observations about the physiology of constrictive pericarditis and cardiac tamponade: "Just as the heart labors when affected by disease within, so it does when oppressed from without by disease of its covering. So it happens when that same covering of the heart fills with an effusion and the walls are compressed with water on every side, so that they cannot dilate to receive the blood, then truly the pulse diminishes until at length it is suppressed by even more water, when syncope, and death itself follows. Just as the accumulation of too much water harms the heart, so too does trouble come when the heart and the pericardium become everywhere adherent...."

Early in the 19th century, Morgagni described cardiac compression by hemopericardium and by pericardial calcification, noted that the apex beat was often absent in patients with extensive pericardial ad-

hesion, and advocated pericardiocentesis via incision for treatment of pericardial tamponade. Corvisart and his student Laennec distinguished adhesive pericarditis from pericardial effusion by physical examination. Romero reported the first successful pericardiotomy to relieve pericardial effusion, and in 1840, Franz Schuh performed the first successful "blind" pericardiocentesis with a trocar to relieve cardiac tamponade. Norman Cheevers of Guy's Hospital in London astutely appreciated the physiology of constrictive pericarditis: "The principal cause of dangerous symptoms ... appears to arise from the occurrence of gradual contraction in the layer of adhesive material which has been deposited around the heart, compressing its muscular tissue and embarrassing its systolic and diastolic movement, but more particularly the latter. The ventricles, having become diminished in capacity, make up for this loss by the rapidity of their contractions...."

In the mid-1800's, Joseph Skoda reported the characteristic physical findings of constrictive pericarditis including the "diastolic heart beat" (pericardial knock), systolic precordial retraction, and sudden diastolic collapse of the cervical veins (prominent venous *y* descent). Kussmaul made the classic bedside observations of neck vein distention in compressive pericardial disorders and pulsus paradoxus, the hallmark of acute cardiac tamponade, which he described as paradoxical because the palpated pulse disappeared during inspiration even though the heart continued to beat. He also described the finding of an inspiratory increase in central venous pressure in constrictive pericarditis, now known as *Kussmaul's sign*. Early in the 20th century, the first pericardiectomy for constrictive pericarditis was performed by Hallopeau.

Even with the tremendous experimental advances made in this century toward understanding the physiology of the normal and diseased pericardium and appreciating the clinical picture of pericardial disease, Sir William Osler's caveat is still applicable: "Even with copious effusion, the onset and course may be so insidious that no suspicion of the true nature of the disease is aroused. . . . Perhaps no serious disease is so frequently overlooked by the practitioner. Postmortem experience shows how often pericarditis is not recognized or goes on to resolution and adhesion without attracting notice."

ANATOMY

The pericardium forms a strong flask-shaped sac with short tubelike extensions that enclose the origins of the aorta and its junction with the aortic arch, the pulmonary artery where it branches, the proximal pulmonary veins, and venae cavae. Fibrous tissue of the pericardium actually blends with adventitia of the great arteries to form very strong attachments. In addition, the pericardium has firm ligamentous attachments anteriorly to the sternum and xiphoid process, posteriorly to the vertebral column, and inferiorly to the diaphragm.[3]

The human pericardium receives its arterial blood supply from small branches of the aorta and internal mammary and musculophrenic arteries. The pericardium is innervated by the vagus, left recurrent laryngeal nerve, and esophageal plexus and also has rich sympathetic innervation from the stellate and first dorsal ganglia and the cardiac, aortic, and diaphragmatic plexuses. The phrenic nerves course over the pericardium en route to the diaphragm. The afferent nerves responsible for pain perception appear to be transmitted via the phrenic nerve entering the spinal cord at C4–C5.[3,4] It appears that the anterior parietal pericardium is pain-sensitive while the lateral and posterior parietal pericardial regions are not.

The pericardium is composed of a fibrous outer layer composed of collagen bundles and elastin fibers and an inner serous membrane composed of a single layer of mesothelial cells. The inner serous layer is intimately attached to the surface of the heart and epicardial fat to form the *visceral pericardium*, and this inner serous membrane reflects back on itself to line the outer fibrous layer to form the *parietal pericardium*. The pericardium has two major serosal tunnels: the transverse sinus, which lies posterior to the great arteries and anterior to the atria and superior vena cava, and the oblique sinus, which lies posterior to the left atrium so that the posterior left atrial wall is actually separated from the pericardial space. The fact that the oblique sinus is usually not fluid-filled in the presence of a pericardial effusion is clinically important in that it explains why an echo-free space denoting an effusion is often not detected behind the left atrium during echocardiography.

The serous visceral pericardium is attached to the parietal pericardium by delicate connective tissue with elastin fibers. The parietal pericardium is composed of collagen fibers interlaced with extensive elastic fibers, which are wavy during childhood and become progres-

sively straighter with age, suggesting that young pericardia are more compliant than those of the elderly. Electron microscopy reveals that exuberant microvilli and long, single cilia project from the serous mesothelium composing the visceral pericardium and the inner lining of the parietal pericardium (Fig. 43–1).[5] The microvilli are believed to increase markedly the surface area available for fluid transport, and both microvilli and cilia provide a specialized surface to permit movement of the pericardial membranes over each other during each cardiac cycle and to permit the pericardium to accommodate changes in cardiac shape during contraction.

The human pericardium normally contains up to 50 ml of clear fluid.[6] The visceral pericardium is believed to be the source of normal pericardial fluid and of excessive fluid in disease states. Normal pericardial fluid appears to be an ultrafiltrate of plasma, since electrolytes are present in pericardial fluid in concentrations compatible with such an ultrafiltrate; protein concentrations are about one-third those of the plasma, and albumin is present in a higher ratio in pericardial fluid reflecting its lower molecular weight.[7] The membrane characteristics of the pericardium tend to favor fluid removal rather than accumulation,[8] which may be a safety factor preventing the development of cardiac tamponade. Current data suggest that drainage of the pericardial space occurs both by the thoracic duct via the parietal pericardium and by the right lymphatic duct via the right pleural space.

FUNCTIONS OF THE PERICARDIUM

The pericardium serves several membrane functions. Its ligamentous attachments help to fix the heart anatomically and prevent excessive motion with changes in body position. The pericardium also reduces friction between the heart and surrounding organs and provides a barrier against the extension of infection and malignancy from contiguous organs to the heart itself. The role of the pericardium in the regulation of the circulation is controversial, since congenital absence or surgical excision of the pericardium is *not* associated with overt disturbances of cardiac function. However, observations in both dogs and man indicate that the pericardium may play a role in (1) the distribution and equalization of hydrostatic forces on the heart, (2) the prevention of acute cardiac dilatation, and (3) diastolic coupling of the two ventricles[7a] (see later).

The normal pericardium is stiff, and the relationship between pressure within the pericardium and total intrapericardial volume, which is the sum of the volume of the heart itself and the reserve volume of the surrounding peri-

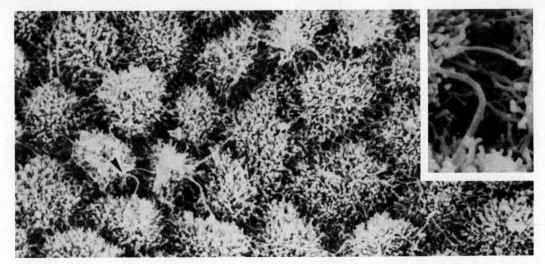

FIGURE 43–1 Scanning electron micrograph of human parietal pericardium. The mesothelial cells are covered with microvilli, and individual long cilia (arrow) are also present. Insert shows cilia at higher magnification. (From Ishihara, T., et al.: Histologic and ultrastructural features of normal human parietal pericardium. Am. J. Cardiol. *46*:744, 1980.)

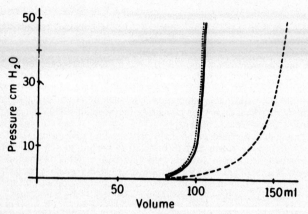

FIGURE 43–2 Pressure-volume curves before (left) and after (right) removal of the pericardium of an isolated dog heart. Solid line is pericardial volume, dotted line is heart volume within the pericardium, and dashed line is heart volume after removal of pericardium. Note that the curve at left is flat initially but becomes extremely steep as total volume within the pericardium increases. After removal of the pericardium (right curve), an increase in heart volume results in a lesser rise in pressure than with the pericardium intact. (From Hort, W.: Herzbentel und Herzgrosse. Arch. Kreislaufforsch. **44**:21, 1964.)

cardial sac, appears as a steep curve when plotted on a graph.[3] Thus, once the pericardium is filled, intrapericardial pressure rises sharply as volume is increased (Fig. 43–2). Normally, the pericardial sac is filled with a thin film of fluid distributed throughout the pericardial space in such a way that the pericardial reserve volume is not exceeded. This permits respiratory and postural changes in cardiac volume and total intrapericardial volume to occur without significant changes in intrapericardial pressure. Normally, pericardial pressure is equal to intrapleural pressure and varies from −5 to +5 cm H_2O during the respiratory cycle.[9] Pericardial pressure is transmitted uniformly throughout the fluid-filled intrapericardial space, thus minimizing the impact of gravitational or inertial forces on the circulation. This is analogous to the hydraulic function of cerebral spinal fluid relative to the cerebral circulation.[10]

Pericardial pressure is also a determinant of the *transmural distending pressure* of the cardiac chambers and contributes to the operation of the Frank-Starling mechanism in the beat-to-beat regulation of stroke volume. The transmural distending pressure of either ventricle is the difference between intracardiac and intrapericardial pressures and is independent of gravity. For example, when left ventricular end-diastolic pressure is +5 mm Hg and intrapericardial pressure is −2 mm Hg, relative to atmosphere, the actual ventricular distending pressure is 5 − (−2) = 7 mm Hg. With the chest closed, the presence of equal transmural pressures at all levels of the heart relative to gravity helps to insure uniform diastolic fiber stretch and operation of the Frank-Starling mechanism.[11]

When the volume of the heart or other contents of the pericardial sac increase and exceed the elastic limits of the pericardium, during diastole the heart is shifted to the steep portion of the curve relating intrapericardial pressure and volume, resulting in marked increases in intrapericardial and intracardiac pressures. However, the difference between the two pressures, i.e., the *transmural pressure*, usually declines. In the extreme case of cardiac tamponade,

in which both intrapericardial and intracardiac pressures are markedly increased, the transmural pressure distending the ventricles may fall precipitously, resulting in decreased ventricular diastolic volumes and preload. Conversely, when a reduction in elevated intracardiac volume occurs, intrapericardial pressure also falls, which promotes ventricular filling. This is exemplified by the changes in intrapericardial pressure and venous return that occur during ventricular ejection in every cardiac cycle. Ventricular ejection is accompanied by abrupt descent of the atrioventricular junction (the "base" of the heart) and a reduction in right atrial pressure, manifest by the x descent* in the right atrial pressure pulse as well as by a decline in intrapericardial pressure. These changes result in a surge of venous return during systole, particularly when ventricular and pericardial pressures are increased.[12] Brecher has shown that the acceleration of venous return during systolic ejection is diminished by opening of the pericardium.[13] These findings, taken together, indicate that changes in intrapericardial pressure modulate the regulation of stroke volume by ventricular preload, i.e., the Frank-Starling mechanism, particularly at higher ventricular and pericardial pressures.

Limitation of Cardiac Distention.   The relatively nondistensible pericardium may help to limit acute distention of the heart.[14,15] This was appreciated as early as 1898 by Bernard, who used a pump to increase pressure in excised hearts with and without the pericardium and noted that hearts unsupported by the pericardium ruptured at lower pressures than did hearts with intact pericardia.[16] More recent studies in dogs have suggested that the pericardium may *restrain* left ventricular filling, so that ventricular volume is greater at any given ventricular pressure with the pericardium removed than with the pericardium intact.[17-20] In addition, acute changes in intracardiac and total intrapericardial volume result in an upward shift of the left ventricular pressure-volume relationship, which is in part mediated by the restraining effect of the pericardium.

Thus, Shirato and Shabetai demonstrated that acute volume loading with dextran in dogs with intact pericardia resulted in an upward shift in the left ventricular pressure-segment length relation, i.e., left ventricular pressure was higher at any given segment length while the reduction of venous return and cardiac volume by means of nitroprusside administration shifted the curves downward toward control levels (see Figure 12–24, p. 429).[21] This occurred because nitroprusside and other vasodilators that decrease right heart filling reduce the total volume occupied by the heart within the pericardial space and thus reduce the restraining of the left ventricle by the pericardium; in turn, this causes a downward shift of the left ventricular pressure-volume relation so that a given left ventricular volume is associated with a lower left ventricular diastolic pressure. After pericardiectomy, volume loading resulted in a rightward shift in the pressure–segment length relation[21a] and, after nitroprusside, a leftward shift along a single

---

*It is recognized that the descent in venous pressure after the *a* wave is usually termed the *x* descent and, after the *c* wave, the *x'* descent. In this chapter, the major systolic venous pressure descent after the *a* and *c* waves will be termed the *x* descent.

curve. When the effect of the pericardium was eliminated by plotting left ventricular *transmural pressure* versus segment length, the points during all interventions also fell along a single curve.

Refsum et al. investigated the role of the pericardium in the mechanism of shifts in the left ventricular pressure-volume relationship by infusing saline both intravenously and into the pericardial sac in closed-chest dogs in which intrapericardial and cardiac volumes were assessed by computed tomography.[22] Acute upward shifts in the left ventricular diastolic pressure-volume relationship during volume loading were due to elevations in intrapericardial pressure induced by increases in total intrapericardial volume.

A restraining effect of the pericardium has also been observed early in the course of chronic volume overloading induced by formation of arteriovenous shunts in dogs prior to enlargement of the pericardium by stretch or hypertrophy, but this restraining effect was not apparent in dogs studied late during the course of chronic volume overload.[23] This finding suggests that chronic left ventricular enlargement and hypertrophy are accompanied by compensatory hypertrophy or stretch of the pericardium and an increase in total intrapericardial volume.

These observations, taken together, suggest that shifts in the left ventricular intracavity pressure-volume relation following volume loading or vasodilator administration are largely due to changes in intrapericardial pressure. However, the pericardium does not affect *intrinsic* myocardial compliance[24] nor does it account for changes in the left ventricular diastolic pressure-volume relationship observed during ischemia.[25]

Ventricular Interdependence.   The pericardium also contributes to *diastolic coupling* between the two ventricles, i.e., to ventricular interdependence. The distention of one ventricle alters the distensibility of the other, even in the absence of the pericardium.[26–29] This effect appears to be mediated in part by shared encircling muscle bands and by the interventricular septum, which tends to bulge into the left ventricle, causing a change in the shape of the left ventricle when the right ventricle is distended.[30–32] In the *absence* of the pericardium, large increases in right ventricular volume and pressure are required to cause an appreciable increase in left ventricular filling pressure (Fig. 43–3).[33,34] In contrast, the presence of an intact pericardium markedly accentuates the coupling between ventricular diastolic pressures.[35–39] When right ventricular volume and pressure are increased with the pericardium intact, right and left ventricular filling pressures are closely correlated and left ventricular volume is smaller than in the absence of the pericardium, when cardiac distensibility is primarily related to properties of the myocardium.[39] This effect of the pericardium on diastolic ventricular interaction is present at normal filling pressures and becomes of increasing importance at high right ventricular filling pressures.[33] The normal pericardium does not appear to contribute importantly to the interaction of the ventricles during systole.[40]

In *summary*, there is experimental evidence that the pericardium limits acute distention of the heart, mediates changes in the relationship between ventricular pressure and volume, and enhances the effect that distention of one ventricle has on the diastolic pressure-volume relations of the contralateral ventricle.

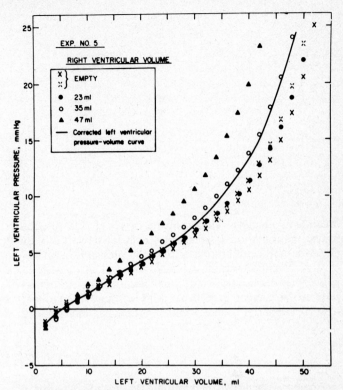

FIGURE 43–3 Left ventricular pressure-volume curves of the canine left ventricle without the pericardium obtained with the right ventricle empty and containing several different volumes. Increases in right ventricular volume result in a higher left ventricular pressure at the same left ventricular volume. This effect is most pronounced over the range of elevated left ventricular pressures and volumes. (From Taylor, R. R., et al.: Dependence of ventricular distensibility on filling of the opposite ventricle. Am. J. Physiol. *213*:711, 1967.)

Functions of the Pericardium in Man.   Although one must be cautious in extrapolating the findings of animal experiments to the intact human heart, there is evidence in man that the restraining effects of the pericardium are clinically relevant. First, in humans after pericardiotomy, there is a downward shift of the left ventricular pressure-volume curve that is increasingly apparent as left ventricular volume increases.[41] In addition, angiotensin, nitroprusside, and nitroglycerin infusions, which alter intracardiac volume, cause acute shifts in the left ventricular diastolic pressure-volume relation[42–44] (Fig. 12–24, p. 429), an effect which probably depends on the presence of the pericardium. Ludbrook demonstrated in humans that the downward shift in the left ventricular pressure-volume curve that occurs during nitroglycerin administration is *not* observed with amyl nitrite, which alters aortic pressure but has no acute effect on intracardiac and intrapericardial volumes (Fig. 43–4).[45] After pericardiotomy and loss of the restraining effect of the pericardium, the human left ventricular pressure-volume curve is *not* altered by nitroprusside administration.[46] These observations indicate that the beneficial effects of interventions such as nitroprusside infusion, in which an augmentation of stroke volume may be observed at a lower ventricular filling pressure, are in part due to an alteration of apparent cardiac distensibility mediated by reducing the restraining effect of the pericardium.[47]

The pericardium may also provide a significant restraining effect on acute cardiac dilatation during acute volume

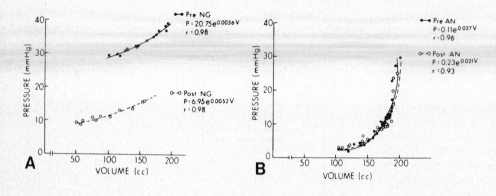

FIGURE 43-4 Left ventricular pressure-volume curves in man (*A*) before and after nitroglycerin (NG) and (*B*) before and after amyl nitrite (AN). Nitroglycerin, which causes venodilation and reduce total intrapericardial volume, shifts the curve downward and leftward. In contrast, the curves before and after amyl nitrite, which causes arterial dilatation, can be superimposed. (From Ludbrook, P. A., et al.: Influence of right ventricular hemodynamics on left ventricular diastolic pressure-volume relations in man. Circulation *59*: 21, 1979, by permission of the American Heart Association, Inc.)

loading in humans. Thus, volume overload due to acute mitral regurgitation is sometimes associated with striking elevation and equilibration of diastolic pressures in all four cardiac chambers similar to that observed in constrictive pericardial disease (p. 1488), but these findings do not appear to be present in patients with chronic volume overload.[48] Similarly, acute right ventricular infarction is sometimes associated with elevation and equilibration of diastolic right and left ventricular pressures[49] that have been shown experimentally to be related to the elevation of intrapericardial pressure.[50] The effect of the pericardium on the coupling between right and left ventricular pressures in man is dramatically illustrated by the pathophysiology of pericardial tamponade (p. 1480).

ACUTE PERICARDITIS

Acute pericarditis is a syndrome due to inflammation of the pericardium characterized by chest pain, a pericardial friction rub, and serial electrocardiographic abnormalities. The incidence of pericardial inflammation detected in several autopsy series ranges from 2 to 6 per cent, whereas pericarditis is diagnosed clinically in only about one out of 1,000 hospital admissions. This suggests that pericarditis is frequently inapparent clinically, although it may occur in the presence of a vast number of medical and surgical disorders (Table 43-1). The most common causes of the syndrome of acute pericarditis include idiopathic or viral pericarditis, uremia, bacterial infection, acute myocardial infarction, tuberculosis, neoplasm, and trauma.[51] All types of pericarditis are more common in men than in women and in adults compared with young children. The relative frequency of causes of pericarditis depend on the clinical setting. Presumed viral or idiopathic pericarditis is common in an outpatient setting, while pericarditis related to trauma, neoplasm, uremia, and postpericardiotomy syndrome is seen more frequently in tertiary hospitals.

The *pathological changes* of acute pericarditis are those of acute inflammation, including the presence of polymorphonuclear leukocytes, increased pericardial vascularity, and deposition of fibrin. Inflammation may also involve the superficial myocardium, and fibrinous adhesions may form between the pericardium and epicardium and between the pericardium and adjacent sternum and pleura. The visceral pericardium may also react to acute injury by exudation of fluid, the character of which is determined by the cause of pericardial inflammation (Table 43-2). The pathological and clinical features of specific etiologies of pericarditis are discussed later in this chapter (Table 43-3). This section will focus on clinical features common to acute pericarditis of many causes.

HISTORY. *Chest pain* is frequently the chief complaint of patients with acute pericarditis; its quality and location are variable. Pain is often localized to retrosternal and left precordial regions and frequently radiates to the trapezius ridge and neck.[52] Occasionally, it may be localized to the epigastrium, mimicking an acute abdomen, or have a dull or oppressive quality, with radiation to the left arm similar to the ischemic pain of myocardial infarction. The pain is often aggravated by lying supine, coughing,

TABLE 43-1 COMMON CAUSES OF PERICARDITIS

Idiopathic
Infectious
   Viral
   Bacterial
   Tuberculous
   Fungal
   Parasitic
Neoplastic
   Primary pericardial tumors
   Metastatic or contiguous spread from extracardiac neoplasms
Radiation injury
Uremia
Rheumatologic diseases
   Rheumatic fever
   Rheumatoid arthritis
   Systemic lupus erythematosus
   Scleroderma
Acute myocardial infarction
Autoimmune cardiac injury
   Dressler's syndrome
   Postpericardiotomy syndrome
Trauma and iatrogenic injury
   Penetrating and nonpenetrating injury
   Cardiac catheterization
   Pacemaker penetration
   Pseudoaneurysm rupture
   Dissecting aortic aneurysm
   Anticoagulants
Drug-induced
   Procainamide
   Hydralazine
   Isoniazid
   Penicillin
   Methysergide
   Daunorubicin
Other
   Myxedema
   Cholesterol pericarditis
   Chylopericardium

TABLE 43–2 ETIOLOGY OF PERICARDIAL EFFUSION

Serous
   Congestive heart failure
   Hypoalbuminemia
   Irradiation
   Viral pericarditis
   Tuberculous pericarditis
   Bacterial pericarditis
  Blood (Hematocrit > 10%)
   Iatrogenic
     Cardiac operation
     Cardiac catheterization
     Trauma (penetrating and nonpenetrating)
     Anticoagulant agents
     Chemotherapeutic agents
   Neoplasm
   Trauma
   Acute myocardial infarction
   Cardiac rupture
   Rupture of ascending aorta or major pulmonary artery
   Coagulopathy
   Uremia
  Lymph or chyle
   Neoplasm
   Iatrogenic
     Cardiothoracic surgery
   Congenital
   Idiopathic ("primary chylopericardium")
   Nonneoplastic obstruction of thoracic duct

Modified from Roberts, W. C., and Ferrans, V. J.: A survey of the causes and consequences of pericardial heart disease. *In* Reddy, P. S., et al. (eds.): Pericardial Disease. New York, Raven Press, 1982, p. 59.

deep inspiration, and swallowing and is eased by sitting up and leaning forward. Sometimes it is noted with each heart beat. The pain associated with pericarditis may arise from inflammation of both the pericardium and the adjacent pleura, accounting for the pleuritic nature of the discomfort. Pericardial pain may also be provoked by stretch of the pericardial sac due to the presence of intrapericardial fluid.

Acute pericarditis may also cause *dyspnea*. This symptom is related in part to the need to breathe shallowly to avoid pericardiopleuritic chest pain. Dyspnea may be aggravated by the presence of fever or by the development of a large pericardial effusion that compresses adjacent bronchi and pulmonary parenchyma. Additional symptoms such as cough, sputum production, or weight loss may be due to an underlying systemic disease such as tuberculosis or uremia.

PHYSICAL EXAMINATION. The *pericardial friction rub* is the pathognomonic physical finding of acute pericarditis. It is a scratching, grating, high-pitched sound, described by Laennec's associate Victor Collin as "the squeak of leather of a new saddle under the rider."[1] Although the sound is believed to arise from friction between the roughened pericardial and epicardial surfaces, a loud pericardial rub may also be heard in the presence of scant or large pericardial effusions.[53] The pericardial friction rub is classically described as having three components that are related to cardiac motion during atrial systole (presystole), ventricular systole, and rapid ventricular filling in early diastole. Spodick's prospective analysis of the pericardial friction rub revealed that the presystolic component is present in about 70 per cent of cases, while a ventricular systolic component is the loudest and most easily heard component, present in almost all cases.[54] The rapid diastolic filling component is detected less frequently and may be slurred into that of atrial contraction, resulting in a biphasic "to-and-fro" rub. In this series, a true three-component rub was detected about half the time and at the lower left sternal border. The single-component rub is the least common but is likely to be the auscultatory finding in patients with atrial fibrillation.

An important feature of the pericardial friction rub is that it is often evanescent and may change in quality from

TABLE 43–3 ETIOLOGICAL AND MORPHOLOGICAL CLASSIFICATIONS OF PERICARDIAL DISEASE

ETIOLOGICAL	MORPHOLOGICAL					
	Fibrinous	*Effusion*	*Fibrous*	*Granulomatous*	*Calcific*	*Cholesterol*
1. Idiopathic	+ +	+	+ +	0	+ +	+ +
2. Infective						
a. Pyogenic	+	+	+	0	0	0
b. Tuberculous	+	+	+ +	+ +	+	+
c. Viral	+ +	+	+	0	0	0
d. Parasitic	+	+	+	+	+	0
e. Fungal	+	+	+	+	+	0
3. Associated with systemic disease						
a. Collagen disease						
(1) Rheumatic fever	+ +	0	0	0	0	0
(2) Rheumatoid arthritis	+	0	+ +	+	0	+
(3) Systemic lupus erythematosus	+	+	+ +	0	0	0
(4) Scleroderma	+	0	+ +	0	0	0
b. Renal disease	+ +	+	+	0	0	0
c. Myxedema	0	+	0	+	+	+ +
d. Sarcoidosis	0	0	0	+ +	0	0
4. Acute myocardial infarction	+ +	0	+	0	0	0
5. Trauma and iatrogenic						
a. Penetrating and nonpenetrating injury	+	+ +	+ +	0	0	+
b. Cardiac catheterization	+ +	+	0	0	0	0
c. Cardiac operation and postpericardiotomy syndrome	+	+	+ +	0	0	0
d. Drugs and hypersensitivity states	+ +	+	0	0	0	0
6. Neoplastic	+	+	0	0	0	0
7. Radiation	+	+	+ +	0	0	0

Modified from Roberts, W. C., and Ferrans, V. J.: A survey of the causes and consequences of pericardial heart disease. *In* Reddy, P. S., et al. (eds.): Pericardial Disease. New York, Raven Press, p. 56.

one examination to the next. Detection of the rub is aided by listening with the stethoscope diaphragm applied firmly to the chest at the lower left sternal border during inspiration and full expiration with the patient sitting up and leaning forward. Occasionally, rubs may be detected with the patient lying supine with arms extended above the head during inspiration or during suspended respiration. If a pericardial rub is not heard on a single examination and acute pericarditis is strongly suspected, this important finding should be sought on repeated examinations in a quiet room.

The single-component pericardial friction rub may be mistaken for a systolic murmur of tricuspid or mitral regurgitation. A pericardial rub may also be confused with the crunch of air in the mediastinum or the artifact of skin scratching against the stethoscope. Pericardial friction rubs may be differentiated from murmurs by (1) the use of exercise to permit detection of a classic three-component rub, (2) the failure of a rub to radiate widely or to vary in timing and duration with inspiration or change in posture in a manner characteristic of regurgitant murmurs, and (3) by the confirmatory finding of typical electrocardiographic changes of pericarditis.

ELECTROCARDIOGRAM. Serial electrocardiograms are extremely helpful in confirming the diagnosis of acute pericarditis. Electrocardiographic changes can occur a few hours or days after the onset of pericardial pain, and the electrocardiographic diagnosis of acute pericarditis is made by detecting the serial appearance of *four stages of abnormalities* of the ST segments and T waves (Fig. 43–5).[55–57] The etiology of these changes is believed to be related to an actual current of injury caused by superficial myocardial inflammation or epicardial injury due to increased pericardial pressure.[58]

Stage I electrocardiographic changes accompany the onset of chest pain and are virtually diagnostic of acute pericarditis. These comprise ST-segment elevation, which, unlike the pattern of ST-segment elevation in acute myocardial infarction, is concave upward and usually present in all leads except aV$_r$ and V$_1$.[58] ST-segment depression may be present in leads aV$_r$ and V$_1$. The T waves are usually *upright* in the leads with ST-segment elevation. Stage II occurs several days later and represents the return of ST segments to baseline, accompanied by T-wave flattening. This change in the ST segments usually occurs *prior* to the appearance of T-wave inversion. In contrast, T waves in acute myocardial infarction often become inverted *before* the ST segments return to baseline. Stage III is characterized by inversion of the T waves so that the T-wave vector becomes directed opposite to the ST-segment vector. T-wave inversion is generally present in most leads and is not associated with the loss of R-wave voltage or the appearance of Q waves. These features help to differentiate this stage of nonspecific T-wave inversion from changes associated with the evolution of transmural or subendocardial myocardial infarction. Stage IV represents the reversion of T-wave changes to normal, which may occur up to weeks or months later. T-wave inversion may occasionally persist indefinitely in patients with chronic pericardial inflammation due to tuberculosis, uremia, or neoplastic pericardial disease.

Electrocardiographic abnormalities appear in about 90 per cent of cases of acute pericarditis, and the finding of typical Stage I changes or a classic evolution of all four stages can be diagnostic even when other clinical features of pericarditis are misleading.[59] All four stages are detected in about 50 per cent of patients with acute pericarditis. In addition, depression of the P-R segment occurs in about 80 per cent of patients with acute pericarditis.[57,59] Depression of the P-R segment occurs during the early stages of ST-segment elevation or T-wave inversion, is usually present in both limb and pericardial leads, and may reflect abnormal atrial repolarization due to atrial inflammation.

Variations of the patterns described above are present in slightly less than 50 per cent of patients with pericarditis and include (1) isolated P-R–segment depression, (2) the absence of one or more stages of the ST-segment and T-wave changes, (3) evolution of Stage I (ST-segment elevation) directly to Stage IV (reversion of T waves to normal), (4) persistence of T-wave inversion, (5) appearance of ST-segment changes in only a few leads, (6) the appearance of marked T-wave inversion before the ST-segments returned to baseline, and (7) the absence of any serial electrocardiographic changes whatsoever.[59,60] Regional ST-segment deviation may be confused with electrocardiographic changes of regional myocardial ischemia.[61]

In addition to the features described above that help to distinguish the ST-segment changes of pericarditis from those of acute myocardial infarction, the changes of Stage I must also be differentiated from the electrocardiographic variant of *normal early repolarization* (p. 232).[61a] This pattern is usually seen in young males, in whom the clinical syndrome of pain and dyspnea suggesting acute pericarditis is absent; P-R–segment depression is occasionally present but is uncommon, and most importantly, *the electrocardiogram does not evolve through a pattern of the return of ST segments to baseline followed by T-wave inver-*

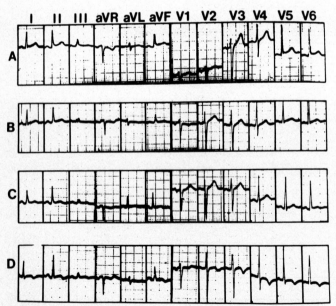

FIGURE 43–5 The four stages of electrocardiographic changes in acute pericarditis. *A*, Stage 1, diffuse ST-segment elevation that is concave upward; *B* and *C*, Stage 2, return of ST segments to baseline with upright T waves; *D*, Stage 3, diffuse T-wave inversion. Stage 4 (not shown) consists of a transition from Stage 3 to the prepericarditis electrocardiographic pattern. (From Spodick, D. H.: Pathogenesis and clinical correlations of the electrocardiographic abnormalities. Cardiovasc. Clin. *8*:201, 1977.)

sion.[62] An ST/ T ratio greater than 0.25 in lead V_6 also appears to discriminate patients with acute pericarditis from those with the normal variant of early repolarization.[63]

Rhythm disturbances occur in approximately one-fifth of patients with acute pericarditis. These disturbances may be related to the proximity of the sinus node and perinodal tissue to the overlying inflamed pericardium,[64] or to actual inflammation of the atria. Sinus tachycardia is common and may be present in the absence of other contributing factors, such as fever or hemodynamic compromise.[65] Profound sinus bradycardia occasionally occurs due to vagal stimulation from inflammation or stretching of the pericardial sac. Intermittent atrial fibrillation, paroxysmal supraventricular tachycardia, and atrial flutter may also occur.[64] Atrioventricular block and bundle branch block are *not* features of acute pericarditis, and these findings suggest the presence of extensive myocardial inflammation, fibrosis, or acute ischemia. Ventricular tachycardia and fibrillation are also extremely rare except in the setting of acute pericarditis complicating acute myocardial infarction.

OTHER LABORATORY FINDINGS. The *chest roentgenogram* is of little diagnostic value in the diagnosis of uncomplicated acute pericarditis. If acute pericarditis is complicated by the appearance of a large pericardial effusion, the chest roentgenogram may show both enlargement and changes in configuration of the cardiac silhouette (Fig. 6–43*A*, p. 176). The chest roentgenogram may provide clues to the underlying etiology of acute pericarditis as in the case of pericarditis secondary to tuberculosis, bacterial pneumonia, or malignancy. The *echocardiogram* is at present the most sensitive and accurate tool in the detection and quantification of pericardial fluid and is discussed on pages 130 to 133. Technetium-99m pyrophosphate scans have also been reported to show either diffuse or regional uptake patterns in one-half to two-thirds of patients with the clinical diagnosis of acute pericarditis,[66,67] and it appears that a positive scan is likely to occur when pericarditis is associated with myocardial inflammation and vascular leakage.[68] Gallium radionuclide scans have also been reported to be useful in detecting acute purulent pericarditis.[69–71]

Acute pericarditis is often associated with nonspecific indicators of inflammation, including leukocytosis and elevation of the sedimentation rate. Cardiac isoenzymes are usually normal, but modest elevation of the MB fraction of creatine phosphokinase may occur in the presence of epicardial inflammation accompanying acute pericarditis.[72,73] For this reason, cardiac isoenzymes can not always be used to differentiate between acute pericarditis and acute myocardial infarction.

Based on the history, physical examination, and clinical setting, some patients may require more extensive diagnostic tests to clarify the possibility of an underlying systemic disease. Because of the serious consequences of missing the diagnosis of tuberculous pericarditis, screening for tuberculosis with a tuberculin skin test and a control skin test to exclude anergy is reasonable for all patients suspected of having acute pericarditis. Other diagnostic tests that may be indicated in individual patients are based on the clinical presentation: (1) blood cultures to exclude associated possible infective endocarditis and bacteremia; (2) acute and convalescent cultures of blood, urine, throat, and feces, if available from the hospital laboratory, to evaluate a sus-

pected viral etiology; (3) fungal serological tests to evaluate a suspected fungal etiology in patients from endemic areas or in immunocompromised patients; (4) ASO titer in children with suspected rheumatic fever; (5) cold agutinins to exclude a mycoplasma etiology; (6) heterophile antibody test to exclude mononucleosis; (7) TSH, T_4, and T_3 to exclude hypothyroidism; (8) BUN and creatinine to exclude uremic etiology; and (9) antinuclear antibody titer (ANA), rheumatoid factor, extractable nuclear antigen and serum complement levels to exclude systemic lupus erythematosus and rheumatoid arthritis or to help assess disease activity in patients with a known collagen vascular disease.

MANAGEMENT. The first step in the management of acute pericarditis consists of establishing whether the pericarditis is related to an underlying problem that requires specific therapy.[74] Nonspecific therapy of an initial episode of pericarditis should include bed rest until pain and fever have disappeared, since activity may cause worsening of symptoms. Observation in the hospital is warranted for almost all patients with acute pericarditis to exclude an associated myocardial infarction or a pyogenic process and to watch for the development of tamponade.

The pain of pericarditis usually responds to nonsteroidal antiinflammatory agents such as aspirin (650 mg orally every 3 to 4 hours) or indomethacin (25 to 75 mg orally four times daily). When pain in severe and does not respond to this therapy within 48 hours, corticosteroids may be employed. If prednisone is used, large doses, such as 60 to 80 mg daily in divided doses, should be given. After 5 to 7 days, if the patient has been free of symptoms for several days, antiinflammatory agents should be tapered. Owing to the adverse consequences of long-term steroid therapy, it is desirable to avoid their use for pain control whenever possible. When long-term steroid administration is needed to control pain and other evidence of inflammation, alternate-day therapy should be attempted. Patients in whom steroids cannot be discontinued may tolerate tapering of steroids and weaning to nonsteroidal antiinflammatory agents. Left stellate ganglion blockade has been used for relief of severe recurrent pericardial pain.

Rarely, total pericardiectomy must be performed in patients with recurrent, disabling pericarditis who cannot be weaned from steroids. Pericardiectomy is usually safe and effective in preventing recurrences of pericardial pain but should only be performed by a surgeon familiar with extensive removal of the pericardium. Antibiotics should be used only to treat documented purulent pericarditis. Anticoagulants should not be administered during the acute phase of pericarditis of any cause. If anticoagulants must be continued owing to the presence of a mechanical prosthetic heart valve, we recommend use of intravenous heparin, which can be promptly reversed with protamine, and both physical examination and echocardiography should be performed at regular intervals to watch closely for the development of a pericardial effusion under pressure.

NATURAL HISTORY. Viral pericarditis, idiopathic pericarditis, post–myocardial infarction pericarditis, or the postpericardiotomy syndrome are usually self-limited; clinical and laboratory signs of inflammation abate after 2 to 6 weeks. The most troublesome complication is the development of recurrent episodes of pericardial inflammation at intervals of weeks or months after the initial episode. Recurrences occur in about one-fourth of patients with an initial episode of acute pericarditis and are most common in viral, idiopathic, rheumatoid, and uremic pericarditis.

Pericarditis can also be complicated by the development of disabling or life-threatening hemodynamic complications due to cardiac compression. These include (1) the development of a pericardial effusion under pressure, resulting in cardiac tamponade; (2) the development of fibrosis and/or calcification of the pericardium, resulting in constrictive physiology; and (3) a combination of both effusive and constrictive pericardial disease.

PERICARDIAL EFFUSION

Pericardial effusion may develop as a response to injury of the parietal pericardium with all causes of acute pericarditis. It may be clinically silent, but if the accumulation of fluid causes intrapericardial pressure to increase, resulting in cardiac compression, the symptoms of cardiac tamponade develop. The development of increased intrapericardial pressure secondary to a pericardial effusion depends on several factors: (1) the absolute volume of the effusion, (2) the rate of fluid accumulation, and (3) the physical characteristics of the pericardium itself. The pericardial space in humans normally contains between 15 and 50 ml of fluid. If additional fluid accumulates slowly, the pericardium stretches; the pericardial sac can accommodate up to 1 to 2 liters without elevation of intrapericardial pressure. However, the normal unstretched pericardial sac can accommodate the *rapid* addition of only 80 to 200 ml of fluid and still remain on the flat portion of the curve relating intrapericardial pressure and volume (Fig. 43–2, p. 1472). If additional fluid is rapidly added to a volume exceeding about 150 to 200 ml, a marked rise of intrapericardial pressure occurs. Intrapericardial pressure may also increase markedly after the accumulation of a smaller amount of fluid if the pericardium is excessively stiff because of fibrosis or tumor infiltration.

PERICARDIAL EFFUSION WITHOUT CARDIAC COMPRESSION

HISTORY. Patients who develop a pericardial effusion without elevation of intrapericardial pressure may have no symptoms whatsoever. Occasionally these patients complain of a constant oppressive dull ache or pressure in the chest, which is probably related to persistent stretching of the pericardial sac. Large pericardial effusions may cause symptoms by mechanical compression of adjacent structures including dysphagia from esophageal compression, cough due to bronchial/tracheal compression, dyspnea from compression of lung parenchyma with subsequent atelectasis, hiccups due to phrenic nerve compression, or hoarseness due to recurrent laryngeal nerve compression. Nausea and a sense of abdominal fullness may be present from pressure on adjacent abdominal viscera.[52]

PHYSICAL EXAMINATION. A small pericardial effusion in the absence of an increase in intrapericardial pressure may result in no specific physical findings, whereas a large effusion may produce several characteristic physical findings. First, the heart sounds may be distant or muffled owing to the interposition of fluid between the chest wall and the cardiac chambers. Compression of the base of the left lung by pericardial fluid produces *Ewart's*

sign, i.e., a patch of dullness on auscultation beneath the angle of the left scapula.[75] Rales may be heard over the lung fields secondary to compression of lung parenchyma. Abnormalities of the arterial pulse, systemic blood pressure, and jugular venous pulse do *not* occur when a large pericardial effusion is present without significant elevation of the intrapericardial pressure.

CHEST ROENTGENOGRAM (see page 174).   Enlargement of the cardiac silhouette usually does not occur until at least 250 ml of fluid have accumulated in the pericardial space. Therefore a normal or unchanged chest roentgenogram does not exclude the presence of a hemodynamically important pericardial effusion. This examination may suggest the presence of a pericardial effusion if there is a rapid increase in the size of the cardiac silhouette in the presence of clear lung fields (see Figure 6–43*A*, p. 176). In some cases the heart may assume a globular or waterbottle shape, blurring the contours along the left cardiac border and obscuring the hilar vessels. The parietal pericardial and epicardial fat layers are normally separated by 1 to 2 mm. The presence of an effusion may result in more marked separation of the pericardial fat lines, apparent on high-quality frontal or lateral chest films in about 25 per cent of patients with pericardial effusions.[76] *Fluoroscopy* may reveal absent or weak pulsations and the absence of any changes in the size and shape of the cardiac silhouette during deep inspiration or the Valsalva maneuver. These findings are especially useful in the cardiac catheterization laboratory when the accumulation of intrapericardial fluid due to possible perforation of the heart by a pacemaker or catheter is suspected.

Venous angiography may reveal a separation of more than 10 mm between the opacified right atrium and the outer border of the cardiac silhouette.[77] Radionuclide scanning with technetium-labeled aggregates of albumin has also been used to label blood within the heart, liver, and lungs simultaneously. The presence of an abnormal unlabeled space between the heart and the adjacent liver and lungs suggests the presence of a pericardial effusion.[78] *Computed tomography* (p. 189) has also been used to image pericardial effusions (Fig. 43–6).[79–82]

ELECTROCARDIOGRAM.   The electrocardiogram may reveal the nonspecific findings of a reduction in QRS voltage and flattening of the T waves as fluid accumulates within the pericardial space.[58,83] Electrical alternans (p. 1484) suggests the presence of a massive pericardial effusion and cardiac tamponade.

ECHOCARDIOGRAPHY (also see page 130). This technique is the most accurate, rapid, and widely used technique for evaluating a pericardial effusion. It is useful in detecting and quantifying an effusion, in following the

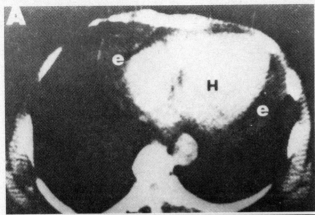

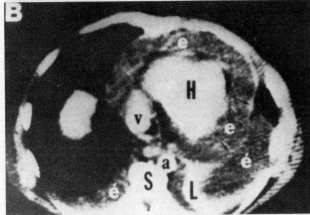

FIGURE 43–6 Computed tomograms of (A) a patient with pericardial effusion alone (e) and (B) a patient with a pericardial effusion (e) that is clearly demarcated from a coexisting pleural effusion (e'). H = heart; L = lung; S = spine; v = inferior vena cava; a = aorta. (From Wong, B. Y. S., et al.: Diagnosis of pericardial effusion by computed tomography. Chest *81*:177, 1982.)

accumulation or resolution of fluid over time, and in assessing the functional status of the cardiac valves and myocardium.[84] Recognition of pericardial fluid depends on the acoustical differences among the pericardium, cardiac muscle, and pericardial fluid. Accumulation of pericardial fluid results in the appearance of an echo-free space between the posterior left ventricular wall and posterior parietal pericardium and between the anterior wall of the right ventricle and adjacent echoes of the parietal pericardium and chest wall (Fig. 43–7).[85] M-mode echocardiography appears to be sufficiently sensitive to detect as little as 20 ml of pericardial fluid.[86]

Although the quantification of pericardial effusions by echocardiography is not precise, several guidelines for assessment are helpful.[86a] Very small effusions are likely to be imaged only posteriorly, with separation of the pericardial and epicardial echoes only in systole. Small- to moderate-sized effusions are likely to be imaged only posteriorly, with the presence of an echo-free space throughout the cardiac cycle. Pericardial effusions of approximately 300 ml can usually be imaged both anteriorly and posteriorly. Moderate-to-large effusions may be associated with excessive swinging motion of the heart and the false-positive appearance of mitral valve prolapse and anterior septal motion. Normally, the echo-free space representing a pericardial effusion disappears behind the left atrium owing to

the absence of fluid in the oblique pericardial sinus. However, in massive effusions, fluid may also collect in the oblique sinus, resulting in an echo-free space behind the left atrium as well as the left ventricle.

M-mode echocardiography is usually adequate to diagnose pericardial effusion, but occasionally the diagnosis may be confused with a left pleural effusion, giant left atrium, pulmonary infiltrate, and retrograde hiatal hernia.[87] Two-dimensional echocardiography (Figs. 43–7, and 5–78, p. 133) is particularly useful in correctly identifying pleural effusions and giant left atria,[88] and in locating a loculated pericardial effusion.[89]

MANAGEMENT. The clinical significance of any pericardial effusion depends on (1) the presence or absence of hemodynamic embarrassment due to increased intrapericardial pressure and (2) the presence and nature of the underlying systemic disease. The use of echocardiography to establish the diagnosis of a pericardial effusion is warranted in suspected cases of acute pericarditis, since presence of an effusion helps to confirm the diagnosis of pericardial disease. Attempts to document the presence of an effusion are also warranted when there is evidence of progressive cardiac enlargement on radiographic examination, since this finding helps to exclude unsuspected myocardial or valvular heart disease as the cause of the

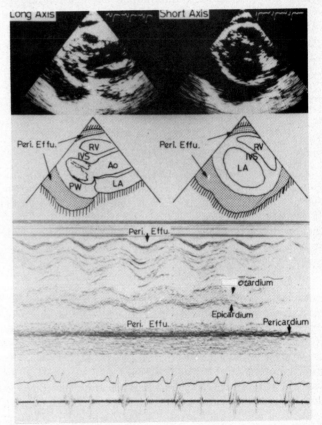

FIGURE 43–7 *Upper panels,* Long- and short-axis views of a large pericardial effusion on a two-dimensional echocardiogram. *Lower panel,* M-mode echocardiogram at the midventricular level showing echo-free spaces that denote anterior and posterior pericardial effusions. Peri. Effu. = pericardial effusion; RV = right ventricle; IVS = interventricular septum; Ao = aorta; PW = left ventricular posterior wall; LA = left atrium. (From Shah, P. M.: Echocardiography in pericardial diseases. *In* Reddy, P. S., et al. [eds.]: Pericardial Disease. New York, Raven Press, 1982, p. 133.)

enlargement. Pericardiocentesis (p. 1486) is *not* indicated unless there is evidence of cardiac compression due to cardiac tamponade or unless analysis of pericardial fluid is essential to establish a diagnosis such as bacterial pericarditis.

CHRONIC PERICARDIAL EFFUSIONS

Chronic pericardial effusions persisting for more than six months may occur in any form of pericardial disease. Often they are surprisingly well tolerated, with no symptoms of cardiac compression, and are discovered when a routine chest roentgenogram discloses an unexpectedly large cardiac silhouette.[90] Chronic pericardial effusions are particularly likely to be found in patients with previous idiopathic or viral pericarditis, uremic pericarditis, and pericarditis secondary to myxedema or neoplasm. The management of chronic pericardial effusion depends in part on the etiology. Stable and apparently idiopathic effusions usually require no specific treatment except for avoidance of anticoagulants.[91] Chronic effusions secondary to tuberculosis, neoplasm, purulent infection, or hemorrhage into the pericardium may progress to cardiac tamponade or pericardial fibrosis, calcification, and constriction. As discussed on page 1505, large chronic effusions secondary to uremia may contribute to intermittent hypotension and instability during dialysis. When chronic pericardial effusion causes serious symptoms, a large subxiphoid pericardiotomy or total pericardiectomy may be warranted.[92,93] In the setting of chronic pericardial effusion, these surgical approaches allow evacuation of loculated fluid, fibrin, or thrombus and sampling of pericardial tissue for culture and histological examination.

PERICARDIAL EFFUSION WITH CARDIAC COMPRESSION: CARDIAC TAMPONADE

An increase in intrapericardial pressure secondary to fluid accumulation within the pericardial space results in cardiac tamponade, which is characterized by (1) an elevation of intracardiac pressures, (2) progressive limitation of ventricular diastolic filling, and (3) a reduction of stroke volume.

PATHOPHYSIOLOGY

As already noted, intrapericardial pressure is normally very close to intrapleural pressure and several mm Hg lower than right and left ventricular diastolic pressures. When the addition of fluid into the pericardial space causes intrapericardial pressure to rise to the level of the right atrial and right ventricular diastolic pressures, the transmural pressure distending these chambers declines to close to zero and cardiac tamponade occurs.[94] The rise of right atrial and intrapericardial pressures is less marked in the presence of hypovolemia, and therefore cardiac tamponade may be masked when hypovolemia is present (Fig. 43–8). Further accumulation of intrapericardial fluid causes both intrapericardial and right ventricular diastolic pressures to rise together to the level of left ventricular diastolic pressure, and subsequently, all three pressures rise together associated with a fall in systemic arterial pressure (Fig. 43–9). If left ventricular diastolic pressure is markedly elevated owing to preexisting left ventricular dis-

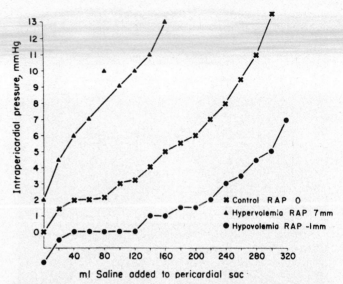

FIGURE 43–8 Pericardial pressure-volume curves obtained by adding saline solution to the pericardial sac in closed-chest anesthetized dogs. The curve is steeper with hypervolemia and less steep with hypovolemia, compared with control, because the heart occupies a greater volume in the pericardial cavity with hypervolemia and a smaller volume with hypovolemia. (From Fowler, N. O.: Physiology of cardiac tamponade and pulsus paradoxus. II. Physiological, circulatory, and pharmacological responses in cardiac tamponade. Mod. Conc. Cardiovasc. Dis. *47*:116, 1978, by permission of the American Heart Association, Inc.)

ease, cardiac tamponade occurs when right ventricular diastolic and pericardial pressures equalize but at a lower level than the left ventricular diastolic pressure.[95]

Equalization of intrapericardial and ventricular filling pressures results in markedly diminished diastolic volumes of both ventricles and a fall in stroke volume. These findings have been observed both in animals subjected to acute experimental tamponade and in humans with acute cardiac

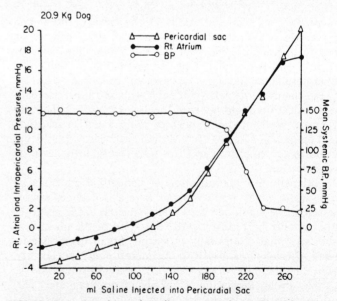

FIGURE 43–9 Experimental cardiac tamponade produced by injection of saline into the pericardial sac of an anesthetized dog. As more than 160 ml is injected, right atrial and intrapericardial pressures rise sharply and equilibrate, and blood pressure (BP) falls abruptly. (From Fowler, N. O.: Physiology of cardiac tamponade and pulsus paradoxus. II. Physiological, circulatory, and pharmacological responses in cardiac tamponade. Mod. Conc. Cardiovasc. Dis. *47*: 115, 1978, by permission of the American Heart Association, Inc.)

tamponade.[95-98] The reduction in stroke volume is initially compensated for by reflex increases in adrenergic tone; both tachycardia and increases in ejection fraction intially help to maintain forward cardiac output.[94,99] The importance of the adrenergic support of the heart is reflected in the finding that when beta-adrenergic blockade is carried out in cardiac tamponade, ejection fraction and stroke volume decline.[98] Systemic vascular resistance increases so that, at first, systemic arterial pressure is maintained at the expense of cardiac output. With severe cardiac tamponade, as cardiac output declines, compensatory mechanisms are no longer sufficient to maintain systemic arterial pressure, and perfusion of vital organs becomes impaired[99]; reduced coronary perfusion causes selective hypoperfusion of the subendocardium.[100,101] The addition of myocardial ischemia during cardiac tamponade could further compromise left ventricular stroke volume. In extreme cardiac tamponade, transmural diastolic ventricular pressures may actually be less than zero, suggesting that ventricular filling occurs by diastolic suction.[102] Sinus bradycardia, mediated by the cardiac depressor branches of the vagus nerve and by the nonvagal mechanism of sinoatrial node ischemia, may also occur during severe cardiac tamponade.[103,104] Profound bradycardia often occurs during severe hypotension and precedes the development of electrical-mechanical dissociation and death.[105]

Cardiac tamponade also alters the dynamics of systemic venous return and cardiac filling. Normally, one surge of systemic venous return occurs during ventricular ejection coincident with the systolic x descent of the venous pressure pulse, and a second surge occurs with the opening of the tricuspid valve in diastole, corresponding to the y descent. In cardiac tamponade, the heart is compressed throughout the cardiac cycle. During ejection, intracardiac volume transiently decreases, resulting in a transient fall in both intrapericardial and right atrial pressures, manifest as the x descent, which is accompanied by a surge of systemic venous return into the right atrium. However, in diastole, the total volume within the pericardial space remains elevated despite opening of the tricuspid valve; intrapericardial pressure remains elevated and equal to right atrial

pressure so that transmural distending pressure is close to zero. As a result, the usual surge of systemic venous return during early diastole is abolished. These events are graphically reflected in the right atrial or systemic venous waveform in cardiac tamponade, in that the systolic x descent is prominent while the diastolic y descent is usually completely absent or attenuated (Fig. 43–10).

Pulsus Paradoxus. Inspiration and the transmission of negative intrathoracic pressure to the pericardial space further alter the dynamics of right and left ventricular filling and are responsible for *pulsus paradoxus*, the inspiratory fall of aortic systolic pressure greater than 10 mm Hg (Fig. 43–11).[106] The finding of weakening of the arterial pulse during inspiration was first recorded in 1854 by Vieordt in a description of purulent pericarditis and was subsequently described by Kussmaul in 1873 as the apparent paradox of the disappearance of the pulse during inspiration despite persistence of the heart beat. It should be emphasized that pulsus paradoxus is in fact an exaggeration of the normal inspiratory decline of left ventricular stroke volume by about 7 per cent and of systemic arterial pressure by 3 per cent.[107]

The complex mechanism of *pulsus paradoxus* in cardiac tamponade has been the subject of considerable controversy.[108] Experimental studies on the effects of inspiration in animals and man have helped to clarify this mechanism. Experiments in humans using radiopaque markers and electromagnetic flowmeters[109,110] have shown that inspiration is normally accompanied by an increase in diastolic dimensions of the right ventricle, a small decrease in left ventricular dimension, and increased velocity of flow from the venae cavae into the right atrium. Pulsus paradoxus in cardiac tamponade appears to result from an exaggeration of these normal findings. Measurement of intracardiac pressures and flow during experimental tamponade[111] and in man during cardiac tamponade[107,112] have demonstrated that inspiration is associated with falls in intrapericardial and right atrial pressures, which results in augmentation of flow from the venae cavae into the right atrium and right ventricle and augmentation of pulmonary artery flow and pulmonary artery systolic pressure. On the left side of the

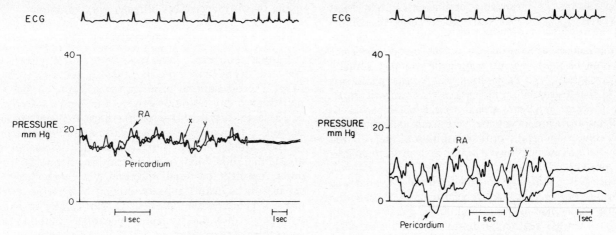

FIGURE 43–10 Right atrial (RA) and pericardial pressure measurements in a patient with cardiac tamponade. *Left panel*, Before pericardiocentesis, RA and pericardial pressures are elevated and equal, and the waveforms show the presence of the systolic x descent and near-absence of the diastolic y descent. *Right panel*, After removal of only 100 ml of pericardial fluid, and before pericardial pressure returns to zero, there is a reduction and separation of RA and pericardial pressures. Note that the RA waveform now shows a prominent diastolic y descent.

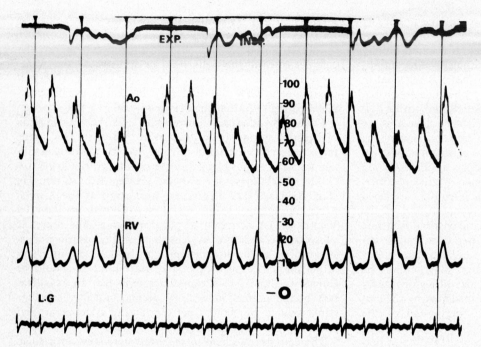

FIGURE 43–11 Recording of aortic (Ao) and right ventricular (RV) pressures in a patient with cardiac tamponade complicated by hypovolemia. *Pulsus paradoxus* is evident as a marked inspiratory decline in aortic systolic and pulse pressures during inspiration (INSP). RV pressure variation is out of phase with aortic pressure. Note that the RV waveform does *not* show a dip-and-plateau configuration. (From Shabetai, R., et al.: The hemodynamics of cardiac tamponade and constrictive pericarditis. Am. J. Cardiol. *26*:480, 1970.)

heart, left atrial and left ventricular diastolic pressures fall, accompanied by a fall in aortic flow and systolic arterial pressure.[107,113] The increase in venous return flow during inspiration results in a marked and exaggerated *increase in right ventricular dimensions* accompanied by a reduction in left ventricular dimensions and flattening and displacement of the septum toward the left ventricle.[114,115] *Thus, pulsus paradoxus in cardiac tamponade is critically dependent on the inspiratory augmentation of systemic venous return and right ventricular filling.*

Shabetai et al. demonstrated clearly that when experimental cardiac tamponade was induced in dogs, pulsus paradoxus did *not* develop when either the right heart was bypassed or right ventricular volume was strictly controlled.[111] These experiments also demonstrated that inspiratory pooling of blood within the lungs or traction on the heart by the diaphragm were *not* essential mechanisms of pulsus paradoxus in cardiac tamponade. Thus, these observations indicate that pulsus paradoxus in cardiac tamponade depends on the inspiratory expansion of right heart filling at the expense of left heart filling. However, competition for a "fixed space" within the pericardium is not the entire mechanism accounting for pulsus paradoxus, since (1) the sum of right and left ventricular volumes actually increases slightly with inspiration; (2) pulsus paradoxus occurs in the absence of an increase in the intrapericardial-pleural pressure gradient, which would be expected to occur if intrapericardial volume were fixed and right ventricular volume increased during inspiration; and (3) the cyclic variations in pulmonary artery and aortic pressures are not precisely 180 degrees out of phase.

Another factor that may contribute to pulsus paradoxus is an inspiratory increase in left ventricular afterload due to an inspiratory rise in transmural aortic pressure.[116] Furthermore, when left ventricular diastolic volume is markedly reduced, the left ventricle may be operating on the steep ascending limb of the Starling curve so that a small inspiratory reduction of left ventricular filling results in marked depression of left ventricular stroke volume and systolic pressure.[117,118] Pulsus paradoxus is occasionally observed in

constrictive pericarditis and restrictive heart disease, and the latter mechanism may account for its presence in these disorders.

Pulsus paradoxus has also been observed in lung disease secondary to emphysema, bronchitis, asthma, acute airway obstruction secondary to tracheal compression, tension pneumothorax, and massive pulmonary embolism.[119–122] Under these circumstances, pulsus paradoxus is probably related both to the transmission of excessively negative intrathoracic pressure during inspiration to the aorta and to exaggerated right heart filling with an associated decrease in left heart filling during inspiration. Pulsus paradoxus may be absent in cardiac tamponade when underlying heart disease causes a marked elevation of left ventricular diastolic pressure so that the two ventricles are unequally compressed,[95] in atrial septal defect when the increase in systemic venous return during inspiration is shared between the two sides of the heart,[123] and in aortic regurgitation when there is a major component of left ventricular filling that is independent of respiratory variation.

ETIOLOGY

Cardiac tamponade may occur with almost any cause of pericarditis and may exist in either an acute or a chronic form. The distribution of etiologies of acute cardiac tamponade in a city hospital between 1963 and 1980 is noted in Table 43–4.[124] In this series the most frequent etiologies of cardiac tamponade were neoplasm and idiopathic or viral pericarditis, followed by pericarditis associated with myocardial infarction, invasive cardiac diagnostic procedures, purulent bacterial infection, and tuberculosis. The use of anticoagulants appears to contribute to the development of acute cardiac tamponade, particularly in patients with pericarditis due to acute myocardial infarction or after cardiac surgery.[124,125]

CLINICAL MANIFESTATIONS

The triad of (1) a decline in systemic arterial pressure; (2) elevation of systemic venous pressure; and (3) a small,

TABLE 43–4 COMMON ETIOLOGIES OF CARDIAC TAMPONADE

DISORDER	%
Malignant disease	32
Idiopathic pericarditis	14
Uremia	9
Acute cardiac infarction (receiving heparin)	9
Diagnostic procedures with cardiac perforation	7.5
Bacterial	7.5
Tuberculosis	5
Radiation	4
Myxedema	4
Dissecting aortic aneurysm	4
Postpericardiotomy syndrome	2
Systemic lupus erythematosus	2
Cardiomyopathy (receiving anticoagulants)	2

Modified from Guberman, B. A., et al.: Cardiac tamponade in medical patients. Circulation 64:633, 1981.

quiet heart was described by the thoracic surgeon Claude S. Beck in 1935.[126] These three features are typical of cardiac tamponade from intrapericardial hemorrhage due to penetrating heart wounds, aortic dissection, and intrapericardial rupture of an aortic or cardiac aneurysm. This syndrome develops when the pericardium is not enlarged or stretched, so that the addition of less than 200 ml of fluid or blood causes intrapericardial pressure to rise abruptly to above 20 to 30 mm Hg. In cases that are not immediately fatal, both cardiac output and arterial pressure fall, accompanied by tachycardia and tachypnea. The patient may be stuporous or agitated and restless, and the additional important finding of pulsus paradoxus may be difficult to appreciate when profound hypotension is present.

Jugular venous pressure is usually markedly elevated, with a typical waveform devoid of a diastolic y descent, but this may be difficult to appreciate at the bedside owing to the presence of tachypnea and the use of accessory respiratory muscles. Precordial heart activity is usually not palpable and heart sounds are distant or inaudible. Cold, clammy extremities and anuria may be present.

Cardiac tamponade is easily confused with other etiologies of shock, such as sepsis or internal hemorrhage. However, systemic venous pressure is not elevated in these conditions (Chap. 18). Therefore, a keen awareness of the possibility of acute cardiac tamponade is essential in patients with a history of accident, trauma, or an invasive cardiac procedure. Cardiac tamponade due to rupture of the heart from acute myocardial infarction may also be confused with cardiogenic shock due to myocardial failure per se, but in the latter condition severe left atrial hypertension with pulmonary edema as well as jugular venous distention are likely to be present. Cardiac tamponade may occasionally be confused with shock due to right ventricular infarction with jugular venous distention and clear lungs. However, the hemodynamics of right ventricular infarction are more like those of constrictive physiology than of tamponade (p. 1505).

Patients in whom cardiac tamponade develops slowly differ from those with cardiac tamponade due to cardiac penetration or rupture. In the setting of more slowly developing cardiac tamponade, patients usually appear acutely ill but not in extremis and the major complaint is usually dyspnea.[124,127] Chest pain of either a pleuritic or an oppressive nature may also be present. In patients with chronic development of tamponade, additional systemic symptoms may include weight loss, anorexia, and profound weakness.

The most common physical finding in a series of medical patients with cardiac tamponade was *jugular venous distention*.[124] In addition to absolute elevation of the systemic venous pressure, a characteristic waveform consisting of a prominent systolic x descent and absent diastolic y descent can often be appreciated at the bedside. Other common physical findings include tachypnea (80 per cent), tachycardia (77 per cent), pulsus paradoxus (77 per cent), pulsus paradoxus with total inspiratory disappearance of the brachial pulse and Korotkoff sounds (23 per cent), pericardial friction rub (29 per cent), hepatomegaly (55 per cent), and diminished heart sounds (34 per cent). It is noteworthy that systolic arterial hypotension, consisting of a systolic pressure less than 100 mm Hg, was present in a minority (36 per cent), and the majority of patients were alert, with warm extremities and preserved urine output.[124]

The finding of *pulsus paradoxus* is critical in making the diagnosis of cardiac tamponade, since most patients with slowly developing cardiac tamponade do not have the classic physical findings of a small, quiet heart and severe hypotension.[124,128] Pulsus paradoxus can be detected on physical examination as an inspiratory decrease in the amplitude of the palpated pulse in the femoral or carotid arteries. Total paradox, i.e., complete disappearance of the palpated pulse during inspiration, occurs during very severe cardiac tamponade or tamponade combined with hypovolemia. The magnitude of the paradoxical pulse can be accurately quantified by means of an intraarterial catheter but may be estimated by cuff sphygmomanometry. The cuff should be inflated 20 mm Hg above systolic pressure and slowly deflated until the Korotkoff sounds are heard only during expiration. The cuff should then be deflated to the point at which Korotkoff sounds are heard equally well in inspiration and expiration. The difference between these pressures is the estimated magnitude of pulsus paradoxus.

Other disorders with systemic venous distention, pulsus paradoxus, and clear lungs that can be confused with cardiac tamponade include obstructive pulmonary disease,[121,122] constrictive pericarditis, restrictive cardiomyopathy,[129] right ventricular infarction,[49] and massive pulmonary embolism.[119,120] Pulsus paradoxus is occasionally noted in shock, but jugular venous distention is usually absent.[130]

The clinical findings may be further modified in patients with so-called *low-pressure cardiac tamponade*[131] who are normotensive and in whom the physical examination is normal except for moderate elevation of jugular venous pressure to about 5 to 15 mm Hg. This syndrome represents an early stage in the development of cardiac tamponade in which accumulation of a pericardial effusion causes intrapericardial pressure to rise to a level of 5 to 15 mm Hg, with equilibration of intrapericardial and right heart diastolic filling pressures. Pericardiocentesis reduces intrapericardial pressure and the separation of right atrial and intrapericardial pressures. Low-pressure cardiac tamponade has been reported in patients with tuberculosis and neoplastic pericarditis and is often associated with severe dehydration.

CHEST ROENTGENOGRAM. There are no roentgenographic features diagnostic of cardiac tamponade. The heart may appear completely normal in size in cardiac tamponade that develops from acute hemopericardium due to cardiac rupture or laceration. On the other hand, if an effusion accumulates more slowly to more than 250 ml, the cardiac silhouette may be enlarged.[127] Other roentgenographic findings may include obscuring of vessels at the hilum, a globular or waterbottle configuration of the heart, clear lungs, and separation of epicardial and pericardial fat pads. These findings suggest the presence of a large pericardial effusion but supply no information about its hemodynamic significance.

ELECTROCARDIOGRAM. The electrocardiographic abnormalities seen in acute cardiac tamponade include those of acute pericarditis and pericardial effusion per se (p. 1476). The development of electrical alternans[132-135] is a more specific indicator of pericardial tamponade and reflects pendular swinging of the heart within the pericardial space (Fig. 43–12).[136-138] Electrical alternans may also occur in constrictive pericarditis, in tension pneumothorax, after myocardial infarction, and with severe cardiac muscle dysfunction. However, the appearance of electrical alternans in a patient with a known pericardial effusion is highly suggestive of cardiac tamponade—a finding that has been confirmed in experimental cardiac tamponade.[139] Electrical alternans of the QRS complex may occur in a 2:1 or 3:1 pattern. Alternans is usually limited to the QRS complex, but alternans of the P wave, QRS complex, and T wave may rarely occur and appears to be limited to extreme cardiac tamponade,[140] often in association with neoplastic or tuberculous effusion. Both the abnormal heart motion within the pericardial sac and electrical alternans disappear when pericardial fluid is aspirated.

ECHOCARDIOGRAM. In patients with jugular venous distention and the possibility of cardiac tamponade, echocardiography is extremely useful and should be performed prior to consideration of pericardiocentesis. In a rare patient who is in extremis from the extremely rapid development of cardiac tamponade, the physician may have to rely on the history and physical findings to make a judgment about the need for pericardiocentesis. If echocardiography is readily available and the patient with suspected cardiac tamponade is not moribund, obtaining an echocardiogram will increase the likelihood of diagnosing

cardiac tamponade correctly. First, the echocardiogram helps to document the presence and magnitude of a pericardial effusion (Figs. 5–74, p. 131, and 5–75 and 5–76, p. 133), the absence of echocardiographic evidence of a pericardial effusion virtually excludes the diagnosis of cardiac tamponade (with the important exception of the postoperative cardiac surgery patient in whom loculated fluid or thrombus may cause cardiac compression). Second, the echocardiogram can rapidly differentiate cardiac tamponade from other causes of systemic venous hypertension and hypotension, including constrictive pericarditis, cardiac muscle dysfunction, and right ventricular infarction. The appearance of dense echoes in the pericardial space or extrinsic to the pericardium suggests the presence of material other than free fluid. Both massive extracardiac hematoma and extrinsic compression of the heart by tumor[141,142] can cause cardiac compression with the physiology of cardiac constriction or cardiac tamponade. When the echocardiogram excludes a pericardial effusion, inappropriate and potentially lethal attempts at pericardiocentesis or pericardiotomy can be avoided.

The echocardiogram can provide additional clues that a pericardial effusion is associated with cardiac tamponade. These important features include a gross reduction in the E-to-F slope and excursion of the anterior mitral valve leaflet,[115] early systolic notching of the anterior right ventricular wall, and sudden posterior motion of the interventricular septum during inspiration.[143] Acute cardiac tamponade has also been shown to be associated with right ventricular diastolic collapse[144] and an exaggerated inspiratory increase and expiratory decrease in right ventricular size.[144,145,145a] The echocardiographic findings of a pericardial effusion, a progressive fall in right ventricular dimensions during expiration, and an inspiratory increase in right ventricular dimensions suggest the diagnosis of cardiac tamponade. However, these changes are not specific,[146] and experimental studies indicate that a single echocardiogram cannot predict the presence or severity of cardiac tamponade.[147]

Radionuclide angiography can also detect right ventricu-

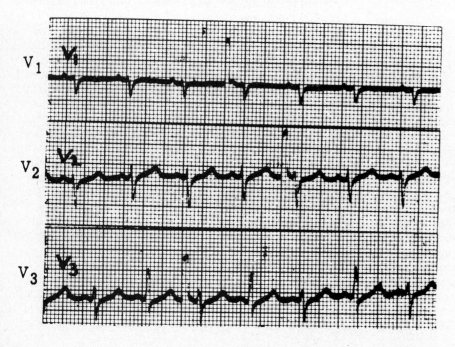

FIGURE 43–12   Electrical alternans (phasic alteration of the amplitude of the R wave) is present in a patient with pericardial effusion and cardiac tamponade. In lead V$_3$, the polarity of the QRS complex also alternates every other beat. (From Goldman, M. J.: Principles of Clinical Electrocardiography, 11th Edition. Los Altos, Lange Medical Publications, 1982, p. 305.)

lar and right atrial compression and compression of the superior vena cava as it enters the pericardium,[148] but these findings, while suggestive of cardiac tamponade, also lack sensitivity and specificity. Therefore it must be emphasized that cardiac tamponade is a clinical not an echocardiographic or a radionuclide diagnosis that is established definitively by documentation of the elevation and equilibration of intrapericardial and right atrial pressures and the reversal of these findings by evacuation of pericardial fluid.

CARDIAC CATHETERIZATION AND ANGIOGRAPHY

Cardiac catheterization is invaluable in establishing the hemodynamic importance of a pericardial effusion. Except in extreme emergencies, situations when the patient is moribund, we prefer to catheterize the right heart and pericardial space in conjunction with pericardiocentesis. Cardiac catheterization (1) provides absolute confirmation of the diagnosis of cardiac tamponade; (2) quantitates the magnitude of hemodynamic compromise; (3) guides pericardiocentesis by documenting that pericardial aspiration is associated with hemodynamic improvement; and (4) permits the detection of coexisting hemodynamic problems including left ventricular failure, right atrial hypertension due to tricuspid valve disease,[149] and effusive-constrictive pericarditis (p. 1496).

Cardiac catheterization typically demonstrates elevation of right atrial pressure with a characteristic prominent systolic x descent and a diminutive or absent y descent. When intrapericardial and right atrial pressures are recorded simultaneously, both are elevated and virtually identical (Fig. 43–10); both pressures fall during inspiration, and intrapericardial pressure may fall slightly below right atrial pressure during systolic ejection at the time of the x descent. If intrapericardial pressure is not elevated, and if right atrial and intrapericardial pressures are not virtually identical, the diagnosis of cardiac tamponade must be reconsidered.

Right ventricular diastolic pressure is elevated and equal to right atrial and intrapericardial pressures and lacks the dip-and-plateau configuration characteristic of constrictive pericarditis. Since right ventricular and pulmonary artery systolic pressures are equal to the pressure developed by the right ventricle plus the intrapericardial pressure, right ventricular and pulmonary artery systolic pressures are usually moderately elevated in the range of 35 to 50 mm Hg. It may be difficult to differentiate right ventricular and pulmonary artery waveforms without the use of fluoroscopy. In the case of severe cardiac compression, right ventricular systolic pressure may be reduced and only slightly higher than right ventricular diastolic pressure.

Usually, the pulmonary capillary wedge pressure and left ventricular diastolic pressure are elevated and equal to intrapericardial pressure when recorded simultaneously. However, in patients with severe underlying left ventricular dysfunction and marked elevation of the left ventricular diastolic pressure prior to the development of pericardial effusion, cardiac tamponade can be present when intrapericardial and right atrial pressures are equal but lower than left ventricular diastolic pressure.[95] Depending on the severity of cardiac compression, left ventricular systolic and aortic pressures may be normal or reduced.

Pulsus paradoxus can be easily documented by intraarterial catheterization and pressure measurement. Simultaneous recording of systemic arterial and right ventricular pressures shows that the inspiratory pressure variation is out of phase (Fig. 43–11). Stroke volume is usually markedly depressed. Cardiac output may be normal, owing to the compensatory effect of tachycardia, or it may be markedly reduced when cardiac tamponade is severe; systemic vascular resistance is usually elevated.

Angiographic studies are not essential if echocardiographic findings suggestive of cardiac tamponade were obtained prior to cardiac catheterization. Right atrial angiography usually demonstrates an abnormal concave appearance of the right atrial heart border and a water density extrinsic to the contrast-filled right atrium due to presence of the pericardial effusion.[150] In an otherwise normal heart, right and left ventricular end-diastolic volumes are usually reduced with normal or increased ejection fractions.

Aspiration of pericardial fluid results initially in the lowering of the identical intrapericardial, right atrial, right ventricular, and left ventricular diastolic pressures, followed by a fall of intrapericardial pressure below right atrial pressure and reappearance of the y descent in the right atrial waveform (Fig. 43–10). Further aspiration causes intrapericardial pressure to fall to a mean level of zero. Since the pressure-volume curve of the pericardium is steep, the initial aspiration of 50 to 100 ml of pericardial fluid usually leads to a striking reduction in intrapericardial pressure, a striking improvement in systemic arterial pressure and cardiac output, and abolition of pulsus paradoxus (Fig. 43–13).

If intrapericardial pressure falls to zero or becomes negative and right atrial pressure remains elevated, *effusive-*

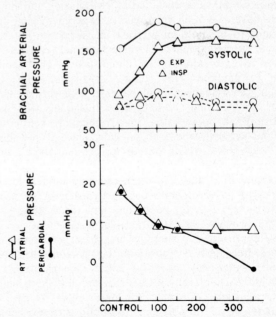

FIGURE 43–13 Hemodynamic changes in a patient with cardiac tamponade during serial 50-ml withdrawals of pericardial fluid. Striking improvement in brachial arterial pressure (*upper panel*) occurs during the initial aspirations. As pericardial fluid is withdrawn, right atrial and intrapericardial pressures (*lower panel*) initially decline together. After pericardial pressure falls below right atrial pressure, right atrial pressure shows no further decline. (From Reddy, P. S., et al.: Cardiac tamponade: Hemodynamic observations in man. Circulation *58*:265, 1978, by permission of the American Heart Association, Inc.)

constrictive pericarditis (p. 1496) should be strongly considered, especially in patients with underlying neoplasm. Other causes of continued elevation of right atrial pressure after successful pericardiocentesis include the coexistence of cardiac tamponade and preexisting left ventricular dysfunction causing, in turn, pulmonary hypertension and right atrial hypertension, tricuspid valve disease, and restrictive cardiomyopathy.

The distinction between cardiac tamponade and the superior vena cava syndrome must always be made in patients with neoplastic disease in whom these lesions may occur singly or together. In patients with obstruction of the superior vena cava, cardiac tamponade may be suspected from the presence of elevated jugular venous pressure and pulsus paradoxus due to respiratory distress. In this condition (without accompanying cardiac tamponade) pressure in the superior vena cava is markedly elevated, with dampened pulsations, and exceeds right atrial and inferior vena cava pressures. If elevation of jugular venous pressure persists after relief of cardiac tamponade in patients with neoplastic disease, obstruction of the superior vena cava, as reflected in a pressure gradient between the superior vena cava and right atrium, should be sought. Superior vena caval obstruction may be amenable to radiation therapy.

PERICARDIOCENTESIS

Hemodynamic support during preparation of the patient for pericardiocentesis or pericardiotomy should include administration of intravenous fluid, blood, plasma, or saline. In experimental cardiac tamponade, administration of norepinephrine and isoproterenol[151] has produced an increase in cardiac output. The vasodilators hydralazine and nitroprusside have also been employed in experimental cardiac tamponade to promote an increase in cardiac output secondary to the reduction of elevated systemic resistance.[152] It is not yet clear whether the administration of vasodilators in conjunction with volume expansion is of any benefit in the management of patients with cardiac tamponade; in fact, it may be hazardous in patients with borderline or frank hypotension. Positive-pressure ventilation should be avoided whenever possible, since it has been shown to depress cardiac output further in patients with cardiac tamponade.[153]

Pericardial fluid under pressure causing tamponade can be evacuated by (1) percutaneous pericardiocentesis using a needle or catheter, (2) pericardiotomy via a subxiphoid pericardial window, or (3) surgical pericardiectomy. Considerable controversy exists regarding the exact indications for pericardiocentesis[154,155] although the procedure has been performed extensively since its initial demonstration in 1840 by the Viennese physician Franz Schuh. The benefits of pericardiocentesis include the rapid relief of cardiac tamponade and the opportunity to obtain accurate hemodynamic measurements before and after pericardial aspiration. The major risk of percutaneous pericardiocentesis is laceration of the heart, coronary arteries, or lung. Prior to the 1970's, pericardiocentesis was usually performed at the bedside without hemodynamic monitoring, few comprehensive means of evaluating its efficacy and hazards were available, and the risk of death or life-threatening complications appeared to be as high as 20 per cent.[155]

Recently, the technique has changed somewhat, and the modern approach is exemplified by the Stanford experience in 123 patients.[156] In the majority of patients, pericardiocentesis was performed by a cardiologist in the cardiac catheterization laboratory using a subxiphoid approach under fluoroscopic guidance with hemodynamic and electrocardiographic monitoring. In this experience, five deaths occurred in association with pericardiocentesis; nonfatal hemopericardium developed in an additional five patients. Pericardiocentesis in this study was successful in obtaining pericardial fluid in 106 of 123 patients. Importantly, *the probability of success in safely obtaining fluid was directly related to the size of the pericardial effusion*, since fluid was obtained in 93 per cent of patients with large effusions located both anteriorly and posteriorly on echocardiogram but in only 58 per cent with a small posterior pericardial effusion. In 23 patients a specific etiological diagnosis was possible from analysis of the pericardial fluid. Cardiac tamponade was successfully relieved by pericardiocentesis in 61 per cent, while the remainder required subsequent surgical drainage owing to either failure to relieve tamponade or recurrence after pericardiocentesis. Surgery was most frequently required in patients with acute traumatic hemopericardium (p. 1533). An unsuspected physiologic cause of increased systemic venous pressure other than simple cardiac tamponade was documented in 40 per cent of the patients studied, including an effusive-constrictive pericarditis in 17 per cent, congestive heart failure in 16 per cent, and coexisting neoplastic superior vena caval obstruction in 5 per cent. Similar experiences with pericardiocentesis have been reported by others.[157–159,159a]

Thus, pericardiocentesis is now safer than it was a decade ago, and the procedure is associated with only about a 0 to 5 per cent risk of developing a life-threatening complication, when performed by an experienced operator in a cardiac catheterization laboratory using the subxiphoid approach. The procedure is most likely to be successful and uncomplicated when performed in patients with clear-cut echocardiographic evidence of a large effusion with an anterior clear space of 10 mm or more (Table 43–5). Cardiac tamponade associated with malignant pericardial effusion or prior radiation therapy can often be managed with pericardiocentesis alone or with a combination of pericardiocentesis, radiation therapy, and local or systemic chemotherapy.[156] This therapeutic approach may be preferable in patients with advanced malignancy when it is desirable to avoid major surgery that is not definitive.

These experiences with pericardiocentesis[156–159] suggest

TABLE 43–5   FACTORS ASSOCIATED WITH OUTCOME OF PERICARDIOCENTESIS

Uncomplicated Pericardiocentesis
  Anterior and posterior pericardial effusion by echocardiography
  Large pericardial effusion: maximum anterior clear space of 10 mm or more by echocardiography
  Malignant pericardial effusion
Complicated Pericardiocentesis
  Small pericardial effusion (<200 ml)
  Posterior pericardial effusion only
  Maximum anterior clear space less than 10 mm by echocardiography
  Loculated effusion
  Traumatic or postsurgical hemopericardium

that the procedure should usually be performed in conjunction with hemodynamic measurements, including right heart and intrapericardial pressures, in order to (1) document the presence of the physiologic changes of cardiac tamponade prior to attempted pericardiocentesis; and (2) to exclude other important coexisting causes of elevated jugular venous pressure, such as effusive-constrictive disease, superior vena caval obstruction, and left ventricular failure. There is rarely justification for performing blind needle pericardiocentesis at the bedside in the absence of optimal hemodynamic monitoring or of a prior echocardiogram documenting the presence of a large anterior and posterior effusion.

Pericardiocentesis is likely to be either complicated or unsuccessful in improving hemodynamics in patients with (1) acute traumatic hemopericardium in which blood enters the pericardial space as rapidly as it can be aspirated, (2) a small pericardial effusion judged to be less than 200 ml in size, (3) absence of an anterior effusion based on echocardiogram, (4) a loculated effusion, or (5) clot and fibrin as well as fluid filling the mediastinal or pericardial space postoperatively. In acute traumatic hemopericardium, needle pericardiocentesis should not be relied upon except as a temporizing measure in an extreme emergency prior to pericardiotomy or pericardial exploration. Hemopericardium secondary to laceration, puncture of the heart, or leaking left ventricular or aortic aneurysm, is likely to recur rapidly after needle drainage, and exploration and repair of the heart or aorta may be necessary.[160] Surgical drainage is also usually preferred in patients with tamponade caused by purulent pericarditis to permit extensive drainage and in patients with suspected or known tuberculous pericarditis to permit bacteriological and histological examination of pericardial biopsy specimens.[161] Management of cardiac tamponade in patients with uremic pericarditis is controversial. Patients may be successfully managed with pericardiocentesis in centers where personnel have had extensive experience with this procedure,[156] while in other centers surgical drainage is the preferred approach.[92,162]

PROCEDURE OF COMBINED CATHETERIZATION AND PERICARDIOCENTESIS

Multiple techniques of pericardiocentesis have been advocated.[163–166] We prefer the following method of combined catheterization and pericardiocentesis, which allows documentation of increased intrapericardial pressure and assessment of hemodynamic improvement after pericardiocentesis.[167] In contrast to traditional bedside sharp-needle pericardiocentesis, this method, utilizes a soft catheter for pericardial aspiration and thus eliminates the prolonged presence of a sharp needle in the pericardial sac, thereby minimizing the risk of cardiac laceration. If possible, pericardiocentesis should be performed in a cardiac procedure laboratory where radiographic and hemodynamic monitoring facilities are optimal and by cardiologists experienced with hemodynamic measurements and the procedure itself. Prior to the procedure, the patient's blood should be typed and cross-matched and the cardiac surgery team alerted.

Pericardiocentesis is performed after the recording of baseline hemodynamic variables and cardiac output. Since the equilibration of right and left ventricular diastolic pressures is an important feature of cardiac tamponade, it is highly desirable to catheterize both sides of the heart and to record right atrial and right ventricular pressures simultaneously with left ventricular pressure. Care should be taken to use equisensitive transducers and to avoid an underdamped catheter-transducer system. It is also useful to record respiratory movements simultaneously with measurements of intraarterial and right atrial pressures to document the extent of arterial pulsus paradoxus and

the presence of a characteristic inspiratory fall in right atrial pressure. Prior to pericardiocentesis, the transducer system that will be used to record intrapericardial pressure should be leveled with the other transducers, calibrated, and connected to a short length of fluid-filled tubing.

Pericardiocentesis is carried out with the patient's *thorax and head tilted up*, which enhances the pooling of the effusion anteriorly and inferiorly. Although multiple sites have been advocated for pericardiocentesis, we strongly prefer the subxiphoid route, since it is extrapleural and avoids the coronary, pericardial, and internal mammary arteries. The skin is shaved, cleansed, and prepared in aseptic fashion, and the skin and subcutaneous tissue are anesthetized with 1 per cent Xylocaine. The skin is pierced with a No. 11 blade, 0.5 cm below and to the left of the xiphoid process, and the subcutaneous tissues are spread with a small curved clamp. A long, 8-inch, thin-walled No. 16 to 18 gauge pointed needle (BD Longdwell, Becton-Dickinson, New Jersey) is attached to a handheld syringe containing 1 per cent lidocaine. The thin-walled needle commonly used for lumbar puncture is *not* adequate because its long sharp bevel poses some hazard. The metal hub of the needle may be attached by a sterile connector to the V lead of an electrocardiographic machine, and the electrocardiogram should be continuously recorded. It is essential that the electrocardiographic apparatus have equipotential grounding with no chance of a current wave that could induce ventricular fibrillation. If this condition cannot be assured, it is safer to omit electrocardiographic monitoring from the needle.

The needle is directed posteriorly until the tip passes posterior to the bony cage. The hub of the needle is then pressed toward the diaphragm and the needle is advanced with a 15-degree posterior tilt, either directly toward the patient's head or toward the right or left shoulder (Fig. 43–14). As the needle is smoothly and slowly advanced, the operator periodically attempts to aspirate fluid and then injects a small amount of lidocaine to clear the needle and to provide anesthesia of the deep tissues. The needle is advanced until the pericardial membrane is felt to "give" and pericardial fluid is aspirated or until ST-segment elevation and ventricular premature beats appear on the electrocardiogram, indicating that the needle has reached the epicardium. In the latter case, the needle is promptly and smoothly withdrawn while the operator attempts to aspirate pericardial fluid un-

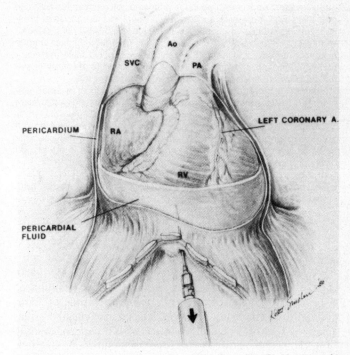

FIGURE 43–14 Pericardiocentesis using the subxiphoid approach, which avoids the major epicardial blood vessels. After the needle enters the pericardial space, a floppy-tip guidewire is passed through the hollow needle, and the needle is exchanged for a flexible catheter with end- and side-holes to facilitate safe and thorough drainage of the pericardial space. (From Shabetai, R.: The Pericardium. New York, Grune and Stratton, 1981, p. 335.)

til the needle lies within the fluid-filled pericardial space and the ECG changes disappear. If fluid cannot be freely aspirated, the needle is slowly withdrawn out of the body, avoiding lateral motion; the needle is flushed and the procedure repeated.

If hemorrhagic fluid is freely aspirated, and it is not clear whether the needle is in the ventricle, atrium, or pericardial space, a few milliliters of contrast medium may be injected under fluoroscopic observation. If the contrast medium instantly swirls and disappears, the needle is within a cardiac chamber; in contrast, the appearance of sluggish layering of contrast medium inferiorly indicates that the needle is correctly positioned. When fluid can be freely aspirated, a soft, floppy-tip guide wire is passed through the hollow needle so that its tip lies within the pericardial space, as confirmed by fluoroscopy. A soft Teflon catheter with multiple sideholes and an end hole (i.e., a Teflon Gensini catheter) is advanced over the guidewire, the guidewire is removed, and a few milliliters of fluid are aspirated. The catheter is then promptly connected to the prepared transducer, and intrapericardial pressure is recorded simultaneously with right atrial and systemic arterial pressure to document the presence of cardiac tamponade.

Fluid samples are then aspirated from the catheter and sent for analysis of protein, amylase, glucose, and cholesterol content; hematocrit and white blood cell count; and bacteriological culture for aerobic and anaerobic bacteria, tuberculosis, and fungi. In most cases, a generous sample of fluid should also be sent in a heparinized container for cytological examination. Right atrial, systemic arterial, and intrapericardial pressures should then be recorded periodically as aliquots of fluid are removed—not only until intrapericardial pressure falls to zero but until no further fluid can be aspirated; intrapericardial pressure may return to normal levels after removal of only 50 to 100 ml of fluid in the presence of an effusion of 1 to 2 liters. When no further fluid can be aspirated or drained, cardiac output and systemic arterial pressure as well as right atrial, right ventricular, and left ventricular pressures should be recorded, the last three simultaneously. The jugular veins should also be examined.

Successful relief of cardiac tamponade is documented by (1) the fall of intrapericardial pressure to levels of −3 and +3 mm Hg, (2) the fall of elevated right atrial pressure and separation between right and left heart filling pressures, (3) augmentation of cardiac output, and (4) disappearance of pulsus paradoxus. The presence of continued elevation and equilibration of right and left ventricular diastolic pressures with the appearance of a *y* descent in the right atrial pressure tracing strongly suggests the presence of a constricting pericardium due to effusive-constrictive pericarditis (p. 1496). Jugular venous distention despite a fall in right atrial pressure should raise the question of coexisting superior vena caval obstruction, particularly in patients with known or suspected malignant disease.

Some cardiologists advocate the routine injection of a small volume of CO_2 or air into the pericardial space to outline the pericardium at the end of the procedure. This procedure has not been shown to be of aid in identifying unsuspected tumor masses,[156] and we do not consider it to be routinely necessary. When the pericardial space is nearly obliterated, there is also the risk of injecting gas into a pleural cavity or cardiac chamber or the production of air tamponade.

It is often desirable to leave the intrapericardial catheter in place for several hours to permit repeated aspiration of fluid if cardiac tamponade recurs or to allow instillation of a nonabsorbable corticosteroid or antineoplastic agent.[168] The catheter may be sutured securely to the skin and attached via a three-way stopcock to a closed drainage bottle with a water seal. If the fluid is hemorrhagic or rich in fibrin, the catheter must be cleared frequently with a few milliliters of fluid. Dilute heparin may be instilled into the catheter to prevent clotting. The catheter should not be left in place for more than 24 to 36 hours because of the risk of introducing infection and producing iatrogenic purulent pericarditis.

Following pericardiocentesis, the majority of patients should be observed for about 24 hours in an intensive care setting for recurrence of cardiac tamponade. It is frequently helpful to obtain an echocardiogram soon after pericardiocentesis to establish the appearance of the heart and pericardium following aspiration. Percutaneous pericardial biopsy is not recommended because of the risk of lacerating the pericardium, pleura, or ventricular wall. If it is essential to obtain a pericardial specimen, the procedure should be performed in the operating room, with direct visualization of the pericardium.

PERICARDIECTOMY AND PERICARDIOTOMY

Surgical evacuation of pericardial fluid under pressure can be accomplished either by an extensive pericardiectomy performed through a formal left thoracotomy or median sternotomy with cardiopulmonary bypass standby or by limited pericardiotomy. *Total pericardiectomy* is indicated when extensive exploration is required. This procedure has the disadvantages of requiring general anesthesia, a long period of convalescence with a painful incision, and attendant postoperative respiratory problems.

An important alternative for patients who do not require extensive pericardial excision is the *subxiphoid limited pericardiotomy*, often called the subxiphoid pericardial window, initially performed in 1829 by Larrey, a surgeon in Napoleon's army.[169] Subxiphoid pericardiotomy can be performed under local anesthesia. After a small longitudinal incision is made below the xiphoid process through the linea alba, the diaphragm and pericardium are dissected away from the sternum, and the diaphragm is retracted inferiorly to permit direct exposure of the anterior pericardium. The pericardium is visualized, a small incision is made in the pericardium, a small segment of pericardium is resected for drainage, and the finger may be inserted blindly into the pericardial sac in an attempt to break down adhesions behind the heart.[170,171] This procedure has advantages over extensive formal pericardiectomy in that it is simpler and shorter, permits both drainage of pericardial fluid and examination of a small pericardial biopsy specimen, and can usually be performed safely in critically ill patients.

Uncommon complications associated with subxiphoid pericardiocentesis include chronic chondritis, pneumothorax, pleural effusions, atelectasis, and wound and pericardial infections.[172] Perioperative mortality ranges from 0 to 22 per cent,[94,170-175] depending largely on the patient's underlying condition and the experience of the operator.

Instillation of intrapericardial steroids has been advocated in recurrent uremic pericardial effusion, and the instillation of various agents, including tetracycline, radioactive gold, radioactive chromic phosphate, antimetabolites, and alkylating agents, has been advocated for patients with neoplastic pericardial effusion after pericardial aspiration. However, no rigorous evaluations of the efficacy of introducing such agents into the pericardium have been carried out.

CONSTRICTIVE PERICARDITIS

Constrictive pericarditis is present when a fibrotic, thickened, and adherent pericardium restricts diastolic filling of the heart. It usually begins with an initial episode of acute pericarditis, which may not be detectable clinically, characterized by fibrin deposition, often with a pericardial effusion. This then slowly progresses to a subacute stage of organization and resorption of the effusion, followed by a chronic stage consisting of fibrous scarring and thickening of the pericardium with obliteration of the pericardial space. In the majority of cases, the visceral and parietal layers become completely fused, but in a few cases, the constricting process is produced primarily by the visceral pericardium (epicardium). Usually, pathological findings are not specific,[176] but the presence of giant cells and caseation suggests underlying tuberculosis. In the chronic stage of constrictive pericarditis, calcium deposition may contribute to thickening and stiffening of the pericardium (Fig. 43–15). Constrictive pericarditis is usually a *symmetrical scarring process* that produces uniform restriction of the filling of all heart chambers. Rare exceptional cases of strictly localized pericardial thickening have been reported, including constricting bands in the atrioventricular groove, surrounding the semilunar valve rings, or in the aortic groove, pulmonary outflow tract, and venae cavae.[177,178]

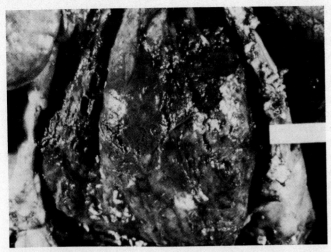

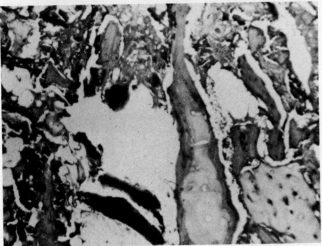

FIGURE 43–15 *Top,* Gross autopsy specimen of the heart from a patient with severe constrictive pericarditis showing encasement of the heart by a markedly thickened and adherent pericardium with dense calcifications. *Bottom,* Photomicrograph ($\times$40) from the same specimen showing extensive calcification with bone and cartilage formation. (From Bloor, C. M.: Cardiac Pathology. Philadelphia, J. P. Lippincott Co., 1978.)

ETIOLOGY. Tuberculosis was formerly a leading cause of constrictive pericarditis, as reported in the classic series of Paul[179] and Andrews.[180] In disadvantaged nations, this is still true, whereas with the advent of anti-tuberculosis therapy this disease now accounts for 20 per cent or less of cases in developed nations.[6] The largest number of cases of constrictive pericarditis today are of unknown etiology. In some cases there is a history of an earlier idiopathic or viral pericarditis.[181] Other non-tubercular causes include chronic renal failure treated with hemodialysis (p. 1505); connective tissue disorders, including rheumatoid arthritis and systemic lupus erythematosus (pp. 1511 and 1512); and neoplastic pericardial infiltration or encasement of the heart due most commonly to lung cancer, breast cancer, Hodgkin's disease, and lymphoma (p. 1507).

Constrictive pericarditis may also occur months to years after mediastinal irradiation, especially following the delivery of more than 4,000 rads to the heart, as may occur during therapy for breast cancer or Hodgkins' disease. It may also develop following the deposition of blood or clot in the pericardial space due to cardiac trauma and following

cardiac surgery or pacemaker implantation (p. 1515). Prior to the advent of penicillin therapy in the 1940's, constrictive pericarditis was a well-known complication of chronic pneumococcal empyema. Today, a wider spectrum of pathological organisms is responsible for constrictive pericarditis, especially after incomplete drainage of purulent pericarditis (p. 1500). Fungal causes include histoplasmosis, which is endemic in the Ohio valley, and coccidioidomycosis in the western United States (p. 1502). Other unusual causes include parasitic infestations including ruptured amebic liver abscess, echinococcal cyst, dracunculosis, and filariasis (p. 1503). Constrictive pericarditis may occasionally follow pericarditis associated with acute myocardial infarction and the postpericardiotomy syndrome. Drugs such as methysergide, hydralazine, and procainamide may induce pericardial inflammation followed by constrictive pericarditis.

Constrictive pericarditis is far less common in *children* than in adults and may rarely occur following a viral syndrome in a child mistakenly thought to have hepatitis or a protein-losing enteropathy.[182] Nontraumatic hemopericardium has been reported in children and young adults with congenital bleeding disorders complicated by a second process such as endocarditis or viral syndrome, and constrictive pericarditis has occurred following pericardial bleeding due to congenital afibrinogenemia.[183] A rare congenital cause of constrictive pericarditis is mulibrey nanism, an autosomal recessive disorder characterized by dwarfism, constrictive pericarditis, abnormal fundi, and fibrous dysplasia of the long bones.[184–186]

Pathophysiology

In classic constrictive pericarditis, a heavily fibrosed or calcified pericardium restricts diastolic filling of all chambers of the heart and determines the diastolic volume of the heart.[99,187] The symmetrical constricting effect of the pericardium results in elevation and equilibration of diastolic pressures in all four cardiac chambers (as well as of pulmonary capillary wedge pressures). In early diastole when intracardiac volume is less than that defined by the stiff pericardium, diastolic filling is unimpeded, and early diastolic filling occurs abnormally rapidly because venous pressure is elevated. Rapid early diastolic filling is abruptly halted when the intracardiac volume reaches the limit set by the noncompliant pericardium.[188]

Instantaneous plots of ventricular volume versus time in patients with constrictive pericarditis have shown that virtually all filling of the ventricle occurs very early in diastole. This abnormal pattern of diastolic filling is reflected in the characteristic dip-and-plateau waveforms in both right and left ventricles (Fig. 43–16). The early diastolic dip corresponds to the period of excessively rapid diastolic filling while the plateau phase corresponds to the period of mid and late diastole when there is little additional ventricular volume expansion. Since the atria are equilibrated with the ventricles in early diastole, the jugular venous waveform and right and left atrial waveforms show a prominent and deep diastolic *y* descent. The systolic *x* descent is usually also present, and the venous waveform may therefore exhibit a characteristic "M" or "W" configuration.

A bimodal pattern of systemic venous return occurs in constrictive pericarditis with an acceleration of systemic

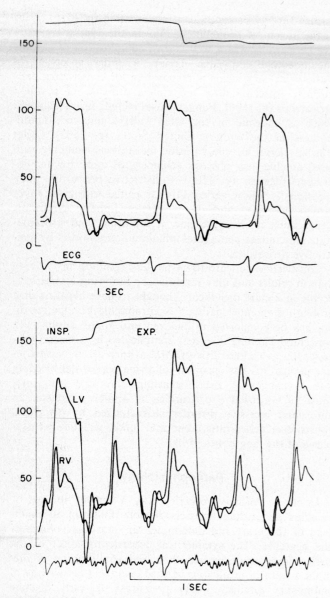

FIGURE 43–16 Simultaneous right ventricular (RV) and left ventricular (LV) pressure recordings in a patient with constrictive pericarditis. *Upper panel*, Equilibration of right and left ventricular diastolic pressures, and a characteristic dip-and-plateau contour of the diastolic waveforms. *Lower panel*, Tachycardia induced by bicycle exercise obscures the diastolic plateau, although diastolic pressures remain equilibrated. (From Shabetai, R.: The Pericardium. New York, Grune and Stratton, 1981, p. 181.)

is the failure of intrathoracic pressure changes during respiration to be transmitted to the pericardial space and intracardiac chambers. As a consequence, during inspiration, systemic venous and right atrial pressure do *not* fall and venous flow into the right atrium does *not* increase, in contrast to the situation in normal subjects and patients with cardiac tamponade (Fig. 43–17). In some patients, systemic venous pressure may actually *increase* with inspiration, i.e., Kussmaul's sign. This finding may occur in other disorders such as chronic right ventricular failure and restrictive cardiomyopathy, in which right atrial and systemic venous pressures are also markedly elevated. However, Kussmaul's sign does *not* occur in acute cardiac tamponade, in which the inspiratory fall in intrathoracic pressure is transmitted to the fluid-filled pericardial space.[189] Pulsus paradoxus is also less common in constrictive pericarditis than in cardiac tamponade, in which the mechanism is thought to be largely the exaggerated increase in right ventricular filling during inspiration at the expense of left ven-

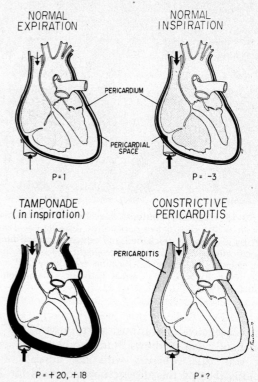

FIGURE 43–17 Schematic illustration of the hemodynamic effects of respiration. In the normal heart (*upper panel*), inspiration results in a fall in intrathoracic and intrapericardial pressure from +1 to −3 mm Hg, which causes an increase in venous return (heavy black arrows) and a slight increase in right ventricular size at the expense of a slight decrease in left ventricular size due to displacement of the interventricular septum from right to left. During cardiac tamponade (*lower left panel*), inspiration causes a fall in the elevated intrapericardial pressure from +20 to +18 mm Hg. Although both the right and left heart volumes are diminished owing to compression by the pericardial effusion, the inspiratory fall in intrapericardial pressure results in an increase in venous return (heavy black arrow), an increase in right heart volume due to septal bulging, and a further decrease in left heart volume. In constrictive pericarditis (*lower right panel*), the inspiratory fall in intrathoracic pressure is not transmitted to the heart, since the pericardial space is obliterated. For this reason, there is minimal or no increase in venous return (light black arrows) during inspiration. (From Shabetai, R.: The Pericardium. New York, Grune and Stratton, 1981, p. 244.)

venous blood flow from the venae cavae into the right atrium during both ventricular systolic ejection and early diastole. The greatest acceleration of venous blood flow occurs during early diastole simultaneous with the *y* descent. This contrasts with the normal filling pattern, in which a bimodal pattern of systemic venous return is also present, but the major surge of venous return occurs during systole. The pattern of systemic venous return in constrictive pericarditis also contrasts with that in cardiac tamponade. Cardiac compression is present throughout diastole in cardiac tamponade, so that the diastolic surge of venous return is blunted and the venous pressure tracing shows an absent diastolic *y* descent and a predominant *x* descent.

Another striking abnormality of constrictive pericarditis

tricular filling. The few cases of constrictive pericarditis in which pulsus paradoxus has been observed may have been due to an inspiratory reduction in left ventricular stroke volume at a time when right ventricular stroke volume was relatively fixed by the constricting pericardium.

Restriction of diastolic filling ultimately results in compensatory renal retention of sodium and water that contributes further to the increase in systemic venous pressure and initially serves to maintain diastolic filling of the ventricles despite pericardial compression. In some cases, the pericardial scar is so dense that diastolic ventricular volumes are reduced. When right and left ventricular preload are substantially reduced, stroke volume and cardiac output fall despite compensatory tachycardia. The presence of reduced cardiac output, tachycardia, and elevated right and left heart filling pressures may simulate myocardial failure, and classic ventricular performance curves may show a reduced left ventricular stroke volume relative to an elevated left ventricular filling pressure. However, it must be emphasized that systolic contraction of the ventricle and the intrinsic contractile state of the myocardium are usually normal or nearly so.[190] Noninvasively obtained systolic time indices,[191,192] invasively obtained isovolumetric indices (V_{max}, dP/dt), and ejection indices (ejection fraction, circumferential shortening) are usually normal.[193] Patients with constrictive pericarditis also demonstrate normal postextrasystolic potentiation of cardiac contraction.[193] In severe cases of constrictive pericarditis, myocardial systolic function may also be depressed.[194] Multiple mechanisms may be responsible, including myocardial atrophy, involvement of the underlying myocardium by inflammation and fibrosis, or compression of superficial coronary arteries in the fibrotic pericardium.[195-197]

Pathophysiological and hemodynamic findings in patients with subacute noncalcific pericarditis of less than one year's duration may differ from those in patients with chronic constrictive pericarditis in whom the pericardium resembles a rigid shell.[198,199] Hancock has suggested that the presence of a thick fluid-fibrin layer in the process of organization leads to relatively *elastic compression of the heart*, which may be compared to "wrapping the heart tightly with rubber bands."[189] The pathophysiological disturbance caused by this nonrigid fibroelastic form of constrictive pericarditis is similar to that in cardiac tamponade, since fibroelastic constriction compresses the heart continuously throughout the cardiac cycle, and respiratory changes in intrathoracic pressure are usually transmitted to the cardiac chambers.[200] Thus, patterns of ventricular filling and waveforms in the subacute form of fibroelastic compression tend to resemble those of cardiac tamponade rather than of constrictive pericarditis, and include a systemic venous waveform with a predominant x descent or equal x and y descents, an inconspicuous early diastolic dip in the ventricular waveform, an inspiratory fall in systemic venous and right atrial pressures, and the presence of pulsus paradoxus (Table 43–6).

Clinical Features

The principal clinical features of severe chronic pericarditis were vividly described by Cheevers of Guy's Hospital in 1842.[200a] In patients in whom systemic venous and right atrial pressures are modestly elevated (10 to 15 mm Hg), left ventricular filling pressure is also usually only modestly elevated. In this setting, symptoms secondary to systemic venous congestion such as edema, abdominal swelling, and discomfort due to ascites and passive hepatic congestion may predominate. Vague abdominal symptoms such as postprandial fullness, dyspepsia, flatulence, and anorexia may also be present. When both right and left heart filling pressures are elevated to the level of 15 to 30 mm Hg, symptoms of pulmonary venous congestion, such as exertional dyspnea, cough, and orthopnea, are present. Pleural effusions and elevation of the diaphragm due to ascites may also contribute to dyspnea. Severe fatigue, weight loss, and muscle wasting suggest the presence of a fixed or reduced cardiac output.

PHYSICAL EXAMINATION. The single most important finding is elevation of jugular venous pressure. If the neck is examined casually, or if the patient is examined supine so that jugular venous pressure is measured above the angle of the jaw, this important clue to the presence of constrictive pericarditis may be missed. A prominent feature of the elevated jugular venous pressure is the rapidly collapsing negative wave of the diastolic y descent.[201,202] In patients in sinus rhythm, both x and y descents can be distinguished; the x descent is synchronous while the diastolic y descent is out of phase with the carotid pulse (see Figure 3–34, p. 63). During a careful examination of the neck veins, both the elevation and abnormal contour of the jugular venous pressure are usually recognized, but these features may be difficult to detect in patients with tachycardia, tachypnea, or arrhythmia. It may also be difficult to distinguish between right heart failure due to tricuspid regurgita-

TABLE 43–6   CLINICAL AND HEMODYNAMIC FEATURES OF COMPRESSIVE PERICARDIAL DISEASE

	CARDIAC TAMPONADE	SUBACUTE "ELASTIC" CONSTRICTION	CHRONIC "RIGID" CONSTRICTION
Duration of symptoms	Hours to days	Weeks to months	Months to years
Chest pain, friction rub	Usual	Recent past	Remote
Pulsus paradoxus	Prominent	Usually prominent	Slight or absent
Kussmaul's sign	Absent	Usually absent	Often present
Early diastolic knock	Absent	Usually absent	Often present
Heart size on chest roentgenogram	Usually enlarged	Usually enlarged	Usually normal, sometimes enlarged
Pericardial calcification	Absent	Rare	Often present
Abnormal P waves or atrial fibrillation	Absent	Absent	Often present
Venous (right atrial) waveform	X or Xy	Xy or XY	XY or xY
Right ventricular dip-plateau waveform	Inconspicuous	Moderately prominent	Prominent
Pericardial effusion	Always present	Often present	Absent

X and Y = prominent x and y descents, respectively; x and y = inconspicuous x and y descents.
Modified from Hancock, E. W.: On the elastic and rigid forms of constrictive pericarditis. Am. Heart J. *100*:917, 1980.

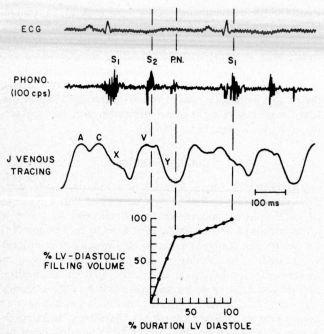

FIGURE 43–18 Electrocardiogram (ECG), phonocardiogram (PHONO), jugular venous pulse tracing, and left ventricular (LV) diastolic filling curve in a patient with constrictive pericarditis and pericardial knock (PN). The pericardial knock occurs simultaneously with the nadir of the diastolic y descent and sudden plateau of the LV filling curve. (From Tyberg, T. I., et al.: Genesis of pericardial knock in constrictive pericarditis. Am. J. Cardiol. 46:570, 1980.)

tion and chronic constrictive pericarditis by neck vein examination at the bedside. The finding of Kussmaul's sign (an inspiratory increase in systemic venous pressure) is difficult to appreciate at the bedside and may be confused with exaggerated amplitude of the venous waves during inspiration.

The arterial pulse may be normal or show a diminished pulse pressure. Severe pulsus paradoxus is uncommon in rigid constrictive pericarditis and rarely exceeds 15 mm Hg unless pericardial fluid under pressure is also present. In some patients the precordium is quiet, while in others there is strikingly visible systolic retraction of the apical impulse. The most impressive abnormality during auscultation is the *diastolic pericardial knock* (see Figure 3–16, p. 51), an early diastolic sound that is often heard along the left sternal border in rigid constrictive pericarditis, infrequently heard in subacute constrictive pericarditis of the fibroelastic variety, and not heard in pure cardiac tamponade.[189] The pericardial knock usually occurs 0.09 to 0.12 second after A_2 and corresponds in timing to the sudden cessation of ventricular filling and the premature diastolic plateau of the diastolic ventricular volume curve (Fig. 43–18).[203,204] The pericardial knock tends to occur earlier and to have a higher acoustic frequency than the typical S_3 gallop sound, and therefore it may be confused with the opening snap of mitral stenosis. Widening of the aortic and pulmonic components of the second heart sound may occur in constrictive pericarditis. This is attributed to a fixed right ventricular stroke volume during inspiration due to pericardial compression as well as the presence of premature aortic valve closure due to a transitory inspiratory decrease in left ventricular stroke volume.[205]

Hepatomegaly is usually present and may be accompanied by ascites. Other evidence of hepatic dysfunction secondary to passive liver congestion and diminished cardiac output may include icterus, spider angiomas, and palmar erythema. In young patients with competent venous valves, edema of the extremities may be noticeably absent in the presence of marked abdominal distention. Older patients with longstanding constrictive pericarditis may have enormous ascites and massive swelling of the scrotum, thighs, and calves. In contrast, the upper torso and arms may show evidence of marked muscle wasting and cachexia.

CHEST ROENTGENOGRAM (See also page 176). The cardiac silhouette may be small, normal, or enlarged. Cardiac enlargement may be apparent due to coexisting pericardial effusion, the contribution of an enormously thickened pericardium, or preexisting cardiac chamber enlargement or hypertrophy. The right superior mediastinum may be prominent due to engorgement of the superior vena cava, and left atrial enlargement is common.[206] Extensive calcification of the pericardium is present in approximately half the patients and raises the possibility of a tubercular etiology. However, this finding is not specific for constrictive pericarditis in that a calcified pericardium is not necessarily a constricted one. Calcification of the pericardium is often detected on the lateral chest film in the atrioventricular groove or along the anterior and diaphragmatic surfaces of the right ventricle. Fluoroscopy may be helpful in distinguishing pericardial calcification from calcium within the wall of a myocardial aneurysm or thrombus or within the mitral or aortic valves, mitral annulus, or coronary arteries. Pleural effusions are present in the majority of patients.[207] Since left atrial pressure is commonly elevated to between 15 to 30 mm Hg, there may be evidence of redistribution of blood flow, while Kerley's B lines or infiltrates suggestive of frank pulmonary edema are rare (Table 43–7).

ELECTROCARDIOGRAM. Electrocardiographic findings include low QRS voltage, generalized T-wave inversion or flattening, and left atrial abnormalities suggestive of P mitrale (Fig. 43–19).[58,199] Atrial fibrillation occurs in less than half the patients with constrictive pericarditis and is thought to be related to longstanding elevation of atrial pressures and atrial enlargement. In a study of constrictive pericarditis in which postmortem specimens were available, Levine noted that atrioventricular block, intraventricular conduction defects, and pseudoinfarction patterns with deep wide Q waves seemed to be related to an extension of calcification into the myocardium and around the coronary arteries, compromising coronary blood flow.[197] An unusual pattern of right ventricular hypertrophy and right-axis deviation may be present in patients with dense pericardial scar overlying the right ventricular outflow tract.[208]

ECHOCARDIOGRAM (See also page 133). One distinct pattern of pericardial thickening in constrictive peri-

TABLE 43–7   RADIOLOGICAL FEATURES OF CONSTRICTIVE PERICARDITIS

Normal heart size	33%
Enlarged heart	67%
Calcified pericardium	43%
Pleural effusion	83%
Pulmonary venous congestion	86%
Left atrial enlargement	85%

Modified from Pulvaneswary, M., et al.: Constrictive pericarditis: Clinical, hemodynamic, and radiologic correlation. Australas. Radiol. 26:53, 1982.

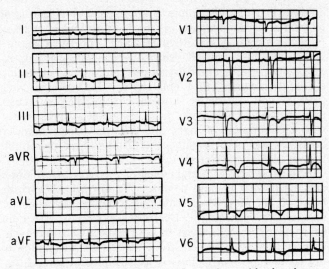

FIGURE 43–19 Electrocardiogram of a patient with chronic constrictive pericarditis showing a wide notched P wave in lead II and diffuse T-wave inversion. (From Spodick, D. H.: Pathogenesis and clinical correlations of the electrocardiographic abnormalities of pericardial disease. Cardiovasc. Clin. *8*:201, 1977.)

carditis consists of two parallel lines representing the visceral and parietal pericardia separated by a clear space of at least 1 mm; another consists of multiple dense echoes (Fig. 43–20).[209] In the absence of a pericardial effusion, it is sometimes difficult to differentiate a thickened pericardium from other causes of thickening of the left ventricular posterior wall, such as myocardial hypertrophy or infiltration. Extreme respiratory variation in the depth of the pulmonic valve *a* wave[210] and premature pulmonic valve opening secondary to a high right ventricular early diastolic pressure may be present,[211] but these changes are also seen in other disorders with high right ventricular early diastolic pressure, such as tricuspid and pulmonic regurgitation. Other echocardiographic abnormalities include reduced motion of the left ventricular posterior wall endocardium of less than 1 mm[212] and abnormal motion of the interventricular septum, evident as systolic flattening and abrupt posterior motion in early diastole, coinciding with the pericardial knock.[213,214] The abnormality in septal motion is not specific and may also occur in bundle branch block, volume overload, and aortic regurgitation in which rapid early diastolic left ventricular filling occurs. The abnormal pattern of rapid early diastolic filling seen in constrictive pericarditis may be reflected in an echocardiographic pattern of abrupt early diastolic posterior motion of the aortic root,[215] and the pattern of a rapid increase in left ventricular dimension in early diastole followed by no change in dimension in mid or late diastole.[216]

About 75 per cent of patients with constrictive pericarditis have at least one of the above findings.[217] The presence of pericardial thickening alone is not diagnostic of constrictive pericarditis, and the likelihood of this diagnosis increases if there is also evidence of an abnormal early rapid diastolic filling pattern and elevation of right ventricular diastolic pressure.

Two-dimensional echocardiography in constrictive pericarditis has been reported to show an immobile and dense appearance of the pericardium, bulging of the interventricular septum into the left ventricle during inspiration, prominent early diastolic filling, and dilatation of the hepatic veins and inferior vena cava.[218]

Other Laboratory Findings. Other abnormal laboratory findings may be present due to chronic elevation of right atrial pressure causing passive congestion of the liver, kidneys, and gastrointestinal tract. These include depressed serum albumin, elevated serum globulin, elevated conjugated and unconjugated serum bilirubin, and abnormal hepatocellular function tests. Protein-losing enteropathy may be evident from the presence of albumin in the stool, and lymphangiectasis on small bowel biopsy.[219,220] Elevated systemic venous pressure may also produce variable degrees of albuminuria as well as pronounced protein loss consistent with the nephrotic syndrome.[221,222] Nonspecific evidence of the presence of chronic disease such as a normocytic and normochromic anemia may be found.

Cardiac Catheterization and Angiography

Cardiac catheterization is useful in the assessment of patients suspected of having constrictive pericarditis (1) to document the presence of elevation and equilibration of diastolic filling pressures, (2) to assess the effects of constrictive pericarditis on stroke volume and cardiac output, (3) to evaluate myocardial systolic function, and (4) to assist in the difficult discrimination between constrictive pericarditis and restrictive cardiomyopathy.

Catheterization of both the right and left ventricles should be performed to permit the simultaneous recording of right and left heart filling pressures. Typical findings include the elevation and virtual identity (within 5 mm Hg) of right atrial, right ventricular diastolic, left atrial (pulmonary capillary wedge), and left ventricular diastolic

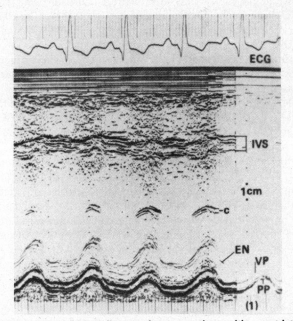

FIGURE 43–20 Echocardiogram from a patient with constrictive pericarditis. Two intense parallel echoes, separated by a small clear space, can be seen posterior to the left ventricular endocardium (EN). At surgery or autopsy, this pattern is usually associated with dense adhesions between the parietal (PP) and visceral (VP) pericardium. ECG = electrocardiogram; IVS = interventricular septum. (From Schnittger, I., et al.: Echocardiography: Pericardial thickening and constrictive pericarditis. Am. J. Cardiol. *42*:388, 1978.)

pressures. Right atrial pressure is characterized by a preserved systolic x descent, a prominent early diastolic y descent, and a and v waves that are small and equal in height and result in the typical "M" or "W" configurations. Both the right and left ventricular diastolic pressures show an early diastolic dip followed by a pressure plateau.[99,167,223] This sign may be obscured by the presence of tachycardia (Fig. 43–16). Care must be taken during pressure recording to use small displacement transducers and to avoid excessive use of connecting tubes or bubbles within the catheters and transducers. Right ventricular and pulmonary artery systolic pressures are usually modestly elevated, in the range of 35 to 40 mm Hg, and rarely exceed 60 mm Hg.

Careful recordings during respiration show that mean right atrial pressure fails to decrease normally or actually rises during inspiration. Since inspiration is associated with the transient pooling of blood within the pulmonary bed and a reduction in right ventricular afterload, inspiration causes a fall in pulmonary artery and right ventricular systolic pressures, pulmonary capillary wedge pressure, and left ventricular diastolic pressure. Because constrictive pericarditis is not associated with marked inspiratory swings in right ventricular filling, pulsus paradoxus is usually absent or less prominent than that observed in cardiac tamponade. Both cardiac output and stroke volume are low-normal or depressed.[167,224] When they are depressed, compensatory tachycardia and elevation of systemic vascular resistance may be found.

The *left ventricular angiogram* usually demonstrates that left ventricular end-systolic and end-diastolic volumes are normal or decreased. In the absence of myocardial fibrosis or inflammation, both isovolumetric and ejection phase indices of systolic function (Chap. 14) are normal.[223,225] Venous angiography may demonstrate superior vena caval dilatation and straightening of the right heart border[226]; pericardial thickening may be detectable. Coronary angiography may demonstrate that the coronary arteries are within the cardiac silhouette rather than on the surface of the heart,[227,228] and rarely diastolic pinching or external compression of the coronary arteries may be detected.[229]

HEMODYNAMIC DIFFERENTIATION AMONG CONSTRICTIVE PERICARDITIS, CARDIAC TAMPONADE, AND RESTRICTIVE CARDIOMYOPATHY.

Although both constrictive pericarditis and tamponade are characterized by elevation and equilibration of right and left ventricular diastolic pressures, several hemodynamic features differ. In contrast to patients with constrictive pericarditis, patients with cardiac tamponade demonstrate (1) marked pulsus paradoxus, (2) a fall in right atrial pressure during inspiration, (3) elevation of intrapericardial pressure, (4) a right atrial pressure tracing with a predominant x descent and an attenuated or absent y descent, and (5) *lack* of a prominent dip-and-plateau pattern in the right and left ventricular pressure pulses.

The findings of cardiac catheterization help to differentiate some but not all patients with *constrictive pericarditis* from those with *restrictive cardiomyopathy* (p. 1422) due to amyloidosis, hemochromatosis, or other causes. In both conditions, right and left ventricular diastolic pressures are elevated, stroke volume and cardiac output are depressed, left ventricular end-diastolic volume is normal or de-

creased, and diastolic filling is impaired.[230] A diagnosis of restrictive cardiomyopathy is more likely when marked right ventricular systolic hypertension is present (pressure > 60 mm Hg), and left ventricular diastolic pressure exceeds right ventricular diastolic pressure at rest or during exercise by more than 5 mm Hg.[231,232] However, in some patients with restrictive cardiomyopathy, hemodynamics may be indistinguishable from constrictive pericarditis, with equilibration of right and left ventricular diastolic pressures and a predominant dip-and-plateau pattern in the ventricular waveforms.[167,232,233]

Angiographically, straightening of the right heart border may be present in both conditions, and thickening of the heart border may be detected due to either pericardial or myocardial thickening.[234] Decreased motion of the right ventricular free wall occurs in both restrictive cardiomyopathy and constrictive pericarditis, while normal motion of the crista supraventricularis is usually present in constrictive pericarditis but not in restrictive cardiomyopathy.[235]

The finding of a depressed left ventricular ejection fraction in the presence of a small heart has been suggested as a discriminating feature of restrictive cardiomyopathy.[234] However, the left ventricular ejection fraction may be normal in some patients with restrictive cardiomyopathy and, conversely, is occasionally reduced in patients with constrictive pericarditis.[232,233] Frame-by-frame analysis of left ventricular filling has been suggested as a method for distinguishing between constrictive pericarditis and restrictive cardiomyopathy.[236] In constrictive pericarditis, early diastolic filling tends to be excessively rapid in contrast to restrictive cardiomyopathy, in which early diastolic filling is slower than normal (Fig. 43–21).

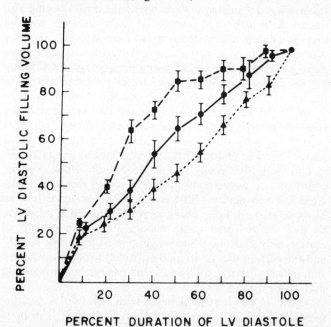

FIGURE 43–21 Composite left ventricular (LV) filling volume curves in normal subjects (solid line, circles), in patients with constrictive pericarditis (dashed line, solid squares), and in patients with restrictive amyloid cardiomyopathy (dotted line, triangles). Early left ventricular filling is exceedingly rapid in patients with constrictive pericarditis, whereas in patients with restrictive cardiomyopathy it is slower than normal. (From Tyberg, T. I., et al.: Left ventricular filling in differentiating restrictive amyloid cardiomyopathy and constrictive pericarditis. Am. J. Cardiol. **47**:791, 1981.)

Endomyocardial biopsy has also proved useful in documenting the presence of amyloidosis in patients in whom constrictive pericarditis and restrictive cardiomyopathy could not be differentiated at cardiac catheterization.[232] However, normal findings on endomyocardial biopsy do not exclude the presence of restrictive cardiomyopathy.[233] Furthermore, a pericardial effusion may rarely coexist with amyloid heart disease.[237,238] In a minority of patients, exploratory thoracotomy with careful examination of both pericardial and myocardial biopsy specimens is warranted to differentiate constrictive pericarditis, a condition that is usually treatable surgically, from restrictive cardiomyopathy, in which treatment is usually expectant.[238]

Diagnosis

Constrictive pericarditis should be suspected in patients with jugular venous distention, unexplained cardiac enlargement, hepatomegaly, systemic edema, or ascites.[202] It must be distinguished from superior vena caval obstruction, nephrotic syndrome, hepatic or intraabdominal disease due to malignancy, and other cardiac causes of right atrial hypertension including restrictive cardiomyopathy, tricuspid stenosis, tricuspid regurgitation, hypertrophic cardiomyopathy, and right atrial myxoma. Supportive, but nondiagnostic clinical features include a history of prior cardiothoracic trauma, acute pericarditis, or prior mediastinal irradiation; on physical examination there may be an early diastolic sound or knock in the absence of cardiac murmurs, and the heart is not massively enlarged. The roentgenogram may show pericardial calcification, and the echocardiogram reveals a thickened pericardium and abnormal diastolic filling patterns. The electrocardiogram may reveal notched P waves, atrial fibrillation, and low QRS voltage.

In the presence of findings suggestive of constrictive pericarditis, right and left heart catheterization with simultaneous pressure measurements should be performed to document the presence of constrictive physiology and to exclude other cardiac causes of right atrial hypertension. Diuresis should be avoided prior to catheterization, since hypovolemia may obscure both the characteristic abnormal waveforms and the elevation and equilibration of right and left heart filling pressures. In patients with a suggestive history but normal hemodynamics, a rapid saline volume challenge should be performed to exclude occult constrictive pericardial disease (p. 1496).

When pericardiocentesis is performed in the catheterization laboratory for cardiac tamponade, right and left heart filling pressures should be meticulously recorded after aspiration to exclude the presence of residual constrictive physiology due to effusive-constrictive pericarditis (p. 1496).

As discussed above, it may be extremely difficult to distinguish patients with constrictive pericarditis from those with restrictive physiology due to amyloidosis,[239–241] hemochromatosis,[242] endomyocardial fibrosis,[243] or eosinophilic endocarditis.[244,245] Both constrictive pericarditis and restrictive cardiomyopathy may show the electrocardiographic changes of atrial fibrillation, left atrial abnormalities, and diffuse low QRS voltage with T-wave flattening. The presence of atrioventricular block and conduction disturbances

simulating myocardial infarction favors the diagnosis of restrictive cardiomyopathy. Echocardiography in some patients with restrictive cardiomyopathy may show abnormal thickening of the ventricular myocardium or a peculiar "sparkling" appearance when amyloidosis is present.[246–248] The simultaneous use of electrocardiography and echocardiography to demonstrate a reduction of the voltage/mass ratio has been described in patients with amyloid restrictive cardiomyopathy in whom diffuse low QRS voltage is associated with increased thickness of the left ventricular wall due to amyloid deposition.[249] As noted above, cardiac catheterization and angiography, often with endomyocardial biopsy, are usually helpful in discriminating constrictive pericarditis from restrictive cardiomyopathy in many patients, but, in a minority, an exploratory thoracotomy may be required.

Management

Constrictive pericarditis is a progressive disease without spontaneous reversal of either pericardial thickening or abnormal symptoms and hemodynamics. A minority of patients may survive for many years with modest jugular venous distention and peripheral edema that is controlled by the judicious use of diet and diuretics. The majority of patients who are symptomatic and come to medical attention, however, become progressively more disabled by weakness, ascites and peripheral edema and subsequently suffer the complications of severe cardiac cachexia. Treatment for constrictive pericarditis is complete resection of the pericardium.

Prior to 1971, surgical mortality from pericardiectomy performed for constrictive pericarditis ranged from 4 to 23 per cent.[250,251] Recent changes in technique have included the use of a median sternotomy, cardiopulmonary bypass to permit greater mobilization of the heart,[252] and performance of pericardiectomy earlier in the course of the disease prior to the appearance of cardiac cachexia and dense pericardial calcification. More recent series have cited an operative mortality of about 4 to 6 per cent,[253–255] and long-term improvement in hemodynamics and symptoms has been reported in about 75 per cent of patients who survive the operation.[253,255–265]

Pericardiectomy should probably not be attempted in patients with very early and mild disease whose symptoms can be completely controlled with the use of a mild diuretic or in very elderly patients with severe liver dysfunction, cachexia, densely calcified pericardium, and massive cardiac enlargement indicative of underlying myocardial damage.[258] Patients with known or suspected tubercular pericarditis should be treated with multidrug anti tuberculosis therapy for two to four weeks prior to operation; if the diagnosis is confirmed, these drugs should be continued for 6 to 12 months after pericardiectomy.

The most common surgical approach for pericardiectomy is via a median sternotomy with cardiopulmonary bypass to permit maximum mobilization of the heart and extensive resection of the pericardium. Complete removal of the parietal pericardium from the phrenic nerve to phrenic nerve is attempted, including freeing up of the atria and venae cavae if obvious constricting bands are present[252,253]; however, care must be taken to avoid laceration of the thin-walled atria and epicardial veins and arteries. If the heart fails to expand and pulsate more vigorously after removal of the parietal pericardium, the possibility of epicardial constriction and the need for visceral pericardiectomy must be considered by the surgeon.

Marked hemodynamic and symptomatic improvement is apparent in some patients immediately after operation. In others, symptomatic improvement and resolution of elevated jugular venous pressure and abnormal filling patterns may be delayed for weeks to months.[253,256,262,263] This delayed or inadequate response to pericardiectomy has been attributed to incomplete pericardial resection,[264] myocardial involvement by the calcified and fibrotic inflammatory process,[265] and epicardial sclerosis.[266]

EFFUSIVE-CONSTRICTIVE PERICARDITIS

Effusive-constrictive pericarditis is the condition of a tense pericardial effusion in the presence of visceral pericardial constriction.[267,268] The hallmark of this condition is continued elevation of right atrial pressure after the aspiration of pericardial fluid and restoration of intrapericardial pressure to zero. This entity may represent a stage in the development of classic constrictive pericarditis. The most common causes of effusive-constrictive pericarditis are the same as for chronic constrictive pericarditis (p. 1489) and include idiopathic or presumed viral pericarditis, tuberculosis, neoplastic infiltration of the pericardium, and mediastinal irradiation.[141,268] *Symptoms* are nonspecific and include atypical chest pain and a heavy sensation over the precordium; in advanced cases, exertional dyspnea may be present.

The *physical findings* usually resemble those of cardiac tamponade, including pulsus paradoxus, a normal or diminished pulse pressure, and jugular venous distention with a predominant *x* descent and an absent *y* descent. The chest roentgenogram usually shows cardiac enlargement consistent with the presence of a pericardial effusion, and the electrocardiogram may show nonspecific ST- and T-wave abnormalities or diffuse low QRS voltage. Both M-mode and wide-angle two-dimensional echocardiograms may show a pericardial effusion sandwiched between thickened pericardial membranes with fibrinous pericardial bands (Fig. 43–22).[269,270]

Although effusive-constrictive pericarditis can be suspected on clinical grounds, the diagnosis is made by recording right heart and intrapericardial pressures both before and after pericardiocentesis. Prior to pericardiocentesis, the physiology of cardiac tamponade may be present (p. 1480) with elevation and equilibration of intrapericardial, right atrial, right ventricular, and left ventricular diastolic pressures. The right atrial pressure tracing usually shows a prominent *x* descent and an inspiratory fall in right heart filling pressure. Pericardiocentesis with restoration of intrapericardial pressure to zero may reduce pulsus paradoxus and improve cardiac output, but it does not restore the hemodynamics entirely to normal. After pericardiocentesis, there is persistent elevation and equilibration of right atrial and right and left ventricular diastolic pressures. The waveforms convert to a pattern like that in constrictive pericarditis, with a prominent *y* descent in the right atrial pressure tracing, a dip-and-plateau pattern in the right ventricular pressure, and the absence of respiratory variation in right heart filling pressures (Fig. 43–23).

Pericardiocentesis may be useful in transiently improving systemic arterial pressure and cardiac output. However, persistent constriction after successful pericardiocentesis indicates the presence of a thickened, constrictive visceral pericardium and the need for further intervention. Treatment consists of total parietal and visceral pericardiectomy[271] and specific therapy for underlying malignancy or tuberculosis, if present.

Occult Constrictive Pericarditis

Bush and coworkers have described a variant of constrictive pericarditis characterized by the presence of significant pericardial disease without overt evidence of cardiac constriction on physical examination or during routine cardiac catheterization.[272,273] The majority of patients have a history of prior acute pericarditis; symptoms are nonspecific and include chronic disabling chest pain, fatigue, and dyspnea. In most patients, the chest roentgenogram reveals borderline cardiomegaly while pericardial calcification is infrequent. The electrocardiogram shows nonspecific ST- and T-wave abnormalities. The echocardiogram is normal in most patients and a minority show either a small pericardial effusion or a filling pattern suggestive of constrictive pericarditis.[272]

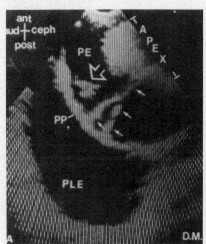

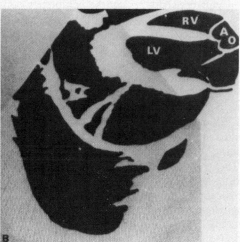

FIGURE 43–22 Two-dimensional echocardiogram (*A*) and schematic diagram (*B*) from a patient with postradiation pericarditis. Dense intrapericardial bands denoting pericardial adhesions (large and small arrows) are present within the pericardial effusion (PE). PP = parietal pericardium; PLE = pleural effusion; RV = right ventricle; AO = aorta; LV = left ventricle. (From Martin, R. P., et al.: Intrapericardial abnormalities in patients with pericardial effusion. Circulation *61*: 568, 1980, by permission of the American Heart Association, Inc.)

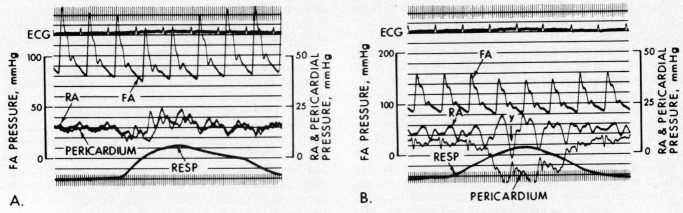

FIGURE 43–23 Femoral arterial (FA), right atrial (RA), and intrapericardial pressure tracings before (A) and after (B) pericardiocentesis in a patient with effusive-constrictive pericarditis. Before pericardiocentesis, right atrial and intrapericardial pressures are elevated and identical, and the y descent is absent from the right atrial waveform. After pericardiocentesis, mean intrapericardial pressure falls to zero, and the right atrial pressure remains elevated and develops a prominent diastolic y descent. (From Mann, T. et al.: Effusive-constrictive hemodynamic pattern due to neoplastic involvement of the pericardium. Am. J. Cardiol. *41*:781, 1978.)

Hemodynamics at rest are normal. However, the rapid infusion of 1,000 ml of prewarmed normal saline over 6 to 8 minutes transforms normal basal hemodynamics into a pattern of constrictive physiology, with elevation and equilibration of right and left ventricular diastolic pressures, the appearance of a prominent y descent in the right atrial pressure tracing, a dip-and-plateau pattern in the right ventricular pressure tracing, and loss of normal respiratory variation in the right atrial pressure pulse. These findings differ from those in normal subjects who usually experience no rise in filling pressures and from patients with myocardial disease in whom right and left ventricular diastolic pressures rise but fail to equilibrate after volume expansion. However, the sensitivity and specificity of volume challenge in the evaluation of patients with atypical chest pain and normal coronary arteries have not been well defined. In particular, the response of patients with atypical chest pain previously treated with beta-adrenergic blocking agents is not known. The likelihood that an abnormal response to volume challenge in patients with atypical chest pain reflects occult constrictive pericarditis is probably improved when there is also a history of remote pericarditis and an abnormal echocardiogram with evidence of pericardial thickening or pericardial effusion.

Total pericardiectomy has been reported in 12 patients with this diagnosis in whom there was histological confirmation of an abnormal pericardium and complete or near-complete resolution of symptoms postoperatively.[273] A few patients who have been restudied by volume challenge after operation no longer demonstrated equilibration of right and left heart filling pressures. It is not clear whether relief of chest pain after pericardiectomy was related to the relief of occult constrictive physiology per se or to relapsing pericarditis.

SPECIFIC FORMS OF PERICARDITIS

VIRAL PERICARDITIS

ETIOLOGY AND PATHOGENESIS. The viruses that most commonly cause acute pericarditis are Coxsackie virus group B and echovirus type 8.[274] Other viruses responsible for acute pericarditis include those which cause mumps, influenza, infectious mononucleosis, poliomyelitis, varicella, and hepatitis B.[275–278] Infectious mononucleosis may cause acute pericarditis with the complications of cardiac tamponade and constrictive pericarditis.[276] Varicella (chickenpox) may be associated with the complications of both severe viral pneumonia and acute pericarditis.[277] *Mycoplasma pneumoniae*, an important cause of adult nonbacterial pneumonia, also rarely causes myopericarditis.[279] There are no clinical features that distinguish acute viral pericarditis from idiopathic pericarditis, and it is likely that many cases of idiopathic pericarditis are due to unrecognized viral infections. The seasonal peak incidence of idiopathic pericarditis is in the spring and fall, which coincides with the increased incidence of enterovirus epidemics.

PATHOLOGY. Viral pericarditis causes inflammation of the visceral and parietal pericardial membranes, with infiltration first of polymorphonuclear leukocytes and then of lymphocytes around small vessels. Fibrin is deposited in the pericardial space, giving the pericardium a shaggy, reddened appearance. The underlying epicardium may also be involved by the inflammatory process. In some cases, the inflammation may result in a serous, serofibrinous, suppurative, or hemorrhagic effusion that may reach a volume of 200 ml, with a predominance of lymphocytes. Serous or serofibrinous effusions usually resolve completely by digestion of fibrin, or they may organize and obliterate the intrapericardial space. Depending on the volume, rate of accumulation, and thickness of the underlying pericardium, a pericardial effusion may result in subacute cardiac tamponade. Both echo and Coxsackie viruses may produce suppurative effusions that resolve by organization, formation of thick adhesions, calcification, and thickening of the pericardium, resulting in constrictive pericarditis.[181,280]

CLINICAL FINDINGS. A prodromal syndrome of an upper respiratory tract infection that may be described as a "cold" or the "flu" within the preceding weeks is frequently reported by patients with viral pericarditis. Clinical features of both viral and idiopathic pericarditis include chest discomfort, fever, pleurisy, cough, dyspnea, and fatigue. The chest pain associated with acute viral or idiopathic pericarditis may be excruciating, and lack of pericardial chest pain is unusual. A pericardial friction rub is present in up to three-fourths of patients and may last up to a week.[281-283] The chest roentgenogram demonstrates a pulmonary infiltrate or pleural effusion in up to 30 per cent of patients, and cardiac enlargement suggestive of a pericardial effusion is present in approximately half the patients.[284]

Viral or idiopathic pericarditis should be suspected in young or otherwise healthy adults with a characteristic prodromal illness and a syndrome of acute pericardial pain. It must be differentiated from pericarditis due to trauma, purulent pericardial infection, myocarditis, and systemic lupus erythematosus. In older patients, pericarditis due to rheumatoid disorders, myocardial infarction, tuberculosis, or neoplasm should be investigated before one presumes a viral etiology. The diagnosis of viral infection is strongly supported by the finding of a greater than fourfold rise in serial neutralizing antibody titers during the initial three weeks of illness.[282] It is rarely productive to attempt to isolate virus from blood, pericardial fluid, pleural fluid, or stool. Pericarditis due to infectious mononucleosis is suggested in the clinical setting of the young patient with high fever, adenopathy, sore throat, and positive heterophile test.

In a patient with a viral illness, the diagnosis of suspected pericarditis is confirmed clinically by the finding of a characteristic pericardial friction rub. Serial electrocardiographic changes of acute pericarditis (p. 1476) are not specific for the etiology of either viral or idiopathic pericarditis; however, the appearance of characteristic electrocardiographic changes may lead to the recognition of pericardial involvement in patients with a viral upper respiratory tract infection. Atrial arrhythmias and sinus tachycardia occur in about one-fourth of patients.[283] Echocardiographic documentation of a pericardial effusion is also evidence of pericardial inflammation in a patient with a viral upper respiratory tract infection and chest pain. Other laboratory findings suggestive of inflammation but not diagnostic of pericarditis include elevation of the sedimentation rate and leukocytosis. Cardiac isoenzymes may be abnormally elevated if there is extensive associated epicarditis or myocarditis.

Acute viral or idiopathic pericarditis is usually a short, dramatic, self-limited illness lasting 1 to 3 weeks. Important complications of acute viral or idiopathic pericarditis include (1) associated myocarditis, (2) recurrent pericarditis, (3) pericardial effusion with cardiac tamponade, and (4) the late development of constrictive pericarditis. Acute myocarditis, which may develop in association with pericarditis due to Coxsackie and echoviruses, may result in acute congestive heart failure, conduction disturbances, and cardiac enlargement that usually resolves completely or rarely leads to the development of a chronic congestive cardiomyopathy. Pericarditis may recur several weeks later in about 15 to 40 per cent of patients, and a small number of patients develop disabling recurrences over months to years that are extremely difficult to manage.[282] These recurrences of pericardial pain may be due to an immunological response to the initial viral injury rather than recurrent viral infections of the pericardium. Acute cardiac tamponade is a rare complication of viral pericarditis that occurs early in the course of acute viral or idiopathic pericarditis due to the rapid accumulation of pericardial fluid under pressure.[281,284,285] Acute pericarditis may appear to resolve and be followed by the insidious appearance of fatigue, edema, and ascites weeks to months later owing to the development of pericardial constriction. Constrictive pericarditis is a long-term complication that occurs in less than 10 per cent of patients with Coxsackie viral pericarditis.[280] Symptoms and abnormal hemodynamics resolve after surgical removal of the visceral as well as parietal pericardium.

MANAGEMENT. Treatment is directed against symptoms, with close observation for the development of cardiac tamponade or myocarditis early in the patient's course. For these reasons, most patients with an initial acute episode of pericarditis should be observed in the hospital. Bed or chair rest is warranted, and the avoidance of excessive motion and exercise helps to relieve pericardial pain and dyspnea. Pericardial pain and fever usually respond to nonsteroidal antiinflammatory agents and occasionally require steroids, as described on page 1477. Patients may be discharged from the hospital when fever and pericardial pain have disappeared and any pericardial effusion that was present has decreased in size. However, patients should be examined at regular intervals over the next few weeks to look for the complications of effusive-constrictive pericarditis and at longer intervals for the development of late constrictive pericarditis. Patients who develop tachyarrhythmias or acute conduction defects suggestive of myocardial involvement warrant close observation and electrocardiographic monitoring.

Recurrent pericarditis may require the reinstitution of antiinflammatory drug therapy with titration to the minimum dose needed to relieve symptoms, followed by gradual tapering of the drug over several weeks to months. Pericardiectomy is rarely needed for relief of severe recurrent pericardial pain in patients who cannot be weaned from steroids or other antiinflammatory drugs[286] or who have more than four recurrent attacks.

TUBERCULOUS PERICARDITIS

ETIOLOGY AND PATHOGENESIS. In industrialized nations, the incidence of tuberculous pericarditis has decreased within the past three decades as a result of effective chemotherapy and public health surveillance. The incidence of tuberculous pericarditis among patients with pulmonary tuberculosis ranges from about 1 to 8 per cent.[287] In earlier decades, tuberculous pericarditis was frequently seen in children and young adults,[288] but today it occurs predominantly in middle-aged and elderly males. The disease continues to be important in immunosuppressed patients and among the underprivileged, including South and

West African blacks, the black poor of the United States, and Asian and African immigrants.[287,289-292]

Tuberculous pericarditis usually develops by retrograde spread from peribronchial, peritracheal, or mediastinal lymph nodes or by early hematogenous spread from the primary tuberculous infection.[288,293,294] Less commonly, the pericardium is involved by the breakdown and contiguous spread of a necrotic tuberculous lesion in the lung, pleura, or spine or by hematogenous spread from distant secondary genitourinary or skeletal infections.[295]

PATHOLOGY. Tuberculous pericarditis usually begins with diffuse fibrin deposits, granuloma formation, and the presence of viable acid-fast bacilli.[294] A pericardial effusion then develops, which may be serous but more often contains some blood with a protein content exceeding 2.5 gm/dl. Although polymorphonuclear leukocytes are present early in the development of the effusion, they are later replaced by lymphocytes, monocytes, and plasma cells. Both complement-fixing antimyolemmal and antimyosin-type antibodies have been demonstrated in about 75 per cent of patients with *acute* tuberculous pericarditis in contrast to the much lower incidence in patients with viral pericarditis or constrictive pericarditis due to all types of tuberculosis, which suggests that cytolysis mediated by antimyolemmal antibodies may contribute to the development of exudative tuberculous pericarditis.[296] A tuberculous pericardial effusion usually develops very slowly and therefore does not cause hemodynamic complications; however, when it accumulates rapidly, even a small effusion may produce cardiac tamponade. As the effusion is absorbed, the pericardium thickens, granulomas proliferate, and a thick coat of fibrin is deposited on the parietal pericardium. At this stage, viable acid-fast bacilli may no longer be present, but caseation may develop and penetrate the myocardium. Finally, fibrous pericarditis develops as the granulomatous reaction is replaced by fibrous tissue and collagen. These changes are followed by the accumulation of cholesterol crystals and the development of pericardial calcification. Constrictive pericarditis develops in almost all patients with tuberculous pericarditis and in about half or less of the patients who receive antituberculosis chemotherapy.[297,298]

CLINICAL MANIFESTATIONS. Tuberculous pericarditis is usually detected clinically either in the effusive stage or late, i.e., after the development of constrictive pericarditis. It usually develops slowly, with nonspecific systemic symptoms such as low-grade fever, malaise, dyspnea, anorexia, weakness, and weight loss. Severe pericardial pain characteristic of viral and idiopathic pericarditis is uncommon in tuberculous pericarditis.[298] A large pericardial effusion usually causes dyspnea and a feeling of heaviness in the chest. Heavy sputum production, cough, and hemoptysis—clues to the presence of cavitary pulmonary tuberculosis—are usually absent.

Abnormalities on *physical examination* usually include fever, dyspnea, and a pericardial friction rub. If the complications of cardiac tamponade or effusive-constrictive pericarditis are present, the physical examination may reveal edema, jugular venous distention, pulsus paradoxus, distant heart sounds, hepatomegaly, and ascites. The *chest roentgenogram* usually shows an enlarged cardiac silhouette, and pleural effusions may be detected in about half

the patients.[282] However, the apices and hila of the lung are usually normal, and pulmonary infiltrates or calcification is present in a minority of the patients. Tuberculous pericarditis may rarely present as a solitary mediastinal mass.[299]

DIAGNOSIS. Tuberculous pericarditis should be suspected in patients with fever and unexplained cardiomegaly, particularly those who are susceptible to tuberculosis, i.e., the underprivileged or immunosuppressed. It is noteworthy that tuberculous pericarditis may develop during chemotherapy for pulmonary tuberculosis.[300] In a minority of patients with pericarditis, a definitive diagnosis of a tuberculous origin may be made by culture or histological demonstration of tuberculosis outside the pericardium (sputum, gastric wash, pleural fluid, liver or bone marrow biopsy). A definitive diagnosis can be made by isolation of the bacillus from the pericardial fluid or pericardial biopsy. It is difficult to establish a definitive bacteriological diagnosis because of the low yield of the bacillus when pericardial fluid is examined by acid-fast stain on microscopy; failure of the bacillus to grow on appropriate media or in guinea pigs, even in patients with known tuberculous pericardial effusion; and the need to observe bacterial cultures for at least eight weeks. The probability of obtaining a definitive diagnosis is greatest if both pericardial fluid and a pericardial biopsy specimen are examined early in the effusive stage.[301] However, it must be emphasized that a negative pericardial biopsy does not exclude tuberculous pericarditis, since in some patients examination of the entire pericardium removed at pericardiectomy or autopsy is required to demonstrate clear-cut evidence of tuberculosis.[302,303]

It may be necessary to make a presumptive clinical diagnosis of tuberculous pericarditis in patients with a large pericardial effusion, a positive tuberculin skin test, and systemic symptoms such as weight loss and anorexia, even when examination of the pericardial fluid and biopsy does not reveal tuberculosis. In such patients, clinical improvement may occur after initiation of antituberculosis chemotherapy. A negative tuberculin skin test may be found in anergic patients. Making a presumptive clinical diagnosis of tuberculous pericarditis requires exquisite judgment, since, on the one hand, treatment should not be withheld from the seriously ill patient, while, on the other, it is not prudent to commit patients with nontuberculous effusions to a prolonged course of multiple-drug antituberculosis therapy.

MANAGEMENT. In the era before antituberculosis chemotherapy, tuberculous pericarditis was rapidly fatal, with a mortality rate greater than 80 per cent; the remaining patients had a protracted course of months to years with a frequently fatal outcome due to miliary tuberculosis or constrictive pericarditis. Since the introduction of early chemotherapy, mortality from acute tuberculous pericarditis has fallen to less than 50 per cent, but the effectiveness of antituberculosis chemotherapy in preventing the development of constrictive pericarditis is controversial.[290,297,298]

Treatment of tuberculous pericarditis includes hospitalization with bed rest and particular attention to findings on physical examination, electrocardiography, and echocardiography that suggest the development of an enlarging pericardial effusion and tamponade. Initial chemotherapy should usually consist of a three-drug regimen, ordinarily oral isoniazid, oral ethambutol, and intramuscular strepto-mycin. The use of corticosteroids has been advocated to reduce pericardial inflammation and enhance resorption of pericardial effusion, but there is no conclusive evidence that steroids reduce the risk of developing tuberculous constrictive pericarditis.[298,304] We believe that corticoste-roids should be reserved for patients with recurrent large effusions or cardiac compression caused by granulation tis-sue who do not respond to antituberculosis drugs alone. In patients with documented cardiac tamponade or with a large pericardial effusion seen on echocardiogram, the effu-sion should be drained initially by percutaneous pericardi-ocentesis with continued catheter drainage. Pericardi-ectomy should be performed after two to four weeks of antituberculosis drug therapy if patients develop large re-current effusions or cardiac compression due to effusive-constrictive disease or constrictive pericarditis.[287,290,304,305] Pericardiectomy should be performed early in the course in patients with clinical and hemodynamic evidence of cardi-ac compression, since mortality is high among patients who undergo pericardiectomy at the late stage of calcific pericardial constriction.

BACTERIAL (PURULENT) PERICARDITIS

Although the clinical spectrum of bacterial purulent pericarditis has changed over the past four decades, mor-tality remains high. Since the introduction of antibiotics in the 1940's, the incidence of bacterial pericarditis detected at autopsy has decreased.[306,307] Prior to 1943, purulent peri-carditis occurred primarily in young, previously healthy males as a complication of pneumococcal pneumonia or empyema, and uncontrolled pleuropulmonary disease due to staphylococci or streptococci.[306] During the antibiotic era, there has been a decline in the incidence of pneumo-coccal and streptococcal pericarditis, although these organ-isms continue to cause life-threatening pericarditis.[307–309] The incidence of hospital-acquired penicillin-resistant staphy-lococcal pericarditis in post-thoracotomy patients has in-creased, and there is a widened spectrum of organisms responsible for bacterial pericarditis including the gram-negative bacilli (Proteus, *E. coli*, Pseudomonas, Klebsiel-la),[307] *Neisseria meningitidis*,[310–313] Salmonella species,[314,315] *Neisseria gonorrhoeae*,[316] *Hemophilus influenzae*,[317] *Pasteu-rella tularensis*,[318] *Streptococcus mitis*,[319] anaerobic organ-isms,[319] and other unusual pathogens.[320–323] Important predisposing factors for the development of purulent peri-carditis include a preexisting sterile pericardial effusion[324] as well as immunodepression due to burns, immunothera-py, lymphoma, or leukemia.[319,325]

The routes of pericardial infection have also changed. Direct pulmonary extension of bacterial pneumonia or em-pyema now accounts for only about 20 per cent of cases of purulent pericarditis.[319] Today, purulent pericarditis tends to occur in adults via (1) contiguous spread from an early postoperative infection after thoracic surgery or trauma, (2) infection related to infective endocarditis, (3) extension from a subdiaphragmatic suppurative source, and (4) he-matogenous spread during bacteremia. In patients with en-docarditis, bacterial pericarditis is common and is detected in about 1 out of 8 patients with endocarditis studied at autopsy and in a higher percentage of those with staphylo-

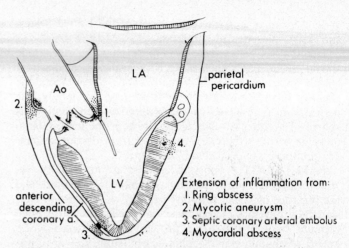

FIGURE 43–24 Schematic representation of the pathogenesis of pericarditis in infective endocarditis. Ao = aorta; LV = left ventri-cle; LA = left atrium. (From Roberts, W. C., and Spray, T. L.: Peri-cardial heart disease: A study of its causes, consequences, and morphologic features. *In* Spodick, D. H. (ed.): Pericardial Diseases. Philadelphia, F. A. Davis Co., 1976, p. 31.)

coccal endocarditis.[307] In such patients, bacterial pericardi-tis may develop by (1) extension from a valve ring abscess, (2) rupture of an aneurysm, (3) extension from a myocar-dial abscess, or (4) septic coronary embolus (Fig. 43–24). An infected myocardial infarction or aneurysm may also be a source for the development of purulent bacterial peri-carditis.[307]

In *children*, bacterial pericarditis is second only to rheu-matic fever as a cause of pericarditis[325]; the most common organisms include *Staphylococcus aureus* followed by *He-mophilus influenzae* and *Neisseria meningitidis*.[317,326–328] Pe-diatric illnesses associated with the development of bacterial pericarditis include pharyngitis, pneumonia, men-ingitis, otitis media, impetigo, endocarditis, and bacterial arthritis. The development of childhood bacterial pericardi-tis carries a high mortality of 36 to 70 per cent, depending on the organism and the risk of extremely rapid early de-velopment of constrictive pericarditis, which has also been reported in infants.[329–331] The high mortality rate in chil-dren appears to be markedly reduced by early diagnosis and combined treatment with parenteral antibiotics and open surgical pericardial drainage.[332,333]

PATHOLOGY. Bacterial pericarditis occurs most commonly by contiguous spread of an intrathoracic infec-tion. In this setting, the initial lesion is an area of acute in-flammation of the parietal pericardium adjacent to the thoracic source. Pericardial fluid may then accumulate and is clear at first, after which bacteria and fibrin appear; the late picture is of grossly purulent fluid with viable organ-isms, a high white blood cell count, and a low glucose content. Usually, bacterial pericarditis is frankly suppura-tive by the time it is detected clinically. The inflammation may result in organization and dense adhesions that cause obliteration of the pericardial space, thickening, and even-tual calcification of the pericardium. In some patients, the inflammation may involve the adjacent sternum, pleura, and diaphragm with formation of dense adhesions between the parietal pericardium and contiguous structures.

CLINICAL FEATURES. Bacterial pericarditis is usu-ally an acute fulminant illness of only a few days' duration. In one series,[319] the mean duration of symptoms prior to hospitalization was only three days. High fevers, shaking chills, night sweats, and dyspnea are common. In most patients the symptom of typical pericardial chest pain is absent. Tachycardia is present in nearly all patients, but a pericardial friction rub is present in less than half. In many cases, the pericarditis remains unsuspected because of the dominant presence of symptoms and signs related to an underlying known infection such as pneumonia or mediastinitis following complicated thoracic surgery or trauma. The appearance of new jugular venous distention and pulsus paradoxus may be the first evidence of pericardial involvement, and these ominous signs reflect the development of cardiac tamponade due to the acute accumulation of suppurative fluid under pressure.[319]

Laboratory findings usually include a leukocytosis with a marked leftward shift. The chest roentgenogram usually shows enlargement of the cardiac shadow and, less commonly, widening of the mediastinum. In the majority of cases, the roentgenogram shows evidence of underlying pneumonia, empyema, or mediastinitis without overt evidence of pericardial involvement. Electrocardiographic changes typically include ST-segment and T-wave changes characteristic of pericarditis in the majority of patients.[309,319] The appearance of electrical alternans suggests the presence of a massive suppurative effusion and raises the possibility of cardiac tamponade. In patients with suspected infective endocarditis, the appearance of a prolonged P-R interval, atrioventricular dissociation, or bundle branch block is strong evidence of extension of infection from the valve ring into the adjacent myocardium—an important predisposing factor for the development of pericarditis, especially in patients with staphylococcal endocarditis.[319]

Pericardial fluid usually shows polymorphonuclear leukocytosis and sometimes frank pus. Pericardial glucose levels are usually depressed and the protein content is elevated[319]; lactate dehydrogenase values may also be markedly elevated.

Purulent bacterial pericarditis should be suspected in a debilitated patient with unexplained high spiking fevers, dyspnea, markedly elevated white blood cell count, and an increase in the size of the cardiac silhouette on chest roentgenogram. The key to the diagnosis, which unfortunately is frequently not made before death, is a high index of suspicion. An echocardiogram should be promptly obtained to look for evidence of a new pericardial effusion and/or loculation of fluid with adhesions. The suspicion of purulent pericardial fluid is an indication to explore the pericardial space. This may be done by percutaneous pericardiocentesis *only* if there is echocardiographic evidence of a large anterior and posterior pericardial effusion that may be safely tapped or, preferably, by a generous subxiphoid pericardial window with thorough pericardial drainage.

Both pericardial fluid and pericardial tissue should be immediately studied by means of Gram-stained, acid-fast, and fungal smears by an experienced examiner. The fluid should then be cultured for aerobic and anaerobic bacteria with appropriate antibiotic sensitivity testing and for fungi and tuberculosis. Meticulous culturing for fungi as well as bacteria is important because of the increasing incidence of fungal pericarditis in patients who have received broad-

spectrum antibiotics in the setting of immunosuppression or recent major surgery.[334] Pericardial fluid should also be examined for white blood cell count and differential, hematocrit, and glucose and protein content. Cultures of blood, sputum, and recent surgical wounds should also be obtained.

Despite the lower incidence of purulent bacterial pericarditis in the antibiotic era, overall survival continues to be extremely poor, averaging about 30 per cent in modern series.[306,319,335] The poor prognosis stems in large part from failure of clinical diagnosis before death. The high mortality from purulent pericarditis can be reduced substantially through the institution of both appropriate parenteral antibiotic therapy and early complete surgical drainage. The survival rate when the disease is recognized early and managed appropriately is about 50 per cent.[306,319,335] Early surgical drainage of the pericardium also helps to prevent the complication of constrictive pericarditis.

In patients treated only with antibiotics without pericardial drainage, the rapid unsuspected development of a large pericardial effusion may result in sudden cardiovascular collapse and death due to cardiac tamponade. In one series, cardiac tamponade developed acutely in 38 per cent of the patients with bacterial endocarditis, provided the initial clue to the presence of purulent pericarditis, and contributed to death in the majority.[319]

A special comment is warranted about pericarditis associated with *meningococcal* infection. The pericardium may become infected early during meningococcal sepsis (in the presence or absence of meningitis) causing purulent pericarditis with cardiac tamponade, with a natural history as described above.[312] In these cases, the pericardial fluid is frankly purulent and viable organisms can usually be isolated. In addition, sterile pericarditis may occur late in the convalescent period in association with arthritis, pleuritis, and ophthalmitis.[319,336,337] This syndrome appears to have an immunological etiology, does not require further antibiotic therapy if the primary infection has been adequately treated, and responds to antiinflammatory agents. A febrile, self-limited polyserositis with pericarditis has also been reported after 2 to 3 weeks of effective treatment of sepsis due to *Staphylococcus aureus*.[338] Acute self-limited pericarditis due to an allergic reaction to penicillin has been described; the presence of marked peripheral eosinophilia provides an important clue that pericarditis is a feature of the drug reaction rather than purulent bacterial pericarditis.[339]

MANAGEMENT. Results of Gram-staining of the pericardial fluid should be used in the selection of antibiotics for initial therapy. If the effusion is purulent but no organisms can be easily identified and tuberculosis is not considered likely, therapy should be initiated with both a semisynthetic antistaphylococcal antibiotic and an aminoglycoside. Dosage should be adjusted in the presence of renal or hepatic dysfunction. Depending on the results of the cultures of the pericardial fluid and blood, antibiotic therapy may then be modified. High concentrations of antibiotics can be achieved in pericardial fluid, so that instillation of antibiotics into the pericardial space is not warranted.[340] However, systemic antibiotics alone are inadequate treatment, and prompt and thorough surgical drainage of the pericardium is essential in almost all patients with bacterial pericarditis.[306,319] Pericardial aspiration of a large anterior and posterior effusion may be extremely helpful in making an initial bacteriological diagnosis and initiating therapy. However, purulent pericardial effusions are likely to recur. Therefore, open drainage, through creation of subxiphoid pericardial window, is usually adequate when the diagnosis is made early and when the pericardial fluid is thin and the pericardium minimally thickened. This procedure is also the preferred route of drainage in severely disabled patients, since it can be performed under local anesthesia and avoids the pleural cavities. In a patient with a thick purulent effusion and dense adhesions with loculation, extensive pericardiectomy is needed to achieve adequate drainage and to prevent late development of constrictive pericarditis.[307,341]

FUNGAL PERICARDITIS

ETIOLOGY AND PATHOPHYSIOLOGY. *Histoplasmosis* is the most common cause of fungal pericarditis.[282,342,343] This diagnosis should be considered in patients suspected of having tuberculous pericarditis who live in the Ohio or Mississippi River Valley or the Western Appalachians, where the fungus is endemic.[343-345] In these areas, histoplasmosis is acquired by inhalation of spores from soil contaminated by infected birds, bats, or chickens. Other fungal infections responsible for pericarditis include coccidioidomycosis, aspergillosis, blastomycosis, and those caused by *Candida albicans* and *Candida tropicalis*.[282,346-348] Coccidioidomycosis pericarditis occurs in patients who have inhaled chlamydospores from soil or dust in areas of the American Southwest, particularly the San Joaquin Valley, and Argentina, where it is endemic.[346,347] Groups at increased risk for the development of fungal pericarditis consequent to disseminated infection include patients addicted to the use of intravenous narcotics and patients who are immunosuppressed or who have received potent broad-spectrum antibiotics.[319,349]

Histoplasmosis pericarditis can develop by direct extension from infected hilar lymph nodes or by hematogenous dissemination from the primary pulmonary focus. The isolation of organisms from pericardial fluid is unusual, which suggests that either too few organisms are present for identification or the pericarditis represents a sterile immune reaction to histoplasmosis antigen in the pericardial space.[343,344] Pericarditis due to fungi other than histoplasmosis may occur as a complication of open heart surgery in adults and children,[350] owing to spread from contiguous infected lymph nodes or pulmonary lesions, or as a result of hematogenous dissemination in patients who are profoundly immunosuppressed with fungal sepsis.

PATHOLOGY. Pericardial fluid may accumulate extremely rapidly and to massive quantities in patients with histoplasmosis.[351] In cases of fungal pericarditis due to agents other than Histoplasma, exudative pericardial effusions tend to accumulate slowly, so that an effusion may be present for months. Fungal pericardial effusions occasionally become organized, with pericardial thickening and the development of a constricting, calcified pericardium.[352]

Histoplasmosis may cause infection of the myocardium and endocardium as well as of the pericardium.[351,353] Similarly, aspergillosis and coccidioidomycosis may cause pericarditis in the context of pulmonary infection, endocarditis,

and myocardial abscess. Therefore, cardiac decompensation in patients with fungal pericarditis may be due both to the presence of cardiac compression from a pericardial effusion or a constrictive pericardium and to an underlying myocardial infection.

CLINICAL FEATURES. Patients with histoplasmosis pericarditis usually develop the disease in the context of an asymptomatic or mild pneumonitis with benign self-limited dissemination to other organs or, rarely, in the setting of severe prolonged disseminated infection.[282,343,345] In the latter situation, disseminated histoplasmosis infection may be evident by fever, anemia, leukopenia, and the syndrome of pneumonitis progressing to pulmonary cavitation, massive hepatomegaly, meningitis, myocarditis, or endocarditis.[351] Marked variability in the severity of histoplasmosis infection is repeatedly observed among patients affected in the same outbreak, but severe disseminated infections are especially likely to occur in young infants and elderly males.

Coccidioidomycosis pericarditis does not occur in the brief self-limited influenza-like form of the infection but is instead a complication of the progressive disseminated form of coccidioidomycosis.[346,347] Blacks, Philippinos, and Chicanos appear to be especially vulnerable to the development of severe and progressive disseminated coccidioidomycosis. These patients are usually chronically ill and debilitated, with fever, weight loss, and the complications of pulmonary infiltrate progressing to cavitary disease with lymphadenopathy, osteomyelitis, and meningitis. In immunocompromised patients, the insidious appearance of symptoms of fungal pericarditis and underlying myocardial infection may initially be overlooked because attention is focused on symptoms related to underlying lymphoma, leukemia, or known valvular endocarditis. In these patients, nonspecific symptoms of fever, chest pain, dyspnea, and malaise may be falsely attributed to the underlying disease.

Physical findings suggestive of cardiac compression (jugular venous distention, hypotension, pulsus paradoxus) may be the first clues to the diagnosis of fungal pericarditis. The chest roentgenogram may show infiltrates, hilar adenopathy or cavitary lesions suggestive of pulmonary fungal infection, or a progressive increase in the size of the cardiac silhouette if a large pericardial effusion develops. However, there are no roentgenographic, electrocardiographic, or echocardiographic features characteristic of fungal pericarditis.

DIAGNOSIS. In patients with evidence of pericarditis, a presumptive clinical diagnosis of *histoplasmosis pericarditis* can be made on the basis of (1) exposure to soil in an endemic area, (2) an elevated complement-fixation titer, (3) a positive Histoplasma skin test, and (4) evidence of characteristic miliary calcifications in the spleen and lung. The Histoplasma skin test should always be performed *after* serological testing to avoid misinterpretation of the latter. Histoplasmosis pericarditis, which occurs in the setting of severe disseminated infection and massive lymphadenopathy, must be differentiated from sarcoidosis, tuberculosis, Hodgkin's disease, and brucellosis. Histological tissue examination and culture are important. In disseminated progressive histoplasmosis, the organism may be isolated from extrapericardial sites such as the bone marrow, exudate from ulcers, or sputum by inoculation on Sabouraud's medium or by guinea pig inoculation with subsequent subculture of the spleen. Histoplasmosis pericarditis may also occur in the absence of progressive disseminated infection. In this latter setting, cultures of pericardial fluid, bone marrow, and pleural fluid are likely to be sterile, and the diagnosis is made by a fourfold or greater rise in complement-fixation antibody titer.[343]

A presumptive diagnosis of *coccidioidomycosis pericarditis* is made in a patient with pericarditis by (1) a history of dust exposure in an endemic area in the American Southwest or South America, (2) a characteristic clinical picture of disseminated coccidioidomycosis involving the lungs and other organs, (3) the appearance of a positive serum precipitin test early in the infection followed by a rising positive complement-fixation antibody titer, and (4) microscopic evidence of the characteristic spherule in biopsy material or exudates. A definitive diagnosis is made by culture identification of the organism on Sabouraud's medium. Coccidioidin skin tests are often negative in the presence of progressive disseminated disease. If pericarditis due to other fungal organisms is suspected, appropriate complement-fixing antibody titers should be measured. Depending on the clinical setting it may be important to obtain pericardial fluid and a pericardial biopsy specimen. The microscopic finding of granulomas alone is nonspecific and may occur in tuberculosis, fungal and parasitic infections, and sarcoid involvement of the pericardium. Therefore, histological documentation of the characteristic appearance of the fungus and subsequent culture identification are important.

MANAGEMENT. Histoplasmosis may cause massive effusions with acute cardiac tamponade.[351,353] Although pericardial calcification and pericardial constriction have been reported in histoplasmosis pericarditis, these are uncommon.[352,354] Intravenous amphotericin B is required only for patients with histoplasmosis pericarditis and severe systemic disease. In nonhistoplasmosis fungal pericarditis, spontaneous remissions do *not* occur; infection progresses until the patient dies either of the underlying disease or of fungal pericardial and myocardial involvement. Drug therapy for pericarditis associated with disseminated coccidioidomycosis, aspergillosis, and blastomycosis consists of prolonged intravenous therapy with amphotericin B. The South American form of blastomycosis may require the addition of a sulfonamide. In many cases of nonhistoplasmosis fungal pericarditis, chronic pericardial fungal infection progresses to severe pericardial constriction or, less commonly, cardiac tamponade.[355] Therefore, depending on the patient's underlying medical condition, pericardiectomy is usually indicated. Intrapericardial instillation of antifungal agents has not proved helpful in these diseases. The marked toxicity associated with prolonged amphotericin B administration underscores the importance of making a definitive diagnosis after histological examination or culture. *Candida pericarditis* associated with fungal sepsis and disseminated infection is treated with amphotericin B, 5-fluorocytosine, and miconazole. Fungal pericarditis occurring in the presence of valvular fungal endocarditis should also be treated by valve replacement.

Pericarditis may also be caused by *Actinomyces israelii* and *Nocardia asteroides,* which are intermediate forms between fungi and bacteria,[356-359] and by parasitic infestations of amebiasis,[360-362] acquired toxoplasmosis,[363,364] and echino-coccosis.[365-367] Very rare causes of parasitic pericarditis include dracunculosis,[368] cysticercosis, and filariasis.[369] These unusual pathogens rarely cause acute cardiac tamponade but may cause chronic constrictive pericarditis (Table 43–8).

PERICARDITIS FOLLOWING ACUTE MYOCARDIAL INFARCTION (See page 1279)

Pericarditis occurs commonly during the first few days after acute myocardial infarction. Although it is recognized clinically in approximately 10 to 15 per cent of patients with acute myocardial infarction, a much higher incidence is detected at autopsy.[370-372] Almost all patients with acute transmural myocardial infarction are found to have evidence of a localized fibrinous pericarditis overlying the infarction at autopsy. Pericarditis occurs following anterior, inferior, and lateral left ventricular infarction and in predominant right ventricular infarction as well. Other forms of pericardial involvement after myocardial infarction include acute pericardial hemorrhage secondary to cardiac rupture (p. 1268) and the late occurrence of Dressler's syndrome (p. 1513).

Pericarditis due to acute myocardial infarction usually involves the deposition of fibrin on the visceral and parietal pericardial surfaces overlying the region of transmural myocardial necrosis. Diffuse postinfarction pericarditis may resolve with the formation of delicate fibrinous adhesions within the pericardial space, obliteration of the pericardial space, or fibrotic pericardial thickening.

CLINICAL FEATURES. Pericarditis is recognized clinically by the appearance of a pericardial friction rub and pericardial chest pain within 12 hours to 10 days after acute myocardial infarction. In most patients with postinfarction pericarditis, a pericardial friction rub and pericardial chest pain appear within four days of infarction.[370,371,373] Appearance of a new friction rub more than 10 days after acute infarction probably represents the onset of Dressler's syndrome (p. 1513) or pericarditis complicating a second infarction. Detection of a pericardial friction rub is an important clue in the diagnosis of pericarditis in patients with postinfarction chest pain. Since pericardial friction rubs are notoriously evanescent, serial auscultatory evaluation of patients in various positions in a quiet room is important for detection. Pericardial rubs with a single systolic component heard near the apex may be confused with a new murmur of mitral regurgitation due to papillary muscle dysfunction or rupture. The pericardial friction rub of postinfarction pericarditis is not associated with any hemodynamic deterioration unless a pericardial effusion under pressure develops, causing cardiac tamponade.

Hemorrhagic cardiac tamponade has been reported in patients with postinfarction pericarditis in the absence of postinfarction rupture of the heart or leakage from a coronary artery.[374] Most, but not all, patients reported to have developed hemorrhagic cardiac tamponade in this context were receiving systemic anticoagulants.[375-378] These observations suggest that systemic anticoagulation contributes to the risk of bleeding into a pericardial effusion in patients with acute pericarditis complicating myocardial infarction.

The electrocardiographic ST-segment and T-wave changes typical of acute pericarditis may be difficult to recognize

TABLE 43–8   UNUSUAL INFECTIOUS CAUSES OF PERICARDITIS

ETIOLOGY	ROUTE OF PERICARDIAL INVOLVEMENT	PATHOLOGY	DIAGNOSIS	MANAGEMENT
Fungi *Actinomyces israelii*	Extension from necrotic foci in mediastinum, lungs, or esophagus; hematogenous spread from necrotic mouth lesion.	1. Anaerobe; causes early mononuclear infiltrate that progresses to necrotic, suppurative lesion with granulomas. 2. May cause pericardial constriction.	1. Clinical evidence of underlying pulmonary or mediastinal infection. 2. Histological demonstration of filamentous acid-fast organisms with sulfur granules or, occasionally, a "ray fungus" colony on pericardial biopsy.	1. Fatal if untreated. 2. High-dose penicillin or tetracycline should be continued for several weeks after apparent cure. 3. Pericardiectomy for pericardial constriction or abscesses.
Nocardia asteroides	Extension from pulmonary focus in immunocompromised or debilitated patients.	1. Aerobe; pathology resembles tuberculosis with granulomas and caseation. 2. May cause pericardial constriction.	1. Histological demonstration of weakly acid-fast, branching filaments.	1. Sulfadiazine or combination of ampicillin and erythromycin. 2. Pericardiectomy for pericardial constriction.
Parasites *Entamoeba histolytica*	Rupture of hepatic abscess through diaphragm.	1. Noninfected serous effusion (20%). 2. Purulent effusion caused by cytolytic damage from parasite enzymes with secondary bacterial infection; pericardial abscesses may develop.	1. Histological demonstration of trophozoites in pericardial biopsy or fluid; "anchovy sauce" appearance of pericardial fluid. 2. Documentation of amebae in other organs *plus* improvement after therapeutic trial.	1. Metronidazole, 500 to 700 mg three times daily for 10 days. 2. Pericardial constriction or abscess requires pericardiectomy.
Toxoplasma gondii	1. Accidental cyst ingestion after exposure to infected animals or following organ transplantation or transfusion (rare). 2. Subsequent trophozoite invasion of nucleated cells.	1. Often involves both myocardium and pericardium. 2. Rupture of inflamed pericardial and epicardial blood vessels with subsequent formation of central necrotic zone with granuloma formation, fibrosis, and calcification.	1. Histological identification of intracellular toxoplasma on pericardial or lymph node biopsies or in spinal fluid. 2. Rising serum antibody titers of dye, complement fixation, or indirect hemagglutination tests.	1. Combination therapy with sulfonamide and 5-p-chlorophenyl-2,4-diamino-6-ethylpyrimidine (Daraprim).
Echinococcus granulosus	1. Ingestion of larvae of dog tapeworms that have passed from duodenum to portal veins as embryos and encyst in myocardium. 2. Pericardial cysts form after rupture of myocardial cysts.	1. Hydatid cysts containing clear fluid with surrounding fibrous shell of giant cells, eosinophils, and fibroblasts.	1. Histological demonstration of scolices in pericardial fluid with Ziehl-Neelsen stain. 2. Positive indirect hemagglutination test.	1. Surgical excision of pericardial cysts with sterilization of cyst contents prior to removal. 2. Indirect cyst aspiration should not be attempted due to risk of constrictive pericarditis following cyst spillage.

in patients with baseline alterations of the ST segment due to prior infarction. However, there are a few useful clues: (1) when pericarditis develops after myocardial infarction, the ST-segment vector may shift leftward and posteriorly from its original position; (2) ST-segment elevation tends to be higher when acute pericarditis complicates transmural myocardial infarction[371]; (3) the *new* appearance of diffuse transient ST-segment elevation or of P-R–segment depression 1 to 4 days after a localized myocardial infarction is suggestive of acute pericarditis; and (4) atrial tachyarrhythmias appear to be more common in patients with pericarditis following infarction.[379,380] However, the appearance of acute postinfarction pericarditis per se does not appear to affect adversely the mortality after acute infarction.[371,373,381]

Postinfarction pericarditis without cardiac compression must be differentiated from acute stress ulcer or gastritis, acute pulmonary embolus, hyperventilation, and, most importantly, recurrent myocardial ischemia. Pericardial pain usually has a typical sharp pleuritic character that becomes intensified in the supine position. In some patients, the pain may have a dull, aching quality and be mistaken for that of myocardial ischemia. Myocardial ischemic pain can usually be differentiated from the pain of postinfarction pericarditis by (1) obvious amelioration of the pain by nitroglycerin and (2) the appearance of new ST-segment and T-wave changes with reciprocal changes.

The development of cardiac tamponade in patients with myocardial infarction may be related to pericardial hemorrhage secondary to pericarditis or to myocardial rupture within the first three days after infarction. Both situations may be associated with cardiovascular collapse, severe hypotension, anuria, jugular venous distention, and an abrupt increase in heart size on the chest roentgenogram. Pericardiocentesis may successfully relieve hemorrhagic cardiac tamponade in patients with postinfarction pericarditis. Massive cardiac hemorrhage secondary to cardiac rupture is usually followed by the rapid development of electromechanical dissociation and death despite successful aspiration of the pericardial space, although survivors have been reported after subacute rupture.[382]

Acute cardiac tamponade secondary to postinfarction pericarditis must also be differentiated from cardiogenic shock without intrapericardial hemorrhage due to an acute ventricular septal defect or mitral regurgitation. The appearance of a new, loud systolic murmur points to an etiology of acute mitral regurgitation or ventricular septal defect, which can be confirmed by findings on echocardiography and cardiac catheterization. In the setting of an inferior myocardial infarction, the appearance of hypotension, pulsus paradoxus, and jugular venous distention may be related to massive right ventricular infarction rather than to cardiac tamponade.[49,50,383,384] Echocardiographic findings of right ventricular enlargement without a significant pericardial effusion, and catheterization findings suggestive of constrictive physiology (right atrial waveform with steep *y* descent) rather than cardiac tamponade (right atrial waveform with attenuated *y* descent) help to differentiate massive right ventricular infarction from cardiac tamponade and prevent inappropriate and possibly disastrous attempts at pericardiocentesis.

MANAGEMENT. Postinfarction pericarditis may produce mild symptoms that require no specific therapy or severe chest pain that persists for several days. If the pain is severe, aspirin or indomethacin will relieve pain within 48 hours in almost all patients.[385] A short course of prednisone may be required in patients whose pain does not improve after a 36-hour trial of nonsteroidal antiinflammatory agents.

There is experimental evidence that indomethacin may increase infarct size[386] and cause coronary vasoconstriction[387] and that indomethacin,[388] ibuprofen,[389] and multiple large doses of corticosteroids[390] interfere with the conversion of the myocardial infarct into a scar, so that marked thinning of the myocardial wall occurs. Although the clinical importance of these experimental findings is not clear, they suggest that steroids and nonsteroidal antiinflammatory drugs should be employed only with caution in patients with acute myocardial infarction. Fortunately, aspirin does not cause any of these adverse effects, and postinfarction pericarditis usually responds well to aspirin. Accordingly, we favor use of this drug.

UREMIC PERICARDITIS (See also page 1757)

ETIOLOGY. Pericarditis is a frequent and serious complication of chronic renal failure. Bright noted the presence of pericarditis in 8 per cent of autopsied patients with chronic renal failure reported in 1836 from Guy's Hospital.[391] Uremic pericarditis was detected in about half the patients with untreated chronic renal failure, although the incidence has decreased slightly in the dialysis era.[392,393]

The etiology of uremic pericarditis is unknown. Viral and bacterial causes have been proposed, but there is no consistent evidence to suggest an infectious origin in the majority of cases of uremic pericarditis.[394] Secondary infections of uremic pericardial effusions occur,[324] and it is unwise to assume that pericarditis in a patient with severe renal disease is simply related to uremia. Excess chronic exposure to toxic catabolic nitrogen metabolites has been suggested as the mechanism responsible for uremic pericarditis. This hypothesis is supported by the observations that uremic pericarditis is rare in patients with acute mild renal failure and that uremic pericarditis often improves with initiation of dialysis in previously untreated patients. However, there is no clear correlation between the development of pericarditis and the levels of blood urea nitrogen, and pericarditis can develop in patients undergoing regular dialysis with near-normal serum creatinine and electrolyte levels.[395,396] Pericarditis appears to be less common in patients undergoing peritoneal dialysis compared with hemodialysis, suggesting the role of an unknown toxin. It has also been proposed that pericarditis in dialysis patients may reflect an immunological response to substances introduced during dialysis. It is possible that etiological factors in nondialyzed patients differ from those in patients undergoing regular dialysis. In the latter group, systemic and regional heparinization during dialysis itself may exacerbate uremic pericarditis by promoting the tendency of vascular pericardial granulation tissue to bleed into the pericardial space.

Acute uremic pericarditis is characterized by the appearance of shaggy, hemorrhagic, fibrinous exudate on both parietal and visceral pericardial surfaces with little acute inflammatory cellular reaction (Fig. 43–25). In some patients, the vascular and friable pericardial surface may bleed, giving rise to hemorrhagic pericardial effusion. If

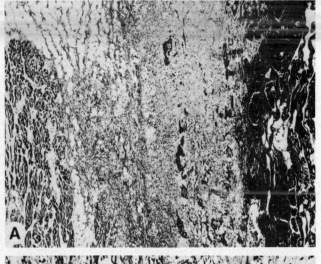

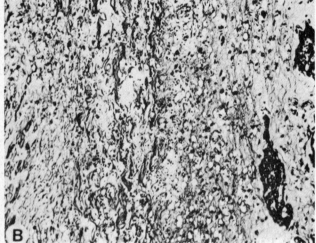

FIGURE 43–25   Micrographs of the epicardium from a patient with uremic pericarditis. *A,* The epicardial surface of fat and underlying muscle cells is covered with a fibrinous and hemorrhagic exudate (×20). *B,* Cardiac muscle cells just beneath the epicardial surface appear to be lysing, and the epicardial surface is covered with granulation tissue composed of blood vessels and fibrous tissue (×70). (From Ferrans, V. J., and Roberts, W. C.: Pathology of pericardial effusion. *In* Reddy, P. S., et al. (eds.): Pericardial Disease. New York, Raven Press, 1982, p. 85.)

the acute pericardial inflammation does not heal, subacute or chronic constrictive pericarditis may develop, coincident with organization of the effusion and formation of thick adhesions within the pericardial space. The pericardium may ultimately become very thick and fibrotic with an onion-peel appearance causing pericardial constriction, although extensive calcification is not common.[397]

CLINICAL FEATURES.   The development of pericarditis in patients undergoing dialysis is of clinical importance, since it may (1) cause disability or life-threatening cardiac tamponade in patients who are otherwise well-compensated on dialysis, (2) compromise the status of patients who are candidates for renal transplantation, and (3) cause hemodynamic complications during routine dialysis. Uremic pericarditis with a large pericardial effusion may first come to clinical attention when an otherwise asymptomatic patient becomes hypotensive and confused upon fluid removal during ultrafiltration. This occurs because volume depletion may cause an abrupt fall in systemic blood pressure when ventricular filling is already compro-

mised by the presence of a large, tense pericardial effusion. The patient's hemodynamic status may be further compromised if a large pericardial effusion coexists with uremic cardiomyopathy (p. 1760) so that a large left ventricular end-diastolic volume is needed to maintain stroke volume and cardiac output.

In addition, some patients develop symptoms of fever and substernal chest pain that is worse in the supine position and increases during inspiration. Patients with a large pericardial effusion may complain of dyspnea, the etiology of which may be difficult to differentiate from pulmonary venous congestion due to underlying myocardial dysfunction or cardiac compression.

The *physical examination* usually discloses tachycardia and a pericardial friction rub.[398] Patients with acute or subacute cardiac tamponade secondary to hemorrhagic effusion may have findings of jugular venous distention, pulsus paradoxus, and hypotension. In patients with a large pericardial effusion, increase in the size of the cardiac silhouette often develops on chest roentgenography, and this must be differentiated from changes in heart size due to myocardial dysfunction and chamber enlargement.

As in other forms of pericarditis, *echocardiography* is extremely useful in documenting the presence or absence of a pericardial effusion, estimating its size, and suggesting the presence of cardiac tamponade[399–401] as well as in detecting evidence of underlying myocardial dysfunction.

Before one makes a presumptive diagnosis of uremic pericarditis, other causes of pericardial effusion should be considered, including purulent pericarditis, neoplastic pericarditis, and pericarditis due to hypothyroidism. New, positive conversion of a tuberculin skin test in the context of the appearance of pericarditis and pericardial effusion should raise the suspicion of tuberculosis in the uremic patient. Cardiac catheterization is recommended in patients who are intolerant of dialysis and who develop dyspnea and hypotension owing to suspected cardiac tamponade. Prior to consideration of pericardiocentesis or pericardiectomy, it is important to document that these clinical findings are indeed related to the hemodynamics of cardiac tamponade (elevation and equilibration of right and left heart filling pressures) rather than to underlying congestive cardiomyopathy, ischemic heart disease, or excessively vigorous ultrafiltration. It must be remembered that pulsus paradoxus may be absent in uremic patients with cardiac tamponade and coexisting left ventricular failure and elevated left ventricular filling pressures.

In the past, uremic pericarditis was a terminal complication of untreated chronic renal failure and was almost uniformly fatal. Now, approximately one-third of dialyzed patients recover from uremic pericarditis without complication while about 20 per cent experience problems of hypotension and arrhythmias and fewer than 10 per cent experience the complications of tamponade and subacute chronic constrictive pericarditis.[396,397,399,402]

MANAGEMENT.   Treatment of uremic pericarditis with a pericardial effusion is controversial, and multiple approaches have been advocated. However, the following principles have emerged: (1) no treatment is required for small, asymptomatic pericardial effusions that can be followed simply by serial echocardiography; and (2) large pericardial effusions in symptomatic patients may resolve after an increase in the frequency of dialysis,[399,403,404] but only half the patients recover with this therapy alone. Fever and a pericardial rub accompanied by a large pericardial effusion may markedly improve with intensification of dialysis combined with a nonsteroidal antiinflammatory drug such as indomethacin.[405-407] The addition of a corticosteroid may also promote an improvement in symptoms and regression of the pericardial effusion in patients who do not respond to dialysis alone, but the complications of long-term steroid administration limit its usefulness in the treatment of recurrent uremic pericarditis. Pericarditis tends to recur when antiinflammatory agents are discontinued, suggesting that these agents only suppress and do not cure the inflammatory process.

Pericardiocentesis followed by instillation of a nonresorbable steroid into the pericardial space has also been advocated,[408,409] but this procedure has been complicated by the development of purulent pericarditis.[410] There are reports of repetitive pericardiocenteses with low morbidity and mortality in uremic patients,[411] but other series have reported a substantial mortality as a consequence of pericardiocentesis.[412] The presence of a friable visceral pericardium increases the risk of cardiac trauma and intrapericardial hemorrhage in uremic pericarditis, and many patients are also compromised by the presence of left ventricular dysfunction. These considerations warrant special caution during the performance of pericardiocentesis in uremic patients and this procedure should probably be carried out only by experienced personnel in an optimal environment, with echocardiographic documentation that a large anterior and posterior effusion is present that can be safely aspirated.

Early pericardiectomy—total, subxiphoid, or limited—in uremic patients with a large pericardial effusion has been advocated to prevent the development of cardiac tamponade and constrictive pericarditis and to allow the procedure to be carried out at a time when the patient is clinically stable.[162,173,412-417] We feel that this approach is excessively aggressive, since many uremic patients with pericardial effusion respond well to medical therapy. Instead, we believe that pericardiectomy should be reserved for patients with pericardial constriction or recurrent cardiac tamponade resistant to antiinflammatory therapy and intensification of dialysis.

We recommend an increased frequency of dialysis combined with the use of a nonsteroidal antiinflammatory agent for the treatment of hemodynamically stable patients with uremic pericarditis. Patients who are hemodynamically unstable with hemodynamic evidence of cardiac tamponade and echocardiographic evidence of a large anterior and posterior effusion may be treated by percutaneous pericardiocentesis with continued catheter drainage of the pericardial sac for 24 to 48 hours. Subxiphoid pericardiotomy is advocated for patients with hemodynamic instability associated with recurrent pericardial effusions following pericardiocentesis or loculated pericardial effusions.

NEOPLASTIC PERICARDITIS

PATHOLOGY. At autopsy, the pericardium is involved in 5 to 10 per cent of patients with malignant neoplasm.[418-422] Lung cancer, breast cancer, leukemia, Hodgkin's disease, and non-Hodgkin's lymphoma account for about 80 per cent of reported cases of malignant pericarditis.[422-431] Other malignancies commonly reported to lead to pericardial involvement include gastrointestinal cancer, sarcomas, and melanoma.[432] Less common causes of malignant pericarditis include systemic mastocytosis, teratoma, and parotid carcinoma.[433-435] *Primary malignancies* of the pericardium are rare and include primarily mesothelioma and, less frequently, malignant fibrosarcoma, angiosarcoma, and benign and malignant teratomas.[436-440]

Metastatic involvement of the pericardium may cause an exudative pericardial effusion with tumor cells in the effusion, thickening and infiltration of the pericardium, and nodular tumor deposits.[441,442] Pericardial metastases *without* associated myocardial metastases are detected in about 75 per cent of cases of cardiac involvement.[431]

Neoplastic pericarditis may cause several syndromes of cardiac compression. Hemorrhagic effusion due to neoplastic infiltration of the pericardium may develop extremely rapidly, causing acute or subacute cardiac tamponade (Fig. 43-26). Pericardial involvement by tumors such as sarcomas, mesotheliomas, and melanomas can also produce a hemorrhagic effusion by erosion of the cardiac chamber or intrapericardial blood vessels, causing acute pericardial distention and abrupt fatal cardiac tamponade. Cardiac tamponade is occasionally the initial presentation of extracardiac malignancy and leukemia.[443-445] Cardiac compression may also occur as a consequence of the development of both a thickened pericardium and a pericardial effusion under pressure (effusive-constrictive pericarditis), or it may be caused by thickening of the pericardium produced by tumor encasement of the heart, causing the physiology of constrictive pericarditis.[141,142,446,447]

CLINICAL FEATURES. Neoplastic pericarditis is often totally asymptomatic and detected only as an incidental finding at autopsy. In other patients, it may cause severe symptoms or fatal complications. Thurber et al. reported that 29 per cent of 189 patients with pericardial metastases detected at autopsy had symptoms referable to the pericardium prior to death, but pericardial involvement was cor-

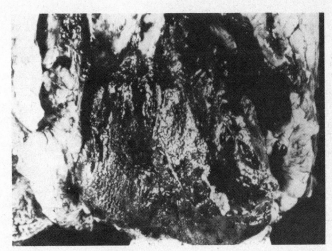

FIGURE 43-26 Gross pathologic specimen of malignant lymphoma metastatic to the heart. The lymphoma has diffusely infiltrated the pericardium and epicardium, resulting in a shaggy hemorrhagic exudate. A mixture of thrombus and blood was present within the pericardial space. (From Bloor, C. M.: Cardiac Pathology. Philadelphia, J. B. Lippincott Co., 1978.)

rectly diagnosed antemortem in only 8.5 per cent.[425] Among those patients with pericardial involvement, it was the direct cause of death in 36 per cent and a contributory factor in 49 per cent. In malignant pericarditis, dyspnea, cough, and chest pain occur frequently, while the physical findings of distant heart sounds and a pericardial friction rub are rarely detected. In many patients, symptoms resulting from pericardial involvement, such as dyspnea, hepatomegaly, and edema, may be incorrectly attributed to the underlying neoplasm, so that malignant pericarditis is not suspected until symptoms and signs of severe cardiac compression appear. Facial swelling, jugular venous distention, pulsus paradoxus, and cardiac tamponade relieved by pericardiocentesis occurred more frequently with neoplastic pericarditis than in patients with an underlying neoplasm and idiopathic or radiation-induced pericarditis.[448]

The *chest roentgenogram* is abnormal in more than 90 per cent of patients with malignant pericarditis and may show cardiac enlargement, mediastinal widening, a hilar mass, or, less commonly, an irregular nodular contour of the cardiac silhouette.[425,448] The *electrocardiogram* is usually abnormal but nonspecific, showing tachycardia, ST- and T-wave changes, low QRS voltage, and occasionally atrial fibrillation. Electrical alternans suggests the presence of a large malignant pericardial effusion under pressure.[449] Electrocardiographic findings rarely seen in pericarditis, such as atrioventricular conduction disturbances, suggest malignant invasion of the myocardium and conduction system.

DIAGNOSIS.   The diagnosis of malignant pericarditis depends on both documentation of pericardial involvement

and substantiation that pericarditis is due to neoplasm. Approximately half the patients with symptomatic pericarditis and neoplastic disease may have *nonmalignant* pericarditis due to prior radiation, idiopathic causes, infection, or an autoimmune disorder.[448] Many patients with advanced neoplastic disease are immunosuppressed as a consequence of their malignancy and/or therapy and are therefore at high risk for tubercular and fungal pericarditis. Acute pericarditis has also been reported as a complication of the intravenous administration of the chemotherapeutic agents adriamycin and daunorubicin.

Echocardiography often provides critical information about the presence and size of a pericardial effusion and the thickness and motion of the pericardium and may suggest the presence of abnormal diastolic filling of the heart due to cardiac compression. Two-dimensional echocardiography may be helpful in the detection of irregular undulating masses that protrude into the pericardial space and suggest the presence of pericardial metastases (Fig. 43–27).[450] Cardiac radionuclide scanning with gallium-67 citrate and technetium-99m pyrophosphate has also been used to detect malignant pericardial effusion,[451,452] but the specificity and sensitivity of these techniques are not established.

As in other forms of pericarditis, pericardiocentesis should be performed in conjunction with cardiac catheterization in patients with a large anterior and posterior pericardial effusion, documented by echocardiography, and suspected cardiac tamponade. Superior vena caval obstruction may coexist with malignant cardiac tamponade and contribute to the development of facial edema and jugular

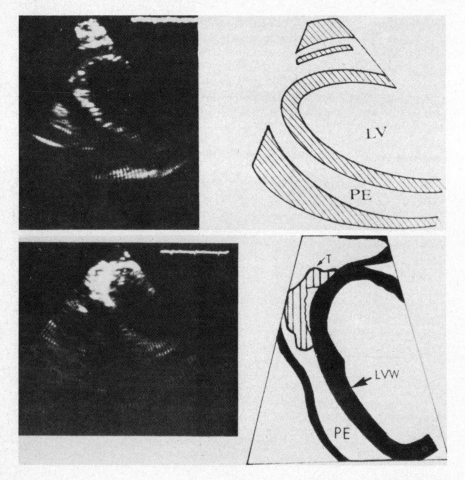

FIGURE 43–27 *Upper panel,* Cross-sectional echogram of an uncomplicated pericardial effusion showing a large clear space that denotes the pericardial effusion (PE) posterior to the left ventricle (LV). *Lower panel,* In contrast, the cross-sectional echogram from a patient with a malignant pericardial effusion shows irregular cauliflower-like masses (T) protruding into the pericardial effusion that represent bulky metastases. (From Chandraratna, P. A. N., et al.: Detection of pericardial metastases by cross-sectional echocardiography. Circulation *63*:167, 1981, by permission of the American Heart Association, Inc.)

venous distention and should be systematically excluded at cardiac catheterization in cancer patients.[156,448,453]

Pericardial fluid obtained at pericardiocentesis is serosanguineous or hemorrhagic in about two-thirds of patients and serous in the remainder. The appearance of the fluid does *not* differentiate between neoplastic, radiation, or idiopathic etiologies. Since treatment strategies differ, it is necessary to carry out a meticulous cytological examination of pericardial fluid in an attempt to differentiate malignant pericarditis from radiation-induced or idiopathic pericarditis. Cytological examination of pericardial fluid is diagnostic of a malignancy in about 85 per cent of cases of malignant pericarditis.[448,454,455] False-negative cytological diagnoses are uncommon in carcinomatous pericarditis but occur more commonly in involvement of the pericardium by lymphoma of mesothelioma.[156,448,456] In patients strongly suspected of neoplastic pericarditis, open pericardial biopsy may be required if the cytological examination of pericardial fluid is negative. If a sufficiently large biopsy specimen is obtained, open pericardial biopsy should provide a histological diagnosis in up to 90 per cent of cases.[454] However, false-negative diagnoses may occur if only a small tissue sample is obtained, and in critically ill patients open pericardial biopsy is not without risk.

In patients with echocardiographic evidence of a thickened pericardium and the physical findings of cardiac compression (jugular venous distention, edema, ascites, and hepatomegaly), cardiac catheterization is useful for documenting the presence of constrictive physiology before a decision is made to proceed with aggressive surgical intervention, i.e., extensive pericardiectomy.

Neoplastic pericarditis with cardiac compression must be differentiated from other causes of jugular venous distention, hepatomegaly, and peripheral edema in cancer patients. The most important of these are (1) underlying left ventricular dysfunction secondary to prior cardiac disease or adriamycin cardiac toxicity, (2) superior vena caval obstruction, (3) malignant hepatic involvement with portal hypertension, and (4) lymphangitic tumor spread in the lungs with secondary pulmonary hypertension.

NATURAL HISTORY. If cardiac tamponade can be avoided or successfully treated, the mere presence of neoplastic pericarditis does not imply that death is imminent. The reported *mean* survival of patients with neoplastic pericarditis ranges from 9 to 13 months.[457] In one series, a Kaplan-Meier analysis indicated a median survival of 4 months.[448] Long-term survival may be seen with neoplastic pericarditis and cardiac tamponade secondary to breast cancer.[458] In one series, 15 patients survived this complication for 1 to 2 years.[456]

MANAGEMENT. Decisions about the management of neoplastic pericardial effusion depend on the underlying condition of the patient, the presence or absence of clinical manifestations related to cardiac compression, and the prognosis and treatment options available for the specific histology and stage of the underlying malignancy. At one extreme are debilitated patients with end-stage malignant disease who have no promising treatment option for the underlying malignancy and a bleak prognosis. In this setting, diagnostic procedures should be as brief and painless as possible, and intervention should be directed toward alleviation of *symptoms* with the goal of improving the quality of

the remaining days or weeks of life. In these patients, pericardiocentesis with catheter drainage is indicated for immediate relief of severe dyspnea, chest pain, or orthopnea. When the general prognosis of the patient is better, several more aggressive treatment options are available, the goals of which are (1) relief of cardiac tamponade, (2) prevention of recurrence of the malignant effusion, and (3) treatment or prevention of constrictive pericardial disease.[459]

In patients with asymptomatic pericardial effusion who have a treatment option of effective chemotherapy or hormonal therapy directed against the underlying malignancy, treatment with systemic agents alone can be attempted while progression of the effusion is observed by means of echocardiography. In patients with cardiac tamponade and large effusions secondary to neoplastic pericarditis, pericardiocentesis with catheter drainage in combination with systemic chemotherapy can be attempted.[156,448,460] If a symptomatic pericardial effusion recurs, more prolonged palliation can be attempted with a subxiphoid pericardiotomy.[461,462] This procedure has the disadvantage of being relatively ineffective when there is extensive tumor encasement of the heart, and pericardial windows may close secondary to the development of adhesions, thereby necessitating more extensive drainage procedures.

Another approach is the instillation of various chemotherapeutic agents or radioisotopes into the pericardial space following pericardiocentesis and catheter drainage. A successful response, i.e., reduction or disappearance of an effusion, is presumably related to sclerosis of the pericardial membranes and obliteration of the pericardial space. Control of recurrent malignant pericardial effusions has been reported with intrapericardial instillation of talc,[460] tetracycline,[463] and antineoplastic agents such as nitrogen mustard, thiotepa, 5-fluorouracil, and methotrexate.[457,459,464–468] Encouraging results have also been claimed after the intrapericardial instillation of radioactive phosphorus (^{32}P), yttrium (^{90}Y), and gold (^{198}Au).[468–471] Side effects of instillation of intrapericardial agents include chest pain, nausea, and fever.

External-beam radiation therapy is an important option for patients with radiosensitive tumors who have not yet received extensive mediastinal or cardiac radiation as a treatment modality.[472] Approximately half the patients with malignant pericarditis due to a variety of primary tumors have responded to this form of treatment.[459,472–475] In one series, malignant pericardial effusion improved significantly in 11 of 16 patients with breast cancer and two of seven patients with lung cancer following 2,500 to 3,000 rads of cardiac radiation, while six of seven patients with malignant pericarditis secondary to leukemia or lymphoma improved with lower doses of cardiac radiation.[474] Extensive surgical pericardiectomy is reserved for patients with symptoms of cardiac compression due to constrictive pericarditis or tumor encasement of the heart who otherwise have a good prognosis (one- to two-year survival) relative to the underlying malignancy.

RADIATION PERICARDITIS

ETIOLOGY. Radiation injury to the heart and pericardium is an important complication of megavoltage radiation therapy used in the treatment of breast carcinoma, Hodgkin's disease, and non-Hodgkin's lymphoma. It is estimated that a threshold dose of around 4,000 rads (1,500 rems) delivered to the heart is required to produce radiation injury to the pericardium.[459,476] In a series of 117 patients with carcinoma of the breast who received radiation therapy, the incidence of radiation-induced cardiac injury was 3.4 per cent,[459] while the incidence of radiation injury to the pericardium in 81 patients who underwent mantle irradiation for Hodgkin's disease was 29 per cent.[477] Pericardial injury may occur during the course of treatment or weeks to months later.[478–482] In one series, 92 per cent of cases presenting with pericardial effusions occurred within 12 months after completion of the course of radiation therapy.[477] However, it is now recognized that radiation pericarditis manifest as chronic pericardial effusion or constrictive pericarditis may become apparent *many years* after radiation therapy.[483–485] Currently employed radiotherapy techniques using subcarinal blocks that shield the heart have helped to decrease the risk of radiation-induced pericardial injury.[486]

PATHOLOGY. Acute radiation pericarditis is associated with fibrin deposition and pericardial fibrosis (Fig. 43–28). The acute inflammatory stage may be accompanied by a pericardial effusion that can be serous, serosanguineous, or hemorrhagic with a high protein and lymphocyte content.[487,488] The inflammation and initial effusion may resolve spontaneously, or the effusion may organize and progress to a stage of dense fibrinous adhesions with gradual obliteration of the pericardial space and thickening of the pericardium, causing a chronic pericardial effusion or a constricting pericardium. Radiation pericarditis is one of the most common causes of effusive-constrictive pericardial disease.[268] Radiation injury represents an important cause of constrictive pericarditis in children, in whom constrictive diseases are otherwise rare.[489]

It is important to recognize that radiation may also injure the heart itself, causing interstitial myocardial fibrosis, valvular thickening, and premature atherosclerosis of the epicardial coronary arteries.[487,490]

CLINICAL FEATURES. The acute form of pericarditis with postradiation pericardial effusion may be transient and asymptomatic, so that the mode of presentation is an increase in heart size seen on the chest roentgenogram. Other patients may present with a syndrome of acute pericarditis consisting of fever, pericardial pain, anorexia, malaise, a pericardial friction rub, and electrocardiographic abnormalities suggestive of this disease. Radiation-induced pericardial effusion may rarely produce fatal cardiac tamponade.[481] In the chronic form of pericardial injury, patients may present more than 20 years after radiation therapy with the insidious onset of fatigue, dyspnea, systemic edema, and jugular venous distention due to the development of constrictive pericarditis.[479,484,485,491,492] The clinical recognition and consequences of this delayed form of pericardial injury have become increasingly important as patients with breast cancer and Hodgkin's disease have prolonged survival and cures.

DIAGNOSIS. Radiation-induced pericarditis with a pericardial effusion is most often confused with pericarditis due to the underlying malignancy. However, patients with malignant pericardial effusion are more likely to present with massive effusions and cardiac tamponade, and cytological examination of pericardial fluid can identify a ma-

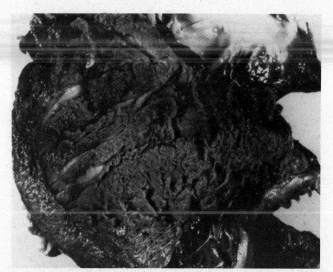

FIGURE 43–28 Gross pathologic specimen of a heart with radiation pericarditis that developed after radiation therapy for lung carcinoma. The surface of the heart is covered with a thick, shaggy, fibrinous pericarditis that was associated with a pericardial effusion. (From Bloor, C. M.: Cardiac Pathology. Philadelphia, J. B. Lippincott Co., 1978.)

lignant origin in about 85 per cent of cases.[448] In some patients, it may be extremely difficult to differentiate between these two entities without resorting to pericardial biopsy and histological examination of the pericardium. When symptoms referable to the pericardium occur years after apparently successful treatment of Hodgkin's disease or lymphoma, the pericarditis is much more likely to be related to radiation injury than to recurrent mediastinal malignancy.

MANAGEMENT. Patients in whom an asymptomatic pericardial effusion develops following radiation therapy may be followed by physical examination and serial echocardiography without the institution of specific therapy. Percutaneous pericardiocentesis should be limited to the treatment of cardiac tamponade or to drainage of a large pericardial effusion when cytological examination is required for management. Systemic corticosteroids may reduce chest pain and the size of the radiation-induced pericardial effusion, and in patients in whom purulent pericarditis is not suspected, a short course of corticosteroids is advised.[493,494] Sometimes pericarditis recurs after withdrawal of corticosteroids.[494,495] Pericardiectomy is required for that small number of symptomatic patients with large recurrent pericardial effusion, severe effusive-constrictive, or constrictive pericarditis. For some patients with constrictive pericarditis the outcome is reported to be excellent after pericardiectomy, while in others the outcome is poor due to persistent visceral pericardial constriction (epicarditis) or underlying myocardial injury.[496,497]

PERICARDITIS RELATED TO HYPERSENSITIVITY OR AUTOIMMUNITY

ACUTE RHEUMATIC FEVER (See also page 1646)

During the 19th century, acute rheumatic fever was believed to be the most common cause of pericarditis, and it was recognized that rheumatic pericarditis could occur independently of overt endocarditis.[498] The condition is now uncommon, but occasionally the development of a pericardial friction rub or effusion is the initial clue to the presence of rheumatic carditis.

Pathophysiology. Rheumatic pericarditis is characterized by fibrin deposition with localized or diffuse fibrous thickening of the pericardium. Osler reported that pericarditis could be accompanied by a fibrinous, serofibrinous, or purulent exudate.[498] The pericardial reaction may resolve spontaneously, and at autopsy there may be little evidence of prior pericardial inflammation in patients who die late from rheumatic heart disease. The development of chronic calcification and constrictive pericarditis, although reported, is very rare.[499]

Clinical Features. Rheumatic pericarditis usually occurs at the onset of the initial episode of acute rheumatic fever and may be asymptomatic or associated with typical pericardial pain and other symptoms of acute rheumatic fever, including fever, malaise, and arthralgias (p. 1648). When present, pericarditis often indicates an extensive pancarditis. The *diagnosis* of rheumatic pericarditis is based on the presence of pericardial chest pain, a pericardial friction rub, or echocardiographic evidence of a pericardial effusion in association with the usual serological and clinical criteria for acute rheumatic fever (p. 1649). In children, the onset of pericarditis, which is otherwise rare in this age group, should prompt a rigorous search for evidence of acute rheumatic fever. In the current era of antibiotic therapy and public hygiene in developed nations where acute rheumatic fever is no longer a common disease, acute rheumatic fever may not be recognized, and the combination of pericarditis, fever, arthralgias, and rash in a child or young adult may be mistaken for a viral exanthem, infectious endocarditis, juvenile rheumatoid arthritis, systemic lupus erythematosus, Henoch-Schönlein purpura, Crohn's disease, or sickle cell crisis.

Management. The treatment of rheumatic pericarditis is that of acute rheumatic fever and includes bed rest and penicillin as well as digoxin if myocardial failure is present. Chest pain associated with rheumatic pericarditis or arthralgias should be treated with aspirin, as described on page 1654. Rarely, corticosteroids are required. Small or moderate-sized pericardial effusions usually resolve spontaneously, and pericardiocentesis should not be performed solely for diagnostic reasons in a patient with documented acute rheumatic fever.

PERICARDITIS ASSOCIATED WITH SYSTEMIC LUPUS ERYTHEMATOSUS (See also page 1661)

Pericarditis usually occurs during flare-ups of disease activity in patients with systemic lupus erythematosus and is rare during quiescent phases of the disease. Pericarditis is detected clinically in about half these patients during the course of their disease, while the prevalence of pericarditis in autopsied patients is as high as 75 per cent.[500-502] The inflammatory process may cause fibrinous or effusive pericarditis with the rare occurrence of pathognomonic hematoxylin bodies in the visceral pericardium.[500] Pericardial fluid may be serous or grossly hemorrhagic with a high protein content, low glucose content, and white cell count below 10,000/mm^2 (composed primarily of polymorphonuclear leukocytes).[501] Pericardial fluid complement levels that are lower than normal serum values have been reported in patients with systemic lupus erythematosus, but caution must be used in interpreting this finding, since total hemolytic complement levels appear to be normally low in pericardial fluid.[501,503] Pericardial effusions may also contain lupus erythematosus cells and immune complexes.[504,505] Cardiac tamponade occurs in less than 10 per cent of patients with systemic lupus erythematosus and clinically recognized pericarditis, while the development of constrictive pericarditis has been reported but is extremely rare.[501,506] Pericarditis due to systemic lupus erythematosus may be accompanied by other cardiac lesions, including verrucous endocarditis,[507] inflammation and necrosis involving the conduction system, and coronary artery vasculitis (p. 1660).[508,509]

Clinical Features. Patients commonly complain of typical pericardial pain, dyspnea, and fever and present with a pericardial friction rub. Diffuse serositis including the presence of unilateral or bilateral pleuritis and pleural effusion is present in about one-fourth of patients.[501,510] The *chest roentgenogram* may show enlargement of the cardiac silhouette, pleural effusions, and parenchymal infiltrates. The roentgenographic findings of new cardiac enlargement and pulmonary venous hypertension due to a pericardial effusion under pressure must be differentiated from congestive heart failure secondary to myocardial dysfunction, a common problem in patients with systemic lupus erythematosus. *Electrocardiographic abnormalities* are those characteristic of acute pericarditis.

Pericarditis should be suspected when patients with systemic lupus erythematosus develop pleuritic chest pain, a pericardial rub, and an enlarging cardiac silhouette on the chest roentgenogram.[510] Since pericarditis usually occurs during periods of active disease, there is typically evidence of increased disease activity on blood tests for complement-fixation levels, antinuclear antibodies, lupus erythematosus cell preparations, and sedimentation rate. The *echocardiogram* may show evidence of a new pericardial effusion, confirming the presence of pericardial inflammation. Since many patients with systemic lupus erythematosus are treated with immunosuppressive corticosteroids and cytotoxic agents, a careful physical examination, blood cultures, and tuberculin skin test should be performed to search for evidence of purulent, fungal, or tuberculous pericarditis. Except when purulent pericarditis is strongly suspected, it is usually not necessary to confirm the clinical diagnosis of systemic lupus erythematosus pericarditis by performing pericardiocentesis. Systemic lupus erythematosus pericarditis can usually be distinguished from viral pericarditis by the absence of a prodromal upper respiratory infection and by the presence of other clinical findings suggestive of active systemic lupus erythematosus.

Management. In the majority of patients, pericarditis subsides when the systemic disease becomes inactive following treatment with corticosteroids or immunotherapy. The unusual complication of cardiac tamponade can ordinarily be treated with pericardiocentesis and usually does not require surgical intervention (i.e., a pericardial window or pericardiectomy). However, since the development of acute cardiac tamponade is unpredictable, patients with systemic lupus erythematosus pericarditis should be hospitalized and under close observation.

RHEUMATOID ARTHRITIS (See also page 1658)

Rheumatoid pericarditis was first described by Charcot, who observed pericardial fibrosis in four of nine autopsied patients.[511] Although pericarditis is detected at autopsy in up to 50 per cent of patients with rheumatoid arthritis, the clinical incidence of symptomatic pericarditis is less than 10 per cent.[501,512-514] Based on echocardiographic criteria for the presence of a pericardial effusion, pericarditis has been detected in 50 per cent of patients with chronic nodular rheumatoid arthritis, in 15 per cent of patients with typical non-nodular rheumatoid arthritis, and in no patients of comparable age with osteoarthritis.[515] Pericarditis tends to appear in patients with other evidence of severe rheumatoid arthritis, including extensive joint deformity, subcutaneous rheumatoid nodules, pneumonitis, and positive serum rheumatoid factor. The development of rheumatoid pericarditis, however, does not appear to correlate with the duration of the arthritis.[512] Rheumatoid pericarditis in adults can cause cardiac tamponade and has become recognized as an important cause of effusive-constrictive pericarditis and constrictive pericarditis.[268,512,516,517] In children with juvenile rheumatoid arthritis, pleuritis, pericarditis, and pneumonitis may occur without evidence of active joint involvement.[518-520]

Pathology. Typical pathological changes in the pericardium described at autopsy are those of nonspecific fibrous thickening of the visceral and parietal pericardium with adhesions and, occasionally, focal deposition of calcium and cholesterol. Rarely, small, necrotic granulomatous nodules are detected on the epicardial surface that are histologically identical to the subcutaneous rheumatoid nodule. Pericardial effusions associated with rheumatoid arthritis pericarditis are usually serous or hemorrhagic, with greater than 5 gm/dl of protein, glucose levels less than 45 mg/dl, and white blood cell counts ranging from 20,000 to 90,000/mm³.[501,512] Pericardial effusion may also contain polymorphonuclear leukocytes with cytoplasmic inclusion bodies characteristic of rheumatoid arthritis. Gamma globulin complexes, positive latex-fixation titers, and low complement levels in the pericardial fluid have also been described.[521] Acute pericarditis may progress to cause diffusely constricting fibrotic pericarditis and can coexist with other cardiac lesions, including granulomatous aortic and mitral valve deformity causing chronic mitral or aortic insufficiency.

Clinical Features. Rheumatoid arthritis is often associated with fever, precordial chest pain, and dyspnea in association with a pericardial friction rub.[521] Pericarditis commonly coexists with an exacerbation of joint inflammation and pleuritis, manifest on the chest roentgenogram as a unilateral or bilateral pleural effusion in about 65 per cent of cases.[521] The electrocardiogram usually shows nonspecific ST-segment and T-wave changes. The presence of atrioventricular block in patients with rheumatoid pericarditis probably reflects rheumatoid myocardial involvement (p. 1660). On echocardiography a pericardial effusion is present in approximately half the patients with nodular rheumatoid arthritis. An effusion may be associated with echocardiographic evidence of mitral valve abnormalities in about 25 per cent of patients.[515,522,523]

Although rheumatoid pericarditis is usually self-limited and benign, cardiac tamponade may develop abruptly in 3 to 25 per cent of patients.[501,512,517] Cardiac tamponade occurs in both adult and juvenile rheumatoid arthritis[518,519,524] and has been reported as a complication of sudden steroid withdrawal.[525] An uncommon but major complication is the rapid onset of subacute constrictive or effusive-constrictive pericarditis.[512,516,517]

Management. Patients with symptomatic pericarditis may be treated with aspirin or other nonsteroidal antiinflammatory agents, as described on page 1477. Pericardiocentesis is indicated for relief of a large anterior-posterior effusion causing cardiac tamponade. Although some authors advocate treatment with corticosteroids,[521] there is no clear evidence that steroids alter the natural history of effusions or prevent the development of the complication of effusive-constrictive pericarditis.[512] In patients with documented effusive-constrictive or constrictive pericarditis, pericardiectomy can provide gratifying hemodynamic and symptomatic improvement.[512,516,517,526,527]

SCLERODERMA PERICARDITIS (See also page 1663)

Pericardial involvement is found at autopsy in about 50 per cent of patients with progressive systemic sclerosis (scleroderma), while pericarditis is detected clinically in about 10 per cent of patients.[501,528-530] While the pathogenesis of scleroderma pericarditis is unknown, it has been suggested that increased collagen formation by fibroblasts, in combination with tissue hypoxia, may result in aberrant collagen metabolism. Histological changes are nonspecific fibrotic pericardial thickening with adhesions and perivascular inflammatory cells. Pericardial effusion was detected by means of echocardiography in 41 per cent of patients with scleroderma, although it had been suspected clinically in only a minority of these.[531]

When present, the pericardial effusion is straw-colored and characterized by a protein content greater than 5 gm/dl, low cell count, and—in contrast to the characteristics of pericardial effusions in systemic lupus erythematosus and rheumatoid arthritis—the *absence* of autoantibodies, low complement levels, and immune complexes.[501] Pericardial involvement is often associated with sclerodermatous infiltration of the heart, causing a restrictive cardiomyopathy.[530]

Scleroderma pericardial disease may present as an acute syndrome resembling viral myocarditis, with fever, chest pain, a pericardial friction rub, and nonspecific electrocardiographic ST- and T-wave changes.[529] Other patients develop a chronic pericardial effusion with symptoms of right and left atrial hypertension, cardiomegaly and pleural effusions on the chest roentgenogram, and low QRS voltage on the electrocardiogram.[501]

There is no definitive treatment for scleroderma pericarditis. Patients with the syndrome of acute pericarditis may be treated with aspirin, as described on page 1477. Rarely, pericardial effusions with cardiac tamponade may develop, necessitating pericardiocentesis.[532] Patients with symptoms and hemodynamic abnormalities due to constrictive pericarditis may require pericardiectomy. It is especially important to perform cardiac catheterization in patients with scleroderma and suspected cardiac tamponade or constrictive pericarditis, since dyspnea and systemic venous hypertension may be related to sclerodermatous cardiac involvement or to pulmonary hypertension with right ventricular failure secondary to pulmonary fibrosis. The development of pericarditis in patients with scleroderma is ominous, since the five-year survival rate is about 25 per cent when isolated pericardial or other cardiac involvement is present and about 75 per cent in patients without heart, lung, or kidney involvement.[533]

PERICARDITIS IN OTHER CONNECTIVE TISSUE DISORDERS

Pericarditis may rarely develop in other connective tissue disorders, including mixed connective tissue disease, Sjögren's syndrome, dermatomyositis, ankylosing spondylitis, Reiter's syndrome, Wegener's granulomatosis, Felty's syndrome, and severe serum sickness.[501,534–536] Pericarditis associated with polyarteritis nodosa may occur in patients who are hepatitis B antigen–positive. It also occurs in disorders of possible autoimmune etiology, including temporal arteritis,[537] inflammatory bowel disease,[538–540] Kawasaki's disease,[541] Still's disease,[542] Whipple's disease,[543] Behçet's disease, and Henoch-Schönlein purpura.[501] Amyloidosis is well known as a cause of infiltrative restrictive myopathy, the hemodynamics of which may mimic constrictive pericarditis (p. 1488), but may also involve the pericardium and cause pericardial effusions.[237,238]

DRUG-RELATED PERICARDITIS

Pericarditis occurs in about 25 per cent of patients with procainamide-related and 2 per cent of those with hydralazine-related development of the systemic lupus erythematosus syndrome.[508,544] In these patients, pericarditis may occasionally be complicated by the development of cardiac tamponade or pericardial constriction.[545–547] Other drugs that may produce pericarditis in association with the drug-induced syndrome of systemic lupus erythematosus include reserpine, methyldopa, isoniazid, and diphenylhydantoin.[502,508,548]

Other drugs appear to produce pericarditis through separate mechanisms. Pericarditis has been reported as a complication of a hypersensitivity reaction with peripheral eosinophilia after administration of penicillin[339] and cromolyn sodium.[549] The mechanisms of drug-induced pericarditis following administration of 6-amino-9-D-psicofuranosylpurine[550] and minoxidil[551,552] are not understood. Pleural and pericardial effusions have also been reported in several patients after administration of dantrolene sodium.[553] Methysergide has been reported to cause constrictive pericarditis as part of a generalized process of mediastinal fibrosis.[554] The anthracycline neoplastic agents doxorubicin and daunorubicin may cause acute pericarditis as well as myocardial inflammation within the first three weeks of drug administration (p. 1690).[555]

Acute drug-related pericarditis usually resolves when the offending drug is discontinued, and improvement may be accelerated by the administration of corticosteroids. The rare development of chronic constrictive pericarditis may be treated by pericardiectomy.

POSTMYOCARDIAL INFARCTION (DRESSLER'S) SYNDROME

Dressler's syndrome is an acute illness with fever, pericarditis, and pleuritis, probably of autoimmune origin, that occurs weeks to months after an acute myocardial infarction.[556] In the majority of the 44 patients described by Dressler in 1959, pericarditis occurred between the 7th and 11th weeks after infarction.[557] Today, a distinction is usually made between simple acute pericarditis, which occurs during the first week after infarction (p. 1503), and Dressler's syndrome, which usually appears two to three weeks after infarction, with a range of one week to several months. Dressler estimated that this syndrome occurred in up to 4 per cent of patients after acute myocardial infarction[557]; however, a recent series from the same hospital indicates that the incidence of Dressler's syndrome has markedly decreased.[558]

The etiology of Dressler's syndrome is unknown. The association of symptoms and the appearance of antimyocardial antibodies has led to the hypothesis that an autoimmune mechanism, with or without a latent viral infection, is the etiology,[559,560] while some workers have concluded that the development of antimyocardial antibodies is not specific for the presence of Dressler's syndrome.[558,561] Leakage of blood into the pericardial space is another proposed mechanism, and the lower current incidence of the syndrome may reflect changing patterns of anticoagulant use in the postinfarction period.[558] It is likely that there are common factors in the pathogenesis of Dressler's syndrome and the postpericardiotomy syndrome (p. 1514), both of which have the following features: (1) an initial insult of endothelial cell injury and entry of blood into the pericardial space; (2) a delayed response after the initial insult, consisting of fever and inflammation of the pericardial surfaces; (3) development of antiheart antibodies; (4) a dramatic response to antiinflammatory agents; and (5) the common occurrence of relapses at intervals as long as two years after the initial episode.

Pathology. The histology of the pericardium usually reveals a nonspecific inflammation with fibrin deposition. In contrast to the acute pericarditis following myocardial infarction in which pericardial inflammation is often patchy, overlying the regions of infarction, the pericarditis in Dressler's syndrome is usually diffuse. A small to moderate-sized serous pericardial effusion may develop, but the incidence of this complication is not known.

Clinical Features. Patients characteristically present with severe malaise, fever, chest pain, and pleurisy.[557,562] The chest pain may be severe enough initially to cause both patient and physician to consider that it is caused by a second myocardial infarction. In other patients, the pain is characterized as a mild, vague discomfort or as pain localized to the substernal, precordial, neck, or back regions with a pleuritic or generalized aching quality. The pain may be severe and unremitting for days to weeks and is not relieved by nitroglycerin. Physical examination often discloses a pericardial friction rub and sometimes a pleural friction rub as well. The chest roentgenogram commonly reveals an enlarged cardiac silhouette secondary to pericardial effusion associated with pleural effusions[557] and, occasionally, transient pulmonary infiltrates. Pericardial effusions too small to be detected on the chest roentgenogram may be detected by echocardiography. Electrocardiographic abnormalities usually consist of serial ST-segment and T-wave changes strongly suggestive of acute pericarditis, but the electrocardiogram may not be helpful in patients with persistent repolarization abnormalities following infarction. Blood tests usually reveal the nonspecific findings of an increased erythrocyte sedimentation rate and peripheral leukocytosis. Tests for antimyocardial antibodies are often positive but are not specific and not widely available or established as a means of confirming the diagnosis.

Dressler's syndrome can usually be discriminated from recurrent myocardial infarction by (1) the characteristics of the chest pain, as described above; (2) the absence of new Q waves on the electrocardiogram; and (3) the absence of a marked rise in the CK-MB band. Small increases in cardiac enzyme levels may occur in pericarditis when the underlying epicardium is involved. Dressler's syndrome must also be distinguished from hemorrhagic pericarditis secondary to chronic systemic anticoagulation, pulmonary embolism and infarction, and progressive cardiac failure.

Management.   A single episode of Dressler's syndrome is usually self-limited, but the syndrome does tend to recur. The initial episode usually warrants hospital admission and observation for the development of pericardial effusion or cardiac tamponade. Oral anticoagulants should be discontinued because of the risk of hemorrhage into a pericardial effusion. As in other patients with acute pericarditis, patients who are severely symptomatic with fever and chest pain usually benefit from treatment with aspirin or a nonsteroidal antiinflammatory agent. Therapeutic failure with these agents is an indication for a trial of corticosteroids, which should be tapered within four weeks followed by substitution with aspirin. Recurrent episodes of Dressler's syndrome may respond only to corticosteroids and occasionally require complete pericardiectomy for relief of intractable pericardial pain or prevention of recurrence.[563] Cardiac tamponade, although uncommon, has been reported[564] and can usually be managed with pericardiocentesis. Constrictive pericarditis is an extremely rare complication of Dressler's syndrome that may be relieved by pericardiectomy.[565,566]

POSTPERICARDIOTOMY SYNDROME

Etiology.   Postpericardiotomy syndrome is identified by the appearance of fever, pericarditis, and pleuritis two to four weeks after a cardiac operation in which the pericardium has been opened and manipulated. This syndrome was first recognized in patients after mitral commissurotomy for rheumatic heart disease, and it was initially believed to represent a reactivation of rheumatic fever.[567] Subsequently it was appreciated that the syndrome could occur following cardiac operations in patients without rheumatic heart disease and that the common denominator appeared to be wide incision and manipulation of the pericardium.[568-570] An identical clinical syndrome has been reported following cardiac perforation by a catheter or transvenous pacemaker, blunt chest trauma, percutaneous diagnostic left ventricular puncture, and epicardial pacemaker implantation.[569] The incidence of postpericardiotomy syndrome following cardiac surgery ranges from 10 to 40 per cent in various series and averages about 30 per cent.[570-573] The observation of a 31 per cent incidence of postpericardiotomy syndrome in patients undergoing cardiac surgery for the Wolff-Parkinson-White syndrome clearly indicates that pericardial damage prior to surgery is *not* a prerequisite for development of the syndrome.[573] Fur-

thermore, pericardial drainage techniques do not appear to affect the frequency of development of the syndrome after cardiac surgery.[574]

Analogous to Dressler's syndrome, the etiology of postpericardiotomy syndrome is hypothesized to be an autoimmune reaction directed against the epicardium in concert with a new or reactivated viral infection.[560,575] Studies by Engle and colleagues have demonstrated that antiheart antibodies appear in the serum of some patients who undergo pericardiotomy and that there is a positive correlation between the level of the titers and the incidence of the syndrome.[572,575] Approximately 70 per cent of patients with the postpericardiotomy syndrome and high antiheart antibody titers also develop a fourfold or higher rise in titer against one or more viral antigens, while in patients without the postpericardiotomy syndrome, a rise in viral titers occurs in only 8 per cent of those with negative antiheart antibody titers and in only 19 per cent of those with low levels of antiheart antibody titers[575]; these findings suggest that viral infection may be a triggering or permissive factor. The postpericardiotomy syndrome is rare in children under 2 years of age who undergo cardiac surgery, a finding that may be related to the short exposure time to viruses or to protective maternal antibodies transmitted via the placenta. The development of pleuritis and pleural effusions is believed to reflect involvement of the pleura adjacent to the inflamed pericardium; involvement of serous membranes distant from the heart is uncommon.

Pathology.   There are no pathognomonic histological features of postpericardiotomy syndrome. The presence of blood in the pericardial space adjacent to an injured epicardium may result in the later development of pericardial adhesions, thickening of the pericardial membranes, and occasionally fibrinous obliteration of the pericardial space, causing pericardial constriction. Pericardial effusions in patients with postpericardiotomy syndrome may be strawcolored, serosanguineous, or frankly hemorrhagic, with a protein content higher than 4.5 gm/dl and a white blood cell count between 3,000 and 8,000/mm³ (composed of both lymphocytes and granulocytes).[576]

Clinical Features.   Patients typically develop an acute illness characterized by fever, malaise, and pleuritic chest pain that usually begins during the second or third postoperative week. In some cases, the fever may reflect a continuation of the more common problem of fever in the first week after operation. The chest pain is typical of acute pericarditis (p. 1474) and often has a pleuritic quality. The physician may not recognize the implication of the chest pain and may inappropriately ascribe it to the surgical incision or the presence of chest tubes. Nonspecific myalgias, arthralgias, and anorexia may also be present.

Physical examination often reveals a pericardial friction rub. It should be noted that the friction rub present in almost all patients during the first few days after cardiac surgery disappears in most patients who do not develop postpericardiotomy syndrome by the end of the first postoperative week. The chest roentgenogram demonstrates bilateral pleural effusions in about two-thirds of patients, pulmonary infiltrates in about one-tenth, and transient enlargement of the cardiac silhouette in half.[573] Electrocardiographic changes include nonspecific ST-segment and T-wave changes and a variety of episodic tachyarrhythmias.

Echocardiography is useful in monitoring the appearance and size of a pericardial effusion, which may be detected in about 40 per cent of patients with the postpericardiotomy syndrome.[577] Thus, the diagnosis of postpericardiotomy syndrome is made on clinical grounds based on recognition of the distinctive features of the syndrome in the postoperative patient. Other causes of postoperative fever, particularly infection, including the viral-induced postperfusion syndrome of atypical lymphocytosis, fever, and hepatosplenomegaly, must be excluded.[578]

Management. The postpericardiotomy syndrome is a self-limited but often prolonged and disabling illness. Fever and severe chest pain are usually relieved by aspirin or nonsteroidal antiinflammatory drugs. Corticosteroids should be reserved for patients in whom fever and chest pain are not relieved within 48 hours by other antiinflammatory agents. Recurrences tend to appear during the first six months after surgery and may occur in up to 50 per cent of patients.

Cardiac tamponade is an important and well-recognized complication of the postpericardiotomy syndrome.[576,579–582] In one large recently reported series of adult patients who survived cardiac surgery, almost 1 per cent developed cardiac tamponade an average of 49 days after surgery, in association with fever, a pericardial friction rub, and pericardial chest pain typical of the postpericardiotomy syndrome.[576] In contrast to the important role of anticoagulation in *early* postoperative bleeding after cardiac surgery, the use of anticoagulants did not appear to be a prerequisite for the development of cardiac tamponade in association with the postpericardiotomy syndrome. Patients at risk for the development of cardiac tamponade tend to have a large pericardial effusion (greater than 500 ml), detected by simple M-mode echocardiography. Cardiac tamponade can be managed conservatively by pericardiocentesis followed by the administration of antiinflammatory agents.[576] Patients with recurrent tamponade require pericardiectomy. Percutaneous pericardiocentesis should not be attempted in patients with echocardiographic evidence of only a posterior effusion, a loculated effusion, or an effusion with dense echoes suggesting the presence of both thrombus and free fluid. Constrictive pericarditis is a complication that may occur months to years after the postpericardiotomy syndrome.[583]

POSTOPERATIVE HEMOPERICARDIUM

Acute cardiac tamponade and pericardial constriction in the *absence* of typical features of the postpericardiotomy syndrome also occur secondary to hemopericardium following cardiac surgery and perforation of the heart during cardiac catheterization, pacemaker insertion, pericardiocentesis, and transthoracic cardiac puncture.[584–586] Although it is a form of traumatic pericarditis, it is included here because of its superficial similarities to the postpericardiotomy syndrome. In some patients, postoperative cardiac tamponade has been successfully managed with pericardiocentesis.[587] However, the development of early and late postoperative tamponade is usually due to the combination of free fluid and organizing thrombus, which requires open surgical drainage of the pericardial space. Localized compression of the left ventricle and right atrium has also been reported as a complication of postoperative cardiac tamponade.[588,589]

Constrictive pericarditis is being recognized increasingly as a complication of cardiac surgery and may occur in patients in whom the pericardium is left open but in situ.[590–594] In a recent review of 5,207 adults who underwent cardiac surgery, 0.2 per cent (11 patients) developed constrictive pericarditis documented by cardiac catheterization an average of 82 days after operation.[595] Important clinical features in these patients included dyspnea, jugular venous distention, pedal edema, and increased roentgenographic heart size, while echocardiographic evidence of pericardial thickening with a posterior pericardial effusion was detected in the majority. In this series, three patients responded to medical therapy with diuretics and antiinflammatory drugs, while the remainder improved after undergoing extensive pericardiectomy and were found to have hemorrhage-induced fibrosis of the pericardium, usually associated with a posterior organized hematoma.[595] Loculated hemorrhage in the posterior pericardial space in association with injury to the pericardium from local hypothermia and povidone-iodine irrigants is postulated to be the triggering stimulus in the development of pericardial inflammation and fibrosis.[592,595]

OTHER FORMS OF PERICARDIAL DISEASE
MYXEDEMA PERICARDIAL DISEASE

Myxedema is frequently associated with a myopathy; pericardial effusion also occurs in up to one-third of patients.[596–599] Since myxedematous patients frequently have ascites, pleural effusions, and uveal edema, it has been suggested that pericardial effusion may be related to a combination of sodium and water retention, slow lymphatic drainage, and increased capillary permeability with protein extravasation.[600] The pericardial fluid is usually clear or straw-colored, with elevated protein and cholesterol concentrations and few leukocytes or red blood cells. Pericardial fluid usually accumulates very slowly and may achieve volumes of 5 to 6 liters. Cholesterol crystals may also be present.[601] Occasionally, the pericardial effusion may resemble a viscous jelly rather than a clear fluid.

Myxedematous pericardial effusions usually do not cause symptoms. Often attention is called to the heart by the finding of marked cardiomegaly on a chest roentgenogram, and a large pericardial effusion is then detected on an echocardiogram.[596] The electrocardiogram often shows nonspecific abnormalities, including low QRS voltage and flattened or inverted T waves due to either myxedematous heart disease or pericardial effusion. The heart rate of myxedematous patients with pericardial effusion has been reported to be even slower than that of myxedematous patients without effusions.[596]

Myxedematous pericardial effusions tend to regress slowly and ultimately disappear over a period of months after patients have been treated with thyroid replacement and have returned to the euthyroid state.[596,599] Cardiac tamponade has been reported, but it is a rare complication.[601–605]

CHOLESTEROL PERICARDITIS

Cholesterol pericarditis results from pericardial injury associated with deposition of cholesterol crystals and a mononuclear cell inflammatory reaction consisting of foam cells, macrophages, and giant cells. The presence of cholesterol crystals in the pericardial space is believed to provoke a chronic inflammatory response that results in effusion and may ultimately lead to the development of constrictive pericarditis. A pericardial effusion that contains cholesterol crystals typically has a glittering "gold" appearance.[601] Cholesterol in the pericardial space may be derived from damaged or necrotic epicardial cells or lysed erythrocytes following hemopericardium.[606,607] The similarities in the lipid and cholesterol contents of pericardial fluid and serum in patients with cholesterol pericarditis suggest that simple transudation may explain the high cholesterol content in the pericardial space.

The management of patients with cholesterol pericarditis includes the detection and treatment of any underlying predisposing condition associated with the development of cholesterol pericarditis, such as tuberculous, rheumatoid, or myxedematous pericarditis or hypercholesterolemia. However, in the majority of cases, cholesterol pericarditis occurs in the absence of a clear underlying disease.[607] Cholesterol pericardial effusions are usually large, but since they develop slowly, they cause cardiac tamponade only occasionally. Pericardiectomy is indicated in the unlikely event of cardiac tamponade as well as in the treatment of massive cholesterol pericardial effusion, which may cause dyspnea and chest pain.[608] The development of constrictive pericarditis requiring pericardiectomy is rare.[609]

CHYLOPERICARDIUM

Chylopericardium consists of the accumulation of a chylous effusion in the pericardial space. Idiopathic chylopericardium is rare, and chylopericardium is usually associated with mechanical obstruction of the thoracic duct or its drainage into the left subclavian vein resulting from (1) surgical or traumatic rupture of the thoracic duct or (2) lymphatic blockage by neoplasms, tuberculosis, or lymphangiectasis.[610] Thoracic duct obstruction with failure of adequate collateral drainage then results in reflux of chyle through lymphatics draining the pericardium. Most patients with chylopericardium are asymptomatic and come to clinical attention when a large, slowly accumulating pericardial effusion is detected on chest roentgenogram or echocardiogram.[610,611] The presence of a connection between a damaged thoracic duct and the pericardial space can be established by lymphangiography[610] and computed tomography[612] as well as by the recovery of ingested Sudan III, a lipophilic dye, from pericardial aspirate.[610]

The pericardial fluid is usually milky white with a high cholesterol and triglyceride content, protein content greater than 3.5 gm/dl, and microscopic fat droplets.[610] Lymphopericardium, which is due to pericardial angiomas as part of a generalized lymphangiectasis, is characterized by clear pericardial fluid.

Cardiac tamponade is rare. The management of symptomatic chylopericardium consists of efforts to reduce the likelihood of recurrence. These include ingestion of a diet rich in medium-chain triglycerides[610] or, if this is unsuccessful, in ligation of the injured thoracic duct, if one is present, above the diaphragm, and parietal pericardiectomy to evacuate chylous fluid and prevent reaccumulation.[610]

TRAUMATIC PERICARDITIS

In addition to penetrating or nonpenetrating cardiac trauma (Chap. 44), other important causes of traumatic pericarditis include rupture of the esophagus into the pericardial space, which may occur from esophageal erosion secondary to esophageal carcinoma or sudden rupture of the esophageal contents into the pericardial space in Boer-

TABLE 43–9   DISORDERS OCCASIONALLY ASSOCIATED WITH PERICARDITIS

Atrial septal defects
Right atrial myxoma
Familial Mediterranean fever
Dego's disease
Gout
Gaucher's disease
Myeloid metaplasia
Silicosis
Scorpionfish (*Scorpaena buttuta*) sting
Pseudomyxoma peritonei

haave's syndrome or as a complication of esophagogastrectomy. Traumatic pericarditis due to esophageal rupture is usually followed by intense erosive pericardial inflammation and infection secondary to the presence of bacteria and foreign bodies (food, salivary amylase, or stomach hydrochloric acid). Esophageal rupture or perforation may also be followed by the development of an esophagopericardial fistula.[613] All these disorders require immediate surgical intervention.[613,614] Pericarditis may also occur secondary to pancreatitis associated with a pericardial effusion with high amylase content and, rarely, the development of cardiac tamponade or a pancreatic-pericardial fistula.[615–617]

Pericardial trauma may also give rise to unusual traumatic syndromes, including cardiovascular collapse following herniation of the heart through a rent in the pericardium, mimicking congenital partial absence of the pericardium[618] with cardiac subluxation,[619] and intrapericardial diaphragmatic hernia.[620,621] Life-threatening cardiac herniation may also occur following radical left pneumonectomy with partial pericardial resection.[622] Herniation of the heart out of the pericardial sac can be diagnosed by thoracoscopy.[623] The rare problem of *traumatic pneumopericardium* may be caused by ulceration of the esophagus with fistula formation to the pericardium, puncture of the pericardium without cardiac laceration during sternal bone marrow aspiration, and artificial ventilation in newborns.[624]

A variety of other diseases have been reported in association with pericarditis (Table 43–9), but it is not clear whether the association is causal or coincidental.[625–632]

PERICARDIAL CYSTS

Pericardial cysts are uncommon and are typically located at the right costophrenic angle.[633] Unusual locations include the left costophrenic angle, hilum, and superior mediastinum at the level of the aortic arch. These anomalies, which come about through abnormal development of mesenchymal tissue during fetal life, are usually unilocular and filled with clear liquid, giving rise to the term "spring-water cysts."[634] Occasionally, the wall of the cyst calcifies.

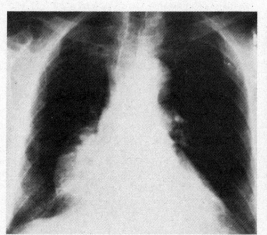
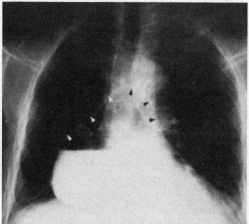

FIGURE 43–29   Chest roentgenogram in a patient with a benign pericardial cyst in a standard upright posteroanterior view. *Left panel,* Typical appearance of the cyst as a density at the lower right heart border. *Right panel,* Appearance after cyst puncture and instillation of contrast media and air. The superior portion of the cyst cavity (arrows) extends medially over the great vessels. (From Peterson, D. T., et al.: Pericardial cyst ten years after pericarditis. Chest 67:719, 1975.)

Pericardial cysts usually do not give rise to symptoms or unusual findings on physical examination. Rarely, chest pain may occur owing to torsion of the cyst.[635] These lesions typically come to medical attention as an unsuspected finding on a chest roentgenogram and must be differentiated from other conditions such as solid tumors, cardiac aneurysms or pseudoaneurysms, and herniation of the omentum or liver through a diaphragmatic defect. In most cases, a cyst can be differentiated from solid tumor or aneurysm by two-dimensional echocardiography or computerized tomography.[636] When a suspected pericardial cyst is present in an unusual location, angiography may occasionally be needed to discriminate a cyst from an aneurysm or pseudoaneurysm. Pericardial cysts located at the right costophrenic angle can be accurately diagnosed and treated by percutaneous aspiration under fluoroscopic guidance (Fig. 43–29).[637] Because long-term followup studies have shown that asymptomatic patients do not develop symptoms or show progressive cyst enlargement, most patients should be managed conservatively, without surgical exploration.[638]

CONGENITAL ABSENCE AND DEFECTS OF THE PERICARDIUM

Congenital absence of the pericardium was first described anatomically by Realdus Columbus in 1559,[2] but its antemortem detection did not occur until 1959.[639] This anomaly usually involves a defect of the left-sided pericardium; total or partial absence of the right-sided pericardium is extremely rare.[640–642]

There is a 3:1 male-to-female predominance among patients with pericardial defects, and about 30 per cent have other congenital anomalies, including atrial septal defect, bicuspid aortic valve, bronchogenic cysts, or pulmonic sequestration.[643,644] Pocock has also suggested an association between congenital absence of the pericardium and mitral valve prolapse.[645]

Total absence of the pericardium is usually associated with no symptoms. Occasionally the patient may complain of chest discomfort and dyspnea. The more common condition of absence of the left pericardium may be associated with no symptoms or with nonexertional chest pain, dyspnea, palpitations, and recurrent pulmonary infections.[644] The etiology of these symptoms is unknown, but they may be related to torsion of the great vessels due to excess mobility of the heart or pleural-epicardial adhesions. The development of empyema, pericarditis, or pleurisy with effusion in these patients is attributed to loss of the anatomical barrier between the heart and the left lung. Absence of the left pericardium is also hypothesized to predispose to the development of post-traumatic mitral regurgitation and ventricular septal defect.[646]

Clinical features include widened splitting of the second heart sound, leftward displacement of the apical impulse, and a systolic murmur at the upper left sternal border that may be related to turbulent blood flow in an unusually mobile heart. Electrocardiographic abnormalities include right-axis deviation due to levoposition of the heart,[641,643] incomplete right bundle branch block, and clockwise displacement of the QRS transition zone of the precordial leads. Tall and peaked P waves in the right precordial leads have also been described.[647]

The standard posteroanterior view of the chest roentgenogram reveals marked leftward displacement of the cardiac silhouette (Fig. 43–30), prominence and clear demarcation of the main pulmonary artery, and interposition of radiolucent lung tissue between the aorta and main pulmonary artery or between the left hemidiaphragm and inferior cardiac border.[640,642] This anomaly must be differentiated from other conditions that cause prominence of the left hilum or pulmonary artery on the standard chest film, including pulmonic valve stenosis, atrial septal defect, idiopathic dilatation of the pulmonary artery, and hilar adenopathy.

M-mode echocardiographic changes in patients with complete absence of the left-sided pericardium are similar to those seen in right ventricular volume overload and include dilatation of the right ventricle and paradoxical anterior motion of the septum in systole.[648] Two-dimensional echocardiography has shown that the anterior movement of the septum toward the transducer in systole is an artifact related to cardiac rotation and exaggerated anterior displacement of the left ventricle.[649] Although the echocardiographic features are not diagnostic, echocardiography adds important supportive evidence to the diagnosis of congenital left-sided pericardial defect and helps to exclude other congenital anomalies, such as pulmonic valve stenosis or atrial septal defect, with which this condition may be confused. Radionuclide perfusion imaging can be used to confirm the diagnosis by the demonstration of a wedge of lung tissue between the heart and left hemidiaphragm[650]; computed tomography can also be used to detect absence of the left pericardium.[651]

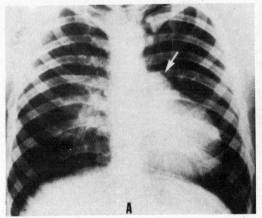

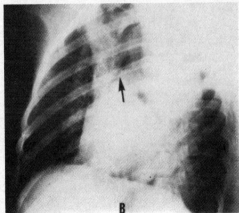

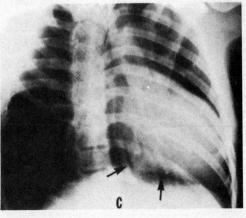

FIGURE 43–30 Chest roentgenograms in a patient with total absence of the left pericardium in posteroanterior (*A*), left anterior oblique (*B*), and right anterior oblique (*C*) views. The heart is shifted leftward, and the pulmonary artery segment is prominent (white arrow). There is a tongue of lung between the aorta and main pulmonary artery (*B*, black arrow) and between the left hemidiaphragm and inferior border of the heart (*C*, black arrows). (From Nassar, W. K., et al.: Congenital absence of left pericardium. Circulation 34:100, 1966, by permission of the American Heart Association, Inc.)

Findings at cardiac catheterization are usually normal. Cardiac angiography with diagnostic left pneumothorax has been used in the past to outline the pericardium, but this procedure is hazardous and is now rarely needed to make the diagnosis of complete absence of the left pericardium if radiological and echocardiographic findings are compatible with the diagnosis. Cardiac catheterization with angiography is indicated only if there is a strong suspicion of associated congenital anomalies requiring surgical correction. Usually no specific therapy is required for management of complete absence of the left-sided pericardium.

Partial left-sided pericardial defects may be complicated by herniation of the left atrial appendage, atrium, or left ventricle through the defect, associated with chest pain, dizziness, syncope, and peripheral emboli.[641,649] Sudden death has been reported secondary to herniation and strangulation of the heart through the defect.[652] Radiological findings are less specific in partial left-sided defects than in complete absence of left pericardium. Pulmonary artery angiography with follow-through of contrast opacification to the left heart is probably the best method for definitively demonstrating herniation of the left atrium or left atrial appendage beyond the left heart border.[653]

The even rarer anomaly of *partial right-sided pericardial defect* may be associated with inspiratory right-sided chest pain secondary to herniation of the right atrium and right ventricle through the defect[654] or herniation of lung into the pericardial cavity.[655] The chest roentgenogram may show an unusual protuberance of the right heart border, and technetium-99m cardiac blood pool imaging may demonstrate that the abnormal contour of the right heart border fills simultaneously with the right atrium.[654] Right atrial angiography in the left anterior oblique projection is helpful in documenting herniation of the right atrium and right ventricle through the pericardial defect. Surgical treatment of partial left- or right-sided pericardial defects is usually indicated to relieve symptoms and prevent cardiac strangulation. The defect may be approached by excision of the atrial appendage, pericardioplasty, or extension of the defect.[641] Attempts to close a large defect may be unsuccessful owing to compression of the heart by the taut pericardium.[654]

References

1. Boyd, L. J., and Elias, H.: Contribution to diseases of the heart and pericardium. Historical introduction. Bull. N. Y. Med. Coll. *18*:1, 1955.
2. Spodick, D. H.: Medical history of the pericardium. The hairy hearts of hoary heroes. Am. J. Cardiol. *26*:447, 1970.
3. Holt, J. P.: The normal pericardium. Am. J. Cardiol. *26*:455, 1970.
4. Spodick, D. H.: Acute Pericarditis. New York, Grune and Stratton, 1959.
5. Ishihara, T., Ferrans, V. J., Jones, M., Boyce, S. W., Kawanami, O., and Roberts, W. C.: Histologic and ultrastructural features of normal human perietal pericardium. Am. J. Cardiol. *46*:744, 1980.
6. Roberts, W. C., and Spray, T. L.: Pericardial heart disease: A study of its causes, consequences and morphologic features. *In* Spodick, D. H. (ed.): Pericardial Diseases. Philadelphia, F. A. Davis, 1976, pp. 11–65.
7. Gibson, A. T., and Segal, M. B.: A study of the composition of pericardial fluid, with special reference to the probable mechanism of fluid formation. J. Physiol. (Lond.) *277*:367, 1978.
7a. Spodick, D. H.: The normal and diseased pericardium: Current concepts of pericardial physiology, diagnosis and treatment. J. Am. Coll. Cardiol. *1*:240, 1983.
8. Pegram, B. L., and Bishop, V. S.: An evaluation of the pericardial sac as a safety factor during tamponade. Cardiovasc. Res. *9*:715, 1975.
9. Morgan, B. C., Guntheroth, W. C., and Dillard, D. H.: The relationship of pericardial to pleural pressure during quiet respiration and cardiac tamponade. Circ. Res. *16*:493, 1965.
10. Avasthey, P., and Wood, E. H.: Intrathoracic and venous pressure relationships during responses to changes in body position. J. Appl. Physiol. *37*:166, 1974.
11. Holt, J. P.: Ventricular end-diastolic volume and transmural pressure. Cardiologia *50*:281, 1967.
12. Holt, J. P., Rhode, E. A., and Kines, H.: Pericardial and ventricular pressure. Cir. Res. *8*:1171, 1960.
13. Brecher, G. A.: Venous Return. New York, Grune and Stratton, 1956.
14. Kuno, Y.: The significance of the pericardium. J. Physiol. *50*:1, 1915.
15. Berglund, E., Sarnoff, S. J., and Isaacs, J. P.: Ventricular function — Role of the pericardium in regulation of cardiovascular hemodynamics. Circ. Res. *3*:133, 1955.
16. Bernard, H. L.: The functions of the pericardium. J. Physiol. *22*:43, 1898.
17. Bartle, S. H., Hermann, H. J., Cavo, J. W., Moore, R. A., and Costenbader, J. M.: Effect of the pericardium on left ventricular volume and function in acute hypervolaemia. Cardiovasc. Res. *2*:284, 1968.
18. Spotnitz, H. M., and Kaiser, G. A.: The effect of the pericardium on pressure-volume relations in the canine left ventricle. J. Surg. Res. *11*:375, 1971.
19. Gibbon, J. H., Jr., and Churchill, E. D.: The mechanical influence of the pericardium upon cardiac function. J. Clin. Invest. *10*:405, 1931.
20. Stokland, O., Miller, M. M., Lekven, J., and Ilebekk, A.: The significance of the intact pericardium for cardiac performance in the dog. Circ. Res. *47*:27, 1980.
21. Shirato, K., Shabetai, R., Bhargave, V., Franklin, D., and Ross, J., Jr.: Alteration of the left ventricular diastolic pressure-segment length relation produced by the pericardium. Circulation *57*:1191, 1978.
21a. Crawford, H. H., Badke, F. R., and Amon, K. W.: Effect of the undisturbed pericardium on left ventricular size and performance during acute volume loading. Am. Heart J. *105*:267, 1983.
22. Refsum, H., Junemann, M., Lipton, M. J., Skioldebrand, C., Carlsson, E., and Tyberg, J. V.: Ventricular diastolic pressure-volume relations and the pericardium. Circulation *64*:997, 1981.
23. LeWinter, M. M., and Pavelec, R.: Influence of the pericardium on left ventricular end-diastolic pressure-segment relations during early and later stages of experimental chronic volume overload in dogs. Circ. Res. *50*:501, 1982.
24. Mirsky, I., and Rankin, J. S.: The effects of geometry, elasticity, and external pressures on the diastolic pressure-volume and stiffness-stress relations. How important is the pericardium? Circ. Res. *44*:601, 1979.
25. Serizawa, T., Carabello, B. A., and Grossman, W.: Effect of pacing induced ischemia on left ventricular diastolic pressure-volume relations in dogs with coronary stenoses. Circ. Res. *46*:430, 1980.
26. Taylor, R. R., Covell, J. W., Sonnenblick, E. H., and Ross, J., Jr.: Dependence of ventricular distensibility on filling of the opposite ventricle. Am. J. Physiol. *213*:711, 1967.
27. Laks, M. M., Garner, D., and Swan, H. J. C.: Volumes and compliances measured simultaneously in the right and left ventricles of the dog. Circ. Res. *20*:565, 1967.
28. Elzinga, G., Van Grondelle, R., Westerhof, N., and Van Den Bos, G. C.: Ventricular interference. Am. J. Physiol. *226*:941, 1974.
29. Santamore, W. P., Lynch, P. R., Meier, G., Heckman, J., and Bove, A. A.: Myocardial interaction between the ventricles. J. Appl. Physiol. *41*:362, 1976.
30. Bemis, C. E., Serur, J. R., Borkenhagen, D., Sonnenblick, E. H., and Urschel, C. W.: Influence of right ventricular filling pressure on left ventricular pressure and dimension. Circ. Res. *34*:498, 1974.
31. Brinker, J. A., Weiss, J. L., Lappe, D. L., Rabson, J. L., Summer, W. R., Permutt, S., and Weisfeldt, M. L.: Leftward septal displacement during right ventricular loading in man. Circulation *61*:626, 1980.
32. Brenner, J. I., and Waugh, R. A.: Effect of phasic respiration on left ventricular dimension and performance in a normal population. Circulation *57*:122, 1978.
33. Spadaro, J., Bing, O. H., Gaasch, W. H., and Weintraub, R. M.: Pericardial modulation of right and left ventricular diastolic interaction. Circ. Res. *48*:233, 1981.
34. Lorell, B. H., Palacios, I., Daggett, W. M., Jacobs, M. L., Fowler, B. N., and Newell, J. B.: Right ventricular distention and left ventricular compliance. Am. J. Physiol. *240*:H87, 1981.
35. Janicki, J. S., and Weber, K. T.: The pericardium and ventricular interaction, distensibility, and function. Am. J. Physiol. *238*:H494, 1980.
36. Bove, A. A., and Santamore, W. P.: Ventricular interdependence. Progr. Cardiovasc. Dis. *23*:365, 1981.
37. Shirato, K., Kanazawa, M., Ishikawa, K., Nakajima, T., and Takishima, T.: The effect of the pericardium on the diastolic properties of the heart. Jpn. Circ. J. *46*:113, 1982.
38. Maruyama, Y., Ashikawa, K., Isoyama, S., Kanatsuke, H., Ino-Oka, E., and Takishima, T.: Mechanical interactions between four heart chambers with and without the pericardium in canine hearts. Circ. Res. *50*:86, 1982.
39. Glantz, S. A., Misbach, G. A., Moores, W. Y., Mathey, D. G., Levken, J., Stowe, D. F., Parmley, W. W., and Tyberg, J. V.: The pericardium substantially affects the left ventricular diastolic pressure-volume relationship in the dog. Circulation *42*:433, 1978.
40. Mangano, D. T.: The effect of the pericardium on ventricular systolic function in man. Circulation *61*:352, 1980.
41. Ringertz, H. G., Misbach, G. A., and Tyberg, J. V.: Effect of the normal pericardium on the left ventricular diastolic pressure-volume relationship. Acta Radiol. *22*:529, 1981.
42. Alderman, E. L., and Glantz, S. A.: Acute hemodynamic interventions shift the diastolic pressure-volume curve in man. Circulation *54*:662, 1976.
43. Brodie, B. R., Grossman, W., Mann, T., and McLaurin, L. P.: Effects of sodium nitroprusside on left ventricular diastolic pressure-volume relations. J. Clin. Invest. *59*:59, 1977.
44. Ludbrook, P. A., Byrne, J. D., Kurnik, P. B., and McKnight, R. C.: Influence of reduction of preload and afterload by nitroglycerin on left ventricular diastolic pressure-volume relations and relaxation in man. Circulation *56*:937, 1977.
45. Ludbrook, P. A., Byrne, J. D., and McKnight, R. C.: Influence of right ventricular hemodynamics on left ventricular diastolic pressure-volume relations in man. Circulation *59*:21, 1979.
46. Wong, C. Y., and Spotnitz, H. M.: Effect of nitroprusside on end-diastolic pressure-diameter relations of the human left ventricle after pericardiotomy. J. Thorac. Cardiovasc. Surg. *82*:350, 1981.
47. Ross, J., Jr.: Acute displacement of the diastolic pressure-volume curve of the left ventricle: Role of the pericardium and the right ventricle. Circulation *59*:32, 1979.
48. Bartle, S. H., and Hermann, H. J.: Acute mitral regurgitation in man. Hemodynamic evidence and observations indicating an early role for the pericardium. Circulation *36*:839, 1967.

49. Lorell, B. H., Leinbach, R. C., Pohost, G. M., Gold, H. K., Dinsmore, R. E., Hutter, A. M., Jr., Pastore, J. O., and DeSanctis, R. W.: Right ventricular infarction. Am. J. Cardiol. 43:465, 1979.

50. Goldstein, J. A., Vlahakes, G. H., Verrier, E. D., Schiller, N. B., Tyberg, J. V., Ports, T. A., Parmley, W. W., and Chatterjee, K.: The role of right ventricular systolic dysfunction and elevated intrapericardial pressure in the genesis of low output in experimental right ventricular infarction. Circulation 65: 513, 1982.

ACUTE PERICARDITIS

51. Sodeman, W. A., and Smith, R. H.: A re-evaluation of the diagnostic criteria for acute pericarditis. Am. J. Med. Sci. 235:672, 1958.

52. Dunn, M., and Rinkenberger, R. L.: Clinical aspects of acute pericarditis. Cardiovasc. Clin. 7-3:131, 1976.

53. Markiewicz, W., Brik, A., Brook, G., Edoute, Y., Monakier, I., Markiewicz, Y.: Pericardial rub in pericardial effusion: Lack of correlation with amount of fluid. Chest 77:643, 1980.

54. Spodick, D. H.: Pericardial rub: Prospective, multiple observer investigation of pericardial friction in 100 patients. Am. J. Cardiol. 35:357, 1975.

55. Spodick, D. H.: Pathogenesis and clinical correlations of the electrocardiographic abnormalities of pericardial disease. Cardiovasc. Clin. 8-3:201, 1977.

56. Hull, E.: The electrocardiogram in pericarditis. Am. J. Cardiol. 7:21, 1961.

57. Spodick, D. H.: Diagnostic electrocardiographic sequences in acute pericarditis: Significance of PR segment and PR vector changes. Circulation 48: 575, 1973.

58. Surawicz, B., and Lasseter, K. C.: Electrocardiogram in pericarditis. Am. J. Cardiol. 26:471, 1970.

59. Spodick, D. H.: Acute pericarditis: ECG changes. Primary Cardiol. 8:78, 1982.

60. Bruce, M. A., and Spodick, D. H.: Atypical electrocardiogram in acute pericarditis: Characteristics and prevalence. J. Electrocardiol. 13:61, 1980.

61. Coffin, C. W., and Scarf, M.: Acute pericarditis simulating coronary artery occlusion. Am. Heart J. 32:515, 1946.

61a. Wanner, W. R., Schaal, S. F., Bashore, T. M., Norton, V. J., Lewis, R. P., and Fulkerson, P. K.: Repolarization variant vs. acute pericarditis. A prospective electrocardiographic and echocardiographic evaluation. Chest 83:180, 1983.

62. Spodick, D. H.: Differential characteristics of the electrocardiogram in early repolarization and acute pericarditis. N. Engl. J. Med. 295:523, 1976.

63. Ginzton, L. E., and Laks, M. M.: The differential diagnosis of acute pericarditis. Circulation 65:1004, 1982.

64. James, T. N.: Pericarditis and the sinus node. Arch. Intern. Med. 110:305, 1962.

65. Dressler, N.: Sinus tachycardia complicating and outlasting pericarditis. Am. Heart J. 72:422, 1966.

66. Olson, H. G., Lyons, K. P., Aronow, W. S., Kuperus, J., Orlando, J. R., and Waters, H. J.: Technetium-99m stannous pyrophosphate myocardial scintigrams in pericardial disease. Am. Heart J. 99:459, 1980.

67. Kadota, K., Matsumori, A., Kambara, H., and Kawai, C.: Myocardial uptake of technetium-99m stannous pyrophosphate in experimental viral myopericarditis. J. Nucl. Med. 20:1047, 1979.

68. Ahmad, M., and Dubiel, J. P.: Tc-99m pyrophosphate myocardial imaging in perimyocarditis. J. Nucl. Med. 22:452, 1981.

69. Martin, P., Devriendt, J., Goffin, Y., and Verhas, M.: Gallium 67 scintigraphy in fibrinous pericarditis associated with bacterial endocarditis. Eur. J. Nucl. Med. 7:192, 1982.

70. Taillefer, R., and Lemieux, R. J., Picard, D., and Dupras, G.: Gallium 67 imaging in pericarditis secondary to tuberculosis in histoplasmosis. Clin. Nucl. Med. 6:413, 1981.

71. Schreiner, D. P., Krishnaswami, V., and Murphy, J. H.: Unsuspected purulent pericarditis detected by gallium-67 scanning: A case report. Clin. Nucl. Med. 6: 411, 1981.

72. Tiefenbrunn, A. J., and Roberts, R.: Elevation of plasma MB creatine kinase and the development of new Q waves in association with pericarditis. Chest 77: 438, 1980.

73. Marmor, A., Grenadir, E., Keidar, A., Edward, S., and Palant, A.: The MB fraction of creatine phosphokinase: An indicator of myocardial involvement in acute pericarditis. Arch. Intern. Med. 139:819, 1979.

74. Hancock, E. W.: Management of pericardial disease. Mod. Conc. Cardiovasc. Dis. 48:1, 1979.

PERICARDIAL EFFUSION

75. Steinberg, I.: Pericarditis with effusion: New observations with a note on Ewart's sign. Ann. Intern. Med. 49:428, 1958.

76. Carsky, E. W., Mauceri, R. A., and Azimi, F.: The epicardial fat pad sign: Analysis of frontal and lateral chest radiographs in patients with pericardial effusion. Radiology 137:303, 1980.

77. Dinsmore, R. E., Miller, A. R., Potsaid, M. S., and Shawdon, H. H.: Cineangiographic patterns in pericardial disease. Am. J. Roentgenol. 86:425, 1966.

78. Mattsson, O.: Scintigraphy of pericardial effusion. Acta Radiol. Diag. 17:737, 1976.

79. Wolverson, M. K., Grider, R. D., Sundaram, M., Heiberg, E., and Johnson, F.: Demonstration of unsuspected malignant disease of the pericardium by computed tomography. C. T. 4:330, 1980.

80. Tomoda, H., Hoshiai, M., Furuya, H., Oeda, Y., Matsumoto, S., Tanabe, T., Tamachi, H., Sasamoto, H., Koide, S., Kuribayashi, S., and Matsuyama, S.: Evaluation of pericardial effusion with computed tomography. Am. Heart J. 99:701, 1980.

81. Wong, B. Y. S., Lee, K. R., and MacArthur, R. I.: Diagnosis of pericardial effusion by computed tomography. Chest 81:177, 1982.

82. Isner, J. M., Carter, B. L., Bankoff, M. S., Konstam, M. D., and Salem, D. N.: Computed tomography in the diagnosis of pericardial heart disease. Ann. Intern. Med. 97:473, 1982.

83. Unverferth, D. V., Williams, T. E., and Fulkerson, P. K.: Electrocardiographic voltage in pericardial effusion. Chest 75:157, 1979.

84. Allen, J. W., Harrison, E. D., Camp, J. C., Bursari, A., Turnier, E., and Lau, F. Y. K.: The role of serial echocardiography in the evaluation and differential diagnosis of pericardial disease. Am. Heart J. 93:560, 1977.

85. Feigenbaum, H.: Echocardiographic diagnosis of pericardial effusion. Am. J. Cardiol. 26:475, 1970.

86. Horowitz, M. S., Schultz, C. S., and Stinson, E. B.: Sensitivity and specificity of echocardiographic diagnosis of pericardial effusion. Circulation 50:239, 1974.

86a. Parameswaran, R., and Goldberg, H.: Echocardiographic quantitation of pericardial effusion. Chest 83:767, 1983.

87. Ratshin, R. A., Smith, M. K., and Hood, W. P., Jr.: Possible false positive diagnosis of pericardial effusion by echocardiography in the presence of large left atrium. Chest 65:112, 1974.

88. Martin, R. P., Rakowski, H., French, J., and Popp, R. L.: Localization of pericardial effusion with wide angle phased array echocardiography. Am. J. Cardiol. 42:904, 1978.

89. Friedman, M. J., Sahn, D. J., and Haber, K.: Two-dimensional echocardiography and B-mode ultrasonography for the diagnosis of loculated pericardial effusion. Circulation 60:1644, 1979.

90. Brown, A. K.: Chronic idiopathic pericardial effusion. Br. Heart J. 28:609, 1966.

91. Bedford, D. E.: Chronic effusive pericarditis. Br. Heart J. 26:499, 1964.

92. Santos, G. H., and Frater, R. W. M.: The subxiphoid approach in the treatment of pericardial effusion. Ann. Thorac. Surg. 23:467, 1977.

93. Hatcher, C. R., Jr., Logue, R. B., Logan, W. D., Jr., Symbas, R. B., Mansour, D. A., and Abbott, O. A.: Pericardiectomy for recurrent pericarditis. J. Thorac. Cardiovasc. Surg. 62:371, 1971.

94. Fowler, N. O.: Physiology of cardiac tamponade and pulsus paradoxus. Physiological, circulatory, and pharmacologic responses in cardiac tamponade. Mod. Conc. Cardiovasc. Dis. 47:115, 1978.

95. Reddy, P. S., Curtiss, E. I., O'Toole, J. D., and Shaver, J. A.: Cardiac tamponade: Hemodynamic observations in man. Circulation 58:265, 1978.

96. Craig, R. J., Whalen, R. E., Behar, V. S., and McIntosh, H. D.: Pressure and volume changes of the left ventricle in acute pericardial tamponade. Am. J. Cardiol. 22:65, 1968.

97. Shabetai, R., Mangiardi, L., Bhargava, V., Ross, J., Jr., and Higgins, C. B.: The pericardium and cardiac function. Progr. Cardiovasc. Dis. 22:107, 1979.

98. Pegram, B. L., Kardon, M. B., and Bishop, V. S.: Changes in left ventricular internal diameter with increasing pericardial pressure. Cardiovasc. Res. 9:707, 1975.

99. Shabetai, R., Fowler, N. O., and Guntheroth, W. G.: The hemodynamics of cardiac tamponade and constrictive pericarditis. Am. J. Cardiol. 26:480, 1970.

100. Wechsler, A. S., Auerbach, B. J., Graham, T. C., and Sabiston, D. C.: Distribution of intramyocardial blood flow during pericardial tamponade: Correlation with microscopic anatomy and intrinsic myocardial contractility. J. Thorac. Cardiovasc. Surg. 68:847, 1974.

101. Frank, M. J., Nadimi, M., Lesniak, L. J., Hilmi, K. I., and Levinson, G. E.: Effects of cardiac tamponade on myocardial performance, blood flow and metabolism. Am. J. Physiol. 220:179, 1971.

102. Brecher, G. A.: Critical review of recent work on ventricular diastolic suction. Circ. Res. 6:554, 1958.

103. Kostreva, D. R., Castaner, A., Pedersen, D. H., and Kampine, J. P.: Nonvagally mediated bradycardia during cardiac tamponade or severe hemorrhage. Cardiology 68:65, 1981.

104. Castaner, A., Kostreva, D. R., and Kampine, J. P.: Changes in autonomic nerve activity during acute cardiac tamponade. Cardiology 66:163, 1980.

105. Friedman, H. S., Gomes, J. A., Tardio, A. R., and Haft, J. I.: The electrocardiographic features of acute cardiac tamponade. Circulation 50:260, 1974.

106. Fowler, N. O.: Cardiac Diagnosis and Treatment. 3rd ed. New York, Harper and Row, 1980, p. 981.

107. Ruskin, J., Bache, R. J., Rembert, J. C., and Greenfield, J. C., Jr.: Pressure-flow studies in man: Effect of respiration on left ventricular stroke volume. Circulation 48:79, 1973.

108. Fowler, N. O.: Physiology of cardiac tamponade and pulsus paradoxus. I. Mechanisms of pulsus paradoxus in cardiac tamponade. Mod. Conc. Cardiovasc. Dis. 47:109, 1978.

109. Goldblatt, A., Harrison, D. C., Glick, G., and Braunwald, E.: Studies on cardiac dimensions in intact, unanesthetized man. II. Effects of respiration. Circ. Res. 13:448, 1963.

110. Wexler, L., Bergel, D. H., Gabe, I. T., Makin, G. S., and Mills, C. J.: Velocity of blood flow in normal human venae cavae. Circ. Res. 23:349, 1968.

111. Shabetai, R., Fowler, N. O., Fenton, J. C., and Masangkay, M.: Pulsus paradoxus. J. Clin. Invest. 44:1882, 1965.

112. Shabetai, R., Fowler, N. O., and Gueron, M.: The effects of respiration on aortic pressure and flow. Am. Heart J. 65:525, 1963.

113. Gabe, I. T., Mason, D. T., Gault, J. H., Ross, J., Jr., Zelis, R., Mills, C. J.,

Braunwald, E., and Schillingford, J. P.: Effect of respiration on venous return and stroke volume in cardiac tamponade. Br. Heart J. *32*:592, 1970.

114. Settle, H. P., Adolph, R. J., Fowler, N. O., Engel, P., Agruss, N. S., and Levenson, N. I.: Echocardiographic study of cardiac tamponade. Circulation *56*:951, 1977.

115. D'Cruz, I. A., Cohen, H. C., Prabhu, R., and Glick, G.: Diagnosis of cardiac tamponade by echocardiography: Changes in mitral valve motion and ventricular dimensions, with special reference to paradoxical pulse. Circulation *52*:460, 1975.

116. McGregor, M.: Current concepts: Pulsus paradoxus. N. Engl. J. Med. *301*: 480, 1979.

117. Friedman, H. S., Sakurai, H., and Lajam, F.: Pulsus paradoxus: A manifestation of a marked reduction of left ventricular end-diastolic volume in cardiac tamponade. J. Thorac. Cardiovasc. Surg. *79*:74, 1980.

118. Robotham, J. L., and Mitzner, W.: A model of the effects of respiration on left ventricular performance. J. Appl. Physiol. *46*:411, 1979.

119. Burdine, J. A., and Wallace, J. M.: Pulsus paradoxus and Kussmaul's sign in massive pulmonary embolism. Am. J. Cardiol. *15*:413, 1965.

120. Cohen, S. I., Kupersmith, J., Aroesty, J., and Rowe, J. W.: Pulsus paradoxus and Kussmaul's sign in acute pulmonary embolism. Am. J. Cardiol. *32*:271, 1973.

121. Rebuck, A. S., and Pengelly, L. D.: Development of pulsus paradoxus in the presence of airways obstruction. N. Engl. J. Med. *288*:66, 1973.

122. Settle, H. P., Jr., Engel, P. J., Fowler, N. O., Allen, J. M., Vassollo, C. L., Hackworth, J. N., Adolph, R. J., and Eppert, D. C.: Echocardiographic study of the paradoxical arterial pulse in chronic obstructive lung disease. Circulation *62*:1297, 1980.

123. Winer, H. E., and Kronzon, I.: Absence of paradoxical pulse in patients with cardiac tamponade and atrial septal defects. Am. J. Cardiol. *44*:378, 1979.

124. Guberman, B. A., Fowler, N. O., Engel, P. J., Gueron, M., and Allen, J. M.: Cardiac tamponade in medical patients. Circulation *64*:633, 1981.

125. Hardesty, R. L., Thompson, M., Lerberg, D. B., Siewers, R. D., O'Toole, J. D., Salerni, R., and Bahnson, H. T.: Delayed postoperative cardiac tamponade: Diagnosis and management. Ann. Thorac. Surg. *26*:155, 1978.

126. Beck, C. S.: Two cardiac compression triads. J.A.M.A. *104*:714, 1935.

127. Symmes, J. C., and Berman, N. D.: Early recognition of cardiac tamponade. Canad. Med. Assoc. J. *116*:863, 1977.

128. Jacobs, J., and Talano, J. V.: Cardiomegaly and paradoxical pulse. Arch. Intern. Med. *138*:1125, 1978.

129. Hetzel, P. S., Wood, E. H., and Burchell, H. B.: Pressure pulses in the right side of the heart in a case of amyloid heart disease and in a case of idiopathic heart failure simulating constrictive pericarditis. Mayo Clin. Proc. *28*:107, 1953.

130. Cohn, J. N., Pinkerson, A. L., and Tristani, F. E.: Mechanism of pulsus paradoxus in clinical shock. J. Clin. Invest. *46*:1744, 1967.

131. Antman, E. M., Cargill, V., and Grossman, W.: Low-pressure cardiac tamponade. Ann. Intern. Med. *91*:403, 1979.

132. Niarchos, A. P.: Electrical alternans in cardiac tamponade. Thorax *30*:228, 1975.

133. McGregor, M., and Baskind, E.: Electrical alternans in pericardial effusion. Circulation *11*:837, 1955.

134. Bashour, F. A., and Cochran, P. W.: The association of electrical alternans with pericardial effusion. Dis. Chest *44*:146, 1963.

135. Littmann, D., and Spodick, D. H.: Total electrical alternation in pericardial disease. Circulation *17*:912, 1958.

136. Feigenbaum, H., Zaky, A., and Grabhorn, L. L.: Cardiac motion in patients with pericardial effusion. A study using reflected ultrasound. Circulation *34*: 611, 1966.

137. Usher, B. W., and Popp, R. L.: Electrical alternans: Mechanism in pericardial effusion. Am. Heart J. *83*:459, 1972.

138. Sbarbaro, J. A., and Brooks, H. L.: Pericardial effusion and electrical alternans: Echocardiographic assessment. Postgrad. Med. *63*:105, 1978.

139. Friedman, H. S., Lajam, F., Calderon, J., Zaman, Q., Marino, N. D., and Gomes, J. A.: Electrocardiographic features of experimental cardiac tamponade in closed-chest dogs. Eur. J. Cardiol. *6*:311, 1977.

140. Spodick, D. H.: Acute cardiac tamponade: Pathologic physiology, diagnosis and management. Progr. Cardiovasc. Dis. *10*:64, 1967.

141. Mann, T., Brodie, B. R., Grossman, W., and McLaurin, L.: Effusive-constrictive hemodynamic pattern due to neoplastic involvement of the pericardium. Am. J. Cardiol. *41*:781, 1978.

142. Wynne, J., Markis, J. E., and Grossman, W.: Extrinsic compression of the heart by tumor masquerading as cardiac tamponade. Cath. Cardiovasc. Diag. *4*:81, 1978.

143. Cosio, F. G., Martinez, J. P., Serrano, C. M., Calzada, C. S., and Alcaire, C. C.: Abnormal septal motion in cardiac tamponade with pulsus paradoxus. Echocardiographic and hemodynamic observations. Chest *71*:787, 1977.

144. Armstrong, W. F., Schilt, B. F., Helper, D. J., Dillon, J. C., and Feigenbaum, H.: Diastolic collapse of the right ventricle with cardiac tamponade: An echocardiographic study. Circulation *65*:1491, 1982.

145. Schiller, N. B., and Botvinick, E. H.: Right ventricular compression as a sign of cardiac tamponade: An analysis of echocardiographic ventricular dimensions and their clinical implications. Circulation *56*:774, 1977.

145a.Kronzon, I., Cohen, M. J., and Winer, H. E.: Contribution of echocardiography to the understanding of the pathophysiology of cardiac tamponade. J. Am. Coll. Cardiol. *1*:1180, 1983.

146. Winer, H., Kronzon, I., and Glassman, E.: Echocardiographic findings in se-vere paradoxical pulse due to pulmonary embolism. Am. J. Cardiol. *40*:808, 1977.

147. Martins, J. B., and Kerber, R. E.: Can cardiac tamponade be diagnosed by echocardiography? Circulation *60*:737, 1979.

148. Uren, R. F., McLaughlin, A. F., and Cormack, J.: Cardiac tamponade: Accurate diagnosis by radionuclide angiography. Aust. N. Z. J. Med. *10*:414, 1980.

149. Shabetai, R., Aravindakshan, V., Danielson, G., and Bryant, L.: Traumatic hemopericardium with tricuspid incompetence. J. Thorac. Cardiovasc. Surg. *57*: 294, 1969.

150. Spitz, H. B., and Holmes, J. C.: Right atrial contour in cardiac tamponade. Radiology *103*:69, 1972.

151. Fowler, N. O., and Holmes, J. C.: Hemodynamic effect of isoproterenol and norepinephrine in acute cardiac tamponade. J. Clin. Invest. *48*:502, 1969.

152. Gascho, J. A., Martins, J. B., Marcus, M. L., and Kerber, R. E.: Effects of volume expansion and vasodilators in acute pericardial tamponade. Am. J. Physiol. *240*:H49, 1981.

153. Moller, C. T., Schoonbee, C. G., and Rosendorff, C.: Hemodynamics of cardiac tamponade during various modes of ventilation. Br. J. Anaesth. *51*:409, 1979.

154. Kotte, J. H., and McGuire, J.: Pericardial paracentesis. Mod. Conc. Cardiovasc. Dis. *20*:102, 1951.

155. Kilpatrick, Z. M., and Chapman, C. B.: On pericardiocentesis. Am. J. Cardiol. *16*:722, 1965.

156. Krikorian, J. G., and Hancock, E. W.: Pericardiocentesis. Am. J. Med. *65*:808, 1978.

157. Wong, B., Murphy, J., Chang, C. J., Hassenein, K., and Dunn, M.: The risk of pericardiocentesis. Am. J. Cardiol. *44*:1110, 1979.

158. Kaiser, E., and Loewenneck, H.: Pericardial puncture. The most favorable anatomical approach. Münch. Med. Wschr. *123*:1697, 1981.

159. Heilerli, B., Anderes, U., and Follath, F.: Diagnosis and therapy of cardiac tamponade. An analysis of 50 patients. Schweiz. Med. Wschr. *111*:735, 1981.

159a.Callahan, J. A., Seward, J. B., Tajik, A. J., Holmes, D. R., Jr., Smith, H. C., Reeder, G.S., and Miller, F. A.: Enhanced safety of two-dimensional echocardiography-directed pericardiocentesis: A technique of choice. J. Am. Coll. Cardiol. *1*:738, 1983.

160. Aron, D. V., Richardson, J. D., Webb, G., Grover, F. L., and Trinkle, J. K.: Subxiphoid pericardial window in patients with suspected traumatic pericardial tamponade. Ann. Thorac. Surg. *23*:545, 1977.

161. Schepers, G. W. H.: Tuberculous pericarditis. Am. J. Cardiol. *9*:248, 1962.

162. Morin, J. G., Mulder, D. S., and Long, R.: Pericardiectomy for uremic tamponade. Canad. J. Surg. *19*:109, 1976.

163. Gotsman, M. S., and Schrire, V.: Pericardiocentesis electrode needle. Br. Heart J. *28*:566, 1966.

164. Glancy, D. L., and Richter, M. A.: Catheter drainage of the pericardial space. Cath. Cardiovasc. Diag. *1*:311, 1975.

165. Lubell, D. K., and Glass, P.: Construction of a simplified pericardiocentesis electrode. Dis. Chest *41*:657, 1962.

166. Owens, W. C., Shaefer, R. A., and Rahimtoola, S. H.: Pericardiocentesis: Insertion of a pericardial catheter. Cath. Cardiovasc. Diag. *1*:317, 1975.

167. Shabetai, R., and Grossman, W.: Profiles in constrictive pericarditis, restrictive cardiomyopathy, and cardiac tamponade. *In* Grossman, W. (ed.): Cardiac Catheterization and Angiography. 2nd ed. Philadelphia, Lea and Febiger, 1980, pp. 358–376.

168. Wei, J. Y., Taylor, G. J., and Aschuff, S. C.: Recurrent cardiac tamponade and large pericardial effusion: Management with an indwelling pericardial catheter. Am. J. Cardiol. *42*:281, 1978.

169. Larrey, D. J.: New surgical procedure to open the pericardium and determine the cause of fluid in its cavity. Clin. Chirurg. *36*:393, 1829.

170. Alcan, K. E., Zabetakis, P. M., Marino, N. D., Franzone, A. J., Michelis, M. F., and Bruno, M. S.: Management of acute cardiac tamponade by subxiphoid pericardiotomy. J.A.M.A. *247*:1143, 1982.

171. Fontenelle, L. J., Cuello, L., and Dooley, B. N.: Subxiphoid pericardial window—A simple and safe method for diagnosing and treating acute and chronic pericardial effusions. J. Thorac. Cardiovasc. Surg. *62*:95, 1971.

172. Fredriksen, R. T., Cohen, L. S., and Mullins, C. B.: Pericardial windows or pericardiocentesis for pericardial effusions. Am. Heart J. *82*:158, 1971.

173. Ribot, S., Frankel, H. J., and Gielchinsky, I.: Treatment of uremic pericarditis. Clin. Nephrol. *27*:127, 1974.

174. Lajos, T. Z., Black, H. E., Cooper, R. G., and Wanka, J.: Pericardial decompression. Ann. Thorac. Surg. *19*:47, 1975.

175. Ibarra, P. C., and Gonzalez, R. L.: Diagnosis and treatment of pericarditis by the subxiphoid approach. Am. J. Surg. *44*:602, 1978.

CONSTRICTIVE PERICARDITIS

176. Agarwal, S., and Chopra, P.: Constrictive pericarditis: A histopathological study of 91 cases. Indian Heart J. *29*:278, 1977. Constrictive Pericarditis

177. Chesler, E., Matha, A. S., Matisonn, R. E., and Rogers, M. N. A.: Subpulmonic stenosis as a result of noncalcific pericarditis. Chest *69*:425, 1976.

178. McGaff, F. J., Haller, J. A., Jr., Leight, L., and Towery, B. T.: Subvalvular pulmonic stenosis due to constriction of the right ventricular outflow tract by a pericardial band. Am. J. Med. *34*:142, 1963.

179. Paul, O., Castleman, B., and White, P. D.: Chronic constrictive pericarditis: A study of 53 cases. Am. J. Med. Sci. *216*:361, 1948.

180. Andrews, G. W. S., Pickering, G. W., and Sellors, T. H.: The aetiology of con-

strictive pericarditis with special reference to tuberculous pericarditis, together with a note on polyserositis. Quart. J. Med. 17:291, 1948.

181. Howard, E. J., and Maier, H.: Constrictive pericarditis following acute Coxsackie viral pericarditis. Am. Heart J. 75:247, 1968.

182. Haycock, G. B., and Jordan, S. C.: Chronic pericardial constriction with effusion in childhood. Arch. Dis. Child. 54:890, 1979.

183. Bonische, C. H., and Jaffe, J. P.: Spontaneous severe constrictive pericarditis in congenital afibrinogenemia: Mechanism, evaluation and successful surgical management. Am. Heart J. 101:503, 1981.

184. Perheentupa, J., Autio, S., Leisti, S., Raitta, C., and Tuuteri, L.: Mulibrey nanism, and autosomal recessive syndrome with pericardial constriction. Lancet 2:351, 1973.

185. Perheentupa, J., Autio, S., Leisti, S., and Raitta, C.: Mulibrey nanism: Dwarfism with muscle, liver, brain and eye involvement. Acta Pediat. Scand. (Suppl.) 206:74, 1970.

186. Voorhees, M. L., Husson, G. S., and Blackman, M. S.: Growth failure with pericardial constriction. The syndrome of mulibrey nanism. Am. J. Dis. Child. 130:1146, 1976.

187. Shabetai, R., Mangiardi, L., Bhargava, V., Ross, J., Jr., and Higgens, C. B.: The pericardium and cardiac function. Progr. Cardiovasc. Dis. 22:107, 1979.

188. Moscovitz, H. L.: Pericardial constriction versus cardiac tamponade. Am. J. Cardiol. 26:546, 1970.

189. Hancock, E. W.: Constrictive pericarditis: Modern view of diagnosis and management. J. Cardiovasc. Med. 41:367, 1980.

190. Lewis, B. S., and Gotsman, M. S.: Left ventricular function in systole and diastole in constrictive pericarditis. Am. Heart J. 86:23, 1973.

191. Armstrong, T. G., Lewis, B. S., and Gotsman, M. S.: Systolic time intervals in constrictive pericarditis and severe primary myocardial disease. Am. Heart J. 85:6, 1973.

192. Khattri, H. N., Bidwei, P. S., Mahapatra, S. S., Sharma, J. K., and Wahi, P. L.: Systolic time intervals in constrictive pericarditis. Indian Heart J. 29:70, 1977.

193. Gaasch, W. H., Peterson, K. L., and Shabetai, R.: Left ventricular function in chronic constrictive pericarditis. Am. J. Cardiol. 34:107, 1974.

194. Harvey, R. M., Ferrer, M. I., Cathcart, R. T., Richards, D. W., and Cournand, A.: Mechanical and myocardial factors in chronic constrictive pericarditis. Circulation 8:695, 1953.

195. Dines, D. E., Edwards, J. E., and Burchell, H. B.: Myocardial atrophy in constrictive pericarditis. Proc. Staff Meet. Mayo Clin. 33:93, 1958.

196. Vogel, J. H. K., Horgan, J. A., and Strahl, C. L.: Ventricular function in chronic constrictive pericarditis: Observations on fiber shortening rate. Cardiol. Digest 6:21, 1971.

197. Levine, H. D.: Myocardial fibrosis in constrictive pericarditis. Electrocardiographic and pathologic observations. Circulation 48:1268, 1973.

198. Kesteloot, H., and Denef, B.: Value of reference tracings in diagnosis and assessment of constrictive epi- and pericarditis. Br. Heart J. 32:675, 1970.

199. Wood, P.: Chronic constrictive pericarditis. Am. J. Cardiol. 7:48, 1961.

200. Hancock, E. W.: On the elastic and rigid forms of constrictive pericarditis. Am. Heart J. 100:917, 1980.

200a. Cheevers, N.: Observations on the disease of the orifice and valves of the aorta. Guy's Hosp. Rep. 7:387, 1842.

201. Gimlette, T. M. D.: Constrictive pericarditis. Br. Heart J. 21:9, 1959.

202. Hancock, E. W.: Constrictive pericarditis. Clinical clues to diagnosis. J.A.M.A. 232:176, 1975.

203. Mounsey, P.: The early diastolic sound of constrictive pericarditis. Br. Heart J. 17:143, 1955.

204. Tyberg, T. I., Goodyer, A. V. N., and Langou, R. A.: Genesis of pericardial knock in constrictive pericarditis. Am. J. Cardiol. 46:570, 1980.

205. Beck, W., Shrire, V., and Vogelpoel, L.: Splitting of the second heart sound in constrictive pericarditis with observations on the mechanism of pulsus paradoxus. Am. Heart J. 64:765, 1962.

206. Plus, G. E., Brower, A. J., and Clagett, O. T.: Chronic constrictive pericarditis: Roentgenologic findings in 35 surgically proved cases. Proc. Staff Meet. Mayo Clin. 32:555, 1957.

207. Heinz, R., and Abrams, H. L.: Radiologic aspects of operable heart disease. IV. Appearances of constrictive pericarditis. Radiology 69:54, 1957.

208. Chesler, E., Mitha, A. S., and Matisonn, R. E.: The ECG of constrictive pericarditis — Pattern resembling right ventricular hypertrophy. Am. Heart J. 91:420, 1976.

209. Schnittger, I., Bowden, R. E., Abrams, J., and Popp, R. L.: Echocardiography: Pericardial thickening and constrictive pericarditis. Am. J. Cardiol. 42:388, 1978.

210. Doi, Y. L., Sugiura, T., and Spodick, D. H.: Motion of pulmonic valve and constrictive pericarditis. Chest 80:513, 1981.

211. Tanaka, C. N., Nishimoto, M., Takeuchi, K., Fukukawa, K., Kawai, S., and Oku, H.: Presystolic pulmonic valve opening in constrictive pericarditis. Jpn. Heart J. 20:419, 1979.

212. Voekel, A. G., Pietro, D. A., Folland, E. D., Fisher, M. L., and Parisi, A. F.: Echocardiographic features of constrictive pericarditis. Circulation 58:871,1978.

213. Gibson, T. C., Grossman, W., McLaurin, L. P., Moos, S., and Craige, E.: An echocardiographic study of the interventricular septum in constrictive pericarditis. Br. Heart J. 38:738, 1976.

214. Candell-Riera, J., Garcia del Castillo, H., Permanyer-Miralda, G., and Soler-Soler, J.: Echocardiographic features of the interventricular septum in chronic constrictive pericarditis. Circulation 57:1154, 1978.

215. Struck, B. L., Fitzgerald, J. W., and Lipton, M.: The posterior aortic wall

echocardiogram: Its relationship to left atrial volume change. Circulation 54:744, 1976.

216. Laurent, F., DeVernejoul, F., Galey, J. J., and Brun, P.: Echocardiography in the evaluation of constrictive pericarditis. Arch. Mal. Coeur 73:85, 1980.

217. Chandraratna, P. A. N., Aronow, W. S., and Imaizumi, T.: Role of echocardiography in detecting the anatomic and physiologic abnormalities of constrictive pericarditis. Am. J. Med. Sci. 283:141, 1982.

218. Lewis, B. S.: Real time two-dimensional echocardiography in constrictive pericarditis. Am. J. Cardiol. 49:1789, 1982.

219. Plauth, W. H., Jr., Waldmann, T. A., Wochner, R. D., Braunwald, N. S., and Braunwald, E.: Protein-losing enteropathy secondary to constrictive pericarditis in childhood. Pediatrics 34:636, 1964.

220. Wilkinson, P., Pinto, B., and Senior, J. R.: Reversible protein-losing enteropathy with intestinal lymphangiectasia, secondary to chronic constrictive pericarditis. N. Engl. J. Med. 273:1178, 1965.

221. Pastor, B. H., and Cahn, M.: Reversible nephrotic syndrome resulting from constrictive pericarditis. N. Engl. J. Med. 262:872, 1960.

222. Daugherty, G. W., Broadbent, J. C., and Brown, A. L., Jr.: Chronic constrictive pericarditis associated with the nephrotic syndrome: Report of case. Proc. Staff Meet. Mayo Clin. 37:283, 1962.

223. Hansen, A. T., Eskildsen, P., and Gotzsche, H.: Pressure curves from the right auricle and the right ventricle in chronic constrictive pericarditis. Circulation 3:881, 1951.

224. Conti, C. R., and Friesinger, G. C.: Chronic constrictive pericarditis, clinical and laboratory findings in 11 cases. Johns Hopkins Med. J. 120:262, 1967.

225. Lewis, B. S., and Gotsman, M. S.: Left ventricular function in systole and diastole in constrictive pericarditis. Am. Heart J. 86:23, 1973.

226. Figley, M. M., and Bagshaw, M. A.: Angiocardiographic aspects of constrictive pericarditis. Radiology 69:46, 1957.

227. Ramsey, H. W., Sbar, S., Elliot, L. P., and Eliot, R. S.: The differential diagnosis of restrictive myocardial myopathy and chronic constrictive pericarditis without calcification: Value of coronary arteriography. Am. J. Cardiol. 25:635, 1970.

228. Alexander, J., Kelley, M. J., Cohen, L. S., and Langou, R. A.: The angiographic appearance of the coronary arteries in constrictive pericarditis. Radiology 131:609, 1979.

229. Goldberg, E., Stein, J., Berger, M., and Berdoff, R. L.: Diastolic segmental coronary artery obliteration in constrictive pericarditis. Cath. Cardiovasc. Diag. 7:197, 1981.

230. Shabetai, R., Fowler, N. O., and Fenton, J. C.: Restrictive cardiac disease. Pericarditis and the myocardiopathies. Am. Heart J. 69:271, 1965.

231. Bhatia, M. D., Grover, D. N., and Roy, S. B.: Haemodynamic effects of exercise in patients with constrictive pericarditis before and after pericardiectomy. Indian Heart J. 29:272, 1977.

232. Swanton, R. H., Brooksby, I. A. B., Davies, M. J., Coltart, D. J., Jenkins, B. S., and Webb-Peploe, M. M.: Systolic and diastolic ventricular function in cardiac amyloidosis. Studies in six cases diagnosed with endomyocardial biopsy. Am. J. Cardiol. 39:658, 1977.

233. Benotti, J. R., Grossman, W., and Cohn, P. F.: Clinical profile of restrictive cardiomyopathy. Circulation 61:1206, 1980.

234. Chew, C., Ziady, G., Raphael, M. J., and Oakley, C. M.: The functional defect in amyloid heart disease. Am. J. Cardiol. 36:438, 1975.

235. Chang, L. W., and Grollman, J. H., Jr.: Angiographic differentiation of constrictive pericarditis and restrictive cardiomyopathy due to amyloidosis. Am. J. Radiol. 130:451, 1978.

236. Tyberg, T. I., Goodyer, A. V. N., Hurst, V. W., Alexander, J., and Langou, R. A.: Left ventricular filling in differentiating restrictive amyloid cardiomyopathy and constrictive pericarditis. Am. J. Cardiol. 47:791, 1981.

237. Broadarick, S., Paine, R. Higa, E., and Carmichael, K. A.: Pericardial tamponade—A new complication of amyloid heart disease. Am. J. Med. 73:133, 1982.

238. Kern, M. J., Lorell, B. H., and Grossman, W.: Cardiac amyloidosis masquerading as constrictive pericarditis. Cath. Cardiovasc. Diag. 8:629, 1982.

239. Gunnar, R. M., Dillon, R. F., Wallyn, R. J., and Elisberg, E. I.: The physiologic and clinical similarity between primary amyloid of the heart and constrictive pericarditis. Circulation 12:827, 1955.

240. Hetzel, P. S., Wood, E. H., and Burchell, H. B.: Pressure pulses in the right side of the heart in a case of amyloid disease and in a case of idiopathic heart failure simulating constrictive pericarditis. Proc. Staff Meet. Mayo Clin. 28:107, 1963.

241. Hoyningen-Huene, C. B. J.: Systemic amyloidosis presenting as constrictive pericarditis. A case studied with cardiac catheterization. Am. Heart J. 67:290, 1964.

242. Wasserman, A. J., Richardson, D. W., Baird, C. L., and Wyso, E. M.: Cardiac hemochromatosis simulating constrictive pericarditis. Am. J. Med. 32:316, 1962.

243. Clark, G. M., Valentine, E., and Blount, S. G.: Endocardial fibrosis simulating constrictive pericarditis. N. Engl. J. Med. 254:349, 1956.

244. Brink, A. J., and Weber, H. W.: Fibroplastic parietal endocarditis with eosinophilia. Loeffler's endocarditis. Am. J. Med. 34:52, 1963.

245. Parrillo, J. E., Borer, J. S., Henry, W. L., Wolff, S. M., and Fauci, A. S.: The cardiovascular manifestations of the hypereosinophilic syndrome. Am. J. Med. 67:572, 1979.

246. Child, J. S., Levisman, J. A., Abbasi, A. S., and MacAlpin, R. N.: Echocardiographic manifestations of infiltrative cardiomyopathy. A report of seven cases due to amyloid. Chest 70:726, 1976.

247. Borer, J. S., Henry, W. L., and Epstein, S. E.: Echocardiographic observations in patients with systemic infiltrative disease involving the heart. Am. J. Cardiol. 39:184, 1977.

248. Child, J. S., Krivokapich, J., and Abbasi, A. S.: Increased right ventricular wall thickness on echocardiography in amyloid infiltrative cardiomyopathy. Am. J. Cardiol. 44:1391, 1979.

249. Carroll, J. D., Gaasch, W. H., and McAdam, K. P. W. J.: Amyloid cardiomyopathy: Characterization by a distinctive voltage/mass ratio. Am. J. Cardiol. 49:9, 1982.

250. Fowler, N. O.: [Chapter 48] In Cardiac Diagnosis and Treatment. 3rd ed. New York, Harper and Row, 1980, pp. 976–1009.

251. Cooley, J. C., Clagett, O. T., and Kirklin, J. W.: Surgical aspects of chronic constrictive pericarditis. A review of 72 operative cases. Ann. Surg. 147:488, 1958.

252. Copeland, J. G., Stinson, E. B., Griepp, R. B., and Shumway, N. E.: Surgical treatment of chronic constrictive pericarditis using cardiopulmonary bypass. J. Thorac. Cardiovasc. Surg. 69:236, 1975.

253. Somerville, W.: Constrictive pericarditis: With special reference to the change in natural history brought about by surgical intervention. Circulation 38 (Suppl. V):102, 1968.

254. Stalpaert, G., Suy, R., Daenen, W., and Nevelsteen, A.: Total pericardiectomy for chronic constrictive pericarditis. Acta Chir. Belg. 80:277, 1981.

255. Wychulis, A. R., Connolly, D. C., and McGoon, D. C.: Surgical treatment of pericarditis. J. Thorac. Cardiovasc. Surg. 62:608, 1971.

256. Collins, H. A., Woods, L. P., and Daniel, R. A., Jr.: Late results of pericardiectomy. Arch. Surg. 89:921, 1964.

257. Fowler, N. O.: Constrictive pericarditis: New aspects. Am. J. Cardiol. 50:1014, 1982.

258. Zucherman, J. F., Rubio, P. A., Guinn, G. A., and Korompai, F. L.: Rational use of operation in pericardial constriction. Int. Surg. 62:204, 1977.

259. Kamaras, J., and Zaborszky, B.: Chronic constrictive pericarditis in children. Cor. Vasa. 23:66, 1981.

260. Kloster, F. E., Crislip, R. L., Bristow, J. D., Herr, R. H., Ritzmann, L. W., and Griswold, H. E.: Hemodynamic studies following pericardiectomy for constrictive pericarditis. Circulation 32:415, 1965.

261. Culliford, A. T., Lipton, M., and Spencer, F. C.: Operation for chronic constrictive pericarditis: Do the surgical approach and degree of pericardial resection influence the outcome significantly? Ann. Thorac. Surg. 29:146, 1980.

262. Viola, A. R.: The influence of pericardiectomy on the hemodynamics of chronic constrictive pericarditis. Circulation 48:1038, 1973.

263. Sawyer, C. G., Burwell, C. S., Dexter, L., Eppinger, E. C., Goodale, W. T., Gorlin, R., Harkin, D. E., and Haynes, F. W.: Chronic constrictive pericarditis. Further consideration of the pathologic physiology of the disease. Am. Heart J. 44:207, 1952.

264. Chambliss, J. R., Jaruszewski, E. J., Brofman, B. L., Martin, J. F., and Feil, H.: Chronic cardiac compression (chronic constrictive pericarditis): A critical study of sixty-one operated cases with followup. Circulation 4:816, 1951.

265. Dalton, J. C., Pearson, R. J., and White, P. D.: Constrictive pericarditis: A review and long-term followup of 78 cases. Ann. Intern. Med. 45:445, 1956.

266. Walsh, T. J., Baughman, K. L., Gardner, T. J., and Bulkley, B. H.: Constrictive epicarditis as a cause of delayed or absent response to pericardiectomy. J. Thorac. Cardiovasc. Surg. 83:126, 1982.

267. Spodick, D. H., and Kumar, S.: Subacute constrictive pericarditis with cardiac tamponade. Dis. Chest 54:62, 1968.

268. Hancock, E. W.: Subacute effusive constrictive pericarditis. Circulation 43:183, 1971.

269. Martin, R. P., Bowden, R., Filly, K., and Popp, R. L.: Intrapericardial abnormalities in patients with pericardial effusion. Circulation 61:568, 1980.

270. Horowitz, M. S., Rossen, R., and Harrison, D. C.: Echocardiographic diagnosis of pericardial disease. Am. Heart J. 97:420, 1979.

271. Rasaretnam, R., and Chanmugam, D.: Subacute effusive-constrictive pericarditis. Br. Heart J. 44:44, 1980.

272. Bush, C. A., Stang, J. M., Wooley, C. G., and Kilman, J.: Occult constrictive pericardial disease. Diagnosis by rapid volume expansion and correction by pericardiectomy. Circulation 56:924, 1977.

273. Kilman, J. W., Bush, C. A., Wooley, C. G., Stang, J. M., Teply, J., and Baba, N.: The changing spectrum of pericardiectomy for chronic pericarditis: Occult constrictive pericarditis. J. Thorac. Cardiovasc. Surg. 74:668, 1977.

SPECIFIC FORMS OF PERICARDITIS

274. Brodie, H. R., and Marchessault, V.: Acute benign pericarditis caused by Coxsackie virus group B. N. Engl. J. Med. 262:1278, 1960.

275. Kleinfeld, M., Milles, S., and Lidsky, M.: Mumps pericarditis: Review of the literature and report of a case. Am. Heart J. 55:153, 1958.

276. Wilson, D. R., Lenkei, S. C., and Patterson, J. F.: Acute constrictive epicarditis following infectious mononucleosis. Circulation 23:257, 1961.

277. Helmly, R. B., Smith, J. O., Jr., and Eisen, B.: Chickenpox with pneumonia and pericarditis. J.A.M.A. 186:870, 1963.

278. Adler, R., Takahashi, M., and Wright, H. T., Jr.: Acute pericarditis associated with hepatitis B infection. Pediatrics 61:716, 1978.

279. Ponka, A.: Carditis associated with Mycoplasma pneumoniae infection. Acta Med. Scand. 206:77, 1979.

280. Cooper, D. K. C., and Sturridge, M. F.: Constrictive pericarditis following Coxsackie virus infection. Thorax 31:472, 1976.

281. Brown, M.D.: Acute benign pericarditis. N. Engl. J. Med. 244:666, 1951.

282. Fowler, N. O., and Manitsas, G. T.: Infectious pericarditis. Progr. Cardiovasc. Dis. 16:323, 1973.

283. Bradley, E. C.: Acute benign pericarditis. Am. Heart J. 67:121, 1964.

284. Connolly, D. C., and Burchell, H. B.: Pericarditis: A ten-year survey. Am. J. Cardiol. 7:7, 1961.

285. Goodman, H. C.: Acute nonspecific pericarditis with cardiac tamponade: A fatal case associated with anticoagulant therapy. Ann. Intern. Med. 48:406, 1958.

286. Blakemore, W. S., Zinsser, H. F., Kirby, C. K., Whitaker, W. B., and Johnson, J.: Pericardiectomy for relapsing pericarditis and chronic constrictive pericarditis. J. Thorac. Cardiovasc. Surg. 39:26, 1960.

287. Larrieu, A. J., Tyers, G. F., Williams, E. H., and Derrick, J. R.: Recent experience with tuberculous pericarditis. Ann. Thorac. Surg. 29:464, 1980.

288. Bellett, S., McMillan, T. M., and Gouley, G. A.: Tuberculous pericarditis: Clinical and pathological study based upon a series of 17 cases. Med. Clin. N. Am. 18:201, 1934.

289. Roy, J. C., Gimei, Y., Condat, J. M., Lokrou, A., Ferrus, P., Soubeyrand, J., and Beda, B. Y.: Pericarditis in adults in Abidjan. Semin. Hop. Paris 57:978, 1981.

290. Desai, H. N.: Tuberculous pericarditis: A review of 100 cases. S. Afr. Med. J. 55:877, 1979.

291. Williams, I. M., and Hetzel, M. R.: Tuberculous pericarditis in South-West London: An increasing problem. Thorax 33:816, 1978.

292. Gooi, H. C., and Smith, J. M.: Tuberculous pericarditis in Birmingham. Thorax 33:94, 1978.

293. Bialock, A., and Levy, S. E.: Tuberculous pericarditis. J. Thorac. Surg. 7:132, 1937.

294. Peel, A. A. F.: Tuberculous pericarditis. Br. Heart J. 10:195, 1948.

295. Auerbach, O.: Pleural, peritoneal, and pericardial tuberculosis. Am. Rev. Tuberc. 61:845, 1950.

296. Maisch, B., Maisch, S., and Kocksiek, K.: Immune reactions in tuberculous and chronic constrictive pericarditis. Am. J. Cardiol. 50:1007, 1982.

297. Schrire, V.: Experience with pericarditis of Groote Schuur Hospital, Cape Town: An analysis of one hundred and sixty cases over a six-year period. S. Afr. Med. J. 33:810, 1959.

298. Hageman, J. H., D'Esopo, N. D., and Glenn, W. W. L.: Tuberculosis of the pericardium: A long-term analysis of forty-four cases. N. Engl. J. Med. 270:327, 1964.

299. Lesar, M. S., Orcutt, J., Wehunt, W. D., and Babcock, T. E.: Pericardial tuberculoma. An unusual cause of mediastinal mass. Radiology 138:309, 1981.

300. Hirasing, R. A., and Van Bel, F.: Tuberculous pericarditis developing during chemotherapy. Eur. J. Resp. Dis. 63:73, 1982.

301. Barr, J. F.: The use of pericardial biopsy in establishing etiologic diagnosis in acute pericarditis. Arch. Intern. Med. 96:693, 1955.

302. Cheitlin, M. D., Serfos, L. J., Sbar, S. S., and Glosser, S. P.: Tuberculous pericarditis: Is limited pericardial biopsy sufficient for diagnosis: Am. Rev. Resp. Dis. 98:287, 1968.

303. Deterling, R. A., Jr., and Humphreys, G. H.: Factors in the etiology of constrictive pericarditis. Circulation 12:30, 1955.

304. Rooney, J. J., Crocco, J. A., and Lyons, H. A.: Tuberculous pericarditis. Ann. Intern. Med. 72:73, 1970.

305. Ortbals, P. W., and Avioli, L. V.: Tuberculous pericarditis. Arch. Intern. Med. 139:231, 1979.

306. Boyle, J. D., Pearce, M. L., and Guz, L. B.: Purulent pericarditis. Review of literature and report of eleven cases. Medicine 40:119, 1961.

307. Klacsmann, P. B., Bulkley, B. H., and Hutchins, G. M.: The changed spectrum of purulent pericarditis. An 86 year autopsy experience in 200 patients. Am. J. Med. 63:666, 1977.

308. Berk, S. L., Rice, P. A., Reynolds, C. A., and Finland, M.: Pneumococcal pericarditis: A persisting problem in contemporary diagnosis. Am. J. Med. 70:247, 1981.

309. Kauffman, C. A., Watanakunakorn, C., and Phair, J. P.: Purulent pneumococcal pericarditis: A continuing problem in the antibiotic era. Am. J. Med. 54:743, 1973.

310. Lukash, W. M.: Massive pericardial effusion due to meningococcic pericarditis. J.A.M.A. 185:598, 1963.

311. Penny, J. L., Grace, W. J., and Kennedy, R. L.: Meningococci pericarditis. Am. J. Cardiol. 18:281, 1966.

312. Herman, R. A., and Rubin, H. A.: Meningococcal pericarditis without meningitis presenting as tamponade. N. Engl. J. Med. 290:143, 1974.

313. Rao, V. S., Rajashekaraian, K. L., Rice, T., Riaz, M., Towne, W., and Kallick, C. A.: Primary meningococcal pericarditis. South. Med. J. 73:1276, 1980.

314. Levin, H. S., and Hosier, D. M.: Salmonella pericarditis. Report of a case and review of the literature. Ann. Intern. Med. 55:817, 1961.

315. Theler, B. D., Noseda, G., Reiner, M., and Keller, H.: Pericarditis and myocarditis in salmonellosis. Schweiz. Med. Wschr. 110:1394, 1980.

316. Vietzke, W. M.: Gonococcal arthritis with pericarditis. Arch. Intern. Med. 117:270, 1966.

317. Benzing, G., III, and Kaplan, S.: Purulent pericarditis. Am. J. Dis. Child. 106:289, 1963.

318. Meredith, H. C., Jr.: Tularemic pericarditis: A report of two cases, including one of constrictive pericarditis. Ann. Intern. Med. 32:688, 1950.

319. Rubin, R. H., and Moellering, R. C., Jr.: Clinical, microbiologic, and therapeutic aspects of purulent pericarditis. Am. J. Med. 59:68, 1975.

320. Callahan, D. L., Morriss, M. J., Kaplan, S. L., and Park, I.: Constrictive pericarditis due to *Streptococcus sanguis*. South. Med. J. *74*:377, 1981.

321. Hanson, G., and Engel, P. J.: Purulent pericarditis caused by beta-hemolytic group C streptococcus. Arch. Intern. Med. *414*:1351, 1981.

322. Lieber, I. H., Rensimer, E. R., and Ericsson, C. D.: Campylobacter pericarditis in hypothyroidism. Am. Heart J. *102*:462, 1981.

323. Rahman, M.: Bacteremia and pericarditis from Campylobacter infection. Br. J. Clin. Pract. *33*:131, 1979.

324. Solomon, C., Roberts, J. E., and Lisa, J. R.: The heart in uremia. Am. J. Pathol. *18*:729, 1942.

325. Nadas, A. S., and Levy, J. M.: Pericarditis in children. Am. J. Cardiol. *7*:109, 1961.

326. Feldman, W. E.: Bacterial etiology and mortality of purulent pericarditis in pediatric patients. Am. J. Dis. Child. *133*:164, 1979.

327. Leggiadro, R. J., and Balsam, D.: *Haemophilus influenzae* sepsis leading to pericarditis despite antimicrobial therapy. Johns Hopkins Med. J. *146*:133, 1980.

328. Wyler, F., Knusli, D., Rutishauser, M., Stocker, F., Weber, J., and Real, F.: Pericarditis purulenta in children. Helv. Paediat. Acta *32*:135, 1977.

329. Jaiyesimi, F., Abioye, A. A., and Antia, A. U.: Infective pericarditis in Nigerian children. Arch. Dis. Child. *54*:384, 1979.

330. Chun, P. K., and Rocchini, A. P.: Occult constrictive pericarditis in infancy. Chest *78*:648, 1980.

331. Vogt, J., Rupprath, G., Divivie, E. R., Dahn, D., and Kunze, E.: Constrictive pericarditis in early infancy. Klin. Paediat. *192*:384, 1980.

332. Cheatham, J. E., Jr., Grantham, R. N., Peyton, M. D., Thompson, W. M., Luckstead, E. F., Razook, J. D., and Elkins, R. C.: *Hemophilus influenzae* purulent pericarditis in children: Diagnostic and therapeutic considerations. J. Thorac. Cardiovasc. Surg. *79*:933, 1980.

333. Stoobant, J., Leanage, R., Deanfield, J., and Taylor, J. F.: Acute infective pericarditis in infancy. Arch. Dis. Child. *57*:73, 1982.

334. Zimmerman, L. E.: Candida and Aspergillus endocarditis. Arch. Parthol. *50*:591, 1950.

335. Gould, K., Barnett, J. A., and Sanford, J. P.: Purulent pericarditis in the antibiotic era. Arch. Intern. Med. *134*:923, 1974.

336. Morse, J. R., Oretsky, M. I., and Hudson, J. A. M.: Pericarditis as a complication of meningococcal meningitis. Ann. Intern. Med. *74*:212, 1971.

337. Pierce, H. I., and Cooper, E. B.: Meningococcal pericarditis: Clinical features and therapy in five patients. Arch. Intern. Med. *129*:918, 1972.

338. Miller, G. C., and Witham, A. C.: Delayed febrile pleuropericarditis after sepsis. Ann. Intern. Med. *79*:194, 1973.

339. Schoenwetter, A. H., and Silber, E. N.: Penicillin hypersensitivity, acute pericarditis and eosinophilia. J.A.M.A. *191*:136, 1965.

340. Tan, J. S., Holmes, J. C., Fowler, N. O., Manitsas, G. T., and Phair, J. P.: Antibiotic levels in pericardial fluid. J. Clin. Invest. *53*:7, 1974.

341. Das, P. B.: Staphylococcal pericarditis and its treatment by early pericardiectomy. Indian Heart J. *29*:90, 1977.

342. Saslaw, S., NorFleet, R. G., and Dapra, D. J.: Acute Histoplasma pericarditis. Arch. Intern. Med. *122*:162, 1968.

343. Picardi, J. L., Kauffman, C. A., Schwarz, J., Holmes, J. C., Phair, J. P., and Fowler, N. O.: Pericarditis caused by *Histoplasma capsulatum*. Am. J. Cardiol. *37*:82, 1976.

344. Young, E. J., Vainrub, B., and Musher, D. M.: Pericarditis due to histoplasmosis. J.A.M.A. *240*:1750, 1978.

345. Kirchner, S. G., Heller, R. M., Sell, S. J., and Altemeier, W. A. III: The radiological features of histoplasma pericarditis. Pediat. Radiol. *7*:7, 1978.

346. Larsen, R., and Scherb, R. E.: Coccidioidal pericarditis. Circulation *7*:211, 1953.

347. Chapman, M. G., and Kaplan, L.: Cardiac involvement in coccidioidomycosis. Am. J. Med. *23*:87, 1957.

348. Gronemeyer, P. S., Weisfeld, A. S., and Sonnenwirth, A. C.: Purulent pericarditis complicating systemic infection with *Candida tropicalis*. Am. J. Clin. Pathol. *77*:471, 1982.

349. Walsh, T. J., and Bulkley, B. J.: Aspergillus pericarditis: Clinical and pathologic features in the immunocompromised patient. Cancer *49*:48, 1982.

350. Walsh, T. J., and Hutchins, G. M.: Postoperative Candida infections in children: Clinicopathologic study of continuing problem of diagnosis and therapy. J. Pediat. Surg. *15*:325, 1980.

351. Dix, J. H., and Gurkaynak, N.: Histoplasmosis with massive pericardial effusion and systemic involvement. J.A.M.A. *182*:687, 1962.

352. Kleger, H. L., and Fisher, E. R.: Fibrocalcific constrictive pericarditis due to *Histoplasma capsulatum*. N. Engl. J. Med. *267*:593, 1962.

353. Prager, R. L., Burney, D. P., Waterhouse, G., and Bender, H. W., Jr.: Pulmonary, mediastinal, and cardiac presentations of histoplasmosis. Ann. Thorac. Surg. *30*:385, 1980.

354. Wooley, C. F., and Hosier, D. M.: Constrictive pericarditis due to *Histoplasma capsulatum*. N. Engl. J. Med. *264*:1230, 1961.

355. Eng, R. J., Sen, P., Browne, K., and Louria, D. B.: Candida pericarditis. Am. J. Med. *70*:867, 1981.

356. Schlossberg, D., Franco-Jove, D., Woodward, C., and Shulman, C.: Pericarditis with effusion caused by *Actinomyces israelii*. Chest *69*:680, 1976.

357. Mohan, K., Dass, S. I., and Kemble, E. E.: Actinomycosis of the pericardium. J.A.M.A. *229*:321, 1974.

358. Causey, W. A., Arnell, P., and Brinker, J.: Systemic Nocardia infection. Chest *65*:360, 1974.

359. Susens, G. P., Al-Shamma, A., Rowe, J. C., Herbert, C. C., Bassis, M. L., and Coggs, G. C.: Purulent constrictive pericarditis caused by *Nocardia asteroides*. Ann. Intern. Med. *67*:1021, 1967.

360. Tyagi, S. K., Anand, I. S., Deodhar, S. D., and Datta, D. V.: A clinical study of amoebic pericarditis. J. Assoc. Physic. India *28*:515, 1980.

361. Bansal, B. C., and Gupta, D. S.: Amoebic pericarditis. Postgrad. Med. J. *47*:678, 1971.

362. Kala, P. C., and Sharma, G. C.: Amoebic pericarditis treated by pericardiectomy. J. Indian Med. Assoc. *74*:194, 1980.

363. Sagrista-Sauleda, J., Permanyer-Miralda, G., Juste-Sanchez, C., De Buen-Sanchez, M. L., Pujadas-Capmany, R., Arcalis-Arce, L., and Soler-Soler, J.: Huge chronic pericardial effusion caused by *Toxoplasma gondii*. Circulation *66*:895, 1982.

364. Feldman, H. A.: Medical progress: Toxoplasmosis. N. Engl. J. Med. *279*:1370, 1968.

365. Chens, W.: Hydatid cysts in the pericardium—A new case and review of the literature. J. Thorac. Cardiovasc. Surg. *30*:56, 1982.

366. Halliday, J. H., Jose, A. D., and Nicks, R.: Constrictive pericarditis following rupture of a ventricular hydatid cyst. Br. Heart J. *25*:821, 1963.

367. DiBello, R.: Cardiac echinococcosis. Late sudden death after surgical treatment. Chest *79*:110, 1981.

368. Kinare, S. G., Parulkar, G. B., and Sen, P. K.: Constrictive pericarditis resulting from dracunculosis. Br. Med. J. *1*:845, 1962.

369. Charon, A., and Sinha, K.: Constrictive pericarditis following filiariasis. Indian Heart J. *25*:213, 1973.

370. Thadani, U., Chopra, M. P., Aber, C. P., and Portal, R. W.: Pericarditis after acute myocardial infarction. Br. Med. J. *2*:135, 1971.

371. Lichstein, E. M., Lieu, H. M., and Gupta, P.: Pericarditis complicating acute myocardial infarction: Incidence of complications and significance of electrocardiogram on admission. Am. Heart J. *87*:246, 1974.

372. Stewart, C. F., and Turner, K. B.: A note on pericardial involvement in coronary thrombosis. Am. Heart J. *15*:232, 1938.

373. Khan, A. J.: Pericarditis of myocardial infarction: Review of the literature with case presentation. Am. Heart J. *90*:788, 1975.

374. Anderson, M. W., Christensen, N. A., and Edwards, J. E.: Hemopericardium complicating myocardial infarction in the absence of cardiac rupture. Arch. Intern. Med. *90*:634, 1952.

375. Aarseth, S., and Lange, H. F.: The influence of anticoagulant therapy on the occurrence of cardiac rupture and hemopericardium following heart infarction. I. A study of 89 cases of hemopericardium. Am. Heart J. *56*:250, 1958.

376. Lange, H. F., and Aarseth, S.: The influence of anticoagulant therapy on the occurrence of cardiac rupture and hemopericardium following heart infarction. II. A controlled study of a selected treated group based on 1,044 autopsies. Am. Heart J. *56*:257, 1958.

377. Miller, R. L.: Hemopericardium with use of oral anticoagulant therapy. J.A.M.A. *209*:1362, 1969.

378. Goldstein, R., and Wolff, L.: Hemorrhagic pericarditis in acute myocardial infarction treated with bishydroxycoumarin. J.A.M.A. *146*:616, 1951.

379. Liberthson, R. R., Salisbury, K. W., and Hutter, A. M., Jr.: Atrial tachyarrhythmias in acute myocardial infarction. Am. J. Med. *60*:956, 1976.

380. Liem, K. L., Durrer, D., and Lie, K. L.: Pericarditis in acute myocardial infarction. Lancet *2*:1004, 1975.

381. Sawaya, J. I., Mujais, S. K., and Armenian, H. K.: Early diagnosis of pericarditis in acute myocardial infarction. Am. Heart J. *100*:144, 1980.

382. Dvorak, K., and Cerny, J.: Long-term survival of subacute cardiac rupture with tamponade in acute myocardial infarction, without surgical intervention (the role of pericardiocentesis). Cor. Vasa. *21*:233, 1979.

383. Jensen, D. P., Goolsby, J. P., Jr., and Oliva, P. B.: Hemodynamic pattern resembling paricardial constriction after acute inferior myocardial infarction with right ventricular infarction. Am. J. Cardiol. *42*:858, 1978.

384. Butman, S., Olson, H. G., Aronow, W. S., and Lyons, K. P.: Remote right ventricular myocardial infarction mimicking chronic pericardial constriction. Am. Heart J. *103*:912, 1982.

385. Berman, J., Haffajee, C. I., and Alpert, J. S.: Therapy of symptomatic pericarditis after myocardial infarction: Retrospective and prospective studies of aspirin, indomethacin, prednisone, and spontaneous resolution. Am. Heart J. *101*:750, 1981.

386. Jugdutt, B. I., Hutchins, G. M., Bulkley, B., Pitt, B., and Becker, L. C.: Effect of indomethacin on collateral blood flow and infarct size in the conscious dog. Circulation *59*:734, 1979.

387. Friedman, P. L., Brugada, P., Kuck, K. H., Bär, F. W. H. M., and Wellens, H. J. J.: Coronary vasoconstrictor effect of indomethacin in patients with coronary artery disease. N. Engl. J. Med. *305*:1171, 1981.

388. Hammerman, H., Kloner, R. A., Schoen, F. J., Brown, E. J., Hale, S., and Braunwald, E.: Indomethacin induced scar thinning following experimental myocardial infarction. Circulation *67*:1290, 1983.

389. Brown, E. J., Kloner, R. A., Schoen, F. J., Hammerman, H., Hale, S., and Braunwald, E.: Scar thinning due to ibuprofen administration following experimental myocardial infarction. Am. J. Cardiol. *51*:877, 1983.

390. Hammerman, H., Kloner, R. A., Schoen, F. J., Brown, E. J., Hale, S., and Braunwald, E.: Scar thinning due to indomethacin administration following experimental myocardial infarction. Clin. Res. *30*:547A, 1982.

391. Bright, R.: Tabular view of the morbid appearance in 100 cases connected with albuminous urine: With observations. Guy's Hosp. Rep. *1*:380, 1836.

392. Wacker, W., and Merrill, J. P.: Uremic pericarditis in acute and chronic renal failure. J.A.M.A. *156*:764, 1954.

393. Skov, P. E., Hansen, H. E., and Spencer, E. S.: Uremic pericarditis Acta Med. Scand. *186*:421, 1969.

394. Osanloo, E., Shalhoub, R. J., Cioffi, R. F., and Parker, R. H.: Viral pericarditis in patients receiving hemodialysis. Arch. Intern. Med. *139*:310, 1979.

395. Bailey, G. L., Hampers, C. L., and Merrill, J. P.: Reversible cardiomyopathy in uremia. Trans. Am. Soc. Artif. Intern. Organs *13*:263, 1967.

396. Shabetai, R.: Uremia, dialysis, and metabolic causes of pericardial disease. *In*: The Pericardium. New York, Grune and Stratton, 1981, pp. 385–389.

397. Lindsay, J., Jr., Crawley, I. S., and Callaway, G. M.: Chronic constrictive pericarditis following uremic hemopericardium. Am. Heart J. *79*:390, 1970.

398. Comty, C. M., Cohen, S. L., and Shapiro, F. L.: Pericarditis in chronic uremia and its sequels. Ann. Intern. Med. *75*:173, 1971.

399. Luft, L. C., Gilman, J. K., and Weyman, A. E.: Pericarditis in the patient with uremia: Clinical and echocardiographic evaluation. Nephron *25*:160, 1980.

400. D'Cruz, I. A., Bhatt, G. R., Cohen, H. C., and Glick, G.: Echocardiographic detection of cardiac involvement in patients with chronic renal failure. Arch. Intern. Med. *138*:720, 1978.

401. Goldstein, D. J., Nagar, C., Srivastava, N., Schacht, R. A., Ferris, F. Z., and Flowers, N. C.: Clinically silent pericardial effusions in patients on long-term hemodialysis. Chest *72*:744, 1977.

402. Morin, J. E., Hollomby, D., Gonda, A., Long, R., and Dobell, A. R. C.: Management of uremic pericarditis: A report of 11 patients with cardiac tamponade and a review of the literature. Ann. Thorac. Surg. *22*:588, 1976.

403. Alfrey, A. C., Goss, J. E., and Ogden, D. A.: Uremic hemopericardium. Am. J. Med. *45*:391, 1968.

404. Masson, J. F., Maes, M. L., and Zilberman, C.: Pericarditis in chronic renal insufficiency treated by periodic hemodialysis. Rev. Med. Intern. *2*:447, 1981.

405. Kwasnik, E. M., Koster, J. K., Lazarus, J. M., Sloss, L. J., Mee, R. B. B., Cohn, L. H., and Collins, J. J.: Conservative management of uremic pericardial effusions. J. Thorac. Cardiovasc. Surg. *76*:629, 1978.

406. Silverberg, S., Oreopoulos, D. G., Wise, D. J., Uden, D. E., Meindok, H., Jones, M., Rapaport, A., and deVeber, G. A.: Pericarditis in patients undergoing long-term hemodialysis and peritoneal dialysis. Am. J. Med. *63*:874,1977.

407. Minuth, A. M. W., Nottebohm, G. A., Eknoyan, G., and Suki, W. N.: Indomethacin treatment of pericarditis in chronic hemodialysis patients. Arch. Intern. Med. *135*:807, 1975.

408. Buselmeir, T. J., Simmons, R. L., Najarian, J. S., Mauer, S. M., Matas, A. J., and Kjellstrand, C. M.: Uremic pericardial effusion. Nephron *16*:371, 1976.

409. Fuller, T. J., Knochel, J. P., Brennan, J. P., Fetner, C. D., and White, M. G.: Reversal of intractable uremic pericarditis by triamcinolone hexacetonide. Arch. Intern. Med. *136*:979, 1976.

410. Feinroth, M. V., Goldstein, E. J., Josephson, A., and Friedman, E. A.: Infection complicating intrapericardial steroid instillation in uremic pericarditis. Clin. Nephrol. *15*:331, 1981.

411. Beaudry, C., Nakamoto, S., and Koloff, W. J.: Uremic pericarditis and cardiac tamponade in chronic renal failure. Ann. Intern. Med. *64*:990, 1966.

412. Singh, S., Newmark, K., Ishikasa, I., Mitra, S., and Berman, L. B.: Pericardiectomy in uremia. The treatment of choice for cardiac tamponade in chronic renal failure. J.A.M.A. *228*:1132, 1974.

413. Engelman, R. M., Levitsky, S., Konchigeri, H. N., Wyndham, C. R. C., Roper, K., and Kurtzman, N. A.: Total pericardiectomy for uremic pericarditis. World J. Surg. *1*:769, 1977.

414. Nickey, W. A., Chinitz, J. L., Flynn, J. J., Adam, A., Kim, K. E., Schwartz, A. B., Onesti, G., and Swartz, C. D.: Surgical correction of uremic constrictive pericarditis. Ann. Intern. Med. *75*:227, 1971.

415. Koopot, R., Zerefos, N. S., and Lavender, A. R.: Cardiac tamponade in uremic pericarditis: Surgical approach and management. Am. J. Cardiol. *32*:846, 1973.

416. Van Baestelaere, W., Verbanck, J., Verschuere, I., Ringoir, S., and Derom, F.: Surgical therapy of uremic pericarditis. Acta Chir. Belg. *80*:293, 1981.

417. Nevelsteen, A., Daenen, W., Suy, R., and Stalpaert, G.: Treatment by limited pericardiectomy. Acta Chir. Belg. *80*:299, 1981.

418. DeLoach, J. F., and Haynes, J. W.: Secondary tumors of the heart and pericardium. Arch. Intern. Med. *91*:224, 1953.

419. Roberts, W. C., Bodey, G. P., and Wertlake, P. T.: The heart in acute leukemia: A study of 420 autopsy cases. Am. J. Cardiol. *21*:388, 1968.

420. Hanfling, S. M.: Metastatic cancer to the heart. Circulation *22*:474, 1960.

421. Young, J. M., and Goldman, I. R.: Tumor metastases to the heart. Circulation *9*:220, 1954.

422. Roberts, W. C., Glancy, D. L., and DeVita, V. T.: Heart in malignant lymphoma (Hodgkin's disease, lymphosarcoma, reticulum cell sarcoma and mycosis fungoides): A study of 196 autopsy cases. Am. J. Cardiol. *22*:85, 1968.

423. Goudie, R. B.: Secondary tumors of the heart and pericardium. Br. Heart J. *17*:183, 1955.

424. Gassman, H. S., Meadows, R., and Baker, L. A.: Metastatic tumors of the heart. Am. J. Med. *19*:357, 1955.

425. Thurber, D. L., Edwards, J. E., and Achor, R. W.: Secondary malignant tumors of the pericardium. Circulation *26*:228, 1962.

426. Cohen, G. U., Perry, T. M., and Evens, J. M.: Neoplastic invasion of the heart and pericardium. Ann. Intern. Med. *42*:1238, 1955.

427. Onuigbo, W. I. B.: The spread of lung cancer to the heart, pericardium, and great vessels. Jpn. Heart J. *15*:235, 1974.

428. Aymard, J. P., Voiriot, P., Witz, F., Colomb, J. N., Lederlin, P., Thibaut, G., Guerci, O., and Herbeuval, R.: Pericarditis as the presenting manifestation of acute monoblastic leukemia. Ann. Med. Intern. *131*:302, 1980.

429. Peterson, C. D., Robinson, W. A., and Kurnick, J. E.: Involvement of the heart and pericardium in the malignant lymphomas. Am. J. Med. Sci. *272*:161, 1976.

430. Jakob, H. G., and Zirkin, R. M.: Hodgkin's disease with involvement of the heart and pericardium. J.A.M.A. *73*:82, 1960.

431. Hagans, J. A.: Hodgkin's granuloma with pericardial effusion. Am. Heart J. *40*:624, 1950.

432. Glancy, D. L., and Roberts, W. C.: The heart in malignant melanoma: A study of 70 autopsy cases. Am. J. Cardiol. *21*:555, 1968.

433. Thomas, D., Dragodanne, C., Frank, R., Prier, A., Chomette, G., and Grosgogeat, Y.: Systemic mastocytosis with myopericardial localization and atrioventricular block. Arch. Mal. Coeur *74*:215, 1981.

434. Arciniegas, E., Hakimi, M., Farooki, Z. Q., and Green, E. W.: Intrapericardial teratoma in infancy. J. Thorac. Cardiovasc. Surg. *79*:306, 1980.

435. Becker, S. N., Reza, M. J., Greenberg, S. H., and Stein, J. J.: Pericardial effusion secondary to mucoepidermoid carcinoma of the parotid gland. A report of an unusual case. Cancer *36*:1080, 1975.

436. Talib, S. H., Chawhan, R. N., Yadov, S. B., Hogade, P. R., and Talib, V. H.: Primary malignant mesothelioma of the pericardium. Indian Heart J. *30*:174, 1978.

437. Harveit, F., Brubakk, O., and Roksted, K.: Pericardial angiomatosis. Acta Med. Scand. *199*:519, 1976.

438. Poole-Wilson, P. A., Farnsworth, A., Braimbridge, M. V., and Pambakian, H.: Angiosarcoma of pericardium. Problems in diagnosis and management. Br. Heart J. *38*:240, 1976.

439. Das, P. B., Fletcher, A. G., and Deodhare, S. G.: Primary mesothelioma of the pericardium. Indian J. Chest Dis. Allied Sci. *18*:262, 1976.

440. Churg, A., Warnock, M. L., and Bensch, K. G.: Malignant mesothelioma arising after direct application of asbestos and fiber glass to the pericardium. Am. Rev. Resp. Dis. *118*:419, 1978.

441. Nakayama, R., Yoneyama, T., and Takatani, O.: A study of metastatic tumors to the heart, pericardium, and great vessels. Incidences of metastases to the heart, pericardium and great vessels. Jpn. Heart J. *7*:227, 1966.

442. Kline, J. K.: Cardiac lymphatic involvement by metastatic tumor. Cancer *29*:799, 1972.

443. Liepman, M. K., and Goodlerner, S.: Surgical management of pericardial tamponade as a presenting manifestation of acute leukemia. J. Surg. Oncol. *17*:183, 1981.

444. Almagro, V. A., Caya, J. G., and Remeniuk, E.: Cardiac tamponade due to malignant pericardial effusion in breast cancer: A case report. Cancer *49*:1929, 1982.

445. Fraser, R. S., Viloria, J. B., and Wang, N. S.: Cardiac tamponade as a presentation of extracardiac malignancy. Cancer *45*:1697, 1980.

446. Donnelly, M. S., Weinberg, D. S., Skarin, A. T., and Levine, H. D.: Sick sinus syndrome with seroconstrictive pericarditis in malignant lymphoma involving the heart: A case report. Med. Pediat. Oncol. *9*:273, 1981.

447. Elguezabal, A., Farry, J. P., and Depace, N. L.: Massive metastatic cardiac tumor encasement with pericardial constriction. J. Med. Soc. N.J. *77*:820, 1980.

448. Posner, M. R., Cohen, G. I., and Skarin, A. T.: Pericardial disease in patients with cancer. Am. J. Med. *71*:407, 1981.

449. Usher, B. W., and Popp, R. L.: Electrical alternans: Mechanism in pericardial effusion. Am. Heart J. *83*:459, 1972.

450. Chandraratna, P. A. N., and Aronow, W. S.: Detection of pericardial metastases by cross-sectional echocardiography. Circulation *63*:197, 1981.

451. Simpson, A.J.: Malignant pericardial effusion diagnosed by combined ^{67}Ga-citrate and ^{99m}Tc-pertechnetate scintigraphy. Clin. Nucl. Med. *3*:445, 1978.

452. Quaife, M. A., Boschult, P., Baltaxe, H. A., Jr., and Dzindzio, B.: Myocardial accumulation of labelled phosphate in malignant pericardial effusion. J. Nucl. Med. *20*:392, 1979.

453. Comyn, D. J.: Cardiac tamponade with superior vena caval obstruction. S. Afr. Med. J. *54*:750, 1978.

454. Zipf, R. E., Jr., and Johnston, W. W.: The role of cytology in the evaluation of pericardial effusion. Chest *62*:593, 1972.

455. King, D. T., and Nieberg, R. K.: The use of cytology to evaluate pericardial effusions. Ann. Clin. Lab. Sci. *9*:18, 1979.

456. Yazdi, H. M., Hajdu, S. I., and Melamed, M. R.: Cytopathology of pericardial effusions. Acta Cytol. J. *24*:401, 1980.

457. Smith, F. E., Lane, M., and Hudgins, D. T.: Conservative management of malignant pericardial effusion. Cancer *33*:47, 1974.

458. Hirsch, D. M., Nydick, I., and Farrow, I. W.: Malignant pericardial effusion secondary to metastatic breast carcinoma: A case of long-term remission. Cancer *19*:1269, 1966.

459. Theologides, A.: Neoplastic cardiac tamponade. Semin. Oncol. *5*:181, 1978.

460. Flannery, E. P., Gregoratos, G., and Corder, M. P.: Pericardial effusion in patients with malignant diseases. Arch. Intern. Med. *135*:976, 1975.

461. Hankins, J. R., Satterfield, J. R., Aisner, J., Wiernik, P. H., and McLaughlin, J. S.: Pericardial window for malignant pericardial effusion. Ann. Thorac. Surg. *30*:465, 1980.

462. Hill, G. J., and Cohen, B. I.: Pleural pericardial window for palliation of cardiac tamponade due to cancer. Cancer *26*:81, 1970.

463. Davis, S., Sharma, S. M., Blumberg, E. D., and Kim, C. S.: Intrapericardial tetracycline for the management of cardiac tamponade secondary to malignant pericardial effusion. N. Engl. J. Med. *299*:1113, 1978.

464. Weisberger, A. S., Levine, B., and Storaasli, L. P.: Use of nitrogen mustard in treatment of serous effusions of neoplastic origin. J.A.M.A. *159*:1704, 1955.

465. Suhrland, L. G., and Weisberger, A. S.: Intracavitary 5-fluorouracil in malignant effusions. Arch. Intern. Med. *116*:431, 1965.

466. Weisberger, A. S.: Direct instillation of nitrogen mustard in the management of malignant effusions. N. Y. Acad. Sci. *68*:1091, 1958.

467. Terpenning, M., Orringer, M., Wheeler, R.: Intrapericardial nitrogen mustard with catheter drainage for the treatment of malignant effusions. Proc. Am. Assoc. Cancer Res. *20*:286, 1979.

468. Mauch, P. E.: Treatment of malignant pericardial effusions. *In* DeVita, V. T., Hellman, S., and Rosenberg, S. A. (eds.): Cancer. Principles and Practice of Oncology. Philadelphia, J. B. Lippincott Co., pp. 1571–1573.

469. Martini, N., Freiman, A. J., Watson, R. C., and Hilaris, B. S.: Intrapericardial instillation of radioactive chromic phosphate in malignant pericardial effusion. Am. J. Roentgenol. *128*:639, 1977.

470. O'Bryan, R. M., Talley, R. W., and Brennan, M. J.: Critical analysis of the control of malignant effusions with radioisotopes. Henry Ford Hosp. Med. J. *16*:3, 1968.

471. Clarke, T. H.: Radioactive colloidal gold Au^{198} in the treatment of neoplastic effusion. Northwest Med. Sch. Quart. Bull. *26*:98, 1952.

472. Bian, S., Brufman, G., Klein, E., and Hochman, A.: The management of pericardial effusion in cancer patients. Chest *71*:182, 1977.

473. Terry, L. N., and Kligerman, M. M.: Pericardial and myocardial involvement in lymphomas and leukemias—the role of radiotherapy. Cancer *25*:1003, 1970.

474. Cham, W. C., Freiman, A. H., and Carstens, P. H. B.: Radiation therapy of cardiac and pericardial metastases. Ther. Radiol. *114*:701, 1975.

475. Lokich, J. J.: The management of malignant pericardial effusion J.A.M.A. *224*:1401, 1973.

476. Steward, J. R., Cohn, K. E., and Fajardo, L. F.: Radiation-induced heart diesease: A study of twenty-five patients. Radiology *89*:302, 1967.

477. Martin, R. G., Ruckdeschel, J. C., Chang, P., Byhardt, R., Bouchard, R. J., and Wiernik, P. H.: Radiation-related pericarditis. Am. J. Cardiol. *35*:216, 1975.

478. Cohn, K. E., Stewart, J. R., Fajardo, L. F., and Hancock, E. W.: Heart disease following radiation. Medicine *46*:281, 1967.

479. Muggia, F. M., and Cassileth, P. A.: Constrictive pericarditis following radiation therapy. Am. J. Med. *44*:116, 1968.

480. Masland, D. S., Rotz, C. T., Jr., and Harris, J. H.: Post-radiation pericarditis with chronic pericardial effusion. Ann. Intern. Med. *68*:97, 1968.

481. Ruckdeschel, J. C., Chang, P., Martin, R. G., Byhardt, R. W., O'Connell, M. J., Sutherland, J. C., and Wiernik, P. J.: Radiation-related pericardial effusions in patients with Hodgkin's disease. Medicine *54*:245, 1975.

482. DiMatteo, J., Vacheron, A., Heulin, A., Meeus, L., DiMatteo, G., Gilles, R., DeLage, F., and de Ratuld, A.: Cardiac complications of thoracic radiotherapy. Arch. Mal. Coeur. *71*:447, 1978.

483. Scott, D. L., and Thomas, R. D.: Late onset constrictive pericarditis after thoracic radiotherapy. Br. Med. J. *1*:341, 1978.

484. Applefeld, M. M., Slawson, R. G., Hall-Craigs, M., Green, D. C., Singleton, R. T., and Wiernik, P. H.: Delayed pericardial disease after radiotherapy. Am. J. Cardiol. *47*:210, 1981.

485. Haas, J.: Symptomatic constrictive pericarditis developing 45 years after radiation therapy to the mediastinum. Am. Heart J. *77*:89, 1969.

486. Carmel, R. J., and Kaplan, H. S.: Mantle irradiation in Hodgkin's disease. Cancer *37*:2813, 1976.

487. Fajardo, L. F., Stewart, J. R., and Cohn, K. E.: Morphology of radiation-induced heart disease. Arch. Pathol. *86*:512, 1968.

488. Glicksman, A. S., and Nickson, J. J.: Acute and late reactions to irradiation in the treatment of Hodgkin's disease. Arch. Intern. Med. *131*:369, 1973.

489. Greenwood, R. D., Rosenthal, A., Cassedy, R., Jaffe, N., and Nadas, A. S.: Constrictive pericarditis in childhood due to mediastinal irradiation. Circulation *50*:1033, 1974.

490. Brosius, F. C., Waller, B. F., and Roberts, W. C.: Radiation heart disease. Am. J. Med. *70*:519, 1981.

491. Steinberg, I.: Effusive-constrictive pericarditis: Two cases illustrating value of angiocardiography in diagnosis. Am. J. Cardiol. *19*:434, 1976.

492. Stroobandt, R., Knieriem, H. J., DeWolf, L., and Joosens, J. V.: Radiation-induced heart disease. Acta Cardiol. *30*:383, 1975.

493. Biran, S.: Corticosteroids in radiation-induced pericarditis. Chest *74*:96, 1978.

494. Keelan, M. H., and Rudders, R. A.: Successful treatment of radiation pericarditis with corticosteroids. Arch. Intern. Med. *134*:145, 1974.

495. Castellino, R. A., Gladstein, E., and Turbow, M. M.: Latent radiation injury of lungs or heart activated by steroid withdrawal. Ann. Intern. Med. *80*:593, 1974.

496. Morton, D. L., Kagan, A. R., Roberts, W. C., O'Brien, K. P., Holmes, E. C., and Adkins, P. C.: Pericardiectomy for radiation-induced pericarditis with effusion. Ann. Thorac. Surg. *8*:195, 1969.

497. Applefeld, M. M., Cole, J. F., Pollock, S. H., Sutton, F. J., Slawson, R. G., Singleton, R. T., and Wiernik, P. H.: The late appearance of chronic pericardial disease in patients treated by radiotherapy for Hodgkin's disease. Ann. Intern. Med. *94*:338, 1981.

498. Osler, W.: The Principles and Practice of Medicine. New York, D. Appleton and Company, 1892, p. 273.

499. Przybojewski, J. Z.: Rheumatic constrictive pericarditis. A case report and review of the literature. S. Afr. Med. J. *59*:682, 1981.

500. Bulkley, B. H., and Roberts, W. C.: The heart in systemic lupus erythematosus and the changes induced in it by corticosteroid therapy. Am. J. Med. *58*:243, 1975.

501. Cohen, A. S., and Canoso, J. J.: Pericarditis in the rheumatologic diseases. *In*

502. Spodick, D. H. (ed.): Pericardial Diseases. Philadelphia, F. A. Davis Co., 1976, pp. 237–255.

502. Cohen, A. S., and Canoso, J. J.: Pericarditis in the rheumatologic diseases. Cardiovasc. Clin. *1*:237, 1976.

503. Kinney, E., Wynn, J., Hinton, D. M., Demers, S. L., O'Neill, M., Parr, G., Ward, S., and Zelis, R.: Pericardial-fluid complement. Normal values. Am. J. Clin. Pathol. *72*:972, 1979.

504. Quismorio, J. P., Jr.: Immune complexes in pericardial fluid in systemic lupus erythematosus. Arch. Intern. Med. *140*:112, 1980.

505. Jacobsen, E. J., and Reza, M. J.: Constrictive pericarditis in systemic lupus erythematosus. Demonstration of immunoglobulins in the pericardium. Arthritis Rheum. *21*:972, 1978.

506. Starkey, R. H., and Hahn, B. H.: Rapid development of constrictive pericarditis in a patient with systemic lupus erythematosus. Chest *63*:448, 1973.

507. Libman, E., and Sacks, B.: A hitherto undescribed form of valvular and mural endocarditis. Arch. Intern. Med. *33*:701, 1924.

508. Perlroth, M. G.: Connective tissue disease and the heart. J.A.M.A. *231*:410, 1975.

509. Homcy, C. J., Liberthson, R. R., Fallon, J. T., Gross, S., and Miller, L. M.: Ischemic heart disease in systemic lupus erythematosus in the young patient: Report of six cases. Am. J. Cardiol. *49*:478, 1982.

510. Collins, R. L., Turner, R. A., Nomeir, A. M., Hunt, R., Johnson, A. M., McLean, R. L., and Watts, L. E.: Cardiopulmonary manifestations of systemic lupus erythematosus. J. Rheumatol. *5*:299, 1978.

511. Charcot, J. M.: Clinical lecture on senile and chronic diseases. London, Sydenham Society, 1981, pp. 172–175.

512. Thadani, U., Iveson, J. M., and Wright, V.: Cardiac tamponade, constrictive pericarditis and pericardial resection in rheumatoid arthritis. Medicine *54*:261, 1975.

513. Gordon, D. A., Stein, J. N., and Broder, I.: Extra-articular features of rheumatoid arthritis: A systemic analysis of 127 cases. Am. J. Med. *54*:445, 1973.

514. Lebowitz, W. B.: The heart in rheumatoid arthritis (rheumatoid disease). A clinical and pathologic study of 22 cases. Ann. Intern. Med. *58*:102, 1963.

515. Kirk, J., and Cosh, J.: The pericarditis of rheumatoid arthritis. Quart. J. Med. *38*:397, 1969.

516. John, J. T., Jr., Hough, A., and Sergent, J. S.: Pericardial disease in rheumatoid arthritis. Am. J. Med. *66*:385, 1979.

517. Burney, D. P., Martin, C. E., Thomas, C. S., Fisher, R. D., and Bender, H. W., Jr.: Rheumatoid pericarditis. Clinical significance and operative management. J. Thorac. Cardiovasc. Surg. *77*:511, 1979.

518. Majeed, H. A., and Kvasnicka, J.: Juvenile rheumatoid arthritis with cardiac tamponade. Ann. Rheum. Dis. *37*:273, 1978.

519. Vukman, R. B., and Fay, G. J.: Juvenile rheumatoid arthritis with pericardial tamponade in an adult. Arch. Intern. Med. *141*:1078, 1981.

520. Yousefadeh, D. K., and Fishman, P. A.: The triad of pneumonitis, pleuritis, and pericarditis in juvenile rheumatoid arthritis. Pediat. Radiol. *8*:147, 1979.

521. Franco, A. E., Levine, H. D., and Hall, A. P.: Rheumatoid pericarditis. Ann. Intern. Med. *77*:837, 1972.

522. Parkash, R., Atassi, A., Poske, R., and Rosen, K. M.: Prevalence of pericardial effusion and mitral valve involvement in patients with rheumatoid arthritis without cardiac symptoms. N. Engl. J. Med. *289*:597, 1973.

523. Nomeir, A., Turner, R., and Watts, E.: Cardiac involvement in rheumatoid arthritis. Ann. Intern. Med. *79*:800, 1973.

524. Yancey, C. L., Doughty, R. A., Cohlan, B. A., and Athreya, B. H.: Pericarditis and cardiac tamponade in juvenile rheumatoid arthritis. Pediatrics *68*:369, 1981.

525. Mathew, P. K.: Pericardial tamponade secondary to sudden steroid withdrawal in chronic rheumatoid arthritis. Chest *75*:532, 1977.

526. Keith, T. A.: Chronic constrictive pericarditis in association with rheumatoid disease. Circulation *25*:477, 1962.

527. Kennedy, W. P. U, Partridge, R. E. H., and Matthews, M. B.: Rheumatoid pericarditis with cardiac failure treated by pericardiectomy. Br. Heart J. *28*:602, 1966.

528. Nassar, W. K., Miskin, M. E., and Rosenbaum, D.: Pericardial and myocardial disease in progressive systemic sclerosis. Am. J. Cardiol. *22*:538, 1968.

529. McWhorter, J. E., and LeRoy, E. C.: Pericardial disease in scleroderma (systemic sclerosis). Am. J. Med. *57*:566, 1974.

530. Bulkley, B. H., Rjdolfi, R. T., Salyer, W. R., and Hutchins, G. M.: Myocardial lesions of progressive systemic sclerosis. Circulation *53*:483, 1976.

531. Smith, J. W., Clements, P. J., Levisman, J., Furst, D., and Foss, M.: Echocardiographic features of progressive systemic sclerosis. Am. J. Med. *66*:28, 1979.

532. Uhl, G. S., and Kippes, G. M.: Pericardial tamponade in systemic sclerosis (schleroderma). Br. Heart J. *42*:345, 1979.

533. Medsger, T. A., Jr., Masi, A. T., and Rodnan, G. P.: Survival with systemic sclerosis (scleroderma). A life-table analysis of clinical and demographic factors in 309 patients. Ann. Intern. Med. *75*:369, 1971.

534. Csonka, G. W., and Oates, J. K.: Pericarditis and electrocardiographic changes in Reiter's syndrome. Br. Med. J. *1*:866, 1957.

535. Goldman, M. J., and Lau, F. Y. K.: Acute pericarditis associated with serum sickness. N. Engl. J. Med. *250*:278, 1954.

536. Shapiro, L., and Buckingham, R. B.: Septic rheumatoid pericarditis complicating Felty's syndrome. Arthritis Rheum. *24*:1435, 1981.

537. Dupond, J. L., and Leconte-des-Floris, R.: Temporal arteritis manifested as an acute febrile pericarditis. J.A.M.A. *247*:2371, 1982.

538. Dawes, P. T., and Atherton, S. T.: Coeliac disease presenting as recurrent pericarditis. Lancet *1*:1021, 1981.

539. Thompson, D. C., Lennard-Jones, J. E., Swarbrick, E. T., and Bown, R.: Pericarditis and inflammatory bowel disease. Quart. J. Med. *48*:93, 1979.

540. Becker, S. A., Wishnitzler, R., Botwin, S., Eliraz, A., and Bass, D. D.: Myopericarditis associated with inflammatory bowel disease. J. Clin. Gastroenterol. *3*:267, 1981.

541. Laane, B. F.: Infantile polyarteritis nodosa or mucocutaneous lymph node syndrome (Kawasaki disease). Arteritis associated with aneurysm, thromboses and rupture of the coronary artery with cardiac tamponade. Tisddkr. Nor. Laegeforen. *101*:1583, 1981.

542. Desablens, B., Lesbre, J. P., Wattebled, R., Herve, M. A., Schurtz, C., DeLobel, J., and Messerschmitt, J.: Adult Still's disease with constrictive pericarditis. Sjögren's syndrome, and varied leucocytic abnormalities. Semin. Hop. Paris *56*:1163, 1980.

543. Vlietstra, R. E., Lie, J. T., Kuhl, W. E., Danielson, G. K., and Roberts, M. K.: Whipple's disease involving the pericardium: Pathologic confirmation during life. Aust. N. Z. J. Med. *8*:649, 1978.

544. Alarçon-Segovia, D.: Drug-induced lupus syndromes. Mayo Clin. Proc. *44*: 664, 1969.

545. Stein, H. B., Dodek, A., Lawson, L., and Rae, A.: Procainamide-induced lupus erythematosus: Report of a case with a large pericardial effusion and fluid analysis. J. Rheumatol. *6*:543, 1979.

546. Goldberg, M. J., Husain, M., Wajszczuk, W. J., and Rubenfire, M.: Procainamide-induced lupus erythematosus pericarditis encountered during coronary artery bypass surgery. Am. J. Med. *69*:159, 1980.

547. Carey, R. M., Coleman, M., and Feder, A.: Pericardial tamponade: A major manifestation of hydralazine-induced lupus syndrome. Am. J. Med. *54*:84, 1973.

548. Harrington, T. M., and Davis, D. E.: Systemic lupus-like syndrome induced by methyldopa therapy. Chest *79*:696, 1981.

549. Slater, E. E.: Cardiac tamponade and peripheral eosinophilia in a patient receiving cromolyn sodium. Chest *73*:878, 1978.

550. Yates, R. C., and Olson, K. B.: Drug-induced pericarditis. Report of three cases due to 6-amino-9-D-psicofuranosylpurine. N. Engl. J. Med. *265*:274, 1961.

551. Bennett, W. M.: Pericardial effusions associated with minoxidil. Lancet *2*:1356, 1977.

552. Houston, M. C., McChesney, J. A., and Chatterjee, K.: Pericardial effusion associated with minoxidil therapy. Arch. Intern. Med. *141*:69, 1981.

553. Petusevsky, M. L., Faling, L. J., Rocklin, R. E., Snider, G. L., Merliss, A. D., Moses, J. M., and Dorman, S. A.: Pleuropericardial reaction to treatment with Dantrolene. J.A.M.A. *242*:2772, 1979.

554. Meeran, M. K., Ahmed, A. H., Parsons, F. M., and Anderson, C. K.: Constrictive pericarditis due to methysergide therapy. S. Afr. Med. J. *50*:1595, 1976.

555. Bristow, M. R., Thompson, P. D., Martin, R. P., Mason, J. W., Billingham, M. E., Harrison, D. C.: Early anthracycline toxicity. Am. J. Med. *65*:823, 1978.

556. Dressler, W.: A postmyocardial infarction syndrome. Preliminary report of a complication resembling idiopathic recurrent benign pericarditis. J.A.M.A. *160*: 1379, 1956.

557. Dressler, W.: The post-myocardial infarction syndrome. A report of forty-four cases. Arch. Intern. Med. *103*:28, 1959.

558. Lichstein, E., Arsura, E., Hollander, G., Greengart, A., and Sanders, M.: Current incidence of post-myocardial infarction (Dressler's) syndrome. Am. J. Cardiol. *50*:1269, 1982.

559. Davies, A. M., and Gery, I.: The role of autoantibodies in heart disease. Am. Heart J. *60*:669, 1960.

560. Van der Geld, H.: Anti-heart antibodies in the post-pericardiotomy and the post–myocardial infarction syndrome. Lancet *2*:617, 1964.

561. Liem, K. L., ten Veen, J. H., Lie, K. I., Feltkamp, T. E. W., and Durrer, D.: Incidence and significance of heart muscle antibodies in patients with acute myocardial infarction and unstable angina. Acta Med. Scand. *206*:473, 1971.

562. Weiser, N. J., Kantor, M., and Russell, H. K.: Post–myocardial infarction syndrome. Circulation *20*:371, 1959.

563. Gibbons, J. A., and Vieweg, W. V.: Dressler's syndrome and angina pectoris relieved by surgery. Chest *77*:431, 1980.

564. Blau, N., Shen, B., and Pittman, D. E.: Massive hemopericardium in a patient with postmyocardial infarction syndrome. Chest *71*:4, 1977.

565. Goldhaber, S. Z., Lorell, B. H., and Green, L. H.: Constrictive pericarditis. A case requiring pericardiectomy following Dressler's postmyocardial infarction syndrome. J. Thorac. Cardiovasc. Surg. *81*:793, 1981.

566. Haiat, R., Desoutter, P., Stolitz, J. P., Chousterman, M., Cattan, P., and Gandjbakhch, I.: Constrictive pericarditis secondary to myocardial infarction. Arch. Mal. Coeur *74*:1349, 1981.

567. Soloff, L. A., Zatuchni, J., Janton, D. H., O'Neill, T. J. E., and Glover, R. P.: Reactivation of rheumatic fever following mitral commisurotomy. Circulation *8*:481, 1953.

568. Engle, M. A., and Ito, T.: The postpericardiotomy syndrome. Am. J. Cardiol. *7*:73, 1961.

569. Peters, R. W., Scheinman, M. M., Raskin, S., and Thomas, A. N.: Unusual complications of epicardial pacemakers. Am. J. Cardiol. *45*:1088, 1980.

570. Engle, M. A., Klein, A. A., Hepner, S., and Enlers, K. H.: The postpericardiotomy and similar syndromes. Cardiovasc. Clin. *7*:211, 1976.

571. Livelli, F. D., Jr., Johnson, R. A., McEnany, M. T., Sherman, E., Newell, J., Block, P. C., and DeSanctis, R. W.: Unexplained in-hospital fever following cardiac surgery: Natural history, relationship to postpericardiotomy syndrome and a prospective study of therapy with indomethacin versus placebo. Circulation *57*:968, 1978.

572. Engle, M. A., Gay, W. A., Jr., Kaminsky, M. E., Zabriskie, J. B., and Senterfit, L. B.: Postpericardiotomy syndrome then and now. Curr. Probl. Cardiol. *3*:1, 1978.

573. Kaminsky, M. E., Rodan, B. A., Osborne, D. R., Chen, J. T. T., Sealy, W. C., and Putman, C. E.: Postpericardiotomy syndrome. Am. J. Radiol. *138*:503, 1982.

574. DeSaulniers, D., Gervais, N., and Rouleau, J.: Does pericardial drainage decrease the frequency of the postpericardiotomy syndrome? Canad. J. Surg. *24*: 265, 1981.

575. Engle, M. A., Ehlers, K. H., O'Loughlin, J. E., Jr., Linday, L. A., and Fried, R.: The postpericardiotomy syndrome: Iatrogenic illness with immunologic and virologic components. *In* Engle, M. A. (ed.): Pediatric Cardiovascular Disease. Cardiovasc. Clin. 1981, pp. 381–391.

576. Ofori-Krakye, S. K., Tyberg, T. I., Geha, A. S., Hammond, G. L., Cohen, L. S., and Langou, R. A.: Late cardiac tamponade after open heart surgery: Incidence, role of anticoagulants in its pathogenesis and its relationship to the postpericardiotomy syndrome. Circulation *63*:1323, 1981.

577. Ikaheimo, M., and Takkunen, J.: Postpericardiotomy syndrome diagnosed by echocardiography. Scand. J. Thorac. Cardiovasc. Surg. *13*:305, 1979.

578. Wheeler, E. O., Turner, J. D., and Scannell, J. G.: Fever, splenomegaly, and atypical lymphocytes. A syndrome observed after cardiac surgery utilizing a pump oxygenator. N. Engl. J. Med. *266*:454, 1962.

579. Berger, R. L., Loveless, G., and Warner, O.: Delayed and latent postcardiotomy tamponade: Recognition and nonoperative treatment. Ann. Thorac. Surg. *12*:22, 1971.

580. McCabe, J. C., Engle, M. A., and Ebert, P. A.: Chronic pericardial effusion requiring pericardiectomy in the postpericardiotomy syndrome. J. Thorac. Cardiovasc. Surg. *67*:814, 1974.

581. King, T. E., Jr., Stelzner, T. J., and Sahn, S. A.: Cardiac tamponade complicating the postpericardiotomy syndrome. Chest *83*:500, 1983.

582. Herzog, D. B., Gilberg, E. M., and Levy, J. M.: Pericardial window complicated by acute congestive heart failure in a patient with chronic pericardial effusion. Pediatrics *57*:967, 1976.

583. Rice, E. P. L., Pifarre, R., and Montoya, A.: Constrictive pericarditis following cardiac surgery. Ann. Thorac. Surg. *31*:450, 1981.

584. Dane, T. E. B., and King, E. B.: Fatal cardiac tamponade and other mechanical complications of central venous catheters. Br. J. Surg. *62*:6, 1975.

585. Foster, C. J.: Constrictive pericarditis complicating an endocardial pacemaker. Br. Heart J. *47*:497, 1982.

586. Schwartz, D. J., Thanavaro, S., Kleiger, R. E., Krone, R. J., Connors, J. P., and Oliver, G. C.: Epicardial pacemaker complicated by cardiac tamponade and constrictive pericarditis. Chest *76*:226, 1979.

587. Lindenau, K. F., Warnke, H., and Bergmann, U.: Cardiac tamponade following open heart surgery. Zentralbl. Chir. *104*:1345, 1979.

588. Jones, M. R., Vine, D. L., Attas, M., and Todd, E. P.: Late isolated left ventricular tamponade. J. Thorac. Cardiovasc. Surg. *77*:142, 1979.

589. Marx, P., Jaffe, C., Laks, H., and Wolfson, S.: Delayed post–cardiac-surgery tamponade producing localized right atrial compression. Cath. Cardiovasc. Diag. *7*:275, 1981.

590. Kanakis, C., Sheikh, A. I., and Rosen, K. M.: Constrictive pericardial disease following mitral valve replacement. Chest *79*:593, 1981.

591. Little, W. C., Primm, R. K., Karp, R. B., and Hood, W. P., Jr.: Clotted hemopericardium with the hemodynamic characteristics of constrictive pericarditis. Am. J. Cardiol. *45*:386, 1980.

592. Marsa, R., Mehta, S., Willis, N., and Bailey, L.: Constrictive pericarditis after myocardial revascularization: Report of three cases. Am. J. Cardiol. *44*:177, 1979.

593. Cohen, M. V., and Greenberg, M. A.: Constrictive pericarditis: Early and late complication of cardiac surgery. Am. J. Cardiol. *43*:657, 1979.

594. Brown, D. F., and Older, T.: Pericardial constriction as a late complication of coronary bypass surgery. J. Thorac. Cardiovasc. Surg. *74*:61, 1977.

595. Kutcher, M. A., King, S. B., Alimurung, B. N., Craver, J. M., and Logue, R. B.: Constrictive pericarditis as a complication of cardiac surgery: Recognition of an entity. Am. J. Cardiol. *50*:742, 1982.

596. Kerber, R. E., and Sherman, B.: Echocardiographic evaluation of pericardial effusion in myxedema. Incidence and biochemical and clinical correlations. Circulation *52*:823, 1975.

597. Kern, R. A., Soloff, L. A., Snope, W. J., and Bello, C. T.: Pericardial effusion: A constant, early, and major factor in the cardiac syndrome of hypothyroidism (myxedema heart). Am. J. Med. Sci. *217*:609, 1949.

598. Kurtzman, R. S., Chepey, J. J., and Otto, D. L.: Myxedema heart disease. Radiology *84*:624, 1965.

599. Hardisty, C. A., Naik, D. R., and Munro, D. S.: Pericardial effusion in hypothyroidism. Clin. Endocrinol. *13*:349, 1980.

600. Parving, H., Hansen, J. M., Nielsen, S. V., Rossing, N., Munck, O., and Lassen, N. A.: Mechanisms of edema formation in myxedema-increased protein extravasation and relatively slow lymphatic drainage. N. Engl. J. Med. *301*:460, 1981.

601. Davis, P. J., and Jacobson, S.: Myxedema with cardiac tamponade and pericardial effusion of "gold paint" appearance. Arch. Intern. Med. *120*:615, 1967.

602. Sharma, S. K., and Bordia, A.: Cardiac tamponade due to pericardial effusion in myxedema. Indian Heart J. *21*:210, 1969.

603. Das, S., Lieberman, A. N., and Schussler, G. C.: Prolonged persistence of a large pericardial effusion and hemodynamic evidence of cardiac tamponade during treatment of myxedema. Clin. Cardiol. *5*:459, 1982.

604. Singh, A., and Krishan, I.: Cardiac tamponade due to massive pericardial effusion in myxedema. Br. J. Med. Prac. *24*:347, 1970.

605. Spitzer, S., Adam, A., and Mason, D.: Myxedema complicated by pericardial tamponade. Penn. Med. *73*:33, 1970.

606. Brawley, R. K., Vasko, J. S., and Marrow, A. G.: Cholesterol pericarditis. Considerations of its pathogenesis and treatment. Am. J. Med. *41*:235, 1966.

607. Rosenbau, D. L., and Yu, P. N.: Idiopathic cholesterol pericarditis with effusion. Am. Heart J. *70*:515, 1965.

608. Ridenhouse, C. E., and Kiphart, R. J.: Idiopathic cholesterol pericarditis treated with pericardiectomy. Ann. Thorac. Surg. *4*:360, 1967.

609. Stanley, R. J., Subramanian, R., and Lie, J. T.: Cholesterol pericarditis terminating as constrictive calcific pericarditis. Follow-up study of patient with 40-year history of disease. Am. J. Cardiol. *46*:511, 1980.

610. Dunn, R. P.: Primary chylopericardium: A review of the literature and an illustrated case. Am. Heart J. *89*:369, 1975.

611. Pollard, W. M., Schuchmann, G. F., and Bowen, T. E.: Isolated chylopericardium after cardiac operations. J. Thorac. Cardiovasc. Surg. *81*:943, 1981.

612. Rankin, R. N., Raval, B., and Finley, R.: Primary chylopericardium: Combined lymphangiographic and CT diagnosis. J. Comput. Assist. Tomog. *4*: 869, 1980.

613. Shahian, D. M., and Kittle, C. F.: Successful management of esophago-pericardial fistula complicating esophagogastrectomy. J. Thorac. Cardiovasc. Surg. *82*:83, 1981.

614. Hardy, G. J., Nicholson, D. M., Murphy, D. A., Johnstone, D. E., and Marrie, T. J.: Polymicrobial purulent pericarditis. Canad. J. Surg. *24*:80, 1981.

615. Mitchell, C. E.: Relapsing pancreatitis with recurrent pericardial and pleural effusions. Ann. Intern. Med. *60*:1047, 1964.

616. Davidson, E. D., Horney, J. T., and Salter, P. P.: Internal pancreatic fistula to the pericardium and pleura. Surgery *85*:478, 1979.

617. Withrington, R., and Collins, P.: Cardiac tamponade in acute pancreatitis. Thorax *35*:959, 1980.

618. King, J. B., and Sapsford, R. N.: Acute rupture of the pericardium with delayed dislocation of the heart: A case report. Injury *9*:303, 1978.

619. Christides, C., Laskar, M., Kim, M., Grousseau-Renaudie, D., and Pouget, X.: Post-traumatic rupture of the pericardium with cardiac luxation associated with myocardial infarction and a rupture of the aortic isthmus. J. Chir. *118*: 505, 1981.

620. Meng, R. L., Straus, A., Milloy, F., Kittle, C. F., and Langston, H.: Intrapericardial diaphragmatic hernia in adults. Ann. Surg. *189*:359, 1979.

621. Larrieu, A. J., Weiner, I., Alexander, R., and Wolma, F. J.: Pericardiodiaphragmatic hernia. Am. J. Surg. *139*:436, 1980.

622. Hasse, J., Perruchoud, A., Wolff, G., and Gradel, E.: Right-to-left atrial shunt in cardiac dislocation following extensive pneumonectomy. Thorac. Cardiovasc. Surg. *27*:330, 1979.

623. Rodgers, B. M., Moulder, P. V., and Delaney, A.: Thoracoscopy: New method of early diagnosis of cardiac herniation. J. Thorac. Cardiovasc. Surg. *78*:623, 1979.

624. Schuhfried, G.: Pneumopericardium in newborns during artificial ventilation. Paediat. Paedol. *14*:135, 1979.

625. Semler, H. J., Brandenburg, R. O., and Kirklin, J. W.: Pericardial disease complicating congenital heart lesions. Ann. Intern. Med. *53*:494, 1960.

626. Yahini, J. H., Goor, D., Kraus, Y., Pauzner, Y. H. M., and Neufeld, H. N.: Atrial septal defect and constrictive pericarditis. Am. J. Cardiol. *17*:718, 1966.

627. Engle, M. A.: Cardiac involvement in Cooley's anemia. Ann. N.Y. Acad. Sci. *119*:694, 1964.

628. Zemer, D., Cabili, S., Revach, M., and Shahin, N.: Constrictive pericarditis in familial Mediterranean fever. Israel J. Med. Sci. *13*:55, 1977.

629. Frenkenfeld, R. H., Waters, C. H., and Steiner, R. C.: Bilateral myxomas of the heart. Ann. Intern. Med. *53*:827, 1960.

630. Pierce, R. N., and Walker-Smith, G. J.: Intrathoracic manifestations of Dego's disease (malignant atrophic papulosis). Chest *73*:79, 1978.

631. Paulley, J. W., Barlow, K. E., and Cutting, P. E. J.: Acute gouty pericarditis. Lancet *1*:21, 1963.

632. Abdun Nur, D., Marcus, C. S., and Russell, F. E.: Pericarditis associated with scorpionfish (*Scorpaena buttata*) sting. Toxicon *19*:579, 1981.

633. Feigin, D. S., Fenoglio, J. J., McAllister, H. A., and Madewell, J. E.: Pericardial cysts: A radiologic-pathologic correlation and review. Radiology *125*:15, 1977.

634. Maier, H. C.: Diverticulum of the pericardium: With observations on mode of development. Circulation *16*:1040, 1957.

635. Mabille, J. P., Pignon, L., Trigalou, D., and Viard, H.: Twisted pedunculated pleuro-pericardial cyst. J. Radiol. (Fr.) *61*:177, 1980.

636. Rogers, C. I., Seymour, E. Q., and Brock, J. G.: Atypical pericardial cyst location: The value of computed tomography. J. Comput. Assist. Tomog. *4*:683, 1980.

637. Klatte, E. C., and Yune, H. Y.: Diagnosis and treatment of pericardial cysts. Radiology *104*:541, 1972.

638. Unverferth, D. V., and Wooley, C. F.: The differential diagnosis of paracardiac lesions: Pericardial cysts. Cath. Cardiovasc. Diag. *5*:31, 1979.

639. Ellis, K., Leeds, N. E., and Himmelstein, A.: Congenital deficiencies in partial pericardium: Review of two new cases including successful diagnosis by plain roentgenography. Am. J. Roentgenol. *82*:125, 1959.

640. Glover, L. B., Barcia, A., and Reeves, T. J.: Congenital absence of the pericardium. Am. J. Roentgenol. *106*:542, 1969.

641. Nasser, W. K.: Congenital absence of the left pericardium. Am. J. Cardiol. *26*: 466, 1970.

642. Bor, I., and Kafke, V.: Aplasia of pericardium. J. Cardiovasc. Surg. *2*:389, 1961.

643. Morgan, J. R., Rogers, A. K., and Forker, A. D.: Congenital absence of the left pericardium. Ann. Intern. Med. *74*:370, 1971.

644. Pisano, D., Angeloni, J., Goldberg, H., and Nakhjavan, F. K.: Congenital absence of the pericardium: Report of a case. J. A.O.A. *80*:407, 1981.

645. Pocock, W. A., Lakier, J. B., and Benjamin, J. D.: Billowing mitral valve syndrome in association with absent left pericardium. S. Afr. Med. J. *52*:813, 1977.

646. Reginao, E., Speroni, F., Riccardi, M., Verunelli, F., and Eufrate, S.: Post-traumatic mitral regurgitation and ventricular septal defect in absence of left pericardium. Thorac. Cardiovasc. Surg. *28*:213, 1980.

647. Inoue, H., Fujii, J., Mashima, S., and Marao, S.: Pseudo right atrial overloading pattern in complete defect of the left pericardium. J. Electrocardiol. *14*:413, 1981.

648. Payvandi, M. N., and Kerber, R. E.: Echocardiography in congenital and acquired absence of the pericardium. An echocardiographic mimic of right ventricular volume overload. Circulation *53*:86, 1976.

649. Nicolosi, G. L., Borgioni, L., Alberti, E., Burelli, C., Maffesanti, M., Marino, P., Slavich, G., and Zanuttini, D.: M-mode and two-dimensional echocardiography in congenital absence of the pericardium. Chest *81*:610, 1982.

650. D'Altoria, R. A., and Caro, J. Y.: Congenital absence of the left pericardium detected by imaging of the lung: Case report. J. Nucl. Med. *18*:267, 1977.

651. Baim, R. S., MacDonald, I. L., Wise, D. J., and Lenkei, S. C.: Computed tomography of absent pericardium. Radiology *135*:127, 1980.

652. Saito, R., and Hotta, F.: Congenital pericardial defect associated with cardiac incarceration: Case report. Am. Heart J. *100*:866, 1980.

653. Rogge, J. D., Mishkin, M. E., and Genovese, P. D.: Congenital partial pericardial defect with herniation of the left atrial appendage. Ann. Intern. Med. *64*: 137, 1966.

654. Minocha, G. K., Falicov, R. E., and Nijensohn, E.: Partial right-sided congenital pericardial defect with herniation of the right atrium and right ventricle. Chest *76*:484, 1979.

655. Moene, R. J., Dekker, A., and van der Harten, H. J.: Congenital right-sided pericardial defect with herniation of part of the lung into the pericardial cavity. Am. J. Cardiol. *31*:519, 1973.

44

TRAUMATIC HEART DISEASE

by Peter F. Cohn, M.D., and Eugene Braunwald, M.D.

THE PROBLEM IN PERSPECTIVE

Unfortunately, traumatic heart disease is often regarded as an uncommon and even esoteric form of heart disease of interest primarily to physicians in the military service. That this is not the case is attested to by the statistics—violent injury accounts for the majority of deaths in persons under 40 years of age,[1] and among these victims cardiac trauma is one of the leading causes of death.[2,3] In recent years, reports of increasing traumatic heart disease in civilians may be attributed to the accelerating mechanization of contemporary life—whether on the farm, in the home, in industry, or on the roads. For example, it has been estimated that almost 20 per cent of over five million instances of bodily injury of at least moderate severity resulting from auto accidents are associated with cardiac trauma.[4] The increasing frequency of physical violence has resulted in a corresponding increase in the incidence of traumatic heart disease. Although all age groups and both sexes are susceptible to traumatic heart disease, *young adult males* are the most frequent victims, since they are more likely to have automobile and motorcycle accidents, incur injuries while performing heavy labor, and be involved in acts of physical violence.

There is, regrettably, no evidence that the frequency of these mishaps is declining or even approaching a plateau. At Boston City Hospital, for example, the annual incidence of penetrating wounds of the heart rose from 2.8 cases during the period from 1956 through 1964 to 8.0 cases from 1965 through 1976.[5] In addition, the incidence of medically related cardiac trauma is also rising, such as increased use of intravascular and intracardiac catheters leading to penetrating injuries of the heart and great vessels, and resuscitative cardiac massage causing a variety of nonpenetrating injuries of these organs.

The two principal, immediate consequences of cardiac injury are *exsanguinating hemorrhage* and *cardiac tamponade*. Effective treatment has resulted in an increasing number of immediate survivors, and later sequelae, including myocardial infarction, aneurysm, pseudoaneurysm, ventricular septal defect, valvular damage, recurrent pericarditis, and constrictive pericarditis, are becoming far more common. Serious cardiac trauma is frequently overlooked in patients with nonpenetrating injury, particularly when other structures such as the thoracic cage and lungs are obviously damaged. Such oversight can be tragic, because the lethal consequences of cardiac injury may suddenly emerge after the more superficial injuries have been attended to. Clearly, a much higher index of suspicion of this possibility is necessary if the increasing magnitude of this problem is to be halted and reversed.

NONPENETRATING CARDIAC INJURY

Nonpenetrating injuries result from the effects of external physical forces, but it is important to recognize that these forces need not be applied directly to the chest, since injuries to the heart and great vessels may also occur with trauma to other parts of the body. Parmley et al. have summarized the mechanisms of nonpenetrating injuries to the heart as follows: (1) direct force against the chest; (2) bidirectional force against the thorax; (3) indirect forces resulting in a marked increase in intravascular pressure, as from sudden compression in the abdomen and lower extremities; (4) decelerative forces; (5) blast forces; (6) concussive forces; and (7) combinations of the above.[6]

The most common cause of nonpenetrating injury in civilian life is probably that directly related to vehicular impact, either by direct compression, usually with the steering wheel squeezing the heart between the sternum and the spine, or by indirect compression.[7,8] Causes of nonpenetrating injuries other than automobile and motorcycle accidents include direct blows to the chest by any kind of blunt object or missile, such as a clenched fist or even various kinds of sporting equipment, as well as by the kicks of animals, falls, and cardiac resuscitative procedures. Fractures of the bony structures of the chest wall are *not* necessary accompaniments of cardiac injury in any of these situations. This point is of critical importance, since *the absence of such obvious injuries following trauma should by no means exclude the possibility of nonpenetrating injury to the heart.* The clinical manifestations may not be apparent for days or even weeks after the accident.[9]

Pathological findings following nonpenetrating cardiac injury usually include some degree of pericarditis, which may be associated with the late development of constriction. Changes in the heart itself range from minute ecchymotic areas in the subepicardium or subendocardium to transmural contusions with edematous, fragmented, or necrotic muscle fibers, surrounded at first by red blood cells and invaded soon thereafter by polymorphonuclear leukocytes. The external appearance of the heart may be misleading in the case of nonpenetrating injury, since large areas of intramural contusion,[10] including involvement of the interventricular septum, may not be apparent. In patients who survive the injury, healing is by scar formation resembling that following acute myocardial infarction, and post-traumatic aneurysms resembling postinfarction aneurysms may develop. The types of cardiac injury resulting from blunt (nonpenetrating) trauma are listed in Table 44–1, the most severe forms being rupture of the aortic or mitral valve and rupture of the interventricular septum or even of the free wall of a cardiac chamber. These injuries are frequently fatal, but fortunately they constitute only a small fraction of all nonpenetrating injuries (Table 44–2).

Pericardium (See also p. 1480)

Injury to the pericardium in blunt trauma may range from contusion to laceration or rupture. Whether the pericardium tears or not, some degree of traumatic pericarditis is found at autopsy or operation in most patients sustaining severe blunt trauma of the chest, especially of the precordial area. Parmley et al. reported pericardial laceration or rupture in 249 of 546 autopsy cases of nonpenetrating trauma to the heart,[6] but it should be noted that this rarely

TABLE 44–1 TYPES OF CARDIAC INJURY FROM BLUNT TRAUMA

A. Myocardium
   1. Contusion
   2. Laceration
   3. Rupture
   4. Septal perforation
   5. Aneurysm, pseudoaneurysm
   6. Hemopericardium, tamponade
   7. Thrombosis, systemic embolism
B. Pericardium
   1. Pericarditis
   2. Postpericardiotomy syndrome
   3. Constrictive pericarditis
   4. Pericardial laceration
   5. Hemorrhage
   6. Cardiac herniation
C. Endocardial structures
   1. Rupture of papillary muscle
   2. Rupture of chordae tendineae
   3. Rupture of atrioventricular and semilunar valves
D. Coronary artery
   1. Thrombosis
   2. Laceration
   3. Fistula

From Jackson, D. H., and Murphy, G. W.: Nonpenetrating cardiac trauma. Mod. Conc. Cardiovasc. Dis. *45*:123, 1976, by permission of the American Heart Association, Inc.

occurs as an isolated lesion (Table 44–2) and is usually associated with cardiac contusion and even more serious cardiac injury. On the basis of a series of experiments in a canine model, in which 14 of 18 dogs receiving sublethal blunt chest trauma developed pericardial rents, DeMuth et al. suggested that a higher frequency of pericardial tears than is generally appreciated occurs in survivors of chest trauma.[11] Herniation of the heart or a portion of it through the defect may result from such injuries.[12] Clinically, a rent in the pericardium can occur as a consequence of blunt trauma, and delayed herniation of the heart through

TABLE 44–2 NONPENETRATING CARDIAC TRAUMA

TYPE AND/OR SITE OF INJURY	NUMBER OF CASES	CASES COMBINED WITH AORTIC RUPTURE	TOTAL
Rupture	273	80	353
Right ventricle	56	10	66
Left ventricle	46	13	59
Right atrium	35	6	51
Left atrium	24	2	26
IV septum	25(20*)	7(4*)	30(24*)
IA septum	18(10*)	5(3*)	25(13*)
Multiple chamber ruptures	69	37	106 128
Contusion/laceration	105	24	
Pericardial laceration	18	18	36
Hemopericardium	13	12	25
Valvular laceration/rupture	1(2†)	0(4†)	1(6†)
Aortic valve	1(1†)	0(2†)	1(3†)
Pulmonic valve	0(4†)	0	0(4†)
Tricuspid valve	0(8†)	0	0(8†)
Mitral valve	0(8†)	0(1†)	0(9†)
Mitral and tricuspid valves	0(1†)	0(1†)	0(2†)
Coronary artery laceration/rupture	0(7†)	1(2†)	1(9†)
Papillary muscle laceration/rupture	1(23†)	0	1(23†)
TOTAL	411	135	546

Numbers in parentheses indicate more significant associated cardiac injuries (tabulated in another column).
*Associated with other sites of cardiac rupture.
†Combined with cardiac rupture or other cardiac injury.
From Parmley, L. F., et al.: Nonpenetrating traumatic injury of the heart. Circulation *18*:371, 1958, by permission of the American Heart Association, Inc.

trauma, and delayed herniation of the heart through the rent may then acutely compromise circulatory function.[13]

CLINICAL FEATURES AND DIAGNOSIS. Clinically, traumatic pericarditis is manifested by the development of a typical pericardial friction rub and ST-T–wave changes on the electrocardiogram characteristic of pericarditis (p. 1475 and 1476). During and immediately following the acute episode, the major problem is not the pericarditis itself, but its most common complications, i.e., hemopericardium and resultant tamponade, discussed on p. 1480. Commonly, the patient is restless, with hypotension, oliguria or anuria, distant heart sounds, and pulsus paradoxus. There is usually diffuse low voltage on the electrocardiogram. Pericardial fluid on the echocardiogram (p. 1484) is a key finding.

TREATMENT AND PROGNOSIS. As a rule, uncomplicated pericarditis simply resolves. Tamponade, however, requires emergency operative treatment, as discussed below. Recurrent pericardial effusions sometimes associated with chest pain and fever, i.e., the so-called postcardiotomy syndrome, occur in a small number of patients. The etiology of this syndrome is not clear (p. 1514). Patients with recurrent effusions usually respond to aspirin or indomethacin, but occasionally glucocorticosteroids are necessary. Constrictive pericarditis occurs as a rare complication of traumatic pericarditis, with or without recurrent effusions.

Myocardium

Early experimental studies stressed the vulnerability of the heart to blunt trauma.[14] A method of producing a standard, graded, isolated injury to the myocardium through the intact chest wall of anesthetized dogs using a captive-bolt handgun or an air pressurized impactor with energy transferred through a metal disc has been described.[15–17] As the power was increased, the degree of injury became correspondingly more severe. The first level of energy produced only arrhythmias, intermediate levels produced varying degrees of hematoma associated with impairment of ventricular function, and the highest level of energy was nearly always fatal. An important and surprising finding was gross pathological change in the hearts of animals that showed no clinically apparent ill effects.

Since the consequences of nonpenetrating injury to the myocardium vary in intensity from mild contusion to cardiac rupture, it is not surprising that clinical manifestations also vary proportionately and that a high index of suspicion is often necessary for their recognition in all but the most obvious cases.[18] In patients with preexisting ischemic, valvular, or myopathic heart disease, the added insult of the myocardial trauma can be more serious than a comparable injury in a normal person.

CONTUSION

Myocardial contusion usually produces no significant symptoms and often goes unrecognized. At times, manifestations of the injury are masked by injury to the chest wall or other organs. The importance of a high index of suspicion of this complication is reflected in the experience at the Charity Hospital in New Orleans.[19] From 1963 to 1970, an average of two patients a year with cardiac con-

tusion were admitted to the surgical service but, with increasing interest in and attention devoted to this problem, an average of eight patients per year were admitted from 1971 through 1973; in many of the latter patients, the diagnosis was not evident immediately but was established 48 hours after admission or even later. Most of the patients were young males involved in automobile accidents. Thus, as is the case with any condition, there is a higher frequency of diagnosis of cardiac contusion associated with increasing awareness of the lesion.

Clinical Features and Diagnosis. The most common symptom of myocardial contusion is precordial pain resembling that of myocardial infarction, but the pain from other sites of chest trauma can confuse the clinical picture.[20] As with myocardial infarction, nitroglycerin and related drugs have little effect in relieving the pain. The *electrocardiogram* probably represents one of the most helpful tools for recognizing this syndrome.[21–23] Either nonspecific ST-T abnormalities or the classic findings of pericarditis are the most common changes noted. Initially, electrocardiographic signs of deeper injury to the myocardium, i.e., pathological Q waves, may be dwarfed by pericardial inflammation; only as the latter subsides does injury to the myocardium become more evident. However, because the possibility of cardiac trauma is not considered, an electrocardiogram is often not recorded immediately on patients with chest injuries and the diagnosis may be missed. Just as in acute myocardial infarction, serial findings, i.e., Q waves and the subsidence of the ST-segment and T-wave abnormalities, are of critical importance.

Since *serum enzyme levels* may be elevated by trauma to noncardiac as well as to cardiac tissue, they too are of limited diagnostic value. With the increasing availability of reliable measurements of the MB band of creatine kinase (CK), the cardiospecific isoenzyme of creatine kinase (p. 1254), the presence or absence of cardiac necrosis can be better documented in patients with blunt trauma.[24] Indeed, with the electrocardiogram and CK-MB as screening tests, the detection of myocardial contusion has increased from 7 to 17 per cent of patients with blunt chest trauma presenting to the Henry Ford Hospital.[25]

Another potentially important diagnostic tool is *radionuclide imaging* (Chap. 11).[26] Myocardial perfusion is reduced in areas of myocardial contusion.[27] Chiu et al. have used technetium-labeled pyrophosphate to demonstrate images of positive uptake that were then correlated with postmortem angiograms showing extravasation of contrast material.[28] Images usually became negative 1 week after the trauma. Contused myocardium was found to concentrate ^{99m}Tc-pyrophosphate in quantities comparable to the level observed in ischemic injury.[29] Scanning following injection of radioactive thallium to detect areas of reduced perfusion and of labeled pyrophosphate to locate areas of recent necrosis may be expected to identify patients with myocardial damage following blunt trauma, to localize this damage, and to indicate the extent of the damage. Radionuclide ventriculography often shows a reduced ventricular ejection fraction in such patients.[30] These tests show changes similar to those observed in patients with acute myocardial infarction (Chap. 11).

A wide variety of *arrhythmias* is common with areas of extensive contusion,[31,32] and ventricular tachycardia that degenerates into ventricular fibrillation represents a frequent cause of death in these patients. The precise mechanism responsible for these arrhythmias has not been defined, but in the dog, increasing frequencies of ventricular premature beats were observed with increasing grades of trauma.[16] In addition, both atrioventricular and intraventricular conduction defects, as well as sinus node dysfunction, are seen.[33-35] In contrast to acute myocardial infarction, cardiac contusion rarely leads to severe heart failure unless severe damage to a valve or rupture of the interventricular septum has occurred. However, moderate impairment of right and/or left ventricular function, as reflected in depressed ejection fractions and ventricular function (myocardial performance) curves, is common.[30,36]

Treatment and Prognosis. Treatment of myocardial contusion has traditionally involved a 4- to 6-week period of bed rest with progressive ambulation thereafter.[7] However, in this era of progressively earlier ambulation for patients with myocardial infarction, a more aggressive approach appears to be reasonable. From the point of view of physical activity, we recommend treating these patients in a manner similar to those with acute myocardial infarction with comparable extent of myocardial damage (p. 1303). Treatment with anticoagulants is contraindicated, however, since it may precipitate or exacerbate intramyocardial or intrapericardial hemorrhage. Atrial fibrillation, when present, usually reverts to sinus rhythm spontaneously, but if it does not, digitalis glycosides may be used to slow the ventricular rate and may also cause reversion to sinus rhythm. Chest pain is best treated with analgesics.

The prognosis for complete or partial recovery is generally excellent, but these patients require careful follow-up, since late complications, ranging from ventricular arrhythmias to cardiac rupture, may occur. Coronary occlusion,[37] sinus of Valsalva–right atrial fistula,[38] and cardiac aneurysms[39] are occasional sequelae, and there is no agreement about whether or not surgical resection of the last-named is required.[40] It is our policy to use the presence of heart failure as an indication for operation of aneurysms analogous to that in patients with postinfarct aneurysms (p. 1374).

Although many analogies can be drawn between the cardiac necrosis caused by trauma and that caused by coronary artery disease, a number of critically important differences must be emphasized. Patients with acute myocardial infarction generally have diffuse, obstructive, gradually progressive coronary artery disease, are frequently middle-aged or elderly, and may have underlying heart disease such as that secondary to prolonged hypertension or diabetes mellitus; patients with traumatic myocardial contusion generally have normal coronary vessels and only a discrete area of myocardial damage;[41] most often, they are young and without underlying cardiovascular illness. Hence, the long-term prognosis in patients with myocardial necrosis secondary to trauma tends to be far better, *if they survive the acute episode.*

RUPTURE

There appear to be two mechanisms of cardiac rupture; (1) acute laceration due to compression of the heart by direct force, and (2) contusion and hemorrhage that proceed to necrosis, softening, and rupture several days following the trauma. Rupture of a cardiac chamber usually, but not always, results in immediate death. However, Bright and Beck reported that 30 of 152 patients with ventricular rupture survived 30 minutes or longer after the initial trauma.[14] It is this minority of patients that must be assessed and treated immediately in the emergency room setting.

Clinical Features and Diagnosis. In the patient who survives the first few minutes of cardiac rupture, the clinical picture of cardiac tamponade described above is common. Although ventricular rupture is far more common than is atrial rupture, the latter occurs particularly following automobile accidents.[42] Rupture of the interventricular septum should be suspected in patients who develop severe congestive heart failure immediately or within several days of the trauma, together with a new holosystolic murmur along the left sternal border; however, trauma to the mitral valve apparatus, which may present with a similar picture clinically, must be excluded. Based on a series of 546 autopsy cases of nonpenetrating injury to the heart, the incidence of rupture of the ventricular septum has been estimated by Parmley et al. to be a little more than 5 per cent, with a similar number of patients experiencing rupture of the atrial septum (Table 44–2).[6] These lesions may occur without other serious cardiac injuries, but occasionally other abnormalities are present, including valve cusp perforations and a variety of intracardiac shunts.[43,44] The predilection for perforation of the ventricular septum is highest at the apex, but any portion of the muscular septum may be involved, and multiple perforations are not uncommon. The diagnosis of ventricular septal defect and of damage to the mitral valve apparatus can be confirmed by means of catheterization, demonstration of an oxygen step-up in the right ventricle, and left ventricular angiography.[45]

Treatment and Prognosis. Patients with external rupture of the heart obviously require emergency operation if they are to have any chance of survival. Although surgery should not be postponed, pericardiocentesis and expansion of the intravascular volume can be carried out while the most rapid preparations possible for operation are undertaken. Successful surgical treatment of external cardiac rupture has been reported in a small number of cases.[4,46] In contrast, patients with rupture of the interventricular septum do not always require emergency operation. Indeed, many defects are small, with minimal left-to-right shunts, and may even heal spontaneously. If heart failure subsequently develops, as occurs in many patients, surgical correction should be carried out promptly and is often successful.[44]

COMPLICATIONS OF CARDIAC RESUSCITATION

In 1960, Kouwenhoven et al. described the technique of closed-chest (external) cardiac massage, and this technique quickly replaced open-chest massage in the management of cardiac arrest.[47] This procedure is generally thought to be safe and simple—so much so that it is included as part of the cardiopulmonary resuscitation technique taught to laymen. What is not sufficiently appreciated is that the procedure itself can often result in serious complications, which may go unrecognized because many of the patients

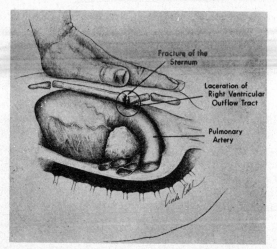

FIGURE 44–1 Schematic diagram showing the mechanism and site of laceration of the right ventricular outflow tract during external cardiac massage. (From Sethi, G.K., et al.: Complications of external cardiac massage. Report of a case of laceration of the right ventricular outflow tract. J. Cardiovasc. Surg. *18*:187, 1977.)

succumb to the cardiac arrest itself.[48] Even at postmortem examination, the complications may be improperly attributed to the underlying cardiac disease.

Rupture of the left ventricle is a more common complication of cardiac massage than rupture of the right ventricle (Figs. 44–1 and 44–2), but rupture of either chamber may occur and may be life-threatening if the patient survives the cardiac dysrhythmia that necessitated massage in the first place. In a series of autopsies on 60 patients in whom external cardiac massage had been carried out, Adelson observed four instances of laceration of the left ventricle and one each of the left atrium and cardiac vein.[49] Since in most instances external resuscitation is performed

for patients with myocardial infarction, it may not always be clear whether the left ventricular rupture preceded or occurred as a consequence of the massage.

Rupture of right ventricular papillary muscles with acute tricuspid regurgitation has also been reported as a complication of closed-chest cardiac massage,[50] as has rupture of the atria[51] and aorta[52] and a variety of noncardiovascular traumatic lesions, such as fracture of the sternum, hemothorax, pneumothorax, and laceration of abdominal organs.[53] Because of the efficacy of cardiopulmonary resuscitation and its increasing use by paramedical personnel and laymen, an increasing number of such complications may be anticipated in the future. This increased incidence will be stemmed only by extensive and repeated educational programs for all individuals likely to employ this technique.

PENETRATING CARDIAC INJURY

Symbas has noted the long medical history of penetrating cardiac wounds, which have been recorded since the time of Hippocrates.[8] Up to the end of the nineteenth century, this type of wound was thought to be invariably fatal.[54]

Penetrating cardiac injuries occurring in civilian life are due to a variety of objects, such as bullets, knives, ice picks, and the like,[55,56] but they may also be due to the inward displacement of ribs or sternal fragments accompanying chest injuries. The chamber most commonly involved in this type of injury is the right ventricle because of its anterior position, followed, in descending order of frequency, by the left ventricle, the right atrium, and the left atrium.[57,58] However, penetrating wounds of the precordium are not the only types of wounds that may result in cardiac injury. Occasionally, wounds of other areas of the

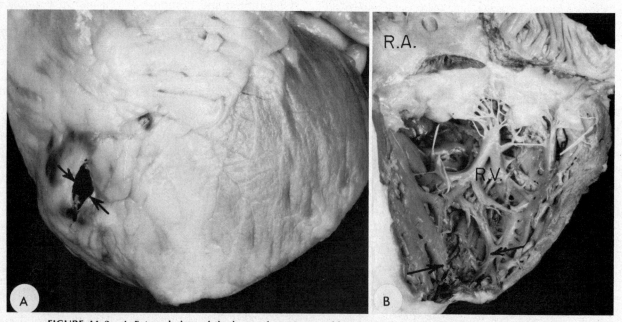

FIGURE 44–2 *A*, External view of the heart of an 85-year-old woman who died of massive pulmonary embolism and in whom closed-chest massage was unsuccessful. There is a laceration (between arrows) at the apex of the right ventricle. *B*, Interior view of the right atrium (RA) and right ventricle (RV). The laceration of the right ventricular apex lies between the arrows. There is also a laceration of the right atrium that did not involve the full thickness of the wall. (From Baldwin, J.J., and Edwards, J.E.: Rupture of right ventricle complicating closed chest massage. Circulation *53*:562, 1976, by permission of the American Heart Association, Inc.)

chest, as well as of the neck and upper abdomen, are associated with penetration of the heart. In addition, intravenous or intracardiac catheters may fracture and become impaled within the walls of a great vessel or cardiac chamber (Chap. 9).[59] Migration of an indwelling venous catheter into the pulmonary artery, which may ultimately lead to perforation of this vessel, is another complication that has increased in frequency with its widespread use in intensive care units.[60] Formerly, thoracotomy was necessary to remove these catheter fragments, but noninvasive snare devices are now available for this purpose.[61]

Perforation of the right ventricle with a transvenous pacing electrode is not uncommon, but tamponade is rare.[62] The postcardiotomy syndrome (p. 1514) however, may occur following such a perforation.[63] During cardiac catheterization, perforation of the thin-walled right atrium or outflow tract of the right ventricle has been reported.[64] Such patients usually require only careful observation, but when tamponade occurs, immediate drainage is mandatory.[65] Dissection of the aorta or arch vessels has been reported as a complication of retrograde arterial catheterization and occasionally is also severe enough to require operative intervention.[66]

Penetrating wounds of the heart often result in laceration of the pericardium, sometimes occurring alone but usually associated with laceration of the myocardium itself. One or more chambers but also the cardiac valves and their accessory structures, as well as the interventricular and interatrial septa, may be perforated. When laceration of the pericardium occurs as an isolated lesion, acute compromise of cardiac function resulting from herniation of the heart may be the presenting manifestation. Occasionally, low-velocity missiles may penetrate the cardiac chambers but may be retained within the myocardium.

The most common penetrating injuries resulting from physical violence are stab and gunshot wounds.[67] The former do not necessarily cause extensive cellular destruction adjacent to the wound; they resemble surgical incisions, and transmural wounds in the thick-walled left ventricle may actually seal quickly without disastrous consequences. In contrast, bullet wounds are associated with bleeding that is not usually self-limited and extensive cellular destruction in and adjacent to the path of the bullet. When a coronary artery is lacerated or perforated, myocardial infarction may ensue.

CLINICAL FEATURES AND DIAGNOSIS. The clinical picture of a penetrating wound of the heart depends on several factors, including the mechanism of injury (i.e., bullet, knife, ice pick), the size of the wound, and the precise location of the structures injured. Pericardial laceration occurring by itself is uncommon and of relatively little significance, unless infection supervenes. Rather, the injuries to underlying cardiac structures usually determine the clinical presentation, course, and choice of treatment. However, the *nature* of the pericardial wound is important, i.e., whether or not the wound is open and allows free drainage of intrapericardial blood. If the pericardium remains open and extravasated blood can pass freely into the pleural cavities or mediastinum, cardiac tamponade will not develop, at least initially, and the presenting signs and symptoms will be those of hemorrhage and hemothorax. On the other hand, if the pericardium does *not*

permit free drainage, because its opening has been obliterated by a blood clot, adjacent lung tissue, or other structures, or because a flap develops in the pericardial rent, immediate exsanguination may be averted, but tamponade may occur minutes or hours later.[68] In some instances, blood accumulates both intra- and extrapericardially.

Whether the hemorrhage is intra- or extrapericardial, its severity can often be surmised from the clinical picture. Traumatic penetrating lesions of the heart are usually associated with injuries to the lungs and other organs, which may predominate at first; a high index of suspicion of cardiac penetration is necessary when patients are evaluated following thoracic or upper abdominal trauma. Though extensive injuries to the pericardium and underlying heart are usually immediately fatal or result in shock, delayed clinical manifestations of cardiac injury as a result of hemorrhage, infection, retained foreign bodies, or arrhythmias may become apparent after the other bodily injuries have been attended to. Failure to give serious consideration to the possibility that *cardiac* damage has occurred in a patient with obvious noncardiac trauma may lead to an unanticipated catastrophe.

Although echocardiography is extremely valuable in the recognition of pericardial effusion (p. 1478) and in the recognition of foreign bodies in the heart,[68a] it is not always readily available in an emergency setting. When agitation, cool and clammy skin, neck vein distention, pulsus paradoxus, and other classic findings of tamponade (considered earlier) are present, the diagnosis can be relatively simple; in patients without such typical findings, the clinical picture may be attributed to blood loss, especially since volume expansion can improve the hemodynamic state at least temporarily.[69] Fallah-Nejad et al. reported a series of 20 cases of penetrating cardiac injuries; the diagnosis was not immediately obvious in 10 patients in whom the signs of cardiac tamponade were either obscured or occurred late.[70] In several of these patients an initial salutary response to a volume load—with restoration of hemodynamics to apparently normal levels—was responsible for the failure to recognize the underlying cardiac injury. Whether or not pericardiocentesis should be performed as a diagnostic test is controversial. If nonclotting blood is obtained, the diagnosis of hemopericardium is confirmed, and the accompanying decompression may constitute effective, albeit temporary, initial treatment. If the pericardiocentesis is negative, however, cardiac tamponade cannot be ruled out. Since, as discussed below, the primary management in any event is thoracotomy, it seems to us pointless to waste valuable time with pericardial aspiration unless there is doubt regarding the diagnosis.

TREATMENT. Successful treatment of penetrating wounds by pericardial aspiration was reported several times during the nineteenth century. Nonetheless, until the first successful cardiorrhaphy,[54] there was great pessimism about survival following penetrating cardiac injury. Today, the definitive treatment of cardiac wounds *accompanied by severe hemorrhage* is immediate thoracotomy and cardiorrhaphy. Although multiple pericardioscenteses are no longer considered a substitute for thoracotomy in the treatment of cardiac wounds associated with cardiac tamponade, there may still be a role for pericardial aspiration *while preparing for operation* (Table 44–3). The availability

TABLE 44–3   MANAGEMENT OF PATIENTS WITH STAB WOUNDS TO
THE HEART

1. Immediate pericardiocentesis
2. Placement of central venous pressure (CVP) catheter to withdraw
   blood and infuse fluids
3. Chest roentgenogram only if condition permits
4. Thoracotomy and repair of bleeding site
5. Wound closure with placement of pericardial drainage tubes
6. Postoperative antibiotic therapy

From Harvey, J. C., and Pacifico, A. D.: Primary operative management: Method
of choice for stab wounds to the heart. South. Med. J. *68*:149, 1975, by permission
of the Southern Medical Journal.

in many hospitals of surgical teams and equipment for cardiopulmonary bypass has permitted the safe and effective
repair of many penetrating injuries of the heart.

Lemos and associates described a 13-year experience
with 121 patients undergoing surgical treatment of cardiac
wounds in Brazil.[71] Gunshot wounds outnumbered stab
wounds, nearly 72 per cent of the patients were in shock
or "pre-shock," and 33 per cent had cardiac tamponade at
the time of presentation to the hospital. Over 40 per cent
of these patients were taken to the operating room within
30 minutes of arrival at the hospital, and an overall mortality of 26 per cent in patients with isolated cardiac
wounds was reported. Harvey and Pacifico noted that
there were no deaths among 24 patients with cardiac stab
wounds who received primary operative management, but
in contrast there were three deaths among 10 patients who
were managed conservatively (including multiple pericardial aspirations).[72] Symbas et al. studied a series of 102 patients with bullet and stab wounds and concluded that
immediate operation is the treatment of choice for tamponade.[73] Szentpetery and Lower concluded in their study of
30 consecutive patients with penetrating wounds that immediate operation is recommended for all penetrating injuries but that pericardiocentesis still has a role in the
emergency relief of tamponade.[74]

Obviously, the decision for or against thoracotomy must
depend, in part, on the setting in which the patient is encountered, the availability and skill of the surgical team,
and facilities for cardiopulmonary bypass, all measured
against the gravity of the clinical picture. Even in hospitals
without the facilities for cardiopulmonary bypass, treatment of penetrating injuries of the heart may be very successful.[67,75] In 34 such patients, of whom 31 were in shock
at the time of operation, there was no immediate mortality, although the late mortality was 23 per cent.

Occasionally, thoracotomy may be performed in moribund patients for whom general anesthesia is unnecessary.
However, every effort must be made to maintain adequate
ventilation. Administration of antibiotics and tetanus prophylaxis should also be instituted as routine measures. Operative treatment includes repair of the pericardium,
myocardium, aorta, and valves as well as of any lacerations of the coronary arteries. At operation, the heart and
great vessels should be thoroughly examined for the presence of multiple wounds. When the bullet has penetrated
the anterior wall of the heart, the posterior wall should always be inspected for an exit wound before the chest is
closed. Many victims of penetrating cardiac injury, young
and otherwise in good health, can withstand relatively
long periods of hypoperfusion without irreversible brain,

renal, or cardiac damage. Therefore, one should err on the
side of aggressive attempts at resuscitation in patients who
arrive moribund in the operating room. Retained foreign
bodies in the heart are less of a problem in civilian than in
military injuries, because shootings in civilian life usually
occur at short range and thus result in through-and-
through wounds.

There is disagreement concerning whether or not retained foreign bodies should be removed. Certainly, if the
projectile is accessible, it should be removed; otherwise, if
small (less than 1 cm in diameter), it can probably be left
in place,[76] although there is some risk of later infection,
pain, aneurysm formation, or migration of the foreign
body.[77,78] In addition, dealing with a patient who is preoccupied with the knowledge that he has a foreign body retained in or close to the heart may present some difficulty;
indeed, anxiety can become excessive, impairing the patient's function more than the physical damage and, occasionally, becoming an indication for reoperation and
extraction of the object. The serious consequences of a foreign body embolus from the left ventricle also encourages
a more aggressive surgical policy toward foreign bodies
lodged in that chamber than in the right ventricle. Foreign
bodies embedded at strategic points in great vessels may
erode the vessel and cause potentially severe hemorrhage
or may embolize. As noted by Mattox et al. in a series of
28 patients with bullet emboli, complications are usually
secondary to associated injuries rather than to removal of
the bullets.[79]

Late complications of penetrating wounds of the heart
are quite common and include post-traumatic pericarditis
and infection as well as arrhythmias, ventricular septal defect, and ventricular aneurysm.

PROGNOSIS.   The outlook following a penetrating
wound depends, first and foremost, on the extent of the injury. Gunshot wounds of the heart are usually immediately fatal, with a slightly lower mortality for stab wounds;
among the latter, knife wounds are more serious than are
ice pick wounds. Wilson and Bassett have estimated that
80 to 90 per cent of patients with *stab* wounds who *reach*
the hospital alive can be saved.[55] In addition, wounds that
cause cardiac tamponade rather than massive extrapericardial hemorrhage are more likely to be successfully corrected. Patients who require 500 ml or less of blood
preoperatively to maintain a satisfactory arterial pressure
exhibited a mortality of 10 per cent, compared with those
requiring more than 1000 ml, in whom mortality was
much higher (36 per cent).[55] Salvage rates are lower in patients with penetrating wounds involving thin-walled structures such as the atria or the pulmonary artery (43 and 67
per cent, respectively), since they rarely seal off spontaneously, whereas injury to the ventricles is associated with
distinctly higher survival (about 85 per cent). The state of
consciousness and the extent of damage to the central nervous system, if any, at the time the patient presents to the
hospital also affect prognosis; Wilson and Bassett reported
that over half of those in coma succumbed compared with
11 per cent of conscious patients.[55] It is clear that delay in
performing the initial thoracotomy also adversely influences the chances for survival.

Rupture of the interventricular septum is often a late
complication of penetrating injury as it is with blunt inju-

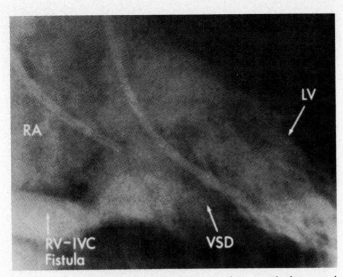

FIGURE 44–3 Angiocardiogram demonstrating ventricular septal defect (VSD) and right ventricular–inferior vena caval (RV-IVC) fistula in a 16-year-old boy who sustained a bullet wound to the chest 3 months earlier. At that time, emergency thoracotomy revealed only an entrance wound of the left ventricle (LV), which was sutured. Three months later, he was readmitted with severe congestive heart failure, and angiography was performed by injecting contrast media into the left ventricle. (From Rayner, A. V. S., et al.: Post-traumatic intracardiac shunts. Report of 2 cases and review of the literature. J. Thorac. Cardiovasc. Surg. *73:*728, 1977.)

ry (Fig. 44–3). Asfaw et al. described 12 patients with stab wounds who presented with cardiac tamponade and who had epicardial and pericardial wounds which were repaired at thoracotomy.[80] Days to years later, septal defects were diagnosed, but only four patients were symptomatic enough to warrant subsequent reoperation for closure of the defect.

INJURIES TO CARDIAC VALVES, PAPILLARY MUSCLES, AND CHORDAE TENDINEAE

Historically, reports of injuries to the cardiac valves and their accessory structures date back to the late nineteenth century. Patients with preexisting valvular heart disease may be at higher risk than those with normal valves for the development of valvular injury following blunt trauma. Parmley et al. reported a 9 per cent incidence of valvular injury in their report of 546 cases of nonpenetrating chest trauma (Table 44–2).[6] Damage to the aortic valve is by far the most common of these lesions (Fig. 44–4). (Parmley's series appears to be an exception in this regard). This is followed, in order, by damage to the mitral and tricuspid valves, presumably owing to the higher pressures generated by blunt trauma to the aorta, as noted by Jackson and Murphy.[4] The aortic valve is probably most vulnerable to damage early in diastole, when the ventricle and aorta are nearly full.[81] Damage to cardiac valves may also occur as a consequence of penetrating wounds of the heart, but, in contrast to the damage caused by nonpenetrating injury, these are rarely solitary lesions. Indeed, sustained damage of the aortic valve should be suspected in any patient without a history of heart disease who presents with a heart murmur after severe blunt trauma to the chest.

CLINICAL FEATURES AND DIAGNOSIS. New,

loud, musical murmurs are characteristic of injury to the valves and their supporting structures. The combination of a high-pitched diastolic blowing murmur with a widened pulse pressure following blunt trauma to the chest suggests rupture of the *aortic valve.* The murmur and the hemodynamic consequences of the rupture may not appear for several days following the trauma. Aortic regurgitation may also occur transiently owing to perivalvular edema or hemorrhage.

Rupture of the *mitral valve* or of a papillary muscle appears to occur as a consequence of sudden obstruction to left ventricular outflow due to blunt injury in early diastole. It is usually associated with the development of precordial pain and a loud, harsh holosystolic murmur that radiates to the apex. Fulminant pulmonary edema quickly develops; those patients with lesser degrees of regurgitation due to torn leaflets or chordae tendineae may remain compensated for longer periods of time, although they may eventually show signs of decompensation.

Rupture of the *tricuspid valve* is rare[82,83] and more benign than mitral valve rupture, with symptoms ranging from fatigue to ascites and edema.[7] Physical findings can be striking, with prominent systolic venous pulsations, hepatic pulsations, and a typical holosystolic murmur with inspiratory accentuation. At cardiac catheterization, "ventricularization" of the atrial pressure, i.e., giant v waves in the right atrial pressure pulse, can be demonstrated. A valve damaged by trauma is flail, and this can be recognized by echocardiography, whereas left-heart catheterization and selective angiocardiography are most useful in assessing the severity and hemodynamic consequences of the injury.

TREATMENT AND PROGNOSIS. The prognosis depends largely on the severity of the regurgitation. Since the lesion usually develops suddenly, the ventricle does not have the opportunity to adapt to this burden, as it does in most forms of chronic valvular regurgitation. Obviously, the baseline condition of the ventricle prior to the trauma and the presence of other injuries occurring simultaneously affect the heart's ability to tolerate the insult. Before the

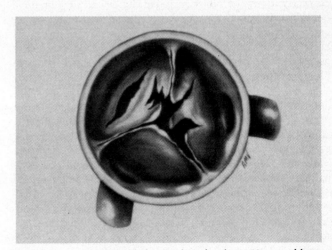

FIGURE 44–4 Diagram of the aortic valve in a 43-year-old man without known aortic valve disease who suffered blunt chest trauma. The diagram illustrates disruption along the base of the noncoronary cusp, laceration of the leading edge of this cusp, and severe laceration of the left coronary cusp. (From McIlduff, J.B., and Foster, E.D.: Disruption of normal aortic valve as a result of blunt chest trauma. J. Trauma *18:*373, 1978.)

development of cardiac surgery, a mean survival of 3½ years was reported in patients with traumatic aortic regurgitation.[84] Even in the current era when effective surgical treatment is possible, survival without the need for operation is not uncommon in patients with mild or moderate regurgitation. With severe left ventricular failure due to a ruptured mitral valve or papillary muscle, however, early surgery is mandatory, and, as in the case for the aortic valve,[85] replacement of the valve is usually preferred over valvuloplasty. It must be appreciated that the diagnosis of acute left ventricular failure may be difficult immediately after serious trauma, because fractured ribs and pulmonary contusions may be blamed for the shortness of breath and dyspnea. When left ventricular failure develops slowly or the lesion is not hemodynamically significant, as with lesser degrees of injury, medical therapy may suffice. Hemorrhage into a papillary muscle may cause late necrosis and delayed rupture, and these patients must be observed carefully.

Post-traumatic *tricuspid* regurgitation appears to have a more benign course, and many patients survive for long periods with supportive treatment. However, when failure does occur, valve replacement is the procedure of choice.

INJURIES TO THE CORONARY ARTERIES

Transmural myocardial infarctions have been reported following blunt trauma, but angiographic confirmation of coronary obstruction is rare, and, when found, its relationship to preexisting coronary atherosclerosis may be difficult to determine. When infarction occurs, it may not be clear whether it results directly from myocardial contusion, from trauma to a coronary artery, or from some combination of these two processes. In many cases of myocardial infarction, preexisting coronary artery disease has been present, and it is reasonable to postulate that the injury dislodges a plaque, which then obstructs the vessel completely.[86] However, it is also possible that a normal coronary artery becomes occluded, by either a traumatically induced intimal tear or hemorrhage. Indeed, coronary arteriography has provided strong evidence that myocardial infarction follows blunt chest trauma in previously asymptomatic persons with normal vessels except for complete obstruction of the vessel supplying the infarcted area (Fig. 44–5).[87,88] The complications of myocardial infarction —arrhythmias, pump failure, and late development of aneurysms—are similar when the lesion has an atherosclerotic basis, and treatment is similar as well. However, it may be anticipated that following survival from the initial episode, the long-term prognosis will be more favorable in patients with traumatic damage of a coronary artery, because the remaining vessels are usually normal.

Left ventricular *aneurysms* and *pseudoaneurysms* following injury to the coronary arteries can lead to rupture, cardiac failure, embolism, or arrhythmia. Operative intervention is indicated, particularly in the presence of a pseudoaneurysm, in which the myocardium has actually ruptured but in which a thrombus, fibrous tissue, and/or pericardium prevent exsanguination, since external rupture —an event which is usually fatal—is likely to occur ultimately if left untreated. Pseudoaneurysm can often be differentiated from true aneurysm by contrast or radionuclide angiography.

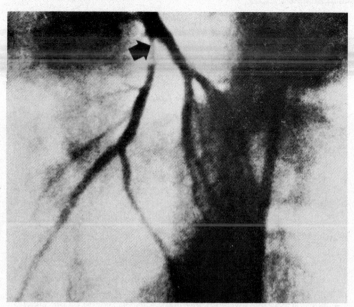

FIGURE 44–5 Left coronary arteriogram in the left anterior oblique position in a 26-year-old man who sustained an anterior wall myocardial infarction following blunt chest trauma. Arteriography performed 6 months later because of recurrent chest pain demonstrated an obstructive lesion in the left anterior descending artery (arrow). (From Jenkins, J.L., and Nishimura, A.: Coronary artery obstruction and myocardial infarction resulting from nonpenetrating chest trauma. Tex. Med. *71*:78, 1975.)

Formation of an *arteriovenous fistula* is an unusual complication of traumatic damage of a coronary artery.[89,90] Injury to the right coronary artery is more commonly followed by an arteriovenous fistula than is injury to the left. The venous side of the fistula may be the coronary sinus, the great cardiac vein, the right atrium, or the right ventricle; in the last instance, the fistula should be termed an "arteriocameral fistula." The murmur in traumatic coronary arteriovenous or arteriocameral fistula is usually loud, widely radiating, and continuous; the electrocardiogram frequently shows transmural myocardial infarction, and the roentgenogram exhibits cardiomegaly with increased pulmonary vascularity. In patients who do not undergo surgical repair, symptoms of congestive heart failure and chest pain are frequent.[91]

In 1969, Rea et al. reviewed 58 patients with *laceration of a coronary artery* due to penetrating injury and added 22 new cases.[92] The overall mortality ranged from 40 per cent with stab wounds to 67 per cent with gunshot wounds. Espada et al. reported nine patients with coronary artery lacerations among a series of 76 penetrating wounds of the heart, including seven patients with stab wounds and two with gunshot wounds.[93] As might be anticipated, the left anterior descending coronary artery is the vessel most commonly involved, and at operation, the treatment of choice is suture-ligation of the cut vessel with coronary artery bypass grafting if the lacerated vessel is large and the lesion is a proximal one. Angiography is not advised in the emergency setting, as it is with nonpenetrating trauma. However, postoperative angiography is useful in localizing the presence of possible residual injuries such as a coronary arteriocameral fistula.

INJURIES TO THE GREAT VESSELS
(See also pp. 1564–1566)

Rupture of the aorta is one of the most common traumatic lesions involving the heart or great vessels. The first case of rupture of the aorta due to *blunt* trauma was reported by Vesalius in 1557,[94] and its relative frequency is reflected in the finding that in one of every six automobile accident victims dying from blunt chest trauma the aorta is ruptured.[95] To a lesser extent, aortic rupture also occurs with falls from heights and other types of crushing injuries. Rupture occurs in the isthmus in 90 per cent of cases. Multiple tears may be present in some patients, and in others the edges of the torn aorta may be separated by several centimeters, producing a mediastinal hematoma or pseudoaneurysm.

It has been estimated that 10 to 20 per cent of patients with ruptured aorta live long enough to be treated successfully under ideal circumstances,[96] which include a high level of awareness of the possibility of aortic rupture in victims of automobile accidents as well as a well-coordinated team approach.[97] As with cardiac injury, rupture of the aorta may be overshadowed by injuries to other organs, and the diagnosis may be overlooked. Patients with aortic rupture often complain of pain in the back in addition to the chest, similar to that in patients with aortic dissection (p. 1550). If the expanding mediastinal hematoma or false aneurysm narrows the aortic lumen, or if the torn intima and media cause partial aortic obstruction, ischemia of the spinal cord and kidneys may ensue. A systolic murmur may be heard in the midscapular region, and widening of the superior mediastinum is visible on the chest roentgenogram (Fig. 44–6).[98]

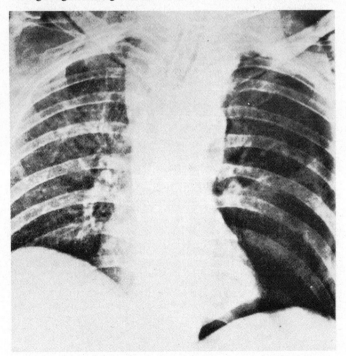

FIGURE 44–6 Chest x-ray demonstrating pronounced widening of the upper mediastinum, tracheal displacement, and left pneumothorax in a 35-year-old man who sustained traumatic rupture of the aorta as a result of an automobile accident. (From Puijlaert, C. B. A. J.: Roentgen diagnosis of traumatic rupture of the aorta. Radiologia Clin. *45*:217, 1976.)

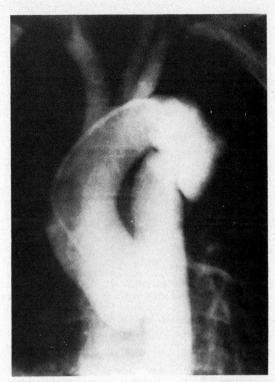

FIGURE 44–7 In a 27-year-old male, acute false and irregular aneurysm of the thoracic aorta just distal to the left subclavian artery. (Reproduced with permission from Andresen, J., and Axelsen, F.: Traumatic rupture of the thoracic aorta. Scand. J. Thorac. Cardiovasc. Surg. *14*:281, 1980.)

A diagnostic triad that occurs in well over half the cases of ruptured aorta consists of (1) increased arterial pressure and pulse amplitude in the upper extremities, (2) decreased pressure and pulse amplitude in the lower extremities, and (3) radiological evidence of widening of the superior mediastinum.[98,99] Chronic rupture of the aorta may be manifested by hoarseness, dysphagia, and cough. The diagnosis can be confirmed by aortography, which should be performed as soon as the nature of the injury is suspected. Aortography is essential for diagnosing and localizing the injury; the entire thoracic aorta and its branches should be visualized so as not to overlook a rupture occurring at an unusual site or multiple sites of rupture (Fig. 44–7).[100]

Penetrating trauma to the great vessels, which is usually the result of bullet or stab wounds, occurs most commonly in conjunction with cardiac wounds. Cardiac tamponade is a frequent complication of injury to the intrapericardial segment of one of the great vessels, but when it is extrapericardial, massive hemothorax is usually the presenting finding. The superior vena cava, trachea, or esophagus or some combination of these structures may be compressed if a large mediastinal hematoma forms as a result of bleeding. Injury to the innominate or carotid arteries may compress these vessels, with resultant neurological signs. An arteriovenous fistula may develop with symptoms of congestive heart failure accompanied by a systolic or, more commonly, a continuous murmur.[101] These fistulous connections may also involve the systemic and pulmonary vessels.[102]

Penetrating injury to the great vessels should be suspected in any patient in whom a projectile traverses the mediastinum and is suggested by radiological evidence of a

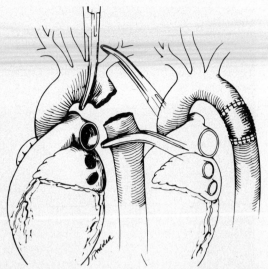

FIGURE 44–8 Method of obtaining vascular control (left) and attaching the woven Dacron graft (right) in patients with transections of the descending aorta secondary to blunt trauma. (From Pickard, L.R., et al.: Transection of the descending thoracic aorta secondary to blunt trauma. J. Trauma *17*:749, 1977.)

widened mediastinum. Aortography should be performed immediately, provided that emergency thoracotomy for shock or tamponade can be deferred briefly. Immediate operation, sometimes using a heparinized shunt between the ascending and descending aorta, should be carried out as soon as the diagnosis of thoracic aortic disruption has been established.[103] At the time of operation, the widest possible exposure is recommended. Pickard et al. described their experience with 22 patients with transection of the descending thoracic aorta secondary to blunt trauma who reached the hospital alive; five patients died shortly after admission, three died in the operating room, three died within 30 days of operation, and one died more than 1 year after the injury.[104] Ten patients were long-term survivors. A Dacron tube graft was utilized to bridge the defect in the majority of patients (Fig. 44–8). Similarly, 29 of 36 patients treated at the Grady Memorial Hospital from 1967 to 1972 for penetrating wounds of the great vessels recovered.[105]

In order to avoid the problem inherent in heparinization, i.e., bleeding from what are often multiple sites of trauma, tears of the descending thoracic aorta may often be repaired without cardiopulmonary bypass by simple aortic cross-clamping, as long as the cross-clamp time is restricted to less than 30 minutes.[106,107] An experienced surgeon can interpose a graft into the aorta with a total occlusion time ranging from 13 to 21 minutes, and ischemic injury to the spinal cord or kidneys should not occur. This technique may be aided by the intravenous administration of nitroprusside, which can maintain proximal aortic systolic pressure below 140 mm Hg.

Antiadrenergic agents such as guanethidine, reserpine, and propranolol, which have been utilized in the treatment of spontaneous dissection of the aorta (p. 1553), may also have a role in treatment of patients with aortic rupture if, for logistical reasons, operation must be deferred.

References

1. Committee on Trauma and Committee on Shock: Accidental death and disability: The neglected diseases of modern society. Washington, D.C., National Academy of Sciences, 1965, p. 5.

2. Cheitlin, M. D.: Cardiovascular trauma, part I (key references). Circulation 65: 1529, 1982.

3. Cheitlin, M. D.: Cardiovascular trauma, part II (key references). Circulation 66: 244, 1982.

4. Jackson, D. H., and Murphy, G. W.: Nonpenetrating cardiac trauma. Mod. Concepts Cardiovasc. Dis. 45:123, 1976.

5. Sherman, M. M., Saini, V. K., Yarnoz, M. D., Ramp, J., Williams, L. F., and Berger, R. L.: Management of penetrating heart wounds. Am. J. Surg. 135: 553, 1978.

6. Parmley, L. F., Manion, W. C., and Mattingly, T. W.: Nonpenetrating traumatic injury of the heart. Circulation 18:371, 1958.

7. Liedtke, A. J., and DeMuth, W. E., Jr.: Nonpenetrating cardiac injuries: A collective review. Am. Heart J. 86:687, 1973.

8. Symbas, P. N.: Cardiac trauma. Am. Heart J. 92:387, 1976.

9. MacKintosh, A. F., and Fleming, H. A.: Cardiac damage presenting late after road accidents. Thorax 36:811, 1981.

10. Allen, R. P., and Liedtke, A. J.: The role of coronary artery injury and perfusion in the development of cardiac contusion secondary to nonpenetrating chest trauma. J. Trauma 19:153, 1979.

11. DeMuth, W. E., Lerner, E. H., and Liedtke, A. J.: Nonpenetrating injury of the heart: An experimental model. J. Trauma 13:639, 1973.

12. Coats, R. R., Sakai, K., and Lam, C. R.: Extensive diaphragmatic rupture—Pericardial rupture from blunt trauma. J. Thorac. Cardiovasc. Surg. 17:223, 1974.

13. King, J. B., and Sapsford, R. N.: Acute rupture of the pericardium with delayed dislocation of the heart: A case report. Injury 9:303, 1978.

14. Bright, E. F., and Beck, C. S.: Nonpenetrating wounds of the heart: Clinical and experimental studies. Am. Heart J. 10:293, 1935.

15. Anderson, A. E., and Doty, D. B.: Cardiac trauma: An experimental model of isolated myocardial contusion. J. Trauma 15:237, 1975.

16. Lau, V.-K., Viano, D.C., and Doty, D. B.: Experimental cardiac trauma—Ballistics of a captive bolt pistol. J. Trauma 21:39, 1982.

17. Stein, P. D., Sabbah, H. N., Viano, D. C., and Vostal, J. J.: Response of the heart to nonpenetrating cardiac trauma. J. Trauma 22:364, 1982.

18. Gay, W.: Blunt trauma to the heart and great vessels. Surgery 91:507, 1982.

19. Jones, J. W., Hewitt, R. L., and Drapanas, T.: Cardiac contusion: A capricious syndrome. Ann. Surg. 181:567, 1975.

20. Saunders, C. R., and Doty, D. B.: Myocardial contusion Surg. Gynecol. Obstet. 144:595, 1977.

21. Watson, J. H., and Bartholomae, W. M.: Cardiac injury due to nonpenetrating chest trauma. Ann. Intern. Med. 52:871, 1960.

22. Potkin, R. T., Werner, J. A., Trobaugh, G. B., Chestnut, C. H., III, Carrico, C. J., Hallstrom, A., and Cobb, L. A.: Evaluation of noninvasive tests of cardiac damage in suspected cardiac contusion. Circulation 66:627, 1982.

23. Katz, S., Gimmon, Z., and Appelbaum, A.: Cardiac contusion in the patient with multiple injuries. Injury 12:180, 1980.

24. Lindsey, D., Navin, T. R., and Finley, P. R.: Transient elevation of serum activity of MB isoenzyme of creatine phosphokinase in drivers involved in automobile accidents. Chest 74:15, 1978.

25. Torres-Mirabal, P., Gruenberg, J. C., Brown, R. S., and Obeid, F. N.: Spectrum of myocardial contusion. Am. Surg. 48:383, 1982.

26. McConnell, B. J., McConnell, R. W., and Guiberteau, M. J.: Radionuclide imaging in blunt trauma. Radiol. Clin. North Am. 19:37, 1981.

27. Ware, R. E., Martin, L. G., Tyras, D. H., Kourias, E., and Symbas, P. N.: Coronary arterial injection of radioactive albumin microspheres in diagnosis of experimental myocardial contusion. Surg. Forum 23:138, 1972.

28. Chiu, C. L., Roelofs, J. D., Go, R. T., Doty, D. B., Rose, E. F., and Christie, J. H.: Coronary angiographic and scintigraphic findings in experimental cardiac contusion. Radiology 116:679, 1975.

29. Downey, J., Chagrasulis, R., Fore, D., and Parmley, L.F.: Accumulation of technetium-99m stannous pyrophosphate in contused myocardium. J. Nucl. Med. 18:1171, 1977.

30. Sutherland, G. R., Calvin, J. E., Driedger, A. A., Holliday, R. L., and Sibbald, W. J.: Anatomic and cardiopulmonary responses to trauma with associated blunt chest injury. J. Trauma 21:1, 1981.

31. Bharati, S., Chervony, A., Gruhn, J., Rosen, K. M., and Lew, M.: Atrial arrhythmias related to trauma to the sinoatrial node. Chest 61:331, 1972.

32. Fox, K. M., Rowland, E., Krikler, D. M., Bentall, H. H., and Goodwin, J. F.: Electrophysiological manifestations on nonpenetrating cardiac trauma. Br. Heart J. 43:458, 1980.

33. Fox, K. M., Rowland, E., Krikler, D. M., Bentall, H. H., and Goodwin, J. F.: Electrophysiological manifestations of nonpenetrating cardiac trauma. Br. Heart J. 43:458, 1980.

34. Brennan, J. A., Field, J. M., and Liedtke, A. J.: Reversible heart block following nonpenetrating chest trauma. J. Trauma 19:784, 1979.

35. Bognolo, D. A., Rabow, F. I., Vijayanagar, R. R., and Eckstein, P. F.: Traumatic sinus node dysfunction. Ann. Emerg. Med. 11:319, 1982.

36. Torres-Mirabal, P., Gruenberg, J. C., Talbert, J. G., and Brown, R. S.: Ventricular function in myocardial contusion: A preliminary study. Crit. Care Med. 10:19, 1982.

37. Wainwright, R. J., Edwards, A. C., Maisey, M. N., and Sowton, E.: Early occlusion and late stricture of normal coronary arteries following blunt chest trauma. Chest 78:796, 1980.

38. DeSa'Neto, A., Padnick, M. B., Desser, K. B., and Steinhoff, N. G.: Right sinus of valsalva–right atrial fistula secondary to nonpenetrating chest trauma. Circulation 60:205, 1979

39. Rheuban, K. S., Tompkins, D. G., Nolan, S. P., Berger, B., Martin, R., and

Schneider, J. A.: Myocardial necrosis and ventricular aneurysm following closed chest injury in a child. J. Trauma 21:170, 1981.

40. Candell, J., Valle, V., Payá, J., Cortadellas, J., Esplugas, E., and Rius, J.: Post-traumatic coronary occlusion and early left ventricular aneurysm. Am. Heart J. 97:509, 1979.

41. Allen, R. P., and Liedtke, A. J.: The role of coronary artery injury and perfusion in the development of cardiac contusion secondary to nonpenetrating chest trauma. J. Trauma 19:153, 1979.

42. Smith, J. M., III, Grober, F. L., Marcos, J. J., Arom, K. V., and Trinkle, J. K.: Blunt traumatic rupture of the atria. J. Thorac. Cardiovasc. Surg. 71:617, 1976.

43. Hines, G. L., Doyle, E., and Acinapura, A. J.: Post-traumatic ventricular septal defect, mitral insufficiency, and multiple coronary cameral fistulas. J. Trauma 17:234, 1977.

44. Rayner, A. V. S., Fulton, R. L., Hess, P. J., and Daicoff, G. R.: Post-traumatic intracardiac shunts. Report of 2 cases and review of the literature. J. Thorac. Cardiovasc. Surg. 73:728, 1977.

45. Pickard, L. R., Mattox, K. L., and Beall, A. C., Jr.: Ventricular septal defect from blunt chest injury. J. Trauma 20:329, 1980.

46. Williams, J. B., Silver, D. G., and Laws, H. L: Successful management of heart rupture from blunt trauma. J. Trauma 21:534, 1981.

47. Kouwenhoven, W. B., Jude, J. R., and Knickerbocker, G. G.: Closed chest cardiac massage. J.A.M.A. 173:1064, 1966.

48. Bodily, K., and Fischer, R. P.: Aortic rupture and right ventricular rupture induced by closed chest cardiac massage. Minn. Med. 62:225, 1979.

49. Adelson, L.: A clinicopathologic study of the anatomic changes in the heart resulting from cardiac massage. Surg. Gynecol. Obstet. 104:513, 1957.

50. Gerry, J. L., Bulkley, B. H., and Hutchins, G. M.: Rupture of the papillary muscle of the tricuspid valve. A complication of cardiopulmonary resuscitation and a rare cause of tricuspid insufficiency. Am. J. Cardiol. 40:825, 1977.

51. Wolfe, W. G., Dudley, A. W., Jr., and Wallace, A. G.: A pathological study of unsuccessful cardiac resuscitation. Arch. Surg. 96:123, 1968.

52. Nelson, D. A., and Ashley, P. F.: Rupture of aorta during closed-chest cardiac massage. J.A.M.A. 193:681, 1965.

53. Clark, D. T.: Complications following closed-chest massage. J.A.M.A. 181:337, 1962.

54. Rehn, L.: Ueber penetrirende Herzwunden und Herznaht. Arch. Klin. Chir. 55:315, 1897.

55. Wilson, R. F., and Bassett, J.S.: Penetrating wounds of the pericardium or its contents. J.A.M.A. 195:513, 1966.

56. Symbas, P. N.: Chest trauma: What injury, what treatment approach? J. Cardiovasc. Med. 6:989, 1981.

57. Jones, E. W., and Helmsworth, J.: Penetrating wounds of the heart. Thirty years' experience. Arch. Surg. 96:671, 1968.

58. Fallahnejad, M., Kutty, A. C. K., and Wallace, H. W.: Secondary lesions of penetrating cardiac injuries. Ann. Surg. 191:228, 1980.

59. Doering, R. B., Stemmer, E. A., and Connolly, J. E.: Complications of indwelling venous catheters with particular reference to catheter embolus. Am. J. Surg. 114:259, 1967.

60. Bernhardt, L. C., Wegner, G. P., and Mendenhall, J. T.: Intravenous catheter embolization to the pulmonary artery. Chest 57:329, 1970.

61. Bloomfield, D. A.: The nonsurgical retrieval of intracardiac foreign bodies — An international survey. Cathet. Cardiovasc. Diagn. 4:1, 1978.

62. Escher, D. J. W.: Types of pacemakers and their complications. Circulation 47:1119, 1973.

63. Kaye, D., Frankl, D., and Arditi, L. I.: Probable postcardiotomy syndrome following implantation of a transvenous pacemaker. Report of the first case. Am. Heart J. 90:627, 1975.

64. Gorlin, R.: Perforations and other cardiac complications. Chapter 6 in Cooperative Study on Cardiac Catheterization. Circulation 47 (Suppl. 3):36, 1968.

65. Morrow, A. G., Reis, R. L., and Ross, J., Jr.: Cardiac tamponade during cardiac catheterization. Management by immediate pericardiostomy and drainage. Am. Heart J. 77:167, 1969.

66. Wellons, H. A., Jr., and Singh, R.: Acute dissecting aortic aneurysm resulting from retrograde brachial arterial catheterization. Successful operative intervention. Am. J. Cardiol. 33:562, 1974.

67. Wilder, J. R., Dhar, N., Khochadkar, A., and Kryger, S.: Penetration injury to the heart. J.A.M.A. 244:2080, 1980.

68. Boyd, T. F., and Strieder, J. W.: Immediate surgery for traumatic heart disease. J. Thorac. Cardiovasc. Surg. 50:305, 1965.

68a. Hassett, A., Moran, J., Sabiston, D. C., and Kisslo, J.: Use of echocardiography for the evaluation and management of penetrating missile wounds of the heart. J. Am. Coll. Cardiol. 1:708, 1983.

69. Cooper, F. W., Jr., Stead, E. A., Jr., and Warren, J. V.: The beneficial effect of intravenous infusions in acute pericardial tamponade. Ann. Surg. 120:822, 1944.

70. Fallah-Nejad, M., Wallace, H. W., Su, C. C., Kutty, A. C., and Blakemore, W. S.: Unusual manifestation of penetrating cardiac injuries. Arch. Surg. 11:1257, 1975.

71. Lemos, P. C. P., Akumura, M., Azeveda, A. C., DePaula, W., and Zerbini, E. J.: Cardiac wounds. Experience based on a series of 121 operated cases. J. Cardiovasc. Surg. 17:1, 1976.

72. Harvey, J. C., and Pacifico, A. D.: Primary operative management. Method of choice for stab wounds to the heart. South. Med. J. 68:149, 1975.

73. Symbas, P. N., Harlaftis, M. D., and Waldo, J. W.: Penetrating cardiac wounds: A comparison of different therapeutic methods. Ann. Surg. 183:377, 1976.

74. Szentpetery, S., and Lower, R. R.: Changing concepts in the treatment of penetrating cardiac injuries. J. Trauma 17:457, 1977.

75. Beach, P. M., Jr., Bognolo, D., and Hutchinson, J. E.: Penetrating cardiac trauma. Experience with 34 patients in a hospital without cardiopulmonary bypass capability. Am. J. Surg. 131:411, 1976.

76. Bland, E. F., and Beebe, G. W.: Missiles in the heart. A twenty-five year follow-up report of World War II cases. N. Engl. J. Med. 274:1039, 1966.

77. Moncada, R., Matuga, T., Unger, E., Freeark, R., and Pizarro, A.: Migratory trauma—cardiovascular foreign bodies. Circulation 57:186, 1978.

78. Alsofrom, D. J., Marcus, N. H., Seigel, R. S., Talbot, W. A., Akl, B. F., Schiller, W. R., and Sklar, D. P.: Shotgun pellet embolization from the chest to the middle cerebral arteries. J. Trauma 22:155, 1982.

79. Mattox, K. L., Beall, A. C., Jr., Ennix, C. L., and DeBakey, M. E.: Intravascular migratory bullets. Am. J. Surg. 137:192, 1979.

80. Asfaw, I., Thoms, N. W., and Arfulu, A.: Interventricular septal defects from penetrating injuries of the heart. A report of 12 cases and review of the literature. J. Thorac. Cardiovasc. Surg. 69:450, 1975.

81. Morritt, G. N., Taylor, N. C., Miller, H. C., and Walbaum, P. R.: Traumatic aortic regurgitation. J. R. Coll. Surg. (Edinb.) 24:87, 1979.

82. Stephenson, L. W., MacVaugh, H., III, and Kastor, J. A.: Tricuspid valvular incompetence and rupture of the ventricular septum caused by nonpenetrating trauma. J. Thorac. Cardiovasc. Surg. 77:768, 1979.

83. Watanabe, T., Katsume, H., Matsukubo, H., Furukawa, K., and Ijichi, H.: Ruptured chordae tendineae of the tricuspid valve due to nonpenetrating trauma. Chest 80:751, 1981.

84. Howard, C. P.: Aortic insufficiency due to rupture by strain of a normal aortic valve. Can. Med. Assoc. J. 19:12, 1928.

85. Kimbler, R. W., Stokes, J. P., and Barnhorst, D. A.: The surgical treatment of traumatic rupture of the aortic valve. Report of a case after blunt trauma. J. Trauma 17:168, 1977.

86. Roberts, W. C., and Maron, B. J.: Sudden death while playing professional football. Am. Heart J. 102:1061, 1981.

87. Pifarre, R., Grieco, J., Garibaldi, A., Sullivan, H. J., Montoya, A., and Bakhos, M.: Acute coronary artery occlusion secondary to blunt chest trauma. J. Thorac. Cardiovasc. Surg. 83:122, 1982.

88. Vlay, S. C., Blumenthal, D. S., Shoback, D., Fehir, K., and Bulkley, B. H.: Delayed acute myocardial infarction after blunt chest trauma in a young woman. Am. Heart J. 100:907, 1980.

89. Anderson, G. P., Adicoff, A., Motsay, G. J., Sako, Y., and Gobel, F. L.: Traumatic right coronary arterial–right atrial fistula. Am. J. Cardiol. 35:439, 1975.

90. Alter, B. R., Wheeling, J. R., Martin, H. A., Margo, J. P., Treasure, R. L., and McGranahan, G. M., Jr.: Traumatic right coronary artery–right ventricular fistula with retained intramyocardial bullet. Am. J. Cardiol. 40:815, 1971.

91. Snyder, J. S., Lindsay, J., Jr., Faris, J. V., and Glasser, S. P.: Traumatic coronary artery fistula. South. Med. J. 71:649, 1978.

92. Rea, W. J., Sugg, W. L., Wilson, L. C., Webb, W. R., and Ecker, R. R.: Coronary artery lacerations: An analysis of 22 patients. Ann. Thorac. Surg. 7:518, 1969.

93. Espada, R., Whisennard, H. H., Mattox, K. L., and Beall, A. C., Jr.: Surgical management of penetrating injuries to the coronary arteries. Surgery 78:755, 1975.

94. Symbas, P. N.: Great vessels injury. Am. Heart J. 93:518, 1977.

95. Greendyke, R. M.: Traumatic rupture of the aorta. Special reference to automobile accidents. J.A.M.A. 195:527, 1966.

96. Spencer, K. L., Guerin, P. F., Blake, H. A., and Bahnson, H. T.: A report of 15 patients with traumatic rupture of the aorta. J. Thorac. Cardiovasc. Surg. 41:1, 1961.

97. Ayella, R. J., Hankins, J. R., Turney, S. Z., and Cowley, R. A.: Ruptured thoracic aorta due to blunt trauma. J. Trauma 17:199, 1977.

98. Puijlaert, C. B. A. J.: Roentgen diagnosis of traumatic rupture of the aorta. Radiologia Clin. 45:217, 1976.

99. Symbas, P. N., Tyras, D. H., Ware, R. E., and Hatcher, C. R., Jr.: Rupture of the aorta. A diagnostic triad. Ann. Thorac. Surg. 15:405, 1973.

100. Kirsh, M. M., Orringer, M. B., Behrendt, D. M., Mills, L. J., Tashjian, J., and Sloan, H.: Management of unusual traumatic ruptures of the aorta. Surg. Gynecol. Obstet. 146:365, 1978.

101. Norman, J. C., Weber, W. J., Wilson, W. S., and Sloan, H.: Post-traumatic fistula of the aorta, pulmonary artery and right ventricle. Ann. Surg. 161:357, 1965.

102. Arom, K. V., and Lyons, G. W.: Traumatic pulmonary arteriovenous fistula. J. Thorac. Cardiovasc. Surg. 70:918, 1975.

103. Akins, C. W., Buckley, M. J., Daggett, W., McIlduff, J. B., and Austen, W. G.: Acute traumatic disruption of the thoracic aorta: A ten-year experience. Ann. Thorac. Surg. 31:305, 1981.

104. Pickard, L. R., Mattox, K. L., Espada, R., Beall, A. C., and DeBakey, M. E.: Transection of the descending thoracic aorta secondary to blunt trauma. J. Trauma 17:749, 1977.

105. Symbas, P. N., Kourias, E., Tyras, D. H., and Hatcher, C. R., Jr.: Penetrating wounds of great vessels. Ann. Surg. 179:757, 1974.

106. Vasko, J. S., Raess, D. H., Williams, T. E., Jr., Kakos, G. S., Kilman, J. W., Meckstroth, C. V., Cattaneo, S. M., and Klassen, K. P.: Nonpenetrating trauma to the thoracic aorta. Surgery 82:400, 1977.

107. Turney, S. Z., Attar, S., Ayella, R., Cowley, R. A., and McLaughlin, J.: Traumatic rupture of the aorta. A five-year experience. J. Thorac. Cardiovasc. Surg. 72:727, 1976.

45

DISEASES
OF THE AORTA

by Eve E. Slater, M.D., and Roman W. De Sanctis, M.D.

THE NORMAL AORTA

Function. Appropriately called by the ancients "the greatest artery," the aorta is admirably suited for its job. This thin but large and remarkably tough vessel must absorb the impact of 2.5 to 3 billion heartbeats in the average lifetime of an individual, while over the same span carrying roughly 200,000,000 liters of blood to the periphery!

Arteries can be categorized as either "conductance" or "resistance" vessels. Conductance vessels are the conduits for blood, and the aorta is the epitome of a conductance vessel. It is composed of three layers: a thin inner tunica intima; a thick tunica media; and a rather thin outer layer, the tunica adventitia. The strength of the aorta resides in its media, which is composed of laminated but intertwining sheets of elastic tissue arranged in a spiral fashion to afford maximum strength. As thin as it is, the wall of the aorta can withstand the experimental pressure of thousands of millimeters of mercury without bursting. In contrast to the peripheral arteries, the aortic media contains very little smooth muscle, although there is a network of some smooth muscle and collagen between the elastic membranes. This tremendous accretion of elastic tissue in the aorta gives it not only great tensile strength but also elasticity, which serves a vital circulatory function. The aortic intima is a thin, delicate layer linked by endothelium and easily traumatized. The adventitia contains mainly collagen but also houses the important vasa vasorum and lymphatics, which nourish the aortic wall.

As ventricular systole develops, part of the force imparted by the contracting ventricle is converted into potential energy stored in the wall of the aorta as it is distended by the bolus of blood ejected into it. In diastole, this potential energy in the stretched aortic wall is transformed into kinetic energy as the resilient aorta decompresses, and the force that is created acts against the column of blood contained within the lumen. With a competent aortic valve proximally, the blood is thus further propelled distally into the arterial bed. The pulse wave itself with its milking effect is transmitted along the aorta to the periphery at a speed of about 5 meters per second. This is much faster than the velocity of the intraluminal blood, which travels only 40 to 50 cm per second. Thus, the aorta plays a major role in keeping the blood circulating after it is delivered into the aorta by the heart.

The systolic pressure developed within the aorta is a function of the volume of blood ejected into the aorta, the compliance or distensibility of the aorta, and the resistance to blood flow. The last is determined primarily by the tone in the peripheral muscular arteries and arterioles and to a slight extent by the inertia of the column of blood in the aorta when systole commences. The aorta and its arterial branches tend to stiffen with age, accounting for the increase in systolic blood pressure as people grow older.

In addition to its conductance and pumping functions, the aorta plays a role in the control of systemic vascular resistance and heart rate. Pressure-responsive receptors analogous to those in the carotid sinus lie in the ascending aorta and the aortic arch and send afferent signals to the vasomotor center in the brain stem by way of the vagus nerves. Raising the aortic pressure causes reflex reduction of vascular resistance and bradycardia, whereas lowering the pressure increases the heart rate.

Anatomic Considerations. The aorta consists of thoracic and abdominal portions. In turn, the thoracic aorta is composed of three segments: the ascending aorta, the aortic arch, and the descending thoracic aorta.

The *ascending aorta* in a normal adult is about 3 cm wide at its origin from the base of the heart and extends 5 to 6 cm cephalad to join the arch. Normally, the ascending aorta lies just to the right of the midline. Its proximal portion is within the pericardial cavity. Nearby structures include the pulmonary trunk in front and the left atrium, right pulmonary artery, and right main stem bronchus behind.

The *arch of the aorta* gives rise to all of the brachiocephalic vessels. It courses slightly leftward in front of the trachea and then proceeds dorsally and inferiorly above the left main stem bronchus to the left of the trachea and esophagus. The arch assumes almost a directly anteroposterior orientation in the superior mediastinum. Other closely related structures are the left phrenic and vagus nerves to the left of the arch; inferiorly lie the bifurcation of the pulmonary trunk and most of the left lung. The left recurrent laryngeal nerve also loops underneath it distally.

The *descending thoracic aorta* is the continuation of the aorta beyond the arch. It lies in the posterior mediastinum to the left of the vertebral column, gradually courses in front of the vertebral column as it descends, occupying a position behind the esophagus, and passes through the diaphragm, usually at the level of the 12th thoracic vertebra.

A small but important segment called the *aortic isthmus* is the point at which the arch and descending thoracic aorta join. This is where coarctations of the aorta are usually located, and it is also the point at which the mobile portion of the aorta—the ascending aorta and arch—becomes relatively fixed to the thorax by the pleural reflections, intercostal arteries, and left subclavian artery. The aorta is especially vulnerable to trauma at this point.

The *abdominal aorta* forms the continuation of the thoracic aorta, giving off the important splanchnic vessels and ending in the aortic bifurcation at the level of the 4th lumbar vertebra.

EXAMINATION OF THE AORTA

Unless the aorta is abnormally enlarged, the only location at which it can be palpated is in the abdomen. The ease with which it can be felt depends largely on the body habitus and on the pulse pressure; it is readily felt in thin individuals. It is quite sensitive to pressure. Auscultation usually is unrevealing in aortic diseases, except for occasional bruits at sites of narrowing of the aorta or its tributary branches. Diseases of the proximal ascending aorta sometimes involve the aortic valve, with resultant aortic regurgitation.

Chest roentgenography and fluoroscopy are valuable and simple procedures for assessing the aorta. Normally, the ascending aorta is not visible on the direct anteroposterior chest roentgenogram. The aortic arch is seen as the aortic "knob" or "knuckle" in the superior mediastinum just to the left of the vertebral column (Fig. 6–1, p. 147). The edge of the descending thoracic aorta can often be recognized to the left of the spine.

On the lateral chest roentgenogram, the proximal ascending aorta can be seen as an indistinct shadow in the middle mediastinum arising from the base of the heart. The ascending aorta and arch are best demonstrated in a left anterior oblique projection—a view that should always be included when disease of the thoracic aorta is suspected (Fig. 6–12, p. 155).

Calcification in the aortic knob is often present, particularly in older people and patients with hypertension. It has little significance. Arteriosclerosis often results in extensive aortic calcification. The location of aortic calcification is useful in the differential diagnosis of aortic disease. For example, syphilis usually causes calcification of the ascending aorta predominantly, whereas arteriosclerotic calcification is ordinarily densest in the arch and the descending thoracic and abdominal aorta. Aneurysms of the abdominal aorta can often be seen radiographically if they are calcified. A lateral film of the abdomen is the most useful view for demonstrating them.

Normally, the aorta tends to elongate and widen slightly with age, a process which is accelerated by hypertension. Aneurysms, of course, appear as localized dilations of the aorta. It is sometimes difficult to distinguish aneurysms from other mediastinal masses. In such cases fluoroscopy may be very helpful by showing the presence or absence of pulsations in the mass.

Angiographic study of the aorta has represented a signal advance in the evaluation of aortic diseases. Aneurysms, aortic dissections, and occlusive disease of the aorta and its arterial branches can usually be readily demonstrated by a contrast study (Fig. 45–7). There is expectation that with technical improvements in digital subtraction angiography, performed by venous injection of contrast material, adequate aortic definition will be possible while obviating the need for catheterization of the aorta.[1]

Ultrasonography has also provided an important adjunct to the diagnosis of aortic diseases. The presence or absence of an abdominal aortic aneurysm can be definitively established by this simple noninvasive technique. In particular, cross-sectional (2-D) echocardiography (p. 135) is extremely accurate in both diagnosing and sizing abdominal aortic aneurysms (Fig. 45–1) and can also provide valuable information about the location and size of aortic root aneurysms.[2-4]

ANTERIOR

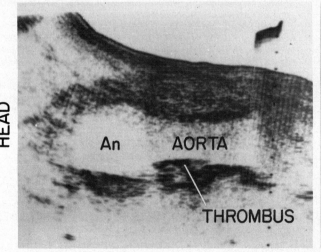 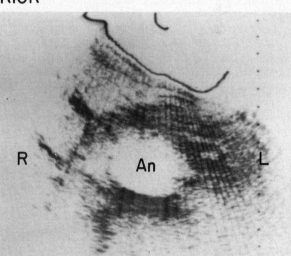

POSTERIOR

FIGURE 45–1 Cross-sectional echocardiograms of an abdominal aortic aneurysm in a 62-year-old man. *Left,* lateral view showing a 5-cm aneurysm (An), with dilatation of the aorta distal to the aneurysm. The widened aorta is visualized down to the aortic bifurcation. Note the thrombus in the wall of the aneurysm. The dense echoes between the aneurysm and skin are made up of subcutaneous fat, muscle, and mesenteric contents. *Right,* Echogram with the ultrasound beam oriented in the anteroposterior direction showing the aneurysm clearly. R and L indicate the patient's right and left sides. The distance between each of the dots aligned vertically on the right in both scans represents 1 cm. (Courtesy of Rob Kirkpatrick, M.D., Department of Radiology, Massachusetts General Hospital, Boston.)

Computed tomographic scanning of the body (CT scan), enhanced by intravenous injection of contrast material, is being used increasingly for noninvasive visualization of the aorta (see Fig. 45–4). CT scans are particularly useful for the diagnosis and sizing of thoracic and abdominal aortic aneurysms and for the diagnosis of aortic dissection and traumatic aneurysms of the aorta.[5,6,6a] In determining the size of abdominal aortic aneurysms, the CT scan is as accurate as ultrasonography, if not more so.

DISEASES OF THE AORTA

Pathogenesis

Although the pathogenesis of diseases of the aorta is discussed in several of the individual subsections, a brief commentary upon those factors which act adversely upon the aorta is appropriate at this point. Diseases of the aorta are either congenital or acquired. Congenital defects in turn are either gross anatomical abnormalities, such as coarctation, right aortic arch, anomalous arterial branches, double aortic arches, and so on, or histological disorders, such as degenerative abnormalities in the aortic wall that predispose to later problems, e.g., cystic medial degeneration in the Marfan syndrome and other inherited connective tissue disorders.

Acquired diseases of the aorta are primarily the result of degenerative changes in the aortic wall. Prominent among the factors which lead to this degeneration are aging, arteriosclerosis, hypertension, and specific infectious, inflammatory, or autoimmune diseases that involve the aorta focally or diffusely. Some of these processes may affect the aortic root, with resultant aortic regurgitation, or the major arterial branches arising from the aorta. Recently, the importance of the velocity at which blood is ejected from the left ventricle (dV/dt) as a major shearing stress on the aortic wall has also been emphasized as promoting aortic dissection.[8]

Arteriosclerosis is especially important in the pathogenesis of aortic aneurysms. There are several current theories, none mutually exclusive, to explain the development of atherosclerosis.[5] These are reviewed in Chapter 34.

Iwatsuki and colleagues have conducted a fascinating series of experiments: The initiation and maintenance of experimentally induced hypertension could be prevented or reversed by the inhibition of collagen cross linkage through administration of β-aminopropionitrile. This suggests that hypertension leads to structural aortic changes which, in turn, initiate an aortic response that serves to perpetuate the hypertensive syndrome.[9]

Indeed, hypertension itself may promote further damage, not only by injuring the endothelium or increasing formation of collagen but also by accelerating medial degeneration in patients with a molecular defect in their structural proteins, i.e., collagen or elastin—which then deteriorate more rapidly when exposed to hemodynamic stress. It appears that some degree of medial degeneration is part of the aging process, but these changes are much more extensive in individuals with hypertension.[10–12] Acute hypertension has also been shown experimentally to decrease blood flow into the vasa vasorum, thereby reducing nutrient flow into the media and resulting in ischemia and weakening of the wall.[13]

The only congenital gross anatomical disease considered in this chapter is pseudocoarctation. *Coarctation* is discussed on pages 887, 973, and 1038. All other conditions discussed either are acquired or result from congenital histological changes in the aortic wall.

ARTERIOSCLEROTIC AORTIC ANEURYSMS

Abdominal Aortic Aneurysms

Approximately three-quarters of all arteriosclerotic aortic aneurysms are confined to the abdominal aorta. Normally, in the adult, the aorta measures 2 cm in diameter at the level of the celiac axis, measures 1.8 cm just below the renal arteries, and continues to taper slightly to the iliac vessels. It is in the area between the renal arteries and the aortic bifurcation that most abdominal aneurysms occur. Clinically significant aneurysms measure 4 cm or more in diameter. (Charles De Gaulle, Albert Einstein, and Robert Frost all succumbed to ruptured abdominal aortic aneurysms.)

Etiology and Pathogenesis. Abdominal aortic aneurysms arise in some areas of dense atherosclerosis. The atherosclerotic process erodes the aortic wall, destroying the medial elastic elements. This causes weakening of the aortic wall and eventually leads to fusiform or, rarely, saccular dilatation of the abdominal aorta. As the aorta widens, tension in the wall of the aorta rises in accordance with Laplace law, which states that tension is proportional to the product of pressure and radius. Further widening results in greater tension, which in turn leads to acceleration in the rate of enlargement of the aneurysm. A vicious circle is thus established which produces dilatation that is often rapidly progressive. Hypertension may also contribute to the pathogenesis of these aneurysms.

Most abdominal aortic aneurysms arise just below the renal arteries and extend to, and sometimes involve, the aortic bifurcation. Only 2 to 5 per cent of abdominal aortic aneurysms are suprarenal, and these usually result from the distal extension of a thoracic aneurysm into the abdomen.[14] As aneurysms expand they may compress contiguous structures. Laminated thrombi frequently form in areas of stagnant flow within the aneurysm. Thrombotic and arteriosclerotic debris may embolize distally[15] (p. 1566) and compromise the circulation of tributary arteries. Finally, the aneurysm may rupture. Of those aneurysms which do rupture, 80 to 90 per cent rupture retroperitoneally, with a mean interval of 24 hours between rupture and death. The remainder rupture into the peritoneal cavity, causing rapid demise from exsanguination.[16]

CLINICAL MANIFESTATIONS. The majority of abdominal aneurysms are asymptomatic and are discovered on routine physical examination or on a routine abdominal roentgenogram.[17] Aneurysms may cause a sense of fullness in the epigastrium. If pain is present, it is usually located in the hypogastrium and lower back. The pain is usually steady, with a gnawing quality, and may last for hours or days at a time. In contrast to musculoskeletal back pain, it is not affected by movement, although patients may be more comfortable in certain positions, such as with the legs drawn up. Some astute asymptomatic patients may suspect an aneurysm by recognizing an abnormal pulsation of the aorta, as when lying down reading a book perched on the abdomen. Expansion and impending rupture are heralded by the development of pain, often of sudden onset, which is characteristically constant and severe and located in the back or lower abdomen, sometimes with radiation into groin, buttocks, or legs. Actual rupture is associated with the abrupt onset of catastrophic abdominal or back pain or both, hypotension, and usually shock. Pain is ordinarily particularly severe in the retroperitoneal area.[18,19]

Many aneurysms can be detected on physical examination, although even large aneurysms may be difficult or impossible to detect in obese individuals. When palpable, a pulsatile mass extending variably from between the xiphoid process to the umbilicus may be appreciated. Owing to difficulty in separating the abdominal aorta from surrounding structures by palpation, the size of an aneurysm tends to be overestimated in the physical examination. Moreover, it may sometimes be difficult to differentiate a tortuous, ectatic aorta from true aneurysmal dilatation. Aneurysms are often sensitive to palpation and may be quite tender if they are rapidly expanding or about to rupture. Aneurysms should always be palpated cautiously, particularly if they are tender.[20]

Associated occlusive arterial disease is sometimes present in the femoral pulses and pulses distally in the legs or feet. Bruits may be heard over the aneurysm or arising from the diseased arteries but are not requisite to the diagnosis. Rarely, an aneurysm may expand in such a way to occlude the inferior vena cava or one of the iliac veins, resulting in venous congestion and edema in one or both legs. Occasionally an arteriovenous fistula may be formed by spontaneous rupture into the inferior vena cava or iliac vein, and a syndrome of high-output cardiac failure results.

Patients who suffer rupture of an abdominal aortic aneurysm are critically ill. Hemorrhagic shock may ensue rapidly and is manifested by hypotension, vasoconstriction, skin mottling, diaphoresis, mental obtundation, and oliguria. Retroperitoneal hemorrhage may be signaled by hematomas in the flanks and groin. Rupture into the abdominal cavity may result in abdominal distention, whereas rupture into the duodenum presents as massive gastrointestinal hemorrhage.

DIAGNOSIS AND SIZING OF ANEURYSMS. Currently, aneurysms may be detected and their size estimated by six methods: (1) physical examination, (2) routine roentgenography, (3) abdominal cross-sectional echocardiography, (4) CT scan, (5) abdominal aortic angiography, and (6) digital subtraction angiography.

Brewster and colleagues have carefully compared the physical examination, routine roentgenography, two-dimensional echocardiography and aortic angiography for sizing abdominal aortic aneurysms.[21] Physical examination is clearly the least accurate. Lateral x-ray examination of the lumbar spine is inexpensive and reliably detects the outline of the aneurysm if its wall is calcified (Fig. 45–2). However, this is not the case in at least one-quarter of all patients with aneurysms; in them, therefore, the lesion cannot be visualized radiographically.[22]

Cross-sectional ultrasound is very accurate and is easily and atraumatically performed (Fig. 45–1). Refinements in ultrasonic techniques have permitted precise determination of the aortic adventitial border. Thus abdominal ultrasound is currently the simplest and best way to detect and size an abdominal aortic aneurysm.

Abdominal aortic angiography is less accurate in predicting size because the full width of an aneurysm may be masked by the presence of nonopacified mural thrombus (Fig. 45–3). Moreover, angiography carries with it a small but definite incidence of complications, including hematoma, localized dissection, infection, embolization, and renal

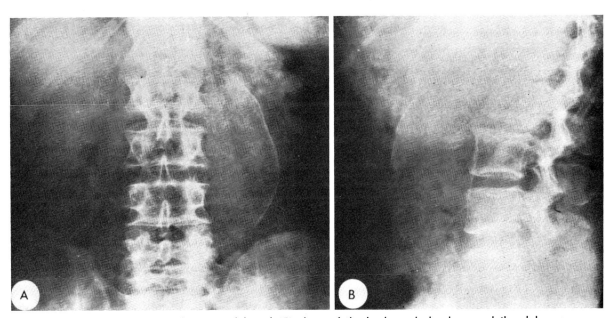

FIGURE 45–2 Anteroposterior (A) and lateral (B) views of the lumbar spinal column and the abdomen, disclosing a soft tissue mass with curvilinear calcification. (From Estes, J. E., Jr.: Abdominal aortic aneurysm: A study of one hundred and two cases. Circulation 2:261, 1950, by permission of the American Heart Association, Inc.)

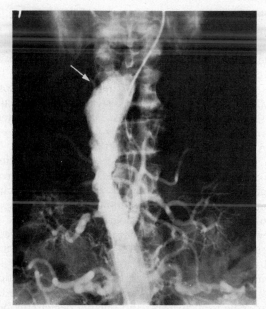

FIGURE 45–3 Abdominal aortogram showing an abdominal aortic aneurysm in a 64-year-old man. The aneurysm measures almost 6 cm in diameter and is wider than it appears because of a laminated thrombus in its wall. A faint rim of calcification outlining the left side of the aneurysm can be seen (arrow). The left renal artery is significantly narrowed. (Courtesy of Christos Athanasoulis, M.D., and Arthur Waltman, M.D., Section of Vascular Radiology, Massachusetts General Hospital, Boston.)

failure. Nevertheless, when angiography is performed in experienced hands, the morbidity from the procedure is minimal, and valuable information is often gleaned from it. Thus, in a survey of 190 patients, angiography of the aorta and distal circulation resulted in only minor complications in 2 per cent; averted an incorrect diagnosis in 11 per cent; revealed extension of the aneurysm above the renal arteries in 5 per cent; showed renal artery stenosis in 22 per cent and atypical renal arterial anatomy in 17 per cent; and delineated significant occlusive vascular disease in 48 per cent and associated aneurysms of the iliac, hypogastric, femoral, and popliteal vessels in 50 per cent.[23] Thus, aortography—if performed by experienced angiographers—is currently recommended for patients in whom there is any question of a correct diagnosis, for hypertensive patients with possible renal arterial disease, when the extent of the aneurysm is unclear, and for patients with suspected associated occlusive or aneurysmal diseases. In fact, at our institution, it is done routinely in most patients under consideration for surgery in order to facilitate perioperative management.

Current experience with CT scanning indicates that it may prove to be as useful as or even more accurate than ultrasound in the diagnosis and measurement of abdominal aortic aneurysms (see Fig. 45–4). CT scanning has additional advantages over ultrasound in that it provides information about the location of the renal arteries in relationship to the aneurysm; it may demonstrate retroperitoneal hemorrhage from an aneurysm; and it provides potentially useful information about other abdominal organs.[5,6] On the other hand, it does involve the use of radiation and is more costly and time-consuming than ultrasound.

Although experience with *digital subtraction angiography* (p. 191) is only now being accumulated, it is hoped that this technique will eventually yield information as detailed as that provided by aortography, while eliminating the need for intraarterial injection.

NATURAL HISTORY. There is a crucial relationship between the size of aneurysms and their natural history, which is why it is so important to determine their width. Half of all aneurysms greater than 6 cm in diameter rupture within 1 year, compared with 15 to 20 per cent of aneurysms less than 6 cm.[24] In a review of 24,000 consecutive autopsies, Darling et al. found that aneurysms 10 cm or larger had a 60 per cent incidence of rupture; those between 7 and 10 cm had a 45 per cent incidence of rupture; and those measuring 4 to 7 cm had a 25 per cent incidence of rupture.[25] The time course of rupture is hard to judge in such studies because so many patients succumb to complications of associated arteriosclerosis elsewhere, especially disease of the cerebrovascular and coronary arteries. However, Szilagyi et al. have computed mean survival for patients with aneurysms of less than 6 cm as 34.1 months, compared with 17.0 months for aneurysms greater than 6 cm.[24]

MANAGEMENT. At present, elective surgery is advised for all abdominal aortic aneurysms 6 cm in diameter or wider, assuming that surgical risks are not prohibitive because of other medical problems. Indeed, on the basis of Darling's studies, aneurysms as small as 4 cm should be resected in otherwise good surgical candidates. In poor-risk patients with aneurysms of 4 to 6 cm, close follow-up is advised with immediate surgery if the aneurysm is expanding or shows signs of impending rupture.

Surgery consists of resection of the aneurysm and insertion of a prosthesis, of which Dacron is the most widely

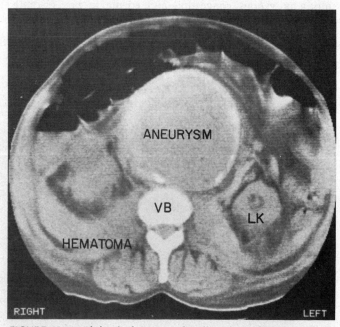

FIGURE 43–4 Abdominal CT scan showing a large, leaking abdominal aortic aneurysm. The aneurysm measures approximately 11 cm in diameter and abuts the vertebral body (VB) posteriorly. The light areas in the periphery of the aneurysm are calcific deposits in the aortic wall. The lower pole of the left kidney is identified (LK), and behind the right kidney is a retroperitoneal hematoma. (Courtesy of Dr. Jack Wittenberg, Department of Radiology, Massachusetts General Hospital, Boston.)

used at present.[26] Sometimes a simple tube graft is all that is necessary, although frequently the operation must be carried distally into one or both iliac vessels in order to excise the aneurysm completely. With large aneurysms, much of the wall of the aneurysm may be left in situ ("intrasaccular" approach of Creech). This reduces the need for extensive dissection, thereby decreasing aortic cross-clamping time, and has significantly diminished the problem of postoperative sexual dysfunction.

Expanding or ruptured abdominal aortic aneurysms are true surgical emergencies. In the case of rupture, patients can sometimes be stabilized by using a compression G-suit, a garment which may diminish the rate of bleeding by exerting counterforce externally against the abdomen. However, operation must be undertaken as soon as possible.[16]

Advances in perioperative management have improved survival rates in patients undergoing surgical resection of abdominal aortic aneurysms. Many of these patients have significant heart disease, and monitoring of the arterial blood pressure, cardiac output, cardiac filling pressures, and urine output may help enormously in their operative management.[27] These measurements provide a valuable guide to volume replacement. So-called "declamping shock" has been virtually eliminated by volume replacement guided by monitored pressures.[28] This term is applied to a syndrome characterized by marked hypotension upon release of the aortic cross clamp at the completion of surgery; the cause is believed to be pooling of blood in the dilated distal vascular bed and release of vasodepressor substances that have accumulated during surgery distal to the aortic clamp. The administration of mannitol and potent loop diuretics such as intravenous furosemide has reduced the frequency of postoperative renal failure.[29] The occurrence of renal failure postoperatively in patients with ruptured abdominal aortic aneurysms has correlated with very poor survival rates.[30] Autotransfusion has led to less frequent occurrence of hepatitis and fewer transfusion reactions.[31] Antibiotic coverage has reduced the frequency of infections. Hypothermia has been better controlled, and better understanding of the clotting system has improved management of hemostasis.[32]

Many patients with abdominal aortic aneurysms are heavy smokers and have serious chronic obstructive lung disease. Such patients have benefited greatly by improvements in postoperative respiratory care. Preoperative preparation of pulmonary patients is also important, and smokers should abstain from tobacco for at least 1 month in advance of surgery.[33]

If there is evidence of carotid artery disease in patients facing elective aneurysm resection, preoperative evaluation and surgery for critical carotid stenoses, if indicated, have resulted in fewer strokes. In occasional patients with severe coronary artery disease, it has proved wise to evaluate the coronary arterial tree angiographically and to perform coronary bypass surgery, if indicated, before subjecting the patient to aneurysm resection.[34] In cases of associated renal artery stenosis with renin-dependent hypertension or severe stenosis jeopardizing renal function, simultaneous renal artery reconstruction is often performed.[35]

OPERATIVE RISK. The risk of operation obviously depends on the general status of the patient and on whether or not the aneurysm has ruptured. Prompt recognition and immediate operation for patients with rupture have markedly improved survival rates. In low-risk patients, the mortality from the elective resection of abdominal aortic aneurysms should be 2 to 7 per cent. With expanding aneurysms, mortality is 5 to 15 per cent, and with rupture, mortality has reached a plateau at approximately 50 per cent, the major determinant of survival being the speed with which surgery is accomplished.[24,29,32,35–39]

Age and preexisting cardiac, pulmonary, cerebrovascular, and/or renal diseases all add to the risk of operation. Nevertheless, resection of nonruptured aneurysms in 63 octogenarian patients was accomplished with a 5 per cent overall mortality in an experienced center, contrasted with a 50 per cent mortality for unoperated-on patients; thus age per se should not be a definite contraindication for surgery in an otherwise healthy patient.[40]

An alternative to aneurysmectomy for very high-risk patients has been reported by Leather et al.[41] This group has combined thrombosis of the aortic aneurysm with right axillary to bilateral femoral artery bypass conduits. Thrombosis of the aneurysm usually followed the interruption of flow below the aortic bifurcation achieved by ligation of the iliac outflow vessels. If the aneurysm did not thrombose within 72 hours, the iliac outflow vessels responsible for continued patency were identified by angiography and were occluded by intraarterial injection of bucrylate. Although the perioperative and late mortality in these patients was high (6 deaths among 15 patients), the deaths were mostly related to associated diseases and not to the operative procedure itself.

The statistics showing better survival with elective resection of aneurysms are impressive. From several reports, the 5-year survival rate is only 5 to 10 per cent in patients with unexcised aneurysms larger than 6 cm, compared with over 50 per cent for those who undergo resection and 80 per cent for the age-matched "normal" population. *Late* survival is unaffected by whether the aneurysm was electively resected, acute, or ruptured.[39] With aneurysms smaller than 6 cm, the 5-year unoperated survival rate is about 50 per cent, as opposed to 60 to 70 per cent for those who undergo resection.[20,42–45]

COMPLICATIONS. The rate of late complications of aneurysmectomy has been reported as 8.5 per cent.[46] These complications include occlusion of the prosthesis (4 per cent), stenosis (0.6 per cent), false aneurysm formation (3 per cent), enteric fistula formation (1 per cent), and infection (3 per cent). Patients with graft occlusion usually have evidence of prior distal vascular disease which impedes aortic runoff. Occlusions occur mainly at the sites of anastomosis, and patients usually develop ischemic symptoms distal to the graft site. These stenoses may be increasingly amenable to correction by balloon catheter angioplasty (p. 297). False aneurysms may be caused by infection, but others arise spontaneously and are seen as expanding masses in the groin, abdomen, or lower back. Enteric fistulas are caused by rupture of the graft into the duodenum, resulting in gastrointestinal hemorrhage, and are associated with a high mortality. This complication can occur anywhere from 1 day to several years after operation, and the diagnosis must be suspected in any patient who has undergone abdominal aneurysmectomy and who presents with melena, hematemesis, hematochezia, or abdominal pain.[47] Recognition is obtained by gastrointestinal series, endoscopy, colonoscopy, or angiography. Infections most commonly are seen as a painful or tender groin mass, with or without a draining sinus. Recommended therapy involves administration of antibiotics, removal of the infected prosthetic material, and reestablishment of the circulation by an alternate route, usually axillofemoral bypass.

Attention has been called to the occasional occurrence of colonic ischemia following aneurysm surgery, caused by the necessary intraoperative sacrifice of the inferior mesenteric artery in patients with concomitantly diseased superior or mesenteric and hypogastric arteries, resulting in inadequate perfusion of the colon.[48,49] This complication is best avoided by paying careful attention to collateral blood flow to the colon, maintaining an inadequate blood pressure during surgery, and handling the distal colon carefully at the time of operation. If necessary, reimplantation of the inferior mesenteric artery can be performed if collateral circulation is inadequate.

THORACIC AORTIC ANEURYSMS

About one-quarter of all arteriosclerotic aneurysms involve the thoracic aorta.[50] Dilatation may occur anywhere along the thoracic aorta—that is, the ascending segment, the arch, or the descending portion; the latter two sites are the more common ones. This contrasts with luetic aneurysms, which are located predominantly in the ascending aorta. Sometimes the entire aorta is ectatic, with localized aneurysms at many sites in both the thoracic and the abdominal aorta. Aneurysms of the descending thoracic aorta not infrequently extend into the abdominal aorta, creating a thoracoabdominal aneurysm.

Pathogenesis. The pathogenesis of arteriosclerotic aneurysms is identical to that of those in the abdominal aorta. The arteriosclerotic process leads to weakening of the aortic wall, medial degeneration, and localized dilatation. Hypertension often coexists and contributes both to the undermining of the strength of the aortic wall and to expansion of the aneurysm. In the thorax, localized saccular aneurysms are somewhat more common than circumferential or fusiform aneurysms. The natural history of thoracic aneurysms differs somewhat from that of abdominal aortic aneurysms in that spontaneous rupture without warning is less common, because evidence of a growing thoracic aneurysm is usually afforded by symptoms caused by the compression of surrounding structures.[51]

CLINICAL MANIFESTATIONS. Thoracic aneurysms are very frequently associated with widespread atherosclerosis, particularly of the renal, cerebral, and cardiac arteries. In fact, the consequences of arterial obliterative disease in these other areas may dominate the clinical picture.

Symptoms and signs of thoracic aneurysms are related to their size and location and are caused primarily by their impingement upon adjacent structures. Thus, tracheal deviation, wheezing, cough, dyspnea, stridor, hemoptysis, recurrent pneumonitis, and intrapulmonary hemorrhage are the direct result of compression of the tracheobrachial tree and contiguous lung, especially the left main stem bronchus, by aneurysms of the descending thoracic aorta. Occasionally, an asymptomatic arch aneurysm will be visible or palpable rising above the suprasternal notch. Hoarseness may follow compression of the recurrent laryngeal nerve. Arch aneurysms sometimes produce a tracheal tug. Dysphagia arises from pressure against the nearby esophagus. The superior vena caval syndrome can develop as a consequence of obstruction of venous return from the superior vena cava or innominate veins.

Pain is due to compression and erosion of adjacent musculoskeletal structures. It is usually steady and boring—occasionally pulsating—and may be extremely severe. The sternum and right thoracic cage may be eroded by large aneurysms of the ascending aorta, and the vertebral column and posterior left ribs by descending thoracic aortic aneurysms. Visible and pulsatile masses are evident when aneurysms reach and begin to erode through the chest wall. Rupture of an aneurysm is heralded by the dramatic onset of excruciating pain, usually in the area where some pain had existed previously.

DIAGNOSIS. Most thoracic aortic aneurysms are readily visible on chest roentgenograms (Fig. 45–5), with fluoroscopy helping to differentiate an aneurysm from other types of mediastinal masses, such as neoplasms. However, some aneurysms are small, especially saccular aneurysms, which may rupture without having been visible on chest roentgenogram (Fig. 45–6).

Aortic angiography is clearly the definitive procedure for outlining an aneurysm, to make a diagnosis and to reveal the anatomical features of the aneurysm (Fig. 45–7). It should be performed in all patients under consideration for surgical repair. CT enhanced by the use of a contrast medium can be used to identify and size aneurysms of both the ascending and the descending thoracic aorta.[6,7] Alternatively, significant aneurysms of either the ascending or the descending thoracic aorta can be defined by cross-sectional echocardiography, but in the thoracic aorta, as contrasted with the abdominal aorta, this technique is not nearly so accurate as the CT scan, especially in the descending thoracic aorta.

NATURAL HISTORY. Data for the true natural history of arteriosclerotic thoracic aortic aneurysms are somewhat scanty, but, as with abdominal aneurysms, ultimate survival is related to the size of the aneurysms. Thoracic aneurysms greater than 6 or 7 cm in diameter are more prone to rupture than smaller ones.[51] Aneurysms that indicate expansion by producing symptoms of compression of surrounding structures are obviously diagnosed and treated earlier than aneurysms at silent sites. As noted, thoracic aneurysms are frequently associated with severe generalized arteriosclerosis, and many patients die of complications of arteriosclerosis before an aneurysm can rupture. When aneurysms do pursue a natural course, it has been found that symptomatic aneurysms are more prone to rupture than asymptomatic ones. In the study of Joyce et al. of 107 patients with thoracic aneurysms—73 per cent of which were arteriosclerotic—a 27 per cent 5-year survival rate for patients with symptomatic aneurysms was reported, as opposed to a 58 per cent 5-year survival rate for those without symptoms.[52] One-third of all deaths were attributed to aneurysm rupture, but over one-half of the mortality was caused by complications of arteriosclerosis unrelated to the aneurysm.

MANAGEMENT. Historically, surgical therapy once consisted of the introduction of long lengths of thrombogenic wire into an aneurysm, with the resultant thrombus

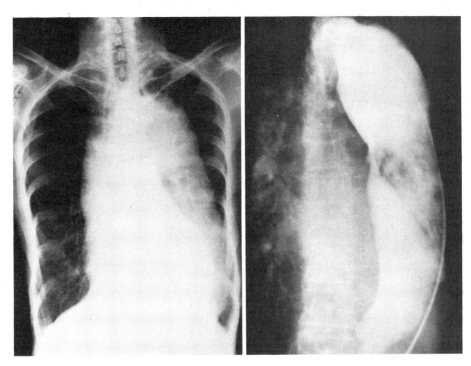

FIGURE 45–5 Large arteriosclerotic aneurysm of the descending thoracic aorta in a 69-year-old man. *Left*, Posteroanterior chest roentgenogram showing the widened aorta. *Right*, The aneurysm is outlined with contrast medium and originates just distal to the aortic arch, extending to the level of the diaphragm. (Courtesy of Robert Dinsmore, M.D., Chief of Cardiac Radiology, Massachusetts General Hospital, Boston.)

buttressing the wall of the aneurysm.[53] Direct wrapping of the aneurysm has also been tried. Currently, surgical excision is the procedure of choice whenever possible and is advised for aneurysms measuring 7 cm or more in diameter in the ascending and descending thoracic aorta. Clearly, even smaller aneurysms should be resected if they are producing symptoms. The aggressiveness with which surgical repair is undertaken depends greatly upon the general condition of the patient. The surgical procedure must be tailored to the specific aneurysm. Saccular aneurysms can sometimes be excised directly without resection of the aorta. Fusiform aneurysms in the ascending and descending thoracic aorta are best resected and replaced with a prosthetic tubular sleeve of appropriate size. Total cardiopulmonary bypass is necessary for the removal of ascending aortic aneurysms, and partial bypass to support the circulation distal to the aneurysm is often advisable in the resection of descending thoracic aortic aneurysms. A temporary shunt (Gott shunt) may be required from the proximal aorta to the aorta beyond the aneurysm to divert blood around the site of the aneurysm while it is being repaired.

Although fusiform aneurysms of the arch have been successfully excised surgically, the risks of operation in this area are high. Arch aneurysmectomy requires not only excision of the aneurysm but also reimplantation of all the brachiocephalic vessels. Perfusion by local cannulation of each of these important arteries is necessary while they are being reimplanted. Alternatively, resection of the aneurysm using profound hypothermia and circulatory arrest, a technique that is becoming increasingly favored by many surgical groups, has been employed successfully.[54,55]

Surgical results have improved considerably in recent years, with most major centers reporting an 80 to 85 per cent survival rate for the elective resection of ascending and descending thoracic aortic aneurysms.[56] Kidd et al. reported the results of operation in 83 patients with arteriosclerotic aneurysms of the ascending aorta operated upon

between 1970 and 1975.[57] There was a 90 per cent early and an 84 per cent late survival rate. In a report on 82 patients with thoracoabdominal aneurysms, the survival rate was 94 per cent.[58]

Major complications of the operation are technical, especially hemorrhage from tearing of the diseased aorta. A

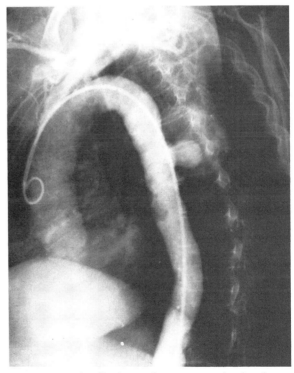

FIGURE 45–6 A localized saccular aneurysm in the descending thoracic aorta is clearly shown in the aortic angiogram of this 62-year-old man. The aneurysm had leaked, and a faint halo caused by the hematoma can be seen surrounding the aneurysm. The routine chest film appeared normal in this patient. (Courtesy of Christos Athanasoulis, M.D., and Arthur Waltman, M.D., Section of Vascular Radiology, Massachusetts General Hospital, Boston.)

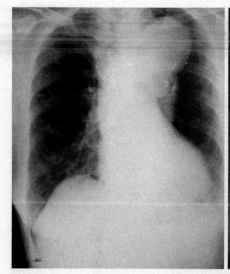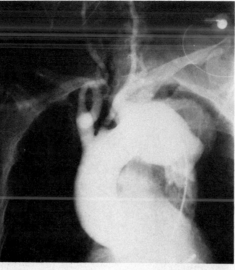

FIGURE 45–7 *Left,* Posteroanterior chest roentgenogram in a 66-year-old woman with an arteriosclerotic aneurysm of the descending thoracic aorta. *Right,* Aortographic appearance in the left oblique anterior projection. The aneurysm arises just at the site of origin of the left subclavian artery. Thrombus is evident in the outer wall of the aneurysm on the angiogram. (Courtesy of Christos Athanasoulis, M.D., and Arthur Waltman, M.D., Section of Vascular Radiology, Massachusetts General Hospital, Boston.)

catastrophic complication of resection of descending thoracic aortic aneurysms is paraplegia from the inadvertent interruption of the arterial blood supply to the spinal cord. This problem has been reduced considerably by maintaining distal aortic perfusion during surgery; by reducing the period of aortic cross clamping; by removal of minimal segments of aorta with the attendant intercostal arteries, especially in the areas of T7 through T9; and by prompt treatment of hypertension in the proximal aorta, which elevates cerebrospinal fluid pressure, thus reducing collateral blood flow to the spinal cord.[55,59–61] Complications of associated arteriosclerosis, such as myocardial infarction, cerebrovascular infarcts, and renal failure, often manifest themselves under the massive physiological stress of surgery.

Many patients with arteriosclerotic aneurysms are heavy smokers, and pulmonary complications are frequent. The left lung may be severely traumatized in resection of large aneurysms of the descending thoracic aorta, a complication which may seriously jeopardize the patient, particularly if there is underlying pulmonary disease.

Widespread aneurysmal dilatation of the aorta often precludes operation, although there are isolated reports of successful surgical replacement of essentially the entire diseased thoracic and abdominal aorta.[62] Associated diseases —especially pulmonary—make any operation impossible in still others. Although it seems logical to reduce blood pressure vigorously in patients with aneurysms and to reduce the velocity of ventricular ejection (p. 1553), the long-term impact of such therapy on retarding the expansion of aneurysms and improving survival is unknown.

AORTIC DISSECTION

Acute aortic dissection is a relatively common catastrophic illness and occurs at the rate of at least 2000 new cases per year in the United States.[63–65] Over the past two decades, great strides have been made in the diagnosis and the medical and surgical treatment of this highly lethal disease. It has been cogently pointed out that the term *dissecting hematoma* describes this entity more accurately than does the more widely used dissecting aneurysm. More

recently, the simpler term *aortic dissection* has gained favor.

Aortic dissection is caused by the sudden development of a tear in the aortic intima, opening the way for a column of blood driven by the force of the arterial pressure to enter the aortic wall, destroying the media and stripping the intima from the adventitia for variable distances along the length of the aorta.[65a] It is uncertain whether the primary event in aortic dissection is rupture of the intima with secondary dissection into the media, or hemorrhage within a diseased media followed by disruption of the subjacent intima and subsequent propagation of the dissection through the intimal tear (Fig. 45–8). However, it is clear that occasional cases of extensive aortic dissection can occur without any identifiable intimal tear.

The manifestations of aortic dissection in any given patient are determined by the path taken by the dissecting hematoma as it progresses through the aorta. Thus, the circulation of any major artery arising from the aorta may be compromised; disruption of the support of the aortic valve by extension into the aortic root may cause aortic incompetence; and finally the dissecting column may rupture through the adventitia anywhere along the aorta, although the two most common sites of rupture are the pericardial space and the left pleural cavity.

CLASSIFICATION. Most schemata for classification of aortic dissection are based upon the fact that over 95 per cent of all dissections arise in one of two locations: (1) the ascending aorta within several centimeters of the aortic valve; and (2) the descending thoracic aorta, usually just beyond the origin of the left subclavian artery at the site of the ligamentum arteriosum.[64] The widely used classification of DeBakey et al. recognizes three groups (Fig. 45–9).[66] Types I and II both begin in the ascending aorta; Type I extends beyond the ascending aorta and arch, whereas Type II is confined to the ascending aorta. Type III originates in the descending thoracic aorta and usually propagates distally for a variable distance; more rarely, it extends retrograde into the arch and ascending aorta. An additional category, Type IV, has recently been proposed to include iatrogenic retrograde dissection due to intraarterial catheterization or cannulation.[67]

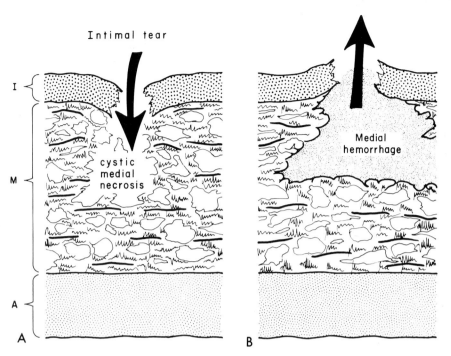

Intimal tear

cystic medial necrosis

Medial hemorrhage

FIGURE 45–8 Proposed mechanisms of initiation of aortic dissection. In both cases, cystic medial necrosis is present. In *A*, an intimal tear is the initial event, allowing aortic blood to enter the media. In *B*, the primary event is hemorrhage into the media, with secondary rupture of the overlying intima. I = intima; M = media; A = adventitia.

Still another classification, based upon approach to therapy and proposed by Daily et al., delineates two types, A and B.[68] Type A includes all proximal dissections and those distal dissections that extend retrograde to the arch and ascending aorta; Type B refers to all other distal dissections without proximal extension.

Since the behavior and management of Types I and II dissections are similar, many investigators, including ourselves, have adopted a simple two-category classification into "proximal" (DeBakey Types I and II) and "distal" (DeBakey Type III) dissections.[69] "Ascending" and "descending" have also been used synonymously with "proximal" and "distal." Proximal dissections occur more frequently than distal dissections in a ratio of almost two to one in autopsy series. However, because proximal dissections are more rapidly lethal, many clinical series report larger numbers of patients with distal than proximal dissection.[69,70]

Occasional other sites of origin are the aortic arch and the abdominal aorta. Furthermore, individual arteries may be the locus of isolated dissection, especially the coronary and carotid arteries.[71,72] The subject of aortic dissection has been discussed in several recent reviews.[63–65]

ETIOLOGY AND PATHOGENESIS. Degeneration of the aortic media is believed to be the pathological prerequisite for the development of aortic dissection.[64,65,65a] Usually, this consists of deterioration of the collagen and elastic tissue, often with cystic changes. This process, termed cystic medial necrosis or degeneration, most often is the result of chronic stress against the aortic wall, such as might occur with longstanding hypertension. Indeed, hypertension is an important contributing factor to aortic dissection and is found in well over half of all cases. It is especially prevalent with distal dissection.

Although some degree of medial degeneration has been shown to be part of the normal aging process in the aorta, these changes are qualitatively and quantitatively much greater in patients with aortic dissection.[11,12] Cystic medial degeneration is an intrinsic feature of the hereditary defects of connective tissue, especially the Marfan (p. 1665) and Ehler-Danlos (p. 1668) syndromes. Indeed, aortic dissection—especially proximal dissection—is a frequent and serious complication of Marfan (see p. 1556) syndrome. However, cystic medial degeneration and aortic dissection may occur in the absence of an associated phenotypic syndrome.[73] Certain congenital cardiovascular abnormalities, especially coarctation of the aorta and bicuspid aortic valves, seem to predispose to aortic dissection.[74,75] A combination of bicuspid aortic valve, cystic medial degeneration, and aortic root dissection in the absence of the Marfan syndrome has been described.[76]

An unexplained relationship exists between pregnancy and aortic dissection. About half of all aortic dissections in women under the age of 40 occur during pregnancy, usually in the last trimester. Isolated coronary artery dissection also usually occurs during pregnancy.

In older patients, dissections occasionally originate by way of perforation through an intimal atheromatous plaque. Trauma almost never causes a classic aortic dissection, although a localized tear in the region of the aortic isthmus is not uncommon following massive chest trauma.[77] Rarely, dissection of the aorta is a complication of other forms of vasculitis, including granulomatous arteritis (p. 1663).

Although strenuous physical exertion and emotional stress have been linked to aortic dissection, such a relationship is not usual. In a series of 124 cases of aortic dissection that we reviewed, we found such a history in only 14 per cent.[69]

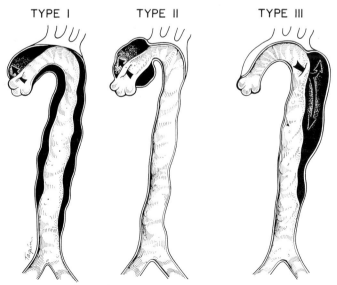

TYPE I   TYPE II   TYPE III

"PROXIMAL" or "ASCENDING"   "DISTAL" or "DESCENDING"

FIGURE 45–9   The DeBakey classification of aortic dissections.

The role played by chemicals toxic to connective tissue in the etiology of dissecting aneurysm in human beings is unknown. It is well known that the seeds of *Lathyrus odoratus* (sweet pea), which contain aminopropionitrile, cause cystic medial degeneration and dissecting aneurysm in rats.[78] We have encountered a proximal dissection in a young man with no other obvious predisposing factors who had a prolonged industrial exposure to dimethyl hydrazine, a connective tissue toxin.[69]

CLINICAL MANIFESTATIONS. Aortic dissection afflicts men more frequently than women in a ratio of approximately two to one and has a peak incidence in the sixth and seventh decades, with a range from childhood well into the nineties.[79] Patients with proximal dissection are on the average somewhat younger.[80] By far the most common presenting symptom of aortic dissection is *severe pain*, which is found in over 90 per cent of cases.[80a] In fact, those patients without pain usually have suffered some disturbance of consciousness as a result of the dissection that renders them unable to perceive pain. Nonetheless, painless dissection can and does occur rarely.[81]

Cataclysmic in onset, the pain of aortic dissection is often as severe at its inception as it ever becomes. This feature contrasts with that of myocardial infarction, where the pain usually has a crescendo-like onset. The pain of dissection may be all but unbearable, forcing the patient to writhe in agony or to pace restlessly in an attempt to gain some measure of relief. Several features of the pain may arouse suspicion of aortic dissection. The quality of the pain as described by the patient is often remarkably appropriate to the actual event. Adjectives such as "tearing," "ripping," and "stabbing" are frequently used. Another characteristic of the pain of aortic dissection is its tendency to migrate from the point of its origin to other sites, following the path of the dissecting hematoma as it extends through the aorta. Vasovagal manifestations, such as a drenching sweat, apprehension, nausea, vomiting, and faintness, are common at the outset.

The location of pain may be of some help in suggesting the site of origin.[69] Pain felt maximally in the anterior thorax is more frequent with proximal dissection, whereas pain that is most severe in the interscapular area is much more common with a distal site of origin. Although pain may be felt simultaneously in the anterior and posterior chest with both proximal and distal dissection, the *absence* of posterior interscapular pain strongly militates against a distal dissection, since over 90 per cent of patients with distal dissection report some back pain. Pain in the neck, throat, jaw, or teeth often occurs in dissections that involve the ascending aorta or arch.

Less common modes of presentation include congestive heart failure with or without associated chest pain, cerebrovascular accidents, syncope, paraplegia, and pulse loss with or without ischemic pain. Heart failure usually results from severe aortic regurgitation secondary to the dissection. The occurrence of syncope in aortic dissection may bear special significance. Syncope without focal neurological signs occurred in 6 of 124 patients in our series. In each case, there was evidence for rupture of the dissection into the pericardial cavity with cardiac tamponade.[69]

DIAGNOSIS. The diagnosis of aortic dissection can often be made with reasonable assurance from the *physical examination* alone. It has been noted that patients with aortic dissection may appear to be in shock; however, the blood pressure when measured is frequently elevated.[82] Over 50 per cent of patients with distal dissection are hypertensive on initial presentation. Hypotension usually results from cardiac tamponade; intrapleural or intraperitoneal rupture; or dissection of the brachiocephalic vessels resulting in "pseudohypotension," i.e., the inability to measure the blood pressure accurately because of occlusion of the brachial arteries.

Those physical findings most typically associated with aortic dissection, namely, pulse deficits, aortic regurgitation, and neurological manifestations, are more characteristic of proximal than distal dissection. Pulse abnormalities, which include the absence, diminution, or reduplication of pulses, occur in approximately one-half of patients with proximal dissection and, most commonly, involve the brachiocephalic vessels. Pulse deficits are much less common in patients with distal dissection and tend to involve the left subclavian and femoral arteries, although the femoral vessels are equally affected by the distal propagation of a proximal dissection. As depicted in Figure 45–10, pulses may be lost either by direct compression of the lumen of an artery by extension of the dissection into it or by blockade due to a flap of intima overlying the vessel orifice. Rarely, intimointimal intussusception may occur.[83] In either case, pulse deficits in aortic dissection may be transitory owing to decompression of the hematoma by distal reentry into the true lumen or by movement of the intimal flap away from the occluded orifice.

Aortic regurgitation is an important feature of proximal dissection and occurs in over 50 per cent in most series.[83a] When aortic regurgitation is present in patients with distal dissection, it most commonly antedates the dissection and results from preexisting dilatation of the aortic root due to severe hypertension or annuloaortic ectasia. The murmur of aortic regurgitation in aortic dissection often has a musical quality and may be heard better along the right than the left sternal border (p. 1111). It may wax and wane, the intensity varying directly with the height of the arterial blood pressure. Depending upon the severity of the regurgitation, other peripheral signs of aortic incompetence may be present, such as collapsing pulses and a wide pulse pressure. There are three mechanisms of aortic regurgitation in proximal dissection (Fig. 45–11): First, the dissec-

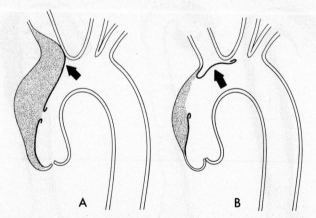

FIGURE 45–10 Two possible mechanisms for the loss of pulses in aortic dissection. In *A*, the dissecting column of blood occludes the origin of the innominate artery. In *B*, a flap of intima obstructs the orifice. Distal reentry may decompress the hematoma, or the intimal flap may move away from the orifice. If either occurs, pulses may be wholly or partially restored.

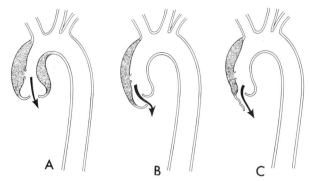

FIGURE 45–11 Mechanisms of aortic regurgitation in proximal dissecting aortic aneurysm. *A*, A circumferential tear pulls the annulus apart, preventing the leaflets from coapting. *B*, With asymmetrical dissection, pressure from the hematoma depresses one leaflet below the line of closure of the other. *C*, The annular support is disrupted, resulting in a flail aortic leaflet and aortic regurgitation.

tion may dilate the aortic root, widening the annulus so that aortic leaflets are unable to coapt in diastole; second, in an asymmetrical dissection, pressure from the dissecting hematoma may depress one leaflet below the line of closure of the others; and third, the annular support of the leaflets or the leaflets themselves may be torn so as to render the valve incompetent.

As noted, patients with proximal dissection sometimes have heart failure, which is almost always due to the sudden onset of severe aortic insufficiency. In rare cases, the congestive failure may be so severe as to mask the murmur and other usual signs of aortic regurgitation. In a few such patients whom we have encountered, the presence of disproportionately bounding pulses in the face of severe heart failure, coupled with a history highly suggestive of aortic dissection, served as a clue to the correct diagnosis.

Neurological deficits associated with aortic dissection include cerebrovascular accidents, ischemic peripheral neuropathy, ischemic paraparesis, and disturbances of consciousness.[84] Each of these is more common with proximal dissection, but deficits in the lower extremities are equally frequent in proximal and distal dissection.

Other occasionally encountered clinical manifestations of aortic dissection include pulsation of one of the sternoclavicular joints,[85] Horner's syndrome due to compression of the superior cervical sympathetic ganglion, vocal cord paralysis and hoarseness from pressure against the left recurrent laryngeal nerve, superior mediastinal syndrome from superior vena caval compression,[86] pulsating neck masses, tracheal or bronchial compression with bronchospasms,[64,87] hemorrhage into the tracheobronchial tree with hemoptysis,[88] hematemesis due to perforation into the esophagus,[89] heart block from retrograde burrowing of a dissection into the interatrial septum and thence down to the AV node,[90] and a continuous murmur due to rupture into the right atrium or ventricle.[91] Pleural effusions result from rupture of the dissection into one of the pleural spaces—usually the left—or simply from an exudative inflammatory reaction around the involved aorta. Additional complications may result from occlusion of important arteries by the dissection. Mesenteric infarction, renal infarction with severe renovascular hypertension, and myocardial infarction (seen in 1 to 2 per cent of patients with proximal dissection) are among the more serious occlusive events. Occasionally,

high fever results presumably from the release of pyrogenic substances from the hematoma or from associated effusions.

Routine laboratory studies are not very helpful in making the diagnosis of aortic dissection. Anemia may develop from significant hemorrhage or sequestration of blood in the false channel. A mild to moderate polymorphonuclear leukocytosis (10,000 to 14,000/mm^3) is common. Lactic acid dehydrogenase (LDH) and bilirubin levels are sometimes elevated because of hemolysis of blood sequestered within the false lumen. Serum glutamic oxaloacetic transaminase (SGOT) and creatine phosphokinase (CPK or CPK-MB) values are usually normal. Disseminated intravascular coagulation has been reported rarely.[92] The electrocardiogram frequently shows left ventricular hypertrophy from preexistent hypertension and usually the absence of acute ischemic changes. The absence of electrocardiographic changes of myocardial ischemia or infarction in a patient with severe chest pain is a helpful point in differential diagnosis from myocardial infarction.

Diagnostic ultrasound (M-mode), in combination with cross-sectional (2-D) echocardiography, is helpful in the detection of a proximal dissection by revealing a widened aortic root, with delineation of the dissecting hematoma[93–95,95a] (Fig. 45–12). CT scan with contrast injection is quite accurate in defining both ascending and descending dissections, provided there is identification of a false lumen to distinguish the dissection from a fusiform aneurysm.[6,7,95–97,95a] Although 2-D echocardiography and CT clearly offer the advantage of noninvasive diagnosis,[95b] angiography is generally required to define the full extent of the dissection, to outline the relationship of the dissection to the major aortic branches, to evaluate aortic valve competency, and to identify the site of the intimal tear. Thus, these noninvasive techniques—especially the CT scan—may be most useful in the long-term follow-up of treated patients with aortic dissection, for evidence of localized aneurysm formation.[98,99] Chest roentgenogram and aortic angiography provide the most substantive laboratory means of initial and definitive diagnosis, respectively. Chest roentgenography almost always reveals an abnormally widened aortic contour.[100] A localized bulge may overlay the site of origin, and the aortic silhouette may be widened wherever the dissection extends. If the aortic knob is calcified, a greater than 1 cm separation of the intimal calcification from the adventitial border (the "calcium sign") is virtually pathognomonic of aortic dissection (Fig. 45–13). Tracheal deviation or a left pleural effusion may be seen. Comparison to previous films is most helpful. On the other hand, it is possible for extensive aortic dissection to occur without radiographic abnormalities.

Fluoroscopy of the aorta may suggest aortic dissection in that pulsations in the abnormally widened aorta are diminished or absent over an area of dissection. This contrasts with the exaggerated pulsations usually seen in a true aneurysm.

The single, most important study in the diagnosis of aortic dissection is *aortic angiography*. Although originally performed by injection of contrast material into the pulmonary artery with aortic opacification following the pulmonary venous phase, retrograde angiography is now the method of choice. The hazards of this approach have proved minimal, provided the catheter is carefully inserted

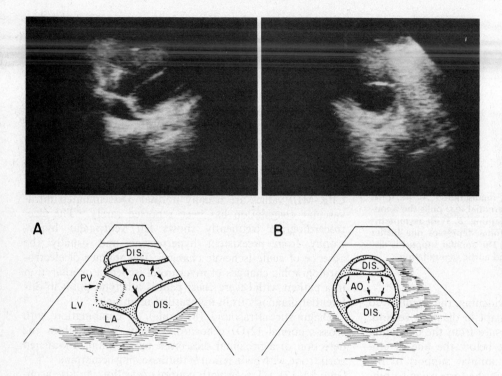

DIS.

PV   AO

LV   DIS.

LA

A

DIS.

AO

DIS.

B

FIGURE 45–12 Cross-sectional echogram of the proximal aorta in a 63-year-old woman with dissection of the proximal aorta occurring 12 years after implantation of a Starr-Edwards aortic valve prosthesis. *A*, Parasternal long-axis recording. *B*, Short-axis recording. The actual recordings are shown above, and diagrammatic representations of the findings are pictured below. The echodense prosthetic valve (PV) is easily seen on the long-axis recording. Surrounding the aorta (AO) is the false channel of the dissection (DIS). (From Weyman, A. E.: Cross-sectional Echocardiography. Philadelphia, Lea and Febiger, 1982.)

and contrast material is not injected into the false channel. Aortic angiography has three objectives: (1) to establish a definite diagnosis, (2) to identify the site of origin of the dissection, and (3) to delineate the extent of the dissection and the distal circulation to vital organs (Fig. 45–14 and 45–15).

One additional feature to be assessed by angiography is the degree to which the false channel is opacified. There is evidence that the prognosis in medically treated patients is

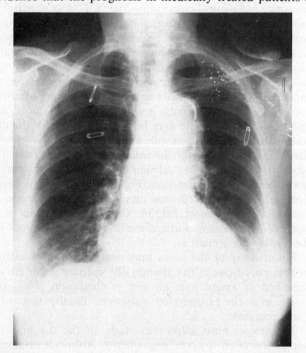

FIGURE 45–13 "Calcium sign" in distal dissection in an 80-year-old woman with longstanding hypertension. Note the marked separation of the calcification in the aortic knob and descending thoracic aorta from the outer wall of the aorta. This distance is normally no greater than 0.5 cm.

better in those with a nonopacified false channel, presumably an indication of thrombus formation in the channel which may serve to buttress the wall of the dissected aorta.[101] Although highly accurate, angiography is not without occasional pitfalls in the detection of aortic dissection. Failure of angiography to show a dissection can occur if there is faint opacification of the false lumen, unusual tearing of the intima, a very small and localized dissection, or equal simultaneous opacification of both channels.[102] Nevertheless, when properly performed and interpreted, angiography provides a definitive diagnosis in almost every case and is well tolerated by even critically ill patients.

MANAGEMENT. Therapy for aortic dissection is directed at halting the progression of the dissecting hematoma, since fatal complications arise not from the intimal tear itself, but rather from the subsequent course taken by the dissection.[102a] Without treatment, aortic dissection is almost always fatal. In a collective review of long-term survival in untreated aortic dissection, more than one-quarter of all patients were dead within 24 hours, more than one-half died within the first week, more than three-quarters died within 1 month, and more than 90 per cent died within 1 year.[103]

The first surgical approach to aortic dissection was the so-called fenestration procedure by which the dissected aorta was incised and a distal communication was created between the true and false channels, thereby decompressing the false lumen.[104,105] Definitive surgical therapy was pioneered by DeBakey and colleagues in the early 1950's.[106] Its principles are to excise the intimal tear; to obliterate the false channel by oversewing aortic edges; to reconstitute the aorta with or without interposition of a synthetic graft; and to restore aortic valve competence by resuspension of the displaced aortic leaflets or by prosthetic valve replacement of the aortic valve in the case of proximal dissection.

In the midst of growing enthusiasm for surgical therapy,

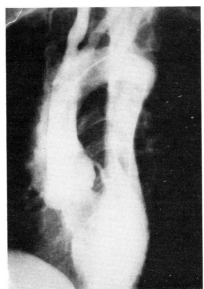
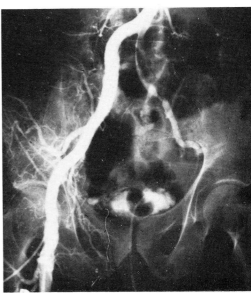

FIGURE 45–14 *Left*, Thoracic aortogram in the left anterior oblique projection showing a dissection beginning in the ascending aorta and spiraling through the aortic arch into the descending aorta. The false lumen can be faintly visualized. *Right*, Angiogram of the distal aorta showing virtual obstruction of the left iliac artery by the dissection. (Courtesy of Christos Athanasoulis, M.D., and Arthur Waltman, M.D., Section of Vascular Radiology, Massachusetts General Hospital, Boston.)

aggressive medical treatment of aortic dissection was first advocated by Wheat, Palmer, and collaborators.[107] They established two goals for pharmacological therapy: (1) reduction of the systolic blood pressure, and (2) diminution of the velocity of left ventricular ejection (dV/dt), which Prokop, Palmer, and Wheat consider a major stress acting upon the aortic wall that contributes to the genesis and propagation of aortic dissection.[8] Originally introduced for patients too ill to withstand surgery, medical therapy now forms the basis for the initial treatment of virtually all patients with aortic dissection prior to definitive diagnosis by angiography and serves as primary long-term therapy in a large additional subset of patients.

Early Emergency Treatment. All patients in whom there is a strong index of suspicion for aortic dissection should be immediately admitted to an intensive care unit, where blood pressure, cardiac rhythm, central venous pressure, urine output, and, when necessary, pulmonary wedge pressure and cardiac output can be monitored. Initial therapeutic goals are the elimination of pain and the reduction of systolic blood pressure to 100 to 120 mm Hg or to the lowest level commensurate with adequate vital organ (cardiac, renal, and cerebral) perfusion. Simultaneously, arterial dV/dt, which reflects the velocity of left ventricular ejection, should be reduced by beta-adrenergic blockade regardless of whether systolic hypertension or pain is present.

For acute reduction of arterial pressure, the potent vasodilator sodium nitroprusside is very effective, mixed as 50 to 100 mg in 500 ml of 5 per cent dextrose in water and infused initially at 25 to 50 μg/min, with dosages varying according to blood pressure response. Side effects include nausea, restlessness, somnolence, hypotension, and cyanide or thiocyanate toxicity, which can develop after more than 48 hours of continuous use (p. 537). Sodium nitroprusside alone can cause an increase in dV/dt, which can potentially contribute to propagation of the dissection.[108] Thus, adequate simultaneous beta-adrenergic blockade is essential when this drug is used.[107a]

If sodium nitroprusside is ineffective or poorly tolerated, the ganglionic blocking agent trimethaphan (Arfonad), mixed as 500 mg to 2.0 gm in 500 ml of 5 per cent glucose

and water, is used. Initial infusion rate is 1 mg/min, titrating the dose against the blood pressure response, which is enhanced by the orthostatic maneuver of elevating the head of the bed. Limitations in the use of this powerful agent include severe hypotension, tachyphylaxis, somnolence, and sympathoplegia with urinary retention, constipation, ileus, and pupillary dilatation. In contrast with sodium nitroprusside, trimethaphan depresses dV/dt, which should provide a relative advantage in the treatment

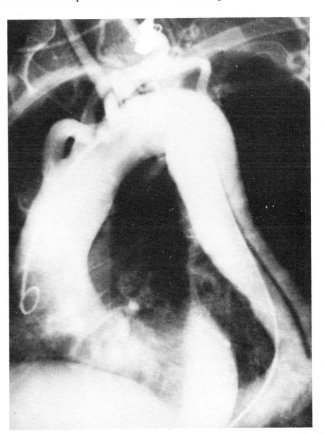

FIGURE 45–15 Left oblique anterior view of the aorta outlined angiographically showing a distal aortic dissection in a 63-year-old man. The true and false channels are clearly seen. The false channel is heavily opacified.

of aortic dissection. However, its unpleasant side effects and rapid tachyphylaxis have relegated this drug to a position of second choice in acute therapy in most centers.

To reduce dV/dt acutely, propranolol should be used in incremental doses of 1 mg intravenously every 5 minutes until there is evidence of satisfactory beta-adrenergic blockade, usually indicated by a pulse rate of 60 to 80 beats/min in the acute setting. A test dose of 0.5 mg intravenously is advised. Maximum initial total dose should not exceed 0.15 mg/kg. Further propranolol should be given intravenously every 4 to 6 hours in order to maintain adequate beta-adrenergic blockade, as reflected in heart rate, usually in dosages somewhat less than the initial amount, i.e., 2 to 6 mg. In chronic stable dissection, propranolol (or an alternative beta blocker) can be started orally, using 20 to 40 mg every 6 hours. Propranolol is contraindicated in the presence of bradycardia, asthma or heart failure. An alternative drug to reduce both blood pressure and dV/dt acutely is reserpine, 1 to 2 mg intramuscularly every 4 to 6 hours. Side effects of reserpine are drowsiness, depression, and peptic ulceration from the stimulation of hydrochloric acid secretion by the stomach. The latter risk can be minimized by concomitant administration of cimetidine, 300 mg intravenously or orally every 6 hours.

Once stabilized, the patient should undergo angiography for a definitive diagnosis. Angiography should be performed within 6 hours after admission, unless a life-threatening complication such as aortic rupture, free aortic regurgitation, cardiac tamponade, or compromise of a vital organ has supervened. If any of these potentially lethal problems arise, then surgery must be undertaken immediately, with angiography performed if possible while the operating room is being readied.

Definitive Subsequent Therapy.   Despite minor variations from center to center, a remarkably consistent approach to definitive therapy of aortic dissection has evolved, based upon experience with surgical and medical treatment over the past decade. Although either medical or surgical therapy can be associated with an extremely successful outcome, it can be generally stated that *surgical results are superior to medical results in proximal dissection*, and, conversely, *medical therapy offers a relative advantage over surgery in most cases of uncomplicated distal dissection*.[109-114] These differences are based largely upon the disparate natural history of proximal and distal disease. Even minute progression of a proximal dissection poses potentially devastating consequences such as pulse loss, aortic regurgitation, neurological compromise, or cardiac tamponade. Thus, immediate surgical repair promises a better outcome. In contrast, patients with distal dissection are for the most part older and have a relatively increased incidence of advanced atherosclerotic or cardiopulmonary disease, thus rendering their surgical risks considerably higher. Medical therapy has proved to be quite effective in this group.

Recent studies report a hospital survival of approximately 60 per cent for patients with acute proximal dissection treated surgically and 80 per cent for those with acute distal dissection treated medically. Hospital survival for patients with chronic dissection treated either surgically — usually because of aortic insufficiency or an enlarging aneurysm — or medically is greater than 80 per cent.[113-116] The somewhat poorer results for surgically treated patients with acute dissection are mostly attributable to complica-tions that have already occurred as a result of the dissection prior to the utilization of definitive therapy.[114] The definitely improved survival in patients with chronic dissection derives from this same principle, i.e., they have already selected themselves out as a group destined to do well because they have survived the initial high mortality that occurs within the first 2 weeks of onset of the dissection.[66,110,112-114] The results of long-term follow-up will be discussed below.

The generally advocated *indications for definitive surgical therapy* are summarized in Table 45–1. Note that occasional patients with proximal dissection who refuse surgery or for whom surgery is contraindicated by age or prior debilitating illness can be treated successfully by medical therapy. Moreover, both early and late medical therapy are usually required in *all* patients, including those treated surgically, to provide stabilization initially and to protect against redissection subsequently.

Surgical Therapy

Although the precise timing of surgery in patients without life-threatening complications is somewhat controversial, prompt repair is generally recommended to obviate even minute progression of the hematoma resulting in further complications. Surgical risk for all patients is obviously increased by age; associated diseases, especially pulmonary emphysema; aneurysm leakage; cardiac tamponade; shock; difficulty with blood pressure control; or vital organ compromise, in particular myocardial infarction or cerebrovascular accident.

As noted, the objectives of definitive surgical therapy are excision of the intimal tear and obliteration of entry into the false lumen by suturing together the edges of the dissected aorta proximally and distally. Aortic continuity is then reestablished either by joining the edges of the aorta directly, or, more commonly, by interposing a prosthetic sleeve graft between the two ends of the aorta (Fig. 45–16). Knowledge of the routes of perfusion of vital organs distal to the surgical site as determined by angiography may be of importance. For example, one or both renal arteries occasionally are found to be fed from the false lumen, in which case the false channel in the distal end of the surgically transected aorta might be left unclosed.[114a]

TABLE 45–1   INDICATIONS FOR DEFINITIVE SURGICAL AND MEDICAL THERAPY IN AORTIC DISSECTION

Surgical
1. Treatment of choice for proximal dissection.
2. Treatment for distal dissection complicated by the following:
   a. Progression with vital organ compromise.
   b. Rupture or impending rupture (saccular aneurysm formation).
   c. Aortic regurgitation.
   d. Inability to control pain or blood pressure medically.
   e. Retrograde extension into the ascending aorta.
   f. Marfan syndrome.

Medical
1. Treatment of choice for uncomplicated distal dissection.
2. Treatment for uncomplicated proximal dissection if the site of origin cannot be clearly identified.*
3. Treatment for stable, isolated arch dissection.
4. Treatment of choice for chronic dissection, i.e., uncomplicated dissection presenting 2 weeks or later after onset.

---

*Some authors advise surgical therapy for all proximal dissections, regardless of site of origin.[113]

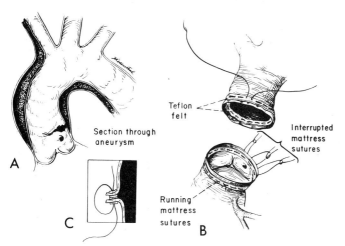

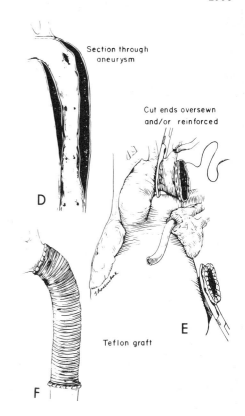

FIGURE 45–16 Several steps in the surgical repair of a proximal (*A, B,* and *C*) and a distal (*D, E,* and *F*) aortic dissection. *A* and *D* show the dissections and the intimal tears. *B,* The aorta has been transected, and the ends of the aorta have been oversewn to obliterate the false lumen and have been buttressed with Teflon felt to prevent the sutures from tearing through the fragile tissue. *C,* The aortic ends are brought together in such a way that the Teflon is again used to reinforce the suture line between the two ends of the aorta or between the aorta and a sleeve graft, if such a graft is necessary for reconstitution of the aorta. *E* shows resection of a distal dissection, with a Teflon graft interposed in *F.* (*D, E,* and *F* reprinted by permission from Austen, W. G., and DeSanctis, R.: Surgical treatment of dissecting aneurysm of the thoracic aorta. N. Engl. J. Med. *272*:1314, 1965.)

When aortic regurgitation complicates aortic dissection, simple decompression of the false channel may be all that is necessary to resuspend the leaflets and restore valvular competence. However, most surgeons have become increasingly aggressive about replacing the aortic valve with a prosthesis if it appears that even moderate aortic regurgitation will be present after the leaflets are decompressed, thus avoiding the high risk of having to replace the aortic valve with a second operation through a diseased aorta at some later date.

For repair of a proximal dissection, full cardiopulmonary bypass is necessary. On occasion, because of extensive dissection of the aorta, it may be difficult to find a safe site for placement of a perfusion cannula. In rare cases, we have had to abandon plans for surgical repair of a proximal dissection for this reason. In the repair of dissections of the descending thoracic aorta, support of the distal circulation may be necessary and can be achieved either by partial left heart bypass or by using a conduit which carries blood from the proximal to the distal aorta, circumventing the site of the dissection.

The actual operative procedure itself, in aortic dissection, is technically demanding. The wall of the diseased aorta is often friable, and the repair must be performed with meticulous care. The use of Teflon felt to buttress the wall and prevent sutures from tearing through the fragile aorta (Fig. 45–16*B*) has represented a significant technical advance. An alternate surgical approach consists of the wrapping of an unstable arch dissection with Dacron.[117] Bleeding, infection, and pulmonary or renal insufficiency constitute the most common early complications of surgical therapy. Spinal cord ischemia with resultant paraplegia due to inadvertent interruption of blood supply from the anterior spinal or intercostal arteries is a rare but dreaded consequence. Late complications include progressive aortic regurgitation if the aortic valve has not been replaced, lo-

calized aneurysm formation, and rarely, redissection at the original site of repair or at an independent secondary site.

Several innovative techniques for high-risk patients have been reported recently. One utilizes an intraluminal sutureless prosthesis for patients with friable thoracic aortic tissue.[118] The other, applied especially to distal, but also to proximal dissection, consists of bypassing the dissected aorta with a Dacron sleeve, ligating the aorta at the site of proximal extension of the dissection, and creating reversal of flow in the distal aorta to perfuse the major arterial branches arising from the dissected segment.[119] Both techniques have been used on only small numbers of patients, and long-term follow-up is lacking.

Medical Therapy. Indications for *definitive medical therapy* are summarized in Table 45–1. Clearly, operation must be performed if there is medical failure, for example, rupture or impending rupture, progression of the dissection with vital organ compromise, aortic regurgitation, or inability to control pain or blood pressure with drugs. Although we prefer medical therapy for low-risk patients with stable distal dissection, some centers advise surgery in this group as well.[113] Unfortunately, controlled studies of medically versus surgically treated patients with distal dissection and comparable surgical risks are lacking.

Although there is not unanimous agreement, medical therapy is still generally recommended for uncomplicated proximal dissection if the site of origin cannot be identified or isolated surgically. Similarly, because of the extreme difficulty of the operation involved with aortic arch dissections, medical therapy is usually advocated in those rare dissections which originate in the arch, with operative intervention reserved for serious complications that might occur on medical treatment.

Medical therapy is advocated for patients with chronic dissection, defined as a stable aortic dissection that has occurred 2 or more weeks prior to presentation, unless, of course, aortic regurgitation related to the dissection becomes hemodynamically significant.

Complications of medical therapy include severe hypotension related to the drugs, with possible precipitation of acute tubular necrosis, cerebrovascular accident, or myocardial infarction, although in a recent report of 52 medically treated patients none of these proved fatal.[114] Some of the drugs may cause somnolence and depression, and the specific side reactions and problems of each particular drug regimen must be anticipated.

Late follow-up of patients leaving the hospital with treated aortic dissection shows an actuarial survival rate comparable to that of individuals without dissection; there are no significant differences between patients with proximal vs. distal dissection, acute vs. chronic dissection, or medical vs. surgical treatment.[114] Thus, initially successful surgical or medical therapy for aortic dissection is sustained on long-term follow-up. Late complications include redissection, regurgitation, and localized saccular aneurysm formation; these occur in fewer than 3 per cent of patients.

Chronic medical therapy to control hypertension and continuous beta-adrenergic blockade is indicated for all patients who have sustained an aortic dissection, regardless of whether they have received definitive surgical or medical therapy. Systolic blood pressure should be controlled at or below a level of 130 to 140 mm Hg, or even lower if tolerated. Preferred agents are those with a negative inotropic as well as hypotensive effect, such as the beta blockers, methyldopa, clonidine, or reserpine, together with a diuretic. Hydralazine or minoxidil increases cardiac output and arterial dV/dt and should be used only in the presence of adequate beta-adrenergic blockade. There is at present insufficient experience using the converting enzyme inhibitors or calcium channel antagonists in aortic dissection to comment upon their use in the treatment of this disease.

Follow-up of patients who have sustained an aortic dissection should include careful and repeated physical examinations; periodic chest roentgenograms, CT scans, 2-D echocardiographic studies, or, where available, high-resolution digital subtraction angiography may also be useful in long-term follow-up for evidence of localized aortic aneurysm formation. The approach to therapy in patients with proximal or distal dissection is summarized in Table 45–2.

ANNULOAORTIC ECTASIA

As aortic valve surgery evolved, it became clear that a significant number of patients with pure aortic regurgitation had this lesion on the basis of idiopathic dilatation of the proximal aorta and the aortic annulus. The term annuloaortic ectasia was first used by Ellis et al. in 1961 to describe this pathological condition.[120] The entity has been subsequently recognized with increasing frequency and makes up about 5 to 10 per cent of the population of patients who currently undergo aortic valve replacement for pure aortic regurgitation.

Etiology and Pathogenesis. The common pathological feature shared by patients with annuloaortic ectasia is that of severe changes of cystic medial necrosis in the wall of the afflicted aorta. Some degree of cystic medial necrosis with annuloaortic ectasia is found in virtually all cases of the Marfan syndrome.[121,122] In fact, it can be severe and is a frequent cause of death from fatal aortic rupture or dissection in Marfan syndrome (p. 1665). In most reported series of patients with annuloaortic ectasia, however, patients with classic Marfan syndrome have been excluded. Careful examination of patients with this condition usually reveals that about one-fourth to one-half have other stigmata of Marfan syndrome, indicating that many of these patients represent a forme fruste of that connective tissue disorder. In a clinicogenetic study of 18 patients with severe aortic regurgitation and dilatation of the ascending aorta but without other evidence of the Marfan syndrome except on pathological examination of the aorta, Emanuel et al. reported that 37.3 per cent of 126 first-degree relatives whom they examined had one or more stigmata of Marfan syndrome.[122a] Thus, it appears clear that many of these patients have primarily the aortic abnormalities of Marfan syndrome without the other manifestations of the disease. In summary, then, patients with annuloaortic ectasia appear to fall into three groups: (1) those with classic Marfan syndrome; (2) those with a forme fruste of the Marfan syndrome; and (3) those with cystic medial necrosis with no obvious underlying cause.

As the media degenerates, the aorta widens. The aortic root is involved, and the annulus dilates, carrying the aortic leaflets apart and eventually making it impossible for these edges to meet in diastole; aortic regurgitation ensues. The diseased aorta may dissect, and this may aggravate the aortic regurgitation.

CLINICAL MANIFESTATIONS. Men predominate over women in virtually all series by a ratio of anywhere between 2 and 8 to 1. Those patients without obvious Marfan syndrome usually are seen in the fourth, fifth, and sixth decades with progressively more severe aortic regurgitation. Patients with the classic Marfan syndrome or a forme fruste are generally younger. Some patients with annuloaortic ectasia experience sudden onset and rapid progression of symptoms, which may be due in part to severe aortic regurgitation secondary to aortic dissection. In the study of Lemon and White, recent aortic root dissection was found in 11 of 25 patients with annuloaortic ectasia who came to surgery.[123] All 11 of these patients had experienced chest pain before operation, although chest pain was also present in several patients with annuloaortic ectasia proven subsequently not to have had an aortic dissection.

The abnormal pulsation of the dilated aorta is sometimes palpable in the chest over the 2nd and 3rd right intercostal spaces, especially if the examination is done with

---

TABLE 45–2 APPROACH TO THE
PATIENT WITH ACUTE AORTIC DISSECTION

Initial

1. Immediate monitoring and stabilization of vital signs, including pulse, blood pressure, cardiac rhythm, central venous pressure, urinary output, and, if necessary, pulmonary capillary wedge pressure.
2. Reduce systolic blood pressure to 100–120 mm Hg or lowest possible level commensurate with adequate organ perfusion. Use *nitroprusside*, 50–100 mg in 500 ml D$_5$W, infuse at 25–50 µg/min; or *trimethaphan*, 500 mg–2 gm in 500 ml D$_5$W, infuse at 1 mg/min and titrate against blood pressure response.
3. Institute beta blockade with propranolol, 1.0 mg IV over 5 min, and repeat until pulse $\leq$ 60 or to a total of 0.15 mg/kg. Repeat dose every 4–6 hours.
4. Once stable, proceed to definite diagnosis by angiography. Decide whether to use medical or surgical therapy.

Subsequent Definitive

1. *Proximal Dissection.* Surgery unless definite contraindication. (If associated with myocardial infarct or cerebrovascular accident, surgical results are poor.)
2. *Distal Dissection.* Medical unless:
   a. Rupture or impending rupture (large dilated and opacified false lumen and/or late development of a saccular aneurysm).
   b. Progression with vital organ compromise.
   c. Aortic regurgitation.
Note: Regardless of the type of dissection or ultimate therapy, medical therapy must be administered both initially and as long-term treatment to control blood pressure and arterial dV/dt and thus diminish the risk of hematoma progression or redissection.

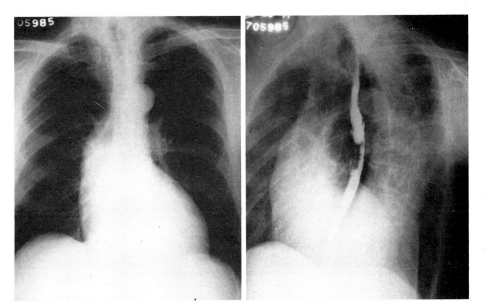

FIGURE 45–17 Posteroanterior (*left*) and left anterior oblique (*right*) chest roentgenograms in a 65-year-old man who had annuloaortic ectasia with severe aortic regurgitation that had developed over a 4-year period. Note the wide ascending aorta.

the patient sitting and in full expiration. We have also seen two patients with annuloaortic ectasia who had pulsation of the right sternoclavicular joint.

There is nothing especially unique to the signs and symptoms of aortic regurgitation in patients with annuloaortic ectasia as opposed to those who have aortic regurgitation from other causes, except for the greater intensity of the diastolic murmur to the right of the sternum in the former group and to the left in patients with a primary valvular abnormality. Lemon and White did find that the two features of an acute or subacute development of symptoms and the presence of chest pain were more frequently found in the group of patients with annuloaortic ectasia than in those with pure aortic valvular regurgitation, presumably on a rheumatic basis.[123] Features of the Marfan syndrome should be sought. They may be obvious, subtle, or absent.

The chest film usually shows a grossly dilated aortic root and ascending aorta (Fig. 45–17), with left ventricular enlargement proportionate to the severity of aortic regurgitation. Calcification in the aortic valve and dilated aorta is usually absent. Echocardiography or CT scan, in addition to showing classic features of aortic regurgitation (p. 115), demonstrates an abnormally widened aortic root. The huge aorta and the aortic regurgitation are easily demonstrated angiographically. Lemon and White identified three types of angiographic aortic enlargement: (1) "pear-shaped" enlargement (56 per cent) (Fig. 45–18); (2) diffuse symmetrical dilatation (27 per cent); and (3) dilatation limited to the sinuses of Valsalva (6 per cent).[123] In our own unpublished experience, aneurysmal dilatation of the sinuses of Valsalva is typically seen in those with Marfan syndrome. The mean maximal aortic diameter in Lemon and White's patients was 7.6 ± 2.7 cm and ranged from

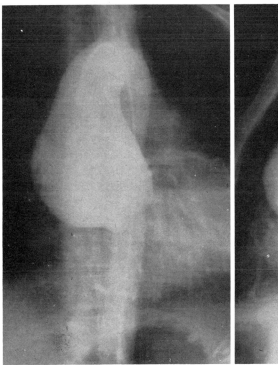

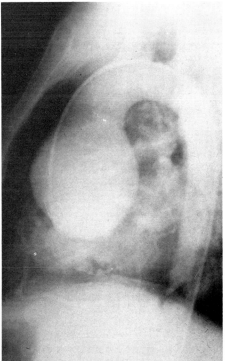

FIGURE 45–18 Anteroposterior (*left*) and lateral (*right*) aortogram in a man with annuloaortic ectasia. The bulbous, pear-shaped aortic root can be easily seen. The left ventricle is opacified consequent to aortic regurgitation. (Courtesy of Christos Athanasoulis, M.D., and Arthur Waltman, M.D., Section of Vascular Radiology, Massachusetts General Hospital, Boston.)

4.8 to 15 cm. This is two to five times the normal aortic diameter. Because dissections are characteristically small, circumscribed, and confined to the ascending aorta, they may not be easy to identify angiographically.

MANAGEMENT. Surgical correction using full cardiopulmonary bypass is usually undertaken for relief of the aortic regurgitation, when the latter is severe and responsible for symptoms of left ventricular failure or when the left ventricle or ascending aorta is increasing in size. However, in addition to replacing the aortic valve, resection of the aneurysmal aorta with insertion of a prosthetic (Dacron or Teflon) graft is generally required. Some surgeons advise sewing an artificial aortic valve to one end of a long prosthetic sleeve and suturing this in place from the aortic annulus at the end to the ascending aorta where it narrows beyond the aneurysm at the other. This reconstruction necessitates reimplantation of the coronary arteries. In fact, with aneurysmal sinuses of Valsalva, the coronary ostia may be carried cephalad by the enlarging sinuses, again necessitating ligation and reimplantation of the coronary arteries or the construction of saphenous vein bypass conduits from the aorta to the ligated coronary arteries. Because of the magnitude of the operation and the frequently friable tissues which make operation difficult, the risks of failure of aortic valve replacement and aneurysm resection are between 10 and 15 per cent in most centers; 5- and 10-year survival rates have been reported at 77 per cent and 57 per cent, respectively.[124] A recent report describing early and late survival for patients with the Marfan syndrome requiring aortic valve replacement and ascending aortic repair revealed no hospital mortality and a late survival rate of 61 per cent.[125] A tentative recommendation for elective repair of the aorta in patients with Marfan syndrome and aortic root diameter greater than 5.5 cm was made.[124]

Although postoperative results in survivors may be excellent, there is a disturbing occurrence of late sudden deaths, mostly from aortic dissection. However, death from progressive heart failure and sudden cardiac deaths also occur.

AORTIC ARTERITIS SYNDROMES

Takayasu's Arteritis

This peculiar arteritis was first noted in 1908 by the Japanese ophthalmologist Takayasu, who described a young woman with cataracts and unusual wreath-like arteriovenous anastoamoses surrounding the optic papillae[126] (Fig. 2–2C, p. 18). In discussing this case, Takayasu's colleagues called attention to two patients with similar ocular findings who also had absent radial pulses. Subsequently, this disease entity has been described by a variety of terms which reflect some of its many features, such as "aortic arch syndrome," "pulseless disease," "reversed coarctation," "occlusive thromboaortopathy," "young female arteritis," as well as Takayasu's arteritis.

DESCRIPTION, PATHOPHYSIOLOGY, AND ETIOLOGY. Although the majority of cases have been reported from Asia and Africa and most large series consist of Orientals, with a heavy predilection for women, this disease occurs worldwide.[127,128]

The basic pathological process is that of marked intimal proliferation and fibrosis and fibrous scarring and degeneration of the elastic fibers of the media, with round cell infiltration of variable intensity. However, fibrosis predominates over cellular reaction. The adventitia and intima become markedly thickened and vasa vasorum are destroyed. In its advanced cicatricial stage, the gross appearance of the aorta strikingly resembles the tree-barking of luetic aortitis. The proliferation process leads to obliterative luminal changes in the aorta and involved arteries. Localized aneurysm formation, poststenotic dilatation, and calcification in the aortic and arterial walls are late complications.[129,130] The process most often involves the arch of the aorta and its major branches, usually with changes that are most marked at the points of origin of the arteries from the aorta. It may present as multisegmental aortic disease with areas of normal wall between affected sites, diffuse involvement of the aorta, or predominantly disease of individual arteries arising from the aorta. The pulmonary arterial tree may also be affected.

Ueno et al. have subdivided the disease into three types, depending upon the sites of involvement (Fig. 45–19).[131] Type I involves primarily the aortic arch and its branches. Type II spares the aortic arch, involving the thoracoabdominal aorta and its branches; Type III combines features of both. More recently, Lupi-Herrera and colleagues have suggested a fourth category, Type IV, in which there is pulmonary arterial involvement.[128] In their series of 107 cases, the incidence of the various types was as follows: Type I, 8 per cent; Type II, 11 per cent; Type III, 65 per cent; and Type IV, 45 per cent (including several patients in the other groups).

A specific etiology for Takayasu's arteritis has not been forthcoming.[132] It has been linked to rheumatic fever, streptococcal infections, rheumatoid arthritis, and other collagen vascular diseases. Although giant cells are occasionally found in pathological specimens of vessels involved by the disease, the entity seems clearly distinct from giant cell arteritis, which affects predominantly patients over the age of 50 and involves mainly medium-sized muscular arteries. Although the aortic scarring of advanced Takayasu's arteritis resembles that of syphilis, nothing else suggests a causal relationship. Some investigators have reported a

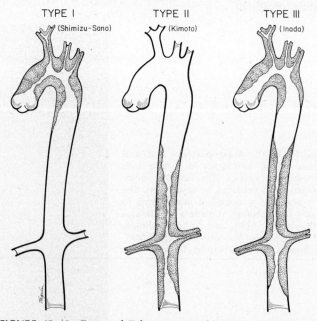

FIGURE 45–19 Types of Takayasu's arteritis. Type I involves primarily the aortic arch and brachiocephalic vessels. Type II affects the thoracoabdominal aorta and particularly the renal arteries. Type III combines features of both Types I and II. Types I and III may be complicated by aortic regurgitation. The eponyms for each type are noted.

strikingly higher incidence of tuberculin skin reactivity to both *Mycobacterium tuberculosis* and atypical mycobacteria in patients with Takayasu's arteritis compared with the general population, raising the possibility of a relationship to tuberculosis.[133] Although antiaortic antibodies have been detected in patients with this disease, their etiologic role is uncertain. Overall, the bulk of evidence favors an autoimmune etiology. It is likely that the arteritis represents the final common pathological expression of a number of different antigenic stimuli in susceptible patients. Recent evidence emphasizes an association between Takayasu's arteritis and certain HLA antigen subtypes.[134,135]

CLINICAL MANIFESTATIONS. The disease affects more women than men, in a ratio of 8.5 to 1. In as many as three-fourths of cases, onset is in the teenage years, although cases beginning in infancy or late middle age have been reported.[128,136,137] More than half the patients with this disease develop an initial systemic illness characterized by symptoms such as fever, anorexia, malaise, weight loss, night sweats, arthralgias, pleuritic pain, and fatigue. Localized pain and tenderness may be noted over affected arteries. This phase subsides, and these patients—as well as those who do not go through this so-called initial "systemic phase"—after a latent period of variable duration show symptoms and signs referable to the obliterative and inflammatory changes in the vessels. These late manifestations include diminished or absent pulses in 96 per cent, bruits in 94 per cent, hypertension in 74 per cent, and heart failure in 28 per cent.[128] The retinopathy originally described by Takayasu is seen in only about 25 per cent and is usually associated with carotid arterial involvement.

The ocular process may lead to retinal detachment and loss of vision.

Patients with Types I and III manifest those findings which are considered to be most typical of this disease, namely "reversed" coarctation of the aorta with absent or diminished upper body pulses and barely detectable blood pressure in the arms, higher pressures in the lower extremities, bruits overlying diseased arteries, manifestations of ischemia at various affected sites, and syncope. Patients with Type II arteritis may have abdominal angina and claudication of the limbs but also tend to develop hypertension because of renal arterial involvement. In fact, hypertension is an extremely important complication of this disease, and it may be difficult to recognize because of the diminished pulsations in the arms. Hypertension appears to arise through several mechanisms, the two most important of which are hemodynamically significant coarctation of the aorta and renal artery stenosis. Decreased aortic capacitance and reduced baroreceptor reactivity may be contributory.[138,139]

Heart failure, when present, is usually seen in very young patients and appears to be a consequence of systemic hypertension. Rarely, aortic regurgitation can also contribute to congestive failure and is due to severe hypertension or to inflammation and scarring of the aortic valve by the inflammatory process.[140] The ostia and proximal segments of the coronary arteries can be affected, resulting in angina or myocardial infarction.[141,142] Rarely, aneurysms are palpable or arteriovenous fistulas occur.[137] Takayasu's arteritis may be a common cause of atypical coarctation syndromes in adults.[130,136,143,144] The frequent ab-

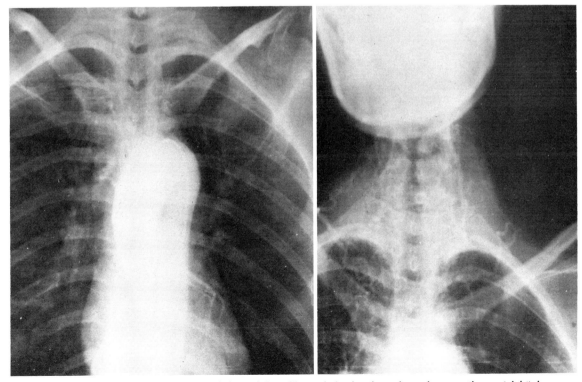

FIGURE 45–20 Thoracic aortogram (*left*) and late films of the head, neck, and upper thorax (*right*) in a 34-year-old Chinese woman with Takayasu's arteritis and no palpable pulses in the upper half of her body. The aortogram shows no direct filling of any of the major arteries arising from the aorta except the coronary arteries. In the delayed film (*right*) collateral channels faintly fill the carotid and vertebral systems.

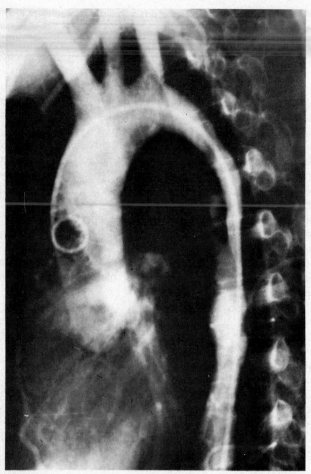

FIGURE 45–21 Aortogram in a 28-year-old Korean man with the clinical features of coarctation of the aorta that proved to be the result of Takayasu's arteritis. Note the typical "rat-tail" angiographic appearance of the descending thoracic aorta.

sence of antecedent systemic symptoms and the more equal sex distribution of this form of the disease have been stressed. It is also believed that Takayasu's arteritis may be responsible for some cases of what appear to be primary pulmonary hypertension.[145,146]

Laboratory abnormalities during the systemic phase are frequent.[133] The sedimentation rate is usually elevated, and a low-grade leukocytosis and mild anemia of chronic disease are common. These return toward normal when the systemic phase resolves. IgG values are almost invariably increased. Other serological abnormalities are common but not specific. These include elevated levels of C-reactive protein, increased antistreptolysin-O titers, and the occasional presence of rheumatoid factor and antinuclear antibodies.

Chest roentgenograms are usually unrevealing, although a rim of calcification is sometimes seen in the walls of the affected arteries. Arteriography reveals typical findings of an irregular intimal surface, with stenosis of the aorta or its tributary arteries, poststenotic dilatations, saccular aneurysms, and even complete occlusion of vessels (Fig. 45–20). Lande and Rossi have described the affected thoracic aorta as having a typical, narrowed, "rat tail" angiographic appearance (Fig. 45–21).[147]

TREATMENT AND PROGNOSIS.   Adrenal corticosteroids are effective in relieving constitutional symptoms in patients with the systemic phase of the disease.[148] Fever,

malaise, and fatigue are often dramatically relieved by steroids, and the sedimentation rate, which is a sensitive indicator of the activity of the disease, falls toward normal. There is also some evidence that corticosteroids may retard progression of arterial narrowing during the active stage of the disease. Anticoagulant drugs, including those of the warfarin family, and drugs that inhibit platelet function, such as aspirin and dipyridamole, are recommended both for treatment of transient ischemic symptoms and for prevention of progression of the disease. Their precise efficacy is not established. *Surgical treatment* of many different types may be needed to deal with late complications of Takayasu's arteritis.[149–151] These include endarterectomy, bypass of obstructed arteries (especially the renal arteries), resection of localized coarctations, excision of saccular aneurysms, and, rarely, aortic valve replacement.

The course of the disease is unpredictable, but slow progression over a period of months to years is usual. Morbidity and mortality depend upon the presence or absence of severe complications, which include retinopathy, secondary hypertension, aortic regurgitation, and aortic or arterial aneurysms. In one series, eventless survival over 7 years was 97 per cent in patients without major complications, compared with 59 per cent in patients with complications.[152] Heart failure and cerebrovascular accidents are common causes of death.

Giant Cell Arteritis

This disease of unknown cause is predominantly a disease of elderly people and characteristically involves medium-sized arteries. However, the aorta and its major branches are affected in about 15 per cent of cases.[153,154] The disease is also referred to as "granulomatous arteritis," "cranial" or "temporal" arteritis, and "arteritis of the aged." It is closely allied to a syndrome characterized by diffuse muscular aching and stiffness called polymyalgia rheumatica.

Pathophysiology and Etiology.   The many names given this disease describe its important features. The characteristic pathological lesion that distinguishes it from other arteritis syndromes is granulomatous inflammation of the media of small- to medium-caliber arteries, about the size of the temporal artery, and especially vessels of the head and neck. In addition to the granulomas, an inflammatory infiltrate is usually found, composed largely of eosinophils, plasma cells, and other mononuclear elements. Endarteritis is not an important feature, but the mural involvement can lead to obstruction of the lumen of involved arteries. Rarely, the aortic wall may be weakened by the granulomatous process, leading to localized aneurysm formation, aortic annular dilatation, and aortic regurgitation. One of the more vivid examples of such aortic involvement by giant cell arteritis is the case report by Austen and Blennerhassett of a young black woman with an aortic aneurysm extending from the aortic valve to the origin of the innominate artery, with wide-open aortic regurgitation from annular dilatation.[155]

Involvement of the aorta and its major tributaries, when it occurs, may coexist with the more classic and prevalent syndromes of temporal arteritis and polymyalgia rheumatica, or, rarely, the aorta may serve as the primary target of this disease.

The etiology of giant cell arteritis is unknown, although the generalized systemic manifestations of the disease and its occasional apparent temporal relationship to prior immunization or a viral illness suggest a possible infectious or autoimmune origin.[156] Klein et al. point out that involvement of the aorta and larger arteries may often arise as corticosteroid therapy for the more classic forms of this disease is being tapered.[153]

CLINICAL MANIFESTATIONS.   Giant cell arteritis typically affects patients over the age of 50 and occurs predominantly in women. The classic presentation is a triad of severe headache, marked malaise, and fever. Other severe constitutional symptoms are common and include anorexia, weight loss, lassitude, myalgias, and night sweats. Headaches are sometimes intense and almost unbearable. Headache typically occurs over involved arteries, usually the temporal arteries, but occasionally the occipital region. The area around the arteries is exquisitely sensitive to pressure, and complaints such as being unable to rest the head comfortably against a pillow are common. Claudication in the jaw muscles while chewing occurs in up to two-thirds of patients and is considered most suggestive of the diagnosis.[157] A serious complication that may occur anywhere in the course of the disease is the onset of blindness from involvement of the ophthalmic artery—blindness that is often irreversible. Visual symptoms ranging from blurring to diplopia and visual loss occur in 25 to 50 per cent of patients.[157] In its milder forms, patients may complain only of generalized muscular aches and pains and unusual fatigue, the syndrome of polymyalgia rheumatica. Blindness in these cases is uncommon.[157]

On rare occasions, consequences of involvement of the aorta or its major tributaries may be the first manifestations of the disease, although more typically, when such involvement occurs, it is part of the more generalized syndrome. However, when aortic or major branch disease is present, the symptoms are similar to those of Takayasu's arteritis and are the result of ischemia in the structures supplied by the involved arteries. Specifically, symptoms may include claudication of either upper or lower extremities, paresthesias, Raynaud's phenomenon, abdominal angina, coronary ischemia, transient cerebral ischemic attacks, and aortic arch and great vessel "steal" syndromes. More rarely, aortic aneurysms, aortic regurgitation, and aortic dissection may occur.[158] Interestingly, renal artery involvement is almost never seen, in contrast with Takayasu's arteritis.[153] Death can occur from aortic rupture or dissection.

On *physical examination*, fever is almost universal and patients appear toxic. Involved vessels are thickened and very tender. Indeed, an experienced examiner can often make the diagnosis of temporal arteritis with virtual certainty at the bedside simply by palpating an indurated, beaded, tender, temporal artery. Pulses may be lost, and bruits may occur over sites of arterial occlusion. Signs of aortic regurgitation are rarely present.

The *laboratory* may be helpful in making the diagnosis. A very high sedimentation rate is virtually a sine qua non for this disease and is a valuable guide to the activity of the process. A moderate normochromic, normocytic anemia is the rule. Acute phase reactants such as alpha$_2$ globulin are increased, and IgG levels also are often elevated.

The *diagnosis* is usually confirmed by biopsy of an involved artery, usually the temporal artery. In cases of larger vessel and aortic involvement, angiography may serve to differentiate arteritis from arteriosclerosis by the following features as described by Klein et al.: (1) long, smooth tapering stenosis alternating with segments of normal or even slightly increased diameter; (2) the absence of irregular ulcerated atheromatous plaques seen in profile; and (3) the more typical anatomical distribution of arteritis to include subclavian, axillary, and brachial arteries.[153]

MANAGEMENT. High-dose steroid therapy, e.g., 60 to 80 mg of prednisone per day, is recommended in all patients with granulomatous arteritis. The intent of therapy is not only to reverse the disease but also to prevent progression, especially in the ophthalmic arteries with resultant blindness. Using constitutional symptoms and the sedimentation rate as a guide, steroids usually can be reduced gradually, and the overall course is one of progressive improvement and eventual complete resolution. However, in many patients, the course of the disease may be protracted for months or years. Very rarely, surgical resection of an expanding aneurysm or replacement of a regurgitant aortic valve is necessary.[132,155,158,159]

Other Arteritis Syndromes

In addition to the aortic inflammation of Takayasu's and giant cell arteritis, isolated aortic regurgitation due to dilatation of the aortic valve ring with associated aortic root involvement may occur during the course of ankylosing spondylitis, psoriatic arthritis, arthritis associated with ulcerative colitis, relapsing polychondritis, and Reiter's syndrome.[160–164] Additionally, it is likely that aortic aneurysms rarely can complicate Behcet's syndrome.[165]

Reported instances of aortitis complicating each of these diseases is rare. For example, it is seen in 1 to 4 per cent of patients with ankylosing spondylitis (p. 1656), and only 15 well-described cases of Reiter's syndrome with aortic regurgitation have been documented (p. 1658). Nevertheless, the symptoms of aortic regurgitation and resultant heart failure may eventually dominate the clinical picture. In each case of arthritis-associated aortitis, the underlying arthritic disease is particularly fulminant and prolonged, and multiple extraarticular features are usually manifest.

Pathological features. These appear to be similar in each of the above diseases. In the early stages of inflammation there is marked dilatation of the aortic valve ring with patchy elastic tissue disruption, an active inflammatory cell infiltrate, and subendothelial fibrosis.[163] These changes are most marked in the aortic root. Later, the proximal ascending aorta develops a picture not unlike that of luetic aortitis, with intimal thickening, coarse, granular plaque formation, and characteristic obliterative endarteritis of the vasa vasorum. The aortic root dilates but usually without frank aneurysm formation. Early, the aortic valve cusps remain essentially normal and later become thickened and retracted, presumably as a result of the incompetence that arises from root dilatation.

The clinical features are those of aortic regurgitation and especially resemble those of annuloaortic ectasia. However, it is worth noting that the course of this disease is variable. Some patients evolve a rapidly progressive course of cardiac decompensation, whereas others have a more indolent and stable natural history. Thus the development of aortic regurgitation does not necessarily signify an irreversible downhill course. There is some evidence that the inflammation of the aortic root may be episodic; worsening of aortic regurgitation may also follow an intermittent course.

Paulus et al. make particular note of the seemingly high incidence of first-degree heart block in their patients with Reiter's syndrome.[163] This block was transient in two of their three patients, and, in one, it antedated the murmur of aortic regurgitation by 3 years. Heart block presumably results from inflammatory infiltrate in the area of the atrioventricular node and can progress to higher grade block. In fact, complete heart block can occur.

Treatment consists of that required for the underlying

arthritis or other disease. Aortic valve replacement should be performed when indicated, although special problems may be encountered in these patients. For example, pulmonary function is often impaired in ankylosing spondylitis as a result of rigidity of the thoracic spine and chest wall. In the rare patient with ulcerative colitis who requires aortic valve replacement, a porcine valve is recommended so that anticoagulation will be unnecessary. In contrast to annuloaortic ectasia, replacement of the ascending aorta itself is almost never necessary.

CARDIOVASCULAR SYPHILIS

Once accounting for between 5 and 10 per cent of all cardiovascular deaths, syphilitic disease of the heart and aorta has become a relative rarity in most major medical centers today owing to the aggressive treatment of lues in its early stages with effective antibiotics. However, the resurgence of syphilis over the past two decades makes it likely that a corresponding increase in the number of cases of cardiovascular syphilis will appear in the future.

Cardiovascular complications occur in approximately 10 to 12 per cent of cases of untreated lues.[166] The latent period may extend from 5 to 40 years after the initial spirochetal infection, with a usual time of 10 to 25 years.

Pathology. The consequences of lues are the direct results of spirochetal infection of the aortic media, thought to occur usually during the secondary phase of the disease, with subsequent inflammation and scarring of the aortic wall. Although the aorta may be invaded anywhere along its course, the most common location—and, in fact, the hallmark of the disease—is the ascending aorta. It is postulated that this area has a proclivity for syphilitic involvement because it is richer in lymphatics than any other portion of the aorta. The muscular and elastic tissues of the media are destroyed by the spirochetal invasion and resultant inflammatory process and are replaced by vascular fibrous tissue. There is an occlusive endarteritis of the vasa vasorum, with perivascular cuffing by plasma cells and lymphocytes.

The aortic wall becomes progressively weakened by the inflammatory process, and it may become calcified. Weakening of the wall leads to the development of aneurysmal dilatation. The overlying intima assumes a furrowed, wrinkled appearance covered with large plaques of a glistening, pearly material. This accounts for the "tree bark" appearance of the involved aorta that is characteristic, but not pathognomonic, of luetic aortitis.

The infection may extend into the aortic root, resulting in aortic regurgitation which is due to dilatation of the aortic annulus and separation of the aortic valve commissures. The support of the leaflets is undermined, and this combination of separation of the leaflets by widening of the annulus and undermining of the support of the cusps leads to progressively more severe aortic regurgitation. The leaflets are often floppy with curling of their edges, although this may be as much a consequence as a cause of the regurgitation. Often with aortic regurgitation there is an associated aneurysm, with calcification in the wall of the aneurysm and the annulus of the valve and base of the leaflets. An obliterative endarteritis may also obstruct the ostia of the two coronary arteries. Unfortunately, the scarring and injury from lues may progress long after the spirochetal organisms have been eradicated, accounting for what is so often a very long latent period before luetic aortitis becomes manifest.

There are four categories of syphilitic heart disease:[167] (1) uncomplicated syphilitic aortitis, (2) syphilitic aortic aneurysm, (3) syphilitic aortic valvulitis with aortic regurgitation, and (4) syphilitic coronary ostial stenosis. From autopsy studies, about one-third of patients with cardiovascular lues are "asymptomatic," meaning that they have postmortem pathological evidence of luetic involvement of the aortic wall without clinical manifestations. About half

have a significant aortic aneurysm, and, of these, one-half to one-third have associated aortic regurgitation. Five to 10 per cent will have essentially pure aortic regurgitation, and 26 per cent will have significant luetic coronary ostial stenosis, often in association with aortic regurgitation or an aortic aneurysm, but occasionally as the only luetic manifestation.[167]

CLINICAL MANIFESTATIONS. Luetic aneurysms can arise anywhere along the aorta, but the most typical location is in the ascending aorta. They are usually saccular but may be fusiform. In the absence of aortic regurgitation, aneurysms may undergo significant enlargement without producing symptoms. Eventually, an aneurysm may expand enough to reach, compress, and even erode contiguous structures, particularly the sternum and anterior right thoracic cage in the case of aneurysms of the ascending aorta. A thrusting, pulsating mass may be seen and palpated. Although luetic aneurysms frequently rupture, they very rarely lead to aortic dissection.

Erosion of the bony structures of the chest wall causes pain at the site of involvement. Ascending aortic aneurysms and those involving the arch may produce a tracheal tug, stridor, and dysphagia. Aneurysms elsewhere may cause symptoms from compression of adjacent structures similar to those of any type of aneurysm located in the same area, such as hoarseness from compression of the left recurrent laryngeal nerve and cough from pressure against the left main stem bronchus in the case of aneurysms of the descending thoracic aorta. Compression of the main pulmonary artery, causing pulmonic stenosis, and rupture of syphilitic aneurysms into a pulmonary artery have been reported rarely.[168]

Although rare, luetic abdominal aortic aneurysms most commonly originate at the level of the 12th thoracic to the 2nd lumbar vertebrae, appearing before age 50, in contrast with arteriosclerotic aneurysms that tend to occur in older patients and are usually located below the level of the renal arteries.[169]

Luetic aortic regurgitation (p. 1106) tends to occur in older patients with luetic cardiovascular disease, presumably because of the longer duration of the disease in these individuals.[170] The earliest auscultatory sign of luetic aortic valve involvement is a tambour-like aortic closure sound. Because of the dilated aortic root, the murmur of luetic aortic regurgitation may be more prominent along the right sternal edge rather than the left, which is usually the case with rheumatic aortic regurgitation. The luetic aortic regurgitant murmur is often musical in quality. Rarely, eversion of one of the aortic cusps—especially the noncoronary leaflet—causes a spectacular, cooing diastolic murmur that is grade 5 or 6 in intensity, with a thrill. It may be heard intermittently and is often mistaken for a systolic murmur because of its loudness and honking quality.

Because there is often considerable calcification in the aortic annulus and stiffness of the base of the aortic leaflets, and because of the usually dilated proximal aorta, a loud systolic ejection murmur, sometimes with a thrill, is often present in luetic aortic valve disease in the absence of any significant aortic stenosis. Also, a loud, slapping, systolic ejection sound is sometimes caused by sudden distention of the dilated aorta by a large volume of blood in early systole.

A few clinical features of luetic aortic regurgitation may

be peculiar to it. Thus an associated aneurysm of the ascending aorta may be felt. Also, because of the concomitant coronary ostial stenosis, angina may be disproportionately severe for the degree of apparent aortic regurgitation. Atrial fibrillation, rare in other types of pure aortic regurgitation, is more frequent in luetic heart disease, perhaps again owing to the occasional occurrence of coronary ostial disease. Otherwise, the bounding pulses, wide pulse pressure, other signs of aortic diastolic runoff, and electrocardiographic evidence of left ventricular hypertrophy do not serve to distinguish luetic from other types of aortic regurgitation of equal severity.

DIAGNOSIS. Usually, there is a history of syphilis, and other manifestations of tertiary lues are found in 10 to 30 per cent of patients with cardiovascular syphilis. Fifteen to 30 per cent of patients have negative routine serological tests (Wasserman, Hinton, Kahn, Venereal Disease Research Laboratories [VDRL], and Kolmer) for syphilis.[171] On the other hand, serological tests directed against a specific treponema antigen, such as the *Treponema pallidum* immobilization (TPI) test or the fluorescent treponemal antibody absorption (FTA-ABS) test are almost invariably positive. The chest roentgenogram may afford extremely valuable clues to the diagnosis of luetic aortitis. The calcification in the ascending aorta proximal to the brachiocephalic vessels is almost always much more extensive than that elsewhere. This is in sharp contrast to arteriosclerosis.

Angiography may delineate the aneurysm (Fig. 45–22) and help to quantify the severity of aortic regurgitation. In patients suspected of having coronary ostial stenosis and in any patient with cardiovascular syphilis in whom surgical correction is contemplated, the coronary artery anatomy—and, particularly, the ostia—should be visualized by angiography if possible. Sometimes, the ostial lesion is so pronounced that it may prove to be impossible to enter the lumen of the affected artery with the catheter.

TREATMENT. All patients with syphilis, including cardiovascular syphilis, who are seen 1 year or more after the initial contact should be given a course of antibiotic therapy aimed at curing the spirochetal infection. Penicillin is still the most effective antibiotic and can be given by either of two schedules: (1) benzathine penicillin G, (Bicillin), 2.4 million units intramuscularly weekly for 3 weeks (total of 7.2 million units), or (2) aqueous procaine penicillin G, 600,000 units intramuscularly daily for 15 days. For patients allergic to penicillin, the recommended therapy is tetracycline, 500 mg orally four times daily for 30 days, or cephaloridine, 0.5 to 1.0 gm intramuscularly daily for 10 days. Although some suggest erythromycin, 500 mg orally four times daily for 30 days, as another alternative to penicillin, this regimen is generally considered to be less effective than the others. The effectiveness of treatment can be monitored by a decrease in VDRL titer, with the desired result being a fourfold reduction in titer in 12 to 24 months.[171,172]

Although a course of antibiotics is recommended in any previously untreated patient with cardiovascular syphilis, even those with a negative serology, there is no good evidence that such treatment reverses, or even halts, the progression of aortitis or aortic regurgitation. In cases of cardiovascular syphilis, cerebrospinal fluid examination should also be performed, and, if positive, this too should be followed to assure the adequacy of therapy. Since the efficacy of antibiotics other than penicillin against syphilis is not well studied beyond 1 year, close follow-up of patients treated with these alternative modes is recommended.

The indications for excision of the luetic aneurysms are similar to those for other thoracic aortic aneurysms (p. 1547): a diameter of 7 cm or larger or an aneurysm of any size that produces symptoms or is expanding rapidly. Since many luetic aneurysms are saccular, aneurysmorrhaphy is occasionally adequate. However, since ongoing aortitis and scarring are possible, it is probably wiser to replace as much as possible of the diseased aorta with a prosthetic graft. Prosthetic replacement of the aortic valve is indicated for significant aortic regurgitation, and the results are as good as in aortic regurgitation of other causes. Since coronary artery disease of syphilis is usually ostial, a localized endarterectomy at the orifices of the coronary arteries may be possible.[173] If an adequate lumen cannot be obtained by endarterectomy, bypass conduits may be necessary.

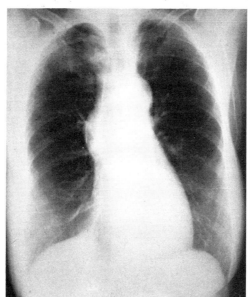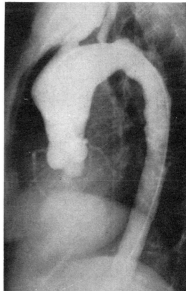

FIGURE 45–22 Films obtained from a 58-year-old woman with leutic aortitis. *Left,* Posteroanterior chest film showing an aneurysm of the ascending aorta with a faint rim of calcification. *Right,* Angiographic appearance of the aneurysm in the lateral view. (Courtesy of Christos Athanasoulis, M.D., and Arthur Waltman, M.D., Section of Vascular Radiology, Massachusetts General Hospital, Boston.)

PSEUDOCOARCTATION

Pseudocoarctation of the aorta is a rare condition resulting from elongation of the aortic arch, with redundancy and kinking of the aorta just distal to the origin of the left subclavian artery at the level of the ligamentum arteriosum.[174,175] Other terms used to describe this entity have included "mild coarctation," "atypical coarctation," or "subclinical coarctation."[176] Etiology is believed to be congenital, with a lack of compression and fusion of certain of the segments of the dorsal aortic root and fourth arch.[177] It is of interest that the incidence and distribution of associated cardiac anomalies parallel those seen in true coarctation. These anomalies include bicuspid aortic valve, sinus of Valsalva aneurysms, ventricular septal defect, and corrected transposition.[178]

Clinical Manifestations. The pressure gradient across the deformed area is usually trivial or absent. Thus, the clinical features of true coarctation—upper extremity hypertension, lower extremity hypotension, and the development of collateral arterial circulation—are absent. Physical findings are often those of the associated lesions, although a murmur is sometimes heard over the aortic kink in the interscapular area. With mild degrees of obstruction, blood pressure in the lower extremities may be slightly reduced, and there may be a subtle pulse lag between the radial and femoral arteries.

The entity can usually be recognized on chest roentgenography. The typical appearance is that of a double rounded density in the left superior mediastinum. Pitfalls in interpretation of the x-ray films are common. The upper density, though relatively translucent, represents the uppermost extension of redundant aorta and is often mistaken for tumor or aneurysm.[179] The lower density is the area of the aorta involved by poststenotic dilatation, and it is often misinterpreted as the aortic knob. Calcification may occur in the area of narrowing. Angiography confirms the diagnosis.

Significance. Problems may arise in pseudocoarctation from the formation of aneurysms by enlargement of the area either proximal or distal to the kink (Fig. 45–23). Associated aneurysms of the left subclavian artery have been reported.[180,181] Rarely, thrombus forms at the site of atheromatous degeneration and calcification in the kinked segment.[182] Complete thrombosis can produce a picture mimicking true coarctation, although collateral arterial circulation is notably absent.[182,183] Thrombus can also propagate directly into tributary vessels or embolize distally. The left subclavian artery is particularly vulnerable because of its proximity to the pseudocoarctation. Infection at the site of aortic narrowing is a rare problem.

Treatment. Therapy is necessary only for complications of pseudocoarctation. In the absence of complications, surgical resection is not indicated.[184] If a bruit or pressure gradient is present over an area of pseudocoarctation, antibiotic prophylaxis for endocarditis should be given before dental or surgical procedures.

AORTIC TRAUMA
(Also see p. 1537)

Blunt Trauma

Aortic injuries are associated with severe blunt trauma, and they are far from rare. In one autopsy series of fatal automobile accidents, rupture of the aorta was found in one-sixth of all victims.[185]

Etiology and Pathogenesis. Aortic trauma most commonly results from injuries associated with sudden high-speed deceleration upon impact, such as that resulting from motor vehicle accidents or severe falls.[185–188] The abrupt deceleration of the body as it crashes to a sudden stop creates enormous shearing forces which act maximally at those points where a highly mobile portion of the aorta joins a fixed segment. Less frequently, pressure or blast injuries may produce rupture of the aorta, believed to be caused by an acute increase in intraaortic pressure generated by the compression of blood contained within the aorta and further increased by the force imparted by cardiac systole.

Although the aorta may be torn anywhere along its length, the most frequent point of rupture, the site of 90 per cent of cases, is in the aortic isthmus at the site of insertion of the ligamentum arteriosum, just distal to the origin of the left subclavian artery. Here, the relatively mobile descending thoracic aorta sweeps dorsally to become fixed to the thoracic cage by the ligamentum arteriosum, the intercostal arteries, and the left subclavian artery. The injury may vary from a miniscule rent in the aortic wall to a complete circumferential transection of all three layers of the aorta. In the series of Parmley et al., 80 per cent of 296 cases of aortic trauma had a circumferential tear.[186] If the aorta is partially transected and the patient survives, a localized saccular aneurysm or pseudoaneurysm may develop subse-

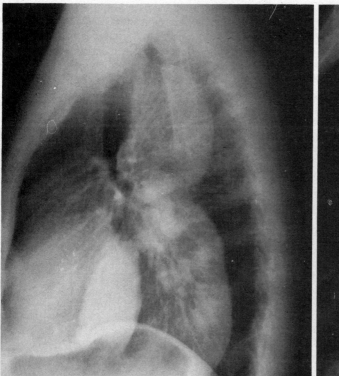
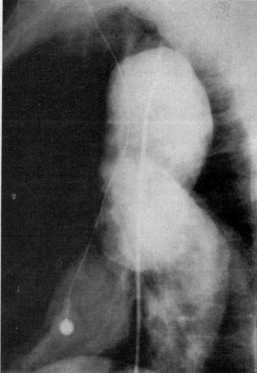

FIGURE 45–23 Pseudocoarctation of the aorta, with aneurysmal dilatation of the aorta proximal and distal to the point of narrowing. *Left,* Lateral chest roentgenogram. *Right,* The aorta is outlined with contrast material.

quently at the site of the tear. Pseudoaneurysms may also form between the two ends of a totally transected aorta.

In addition to the aortic isthmus, which is the locus of 90 per cent of all aortic injuries, other areas of injury include the supravalvular portion of the ascending aorta; the innominate artery, which may be avulsed from the aorta; the aortic arch; other portions of the descending thoracic aorta; the abdominal aorta; and combinations of these.

CLINICAL MANIFESTATIONS. The diagnosis of aortic trauma is often obscured by the presence of other serious injuries, such as central nervous system damage, visceral injury, and multiple systemic fractures. About two-thirds of patients with aortic rupture have clear-cut evidence of other thoracic trauma, such as chest or cardiac contusions, rib or vertebral fractures, pulmonary contusions, and hemorrhagic pleural effusions. The remaining one-third are surprisingly free of overt evidence of chest-wall injury.[187]

Few symptoms are directly attributable to the aortic trauma per se. Pressure from a localized hematoma can cause dyspnea and stridor from tracheal or bronchial compression, dysphagia from esophageal compression, or superior vena caval syndrome from caval compression. Although it is uncommon, the syndrome of so-called "acute coarctation" with upper extremity hypertension, reduced blood pressure in the lower extremities, a systolic murmur over the precordium or in the interscapular area, and a palpable radial-femoral pulse lag is virtually classic for the diagnosis.[189] An interscapular systolic bruit may be heard. Otherwise, the physical examination is quite unrevealing. Localized aneurysms developing in the aortic isthmus late after trauma may cause hoarseness, cough, and dysphagia from compression of the adjacent recurrent laryngeal nerve, bronchus, and esophagus.

DIAGNOSIS. Because the diagnosis is so frequently overshadowed by the presence of other severe injuries, rupture of the aorta is often overlooked. *A high index of suspicion is crucial, and evidence of aortic trauma should be sought in any patient with severe bodily injuries.* In the absence of classic physical findings, a common situation, the diagnosis is best suspected from the chest roentgenogram, which, if properly performed and interpreted, is abnormal in over 90 per cent of patients with traumatic aortic rupture; the most important radiologic abnormality is widening of the mediastinum.[190–192] Marsh and Sturm have delineated criteria for rupture of the aorta based upon a 40-degree anteroposterior supine chest film. The numbers on Figure 45–24 correspond to these criteria: (1) mediastinum measuring greater than 8 cm at the level of the aortic knob; (2) shift of trachea toward the right; (3) blurring of the normally sharp outline of the aorta; (4) obliteration of the medial aspect of the apex of the upper lobe of the left lung; (5) opacification of the clear space between the aorta and pulmonary artery; and (6) depression of the left main stem bronchus below 40 degrees.[193] Ayella et al. have emphasized the need for a true erect anteroposterior chest film, with the patient tilted a few degrees forward from the vertical axis to facilitate recognition of a widened mediastinum.[188] Additionally, the presence of a left apical cap due to mediastinal bleeding that extends into the left extrapleural apical space should prompt further search for traumatic aortic rupture.[194] CT with contrast injection may confirm the diagnosis and should be performed as expeditiously as possible in a stable patient who has sustained se-

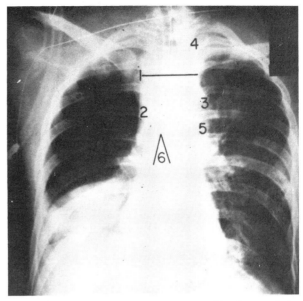

FIGURE 45–24 Aortic trauma. Roentgenographic characteristics of rupture of the proximal descending thoracic aorta in the supine anteroposterior projection (film-to-tube distance = 40 inches). See text for key to numbers. (From Marsh, D. G., and Sturm, J. T.: Traumatic aortic rupture: Roentgenographic indications for angiography. Ann. Thorac. Surg. *21:*337, 1976.)

vere chest trauma.[7] Should the diagnosis remain in question or if the patient is unstable the threshold for performing angiography in suspected cases should be low (Fig. 45–25).

COURSE AND PROGNOSIS. Approximately 80 per cent of patients with aortic rupture die instantly, although usually from other injuries, such as massive hemorrhage from other sites, trauma to other vital organs, or brain damage. Of those who survive the initial event, death often occurs from progressive hemorrhage at the site of the aortic tear within the first week. However, even with complete transection of the aorta, patients may be remarkably stable. About 2 to 5 per cent of patients with partial tears of the aorta go on to develop a localized aneurysm or pseudoaneurysm over a period of months or years, usually anterior to the aortic isthmus. This may either remain stable or ultimately expand. Such traumatic aneurysms frequently calcify or may become infected.[195,196]

TREATMENT. The treatment of aortic trauma is operative repair, which should be undertaken as soon as possible once the condition is recognized. Occasionally, other serious injuries make it necessary to delay operation in order to stabilize the patient, but even in the face of other severe trauma, surgery should be performed if there is evidence of progressive hemorrhage from the aorta. Rupture of the aorta is usually treated by resecting the torn segment of the aorta and inserting an interposed prosthetic graft into the two ends of the aorta. It may be necessary to support the distal circulation with a pump oxygenator or conduit bypass from the proximal to the distal aorta around the rupture in order to avoid ischemic damage to the spinal cord, abdominal viscera, and kidneys. Prompt recognition and operation for a ruptured aorta has resulted in survival of 75 to 80 per cent of patients with this injury who reach the hospital alive.[188]

In cases of localized saccular aneurysms developing late after trauma, surgical excision is advised if the patient is

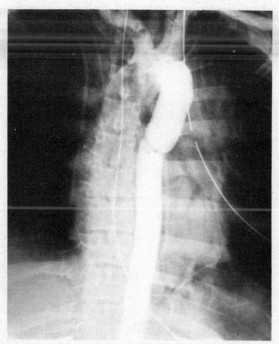

FIGURE 45–25   Thoracic aortogram in a 26-year-old man injured in a motor vehicle accident, showing traumatic transection of the aorta. The site of the tear can be clearly seen. (Courtesy of Robert Dinsmore, M.D., Massachusetts General Hospital, Boston.)

an otherwise reasonable operative candidate. The long-term follow-up of patients with such lesions indicates that about half of the aneurysms slowly expand and may even rupture. Surgery is curative and can be undertaken at a small risk (1 to 3 per cent).

Penetrating Trauma

Penetrating trauma of the aorta or any of its major arterial trunks is caused by puncture or laceration by missiles or knives, particularly bullet and stab wounds. Massive hemorrhage, often leading to rapidly fatal exsanguination, is common. The consequences of the trauma depend upon the site and severity of perforation. Thus, perforation of the aorta within the pericardial sac may lead to cardiac tamponade. Perforation of the aorta elsewhere may cause massive hemorrhage, with compression of surrounding structures by the hematoma, such as the vena cava, tracheobronchial tree, and esophagus. Occlusion of a lacerated artery itself or of adjacent vessels may occur, producing focal signs and symptoms such as loss of the right carotid and brachial pulses, with right hemispheric neurological signs in the case of occlusion of the innominate artery. Occasionally, simultaneous penetration of an adjacent artery and vein may cause an arteriovenous fistula, with a resultant continuous murmur, wide pulse pressure, and increased cardiac output.

MANAGEMENT.   Immediate surgical repair should be undertaken in any patient suspected of having a penetrating wound of the aorta, i.e., one with a missile or stab wound of the chest associated with a wide mediastinum on roentgenogram. If the patient's condition allows it, emergency angiography can usually pinpoint the site of perforation. However, in most patients who survive to reach the hospital, immediate operation for closure of the wound and evacuation of the hematoma is necessary. Similarly, laceration or penetrating wounds of arteries require urgent surgical correction.

AORTIC THROMBOEMBOLIC DISEASE

Aortic Embolism

Between 10 and 25 per cent of peripheral arterial emboli affect the aortic bifurcation, resulting in what are termed "saddle emboli." At least 90 per cent of these emboli originate within the chambers of the left side of the heart; 5 per cent come from the aorta itself, usually from thrombus overlying an arteriosclerotic plaque; and the remainder came from undetermined sites.[197] Rarely, paradoxical systemic embolism from the venous circulation occurs through a patent foramen ovale or atrial septal defect. Conditions that predispose to peripheral embolism are myocardial infarction with mural thrombus, ventricular aneurysm, prosthetic valves, congestive cardiomyopathy, and atrial fibrillation, especially in patients with rheumatic mitral stenosis. So-called "marantic endocarditis" is occasionally encountered in chronically ill patients, especially those with malignant disease, and consists of sterile intracardiac thrombi that may dislodge and travel to distal sites. Other less frequent conditions that serve to cause arterial emboli are left atrial myxomas and acute and subacute bacterial endocarditis. Emboli in endocarditis are usually small, although large emboli are seen in acute bacterial endocarditis and fungal (*Candida*) endocarditis. An increased tendency to thromboembolism is encountered in women taking contraceptive pills and estrogens, in patients with malignant diseases, particularly carcinoma of the pancreas, and, rarely, in patients with antithrombin III deficiency.[198]

CLINICAL MANIFESTATIONS.   Aortic bifurcation embolism is heralded by the sudden onset of excruciating pain in both legs. The pain usually extends distally from the midthigh area, but can also involve the buttocks, lumbosacral area, and perineum. Associated with the intense pain are numbness, symmetrical weakness, and paresthesias. Schatz and Stanley have summarized in alliteration this classic presentation as "*p*ain, *p*aralysis, *p*aresthesias, *p*ulselessness, and *p*allor."[199]

Examination reveals cold, pale extremities which are cyanotic and often exhibit a mottled, reticulated, reddish-blue appearance. These changes may progress to the blue-black color of gangrene, beginning first in the toes and extending proximally. Pulses are absent below the abdominal aorta. Initially sluggish, capillary filling is ultimately absent. Signs of ischemic neuropathy are present and include diminished or absent deep tendon reflexes, symmetrical weakness, and loss of all modalities of sensation, usually with demarcation at the level of the midthigh. If ischemia persists long enough, there may be myonecrosis with the release of products of muscle breakdown into the bloodstream, causing shock, hypotension, hyperkalemia, myoglobinuria, and acute tubular necrosis. Sepsis may add a serious further dimension to an already desperate problem. If perfusion is not reestablished within a few hours, death is almost inevitable.

The *differential diagnosis* includes acute aortic thrombosis from arteriosclerotic disease and dissecting aortic aneurysm. With thrombosis, there is usually a history of prior claudication, and an embolic source is lacking. With aortic dissection, a history of severe chest or back pain and an abnormal aortic contour on chest x-ray film usually provide distinguishing features.

The diagnosis is confirmed by angiography. However, most investigators advise prompt surgical intervention without angiography if the diagnosis is strongly suspected in order to avoid the loss of valuable time that could lead to irreversible ischemic damage to the limbs.

THERAPY. Most emboli can be removed by using Fogarty balloon-tipped catheters inserted through a transfemoral arterial approach under local anesthesia. In addition to retrieving the embolic material, passage of the Fogarty catheters into the distal arterial bed may result in the removal of any thrombus that may have formed as a result of the stagnant flow beyond the embolus. If the embolus cannot be retrieved with Fogarty catheters, removal by direct transabdominal aortotomy is necessary. Operative mortality ranges from 15 to 30 per cent, with death due to the underlying cardiac disease; limb salvage is estimated at 80 to 90 per cent in most series.[200] Anticoagulation with constant intravenous heparin is instituted upon completion of the operation and continued until therapeutic levels are achieved with one of the warfarin sodium family of drugs. Depending upon the clinical situation, long-term anticoagulant therapy using warfarin or antiplatelet agents may be required. Using the transfemoral approach, surgery can be carried out with a low mortality even in patients whose other disease makes them poor operative risks. Limbs are almost uniformly salvaged if operation is undertaken promptly. All embolic debris should be cultured and examined microscopically. Left atrial myxomas are sometimes first recognized by the pathological examination of embolic specimens.

Aortic Thrombosis

Rarely, primary thrombosis of the distal abdominal aorta may be seen as a result of atheromatous disease or in rare patients with deficiency in antithrombin III. In such patients, treatment is generally surgical, although an occasional case of successful balloon catheter dilation has been reported.[198,201]

Atheromatous Emboli

Embolism of atheromatous debris from the disruption of arteriosclerotic plaques in the aorta or its major arterial trunks has been noted with increasing frequency. Usually, such embolism takes the form of showers of microemboli, measuring between 150 and 600 μm in size, into small arterial branches—an entity that is also termed "cholesterol embolism." However, the obstruction of large arteries by embolic arteriosclerotic material may also occur. By far the most common cause of cholesterol embolism is surgery which involves the manipulation of an atherosclerotic aorta.[15] Thus, atheromatous embolism into the renal and splanchnic vascular beds is common after major abdominal vascular procedures, particularly the resection of abdominal aortic aneurysms. Embolism of atheromatous material also occurs as an occasional complication of intra-arterial cannulation, cardiac catheterization, and cardiopulmonary bypass. In addition to these iatrogenic causes, however, spontaneously occurring cholesterol embolism is encountered, particularly from the aorta into the femoral-popliteal system. Recent studies have suggested a causal relationship between cholesterol embolism and anticoagu-

lant therapy, especially long-term anticoagulation with warfarin sodium–type drugs. Presumably, anticoagulation promotes hemorrhage into plaques, leading to their disruption, or prevents the formation of protective thrombus over ulcerated plaques. Finally, atheromatous embolism has followed blunt trauma to the aorta.[202]

CLINICAL MANIFESTATIONS. The consequences of cholesterol embolism depend upon the vascular bed involved as well as the extent to which the small arterial vessels are occluded. Two important complications of cholesterol embolism following abdominal aortic surgery are pancreatitis and renal failure from diffuse microinfarction of the pancreas and kidneys, respectively.[14,203] Renal failure may be severe and irreversible[204] (p. 1752). Occasionally, cholesterol embolism has been implicated as a cause of severe renovascular hypertension.[205] Gastrointestinal hemorrhage from microinfarction of abdominal viscera is also encountered.[206] Showers of atheromatous emboli may affect the cerebral circulation, producing either focal neurological defects or a diffuse encephalopathic picture. In such cases, shiny cholesterol particles are sometimes visible in the retinal arteries.[203]

Spontaneously occurring cholesterol embolism in the lower extremities is manifested by bilateral pain, livedo reticularis, and purpuric and ecchymotic lesions in the lower legs, feet, and toes. These manifestations may be paroxysmal as emboli intermittently dislodge from their sites of origin. Skin necrosis and ischemic gangrene are common, especially in the toes ("purple toe syndrome"). In the face of this clinical evidence of severe ischemia, arterial pulses are characteristically well preserved unless there is coincidental peripheral vascular disease.

The clinical picture may mimic that of a vasculitis or septic embolism from neisserial organisms—especially meningococcemia—or bacterial endocarditis. The absence of fever and other signs of systemic illness and the localized distribution of the lesions serve to distinguish cholesterol embolism from these other entities. The diagnosis has been made by muscle biopsy, which may show cholesterol particles in the arterioles.[204]

THERAPY. For the most part, there is no specific treatment for cholesterol microembolism. Careful attention to the prevention of necrosis and infection in the involved extremities is important. Although the amputation of gangrenous digits is occasionally necessary, the ultimate prognosis for recovery is quite good, unless embolism is frequent and recurrent. Pancreatitis often subsides, even though it may be severe. Renal failure may be irreversible.

The use of anticoagulants in the prevention of further embolism is controversial, with some investigators advocating that they be given and others contending that they promote further atheromatous emboli.[203,207] Overall, it appears that they are not of much value.

In instances of recurrent atheromatous embolism, it may be possible to pinpoint the source of the cholesterol particles by angiography and perform an endarterectomy or an excision of the involved segment with replacement with a prosthetic graft.

AORTIC BACTERIAL INFECTIONS

The term "infected aneurysm" has gradually replaced the original designation of "mycotic aneurysm" used by

Osler to define any localized dilation caused by sepsis in the wall of the aorta or any artery and thus to avoid confusion with infections of truly fungal origin. Infection can cause virtually any kind of aneurysmal dilatation, including fusiform, saccular, and false aneurysms. Rupture into the venous system may cause arteriovenous fistulas. Alternatively, infection may arise within preexisting arteriosclerotic aneurysms. Infected aortic aneurysms are rare, with only 1.2 cases per year recently being reported from a large general hospital.[208] Rarely, tuberculosis can infect the aorta, but, as of 1965, only 110 cases of tuberculous aortitis had been reported in the world's literature.[209]

Pathogenesis. Vascular infection may arise by any of three different mechanisms. First, septic emboli from bacterial endocarditis or diffuse bacteremia may infect normal or diseased tissue. This mechanism of infection has become less frequent owing to the widespread use of effective antibiotics for the control of septicemia. Second, there may be contiguous spread from adjacent abscesses, infected lymph nodes, empyema, and so on. This is the usual cause for tuberculous vascular involvement. Third, sepsis may be introduced directly from an external source, such as trauma, intravenous injections, or surgery. The incidence of this type of infection is increasing because of more frequent motor vehicle accidents, the widespread use of intravenous narcotics by drug addicts, and the performance of more intravascular procedures which may produce a portal for infection, such as cardiac catheterization and intraaortic balloon counterpulsation. With this type of sepsis, the peripheral arteries are obviously more frequently involved than the aorta per se.

Although virtually any organism may infect the arterial tree, certain bacteria seem to have a proclivity for this type of infection. In particular, this is true of the *Salmonella* group, which tends to infect arteriosclerotic aneurysms.

CLINICAL MANIFESTATIONS. Most patients with infected aortic aneurysms are febrile; the height of the fever depends upon the severity of infection, the organism, and the site of the infection. Extremely high fever and rigors are common. Symptoms may arise from localized expansion of an infected aneurysm, such as dysphagia from esophageal compression and pain in areas contiguous to the infected sac. If palpable, infected aneurysms are almost always tender. A tender and pulsatile mass in a febrile patient should be considered an infected aneurysm until proved otherwise. Jarrett et al. have suggested that infected aortic aneurysms can be differentiated from sterile ones by the presence of fever, relative preponderence in women, tenderness, lack of calcification, and a tendency for early vertebral erosion.[208] With tuberculous involvement, evidence is almost always seen on chest x-ray film.[210] This, coupled with a pulsating mass lesion, should elicit the correct diagnosis.

Sepsis in more peripheral arteries presents most commonly as fever with a palpable, painful, pulsating mass. Symptoms of compression of contiguous structures may also be present, such as arterial regurgitation or a neuropathy.[211] Small abscesses in the distribution of the artery are often seen in staphylococcal infections.

Leukocytosis, elevated sedimentation rate, and positive blood cultures are present in most cases. Commonly reported organisms are *Staphylococcus aureus* and *Salmonella* species; other gram-positive and gram-negative organisms, such as pneumococcus, *Pseudomonas*, and anaerobes, are found less frequently. Rarely, fungal infections with *Candida* or *Aspergillus* may occur. Localization of suspected infected aneurysms in a patient with sepsis can be aided by angiography. Valuable information can sometimes be obtained from ultrasound, gallium, and CT scans.

The natural history of infected aneurysms is that of progressive expansion, thinning of the aneurysm wall, and eventual rupture. Jarrett et al. found a more rapid progression in patients with gram-negative infections.[208]

THERAPY. Treatment is always surgical excision, combined with appropriate antibiotic or antituberculous chemotherapy. Wide excision of infected tissue is advised.[208,212] Usually a prosthetic tube graft must be inserted if the aorta or a major artery is involved. Early recognition and therapy clearly alter the outcome favorably.

AORTIC TUMORS

A review cites 21 cases of primary aortic tumors recorded in the world's literature.[213] Clearly secondary tumors can arise from direct extension and invasion from adjacent lung or abdominal neoplasms or from embolic spread. Histological types include fibrosarcoma (most commonly), fibromyxosarcoma, myxosarcoma, fibromyxoma, angiosarcoma, malignant fibrous histocytoma, and leiomyosarcoma.

In the 21 cases of primary aortic tumors, the age of the patients ranged from infancy to 70 years with a mean of 53 years; sex distribution was equal. Presentation in over half of the cases was pain with proximal hypertension due to the acquired coarctation, decreased femoral pulses, fever, claudication, and, occasionally, bruits. Diagnosis is made by the usual noninvasive or angiographic techniques, with the irregular appearance of the lumen and lack of enlargement of the outer diameter of the aorta being key features.

References

1. Buonocore, E., Meaney, T. F., Borkowski, G. P., Pavlicek, W., and Gallagher, J.: Digital subtraction angiography of the abdominal aorta and renal arteries. Radiology 139:281, 1981.
2. Ferrucci, J. T., Jr.: Body ultrasonography. N. Engl. J. Med. 300:538, 590, 1979.
3. DeMaria, A. N., Bommer, W., Neumann, A., Weinert, L., Bogren, H., and Mason, D. T.: Identification and localization of aneurysms of the ascending aorta by cross-sectional echocardiography. Circulation 59:755, 1979.
4. Meyer, J. F., and Wall, H. N., Jr.: Ultrasonic evaluation of the aorta. In Lindsay, J., Jr., and Hurst, J. W. (eds.): The Aorta. New York, Grune and Stratton, 1979, p. 345.
5. Eriksson, I., Hemmingsson, A., and Lindgren, P. G.: Diagnosis of abdominal aortic aneurysms by aortography, computer tomography and ultrasound. Acta Radiol. [Diagn.] 21:209, 1980.
6. Godwin, J. D., Herfkens, R. H., Skioldebrand, C. G., Federle, M. P., and Lipton, M. J.: Evaluation of dissections and aneurysms of the thoracic aorta by conventional and dynamic CT scanning. Radiology 136:125, 1980.
6a. Moncada, R., Demos, T. C., and Churchill, R.: Detecting disease of the aorta by computed tomography. J. Cardiovasc. Med. 8:186, 1983.
7. Egan, T. J., Neiman, H. L., Herman, R. J., Malave, S. R., and Sanders, J. H.: Computed tomography in the diagnosis of aortic aneurysm dissection of traumatic injury. Radiology 136:141, 1980.
8. Prokop, E. K., Palmer, R. F., and Wheat, M. W., Jr.: Hydrodynamic forces in dissecting aneurysms. In vitro studies in a Tygon model and in dog aortas. Circ. Res. 27:121, 1970.
9. Iwatsuki, K., Cardinale, G. J., Spector, S., and Udenfriend, S.: Reduction of blood pressure and vascular collagen in hypertensive rats by β-aminopropionitrile. Proc. Natl. Acad. Sci. USA 74:360, 1977.
10. Saruk, M., and Eisenstein, R.: Aortic lesion in Marfan syndrome—The ultrastructure of cystic medial degeneration. Arch. Pathol. Lab. Med. 101:74, 1977.
11. Schlatmann, T. J. M., and Becker, A. E.: Histologic changes in the normal aging aorta. Am. J. Cardiol. 39:13, 1977.
12. Schlatmann, T. J. M., and Becker, A. E.: Pathogenesis of dissecting aneurysm of the aorta. Am. J. Cardiol. 39:21, 1977.
13. Heistad, D. D., Marcus, M. L., Law, E. G., Armstrong, M. L., Ehrhardt, J. C., and Abboud, F. M.: Regulation of blood flow to the aortic media in dogs. J. Clin. Invest. 62:133, 1978.
14. Crane, C.: Arteriosclerotic aneurysm of the abdominal aorta. Some pathologic and clinical correlations. N. Engl. J. Med. 253:954, 1955.
15. Thurlbeck, W. M., and Castleman, B.: Atheromatous emboli to the kidneys after aortic surgery. N. Engl. J. Med. 257:442, 1957.
16. Darling, R. C.: Ruptured arteriosclerotic abdominal aortic aneurysms. Am. J. Surg. 119:397, 1970.
17. Weintraub, A. M., and Gomes, M. N.: Clinical manifestations of abdominal aortic aneurysm and thoracoabdominal aneurysm. In Lindsay, J., Jr., and Hurst, J. W. (eds.): The Aorta. New York, Grune and Stratton, 1979, p. 131.
18. Moore, H. D.: Abdominal aortic aneurysms. J. Cardiovasc. Surg. 17:47, 1976.
19. McGregor, J. C.: Unoperated ruptured abdominal aortic aneurysms: A retro-

spective clinicopathologic study over a 10-year period. Br. J. Surg. 63:113, 1976.

20. Hertzer, N. R., and Beven, E. G.: Abdominal aortic aneurysm. Postgrad. Med. 61:72, 1977.

21. Brewster, D. C., Darling, R. C., Raines, J. K., Sarno, R., O'Donnell, T. F., Ezpeleta, M., and Athanasoulis, C.: Assessment of abdominal aortic aneurysm size. Circulation 56:164, 1977.

22. Retief, P. J., and Loubser, J. S.: Diagnosis and treatment of abdominal aortic aneurysm. A report of 82 cases. S. Afr. Med. J. 56:67, 1979.

23. Brewster, D. C., Retana, A., Waltman, A. C., and Darling, R. C.: Angiography in the management of aneurysms of the abdominal aorta. Its value and safety. N. Engl. J. Med. 292:822, 1975.

24. Szilagyi, D. E., Smith, R. F., DeRusso, F. J., Elliott, J. P., and Sherrin, F. W.: Contribution of abdominal aortic aneurysmectomy to prolongation of life. Ann. Surg. 164:678, 1966.

25. Darling, R. C., Messina, C. R., Brewster, D. C., and Ottinger, L. W.: Autopsy study of unoperated abdominal aortic aneurysms. The case for early resection. Circulation 56(Suppl. II):161, 1977.

26. Linton, R. R.: Atlas of Vascular Surgery. Philadelphia, W. B. Saunders Co., 1973, pp. 266–269.

27. Attia, R. R., Murphy, J. D., Snider, M., Lappas, D. G., Darling, R. C., and Lowenstein, E.: Myocardial ischemia due to infrarenal aortic cross-clamping during aortic surgery in patients with severe coronary artery disease. Circulation 53:961, 1976.

28. Bush, H. L., Jr., LoGerfo, F. W., Weisel, R. D., Mannick, J. A., and Hechtman, H. B.: Assessment of myocardial performance and optimal volume loading during elective abdominal aortic resection. Arch. Surg. 112:1301, 1977.

29. Thompson, J. E., Hollier, L. H., Patman, R. D., and Persson, A. V.: Surgical management of abdominal aortic aneurysms: Factors influencing mortality and morbidity — A 20-year experience. Ann. Surg. 181:654, 1975.

30. Cullen, D. J., Ferrara, L. C., Briggs, B. A., Walker, P. F., and Grehert, J.: Survival, hospitalization charges and follow-up results in critically ill patients. New Engl. J. Med. 294:982, 1976.

31. Brener, B. J., Raines, J. K., and Darling, R. C.: Intraoperative autotransfusion in abdominal aortic resections. Arch. Surg. 107:78, 1973.

32. Levin, P. M., Shore, E. H., Treiman, R. L., and Foran, R. F.: Ruptured abdominal aortic aneurysms. Surgical treatment. West. J. Med. 123:431, 1975.

33. Spencer, F. C.: Diseases of great vessels. In Schwartz, S. I., and Shires, T.: Principles of Surgery. 3rd ed. New York, McGraw-Hill Book Co., 1979, p.883.

34. Young, A. E., and Couch, N. P.: Coronary artery disease and aortic aneurysm surgery. Lancet 1:1005, 1977.

35. Brewster, D. C., Bluth, J., Darling, R. C., and Austen, W. G.: Combined aortic and renal artery reconstruction. Am. J. Surg. 131:457, 1976.

36. Crawford, E. S., Saleh, S. A., Babb, J. W., III, Glaeser, D. H., Vaccaro, P. S., and Silvers, A.: Infrarenal abdominal aortic aneurysm: Factors influencing survival after operation performed over a 25-year period. Ann. Surg. 193:699, 1981.

37. Ottinger, L. W.: Ruptured arteriosclerotic aneurysm of the abdominal aorta: Reducing mortality. J.A.M.A. 233:147, 1975.

38. Darling, R. C., and Brewster, D. C.: Elective treatment of abdominal aortic aneurysms. World J. Surg. 4:661, 1980.

39. Fielding, J. W. L., Black, J., Ashton, F., Slaney, G., and Campbell, D. J.: Diagnosis and management of 528 abdominal aortic aneurysms. Br. Med. J. 283:355, 1981.

40. O'Donnell, T. F., Darling, R. C., and Linton, R. R.: Is 80 years too old for aneurysmectomy? Arch. Surg. 111:1250, 1976.

41. Leather, R. P., Shah, D., Goldman, M., Rosenberg, M., and Karmody, A. M.: Nonresective treatment of abdominal aortic aneurysms. Use of acute thrombosis and axillofemoral bypass. Arch. Surg. 114:1402, 1979.

42. Baker, A. G., and Roberts, B.: Long-term survival following abdominal aortic aneurysmectomy. J.A.M.A. 212:445, 1970.

43. DeWeese, J. A., Blaisdell, F. W., and Foster, J. H.: Optimal resources for vascular surgery. Circulation 46:305, 1972.

44. Hicks, G. L., Eastland, M. W., and DeWeese, J. A.: Survival improvement following aortic aneurysm resection. Ann. Surg. 181:863, 1975.

45. Soreide, O., Lillestol, J., Christensen, O., Gromsgaard, L., Myhre, H. O., Solheim, K., and Trippestad, A.: Abdominal aortic aneurysms: Survival analysis of four hundred thirty-four patients. Surgery 91:188, 1982.

46. Thompson, W. M., Johnsrude, I. S., Jackson, D. C., Older, R. A., and Wechsler, A. S.: Late complications of abdominal aortic reconstructive surgery: Roentgen evaluation. Ann. Surg. 185:326, 1977.

47. Kierman, P. D., Pairolero, P. C., Hubert, J. P., Jr., Mucha, P., Jr., and Wallace, R. B.: Aortic graft-enteric fistula. Mayo Clin. Proc. 55:731, 1980.

48. Ottinger, L. W., Darling, R. C., Nathan, M. J., and Linton, R. R.: Left colon ischemia complicating aorto-iliac reconstruction. Causes, diagnosis, management and prevention. Arch. Surg. 105:841, 1972.

49. Ernst, C. B., Hagihara, P. F., Daugherty, M. E., Sachatello, C. R., and Griffen, W. O.: Ischemic colitis incidence following abdominal aortic reconstruction. A prospective study. Surgery 80:417, 1976.

50. Lindsay, J., Jr.: Thoracic aneurysms. In Lindsay, J., Jr., and Hurst, J. W. (eds.): The Aorta. New York, Grune and Stratton, 1979, p. 121.

51. Crisler, C., and Bahnson, H. T.: Aneurysm of the aorta. Curr. Probl. Surg. 1–64, 1972.

52. Joyce, J. W., Fairbairn, J. F., Kincaid, O. W., and Juergens, J. L.: Aneurysms of the thoracic aorta — A clinical study with special reference to prognosis. Circulation 29:176, 1964.

53. Altman, P., and Voorhees, A. B.: Aneurysm of the aorta treated by wiring. Case report of a 38-year survival. Ann. Surg. 184:738, 1976.

54. Griepp, R. B., Stinson, E. B., Hollingsworth, J. F., and Buehler, D.: Prosthetic replacement of the aortic arch. J. Thorac. Cardiovasc. Surg. 70:1051, 1975.

55. Culliford, A. T., Ayvaliotis, B., Shemin, R., Colvin, S. B., Isom, O. W., and Spencer, F. C.: Aneurysms of the ascending aorta and transverse arch: Surgical experience in 80 patients. J. Thorac. Cardiovasc. Surg. 83:701, 1982.

56. Symbas, P. N.: Treatment of thoracic surgical aortic diseases. In Lindsay, J., Jr., and Hurst, J. W. (eds.): The Aorta. New York, Grune and Stratton, 1979, p. 259.

57. Kidd, J. N., Reul, G. J., Cooley, D. A., Sandiford, F. M., Kyger, E. R., and Wukasch, D. C.: Surgical treatment of aneurysms of the ascending aorta. Circulation 54(Suppl. III):118, 1976.

58. Crawford, E. S., Snyder, D. M., Cho, G. C., and Roehm, J. O. F., Jr.: Progress in treatment of thoracabdominal and abdominal aortic aneurysms involving celiac, superior mesenteric, and renal Ann. Surg. 188:404,1978.

59. Crawford, E. S., and Rubio, P. A.: Reappraisal of adjuncts to avoid ischemia in the treatment of aneurysms of descending thoracic aorta. J. Thorac. Cardiovasc. Surg. 66:693, 1973.

60. Wakabayashi, A., and Connolly, J. E.: Prevention of paraplegia associated with resection of extensive thoracic aneurysms. Arch. Surg. 111:1186, 1976.

61. Stallone, R. J., Iverson, L. I. G., and Young, J. N.: Descending thoracic aortic aneurysm: A 10 year surgical experience. Am. J. Surg. 142:106, 1981.

62. Mannick, J. A.: Surgical treatment of aneurysms of the abdominal and thoracic aorta. Prog. Cardiovasc. Dis. 16:69, 1973.

63. Wheat, M. W., Jr.: Acute dissecting aneurysms of the aorta: Diagnosis and treatment — 1979. Am. Heart J. 99:373, 1980.

64. Roberts, W. C.: Aortic dissection: Anatomy, consequences, and causes. Am. Heart J. 101:195, 1981.

65. Doroghazi, R. M., and Slater, E. E. (eds.): Aortic Dissection. New York, McGraw-Hill Book Co., 1983.

65a. Wheat, M. W., Jr.: Pathogenesis of aortic dissection. In Aortic Dissection. Doroghazi, R. M., and Slater, E. E. (eds.): New York, McGraw-Hill Book Company, 1983, p. 55.

66. DeBakey, M. E., Henly, W. S., Cooley, D. A., Morris, G. C., Jr., Crawford, E. S., and Beall, A. C.: Surgical management of dissecting aneurysms of the aorta. J. Thorac. Cardiovasc. Surg. 49:130, 1965.

67. Sethi, G. K., Hughes, R. K., and Takaro, T.: Dissecting aortic aneurysms. Ann. Thorac. Surg. 18:201, 1974.

68. Daily, P. O., Trueblood, H. W., Stinson, E. B., Wuerflein, R. D., and Shumway, N. E.: Management of acute aortic dissection. Ann. Thorac. Surg. 10:237, 1970.

69. Slater, E. E., and DeSanctis, R. W.: The clinical recognition of dissecting aortic aneurysm. Am. J. Med. 60:625, 1976.

70. Leonards, J. C., and Hasleton, P. S.: Dissecting aortic aneurysms: A clinicopathological study. Q. J. Med. 48:55, 1979.

71. Bulkley, B. H., and Roberts, W. C.: Dissecting aneurysm (hematoma) limited to coronary artery. Am. J. Med. 55:747, 1973.

72. Hochberg, F. H., Bean, C., Fisher, C. M., and Roberson, G. H.: Stroke in a 15-year-old girl secondary to terminal carotid dissection. Neurology 25:725, 1975.

73. Loeppky, C. B., Alpert, M. A., Hamel, P. C., Martin, R. H., and Saab, S. B.: Extensive aortic dissection from combined-type cystic medial necrosis in a young man without predisposing factors. Chest 79:116, 1981.

74. Fukuda, T., Tadavarthy, S. M., and Edwards, J. E.: Dissecting aneurysm of aorta complicating aortic valvular stenosis. Circulation 53:169, 1976.

75. Gore, I., and Seiwert, V. J.: Dissecting aneurysm of the aorta: Pathologic aspects. Arch. Pathol. 53:121, 1952.

76. McKusick, V. A., Logue, R. B., and Bahnson, H. T.: Association of aortic valvular disease and cystic medial necrosis of the ascending aorta; report of four instances. Circulation 16:188, 1957.

77. Faraci, R. M., and Westcott, J. L.: Dissecting hematoma of the aorta secondary to blunt chest trauma. Diagn. Radiol. 123:569, 1977.

78. Ponseti, I. V., and Baird, W. A.: Scoliosis and dissecting aneurysm of the aorta in rats fed with Lathyrus odoratus seeds. Am. J. Pathol. 28:1059, 1952.

79. Fikar, C. R., Amrhein, J. A., Harris, J. P., and Lewis, E. R.: Dissecting aortic aneurysm in childhood and adolescence. Clin. Pediatr. 20:578, 1981.

80. Hirst, A. E., Jr., Johns, V. J., Jr., and Kime, S. W., Jr.: Dissecting aneurysm of the aorta. A review of 505 cases. Medicine 37:217, 1958.

80a. Slater, E. E.: Aortic dissection: Presentation and diagnosis. In Doroghazi, R. M., and Slater, E. E. (eds.): Aortic Dissection. New York, McGraw-Hill Book Company, 1983, p. 61.

81. Cohen, S., and Littman, D.: Painless dissecting aneurysm of the aorta. N. Engl. J. Med. 271:143, 1964.

82. Lindsay, J., Jr., and Hurst, J. W.: Clinical features and prognosis in dissecting aneurysm of the aorta. A reappraisal. Circulation 35:880, 1967.

83. Symbas, P. N., Kelly, T. F., Vlasis, S. E., Drucker, M. H., and Arensberg, D.: Intimo-intimal intussusception and other unusual manifestations of aortic dissection. J. Thorac. Cardiovasc. Surg. 79:926, 1980.

83a. Hirst, A. E., and Gore, I.: The etiology and pathology of aortic regurgitation. In Doroghazi, R. M., and Slater, E. E. (eds.): Aortic Dissection. New York, McGraw Hill Book Company, 1983, p. 13.

84. Weisman, A. D., and Adams, R. D.: Neurological complications of dissecting aortic aneurysm. Brain 67:69, 1944.

85. Logue, R. B., and Sikes, C.: New sign in dissecting aneurysm of the aorta. Pulsation of sternoclavicular joint. J.A.M.A. 148:1209, 1952.

86. Riley, D. J., Liv, R. T., and Saxanoff, S.: Aortic dissection: A rare cause of the superior vena cava syndrome. J. Med. Soc. N. J. *78*:187, 1981.

87. Buja, M. L., Ali, N., and Roberts, W. C.: Stenosis of the right pulmonary artery: A complication of acute dissecting aneurysm of the ascending aorta. Am. Heart J. *83*:89, 1972.

88. McCarthy, C., Dickson, G. H., Besterman, E. M. M., Bromley, L. L., and Thompson, A. E.: Aortic dissection with rupture through ductus arteriosus into pulmonary artery. Br. Heart J. *34*:284, 1972.

89. Roth, J. A., and Parekh, M. A.: Dissecting aneurysms perforating the esophagus. N. Engl. J. Med. *299*:776, 1978.

90. Thiene, G., Rossi, L., and Becker, A. E.: The atrioventricular conduction system in dissecting aneurysm of the aorta. Am. Heart J. *98*:447, 1979.

91. Morris, A. L., and Barwinsky, J.: Unusual vascular complications of dissecting thoracic aortic aneurysm. Cardiovasc. Radiol. *1*:95, 1978.

92. ten Cate, J. W., Timmers, H., and Becker, A. E.: Coagulopathy in ruptured or dissecting aortic aneurysms. Am. J. Med. *59*:171, 1975.

93. Matsumoto, M., Matsuo, H., Ohara, T., Yoshioka, Y., and Abe, H.: A two-dimensional echoaortocardiographic approach to dissecting aneurysms of the aorta to prevent false positive diagnoses. Radiology *127*:491, 1978.

94. Victor, M. F., Mintz, G. S., Kotler, M. N., Wilson, A. R., and Segal, B. L.: Two dimensional echocardiographic diagnosis of aortic dissection. Am. J. Cardiol. *48*:1155, 1981.

95. Larde, D., Belloir, C., Vasile, N., Frija, J., and Ferrane, J.: Computed tomography of aortic dissection. Radiology *136*:147, 1980.

95a. Perez, J. E.: Noninvasive diagnosis: Computed tomography and ultrasound. *In* Doroghazi, R. M., and Slater, E. E. (eds.): Aortic Dissection. New York, McGraw-Hill Book Company, 1983, p. 133.

95b. Smith, D. C., and Jang, G. C.: Radiological diagnosis and aortic dissection. *In* Doroghazi, R. M., and Slater, E. E. (eds.): Aortic Dissection. New York, McGraw Hill-Book Company, 1983, p. 71.

96. Heiberg, E., Wolverson, M., Sundaram, M., Connors, J., and Susman, N.: CT findings in thoracic aortic dissection. Am. J. Radiol. *136*:13, 1981.

97. Moncada, R., Salinas, M., Churchill, R., Love, L., Reynes, C., Demos, T. C., Gunnar, R. M., and Pifarre, R.: Diagnosis of dissecting aortic aneurysm by computed tomography. Lancet *1*:238, 1981.

98. Turley, K., Ullyot, D. J., Godwin, J. D., Wilson, J. M., Lipton, M., Carlsson, E., and Ebert, P. A.: Repair of dissection of the thoracic aorta. Evaluation of false lumen utilizing computed tomography. J. Thorac. Cardiovasc. Surg. *81*:61, 1981.

99. Godwin, J. D., Turley, K., Herfkens, R. J., and Lipton, M. J.: Computed tomography for follow-up of chronic aortic dissections. Radiology *139*:655, 1981.

100. Earnest, F., IV, Muhm, J. R., and Sheedy, P. F., II: Roentgenographic findings in thoracic aortic dissection. Mayo Clin. Proc. *54*:43, 1979.

101. Dinsmore, R. E., Willerson, J. T.,, and Buckley, M. J.: Dissecting aneurysm of the aorta. Aortographic features affecting prognosis. Diagn. Radiol. *105*:567, 1972.

102. Shuford, W. H., Sybers, R. G., and Weens, H. S.: Problems of the aortographic diagnosis of dissecting aneurysms of the aorta. N. Engl. J. Med. *280*:225, 1969.

102a. Collins, J. J., Jr., Koster, J. K., Jr., Cohn, L. H., and VanDevanter, S. H.: Common aortic aneurysms: When to intervene. J. Cardiovas. Med. *8*:245, 1983.

103. Anagnostopoulos, C. E., Prabhakar, M. J. S., and Kittle, C. F.: Aortic dissections and dissecting aneurysms. Am. J. Cardiol. *30*:263, 1972.

104. Gurin, D., Bulmer, J. W., and Derby, R.: Dissecting aneurysms of the aorta. Diagnosis and operative relief of acute arterial obstructions due to this course. N.Y. State J. Med. *35*:1200, 1935.

105. Shaw, R. W.: Acute dissecting aortic aneurysms: Treatment by fenestration of the internal wall of the aneurysm. N. Engl. J. Med. *253*:331, 1955.

106. DeBakey, M. E., Cooley, D. A., and Creech, O., Jr.: Surgical considerations of dissecting aneurysm of the aorta. Ann. Surg. *142*:586, 1955.

107. Wheat, M. W., Jr., Palmer, R. F., Bartley, T. D., and Seelman, R. C.: Treatment of dissecting aneurysms of the aorta without surgery. J. Thorac. Cardiovasc. Surg. *50*:364, 1965.

107a. Wheat, M. W.: Intensive drug therapy. *In* Doroghazi, R. M., and Slater, E. E. (eds.): Aortic Dissection. New York, McGraw-Hill Book Company, 1983, p. 165.

108. Palmer, R. F., and Lasseter, K. C.: Nitroprusside and aortic dissecting aneurysm (letter). N. Engl. J. Med. *294*:1403, 1976.

109. Anagnostopoulos, C. E., Athanasuleas, C. L., Garrick, T. R., and Paulissian, R.: Acute Aortic Dissections. Baltimore, University Park Press, 1975.

110. Appelbaum, A., Karp, R. B., and Kirklin, J. W.: Ascending versus descending aortic dissections. Ann. Surg. *183*:296, 1976.

111. Reul, G. J., Jr., Cooley, D. A., Hallman, G. L., Reddy, S. B., Kyger, E. R., III, and Wukasch, D. C.: Dissecting aneurysm of the descending aorta—Improved surgical results in 91 patients. Arch. Surg. *110*:632, 1975.

112. Kidd, J. N., Reul, G. J., Jr., Cooley, D. A., Sandiford, F. M., Kyger, E. R., III, and Wukasch, D. C.: Surgical treatment of aneurysms of the ascending aorta. Cardiovasc. Surg *54*(Suppl.):118, 1976.

113. Miller, D. C., Stinson, E. B., Oyer, P. E., Rossiter, S. J., Reitz, B. A., Griepp, R. B., and Shumway, N. E.: The operative treatment of aortic dissections: Experience with 125 patients over a sixteen year period. J. Thorac. Cardiovasc. Surg. *78*:365, 1979.

114. Doroghazi, R. M., Slater, E. E., Austen, W. G., Buckley, M. J., and DeSanctis, R. W.: Long-term survival for 163 patients with treated aortic dissection. Am. J. Cardiol. (In press.)

114a. Miller, D. C.: Surgical management of aortic dissections: Indications, perioperative management and long-term results. *In* Doroghazi, R. M., and Slater, E. E. (eds.): Aortic Dissection. New York, McGraw-Hill Book Company, 1983, p. 193.

115. Vecht, R. J., Besterman, E. M. M., Bromley, L. L., Eastcott, H. H. G., and Kenyon, J. R.: Acute dissection of the aorta: Long-term review and management. Lancet *1*:110, 1980.

116. Cachera, J. P., Vouhe, P. R., Loisance, D. Y., Menu, P., Poulain, H., Bloch, G., Vasile, N., Aubry, P., and Galey, J. J.: Surgical management of acute dissections involving the ascending aorta. J. Thorac. Cardiovasc. Surg. *82*:576, 1981.

117. Kolff, J., Bates, R. J., Balderman, S. C., Shenkoya, K., and Anagnostopoulos, C. E.: Acute aortic arch dissection: Re-evaluation of the indications for medical and surgical therapy. Am. J. Cardiol. *39*:727, 1977.

118. Lemole, G. M., Strong, M. D., Spagna, P. M., and Karmilowicz, N. P.: Improved results for dissecting aneurysms: Intraluminal sutureless prosthesis. J. Thorac. Cardiovasc. Surg. *83*:249, 1982.

119. Carpentier, A., Deloche, A., Fabiani, J. N., Chauvaud, S., Relland, J., Nottin, R., Vouhe, P., Massoud, H., and Dubost, C.: New surgical approach to aortic dissection: Flow reversal and thromboexclusion. J. Thorac. Cardiovasc. Surg. *81*:659, 1981.

120. Ellis, P. R., Cooley, D. A., and DeBakey, M. E.: Clinical consideration and surgical treatment of annulo-aortic ectasia. J. Thorac. Cardiovasc. Surg. *42*:363, 1961.

121. Lindsay, J., Jr.: The Marfan syndrome and idiopathic cystic medial degeneration. *In* Lindsay, J., Jr., and Hurst, J. W. (eds.): The Aorta. New York, Grune and Stratton, 1979, p. 263.

122. Pyeritz, R. E., and McKusick, V. A.: The Marfan syndrome: Diagnosis and management. N. Engl. J. Med. *300*:772, 1979.

122a. Emanuel, R., Ng, R.A.L., Marcomichelakis, J., Moores, E. C., Jefferson, K. E., Macfaul, P. A., and Withers, R.: Formes frustes of Marfan's syndrome presenting with severe aortic regurgitation. Clinicogenetic study of 18 families. Br. Heart J. *39*:190, 1977.

123. Lemon, D. K., and White, C. W.: Anuloaortic ectasia: Angiographic, hemodynamic and clinical comparison with aortic valve insufficiency. Am. J. Cardiol. *41*:482, 1978.

124. Miller, D. C., Stinson, E. B., Oyer, P. E., Moreno-Cabral, R. J., Reitz, B. A., Rossiter, S. J., and Shumway, N. E.: Concomitant resection of ascending aortic aneurysm and replacement of the aortic valve. J. Thorac. Cardiovasc. Surg. *79*:388, 1980.

125. McDonald, G. R., Schaff, H. V., Pyeritz, R. E., McKusick, V. A., and Gott, V. L.: Surgical management of patients with the Marfan syndrome and dilatation of the ascending aorta. J. Thorac. Cardiovasc. Surg. *81*:180, 1981.

126. Takayasu, M.: Case with unusual changes of the central vessels in the retina. Acta Soc. Ophthalmol. Jap. *12*:554, 1908.

127. McKusick, V.: A form of vascular disease relatively frequent in the Orient. Am. Heart J. *63*:57, 1962.

128. Lupi-Herrera, E., Sanchez-Torres, G., Marcushamer, J., Mispireta, J., Horowitz, S., and Espino Vela, J.: Takayasu's arteritis. Clinical study of 107 cases. Am. Heart J. *93*:94, 1977.

129. Lande, A., and LaPorta, A.: Takayasu arteritis—An arteriographic-pathological correlation. Arch. Pathol. Lab. Med. *100*:437, 1976.

130. Lande, A.: Takayasu's arteritis and congenital coarctation of the descending thoracic and abdominal aorta. A critical review. Am. J. Roentgenol. *127*:227, 1976.

131. Ueno, A., Awane, G., and Wakahayachi, A.: Successfully operated obliterative brachiocephalic arteritis (Takayasu) associated with the elongated coarctation. Jap. Heart J. *8*:538, 1967.

132. Lande, A., Bard, R., Bole, P., and Guarnaccia, M.: Aortic arch syndrome (Takayasu's arteritis). Arteriographic and surgical considerations. J. Cardiovasc. Surg. *19*:507, 1978.

133. Nakao, K., Ikeda, M., Kimata, S., Nhtani, H., Miyahara, M., Ishimi, Z., Hashiba, K., Takeda, Y., Ozawa, T., Matsushita, S., and Kuramochi, M.: Takayasu's arteritis—Clinical report of eighty-four cases and immunological studies of seven cases. Circulation *35*:1141, 1967.

134. Numano, F., Isohisa, I., Maezawa, H., and Juji, T.: HL-A antigens in Takayasu's disease. Am. Heart J. *98*:153, 1979.

135. Volkman, D. J., Mann, D. L., and Fauci, A. S.: Association between Takayasu's arteritis and a B-cell alloantigen in North Americans. N. Engl. J. Med. *306*:464, 1982.

136. Inada, K., Shimizu, H., and Yokoyama, T.: Pulseless disease and atypical coarctation of the aorta with special reference to their genesis. Surgery *52*:133, 1962.

137. Gronemeyer, P. S., and deMello, D. E.: Takayasu's disease with aneurysm of right common iliac artery and iliocaval fistula in a young infant: Case report and review of the literature. Pediatrics *69*:626, 1982.

138. Swinton, N. W., and Cook, G. A.: Systolic hypertension and cardiac mortality of Takayasu's aortoarteritis. Angiology *27*:568, 1976.

139. Takishita, A., Tanaka, S., Orita, G., Kanaide, H., and Nakamura, M.: Baroflex sensitivity in patients with Takayasu's aortitis. Circulation *55*:803, 1977.

140. Akikusa, B., Kondo, Y., and Muraki, N.: Aortic insufficiency caused by Takayasu's arteritis without usual clinical features. Arch. Pathol. Lab. Med. *105*:650, 1981.

141. Pasternac, A., Lesperance, J., Grondin, P., and Cantin, M.: Primary arteritis in Takayasu's disease. A case studied by selective coronary arteriography. Am. J. Roentgenol. *128*:488, 1977.

142. Cipriano, P. R., Silverman, J. F., Perlroth, M. G., Griepp, R. B., and Wexler, L.: Coronary arterial narrowing in Takayasu's aortitis. Am. J. Cardiol. *39*:744, 1977.

143. Sen, P. K., Kinare, S. G., Engineer, S. D., and Parulkar, G. B.: The middle aortic syndrome. Br. Heart J. *25*:610, 1963.

144. Slater, E. E., and Fallon, J. T.: Upper extremity hypertension in a 28-year-old Korean man. Case Records of the Massachusetts General Hospital. N. Engl. J. Med. *299*:1002, 1978.

145. Lande, A., and Bard, R.: Takayasu's arteritis. An unrecognized cause of pulmonary hypertension. Angiology *27*:114, 1974.

146. Lupi, H. E., Sanchez, T. G., Horwitz, S., and Gutierrez, F. E.: Pulmonary artery involvement in Takayasu's arteritis. Chest *67*:69, 1975.

147. Lande, A., and Rossi, P.: The value of total aortography in the diagnosis of Takayasu's arteritis. Radiology *114*:287, 1975.

148. Bonventre, M. V.: Takayasu's disease revisited. N.Y. State J. Med. *74*:1960, 1974.

149. Sunamori, M., Hatano, R., Yokokawa, T., Tsukuura, T., Sakamoto, T., Suzuki, T., Murakami, T., Yokoawa, M., and Numano, F.: Aortitis syndrome due to Takayasu's disease. A guideline for the surgical indication. J. Cardiovasc. Surg. *17*:443, 1976.

150. Bloss, R. S., Duncan, J. M., Cooley, D. A., Leatherman, L. L., and Schnee, M. J.: Takayasu's arteritis: Surgical considerations. Ann. Thorac. Surg. *27*:574, 1979.

151. Hallett, J. W., Jr., Brewster, D. C., Darling, R. C., and O'Hara, P. J.: Coarctation of the abdominal aorta: Current options in surgical management. Ann. Surg. *191*:430, 1980.

152. Ishikawa, K.: Survival and morbidity after diagnosis of occlusive thromboaortopathy (Takayasu's disease). Am. J. Cardiol. *47*:1026, 1981.

153. Klein, R. G., Hunder, G. G., Stanson, A. W., and Sheps, S. G.: Large artery involvement in giant cell (temporal) arteritis. Ann. Intern. Med. *83*:806, 1975.

154. Hamrin, B.: Polymyalgia arteritica. Acta Med. Scand. (Suppl.)*533*:1, 1972

155. Austen, W. G., and Blennerhassett, M. B.: Giant cell aortitis causing an aneurysm of the ascending aorta and aortic regurgitation. N. Engl. J. Med. *272*:80, 1965.

156. Ghose, M. K., Shensa, S., and Lerner, P. I.: Arteritis of the aged (giant cell arteritis) and fever of unexplained origin. Am. J. Med. *60*:429, 1976.

157. Huston, K. A., and Hunder, G. G.: Giant cell (cranial) arteritis: A clinical review. Am. Heart J. *100*:99, 1980.

158. Salisbury, R. S., and Hazleman, B. L.: Successful treatment of dissecting aortic aneurysm due to giant cell arteritis. Ann. Rheum. Dis. *40*:507, 1981.

159. Soorae, A. S., McKeown, F., and Cleland, J.: Aortic valve replacement for severe aortic regurgitation caused by idiopathic giant cell aortitis. Thorax *35*:60, 1980.

160. Davidson, P., Bagenstoss, A. H., Slocumb, C. H., and Daugherty, G. W.: Cardiac and aortic lesions in rheumatoid spondylitis. Proc. Mayo Clin. *36*:427, 1963.

161. Zvaifler, N. J., and Weintraub, A. M.: Aortitis and aortic insufficiency in chronic rheumatic disorders. A reappraisal. Arthritis Rheum. *6*:241, 1963.

162. Pearson, C. M., Kroening, R., Verity, M. A., and Getzen, J. H.: Aortic insufficiency and aortic aneurysm in relapsing polychondritis. Trans. Assoc. Am. Phys. *80*:71, 1967.

163. Paulus, H. E., Pearson, C. M., and Pitts, W.: Aortic insufficiency in five patients with Reiter's syndrome. A detailed clinical and pathologic study. Am. J. Med. *53*:464, 1972.

164. Muna, W. F., Roller, D. H., Craft, J., Shaw, R. K., and Ross, A. M.: Psoriatic arthritis and aortic regurgitation. J.A.M.A. *244*:363, 1980.

165. Little, A. G., and Zarins, C. K.: Abdominal aortic aneurysm and Behçet's disease. Surgery *91*:359, 1982.

166. Kampmeier, R. H.: Manifestations of late syphilis. South. Med. Bull. *53*:17, 1965.

167. Heggtveit, H. A.: Syphilitic aortitis. A clinicopathologic autopsy study of 100 cases, 1950 to 1960. Circulation *29*:346, 1964.

168. Carter, C. H., Agostas, W. N., Sydenstricker, V. P.: Rupture of an aortic aneurysm into the pulmonary artery. A case report. Circulation *5*:449, 1952.

169. Kampmeier, R. H.: Aneurysm of the abdominal aorta. A study of 73 cases. Am. J. Med. Sci. *192*:97, 1936.

170. Prewitt, T. A.: Syphilitic aortic insufficiency. Its increased incidence in the elderly. J.A.M.A. *211*:637, 1970.

171. Sparling, A. F.: Diagnosis and treatment of syphilis. N. Engl. J. Med. *284*:642, 1971.

172. Centers for Disease Control: Syphilis Recommended Treatment Schedules, 1976. The Venereal Disease Control Advisory Committee. Ann. Intern. Med. *85*:94, 1976.

173. Beck, W., Barnard, C. N., and Schrire, V.: Syphilitic obstruction of coronary ostia successfully treated by endarterectomy. Br. Heart J. *27*:911, 1965.

174. Steinberg, I.: Anomalies (pseudocoarctation) of the arch of the aorta—Report of 8 new and review of 8 previously published cases. Am. J. Roentgenol. *88*:73, 1962.

175. Brinsfield, D. E., Shuford, W. M., Plauth, W. H., Jr., and Sybers, R. G.: Congenital anomalies of the aorta. *In* Lindsay, J., Jr., and Hurst, J. W. (eds.): The Aorta. New York, Grune and Stratton, 1979, p. 271.

176. Keller, H. I., and Cheitlin, M. D.: The occurrence of mild coarctation of the aorta (pseudocoarctation) and coarctation in one family. Am. Heart J. *70*:115, 1965.

177. Lavin, N., Mehta, S., Liberson, M., and Pouget, J. M.: Pseudocoarctation of the aorta. An unusual variant with coarctation. Am. J. Cardiol. *24*:584, 1969.

178. Lajos, T. Z., Meckstroth, C. V., Klassen, K. P., and Sherman, N. J.: Pseudocoarctation of the aorta. A variant or an entity? Chest *58*:571, 1970.

179. Griffen, J. F.: Congenital kinking of the aorta (pseudocoarctation). N. Engl. J. Med. *271*:726, 1964.

180. Turner, A. F., Swenson, B. E., Jacobson, G., and Kay, J. H.: Kinking or buckling of the aorta. Case report with complication of aneurysm formation. Am. J. Roentgenol. *97*:411, 1966.

181. Bahabozorgui, S., Bernstein, R. G., and Frater, R. W. M.: Pseudocoarctation of the aorta associated with aneurysm formation. Chest *60*:616, 1971.

182. Bland, E. F., and Castleman, B.: Vascular collapse in a woman with an unusual calcified ring in the aortic arch. N. Engl. J. Med. *280*:1466, 1969.

183. Steinberg, I.: Calcified and dilated ascending aorta due to atheromatous occlusive disease simulating coarctation of the aorta: A report of a case and theory of pathogenesis. Am. J. Roentgenol. *98*:840, 1966.

184. Prian, G. W., Kinard, S. A., Read, C. T., and Diethrich, E. B.: Pseudocoarctation: Diagnosis, etiology, natural history with emphasis on timing and technique of surgical correction. Vasc. Surg. *6*:198, 1972.

185. Greendyke, R. M.: Traumatic rupture of aorta: Special reference to automobile accidents. J.A.M.A. *195*:527, 1966.

186. Parmley, L. F., Mattingly, T. W., Manion, W. C., and Jahnke, E. J.: Nonpenetrating traumatic injury of the aorta. Circulation *17*:1086, 1958.

187. Fleming, A. W., and Green, D. C.: Traumatic aneurysms of the thoracic aorta: Report of 43 patients. Ann. Thorac. Surg. *18*:91, 1974.

188. Ayella, R. J., Hankins, J. R., Turney, S. Z., and Cowley, R. A.: Ruptured thoracic aorta due to blunt trauma. J. Trauma *17*:199, 1977.

189. Malm, J. R., and Deterling, R. A.: Traumatic aneurysm of the thoracic aorta simulating coarctation: A case report. J. Thorac. Cardiovasc. Surg. *40*:271, 1960.

190. Kirsh, M. M., Behrendt, D. M., Orringer, M. B., Gago, O., Gray, L. A., Mills, L. J., Walter, J. F., and Sloan, H.: The treatment of acute traumatic rupture of the aorta. A 10-year experience. Ann. Surg. *184*:308, 1976.

191. Bodily, K., Perry, J. F., Strate, R. G., and Fischer, R. P.: The salvageability of patients with post-traumatic rupture of the descending thoracic aorta in a primary trauma center. J. Trauma *17*:754, 1977.

192. Jang, G. C., Brody, W. R., and Dinsmore, R. E.: Radiologic diagnosis or aortic disease. *In* Lindsay, J., Jr., and Hurst, J. W. (eds.): The Aorta. New York, Grune and Stratton, 1979, p. 295.

193. Marsh, D. G., and Sturm, J. T.: Traumatic aortic rupture: Roentgenographic indications for angiography. Ann. Thorac. Surg. *21*:337, 1976.

194. Simeone, J. F., Deren, M. M., and Cagle, F.: The value of the left apical cap in the diagnosis of aortic rupture. Diagn. Radiol. *139*:35, 1981.

195. Bennett, D. E., and Cherry, J. K.: The natural history of traumatic aneurysms of the aorta. Surgery *61*:516, 1967.

196. Schwartz, M. L., Fisher, R., Sako, Y., Castaneda, A. R., Grage, T. B., and Nicoloff, D. M.: Post-traumatic aneurysms of the thoracic aorta. Surgery *78*:589, 1975.

197. Heiskell, C. A., and Conn, J., Jr.: Aortoarterial emboli. Am. J. Surg. *132*:4, 1976.

198. Shapiro, M. E., Rodvien, R., Bauer, K. A., and Salzman, E. W.: Acute aortic thrombosis in antithrombin III deficiency. J.A.M.A. *245*:1759, 1981.

199. Schatz, I. J., and Stanley, J. C.: Saddle embolus of the aorta. J.A.M.A. *235*: 1262, 1976.

200. Thompson, J. E., and Garrett, W. V.: Peripheral-arterial surgery. N. Engl. J. Med. *302*:491, 1980.

201. Tegtmeyer, C. J., Wellons, H. A., and Thompson, R. N.: Balloon dilation of the abdominal aorta. J.A.M.A. *244*:2636, 1980.

202. Hertzer, N. R.: Peripheral atheromatous embolization following blunt abdominal trauma. Surgery *82*:244, 1977.

203. Perdue, G. D., and Smith, R. B.: Atheromatous microemboli. Ann. Surg. *169*:954, 1969.

204. Carvajal, J. A., Anderson, R., Weiss, L., Grisiner, J., and Berman, R.: Atheroembolism. An etiologic factor in renal insufficiency, gastrointestinal hemorrhages and peripheral vascular diseases. Arch. Intern. Med. *119*:593, 1967.

205. Handler, F. P.: Clinical and pathologic significance of atheromatous embolization, with emphasis on an etiology of renal hypertension. Am. J. Med. *20*:366, 1956.

206. Anderson, W. R., Richards, A. M., and Weiss, L.: Hemorrhage and necrosis of the stomach and bowel due to atheroembolism. A correlative study of atheromatous emboli to the gastrointestinal tract in humans and experimental animals. Am. J. Clin. Pathol. *48*:30, 1967.

207. Moldveen-Geronimus, M., and Merriam, J. C.: Cholesterol embolization. From pathological curiosity to clinical entity. Circulation *35*:946, 1967.

208. Jarrett, F., Darling, R. C., Mundth, E. D., and Austen, W. G.: Experience with infected aneurysms of the abdominal aorta. Arch. Surg. *110*:1281, 1975.

209. Silbergleit, A., Arbulu, A., Defever, B. A., and Nedwicki, E. G.: Tuberculous aortitis. Surgical resection of ruptured abdominal false aneurysm. J.A.M.A. *193*:83, 1965.

210. Felson, B., Akers, P. V., Hall, G. S., Schreiber, J. T., Greene, R. E., and Pedrosa, C. S.: Mycotic tuberculous aneurysm of the thoracic aorta. J.A.M.A. *237*:1104, 1977.

211. Feinsod, F. M., Norfleet, R. G., and Hoehn, J. L.: Mycotic aneurysm of the external iliac artery. A triad of clinical signs facilitating early diagnosis. J.A.M.A. *238*:245, 1977.

212. Anderson, C. B., Butcher, H. R., and Ballinger, W. F.: Mycotic aneurysms. Arch. Surg. *109*:712, 1974.

213. Chen, K. T. K.: Primary malignant fibrous histiocytoma of the aorta. Cancer *48*:840, 1981.

46

COR PULMONALE AND PULMONARY THROMBOEMBOLISM

by E. Regis McFadden, Jr., M.D., and Eugene Braunwald, M.D.

According to the World Health Organization, the chronic form of cor pulmonale is composed of some combination of hypertrophy and dilatation of the right ventricle secondary to pulmonary hypertension; the latter is caused by disease of the pulmonary parenchyma and/or pulmonary vascular system between the origins of the main pulmonary artery and the entry of the pulmonary veins into the left atrium.[1] Acute cor pulmonale is defined as acute right heart strain or overload resulting from the pulmonary hypertension usually due to massive pulmonary embolism.[2] Cor pulmonale includes many disease states with diverse etiologies, pathophysiological mechanisms, and clinical characteristics which have in common only a disturbance of the pulmonary circulation. This chapter focuses on those conditions (with the exclusion of primary pulmonary hypertension, Chap. 25) which act directly on the pulmonary vessels, both acutely and chronically, and those which produce pulmonary hypertension by acting primarily on the gas-exchanging, neuromuscular, and ventilatory control functions of the respiratory system.

ANATOMICAL AND PATHOPHYSIOLOGICAL CORRELATES

Right Ventricular Anatomy

In the first 3 months of life in infants born at, or near, sea level, the right ventricle is larger and heavier and has a greater end-diastolic volume than the left.[3-7] With advancing age, the left ventricle becomes dominant, and in the adult, the right ventricular wall is relatively thin and has a crescentic configuration on cross section. However, in high-altitude dwellers, the situation is different. The degree of right ventricular preponderance, both at birth and for the first 3 months of life, is greater than that seen in low-altitude residents, and the normal regression in size is so delayed that the right ventricular enlargement can persist through the first decade.[6] In native adults living above 12,000 feet, 93 per cent of the hearts in a necropsy series showed some degree of right ventricular enlargement.[8] These morphological findings have a close relationship with the hemodynamic characteristics of individuals at high altitudes and can be related to the degree of pulmonary arterial hypertension.[9]

Several methods are used to ascertain the characteristics, presence, and severity of right ventricular hypertrophy; the two traditional methods involve the measurement of ventricular weight and wall thickness. Many investigators believe that wall thickness determinations are not sufficiently precise. Fulton et al. have provided weight criteria that are used widely.[10] In their technique, the right ventricle is dissected free, and the septum is weighed together with the left ventricle. Right ventricular weight can then be described in absolute terms or as a ratio of the left ventricle (LV) plus the septum (S), i.e., (LV + S)/RV. Using these criteria, a heart is considered normal only if the total ventricular weight is less than 250 gm, the free wall of the right ventricle weighs less than 65 gm, and the ratio of (LV + S)/RV is between 2.3:1 and 3.3:1. If left ventricular hypertrophy is also present, the ratio may be within normal limits or even raised. Using this method, Mitchell and colleagues found that the upper limits of normal (as defined by the mean plus 2 standard deviations) in men 40 or more years of age at death were 69 gm for the right ventricle and 203 gm for the left ventricle plus septum. These observers also noted that in their study right ventricular thickness was a relatively poor index of hypertrophy.[11]

Others have determined muscle fiber size morphometrically and found the distribution of myocardial fiber diameters to be uniform, with a distinct bell-shaped distribution noted for the right ventricle, left ventricle, and septum.[12] In cases of pure right ventricular hypertrophy, the distribution always shifted so that the mean diameter of the muscle fibers from the right ventricle exceeded that of the septum or normal left ventricle.

Right Ventricular Function

Because right ventricular hypertrophy occurs most commonly in association with longstanding elevations in pulmonary arterial pressures, an analogy has often been made between the left ventricle in systemic hypertension and the right ventricle in pulmonary hypertension. Since there is no fundamental difference in either the configuration or the pumping action of the two ventricles before birth, the differences that exist in the adult have been attributed to the flow resistance in the respective circulations.[13] As already noted, the normal adult right ventricle has thin walls and a crescent shape; its pumping action is akin to that of a bellows working in series with a low-pressure circuit, in contrast to the concentric contraction of the left ventricle. The right ventricle is more compliant,[14] and in comparison with the left it is better able to handle an increase in a volume than a pressure load. The evidence in support of this statement is derived in the main from animal data[15-18] (Fig. 46–1), which contrasts the effects of increasing preload and afterload on right and left ventricular function. In the left-hand panel, stroke volume is plotted as a function of various afterloads that were produced by actively constricting the main pulmonary artery and aorta in the dog.[15,16] Small increments in pulmonary artery pressure are associated with sharp decreases in right ventricular stroke volume. In contrast, the left ventricle, which normally works against high initial pressures, continues to maintain stroke volume despite substantial increases in systemic arterial pressure.

The right-hand portion of this figure demonstrates the effects of increasing preload. These ventricular function curves (Chap. 12) were obtained by volume infusions into the atria of dogs.[17,18] Note the marked differences in the respective ventricular stroke work that occur as right and left atrial pressures are increased. For a fourfold elevation in filling pressure (i.e., from 5 to 20 cm H_2O), the increase in left ventricular work was approximately five times that of the right.

In response to chronic pressure loads, significant changes develop in the configuration, mass, and functional characteristics of the right ventricle. The rate at which these occur in man and the magnitude of the pressures needed to produce them are unknown. However, animal studies indicate that alterations in structure and function can be quite rapid following experimental outflow tract obstruction. Spann et al. observed a 71 per cent increase in right ventricular weight in cats 2 days after the pulmonary artery was banded, and within a month weight had risen to 2.5 times the normal value.[19] This increase was not from an elevation in cardiac tissue water, since the wet to dry weight ratios were not significantly different from normal. It is doubtful that the response is as rapid in man.

The lumen of the main pulmonary artery can be reduced by 60 to 80 per cent before aortic pressure declines.[20-22] Because these experiments ignored the effects of neurohumoral compensations that support the systemic circulation, the impression has arisen that the acute right ventricular response is an abrupt, all-or-none event. However, as suggested in Figure 46–1, right ventricular decompensation is really a continuum.[15,18] At right ventricular systolic pressures of 60 to 80 mm Hg, right ventricular dilatation and failure occur with systemic hypotension and hypoperfusion.[23] The rate and/or absolute level of outflow tract obstruction at which these alterations develop can be greatly amplified or attenuated by respectively decreasing or increasing right coronary artery blood flow[23] (Fig. 46–2). The relative role played by changes in coronary blood flow in acute right heart failure secondary to massive thromboembolism in humans has yet to be determined.

Pulmonary Vascular Anatomy

Development. Embryologically, the primitive main pulmonary artery and its main right and left branches are derived from the aortic sac, whereas the peripheral pulmonary arteries arise from a network of vessels around the bronchial bud.[24] Each pulmonary artery forms a close relationship with a stem bronchus and provides an arterial partner for each new airway ramification. This branching pattern of airways and arteries is complete all the way out to the preacinar region by week 16 of intrauterine life, and further growth occurs only in dimensions.[25]

At birth the alveolar region is represented by primitive air sacs, and during early childhood the acini grow rapidly by budding new alveoli from respiratory bronchioli, alveolar ducts, and more distal air spaces.[26,27] New arteries and veins continue to develop up to the 18th month of life and then increase in size with further age.[26] These vessels follow the course of the alveoli and not the airway. By the age of

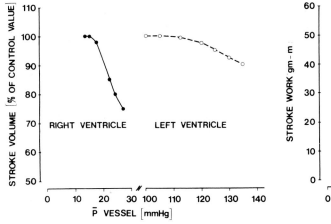

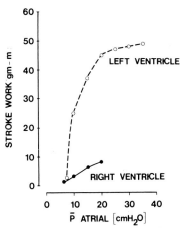

FIGURE 46–1 Effects of increasing preload and afterload on right and left ventricular function. The data in the left panel were obtained by constricting the main pulmonary artery and aorta in dogs. The right panel demonstrates the effect of increasing preloads.

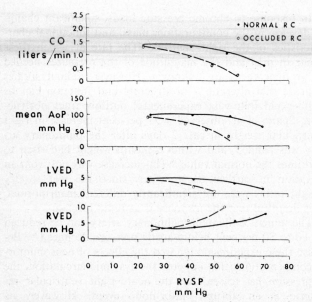

FIGURE 46–2 Hemodynamic responses to increasing levels of right ventricular systolic stress induced by incremental pulmonary artery obstruction before (solid lines) and after (broken lines) right coronary artery (RC) occlusion. CO = cardiac output; AoP = mean aortic pressure; LVED = left ventricular end-diastolic pressure; RVED = right ventricular end-diastolic pressure; RVSP = right ventricular systolic pressure. (From Brooks, H., et al.: Performance of the right ventricle under stress: Relation to right coronary flow. J. Clin. Invest. *50:*2176, 1971.)

8 years the number of alveoli and blood vessels reaches that of the adult.[26]

It has been traditionally held that the branching pattern and course of the airways and pulmonary arteries always parallel each other, at least within the alveolar region. However, Elliot and Reid have described an irregular branching pattern from the hilum to the level of the capillaries with so-called "axial" or "conventional" arteries following the airways and supernumerary arteries, which are side branches arising from the main arteries but without a corresponding airway.[28] Two types of supernumerary vessels have been recognized: aberrant and accessory. An *aberrant* artery arises independently of any airway but then joins one downstream and branches with it. An *accessory* artery branches independently of any airway and usually enters the periphery of a respiratory unit. The function of these vessels is unknown.

Wall Structure. In keeping with its embryological derivation, the main pulmonary artery and the first five generations are elastic in nature but less so than the aorta and major systemic arteries.[29] These vessels are over 3000 μm in diameter in the adult. In the axial pathway, the next three generations are said to be transitional.[30] They have fewer internal and external elastic laminae and range in size from 2000 to 3000 μm. The remainder of the artery is then divided into muscular, partially muscular, and nonmuscular segments.[31]

Muscular arteries have a continuous muscle coat limited by both internal and external elastic laminae. These arteries form the majority of vessels in the lung and are found in a diameter range of 30 to 2000 μm in the adult. The medial muscle coat is very thin compared with the arterioles in the systemic circulation. These vessels give way to partially muscular arteries in which the muscle is arranged in a spiral so that in cross section it appears as a crescent, with the rest of the wall being like a capillary. These vessels are between 30 to 250 μm in external diameter. Nonmuscular arteries are larger than capillaries and range from 30 to 75 μm in diameter in adults.

Although there is great variation in the sizes of arteries that accompany conducting airways such as lobar bronchi, those that follow the respiratory bronchi and alveolar ducts are muscular or partially so.[28-30] The implications for function of these observations are severalfold. It is known that gas exchange occurs in respiratory bronchi and alveolar ducts through the arteries that accompany these structures.[32] When this information is coupled with the fact that hypoxia acts directly to constrict muscular arteries,[32,33] it is apparent that this area of the lung has the propensity for active control of pulmonary blood

flow. Further, since the spiral of muscle in the partially muscular arteries is directly contiguous with the muscle encircling the larger vessels, retrograde propagation of the hypoxic stimulus can occur in the intracellular pathways of the muscle syncytium,[34] and a wider and more severe response can develop.

Innervation. In further contrast to the peripheral circulation, it has proved difficult to demonstrate a nerve supply in the pulmonary circulation. Evidence suggests that although both adrenergic and cholinergic fibers are present, they are sparse in comparison with those of systemic vessels of similar size, and their distribution tends to be concentrated in the larger vessels at the hilum.[31,35]

In summary, the structure of the pulmonary circulation is in keeping with its hemodynamics. The thin-walled, sparsely innervated vessels which contain relatively small amounts of smooth muscle do not favor the development of marked vasomotor responses, and, indeed, vasoconstriction alone is not sufficient to overload the right ventricle to the point of producing acute cor pulmonale.[36] Consequently, mechanical occlusion of the pulmonary circulation can be inferred when there is acute cor pulmonale, and structural alterations in the pulmonary vascular bed must be present in the chronic form.

Physiology of the Pulmonary Circulation
(See also Chapter 25)

The physiology of the pulmonary circulation is unique from several standpoints. Most of this vascular bed is contained within the parenchyma of the lung, and thus the vessels are subjected to external distending and compressive forces which can act independently of any intrinsic properties of the vessels themselves. In addition, the pulmonary circulation is in series with a pump capable of developing only low pressures, yet it must accommodate the entire cardiac output under all states of physical activity. Consequently, it must adjust to wide variations in blood flow without much change in pressure so as not to overload the right ventricle. This section will deal with the pressure, flow, and volume relationships of the pulmonary circulation as they interrelate with the mechanical and gas-exchanging properties of the lungs.

PRESSURE-VOLUME RELATIONSHIPS. Historically, it has been thought that the pulmonary circulation is highly distensible and that the vessels dilate to accommodate increases in cardiac output and, in this manner, prevent an increase in pulmonary artery pressure in high-flow states.[37,38] However, actual measurements of the compliance of the pulmonary vessels have shown that this vascular bed is significantly stiffer than its systemic counterpart[39,40] (Fig. 46–3), and only small increments in blood volume can be accepted by the large pulmonary vessels.[41-44] It has subsequently been demonstrated that a major mechanism to accommodate increased blood volume is the recruitment of previously unperfused vessels.[39,45] Morphological evidence suggests that both recruitment and distention occur with an increase in pulmonary blood flow and that the transmural pressures to which the vessel is subjected are what determines which one predominates.[46] In superior portions of the lung where the vessels are collapsed or where alveolar pressure is greater than pulmonary venous pressure, recruitment appears to be the major mechanism. Distention is more important when pulmonary venous pressure is greater than alveolar pressure (see below).[31]

PRESSURE-FLOW RELATIONSHIPS. Evaluation of the pressure-flow relationships of the pulmonary circulation in normal humans at any fixed lung volume demonstrates a hyperbolic configuration in which large changes in pulmonary blood flow are associated with small eleva-

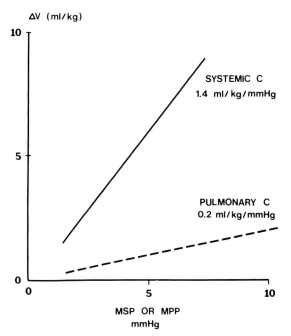

FIGURE 46–3 Comparison of compliances of pulmonary and systemic vascular beds. MSP = mean systemic pressure; MPP = mean pulmonary pressure; C = compliance; ΔV = change in volume. (Redrawn from Guyton, A. C.: Circulatory Physiology: Cardiac Output and Its Regulation. Philadelphia, W. B. Saunders Co., 1963.)

sponse to the transmural pressures to which they are exposed.

Because the pulmonary vessels are within the substance of the lung, their dimensions reflect the forces exerted upon them by the pulmonary parenchyma. At low lung volumes, the extraalveolar vessels tend to collapse because radial traction no longer supports them. Simultaneously, the alveolar vessels are pulled open by the increased recoil forces generated by the tendency of the alveoli to become smaller. As the lung is inflated to volumes above functional residual capacity, the larger vessels tend to be pulled open, but there is now a progressive increase in the resistance of the small vessels as they are squeezed and lengthened by enlarging alveoli. In addition to this deformation, alterations in alveolar pressure can also dynamically influence the lumens of small vessels. When alveolar pressure is positive, as it is during expiration or with the Valsalva maneuver, vessels are compressed. Alternatively, with negative pressure, as with inspiration or the Mueller maneuver, small vessels are subjected to a proportional distending pressure. With this information, it is relatively easy to appreciate that alveolar pressure can play a critical role in determining the distribution of pulmonary blood flow and, accordingly, gas exchange.

DETERMINANTS OF PULMONARY GAS EXCHANGE

Distribution of Pulmonary Blood Flow

In the normal upright human, blood flow per unit volume of lung steadily increases from the apex to the base, with flow at the apex being virtually nil.[47,48] This distribution is affected by changes of posture and by exercise. When a subject is in the supine position, apical blood flow increases but the basal flow remains virtually unchanged, with the result that the distribution from apex to base becomes almost uniform. In this posture, however, flow in the posterior or dependent regions exceeds that in the anterior parts. During mild exercise, flow to both the upper and the lower zones increases but more to the upper, so that flow becomes more evenly distributed.

tions in pulmonary artery pressure (Fig. 46–4A). The net result is that as flow increases, pulmonary vascular resistance decreases (Fig. 46–4B).[36] Consequently, irrespective of whether distention or recruitment occurs, both mechanisms subserve the necessity of maintaining a low pressure circuit during situations of increased blood flow.

If one examines pulmonary vascular resistance as a function of lung volume, a U-shaped curve is found (Fig. 46–4C).[43] At the extremes of lung volume of full inflation and deflation, vascular resistance is high, and it reaches its nadir at about the resting end-expiratory position (i.e., at functional residual capacity). These findings can be explained by considering the geometry assumed by the alveolar and intrapulmonic but extraalveolar vessels in re-

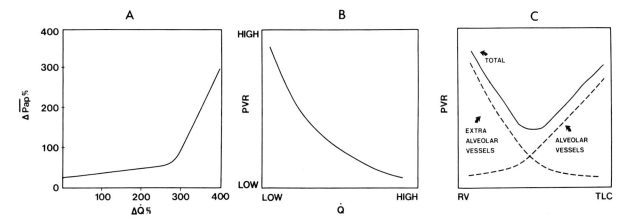

FIGURE 46–4 Some aspects of pulmonary vascular physiology. *A,* Pressure-flow relationship. *B,* Resistance-flow relationship. *C,* Pulmonary vascular resistance as a function of lung volume for the total system and for extraalveolar and alveolar vessels. ΔPAP = per cent change of mean pulmonary artery pressure from control; ΔQ = per cent change in cardiac output; 100 = normal cardiac output; RV = residual volume; TLC = total lung capacity.

West and colleagues[47-50] and Permutt and Riley[51] have independently demonstrated that the pressure-flow relationships through the lung can be analogous to those of a "waterfall" or Starling resistor. The basic point of these studies is that the effective pressure drop in the pulmonary vasculature is not always the difference between inflow (pulmonary artery) and outflow (left atrial) pressures but often is between the inflow pressure and the closing pressure of small vessels downstream.

In normal human lungs pulmonary arterial and venous pressures both increase from superior to dependent regions because of hydrostatic effects resulting from gravity acting on the blood.[49-52] However, alveolar pressures remain essentially constant throughout the lung. Alveolar pressure exceeds venous pressure at a more dependent portion of the lung than does arterial pressure. This results in distribution of blood flow to three major areas (Fig. 17–4, p. 564). In the most superior area (zone I) no flow occurs because alveolar pressure exceeds pulmonary arterial pressure. Presumably, this is because thin-walled collapsible vessels are directly exposed to alveolar pressure. In humans, the pulmonary artery pressure is sufficiently high to bring blood to the apex of the lung so that no zone I is present under normal conditions. It can develop, however, if pulmonary artery pressure falls or if alveolar pressure is elevated, as it is in obstructive airway disease. In the middle zone (zone II), arterial pressure exceeds alveolar pressure, but the latter is greater than venous pressure. Here, flow through the capillaries is proportional to the difference between arterial and alveolar pressure. In the lowest zone, zone III, venous pressure exceeds alveolar pressure, the vessels are held open, and flow is determined in the usual way by the arterial-venous pressure difference. Hughes and associates[53] and West et al.[54] have also observed a small zone of reduced flow at the very base of the lung and have attributed this to a possible increase in the interstitial pressure as a consequence of the reduced expansion of the lung parenchyma in the lower zone. This has, therefore, been called zone IV. There is still some uncertainty about the cause of the reduced flow in this area, but the concept of reduction in flow caused by an increased interstitial pressure is almost certainly important in mitral stenosis and may be responsible for the reduction in basilar blood flow observed in that condition.

Distribution of Ventilation

The distribution of ventilation, like that of perfusion, decreases from base to apex in the normal lung, but the rate of change is only about one third that seen with blood flow[47] (Fig. 46–5). Here, too, gravity plays a role, and changes in posture have an influence. Thus, when normal subjects lie supine, the difference in ventilation between the anatomical upper and lower zones is abolished,[47] and in the inverted lung, the apex ventilates better than the base, so the normal pattern is reversed.

Evaluation of the relative rates of expansion of the upper and lower zones in the upright position reveals different patterns of distribution, depending upon the lung volume from which inspiration is initiated.[55-57] As a consequence of the effect of gravity and the shape of the pressure-volume curve of the lung, when a normal subject takes a breath from functional residual capacity (FRC), ventilation is preferentially distributed to the dependent lung zones. Since blood flow in the resting state is also preferentially distributed to this area, this matching of ventilation to perfusion in different body positions insures efficient gas exchange under a variety of physiological conditions.

If breathing takes place at lung volumes lower than FRC, the distribution of ventilation is quite different. Because of closure of dependent airways, the most inferior portions of the lung do not ventilate, and all of the inspired gas goes preferentially to the upper zones. The phenomenon of airway closure at low lung volumes has major physiological significance and can produce substantial alterations in ventilation-perfusion relationships and arterial hypoxia.[58,59]

Ventilation-perfusion Ratios

Ventilation-perfusion $(\dot{V}_A/\dot{Q})$ ratios are important because they are the determinants of the gas exchange that occurs in any part of the lung, and thereby they affect the overall efficiency of the lungs in taking up oxygen and eliminating carbon dioxide.[47,60-62] The partial pressure of oxygen in the alveolar gas (and therefore in the end-capillary blood) is set by a balance between the rate of removal by the blood and its rate of replenishment by ventilation. If ventilation is gradually reduced and perfusion maintained to an alveolus, oxygen tension falls and carbon dioxide tension rises. The limit is reached when the unit is not ventilated at all, and the pulmonary venous oxygen and carbon dioxide will be those of mixed venous blood. This is a $\dot{V}_A/\dot{Q}$ relationship of zero and corresponds to the situation in which there is a true anatomical pulmonary arteriovenous shunt, e.g., a pulmonary arteriovenous fistula or a functional one such as produced by atelectasis. By contrast, if perfusion to a normally ventilating alveolus is gradually reduced, the oxygen tension in the venous blood draining this alveolus rises and the partial pressure of carbon dioxide falls. The limit now occurs when the unit is unperfused. This is a $\dot{V}_A/\dot{Q}$ of infinity and is seen in situations in which blood supply is disrupted, such as by pulmonary emboli or other disease in which occlusion of the pulmonary arterial circulation occurs. Between these two

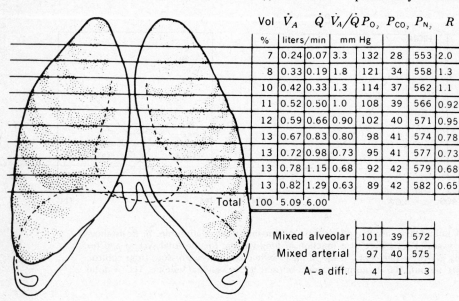

Vol	$\dot{V}_A$	$\dot{Q}$	$\dot{V}_A/\dot{Q}$	P_{O_2}	P_{CO_2}	P_{N_2}	R
%	liters/min			mm Hg			
7	0.24	0.07	3.3	132	28	553	2.0
8	0.33	0.19	1.8	121	34	558	1.3
10	0.42	0.33	1.3	114	37	562	1.1
11	0.52	0.50	1.0	108	39	566	0.92
12	0.59	0.66	0.90	102	40	571	0.95
13	0.67	0.83	0.80	98	41	574	0.78
13	0.72	0.98	0.73	95	41	577	0.73
13	0.78	1.15	0.68	92	42	579	0.68
13	0.82	1.29	0.63	89	42	582	0.65
Total 100	5.09	6.00					

	P_{O_2}	P_{CO_2}	P_{N_2}
Mixed alveolar	101	39	572
Mixed arterial	97	40	575
A-a diff.	4	1	3

FIGURE 46–5 Regional differences in alveolar ventilation ($\dot{V}_A$) and perfusion ($\dot{Q}$) in the normal upright lung. Vol = lung volume; $\dot{V}_A/\dot{Q}$ = ventilation-perfusion ratios; P_{O_2} = partial pressure of oxygen; P_{CO_2} = partial pressure of carbon dioxide; P_{N_2} = partial pressure of nitrogen; R = respiratory exchange ratio; A-a diff. = alveolar-arterial differences. (From West, J. B.: Disturbances of respiratory function. In Petersdorf, R. G., et al. (eds.): Harrison's Principles of Internal Medicine. 10th ed. New York, McGraw-Hill Book Co., 1983.)

extreme examples, a wide range of $\dot{V}_A/\dot{Q}$ abnormalities is possible.

The alveoli hypoventilated in relation to their perfusion (i.e., low $\dot{V}_A/\dot{Q}$ ratio) cause hypoxemia, and their presence has the same effect as mixing venous and arterial blood. This is termed venous admixture or wasted blood and is evaluated clinically by determining the oxygen tension difference between ideal alveolar gas and arterial blood. Normally, venous admixture or "shunt effect" is only about 2 to 3 per cent of cardiac output,[63-65] but in severe disease it may rise to 30 per cent or more. The normal alveolar-arterial difference of oxygen (A-aDO$_2$) is 20 mm Hg or less.[63-65]

The alveoli which are hyperventilated in relation to their perfusion (i.e, high $\dot{V}_A/\dot{Q}$ ratio) mainly affect CO$_2$ elimination. They behave as if part of the inspired gas bypassed the alveoli, so this effect has been called "wasted ventilation" or an increase in "physiological dead space." It is evaluated by comparing mixed expired and arterial CO$_2$, using the Bohr equation. Normally the physiological dead space is less than 30 per cent of the tidal volume.[65,66] In severe lung disease it can rise to 50 per cent or more. Every pathological condition that directly affects the pulmonary parenchyma or its vascular bed results in mismatched ventilation and blood flow. Consequently, this abnormality is by far the most common cause of arterial hypoxemia in disease states. Both venous admixture and physiological dead space are typically increased in chronic obstructive and infiltrative lung diseases. In pulmonary thromboembolism an increase in dead space predominates.

In many pulmonary parenchymal diseases, blood supply to poorly ventilating areas tends to be reduced, so that the $\dot{V}_A/\dot{Q}$ ratios are not as low as they would otherwise be. One reason for this is that the local pathological process tends to disturb both ventilation and perfusion by its mechanical effects. Another is local hypoxic vasoconstriction, which shunts blood away from the involved alveoli.[32,33,67-69] In the case of thromboembolic phenomena, the regional decreases in CO$_2$ concentration that occur cause local increases in the resistance of small airways and thus reduce ventilation to the affected region.[70]

Other Causes of Abnormal Arterial Blood Gases

In addition to $\dot{V}_A/\dot{Q}$ inequalities, there are four other causes of arterial hypoxemia: (1) anatomical right-to-left intracardiac or intrapulmonary shunts (Chaps. 29 and 30); (2) reductions in the inspired concentration of O$_2$; (3) defects in the diffusion of O$_2$ from the alveolus to the blood; and (4) alveolar hypoventilation.

Although it was originally thought that measurements of the *diffusing capacity* of the lung for oxygen demonstrated a specific impairment in molecular O$_2$ transfer across a thickened membrane (i.e., alveolar capillary block),[71] it is now appreciated that single breath tests of diffusing capacity that employ carbon monoxide are profoundly influenced by three variables: (1) the surface area available for diffusion, (2) the volume of blood within the capillaries, and (3) the rate of combination of CO and hemoglobin.[72] Other factors, such as the molecular path for diffusion and the stratified heterogeneity of gas mixtures, also play a role.[73] In addition to the above, steady-state methods are also influenced by regional $\dot{V}_A/\dot{Q}$ relationships.[72] Thus, these techniques do not measure the thickness of the alveolar-capillary membrane, and in any disease associated with a loss of elastic recoil (loss of surface area through disruption of alveolar walls), marked $\dot{V}_A/\dot{Q}$ heterogeneities or loss of capillary bed will be associated with a reduced "diffusing capacity." Even so, the effect that this has on gas exchange is, at most, small.[74]

Alveolar hypoventilation is a condition in which insufficient gas ex-

change occurs to meet metabolic demands. It can result from many causes: severe $\dot{V}_A/\dot{Q}$ inequalities; reduced drive from the respiratory center so that the patient "will not breathe"; failure of the patient's respiratory system to act on the information sent from the central nervous system because of severe intrinsic pulmonary disease; or abnormalities of the neuromuscular apparatus of the chest wall or diaphragm.[75] In the latter cases the patient "cannot breathe." Regardless of cause, the cardinal features of the arterial blood are hypoxemia and hypercapnia, and both must be present to establish the diagnosis. The various diseases associated with alveolar hypoventilation and the mechanisms by which it comes about in each are discussed as examples of chronic cor pulmonale later in this chapter.

Effects of Alveolar Gas Tensions on the Pulmonary Circulation

The most potent stimulus for the development of pulmonary vasoconstriction is alveolar hypoxia.[31,33,67,68,76] Although acute vasoconstriction appears when the alveolar pO$_2$ is 60 mm Hg or lower, this response is found only in approximately two-thirds of normal subjects.[77] It is speculated that the subjects who respond to hypoxemia with pulmonary vasoconstriction are those who would be prone to develop chronic cor pulmonale if they developed a disease that interfered with effective alveolar ventilation.[78]

Acidosis also has been shown to produce significant increases in pulmonary vascular resistance as well as to act synergistically with hypoxia.[79] In contrast, an increase in arterial pCO$_2$ seems to exert no direct effect. Instead it seems to operate by way of the increase in hydrogen ion concentration that it induces. The interaction of hypoxia and acidemia is clinically important; these two conditions frequently coexist, and their interplay follows a predictable pattern (Fig. 46-6). At minor degrees of oxygen unsaturation, pulmonary artery pressure is relatively insensitive to hydrogen ion concentration, whereas it is extremely sensitive at high levels of unsaturation.[79] On the other hand, when the pH is high, the pressor effect of hypoxia is blunted.

Although the localization of the pulmonary vascular pressor response within the lung is still controversial, most studies indicate that it occurs in partially muscular arteries

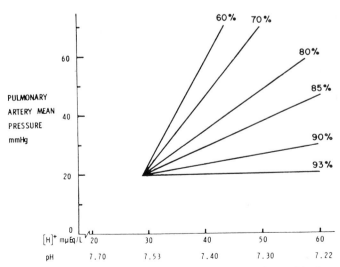

FIGURE 46-6 Relationship of arterial oxygen saturation and hydrogen ion concentration to pulmonary artery pressure. (From Enson, Y., et al.: The influence of hydrogen ion concentration and hypoxia on the pulmonary circulation. J. Clin. Invest. *43*:1146, 1964.)

less than 200 μm in diameter.[67,69,80,81] The mechanism by which hypoxia causes pulmonary arterial smooth muscle to constrict is unclear.[68]

However, the available information points toward two major alternatives: an indirect effect by which hypoxia might cause certain cells in the pulmonary parenchyma to release vasoactive substances (e.g., histamine from mast cells) or a direct effect of hypoxia on pulmonary arterial smooth muscle. Other influences may enhance hypoxic pulmonary vasoconstriction. For example, it is possible that extrapulmonic reflexes or the adrenergic neurotransmitter norepinephrine may augment the pressor response.

PULMONARY THROMBOEMBOLISM AND ACUTE COR PULMONALE

Incidence

It has been estimated that approximately 650,000 patients are afflicted annually with symptomatic pulmonary emboli.[82] Approximately one-fourth of these are fatal (Fig. 46–7). The incidence of pulmonary emboli in autopsy series has been reported to vary from 10 to 64 per cent.[83–86] This large range can be explained by the criteria used to establish the diagnosis and the patient populations studied. In unselected autopsies of adults with grossly visible thromboemboli as the endpoint, the usual figure quoted is around 10 per cent.[83,84] In older patients, particularly those with chronic lung or heart diseases or both, figures of 30 per cent or more are common.[85] However, when subtle pathological effects such as traces of emboli and healed residue are diligently sought in addition to visible thromboemboli, the incidence of pulmonary embolism reportedly can exceed 60 per cent.[86] A large fraction of these emboli, however, are of little clinical significance.

In contrast, the incidence of acute cor pulmonale, fatal pulmonary emboli, or a combination of the two is unknown. Estimates range from 0.1 to 1 per cent of all postsurgical patients.[87,88] Acute pulmonary embolism may be the most common form of acute lung disease among hospitalized patients[89] and, in some series, has been found to be the most common cause of sudden unexpected death in this population[90] (p. 776). Since the diagnosis was not suspected clinically in many of the above studies, the notion has arisen that pulmonary embolism is a very common, but clinically silent, disorder. Although this is undoubtedly true in populations who are chronically ill, bedridden, or postsurgical, the true prevalence of pulmonary embolism in a previously normal population is unknown; this condition may be grossly overdiagnosed in such individuals.[91]

Etiology

From both clinical and pathophysiological standpoints, the preponderant cause of acute cor pulmonale is the rapid obstruction of the pulmonary circulation by thrombi embolized from distant sources.[92] These may be massive and produce partial or complete occlusion of major arteries, or they may be extensive with multiple obstructions of small arterioles. By far the most common source of emboli is the deep veins of the legs,[93–95] and the incidence of lower extremity thrombosis among patients with thromboemboli ranges from 80 to 100 per cent.[96,97] It has been shown convincingly that when thrombi are present in the legs there will be clinical evidence of their presence in only about 50 per cent of cases.[95] Havig performed a complete dissection of the whole lower venous tree, including the plantar and iliac veins, in 80 per cent of the patients who died in a major hospital in Oslo and demonstrated that deep vein thrombosis may start independently at all levels of the venous tree but usually begins in the large venous sinuses of the calf and plantar muscles and in the valve pockets of the axial calf and thigh veins.[98] There is some suspicion that a clot formed in the thigh area is more prone to embolize than is one in a calf.[99]

Three factors are usually listed as fostering the development of venous thrombosis: stasis or slowing of blood in the extremities, damage to the vessel wall, and alterations in the coagulating mechanism of the blood.[92] Of these three, the last is the least well documented, and only a congenital deficiency of antithrombin III has been shown to correlate with excessive thrombotic risk.[100] By far the most common clinical problem is stasis, and it is encountered in many contexts, such as bed rest in the postoperative period and in the presence of congestive heart failure, as well as prolonged periods of sitting during ground or air travel.

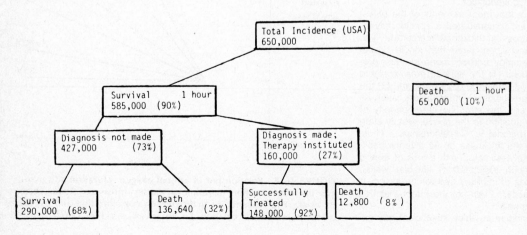

FIGURE 46–7 Diagrammatic representation showing estimated total annual incidence of patients with symptomatic pulmonary emboli in the United States (top box). The outcome in each category (number of patients and per cent) is shown in descending order from top to bottom. (Reproduced with permission from Bell, W. R., and Simon, T. L.: Am. Heart J. *103*: 239, 1982.)

Since the clinical signs and symptoms of venous thrombosis are frequently slight or absent, various laboratory approaches have been devised to facilitate the diagnosis.

Radiofibrinogen techniques rely upon the incorporation of labeled fibrinogen into the thrombus. Once this has occurred, the thrombus is detectable by surface counting. This technique has been used in two circumstances with slightly differing results. When employed *before* thrombus formation has occurred in high-risk groups of patients, it has proved to be a highly sensitive and reliable method of early detection and follow-up.[101,102] However, when used *after a* thrombus has formed, it will detect the presence of the clot only 60 to 80 per cent of the time.[103]

Impedance phlebography and Doppler ultrasound methods measure the speed with which blood leaves the legs. Both involve mechanical obstruction to venous outflow to induce a pooling of blood in the veins, followed by release and monitoring of the flow generated. Impedance phlebography relies upon calf resistance, whereas the Doppler method records frequency shifts in the ultrasound signal.[97,103] These techniques rarely produce false-positive results, but both have a significant incidence of false-negative results because they are relatively insensitive, requiring moderate to marked venous obstruction for best measurements.[92,97]

Although it is generally considered that the legs should be considered the source of an embolus in the absence of other clearly recognizable loci of thrombi, such as the right side of the heart or pelvic veins, it is important to recognize that emboli can also arise from axillary, hepatic portal, and renal veins.[104-106] Renal vein embolus is often associated with distinct symptom complexes characterized by evanescent pulmonary infiltrates in conjunction with the nephrotic syndrome. Other occlusive matter, such as amniotic fluid released during cesarean section or prolonged and difficult labor,[107] bone marrow particulates following trauma or cardiopulmonary resuscitation,[108] fat emboli following trauma,[109] air emboli or insufflation from open wounds in the neck or by intravenous introduction,[110] and tumor emboli[111] have also been implicated, on occasion, in the production of acute cor pulmonale. Still less common but quite dramatic forms of acute cor pulmonale have been encountered in massive pneumothorax, massive atelectasis, mediastinal emphysema, blast injuries, and, rarely, with rupture of an aortic aneurysm into the pulmonary artery.[112]

Pathophysiology

Since pulmonary embolism is a common disorder that has been intensively investigated, one would anticipate that it would be possible to describe its pathophysiology with great precision. Unfortunately, this is not the case, and a number of mechanisms have been proposed to explain the hemodynamic impact with its attendant cardiopulmonary and systemic sequelae.[92] Part of the reason for this is that in the past relatively little in the way of detailed investigation has been performed in acutely ill patients, and the cardiopulmonary alterations are often transient. Therefore, most concepts have been based upon acute, controlled animal studies. Here, too, difficulties have arisen because data have been derived from different species, and occlusions have been produced by ligatures or embolic material that

has varied from inert beads and starch granules to clots formed in vivo.

ROLES OF VASCULAR OBSTRUCTION AND NEUROHUMORAL FACTORS. Obstruction of the pulmonary circulation is the sine qua non for the development of the acute, severe, pulmonary hypertension that occurs with emboli, but debate rages over whether it is the sole factor. Quantitatively, it has been recognized since early in this century that mechanical occlusion of 60 to 80 per cent of the lumen of the main pulmonary artery is necessary before the right ventricle dilates and fails.[15,113-115] Hyland and colleagues extended these observations by injecting polystyrene spheres, glass beads, or aged blood clots of precisely graded size into the right atria of dogs to occlude selectively the pulmonary arteries from lobar branches down to small precapillary vessels.[116] They found that irrespective of the material embolized, the majority of vessels at each level had to be obstructed before hypertension appeared. They therefore concluded that mechanical obstruction rather than vasoconstriction was the mechanism underlying the development of pulmonary hypertension. McIntyre and Sasahara reached similar conclusions in humans by observing a linear relationship between the extent of vascular obstruction, as measured during angiography, and mean pulmonary arterial pressure in patients free of cardiopulmonary disease prior to an embolic episode[117] (Fig. 46-8). However, this relationship did not exist in patients with heart or lung disease.[118]

Although mechanical obstruction is obviously quite important, this mechanism is irreconcilable with the observation that total occlusion of either the right or the left main pulmonary artery by a balloon is entirely innocuous in normal humans and produces only minor changes in pulmonary artery pressure.[70,119] Yet, in the study of McIntyre and Sasahara cited above, obstruction of 30 per cent of the

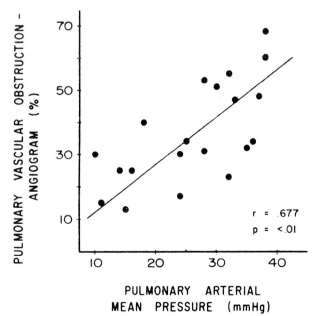

FIGURE 46–8 Relationship between percentage of angiographic obstruction and mean pulmonary artery pressure in patients free of cardiopulmonary disease prior to pulmonary embolization. (From McIntyre, K. M., and Sasahara, A. A.: Hemodynamic response to pulmonary embolism in patients free of prior cardiopulmonary disease. Am. J. Cardiol. 28:228, 1971.)

pulmonary vasculature with emboli was associated with significant symptomatology, mean pulmonary artery pressures in excess of 30 mm Hg, and an elevation of total pulmonary resistance.[117] Consequently, since the full, acute syndrome occurs when much less than half of the vascular bed is occluded, *mechanical obstruction alone does not completely define the circulatory effects of embolization.*[117,118,120-124] Further, the mechanical theory does not readily explain the abnormalities that also occur in lung mechanics and gas exchange. Therefore, reflex neural and humoral factors must also be considered as participating in the genesis of the clinical picture.

Powerful evidence for humoral activity is derived from the work of Halmagyi et al.[125] In cross circulation experiments in sheep, these investigators demonstrated that pulmonary embolism induced in the donor simultaneously produced a rise in pulmonary artery pressure and a fall in lung compliance in both the donor and the recipient. The transmitted effects could be reversed in the recipient by interrupting the cross circulation and inflating the lung.

The injection of barium sulfate into the pulmonary circulation, in addition to increasing pulmonary vascular resistance,[126] constricts alveolar ducts and terminal bronchi with resultant marked decreases in pulmonary compliance.[127] These physiological effects are indistinguishable from those observed following pulmonary arterial infusions of collagen[128] or thrombin,[128] and it appears that the common denominator underlying these diverse agents is platelet aggregation with release of their potent vaso- and bronchoactive contents.[126,128-131] These observations have direct bearing on the pathogenesis of macroembolization.

Even though the precise pathophysiological sequence has not been worked out, morphological and pharmacological evidence suggests that in vivo autologous thromboemboli contain traces of thrombin and its precursors that cause aggregation of platelets on the embolus and release of their contents.[132] Emboli recovered from the lungs of dogs have been shown to have a coating of fibrin, leukocytes, and degranulated platelets that were not present at their site of formation in the limbs.[133] If platelet adhesion is prevented by platelet aging or washing the clot or by pretreatment with indomethacin,[131] or if thrombin formation is blocked by heparin,[132,134] the cardiopulmonary consequences of emboli are aborted. Similar findings occur if the products released from platelets are counteracted by administration of specific antagonists[129,134,135] or if emboli are produced in thrombocytopenic animals.[132] Thus, it appears that humoral agents released from platelets, such as histamine, serotonin, and the prostaglandins, pass into the pulmonary circulation after impaction of emboli and may be responsible for contraction of vascular and bronchial smooth muscle.

In addition to constriction of alveolar ducts and respiratory bronchioles, bronchoconstriction also occurs in airways up to 3 mm in diameter following embolization.[136] Since the terminal bronchioles and alveolar ducts are the only airways believed to be perfused by the pulmonary circulation,[137] constriction of these larger airways must be accomplished in some other way. It is possible that after release, the agents may diffuse locally, producing concentration gradients along the airway walls or in adjacent tissues. Alternatively, recirculation via the bronchial circulation could constrict airways. It is important to recognize, however, that local amplification of the biochemical response is also possible. For example, plasmin activated via the fibrinolytic pathway can initiate enzymatic reactions that can generate anaphylatoxins, which in turn can cause tissue mast cells to release their potent vasoactive and bronchoconstricting chemicals. This reaction would be expected to be intense but relatively short-lived, since the inhibitors of these compounds are also present or can be generated locally—a circumstance that also fits with the time course of the clinical sequelae of emboli.

It is apparent that the ingredients for severe, regional, and systemic effects are present. Bronchoconstriction and closure of distal lung units in embolized and nonembolized areas can produce wheezing and dyspnea as well as local ventilation-perfusion imbalances that can explain the *arterial hypoxemia* so commonly encountered in pulmonary embolism. *Hyperpnea* and *tachypnea* can also occur from summation of the stimuli of anxiety, systemic hypotension, reflex stimulation of lung afferents, and arterial hypoxemia if severe enough. The resulting hyperventilation gives rise to hypocapnia, which can aggravate airway smooth muscle contraction. All the effects need not be purely local, for at least one biological amine that figures prominently in the reaction (histamine) has been demonstrated to be a potent stimulant of vagal afferent discharges,[138] and it is likely that other agents released or generated may also activate vagal reflexes.[131]

HEMODYNAMIC RESPONSES. Because patients with pulmonary emboli are often so acutely ill, relatively few data on the human dynamics of this condition were available until recently. However, with publication of results of the second phase of the Urokinase–Pulmonary Embolism Trial,[124] it became possible to piece these voluminous data together with previous studies of smaller numbers of patients[117,118,123,139,140] to gain both general and specific insights.

In this national cooperative study,[124] complete hemodynamic measurements were obtained prior to treatment in 143 patients with angiographically proved thromboemboli. The most common abnormalities noted were arterial hypoxemia and right ventricular systolic pressures greater than 25 mm Hg. In decreasing order of frequency were elevations in total pulmonary resistance (> 200 dynes-sec-cm^{-5}), right ventricular end-diastolic pressure (> 6 mm Hg), mean pulmonary artery pressure (> 20 mm Hg), and mean right atrial pressure (> 6 mm Hg). Decreases in cardiac index (< 2.7 liter/min/meter^2) paralleled the changes in mean right atrial pressure. Comparisons of the extent of the embolism with the hemodynamic response indicate that those patients with massive embolism (defined as obstruction of two or more lobar arteries) had more marked abnormalities (Fig. 46–9). In patients with massive obstruction, mean right atrial, right ventricular systolic and end-diastolic, and mean pulmonary artery pressures were all higher and cardiac index and arterial oxygen tensions were lower than in patients with submassive obstruction. However, despite the statistical significance of these findings, considerable overlap was seen in the values for individuals in the submassive and massive groups as well as in the normal range. In addition, this type of analysis did not take into consideration the state of cardiopulmonary function before the insult.

When the latter is taken into account, the most fre-

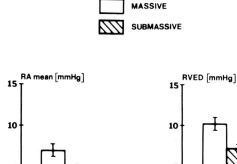

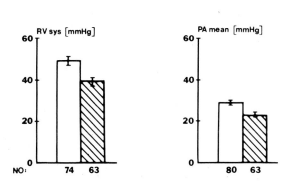

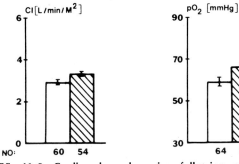

FIGURE 46–9 Cardiac hemodynamics following massive and submassive pulmonary emboli. The heights of the bars represent mean values, and the brackets are standard errors of the mean. The numbers below each graph indicate the size of the population studied. RA mean = right atrial mean pressure; RVED = right ventricular end-diastolic pressure; RV sys = right ventricular systolic pressure; PA mean = mean pulmonary artery pressure; CI = cardiac index; pO_2 = arterial oxygen tension. (Redrawn from National Cooperative Study: The urokinase pulmonary embolism trial. Circulation 47 (Suppl. II):1, 1973, by permission of the American Heart Association, Inc.)

quently observed postembolic abnormality in patients free of prior cardiac or pulmonary disease is *arterial hypoxemia*.[117,124,141] This usually occurs as the only manifestation of embolism when 25 per cent or less of the vasculature is obstructed.[117] Consequently, in the absence of other diseases that can produce hypoxemia, this finding is of great clinical value.[141]

A normal PaO_2 does not exclude the diagnosis.[87,124] In the urokinase trial, approximately 12 per cent of the patients had a PaO_2 of 80 mm Hg or more.[124] Use of the alveolar-arterial gradient for oxygen (A-aDO_2) is much more discriminatory, and, although no formal studies exist, it will probably always be abnormal in patients with significant

pulmonary embolization. For example, if the PaO_2 were 85 mm Hg and the $PaCO_2$ were 30 mm Hg, with the patient breathing room air at sea level, the A-aDO_2 would be abnormally elevated to at least 28 mm Hg. This value can be calculated from an abbreviated version of the alveolar air equation:

$$PAO_2 = PIO_2 - \frac{PaCO_2}{RQ}$$

where PAO_2 = alveolar O_2 tension
PIO_2 = inspired O_2 tension (fractional concentration multiplied by the barometric pressure minus water vapor)
$PaCO_2$ = arterial CO_2 tension
RQ = respiratory quotient

In this case, PIO_2 is equal to $0.21 \times (760 - 47)$, or 150 mm Hg. Since in practice RQ is tedious to measure, for clinical purposes one can assume a steady-state value of 0.8. This would be the lower limit if the patient were not retaining CO_2, because unsteady-state conditions other than this would tend to produce values of 1 or more and so further reduce the $PaCO_2/RQ$ ratio. Thus,

$$PAO_2 = 150 - \frac{30}{0.8}$$

$$A\text{-}aDO_2 = PAO_2 - PaO_2$$
$$= 113 - 85$$
$$= 28$$

If RQ were 1, then A-aDO_2 would be even more abnormal, i.e., 35 mm Hg. Thus, even though the absolute arterial oxygen tension is normal, gas exchange can still be abnormal.

The next most frequent derangement is *pulmonary hypertension*. It has been observed in approximately 70 per cent of the patients in several series[117,120,123,139] and can be expected to occur after 25 to 35 per cent of the vasculature has been obstructed in a previously normal vascular bed. A mean pulmonary artery pressure exceeding 40 mm Hg, even in the face of massive obstruction, seems to be the maximum pressureload that a previously normal right ventricle can generate.[117,123,139] Thus, pressures at such levels suggest massive obstruction, chronic recurrent embolization, or other causes of prior pulmonary artery hypertension.[117,118]

Elevation in right atrial mean pressure can be expected in approximately 50 per cent of cases, and it bears a direct relationship to the degree of pulmonary hypertension. In one study, right atrial mean pressure was always elevated whenever mean pulmonary artery pressure exceeded 30 mm Hg.[117] Thus, neck vein distention following a pulmonary embolus in a person without previous pulmonary hypertension signifies massive embolization.

In the absence of cardiac failure, the cardiac index is typically elevated in response to pulmonary emboli.[117,124,139] When depression of output occurs, it is virtually always in association with massive obstruction. It has been suggested that one of the mechanisms for cardiac depression is the mechanical compromise of right coronary artery blood flow.[23] However, this seems unlikely as there is now abundant evidence that perfusion of both coronary beds reflexly increases following pulmonary embolization.[142-145]

In patients with prior heart or lung disease, or both, the consequences of pulmonary emboli are markedly different. In general, for any degree of obstruction, the hemodynamic abnormalities are significantly greater than in previously normal individuals who suffer an embolus.[118] Mean pulmonary artery pressures of 40 mm Hg or more are common in this group, and elevations in right atrial pressures and depressions of cardiac index are the rule rather than the exception.[118,124] These patients are also more likely to develop acute left ventricular or global heart failure;[146] massive obstruction with survival is extremely uncommon.

Clinical Manifestations

SIGNS AND SYMPTOMS. The largest antemortem collection of the presenting signs and symptoms of patients with confirmed pulmonary emboli is summarized in Tables 46–1 and 46–2.[121,122] These 327 patients had been included in either the Urokinase–Pulmonary Embolism Trial[124] or the Urokinase-Streptokinase Embolism Trial,[121] and of them, 215 were free of preexisting cardiac or pulmonary disease prior to embolization[122] (Table 46–2). These data support the general clinical impression that no single symptom or combination of symptoms is diagnostic of pulmonary embolism.[89,118,147] Chest pain and dyspnea, found in over 85 per cent of the patients, were the most frequent symptoms. (In three-fourths of the group, the pain was pleuritic in nature.) Apprehension and cough were seen in 50 to 60 per cent of the patients. Hemoptysis, diaphoresis, and syncope were present in only a minority. When the extent of the embolization was examined in relation to symptoms, apprehension and syncope occurred with signficantly greater frequency in those with massive emboli, whereas pleuritic chest pain and hemoptysis were more common in patients with less extensive involvement. Quite similar patterns were noted in those without antecedent cardiopulmonary disease (Table 46–2). Dyspnea and cough tended to be prodromal, often noted by the patient as early as 5 or more days before the diagnosis was established. Chest pain tended to develop 3 to 4 days before definitive work-up, and the symptoms of apprehension, diaphoresis, and syncope were acute, usually occurring within 36 hours or less of presentation.

Tachypnea was the most common sign. Rales, an increased pulmonic component of the second heart sound, tachycardia, and fever were the next most frequent physical findings. Gallop rhythms, diaphoresis, and phlebitis

TABLE 46–1   INCIDENCE OF SYMPTOMS AND SIGNS IN 327 PATIENTS WITH THROMBOEMBOLISM

	TOTAL SERIES n = 327 (%)	MASSIVE EMBOLI n = 197 (%)	SUBMASSIVE EMBOLI n = 130 (%)
Symptoms			
Chest pain	88	85	82
Dyspnea	84	85	82
Apprehension	59	65	50
Cough	53	53	52
Hemoptysis	30	23	40
Diaphoresis	27	29	23
Syncope	13	20	4
Signs			
Tachypnea (resp. > 16/min)	92	95	87
Rales	58	57	60
Increased pulmonic 2nd sound	53	58	45
Tachycardia (pulse > 100/min)	44	48	38
Fever (temp. > 37.8°C)	43	43	42
Gallop	34	39	25
Diaphoresis	36	42	27
Phlebitis	32	36	26
Edema	24	23	25
Murmur	23	27	16
Cyanosis	19	25	9

From Bell, W. R., et al.: The clinical features of submassive and massive pulmonary emboli. Am. J. Med. 62:355, 1977.

TABLE 46–2   INCIDENCE OF SYMPTOMS AND SIGNS IN 214 PATIENTS WITH THROMBOEMBOLISM WITHOUT PREEXISTING CARDIAC OR PULMONARY DISEASE

	TOTAL SERIES n = 214 (%)	MASSIVE EMBOLI n = 145 (%)	SUBMASSIVE EMBOLI n = 69 (%)
Symptoms			
Chest pain	74	67	85
Dyspnea	84	86	78
Apprehension	63	70	50
Cough	50	48	55
Hemoptysis	28	23	35
Diaphoresis	36	44	20
Syncope	13	17	4
Signs			
Tachypnea (resp. > 20/min)	85	87	81
Rales	56	55	56
Increased pulmonic 2nd sound	57	62	47
Tachycardia (pulse > 100/min)	58	66	42
Fever (temp. > 37.8°C)	50	50	51
Diaphoresis	36	44	20
Phlebitis	41	39	47
Cyanosis	18	24	3

From Stein, P. D., et al.: History and physical examination in acute pulmonary embolism in patients without preexisting cardiac or pulmonary disease. Am. J. Cardiol. 47:218, 1981.

were each found in approximately one-third of the population, whereas edema, murmurs, and cyanosis were each noted in one-fourth or less. An accentuated pulmonic second sound, third and fourth heart sounds, murmurs, and cyanosis all occurred more frequently in those patients who had suffered massive rather than submassive embolization. Again, the patterns observed in the patients who were previously well mirrored those noted in this group as a whole.

The "classic triads" of hemoptysis, cough, and diaphoresis; hemoptysis, chest pain, and dyspnea; or dyspnea, chest pain, and apprehension were uncommon. The same lack of specificity was found in signs. Although tachypnea occurred in over 90 per cent of the population, its presence or absence, as that of hypoxemia, does not establish or eliminate the diagnosis. The combination of elevated heart rate, respiration, and temperature (Allen's sign) was present in only 23 per cent of patients. In the patients without preexisting heart or lung disease, the presenting symptoms were (1) pleuritic pain without hemoptysis (41 per cent); (2) pulmonary infarction with hemoptysis (25 per cent); (3) uncomplicated embolism with only dyspnea (10 per cent); and (4) circulatory collapse with shock (10 per cent) and syncope (9 per cent). Three per cent had nonpleuritic chest pain with dyspnea, and 0.5 per cent showed deep venous thrombosis with tachypnea. Thus, regardless of their varying degree of sensitivity, the symptoms and signs of pulmonary embolism are quite nonspecific.

With usual medical treatment, the clinical parameters clear progressively. Within a week after heparin therapy was initiated in the National Cooperative Trial,[124] the complaints of dyspnea, chest pain, and apprehension had cleared in 78, 74, and 85 per cent of the patients, respectively. However, cough resolved more slowly: 2 weeks after embolization, 48 per cent of the patients still had this complaint. Generally, the signs cleared more slowly than did the symptoms. Although diaphoresis disappeared in 83 per cent of the patients within 1 week, 62 and 63 per cent still had rales and an accentuated pulmonic component of the second heart sound, respectively.

In addition to the usual symptom complex associated with embolization, variant clinical expressions also occur. Thus, Israel and Goldstein[89] and Potts and Sahn[148] have described a total of 14 patients in whom abdominal pain was the predominant symptom. In 8 of the patients, these complaints were so severe that the correct diagnosis was delayed while attention was diverted to what appeared to be acute surgical abdomens. Another infrequent but perplexing manifestation is acute bronchospasm. Although many patients with recent emboli characteristically develop airway obstruction,[149] this is usually detectable only by appropriate pulmonary function tests. Occasionally, however, this airflow obstruction is so severe that acute wheezing develops, and the patient initially is thought to have bronchial asthma.[150–152] Pulmonary embolism may also masquerade as coronary insufficiency.[153]

ELECTROCARDIOGRAM (see also p. 212). Like the signs and symptoms of acute pulmonary embolization, the electrocardiographic alterations are highly variable and in the majority of instances are nondiagnostic[124,141,154–156] (Chap. 7). The types of changes observed in a large series of patients and their frequency distribution are summarized in Table 46–3.[124] In this study the pretreatment electrocardiograms were entirely normal in only 13 per cent of patients. Rhythm disturbances were present in 11 per cent, with premature ventricular beats the most common. Conduction disturbances were found in 65 per cent of the patients, ST-T changes in 64 per cent, and T-wave inversion in 40 per cent. The electrocardiographic manifestations of acute cor pulmonale ($S_1Q_3T_3$, complete or incomplete right bundle branch block, P-pulmonale, or right axis deviation) were uncommon. Patients with prior cardiopulmonary disease had a greater frequency of arrhythmias, conduction disturbances, and QRS changes, whereas patients with massive emboli had more QRS, ST-T segment, and T-wave

changes. These findings are in general agreement with those of other investigations[141,154] and indicate that the electrocardiogram is not specific in pulmonary embolus and not particularly helpful in establishing the diagnosis. Moreover, it is insensitive to the rate of resolution of the emboli.

Even though the results of the studies described above are disappointing from a diagnostic standpoint, some data suggest that the hemodynamic variables are altered in a characteristic fashion (Figs. 7–16, p. 213, and 46–10) when the electrocardiogram is conclusive for, or suggestive of, acute right-heart strain in patients without cardiopulmonary disease prior to embolization. Such electrocardiograms were observed only when the mean pressures in the pulmonary artery and right atria exceeded 30 and 8 mm Hg, respectively; the total pulmonary resistance was greater than 500 dynes-sec-cm^{-5}; cardiac index was depressed; and the degree of pulmonary vascular obstruction exceeded 40 per cent.[154] Thus in the patients whose electrocardiograms were diagnostic of, or consistent with, right-heart strain, the clinical picture indicated that a cardiopulmonary catastrophe had occurred. Consequently, although the electrocardiogram can be of little value in arousing the clinical suspicion of pulmonary embolism per se, it may be useful in distinguishing between the two most frequent cardiopul-

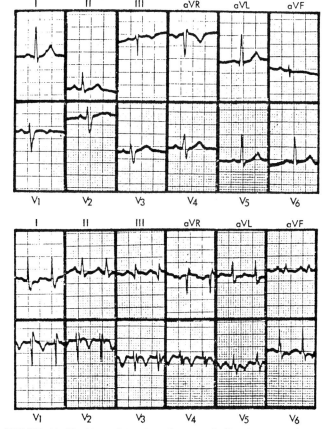

FIGURE 46–10 Normal (*top*) and postembolic (*bottom*) electrocardiograms in a 26-year-old patient who underwent arthrotomy of the knee. The bottom tracing shows the diagnostic features of acute right ventricular strain. Changes include acute development of a prominent S1, Q3 pattern with incomplete right bundle branch block, tachycardia (150 beats/min), and an axis shift from 0 to +30 degrees. (From McIntyre, K. M., et al.: Relation of the electrocardiogram to hemodynamic alterations in pulmonary embolism. Am. J. Cardiol. *30*:205, 1972.)

TABLE 46–3 ELECTROCARDIOGRAPHIC ABNORMALITIES IN 131 PATIENTS WITH PULMONARY EMBOLISM

	PER CENT OF PATIENTS
Rhythm Disturbances	
Premature beats	11
Atrial	3
Ventricular	9
Atrial fibrillation	3
QRS Abnormalities	65
Right axis	5
Left axis	12
Incomplete right bundle branch block	5
Complete right bundle branch block	11
Right ventricular hypertrophy	5
$S_1 S_2 S_3$ pattern	9
$S_1 Q_3 T_3$ pattern	11
ST-T Abnormalities	64
T-wave inversion	40
ST-T segment depression	33
ST-T segment elevation	11

From National Cooperative Study: Urokinase–Pulmonary Embolism Trial. Circulation *47* (Suppl. II): 1, 1973, by permission of the American Heart Association, Inc.

monary catastrophes: acute myocardial infarction and acute massive pulmonary embolism.

ABNORMALITIES IN RESPIRATORY FUNCTION.

As described earlier in this chapter, acute pulmonary embolization in experimental animals has been shown to affect airways as well as blood vessels in both embolized and nonembolized areas. Consequently, both the mechanical and the gas-exchanging properties of the lungs are disturbed. Functionally, this produces tachypnea, hypoxemia, increased arterial-alveolar differences for oxygen and carbon dioxide, elevated physiological dead space, diminished lung compliance, increased airway resistance, and a fall in lung volume.[125-127,131,134,157-161] Many of these alterations in lung function result from closure of dependent airways and constriction of small bronchi, respiratory bronchioles, and alveolar ducts. The net effect is a disruption of normal ventilation-perfusion relationships so that gas exchange is impaired.

In humans, the acute effects of embolization per se are considerably less clear because the interpretation of the various functional abnormalities that have been described is limited by such factors as time of study and patient selection. For example, very few studies of mechanical lung function have been performed close in time to an embolic episode. Sasahara and colleagues reported reductions in vital capacity and forced expiratory volumes in 80 per cent or more of a large group of patients, two-thirds of whom were studied within a week of the suspected embolism.[149] These abnormalities improved acutely in some patients following heparin treatment, thereby suggesting an element of bronchospasm via the release of platelet products. However, most of the patients in this study had preexisting heart or lung disease or both, making it impossible to sort out the relative contributions of each disease process.

Alveolar gas exchange has been studied frequently in the acute embolic period, presumably because these techniques do not require extensive manipulation of severely ill persons, and the data are often directly useful in patient care. As in animal studies, a number of investigations have demonstrated hypoxemia, tachypnea, mismatched $\dot{V}_A/\dot{Q}$ ratios, reduced diffusing capacities, and widened arterial-alveolar gradients for CO_2.[149,162-168] The last finding stems from ventilation coming from high $\dot{V}_A/\dot{Q}$ areas of the lung, which dilutes the CO_2 concentration in the expired alveolar air and was originally proposed as a useful procedure to diagnose pulmonary embolism.[163,164] Although a sensitive test, it is time-dependent (i.e., apt to be abnormal in the immediate postembolic period and not hours or days later) and nonspecific in that any focal abnormality in $\dot{V}_A/\dot{Q}$ will produce it. Hence it has been superseded by other diagnostic procedures.

The fall in diffusing capacity has been explained by a reduction in the functional area of pulmonary capillaries by the embolization. Daum investigated the membrane and blood components of pulmonary diffusion and could account for all of the measured resistance to O_2 transfer by a reduction in capillary blood volume.[167] Thus, this is not an impairment of diffusion in the sense of an "alveolar capillary" block.

The chief mechanism at work in producing hypoxemia appears to be widespread regional inequalities in $\dot{V}_A/\dot{Q}$ ratios of various magnitudes that are scattered throughout the lungs. Wilson and coworkers have suggested that the immediate cause of hypoxemia in patients with no previous heart or lung disease is related to venous admixture but that the persistence of hypoxemia beyond the acute phase resulted from right-to-left shunting secondary to atelectasis.[168] The reason why the latter should develop is unknown, but some data indicate that surfactant formation (and hence alveolar stability) is reduced by temporarily interrupting pulmonary arterial supply to an area of the lung.[169]

The long-term effects of emboli on lung function in patients who were previously normal are frequently quite subtle at rest and consist of mild reductions in vital capacity, arterial oxygen tension, and diffusing capacities.[170] With exercise, wasted ("dead space") ventilation often increases abnormally or fails to fall if elevated initially, and hypoxemia worsens.[171,172] Because of these findings and the often vague clinical complaints associated with small embolic episodes, performance of detailed studies of gas exchange, both at rest and during physical exertion, in patients suspected of having occlusive pulmonary vascular disease can be quite rewarding in suggesting the diagnosis.

RADIOGRAPHIC ABNORMALITIES

(see also Chap. 6). Before considering the roentgenographic manifestations of pulmonary thromboembolism, it must be noted that the majority of episodes confirmed by angiography show no abnormalities on plain chest radiographs.[173,174] When changes are present, however, they may be distinctive and can strongly suggest the diagnosis. The four manifestations of embolization *without infarction* are oligemia, change in vessel size, alterations in size and configuration of the heart, and loss of lung volume.

Loss of lung volume, as manifested, for example, by an elevated diaphragm, is the most common radiographic sign of pulmonary embolism. It has been observed in as many as 41 per cent of the patients in one large series.[124] In contrast, local pulmonary oligemia occurs infrequently and only with occlusion of large vessels. Although this finding has been confirmed as a valid sign of embolization,[175,176] it is seldom of sufficient degree to be convincing.[174,177] Oligemia is more often detected when a whole lung, or a major part of it, is deprived of its pulmonary arterial circulation (Fig. 46-11). In these circumstances, the unilateral oligemia contrasts markedly with the pleonemia of the other lung.[178] Generalized pulmonary oligemia is almost invariably the result of widespread obstruction of smaller pulmonary arteries from recurrent embolization. This finding is nearly always associated with the signs of pulmonary hypertension (see below). Enlargement of a major hilar artery is an important radiographic sign.[177,179-181] This is particularly valuable diagnostically when serial roentgenograms reveal progressive enlargement of the affected vessel[179] (Fig. 46-11). Equally important to the increase in size is the abrupt tapering of an occluded vessel (knuckle sign).[176] These alterations were found in 23 per cent of the patients in the National Cooperative Urokinase Trial, whereas focal oligemia was recorded in only 15 per cent.[124]

The postembolic cardiac changes consist of cardiac enlargement due to dilatation of the right ventricle, increase in size of the main pulmonary artery, and increase in the size and rapidity of tapering of the hilar vessels.[179] Dilatation of the azygous vein and of the superior vena cava, reflecting right-sided heart failure, may also be found. Cardiac changes are the least common roentgenographic

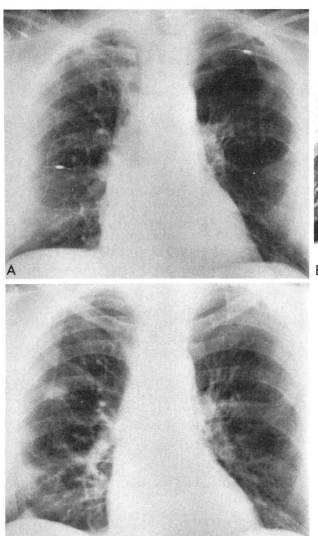

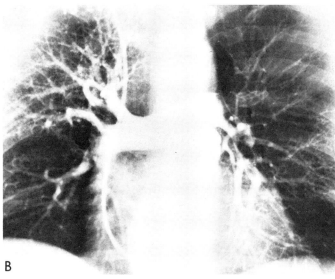

FIGURE 46–11 *A*, Enlarged left main pulmonary artery and oligemia of the left upper lobe. *B*, A large filling defect with absence of perfusion to the left upper lobe and with segmental defects in the left lower lobe. *C*, Chest radiograph after recovery, demonstrating normal vascular markings in previously affected areas.

manifestations of embolization[124] and are the most difficult ones to recognize in acutely tachypneic patients who have undergone bedside evaluations.[174]

Pulmonary Infarction. The roentgenographic changes in embolism with infarction are basically the same as those described above except that oligemia is replaced by parenchymal consolidation. The latter can be produced by either hemorrhage or true infarction with tissue necrosis, and radiographic techniques cannot differentiate the two. There is considerable difference of opinion about what percentage of emboli results in infarction of lung parenchyma, but postmortem findings indicate that as few as 10 to 15 per cent do so.[86,182] Infarction tends to occur in situations in which either the pulmonary venous drainage or the bronchial circulation has been compromised by a preexisting disease process, particularly congestive failure, malignancy, or chronic lung disease.[183–185] The reasons for this are not entirely clear, but it appears that after an embolus the viability of the pulmonary tissue is determined at least in part by the integrity of the bronchial circulation, the magnitude of the obstruction, and the site of the embolization.

The time interval between an embolic episode and the development of a radiographic density varies greatly. A pulmonary infiltrate may occur within 10 to 12 hours[175] or as late as a week after the occlusion.[175,186] As with the other

clinical manifestations of embolization, the "classic" configuration of an infarct as a truncated cone is uncommon.

The time of resolution of the pulmonary infiltrates is variable and is a reliable indicator of the nature of the consolidation process. Hemorrhage may clear within 7 to 10 days or less, often without residuum.[187] By contrast, resolution of an infarct averages 20 days[174] and may take as long as 5 weeks. Serial chest films frequently show these consolidations evolving into atelectatic streaks or pleural thickening. Rarely, an infarcted area undergoes liquefaction and cavitation.[188–192] This can occur in the absence of sepsis or pulmonary infection and in extremely rare instances can result in the development of a bronchopleural fistula.[192] Pleural effusion is as common as parenchymal consolidation as a roentgenographic manifestation of thromboembolic disease, and usually indicates that infarction has occurred.[193] The amount of fluid varies. It is frequently small but on occasion may be abundant. It usually develops and absorbs synchronously with the infarction, though it may appear later and clear sooner.[174]

Diagnosis

As already indicated, the bedside diagnosis of pulmonary thromboembolism is unreliable because the clinical features of the disorder are varied and nonspecific. Szucs et al. assessed the sensitivity of certain laboratory tests in a prospective study of patients with angiographically documented acute pulmonary embolism.[141] Electrocardiographic evidence of right-heart strain occurred in 18 per cent; each had massive pulmonary embolism. Nonspecific chest roentgenographic abnormalities (infiltrates, effusion, or elevated diaphragm) occurred in 71 per cent. Lactic dehydrogenase was increased in 83 per cent of the patients, but serum glutamic oxaloacetic transaminase and bilirubin determinations were of little value. Arterial oxygen tensions, measured while the patient breathed room air, were decreased (≤ 80 mm Hg) in all patients. Thus, although diagnostic strategies of various accuracy have been proposed,[110,194] the most definitive procedures available are photoscanning and selective pulmonary angiography.

VENTILATION-PERFUSION SCINTIGRAPHY (also see pp. 388 to 392). The use of perfusion scanning in the assessment and diagnosis of pulmonary embolism was first described by Wagner and associates in 1964 and allows for determinations of the distribution of pulmonary blood flow in vessels as small as 50 μm.[195] Consequently, this procedure is very sensitive, but it lacks specificity. Although a normal scan provides convincing evidence for the absence of pulmonary emboli,[147,196] an abnormal scan can be ambiguous diagnostically because it can be produced by any condition that alters regional blood flow.[197] This is exemplified by a recent report of scan abnormalities in 88 per cent of 59 patients *without* angiographic demonstration of embolism.[198] The converse is even more disturbing. Bell and Simon observed 18 patients who were reported by scan to have a low probability of emboli, yet 10 had massive and 7 submassive emboli on angiography.[199]

Because of observations like these, various indices have been proposed to improve the scintigraphic definition of pulmonary embolism. The most common are (1) the size and distribution of perfusion abnormalities,[196,198] (2) the relationship between regional perfusion and ventilation,[199,200] (3) comparison of perfusion patterns after variable time intervals,[201,202] and (4) correlation with the conventional chest film.[197,198] Analysis of the relative value of the first three factors in patients with angiographically proved emboli indicates that a large perfusion defect and a $\dot{V}_A/\dot{Q}$ mismatch correlate strongly with pulmonary embolism.

McNeil et al.[192] and others[196,198] have found that lung or lobar defects on scan are likely to be the result of vascular obstruction. This is the so-called high-probability scan.[198] In this study, 80 per cent of lobar defects were associated with emboli, whereas segmental or subsegmental defects alone showed only a 30 per cent association. Thus, perfusion patterns per se are only fair discriminants. The addition of a ventilation scan (also discussed in Chapter 11) to look for $\dot{V}_A/\dot{Q}$ mismatches in the nonperfused area considerably strengthens the diagnostic capabilities.[197,198,200] In patients with multiple segmental and lobar perfusion defects and normal ventilation, the possibility of pulmonary embolism being shown by angiography is said to exceed 90 per cent.[203,204] A matched loss of perfusion and ventilation is not usually observed with embolization; thus, when found, it suggests other pathological processes such as chronic lung disease or heart failure. However, atelectasis, which may occur in embolization, with or without infarction, is associated with both abnormal ventilation and perfusion.

In addition, it is doubtful whether a ventilation scan can exclude the diagnosis of pulmonary embolism in patients with obstructive airway disease or extensive parenchymal disease, since these diseases reduce the likelihood of finding a defect on a perfusion scan without an associated abnormality on the ventilation scan.

Sequential examinations reveal that scanning is most useful early in the disease. In the absence of recurrent emboli, the reliability of the scan diminishes rapidly as perfusion improves, finally returning to normal or to a pattern of diagnostic uncertainty.[139,197,201,202,205] Thus in the absence of other, quickly reversible, pathological conditions (asthma, pneumonia, congestive heart failure), a changing perfusion pattern suggests the presence of pulmonary embolus. Conversely, a fixed pattern is unlikely to represent embolic sequelae. A word of caution, however, in interpreting sequential scans is in order. Several observers[206,207] have described the appearance and disappearance of perfusion shifts in serial lung scans in angiographically patent vessels. Investigations failed to reveal new embolization, and it was concluded that the resolution of thromboemboli caused physiological redistribution of perfusion secondary to changes in relative impedance to flow in different areas of the lung.

A fourth way of increasing the specificity of the perfusion scan is to utilize the chest roentgenogram. The predictability of pulmonary embolism in high probability scans may be increased further if the chest film shows at least one of the following features of pulmonary embolism: infiltrate, pleural effusion, atelectasis, and elevated hemidiaphragm. If two features are present, the predictive value approaches 100 per cent.[197,198]

PULMONARY ANGIOGRAPHY. Selective pulmonary arteriography (the injection of contrast material into pulmonary artery branches which supply a segment or lobe) is considered to be the most specific test available for the detection of pulmonary embolism.[124,198,205,208,209] The absolute accuracy of pulmonary arteriography is difficult to assess, since small emboli may undergo rapid lysis[205] and an immediate postmortem examination is a rare event in humans. Unlike scanning procedures, which are maximally useful in detecting small emboli, angiography is seldom of value when the obstructed vessels are 2 mm or less in diameter.[177,205]

The most dependable roentgenographic signs are actual cut-offs (Fig. 46–11) or filling defects in the larger arteries or segmental vessels (Fig. 46–12).[176,177,198,208] Other findings that may suggest the diagnosis include local segmental hypovascularity; absent, diminished, or delayed arterial and venous flow; tortuous sequential vessels; alteration in the caliber of arteries proximal or distal to an embolus; and loss of volume of the affected lung segments.[176,177,198,208]

In their study of the criteria of the angiographic diagnosis of acute pulmonary embolism, Stein and colleagues emphasized the importance of evaluating the presence of other disease that might affect the pulmonary vasculature and thereby alter the angiographic pattern.[210] These observers noted that filling defects, vessel cut-offs, and pruning of the peripheral vessels occur only in pulmonary embolism. However, if oligemia and asymmetry of blood flow are used as the criteria, the possibility of false-positive diagnosis exists in that these abnormalities can be found in association with chronic lung disease or congestive heart

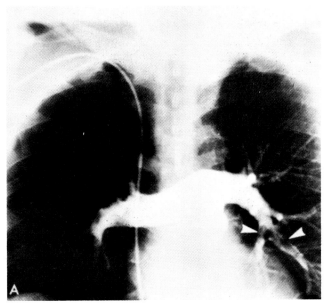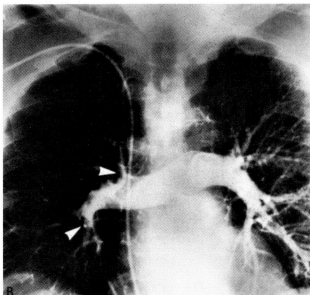

FIGURE 46–12   Multiple bilateral filling defects (arrows).

failure in the absence of intrinsic vascular occlusion.

Pulmonary arteriography in experienced hands is a relatively safe procedure. In five separate series involving almost 2600 patients, only six deaths related to pulmonary arteriography occurred; all of these occurred in patients with severe underlying embolic disease or pulmonary hypertension.[124,198,204,208,211] Nonfatal complications have been reported in approximately 4 per cent of patients.[208,211] Half of these related to the catheterization (cardiac perforation and arrhythmia) and the other half related to the contrast material (bronchospasm and anaphylaxis).

LABORATORY DIAGNOSIS. The triad of increased LDH, normal SGOT, and increased bilirubin has been reputed to be indicative of pulmonary embolism and infarction and useful in differentiation from myocardial infarction or pneumonia.[212] Subsequent investigation has not confirmed the original enthusiasm for its value, and several studies have found enzyme levels to be of little if any value in diagnosis.[124,141,213] As with other diagnostic procedures, variations in reported results may reflect different time intervals between the embolic episode and performance of the test, and different patient populations. Recently, interest has been generated in measurements of fibrin split products in patients with suspected embolism.[214] The data available thus far suggest that this test is sensitive, but its specificity needs further assessment.

Treatment (See Table 46–4)

The management of pulmonary embolism is determined importantly by the degree to which the circulation has been compromised.[215] Since most emboli resolve in time, the goals of treatment with the available agents are simple and twofold: to sustain life and to prevent recurrence. The studies of Barritt and Jordan[216] and others[217] have clearly

TABLE 46–4   TREATMENT REGIMENS IN PULMONARY EMBOLISM (PE)

1. Submassive PE	2. Massive PE	3. Anticoagulants Contraindicated
a. Heparin 70 μ/kg IV simultaneously with infusion of 20–25 μ/kg/hr IV regulated to keep APTT between 60–80 sec or Lee-White CT between 20–40 min for 7–10 days or b. Heparin, 55–70 μ/kg every 4 hr IV 7–10 days	a. Heparin 10,000 units IV simultaneously with infusion of 25 μ/kg/hr IV for 7–10 days regulated by laboratory test or b. Heparin, 7000–10,000 units every 4 hr IV for 24–48 hours followed by 55–75 μ/kg every 4 hours for 7–9 days or c. Streptokinase, 250,000 units IV for 30 minutes followed by 100,000 μ/hr for 24 hr; or urokinase, 4400 CTA μ/kg for 10 minutes followed by 4400 CTA μ/kg/hr for 12–24 hr. During thrombolytic therapy, the thrombin time should be 2–7× baseline. At completion of thrombolytic infusion when thrombin time is less than 2× baseline (3–4 hr later), start heparin therapy as in 2a or b.	Vena caval of ligation, umbrella or balloon, for life-threatening embolus; plication for other cases

Long-term therapy
a. Warfarin to keep prothrombin 8–25% activity, overlap 3–5 days with heparin and continue at least 12 weeks; further therapy guided by status of predisposing conditions

b. Heparin, 5000 units every 8–12 hr or subcutaneously for a minimum of 12 weeks

APTT = activated partial thromboplastin time; CT = clotting time. (Reproduced with permission from Bell, W. R., and Simon, T. L.: Am. Heart J. *103*:239, 1982.)

shown a significant reduction in mortality after pulmonary embolism, from approximately 25 to 5 per cent, among patients treated with anticoagulants. Therapy with heparin is adequate in most instances.[218]

In the absence of contraindications to anticoagulants, the current recommendation is 10,000 units of heparin intravenously in a single injection when pulmonary embolism is first suspected and diagnostic studies are not complete. After confirmation, heparin should be continued in amounts adequate to prevent platelet-thrombin interaction:[219,220] 5000 to 7500 units every 4 hours by intravenous administration, or, preferably, 1000 units per hour by constant infusion. Two controlled trials have shown continuous heparin therapy to be significantly safer from hemorrhagic complications,[221,222] but there is some suggestion that recurrent thromboembolism may be more prevalent with this approach.[223] The need for clotting time or partial thromboplastin time determinations to monitor the dose has been debated in the past; properly performed, these tests are helpful in reducing the incidence of hemorrhagic complications.[124] Heparin should be continued until the patient's cardiopulmonary status has stabilized and any evidence of venous thrombosis has resolved, which requires about 8 days.

Oral anticoagulants are usually instituted when the heparin is being tapered and the patient begins ambulation. No guidelines for duration of oral anticoagulation have been available, and most authorities recommend 3 to 6 months.[212] One randomized trial in which patients were treated for either 6 weeks or 6 months concluded that there was no benefit from oral anticoagulants administered for longer than 6 weeks in patients experiencing a single episode of phlebitis or pulmonary embolism or both.[224] In this study, the indications for therapy for 6 months were a past history of venous thromboembolism, a recurrent thrombotic tendency, or continuing predisposing cause. If the embolization is small and is the result of a specific predisposing factor that has subsequently resolved, anticoagulation, of course, may be discontinued sooner.

Although heparin is the cornerstone of therapy, it has the disadvantage of not being thrombolytic. The value of two thrombolytic agents, streptokinase and urokinase, has been extensively investigated. Urokinase has received most

attention because it is not antigenic or pyrogenic, and its administration does not appear to require precise dosage or complex laboratory controls. The experience gained indicates that patients with acute pulmonary emboli who receive lytic therapy gain a short-lived advantage over those given heparin.[124,125] There is greater resolution of the emboli and hemodynamic improvement in the first 24 hours with thrombolytic therapy, particularly in patients with massive emboli, but this difference quickly disappears. Controlled trials have not shown any significant differences in mortality rates between the two therapeutic approaches. The available data suggest that thrombolytic therapy may prove valuable in treating patients with massive pulmonary embolism with hemodynamic compromise who were previously considered candidates for emergency pulmonary embolectomy.

Aside from pulmonary embolectomy, the surgical approaches to pulmonary embolism are also designed to prevent recurrent episodes. Accumulated experience has shown that either clipping or tying the inferior vena cava or interrupting flow with an "umbrella" directly below the renal veins is the procedure of choice (Fig. 46–13).[226–228] The patients most likely to need this therapy are those with contraindications to anticoagulants or those in whom recurrent emboli develop despite well-controlled anticoagulation.[219,227] As noted, the recognition of a recurrence during the acute phase of pulmonary embolism is a difficult clinical problem that requires angiography for confirmation; it can be hazardous to rely only on clinical findings or lung scans.[206,207] Even surgical procedures are not absolutely effective, and recurrences can occur[227,229] because sizable collateral channels develop through which embolization may recur with the passage of time and thrombi may form proximal to the site of caval manipulation.

Pulmonary embolectomy appears to be useful in very selective instances. The procedure requires cardiopulmonary bypass and carries with it a very high mortality, often exceeding 50 per cent.[230–232] Currently, indications for surgery are massive embolization with shock which fails to respond to vigorous medical therapy with isoproterenol, oxygen, and heparin.[220,233]

The most recent trend in the approach to pulmonary embolism is the prevention of its occurrence in high-risk

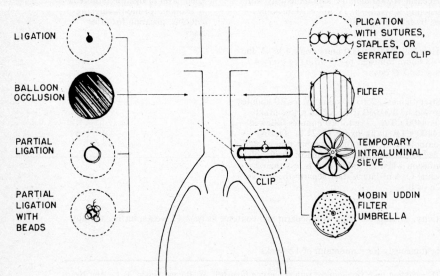

FIGURE 46–13 The various methods and devices used in the inferior vena cava to arrest emboli of lethal size. (From Gardner, A. M. N.: Inferior vena cava interruption in the prevention of fatal pulmonary embolism. Am. Heart J. *95*:679, 1978.)

groups. One of the most efficient ways of achieving this goal is to prevent the development of venous thrombosis in the lower extremities by early ambulation.[234] In those patients in whom this approach is not feasible, the classic study of Sevitt and Gallagher has clearly established the role of prophylactic anticoagulation as a useful alternative.[235] The most favored approach at present is to administer small doses of heparin (5000 units of high-potency heparin) every 12 hours to patients 40 years of age or older who are to undergo thoracoabdominal or gynecological surgery under general anesthesia. Data regarding prevention of deep venous thrombosis and pulmonary embolization in patients treated with this regimen are quite persuasive.[236,237] However, this approach does have limitations, and it has not been found to be very effective in patients with hip fracture or in those undergoing prostatic surgery.[238]

Prognosis

The natural history of pulmonary thromboembolism is not completely known. Available data indicate that considerably less than 10 per cent of all emboli are lethal in the acute phase,[88,182,239,240] and in those that are, 75 per cent of the deaths occur within 60 minutes of the onset of symptoms, with the remaining 25 per cent occurring within the next 48 hours.[241,242] Consequently, death in those who survive the acute insult long enough to be diagnosed and placed on therapy is a relatively rare event.[232,242]

Experimental studies in dogs have demonstrated that resolution of pulmonary vascular obstruction by fresh autologous blood clots begins within hours of embolism, and small emboli are lysed so rapidly that little or no evidence of their presence is detectable 5 to 13 days later, even with careful histological examination.[243] In humans, resolution appears to be slower. There is usually minimal angiographic and hemodynamic resolution of the vascular obstruction in the first 7 days following embolization, and complete clearing usually takes many weeks.[139] In one study in which serial lung scans were used, 15 per cent of patients showed complete resolution at 2 weeks, and 30 per cent required a month.[201] In the National Cooperative Urokinase Trial, lung scans had improved by only 50 per cent at 14 days, and prominent residual scan defects remained for 3 months.[124] In fact, 16 per cent of the patients had not completely cleared their defects in a year.

The factors that determine which patients will experience complete resolution and which will have persistent unresolved embolism have not been delineated. Similarly, the frequency of chronic cor pulmonale due to unresolved or recurrent embolism is not known. Paraskos and associates evaluated 50 patients with documented acute pulmonary embolism 1 to 7 years after the acute episode.[202] Their findings demonstrate that the vast majority of patients will return to their usual state of health and that unresolved embolism is an uncommon event. In this study, the most important factor influencing long-term survival was the presence of preexisting heart disease, especially left ventricular failure. The frequency of cor pulmonale or recurrent pulmonary embolism was less than 1 per cent. Thus the long-term prognosis in patients previously in good health appears to be quite good.

CHRONIC COR PULMONALE

Incidence

Because of its association with chronic lung disease, chronic cor pulmonale is believed to be a common type of heart disease.[1,76,244] Although precise figures on prevalence are lacking, it is possible to appreciate the potential magnitude of the problem by recognizing that chronic bronchitis and emphysema are its most common causes and that these two diseases result in approximately 30,000 deaths per year.[245] In one study in England, cor pulmonale was responsible for 30 to 40 per cent of all clinical cases of heart failure, of a total of 487 cases of cardiac disease,[246] and in the United States 10 to 30 per cent of hospital admissions for congestive heart failure are due to cor pulmonale.[247] Most patients are 45 years of age or older, and men are affected more frequently than women.

Etiology

There are many causes of cor pulmonale. Any disease that affects ventilatory mechanics, gas exchange, or the vascular bed either directly, through intrapulmonic events, or indirectly, via its effect on ventilatory control or the neuromuscular apparatus of respiration, may cause cor pulmonale. Since this is true of essentially all primary pulmonary disorders, the development of cor pulmonale simply indicates that the primary disease was sufficiently advanced to raise pulmonary artery pressure, cause right ventricular hypertrophy, and impair right ventricular function. Fortunately, most disorders affect too little of the lungs or are too circumscribed in their effects on gas exchange to initiate the train of events that leads to right ventricular hypertrophy and failure. A list of the various disease categories commonly associated with cor pulmonale, along with some specific examples of each process, is presented in Table 46–5.

Pathophysiology

Factors Contributing to the Development of Pulmonary Hypertension. The most important pathogenetic mechanisms that produce abnormalities in right ventricular structure and function are pulmonary hypertension and abnormal concentrations of blood gases that directly modify myocardial performance.[247a] As noted above (p. 1574), the normal pulmonary circulation is a low-resistance system with considerable reserve; therefore, substantial reductions in the size of the effective vascular bed must occur before pulmonary hypertension develops and becomes sustained. The pathogenetic sequence is unknown, and probably a number of mechanisms interact to produce pulmonary hypertension. Any theory regarding the development of cor pulmonale must take into account the effects

**TABLE 46–5   DISEASE CATEGORIES ASSOCIATED
WITH CHRONIC COR PULMONALE**

Disorders of Pulmonary Parenchyma and Intrathoracic Airways

Chronic obstructive pulmonary disease
Chronic suppurative lung disease
Restrictive lung disease

Disorders of the Neuromuscular Apparatus and Chest Wall

Myopathic
Neurological
Thoracic deformity

Inadequate Ventilatory Drive

Obesity-hypoventilation syndromes
Primary alveolar hypoventilation
Sleep apnea syndromes (central)
Chronic mountain sickness

Upper Airway Obstruction

Pharyngeal-tracheal obstruction
Sleep apnea (obstructive)

Pulmonary Vascular Disorders

Multiple pulmonary emboli
Primary pulmonary hypertension
Miscellaneous

of the anatomical loss of vessels, i.e., anatomical restriction of the pulmonary vascular bed, pulmonary arteriolar constriction, increased blood viscosity, and increased blood flow, although their relative roles have not been clearly defined.[244]

It has long been thought that the essential pathology in chronic cor pulmonale is a *physical loss of vessels*, leading to a restricted vascular bed. Although it is certainly true that this mechanism contributes to the pulmonary hypertension seen in vascular occlusion resulting from multiple pulmonary emboli, aplasia, or extensive excision of lung tissue,[36,76,248] other factors also must be considered since emphysema, a disease in which alveolar vessels are widely destroyed, is typically associated with resting pulmonary

hypertension and cor pulmonale only late in its course.[249,250] Thus, a decrease in the anatomical extent of the pulmonary vascular bed does not play a major role in the development of pulmonary hypertension unless the reduction is extreme. However, other processes (i.e., a constricted vascular bed) can *decrease the effective cross-sectional area without a loss of vessels*. The effective area can be reduced by arteriolar constriction secondary to alveolar hypoxemia and acidosis[32,33,67–70,76–80] and by the pathological changes responsible for pulmonary hypertension[251–254] (Chap. 25).

The potent vasoconstricting influence resulting from alveolar hypoxia (Fig. 46–14) is shared by the disease entities responsible for chronic cor pulmonale and listed in Table 46–5. The resulting pulmonary hypertension, when persistent, can make the vessels rigid and reduce their lumina by producing intimal thickening, inflammatory changes, and medial hypertrophy.[251–255]

Intimal thickening, regardless of its mechanism, often has a patchy distribution and is a frequent postmortem finding in patients beyond the age of 40 years who were free of pulmonary hypertension during life.[255] Therefore, the extent must be great to account for the perpetuation or worsening of pulmonary hypertension. The reversibility of this process is unknown, but when intimal thickening is produced by fibrosis, it is presumably permanent. Inflammatory changes vary from cellular infiltrates to fibrinoid necrosis and fibrosis. Most often these types of alterations are found in diffuse inflammatory lung lesions or with systemic illness with vasculitis; however, they have been noted secondary to pulmonary hypertension of any cause[252,255,256] (Chap. 25). Hypertrophy and hyperplasia of the smooth muscle in the media of the arterioles are regular findings in long-standing pulmonary hypertension and have been found to be reversible to some extent.[251–253]

An *increase in the viscosity of blood* has been shown experimentally to raise pulmonary vascular resistance[257] (p. 824). Viscosity is generally elevated as a result of chronic

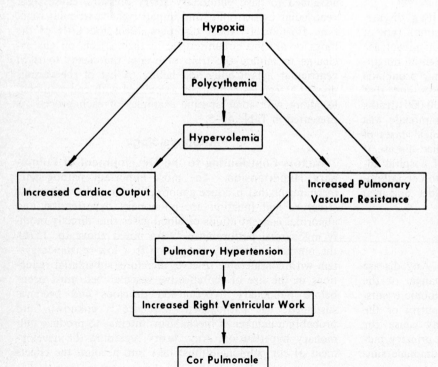

FIGURE 46–14 Schematic representation of the pathogenetic consequences of chronic hypoxia, regardless of cause, that culminate in cor pulmonale. (Reproduced with permission from Murray, J. F.: Respiration. In Pathophysiology—The Biological Principles of Disease. Smith, L. H., Jr., and Thier, S. O. (eds.): W. B. Saunders Co., Philadelphia, 1981, 1871 pp.)

hypoxemia stimulating red cell production through erythropoietin release. It represents an adaptation in that it provides the body with an increased oxygen-carrying capacity. However, the compensatory mechanism is useful only up to a point because the high hematocrit can interfere with blood flow in the capillaries and offset any potential benefits. The mechanism by which this occurs is complex. Blood is a non-Newtonian fluid, and its viscosity is an inverse function of shear rate, which varies with flow.[258] With high hematocrits the shear rates are low, and as the blood flow slows in the capillaries, viscosity increases even further, requiring a greater driving pressure. These considerations have served as the rationale for phlebotomy in selected patients with cor pulmonale.

The final factor that has been proposed as contributing to pulmonary hypertension is an *increase in pulmonary blood flow.* Extensive intimal hypertrophy and pathological medial necrosis have been created in the pulmonary circulation of animals by anastomosing a pulmonary artery either to the aorta or to one of its main branches.[259] Although studies demonstrate that bronchial artery-pulmonary vasculature collateral channels develop in chronic obstructive pulmonary disease,[260,261] these channels are seldom of quantitative significance except in the case of bronchiectasis.[261] As discussed below, increased cardiac outputs can raise pulmonary pressures in patients with both constricted and restricted vascular beds.

It is not clear how the above-described pathogenetic mechanisms interrelate in the development of pulmonary hypertension. It is easy to appreciate that the loss of vessels and diffuse constriction of the arterioles with its attendant pathological changes in their walls and lumina can combine to cause a reduction of the pulmonary vascular bed, which in turn causes an increase in pulmonary vascular resistance. However, these changes need not be manifest at rest as an elevated pulmonary artery pressure. As shown in Figure 46–4, the normal pulmonary vascular bed has the ability to accept large increases in flow without increasing pressure, probably through the recruitment of parallel vascular channels. In the case of a restricted vascular bed, this reserve is lost and the patients act as though they were starting at the bend of the normal pressure-flow relationship (Fig. 46–15).

Under these circumstances pressure can rise dramatically with exercise or any other condition that causes cardiac output to increase. With time and progression of the underlying disease as the secondary changes in the vessels develop, further reducing pulmonary vascular reserve, pulmonary artery pressure becomes elevated, even at rest. Now the pressure-flow relationship (Fig. 46–4A) is shifted upward and to the left as in a constricted bed, so that small increments in flow produce large increases in pressure over the entire range of cardiac outputs. It may be inferred that small increases in output are accompanied by large increases in work. Increases in viscosity and collateral blood flow worsen the situation by further increasing pulmonary artery pressure.

The data to support this general picture are derived from observations on the response to exercise of patients with chronic bronchitis (constricted vascular bed) and emphysema (restricted vascular bed).[262–264] In the former, pulmonary diffusing capacity *increases normally* with increases in cardiac output with exercise, and the work capacity of

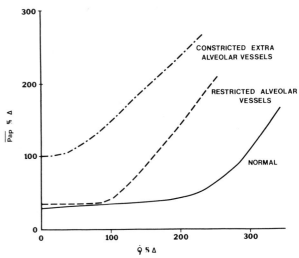

FIGURE 46–15 Pressure-flow relationship of normal, restricted, and constricted pulmonary vascular beds. The vertical axis indicates the percentage of change in mean pulmonary artery pressure (PAP % Δ), whereas the horizontal scale shows the percentage of change in cardiac output (Q̇ % Δ). In both instances 100% = normal, basal level.

these patients is limited by their state of pulmonary mechanics and resulting gas exchange. It appears that the ability to dilate extraalveolar vessels normally and recruit alveolar vessels intact, although pulmonary artery pressure rises. Conversely, in patients with emphysema without resting pulmonary hypertension, diffusing capacity *does not increase normally* with exercise. The work capacity of these patients is limited by insufficient effective alveolar-capillary surface rather than by cardiac output or ventilation, and recruitment of alveolar vessels is severely curtailed.[262]

RIGHT VENTRICULAR DYNAMICS. The hemodynamic findings in cor pulmonale depend to some extent on the cause and duration of the underlying pathological process. Patients with relatively mild obstructive lung disease without severe hypoxemia generally have normal mean right atrial and right ventricular end-diastolic pressures, normal or low cardiac outputs, normal or slightly elevated pulmonary artery pressures, and slightly elevated pulmonary vascular resistances at rest.[264–272,272a,272b] Right ventricular ejection fractions, as determined by radionuclide techniques, tend to be normal.[270,271] With exercise, pulmonary artery pressure rises further, right ventricular stroke work increases (Fig. 46–16), and right ventricular ejection fractions fall.[270,271] Relating end-diastolic pressure to stroke work suggests that these patients operate on an extension of the normal right ventricular function curve.[269] This set of findings need not be accompanied by clinical or electrocardiographic evidence of right ventricular hypertrophy.[264] However, acute right ventricular failure can develop in these patients if respiratory failure is precipitated by a pulmonary infection.

Progression of the airway obstruction tends to accentuate these findings. As the ventilatory impairment worsens, the hemodynamic alterations follow suit. At the stage when severe chronic hypoxemia develops, usually in association with chronic hypercapnia, there is moderate pulmonary hypertension at rest, which becomes more severe during exercise in association with abnormal right ventricular filling pressures and function.[269–271] Cardiac output tends to be normal or slightly elevated at rest but increases little with exercise while air is being breathed; oxy-

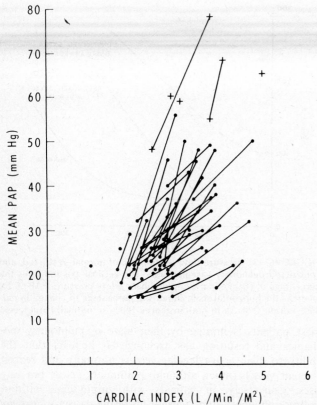

FIGURE 46–16 Relationship between mean pulmonary artery pressure (PAP) and cardiac index at rest and during exercise in patients with chronic obstructive lung disease. Crosses (+) indicate patients with arterial oxyhemoglobin saturation of less than 80 per cent. Resting and exercise values are connected by solid lines. (Reprinted with permission from Burrows, B., et al.: Patterns of cardiovascular dysfunction in chronic obstructive lung disease. N. Engl. J. Med. *286*: 912, 1972.)

gen administration, however, may improve the right ventricular ejection fraction.[271] Mean pulmonary artery pressures can reach levels of 60 to 80 mm Hg, and these patients are likely to show the clinical and electrocardiographic changes usually ascribed to cor pulmonale. Failure of the right ventricle is associated with an expanded circulating blood volume. However, in contrast to left ventricular failure, the pulmonary blood volume/total volume ratio remains essentially normal (approximately 1 to 10) even though red cell mass may be considerably increased.[273] Both circulating plasma volume and lung water increase,[273, 274] and both have been shown to decrease as pulmonary artery pressure is lowered with therapy.

LEFT VENTRICULAR DYNAMICS. Abnormally elevated pulmonary venous pressures, with or without overt left ventricular failure, invariably produce alterations in pulmonary mechanics and gas exchange, even in patients with normal lungs (Chapter 54). Consequently, left ventricular dysfunction could have deleterious effects in cor pulmonale. Controversy persists about whether the combined pulmonary–right ventricular pathologic condition in these patients produces the left ventricular disease, or whether the latter results from independent causes.

The view that disorders of the right ventricle may result in left ventricular disease has gained support from several sources. Animal experiments have shown that (1) right

ventricular failure following banding of the pulmonary artery leads to similar morphological and biochemical changes in both cardiac chambers and to reduced contractility of the left ventricle,[275–277] (2) in both isolated hearts and intact animals alterations in right ventricular compliance or dimensions also change the mechanical properties of the left ventricle,[14,278,279] and (3) cattle with severe pulmonary hypertension at high altitude have increased left ventricular end-diastolic pressures.[280] Although these observations are provocative, their relevance to human disease is uncertain.

Autopsy studies have shown that left ventricular hypertrophy occurs in some patients with cor pulmonale,[281–283] and left ventricular dysfunction of varying degrees has been observed in vivo.[283–285] In all of these investigations, none of the usual etiologies of left ventricular disease were apparent. Thus, it appears that the structure and function of the left ventricle can become abnormal in association with the pathogenetic mechanisms underlying cor pulmonale. However, this is probably a very uncommon occurrence and the weight of current evidence indicates that cor pulmonale need not seriously affect left ventricular performance.[264,269,282,286–292] When abnormalities have been found, they could be explained either by a reduction in right ventricular stroke volume causing diminished left-sided filling or by independent disease processes such as coronary arteriosclerosis.[292] However, given the heterogeneity of the population with cor pulmonale and the variance of its natural history, the controversy will undoubtedly continue.[291]

Clinical Manifestations

As with other aspects of cor pulmonale, the clinical, radiological, therapeutic, and prognostic features are strongly influenced by the underlying disease process responsible for the pulmonary hypertension. For this reason, the subsequent presentation deals with many of these parameters as they specifically apply to the various disease categories listed in Table 46–5. Without doubt, the diseases that affect the pulmonary parenchyma, the intrathoracic airways, or both account for the vast majority of the cases of cor pulmonale. Within this category, the most common cause is chronic obstructive lung disease.

CHRONIC OBSTRUCTIVE PULMONARY DISEASE (COPD). COPD consists of chronic bronchitis, emphysema, and bronchial asthma. However, atopic asthma does *not* produce chronic cor pulmonale[250] and intrinsic, or nonatopic, asthma is often a variant of chronic bronchitis; in this chapter, COPD is used to denote chronic bronchitis and emphysema exclusively.

In most patients with COPD, chronic bronchitis and emphysema coexist, but cor pulmonale is restricted to those with functionally significant airway disease with or without emphysema.[250] This admixture has given rise to a great deal of confusion in terminology in the literature, and until the matter was sorted out by Burrows and colleagues[293] and Mitchell and Filley,[294] the terms bronchitis and emphysema were frequently considered to be synonymous. Additional observations uncovered fundamental differences in the clinical, physiological, and pathological features of the two conditions and laid the groundwork for a better understanding of these diseases.[75,262,293,295,296]

On the basis of this information, it is possible to think

TABLE 46–6 COMPARISON OF THE CLINICAL AND PHYSIOLOGICAL FEATURES OF EMPHYSEMA AND CHRONIC BRONCHITIS

	EMPHYSEMA	CHRONIC BRONCHITIS
Synonyms	Pink puffer	Blue bloater
	Fighter	Nonfighter
Signs and Symptoms		
Cough and sputum	Scant	Marked
Dyspnea at rest	Marked	Usually absent
Recurrent chest infections	Unusual	Frequent
Cyanosis	No	Yes
Edema	No	Yes
Increased AP diameter of thorax	Marked	Mild
Hyperresonance to percussion	Marked	Mild
Pulmonary Gas Exchange		
Hematocrit	Normal	Elevated
P_aO_2	Slight reduction	Marked reduction
P_aCO_2	Low or normal	Elevated
Diffusing capacity	Markedly decreased	Normal or slightly reduced
Pulmonary Mechanics		
Expiratory flow rates	Reduced	Reduced
Elastic recoil	Markedly reduced	Normal or slightly reduced
Lung volumes	Marked hyperinflation	Mild hyperinflation
Pulmonary Circulation		
Pulmonary hypertension at rest	None or mild	Marked
with exercise	Moderate	Marked
Right heart failure	Terminal	Repeated

of COPD as a continuum, with chronic bronchitis at one extreme and emphysema at the other and the majority of patients having features of both conditions. The distinctions between the two groups are presented in Table 46–6. In the chronic bronchitis variety ("blue bloater," "nonfighter"), chronic cough with sputum production, frequently recurring chest infection, secondary erythrocytosis, and repeated bouts of right heart failure are common. Physiologically, the patients have hypoxemia and hypercapnia at rest, normal diffusing capacities, and elevated residual volumes, functional residual capacities, and airway resistances, with relatively normal values for total lung capacity and pulmonary compliance. Maximum flow rates and forced expiratory volumes are abnormally depressed. Chest radiographs show hyperinflated lungs, increased lung markings, and cardiomegaly.

The basic abnormality is widespread but regionally unequal airway obstruction that results in mismatched $\dot{V}_A/\dot{Q}$ relationships. In regions of low $\dot{V}_A/\dot{Q}$ ratios, pulmonary arterial constriction on the basis of hypoxia, hypercapnia, and/or acidosis occurs. With progression, net alveolar hypoventilation develops, the vascular bed becomes constricted, and resting pulmonary hypertension ensues.

In the emphysematous type ("pink puffer," "fighter"), dyspnea is the predominant symptom, and cough and sputum are considerably less prominent. Erythrocytosis is uncommon, and right heart failure tends to occur as a terminal event. In keeping with the hyperventilation, the alveolar-arterial gradient for oxygen is abnormally elevated, but arterial oxygen tension is usually normal or only slightly depressed; hypocapnia is common. Standard spirometric indices cannot differentiate this group from those with chronic bronchitis, as the degree of obstruction as measured by this technique is similar. However, the pink puffer has abnormally low diffusing capacities, enormous

lung volumes, and very high values for pulmonary compliance. Roentgenograms of the chest reveal marked hyperinflation with flattened diaphragms, oligemia of the peripheral lung fields, and a small heart. With the onset of cor pulmonale, the prominence of the vascular markings increases, but right ventricular enlargement may be difficult to appreciate.

Although there is some airway disease in this condition, the primary pathological defect is widespread destruction of alveolar septa. As a result, the surface area for gas exchange is lost more or less in proportion to alveolar vessels, and arterial gas tensions can be reasonably well maintained for a period of time by increasing ventilation. However, the destruction of the parenchyma results in loss of lateral traction of small airways so that they narrow and collapse. Then the regional distribution of inspired air becomes more impaired, with resultant worsening of the abnormalities in $\dot{V}_A/\dot{Q}$ ratios. These patients initially have a restricted vascular bed, with normal pulmonary artery pressures at rest. As their disease process worsens with airway disease and further deterioration of gas exchange, secondary changes in the vasculature occur and resting pulmonary artery hypertension and cor pulmonale develop.

The *clinical manifestations* of cor pulmonale with heart failure are increasing dyspnea; episodes of paroxysmal cough, occasionally with syncope; and fluid retention with pitting edema and sometimes ascites. The distended neck veins exhibit prominent *a* and *v* waves and do not collapse with inspiration. Central cyanosis and an enlarged, tender liver are often present. Right ventricular hypertrophy is indicated by a palpable parasternal or subxiphoid heave. On auscultation, an S3 gallop, accentuated by inspiration, and a loud pulmonic second sound are frequently present. A holosystolic murmur along the lower left parasternal edge, accentuated by inspiration, usually indicates tricuspid regurgitation. These cardiac findings can be evanescent and can develop quickly when acute respiratory failure is superimposed on COPD. Examination of the lungs reveals diffuse inspiratory and expiratory rhonchi and wheezes. If acute respiratory failure is present in addition, papilledema, confusion, a hyperkinetic circulation, and asterixis may also be present.

Fundamental *treatment* of cor pulmonale in COPD is to relieve pulmonary hypertension by improving gas exchange.[297] This is accomplished by reducing bronchial smooth muscle constriction, promoting drainage of retained secretions, treating respiratory tract infections, and providing supplemental oxygen. The first two goals can be achieved simultaneously with the use of bronchodilators. In addition to relieving smooth muscle spasm, the sympathomimetics also increase mucociliary transport.[298] The net effect of these measures is the reduction of airway obstruction and the improvement of the regional distribution of inspired air and, through that, $\dot{V}_A/\dot{Q}$ relationships. Methylxanthines provide benefits above and beyond the usual bronchodilatation, for this class of compounds may produce favorable hemodynamic effects as well. In one study the intravenous administration of aminophylline in patients with cor pulmonale was shown to reduce mean pulmonary artery and right and left ventricular end-diastolic pressures significantly without inducing a change in the cardiac index,[299] and in another, right and left ventricular ejection fractions were increased.[300]

The beneficial effects of controlled oxygen therapy are well established in several circumstances. In acute respiratory failure, supplemental O_2 results in prompt and often dramatic improvement in pulmonary hemodynamics[264,265] (Fig. 46–17). In patients with progressive right ventricular hypertrophy or recurrent heart failure from cor pulmonale associated with severe hypoxemia ($PaO_2 < 50$ mm Hg) and severe pulmonary hypertension, marked improvement has been found when O_2 was administered for 15 or more

hours per day.[301,302] However, a multicenter controlled trial showed that continuous O_2 for 24 hours a day provided the optimal therapy.[303] Such treatment appears to be safe, and some data suggest that it leads to prolonged survival.[304] However, if chronic O_2 therapy is being contemplated, it is *mandatory* to demonstrate that the supplemental O_2 does not result in worsening of alveolar hypoventilation with progressive hypercapnia.

The indications for the use of ancillary therapeutic measures such as phlebotomy, diuretics, and cardiac glycosides are considerably less clear. In the case of phlebotomy, most studies, including a recent double-blind investigation, have demonstrated an improvement in the subjective complaints related to vascular engorgement but no evidence of improvement in pulmonary gas exchange, mechanics, or hemodynamics.[305,306] Diuretics are commonly used for cor pulmonale with failure, and, although there is little question of their effectiveness in relieving fluid retention, there are scant data to demonstrate that they improve pulmonary hemodynamics or gas exchange in the absence of left ventricular decompensation. Nobel et al. reported an improvement in arterial blood gases with furosemide, but each of their four patients was given O_2 and other therapy concomitantly.[307] Attempts to reduce pulmonary artery pressures with vasodilators have led to conflicting results.[308,309]

The use of digitalis glycosides in patients with cor pulmonale is quite controversial. Digitalis apparently is effective in raising cardiac output in patients with cor pulmonale at rest but only at the expense of concomitant increases in pulmonary artery pressures. The subject has been reviewed, and the consensus is that there is no clearcut evidence that cardiac glycosides are of substantial benefit unless left ventricular failure coexists.[310,311]

The *prognosis* of cor pulmonale in patients with COPD is difficult to state with certainty, for it is inextricably linked to the underlying disorder. When cor pulmonale de-

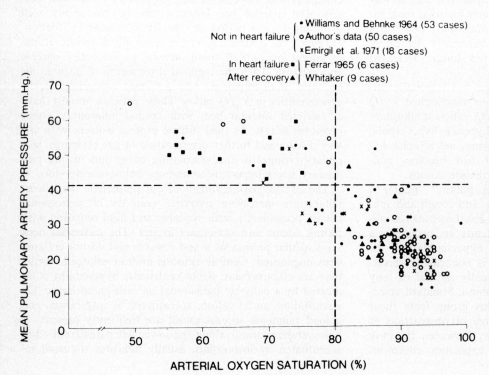

FIGURE 46–17 Relationship of resting mean pulmonary artery pressure to arterial oxygen saturation in 136 cases of chronic obstructive pulmonary disease. Solid squares represent data obtained in patients in heart failure; solid triangles, data from same subjects after recovery. The dashed lines are drawn at arbitrary points to indicate the relative risks of severe pulmonary hypertension (i.e., mean pulmonary artery pressure > 40 mm Hg) in patients with arterial O_2 saturation values greater than, or less than, 80 per cent. (From Burrows, B.: Arterial oxygenation and pulmonary hemodynamics in patients with chronic airways obstruction. Proceedings of Conference on Scientific Basis of Respiratory Therapy. Am. Rev. Respir. Dis. *110*:64, 1974.)

velops in patients with emphysema, life expectancy is quite short, yet patients with bronchitis usually tolerate three to five such episodes before ultimately succumbing to their disease. Although long-term survival has been reported following the onset of cor pulmonale with heart failure, the 2- to 3-year survival rate ranges from 33 to 50 per cent,[312–315] but it may be improving with continuous O_2 therapy.

CHRONIC SUPPURATIVE PULMONARY DISEASE. The two prime examples of chronic suppurative disease associated with chronic cor pulmonale are bronchiectasis and cystic fibrosis.

Bronchiectasis. This chronic inflammatory disease is characterized clinically by cough and the production of copious amounts of purulent sputum and pathologically by cylindrical and saccular dilatation of airways.[316,317] In the majority of patients one can elicit a history of pneumonia developing as a complication of measles, pertussis, or some other contagious disease of childhood. It is thought that bacterial pneumonia and associated atelectasis are responsible for the destruction and dilatation of the bronchial walls. A small percentage of cases are associated with congenital defects such as Kartagener triad (p. 1618) and either congenital or acquired defects in immune mechanisms. Cor pulmonale develops in far-advanced cases in which destruction of lung tissue and fibrosis are extensive. The mechanism for pulmonary hypertension is believed to be capillary loss, hypoxia, and increased bronchial-pulmonary collateral blood flow. Formerly this was a relatively common affliction, but bronchiectasis has decreased considerably in incidence since the advent of the antibiotic era.

Cystic Fibrosis. This genetic defect is characterized by the secretion from exocrine glands of thick, tenacious mucus in which the mucopolysaccharide content is relatively insoluble and easily denatured. The lungs are involved to some extent in virtually all patients with the disease, and the thick mucus throughout the tracheobronchial tree partially or completely obstructs air passages, giving rise to focal atelectasis, pneumonia, bronchiectasis, and abscess formation.[318] Cor pulmonale is an important feature in the natural history, and it contributes to 70 per cent of the deaths.[319] An echocardiographic scoring system has been devised that provides a method for assessing the progression of the cardiac involvement in patients with cystic fibrosis and for evaluating prognosis.[320] Physiological studies have suggested that hypoxia is the principal stimulus to the production of pulmonary hypertension,[321] and pathological data have supported this by demonstrating that the thickening of the medial muscle layer is proportional to the degree of right ventricular hypertrophy.[322] In the past, the development of cardiac failure usually presaged death within a few months. In recent years, however, the prognosis has been improving, and a number of patients have survived for considerable periods.[323] These patients have been maintained on a vigorous, comprehensive, pulmonary care program with postural drainage, antibiotics, and bronchodilators.

RESTRICTIVE LUNG DISEASES. This category encompasses a multitude of diseases which have in common a loss of functioning pulmonary parenchyma with restriction of the pulmonary vascular bed. The latter results from a physical loss of vessels as well as from intrinsic abnormalities in the lumina and walls of those remaining. Essentially, five processes alone or in combination can

produce this effect: (1) diffuse interstitial, (2) diffuse alveolar, (3) mixed alveolar-interstitial, (4) chest wall and pleural, and (5) extensive resection of lung tissue with disease in the residual parenchyma. Specific examples of the first three categories are sarcoidosis, radiation fibrosis, connective tissue disorders with primary or secondary lung involvement, fibrosing alveolitis, alveolar proteinosis, pneumoconiosis, and progressive massive fibrosis. The prototypes for the fourth and fifth categories are thoracoplasty for chronic tuberculosis and surgical resections for granulomatous disease or bronchiectasis.

Pulmonary parenchymal disease, especially when complicated by fibrosis of tissue and secondary vascular changes, can lead to severe pulmonary hypertension. As with the other conditions with a restricted vascular bed, the pulmonary hypertension is initially confined to circumstances in which the cardiac output is elevated. As the vascular bed becomes further restricted and the vessels stiffen, pulmonary hypertension persists at rest and intensifies with increased blood flow. As long as hypoxemia remains mild, pulmonary hypertension is modest, but cor pulmonale develops with respiratory failure. Fortunately, the sequence is not inevitable in most patients with these problems. If the pathological process stabilizes, as is often the case, the patient is left with modest pulmonary hypertension at rest, which is usually well tolerated.[76]

In these diseases, the lungs are stiff, with reduced volumes, and minute ventilations are high, with or without an elevated alveolar ventilation. Arterial O_2 and CO_2 tensions are usually moderately disturbed at rest, but severe hypoxemia may develop with exercise. The diffusing capacity is low and fails to increase normally as cardiac output is increased. In contrast to the chronic obstructive syndromes, a poor correlation exists between arterial blood gases and pulmonary artery pressure,[324] and there seems to be a parallel deterioration in pulmonary mechanics and hemodynamics.[325] As a general rule, when the vital capacity is greater than 80 per cent of normal, hemodynamics are normal. When vital capacity lies between 50 and 80 per cent, vascular resistance is increased and pulmonary artery pressure in the resting state is at the upper limits of normal. When vital capacity is below 50 per cent, pulmonary hypertension is present at rest. The role of hypoxic vasoconstriction in these patients has been difficult to clarify. Experimental evidence indicates that the ability of the pulmonary vasculature to respond to alveolar hypoxia is abnormal in diseased regions, so that when hypoxia does occur, blood is shifted toward the affected areas, thus worsening net gas exchange.[326] In any event, the development of severe hypoxemia and carbon dioxide retention heralds the onset of right ventricular failure, which is usually seen late in the course.

In keeping with the pathophysiology, the prominent symptoms of restrictive lung disease are tachypnea at rest and severe dyspnea on exertion. Fine inspiratory rales are found, along with the previously mentioned signs of pulmonary hypertension and right ventricular hypertrophy and/or failure. Early in the course of patients with pulmonary fibrosis, glucocorticoids or immunosuppressive drugs may be helpful if noninfectious inflammatory processes are believed present. In the late stages with extensive pulmonary fibrosis, these modalities are unsuccessful; all that can be offered is continuous O_2 therapy, diuretics, and cardiac glycosides. Although many of the diseases in this category progress slowly, once cor pulmonale develops the prognosis is grim.

DISORDERS OF THE NEUROMUSCULAR APPARATUS AND CHEST WALL.

These disorders have in common the mechanical failure of the bellows apparatus, through weakness or paralysis of the respiratory muscles or through distortion of the geometry of the thorax. Several factors contribute to the development of cor pulmonale.

Failure of the Neuromuscular Apparatus. Respiratory muscle weakness can result from generalized diseases of muscles such as myopathic infiltrating diseases or muscular dystrophy, but it more commonly follows a neurological disorder, such as a cord lesion at or below the third cervical vertebra, amyotrophic lateral sclerosis, myasthenia gravis, poliomyelitis, Guillain-Barré syndrome, and so on.[327] In all of these diseases, the primary derangement is *generalized alveolar hypoventilation* from mechanical impedance to the movement of the rib cage, diaphragm, or both. The lungs and airways are usually not diseased, although they can become so with retained secretions and multiple aspirations. Although acute respiratory failure is common in these diseases, for cor pulmonale to develop in response to the hypoxic and hypercapneic stimuli the disorder must be chronic; consequently, this complication tends to be seen more often with cord lesions than with the other conditions just noted. Mechanical ventilatory support is the only treatment for the hypoventilation; a cuirass type of respirator is effective in these patients. Along with this, vigorous bronchial toilet facilitates the impaired handling of secretions that frequently coexists.

Bilateral diaphragmatic paralysis is an uncommon but insidious and frequently missed cause of cor pulmonale.[328] In the upright position ventilation is reasonably normal, but with assumption of the supine position gas exchange deteriorates. The diagnosis may be suspected in the patient with supine breathlessness, a disturbed sleep pattern, paradoxical (i.e., inward) motion of the abdomen on inspiration, and a low vital capacity in the erect position. Treatment consists of assisting ventilation during sleep. This can easily be accomplished under most circumstances with a rocking bed. When this is inadequate, electrical pacing of the diaphragm may be used.[329] Occasionally, diaphragmatic fatigue can contribute to the respiratory failure of COPD.[330]

Chest-Wall Disorders. The common congenital or acquired abnormalities that distort the geometry of the thoracic cage are kyphoscoliosis, pectus excavatum, pectus carinatum, and ankylosing spondylitis; only kyphoscoliosis is associated with cor pulmonale.[331] Kyphosis refers to any posterior angulation of the spine, and scoliosis consists of a lateral displacement with at least one compensatory curve in the opposite direction. Of these two processes, a kyphotic angle exceeding 100 degrees or an angle of scoliosis in excess of 120 degrees may be associated with cor pulmonale.[332] Such marked structural abnormalities of the thorax lead to abnormal positioning and functioning of the respiratory muscles, compression of the lung and pulmonary vasculature, and abnormal gas exchange.[332,333] In addition, it has been suggested that scoliosis interferes with the growth and development of alveoli and pulmonary arteries;[334] dyspnea is the major symptom of these disorders.

Therapy is directed toward avoiding complicating infec-

tions; episodes of acute respiratory failure are treated with mechanical ventilation. Surgical improvement of the thoracic deformity is not often associated with a commensurate change in cardiorespiratory function.[335]

INADEQUATE VENTILATORY DRIVE. The common denominator in this category is a depressed output from the respiratory center, with resultant generalized alveolar hypoventilation. Cor pulmonale is then the result of chronic hypoxemia and hypercapnia.

Obesity-Hypoventilation Syndrome. The association of extreme obesity with alveolar hypoventilation was originally made by Sir William Osler; Burwell et al. subsequently coined the term "pickwickian syndrome" to describe the combination of obesity, somnolence, plethora, and edema.[336] Despite many investigations, the pathogenesis of the hypoventilation in this syndrome remains obscure.[337] Excessive reduction of chest-wall compliance and muscle weakness secondary to obesity may account for part, but many extremely obese individuals with these defects do not hypoventilate. These patients may have abnormally low ventilatory responses to hypercapneic and anoxic stimulation, which improve with treatment.[338,339] Consequently, hyposensitivity of the respiratory center, whether acquired or preexistent, is probably a background factor.

The primary *treatment* of this disorder consists of weight reduction. The respiratory stimulant progesterone and its congeners have been shown to increase alveolar ventilation so that hypoxemia, hypercapnia, and cor pulmonale all improve substantially.[339,340] This may prove to be a useful adjunct until weight is reduced. If the respiratory and cardiac failure are life-threatening, ventilatory assistance may be required.

Some obese patients have periodic respirations, particularly during sleep. This sleep apnea syndrome is discussed next.

Sleep Apnea Syndromes. After the description of the Pickwickian syndrome, variant manifestations such as periodic respirations and hypersomnia were recognized, and it soon became apparent that many of the clinical and pathophysiological changes were secondary to abnormal respiratory patterns during sleep.[341] Three types of patterns have been recorded: (1) central apnea, in which airflow stops in conjunction with cessation of all respiratory muscle effort; (2) obstructive apnea, in which upper airway obstruction causes airflow to cease despite continuing or increasing efforts of the inspiratory muscles (the obstruction is believed to result from relaxation or discoordination of the buccal and pharyngeal muscles); and (3) mixed apnea, in which airflow and respiratory effort stop early in the episode, followed by a resumption of unsuccessful respiratory effort.[341,342] Irrespective of the mechanism, if the apneic periods are prolonged or repetitive, hypoventilation with hypoxemia, hypercapnia, and pulmonary hypertension develop, at first with sleep and then gradually when the patient is awake. Pulmonary capillary wedge pressures may also increase during periods of apnea.[343] The clinical symptomatology differs depending on the type, frequency, and intensity of the abnormal, sleep-related respiratory pattern.

The common clinical manifestations are loud snoring, abnormal behavior during sleep (somnambulism, tremors, or myoclonus), altered states of consciousness, nocturnal enuresis, morning headache, daytime hypersomnolence, and hypnagogic hallucinations. Most of these stem from the fact that the patient rarely reaches the deep stages of sleep because of hypoxic arousal and so is chronically sleep-deprived. The majority of patients with sleep apnea are *not obese* and ventilate normally when awake. Patients with obstructive apnea tend to have less severe hypoventilation and fewer hemodynamic abnormalities than patients with the other varieties. Treatment of central apnea consists of nocturnal diaphragmatic pacing;[329,344] tracheostomy is indicated in the obstructive variety.[345] If the latter type occurs in an obese patient, weight reduction may obviate the need for a permanent tracheal cannula. In the mixed group—those with combined central and obstructive etiologies—combined tracheostomy and diaphragmatic pacing are currently recommended.[344] Nocturnal O_2 therapy may be helpful in some patients by reducing the duration of the apneic periods and decreasing the related arrhythmias.[346]

Primary Alveolar Hypoventilation. Generalized alveolar hypoventilation in the absence of obesity or intrinsic disease of the lungs, chest wall, or neuromuscular apparatus has been ascribed to a failure of the autonomic control of ventilation. Most cases are acquired and are seen following encephalitis, brain stem surgery, meningitis, and the like, but congenital occurrence has been reported.[85,347] In this rare disease, the respiratory center does not respond to its chemical stimuli, and the patient has a flat or markedly depressed ventilatory–carbon dioxide response curve. However, an affected patient can improve alveolar ventilation and restore the arterial oxygen and carbon dioxide to normal by voluntary hyperventilation. This syndrome has been called *Ondine's curse.* The pathogenesis and treatment are similar to that outlined for other forms of generalized alveolar hypoventilation. An interesting therapeutic development is long-term pacing of the diaphragm by means of electrical stimulation of the phrenic nerves.[329]

Chronic Mountain Sickness. Some acclimatized residents of high altitudes suffer a transient loss of their adaptation after short stays at sea level and, upon return to altitude, develop acute pulmonary edema with circulatory and electrocardiographic changes similar to those seen in acute cor pulmonale[348] (p. 568). Some persons remaining at high altitude lose their acclimatization and develop signs and symptoms of generalized alveolar hypoventilation with chronic cor pulmonale. This syndrome is variously called *chronic mountain sickness, soroche,* or *Monge disease.*[349,350] The mechanism for the hypoventilation is unknown, but Severinghaus et al. have postulated that it is due to an adaptation or desensitization of the hypoxic chemoreceptors in the carotid body to chronic hypoxia.[351] The only treatment is removal of the patient to sea level, where pulmonary artery pressure falls acutely. With prolonged residence polycythemia disappears, and there is believed to be some involution of the structural changes of the pulmonary vessels.

UPPER AIRWAY OBSTRUCTION. Obstruction of the upper airways may be responsible for an inadequate ventilatory drive, global alveolar hypoventilation, and cor pulmonale. For the most part this occurs in children, especially black children, who have enlarged tonsils and adenoids.[352] Other causes include vascular ring (p. 1013), macroglossia, micrognathia, laryngotracheomalacia, laryn-

geal web, Crouzon disease, Hurler syndrome, and severe Pierre Robin syndrome,[353,354] but it can also develop with obstruction during sleep in both children and adults.[344] The mechanism for the hypoventilation is not at all clear. It has been suggested that an abnormally reactive pulmonary vascular bed, a defect in the central control of respiration, and an interference with normal sleep physiology, as in the sleep apnea syndrome, may play a part. There is little direct evidence for the first mechanism. However, it is known that ventilatory responsiveness to carbon dioxide is blunted in these patients and that it does not return to normal following therapy.[355]

The clinical features may mimic asthma, but more often the patients display somnolence, respiratory stridor, and recurrent respiratory tract infections. Treatment consists of surgical removal of the obstruction.

PULMONARY VASCULAR DISORDERS (see also Chap. 25). This category consists of diseases that primarily affect the pulmonary vasculature, with minimal or no parenchymal involvement. These diseases represent the most straightforward pathogenetic sequence in which pulmonary hypertension and right ventricular overloading are consequences of a progressive increase in pulmonary vascular resistance resulting from gradual obliteration of the blood vessels. In addition to their pathophysiology, these diseases also share in common the symptom of dyspnea and strikingly high pulmonary artery pressures, despite the fact that both vital capacity and pulmonary gas exchange may be only minimally impaired.[356] The latter is frequently of considerable diagnostic importance.

Multiple Pulmonary Emboli. Chronic thromboembolic disease occurs in two fashions. In the first, an obvious onset of the disease in the form of pleurisy or pulmonary infarction is followed by a protracted course characterized by step-wise impairment from acute attacks of dyspnea. In the second, patients tend to develop pulmonary hypertension and cor pulmonale slowly and silently without any antecedent gross pulmonic event.[248] Tachypnea, persisting during sleep, is an outstanding clinical feature of both varieties. Nonspecific symptoms such as tiredness, tachycardia, atypical chest pain, cough, and episodes of fever may also be part of the picture. Plain chest films may be of value in making the diagnosis if locally reduced vascular markings are found, but the diagnostic mainstay is pulmonary angiography. The prognosis is poor without early diagnosis. Treatment consists of preventing further embolization with anticoagulants or vena caval interruption or rarely by surgical evaluation of emboli in the pulmonary arterial bed.

Other Causes of Pulmonary Hypertension. *Schistosomiasis* is endemic in many parts of the world. Pulmonary hypertension is produced by ova emboli released by female worms lodged in pelvic or mesenteric veins.[357]

Sickle cell anemia can produce pulmonary hypertension through several mechanisms. The major one is extensive occlusion and microinfarction due to aggregation and sickling of the red blood cells in the pulmonary circulation (Chap. 49). Contributing factors are increased collateral blood flow and hyperviscosity.[358,359]

Pulmonary and/or systemic arteritis (Chap. 48) can be associated with the development of pulmonary hypertension. Most often this occurs in conjunction with collagen-vascular diseases such as scleroderma, lupus erythematosus, and rheumatoid arthritis. Usually there is pulmonary fibrosis in addition to the arteritis, but occasionally cor pulmonale can develop in its absence.[256]

Pulmonary venoocclusive disease is a rare disorder in which there is gradual obliteration of the pulmonary veins and venules (Chap. 25).[360] It tends to affect children and young adults, and its etiology is unknown. Chest radiographs show Kerley B lines and may help differentiate this disease from other entities like primary pulmonary hypertension and recurrent pulmonary emboli, but the diagnosis rests on lung biopsy.[361] The morphological picture shows narrowing and occlusion of small veins by organized thrombi. Nodular areas of congestion, interstitial fibrosis, and pneumonitis are regularly present as well. Anticoagulants do not seem to be of benefit, but successful treatment with immunosuppressive drugs has been reported.[362]

Electrocardiographic Findings (Table 46–7)

In the past, the use of the electrocardiogram to make the diagnosis of cor pulmonale has centered largely, if not exclusively, upon the demonstration of right ventricular hypertrophy. The classic criteria of a shift of the mean QRS axis to the right (right axis deviation greater than $+$ 110 degrees), an R:S ratio in V_1 greater than 1, and an R:S ratio in V_6 of less than 1 were derived from patients with congenital heart disease[363,364] and have proved to be relatively poor criteria of cor pulmonale in patients with

---

TABLE 46–7 ELECTROCARDIOGRAPHIC CHANGES IN COR PULMONALE

ECG Criteria for Cor Pulmonale without *Obstructive Disease of the Airways**

1. Right-axis deviation with a mean QRS axis to the right of $+$ 110°
2. R/S amplitude ratio in $V_1 > 1$
3. R/S amplitude ratio in $V_6 < 1$
4. Clockwise rotation of the electrical axis
5. P-pulmonale pattern
6. S_1Q_3 or $S_1S_2S_3$ pattern
7. Normal-voltage QRS

ECG Changes in Chronic Cor Pulmonale with *Obstructive Disease of the Airways†*

1. Isoelectric P waves in lead I or right-axis deviation of the P vector
2. P-pulmonale pattern (an increase in P-wave amplitude in II, III, aV_f)
3. Tendency for right-axis deviation of the QRS
4. R/S amplitude ratio in $V_6 < 1$
5. Low-voltage QRS
6. S_1Q_3 or $S_1S_2S_3$ pattern
7. Incomplete (and rarely complete) right bundle branch block
8. R/S amplitude ratio in $V_1 > 1$
9. Marked clockwise rotation of the electrical axis
10. Occasional large Q wave or QS in the inferior or midprecordial leads, suggesting healed myocardial infarction

---

*Any one of the first three criteria suffices to raise suspicion of right ventricular hypertrophy. The diagnosis becomes more certain if two or more of these findings are present (2 and 7). The last four criteria commonly occur in cor pulmonale secondary to primary alveolar hypoventilation interstitial disease of the lung, or pulmonary vascular disease.

†The first seven criteria are suggestive but nonspecific; the last three are more characteristic of cor pulmonale in obstructive disease of the airways.

Reproduced with permission from Holford, F. D.: The electrocardiogram in lung disease. *In* Fishman, A. P. (ed.): Pulmonary Diseases and Disorders. New York, McGraw-Hill, 1980, p. 140.

---

chronic obstructive lung disease.[365,366] The reason is that right ventricular hypertrophy per se is a late manifestation in these syndromes and occurs only after repeated dilatation of the ventricle.[156]

Kilcoyne and associates studied 200 patients with chronic obstructive lung disease and were able to demonstrate that when the arterial oxygen saturation fell below 85 per cent and mean pulmonary pressure was 25 mm Hg or greater, one or more of the following changes would develop in the electrocardiogram: (1) a rightward shift of the mean QRS axis of 30 degrees or more from its previous position; (2) inverted, biphasic, or flattened T waves in the right precordial leads; (3) depressed ST segments in leads II, III, and aV_f; and (4) incomplete or complete right bundle branch block.[366] With an increase in arterial saturation, these alterations disappeared. The T-wave changes in the right precordial leads and the axis shifts to the right occurred with only modest elevations of pulmonary artery pressure, but if these elevations became more severe, and if recurrences were frequent, then the rightward rotation of the QRS axis and the T-wave changes in the right precordial leads tended to become persistent. If pulmonary function were not improved, true right-axis deviation (a frontal plane axis greater than $+90$ degrees) and increased R-wave voltage in the right precordial leads developed. Once the latter occurred, the electrocardiogram was less likely to mirror any physiological variability, as reversion of the increased voltage to normal rarely occurred after improvement in arterial blood gases.

Other studies have suggested that clockwise rotation, right-axis deviation, a qR pattern in aV_r, and electrocardiographic evidence of right atrial enlargement, in that order, would also point to right ventricular hypertrophy in patients with chronic cor pulmonale (Chap. 7).[367] Occasionally in chronic obstructive lung disease the mean QRS axis may be directed posteriorly, superiorly, and to the right so that there is apparent left-axis deviation in the standard limb leads.[368] This pattern, along with low voltage, is most often associated with emphysema.[369]

Electrocardiographic features of prognostic importance in severe chronic bronchial obstruction have been outlined by Kok-Jensen.[370] In a study of 288 patients, survival was found to be very poor in patients with a QRS axis of $+90$ to $+180$ degrees and an amplitude of the P wave in lead II of 0.20 mV or more; only 37 and 42 per cent, respectively, of the patients with these changes were alive after 4 years.

References

1. Chronic cor pulmonale: Report of an expert committee. Wld. Hlth. Org. Tech. Rep. Ser. *213*:1, 1961.
2. McGinn, S., and White, P. D.: Acute cor pulmonale resulting from pulmonary embolism, J.A.M.A. *104*:1473, 1935.
3. Lewis, T.: Observations upon ventricular hypertrophy with especial reference to preponderance of one or other chamber. Heart *5*:367, 1914.
4. Emery, J. L., and Mithal, A.: Weight of cardiac ventricles at and after birth. Br. Heart J. *23*:313, 1961.
5. Keen, E. N.: The post-natal development of the human cardiac ventricles. J. Anat. *89*:484, 1955.
6. Arias-Stella, J., and Recavarren, S.: Right ventricular hypertrophy in native children living at high altitude. Am. J. Pathol. *41*:55, 1962.
7. Mathew, R., Thilenius, O. G., and Arcilla, R. A.: Comparative response of right and left ventricles to volume overload. Am. J. Cardiol. *38*:239, 1976.
8. Recavarren, S., and Arias-Stella, J.: Right ventricular hypertrophy in people born and living at high altitudes. Br. Heart J. *26*:806, 1964.
9. Penaloza, D., Sime, F., Banchero, N., Gamboa, R., Cruz, J., and Martico-

Rena, E.: Pulmonary hypertension in healthy men born and living at high altitudes. Am. J. Cardiol. *11*:150, 1963.

10. Fulton, R. M., Hutchinson, E. C., and Jones, A. M.: Ventricular weight in cardiac hypertrophy. Br. Heart J. *14*:413, 1952.

11. Mitchell, R. S., Stanford, R. E., Silvers, G. W., and Dart, G.: The right ventricle in chronic airway obstruction: A clinicopathologic study. Am. Rev. Respir. Dis. *114*:147, 1976.

12. Ishikawa, S., Fattal, G. A., Popiewicz, J., and Wyatt, J. P.: Functional morphometry of myocardial fibers in cor pulmonale. Am. Rev. Respir. Dis. *105*:358, 1972.

13. Brecher, G. A., and Galletti, P. M.: Functional anatomy of cardiac pumping. *In* Hamilton, A. F., and Dow, P. (eds.): Handbook of Physiology; Circulation. Vol. II. Washington, D.C., American Physiological Society, 1963, p. 759.

14. Laks, M. M., Garner, D., and Swan, H. J. C.: Volumes and compliances measured simultaneously in the right and left ventricles of the dog. Circ. Res. *20*:565, 1967.

15. Abel, F. L., and Waldhausen, J. A.: Effects of alterations in pulmonary vascular resistance on right ventricular function. J. Thorac. Cardiovasc. Surg. *54*:886, 1967.

16. Abel, F. L.: Effects of alterations in peripheral resistance on left ventricular function. Proc. Soc. Exp. Biol. Med. *120*:52, 1965.

17. de V. Cotten, M., and Maling, H. M.: Relationships among stroke work, contractile force and fiber length during changes in ventricular function. Am. J. Physiol. *189*:580, 1957.

18. Sarnoff, S. J., and Berglund, E.: Ventricular function. I. Starling's law of the heart studied by means of simultaneous right and left ventricular function curves in the dog. Circulation *9*:706, 1954.

19. Spann, J. R., Buccino, R. A., Sonnenblick, E. H., and Braunwald, E. B.: Contractile state of cardiac muscle obtained from cats with experimentally produced ventricular hypertrophy and heart failure. Circ. Res. *21*:341, 1967.

20. Haggart, G. E., and Walker, A. M.: The physiology of pulmonary embolism as disclosed by quantitative occlusion of the pulmonary artery. Arch. Surg. *6*:764, 1923.

21. Gibbond, J. H., Hopkinson, M., and Churchill, E. D.: Changes in the circulation produced by gradual occlusion of the pulmonary artery. J. Clin. Invest. *11*:543, 1932.

22. Fineberg, M. H., and Wiggens, C. J.: Compensation and failure of the right ventricle. Am. Heart J. *11*:255, 1936.

23. Brooks, H., Kirk, E. S., Vokonas, P. S., Urschel, C. W., and Sonnenblick, E. H.: Performance of the right ventricle under stress: Relation to right coronary flow. J. Clin. Invest. *50*:2176, 1971.

24. Krahl, V. E.: Anatomy of the mammalian lung. *In* Fenn, O. W., and Rahn, H. (eds.): Handbook of Physiology; Respiration. Vol. I. Washington, D.C., American Physiological Society, 1964, p. 224.

25. Hislop, A., and Reid, L.: Intrapulmonary arterial development during fetal life—branching pattern and structure. J. Anat. *113*:35, 1972.

26. Davies, G. M., and Reid, L.: Growth of the alveoli and pulmonary arteries in childhood. Thorax *25*:669, 1970.

27. Boyden, E. A., and Tompsett, D. H.: The changing patterns in the developing lungs of infants. Acta Anat. *61*:164, 1965.

28. Elliott, F. M., and Reid, L.: Some new facts about the pulmonary artery and its branching pattern. Clin. Radiol. *16*:193, 1965.

29. Hislop, A., and Reid, L.: Pulmonary arterial development during childhood; Branching pattern and structure. Thorax *28*:129, 1973.

30. Reid, L.: Morphology of pulmonary circulation in health and disease. Kongr. Ber. Wiss. Tag. Norddtsch. Lung. Bronchialhk. *14*:333, 1975.

31. Fishman, A. P.: Regulation of the pulmonary circulation. *In* Fishman, A. P. (ed.): Pulmonary Diseases and Disorders. New York, McGraw-Hill Book Co., 1980, p. 397.

32. Staub, N. C., and Storey, W. F.: Relation between morphological and physiological events in lung using rapid freezing. J. Appl. Physiol. *17*:381, 1962.

33. von Euler, U. S., and Liljestrand, G.: Observations on the pulmonary arterial blood pressure in the cat. Acta Physiol. Scand. *12*:301, 1946.

34. Barr, L.: Smooth muscle as an electrical syncytium. *In* Fishman, A. P., and Hecht, H. H. (eds.): The Pulmonary Circulation and the Interstitial Space. Chicago, University of Chicago Press, 1969, p. 161.

35. Hebb, C.: Motor innervation of the pulmonary blood vessels of mammals. *In* Fishman, A. P., and Hecht, H. H. (eds.): The Pulmonary Circulation and the Interstitial Space. Chicago, University of Chicago Press, 1969, p. 195.

36. Fishman, A. P.: Dynamics of the pulmonary circulation. *In* Hamilton, W. F., and Dow, P. (eds.): Handbook of Physiology; Circulation. Vol. II, Washington, D. C., American Physiological Society, 1963, p. 1667.

37. Bard, P.: The pulmonary circulation and respiratory variations in the systemic circulation. *In* Bard, P. (ed.): Medical Physiology. St. Louis, Mosby, 1961, p. 231.

38. Brofman, B. L., Charms, B. L., Kohn, P. M., Elder, J., Newman, R., and Rizika, M.: Unilateral pulmonary artery occlusion in man. Control Studies. J. Thorac. Surg. *34*:206, 1957.

39. Guyton, A. C.: Circulatory Physiology: Cardiac Output and Its Regulation, Philadelphia, W. B. Saunders Co., 1963.

40. Maseri, A., Caldini, P., Howard, P., Joshi, R. C., Permutt, S., and Zierler, K. L.: Determinants of pulmonary vascular volume—recruitment versus distensibility. Circ. Res. *31*:218, 1972.

41. Lanari, A., and Agrest, A.: Pressure-volume relationship in the pulmonary vascular bed. Acta Physiol. Lat. Am. *4*:116, 1954.

42. Caro, C. G.: Extensibility of blood vessels in isolated rabbit lung. J. Physiol. (Lond.) *178*:193, 1965.

43. Howell, J. B. L., Permutt, S., Proctor, D. F., and Riley, R. L.: Effect of inflation of the lung on different parts of the pulmonary vascular bed. J. Appl. Physiol. *16*:71, 1961.

44. Engelberg, J., and DuBois, A. B.: Mechanics of pulmonary circulation in isolated rabbit lungs. Am. J. Physiol. *186*:401, 1959.

45. Maseri, A., Caldini, P., Permutt, S., and Zierler, K. L.: Pressure volume relationship in the pulmonary circulation. *In* Widimsky, J., Daum, S., and Herzog, H. (eds.): Progress in Respiration Research. Vol. 5. Basel, S. Karger, 1970, p. 53.

46. Glazier, J. B., Hughes, J. M. B., Maloney, J. E., and West, J. B.: Measurements of capillary dimensions and blood volume in rapidly frozen lungs. J. Appl. Physiol. *26*:65, 1969.

47. West, J. B.: Ventilation/Blood Flow and Gas Exchange. 2nd ed. Philadelphia, F. A. Davis Co., 1970.

48. West, J. B.: The use of radioactive materials in the study of lung function. *In* Fishman, A. P. (ed.): Pulmonary Diseases and Disorders. New York, McGraw-Hill Book Co., 1980, p. 378.

49. West, J. B., Dollery, C. T., and Nelmark, A.: Distribution of blood flow in isolated lungs: Relation to vascular and alveolar pressures. J. Appl. Physiol. *19*:713, 1964.

50. West, J. B., and Dollery, C. T.: Distribution of blood flow and the pressure-flow relations of the whole lung. J. Appl. Physiol. *20*:175, 1965.

51. Permutt, S., and Riley, R. L.: Hemodynamics of collapsible vessels with tone: The vascular waterfall. J. Appl. Physiol. *18*:924, 1963.

52. West, J. B., and Dollery, C. T.: Distribution of blood flow and ventilation-perfusion ratio in the lung, measured with radioactive CO_2. J. Appl. Physiol. *15*:405, 1960.

53. Hughes, J. M. B., Glazier, J. B., Maloney, J. E., and West, J. B.: Effect of interstitial pressure on pulmonary blood flow. Lancet *1*:192, 1967.

54. West, J. B., Dollery, C. J., and Heard, B. E.: Increased pulmonary vascular resistance in the dependent zone of the isolated dog lung caused by perivascular edema. Circ. Res. *17*:191, 1965.

55. Kaneko, K., Milic-Emili, J., Dolovich, M. B., Dawson, A., and Bates, D. V.: Regional distribution of ventilation and perfusion as a function of body position. J. Appl. Physiol. *16*:465, 1961.

56. Milic-Emili, J., Henderson, J. A. M., Dolovich, M. B., Trop, D., and Kaneko, K.: Regional distribution of inspired gas in the lung. J. Appl. Physiol. *21*:749, 1966.

57. Klocke, R. A.: Intrapulmonary distribution of air and blood. *In* Fishman, A. P. (ed.): Pulmonary Diseases and Disorders. New York, McGraw-Hill Book Co., 1980, p. 373.

58. LeBlanc, P., Ruff, F., and Milic-Emili, J.: Effect of age and body position on airway closure in man. J. Appl. Physiol. *28*:448, 1970.

59. Craig, D. B., Wahba, W. M., Don, H. F., Coutre, J. G., and Becklake, M. R.: Closing volume and its relationship to gas exchange in seated and supine position. J. Appl. Physiol. *31*:717, 1971.

60. Farhi, L. E.: Ventilation-perfusion relationship and its role in alveolar gas exchange. *In* Caro, C. (ed.): Recent Advances in Respiratory Physiology. London, W. H. Arnold, 1965.

61. Rahn, H., and Farhi, L. E.: Ventilation, perfusion, and gas exchange—the $\overset{\bullet}{V}$a/Q concept. *In* Fenn, W. O., and Rahn, H. (eds.): Handbook of Physiology: Respiration. Vol. 1. Washington, D.C., American Physiological Society, 1964, p. 735.

62. West, J. B.: Ventilation-perfusion inequality and overall gas exchange in computer models of the lung. Respir. Physiol. *7*:88, 1969.

63. Lenfant, C.: Measurements of ventilation-perfusion distribution with alveolar-arterial differences. J. Appl. Physiol. *18*:1090, 1963.

64. Filley, G. F., Gregorie, F., and Wright, G. W.: Alveolar and arterial oxygen tensions and the significance of the alveolar-arterial oxygen tension differences in normal man. J. Clin. Invest. *33*:517, 1954.

65. Raine, J. M., and Bishop, J. M.: A-a difference in O_2 tension and physiologic dead space in normal man. J. Appl. Physiol. *18*:284, 1963.

66. Severinghaus, J. W., and Stupfel, M.: Alveolar dead space as an index of distribution of blood flow in pulmonary capillaries. J. Appl. Physiol. *10*:335, 1957.

67. Fishman, A. P.: Respiratory gases in the regulation of the pulmonary circulation. Physiol. Rev. *41*:214, 1961.

68. Fishman, A. P.: Hypoxia and its effects on the pulmonary circulation. Circ. Res. *38*:221, 1976.

69. Bergofsky, E. H.: Mechanisms underlying vasomotor regulation of regional pulmonary blood flow in normal and disease states. Am. J. Med. *57*:378, 1974.

70. Swenson, E. W., Finley, T. N., and Guzman, S. V.: Unilateral hypoventilation in man during temporary occlusion of one pulmonary artery. J. Clin. Invest. *40*:828, 1961.

71. Austrian, R., McClement, J. H., Renzetti, A. D., Jr., Donald, K. W., Riley, R. L., and Cournand, A.: Clinical and physiologic features of some types of pulmonary diseases with impairment of alveolar-capillary diffusion. The syndrome of "alveolar-capillary block." Am. J. Med. *11*:667, 1951.

72. Bates, D. V., Macklem, P. T., and Christie, R. V.: Respiratory Function in Disease, 2nd Ed. Philadelphia, W. B. Saunders Co., 1971, p. 75.

73. Engel, L. A., and Macklem, P. T.: Gas mixing and distribution in the lung. *In* Widdicombe, J. G. (ed.): Respiratory Physiology II. International Review of Physiology, Vol. 14. Baltimore, University Park Press, 1977, p. 37.

74. Rahn, H., and Fenn, W. O.: A Graphical Analysis of the Respiratory Gas Exchange. Washington, D.C., American Physiological Society, 1962.

75. Sykes, M. K., McNicol, M. W., and Campbell, E. J. M.: Respiratory Failure. Oxford, Blackwell Scientific Publications, 1971, p. 56ff.

76. Fishman, A. P.: Cor pulmonale. Am. Rev. Respir. Dis. *114*:775, 1976.

77. Fowler, K. T., and Read, J.: Effect of alveolar hypoxia on zonal distribution of pulmonary blood flow. J. Appl. Physiol. *18*:244, 1963.

78. Lindsay, D. A., and Reed, J.: Pulmonary vascular responsiveness in the prognosis of chronic obstructive lung disease. Am. Rev. Respir. Dis. *105*:242, 1972.

79. Enson, Y., Guintini, C., Lewis, M. L., Morris, T. Q., Ferrer, I. M., and Harvey, R. M.: The influence of hydrogen ion concentration and hypoxia on the pulmonary circulation. J. Clin. Invest. *43*:1146, 1964.

80. Bergofsky, E. H., Haas, F., and Procelli, R. J.: Determination of the sensitive vascular sites from which hypoxia and hypercapnia elicit rises in pulmonary arterial pressure. Fed. Proc. *27*:1420, 1968.

81. Aviado, D. M.: The Lung Circulation. Vol. 1. London, Pergamon Press, 1965.

PULMONARY THROMBOEMBOLISM

82. Bell, W. R., and Simon, T. L.: Current status of pulmonary thromboembolic disease: Pathophysiology, diagnosis, prevention, and treatment. Am. Heart J. *103*:239, 1982.

83. Parker, B. M., and Smith, J. R.: Pulmonary embolism and infarction: Review of physiologic consequences of pulmonary arterial obstruction. Am. J. Med. *24*:402, 1958.

84. Allison, P. R., Dunnill, M. S., and Marshall, R.: Pulmonary embolism. Thorax *15*:273, 1960.

85. Moran, T.: Autopsy incidence of pulmonary embolism in coronary heart disease. Ann. Intern. Med. *32*:949, 1956.

86. Freiman, D. G., Suyemoto, J., and Wessler, S.: Frequency of pulmonary thromboembolism in man. N. Engl. J. Med. *272*:1278, 1965.

87. Dexter, L., and Dalen, J. E.: Pulmonary embolism and acute cor pulmonale. *In* Hurst, J. W. (ed.): The Heart. 4th ed. New York, McGraw-Hill Book Co., 1974, p. 1472.

88. Poe, N. D., Dore, E. K., Swanson, L. A., and Taplin, G. V.: Fatal pulmonary embolism. J. Nucl. Med. *10*:28, 1969.

89. Israel, H. L., and Goldstein, F.: The varied clinical manifestations of pulmonary embolism. Ann. Intern. Med. *47*:202, 1957.

90. McIntyre, K. M., and Levine, H. J.: Cardiac arrest and resuscitation. *In* Spitzer, S., Oaks, W. W., and Moyer, J. (eds.): Emergency Medical Management. New York, Grune and Stratton, 1971, p. 4.

91. Robin, E. D.: Overdiagnosis and overtreatment of pulmonary embolism: The Emperor may have no clothes. Ann. Intern. Med. *87*:775, 1977.

92. Fishman, A. P.: Pulmonary thromboembolism. Pathophysiology and clinical features. *In* Fishman, A. P. (ed.): Pulmonary Diseases and Disorders. New York, McGraw-Hill Book Co., 1980, p. 809.

93. Sevitt, S.: Venous thrombosis and pulmonary embolism. Am. J. Med. *33*:703, 1962.

94. Byrne, J. J., and O'Neil, E. E.: Fatal pulmonary emboli: A study of 130 autopsy proven fatal emboli. Am. J. Surg. *83*:47, 1952.

95. Kistner, R. L., Ball, J. J., Nordyke, R. A., and Freedman, G. G.: Incidence of pulmonary embolism in the course of thrombophlebitis of the lower extremities. Am. J. Surg. *124*:169, 1972.

96. Sharma, G. V. R. K., O'Connell, D. C., Wheeler, H. B., Belko, J. S., and Sasahara, A. A.: Deep venous thrombosis as a diagnosis clue to pulmonary embolism. Am. J. Cardiol. *33*:170, 1974.

97. Young, A. E., Henderson, B. A., Phillips, D. A., and Couch, N. P.: Impedance plethysmography: Its limitations as a substitute for phlebography. Cardiovasc. Radiol. *1*:233, 1978.

98. Havig, O.: Deep vein thrombosis and pulmonary embolism. Acta Chir. Scand. (Suppl.) *478*:1, 1977.

99. Moser, K. M., and LeMoine, J. R.: Is embolic risk conditioned by location of deep venous thrombosis? Ann. Intern. Med. *94*:439, 1981.

100. Rosenburg, R. D.: Hypercoagulability and Methods for Monitoring Anticoagulant Therapy. Washington, D.C., U.S. Department of Health, Education and Welfare, Publication No. (NIH) 76-866, 1976.

101. Kakkar, V. V., and Corrigan, T. P.: Detection of deep venous thrombosis: Survey and current states. Progn. Cardiovasc. Dis. *17*:207, 1974.

102. O'Brien, J. R.: Detection of thrombosis with ^{125}iodine-fibrinogen. Lancet *2*:396, 1970.

103. Moser, K. M., Branch, B. B., and Dolan, G. F.: Comparison of venography, impedance plethysmography and radiolabelled fibrinogen in clinically suspected deep venous thrombosis of the lower extremities. J.A.M.A. *237*:2195, 1977.

104. Falicov, R. E., Resnekov, L., and Petasnick, J.: Progressive pulmonary vascular obstruction and cor pulmonale due to repeated embolism from axillary vein thrombosis. Ann. Intern. Med. *73*:429, 1970.

105. Pollak, V. E., Kark, R. M., Pirani, C. L., Shafter, H. A., and Muehrcke, R. C.: Renal vein thrombosis and the nephrotic syndrome. Am. J. Med. *21*:496, 1956.

106. Senior, R. M., Britton, R. C., Turino, G. M., Wood, J. A., Langer, G. A., and Fishman, A. P.: Pulmonary hypertension associated with cirrhosis of the liver and with portacaval shunts. Circulation *38*:88, 1968.

107. Peterson, E. P., and Taylor, H. B.: Amniotic fluid embolism: An analysis of 40 cases. Obstet. Gynecol. *35*:787, 1970.

108. Rogel, S., Rosenmann, E., and Rachmilewitz, E. A.: Multiple pulmonary infarctions caused by bone marrow emboli. N. Engl. J. Med. *272*:732, 1965.

109. Dines, D. D., Linscheid, R. L., and Didier, E. P.: Fat embolism syndrome. Mayo Clin. Proc. *47*:237, 1972.

110. Deal, C. W., Fielden, B. P., and Monk, I.: Hemodynamic effects of pulmonary air embolism. J. Surg. Res. *11*:533, 1971.

111. Winterbauer, R. H., Elfenbein, I. B., and Ball, W. C., Jr.: Incidence and clinical significance of tumor embolization to the lungs. Am. J. Med. *45*:271, 1968.

112. Ingram, R. H., Jr.: Cor pulmonale with diseases affecting the pulmonary circulation. *In* Practice of Medicine. Vol. 6. Hagerstown, Md., Harper Medical, Harper and Row, 1971, p. 2.

113. Fineberg, M. H., and Wiggers, C. J.: Compensation and failure of the right ventricle. Am. Heart J. *11*:255, 1936.

114. Haggart, G. E., and Walker, A. M.: The physiology of pulmonary embolism as disclosed by quantitative occlusion of the pulmonary artery. Arch. Surg. *6*:764, 1923.

115. Gibbon, J. H., Hopkins, M., and Churchill, E. D.: Changes in the circulation produced by gradual occlusion of the pulmonary artery. J. Clin. Invest. *11*:543, 1932.

116. Hyland, J. W., Smith, G. T., McGuire, L. B., Harrison, D. C., Haynes, F. W., and Dexter, L.: Effect of selective embolization of various sized pulmonary arteries in dogs. Am. J. Physiol. *204*:619, 1963.

117. McIntyre, K. M., and Sasahara, A. A.: Hemodynamic response to pulmonary embolism in patients free of prior cardiopulmonary disease. Am. J. Cardiol. *28*:228, 1971.

118. McIntyre, K. M., Sasahara, A. A., and Sharma, G. V.: Pulmonary thromboembolism: Current concepts. Adv. Intern. Med. *18*:199, 1972.

119. Brandfonbrenner, M., Turino, G. M., Himmelstein, A., and Fishman, A. P.: Effects of occlusion of one pulmonary artery on pulmonary circulation in man. Fed. Proc. *17*:19, 1958.

120. McDonald, I. G., Hirsh, J., Hale, G. S., and O'Sullivan, E. F.: Major pulmonary embolism; A correlation of clinical findings, hemodynamics, pulmonary angiography, and pathological physiology. Br. Heart J. *34*:356, 1972.

121. Bell, W. R., Simon, T. L., and DeMets, D. L.: The clinical features of submassive and massive pulmonary emboli. Am. J. Med. *62*:355, 1977.

122. Stein, P. D., Willis, P. W., and DeMets, D. L.: History and physical examination in acute pulmonary embolism in patients without preexisting cardiac or pulmonary disease. Am. J. Cardiol. *47*:218, 1981.

123. Miller, G. A. H., and Sutton, G. C.: Acute massive pulmonary embolism. Clinical and haemodynamic findings in 23 patients studied by cardiac catheterization and pulmonary arteriography. Br. Heart J. *32*:518, 1970.

124. National Cooperative Study: The urokinase-pulmonary embolism trial. Circulation *47*(Suppl. II):1, 1973.

125. Halmagyi, D. F., Starzecki, B., and Horner, G. J.: Humoral transmission of cardiorespiratory changes in experimental lung embolism. Circ. Res. *14*:546, 1964.

126. Bo, G., Hognestad, J., and Vaage, J.: The role of blood platelets in pulmonary responses in microembolization with barium sulfate. Acta Physiol. Scand. *90*:244, 1974.

127. Nadel, J. A., Colebatch, H. J. H., and Olsen, C. R.: Location and mechanism of airway constriction after barium sulfate microembolism. J. Appl. Physiol. *19*:387, 1964.

128. Bo, G., and Hognestad, J.: Effects on the pulmonary circulation of suddenly induced intravascular aggregation of blood platelets. Acta Physiol. Scand. *85*:523, 1972.

129. Swendenborg, J.: Thrombin-induced vasoconstriction in the pulmonary circulation. Scand. J. Clin. Lab. Invest. *27*:321, 1971.

130. Stein, M., and Thomas, D. P.: Role of platelets in the acute pulmonary responses to endotoxin. J. Appl. Physiol. *23*:47, 1967.

131. Vaage, J.: Vagal reflexes in the bronchoconstriction occurring after induced intravascular platelet aggregation. Acta Physiol. Scand. *97*:94, 1976.

132. Thomas, D. P., Gurewich, V., and Ashford, T. P.: Platelet adherence to thromboemboli in relation to the pathogenesis and treatment of pulmonary embolism. N. Engl. J. Med. *274*:953, 1966.

133. Wessler, S., Reiner, L., Freiman, D. G., Reimer, S. M., and Lertzman, M.: Serum-induced thrombosis: Studies of its induction and evolution under controlled conditions *in vivo*. Circulation *20*:864, 1959.

134. Thomas, D., Stein, M., Tanabe, G., Rege, V., and Wessler, S.: Mechanism of bronchoconstriction produced by thromboemboli in dogs. Am. J. Physiol. *206*:1207, 1964.

135. Rosoff, C. B., Salzman, E. M., and Gurewich, V.: Reduction of the platelet serotonin and the response to pulmonary emboli. Surgery *70*:12, 1971.

136. Clarke, S. W., Graf, P. D., and Nadel, J. A.: *In vivo* visualization of small airway constriction after pulmonary microembolism in cats and dogs. J. Appl. Physiol. *29*:646, 1970.

137. Von Hayek, H.: The Human Lung. New York, Hafner, 1960.

138. Nadel, J. A.: Mechanisms of airway response to inhaled substances. Arch. Environ. Health *16*:171, 1968.

139. Dalen, J. E., Banas, J. S., Brooks, H. L., Evans, G. L., Paraskos, J. A., and Dexter, L.: Resolution rate of acute pulmonary embolism in man. N. Engl. J. Med. *280*:1194, 1969.

140. Tibbutt, D. A., Davies, J. A., Anderson, J. A., Fletcher, E. W. L., Hamill, J., Holt, J. M., Thomas, M. L., Lee, G. D. J., Miller, G. A. H., Sharp, A. A., and Sutton, G. C.: Compression by controlled clinical trial of streptokinase and heparin in the treatment of life-threatening pulmonary embolism. Br. Med. J. *1*:343, 1974.

141. Szucs, M. M., Brooks, H. L., Grossman, W., Banas, J. S., Meister, S. G., Dexter, L., and Dalen, J. E.: Diagnostic sensitivity of laboratory findings in acute pulmonary embolism. Ann. Intern. Med. *74*:161, 1971.

142. Stein, P. D., Alshabkhoun, S., Hawkins, H. F., Hyland, J. W., and Jarret, C. E.: Right coronary blood flow in acute pulmonary embolism. Am. Heart J. 77:356, 1969.

143. Vatner, S. F., and Van Citters, R. L.: Effects of acute pulmonary embolism on coronary dynamics in the conscious dog. Am. Heart J. 83:50, 1972.

144. Symbas, P., and Bonanno, J. A.: Coronary blood flow in acute experimental pulmonary embolization. J. Surg. Res. 10:377, 1970.

145. Stein, P. D., Alshabkhoun, S., Hatem, C., Pur-Shahriari, A. A., Haynes, W., Harken, D. E., and Dexter, L.: Coronary artery blood flow in acute pulmonary embolism. Am. J. Cardiol. 21:32, 1968.

146. Dexter, L.: Clinical aspects of pulmonary embolism and their relation to pathophysiology. Bull. Physio-Pathol. Respir. 6:21, 1970.

147. Romhitt, D. W., Holmes, J. C., and Fowler, N. O.: Mimicry in pulmonary embolism. Geriatrics 27:73, 1972.

148. Potts, D. E., and Sahn, S. A.: Abdominal manifestations of pulmonary embolism. J.A.M.A. 235:2835, 1976.

149. Sasahara, A. A., Cannilla, J. E., Morse, R. L., Sidd, J. J., and Tremblay, G. M.: Clinical and physiologic studies in pulmonary thromboembolism. Am. J. Cardiol. 20:10, 1967.

150. Windebank, W. J., Boyd, G., and Moran, F.: Pulmonary thromboembolism presenting as asthma. Br. Med. J.: 1:90, 1973.

151. Webster, J. R., Saadeh, G. B., Eggum, P. R., and Suker, J. R.: Wheezing due to pulmonary embolism. Treatment with heparin. N. Engl. J. Med. 274:931, 1966.

152. Olazabal, F., Roman-Irizarry, L. A., Oms, J. D., Conde, L., and Marchand, E. J.: Pulmonary emboli masquerading as asthma. N. Engl. J. Med. 278:999, 1968.

153. Shaw, R. A., Schonfeld, S. A., and Whitcomb, M. E.: Pulmonary embolism presenting as coronary insufficiency. Arch. Intern. Med. 141:651, 1981.

154. McIntyre, K. M., Sasahara, A. A., and Littman, D.: Relation of the electrocardiogram to hemodynamic alterations in pulmonary embolism. Am. J. Cardiol. 30:205, 1972.

155. Webber, D. M., and Phillips, J. H.: A re-evaluation of electrocardiographic changes accompanying acute pulmonary embolism. J. Med. Sci. 251:381, 1966.

156. Holford, F. D.: The electrocardiogram in lung diseases. In Fishman, A. P. (ed.): Pulmonary Diseases and Disorders. New York, McGraw-Hill Book Co., 1980, p. 139.

157. Levy, S. E., Stein, M., Totten, R. S., Bruderman, I., Wessler, S., and Robin, E. D.: Ventilation perfusion abnormalities in experimental pulmonary embolism. J. Clin. Invest. 44:1699, 1965.

158. Julian, D. G., Travis, D. M., Robin, E. D., and Crump, C. H.: Effect of pulmonary artery occlusion upon end-tidal CO_2 tension. J. Appl. Physiol. 15:87, 1960.

159. Fisher, S. R., Duranceau, A., Floyd, R. D., and Wolfe, W. G.: Comparative changes in ventilatory dead space following micro and massive pulmonary emboli. J. Surg. Res. 20:195, 1976.

160. Levy, S. E., and Simmons, D. H.: Redistribution of alveolar ventilation following pulmonary thromboembolism in the dog. J. Appl. Physiol. 36:60, 1974.

161. Levy, S. E., and Simmons, D. H.: Mechanism of arterial hypoxemia following pulmonary thromboembolism in dogs. J. Appl. Physiol. 39:41, 1975.

162. Colp, C. R., and Williams, M. H., Jr.: Pulmonary functions following pulmonary embolization. Am. Rev. Respir. Dis. 85:799, 1962.

163. Robin, E. D., Forkner, C. E., Bromberg, P. A., Croteau, J. R., and Travis, D. M.: Alveolar gas exchange in clinical pulmonary embolism. N. Engl. J. Med. 262:283, 1960.

164. Robin, E. D., Julian, D. G., Travis, D. M., and Crump, C. H.: A physiologic approach to the diagnosis of acute pulmonary embolism. N. Engl. J. Med. 260:586, 1959.

165. Bass, H., Heckscher, T., and Anthonisen, N. R.: Regional pulmonary gas exchange in patients with pulmonary embolism. Clin. Sci. 33:355, 1967.

166. Stanek, V., Widimsky, J., and Jebavy, P.: Respiratory function in recurrent pulmonary embolism. Respiration 30:223, 1973.

167. Daum, S.: The diffusing capacity of the lungs in pulmonary embolism. Respiration 26:8, 1969.

168. Wilson, J. E., III, Pierce, A. K., Johnson, R. L., Jr., Winga, E. R., Harrell, W. R., Curry, G. C., and Mullins, C. B.: Hypoxemia in pulmonary embolism, a clinical study. J. Clin. Invest. 50:481, 1971.

169. Morgan, T. E., and Edmunds, L. H., Jr.: Pulmonary artery occlusion. III. Biochemical alterations. J. Appl. Physiol. 22:1012, 1967.

170. Kafer, E. R.: Respiratory function in pulmonary thromboembolic disease. Am. J. Med. 47:904, 1969.

171. Jones, N. L., and Goodwin, J. F.: Respiratory function in pulmonary thromboembolic disorders. Br. Med. J. 1:1089, 1965.

172. Nadel, J. A., Gold, W. M., and Burgess, S. H.: Early diagnosis of chronic pulmonary vascular obstruction. Value of pulmonary function tests. Am. J. Med. 44:16, 1968.

173. Williams, J. R., and Wilcox, W. C.: Pulmonary embolism: Roentgenographic and angiographic considerations. Am. J. Roentgenol. 89:333, 1963.

174. Figley, M. M., Gerdes, A. J., and Ricketts, H. J.: Radiographic aspects of pulmonary embolism. Semin. Roentgenol. 2:389, 1967.

175. Fleischner, F. G.: Roentgenology of the pulmonary infarct. Semin. Roentgenol. 2:61, 1967.

176. Lamas, R., and Swenson, E. W.: Diagnostic clues in pulmonary thromboembolism evaluated by angiographic and ventilation blood flow studies. Thorax 20:327, 1965.

177. Weiner, S. N., Edelstein, J., and Charms, B. L.: Observations on pulmonary embolism and the pulmonary angiogram. Am. J. Roentgenol. 98:859, 1966.

178. Fleischner, F. G.: Unilateral pulmonary embolism with increased compensatory circulation through the unoccluded lung: Roentgen observations. Radiology 73:591, 1959.

179. Fleischner, F. G.: Pulmonary embolism. Clin. Radiol. 13:169, 1962.

180. Chrispin, A. R., Goodwin, J. F., and Steiner, R.: The radiology of obliterative pulmonary hypertension and thromboembolism. Br. J. Radiol. 36:705, 1963.

181. Teplick, J. G., Haskin, M. E., and Steinberg, S. B.: Changes in the main pulmonary artery segment following pulmonary embolism. Am. J. Roentgenol. 92:557, 1964.

182. Smith, G. T., Dammin, G. J., and Dexter, L.: Postmortem arteriographic studies of the human lung in pulmonary embolization. J.A.M.A. 188:143, 1964.

183. Dalen, J. E., Haffajee, C. I., Alpert, J. S., Howe, J. P., III, Ockene, I. S., and Paraskos, J. A.: Pulmonary embolism, pulmonary hemorrhage, and pulmonary infarction. N. Engl. J. Med. 296:1431, 1977.

184. Tsao, M. S., Schraufnagel, D., and Wang, N.-S.: Pathogenesis of pulmonary Infarction. Am. J. Med. 72:599, 1982.

185. Ellis, F. H., Jr., Grindlay, J. H., and Edwards, J. E.: The bronchial arteries. II. Their role in pulmonary embolism and infarction. Surgery 31:167, 1952.

186. Stein, G. N., Chen, J. T., Goldstein, F., Israel, H. L., and Finkelstein, A.: The importance of chest roentgenography in the diagnosis of pulmonary embolism. Am. J. Roentgenol. 81:255, 1959.

187. Castleman, B.: Pathologic observations on pulmonary infarction in man. In Sasahara, A. A., and Stein, M. (eds.): Pulmonary Embolic Disease. New York, Grune and Stratton, 1965, p. 86.

188. Vidal, E., LeVeen, H. H., Yarnoz, M., and Piccone, V. A., Jr.: Lung abscess secondary to pulmonary infarction. Ann. Thorac. Surg. 6:557, 1971.

189. Scharf, J., Nahair, A. M., Munk, J., and Lichtig, C.: Aseptic cavitation in pulmonary infarction. Chest 59:456, 1971.

190. Levin, L., and Kernohan, J. W.: Pulmonary abscess secondary to bland pulmonary infarction. Dis. Chest. 14:218, 1948.

191. Chester, E. M., and Krause, G. R.: Lung abscess secondary to aseptic pulmonary infarction. Radiology 39:647, 1942.

192. McFadden, E. R., Jr., and Luparello, F.: Bronchopleural fistula complicating massive pulmonary infarction. Thorax 24:500, 1969.

193. Fraser, R. G., and Paré, J. A. P.: Diagnosis of Diseases of the Chest. Vol. 2. Philadelphia, W. B. Saunders Co., 1970.

194. McNeil, B. J.: A diagnostic strategy using ventilation-perfusion studies in patients suspect for pulmonary embolism. J. Nucl. Med. 17:613, 1976.

195. Wagner, H. N., Jr., Sabiston, D. C., Jr., McAfee, J. G., Tow, D. E., and Stern, H. S.: Diagnosis of massive pulmonary embolism in man by radioisotope scanning. N. Engl. J. Med. 271:377, 1964.

196. Gilday, D. L., Poulouse, K. P., and Deland, F. H.: Accuracy of detection of pulmonary embolism by lung scanning correlated with pulmonary angiography. Am. J. Roentgenol. Radium Ther. Nucl. Med. 115:732, 1972.

197. McNeil, B. J., Holman, L., and Adelstein, S. J.: The scintigraphic definition of pulmonary embolism. J.A.M.A. 227:753, 1974.

198. Moses, D. C., Silver, T. M., and Bookstein, J. J.: The complementary roles of chest radiography, lung scanning and selective pulmonary angiography in the diagnosis of pulmonary embolism. Circulation 49:179, 1974.

199. Bell, W. R., and Simon, T.: A comparative analysis of pulmonary perfusion scans with pulmonary angiograms. Am. Heart J. 92:700, 1976.

200. DeNardo, C. L., Goodwin, D. A., Ravasini, R., and Dietrich, P. A.: The ventilatory lung scan in the diagnosis of pulmonary embolism. N. Engl. J. Med. 282:1334, 1970.

201. Tow, D. E., and Wagner, H. N., Jr.: Recovery of pulmonary arterial blood flow in patients with pulmonary embolism. N. Engl. J. Med. 276:1053, 1967.

202. Paraskos, J. A., Aldestein, S. J., Smith, R. E., Rickman, F. D., Grossman, W., Dexter, L., and Dalen, J.: Late prognosis of acute pulmonary embolism. N. Engl. J. Med. 289:55, 1973.

203. McNeil, B. J.: A diagnostic strategy using ventilation-perfusion studies in patients suspect for pulmonary embolism. J. Nucl. Med. 17:613, 1976.

204. Cheely, R., McCartney, W. H., Perry, J. R., Delaney, D. J., Bustad, L., Wynia, V. H., and Griggs, T. R.: The role of non-invasive tests versus pulmonary angiography in the diagnosis of pulmonary embolism. Am. J. Med. 70:17, 1981.

205. Moser, K. M., Harsanyi, P., Rius-Garriga, G., Guisan, M., Landis, G. A., and Miale, A.: Assessment of pulmonary photoscanning and angiography in experimental pulmonary embolism. Circulation 39:663, 1969.

206. Isawa, T., Wasserman, K., and Taplin, G. V.: Variability of lung scans following pulmonary embolization. Am. Rev. Respir. Dis. 101:207, 1970.

207. Moser, K. M., Longo, A. M., Ashburn, W. L., and Guisan, M.: Spurious scintiphotographic recurrence of pulmonary emboli. Am. J. Med. 55:434, 1973.

208. Dalen, J. E., Brooks, H. C., Johnson, L. W., Meister, S. G., Szücs, M. M., Jr., and Dexter, L.: Pulmonary angiography in acute pulmonary embolism: Indications, techniques, and results in 367 patients. Am. Heart J. 81:175, 1971.

209. Sasahara, A. A., Stein, M., Simon, M., and Littman, D.: Pulmonary angiography in the diagnosis of thromboembolic disease. N. Engl. J. Med. 270:1075, 1964.

210. Stein, P. D., O'Connor, J. F., Dalen, J. E., Pur-Shahriari, A. A., Hoppin, F. G., Jr., Hammond, D. T., Haynes, F. W., Fleischner, F. G., and Dexter, L.: The angiographic diagnosis of acute pulmonary embolism: Evaluation of criteria. Am. Heart J. 73:730, 1967.

211. Mills, S. R., Jackson, D. C., Older, R. A., Heaston, D. K., and Moore, R. V.: The incidence, etiologies, and avoidance of complications of pulmonary angiography in a large series. Diagn. Radiol. 136:295, 1980.

212. Wacker, W. E., Rosenthal, M., Snodgrass, P. J., and Amador, E.: A triad for the diagnosis of pulmonary embolism and infarction. J.A.M.A. 178:8, 1961.

213. Schonell, M. E., Crompton, G. K., Forshall, J. M., and Whitby, L. G.: Failure to differentiate pulmonary infarction from pneumonia by biochemical tests. Br. Med. J. *1*:1146, 1966.

214. Bynum, L., Crotty, C. M., and Wilson, J. E., III: Diagnostic value of tests of fibrin metabolism in patients predisposed to pulmonary embolism. Arch. Intern. Med. *139*:283, 1979.

215. Moser, K. L.: Pulmonary thromboembolism. *In* Petersdorf, P., et al. (eds.): Harrison's Principles of Internal Medicine. 10th ed. New York, McGraw-Hill Book Co., 1983, p. 1248.

216. Barritt, D. W., and Jordan, S. C.: Anticoagulant drugs in the treatment of pulmonary embolism. A controlled trial. Lancet *1*:1309, 1960.

217. Kernahan, R. J., and Todd, C.: Heparin therapy in thromboembolic disease. Lancet *1*:621, 1966.

218. Colman, R. W.: Prophylaxis and treatment of thromboembolism based on pathophysiology of clotting mechanisms. *In* Fishman, A. P. (ed.): Pulmonary Diseases and Disorders. New York, McGraw-Hill Book Co., 1980, p. 827.

219. Deykin, D.: Current status of anticoagulant therapy. Am. J. Med. *72*:659, 1982.

220. Sasahara, A. A.: Therapy for pulmonary embolism. J.A.M.A. *229*:1975, 1974.

221. Glazier, R. L., and Crowell, E. B.: Randomized prospective trial of continuous vs. intermittent heparin therapy. J.A.M.A. *236*:1365, 1976.

222. Salzman, E. W., Deykin, D., Mayer-Shapiro, R., and Rosenberg, R.: Management of heparin therapy: Controlled prospective trial. N. Engl. J. Med. *292*:1046, 1975.

223. Wilson, J. E., Bynum, L. J., and Parkey, R. W.: Heparin therapy in venous thromboembolism. Am. J. Med. *70*:808, 1981.

224. O'Sullivan, E. F.: Duration of anticoagulant therapy in venous thromboembolism. Med. J. Aust. *2*:1104, 1972.

225. Sharma, G. V. R. K., Cella, G., Parisi, A. F., and Sasahara, A. A.: Thrombolytic therapy. N. Engl. J. Med. *306*:1268, 1982.

226. Donaldson, M. C., Wirthlin, L. S., and Donaldson, G. A.: Thirty-year experience with surgical interruption of the inferior vena cava for prevention of pulmonary embolism. Ann. Surg. *191*:367, 1980.

227. Silver, D., and Sabiston, D. C.: The role of vena caval interruption in the management of pulmonary embolism. Surgery *77*:1, 1975.

228. Mobin-Uddin, K., Callard, G. M., Bolooki, H., Rubinson, R., Michie, D., and Jude, J. R.: Transvenous caval interruption with umbrella filter. N. Engl. J. Med. *286*:55, 1972.

229. Gurewich, U., Thomas, D. P., and Rabinov, K. R.: Pulmonary embolism after ligation of the inferior vena cava. N. Engl. J. Med. *274*:1350, 1966.

230. Cooley, D. A., and Beall, A. C.: Embolectomy for acute massive pulmonary embolism. Surg. Gynecol. Obstet. *126*:805, 1968.

231. Warren, R.: The current status of pulmonary embolectomy. *In* Sasahara, A. A., and Stein, M. (eds.): Pulmonary Embolic Disease. New York, Grune and Stratton, 1965, p. 283.

232. Alpert, J. S., Smith, R. E., Ockene, I. S., Askenazi, J., Dexter, L., and Dalen, J. E.: Treatment of massive pulmonary embolism: The role of pulmonary embolectomy. Am. Heart J. *89*:413, 1975.

233. McDonald, I. G., Hirsh, J., Hale, G. S., Cade, J. F., and McCarthy, R. A.: Isoproterenol in massive pulmonary embolism: Hemodynamic and clinical effects. Med. J. Aust. *2*:201, 1968.

234. Miller, R. R., Lies, J. E., Carretta, R. F., Wampold, D. B., DeNardo, G. L., Krans, J. F., Amsterdam, E. A., and Mason, D. T.: Prevention of lower extremity venous thrombosis by early mobilization. Confirmation in patients with acute myocardial infarction by ¹²⁵I-fibrinogen uptake and venography. Ann. Intern. Med. *84*:700, 1976.

235. Sevitt, S., and Gallagher, N. G.: Prevention of venous thrombosis and pulmonary embolism in injured patients. Lancet *2*:981, 1959.

236. Kakkar, U. V., Corrigan, T. P., and Fossard, D. P.: Prevention of fatal postoperative embolism by low dose heparin: An international multicenter trial. Lancet *2*:45, 1975.

237. Wessler, S., and Yin, E. T.: Theory and practice of minidose heparin in surgical patients: A status report. Circulation *47*:671, 1973.

238. Evarts, M., and Alfide, J.: Thromboembolism after total hip reconstruction: Failure of low doses of heparin in prevention. J.A.M.A. *225*:515, 1973.

239. Horowitz, R. E., and Tatter, D.: Lethal pulmonary embolism. *In* Sherry, S., Brinkhous, K. M., and Genton, E. (eds.): Thrombosis. Washington, D.C., National Academy of Sciences, 1961, p. 9.

240. Howe, M., Sevitt, S., and Thomas, D. P.: Venous Thrombosis and Pulmonary Embolism. Cambridge, Harvard University Press, 1970.

241. Donaldson, G. A., Williams, C., Scannell, J. G., and Shaw, R. S.: Reappraisal of application of the Trendelenburg operation to massive fatal embolism. N. Engl. J. Med. *268*:171, 1963.

242. Alpert, J. S., Smith, R., Carlson, J., Ockene, I. S., Dexter, L., and Dalen, J. E.: Mortality in patients treated for pulmonary embolism. J.A.M.A. *236*:1477, 1976.

243. Austin, J. H. M., Wilner, G. D., and Dominguez, C.: Natural history of pulmonary thromboemboli in dogs. Radiology *116*:519, 1975.

CHRONIC COR PULMONATE

244. Fishman, A. P.: Cor pulmonale. *In* Fishman, A. P. (ed.): Pulmonary Diseases and Disorders. New York, McGraw-Hill Book Co., 1980, p. 853.

245. Respiratory Disease. Task force report on prevention, control and education. Washington, D.C., U.S. Department of Health Education and Welfare, Public Health Service, National Institute of Health, 1977, p. 83.

246. Stuart-Harris, C. H., Twidle, R. H. S., and Clifton, M. A.: Hospital study of congestive heart failure with special reference to cor pulmonale. Br. Med. J. *2*:201, 1959.

247. Inter-Society Commission for Heart Disease Resources: Primary prevention of pulmonary heart disease. Circulation *41*:A-17, 1970.

247a. Berbel, L. N., and Miro, R. E.: Pulmonary hypertension in the pathogenesis of cor pulmonale. Cardiovasc. Rev. *4*:359, 1983.

248. Wilhelmsen, L., Selander, S., Sonderholm, B., Paulin, S., Varnauskas, E., and Werko, L.: Recurrent pulmonary embolism. Medicine *42*:335, 1963.

249. Hicken, P., Brewer, D., and Heath, D.: The relationship between the weight of the right ventricle of the heart and the internal surface area and number of alveoli in the human lung in emphysema. J. Pathol. Bacteriol. *92*:529, 1966.

250. Thurlbeck, W. M., Henderson, J. A., Fraser, R. G., and Bates, D. V.: Chronic obstructive lung disease. A comparison between clinical, roentgenologic, functional and morphologic criteria in chronic bronchitis, emphysema, asthma and bronchiectasis. Medicine *48*:81, 1970.

251. Edwards, J. E.: Pathology of chronic pulmonary hypertension. Pathol. Annu. *9*:1, 1974.

252. Wagenvoort, C. A., and Wagenvoort, N.: Hypoxic pulmonary vascular lesions in man at high altitude and in patients with chronic respiratory disease. Pathol. Microbiol. *39*:276, 1973.

253. Semmens, M., and Reid, L.: Pulmonary arterial muscularity and right ventricular hypertrophy in chronic bronchitis and emphysema. Br. J. Dis. Chest. *68*:253, 1974.

254. Oppenheimer, E. H., and Esterly, J. R.: Medial mucoid lesions of the pulmonary artery in cystic fibrosis, pulmonary hypertension, and other disorders. Lab. Invest. *30*:411, 1974.

255. Wagenvoort, C. A., Heath, D., and Edwards, J. E.: The Pathology of the Pulmonary Vasculature. Springfield, Ill., Charles C Thomas, 1964.

256. Clausen, K. P., and Geer, J. C.: Hypertensive pulmonary arteritis. Am. J. Dis. Child. *118*:718, 1969.

257. Roos, A.: Poiseuille's law and its limitation in vascular systems. *In* Grover, R. F. (ed.): Progress in Research in Emphysema and Chronic Bronchitis. Basel, Karger, 1963, p. 32.

258. Wells, R. E., and Merrill, E. W.: Influence of flow properties of blood upon viscosity hematocrit relationships. J. Clin. Invest. *41*:1591, 1962.

259. Saldana, M. A., Harley, R. A., Liebow, A. A., and Carrington, C. B.: Experimental extreme pulmonary hypertension and vascular disease in relation to polycythemia. Am. J. Pathol. *52*:935, 1968.

260. Balchum, O. J., Jung, R. C., Turner, A. F., and Jacobson, G.: Pulmonary artery to vein shunts in obstructive pulmonary disease. Am. J. Med. *43*:178, 1967.

261. Boushy, S. F., North, L. B., and Trice, J. A.: The bronchial arteries in chronic obstructive pulmonary disease. Am. J. Med. *46*:506, 1969.

262. Marcus, J. H., McLean, R. L., Duffell, G. M., and Ingram, R. H.: Exercise performance in relation to the pathophysiologic type of chronic obstructive pulmonary disease. Am. J. Med. *49*:14, 1970.

263. Harris, P., Segal, N., and Bishop, J. M.: The relation between pressure and flow in the pulmonary circulation in normal subjects and in patients with chronic bronchitis and mitral stenosis. Cardiovasc. Res. *2*:73, 1968.

264. Burrows, B., Kettel, L. J., Niden, A. H., Rabinowitz, M., and Diener, C. F.: Patterns of cardiovascular dysfunction in chronic obstructive lung disease. N. Engl. J. Med. *286*:912, 1972.

265. Whitaker, W.: Pulmonary hypertension in congestive heart failure complicating chronic lung disease. Q. J. Med. *23*:57, 1954.

266. Ferrer, M. I.: Disturbances in the circulation in patients with cor pulmonale. Bull. N.Y. Acad. Med. *41*:942, 1965.

267. Williams, J. F., and Behnke, R. H.: The effect of pulmonary emphysema upon cardiopulmonary hemodynamics at rest and during exercise. Ann. Intern. Med. *60*:824, 1964.

268. Emirgil, C., Sobol, B. J., Herbert, W. H., and Trout, K. W.: Routine pulmonary function studies as a key to the status of the lesser circulation in chronic obstructive pulmonary disease. Am. J. Med. *50*:191, 1971.

269. Khaja, F., and Parker, J. D.: Right and left ventricular performance in chronic obstructive lung disease. Am. Heart J. *82*:319, 1971.

270. Berger, H. S., Matthay, R. A., Loke, J., Marshall, R. C., Gottschalk, A., and Zaret, B. L.: Assessment of cardiac performance with quantitative radionuclide angiocardiography: Right ventricular ejection fraction with reference to findings in chronic obstructive pulmonary disease. Am. J. Cardiol. *41*:897, 1978.

271. Olvey, S. K., Redufo, L. A., Stevens, P. M., Deaton, W. J., and Miller, R. R.: First pass radionuclide assessment of right and left ventricular ejection fraction in chronic pulmonary disease. Effect of oxygen upon exercise response. Chest *78*:4, 1980.

272. Stein, P. D., Sabbah, H. N., Anbe, D. T., and Marzilli, M.: Performance of the failing and non-failing right ventricle of patients with pulmonary hypertension. Am. J. Cardiol. *44*:1050, 1979.

272a. Kawakami, Y., Kishi, F., Yamamoto, H., and Miyamoto, K.: Relation of oxygen delivery, mixed venous oxygenation and pulmonary hemodynamics to prognosis in chronic obstructive pulmonary disease. N. Engl. J. Med. *308*:1045, 1983.

272b. Bergofsky, E. H.: Tissue oxygen delivery and cor pulmonale in chronic obstructive pulmonary disease. N. Engl. J. Med. *308*:1092, 1983.

273. Samet, P., Fritts, H. W., Jr., Fishman, A. P., and Cournand, A.: The blood volume in heart disease. Medicine *36*:211, 1957.

274. Turino, G. M., Edelman, N. H., Richards, E. C., and Fishman, A. P.: Extravascular lung water in cor pulmonale. Bull. Physiol. Pathol. Respir. *4*:47, 1968.

275. Chidsey, C. A., Kaiser, G. A., Sonnenblick, E. H., Spann, J. F., and Braun-

PART
IV

HEART DISEASE AND DISEASES OF OTHER ORGAN SYSTEMS

47 GENETICS AND CARDIOVASCULAR DISEASE

by Joseph L. Goldstein, M.D., and Michael S. Brown, M.D.

GENERAL PRINCIPLES OF CARDIOVASCULAR GENETICS

As with diseases affecting other body systems, genetic factors play a significant role in the pathogenesis of most diseases of the heart. In some disorders, such as the Marfan syndrome and familial hypercholesterolemia, the genetic effects are relatively clearly discernible and easy to analyze. In other diseases, such as most forms of congenital heart disease, the role of hereditary factors, although demonstrable, is less clear-cut, and the fundamental genetic mechanisms remain obscure.

In this chapter, we first review the general principles of hereditary disease as they apply to the major forms of heart disease. This is followed by a discussion of those disorders of the cardiovascular system for which a clear-cut genetic etiology has been demonstrated. In discussing a disorder, we have placed the major emphasis on the genet-

ic aspects rather than on the clinical features, which are discussed elsewhere in this book.

MOLECULAR BASIS OF GENE EXPRESSION. All hereditary information is transmitted from parent to offspring through the inheritance of deoxyribonucleic acid (DNA). *DNA* is a linear polymer composed of purine and pyrimidine bases, the sequence of which ultimately determines the sequence of amino acids in every protein molecule made by the body. The four types of bases in DNA are arranged in groups of three, each group forming a code word or codon that signifies a particular amino acid. A *gene* represents the sequence of bases in DNA that codes for the amino acid sequence of a single polypeptide chain of a protein molecule.[1] The gene is the basic unit of heredity that is transmitted to each offspring during the formation of sperm and ova. The recent discovery that genes are not continuous sequences of DNA but consist of coding sequences (exons) interrupted by intervening sequences (introns) has led to a new view of gene expression that is beyond the scope of this chapter (for review, see reference 1).

It is estimated that the amount of DNA in the nucleus of each human cell is sufficient to code for several million genes. The genes are arranged in linear sequence organized into rod-shaped bodies called *chromosomes*. Each human cell contains 46 chromosomes, arranged in 23 pairs, one member of each pair having been derived from each of the individual's parents. Thus, each individual inherits two copies of each chromosome and hence two copies of each gene. The site at which a gene is located on a particular chromosome is termed the *genetic locus*. When a gene occupying a genetic locus exists in two or more different forms, these alternate forms of the gene are referred to as *alleles*.

A given gene always resides at a specified genetic locus on one particular chromosome. For example, the genetic locus for the human Rh blood group is on chromosome No. 1; at this chromosomal site in each individual there are two Rh genes, one on chromosome No. 1 derived from the mother and the other on chromosome No. 1 derived from the father. When both genes at the same genetic locus are identical, the individual is a *homozygote*. When the two genes differ (i.e., two alleles are present at the locus), the individual is a *heterozygote*. Each individual is homozygous at some loci and heterozygous at others.

Considerable progress has been made in recent years in delineating the human gene map. The chromosomal location of more than 350 genes is now known.[2]

MUTATION AS THE ORIGIN OF GENETIC DISEASE. A *mutation* is a stable, heritable alteration in DNA. Although the causes of mutation in human beings are largely unknown, a variety of environmental agents, such as radiation, viruses, and chemicals, are among the factors that are implicated.

Mutations can involve a visible alteration in the structure of a chromosome, such as a deletion or translocation of a portion of a chromosome, or they can involve a minute change in one of the purine or pyrimidine bases of a single gene. Most commonly, such "point" mutations consist of the substitution of one base for another, thus changing the meaning of the codon containing that base; hence, their designation as *missense mutations*. Of all of the human mutations so far elucidated, the vast majority involve such single-base changes. These missense mutations cause the substitution of one amino acid for another in the protein specified by the mutant gene. Such substitution can have little effect on the function of the protein, or it can totally eliminate all function. If the protein that is involved happens to be an enzyme, the loss of function may produce a metabolic disease.

CELLULAR MECHANISM BY WHICH MUTANT GENES PRODUCE DISEASES. Critical to the modern understanding of heredity is the concept that the only information transmitted from generation to generation is the sequence of bases in DNA and that these sequences, in turn, specify only the primary structure of RNA and protein molecules. All other chemical reactions within a cell—such as the synthesis of complex lipids and carbohydrates, the formation of membranes and other cellular organelles,

the accumulation and partitioning of inorganic ions, and so on—occur as a secondary consequence of the action of specific proteins. Many of these proteins are enzymes that catalyze the biochemical conversion of one molecule into another. Others are structural proteins, such as collagen and elastin, and still others are regulatory proteins that dictate how much of each enzyme and each structural protein is to be made.

Since proteins are the cellular molecules the structures of which are encoded by genes, mutations in genes exert their deleterious effects by altering the structure of enzymes, structural proteins, or regulatory proteins. Thus, in a disease like Pompe disease (Type II glycogen storage disease), massive accumulation of glycogen in the heart is due not to a primary structural abnormality in the polysaccharide glycogen but to a structural abnormality in a protein, acid maltase, a lysosomal enzyme that is required to degrade glycogen.

GENETIC HETEROGENEITY. This exists when two or more mutations can produce a similar clinical syndrome. It is now believed that most, if not all, hereditary diseases, when carefully analyzed, will be shown to be genetically heterogeneous.[3]

Genetic heterogeneity may result from the existence of mutations at a single genetic locus (allelic mutations) or from mutations at different genetic loci (nonallelic mutations). In some cases of heterogeneity, not merely does the genetic locus differ but the mode of inheritance will also differ. For example, atrial septal defect can be inherited by an autosomal dominant mechanism in some families and by a multifactorial mechanism in other families.

CATEGORIES OF GENETIC DISORDERS AFFECTING THE CARDIOVASCULAR SYSTEM

Genetic diseases of the cardiovascular system, like all genetic disorders, generally fall into one of three categories:

1. *Chromosomal disorders* involve the lack, excess, or abnormal arrangement of one or more chromosomes, producing excessive or deficient genetic material and affecting many genes.

2. *Mendelian* or *single-gene disorders* are determined primarily by a single mutant gene that is transmitted to offspring in a predictable way. As a result, these disorders display simple (mendelian) inheritance patterns which can be classified into autosomal dominant, autosomal recessive, or X-linked types.

3. *Multifactorial disorders* are caused by an interaction of multiple genes and multiple exogenous or environmental factors. Although many of these multifactorial disorders, such as coronary artery disease (CAD) and most types of congenital heart disease, "run in families," the inheritance pattern is complex and unpredictable. In general, the risk to relatives is much less than that seen in the single-gene disorders. As discussed below, each of these three categories of genetic disease presents different problems with respect to causation, prevention, diagnosis, genetic counseling, and treatment.

Chromosomal Disorders

As noted, the number of chromosomes in normal individuals is 46, of which 44 represent the 22 pairs of *auto-

somes and the other 2 are the *sex chromosomes*. Females have 2 X chromosomes (XX) and males have 1 X chromosome and 1 Y chromosome (XY). Each of the 22 pairs of autosomes and the 2 sex chromosomes can be identified microscopically on the basis of size, location of the centromere (which divides the chromosome into arms of equal or unequal length), and unique banding pattern (which is determined after treatment with special dyes and proteolytic enzymes).

Of the two most common chromosomal disorders causing heart disease, one results from an extra chromosome and the other results from a deficiency of one chromosome. Trisomy 21 (Down syndrome or mongolism) is characterized by the presence of three rather than two copies of chromosome 21, and the common form of Turner syndrome is characterized by the presence of one X chromosome rather than two X's or an X and a Y. The abnormality in both of these disorders appears to arise through *nondisjunction*, either during meiosis in one parent (i.e., in spermatogenesis or oogenesis) or in the first mitotic cleavage of the zygote. In meiotic nondisjunction, a pair of chromosomes does not separate normally so that both members of the pair (or none) pass into one gamete. When an additional copy of the chromosome is added during fertilization, three copies of the same chromosome (or only one) are in the new zygote instead of the pair found in normal persons.

The detected frequency of chromosomal aberrations among unselected newborn infants is 1 in 200 (0.5 per cent), whereas among first trimester spontaneous abortions the frequency of chromosomal defects is as high as 50 per cent. Thus, the vast majority of chromosomal abnormalities are lost in early fetal life. In most instances chromosomal disorders occur as new mutations; both parents are usually normal, and the risk of recurrence to relatives is usually low.

Single-gene Disorders

Disorders caused by the transmission of a single mutant gene show one of three simple (or mendelian) patterns of inheritance: (1) autosomal dominant, (2) autosomal recessive, or (3) X-linked. The distinction between "dominant" and "recessive" must be understood as one of convenience in pedigree analysis rather than as necessarily implying a fundamental difference in genetic mechanism. The term *dominant* implies that a mutation will be clinically manifest when an individual has a single dose of this mutation (or is *heterozygous* for it), whereas the term *recessive* implies that a double dose (or *homozygosity*) is required for clinical detection. Genes themselves are never dominant or recessive; their effects, however, produce clinical patterns that are classified as dominant or recessive.

The demonstration that a particular syndrome shows one of the three mendelian patterns of inheritance implies that its pathogenesis, no matter how complex, is due to an abnormality in a single protein molecule. For example, in the Marfan syndrome, all the clinical manifestations, which include such seemingly unrelated disturbances as ectopia lentis, scoliosis, arachnodactyly, and dissecting aneurysm, are the physiological consequences of a single abnormal protein that is encoded by a single abnormal gene. In many mendelian disorders, especially in those with dominant inheritance, it is not yet possible to demonstrate directly the protein that is primarily altered by the mutation. In such cases, only the distal physiological effects of the mutation are recognizable. Nevertheless, it is safe to assume that a single primary defect exists whenever a disease is transmitted by a single gene mechanism and that the various manifestations of the disease can all be related to the mutational event by a more or less complicated "pedigree of causes."

AUTOSOMAL DOMINANT DISORDERS. Dominant diseases are those manifest in the heterozygous state, i.e., when only one abnormal gene (*mutant allele*) is present and the corresponding partner allele on the homologous chromosome is normal. The gene responsible for an autosomal dominant disorder is located on 1 of the 22 autosomes; thus, both males and females can be affected. Since alleles segregate independently at meiosis, there is a one in two chance that the offspring of an affected heterozygote will inherit the mutant allele and, similarly, a one in two chance of his or her inheriting the normal allele.

The following features are characteristic of autosomal dominant inheritance: (1) Each affected individual has an affected parent (unless the condition arose by a new mutation in the individual or is mildly expressed in the affected parent); (2) an affected individual will bear, on the average, both normal and affected offspring in equal proportions; (3) normal children of an affected individual will have only normal offspring; (4) men and women are affected in equal proportion; (5) each sex is equally likely to transmit the condition to male and female offspring, with male-to-male transmission occurring; and (6) vertical transmission of the condition through successive generations occurs, especially when the trait does not impair reproductive capacity.

Although half the offspring of an individual with an autosomal dominant condition will inherit the disease, it is not necessarily true that each affected person must have an affected parent. In every autosomal dominant disease a certain proportion of affected persons owe the disorder to a new mutation rather than to an inherited mutation. The parent in whose germ cells the new mutation arose will be clinically normal. Likewise, the siblings of the affected individual will be normal, since the mutation will affect only a single germ cell. However, the affected individual will transmit the disease and half of his or her children will be affected.

The proportion of patients with dominant disorders who represent new mutations is inversely proportional to the effect of the disease on *biological fitness*. Biological fitness refers to the ability of an affected individual to produce children who survive to adult life and reproduce. In the extreme case, if a dominant mutation produces absolute infertility, then all observed cases would of necessity represent new mutations, and it would be impossible to prove the genetic transmission of the trait. In less severe disorders, as in the Marfan syndrome, the cardiac disease reduces biological fitness to about 85 per cent of normal, and the proportion of cases due to new mutations is about 15 per cent.

Before concluding that a dominant disorder in a given patient with unaffected parents is the result of a new mutation, two other considerations are important: (1) the possibility that the gene may be carried by one parent in whom the disease is of low expressivity (discussed below), and (2) the possibility that extramarital paternity may have occurred, which is found in about 3 to 5 per cent of randomly studied children in the United States.

Most autosomal dominant disorders show two characteristic features that are not usually seen in recessive syndromes: (1) *delayed age of onset*, and (2) *variability in clinical expression*. Delayed age of onset is seen in such disorders as myotonic dystrophy (p. 1708) and hypertrophic obstructive cardiomyopathy (p. 1409). These disorders typically do not become manifest clinically until adult life, even though the mutant gene is present from the time of conception. Variability in clinical expression is illustrated dramatically by the Holt-Oram syndrome (discussed below). Patients in the same family inheriting the same abnormal gene may manifest any one of the following: (1) atrial septal defect and a skeletal abnormality of the upper extremity, (2) only atrial septal defect, or (3) only a skeletal abnormality of the upper extremity. This diversity in clinical manifestations makes it difficult to recognize that each family member suffers from the same genetic abnormality.

Since dominant mutations involve a type of gene product that in a 50 per cent deficiency is capable of producing clinical symptoms in heterozygotes, the responsible mutations are likely to involve abnormalities in two classes of proteins: (1) those that regulate complex metabolic pathways, such as membrane receptors and rate-limiting enzymes in pathways under feedback control, and (2) key structural proteins, such as those involved in connective tissue formation. At present, however, the basic biochemical defects have been identified in only a handful of the known autosomal dominant disorders.

Examples of autosomal dominant disorders that involve the cardiovascular system include the Holt-Oram syndrome, the Noonan syndrome, the Marfan syndrome, hypertrophic obstructive cardiomyopathy, and familial hypercholesterolemia.

AUTOSOMAL RECESSIVE DISORDERS. Autosomal recessive conditions are clinically apparent only in the homozygous state, i.e., when both alleles at a particular genetic locus are mutant alleles. The gene responsible for an autosomal recessive disorder is located on 1 of the 22 autosomes; thus, both men and women can be affected.

The following features are characteristic of autosomal recessive inheritance: (1) the parents are clinically normal; (2) only siblings are affected and vertical transmission does not occur; and (3) men and women are affected in equal proportions.

The relative infrequency of recessive genes in the population and the requirement that two abnormal genes be present for clinical expression combine to create special conditions for autosomal recessive inheritance: (1) If a husband and a wife are both carriers for the same autosomal recessive gene, 25 per cent of the children will be normal, 50 per cent will be heterozygous carriers, and 25 per cent will be homozygous and affected with the disease; (2) if an affected individual marries a heterozygote (as may occur with consanguineous marriage), half the children will be affected, and a pedigree simulating dominant inheritance would result; (3) if two individuals with the same recessive disease marry, all of their children will be affected; and (4) the more infrequent the mutant gene in the population, the stronger the likelihood that affected individuals will be the product of consanguineous matings.

In general, consanguinity is an infrequent finding clinically in most families with recessive diseases in the United States. This is because the background rate for consanguinity in the general population is very low. Thus, in most of the United States (as opposed to areas with relative geographical isolation, such as northern Norway, Switzerland, and so on), a disorder must be extremely rare before it is associated with an important frequency of consanguinity. For example, consanguinity is expected in a large proportion of families having children with very rare disorders such as the Kartagener syndrome and mulibrey nanism.

The clinical picture in autosomal recessive disorders tends to be more uniform than that of dominant diseases, and onset often occurs early in life. As a general rule, recessive disorders are more commonly diagnosed in children, whereas dominant diseases are more frequently encountered in adults.

Inasmuch as only one of four children in a sibship is expected to be affected with a recessive disease, multiple cases in a family may not occur. This is especially true in a society in which small families are common. Consider, for example, 16 families in which both parents are heterozygous for the same recessive disorder. If each family has 2 children, 9 of the families will have no affected children, 6 will have 1 affected and 1 normal child, and only 1 of the 16 families will have 2 affected children. Thus, in the United States, physicians will usually see sporadic or isolated cases of a recessive disorder without an affected sibling to alert them to the possibility of a genetic etiology. Fortunately, because of the relatively uniform clinical picture of recessive disorders and because most can be diagnosed by biochemical tests, the correct diagnosis can usually be made even when no other members of a family are clinically affected.

The basic biochemical lesions underlying many autosomal recessive disorders have been identified. Of the three types of proteins in which mutations could occur (i.e., enzymes, structural proteins, and regulatory proteins), the most easy to study have been the enzymes. A mutation that destroys the catalytic activity of an enzyme generally does not impair the health of a heterozygote (i.e., an individual who has one mutant allele specifying a functionless enzyme and one normal allele on the partner chromosome specifying a normal enzyme). In this situation each cell in the body usually produces about 50 per cent of the normal number of active enzyme molecules. However, metabolic regulatory mechanisms avert any clinical consequences of this 50 per cent deficiency, and so heterozygotes are usually clinically normal. On the other hand, when an individual inherits functionless alleles at both loci specifying an enzyme, the reduction in enzyme activity is too great for any compensatory mechanism to overcome, and a disease results. Thus, heterozygotes for homocystinuria, in which patients have half the normal activity of cystathionine synthase, are clinically asymptomatic because the body compensates for the half-normal level of the enzyme by raising the homocystine concentration approximately two-fold. Under these conditions a normal amount of homocystine can be metabolized and no symptoms occur. On the other hand, the homozygote for homocystinuria has such a severe reduction in cystathionine synthase activity that enormous levels accumulate within the blood and tissues, causing thrombotic events at a young age.

Examples of autosomal recessive disorders involving the heart include Pompe disease (pp. 1051 and 1622), the Kartagener syndrome (p. 1618), homocystinuria, and the Jervell and Lange-Nielsen syndrome (p. 1626).

X-LINKED DISORDERS. The genes responsible for one class of disorders are located on the X chromosome, and thus the clinical risk and severity of the disease are different for the two sexes. Since a woman has two X chromosomes, she may be either heterozygous or homozygous for the mutant gene, and the trait may therefore demonstrate either recessive or dominant expression. Men, on the other hand, have only one X chromosome, so they can be expected to display the full syndrome whenever they inherit the gene, regardless of whether the gene behaves as a recessive or as a dominant trait in a woman. Thus, the terms *X-linked dominant* or *X-linked recessive* refer only to the expression of the gene in women.

An important feature of all X-linked inheritance is the absence of male-to-male (i.e., father-to-son) transmission of the trait. This follows from the fact that a man must always contribute his Y chromosome to his sons; hence, he can never contribute his X chromosome. On the other hand, a man contributes his X chromosome to all of his daughters.

The characteristic features of X-linked recessive inheritance are as follows: (1) In contrast to the vertical transmission in dominant traits (parents and children affected) and the horizontal transmission in autosomal recessive traits (siblings affected), the pedigree pattern in X-linked recessive traits tends to be oblique because of the occurrence of the trait in the sons of normal carrier sisters of affected males (uncles and nephews affected); (2) male offspring of carrier women have a 50 per cent chance of being affected; (3) all female offspring of affected males are carriers; (4) affected males do not transmit the trait to any offspring; and (5) affected homozygous females occur only when an affected male marries a carrier female.

Examples of X-linked recessive disorders involving the heart include Duchenne muscular dystrophy (p. 1704), Fabry disease (p. 1425), and the Hunter syndrome.

Multifactorial Genetic Diseases

Most of the common diseases of the heart, such as coronary artery disease and congenital heart disease, have long been known to "run in families." They fit best into the category of *multifactorial genetic diseases.* The genetic element in these disorders rarely manifests itself in an all-or-none fashion as it does in the single-gene disorders and in chromosomal aberrations. Instead, the interaction of multiple genes with multiple environmental factors produces the familial aggregation.[4]

In the multifactorial genetic diseases, there is a *polygenic component* consisting of multiple genes that interact in a cumulative fashion. An individual inheriting the right combination of these genes passes beyond a "threshold of risk," at which point an *environmental component* determines whether or not and to what extent he or she is clinically affected. For another individual in the same family to express the same syndrome, he must inherit the same or a very similar combination of genes. Since the first-degree relatives of an affected individual (i.e., parents, siblings, and offspring) each share half his genes, they are all at increased risk of exhibiting the same polygenic syndrome. Second-degree relatives (uncles, aunts, and grandparents) share on the average one-fourth of an individual's genes ($\frac{1}{2}$)^2, and third-degree relatives (cousins) share one-eighth ($\frac{1}{2}$)^3. Thus, as the degree of relation becomes more distant, the likelihood of a relative inheriting the same combination of genes becomes less. Moreover, the chance of any relative inheriting the right combination of risk genes decreases as the number of genes required for the expression of a given trait increases.

Since the precise number of genes responsible for polygenic traits is unknown, one cannot calculate the precise risk of inheritance for a relative of an affected individual. Rather, one must rely on empirical risk figures (i.e., a direct tally of the proportion of affected relatives in previously reported families). In contrast to the single-gene disorders, in which 25 or 50 per cent of the first-degree relatives of an affected proband are at genetic risk, multifactorial genetic disorders generally affect no more than 5 to 10 per cent of first-degree relatives. Moreover, in contrast to mendelian traits, the recurrence risk of multifactorial conditions varies from family to family, and its estimation is significantly influenced by two factors: (1) the number of affected persons already present in the family, and (2) the severity of the disorder in the index case. The larger the number of affected relatives and the more severe their disease, the higher the risk to other relatives.

The hypothesis of a polygenic component in the inheritance of multifactorial diseases has been given a sound basis in recent years by the demonstration that at least one-third of all gene loci harbor different alleles that vary among individuals. Such a large degree of variation in normal genes, such as those that specify blood groups and the HLA system, undoubtedly provides the substratum for variations in genetic predisposition with which environmental factors can interact. Such variation among a normal gene is termed a *polymorphism.* An important observation of recent years has been the finding that certain alleles at the HLA loci predispose individuals to certain specific diseases. For example, if one inherits the B-27 allele at the HLA-B locus, one has a 120-fold greater chance for developing ankylosing spondylitis than an individual who lacks this allele. Ankylosing spondylitis remains a multifactorial disease, however, because its development clearly requires one or more other factors in addition to the B-27 allele. Thus, fewer than 15 per cent of people who inherit this allele develop this disease.

Multifactorial disorders are heterogeneous in the sense that the relative contribution of the polygenic factors ("risk genes") and environmental factors to the etiology will vary greatly from patient to patient. However, it is important to remember that among common phenotypes that are largely multifactorial, there will often be a small proportion in whom the phenotype is created by major mutant genes. For example, although coronary artery disease is usually of multifactorial etiology, about 5 per cent of subjects with premature myocardial infarctions are heterozygotes for familial hypercholesterolemia, a single-gene disorder that produces atherosclerosis in the absence of any other predisposing factor.[5] Similarly, in a small proportion of patients with other common cardiovascular diseases such as atrial septal defect, the condition is not multifactorial but determined by a single gene, as in the Holt-Oram syndrome.

GENE ACTION AND THE CARDIOVASCULAR SYSTEM

The existence of a gene affecting a specific cardiac function is frequently inferred from genetic analysis of pedigrees showing mendelian inheritance of a heart disorder. The function of the gene is deduced by analysis of the defect produced in family members who carry a mutant allele. Since at least 50 simply inherited disorders of the heart and vasculature are currently recognized (composing about 5 per cent of all mendelian disorders currently known to exist in humans),[6] there must be at least 50 genes and hence 50 protein molecules that affect cardiac function in a major way. Mutation of these genes produces cardiac dysfunction, which can be manifest clinically at several levels, including congenital cardiac malformations, derangement of the connective tissue elements of the heart and vascular system, cardiomyopathies, cardiac arrhythmias and conduction defects, pericarditis, cardiac tumors, and coronary artery disease. The nature of the proteins specified by these 50 critical genes is generally unknown.

The single-gene–determined disorders of the heart may potentially provide investigative models for unraveling the complexities of cardiovascular physiology and biochemistry. Most significant has been the use of the familial hypercholesterolemia syndrome to delineate a mechanism by which human cholesterol metabolism is regulated.[7] Inasmuch as several mendelian disorders that affect cardiac muscle structure (such as hypertrophic obstructive cardiomyopathy) are now recognized, it is predictable that the elucidation of the basic defect in each of them will provide biochemical information necessary to define the basis of human structural abnormalities, such as cardiac hypertrophy.

GENETIC COUNSELING IN CARDIOLOGY

THE FAMILY HISTORY

When caring for a patient with a possible genetic disorder involving the heart, the physician begins by taking a careful *family history* and by carrying out a *family evaluation*. The first step involves obtaining certain information on the *proband* or *index case* (i.e., the clinically affected person who has brought the family to attention) and on each of the patient's *first-degree relatives* (i.e., the parents, sibs, and offspring of the proband). This information includes the given name, surname, and maiden name; birth date or current age; age at death, whether an autopsy was performed, and cause of death; and presence of any disease or defect. Ideally, the family history should also include the name and address of the individuals' physicians and the hospitals to which they were admitted.

The second step includes asking six questions designed to survey the family for the presence of disease:

1. Is there any relative with an identical or similar trait?

2. Is there any relative with a trait that is absent in the proband but that is known to occur in some patients with the same disease? This question requires that the physician have some knowledge about the manifestations of the disease in question. For example, when obtaining the family history from a proband with dissecting aneurysm possibly caused by the Marfan syndrome, one should ask about the occurrence of eye abnormalities, cardiac abnormalities, and skeletal abnormalities in the proband's relatives.

3. Is there any relative with a trait that is recognized to be genetically determined? The purpose of this question is to ascertain the occurrence of hereditary disease in the family even though the patients may not consider themselves to be involved.

4. Is there any relative with an unusual disease, or has any relative died of a rare condition? The purpose of this question is to identify a condition that might be genetically determined though not recognized as such by the patient. In addition, this question may help to identify conditions in relatives that might be etiologically related to the patient's problem. For example, a patient with a cardiac tumor should be suspected of having underlying tuberous sclerosis if he or she has a brother with adenoma sebaceum and mental retardation, both of which can be manifestations of the tuberous sclerosis gene.

5. Is there any consanguinity in the family? Not only should this inquiry be made directly, but, in addition, one should ask whether common last names appear in the families of husband and wife. Consanguineous marriage may be the source of a rare autosomal recessive syndrome, such as Pompe disease, and sometimes its presence in the family may not be known by the proband.

6. What is the ethnic origin of the family? Persons of certain ethnic origins have an increased chance of certain genetic diseases. Mulibrey nanism (p. 1626) is one example of a familial heart disease that occurs with increased frequency in a specific ethnic group, the Finns.

The third step involves an examination of available family members, both those affected and those believed to be unaffected.

RETROSPECTIVE GENETIC COUNSELING

The prevention of hereditary cardiac diseases requires the identification of matings that are capable of producing defective offspring. These may be matings in which one of the two individuals is carrying a dominant or X-linked gene mutation or matings in which both individuals are carriers of a deleterious recessive gene. Such individuals are usually identified through an affected child or near relative, in which case retrospective genetic counseling can be provided.

When advising family members about the risk of transmitting a disorder that has already affected someone in the family, the first step is to be certain of the *correct diagnosis* —in particular, to make certain that the problem in question is really of genetic origin. This is especially important in cardiac disorders that may have both genetic and nongenetic causes. For example, some cases of patent ductus arteriosus are caused by a multifactorial genetic mechanism, whereas others are caused by rubella (p. 942).

Second, if the disease has a hereditary element, one must consider the possibility of *genetic heterogeneity,* a situation in which clinically similar genetic disorders show varying patterns of inheritance. For example, there are two types of atrial septal defect that resemble each other closely: a rare form showing autosomal dominant inheritance, as in the Holt-Oram syndrome (p. 1030 and 1616), and a common form having a multifactorial etiology.

To estimate the *recurrence risk,* one must consider what is known of the genetic mechanisms determining the relevant disorder. When more than one genetic mechanism exists, or when environmental factors can cause clinically indistinguishable traits, then the *relative probabilities* of the different mechanisms operating in the particular family are computed. For conditions determined by simple mendelian inheritance, there is no difficulty in predicting the probability of an offspring being affected, provided the genotypes of the parents can be recognized. Identification of the parental genotype is easiest for autosomal recessive and X-linked disorders, since the basic lesions in these two forms of mendelian inheritance usually involve simple enzyme deficiencies for which biochemical tests are now available.

Identification of the parental genotype is considerably more difficult for autosomal dominant disorders, since the basic defect is known for only a few. Thus, diagnosis of the heterozygote for a dominant disorder depends almost exclusively on the clinical evaluation and a careful pedigree analysis. In counseling a family in which one relative is affected with a dominant disorder, it is important that appropriate clinical examination of all first-degree relatives and appropriately selected distant relatives be carried out. If relatives appear unaffected, one must constantly consider the possibility that the clinical symptoms may be masked by *delayed age of onset* and *variability in expression.* When no relatives are affected, the possibility of a new dominant mutation must be entertained. The probability of a case of an autosomal dominant disorder being the result of a new mutation is inversely proportional to the reproductive fitness of the disorder.

In advising families about multifactorial genetic diseases in which the inheritance pattern is not clear-cut, such as premature coronary artery disease, the physician must resort to empirical risk estimates that have been derived from retrospectively assembled data (see Chap. 35).

Once the parental genotypes are determined, the genetic prognosis is usually presented in terms of probability that a given couple will produce an affected offspring. The physician providing genetic counseling must make certain that the couple understands not only the meaning of such absolute risk figures but also the severity of the disease and the variability in clinical expression. In other words, in dealing with a disorder such as the Noonan syndrome, it is important not only that the parents realize that they have a 50 per cent risk of producing a child with this disorder but also that they know that a certain proportion of patients with the disorder have severe disease, a certain proportion have mild disease, and so on. They should also have an understanding of the potential impact of the disease on their family. Thus, a disease that is lethal at birth might be classified by some as more "severe" than one that is lethal at age 16, but the latter is likely to have a much more profound impact on the family.

Although different families initially react in different ways to the same risk, most couples who seek genetic advice can be expected to take a responsible course of action that is based on the information quoted. Thus, the physician avoids giving direct advice to the couple concerning whether they "should" or "should not" have children. For serious genetic disease, it has been observed that when the recurrence risk is high, i.e., equal to or greater than 1 in 10, most parents are deterred from planning further children. When the risks are low, i.e., less than 1 in 10, most parents continue with additional pregnancies.[8]

PRENATAL DIAGNOSIS

The use of transabdominal amniocentesis permits diagnosis of certain genetic diseases at an early enough stage to terminate the pregnancy to prevent the birth of a defective child. This procedure allows high-risk couples the opportunity to have unaffected children, provided they are willing to have the pregnancy terminated in the event that an abnormal fetus is detected.[1,9]

TABLE 47–1   GENETIC DISORDERS AFFECTING THE HEART FOR WHICH PRENATAL DIAGNOSIS IS FEASIBLE

DISORDER	EXPRESSION IN CULTURED AMNIOTIC FLUID CELLS	DETECTABLE ABNORMALITY
Down syndrome	Yes	Trisomy 21 or unbalanced 14/21 translocation by karyotype
Ellis–van Creveld syndrome	No	Visualization of bilateral polydactyly by fetoscopy
Duchenne muscular dystrophy	No	Decreased level of creatine phosphokinase (CPK) in fetal blood
Myotonic dystrophy	No	Gene for *myotonic dystrophy* closely linked with *secretor* gene, the product of which is present in amniotic fluid
Ehlers-Danlos, Type IV	Yes	Deficient synthesis of Type III collagen
Homocystinuria	Yes	Deficiency of cystathionine synthase
Pompe disease	Yes	Deficiency of lysosomal acid maltase
Homozygous familial hypercholesterolemia	Yes	Deficiency of receptors for low-density lipoprotein
Cholesteryl ester storage disease	Yes	Deficiency of lysosomal acid lipase
Fabry disease	Yes	Deficiency of α-galactosidase A
Mucopolysaccharidoses		
Type I-H, Hurler syndrome	Yes	Deficiency of α-L-iduronidase
Type I-S, Scheie syndrome	Yes	Deficiency of α-L-iduronidase
Type I-H/S, Hurler-Scheie compound	Yes	Deficiency of α-L-iduronidase
Type II, Hunter syndrome	Yes	Deficiency of sulfoiduronide sulfatase
Type IV, Morquio syndrome	Yes	Deficiency of N-acetylhexosamine sulfate sulfatase
Type VI, Maroteaux-Lamy syndrome	Yes	Deficiency of arylsulfatase B
Mucolipidosis, Type III	Yes	Deficiency of N-acetylglucosamine-1-phosphotransferase

Prenatal diagnosis usually requires obtaining amniotic fluid at week 16 of gestation, centrifuging the fluid to obtain fetal amniotic cells, and culturing the fetal cells in vitro. The culture process requires about 3 weeks. By this means the karyotype of the fetus can be determined to ascertain fetal sex and to detect various chromosomal aberrations, such as Down syndrome. Moreover, many inborn errors of metabolism can be detected by suitable assays of specific enzyme activities in the cultured fetal cells.

In addition to the use of amniotic cells for prenatal diagnosis, other methods, such as fetoscopy and radiology, can be employed. For example, the Ellis–van Creveld syndrome can be diagnosed in utero by visualization of bilateral polydactyly. Moreover, fetal blood sampling for measurement of the level of creatine phosphokinase (CPK) can be used in the prenatal diagnosis of muscular dystrophy. Table 47–1 lists those genetic disorders affecting the cardiovascular system for which prenatal diagnosis is currently feasible.

GENETICS OF SPECIFIC FORMS OF CARDIOVASCULAR DISEASE

CONGENITAL HEART DISEASES
(See also Chaps. 29 and 30)

Chromosomal Disorders

Approximately 5 per cent of all congenital heart malformations can be traced to a chromosomal aberration.[10] Virtually all cases of a congenital heart malformation associated with a chromosomal defect occur as part of a multiple malformation syndrome. Congenital heart disease is a characteristic feature of most chromosomal disorders, such as trisomy 13, trisomy 18, trisomy 21 (Down syndrome), deletion of the short arm of chromosome 4, deletion of the long arm of chromosome 13, deletion of the long arm of chromosome 18, and Turner syndrome (XO). A chromosomal syndrome that does *not* show an increased frequency of congenital heart disease is the Klinefelter syndrome (XXY). A discussion follows of the two chromosomal syndromes that most commonly cause congenital heart disease, Down syndrome and Turner syndrome.

DOWN SYNDROME.   The trisomy 21 form of Down syndrome (mongolism) is the most common human chromosomal aberration, occurring in approximately 1 in every 600 neonates. Congenital heart disease, which is found in as many as 50 per cent of patients with this disorder, constitutes a major source of morbidity and mortality.[11–14]

The two most common cardiac lesions in Down syndrome are ventricular septal defect and endocardial cushion defect. Among patients with the complete form of endocardial cushion defect, those with Down syndrome account for about 50 per cent.[14] Secundum atrial septal defect, tetralogy of Fallot, and isolated patent ductus arteriosus are also observed in patients with Down syndrome. Transposition of the great arteries and coarctation of the aorta are rarely seen. Most patients having Down syndrome with congenital heart disease have a single lesion. However, as many as 30 per cent of those with heart disease may have multiple cardiac defects.[13]

The decision to repair surgically a congenital heart lesion in a patient with Down syndrome is often a complicated one. Factors to be considered include the seriousness of the defect; whether the patient is living at home or with relatives or is institutionalized; and the patient's degree of cooperation. Although it is generally believed that patients with Down syndrome are poor operative candidates because of their increased susceptibility to infections, recent surgical follow-up studies suggest that their postoperative mortality is no higher than that of a non–Down syndrome population with similar cardiac lesions.[11,15]

The most important factor in preventing the birth of a child with the trisomy 21 form of Down syndrome is maternal age. A marked increase in incidence occurs in children born to older mothers,[16,17] as shown in Table 47–2.

The recurrence risk to a couple who has had one child with the trisomy 21 form of Down syndrome is 2 per cent, i.e., there is a 1 in 50 chance that the next child will also have the trisomy 21 form of Down syndrome.[16] The recurrence risk is 2 per cent regardless of whether the mother is young (age 20) or old (age 45).[16] All women who are 36 years of age and older and all women who have had one child with trisomy 21 Down syndrome should have each of their subsequent pregnancies monitored by amniocentesis for a prenatal diagnosis.

The trisomy 21 aberration accounts for virtually all cases of Down syndrome born to women above age 30 and for 90 per cent of all cases born to women below age 30. The remaining 10 per cent of patients with Down syndrome born to women below age 30 have a translocation form. On karyotype analysis, such patients have the normal number of 46 chromosomes, including 2 normal chromosomes No. 21, 1 normal chromosome No. 14, and an unpaired large chromosome that represents an extra chromosome No. 21 that is joined to 1 chromosome No. 14. There are no clinical differences between children with the trisomy 21 form of Down syndrome and those with the translocation form.

Karyotypes of the parents of children with the translo-

TABLE 47–2   RISK OF HAVING A CHILD WITH DOWN SYNDROME AS A FUNCTION OF MATERNAL AGE

MATERNAL AGE	ESTIMATED RISK
< 20 years	1 in 1800
20–29 years	1 in 1200
30–34 years	1 in 750
35–39 years	1 in 250
40–44 years	1 in 80
≥ 45 years	1 in 25

cation form of Down syndrome exhibit one of the following:

1. In about 90 per cent of cases, both parents have normal karyotypes, so the translocation is assumed to have originated during gametogenesis, and the risk of recurrence is no more than 2 per cent to subsequent children.

2. In 10 per cent of cases one of the parents will have an abnormal karyotype consisting of 45 chromosomes with 1 normal chromosome No. 14, 1 normal chromosome No. 21, and a large chromosome that contains fused copies of both the 14 and 21 chromosomes.

About 5 to 20 per cent of the live-born offspring of an individual who is a "balanced" translocation carrier for the 14/21 chromosome will have Down syndrome, depending on whether the father (5 per cent) or the mother (20 per cent) carries the "balanced" translocation.[16] Other types of translocation occur, but these are much less frequent. Overall, the inherited translocation form of Down syndrome is extremely rare, especially compared with the trisomy 21 form of the disorder. Nevertheless, it is important to identify all such cases so that the pregnancies of all family members who are translocation carriers can be appropriately monitored by amniocentesis.

TURNER SYNDROME (see also p. 1038).   Turner syndrome is characterized by the occurrence in a phenotypic female of the following clinical features: shortness of stature, amenorrhea due to gonadal dysgenesis, shield-shaped chest, pigmented nevi, webbing of the neck, cubitus valgus, shortening of metacarpals and metatarsals, renal abnormalities, and cardiovascular abnormalities. In about 60 per cent of patients with these clinical features, all the cells in the body will be deficient in one of the two X chromosomes (45,X form). The remaining 40 per cent of patients include individuals who have a mixture of cells, some of which show the 45,X karyotype and some of which show the normal karyotype (45,X/46,XX mosaicism), and individuals whose cells show structural abnormalities in one of the two X chromosomes (such as a single isochromosome X or a single ring X chromosome). Patients with the 45,X/46,XX form of Turner syndrome are often less severely clinically involved and may be nearly normal.

Most fetuses with the 45,X form of Turner syndrome die in utero and are aborted spontaneously. Recent studies indicate that the 45,X chromosomal abnormality occurs in as many as 5 per cent of all spontaneous abortions and in about 1 in 2500 female live births.[18]

Cardiovascular abnormalities occur in 35 to 50 per cent of all patients with the 45,X form of Turner syndrome.[19-22] Coarctation of the aorta is by far the most common abnormality that is encountered, accounting for 70 per cent of all cardiac anomalies. Other congenital malformations are occasionally seen, including bicuspid aortic valve, hypertrophic obstructive cardiomyopathy, ventricular septal defect, prolapse of the mitral valve, and dextrocardia.[19-23] Stenosis of the pulmonic valve is rarely, if ever, seen in Turner syndrome. This is in striking contrast to findings in the superficially similar Noonan syndrome, in which coarctation of the aorta is rarely encountered and stenosis of the pulmonic valve is the cardinal cardiac manifestation[22] (discussed below).

Patients with Turner syndrome caused by an isochromosome X or a ring X differ clinically from patients with the 45,X karyotype in that webbing of the neck and coarctation of the aorta are absent.[19,21] In patients with mosaic Turner syndrome, coarctation of the aorta occurs, but its frequency is considerably less than in the 45,X patients.

Adults with Turner syndrome are prone to systemic hypertension. This association between Turner syndrome and hypertension occurs in the absence of coarctation of the aorta and appears to be unrelated to the karyotypic abnormality.[19] The mechanism underlying the hypertension has not been defined.

Family studies have revealed a high frequency of both diabetes mellitus and thyroid autoantibodies in the chromosomally normal relatives of patients with Turner syndrome.[19] These findings have suggested that a genetic tendency to autoantibody formation in parents may predispose to the occurrence of chromosomal abnormalities in their offspring.

Elevated maternal age does not appear to predispose to offspring with Turner syndrome, unlike Down syndrome. Once a couple has had one child with Turner syndrome, the recurrence risk to subsequent offspring is virtually zero.

Single-gene Disorders

At least eight forms of congenital heart disease are now recognized to be caused by single-gene mutations. Together, these eight disorders account for about 5 per cent of all forms of congenital heart disease. In six of these disorders, the responsible mutation causes a multisystem syndrome of which congenital heart disease is only one component. Each of these mutations presumably disrupts the function of a single protein the action of which is necessary for several developmental events, including normal embryogenesis of the heart. Virtually nothing is known of how these mutant genes act at the molecular and cellular level.

The identification of any one of these eight single-gene disorders in a given individual enables the cardiologist to apply knowledge of the genetics of the syndrome to the identification of further cases in the same family and to provide genetic counseling to appropriate family members.

NOONAN SYNDROME (see also p. 986).   The eponym Noonan syndrome describes a common clinical entity characterized by shortness of stature, mild mental retardation, a unique facial appearance (Fig. 47–1), webbing of the neck, cryptorchidism, renal anomalies, and congenital heart disease.[24-29] Skeletal deformities are also frequent, including scoliosis and pectus carinatum. Affected individuals superficially resemble patients with Turner syndrome in that shortness of stature, webbing of the neck, cubitus valgus, skeletal anomalies, renal abnormalities, and congenital heart disease are present in both disorders. Because of these clinical similarities, Noonan syndrome has frequently been referred to in the literature as male "Turner syndrome," "Turner phenotype with normal chromosomes," and XX and XY "Turner phenotype."[24-28]

However, several striking genetic and clinical differences between Noonan syndrome and Turner syndrome clearly separate these two disorders as distinct entities. (1) In contrast to Turner syndrome, in Noonan syndrome both males and females are affected and the karyotype in both

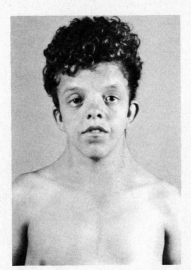

FIGURE 47–1 Eighteen-year-old boy with the Noonan syndrome. The facial abnormalities consist of curly hair, epicanthal folds, ptosis of eyelids, hypertelorism, strabismus, small chin, and low-set ears with abnormal auricles. Webbing of the neck is also evident.

males and females are affected and the karyotype in both sexes is normal;[24-28] (2) coarctation of the aorta, which rarely occurs in Noonan syndrome, is the most frequent cardiac lesion in Turner syndrome; conversely, *pulmonic stenosis*, which does not occur in Turner syndrome, is the most common cardiac lesion in Noonan syndrome;[23-31] and (3) Noonan syndrome is determined by a single mutant gene inherited as an autosomal dominant trait.[25,27,28,32-34]

Approximately 50 per cent of patients with Noonan syndrome have congenital heart disease.[29] The most common lesion is valvular pulmonary stenosis, occurring in about 60 per cent of those patients who have a congenital cardiac malformation. The stenotic pulmonic valve is frequently dysplastic. Characteristically, the annulus is of normal size, but the cusps are thickened and immobile.[23-31] The electrocardiogram is often different from the pattern usually seen in pulmonary valve stenosis: Left anterior hemiblock is common, and a deep S wave is frequently present in the precordial leads.[11,23]

Atrial septal defect and hypertrophic cardiomyopathy occur in about 20 per cent of patients with Noonan syndrome who have congenital heart disease. The cardiomyopathy frequently produces an eccentric hypertrophy of the left ventricle that can easily be missed during cardiac catherization limited to the right side of the heart.[35-38] Although the majority of patients show a single heart defect, some show a combination of pulmonary stenosis and either atrial septal defect or hypertrophic cardiomyopathy.

In addition to anomalies of the heart itself, abnormalities of the systemic arteries have been reported in patients with Noonan syndrome. These include fistulas of the coronary arteries, peripheral pulmonic stenosis, anomalous pulmonary venous septum, hemangiomas, peripheral lymphedema, and intestinal lymphangiectasis.[31]

Patients with Noonan syndrome undergoing cardiac surgery are particularly vulnerable to several complications: (1) technical difficulties because of the dysplastic nature of the pulmonic valve, sometimes necessitating total valve replacement—a formidable problem in infants and young children; (2) difficulty in establishing outflow drainage during total cardiopulmonary bypass because of the systemic venous anomalies; (3) increased risk of malignant hyperpyrexia during general anesthesia; and (4) development of persistent chylothorax because of pulmonary lymphangiectasis.[31]

The evidence for a genetic etiology of Noonan syndrome is provided by its occurrence in multiple siblings and in multiple generations of the same family. Family studies are consistent with autosomal dominant inheritance of a single mutant gene.[25,27,28,32-34] Figure 47-2 shows a pedigree of a family with Noonan syndrome: The mutant gene segregated through three generations, and one affected woman had affected children with two different husbands. As with most autosomal dominant traits, the Noonan syndrome gene shows a marked variation in its clinical expression; some affected individuals show only minor abnormalities (such as epicanthal folds and low-set ears), whereas others in the same family show the full syndrome with severe congenital heart disease.

Although male-to-male transmission of the mutant gene has been documented in several pedigrees,[32-34] most affected men, unlike affected women, show a deficiency in the number of offspring. This deficiency can be attributed to two factors: (1) Males appear to have a higher frequency of severe cardiac lesions than do females and therefore have less chance of surviving to reproductive age, and (2) about 75 per cent of affected males have bilateral cryptorchidism, whereas the affected females appear to have normal gonadal function.[24-34] This striking diminution in reproductive fitness in males with Noonan syndrome is consistent with the clinical observation that as many as 50 per cent of all cases of Noonan syndrome are sporadic cases. Such sporadic cases presumably represent new mutations.

It has been only fourteen years since Noonan syndrome was recognized as a distinct clinical and genetic entity separate from Turner syndrome. Nevertheless, in this short time more than 500 cases of Noonan syndrome have been reported. It has been estimated that the disorder may occur more frequently than 1 in 1000 persons in the population.[39] The basic defect underlying Noonan syndrome is

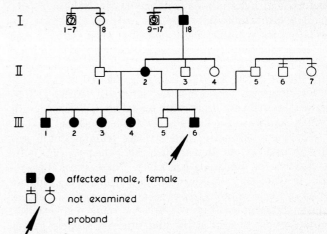

FIGURE 47–2 Pedigree of a family with the Noonan syndrome, showing autosomal dominant transmission of the trait through three generations. Note that II-2 had affected children by two different husbands. (From Baird, P. A., and De Jong, B. P.: Noonan's syndrome [XX and XY Turner phenotype] in three generations of a family. J. Pediatr. *80*:110, 1972.)

unknown. If it follows the pattern of other extremely common genetic diseases, it will ultimately be found to be genetically heterogeneous in that several different mutations will be able to cause a similar clinical syndrome.

In view of the high frequency of Noonan syndrome, the cardiologist should have a high index of suspicion of this disorder whenever a patient with congenital pulmonic stenosis is encountered. Attribution of this lesion to Noonan syndrome may be difficult, especially since 50 per cent of the cases may represent new mutations and thus exhibit a negative family history. The diagnosis is made even more difficult because many of the patients with documented Noonan syndrome have only mild facial abnormalities. Webbing of the neck and associated skeletal abnormalities may be absent. The invariant associated lesion is shortness of stature, so the physician should consider the presumptive diagnosis of Noonan syndrome whenever a patient with pulmonic stenosis and short stature is seen. In these cases, all first-degree relatives should be examined for the presence of mild facial abnormalities of the Noonan type as well as for occult cardiac lesions, especially pulmonic stenosis. The importance of making the diagnosis of Noonan syndrome lies in the ability of the physician to advise the patient that half of his or her children will be similarly affected.

LEOPARD SYNDROME.   The LEOPARD syndrome is a rare, single gene–determined complex of congenital malformations affecting the cardiovascular system, the skin, the inner ear, and somatic and sexual development.[40–42] The cardinal features of the disorder are embodied in the mnemonic device LEOPARD: *L*, lentigenes; *E*, electrocardiographic conduction defects; *O*, ocular hypertelorism; *P*, pulmonic valve stenosis; *A*, abnormalities of genitals; *R*, retardation of growth, and *D*, deafness, sensorineural.[40]

Cardiac abnormalities, a common feature of the disorder, consist of anatomical malformations as well as electrocardiographic conduction defects. Stenosis of the pulmonic valve appears to be the most frequently encountered cardiac lesion. It may exist as an isolated anomaly, or it may be combined with aortic stenosis. Other cardiac defects that have been reported include endocardial fibroelastosis and hypertrophic cardiomyopathy.[40–44] The cardiac disease characteristically appears early in childhood and usually runs a progressive course. The most common electrocardiographic defects include prolonged P-R interval, left anterior hemiblock, widening of the QRS, and complete heart block. The functional significance of these electrocardiographic abnormalities is highly variable from patient to patient, being well tolerated in some or sufficiently serious to produce sudden death in others.

The most distinctive and striking feature of the syndrome, and the one that is diagnostic when present, is the occurrence of numerous lentigenes. These small (up to 5 mm in diameter), dark-brown spots, which spare only the mucosal surfaces, are most concentrated over the neck and upper extremities (Fig. 47–3). In some patients, the lentigenes are present at the time of birth, whereas in others they appear shortly after birth. In all patients, the number increases with age. Lentigenes differ from freckles in several respects: (1) They appear before age 5, whereas freckles usually appear at 6 to 8 years of age; (2) they do not increase in numbers with exposure to sunlight, whereas

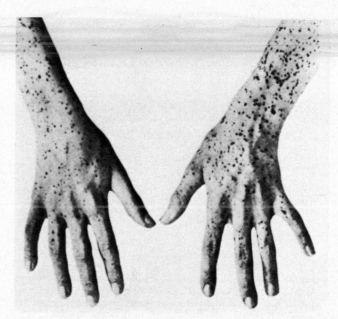

FIGURE 47–3 Skin of a 16-year-old boy with the LEOPARD syndrome covered with numerous deeply pigmented lentigines. (From Polani, P. E., and Moynahan, E. J.: Progressive carciomyopathic lentiginosis. Q. J. Med. *41*:205, 1972.)

freckles do; and (3) microscopically, the quantity of melanocytes and the distribution of melanin in the pigmented and adjacent nonpigmented skin differ.[40]

The LEOPARD syndrome is inherited as an autosomal dominant trait. The clinical findings are highly variable from patient to patient, both within the same family as well as between affected individuals from different families. The most frequently encountered manifestations of the mutant gene are those relating to the cardiovascular system, occurring in at least 95 per cent of affected subjects. About 80 per cent have lentigenes. Deafness and abnormalities of genitals (hypospadias and undescended testes in the male) occur in about 20 per cent of patients.

The population frequency of the gene causing the LEOPARD syndrome is very low. Nothing is currently known about the relative proportion of cases arising from familial transmission of the mutant gene versus those arising from new mutations. Moreover, nothing is known regarding the biochemical action of the mutant gene.

HOLT-ORAM SYNDROME (see also p. 1030).   Although atrial septal defect almost always occurs as a sporadic disorder, there are occasional families in which the pedigree pattern suggests the operation of a single mutant gene. The Holt-Oram syndrome and familial atrial septal defect with prolonged atrioventricular (AV) conduction are two examples of rare autosomal dominant disorders that are hidden among the more common sporadic cases of atrial septal defect.

The cardinal clinical manifestation of the Holt-Oram syndrome is the occurrence of an upper limb deformity in a patient with congenital heart disease.[45–50] Atrial septal defect of the secundum type is the most frequently encountered congenital heart malformation in affected individuals. This is usually accompanied by one or more electrocardiographic abnormalities, such as first-degree atrioventricular block, right bundle branch block, or bradycardia. Ventricular septal defect is the second most commonly encountered congenital heart lesion. Although virtually any form of congenital heart disease has been reported to occur in the syndrome, 70 per cent of affected individuals have either an atrial septal defect or a ventricular septal defect.

Many different upper limb deformities have been observed in association with the congenital heart disease in the Holt-Oram syndrome.[51] These limb deformities are typically bilateral but not necessarily symmetrical. If asymmetry is present, the skeletal lesions are usually more severe on the left side.[47] The most characteristic anomaly involves the thumbs. They may be absent, hypoplastic, triphalangeal, or finger-like. The last-named anomaly is referred to as "digitalization of the thumbs." The radius and the forearm are variably involved, the defects ranging in different patients from absent or hypoplastic radii to phocomelia.

Although deformities of the thumb are the best known features of the Holt-Oram syndrome, they do not occur in every case, nor are they pathognomonic.[51] Bilateral thumb abnormalities may also occur in the Diamond-Blackfan syndrome, in Fanconi anemia, or in thalidomide embryopathy. The most frequently encountered and specific upper limb abnormalities—namely, the presence of an abnormal scaphoid bone and/or accessory carpal bones—are detected on radiographs of the wrists. Various abnormalities also occur in the shoulder. The most common finding is a rotation of the scapula. Deformities of the humeral head and accessory ossicles around the shoulder have also been frequently noted.[51]

As in many dominantly inherited syndromes, individuals inheriting the Holt-Oram gene show varying degrees of clinical involvement. Intrafamilial variability appears to be as great as interfamilial variability.[52] The penetrance of the Holt-Oram gene is nearly 100 per cent, i.e., all individuals who inherit the gene manifest one or more clinical abnormalities, provided that appropriate studies, including wrist radiographs and electrocardiograms, are performed.[49] In about 60 per cent of cases, one of the parents is affected. The other 40 per cent of cases occur sporadically and apparently represent new mutations occurring in the germ cells of one of the parents.[47] Although the biochemical action of the mutant gene has not been defined, it presumably acts by disrupting a critical embryonic event common to the formation of the upper limbs and the heart.

The population frequency of the Holt-Oram syndrome has not been determined. However, the disorder is probably greatly underdiagnosed, with most cases being mistakenly considered as "garden-variety" atrial septal defects. The importance of separating the patient with the Holt-Oram syndrome from those cases of atrial septal defect that are not determined by a single-gene mechanism cannot be overemphasized. If the patient has Holt-Oram syndrome, then 50 per cent of the first-degree relatives (i.e., offspring, siblings, and parents) will be affected. In contrast, if a patient has a sporadic type of atrial septal defect, only about 3 per cent of the first-degree relatives would be affected. Thus, genetic counseling is quite different in these two situations.

FAMILIAL ATRIAL SEPTAL DEFECT WITH PROLONGED AV CONDUCTION. The syndrome of atrial septal defect with prolonged AV conduction represents a second example (the first being the Holt-Oram syndrome) of a single-gene–determined form of atrial septal defect.

Pedigree studies of at least 20 large families leave little doubt about the autosomal dominant inheritance of this disorder.[53-56] The mutant gene shows a high degree of penetrance, and there is surprisingly little pleiotropy. That is, the mutant gene appears to cause only atrial septal defect and an abnormality of the AV conduction system. The latter is manifest clinically as either first- or second-degree heart block. Rarely, complete heart block occurs.

In the absence of a biochemical marker for the mutant gene, the diagnosis can be made only through careful clinical examination of family members of suspected cases. "Garden-variety" atrial septal defect can be excluded both by a family pedigree showing dominant inheritance and by electrocardiographic evidence of AV conduction block. The Holt-Oram syndrome can be ruled out by a normal clinical and radiological examination of the upper extremities.

ELLIS–VAN CREVELD SYNDROME. The Ellis–van Creveld syndrome constitutes a rare form of congenital heart disease that is inherited as an autosomal recessive trait. Affected individuals manifest abnormalities not only of the heart but also of the skeletal system, the nails, and the mouth.[57-59]

Congenital heart disease occurs in 50 to 60 per cent of patients and frequently causes deaths in infancy. The most common cardiac lesion involves the atrium, producing either a single atrium or a large atrial septal defect. The atrial lesion may occur alone, or it may be associated with another cardiac defect, such as aortic atresia, hypoplastic ascending aorta, or hypoplastic left ventricle.

The skeletal findings in the Ellis–van Creveld syndrome are characteristic. The patients have an abnormally small stature that is present from the time of birth. They exhibit a particularly striking shortening in the distal parts of the extremities. Bilateral polydactyly and fusion of the carpal bones are also present. Additional findings include the presence of hypoplastic nails and several oral abnormalities, including labiogingival adherences, accessory frenula, and hypodontia.

About half of affected individuals die in early infancy as a result of cardiorespiratory problems. The majority of survivors have normal intelligence. Eventual adult stature is in the range of 45 to 60 inches (115 to 150 cm).

Although the Ellis–van Creveld syndrome is an extremely rare disorder in the general population, it occurs with high frequency in certain isolated groups. As a result, the genetics of the disease have been well delineated.[58] The following observations support an autosomal recessive inheritance pattern: (1) The disorder occurs with equal frequency in males and females; (2) only siblings are affected in a given family; and (3) about one-third of all cases result from parental consanguinity. Most cases of the disorder in the United States occur in the Old Order Amish, an inbred religious isolate in Lancaster County, Pennsylvania, in which 13 per cent of the population carries the mutant gene.[58]

The underlying biochemical defect responsible for the Ellis–van Creveld syndrome has not yet been identified. Nonetheless, since affected individuals always manifest bilateral polydactyly of the hands, it is possible to make a prenatal diagnosis in pregnancies at risk by inspecting the fetus in utero, using fetoscopy to determine whether or not polydactyly is present.[60]

FAMILIAL SUPRAVALVULAR AORTIC STENOSIS (see also p. 981).

Supravalvular aortic stenosis can occur as an isolated congenital anomaly and as a component of two different clinical entities: (1) as a nonfamilial syndrome resulting from fetal hypercalcemia and characterized by elfin facies (antiverted nostrils, patulous lips, and small chin), mental retardation, dental anomalies, and congenital supravalvular aortic stenosis;[61] and (2) a familial syndrome transmitted as an autosomal dominant trait and characterized by the presence of pulmonary and systemic arterial stenoses in the *absence* of mental retardation and elfin facies.[62-65] Although these two syndromes are often discussed in textbooks as representing a "spectrum of the same disease," they are clinically and genetically distinct disorders. Since the first syndrome is not transmitted by a single-gene mechanism but rather results from excessive exposure or excessive hypersensitivity of fetal tissues to vitamin D, it will not be discussed further.

Patients with familial supravalvular aortic stenosis can exhibit a wide range of arterial abnormalities. Although supravalvular aortic stenosis is the "typical" lesion, many affected individuals have stenosis of the pulmonary artery (peripheral or supravalvular), brachiocephalic arterial stenosis, hypoplasia or coarctation of the descending aorta, and dilatation and tortuosity of the coronary arteries. Like most dominant traits, the mutant gene is variably expressed even among affected persons in the same family.

Most patients initially come to attention because of an asymptomatic heart murmur. Clinical signs of dyspnea, angina pectoris, syncope, or claudication do not usually begin until after age 20 years. Those patients who manifest coarctation of the descending aorta may show signs of hypertension. Since affected individuals are at risk for bacterial endocarditis and should receive antibiotics at appropriate times, it is important to identify all affected relatives as early in life as possible.

KARTAGENER SYNDROME. Kartagener syndrome consists of the triad of sinusitis, bronchiectasis, and situs inversus with dextrocardia.[66-69] The disorder is inherited as an autosomal recessive trait; males and females are affected with equal frequency. In addition to the classic triad mentioned above, affected males are infertile as a result of immobile spermatozoa.

Since individuals with Kartagener syndrome are homozygous for a mutant gene, the clinical course is remarkably uniform among affected persons. These individuals initially come to attention as infants because of mucopurulent nasal discharge and repeated bouts of upper respiratory infections, otitis media, and pneumonia. By the preschool years, most patients exhibit persistent sinusitis, chronic bronchitis, and bronchiectasis. As many as 90 per cent of affected individuals have complete situs inversus, a mirror image reversal of internal organs due to a sinistral instead of a dextral rotation of the viscera occurring between days 10 and 15 of gestation.

In most affected individuals, dextrocardia is the only cardiac manifestation. Occasionally, one or more associated cardiac anomalies are present, such as transposition of the great arteries and trilocular or bilocular heart.

Kartagener syndrome occurs in about 1 person in 68,000. Of all persons with bronchiectasis, about 1.4 per cent have Kartagener syndrome, and of all persons with situs inversus, about 15 per cent have Kartagener syndrome.[70] The occurrence of this disorder in multiple siblings, male as well as female; the absence of any manifestations in the parents or in the children of affected individuals; and the presence of a higher than average frequency of consanguinity among the parents of affected individuals all support an autosomal recessive mode of inheritance.

The nature of the primary genetic defect in the Kartagener syndrome has recently been elucidated by electron microscopic investigation of a ciliated mucosal biopsy or of an ejaculate. These studies show that the nonmotile cilia and sperm obtained from affected individuals are structurally normal in most respects. However, the so-called dynein arms are abnormal.[66,70] Dynein arms are protein structures that normally form temporary cross bridges between adjacent microtubules in cilia and sperm tails (Fig. 47–4). The dynein arms play a role analogous to that of myosin in muscle in that they allow the sliding of the microtubules upon each other to generate movements of cilia and sperm.

Several different mutations can produce the Kartagener syndrome. In all cases the mutant gene disrupts the synthesis either of the dynein protein itself or of a protein that binds dynein to the microtubules,[66,70] causing any one of several types of morphological abnormalities in the ciliary axoneme: missing dynein arms (Fig. 47–4), abnormally short dynein arms, short spokes with no central sheath, missing central microtubules, or displacement of one of the nine peripheral microtubular doublets. The presence of any one of these abnormalities in the ciliary axoneme can presumably produce immobility of sperm and respiratory cilia, accounting for the clinical findings of infertility, sinusitis, and bronchiectasis. The molecular basis of the situs inversus is less certain, but it is reasonable to suppose that a malrotation of the visceral tissues occurs in the embryo when the ciliary movements of visceral epithelia do not occur.

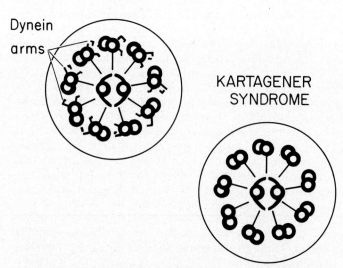

FIGURE 47–4 Schematic drawing of electron micrographs of cross sections through spermatozoa (or respiratory cilia), showing the location of dynein arms in normal cells and their absence in cells from a patient with the Kartagener syndrome. Normal motile spermatozoa and respiratory cilia possess nine micro-tubular doublets, each of which contains two dynein arms.

FAMILIAL PRIMARY PULMONARY HYPERTENSION (see also p. 839).

Primary pulmonary hypertension is a disorder characterized by increased arterial pressure in the pulmonary circulation caused by changes that appear to be intrinsic to the pulmonary vasculature. Although most cases are sporadic, a familial form also occurs.[71-76] The mode of inheritance appears to be autosomal dominant. Many large pedigrees showing vertical transmission through three generations have been reported.[71-76] Onset of symptoms occurs from early childhood to middle age. Except for a history of family involvement, affected individuals show no unique clinical features that allow them to be distinguished from patients with nongenetic forms of primary pulmonary hypertension. However, the presence of the disorder in a man should be a clue to the familial form, since the nongenetic forms occur much more frequently in women than in men.

Multifactorial Disorders

The chromosomal abnormalities and single-gene disorders that produce congenital heart disease account for no more than 5 to 10 per cent of all cases of congenital heart disease.[10] The remaining "garden-variety" cases are believed to result from developmental defects involving multiple genes and possibly environmental factors. Hence, the genetic predisposition in most cases of congenital heart disease is multifactorial.[77-79]

In general, congenital heart defects produced by chromosomal errors (as in Down syndrome) and by single-gene mutations (as in Noonan syndrome and Kartagener syndrome) are a part of a multisystem disorder. On the other hand, congenital heart defects with multifactorial inheritance typically occur as discrete lesions that are not part of a multisystem disorder.

As in other disorders showing multifactorial inheritance, the recurrence risk to first-degree relatives of a patient with a "garden-variety" type of congenital heart disease is considerably less than the 25 to 50 per cent risk that occurs in single-gene disorders. Although the relative risk to the siblings and offspring of such a patient is 3 to 40 times the estimated population frequency, the overall absolute risk for these first-degree relatives is low, in the range of 1 to 4 per cent.[77,80] Table 47–3 lists the expected recurrence

risk for siblings and offspring of patients with the 14 most common forms of congenital heart disease. Although these empirical data are useful in the genetic counseling of families that have had only one child with a congenital heart lesion, they do not apply in families with more than one affected person. When two first-degree relatives are affected, the recurrence risk is subsequent offspring doubles or triples; with three affected, the risks reach 10 to 20 per cent. When the first case is diagnosed in a given family, it is not possible to predict whether that family is at risk for multiple occurrences of congenital heart disease.

HEREDITARY DISORDERS OF CONNECTIVE TISSUE
Single-gene Disorders

The hereditary disorders of connective tissue are a group of diseases in which the predominant pathologic condition involves either the fibrous elements (such as collagen and elastin) or the nonfibrous elements (such as the mucopolysaccharide ground substance) of connective tissue throughout the body.[81] Since collagen, elastin, and mucopolysaccharides are all essential components of arteries and heart valves, it is not surprising that mutations affecting either the structure or the metabolism of these macromolecules would produce abnormalities in cardiac function. We now recognize 17 different hereditary connective tissue disorders in which cardiac involvement is a prominent feature. Each of these disorders is determined by a single-gene mechanism. The major clinical and genetic aspects of these disorders are summarized in Table 47–4.

As evident from this table, four types of cardiovascular disease—premature coronary artery disease, aortic regurgitation, mitral regurgitation, and abnormalities in the peripheral arteries—occur with high frequency in patients with the hereditary disorders of connective tissue. Of the 17 disorders listed in Table 47–4, 7 cause premature coronary artery disease (alkaptonuria, homocystinuria, pseudoxanthoma elasticum, idiopathic arterial calcification of infancy, Hurler syndrome, Hurler-Scheie compound, and Hunter syndrome), and 9 cause aortic or mitral regurgitation or both (Marfan syndrome, familial mitral valve prolapse syndrome, osteogenesis imperfecta, Hurler syndrome,

TABLE 47–3 EMPIRICAL RECURRENCE RISKS FOR SIBLINGS AND OFFSPRING OF PROBANDS WITH CONGENITAL HEART LESIONS

ABNORMALITY IN PROBAND	RISK TO SIBLINGS Number Affected/ Total Number	Per Cent	RISK TO OFFSPRING Number Affected/ Total Number	Per Cent
Ventricular septal defect	28/672	4.2	7/174	4.0
Patent ductus arteriosus	18/516	3.5	6/139	4.3
Tetralogy of Fallot	11/366	3.0	6/141	4.2
Atrial septal defect	11/380	2.9	5/199	2.7
Pulmonic stenosis	10/375	2.7	4/111	3.6
Aortic stenosis	8/361	2.2	4/103	3.9
Coarctation of aorta	5/281	1.8	7/253	2.7
Transposition of great vessels	4/229	1.7		
Atrioventricular canal	4/151	2.6		
Tricuspid atresia	1/98	1.0		
Ebstein anomaly	1/105	1.0		
Truncus arteriosus	1/86	1.2		
Pulmonic atresia	1/80	1.3		
Hypoplastic left heart	8/370	2.2		

(Modified from Nora, J. J., and Nora, A. H.: Circulation *57*:205–213, 1978; Nora, J. J., McGill, C. W., and McNamara, D. G.: Teratology *3*:325–330, 1970; and Nora, J. J., Dodd, P. F., Hattwick, M. A. W., et al.: J.A.M.A. *209*:2052–2053, 1969.)

TABLE 47–4   HEREDITARY DISORDERS OF CONNECTIVE TISSUE WITH CARDIOVASCULAR INVOLVEMENT

DISORDER	MAJOR CLINICAL MANIFESTATIONS *Cardiovascular*	*Noncardiovascular*	CARDIOVASCULAR INVOLVEMENT IN AFFECTED SUBJECTS *(Per Cent)*	TYPICAL AGE OF ONSET OF CARDIOVASCULAR ABNORMALITY	PRIMARY BIOCHEMICAL DEFECT	MECHANISM OF INHERITANCE	REFERENCES
Marfan syndrome	Aortic aneurysm and rupture, mitral regurgitation	Ectopia lentis, gracile habitus, arachnodactyly	50–70	Young adult	Not known	Dominant	81–83
Familial midsystolic click syndrome	Late systolic murmur, midsystolic clicks, abnormal EKG, mitral valve prolapse	None	100	Young adult	Not known	Dominant	84–87
Osteogenesis imperfecta	Aortic regurgitation	Multiple fractures, blue sclerae, otosclerosis, and deafness	Rare	Adult	Not known	Dominant	81
Ehlers-Danlos Type IV*	Rupture of aorta and other large arteries	Severe bruisability, rupture of bowel, minimal joint laxity	>95	Young adult	Deficient synthesis of Type III collagen	Dominant	81, 88–91
Cutis laxa, recessive form	Peripheral pulmonic stenosis, arterial aneurysms	Pendulous skin, hernias, severe emphysema	50	Infancy	Not known	Recessive	92
Alkaptonuria	Calcific aortic stenosis, generalized atherosclerosis	Black urine, pigmentation of cartilage, degenerative joint changes	50–75	Adult	Deficiency of homogentisic acid oxidase	Recessive	81
Homocystinuria*	Arterial and venous thrombosis, myocardial infarction, pulmonary embolism	Ectopia lentis, osteoporosis, mental retardation	>95	Young adult	Deficiency of cystathionine synthase	Recessive	81, 93–96
Pseudoxanthoma elasticum	Coronary artery disease, claudication, hypertension	Peau d'orange skin, retinal angioid streaks, gastrointestinal bleeding	50	Young adult	Not known	Dominant and recessive forms	81, 97–101
Idiopathic arterial calcification of infancy	Death from myocardial infarction in first 5 months of life, generalized calcification of peripheral arteries	None	100	Neonates	Not known	Recessive	102, 103
Mucopolysaccharidoses*					Abnormal degradation of mucopolysaccharidoses		81, 104, 105

Hurler-Scheie compound, Hunter syndrome, Morquio syndrome, Maroteaux-Lamy syndrome, and Type III mucolipidosis).

The Marfan syndrome and familial mitral valve prolapse syndrome are relatively common and are frequently encountered by cardiologists. Their genetic aspects are discussed here in detail. The 15 other inborn disorders listed in Table 47–4 are rare, each having a population frequency of 1 in 40,000 to 100,000 persons, and are not considered further in this chapter. Pertinent references in the literature are provided in the table.

MARFAN SYNDROME (see also p. 1665). Marfan syndrome is a generalized disorder of connective tissue that is inherited as an autosomal dominant trait. The cardinal manifestations consist of abnormalities of the eye (high-grade myopia and ectopia lentis), of the skeletal system (gangling habitus, arachnodactyly, pectus excavatum, and pectus carinatum), and of the cardiovascular system. In individual patients, all manifestations may not be present.[81]

Cardiac abnormalities occur in at least 60 per cent of affected adults.[81–83] The major cardiovascular lesion in adults is a dilatation of the aortic ring, the sinuses of Valsalva,

and the ascending thoracic aorta. Stretching of the aortic valve leads ultimately to aortic regurgitation, aortic dissection (Chap. 44), or both.

Among 505 unselected cases of aortic dissection, 74 occurred in patients under age 40. Twelve of these younger patients (16 per cent) had Marfan syndrome.[108] Aortic dissection is the most serious complication. Together with the other aortic valve abnormalities, it represents the leading cause of death. Most of the patients are young (in the early 30's) and in good health when dissection occurs.[109] In patients with Marfan syndrome, it has been suggested that propranolol may be useful in preventing aortic dissection by reducing dP/dt to low-normal levels.[110] Pregnancy greatly increases the risk of aortic dissection and rupture and hence poses a serious risk to life.[111,112] Although the basic defect leading to the weakening of the aortic wall is unknown, histological studies show a striking loss of elastic fibers in the media of the damaged aortic segment.[81]

Mitral regurgitation is a frequently encountered cardiac abnormality in affected adults.[81–83] The mitral regurgitation is usually due to redundant cusps and chordae tendineae, producing a "floppy" prolapsed mitral valve (p. 1089). Cineangiography usually shows retroversion of a redun-

TABLE 47–4 HEREDITARY DISORDERS OF CONNECTIVE TISSUE WITH CARDIOVASCULAR INVOLVEMENT Continued

DISORDER	MAJOR CLINICAL MANIFESTATIONS Cardiovascular	MAJOR CLINICAL MANIFESTATIONS Noncardiovascular	CARDIOVASCULAR INVOLVEMENT IN AFFECTED SUBJECTS (Per Cent)	TYPICAL AGE OF ONSET OF CARDIOVASCULAR ABNORMALITY	PRIMARY BIOCHEMICAL DEFECT	MECHANISM OF INHERITANCE	REFERENCES
					due to:		
Type 1-H Hurler syndrome*	Aortic and mitral regurgitation, coronary artery disease, cardiomyopathy	Corneal clouding, coarse features, mental retardation, early death	50–75	Before age 2	Deficiency of α-L-iduronidase (I-H allele)	Recessive	81, 104, 105
Type I-S, Scheie syndrome	Aortic regurgitation	Stiff joints, normal intelligence, corneal clouding	>95	Adult	Deficiency of α-L-iduronidase (I-S allele)	Recessive	81, 104, 105
Type I-H/S, Hurler-Scheie compound*	Aortic and mitral regurgitation	Phenotype intermediate between Hurler and Scheie syndromes	>95	Young adult	Deficiency of α-L-iduronidase (I-H and I-S alleles)	Recessive; genetic compound of Type I-H and I-S alleles	81, 104, 105
Type II, Hunter syndrome (severe)*	Aortic and mitral regurgitation, coronary artery disease, cardiomyopathy	No corneal clouding; milder course than in Type I-H, but death before age 15	>95	Childhood	Deficiency of sulfoiduronide sulfatase (severe allele)	X-linked	81, 104, 105
Type II, Hunter syndrome (mild)*	Aortic and mitral regurgitation, coronary artery disease	Survival to 30's and 50's, fair intelligence	>95	Young adult	Deficiency of sulfoiduromide sulfatase (mild allele)	X-linked	81, 104, 105
Type IV, Morquio syndrome*	Aortic regurgitation	Severe bone changes with gibbus and dwarfism, corneal clouding, normal intelligence	>75	Young adult	Deficiency of N-acetylhexosamine sulfate sulfatase	Recessive	81, 104, 105
Type VI, Maroteaux Lamy syndrome*	Aortic and mitral regurgitation	Corneal clouding, severe osseous changes, normal intelligence	>95	Childhood	Deficiency of arylsulfatase B	Recessive	81, 104, 105
Mucolipidosis, Type III, (pseudo-Hurler polydystrophy)*	Aortic and mitral regurgitation	Claw hand and stiff joints, coarse facies, kyphoscoliosis, corneal clouding, carpal tunnel syndrome, low normal intelligence	>95	Young adult	Deficiency of N-acetylglucosamine-1-phosphotransferase	Recessive	81, 106, 107

*Prenatal diagnosis is possible.

dant posterior mitral valve leaflet with regurgitation occurring in late systole. These patients typically manifest a late systolic murmur with or without mid- to late systolic clicks. In some patients the mitral regurgitation is severe and functionally significant. On the basis of echocardiographic findings, mitral prolapse may be more common than aortic regurgitation. Massive calcification of the mitral annulus is occasionally seen.[113] Less common complications include cystic disease of the lung, recurrent spontaneous pneumothorax, and bacterial endocarditis, which may be superimposed on minor changes of the heart valves.[81]

The cardiac manifestations of Marfan syndrome are more subtle and less severe in children than in adults.[83] The most common cardiac lesion in the pediatric age group is an isolated mitral regurgitation that is usually asymptomatic but can be very severe. In contrast to Marfan adults, affected children rarely manifest signs of aortic root disease. However, when aortic regurgitation is present, the patients show a rapidly deteriorating course. The overall mortality in one large study of children with Marfan syndrome was as high as 14 per cent.[83]

Although the basic defect has not been identified, the genetics of Marfan syndrome are well understood.[81] The disorder is inherited as an autosomal dominant trait with marked variability in clinical expression. In about 85 per cent of cases, one of the parents is affected. The other 15 per cent of cases occur sporadically and apparently represent new mutations occurring in the germ cells of one of the parents.[114] The average age of the fathers of those with sporadic cases is 7 years higher than that of the fathers of those having inherited cases. These data suggest that the new mutations occur in the father's germ cells and that their frequency increases with paternal age.[114]

Relatives at 50 per cent risk for having Marfan syndrome frequently request that studies be performed on them to determine whether they have it and are thus a risk of passing the mutant gene to their children. This may pose a problem for the physician, since some affected patients are asymptomatic and show no obvious features of the syndrome. Nevertheless, subtle manifestations can be detected in a high proportion of asymptomatic Marfan syndrome patients by performing three studies: echocardiography (looking for prolapse of the mitral valve and aortic root dilation), anthropometrical evaluation (measuring the upper and lower body segments), and ophthalmological examination (searching for ectopia lentis).[115,116]

FAMILIAL MITRAL VALVE PROLAPSE SYNDROME (see also p. 1089). Familial mitral valve prolapse syndrome is an autosomal dominant disorder characterized by ballooning or prolapse of the posterior mitral valve leaflet, which produces a midsystolic click and a late systolic murmur.[84-87] Since the initial delineation of the syndrome in 1963, myriad reports have appeared in the literature describing patients with this disorder. However, most of these reports have failed to take into account that prolapse of the mitral valve per se is etiologically a heterogeneous entity and that the dominantly inherited syndrome constitutes only one of its many causes.

A syndrome virtually identical to familial mitral valve prolapse syndrome has also been described in patients with Marfan syndrome, Turner syndrome, Ehlers-Danlos syndrome, hypertrophic obstructive cardiomyopathy, acute rheumatic fever, and coronary artery disease; following mitral commissurotomy; and in association with ruptured chordae tendineae and secundum atrial septal defect.[84,85] In these last-named disorders, prolapse of the mitral valve is considered a secondary phenomenon that results from a variety of abnormalities involving the mitral leaflets, chordae tendineae, papillary muscles, or mitral annulus. The clinical significance of the valvular dysfunction is usually subordinate to that of the primary disease process.

In contrast to the secondary causes of prolapse of the mitral valve, in familial mitral valve prolapse syndrome, the pathologic condition of the mitral valve almost always consists of a myxomatous degeneration.[84,85] Microscopy of involved leaflets shows replacement of the central fibrous tissue by metachromatically staining, loose, myxomatous material accompanied by fibroelastic thickening of the adjacent endocardium.[84]

A large degree of clinical variability appears in families affected with familial mitral valve prolapse syndrome. Affected females more often show clinical signs than do affected males. Symptoms of prolapse of the mitral valve can develop at any age and can range from mild to severe. Common presentations include palpitations, presyncope, syncope, chest pain, dyspnea, and/or fatigue.[84,85] The palpitations are usually due to atrial or ventricular arrhythmias. Sudden death is presumably due to ventricular arrhythmias. The major auscultatory findings typically consist of a nonejection click in midsystole or a late systolic murmur heard best at the cardiac apex or both.[84,85] Diagnosis can be confirmed by echocardiography or ventricular cineangiography. The major complications of the syndrome include bacterial endocarditis, severe mitral insufficiency, and life-threatening arrhythmias.[84,85]

The population frequency of the primary form of prolapse of the mitral valve has been reported to be as high as 6 to 17 per cent among apparently healthy young women.[117,118] These estimates, if correct, place prolapse of the mitral valve among the commonest of all cardiac abnormalities. Although an autosomal dominant mechanism appears to account for mitral valve prolapse in certain families,[84-87] the exact proportion of patients with the primary syndrome who owe their disease to a single mutant gene is unknown. Genetic studies designed to answer this question are made difficult by the presence of silent or asymptomatic prolapse in some subjects who are known to possess the abnormal gene.

CARDIOMYOPATHIES

Single-gene Disorders

At least ten single-gene–determined forms of cardiomyopathy are currently recognized. In some of these disorders, the myocardial disease dominates the clinical picture, as in Pompe disease, familial hypertrophic obstructive cardiomyopathy, and familial cardiomyopathy. In some, the cardiomyopathy occurs as part of a generalized metabolic disease, as in hemochromatosis and familial amyloidosis. In others, the cardiomyopathy occurs as part of a neuromyopathic syndrome, as in myotonic dystrophy, Duchenne muscular dystrophy, and Friedreich ataxia.

POMPE DISEASE (TYPE II GLYCOGEN STORAGE DISEASE) (see also p. 1051). Pompe disease is a rare inborn error of glycogen metabolism that results from an absence of the lysosomal enzyme acid α-1,4-glucosidase.[119] Once synthesized in cells, glycogen is degraded by several mechanisms, one of which involves a nonlysosomal phosphorylytic pathway that converts glycogen to glucose-6-phosphate. The other pathway involves hydrolysis of the glycogen to glucose within lysosomes. In the absence of the lysosomal acid maltase, large amounts of glycogen accumulate within lysosomes of tissues throughout the body including the heart. Since the nonlysosomal phosphorylytic pathway of glycogen breakdown is normal in Pompe disease, carbohydrate metabolism is normal and hypoglycemia does not occur.

The massive accumulation of glycogen in body tissues in Pompe disease leads to a characteristic clinical picture that becomes apparent within the first few months of life. Affected infants typically manifest feeding difficulty, inadequate weight gain, respiratory difficulty, hypotonia, atrophy of subcutaneous fat, enlarged tongue, and congestive heart failure.[119] Death from cardiac failure invariably occurs within the first year of life. The cardiomyopathy of Pompe disease is characterized by the absence of significant heart murmurs, the presence of massive cardiomegaly on chest roentgenograms, and the presence of several distinctive electrocardiographic findings. The latter include a short P-R interval (0.05 to 0.09 sec) and huge QRS complexes.[120]

Pompe disease is inherited as an autosomal recessive trait. The gene coding for lysosomal acid α-1,4-glucosidase is located on chromosome 17.[122] Because the disorder is quite rare (occurring with a population frequency of less than 1 in 100,000 persons[121]), about 20 per cent of affected cases are associated with parental consanguinity. As in most recessive disorders, the heterozygous parents manifest no detectable clinical abnormalities. Inasmuch as the lysosomal acid α-1,4-glucosidase enzyme is normally present in cultured amniotic fluid cells, prenatal diagnosis of homozygous affected fetuses is feasible and has successfully been carried out in couples who have a 25 per cent recurrence risk for having a second child with Pompe disease.[123]

FAMILIAL HYPERTROPHIC OBSTRUCTIVE CARDIOMYOPATHY (see also p. 1409). Familial hypertrophic obstructive cardiomyopathy is determined by an autosomal dominant mechanism. Recent studies of both the asymptomatic and the symptomatic relatives of patients with clinically apparent cases have demonstrated that asymmetrical septal hypertrophy, often without outflow obstruction, represents the most constant and characteristic feature of this disorder.[124,125] Asymmetrical septal hypertrophy is detected by echocardiography and is defined as the presence of a ventricular septum that is at least 30 per cent thicker than the posterobasal wall of the left ventricle.[124]

The mutant gene appears to be fully penetrant; that is, virtually all individuals who inherit the gene show asymmetrical septal hypertrophy. Nevertheless, the resulting clinical manifestations are variable from patient to patient.[124,125] In full-blown cases of hypertrophic obstructive cardiomyopathy, the asymmetrical septal hypertrophy progresses to ventricular outflow tract obstruction, and this, in turn, leads to the clinical findings of dyspnea, fatigability, angina, syncope, palpitations due to arrhythmias, and sudden death.[126] Patients with the complete syndrome, who typically come to medical attention between the ages of 20 and 30 years, probably represent no more than 20 per cent of all individuals affected with familial hypertrophic obstructive cardiomyopathy.[124] The other 80 per cent of subjects who have inherited the mutant gene show echocardiographic evidence of asymmetrical septal hypertrophy but manifest no clinical abnormalities (about 20 per cent of gene carriers) or show nonspecific electrocardiographic and auscultatory findings that are nondiagnostic (60 per cent of gene carriers).[124]

Many large pedigrees with familial hypertrophic obstructive cardiomyopathy have been reported in the literature, providing abundant evidence for autosomal dominant transmission.[126-129] The most impressive pedigree to date is that of a French-Canadian kindred in which the genealogical survey was extended to the original emigrant from France in the 1600's.[128] In family studies, echocardiography has demonstrated that 93 per cent of probands have an affected parent,[124] thus implying that no more than 7 per cent of cases of hypertrophic obstructive cardiomyopathy represent new mutations. This estimate agrees well with estimates of the limited extent to which this disorder reduces reproductive fitness.

A subgroup of families with unusually frequent premature deaths (termed "malignant" hypertrophic cardiomyopathy) has recently been identified.[129] Of the 69 first-degree relatives in these 8 families, 41 had clinical evidence of hypertrophic cardiomyopathy and 32 (78 per cent of those affected) died of heart disease before 50 years of age. Sudden and unexpected death occurred in 23 of the 32 patients.

The basic biochemical defect is unknown. Discovery of the mechanism of action of the mutant gene will undoubtedly provide insight into the biochemical and cellular basis of ventricular hypertrophy.

FAMILIAL CARDIOMYOPATHY (see also p. 1400). The designation familial cardiomyopathy is used to refer to an ill-defined and undoubtedly heterogeneous group of entities having the common denominators of cardiomegaly, congestive cardiomyopathy, and familial occurrence, suggestive of autosomal dominant inheritance. The major clinical manifestations of familial cardiomyopathy include cardiomegaly, congestive heart failure, arrhythmias, syncope, and sudden death. Angina pectoris and embolic episodes are also frequently noted. Electrocardiographic abnormalities, which include rhythm disturbances, left ventricular hypertrophy, intraventricular conduction defects, abnormal Q waves, and the Wolff-Parkinson-White pattern, are often present in affected individuals many years prior to signs of clinical deterioration.[130-135]

The prognosis is highly variable from person to person. Some affected individuals remain asymptomatic except for electrocardiographic abnormalities. Others die of intractable heart failure or of arrhythmias as young adults.[131] Histological examination of affected hearts typically reveals diffuse fibrosis with severe hypertrophy of the remaining muscle fibers.[130-135]

Although the autosomal dominant inheritance of familial cardiomyopathy is beyond doubt in certain pedigrees, there are no unique clinical manifestations of the mutant gene. Thus, in the patient who has a congestive cardiomyopathy and whose family history is not informative, it is difficult to know whether there is a 50 per cent risk of transmitting the disorder to children or whether the cardiomyopathy has a nongenetic etiology.

IDIOPATHIC HEMOCHROMATOSIS (see also p. 1425). Idiopathic hemochromatosis is a hereditary multisystem disorder characterized by the deposition of iron in the liver, pancreas, skin, and heart.[136,137] Clinical manifestations consist of cirrhosis, diabetes mellitus, hyperpigmentation, hypogonadism, cardiomyopathy, and a high incidence of hepatoma. The clinical manifestations are delayed for many years until iron overload has caused significant tissue damage and organ failure. The average diet in America allows a maximal routine iron balance of about 4 mg/per day in males.[137] The average age of overt clinical presentation is usually 40 years or older. Diagnosis is confirmed by the finding of an elevated serum iron concentration ($>$ 180 μg per cent), an elevated transferrin saturation ($>$ 80 per cent), an elevated serum ferritin level ($>$ 900 ng/ml), and an increase in the hepatic iron content ($>$ 600 μg/100 mg dry weight) in the absence of known causes of exogenous iron overload.

The major cardiac findings are rhythm and conduction disturbances and biventricular congestive heart failure, which occur separately or together.[136] The commonest arrhythmias are ventricular extrasystoles, paroxysmal atrial tachycardia and fibrillation, and atrioventricular block. The clinical manifestations of congestive failure include dyspnea, edema, ascites, and a large, globular cardiac silhouette on chest roentgenograms. Rarely, hemochromatosis simulates constrictive pericarditis (presumably because of the decrease in myocardial compliance caused by the iron infiltration of the myocardium), and in such patients a small or normal-sized heart is seen.

Cardiac manifestations are the presenting feature in only 15 per cent of cases, but approximately one-third of patients with hemochromatosis die from congestive heart failure.[137] Cardiac abnormalities are particularly prominent in young patients. Death usually follows within 1 year of onset. A program of repeated phlebotomy may alleviate congestive failure and increase survival in individual patients.

Idiopathic hemochromatosis has long been recognized to be an inherited disorder, yet its genetics remained, until recently, a controversial subject.[138,139] The difficulty in delineating the precise mode of inheritance arose for several reasons. First, the basic biochemical defect that causes excessive iron absorption from the intestine has not been defined, and thus no unequivocal method for identifying the genotype of affected individuals is available. Second, the phenotypic expression of the disease is highly variable and is greatly influenced by age, sex (the full-blown syndrome is 10 times more common in men than in women), and environmental factors that cause liver damage and promote iron absorption (such as alcoholism, hepatitis, and chronic malnutrition).

In some families parents are free of any evidence of disease, whereas one or more of their offspring become ill as middle-aged adults; this suggests classic autosomal recessive inheritance.[140,141] In other families, three successive generations have been involved, suggesting autosomal dominant inheritance.[142] Recent studies, however, have pointed out that the vertical transmission of full-blown cases of hemochromatosis is rare, even though it is not unusual to find minor derangements of iron metabolism in the children, siblings, and parents of affected individuals.[137] The most reasonable genetic hypothesis is that the overt cases represent individuals who are homozygous for an abnormal gene, and the individuals with minor abnormalities in iron metabolism are heterozygous carriers.[137]

The genetic hypothesis of autosomal recessive inheritance has recently been clarified by studies of HLA genotype in affected individuals and their relatives.[141-147] The gene causing hemochromatosis is situated close to the HLA-A locus on the short arm of chromosome 6. The gene is present in the heterozygous state in 8 to 10 per cent of Caucasian populations, with 1 in 333 individuals in the population being homozygotes.

Because of the close linkage between the hemochromatosis gene and the HLA loci, siblings with overt hemochromatosis usually have identical HLA alleles on both maternal and paternal chromosomes, i.e., they have the same HLA haplotypes. The most common haplotype in kindreds with hemochromatosis involves the A-3 allele and the B-14 allele (haplotype: HLA-A-3, B-14). However, other haplotypes also occur, thus indicating that the genetic locus for hemochromatosis is clearly distinct from any of the HLA loci. Among the affected homozygotes who have the HLA-A-3 alleles, 30 per cent are homozygous for the A-3 allele, and the remaining 70 per cent are heterozygous for the A-3 allele.[137]

The reason for the association between the HLA-A-3 allele and the hemochromatosis gene is unknown. This linkage possibly suggests a common ancestral origin of the hemochromatosis gene for all affected individuals who carry the HLA-A-3 allele. For example, a mutation leading to enhanced iron absorption may have arisen adjacent to the HLA-A locus on chromosome 6 of an individual who by chance carried the A-3 allele. Because of tight linkage, the two genes have not been separated by recombination over the years, thus explaining the high frequency of HLA-A-3 alleles among affected patients.

Removal of iron by repeated venesections (weekly for 3 years and every 3 to 4 months thereafter) or treatment with an iron chelating agent desferrioxamine or both prolongs survival, cures the cardiomyopathy, and may arrest the cirrhosis. Thus, it is incumbent upon the physician who diagnoses a patient with idiopathic hemochromatosis to identify all affected homozygotes among the siblings. This can be done by HLA typing in conjunction with in-

vestigation of plasma iron levels, ferritin levels, and total iron-binding capacity.[137] Prophylactic venesections in asymptomatic homozygotes should prevent clinical expression of the disorder.

FAMILIAL AMYLOIDOSIS (see also p. 1423).   Amyloid can affect the heart in several ways, including infiltration of the myocardium, infiltration of the walls of the coronary arteries, and deposition in the valves.[148] In most patients with cardiac amyloidosis, the condition does not appear to be inherited. Rather, it is associated with a systemic disorder, such as multiple myeloma, tuberculosis, or chronic osteomyelitis, or it occurs in a relatively high proportion of elderly people in the form of senile cardiac amyloidosis which is localized exclusively to the heart.[148,149] On the other hand, a dominantly inherited form of primary systemic amyloidosis has been reported in several families.[150,151] The predominant clinical feature in these families is cardiac involvement, which appears in the fifth decade of life as a restrictive cardiomyopathy, producing congestive heart failure and progressing to death in 3 to 6 years.

MYOTONIC DYSTROPHY (See also p. 1708).   Myotonic dystrophy (Steinert disease) is a multisystem disorder inherited as an autosomal dominant trait.[152] The characteristic clinical features include the presence of myotonia (especially in the hands), atrophy of the muscles of the face and the sternocleidomastoids (causing the expressionless "myopathic facies"), bilateral cataracts, frontal baldness, testicular atrophy, infertility or menstrual irregularities, hyperinsulinemia, hypercatabolism of immunoglobulins, and cardiac abnormalities.

The manifestations of the cardiac disease vary from asymptomatic electrocardiographic abnormalities to overt rhythm and conduction disturbances with heart failure. Abnormal electrocardiographic patterns have been reported in over 50 per cent of affected patients.[153-156] These abnormalities include sinus bradycardia, left-axis deviation, low-voltage T waves, atrial flutter and fibrillation, and AV conduction disturbances that vary from an innocuous prolonged P-R interval to complete AV block with Stokes-Adams attacks. In general, the systemic disease, which begins in the early 20's, is present for several years before cardiac manifestations become overt. Occasionally, however, the rhythm disturbances, conduction defects, or heart failure may become the chief presenting problem and dominate the clinical picture.

The best methods for identifying asymptomatic subjects at 50 per cent risk for ultimately developing the full-blown syndrome are slit-lamp examination (for lens changes), electromyography (for myotonic discharge), and measurement of serum immunoglobulins (for low IgG levels).[157] About 25 per cent of index subjects with myotonic dystrophy owe their disease to a new mutation.[157]

The gene causing myotonic dystrophy is linked to the gene *secretor*, which determines the secretion of the ABO blood group substances into blood fluids, including saliva and amniotic fluid.[158] This linkage relation makes it possible, in selected families, to perform amniocentesis for determination of secretor status of the fetus and thereby predict inheritance of the gene for myotonic dystrophy.[159]

DUCHENNE MUSCULAR DYSTROPHY (see also p. 1704).   As this disorder is inherited as an X-linked recessive trait, it occurs almost exclusively in males. It characteristically begins during the first 5 years of life. Initial involvement of the pelvic girdle muscles causes lumbar lordosis, a clumsy waddling gait, and pseudohypertrophy of the calves. Progression to other muscles is rapid, and most affected boys are confined to a wheelchair or bed by age 10 years.[160]

The severe and widespread nature of the skeletal muscle impairment generally overshadows the myocardial involvement, which is present in almost all cases. The electrocardiogram is characteristic in that a tall R wave in lead V_1 and deep Q waves in leads I, aV_1, and V_{5-6} are said to occur in no other form of muscular dystrophy.[161] In the majority of patients with Duchenne muscular dystrophy, the distinctive electrocardiogram is the only evidence of cardiac involvement. However, progressive heart failure may develop after years of cardiac stability, and a variety of arrhythmias occur, including labile sinus tachycardia, paroxysmal ventricular tachycardia, and atrial flutter.[161] At autopsy, the heart is not enlarged or hypertrophic. The cardinal pathological findings consist of left ventricular fibrosis and an arteriopathy involving small intramural coronary arteries.[161]

Although the underlying biochemical defect remains obscure, early skeletal muscle damage can be detected by release of the muscle enzyme creatine phosphokinase (CPK) into the serum, thus providing a useful diagnostic test for affected boys. Two-thirds of heterozygous carrier women also have elevated serum CPK levels, making this test useful in genetic counseling.[162] About one-sixth of asymptomatic carrier women show the distinctive electrocardiogram that is seen in affected boys.[163,164]

The sisters of affected boys often seek genetic counseling and carrier testing before planning their families. Recent studies have demonstrated the potential usefulness of measurements of CPK levels in fetal plasma as an accurate method for prenatal diagnosis of the disorder.[165] However, obtaining fetal blood samples is difficult, and the procedure is performed in very few centers.[165]

FRIEDREICH ATAXIA (see also p. 1711). Friedreich ataxia is a familial neuromuscular disorder, inherited as an autosomal recessive trait and characterized clinically by spinocerebellar ataxia, loss of deep tendon reflexes, skeletal deformities, and cardiomyopathy.[166] The one distinctive clinical sign is "Friedreich foot" (Fig. 50–13, p. 1712), a bilateral deformity characterized by *pes cavus* with hammertoes.

Electrocardiographic abnormalities have been found in over 90 per cent of cases and are present in young children close to the time of onset of the neurological disorder.[166–169] The most frequent electrocardiographic change is inversion of the T waves, especially in the left precordial leads but also in leads I, II, and aV_f. Labile sinus tachycardia is common, and rhythm disturbances, especially atrial fibrillation and paroxysmal supraventricular tachycardia, develop in late stages of the disease. Findings suggestive of biventricular hypertrophic obstructive cardiomyopathy have also been reported.[170,171] At autopsy, the heart shows muscle fiber hypertrophy, interstitial fibrosis, and obliterative disease of small intramural coronary arteries.[169]

The parents of affected patients, who are obligate heterozygotes, do not typically have clinically significant cardiac disease but occasionally may show electrocardiographic abnormalities and asymmetrical septal hypertrophy by echocardiography.[172]

Multifactorial Disorders

ENDOCARDIAL FIBROELASTOSIS (see also p. 1049). Endocardial fibroelastosis is a disease of infancy and early childhood characterized by thickening of the endocardium, especially of the left ventricle, with resulting cardiac hypertrophy and congestive heart failure. The primary form of the condition occurs in the absence of any other congenital cardiac abnormalities.[173,174] Like Pompe disease, primary endocardial fibroelastosis causes congestive heart failure and early death in infancy in the absence of cyanosis or significant murmurs.

The incidence of primary endocardial fibroelastosis in the United States is relatively high: 1 case in 5000 to 6000 live births.[175] The occurrence of the disorder among male and female siblings in certain families suggests that one form of endocardial fibroelastosis is due to autosomal recessive inheritance of a mutant gene.[175–177] In addition, an X-linked form of endocardial fibroelastosis has also been described. However, the majority of cases occur sporadically, and, when all family data are subjected to genetic analysis, the proportion of affected siblings is about 7 per cent, a number that is significantly below the expected 25 per cent for simple autosomal recessive inheritance.[176–178] The simplest hypothesis and the one most consistent with available data is that primary endocardial fibroelastosis is heterogeneous in etiology, some cases having a nongenetic cause, some cases being due to autosomal recessive or X-linked recessive inheritance, and most cases having a multifactorial etiology.[176–178]

The biochemical basis of one form of autosomal recessively inherited endocardial fibroelastosis has recently been traced to a severe deficiency of plasma and tissue carnitine.[179] This discovery was made in a family in which cardiomyopathy developed in four of five children, three of whom died suddenly and were found at autopsy to have endocardial fibroelastosis. Study of the surviving affected member of the kindred and autopsy of one of the deceased siblings revealed a 90 to 95 per cent reduction in the carnitine level in plasma, heart and skeletal muscle, and liver. Treatment of the affected child with oral L-carnitine improved myocardial function and reduced the cardiomegaly. The enzymatic basis for the carnitine deficiency in this family is not known. Although other patients with generalized carnitine deficiency have been described, their major clinical manifestation typically consists of progressive skeletal myopathy rather than cardiomegaly.[180] Further studies will be necessary to determine what proportion of patients with nonfamilial and familial forms of endocardial fibroelastosis owe their disease to carnitine deficiency.

CARDIAC ARRHYTHMIAS AND CONDUCTION DEFECTS
Single-gene Disorders

In addition to the familial cardiomyopathies that may occur with arrhythmias or conduction defects, a number of familial syndromes that primarily affect the pacemaking and conducting tissues of the heart have been described. Although familial aggregation has been reported for virtually every type of cardiac arrhythmia and conduction defect, in most cases the available genetic data are insufficient to determine whether the defect in a given family results from a single-gene mutation or a multifactorial genetic mechanism. Evidence for a single-gene mechanism is compelling, however, in several distinct syndromes.

JERVELL AND LANGE-NIELSEN SYNDROME (see also p. 781). This disorder is characterized by congenital deafness, syncope, prolonged Q-T interval, and sudden death.[181-184] Affected individuals are seen typically in childhood with congenital high-tone perceptive deafness, which is bilateral and severe, and fainting spells precipitated by exertion or nervousness. The electrocardiogram shows a prolonged Q-T interval and large T waves. The syncopal attacks are believed due to episodic ventricular arrhythmias or Stokes-Adams attacks. Administration of digitalis can reduce the Q-T interval and diminish the frequency of syncopal attacks. Since syncopal attacks are usually provoked by exercise, fear, or anger, affected children should be protected from physical and mental stress. At autopsy, histological abnormalities in the artery to the sinus node and to the AV node have been demonstrated.

The cardiac and auditory abnormalities appear to represent a pleiotropic expression of a single gene abnormality, which is inherited by an autosomal recessive mechanism.[185] The incidence of consanguinity among the parents of affected subjects is increased.[182] Although the heterozygotes are clinically normal, their electrocardiograms may show a mildly prolonged Q-T interval.[182] The overall incidence of homozygous affected individuals among all deaf children is about 1 case in 100, whereas among the general population it is about 1 case in 300,000 persons.[182,185]

ROMANO-WARD SYNDROME (see also p. 781). Romano-Ward syndrome is similar to Jervell and Lange-Nielsen syndrome in that affected individuals show a prolonged Q-T interval and an abnormal configuration of T waves on their electrocardiograms and are prone to ventricular fibrillation and sudden death.[186-190] The two syndromes are clinically and genetically distinct: Deafness is not a feature of Romano-Ward syndrome, and Romano-Ward syndrome is inherited as an autosomal dominant trait.

Patients are usually healthy except for episodes which may take one of three forms: (1) transient attacks of palpitation, numbness, or anginal chest pain without loss of consciousness; (2) sudden loss of consciousness, usually precipitated by exertion or emotional stress; or (3) sudden death. The disorder is predominantly a childhood illness, with onset usually before age 3 years. However, as in most autosomal dominant disorders, a marked variation in the degree of clinical expression occurs, and some affected subjects do not show clinical signs until age 30 years. In general, the later the age of onset, the milder the disease and the less the threat of sudden death. The molecular basis for the underlying abnormality is not known.

FAMILIAL HEART BLOCK (see also page 1014). At least two genetically distinct causes of heart block are currently recognized—one with a congenital onset and one with an adult onset. The congenital disorder is seen either at the time of birth or in early childhood as severe bradycardia due to complete AV block. The prognosis for the congenital form of familial heart block is extremely poor.

Most affected individuals die in the neonatal period. Autopsy of several cases has revealed an absence of the AV node as well as an absence of myocardial fibers in the lower part of the interatrial septum.[191,192]

Early studies suggested that congenital heart block was inherited as an autosomal recessive trait.[191,192] However, recent reports have shown that a large proportion of infants previously diagnosed as having the autosomal recessive form of congenital heart block are offspring of mothers who have systemic lupus erythematosus. The placental transfer of maternal immune complexes is presumed to cause damage to the fetal cardiac conduction system in utero.[193-195] In one study of congenital heart block, 14 of 22 affected children had been born to 11 mothers who had clinical or laboratory evidence of lupus.[194] Congenital heart block may thus represent a familial disease that is not genetic. The clinician should suspect the presence of lupus or a related collagen vascular disease in any mother who gives birth to an infant with congenital heart block.

Familial heart block of adult onset appears to be inherited as an autosomal dominant disorder with varying expressivity.[196-199] Affected individuals typically are seen between the ages of 30 and 50 years with one of the following conduction abnormalities: right bundle branch block alone, left-axis deviation alone, right bundle branch block and left-axis deviation, or complete heart block. Patients may also show atrial fibrillation, atrial flutter, or bidirectional tachycardia. It must be emphasized that affected individuals in the same family characteristically manifest different electrocardiographic patterns. The electrocardiogram in the adult form of familial heart block tends to show a wider QRS complex than is found in the congenital form of familial heart block. Left untreated without a pacemaker, most patients with the adult form of familial heart block ultimately develop syncopal episodes or die suddenly—hence the need for the physician to examine and treat asymptomatic relatives who are at 50 per cent genetic risk.

WOLFF-PARKINSON-WHITE SYNDROME (see also p. 712). The electrocardiographic features of this syndrome are the presence of a short P-R interval and a prolonged QRS, the latter being specifically characterized by a slurred upstroke of the R wave called a delta wave. Patients with Wolff-Parkinson-White (WPW) syndrome are especially prone to paroxysmal supraventricular tachycardia. Although the majority of patients with WPW syndrome do not have a familial disorder, a familial occurrence has been reported on numerous occasions.[200,201] In certain families, WPW syndrome occurs as a dominantly inherited disorder with no associated cardiac defects, whereas in other families it can occur in association with a dominantly inherited form of familial cardiomyopathy.[202]

CONSTRICTIVE PERICARDITIS
(See also Chap. 43)

MULIBREY NANISM. Mulibrey nanism is a rare autosomal recessive disorder in which constrictive pericarditis is one of the cardinal manifestations. Described for the first time in 1973, the syndrome was given the name mulibrey nanism to symbolize some of these protean features.

Mulibrey stands for *mu*scle, *li*ver, *br*ain, and *eyes*; nanism is derived from the Greek word for dwarf, *nanos*.[203,204] A more appropriate name would be "constrictive pericarditis with dwarfism" to emphasize the two most prominent and consistent features of the syndrome.

Growth failure is evident at the time of birth and is progressive. Affected infants show a triangular face often with hypocephaloid skull, muscular hypotonia, a peculiar squeaky voice, and yellowish dots and pigment dispersion in the ocular fundus. Of 28 patients described in the literature, 25 have shown clinical signs of pericardial constriction, as manifested by prominent neck veins, elevated right-heart pressures on cardiac catherization, and hepatomegaly.[203-208] About 30 per cent of the affected patients so far reported have had ascites, peripheral edema, and proven pericardial constriction necessitating treatment by pericardiotomy.[203-208] Microscopic examination shows a thickened pericardium with calcium deposits but without evidence of active inflammation.[208]

Twenty-four of the 28 reported cases have come from a sparsely settled area of Finland.[203,204] Two cases have been reported in Canadians,[206] one case in an American,[208] and one case in an Egyptian.[207] All the familial cases have been limited to siblings, and most of the single cases (three of the Finnish patients, the American patient, and the Egyptian patient) have been born to consanguineous parents. These observations strongly support autosomal recessive inheritance. The pathogenesis of this unique disorder is completely unknown.

CARDIAC TUMORS
(See also Chap. 42)

The two most common primary tumors of the heart, myxomas and rhabdomyomas, can occur with or without familial involvement. The nonfamilial cases could represent (1) the occurrence of nongenetic cases, (2) the sporadic occurrence of tumors owing to new single-gene mutations, or (3) the occurrence of only one homozygote in a sibship as in autosomal recessive inheritance. In general, patients with nonfamilial tumors tend to have a single tumor, whereas those with tumors of a genetic origin tend to have multiple tumors.

INTRACARDIAC MYXOMA (see also p. 1460). Most cases of intracardiac myxoma occur as sporadic cases without familial involvement. However, since 1971 at least five families with multiple affected members have been reported.[209-214] In three of the families, only siblings have been affected, suggesting autosomal recessive inheritance.[209-212] However, in two families autosomal dominant inheritance was suggested by the occurrence of myxomas in both a parent and one or more siblings.[213,214] Affected individuals typically come to attention between the ages of 20 and 40 years because of syncope or signs of systemic embolization. The unique feature of the familial myxoma syndrome, as distinct from the more common nonfamilial tumor, is the presence of multiple tumors that are frequently in atypical locations, such as the pulmonic valve and the right ventricle.

RHABDOMYOMA (see also p. 1461). At least 50 per cent of patients with a single rhabdomyoma of the heart and probably all patients with multiple cardiac rhabdomyomas have tuberous sclerosis.[215] This autosomal dominant disorder is characterized clinically by the following features: adenoma sebaceum of the skin, mental retardation, epilepsy, intracranial calcifications, cutaneous findings (shagreen patches, periungual fibromas, depigmented cutaneous areas), honeycomb lung, gliomas of the brain, retinal phakomas, mixed mesodermal tumors of the kidney, and multiple cardiac rhabdomyomas.[216,217] As in most autosomal dominant disorders, a wide range of variability in clinical expression from patient to patient occurs.

The most common clinical manifestations, present in at least 60 per cent of affected individuals, are adenoma sebaceum, epilepsy, mental retardation, shagreen patches, and depigmented cutaneous areas.[216,217] Multiple rhabdomyomas, although highly specific for tuberous sclerosis, are a relatively infrequent manifestation, with no more than 5 per cent of affected individuals developing clinically significant cardiac tumors. Although the rhabdomyomas can occur at any age, they typically come to clinical attention in the neonatal period.[215] The typical patient with rhabdomyomas either shows signs of cardiac failure in the first few days of life or has severe arrhythmias.[215] Some rhabdomyomas may undergo neoplastic change to rhabdomyosarcoma.

CORONARY ARTERY DISEASE
(See also Chap. 35)

Evidence that genetic factors contribute to the pathogenesis of coronary atherosclerosis is based on observations of four types: (1) differences in prevalence among genetically different groups living under similar environmental circumstances;[218] (2) familial aggregation in which first-degree relatives of index coronary patients less than 60 years of age show a five- to sevenfold increased risk of death from myocardial infarction, compared with controls;[219,220] (3) higher concordance for myocardial infarction in identical twins as opposed to fraternal twins (for female twin pairs: 44 per cent concordance for monozygotic twins and 14 per cent for dizygotic twins);[221] and (4) association with one or more genetically determined risk factors, such as hypercholesterol-emia, hypertriglyceridemia, diabetes mellitus, hypertension, obesity, personality type, and distribution of coronary vasculature.[222-224,224a]

In most families that seem genetically predisposed to coronary artery disease by history, the nature of the genetic factors underlying this predisposition is obscure. Most patients with coronary artery disease have inherited multiple predisposing genes that interact with multiple environmental factors to produce the disease. In these patients atherosclerosis does not have a single cause. Yet treatment of one of the predisposing factors, such as mild hypertension, hypercholesterolemia, or smoking, will likely slow the progression of the disease.

TABLE 47–5   SINGLE GENE DISORDERS THAT PREDISPOSE TO PREMATURE CORONARY ARTERY DISEASE

DISORDER	TYPICAL AGE FOR MYOCARDIAL INFARCTION	PRIMARY BIOCHEMICAL DEFECT	MECHANISM OF INHERITANCE	ESTIMATED POPULATION FREQUENCY	REFERENCES
Familial hypercholesterolemia		Defective cell surface receptor for plasma LDL	Dominant		7, 225–227
Heterozygous form	Adult			1 in 500	
Homozygous form*	Childhood			1 in 1,000,000	
Multiple lipoprotein-type hyperlipidemia					
(Familial combined hyperlipidemia	Adult	Not known	Dominant	1 in 200	225, 227
Familial hypertriglyceridemia	Adult	Not known	Dominant	1 in 300	225, 227
Familial dysbetalipoproteinemia	Adult	Deficiency of Apo E-III	Recessive	1 in 40,000	225, 227
Hurler syndrome, Type I-H mucopolysaccharidosis*	Childhood	Deficiency of α-L -iduronidase	Recessive	1 in 40,000	81,104
Hunter syndrome, Type II mucopolysaccharidosis*	Childhood	Deficiency of sulfoiduronide sulfatase	X-linked	1 in 30,000	81,104
Homocystinuria*	Young adult	Deficiency of cystathionine synthase	Recessive	1 in 75,000	81, 93–95
Pseudoxanthoma elasticum	Young adult	Not known	Dominant and recessive	1 in 100,000	81, 101
Alkaptonuria	Adult	Deficiency of homogentisic acid oxidase	Recessive	1 in 100,000	81
Werner syndrome	Adult	Not known	Recessive	1 in 500,000	228, 229
Fabry disease*	Young adult	Deficiency of α-galactosidase A	X-linked	1 in 40,000	230, 231
Cholesteryl ester storage disease*	Young adult	Deficiency of lysosomal acid lipase	Recessive	1 in 1,000,000	232
Arterial calcification of infancy	Neonates	Not known	Recessive	1 in 1,000,000	102, 103

*Prenatal diagnosis is possible.

In some patients coronary artery disease is produced by a single abnormal gene that has a major effect. At least 13 different single-gene disorders, and hence at least 13 different mutant genes, are known to predispose to premature coronary artery disease (Table 47–5). The most common of these single-gene disorders are those that produce hyperlipidemia. At least 20 per cent of consecutively studied survivors of acute myocardial infarction manifest one of these common autosomal dominant forms of familial hyperlipidemia: familial hypercholesterolemia, familial hypertriglyceridemia, or multiple lipoprotein–type hyperlipidemia.[225] The other monogenic hyperlipidemia that predisposes to coronary artery disease, familial dysbetalipoproteinemia (Type 3 hyperlipidemia), is much less common, occurring in only about 1 in 500 unselected survivors of myocardial infarction.[225] These four monogenic forms of hyperlipidemia are discussed in the next section.

In addition to the familial hyperlipidemias, at least nine inborn errors of metabolism are seen, in which coronary narrowing and occlusion are often part of the clinical syndrome, e.g., Hunter syndrome, Hurler syndrome, homocystinuria, alkaptonuria, pseudoxanthoma elasticum, Werner syndrome, idiopathic arterial calcification of infancy, cholesteryl ester storage disease, and Fabry disease (Table 47–5). The mechanism for the coronary occlusion differs for each disorder and is directly related to the action of the particular gene. For example, in the Hunter and Hurler syndromes (p. 1670), mucopolysaccharides accumulate in the coronary vessels, whereas in Fabry disease, glycolipids accumulate (p. 1425). Seven of these inborn errors are inherited as autosomal recessive traits (Table 47–5). Although the homozygous form of each condition occurs rarely, with incidences ranging from 1 to 40,000 (homocystinuria) to 1 in 500,000 (Werner syndrome), the estimated combined frequency for the heterozygous carriers of these seven genes is quite significant, involving somewhere between 1 in 30 and 1 in 100 persons in the population. It will therefore be important to determine whether any of the genes for these seven inborn errors can significantly predispose its heterozygous carriers to develop premature coronary atherosclerosis. No such data are currently available.

Single-gene Disorders Causing Hyperlipidemia and Premature Atherosclerosis

Four monogenic diseases exist in which hyperlipidemia results from a discrete inborn error of metabolism affecting the synthesis, degradation, or structure of a plasma lipoprotein. Each of these single-gene diseases predisposes to coronary atherosclerosis. Together, these diseases are responsible for about 20 per cent of myocardial infarctions that occur before the age of 60.[225] To provide a conceptual background for discussion of these disorders, a brief explanation of normal lipoprotein transport is necessary (for review, see references 233 and 234).

The plasma lipoproteins are globular particles of high molecular weight that transport triglycerides and cholesteryl esters. Each lipoprotein contains a nonpolar core in which cholesteryl ester and triglyceride molecules are packed to form an oil droplet (Fig. 47–5). Surrounding the core is a polar surface coat composed predominantly of phospholipids and unesterified cholesterol. Each lipoprotein also contains specific proteins (termed *apoproteins*) that bind to enzymes or transport proteins, directing the lipoprotein to its sites of metabolism.

The lipoproteins of human plasma can be divided into five major classes, which are discussed in detail in Chapter

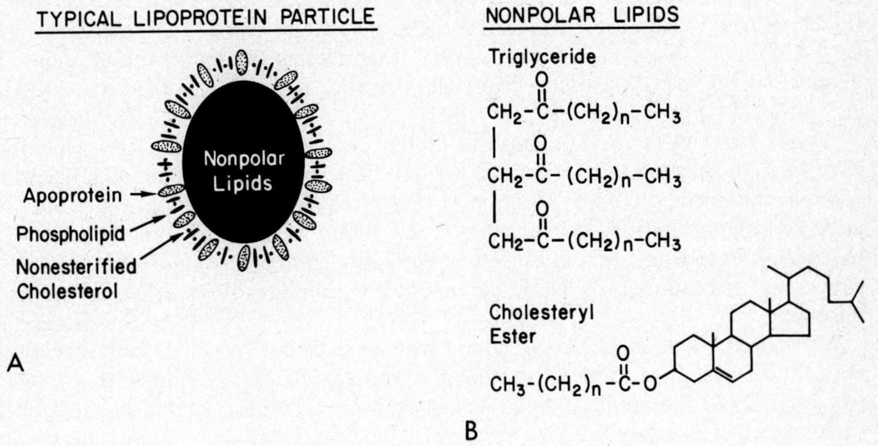

FIGURE 47–5 *A*, Diagrammatic representation of the structure of a typical plasma lipoprotein particle. The *core* of the spherical lipoprotein particle is composed of two nonpolar lipids, triglyceride and cholesteryl ester, which are present in different lipoproteins in varying amounts. The nonpolar core is surrounded by a *surface coat* composed primarily of phospholipids. Apoproteins are exposed at the surface and extend into the core. Variable amounts of unesterified cholesterol are interdigitated with the phospholipids of the surface coat. The quantitative composition of each of the different classes of lipoprotein particles in human plasma is discussed in Chapter 34 (see Fig. 34-3). *B*, Structures of the two nonpolar lipids, triglyceride and cholesteryl ester. In order for these nonpolar lipids to be assimilated into tissues, the ester bonds between the fatty acids and either glycerol (triglycerides) or cholesterol (cholesteryl esters) must be broken by lipoprotein lipase and the lysosomal cholesteryl esterase, respectively.

35. As shown in Table 35–3, p. 1210, each of these five lipoprotein classes differs from the others in the relative proportion of cholesteryl ester and triglyceride in the core, in the nature of its apoproteins, and in density, size, and electrophoretic mobility.[235]

A model showing the salient features of plasma lipoprotein transport is illustrated in Figure 47–6. Lipoproteins transport lipids that are absorbed from the intestine as well as those that are synthesized within the body.[233,234] Within the intestine, cholesterol and triglycerides are incorporated into large lipoprotein particles called *chylomicrons*. After they enter the bloodstream, the chylomicrons bind to an enzyme, *lipoprotein lipase*, which is adherent to capillary walls in adipose tissue and muscle. This enzyme hydrolyzes the triglycerides of the chylomicrons. The liberated fatty acids enter the underlying adipocytes or muscle cells, where they are either reesterified to triglycerides for storage or oxidized for energy.

After the triglycerides are removed, the remainder of the chylomicron dissociates from the capillary wall and reenters the circulation, where it is now designated as a *chylomicron remnant*. The chylomicron remnant is relatively poor in triglyceride and enriched in cholesteryl esters. It is also enriched in an important protein called *apoprotein E.* Chylomicron remnants travel to the liver, where they are taken up with great efficiency as a result of the binding of the apoprotein E to receptors on the surface of hepatocytes. Overall, the two-step pathway of chylomicron metabolism delivers dietary triglyceride to adipose tissue and muscle and dietary cholesterol to the liver.[233,234]

In the liver the metabolism of dietary fat and endogenously synthesized fat is coordinated to supply needed amounts of fuel and cholesterol to body tissues despite fluctuations in dietary intake. To supply cholesterol and triglcerides to body tissues, the liver incorporates them into *very low-density lipoproteins (VLDL)*.

VLDL particles are triglyceride-rich and thus resemble chylomicrons, although they are smaller in size. The triglycerides of VLDL are removed through interaction with lipoprotein lipase. The cholesteryl ester–rich remnant of VLDL metabolism is released from the endothelial wall and reenters the circulation, where it is designated *intermediate-density lipoprotein (IDL)*. Although it is similar in structure to the chylomicron remnant, the IDL particle

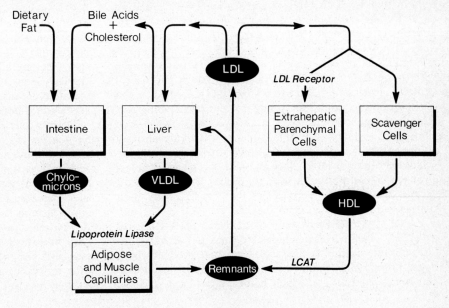

FIGURE 47–6 Model for plasma lipoprotein transport in humans. The details of this model are discussed in the text. VLDL=very low-density lipoprotein; LDL=low-density lipoprotein; HDL=high-density lipoprotein; LCAT=lecithin: cholesterol acyltransferase.

has a different fate. Instead of being taken up by the liver, the IDL particle remains in the circulation, where the last traces of triglyceride are removed, and the particle is converted into *low-density lipoprotein (LDL)*. During this conversion, all of the apoproteins leave the particle, with the exception of apoprotein B.

About two-thirds to three-fourths of the cholesterol in normal human plasma is contained within LDL particles. LDL is the particle whose elevation is most frequently related to atherosclerosis. When patients are found to have hypercholesterolemia, this is almost always due to an elevation in the number of LDL particles per milliliter of plasma.

In normal humans LDL circulates with a half-time of about 1.5 days. It is metabolized in liver and extrahepatic tissues. LDL is metabolized by at least two pathways. One pathway involves specific *LDL receptors*, which are located on the surface of liver and extrahepatic cells. The receptor recognizes the *apoprotein B* component of LDL. Binding leads to the uptake and degradation of LDL through a process called *receptor-mediated endocytosis*. This process liberates cholesterol, which all cells need for synthesis of new plasma membranes and which specialized cells need for synthesis of steroid hormones and bile acids.[234]

In normal humans the LDL receptor mediates the degradation of one-third to two-thirds of the LDL particles that are metabolized each day. The remainder of LDL is degraded by receptor-independent pathways. Some of this degradation is believed to occur in macrophages and cells of the reticuloendothelial system, which degrade all plasma proteins. In contrast to the receptor-mediated pathway, which supplies cholesterol to cells for specific metabolic purposes, the *scavenger cell pathway* functions primarily to clear plasma of excess proteins.[233,234,236]

As the membranes of parenchymal cells and scavenger cells undergo turnover and as cells die and are renewed, cholesterol is released into the plasma, where it binds to *high-density lipoprotein (HDL)*. When it leaves the tissues, cholesterol is in an unesterified form. For transport in plasma, the cholesterol must be esterified; that is, a fatty acid must be attached in ester linkage to the cholesterol. This esterification reaction occurs in the plasma. The cholesterol that binds to HDL is acted upon by a circulating enzyme called *lecithin:cholesterol acyltransferase (LCAT)*. The cholesteryl esters that are formed by this enzyme are quickly transferred to VLDL and LDL particles in plasma.[237] This completes a cycle by which extrahepatic cells take up cholesterol from LDL and then return cholesterol to new particles of LDL as they are being formed in the plasma. This continuous cycling of cholesterol into and out of tissues accounts for a large fraction of the plasma cholesterol in humans.[234] This explains why acute changes in dietary cholesterol have relatively small effects on the plasma cholesterol level, since most of the plasma cholesterol represents molecules that are cycling into and out of various tissues and not molecules that have recently been synthesized or absorbed from the diet.[234]

FAMILIAL HYPERCHOLESTEROLEMIA (see also p. 1214). Familial hypercholesterolemia is the outstanding example of a single-gene mutation that produces both hypercholesterolemia and atherosclerosis. It is an autosomal dominant trait for which homozygotes exist. Hetero-

zygotes for familial hypercholesterolemia number about 1 in 500 persons in the population, making this disease one of the most common disorders that is caused by a single mutant gene. Homozygotes for familial hypercholesterolemia are rare; they occur at a frequency of 1 in one million.[7,227]

The inherited defect in familial hypercholesterolemia lies in the gene for the cell-surface LDL receptor. Heterozygotes inherit one mutant gene for the receptor and one normal gene. Their cells are able to produce half the normal number of receptors. Homozygotes inherit two copies of the mutant gene. Their cells can produce few, if any, LDL receptors. The heterozygous and homozygous forms of the disease differ in severity. Heterozygotes have 2- to 3-fold elevations of plasma LDL, whereas homozygotes have 6- to 10-fold elevations. Heterozygotes develop myocardial infarctions typically in their 30's and 40's, whereas homozygotes usually develop mycardial infarctions before the age of 20.

Clinical Features

Heterozygous Familial Hypercholesterolemia. At the time of birth, these individuals have two- to three-fold elevation in the LDL-cholesterol level, which persists throughout life.[238] This hypercholesterolemia leads to cholesterol deposition in arteries (producing atheromas) and in tendons (producing xanthomas).

A number of studies have carefully documented the incidence of premature coronary artery disease in heterozygotes. In England, Slack found that the mean onset of coronary artery disease was 43 years for heterozygous men and 53 years for heterozygous women.[239] Eighty-five per cent of the affected males and 58 per cent of the affected females had sustained a myocardial infarction by age 60. In Denmark, Jensen et al. found that the incidence of coronary artery disease among heterozygotes over a 20-year period (32 per cent) was 25 times greater than among unaffected relatives (1.3 per cent).[240]

In the United States, familial hypercholesterolemia heterozygotes constitute about 5 per cent of all patients who have a myocardial infarction.[225] Stone et al. found that the cumulative probability of coronary artery disease by age 40 in male heterozygotes was 16 per cent.[241] By age 60 it had risen to 52 per cent, as opposed to 12.7 per cent in unaffected men. Female heterozygotes showed an incidence of coronary artery disease of 33 per cent by age 60, compared with only 9 per cent in unaffected females. Thus, despite the presence of the same genetic abnormality and similarly elevated plasma LDL levels, heterozygous women manifest coronary artery disease less often and at a later age than do heterozygous men.

Despite this marked increase in the frequency of coronary artery disease, familial hypercholesterolemia heterozygotes do *not* appear to have an increased frequency of cerebral vascular disease or of hypertension. The incidence of peripheral vascular disease is possibly elevated in familial hypercholesterolemia heterozygotes, but not in so striking a fashion as the incidence of coronary artery disease. In contrast, patients with familial dysbetalipoproteinemia have an increased incidence of both coronary artery disease and peripheral vascular disease (see below). Patients with dysbetalipoproteinemia accumulate IDL particles in plasma, whereas familial hypercholesterolemia patients ac-

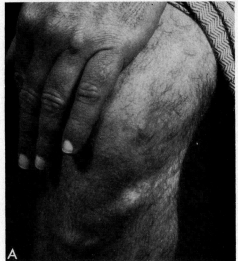

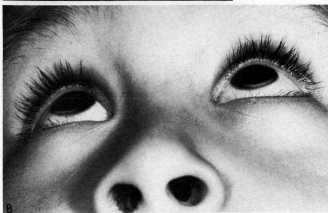

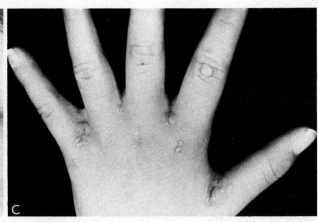

FIGURE 47-7 Forms of xanthomas and other lipid deposition frequently seen in patients with familial hypercholesterolemia. Tendon xanthomas (*A*) and arcus corneae (*B*) occur in both heterozygotes and homozygotes. Cutaneous planar xanthomas (*C*), which usually have a bright orange hue, occur in homozygotes and not in heterozygotes.

cumulate LDL particles. It is possible that the LDL particles have a greater toxicity for coronary arteries than for peripheral arteries, whereas IDL particles are equally toxic for both types of vessels.

Familial hypercholesterolemia heterozygotes also have tendon xanthomas, which are nodular swellings that may involve the Achilles tendon and various tendons about the knee, elbow, and dorsum of the hand (Fig. 47–7*A*). Like the atheromas, the xanthomas consist of massive deposits of cholesterol, apparently derived from the deposition of LDL particles. The cholesterol is located as amorphous extracellular deposits as well as vacuoles within scavenger cells (macrophages) that have invaded the lesion. The latter becomes so swollen with lipid droplets that they are termed foam cells.

In familial hypercholesterolemia heterozygotes, cholesterol deposits are also formed in the soft tissue of the eyelid, producing xanthelasma, and within the cornea, producing arcus cornae (Fig. 47–7*B*). Whereas tendon xanthomas are diagnostic of familial hypercholesterolemia, xanthelasma and arcus corneae are not specific. The latter also occur in many adults with normal plasma lipid levels. The incidence of tendon xanthomas in familial hypercholesterolemia increases with age, but no more than 75 per cent of affected heterozygotes display this sign.[227]

Homozygous Familial Hypercholesterolemia. Homozygotes have marked elevations in the plasma level of LDL from birth, the plasma cholesterol level usually being six-

to eightfold above normal. A unique type of planar cutaneous xanthoma is often present at birth and always develops within the first 6 years of life.[227,242] These yellow xanthomas occur at points of trauma, such as over the knees, elbows, and buttocks. They almost always occur in the interdigital webs of the hands, particularly between the thumb and index finger (Fig. 46–7*C*). Tendon xanthomas, arcus corneae, and xanthelasma also occur in homozygotes.

Coronary artery atherosclerosis in homozygotes is rapidly progressive. Angina pectoris, myocardial infarction, or sudden death occur commonly in homozygotes between the ages of 5 and 30. One homozygote is even recorded as having had an acute myocardial infarction as early as 18 months of age. Very few homozygotes survive past age 30.[9,227]

In homozygotes, severe atherosclerosis occurs not only in the coronary arteries but also in the thoracic and abdominal aorta as well as in the major pulmonary arteries.[227,243] Microscopic examination of the coronary and pulmonary arterial lesions in these children and young adults shows typical atherosclerotic plaques as well as a striking intimal infiltration of xanthomatous foam cells and cholesterol clefts that are reminiscent of the histological appearance of a tendon xanthoma.[243,244] Atheromatous and xanthomatous involvement of the aortic valve is another characteristic cardiac manifestation observed in the homozygote. The deposition of cholesterol frequently produces significant aortic stenosis, which in turn causes congestive heart failure.[243,243a,245] In at least six homozygotes, necropsy has confirmed the presence of an aortic valve lesion, and in several of these cases histological studies have demonstrated cholesterol clefts and foam cells in the aortic valve cusps, at the same time excluding an associated rheumatic valvulitis or congenital bicuspid valve.[227,243]

Xanthomatous plaquing and thickening of the endocardial surfaces of the mitral valve and endocardium have also been observed in the homozygote and may explain the clinical findings of mitral regurgitation and mitral stenosis that are occasionally reported.[243] Since the homozygote often has painful joints, a persistently elevated sedimentation rate (due to the high plasma LDL level), and cardiac murmurs, a misdiagnosis of acute rheumatic fever may easily be made.[246] Diffuse xanthomatous infiltration of the myocardium is occasionally mentioned as another pathological lesion in the homozygote,[243] but this has not been well-documented.

In contrast to the disorders causing hypertriglyceridemia, in familial hypercholesterolemia, obesity and diabetes mellitus do not occur with increased frequency in either the homozygote or the heterozygote. A slender body habitus is the general rule.

Pathogenesis. The primary defect in familial hypercholesterolemia resides in the gene for the LDL receptor (Fig. 47–5). Three types of mutant alleles at the LDL receptor locus have been described.[247,248] The most common mutant allele—designated R^{b^0}, or receptor-negative—specifies a gene product that is nonfunctional. Second in frequency is a mutant allele—designated R^{b^-}, or receptor-defective—that produces a receptor possessing only 1 to 10 per cent of normal LDL-binding activity. The third type of mutant allele, which is very rare, produces the so-called internalization defect; it is designated R^{b^+,i^0} and produces a receptor that binds LDL normally but is unable to transport the receptor-bound lipoprotein into the cell. The cells of phenotypic homozygotes show total or nearly total inability to bind or take up LDL; they possess two mutant alleles at the LDL receptor locus. The cells of heterozygotes are able to bind and take up LDL at one-half the normal rate;[247] they have one normal allele and one of the three mutant alleles at the LDL receptor locus. LDL catabolism is blocked, and the level of LDL in plasma rises in a manner that is inversely proportional to the reduction in LDL receptors.[236,249] In homozygotes an increased production of LDL has also been noted.[250,251] In familial hypercholesterolemia homozygotes, a large fraction of circulating LDL is secreted directly from the liver into the plasma, in contrast to normal individuals, in whom all plasma LDL appears to be derived from VLDL.[252] This combination of an overproduction and reduced catabolism of LDL is responsible for the high LDL levels in affected patients.[236,249]

The LDL level rises six- to eightfold above normal in homozygotes and two- to threefold above normal in heterozygotes. The elevated LDL level causes an increase in the uptake of LDL by scavenger cells, which do not utilize the LDL receptor in both types of subjects, and, as a consequence, LDL-cholesterol accumulates in these macrophage-like cells at various sites in the body, such as in tendon, producing xanthomas. The accelerated coronary atherosclerosis characteristic of familial hypercholesterol-

emia also results from the high LDL levels that penetrate the artery wall following endothelial damage. The large quantities of LDL that infiltrate the artery wall present a load of lipoproteins that is greater than can be cleared from the interstitial space by the scavenger cells, ultimately resulting in atherosclerosis (Chap. 34). There is also evidence that the high LDL levels may enhance the growth of the atherosclerotic plaques by accelerating the aggregation of platelets at sites of endothelial injury.[253]

Diagnosis. The finding of an isolated elevation of plasma cholesterol with a normal concentration of plasma triglycerides suggests the diagnosis of heterozygous familial hypercholesterolemia. Such an elevation in plasma cholesterol is due to an isolated elevation in the plasma concentration of LDL (Type IIA hyperlipoproteinemia) in nearly all cases. However, it must be appreciated that most individuals with Type IIA hyperlipoproteinemia have, rather than familial hypercholesterolemia, a form of polygenic hypercholesterolemia that puts them on the upper end of the bell-shaped curve for the general population.[227] As noted below, Type IIA hyperlipoproteinemia may be caused by the disease multiple lipoprotein–type hyperlipidemia. As shown in Table 35–8, p. 1213, hypothyroidism and nephrotic syndrome, can also cause Type IIA hyperlipoproteinemia.

Among individuals with a Type IIA lipoprotein pattern, those with heterozygous familial hypercholesterolemia can usually be distinguished from those with polygenic hypercholesterolemia and multiple lipoprotein–type hyperlipidemia. In familial hypercholesterolemia, the plasma cholesterol level tends to be higher than in the other two disorders. Thus, a plasma cholesterol level in the range of 350 to 400 mg/dl is much more suggestive of heterozygous familial hypercholesterolemia than of the other disorders. However, cholesterol levels of 285 to 350 mg/dl are not diagnostic and may be observed in many patients with heterozygous familial hypercholesterolemia as well as with other disorders. Tendon xanthomas do not occur typically in patients with forms of hyperlipidemia other than familial hypercholesterolemia. Other family members should be surveyed when the diagnosis is in doubt. The penetrance of the gene is extremely high in familial hypercholesterolemia, with 50 per cent of first-degree relatives showing an elevated plasma cholesterol level. Hypercholesterolemia in childhood is characteristic of familial hypercholesterolemia but not of the other aforementioned disorders.[227,233]

A small fraction, approximately 10 per cent, of heterozygotes with familial hypercholesterolemia have, in addition to the raised cholesterol level, an elevated plasma triglyceride level (Type IIB pattern). This condition is difficult to differentiate from multiple lipoprotein–type hyperlipidemia. However, the presence of a tendon xanthoma or a hypercholesterolemic child in the family favors the diagnosis of heterozygous familial hypercholesterolemia.

The diagnosis of *homozygous familial hypercholesterolemia* can readily be established. Often a dermatologist is the first to see these patients in childhood because of obvious cutaneous xanthomas. Occasionally, the development of angina pectoris due to premature coronary atherosclerosis or a syncopal episode caused by xanthomatous aortic stenosis are the presenting features. A cholesterol level greater than 600 mg/dl with a normal triglyceride level in a nonjaundiced child suggests this diagnosis. Both parents should have heterozygous familial hypercholesterolemia with moderately elevated cholesterol levels.

The diagnosis of both heterozygotes and homozygotes with familial hypercholesterolemia can be established in specialized laboratories by direct measurement of the number of LDL receptors on freshly isolated blood lymphocytes[254] or cultured skin fibroblasts.[226] The finding of an absence of LDL receptors on cultured amniotic fluid cells has permitted the diagnosis of homozygous familial hypercholesterolemia in utero.[255]

Treatment. Every effort should be made to lower the plasma LDL level into the normal range, since atherosclerosis in this disorder is a consequence of the longstanding elevation of plasma LDL levels. Patients should be placed on a diet that is low in cholesterol and saturated fats and high in polyunsaturated fats (p. 1225); this usually results in a 10 to 15 per cent drop in the plasma cholesterol level.[227,256]

When dietary therapy fails to lower the cholesterol levels to the normal range, bile acid–binding resins, such as cholestyramine or colestipol (p. 1226), should be added to the regimen. These resins trap the bile acids that are secreted by the liver into the intestine and transport them into the feces. The initial result of this treatment is a dramatic loss of cholesterol from the body, since the body responds to bile acid depletion by converting additional cholesterol into bile acids. However, subjects with familial hyperlipoproteinemia respond to this loss of cholesterol stores with a compensatory enhancement of cholesterol synthesis by the liver, which ultimately limits the long-term success of this therapy. However, the addition of nicotinic acid may help to block this compensatory increase in hepatic cholesterol synthesis.[227,256] The extent of reduction in plasma cholesterol level that is usually achieved in heterozygotes is in the range of 25 per cent with the combination of diet and bile acid–binding resins, and nicotinic acid allows the addition of a further lowering of the cholesterol levels. Gastrointestinal bloating, cramps, and constipation are the major side effects of bile acid–binding resins, whereas hepatotoxicity, flushing, and headaches are the major side effects of nicotinic acid. Partial ileal bypass has the same functional effect as bile acid–binding resins, i.e., it causes a loss of bile acids in the stool and results in a moderate to marked lowering of plasma cholesterol level in heterozygotes. This operation may be indicated in patients in whom drug therapy is not tolerated.

A reduction of serum cholesterol is much more difficult to achieve in homozygotes than heterozygotes, since combination therapy consisting of diet, a bile acid–binding resin, and nicotinic acid has little effect[227,256] and ileal bypass is uniformly ineffective.[257] Portacaval anastomosis, has been effective in several children,[251,258] but must still be regarded as an experimental procedure. Plasma exchanges at monthly intervals using a continuous-flow blood cell separator will lower the cholesterol in all homozygotes[259] to about 300 mg/dl; it then gradually rises over the ensuing 4 weeks to the pretreatment level of 600 to 900 mg/dl. Plasma exchange is the treatment of choice for familial hypercholesterolemia homozygotes when facilities for carrying out this procedure on a monthly basis are available.

FAMILIAL HYPERTRIGLYCERIDEMIA (see also p. 1215)

Clinical Features. Patients with this common autosomal dominant disorder, in which the concentration of VLDL is elevated in the plasma, do not usually exhibit hypertriglyceridemia until puberty or early adulthood. The fasting plasma triglyceride level then tends to be moderately elevated and in the range of 200 to 500 mg/dl (Type IV lipoprotein pattern). Obesity, hyperglycemia, hyperinsulinemia, hypertension, and hyperuricemia occur frequently in these patients.[234,260] Xanthomas are *not* a characteristic feature.

Patients with familial hypertriglyceridemia exhibit an increased incidence of atherosclerosis; affected patients constituted 5 per cent of all patients with myocardial infarction in one study.[225] It is not certain that the hypertriglyceridemia per se accounts for the increased atherosclerosis, since many patients with this condition have diabetes, obesity, and hypertension[261] and each of these features by itself may predispose to atherosclerosis.

Patients with familial hypertriglyceridemia with mild to moderate elevations of VLDL can develop a severe exacerbation when exposed to a variety of precipitating factors, such as excessive consumption of alcohol, poorly controlled diabetes, ingestion of birth control pills containing estrogen, and the development of hypothyroidism.[261] The plasma triglyceride level in affected patients can rise to values in excess of 1000 mg/dl in response to any of these stimuli, and large triglyceride-laden particles with the characteristics of chylomicrons appear in the plasma. Such patients develop *mixed hyperlipidemia*, with an elevation in the concentration of both VLDL and chylomicrons (Type V lipoprotein pattern) during these exacerbations. Patients may develop eruptive xanthomas and pancreatitis whenever the concentration of chylomicrons rises to high levels. The chylomicron-like particles disappear from the plasma, and the patient returns to the basal condition, in which the concentration of triglycerides is moderately elevated when the exacerbating condition is treated.

Some of the members in certain families with the so-called "familial Type V hyperlipidemia" exhibit a severe mixed hyperlipemia even in the absence of known exacerbating factors. Only the mild form of the disease, with moderate hypertriglyceridemia and no hyperchylomicronemia (Type IV pattern), may be present in other affected individuals in the same family.[234,260]

Pathogenesis. Familial hypertriglyceridemia is transmitted as an autosomal dominant trait, implying a mutation of a single gene. This disorder appears to be genetically heterogeneous in that patients from different families may have different mutations accounting for the hypertriglyceridemia phenotype.[234,260] No abnormalities of lipoprotein structure have thus far been identified. Some patients have an elevated production rate for VLDL, especially when they ingest diets that are high in carbohydrate. Although many of these patients suffer from obesity and diabetes mellitus, other individuals with obesity and diabetes mellitus also overproduce VLDL but have normal plasma VLDL levels. This observation suggests that inability to catabolize the triglycerides of VLDL represents the underlying defect in patients with familial hypertriglyceridemia. Hypertriglyceridemia results when VLDL production rates become elevated owing to obesity or diabetes.[234,260] However, lipoprotein lipase activity in plasma following the administration of heparin is generally normal.

Diabetes and obesity tend to increase VLDL production and hence to exacerbate hypertriglyceridemia in this syndrome, but the increased prevalence of these conditions is believed to be fortuitous. There is evidence that hypertriglyceridemia and diabetes are inherited by independent mechanisms.[262] However, the hypertriglyceridemia is much more severe when an individual inherits both the gene or genes for diabetes and the gene for hypertriglyceridemia, and such a person is more likely to come to medical attention. Similarly, an individual of normal weight with familial hypertriglyceridemia will usually have mild hypertriglyceridemia and will be less likely to come to medical attention. However, if such an individual becomes obese, the hypertriglyceridemia will worsen, and a diagnosis is more likely to be made.[234]

Diagnosis. A moderate elevation in plasma triglyceride level, together with a normal cholesterol level, suggests the possibility of familial hypertriglyceridemia. Plasma electrophoresis shows an increase in the pre-beta fraction (Type IV lipoprotein pattern). In the occasional patient who exhibits severe hypertriglyceridemia with an elevation of chylomicrons and VLDL (Type V lipoprotein pattern), the plasma shows a creamy supernatant layer (chylomicrons) and a cloudy infranatant layer (VLDL) after overnight storage in the refrigerator.[234,260]

No simple test currently exists to determine whether an individual who has an elevation in VLDL levels with or without an elevation in chylomicrons has familial hypertriglyceridemia or hypertriglyceridemia due to some other genetic or acquired cause, such as multiple lipoprotein-type hyperlipidemia or sporadic hypertriglyceridemia. However, half of the first-degree relatives of patients with typical cases of familial hypertriglyceridemia exhibit hypertriglyceridemia, and no relatives with isolated hypercholesterolemia should be found. When the latter is present, the diagnosis of multiple lipoprotein-type hyperlipase is suggested.

Treatment. It is essential, first of all, to control all of the exacerbating conditions, including obesity. The diet should be restricted in calories, saturated fat, and alcohol. Diabetes mellitus and hypothyroidism, if present, should be treated vigorously; oral contraceptives should be avoided. However, if the above measures fail, clofibrate is usually effective[234,260] (p. 1226).

MULTIPLE LIPOPROTEIN–TYPE HYPERLIPIDEMIA (FAMILIAL COMBINED HYPERLIPIDEMIA). In this common disorder, inherited as an autosomal dominant trait, affected individuals in a single family characteristically show one of three different lipoprotein patterns: hypercholesterolemia (Type IIA), hypertriglyceridemia (Type IV), or both hypercholesterolemia and hypertriglyceridemia.[225,234] In this condition, hyperlipidemia is not usually present in affected patients in childhood but begins to appear at puberty and continues thereafter. The lipid elevations are often mild, and they change over time in affected individuals, often exhibiting a mildly elevated cholesterol level at one examination and/or a mildly elevated triglyceride level at another. An elevation in the incidence of myocardial infarction in affected women as well as men is characteristic, and there is usually a strong family history of premature coronary artery disease. Indeed, patients with multiple lipoprotein–type hyperlipidemia

constitute about 10 per cent of all patients who have a myocardial infarction.[225] Xanthomas are not a feature of this condition. Although the incidence of obesity, hyperuricemia, and glucose intolerance is increased in affected individuals, especially those with hypertriglyceridemia, this association is not so striking as the one found with familial hypertriglyceridemia.

Pathogenesis. Since the disease is transmitted within families as an autosomal dominant trait, a mutation in a single gene is probably responsible. As would be expected with this mode of inheritance, about half of the first-degree relatives of an affected individual also have hyperlipidemia.[225,263-267] A key feature of this condition is the great variability of blood lipids among affected individuals in the same family and, as already pointed out, in the same individual at different times. About one-third of relatives of those individuals with hyperlipidemia will have hypercholesterolemia (Type IIA lipoprotein pattern), one-third will have hypertriglyceridemia (Type IV), and the remainder both hypercholesterolemia and hypertriglyceridemia (Type IIB). The plasma lipid levels tend to hover at the 95th percentile for the population. The variability of lipoprotein phenotypes that constitutes the characteristic feature of this condition is illustrated in Figure 47–8, which shows the pedigrees of four large families affected by this disorder.

It has been postulated that affected individuals have an elevated secretion rate for VLDL from the liver[225], and that this overproduction of VLDL may manifest itself alternatively as an elevation in plasma VLDL levels (hypertriglyceridemia), an elevation in LDL levels (hypercholesterolemia), or both, depending on the interplay of factors governing the efficiency of conversion of VLDL to LDL and the efficiency of catabolism of LDL. As in familial hypertriglyceridemia, the hyperlipidemia is worsened by diabetes, alcoholism, and hypothyroidism.

Diagnosis. There are no clinical or laboratory methods that indicate whether an individual with hyperlipidemia has the multiple lipoprotein–type disorder, since type IIA, IIB, and IV lipoprotein patterns can each occur in patients with several diseases (Table 35–8, p. 1213). However, this disorder should be suspected in any individual whose hyperlipoproteinemia is mild, whose lipoprotein type changes with time, and among whose relatives multiple abnormal lipoprotein types occur (Fig. 47–8). Tendon xanthomas in the patient or relatives or the finding of hypercholesterolemia in a relative under the age of 10 years, both of which suggest the diagnosis of heterozygous familial hypercholesterolemia , exclude the diagnosis of multiple lipoprotein–type hyperlipidemia.

Treatment. Weight reduction, restriction of dietary saturated fat and cholesterol, and avoidance of alcohol and oral contraceptives are useful general measures. In addition, clofibrate is effective when the triglyceride level is elevated with or without hypercholesterolemia, while a bile acid-binding resin usually lowers an elevated cholesterol level. However, the lowering of cholesterol levels with such a drug may be accompanied by an increase in triglyceride levels that tends to negate its beneficial effects.

FAMILIAL DYSBETALIPOPROTEINEMIA (TYPE III HYPERLIPOPROTEINEMIA) (see also p. 1215). The expression of this disorder, which is transmitted by a single-gene mechanism, requires the presence of contribu-

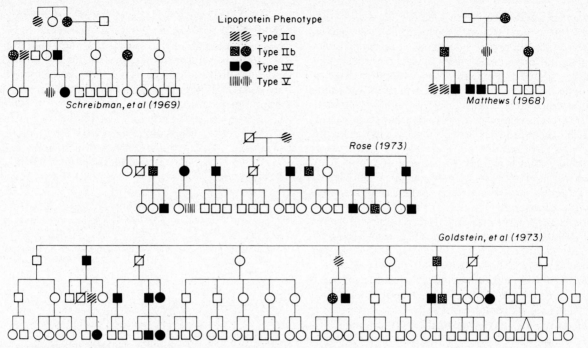

FIGURE 47–8 Pedigrees of four large families showing the characteristics of multiple lipoprotein-type hyperlipidemia. (Adapted from data contained in references 225 and 264 to 266.)

tory environmental or genetic factors.[234,268] The plasma concentrations of cholesterol and triglycerides are both elevated because of the accumulation in plasma of remnant-like particles derived from the partial catabolism of VLDL and chylomicrons.

Clinical Features. Hyperlipidemia or any of the other clinical features of the disease are usually not manifest until after the age of 20 years. Two types of cutaneous xanthomas are characteristic of familial dysbetalipoproteinemia: xanthomata striata palmaris, which appear as orange or yellow discolorations of the palmar and digital creases, and tuberous or tuberoeruptive xanthomas, which are bulbous cutaneous xanthomas that may vary from pea- to lemon-sized and are characteristically located over the elbows and knees. Xanthelasmas of the eyelids also occur, but these are not unique to this disorder (p. 16). Patients with clinical manifestations of dysbetalipoproteinemia are often found to have hypothyroidism, obesity, or diabetes mellitus.[234,268,269]

Clinically, this condition is characterized by severe atherosclerosis involving the coronary arteries, the internal carotids, and the abdominal aorta and its branches. Forty-three per cent of the nearly 50 patients described by Morganroth et al.[268] had detectable vascular disease, and in the one-third who had coronary artery disease the mean age of onset was 38 years in men and about a decade later in women. Peripheral vascular disease, manifest mainly as claudication, was also found in about one-third, again appearing earlier in men than in women; cerebrovascular disease occurred in 5 of their 47 patients. Except for homozygous familial hypercholesterolemia, familial dysbetalipoproteinemia probably results in as high a risk of premature vascular disease as any form of hyperlipidemia. This diagnosis should be considered in any patient who has hyperlipidemia and peripheral vascular disease.

Pathogenesis. This form of hyperlipidemia is caused by the accumulation of relatively large lipoprotein particles that contain both triglycerides and cholesteryl esters and that resemble the remnants that are normally produced from the catabolism of VLDL and chylomicrons through the action of lipoprotein lipase (Fig. 47–5). These remnant particles are rapidly taken up by the liver of normal subjects, and hence they are barely detectable in plasma. However, the uptake of remnants by the liver is blocked in patients with familial dysbetalipoproteinemia, leading to the accumulation of high levels of these lipoproteins in plasma and deposition in tissues, producing xanthomas and atherosclerosis.[234,268]

Patients with familial dysbetalipoproteinemia are homozygous for a mutant gene specifying apoprotein E, a normal constituent of VLDL and chylomicron remnants.[270] The normal function of apo E is to bind to hepatic lipoprotein receptors, an event which is necessary for the rapid hepatic uptake of IDL and chylomicron remnants.[235] The apo E gene is polymorphic in the population. The three common alleles are designated ϵ^2, ϵ^3, ϵ^4.[268,271] The ϵ^3 and ϵ^4 alleles code for proteins that function normally. The protein specified by the ϵ^2 allele is nonfunctional. It does not bind to hepatic receptors.[272]

About 1 per cent of Caucasian individuals are homozygous for the ϵ^2 allele. However, only 1 in 100 of these homozygous individuals (or 1 in 10,000 of the general population) has clear-cut familial dysbetalipoproteinemia.[268] The vast majority of ϵ^2 homozygotes are able to compensate somehow for their defective protein. They have very slight elevations in the concentration of IDL and chylomicron remnants in plasma and are asymptomatic. The reason why 1 per cent of the ϵ^2 homozygotes cannot compensate for their defect and develop severe dysbetalipoproteinemia is not known. In some families the expression of dysbetalipoproteinemia appears to require two factors: (1) homozygosity for the ϵ^2 allele and (2) the independent inheritance of another form of genetic hyperlipidemia, such as familial combined hyperlipidemia or familial hypercholesterolemia.[273] When either of these dominant traits is present together with ϵ^2 homozygosity, the disease is expressed as familial dysbetalipoproteinemia. Other subjects with symptomatic dysbetalipoproteinemia who are ϵ^2 homozygotes apparently have the clinical expression brought on by hypothyroidism or by diabetes mellitus.[268,269]

Diagnosis. Approximately 80 per cent of symptomatic patients with familial dysbetalipoproteinemia exhibit palmar or tuberous xanthomas. The diagnosis is also suggested when a moderate elevation in the plasma concentration of both cholesterol and triglyceride occurs in such a way that the absolute concentrations of cholesterol and triglyceride are nearly equal (e.g., the plasma cholesterol and triglyceride levels are both about 300 mg/dl). However, this finding is not a uniform one, since when the disease is in exacerbation, the plasma triglyceride level tends to rise much higher than the cholesterol level.

The diagnosis is strongly supported by the finding of a so-called "broad beta" band on lipoprotein electrophoresis (Type III pattern), which results from the presence of the remnant particles that migrate between beta- and pre–beta-lipoproteins and cause a distinctive smear of this region of the electrophoretogram. Two procedures that require specialized laboratories can be used to establish the diagnosis firmly. When the chemical composition of the VLDL is measured in plasma subjected to ultracentrifugation, the VLDL fraction contains the normal remnant particles and has a relatively high ratio of cholesterol to triglyceride.[234,260,268] The diagnosis can be confirmed by the finding of homozygosity for expression of the ϵ^2 allele after isoelectric focusing of the proteins extracted from the remnant particles.[260,268]

Treatment. A trial of l-thyroxine should be instituted if a careful search reveals any evidence of hypothyroidism. A dramatic lowering of lipid levels occurs when hypothyroidism is treated. In addition, vigorous treatment of obesity and diabetes mellitus is indicated. However, if these measures are not successful, treatment with clofibrate is indicated and usually results in a dramatic and sustained reduction in plasma lipid levels.[256,260]

HYPERTENSION

The genetics of essential hypertension are discussed on page 863. In brief, the current view is that blood pressure shows a continuous distribution, that multiple genes and multiple environmental factors act in concert to determine the level of one's blood pressure, just as the determination of intelligence and skin color is multifactorial, and that essential hypertension represents the upper end of the blood pressure distribution. Thus, the etiology of hypertension in the vast majority of patients will not be traceable to the operation of a single mutant gene. However, the physician should be aware that there are a number of rare monogenic disorders in which hypertension is a part of the clinical syndrome. These rare disorders, which often masquerade under the umbrella of essential hypertension, are listed in Table 47–6.

References

1. Stanbury, J. B., Wyngaarden, J. B., Fredrickson, D. S., Goldstein, J. L., and Brown, M. S.: The Metabolic Basis of Inherited Disease. 5th ed. New York, McGraw-Hill Book Co., 1983, pp. 3, 61.
2. McKusick, V. A.: The anatomy of the human genome. Am. J. Med. *69*:267, 1980.
3. Harris, H.: The Principles of Human Biochemical Genetics, 3rd ed. Amsterdam, North-Holland Publishing Co., 1980.
4. Vogel, F., and Motulsky, A. G.: Human Genetics: Problems and Approaches. Berlin, Springer-Verlag, 1979.
5. Goldstein, J. L.: Genetic aspects of hyperlipidemia in coronary heart disease. Hosp. Pract. *8*:53–65, 1973.
6. McKusick, V. A.: Mendelian Inheritance in Man. 4th ed. Baltimore, Johns Hopkins University Press, 1975.
7. Goldstein, J. L., and Brown, M. S.: The LDL receptor defect in familial hypercholesterolemia: Implications for pathogenesis and therapy. Med. Clin. North Am. *66*:335, 1982.
8. Carter, C. O., Roberts, J. A. F., Evans, K. A., and Buck, A. R.: Genetic clinic, Lancet *1*:281, 1971.
9. Epstein, C. J., and Golbus, M. S.: Prenatal diagnosis of genetic diseases. Am. Sci. *65*:703, 1977.
10. Nora, J. J., and Nora, A. H.: Recurrence risks in children having one parent with a congenital heart disease. Circulation *53*:701, 1976.
11. Noonan, J. A.: Syndromes associated with cardiac defects. In Engle, M. A. (ed.): Pediatric Cardiovascular Disease II. Philadelphia, F. A. Davis Co., 1981, p. 97.
12. Tandon, R., and Edwards, J. E.: Cardiac malformations associated with Down's syndrome. Circulation *47*:1349, 1973.
13. Park, S. C., Mathews, R. A., Zuberbuhler, J. R., Rowe, R. D., Neches, W. H., and Lenox, C. C.: Down syndrome with congenital heart malformation. Am. J. Dis. Child. *131*:29, 1977.
14. Greenwood, R. D., and Nadas, A. S.: The clinical course of cardiac disease in Down's syndrome. Pediatrics *58*:893, 1976.
15. Katlic, M. R., Clark, E. B., Neill, C., and Haller, J. A., Jr.: Surgical management of congenital heart disease in Down's syndrome. J. Thorac. Cardiovasc. Surg. *74*:204, 1977.
16. Mikkelsen, M., and Stene, J.: Genetic counseling in Down's syndrome. Hum. Hered. *20*:457, 1970.
17. Hook, E. B.: Estimates of maternal age-specific risks of a Down-syndrome birth in women aged 34–41. Lancet *2*:33, 1976.
18. Gerald, P. S.: Sex chromosome disorders. N. Engl. J. Med. *294*:706, 1976.
19. Engel, E., and Forbes, A. P.: Cytogenetic and clinical findings in 48 patients with congenitally defective or absent ovaries. Medicine *44*:135, 1965.
20. Schmid, W., Naef, E., Murset, G., and Prader, A.: Cytogenetic findings in 89 cases of Turner's syndrome with abnormal karyotypes. Humangenetik *24*:93, 1974.
21. Palmer, C. G., and Reichmann, A.: Chromosomal and clinical findings in 110 females with Turner syndrome. Hum. Genet. *35*:35, 1976.
22. Nora, J. J., Torres, F. G., Sinha, A. K., and McNamara, D. G.: Characteristic cardiovascular anomalies of XO Turner syndrome, XX and XY phenotype and XO/XX Turner mosaic. Am. J. Cardiol. *25*:639, 1970.
23. Van Der Hauwaert, L. G., Fryns, J. P., Dumoulin, M., and Logghe, N.: Cardiovascular malformations in Turner's and Noonan's syndrome. Br. Heart J. *40*:500, 1978.
24. Noonan, J. A.: Hypertelorism with Turner phenotype. Am. J. Dis. Child. *116*:373, 1968.
25. Collins, E., and Turner, G.: The Noonan syndrome—a review of the clinical and genetic features of 27 cases. J. Pediatr. *83*:941, 1973.
26. Nora, J. J., Nora, A. H., Sinha, A. K., Spangler, R. D., and Lubs, H. A.: The Ullrich-Noonan syndrome (Turner phenotype). Am. J. Dis. Child. *127*:48, 1974.
27. Levy, E. P., Pashayan, H., Fraser, F. C., and Pinsky, L.: XX and XY Turner phenotypes in a family. Am. J. Dis. Child. *120*:36, 1970.
28. Nora, J. J., and Sinha, A. K.: Direct familial transmission of the Turner phenotype. Am. J. Dis. Child. *116*:343, 1968.
29. Nora, J. J., Lortscher, R. H., and Spangler, R. D.: Echocardiographic studies

TABLE 47–6   SINGLE-GENE DISORDERS THAT PREDISPOSE TO HYPERTENSION

DISORDER	MECHANISM OF INHERITANCE
Polycystic kidney disease	Dominant
Alport syndrome	Dominant
Medullary thyroid carcinoma with pheochromocytoma	Dominant
Acute intermittent porphyria	Dominant
Neurofibromatosis	Dominant
Pseudoxanthoma elasticum	Dominant and recessive
Riley-Day syndrome (dysautonomia)	Recessive
Adrenogenital syndrome, 17-hydroxylase deficiency	Recessive
Fabry disease	X-linked

of left ventricular disease in Ullrich-Noonan syndrome. Am. J. Dis. Child. *129*:1417, 1975.

30. Caralis, D. G., Char, F., Graber, J. D., and Voigt, G. C.: Delineation of multiple cardiac anomalies associated with the Noonan syndrome in an adult and review of the literature. Johns Hopkins Med. J. *134*:346, 1974.

31. Pearl, W.: Cardiovascular anomalies in Noonan's syndrome. Chest *71*:677, 1977.

32. Qazi, Q. H., Arnon, R. G., Paydar, M. H., and Mapa, H. C.: Familial occurrence of Noonan syndrome. Am. J. Dis. Child. *127*:696, 1974.

33. Bolton, M. R., Pugh, D. M., Mattioli, L. F., Dunn, M. I., and Schimke, R. N.: The Noonan syndrome: A family study. Ann. Intern. Med. *80*:626, 1974.

34. Baird, P. A., and De Jong, B. P.: Noonan's syndrome (XX and XY Turner phenotype) in three generations of a family. J. Pediatr. *80*:110, 1972.

35. Nghiem, Q. X., Toledo, J. R., Schreiber, M. H., Harris, L. C., Lockhart, L. L., and Tyson, K. R. T.: Congenital idiopathic hypertrophic subaortic stenosis associated with a phenotypic Turner's syndrome. Am. J. Cardiol. *30*:683, 1972.

36. Phornphutkul, C., Rosenthal, A., and Nadas, A. S.: Cardiomyopathy in Noonan's syndrome. Br. Heart J. *35*:99, 1973.

37. Tanimura, A., Hayashi, I., Adachi, K., Nakashima, T., Ota, K., and Toshima, H.: Noonan syndrome with hypertrophic obstructive cardiomyopathy. Acta Pathol. Jpn. *27*:225, 1977.

38. Ehlers, K. H., Engle, M. A., Levin, A. R., and Deely, W. J.: Eccentric ventricular hypertrophy in familial and sporadic instances of 46 XX, XY Turner phenotype. Circulation *45*:639, 1972.

39. Summitt, R. L.: Turner syndrome and Noonan's syndrome. J. Pediatr. *75*:729, 1969.

40. Gorlin, R. J., Anderson, R. C., and Blaw, M.: Multiple lentigenes syndrome. Am. J. Dis. Child. *117*:652, 1969.

41. Seuanez, H., Mane-Garzon, F., and Kolski, R.: Cardio-cutaneous syndrome (the "LEOPARD" syndrome). Review of the literature and a new family. Clin. Genet. *9*:266, 1976.

42. Polani, P. E., and Moynahan, E. J.: Progressive cardiomyopathic lentiginosis. Q. J. Med. *41*:205, 1972.

43. Hopkins, B. E., Taylor, R. R., and Robinson, J. S.: Familial hypertrophic cardiomyopathy and lentiginosis. Aust. NZ. J. Med. *5*:359, 1975.

44. Somerville, J., and Bonham-Carter, R. E.: The heart in lentiginosis. Br. Heart J. *34*:58, 1972.

45. Holt, M., and Oram, S.: Familial heart disease with skeletal malformations. Br. Heart J. *22*:236, 1960.

46. Massumi, R. A., and Nutter, D. O.: The syndrome of familial defects of heart and upper extremities (Holt-Oram syndrome). Circulation *34*:65, 1966.

47. Smith, A. T., Sack, G. H., and Taylor, G. J.: Holt-Oram syndrome. J. Pediatr. *95*:538, 1979.

48. Cascos, A. S.: Genetics of atrial septal defect. Arch. Dis. Child. *47*:581, 1972.

49. Gladstone, I., and Sybert, V. P.: Holt-Oram syndrome: Penetrance of the gene and lack of maternal effect. Clin. Genet. *21*:98, 1982.

50. Brans, Y. W., and Lintermans, J. P.: The upper limb–cardiovascular syndrome. Am. J. Dis. Child. *124*:779, 1972.

51. Poznanski, A. K., Stern, A. M., and Gall, J. C., Jr.: Skeletal anomalies in genetically determined congenital heart disease. Radiol. Clin. North Am. *9*:435, 1971.

52. Kaufman, R. L., Rimoin, D. L., McAlister, W. H., and Hartmann, A. F.: Variable expression of the Holt-Oram syndrome. Am. J. Dis. Child. *127*:21, 1974.

53. Bizarro, R. O., Callahan, J. A., Feldt, R. H., Kurland, L. T., Gordon, H., and Brandenburg, R. O.: Familial atrial septal defect with prolonged atrioventricular conduction. Circulation *41*:677, 1970.

54. Emanuel, R., O'Brien, K., Somerville, J., Jefferson, K., and Hegde, M.: Association of secundum atrial septal defect with abnormalities of atrioventricular conduction or left axis deviation. Br. Heart J. *37*:1085, 1975.

55. Bjornstad, P. G.: Secundum-type atrial septal defect with prolonged PR interval and autosomal dominant mode of inheritance. Br. Heart J. *36*:1149, 1974.

56. Pease, W. E., Nordenberg, A., and Ladda, R. L.: Familial atrial septal defect with prolonged atrioventricular conduction. Circulation *53*:759, 1976.

57. da Silva, E. O., Janovitz, D., and de Albuquerque, S. C.: Ellis–van Creveld syndrome: Report of 15 cases in an inbred kindred. J. Med. Genet. *17*:349, 1980.

58. McKusick, V. A., Egeland, J. A., Eldridge, R., and Krusen, D. E.: Dwarfism in the Amish. I. The Ellis–van Creveld syndrome. Bull. Johns Hopkins Hosp. *115*:306, 1964.

59. Blackburn, M. G., and Belliveau, R. E.: Ellis–van Creveld syndrome. Am. J. Dis. Child. *122*:267, 1971.

60. Mahoney, M. J., and Hobbins, J. C.: Prenatal diagnosis of chondroectodermal dysplasia (Ellis–van Creveld syndrome) with fetoscopy and ultrasound. N. Engl. J. Med. *297*:258, 1977.

61. Becroft, D. M. O., and Chambers, D.: Supravalvular aortic stenosis–infantile hypercalcaemia syndrome: *In vitro* hypersensitivity to vitamin D_2 and calcium. J. Med. Genet. *13*:223, 1976.

62. Kahler, R. L., Braunwald, E., Plauth, W. H., Jr., and Morrow, A. G.: Familial congenital heart disease. Am. J. Med. *40*:384, 1966.

63. McDonald, A. H., Gerlis, L. M., and Somerville, J.: Familial arteriopathy with associated pulmonary and systemic arterial stenoses. Br. Heart J. *31*:375, 1969.

64. Johnson, L. W., Fishman, R. A., Schneider, B., Parker, F. B., Jr., Husson, G., and Webb, W. R.: Familial supravalvular aortic stenosis. Chest *70*:494, 1976.

65. Eisenberg, R., Young, D., Jacobson, B., and Boito, A.: Familial supravalvular aortic stenosis. Am. J. Dis. Child. *108*:341, 1964.

66. Afzelius, B. A., and Mossberg, A.: The immotile-cilia syndrome including Kartagener's syndrome. *In* Stanbury, J. B., Wyngaarden, J. B., Fredrickson, D. S., Goldstein, J. L., and Brown, M. S. (eds.): The Metabolic Basis of Inherited Disease. 5th ed. New York, McGraw-Hill, 1983, p. 1986.

67. Holmes, L. B., Blennerhassett, J. B., and Austen, K. F.: A reappraisal of Kartagener's syndrome. Am. J. Med. Sci. *255*:13, 1968.

68. Hartline, J. V., and Zelkowitz, P. S.: Kartagener's syndrome in childhood. Am. J. Dis. Child. *121*:349, 1971.

69. Miller, R. D., and Divertie, M. B.: Kartagener's syndrome. Chest *62*:130, 1972.

70. Afzelius, B. A.: A human syndrome caused by immotile cilia. Science *193*:317, 1976.

71. Melmon, K. L., and Braunwald, E.: Familial pulmonary hypertension. N. Engl. J. Med. *269*:770, 1963.

72. Kingdon, H. S., Cohen, L. S., Roberts, W. C., and Braunwald, E.: Familial occurrence of primary pulmonary hypertension. Arch. Intern. Med. *118*:422, 1966.

73. Kuhn, E., Schaaf, J., and Wagner, A.: Primary pulmonary hypertension, congenital heart disease and skeletal anomalies in three generations. Jpn. Heart J. *4*:205, 1963.

74. Parry, W. R., and Verel, D.: Familial primary pulmonary hypertension. Br. Heart J. *28*:193, 1966.

75. Rogge, J. D., Mishkin, M. E., and Genovese, P. D.: The familial occurrence of primary pulmonary hypertension. Ann. Intern. Med. *65*:672, 1966.

76. Thompson, P., and McRae, C.: Familial pulmonary hypertension. Evidence of autosomal dominant inheritance. Br. Heart J. *32*:758, 1970.

77. Nora, J. J., McGill, C. W., and McNamara, D. G.: Empiric recurrence risks in common and uncommon congenital heart lesions. Teratology *3*:325, 1970.

78. Neill, C. A.: Genetics of congenital heart disease. Annu. Rev. Med. *24*:61, 1973.

79. Child, A. H., and Dennis, N. R.: The genetics of congenital heart disease. Birth Defects: Original Article Series *13*:85, 1977.

80. Nora, J. J., Dodd, P. F., McNamara, D. G., Hattwick, M. A. W., Leachman, R. D., and Cooley, D. A.: Risk to offspring of parents with congenital heart defects. J.A.M.A. *209*:2052, 1969.

CONNECTIVE TISSUE DISORDERS

81. McKusick, V. A.: Heritable Disorders of Connective Tissue. 4th ed. St. Louis, C. V. Mosby Co., 1972.

82. Hirst, A.E., Jr., and Gore, I.: Marfan's syndrome: A review. Prog. Cardiovasc. Dis. *16*:187, 1973.

83. Phornphutkul, C., Rosenthal, A., and Nadas, A. S.: Cardiac manifestations of Marfan syndrome in infancy and childhood. Circulation *47*:587, 1973.

84. Wigle, E. D., Rakowski, H., Ranganathan, N., and Silver, M. D.: Mitral valve prolapse. Annu. Rev. Med. *27*:165, 1976.

85. Devereux, R. B., Perloff, J. K., Reichek, N., and Josephson, M. E.: Mitral valve prolapse. Circulation *54*:3, 1976.

86. Cooper, M. J., and Abinader, E. G.: Family history in assessing the risk for progression of mitral valve prolapse. Am. J. Dis. Child. *135*:647, 1981.

87. Hunt, D., and Sloman, G.: Prolapse of the posterior leaflet of the mitral valve occurring in eleven members of a family. Am. Heart J. *78*:149, 1969.

88. Barabas, A. P.: Heterogeneity of the Ehlers-Danlos syndrome: Description of the three clinical types and a hypothesis to explain the basic defect(s). Br. Med. J. *2*:612, 1967.

89. McKusick, V. A.: Multiple forms of the Ehlers-Danlos syndrome. Arch. Surg. *109*:475, 1974.

90. Pope, F. M., Martin, G. R., and McKusick, V. A.: Inheritance of Ehlers-Danlos type IV syndrome. J. Med. Genet. *14*:200, 1977.

91. Imahori, S., Bannerman, R. M., Graf, C. J., and Brennan, J. C.: Ehlers-Danlos syndrome with multiple arterial lesions. Am. J. Med. *47*:967, 1969.

92. Beighton, P.: The dominant and recessive forms of cutis laxa. J. Med. Genet. *9*:216, 1972.

93. Schimke, R. N., McKusick, V. A., Huang, T., and Pollack, A. D.: Homocystinuria. J.A.M.A., *193*:87, 1965.

94. James, T. N., Carson, N. A. J., and Froggatt, P.: De Subitaneis Mortibus IV. Coronary vessels and conduction system in homocystinuria. Circulation *49*:367, 1974.

95. McCully, K. S.: Vascular pathology of homocysteinemia: Implications for the pathogenesis of arteriosclerosis. Am. J. Pathol. *56*:111, 1969.

96. Fleisher, L. D., Longhi, R. C., Tallan, H. H., Beratis, N. G., Hirschhorn, K., and Gaull, G. E.: Homocystinuria: Investigations of cystathionine synthase in cultured fetal cells and the prenatal determination of genetic status. J. Peditr. *85*:677, 1974.

97. Altman, L. K., Fialkow, P. J., Parker, F., and Sagebiel, R. W.: Pseudoxanthoma elasticum: An underdiagnosed genetically heterogeneous disorder with protean manifestations. Arch. Intern. Med. *134*:1048, 1974.

98. Pope, F. M.: Autosomal dominant pseudoxanthoma elasticum. J. Med. Genet. *11*:152, 1974.

99. Wilhelm, K., and Paver, K.: Sudden death in pseudoxanthoma elasticum. Med. J. Aust. *2*:1363, 1972.

100. Schachner, L., and Young. D.: Pseudoxanthoma elasticum with severe cardiovascular disease in a child. Am. J. Dis. Child. *127*:571, 1974.

101. Bete, J. M., Banas, J. S., Jr., Moran, J., Pinn, V., and Levine, H. J.: Coronary artery disease in an 18 year old girl with pseudoxanthoma elasticum: Successful surgical therapy. Am. J. Cardiol. *36*:515, 1975.

102. Moran, J. J.: Idiopathic arterial calcification of infancy: A clinicopathologic study. Pathol. Annu. *10*:393, 1975.

103. Barson, A. J., Campbell, R. H. A., Langley, F. A., and Milner, R. D. G.: Idiopathic arterial calcification of infancy without intimal proliferation. Virchows Arch. Pathol. Anat. *372*:167, 1976.

104. Schieken, R. M., Kerber, R. E., Ionasescu, V. V., and Zellweger, H.: Cardiac manifestations of the mucopolysaccharidoses. Circulation *52*:700, 1975.

105. McKusick, V. A., and Neufeld, E. F.: The mucopolysaccharide storage diseases. *In* Stanbury, J. B., Wyngaarden, J. B., Fredrickson, D. S., Goldstein, J. L., and Brown, M. S. (eds.): The Metabolic Basis of Inherited Disease. 5th ed. New York, McGraw-Hill Book Co., 1983, p. 751.

106. Kelly, T. E., Thomas, G. H., Taylor, H. A., Jr., McKusick, V. A., Sly, W. S., Glaser, J. H., Robinow, M., Luzzatti, L., Espiritu, C., Feingold, M., Bull, M. J., Ashenhurst, E. M., and Ives, E. J.: Mucolipidosis III (pseudo-Hurler polydystrophy): Clinical and laboratory studies in a series of 12 patients. Johns Hopkins Med. J. *137*:156, 1975.

107. Neufeld, E. F., and McKusick, V. A.: Disorders of lysosomal enzyme synthesis and localization: I-cell disease and Pseudo-Hurler polydystrophy. *In* Stanbury, J. B., Wyngaarden, J. B., Fredrickson, D. S., Goldstein, J. L., and Brown, M. S. (eds.): The Metabolic Basis of Inherited Disease. 5th ed. New York, McGraw-Hill Book Co., 1983, p. 778.

108. Hirst, A. E., Jr., Johns, V. J., Jr., and Kime, S. W., Jr.: Dissecting aneurysm of the aorta: A review of 505 cases. Medicine *37*:217, 1958.

109. Murdoch, J. L., Walker, B. A., Halpern, B. L., Kuzma, J. W., and McKusick, V. A.: Life expectancy and causes of death in the Marfan syndrome. N. Engl. J. Med. *286*:804, 1972.

110. Halpern, B. L., Char, F., Murdoch, J. L., Horton, W. B., and McKusick, V. A.: A prospectus on the prevention of aortic rupture in the Marfan syndrome with data on survivorship without treatment. Johns Hopkins Med. J. *129*:123, 1971.

111. Elias, S., and Berkowitz, R. L.: The Marfan syndrome and pregnancy. Obstet. Gynecol. *47*:358, 1976.

112. Sutinen, S., and Piiroinen, O.: Marfan syndrome, pregnancy, and fatal dissection of aorta. Acta Obstet. Gynecol. Scand. *50*:295, 1971.

113. Grossman, M., Knott, A. P., Jr., and Jacoby, W. J., Jr.: Calcified annulus fibrosis with mitral insufficiency in the Marfan syndrome. Arch. Intern. Med. *121*:561, 1968.

114. Murdoch, J. L., Walker, B. A., and McKusick, V. A.: Parental age effects on the occurrence of new mutations for the Marfan syndrome. Ann. Hum. Genet. *35*:331, 1972.

115. Emanuel, R., Ng, R. A. L., Marcomichelakis, J., Moores, E. C., Jefferson, K. E., Macfaul, P. A., and Withers, R.: Formes frustes of Marfan's syndrome presenting with severe aortic regurgitation. Clinicogenetic study of 18 families. Br. Heart J. *39*:190, 1977.

116. Payvandi, M. N., Kerber, R. E., Phelps, C. D., Judisch, G. F., El-Khoury, G., and Schrott, H. G.: Cardiac, skeletal and ophthalmologic abnormalities in relatives of patients with the Marfan syndrome. Circulation *55*:797, 1977.

117. Procacci, P. M., Savran, S. V., Schreiter, S. L., and Bryson, A. L.: Prevalance of clinical mitral-valve prolapse in 1169 young women. N. Engl. J. Med. *294*:1086, 1976.

118. Markiewicz, W., Stoner, J., London, E., Hunt, S. A., and Popp, R. L.: Mitral valve prolapse in one hundred presumably healthy young females. Circulation *53*:464, 1976.

CARDIOMYOPATHIES

119. Howell, R. R., and Williams, J. C.: The glycogen storage diseases. *In* Stanbury, J. B., Wyngaarden, J. B., Fredrickson, D. S., Goldstein, J. L., and Brown, M. S. (eds.): The Metabolic Basis of Inherited Disease. 5th ed. New York, McGraw-Hill Book Co., 1983, p. 119.

120. Ehlers, K. H., Hagstrom, J. W. C., Lukas, D. S., Redo, S. F., and Engle, M. A.: Glycogen-storage disease of the myocardium with obstruction to left ventricular outflow. Circulation *25*:96, 1962.

121. Ockerman, P. A.: Incidence of glycogen storage disease in Sweden. Paediatr. Scand. *61*:533, 1972.

122. D'Ancona, G. G., Wurm, J., and Croce, C. M.: Genetics of type II glycogenesis: Assignment of the human gene for acid α-glucosidase to chromosome 17. Proc. Natl. Acad. Sci. USA. *76*:4526, 1979.

123. Butterworth, J., and Broadhead, D. M.: Diagnosis of Pompe's disease in cultured skin fibroblasts and primary amniotic fluid cells using 4-Methyl-lumbelliferyl-α-D-glucopyranoside as substrate. Clin. Chim. Acta *78*:335, 1977.

124. Clark, C. E., Henry, W. L., and Epstein, S. E.: Familial prevalance and genetic transmission of idiopathic hypertrophic subaortic stenosis. N. Engl. J. Med. *289*:709, 1973.

125. Bjarnason, I., Jonsson, S., and Hardarson, T.: Mode of inheritance of hypertrophic cardiomyopathy in Iceland. Br. Heart J. *47*:122, 1982.

126. Braunwald, E., Lambrew, C. T., Rockoff, S. D., Ross, J., Jr., and Morrow, A. G.: Idiopathic hypertrophic subaortic stenosis. I. A description of the disease based on an analysis of 64 patients. Circulation *30*(Suppl. 4):3, 1964.

127. Horlick, L., Petkovich, N. J., and Bolton, C. F.: Idiopathic hypertrophic subvalvular stenosis. A study of a family involving four generations. Clinical, hemodynamic and pathologic observations. Am. J. Cardiol. *17*:411, 1966.

128. Pare, J. A. P., Fraser, R. G., Pirozynski, W. J., Shanks, J. A., and Stubington, D.: Hereditary cardiovascular dysplasia. A form of familial cardiomyopathy. Am. J. Med. *31*:37, 1961.

129. Maron, B. J., Lipson, L. C., Roberts, W. C., Savage, D. S., and Epstein, S. E.: "Malignant" hypertrophic cardiomyopathy: Identification of a subgroup of families with unusually frequent premature death. Am. J. Cardiol. *41*:1133, 1978.

130. Perloff, J. K.: The cardiomyopathies—current perspectives. Circulation *44*:942, 1971.

131. Kariv, I., Kreisler, B., Sherf, L., Feldman, S., and Rosenthal, T.: Familial cardiomyopathy. Am. J. Cardiol. *28*:693, 1971.

132. Whitfield, A. G. W.: Familial cardiomyopathy. Q. J. Med. *30*:119, 1961.

133. Ross, R. S., Bulkley, B. H., Hutchins, G. M., Harshey, J. S., Jones, R. A., Kraus, H., Liebman, J., Thorne, C. M., Weinberg, S. B., Weech, A. A., and Weech, A. A., Jr.: Idiopathic familial myocardiopathy in three generations: A clinical and pathologic study. Am. Heart J. *97*:170, 1978.

134. Csanady, M., and Szasz, K.: Familial cardiomyopathy. Cardiology *61*:122, 1976.

135. Boyd, D. L., Mishkin, M. E., Feigenbaum, H., and Genovese, P. D.: Three families with familial cardiomyopathy. Ann. Intern. Med. *63*:386, 1965.

136. Finch, S. C., and Finch, C. A.: Idiopathic hemochromatosis, an iron shortage disease. Medicine *34*:381, 1955.

137. Bothwell, T. H., Charlton, R. W., and Motulsky, A. G.: Idiopathic hemochromatosis. *In* Stanbury, J. B., Wyngaarden, J. B., Fredrickson, D. S., Goldstein, J. L., and Brown, M. S. (eds.): The Metabolic Basis of Inherited Disease. 5th ed. New York, McGraw-Hill Book Co., 1983, p. 1269.

138. Edwards, C. Q., Carroll, M., Bray, P., and Cartwright, G. E.: Hereditary hemochromatosis. N. Engl. J. Med. *297*:7, 1977.

139. Crosby, W. H.: Hemochromatosis: The unsolved problems. Semin. Hematol. *14*:135, 1977.

140. Saddi, R., and Feingold, J.: Idiopathic haemochromatosis: An autosomal recessive disease. Clin. Genet. *5*:234, 1974.

141. Simon, M., Alexandre, J-L., Bourel, M., le Marec, B., and Scordia, C.: Heredity of idiopathic haemochromatosis: A study of 106 families. Clin. Genet. *11*:327, 1977.

142. Rowe, J. W., Wands, J. R., Mexey, E., Waterbury, L. A., Wright, J. R., Tobin, J., and Andres, R.: Familial hemochromatosis: Characteristics of the precirrhotic stage in a large kindred. Medicine *56*:197, 1977.

143. Scheinberg, I. H.: The genetics of hemochromatosis. Arch. Intern. Med. *132*:126, 1973.

144. Simon, M., Bourel, M., Fauchet, R., and Genetet, B.: Association of HLA-A3 and HLA-B14 antigens with idiopathic hemochromatosis. Gut *17*:332, 1976.

145. Bomford, A., Eddleston, A. L. W. F., Kennedy, L. A., Batchelor, J. R., and Williams, R.: Histocompatibility antigens as markers of abnormal iron metabolism in patients with idiopathic haemochromatosis and their relatives. Lancet *1*:327, 1977.

146. Feller, E. R., Pont, A., Wands, J. R., Carter, E. A., Foster, G., Kourides, I. A., and Isselbacher, K. J.: Familial hemochromatosis. N. Engl. J. Med. *29*:1422, 1977.

147. Simon, M., Alexandre, J. L., Rauchet, R., Genetet, B., and Bourel, M.: The genetics of hemochromatosis. Prog. Med. Genet. *4*(new series):135, 1980.

148. Kyle, R. A., and Bayrd, E.D.: Amyloidosis: Review of 236 cases. Medicine *54*:271, 1975.

149. Andrade, C., Araki, S., Block, W. D., Cohen, A. S., Jackson, C. E., Kuroiwa, Y., McKusick, V. A., Nissism, J., Sohar, E., and Van Allen, M. W.: Hereditary amyloidosis. Arthritis Rheum. *13*:902, 1970.

150. Frederiksen, T., Gotzsche, H., Harboe, N., Kraer, W., and Mellemgaard, K.: Familial primary amyloidosis with severe amyloid heart disease. Am. J. Med. *33*:328, 1962.

151. Harrison, W. H., Jr., and Derrick, J. R.: Atrial standstill. A review and presentation of two new cases of familial and unusual nature with reference to epicardial pacing in one. Angiology *20*:610, 1969.

152. Harper, P. S.: Congenital myotonic dystrophy in Britain. Arch. Dis. Child. *50*:505, 1975.

153. Church, S. C.: The heart in myotonia atrophica. Arch. Intern. Med. *119*:176, 1967.

154. Griggs, R. C., David, R. J., Anderson, D. C., and Dove, J. T.: Cardiac conduction in myotonic dystrophy. Am. J. Med. *59*:37, 1975.

155. Salomon, J., and Easley, R. M.: Cardiovascular abnormalities in myotonic dystrophy. Chest *64*:135, 1973.

156. Tanaka, N., Tanaka, H., Takeda, M., Niimura, T., Kanehisa, T., and Terashi, S.: Cardiomyopathy in myotonic dystrophy. A light and electron microscopic study of the myocardium. Jpn. Heart J. *14*:202, 1973.

157. Bundey, S., Carter, C. O., and Soothill, J. F.: Early recognition of heterozygote for the gene for dystrophia myotonica. J. Neurol. Neurosurg. Psychiatry *33*:279, 1970.

158. Renwick, J. H., Bundey, S. E., Ferguson-Smith, M. A., and Izatt, M. M.: Confirmation of linkage of the loci for myotonic dystrophy and ABH secretion. J. Med. Genet. *8*:407, 1971.

159. Schrott, H. G., Karp, L., and Omenn, G. S.: Prenatal prediction in myotonic dystrophy: Guidelines for genetic counseling. Clin. Genet. *4*:38, 1973.

160. Zundel, W. S., and Tyler, F. H.: The muscular dystrophies. N. Engl. J. Med. *10*:537, 596, 1965.

161. Perloff, J. K., Roberts, W. C., De Leon, A. C., Jr., and O'Doherty, D.: The distinctive electrocardiogram of Duchenne's progressive muscular dystrophy. Am. J. Med. *42*:179, 1967.

162. Moser, H., and Emery, A. E. H.: The manifesting carrier in Duchenne muscular dystrophy. Clin. Genet. *5*:271, 1974.

163. Mann, O., DeLeon, A. C., Jr., Perloff, J. K., Simanis, J., and Horrigan, F. D.:

Duchenne's muscular dystrophy: The electrocardiogram in female relatives. Am. J. Med. Sci. *255*:376, 1968.

164. Emery, A. E. H.: Abnormalities of the electrocardiogram in female carriers of Duchenne muscular dystrophy. Br. Med. J. *2*:418, 1969.

165. Mahoney, M. J., Haseltine, F. P., Hobbins, J. C., Banker, B. Q., Caskey, C. T., and Golbus, M. S.: Prenatal diagnosis of Duchenne's muscular dystrophy. N. Engl. J. Med. *297*:968, 1977.

166. Boyer, S. H., IV, Chisholm, A. W., and McKusick, V. A.: Cardiac aspects of Friedreich's ataxia. Circulation *25*:493, 1962.

167. Thoren, C.: Cardiomyopathy in Friedreich's ataxia. Acta Paediatr. *153* (Suppl.):9, 1964.

168. Hewer, R. L.: Study of fatal cases of Friedreich's ataxia. Br. Med. J. *3*:649, 1968.

169. Perloff, J. K.: Cardiomyopathy associated with heredofamilial neuromyopathic diseases. Mod. Concepts Cardiovasc. Dis. *40*:23, 1971.

170. Smith, E. R., Sangalang, V. E., Heffernan, L. P., Welch, J. P., and Flemington, C. S.: Hypertrophic cardiomyopathy: The heart disease of Friedreich's ataxia. Am. Heart J. *94*:428, 1977.

171. Ruschhaupt, D. G., Thilenius, O. G., and Cassels, D. E.: Friedreich's ataxia associated with idiopathic hypertrophic subaortic stenosis. Am. Heart J. *84*:95, 1972.

172. Maione, S., Giunta, A., Mansi, D., Filla, A., Serino, A., Teti, G., de Falco, F. A., and Campanella, G.: Cardiac abnormalities in Friedreich's ataxia patients and first-degree relatives: Evidence of hypertrophic cardiomyopathy in obligate heterozygotes. Acta Neurol. (Naples) *35*:354, 1980.

173. Folger, G. M., Jr.: Endocardial fibroelastosis. Clin. Pediatr. *10*:246, 1971.

174. Mitchell, S. C., Froehlich, L. A., Banas, J. S., Jr., and Gilkeson, M. R.: An epidemiologic assessment of primary endocardial fibroelastosis. Am. J. Cardiol. *18*:859, 1966.

175. Vestermark, S.: Primary endocardial fibroelastosis in siblings. Acta Paediatr. *51*:94, 1962.

176. Hunter, A. S., and Keay, A. J.: Primary endocardial fibroelastosis. Arch. Dis. Child. *48*:66, 1973.

177. Westwood, M., Harris, R., Burn, J. L., and Barson, A. J.: Heredity in primary endocardial fibroelastosis. Br. Heart J. *37*:1077, 1975.

178. Chen, S., Thompson, M. W., and Rose, V.: Endocardial fibroelastosis: Family studies with special reference to counseling. J. Pediatr. *79*:385, 1971.

179. Tripp, M. E., Katcher, M. L., Peters, H. A., Gilbert, E. F., Arya, S., Hodach, R. J., and Shug, A. L.: Systemic carnitine deficiency presenting as familial endocardial fibroelastosis. N. Engl. J. Med. *305*:385, 1981.

180. Engel, A. G., and Angelini, C.: Carnitine deficiency of human skeletal muscle with associated lipid storage myopathy: A new syndrome. Science *179*:899,1973.

181. Jervell, A., and Lange-Nielsen, F.: Congenital deaf-mutism, functional heart disease with prolongation of Q-T interval and sudden death. Am. Heart J. *54*:59, 1957.

182. Jervell, A.: Surdocardiac and related syndromes in children. Adv. Intern. Med. *17*:425, 1971.

183. Schwartz, P. J., Periti, M., and Malliani, A.: The long Q-T syndrome. Am. Heart J. *89*:378, 1975.

184. Denes, P.: Congenital and acquired syndrome of a long Q-T interval. Chest *71*:126, 1977.

185. Fraser, G. R., Froggatt, P., and Murphy, T.: Genetical aspects of the cardioauditory syndrome of Jervell and Lange-Nielsen (congenital deafness and electrocardiographic abnormalities). Ann. Hum. Genet. *28*:133, 1964.

186. Romano, C.: Congenital cardiac arrhythmia. Lancet *1*:658, 1965.

187. Ward, O. C.: A new familial cardiac syndrome in children. J. Irish Med. Assoc. *54*:103, 1964.

188. Itoh, S., Munemura, S., and Satoh, H.: A study of the inheritance pattern of Romano-Ward syndrome. Clin. Pediatr. *21*:20, 1982.

189. Van Der Straaten, P. J. C., and Bruins, C. L. D.: A family with heritable electrocardiographic QT-prolongation. J. Med. Genet. *10*:158, 1973.

190. Moothart, R. W., Pryor, R., Hawley, R. L., Clifford, N. J., and Blount, S. G., Jr.: The heritable syndrome of prolonged Q-T interval, syncope, and sudden death. Chest *70*:263, 1976.

191. Sarachek, N. S., and Leonard, J. J.: Familial heart block and sinus bradycardia. Am. J. Cardiol. *29*:451, 1972.

192. Crittenden, I. H., Latta, H., and Ticinovich, D. A.: Familial congenital heart block. Am. J. Dis. Child. *108*:104, 1964.

193. Winkler, R. B., Nora, A. H., and Nora, J. J.: Familial congenital complete heart block and maternal systemic lupus erythematosus. Circulation *56*:1103, 1977.

194. McCue, C. M., Mantakas, M. E., Tingelstad, J. B., and Ruddy, S.: Congenital heart block in newborns of mothers with connective tissue disease. Circulation *56*:82, 1977.

195. Chameides, L., Truex, R. C., Vetter, V., Rashkind, W. J., Galioto, Jr., F. M., and Noonan, J. A.: Association of maternal systemic lupus erythematosus with congenital complete heart block. N. Engl. J. Med. *297*:1204, 1977.

196. Kennel, A. J., Callahan, J. A., Maloney, J. D., and Zajarilas, A.: Adult-onset familial infra-Hisian block. Am. Heart J. *102*:1447, 1981.

197. Vallianos, G., and Sideris, D. A.: Familial conduction defects. Cardiology *59*:190, 1974.

198. Amat-Y-Leon, F., Racki, A. J., Denes, P., Ten Eick, R. E., Singer, D. H., Bharati, S., Lev, M., and Rosen, K. M.: Familial atrial dysrhythmia with A-V block, Circulation *50*:1097, 1974.

199. Esscher, E., Hardell, L.-I., and Michaelsson, M.: Familial, isolated, complete right bundle-branch block. Br. Heart J. *37*:745, 1975.

200. Harnischfeger, W. W.: Hereditary occurrence of the pre-excitation (Wolff-Parkinson-White) syndrome with re-entry mechanism and concealed conduction. Circulation *19*:28, 1959.

201. Schneider, R. G.: Familial occurrence of Wolff-Parkinson-White syndrome. Am. Heart J. *78*:34, 1969.

202. Massumi, R. A.: Familial Wolff-Parkinson-White syndrome with cardiomyopathy. Am. J. Med. *43*:951, 1967.

203. Perheentupa, J., Autio, S., Leisti, S., Raitta, C., and Tuuteri, L.: Mulibrey nanism, an autosomal recessive syndrome with pericardial constriction. Lancet *2*:351, 1973.

204. Perheentupa, J., Autio, S., Leisti, S., Raitta, C., and Tuuteri, L.: Mulibrey nanism: Review of 23 cases of a new autosomal recessive syndrome. Birth Defects: Original Article Series *11*:3, 1975.

205. Tuuteri, L., Perheentupa, J., and Rapola, J.: The cardiopathy of mulibrey nanism, a new inherited syndrome. Chest *65*:628, 1974.

206. Cumming, G. R., Kerr, D., and Ferguson, C. C.: Constrictive pericarditis with dwarfism in two siblings (mulibrey nanism). J. Pediatr. *88*:569, 1976.

207. Thoren, C.: So-called mulibrey nanism with pericardial constriction. Lancet *2*:731, 1973.

208. Voorhess, M. L., Husson, G. S., and Blackman, M. S.: Growth failure with pericardial constriction. Am. J. Dis. Child. *130*:1146, 1976.

209. Krause, S., Adler, L. N., Reddy, P. S., and Magovern, G. J.: Intracardiac myxoma in siblings. Chest *60*:404, 1971.

210. Liebler, G. A., Magovern, G. J., Park, S. B., Cushing, W. J., Begg, F. R., and Joyner, C. R.: Familial myxomas in four siblings. J. Thorac. Cardiovasc. Surg. *71*:605, 1976.

211. Heydorn, W. H., Gomez, A. C., Kleid, J. J., and Haas, J. M.: Atrial myxoma in siblings. J. Thorac. Cardiovasc. Surg. *65*:484, 1973.

212. Farah, M. G.: Familial atrial myxoma. Ann. Intern. Med. *83*:358, 1975.

213. Siltanen, P., Tuuteri, L., Norio, R., Tala, P., Ahrenberg, P., and Halonen, P. I.: Atrial myxoma in a family. Am. J. Cardiol. *38*:252, 1976.

214. Powers, J. C., Falkoff, M., Heinle, R. A., Nanda, N. C., Ong, L. S., Weiner, R. S., and Barold, S. S.: Familial cardiac myxoma: Emphasis on unusual clinical manifestations. J. Thorac. Cardiovasc. Surg. *77*:782, 1979.

215. Tsakraklides, V., Burke, B., Mastri, A., Runge, W., Roe, E., and Anderson, R.: Rhabdomyomas of heart. Am. J. Dis. Child. *128*:639, 1974.

216. Lagos, J. C., and Gomez, M. R.: Tuberous sclerosis: Reappraisal of a clinical entity. Mayo Clin. Proc. *42*:26, 1967.

217. Nevin, N. C., and Pearce, W. G.: Diagnostic and genetical aspects of tuberous sclerosis. J. Med. Genet. *5*:273, 1968.

CORONARY ARTERY DISEASE

218. Epstein, F. H.: Risk factors in coronary heart disease—environmental and hereditary influences. Isr. J. Med. Sci. *3*:594, 1967.

219. Slack, J., and Evans, K. A.: The increased risk of death from ischaemic heart disease in first degree relatives of 121 men and 96 women with ischaemic heart disease. J. Med. Genet. *3*:239, 1966.

220. Rissanen, A. M., and Nikkila, E. A.: Coronary artery disease and its risk factors in families of young men with angina pectoris and in controls. Br. Heart J. *39*:875, 1977.

221. Harvald, B., and Hauge, M.: Coronary occlusion in twins. Acta. Genet. Med. Gemellol. (Roma) *19*:248, 1970.

222. Epstein, F. H., and Ostrander, L. D., Jr.: Detection of individual susceptibility toward coronary disease. Prog. Cardiovasc. Dis. *13*:324, 1971.

223. Kannel, W. B., Castelli, W. P., Gordon, T., and McNamara, P. M.: Serum cholesterol, lipoproteins, and the risk of coronary heart disease. Ann. Intern. Med. *74*:1, 1971.

224. Bloor, C. M.: Hereditary aspects of myocardial infarction. Circulation *39, 40* (Suppl. 4):130, 1969.

224a.Neufeld, H. N., and Goldbourt, U.: Coronary heart disease: Genetic aspects. Circulation *67*:943, 1983.

225. Goldstein, J. L., Schrott, H. G., Hazzard, W. R., Bierman, E. L., and Motulsky, A. G.: Hyperlipidemia in coronary heart disease. II. Genetic analysis of lipid levels in 176 families and delineation of a new inherited disorder, combined hyperlipidemia. J. Clin. Invest. *52*:1544, 1973.

226. Brown, M. S., and Goldstein, J. L.: Familial hypercholesterolemia: A genetic defect in the low-density lipoprotein receptor. N. Engl. J. Med. *294*:1386, 1976.

227. Goldstein, J. L., and Brown, M. S.: Familial hypercholesterolemia. *In* Stanbury, J. B., Wyngaarden, J. B., Fredrickson, D. S., Goldstein, J. L., and Brown, M. S. (eds.): The Metabolic Basis of Inherited Disease. 5th ed. New York, McGraw-Hill Book Co., 1983, p. 672.

228. Epstein, C. J., Martin, G. M., Schultz, A. L., and Motulsky, A. G.: Werner's syndrome: A review of its symptomatology, natural history, pathologic features, genetics and relationship to the natural aging process. Medicine *45*:177, 1966.

229. Zackai, A. H., Weber, D., and Noth, R.: Cardiac findings in Werner's syndrome. Geriatrics *29*:141, 1974.

230. Duncan, C., and McLeod, G. M.: Angiokeratoma corporis diffusum universale (Fabry's disease). Aust. Ann. Med. *1*:58, 1970.

231. Becker, A. E., Schoorl, R., Balk, A. G., and van der Heide, R. M.: Cardiac manifestations of Fabry's disease. Am. J. Cardiol. *36*:829, 1975.

232. Beaudet, A. L., Ferry, G. D., Nichols, B. L., Jr., and Rosenberg, H. S.: Cholesterol ester storage disease: Clinical, biochemical, and pathological studies. J. Pediatr. *90*:910, 1977.

233. Havel, R. J., Goldstein, J. L., and Brown, M. S.: Lipoproteins and lipid trans-

port. *In* Bondy, P. K., and Rosenberg, L. E. (eds.): Diseases of Metabolism. 8th ed. Philadelphia, W. B. Saunders Co., 1980, p. 393.

234. Brown, M. S., Kovanen, P. T., and Goldstein, J. L.: Regulation of plasma cholesterol by lipoprotein receptors. Science *212*:628–635, 1981.

235. Jackson, R. L., Morisett, J. D., and Gotto, A. M., Jr.: Lipoprotein structure and metabolism. Physiol. Rev. *56*:259, 1976.

236. Goldstein, J. L., and Brown, M. S.: Familial hypercholesterolemia: Pathogenesis of a receptor disease. Johns Hopkins Med. J. *143*:8, 1978.

237. Glomset, J. A., and Norum, K. R.: The metabolic role of lecithin-cholesterol acyltransferase: Perspectives from pathology. Adv. Lipid Res. *11*:1, 1973.

238. Kwiterovich, P. O., Jr., Levy, R. I., and Fredrickson, D. S.: Neonatal diagnosis of familial type-II hyperlipoproteinemia. Lancet *1*:118, 1973.

239. Slack, J.: Risks of ischaemic heart disease in familial hyperlipoproteinaemic states. Lancet *2*:1380, 1969.

240. Jensen, J., Blankenhorn, D. H., and Kornerup, V.: Coronary disease in familial hypercholesterolemia. Circulation *36*:77, 1967.

241. Stone, N. J., Levy, R. I., Fredrickson, D. S., and Verter, J.: Coronary artery disease in 116 kindred with familial type-II hyperlipoproteinemia. Circulation *49*:476, 1974.

242. Khachadurian, A. K., and Uthman, S. M.: Experiences with the homozygous cases of familial hypercholesterolemia. Nutr. Metab. *15*:132, 1973.

243. Goldstein, J. L.: The cardiac manifestations of the homozygous and heterozygous forms of familial type II hyperbetalipoproteinemia. Birth Defects: Original Article Series *8*:202, 1972.

243a.Forman, M. B., Kinsley, R. H., DuPlessis, J. P., Dansky, R., Milner, S., and Levin, S. E.: Surgical correction of combined supravalvular and valvular aortic stenosis in homozygous familial hypercholesterolaemia. S. Afr. Med. J. *61*:579, 1982.

244. Buja, L. M., Kovanen, P. T., and Bilheimer, D. W. : Cellular pathology of homozygous familial hypercholesterolemia. Am. J. Pathol. *97*:327, 1979.

245. Allen, J. M., Thompson, G. R., Myant, N. B., Steiner, R., and Oakley, C. M.: Cardiovascular complications of homozygous familial hypercholesterolaemia. Br. Heart J. *44*:361, 1980.

246. Glueck, C. J., Levy, R. I., and Fredrickson, D. S.: Acute tendinitis and arthritis: A presenting symptom of familial type II hyperlipoproteinemia. J.A.M.A. *206*:2895, 1969.

247. Goldstein, J. L., Brown, M. S., and Stone, J. J.: Genetics of the LDL receptor: Evidence that the mutations affecting binding and internalization are allelic. Cell. *12*:629, 1977.

248. Brown, M. S., and Goldstein, J. L.: Familial hypercholesterolemia: Model for genetic receptor disease. Harvey Lect. Vol. 73, 1977–78.

249. Goldstein, J. L., and Brown, M. S.: Atherosclerosis: The low density lipoprotein receptor hypothesis. Metabolism *26*:1257, 1977.

250. Bilheimer, D. W., Stone, N. J., and Grundy, S. M.: Metabolic studies in familial hypercholesterolemia: Evidence for a gene-dosage effect *in vivo*. J. Clin. Invest. *64*:524, 1979.

251. Bilheimer, D. W., Goldstein, J. L., Grundy, S. M., and Brown, M. S.: Reduction in cholesterol and low density lipoprotein synthesis after portavacal shunt surgery in a patient with homozygous familial hypercholesterolemia. J. Clin. Invest. *56*:1420, 1975.

252. Soutar, A. K., Myant, N. B., and Thompson, G. R.: Simultaneous measurement of apolipoprotein B turnover in very-low- and low-density lipoproteins in familial hypercholesterolaemia. Atherosclerosis *28*:247, 1977.

253. Ross, R., and Glomset, J. A.: The pathogenesis of atherosclerosis. N. Engl. J. Med. *295*:369, 420, 1976.

254. Bilheimer, D. W., Ho, Y. K., Brown, M. S., Anderson, R. G. W., and Gold-

stein, J. L.: Genetics of the low density lipoprotein receptor: Diminished receptor activity in lymphocytes from heterozygotes with familial hypercholesterolemia. J. Clin. Invest. *61*:678, 1978.

255. Brown, M. S., Kovanen, P. T., Goldstein, J. L., Vandenberghe, K., Pryns, J. P., Eeckels, R., Van Den Berghe, H., and Cassiman, J. J.: Prenatal diagnosis of homozygous familial hypercholesterolaemia. Lancet *1*:526, 1978.

256. Kane, J. P., and Malloy, M. J.: Treatment of hypercholesterolemia. Med. Clin. North Am. *66*:537, 1982.

257. Thompson, G. R., and Gotto, A. M.: Ileal bypass in the treatment of hyperlipoproteinaemia. Lancet *2*:35, 1973.

258. Starzl, T. E., Putnam, C. W., Chase, H. P., and Porter, K. A.: Portacaval shunt in hyperlipoproteinaemia. Lancet *2*:940, 1973.

259. Thompson, G. R., Lowenthal, R., and Myant, N. B.: Plasma exchange in the management of homozygous familial hypercholesterolaemia. Lancet *1*:1208, 1975.

260. Havel, R. J. (ed.): Symposium on lipid disorders. Med. Clin. North Am. Vol. 66, 1982, pp. 317–550.

261. Schonfeld, G., and Kudzma, D. J.: Type IV hyperlipoproteinemia. Arch. Intern. Med. *132*:55, 1973.

262. Brunzell, J. D., Schrott, H. H., Motulsky, A. G., and Bierman, E. L.: Myocardial infarction in the familial forms of hypertriglyceridemia. Metabolism *25*:313, 1976.

263. Nikkila, E. A., and Aro, A.: Family study of serum lipids and lipoproteins in coronary heart-disease. Lancet *1*:954, 1973.

264. Rose, H. G., Kranz, P., Weinstock, M., Juliano, J., and Haft, J. I.: Inheritance of combined hyperlipoproteinemia: Evidence for a new lipoprotein phenotype. Am. J. Med. *54*:148, 1973.

265. Matthews, R. J.: Type III and IV familial hyperlipoproteinemia: Evidence that these two syndromes are different phenotypic expressions of the same mutant gene(s). Am. J. Med. *44*:188, 1968.

266. Schriebman, P. H., Wilson, D. E., and Arky, R. A.: Familial type IV hyperlipoproteinemia. N. Engl. J. Med. *287*:981, 1969.

267. Glueck, C. J., Fallat, R., Buncher, C. R., Tsang, R., and Steiner, P.: Familial combined hyperlipoproteinemia: Studies in 91 adults and 95 children from 33 kindreds. Metabolism *22*:1403, 1973.

268. Brown, M. S., Goldstein, J. L., and Fredrickson, D. S.: Familial type 3 hypercholesterolemia (dysbetalipoproteinemia). *In* Stanbury, J. B., Wyngaarden, J. B., Fredrickson, D. S., Goldstein, J. L., and Brown, M. S. (eds.): The Metabolic Basis of Inherited Disease. 5th ed. New York, McGraw-Hill Book Co., 1983, p. 655.

269. Hazzard, W. R., and Bierman, E. L.: Aggravation of broad-beta disease (Type 3 hyperlipoproteinemia) by hypothyroidism. Arch. Intern. Med. *130*:822, 1972.

270. Utermann, G., Hees, M., and Steinnet, A.: Polymorphism of apolipoprotein E and occurrence of dysbetalipoproteinaemia in man. Nature *269*:604, 1977.

271. Zannis, V. I., and Breslow, J. L.: Human very low density lipoprotein apolipoprotein E isoprotein polymorphism is explained by genetic variation and posttranslational modification. Biochemistry *20*:1033, 1981.

272. Schneider, W. J., Kovanen, P. T., Brown, M. S., Goldstein, J. L., Utermann, G., Weber, W., Havel, R. J., Kotite, L., Kane, J. P., Innerarity, T. L., and Mahley, R. W.: Familial dysbetalipoproteinemia. Abnormal binding of mutant apoprotein E to low density lipoprotein receptors of human fibroblasts and membranes from liver and adrenal of rats, rabbits, and cows. J. Clin. Invest. *68*:1075, 1981.

273. Utermann, G., Vogelberg, K. H., Steinmetz, A., Schoenborn, W., Pruin, N., Jaeschke, M., Hees, M., and Canzler, H.: Polymorphism of apolipoprotein E. II. Genetics of hyperlipoproteinemia type III. Clin. Genet. *15*:37, 1979.

48 RHEUMATIC AND HERITABLE CONNECTIVE TISSUE DISEASES OF THE CARDIOVASCULAR SYSTEM

by Gene H. Stollerman, M.D.

Two groups of diseases that affect connective tissues are the so-called rheumatic diseases and the heritable disorders of connective tissues. *The rheumatic diseases* have many clinical features in common and are often classified together because they produce acute and/or chronic arthritis associated with a variety of systemic inflammatory manifestations. Pathologically, they are characterized by diffuse vascular lesions with varying degrees of exudation and fibrosis, and seem to be associated with hyperimmune phenomena. The etiologies of some of the syndromes have been established as complications of well-recognized infections; however, several of the rheumatic diseases remain obscure in regard to both etiology and pathogenesis. They all involve the heart differently and to varying degrees, as would be expected considering the variety of connective tissue structures that make up the heart's "skeleton"—its valve rings, valves, septa, and pericardial sac and the myocardial interstitium, through which courses its rich blood supply.

The *heritable disorders of connective tissue* are rare, genetically determined biochemical lesions of collagen, elastic tissue, or the mucopolysaccharides. In all, structural lesions are produced when the stresses of cardiac action "wear out" the defective cardiac skeleton.

RHEUMATIC DISEASES

RHEUMATIC FEVER (RF)

Rheumatic fever (RF) is frequently classified as a connective tissue disease because its anatomic hallmark is damage to collagen fibrils and to the ground substance of connective tissue (especially in the heart). Of major clinical importance is the presence of potentially lethal myocarditis during the acute attack or, more commonly, the fibrosis of the heart valves, which leads to the crippling hemodynamics of chronic rheumatic heart disease.

Epidemiology of Rheumatic Fever

The relation between the epidemiology of RF and that of streptococcal infection has been reviewed extensively.[1] The current confusion concerning the epidemiology of RF stems from the dramatic decline in incidence and prevalence of the disease despite the fact that group A streptococcal pharyngitis still appears to be common among populations in which RF has become rare.

THE CHANGING PATTERN OF RHEUMATIC FEVER: INCIDENCE, PREVALENCE AND MORTALITY

Since Halsey's study in 1921[2] virtually all those who study this disease have been impressed with the diminishing frequency and severity of acute rheumatic fever (ARF), particularly in the relatively affluent populations of North America and Europe (Fig. 48–1). Reasons for this decline are uncertain but are undoubtedly multiple. Certainly antibiotics for the treatment and prevention of streptococcal infection have been a factor, as demonstrated particularly in military populations.[3,4] However, the incidence and death rate from the disease were decreasing before the introduction of antibiotics. Changes in the virulence and serotypes of group A streptococci have been noteworthy (see below). Improved social conditions, such as better housing and slum clearance, have contributed to the decline, since crowding because of inadequate housing is probably the chief reason for the magnified risk of streptococcal infection and ARF in certain ethnic and disadvantaged populations. Improvement in the delivery of health care in defined populations may also be significant.[5]

The prevalence of rheumatic heart disease among American school children has dropped sharply in recent years, so that the number of cases of congenital heart disease now exceeds those of rheumatic heart disease in these populations.[6] When analyzed separately, the death rate from ARF has been noted to have fallen more sharply than that for rheumatic heart disease.[7] Notwithstanding its decline, rheumatic heart disease still constitutes the leading cause of death from heart disease in the 5-to 24-year-old age

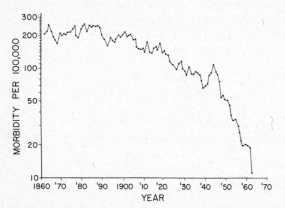

FIGURE 48–1 Reported rheumatic fever incidence in Denmark, 1862–1962. From the Public Health Board of Denmark, Copenhagen, Denmark. (From Stollerman, G. H.: Rheumatic Fever and Streptococcal Infection. New York, by permission of Grune and Stratton, 1975.)

group in most parts of the world and continues to be a serious public health problem.[8]

FACTORS IN THE ATTACK RATE OF RHEUMATIC FEVER

Quantitative Factors. One factor is the severity of the antecedent pharyngeal streptococcal infection. The clearest relationship of group A streptococcal infection to RF is found in military populations subject to epidemic streptococcal sore throat. In patients with frank, exudative streptococcal pharyngitis caused by certain common prevalent pharyngeal strains of virulent group A streptococci, RF followed at a fairly predictable attack rate (approximately 3 per cent) regardless of the age, race, or ethnic group studied and regardless of the year or season in which the study was made.[3] The major variables which seem to be related to this attack rate in such studies are the magnitude of the immune response to the antecedent streptococcal infection[9] and the duration of convalescent carriage of the organism.[10] Weak antistreptolysin O (ASO) responses are associated with ARF attack rates considerably less than 1 per cent, whereas strong responses are associated with rates well in excess of 5 per cent. In fact, in some studies in which patients with still more vigorous responses are selected, the attack rate may equal 10 per cent.[3] If the infecting organism in the pharynx was not eradicated during convalescence, treatment of streptococcal pharyngitis failed to reduce the attack rate of rheumatic fever.

In contrast to the military studies, reports from civilian medical practice suggest that RF may occur less frequently following endemic, sporadic streptococcal disease.[11-14]

Qualitative Factors. Variations in the "rheumatogenicity" of group A streptococcal strains may constitute one factor influencing the attack rate of RF. In several laboratories where regular serotyping of group A streptococci isolated from pharyngeal infections is performed with available antisera prepared against known M-protein serotypes, the frequency of identification of such strains has decreased. Furthermore, the prevalence of several of the major M types notorious for causing epidemic RF (e.g., types 5, 14, and 24) has apparently declined,[13] and attention has shifted to the study of "new" M types among both pharyngeal strains and "skin" strains.[15] The issue of whether there are "nonrheumatogenic group A streptococci"[16] has been sharpened by the clear demonstration that group A streptococcal pyoderma, with or without complicating acute glomerulonephritis (AGN), does not cause ARF.[17] These skin infections are nonrheumatogenic.[18] Since the pharyngeal route of infection is now an accepted requirement for the pathogenesis of ARF (see below), the question of whether such pyoderma strains can cause RF when they produce pharyngitis is of particular interest. Studies in Memphis have clearly shown seasonal epidemiological separation of ARF and AGN.[19] Populations in the southern United States in which pyoderma and ARF both occur show large numbers of cases of AGN in summer when streptococcal pyoderma is prevalent and when ARF is virtually absent. In the fall, when school begins again, AGN and pyoderma decline rapidly and ARF appears abruptly. In Trinidad, where both AGN and ARF are concurrent in the same population with little seasonal variation, cyclical epidemics of AGN have been reported[20] but without parallel changes in the incidence of ARF. A study of the streptococcal strains in this population show a clear distinction between the serotypes associated with AGN and those associated with ARF.[21]

The studies of Widdowson et al. suggest that RF is associated with infections due to virulent strains capable of causing strong type-specific immune responses to M protein and other streptococcal antigens.[22] Such strains belong to the classic M serotypes known to cause ARF.[23,24]

GEOGRAPHY AND CLIMATE

The relationship of RF to the intensity and severity of streptococcal disease is the same in the tropics as in the temperate climates.[25] The clinical features of RF are also alleged to vary in different climates. In warm climates, there is a reported disparity between the high frequency of acute rheumatic carditis and the apparently low frequency of other manifestations of ARF. Sanyal et al. have recently reviewed the disparate studies from India which have emphasized, on the one hand, the absence or paucity of acute rheumatic manifestations in the population and, on the other, a very high incidence of severe carditis.[26] However, when *prospective* studies were made in a general pediatric department in which *all patients suspected of having ARF were admitted* and *recurrent attacks were excluded*, the frequency of the clinical manifestations of rheumatic fever were the same in New Delhi, India, as in the studies in the United States.

HOST FACTORS

Acquired Susceptibility Through Infections. Since ARF develops in a relatively small percentage of patients following even the most virulent streptococcal infection, the issue of host predisposition is often raised. Once RF is acquired, its activation following streptococcal infection is many times greater in rheumatic subjects than in the general population. The recurrence rate per infection, which is as high as 50 per cent during the first year, decreases sharply until 4 to 5 years after the attack, when it levels off at approximately 10 per cent[27,28] and never seems to fall much lower.[29] Although the persistently higher attack rate in individuals having had RF may suggest some degree of genetic predisposition,[30] the diminishing recurrence rate per infection appears to be acquired. An alternative explanation would be that an acquired sensitization persists virtually throughout life.

Age, Sex, and Race. Like streptococcal sore throat, ARF occurs most commonly in the young school-age child and very rarely in early infancy. It is estimated that 40 per cent of streptococcal infections in pediatric populations occur in children 2 to 6 years of age,[31] suggesting that repeated streptococcal infections and sensitization of the host are prerequisite to the development of RF.[32] No true differencs in sex, race, or ethnic group susceptibility have been established. Crowded living conditions account for whatever apparent increased susceptibility has been reported.

Etiology of Reumatic Fever

The four lines of evidence establishing the group A streptococcus as the sole agent causing initial and recurrent attacks of RF (described below) are of necessity indirect, because group A streptococci cannot be recovered from the lesions of RF and no satisfactory experimental model of the disease has been demonstrated.

Clinical Evidence. Although the frequency with which septic sore throat preceded ARF has been recognized for over 100 years, inconsistencies in this relationship have been pointed out repeatedly.[33,34] Almost one-third of patients with ARF deny the occurrence of antecedent sore throat. Throat and blood cultures in such patients show that the former is frequently negative and the latter virtually always sterile at the onset of the rheumatic attack. Recurrences of RF appeared even more mysterious when antecedent streptococcal sore throat was unrecognized and particularly when the chronicity of a rheumatic attack and the hemodynamic complications of rheumatic heart disease made it difficult to distinguish continued versus reactivated rheumatic carditis. On clinical grounds alone, therefore, it is difficult to establish the group A streptococcus as the sole etiological agent.

Epidemiological Evidence. The environmental, bacterial, and host factors which appear to play a role in the development of RF are important primarily because they are related to the incidence of preceding streptococcal infection. Thus, such factors as latitude, altitude, crowding, dampness, economic factors, and age all affect the incidence of RF because they are related to the incidence and severity of streptococcal infections in general (see above). Careful military epidemiological studies over a period of 20 years show a clear sequential relationship between outbreaks of streptococcal pharyngitis and RF.[35]

Immunological Evidence. Initial (primary) or recurrent (secondary) RF does not occur without a streptococ-

cal antibody response.[36] Furthermore, the magnitude of the antibody response is a major variable determining the attack rate of RF following streptococcal pharyngitis.[9] This is true for both primary and secondary attacks.[27] Indeed, the streptococcal immune response is an important criterion for the diagnosis of RF (see below).

Prophylactic Evidence. The final and perhaps most convincing evidence is the prevention of both initial and recurrent attacks of RF by, in the former case, penicillin therapy and, in the latter, continuous chemoprophylaxis against streptococcal infections. Completely effective prophylaxis of streptococcal infections in rheumatic subjects allows us to conclude that RF cannot be reactivated by any other infection, illness, or trauma.[27,36]

Pathogenesis of Rheumatic Fever

Despite the elusiveness of the pathogenesis of RF, there are a few well-established requirements for the development of this postinfectious sequel: (1) the presence of the group A streptococcus, (2) a streptococcal antibody response indicative of actual recent infection, (3) persistence of the organism in the pharynx for a sufficient period of time, and (4) location of the infection in the throat.

Site of Infection. The possible role of lymphatic connections between the pharynx and the heart has been considered. The embryological derivation of the heart links it structurally with the neck in its vascular, lymphatic, and nervous supply. Impressive connections between tonsils and the heart in human beings have been demonstrated by injections of lymphatic channels in cadavers.[18]

Strain of Group A Streptococcus. The quantitative factor of severity of streptococcal infection bears a general relationship to the attack rate of RF. Although a constant attack rate of RF was shown to occur in military epidemics regardless of the M serotype of the infecting strain, these epidemics were caused by a relatively small number of M serotypes that are now well recognized as the most common and dangerous rheumatogenic pharyngeal strains but are not as commonly isolated as they were previously.

Direct Invasion by Group A Streptococci. Because of the sterility of joint and cerebrospinal fluid (in chorea), most attention has centered on a few reports of group A streptococci cultured from heart valves in acute rheumatic endocarditis.[37,38] Although repetition and extension of this work were hampered by the discovery of antibiotics, most investigators believe that these early reports were the results of either contamination at the time of autopsy or agonal or postmortem dissemination and proliferation of streptococci.[39] Attempts to cure RF by intensive antibiotic therapy have not been successful.

The Role of Toxins. Despite the popularity of the concepts of hyperimmunity and autoimmunity in the pathogenesis of RF (see below), none of the antibodies described to date, including those reactive with the heart, has been shown to be cytotoxic. A direct toxic effect, therefore, of some streptococcal product, particularly on the heart, has not yet been ruled out as a pathogenetic mechanism.[1,30]

IMMUNOLOGICAL THEORIES

The most popular pathogenic theory is that RF results from some type of hyperimmune reaction due either to bacterial allergy or autoimmunity. This view is supported by strong evidence, since RF patients are, in general, the population most intensively hyperimmune to all streptococcal products.

The mean antibody titer to virtually every streptococcal antigen that has been studied is increased in patients during the acute stage of RF. Yet no humoral mechanism of tissue injury has been defined. The latent period between streptococcal infection and the onset of RF resembles that of serum sickness, but several features of RF differentiate it from the immune complex diseases with their associated vascular lesions (see The Vasculitis Syndromes, below). The latent period of ARF does not decrease with repeated recurrences, as with repeated bouts of serum sickness. Angioneurotic edema and vasculitis rashes are not a feature of the disease. Complement levels are increased rather than decreased, and autoantibodies associated with immune complex disease (e.g., rheumatoid factor, anti-DNA, and others) are not present. Although low-grade microscopic hematuria may occur, frank lesions of glomerulonephritis are absent. Careful recent studies have identified circulating immune complexes, but they are of small size and not high titer and quickly disappear after the acute stage of polyarthritis.[40] Whether or not they actually cause arthritic inflammation is conjectural.

Much interest has been shown in the possible mechanism of cell-mediated cytotoxic reactions to various streptococcal antigens, particularly as a possible cause of rheumatic carditis. Although cell-mediated responses to some streptococcal antigens have been shown to be blunted during ARF, most reactions are normal or exaggerated. The specificity of these phenomena for the acute rheumatic process is uncertain, although a recent study suggests that some extracellular purified streptococcal products show diminished reactivity with lymphocytes of patients with rheumatic heart disease compared with those of control subjects.[41]

AUTOIMMUNITY. It has been known for many years that the serum of some patients with ARF contains autoantibodies to heart tissues, and numerous reports using a variety of techniques, mostly immunofluorescence, have confirmed this finding.[42-44] Anti-heart antibodies are gamma globulins with specificity for cardiac components reacting primarily with the sarcolemma. Their binding is also associated with deposition of large amounts of complement component C3. Anti-heart antibodies occur more frequently in RF patients who develop carditis than in those who escape it. The frequency of the appearance of such antibodies is very high in patients who have undergone mitral commissurotomy. These antibodies can be adsorbed by the patient's own atrial tissue and therefore are probably autoantibodies. Massive deposits of gamma globulin have also been identified in the hearts of children who died of rheumatic carditis. The role of such antibodies in the pathogenesis of rheumatic fever has been clouded by the growing understanding of autoantibody formation and complement activation as a general response to tissue injury. Cardiac damage by rheumatic, traumatic, or ischemic heart lesions leads to biochemical changes manifested by the production of autoantibody.[45] Thus, myocardial infarction and postpericardiotomy syndromes have been associated with the production of anti-heart antibodies and/or deposition of complement. It is therefore possible that anti-heart antibodies in rheumatic carditis are the *result* rather than the *cause* of tissue injury.

CROSS REACTIONS BETWEEN STREPTOCOCCI AND HUMAN HEART AND OTHER ORGANS. In the early 1960's Kaplan and his associates demonstrated that rabbit antisera against certain group A streptococci react with human heart preparations in the immunofluorescent test.[46,47] Since then, many additional immunological

cross reactions have been described between streptococci and human tissues[48-62] (Fig. 48–2). The immunological details of these reactions and their possible relation to the pathogenesis of RF have been reported and reviewed in detail elsewhere.[1,30,53]

The relationship between anti-heart antibodies in RF and the development of rheumatic heart disease is not clear, and therefore there is no firm evidence for a causal relationship between such cross reactions and the development of rheumatic carditis, however attractive this hypothesis may be.

HOST FACTORS

Genetic Predisposition. The frequent observation of strong familial histories of RF despite the lack of evidence of clear genetic factors predisposing to RF has been puzzling. Only a few adequate studies in identical twins have shown a relatively low concordance of RF (less than 20 per cent), actually considerably lower than that found in some other infections, such as tuberculosis or poliomyelitis.[63] Furthermore, the incidence of ARF is remarkably similar in every human race or ethnic group exposed to rheumatogenic streptococcal disease. It has not been possible, therefore, to define any clear genetic predisposition to the disease, and familial clustering may reflect the factor of infection rather than host predisposition. Although haplotype distributions in rheumatic hosts have not been consistently correlated, there is a suggestion of prominence of HLA-B5, particularly in patients with polyarthritis who are found to have circulating immune complexes.[40]

Immune Response of RF Patients. All antibodies to streptococcal antigens that have been studied have been consistently increased in RF patients compared with patients who have uncomplicated streptococcal pharyngitis.[64] Patients with inactive rheumatic heart disease, however, have depressed cell-mediated responses to some purified streptococcal antigens.[41] RF patients respond normally to other antigens, such as diphtheria toxoid.[65] Conventional immunology would interpret the increased streptococcal immune response to mean that the antecedent streptococcal infection of RF must be of a greater magnitude antigenically than nonrheumatogenic streptococcal infections. Alternatively, or in addition, the rheumatic host may be hyperimmune because of more frequent or more severe streptococcal infections. The depressed cellular immune response to certain purified streptococcal antigens[41] is noteworthy, but the implications with regard to pathogenesis are not clear.

Pathology of Rheumatic Fever

There is often considerable disparity between the severity of the clinical manifestations of RF and the extent of the morbid anatomical changes it produces. Sydenham's chorea, cardiac atrioventricular conduction blocks, and erythema marginatum all appear to be related more to functional disturbances than to visible lesions. In contrast, the persistent focal inflammatory lesions of the myocardium, such as the *Aschoff nodule,* do not always correlate with clinical manifestations of active carditis and have led to differences between pathologists and clinicians with regard

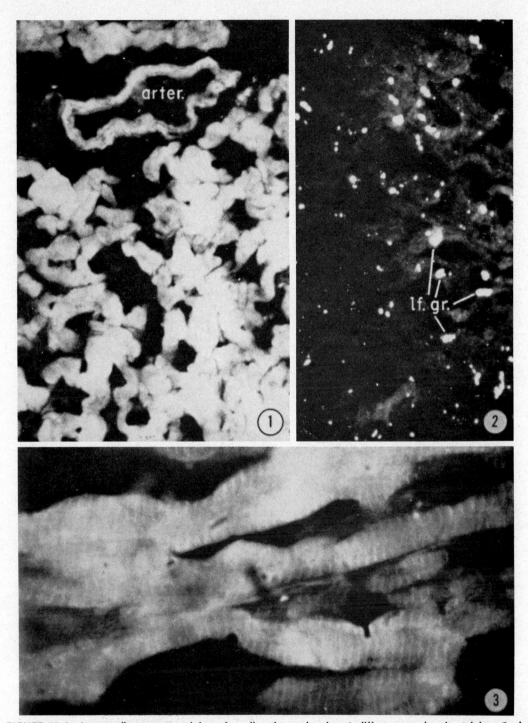

FIGURE 48–2 Immunofluorescent staining of cardiac tissue showing *1,* diffuse sarcoplasmic staining; *2,* absence of specific fluorescence in control section treated with rabbit antiserum free of heart antibody; and *3,* cross-striational staining pattern of left atrial muscle from a patient with rheumatic heart disease. (From Zabriskie, J. B., and Freimer, E. H.: An immunological relationship between the group A streptococcus and mammalian muscle. J. Exp. Med. *124*:661, 1966.)

to the definition of rheumatic activity. In general, however, the acute phase of RF is characterized by diffuse exudative and proliferative inflammatory reactions in the heart, joints, and skin. Small blood vessels and arterioles are commonly involved, but unlike the arteritis of some other connective tissue diseases, thrombotic lesions are not seen.

The term *fibrinoid degeneration* describes the basic structural changes in the collagen of connective tissues.[66,67] The fibrinoid substance resembles and stains like fibrin and is a feature of the earli-

est phase of the myocardial lesions. The collagen fibers in these mucoid areas become swollen and eosinophilic, forming a meshwork of rigid, waxlike fibers. This exudative-degenerative phase[68,69] lasts for 2 to 3 weeks, following which the most characteristic lesion of RF develops—the myocardial *Aschoff nodule.*[70] The proliferative and healing phase then follows and may persist for many months or even years.[71]

In the early stage of development of the Aschoff nodule,[72] lymphocytes collect around and between the eosinophilic material followed soon after by large and sometimes multinucleated cells with ragged basophilic cytoplasm.[72] Many of these cells have a characteristic *owl-*

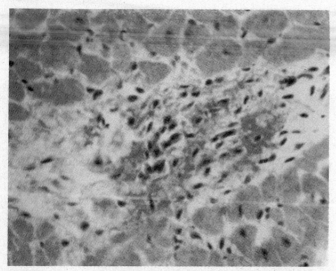

FIGURE 48–3 Early reticular Aschoff body. Note the rigid eosinophilic fibers and clumps of material. The cells are small and elongated (H and E, ×240). (From Lannigan, R.: Cardiac Pathology. London, Butterworth and Co., 1966.)

eye nucleus, which contains a heavy eccentric chromatin dot with fine fibrils radiating to the nuclear membrane (Fig. 48–3). Gradual healing of Aschoff nodules leaves a fibrous scar. Aschoff nodules are virtually pathognomonic of RF with or without collagen fibrinoid lesions.[76]

Ironically, the only lesion pathognomonic of RF is vague with regard to its origin, functional impact on the heart, and relation to the course and severity of the rheumatic attack.[72-78] Aschoff nodules do not seem to account for the acute dilatation of the heart in first attacks of severe carditis. The persistence of Aschoff nodules for many years after a rheumatic attack has been well recognized by pathologists. Biopsies of the left atrial appendage obtained during mitral valve surgery for mitral stenosis have shown persistence of Aschoff nodules in patients who no longer have clinical or laboratory evidence of rheumatic activity[79-81] and who have no recent evidence of streptococcal infection.[82] The persistence of Aschoff nodules seems to be correlated, however, with progressive fibrosis and stenosis of the mitral valve. One series[80,81] showed such lesions in 21 per cent of 191 surgically excised left atrial appendages in patients with mitral stenosis. In the same series, of 91 patients with pure mitral regurgitation, Aschoff nodules were present in the left atrial appendage of only 1 patient.

CARDIAC LESIONS

On gross inspection of the heart, a pancarditis is almost always evident, with fresh exudative pericardial lesions, dilatation of the heart, and verrucous endocardial lesions on the valves.[1,83]

Pericarditis (see also p. 1510). Both layers of the pericardium are thickened and covered with a fibrinous exudate, and serosanguineous pericardial fluid may be present. Mucoid edema occurs early. The deposition of eosinophilic, fibrin-staining material present in other layers of the heart is also seen in the pericardium. With healing, fibrosis and adhesions develop which partially or completely obliterate the pericardial sac, but constrictive pericarditis does *not* occur.

Myocarditis. In addition to the Aschoff bodies, a diffuse cellular infiltrate is present in interstitial tissues. The cells are usually lymphocytes, but polymorphonuclear leukocytes, histiocytes, and eosinophils may also be present. Exudate may be associated with damaged muscle. This interstitial myocarditis may be more important than the nodular Aschoff bodies in producing heart failure. Myo-

cardial fibers are also damaged, and the greatest damage occurs in the vicinity of Aschoff nodules and around blood vessels,[84,85] leading to loss of striations, fatty degeneration, and vacuolation. Myocytolysis and complete loss of fibers may be noted in some areas,[72] and giant cell formation may occur in damaged fibers.

The Conduction System. Despite the high frequency of prolonged atrial ventricular conduction in ARF, visible changes in the bundle of His are seen in the minority of autopsy cases of ARF.[86] The evanescence of heart block and its easy reversibility in most cases by the administration of atropine fit the concept that a functional defect rather than a structural lesion is responsible for this conduction defect.

Endocarditis. The verrucous lesions at the valve edge appear as a mass of eosinophilic material staining as fibrin. At the base and edges of the valve, the cells line up in palisades at right angles to the base and often have elongated Aschoff-type nuclei. As the lesions progress, granulation tissue develops and vascularization and progressive fibrosis take place (Fig. 48–4). The changes involve the annulus as well as the cusps and chordae tendineae, which, as a result of scarring, thicken and shorten.

Arteritis in Coronary Arteries and Other Vessels. Coronary arteritis has been well described in RF for the past 80 years,[87,88] and many pathologists have considered these lesions important in producing myocardial damage in RF. Yet, despite such descriptions, thrombosis of large coronary vessels is very rare in ARF.

RHEUMATIC VALVULAR DEFORMITIES (See also Chap. 32)

Mitral Regurgitation. Incompetence or regurgitation may result from shortening of one or both cusps, from shortening and fusing of chordae and papillary muscles, or from dilatation of the valve ring. By far, the most common clinically apparent lesion of rheumatic heart disease is mitral regurgitation, and such lesions often occur subclinical-

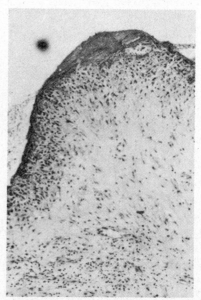

FIGURE 48–4 Rheumatic vegetation showing a layer of dense eosinophilic material and a cellular reaction beneath. The cusp also shows a diffuse cellular infiltrate (H and E, ×60). (From Lannigan, R.: Cardiac Pathology. London, Butterworth and Co., 1966.)

ly when extracardiac symptoms of ARF are absent. Dilatation of the valve ring occurs in active carditis more frequently as a result of acute dilatation of the left ventricle. Marked mitral regurgitation also occurs, however, without acute left ventricular dilatation when the valve cusps and the musculotendinous structures are severely swollen and disorganized by the rheumatic process without coexisting severe myocarditis. In cases of severe regurgitation the degree of stenosis is only moderate, but the same kinds of deformities may be seen in ring, cusps, chordae, and papillary muscles as those described for mitral stenosis. Characteristically, the posterior cusp of the mitral valve is most heavily involved (Fig. 48–5A).

Mitral Stenosis.   This lesion occurs with varying degrees of mitral regurgitation. When stenosis is severe, regurgitation may be relatively unimportant, and the main hemodynamic problem is obstruction to blood flow during diastole. The gross changes in the mitral valve are variable. The cusps may fuse, leaving an ovoid opening, but the cusps themselves may remain thin and pliable. In other instances the cusps become thick, rigid, or even calcified. A "funnel-shaped valve" with its opening at the apex may result when fusion of the cusps occurs with shortening and thickening of the chordae tendineae and papillary muscles. A "buttonhole" mitral valve is formed when shortening of the chordae is less marked and a diaphragm effect, with an oval or slitlike opening, results. The degree of involvement of the chordae and papillary muscles is of great importance in determining the degree of valve dysfunction. The valve ring as well as the cusps contributes to the stenosis with thickening, rigidity, and calcification. Thus, the commissures, cusps, and chordae may all be involved in varying combinations, resulting in much variation in both hemodynamics and physical signs.

Aortic Valve Deformities.   The most common aortic lesion is a combination of stenosis and regurgitation. Pure aortic stenosis is relatively uncommon, but a minimal degree of aortic regurgitation occurs frequently in mild rheumatic involvement. In most cases of symptomatic rheumatic aortic disease, both stenosis and regurgitation occur, but one or the other may be functionally predominant. Deformity of the valve results from fusion of the cusps at the commissures, rigidity and shortening of the cusps alone, or combinations of both processes with calcification superimposed (Fig. 48–5B).

Tricuspid Valve Deformities.   These almost always exist in association with mitral and aortic lesions and occur in approximately 10 per cent of patients with chronic rheumatic heart disease.[83] Gross and Friedberg found that inflammatory lesions were common in the tricuspid and pulmonary valves in RF, but resulting deformities were uncommon.[86]

Pulmonary Valve Deformities.   Pulmonary valve deformities are rarest of all. When they occur, stenosis is more usual than is incompetence. The pathological changes in the pulmonary valve are similar to those in the aortic valve.

Progressive Pathological Changes in Healed Rheumatic Heart Disease.   There are manifestations of progressive changes and continued inflammation that seem unrelated to the original rheumatic process. Disruption of red blood cells ("cardiac hemolytic anemia") can result from valvular defects;[89] platelet turnover and destruction have recently been proved to be excessive in rheumatic heart disease,[90] and resultant thrombosis and fibrosis can occur along with calcification. Recurrent congestive heart failure may cause fatty changes in the myocardium and progressive fibrosis. The endocardium, especially the left atrium in mitral valvular deformity, is prone to develop organized thrombi, to stretch and dilate progressively, and to develop chronic inflammatory changes that are not exudative or clearly rheumatic at all.

EXTRACARDIAC LESIONS

Joints.   Swelling and edema of the articular and periarticular structures with serous effusion into the joint space occur without ero-

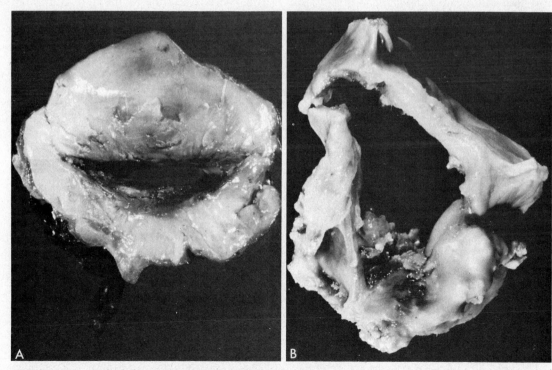

FIGURE 48–5   Excised rheumatic valve. *A*, "Fishmouth" mitral valve. *B*, Aortic valve fixed in open position. (Courtesy of Dr. James W. Pate. From Stollerman, G. H.: Rheumatic Fever and Streptococcal Infection. New York, by permission of Grune and Stratton, 1975.)

sion of the joint surface or pannus formation. The synovial membrane is reddened and thickened and covered with fibrinous exudate. Histologically there is marked edema, engorgement and dilation of blood vessels, and diffuse and focal infiltrates of lymphocytes and polymorphonuclear leukocytes, the latter more numerous initially. Later, focal fibrinoid lesions with histiocytic granulomas may appear,[69,91] but these lesions heal also without residua.

Subcutaneous Nodules. A central zone of fibrinoid necrotic material is surrounded by histiocytes and fibroblasts, and lymphocytes and polymorphonuclear leukocytes collect around small vessels. The structure resembles Aschoff bodies and may heal very rapidly, leaving no apparent scars.

Chorea. Considerable confusion exists concerning the pathology of Sydenham's chorea because (1) few patients die of "pure" chorea, (2) those who die of severe carditis may have inflammatory lesions of the central nervous system without chorea,[92] (3) no single site is consistently involved, (4) Aschoff bodies are not found in the brain,[93,94] and (5) it has not been possible to correlate clinical findings with pathologic changes. Changes found in the central nervous system include arteritis, cellular degeneration, perivascular round cell infiltration, and occasional petechial hemorrhages, but on the whole these are not impressive and are scattered throughout the cortex, cerebellum, and basal ganglia.[95,96]

Rheumatic Pneumonitis. Because this finding occurs with severe carditis only, there has been argument about whether the pulmonary lesion is a rheumatic manifestation or a complication of heart failure. The usual finding is a grossly hemorrhagic lung due to lesions that resemble small infarctions. Fibrin and hemosiderin are deposited in the alveoli, and a hyaline membrane is characteristic. Aschoff bodies are absent, but serous or serofibrinous pleural exudates may occur.

Clinical Manifestations of Rheumatic Fever

The signs and symptoms of ARF vary greatly and are determined by the systems involved, the severity of the lesions and when they appear in the course of the disease, and the stage of the disease when the patient is first observed by the physician. Certain manifestations that follow streptococcal infections (with a frequency far exceeding chance) occur simultaneously, in close succession, or singly. They have been called *major manifestations* and consist of carditis, arthritis, chorea, subcutaneous nodules, and erythema marginatum. The word "major" refers to their importance as diagnostic criteria and not to their importance in the severity of the process or its activity, or to the prognosis.

Minor manifestations of ARF are frequently present and helpful in recognizing the disease. They are too nonspecific, however, to be of major importance in diagnosis. Minor manifestations include such findings as fever, arthralgia, acute phase reactants in the blood, heart block, and a history of previous ARF or rheumatic heart disease.

Antecedent Streptococcal Infection. Evidence for an antecedent streptococcal infection may not be apparent. As many as one-third of patients do not remember having had any illness in the preceding month.[33] Furthermore, in patients with previous RF who were followed prospectively for recurrences, asymptomatic streptococcal infections accounted for 54[27] to 70 per cent[29] of recurrences of RF. The average interval between onset of symptoms of pharyngitis and the symptoms of RF (the latent period) was 18.6 days in one prospective study[97] but may be as short as 1 week or as long as 5 weeks. The latent period is no shorter in patients with previous RF than in those without.

Arthritis. This manifestation occurs in about three-fourths of patients during the acute stage of the disease. In general, joint involvement becomes more common with in-

creasing age of the patient, a trend related to the concomitant decrease in the incidence of carditis and chorea.[98-101]

The arthritis of RF usually involves the large joints, particularly the knees, ankles, elbows, and wrists. Almost any joint, however, may be affected. In the classic attack, several joints are involved in quick succession, each for a brief period of time, resulting in the typical picture of migratory polyarthritis. Each joint remains inflamed for usually no more than a week before it begins to subside, and the inflammation usually abates spontaneously in 2 or 3 weeks. The course of the entire bout of polyarthritis is usually severe for a week in approximately two-thirds of patients and for an additional week or two in the remainder, but by the end of 4 weeks, it will have subsided, with rare exceptions. Flare-ups may occur, however, in a small percentage of patients treated with antirheumatic therapy for 4 to 6 weeks but rarely after a second 6-week course of antirheumatic treatment. Unlike rheumatoid arthritis, RF does not cause permanent joint deformities except for the so-called Jaccoud type of deformity of the metacarpophalaneal joints.[101-103,103a] Acute polyarthritis rarely occurs more than 35 days after the onset of the streptococcal infection, and for that reason, it is almost always associated with a rising or peak titer of streptococcal antibodies. This fact aids in identifying an isolated bout of polyarthritis as rheumatic or in *excluding* RF as an etiology for a given bout of polyarthritis when streptococcal antibodies are not increased.

CARDITIS

Variations in Onset and Course. The most important manifestation of ARF is carditis, which, in its most severe form, causes death from acute cardiac failure. More commonly, however, carditis is less intense, and the predominant effect is scarring of the heart valves. In contrast to the seriousness of its prognosis, rheumatic carditis most often causes no symptoms of its own and is usually diagnosed in the course of the examination of a patient with arthritis or chorea, which directs the physician's attention to the heart, where murmurs are detected. Carditis, therefore, does not come to medical attention if other symptoms of rheumatic fever are absent or if the carditis is not severe enough to cause heart failure, prolonged or severe fever, or the pain of pericarditis. Patients with undiagnosed carditis may later prove to have rheumatic heart disease and usually give no history of a previous rheumatic attack.

Cardiac involvement may often occur in the mildest form of the disease. The incidence of carditis in initial attacks of RF varies from 40 to 51 per cent in reports from the United States and Canada.[102-108] Murmurs indicative of carditis are usually present during the first week of the illness in about three-fourths of all patients in whom carditis is eventually diagnosed.[105] By the second or third week, murmurs will become manifest in 85 per cent of those in whom they will eventually develop.

In another form of its presentation, particularly in children under 6 years of age, carditis begins more insidiously, with only slight or no fever and with vague or absent joint pains. Constitutional symptoms are prominent, however, and anorexia, fatigue, and pallor may progress to shortness of breath and chest pain. The child will then appear wan and chronically ill. Signs of carditis are unequivocal and often include incipient or overt health failure. Such patients usually have serious cardiac involvement.

Acute heart failure in a young patient who has had rheumatic heart disease previously but who has been well compensated should always be suspected as a recurrence of acute rheumatic carditis. Young hearts with rheumatic disease rarely fail because of hemodynamic handicaps alone except when the latter are severe and protracted.

Clinical Signs and Criteria. The four major criteria for the clinical diagnosis of rheumatic carditis are (1) an organic heart murmur or murmurs not previously present, (2) enlargement of the heart, (3) congestive heart failure, and (4) pericardial friction rubs or signs of effusion. If any one of these is unequivocal in a patient with active RF, the diagnosis of carditis is justified.

Murmurs of Acute Rheumatic Carditis. Organic murmurs are almost invariably present. They may not be heard when the heart rate is too rapid, when cardiac output is very low in severe congestive heart failure, when they are obscured by a loud pericardial rub, or, rarely, when there is marked pericardial effusion. Otherwise, the signs of endocarditis are always associated with those of involvement of other layers of the heart.

Apical Systolic Murmur. The mitral valve is the most common site of rheumatic inflammation—about three times as frequently involved as the aortic valve. Inflammation ("valvulitis") causing edema, thickening, and verrucae leads to mitral regurgitation early in the course of the disease and often with mild cardiac involvement. The systolic murmur is heard best at the apex, usually grade 3 or more on a scale of 6 in intensity, and, most important, it has a high-pitched blowing quality.

The difference between functional or innocent apical murmurs and mitral regurgitation is difficult to describe, since it is based mainly on the subjective perception of what is the "pure blow" of regurgitation and what are the low-pitched musical overtones of the functional "vibratory" murmur. Moreover, some children will present with both kinds of murmurs. Furthermore, an unusually loud functional murmur accentuated by fear, pain, and excitement may be incorrectly interpreted as a "changing organic murmur" when antirheumatic treatment quiets the patient and reduces the intensity and quality of the murmur's overtones, whereas the organic blow under such conditions is still clearly heard. The latter may also disappear, but it does so gradually over a period of weeks or months.

Apical Mid-diastolic Murmur (Carey-Coombs Murmur). This murmur begins directly after the onset of the third heart sound and ends before the first heart sound. The mid-diastolic murmur is often transient, low-pitched, and easily missed. The presence of this murmur makes the diagnosis of "mitral valvulitis" more definite, confirms the significance of the apical systolic murmur, and adds to the seriousness of the prognosis for permanent valve injury. The mid-diastolic murmur is easy to confuse with the normal third heart sound heard so commonly in children, especially during increased cardiac output. It is, in fact, an extension and exaggeration of the third heart sound into a murmur and should not be mistaken for the rumbling murmur of mitral stenosis.

Aortic Diastolic Murmur. This murmur may appear early in the course of the disease as an expression of aortic valvulitis and may occur alone or with mitral valvulitis. The aortic diastolic blow may be audible only intermittently, depending, again, on cardiac output. The murmur is a soft, high-pitched, decrescendo blow heard immediately after the second heart sound. A diastolic cooing or crying "sea gull" murmur is rarely heard but can be present evanescently in the aortic valvulitis of acute carditis. Basal systolic murmurs, which are sometimes heard in children with first attacks of acute carditis, are physiologic sounds associated with the ejection of blood into the great vessels. They are functional murmurs of short ejection quality and should not be confused with aortic stenosis—a late sequel.

Cardiac Enlargement and Failure. The most reliable clinical expression of rheumatic myocarditis from the standpoint of diagnosis and prognosis is *dilatation*, particularly of the left atrium and ventricle. Heart size should be carefully measured both clinically and radiographically. In the presence of significant heart murmurs, the degree of enlargement generally reflects the severity of carditis. In two carefully performed cooperative studies designed to evaluate treatment of rheumatic carditis, cardiomegaly occurred in a little more than half the children who developed carditis.

Congestive heart failure is the least common but most serious manifestation of rheumatic carditis. It is reported in 5 to 10 per cent of first attacks of rheumatic carditis. It is more common, however, to encounter severe and fatal heart failure as a manifestation of a *rheumatic recurrence* than of a primary attack. S3 and S4 gallops often accompany congestive failure. Combined with mitral regurgitation due to the valvulitis, these may cause the rocking, chaotic apical impulses that are so characteristic on palpation and so ominous in significance. Chest x-ray evidence of vascular congestion and patchy edema may be more striking than the physical signs and almost always raises the suspicion of rheumatic pneumonitis or pulmonary arteriolar vasculitis and infarction as a differential diagnosis. It may be impossible to exclude the presence of all three complications, since all may occur in the severest forms of RF.

Signs of heart failure may occur during the course of any attack of active carditis, so that patients should be examined frequently and carefully for this complication. The tachypnea and hyperpnea caused by salicylism should not be mistaken for left ventricular failure, nor should enlargement of the liver, so commonly a consequence of the fatty infiltration caused by corticosteroids, be confused with right ventricular failure.

Pericarditis. Pericarditis occurs in approximately 5 to 10 per cent of most large series of ARF.[102,105] Occasionally, pericardial reaction and effusion will be more striking and prominent than the degree of myocarditis (Fig. 48–6). In such cases the regression in apparent heart size and the rate of healing of the attack can be rapid. Conversely, the pericarditis may be a relatively minor aspect of a profound case of heart failure due to severe myocarditis. One rarely sees tamponade without severe heart failure as well.

Arrhythmias. Delayed atrioventricular (AV) conduction, as reflected in prolongation of the P-R interval, occurs with similar frequency to the polyarthritis of ARF,

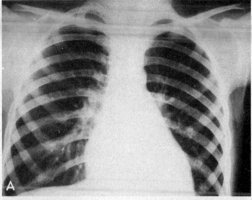

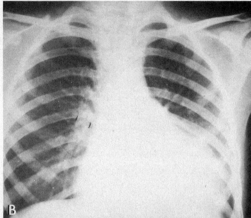

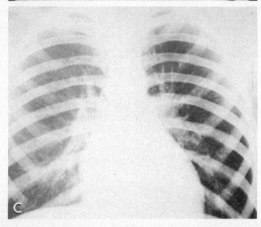

FIGURE 48–6   Pericarditis with effusion during acute rheumatic fever. A, Chest x-ray of a 9-year-old boy at onset of acute rheumatic polyarthritis and carditis. B, Chest x-ray one week later when a pericardial friction rub was heard. C, Chest x-ray about two weeks later when symptoms had subsided. (From Stollerman, G. H.: Rheumatic Fever and Streptococcal Infection. New York, by permission of Grune and Stratton, 1975.)

whether or not clear evidence of carditis is present. The prolongation of AV conduction is easily reversed with atropine,[109] suggesting that this feature is usually due to functional effects of the disease on AV conduction rather than to inflammation and fibrosis of the conduction system. Prolongation of AV conduction may lead to second-degree and, rarely, even third-degree block.[110] The latter is usually of brief duration and reverts spontaneously. Interference and dissociation phenomena are also characteristic of occasional nodal rhythms. Atrial fibrillation is rarely caused by acute rheumatic carditis in contrast to its fre-

quency in patients with longstanding mitral valvular disease with atrial enlargement and chronic atrial subendocardial inflammation.

EXTRACARDIAC MANIFESTATIONS

Subcutaneous Nodules. These are a major manifestation of ARF.[111,112] However, they are not pathognomonic of RF, since they occur in rheumatoid arthritis and systemic lupus erythematosus as well. They rarely occur as an isolated manifestation and are associated most often with severe carditis, appearing usually several weeks after its onset.[113]

Nodules are round, firm, painless subcutaneous lesions varying in size from approximately 0.5 to 2.0 cm. The skin over them is freely movable and not inflamed. They are located over bony surfaces or prominences and over tendons, particularly the extensor of the fingers and toes and flexors of the wrists and ankles. They occur in crops and vary in number from one to usually three or four dozen; when numerous, they tend to be symmetrical (Fig. 48–7). Nodules are evanescent, disappearing sometimes within several days but usually lasting a week or two and rarely more than a month. They tend, therefore, to be much smaller and less persistent than rheumatoid nodules.

Erythema Marginatum. This is a less common feature of RF but is so characteristic that it has taken its rightful place among the five major diagnostic manifestations of the disease. However, it cannot be considered pathognomonic of ARF because it has been reported in sepsis, in drug reactions, in patients with glomerulonephritis, and in children in whom no etiological factor can be identified.[114]

Erythema marginatum appears as a bright-pink smoke ring spreading serpiginously through a pale skin. It is nonpruritic, nonpainful, and neither indurated nor raised. It blanches completely on pressure and is evanescent. The individual lesions usually appear on the trunk and the proximal parts of the extremities but not on the face (Fig. 48–8); they rarely extend distally beyond the elbows or knees. Erythema marginatum may recur intermittently for months, uninfluenced by antirheumatic agents, and when all other signs of rheumatic activity are gone, one can allow the patient to begin to ambulate without fear of a relapse.

Chorea (Sydenham's Chorea, St. Vitus' Dance). This neurological disorder characterized by involuntary, purposeless, rapid movements, muscular weakness, and emotional lability, may be associated with other manifestations of ARF, but it also may appear as the sole expression of the disease—so-called "pure chorea." After puberty it is present exclusively in women, and even in them it declines rapidly after adolescence. Chorea has decreased strikingly in frequency compared with arthritis and carditis.

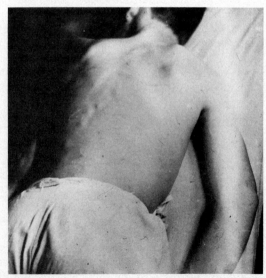

FIGURE 48–7   Subcutaneous nodules along the spinous processes. (From Stollerman, G. H.: Rheumatic Fever and Streptococcal Infection. New York, by permission of Grune and Stratton, 1975.)

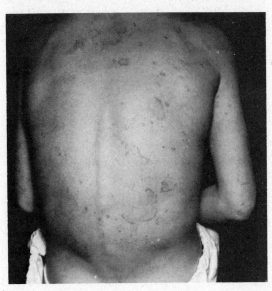

FIGURE 48–8   Erythema marginatum. (Courtesy of Dr. Benedict F. Massell.)

The movements of chorea are abrupt and erratic, not rhythmical or repetitive. In even the most violent attacks, all choreiform movements disappear during sleep and are less violent during rest and sedation. The patient cannot maintain a steady expression but grimaces, grins, frowns, and pouts in rapid succession. The tongue, when protruded, resembles "a bag of worms," may dart in and out, and may contribute to the typical choreiform speech, which is halting, staccato, explosive, and jerky. Handwriting may become clumsy or impossible to read and can be studied serially as a measure of healing; the muscular weakness may be severe enough to resemble a palsy. The electroencephalogram frequently shows abnormally slow waves.[115]

Emotional lability creates personality changes that often herald the onset of a bout of chorea. The patient may become fidgety, restless, cantankerous, and uncooperative.

Chorea may last from 1 week to more than 2 years but usually about 8 to 15 weeks, with a mean of 13.7.[116] Chorea is never seen simultaneously with arthritis but often coexists with carditis. When chorea appears alone, however, the other minor clinical and laboratory signs of ARF may be entirely absent. The erythrocyte sedimentation rate and C-reactive protein may be normal. Even more confusing, in such cases the ASO and other streptococcal antibody titers may not be increased because chorea appears only after a relatively long latent period (as long as 1 to 6 months) following the antecedent streptococcal infection, and after the longest latent period, both the acute phase reactants and the streptococcal antibody titers may have returned to normal.[117,118]

Fever. Some degree of fever accompanies almost all rheumatic attacks at their onset. Temperature usually ranges from 101° to 104°F (38.4° to 40°C), is rarely higher, and has no characteristic pattern. In the usual attack, fever decreases in approximately a week without antipyretic treatment and may become low-grade for another week or two. It rarely lasts for more than several weeks. When antirheumatic agents are used, however, a "rebound" of fever may occur after 4 to 6 weeks of treatment, but it usually subsides spontaneously within a few days except in unusually persistent attacks.

Abdominal Pain. The abdominal pain of RF, which occurs in fewer than 5 per cent of patients with ARF,[119] resembles that seen in other conditions in which acute microvascular mesenteric disease occurs, such as sickle cell crises, sepsis, endotoxin or anaphylactic shock, transfusion reactions, and anaphylactoid purpura.

Epistaxis. In the past, the incidence of epistaxis was reported from as high as 48 per cent in the early 1930's[120] to a low of 4 to 9 per cent in the late 1950's,[99] and perhaps it is even less frequent now.

Rheumatic Pneumonia. When the rheumatic process causes severe carditis, rheumatic inflammation also appears in the lung and cannot be distinguished from patchy pulmonary edema, segmental, platelike atelectatic lesions of pulmonary embolism, or thromboses from vasculitis.[121]

LABORATORY FINDINGS IN RHEUMATIC FEVER

Although there are no pathognomonic tests for RF, laboratory findings are helpful in two major ways: (1) in establishing the antecedent streptococcal infection and (2) in documenting the presence or persistence of an inflammatory process.

ANTECEDENT STREPTOCOCCAL INFECTION. The diagnosis of recent streptococcal infection can be made only tentatively by throat culture but definitely by antibody determinations. Throat cultures are usually negative by the time RF appears. When they are positive, one still cannot be certain whether the organism isolated represents convalescent carriage of the antecedent infection or an intercurrent acquisition of a different strain. Streptococcal antibodies are therefore more useful because they reach a peak titer shortly after the onset of ARF and indicate true infection rather than transient carriage.

ANTIBODIES. The specific antibodies used to diagnose streptococcal infections are primarily antistreptolysin O, antihyaluronidase, antistreptokinase, anti-NADase (anti-DPNase), and anti-DNAse B. Antistreptolysin O has been the most extensively used test and is generally available in hospitals in the United States.[122]

ASO titers vary with age, geographical area, and other factors influencing the frequency of streptococcal infection.[123] Titers of 200 to 300 units/ml are common in healthy children 6 to 14 years of age who live in crowded cities in the temperate zone of the United States.

The chances of detecting a significant antibody response is greatest 2 to 3 weeks after the onset of ARF, which is 4 to 5 weeks after the antecedent streptococcal infection. Thereafter, antibody titers fall off rapidly in the next few months, and after 6 months the decline levels off slowly. For this reason, evidence of increased streptococcal antibodies should be present in all patients at the onset of the rheumatic attack if such onset is well defined. Acute polyarthritis always occurs within a latent period of no more than 4 to 5 weeks after the antecedent streptococcal infection and therefore at or near the peak of the antibody response.

Anti-DNAse B,[124] together with the ASO, has become most generally recommended for diagnosis, with antihyaluronidase a useful third. Recently a product has been marketed which is a concentrate of a variety of extracellular streptococcal antigens made from supernates of broth cultures (antistreptozyme [ASTZ] test). Sheep cells sensitized with this concentrate will agglutinate in the presence of streptococcal antibodies that have not yet been defined. This slide agglutination test is a very sensitive measure of the streptococcal immune response.[125,126] The greatest value of the ASTZ test is in helping to rule out RF, particularly in the diagnosis of isolated polyarthritis when low titers reflect the absence of recent streptococcal disease.

ACUTE PHASE REACTANTS. Acute phase reactants include leukocyte counts, erythrocyte sedimentation rate (ESR), C-reactive protein (CRP), serum mucoprotein, serum hexosamine, serum protein electrophoresis, and several others. The two tests that have gained widest use are the CRP and the ESR. These tests are, of course, not specific for RF, but they are almost always abnormal during the active rheumatic process if it is not suppressed by antirheumatic drugs. "Pure" chorea and, occasionally, persistent erythema marginatum are exceptions. When rheumatic manifestations are obvious, as in the presence of fever and polyarthritis, CRP and ESR are of little value because inflammation is already apparent. During treatment, however, they are quite useful, particularly CRP, in measuring the effectiveness of suppression of the inflammatory process.[127] Particularly when treatment has been discontinued or dosages of antirheumatic agents have been reduced, CRP is very efficient in monitoring the patient for relapse of continued rheumatic inflammation ("rebounds") and in establishing when the active phase of rheumatic inflammation has abated. When ESR and CRP remain normal a few weeks after antirheumatic treatment has been discontinued, the attack will be over unless chorea appears. Even then, however, there will be no exacerbation of the systemic inflammatory component of the attack. Congestive heart failure may cause confusion with both tests. CRP may become positive in pulmonary edema or severe left heart failure of any cause, and the ESR may be slowed by cardiac decompensation.

ANEMIA. The anemia of RF is the normocytic normochromic anemia of chronic inflammation and is of mild to moderate degree.[128] Suppression of inflammation usually corrects the anemia partially or completely, and corticosteroids are particularly potent in this regard. Anemia is a good index of the severity and chronicity of RF.

ELECTROCARDIOGRAPHIC FINDINGS. The electrocardiogram in RF has no characteristic pattern, and the diagnosis of rheumatic carditis should never be made on the basis of electrocardiographic changes alone. Too often the diagnosis of carditis has been made incorrectly when a doubtful systolic murmur has been associated with a prolonged P-R interval or nonspecific ST-T changes. Neither the course of the acute rheumatic attack nor the subsequent development or valvular or myocardial damage can be predicted from the electrocardiographic changes.[104,129,130] Patients with ECG changes but with no other signs of carditis recover completely without the stigmata of rheumatic heart disease.[131]

Diagnosis of Rheumatic Fever

JONES CRITERIA. When T. Duckett Jones formulated his criteria for the diagnosis of ARF in 1944,[132] there was an immediate recognition of their value and considerable consensus about their use. These criteria were adopted in modified form in 1955 by the American Heart Association's Council on Rheumatic Fever and Congenital Heart Disease and were further revised by the same Council's committee in 1965.[133] The current criteria (Table 48–1) emphasize the importance of establishing the presence of the antecedent streptococcal infection by demonstration of increased streptococcal antibodies. If supported by such evidence, two major (or one major and two minor) manifestations indicate a high probability of ARF. However, because virtually all patients with Sydenham's chorea are rheumatic subjects, the diagnosis can be made even when chorea is the sole manifestation.

POLYARTHRITIS. Because of the numerous causes of polyarthritis, the diagnosis of RF is weakest when this manifestation appears alone, and particularly in the adolescent or adult population in which other arthritides are common.

TABLE 48–1 JONES CRITERIA (REVISED)

MAJOR MANIFESTATIONS	MINOR MANIFESTATIONS
Carditis	Fever
Polyarthritis	Arthralgia
Chorea	Previous rheumatic fever or rheumatic heart
Erythema marginatum	disease
Subcutaneous nodules	Elevated ESR or positive CRP
	Prolonged P-R interval

Plus supporting evidence of preceding streptococcal infection: history of recent scarlet fever; positive throat culture for group A streptococcus; increased ASO titer or other streptococcal antibodies.

From Jones Criteria (revised) for guidance in the diagnosis of rheumatic fever. Circulation 32:664, 1965, by permission of the American Heart Association, Inc.

It is helpful to classify polyarthritis pathophysiologically and in the sequence of therapeutic priorities. For this reason, one should consider the following conditions in the differential diagnosis.

DIFFERENTIAL DIAGNOSIS OF POLYARTHRITIS

Bacteremias. In terms of the importance and urgency of diagnosis, it is essential to rule out bacterial infections in all cases of acute polyarthritis. Pneumococcal, meningococcal, gonococcal, streptococcal, and staphylococcal bacteremias should be excluded by obtaining blood for appropriate cultures before antibiotic therapy is initiated. When gonococcal polyarthritis cannot be excluded by cultures of the joints or blood (in the majority of cases), a therapeutic trial of penicillin should be used because a prompt response (within 24 to 48 hours) is almost invariable.[134,135]

Infective endocarditis must also be considered whenever a patient with rheumatic heart disease develops unexplained fever and arthritis[136,137] (Chap. 33).

Osteomyelitis. Especially when pain is referred to the hip, osteomyelitis can be difficult to exclude. Should the diagnosis be suspected, it is best to start treatment as soon as blood cultures are made and without waiting for the results.

Viremias. *Type B hepatitis* and other viruses that can cause rather prolonged viremias (Epstein-Barr virus and cytomegalovirus) can produce a serum sickness syndrome presumably by the formation of circulating immune complexes.

Rubella. The frequency with which rubella produces arthritis, particularly in adult women, has been increasingly appreciated,[138] especially where rubella vaccine is used extensively.[139] When the evanescent rash is either not noticed or not present and the characteristic suboccipital and retrocervical lymphadenopathy goes unnoticed, the presenting picture of arthritis can simulate RF closely.

Immune Complex Disease. A history of receiving animal sera may provide the necessary clue. When penicillin is given to treat streptococcal pharyngitis, however, the situation may be very confusing. Urticaria or angioneurotic edema points to *serum sickness*, as does evidence of acute glomerulonephritis and a fall in serum complement. Low levels of streptococcal antibodies may be the only reliable differential diagnostic feature if other clues of serum sickness are absent.

Sickle Cell Anemia and Other Hemoglobinopathies. Sickle cell disorders have many signs and symptoms that resemble ARF and other diffuse vascular diseases because they are, in fact, associated with microvascular thrombosis and inflammation (Chap. 49). Joint pain, abdominal pain, heart murmurs, cardiac enlargement, and fever all simulate ARF very closely.[140-142]

Rheumatoid Arthritis. When it begins with acute migratory polyarthritis involving the large joints, rheumatoid arthritis imitates ARF. Involvement of many small joints, particularly of the hands and feet, is more characteristic of rheumatoid arthritis, but such involvement may appear later in the course of the disease when it has become low-grade and chronic, with characteristic "morning stiffness" and fusiform swelling of the fingers. A macular rash, lymphadenopathy, and splenomegaly are also more characteristic of rheumatoid arthritis. The chronic course of rheumatoid arthritis may ultimately be the distinguishing features as well as the eventual joint deformities when granulation tissue develops to form the characteristic pannus in the synovia of rheumatoid joints. Streptococcal antibody titers are helpful in differential diagnosis only when they are not increased fortuitously in rheumatoid arthritis[143]

Lymphomas and Granulomas. Leukemia causes fever and acute polyarthritis quite often—10 per cent of cases in some series.[144] Confusion arises because arthritis can appear before the peripheral blood shows leukemic cells. Other lymphomas such as Hodgkin's disease and benign granulomas such as sarcoidosis can also cause hyperimmune phenomena and arthritis.

CARDITIS

Functional ("Innocent") Murmurs. When functional or organic murmurs are typical, there is little problem for the experienced physician. At times, however, a nondescript murmur, especially in an obese or heavy-chested person, may defy sharp distinctions, and repeated examinations and other studies may be required. Such murmurs are often classified as "doubtful" or "questionable" when no other decision can be made.

Myocarditis. In its severe and chronic form, myocarditis due to other diseases may be impossible to distinguish from chronic rheumatic carditis if the heart is dilated and mitral regurgitation is prominent. This situation occurs when patients with ARF have heart failure with no associated extracardiac manifestations to provide clues. In rheumatic carditis, as the patient recovers cardiac compensation, the valvular lesions persist, and the murmurs become, if anything, louder, whereas the reverse is true in viral and other forms of myocarditis.

Pericarditis. Although rheumatic carditis does not produce an isolated pericarditis, at the onset of RF, however, pericarditis may appear before valvulitis and myocarditis are evident. Although many causes of pericarditis can be listed (Chap. 43), primary viral pericarditis most often enters the differential diagnosis in children.[145,146]

Congenital Heart Disease. This is rarely a diagnostic problem except when the cardiac murmur is first discovered during a febrile illness, especially if the heart is overactive and early signs of congestive heart failure are present. Congenital defects of the mitral valve (p. 985) cause the greatest problem,[147] especially when it is an isolated defect. Children who have severe mitral regurgitation with a large failing heart and poor development may present a picture indistinguishable from chronic severe carditis.

Chorea. When chorea is the only manifestation of ARF, the diagnosis depends entirely on the clinician's ability to recognize this manifestation, and appropriate care must be taken to avoid misdiagnosis. Multiple tics or habit spasms in a hyperactive child may pose a problem.

Course, Prognosis, and Natural History of Rheumatic Fever

The clinical course of RF can be quite variable, but in general there is a characteristic sequence of the major manifestations and usually a predictable duration. The latent period between streptococcal infection and the onset of ARF is shortest in arthritis and erythema marginatum and longest in chorea, with that of carditis and subcutaneous nodules in between. The usual duration of a rheumatic attack is rarely longer than 3 months. When severe carditis is present, clinical rheumatic activity may continue for 6 months or more. In fewer than 5 per cent of patients, ARF may remain active for more than 6 months.[148] These cases are classified as "chronic" rheumatic fever.

Carditis. Of the patients in whom carditis develops, murmurs occur during the first week of illness in 76 per cent. In 93 per cent of patients there is evidence of carditis in the first 3 months. Age of onset and severity of carditis influence its chronicity. Before the age of 3 years, 92 per cent of patients in one study[149] and 90 per cent in another[150] had carditis. The incidence of carditis decreased to 50 per cent in the 3- to 6-year age group and to 32 per cent in the 14- to 17-year age group[99] in first attacks. Carditis occurs occasionally after the age of 25 in what are apparently first attacks of ARF. When carditis is mild or evidence for it is borderline, it usually disappears rapidly. Severe carditis prolongs the attack. When severe carditis subsides, low-grade fever and tachycardia often continue, cardiac enlargement usually persists, and new murmurs may appear. Congestive heart failure may occur at any time while carditis is still active.

The mean duration of rheumatic activity is shorter when no suppressive drugs are given.[151] Rheumatic activity appears prolonged when "rebounds" of activity occur after withdrawal of antirheumatic drugs. Suppressive therapy "masks" the inflammation but does not terminate the process and may actually prolong it. The majority of prolonged attacks occur in patients who have had one or more previous attacks, and the incidence of chronic RF increases with the number of recurrences. When antirheumatic therapy is withdrawn and no "rebound" of rheumatic activity is noted for 8 weeks or more, the attack is over and will not be reactivated without a new streptococcal infection.

PROGNOSIS. The data are now conclusive that RF does not recur when streptococcal disease is prevented. The prognosis is at present excellent for the rheumatic subject who escapes carditis during an initial attack of RF. In one 5-year follow-up, rheumatic heart disease did not develop when the acute attack was not accompanied by the appearance of organic heart murmurs.[130] In the United Kingdom–United States Cooperative Study on the treatment of RF,[103,104] similar patients without carditis (defined as the absence of organic murmurs) during the acute attack showed virtually no evidence of late or insidious development of rheumatic heart disease. The percentage of this group of patients with "no carditis" who subsequently had normal hearts was 96 at 5 years and 94 at 10 years. The prognoses become poorer with the increasing severity of initial carditis, so that the percentage of those with congestive heart failure during the acute attack showing complete healing was 30 at 5 years and 40 at 10 years. It is apparent that the healing rate of rheumatic carditis is remarkably high if recurrences are prevented.

Prospective cooperative studies[104] have shown, at 5 years, that the frequency of mitral stenosis was equally distributed between the sexes and was related to the severity of the initial attack of carditis. In fact, a large percentage of the deaths within 5 years were due to such severe mitral valvular deformity. The analysis at 10 years, however, showed the emergence of another group—those whose initial mitral lesion had been relatively mild and who showed slow, progressive obstruction without evidence of recurrent RF or streptococcal disease. This group consisted of predominantly female subjects. It is apparent, therefore, that host factors, as yet undefined, influence the course of valvular sclerosis once mitral deformity has occurred and that progression of rheumatic heart disease may be related to more than the rheumatic inflammation itself. In addition, the tendency of stenotic mitral valves that have been fractured or incised surgically to restenose without evidence of recurrent or active RF is quite apparent in several long-term follow-up studies.[152]

Recurrences of Rheumatic Fever. First attacks of RF in the general population following epidemic streptococcal pharyngitis average 3 per cent, whereas such infections in patients with a history of recent RF may produce a secondary attack rate as high as 65 per cent.[27] Two main explanations for this propensity to recurrences of the rheumatic host are (1) that patients who develop RF differ from the general population in a genetic, congenital, or constitutional manner and that this difference *antedates* the first attack of the disease; and (2) that the first attack *causes* the susceptibility of the patient to further attacks. In the Irvington House study,[153] rheumatic attack rate per infection (R/I) in children decreased from 23 to 11 per cent between the first and fifth year after a rheumatic attack.[28] In adults with rheumatic heart disease, this rate was 4.8 per cent 10 or more years after the last attack.[29] Recurrence rates decline, therefore, with the length of time elapsed since the last attack.

A second factor that clearly increases the chance that a streptococcal infection will be followed by a rheumatic attack is the presence of residual rheumatic heart disease. In the Irvington House studies, the recurrence rate in children with rheumatic heart disease and cardiomegaly was 43 per cent; in patients with rheumatic heart disease and no cardiomegaly, 27 per cent; and in patients without apparent residual heart disease, 10 per cent.[28]

A third factor influencing the R/I is the magnitude of the immune response to the antecedent streptococcal disease as reflected in the increase of ASO titer.

The natural history of RF can now be predicted rather accurately once an initial rheumatic attack abates and a period of convalescence enables an assessment of the degree of healing of carditis. If cardiac healing is complete, prevention of recurrences should guarantee freedom from rheumatic heart disease. Persistence of even a mild degree of mitral regurgitation, although usually quite compatible with normal longevity if rheumatic recurrences and infective endocarditis are avoided, must be observed continuously because of the small but significant percentage of patients in whom mitral stenosis evolves despite careful, continuous antistreptococcal prophylaxis. Such patients, however, constitute but a small percentage of the large numbers of patients with mild rheumatic heart disease whose lesions remain relatively static if rheumatic recurrences are prevented.[154,155] In patients with hemodynamically significant valvular lesions, prognosis should be related principally to the magnitude of the physiological defect. In such patients, of course, recurrent rheumatic carditis is most serious, and these hosts are at greatest risk if streptococcal reinfection is permitted to occur.

Treatment of Rheumatic Fever

GENERAL MANAGEMENT. In any given case of RF, this depends upon the manifestations and severity of the attack. Patients should remain in bed for the duration of the acute and febrile portion of the illness until clinical and laboratory evidence of inflammation abates.

The administration of antiinflammatory or suppressive therapy should ordinarily be delayed until the disease process is clearly expressed in order to establish the diagnosis. Aspirin or corticosteroids administered prematurely to a patient with arthralgia or early monoarticular arthritis and fever may mask the disease process and cause diagnostic

confusion. Furthermore, in isolated polyarthritis a trial of penicillin therapy is often essential to eliminate the diagnosis of septic arthritis, especially gonococcemia (see above), and the therapeutic response to the antibiotic must be carefully evaluated.

Once the diagnosis is established, treatment can begin, usually with a *course of penicillin* adequate to eradicate residual group A streptococci that may be difficult to isolate. Massive penicillin treatment has been used by some investigators in an attempt to alter the frequency of cardiac damage but without success.[156] The usual course of penicillin consists of a single injection of 1.2 million units of benzathine penicillin intramuscularly, or 600,000 units of procaine penicillin intramuscularly, daily for 10 days. This is followed by continuous (secondary) prophylaxis (see below). The risk of contracting a new streptococcal infection may be especially high in hospital environments, and therefore prophylaxis should not be delayed until discharge from the hospital. Prophylaxis during hospitalization is a good way to observe patients for side effects from the medication and to educate them regarding its future use.

ANTIRHEUMATIC THERAPY. The selection of an antirheumatic agent is not critical to the outcome of most attacks of RF.[102–104,107,108,157,158] Corticosteroids and salicylates can be regarded as valuable symptomatic and supportive therapy, but they are not curative and may actually prolong the course of the disease. However, both steroids and salicylates control the toxic manifestations of the disease; contribute to the comfort of the patient; and combat anemia, anorexia, and other constitutional symptoms. In severe rheumatic carditis associated with heart failure, such nonspecific antiinflammatory effects may reduce the burden on the heart and occasionally may tilt the balance in favor of the survival of a critically ill patient. Corticosteroids are often more potent than salicylates in suppressing acute exudative inflammation, and some patients in whom salicylates fail to control the disease respond quickly to relatively large doses of corticosteroids. The effect of such doses on the course of chronic rheumatic carditis is disappointing, however, and their use in early cases of acute carditis has not been proved to decrease residual heart disease. Prolonged use of large doses beyond the period of time required to bring acute manifestations under control is not justified.

Patients with mild arthritis or arthralgia and no carditis may be treated with analgesics only, such as codeine, as needed. Two goals will be thus accomplished: First, the diagnosis may be made more certain by the appearance of definite arthritis in some of the initially questionable cases; and second, the duration of hospitalization or of close observation at home will be decreased because many of the patients will get well in 2 or 3 weeks; moreover, one will not have to worry about, and deal with, posttherapeutic rebounds.

Most current general policy is to administer salicylates when no clear evidence of carditis exists. If signs and symptoms are not adequately suppressed by salicylates, corticosteroids should be substituted. Patients with mild carditis are often given corticosteroids, but without the conviction that these are superior to salicylates. Those with severe carditis are usually treated promptly with corticosteroids, particularly if heart failure is evident, and with the precaution of adequate doses of diuretics and restriction of salt intake to combat sodium retention.

Since neither corticosteroids nor salicylates shorten the course of RF, the duration of therapy must be estimated according to the expected course of the attack. Approximately 75 to 80 per cent of most attacks will subside clinically within about 6 weeks. About 90 per cent will subside in about 12 weeks. Despite the form of therapy used, about 5 per cent of attacks will persist with clinically overt rheumatic manifestations for more than 6 months. The duration of treatment, therefore, can be tailored to the severity of the illness. For example, one might treat a mild attack for 4 weeks, tapering off the dosage of the antirheumatic agent during the ensuing 2 weeks.

It is important to reduce the dose of corticosteroids gradually over a period of about 2 weeks and to recognize that abrupt cessation of treatment leaves the patient in a state of temporary adrenal insufficiency resulting from suppression of endogenous adrenocortical activity during prolonged hormone therapy. For this reason the relapse of ARF following abrupt termination of hormone therapy may be more serious than the initial manifestation of the disease before treatment was started. It has been the policy of some to follow the gradual withdrawal of hormone therapy by administration of salicylates for several weeks or months to assure suppression of inflammation until recovery of normal adrenocortical function occurs.

When treatment of ARF is initiated with salicylates, a dose of 6 to 9 gm of acetylsalicylic acid per day is administered to patients weighing 70 kg or more, and proportionately smaller doses are given to patients weighing less. This is administered in divided doses every 4 hours. The initial doses of acetylsalicylic acid should be continued until a satisfactory clinical response is obtained, that is, until there is complete relief of symptoms and signs of arthritis and the temperature has returned to a normal range. Thereafter the dose may be reduced to two-thirds the initial value and may be maintained until all laboratory manifestations of inflammatory disease have returned to normal. For the remainder of the course of therapy, the dose may be reduced to half the initial daily dose. Should clinical or laboratory evidence of relapse occur when doses are reduced, it is advisable to return to the previous higher dose that suppressed the process.

Toxic manifestations are common with the use of larger doses of salicylates, and these may force a reduction in the dose before the response is adequate. If control of the inflammatory state is not sufficient with lower, subtoxic doses, substitution or addition of another agent should be considered.

An initial dose of prednisone of 40 to 60 mg/day in divided doses for adults and children alike may be started and varied according to the patient's response. With other analogs, such as triamcinolone and dexamethasone, the dose is based on their potency relative to prednisone.

Rebounds of Rheumatic Activity. Clinical or laboratory evidence of rheumatic activity may reappear when suppressive antirheumatic therapy is discontinued. Such reactivation has been termed a "rebound" and should clearly be distinguished from a recurrence. Spontaneous rebounds do not occur more than 5 weeks after complete cessation

of all antirheumatic therapy; by far the majority occur within 2 seeks, but most occur within a few days or while reducing dosage.

Mild rebounds may be characterized only by fever, arthralgia, or mild arthritis; some patients may have only laboratory evidence of relapse, such as reappearance of C-reactive protein in blood and reelevation of erythrocyte sedimentation rate. Murmurs which had disappeared may again be heard. In patients with carditis, rebounds may be severe and a flare-up of pericarditis or congestive heart failure may occur—sometimes more severely than during the initial period of treatment. Mild rebounds subside spontaneously within a week or two and do not require medication.

Treatment of Chorea. This is nonspecific and consists of tranquilization and sedation. For complete details the reader is referred elsewhere.[1,159–161]

Prevention of Rheumatic Fever

The most effective preventive measures against RF are probably socioeconomic. The almost total absence of the disease in the affluent sections of the cities of the western world suggests that spacious housing and noncrowding are at least as important as good diagnosis and treatment of streptococcal sore throat in the prevention of rheumatic attacks. Nevertheless, the natural history of RF can be dramatically altered in several ways by the use of antimicrobials. Mass penicillin prophylaxis can halt epidemics of streptococcal sore throat. Adequate penicillin treatment of acute streptococcal sore throat will abort an initial attack and, less often, rheumatic recurrences. Continuous administration of sulfadiazine or penicillin will prevent recurrent attacks in rheumatic subjects.

SECONDARY PROPHYLAXIS. The term secondary prophylaxis is used to describe protection against rheumatic recurrences by means of continuous chemoprophylaxis.[162] After a diagnosis of RF is established, residual streptococci which may or may not be detectable on throat cultures should be eradicated by a therapeutic course of penicillin as described below for primary prevention.

The most effective form of continuous prophylaxis is a single monthly intramuscular injection of 1.2 million units of benzathine penicillin G.[163–165] An attack rate of less than 1 recurrence per 250 patient-years was documented in patients using this form of prophylaxis in the extensive studies reported by the Irvington House group.[164] This method does not depend upon the patient's fidelity to an oral regimen nor upon the vagaries of absorption from the gastrointestinal tract. It also imposes closer surveillance upon the patient by the managing physician. Studies on the use of intramuscular benzathine penicillin for mass prophylaxis in military populations have suggested that streptococcal infections rarely occur before 3 weeks after an injection of 1.2 million units of this respository penicillin salt. When they occur after this period in rheumatic subjects, the subsequent injection at 4 weeks probably serves as adequate therapy of the infection. Although the reaction rate is somewhat higher for all injectable forms of penicillin, regardless of kind,[166] than with oral penicillin, reactions are very rare after the first months of prophylaxis. In patients who are at highest risk to sustain rheumatic recurrences, especially those with rheumatic heart disease and recent RF, monthly injections of benzathine penicillin are undoubtedly the preferred form of prophylaxis.

Oral prophylaxis is less reliable than repository penicillin prophylaxis. In the Irvington House studies, a recurrence rate of almost 1 per 25 patient-years (10 times that of intramuscular benzathine penicillin) was observed in patients on oral medication.[164] The recommended dosages for oral sulfadiazine prophylaxis are 0.5 gm once daily for patients weighing less than 27 kg (60 lb) and 1 gm once a day for patients weighing more than 27 kg. For oral penicillin prophylaxis, the recommended dose is 200,000 to 250,000 units daily. Even when oral penicillin is administered twice daily no superiority over sulfadiazine has been demonstrated.[167]

Strains of streptococci resistant to sulfonamide have appeared with mass sulfonamide prophylaxis in military populations but have not been a problem in secondary prophylaxis of rheumatic subjects. Reaction rates are low with both oral medications and are rare after the first months of prophylaxis. For the rare patient who is sensitive to both sulfadiazine and penicillin, oral erythromycin may be substituted in a dose of 250 mg twice daily.[168]

It has been difficult to establish a general recommendation concerning the duration of prophylaxis because of the number of variables that influence the attack rate of recurrences following streptococcal infections (see Natural History, above). Although risks of recurrences decline with age and with increased interval from the last rheumatic attack, a relatively high recurrence rate per infection persists for a very long time—5 to 10 years or more. Exceptions to instituting or maintaining prophylaxis should be made in adults only and then only after assessing the risk of high exposure to streptococcal infection (e.g., working with school-age children, in military service, in medical or allied health positions). Patients with significant degrees of rheumatic heart disease or with a history of repeated recurrences (including chorea) or those having had a recent attack require most careful consideration before discontinuation of prophylaxis, a decision that must be regarded as a calculated risk.

Primary Prophylaxis.   The term primary prophylaxis is applied to the prevention of first attacks of RF by treatment of the preceding streptococcal pharyngitis. In military populations with a high frequency of severe streptococcal pharyngitis, penicillin therapy reduced the attack rate of RF from 3.0 to 0.3 per cent.[169] The application of primary prevention to civilian populations, particularly children with sporadic or endemic streptococcal infections, has been more difficult because of the problem of differentiating viral pharyngitis in carriers of group A streptococci from current streptococcal infection and because frequent streptococcal exposure in children tends to keep streptococcal antibody titers elevated (see Epidemiology, above). Throat cultures are helpful, therefore, in eliminating the need for intensive penicillin therapy in patients with nonstreptococcal infection.

Effective therapy demands eradication of the infecting organism, which requires 10 days of consistent treatment if penicillin is administered orally. Many patients fail to extend such treatment beyond the first few days if acute symptoms of streptococcal infection subside. A single intramuscular injection of benzathine penicillin G (600,000 units in children under 27 kg [60 lb] and 1.2 million units in those over 27 kg) is the treatment of choice.[165] If given orally, penicillin G (200,000 or 250,000 units three to four times daily) is recommended. For those sensitive to penicillin, erythromycin (250 mg four times a day or 40 mg/kg per day in younger children) may be substituted.

Mass Antibiotic Prophylaxis.   This type of prophylaxis is effective in populations in which streptococcal pharyngeal infections are epidemic.[170-173] This approach may be indicated occasionally in civil-

ian or institutional epidemics, especially if several cases of RF occur within a few weeks. Mass intramuscular administration of 1.2 million units of benzathine penicillin G to all members of the affected population has been extremely effective.[4]

Immunization with Streptococcal Vaccines.   Although no vaccine is currently available for general distribution, considerable progress has been made on the purification and immunology of streptococcal M proteins and holds promise for future streptococcal vaccine development.[24,174,175,176]

SERONEGATIVE SPONDYLOARTHROPATHIES

COMMON CLINICAL FEATURES AND NOSOLOGY.   A group of rheumatological syndromes has been classified under the heading of seronegative spondyloarthropathies because they have clinical features in common and some pathological lesions, including those of the heart, that are identical.[177,178] They are distinguished from rheumatoid arthritis by the *absence of the characteristic serological changes* of the latter (e.g., increased rheumatoid factor); by the predilection of the arthritis for the sacroiliac, lumbosacral, and apophyseal joints of the spine; by the marked predominance in men over women; and by the extraarticular manifestations of iritis and of aortic regurgitation due to a characteristic lesion at the root of the aorta. The group of syndromes includes ankylosing spondylitis (AS), Reiter's disease (RD), psoriatic arthritis, the intestinal arthropathies, and Behçet's syndrome. Two of the major syndromes, AS and RD, have been associated with dysentery and urethritis. Although the causative agents are usually not apparent, dysentery due to specific bacteria (*Yersinia enterocolitica, Shigella,* and *Salmonella*) has produced most of the features of these syndromes.[178-180] Urethritis due to *Chlamydia trachomatis* has also been implicated as one of the causes of Reiter's syndrome,[181] but in most cases the etiological agent has not been identified.

HISTOCOMPATIBILITY ANTIGEN B27.   The concept of a genetically determined aberrant host response to a variety of infectious agents that can invade the bowel or genitourinary tract has emerged from the demonstration of the striking association of the seronegative spondyloarthropathies with the histocompatibility antigen HLA-B27.[178,179] This membrane antigen occurs with a frequency of approximately 4 to 8 per cent in the normal population, whereas over 90 per cent of patients with either AS or Reiter's disease with spondyloarthropathy are B27-positive. When spondyloarthropathy complicates inflammatory bowel disease, the association with B27 is greater than 80 per cent, and 50 per cent of psoriatic patients with spondylitis are B27-positive. So far, 50 per cent of patients with anterior uveitis have this antigen. When an outbreak of a specific form of dysentery has permitted careful prospective studies, patients with the B27 antigen have had a much greater tendency to develop any form of arthritis than those lacking this antigen. The more specific features of the syndrome such as spondyloarthropathy, iritis, and cardiac involvement have been confined primarily to those who are B27-positive.

Ankylosing Spondylitis

CARDIAC PATHOLOGY.   Several excellent prospective studies have documented the form of cardiac and aortic disease peculiar to ankylosing spondylitis (AS), consisting of the following: dilatation of the aortic valve ring; fibrous thickening, scarring, and variable focal inflammatory lesions of the aortic valve cusps, which sag into the ventricular cavity; dilatation of the sinuses of Valsalva; focal degenerative changes of elastic and muscle fibers of the aortic media; and patchy inflammatory lesions in all layers of the aorta, predominantly in the region adjacent to the aortic valve ring.[182-184] The lesions resemble those of syphilis except that in AS they remain close to the valve ring and do not affect the rest of the aorta. In addition, the basal rather than the distal portion of the aortic cusps is thickened in AS and the dense adventitial scarring extends into the endocardium in the immediate subaortic region. This extension may involve the base of the anterior mitral leaflet and the upper portion of the ventricular septum (Fig. 48–9A).

Aortic regurgitation results from thickening and shortening of the cusps and from their displacement caudally by the mass of fibrous tissue behind the commissures and by dilatation of the aortic valve root consequent to the destruction of elastic tissue (Fig. 48–9B). Mitral regurgitation is infrequent and usually insignificant but can result from dilatation of the left ventricle and from fibrous thickening of the basal portion of the anterior mitral leaflet.[185] The frequent heart block and conduction defects of AS are due to the extension of fibrosis into the muscular septum and destruction of the bundle of His and proximal bundle branches.[184-187]

The lesions of the myocardium are rather nonspecific, consisting of fibrosis, perivascular lymphocytic infiltration, and increased mucinous ground substance. Cardiac enlargement without any apparent cause and hypertrophy and dilatation of the left ventricle are often described, however, and the pathological findings are not commensurate with the clinical manifestations of cardiomyopathy noted in one report[188] nor with the frequency of the cardiac enlargement often described.[182]

Chronic fibrous obliteration of the pericardial cavity has been found at autopsy, but pericarditis is not a prominent clinical feature of the disease. Pericardial rubs and chest pain have been described, however, during more severe, acute, toxic episodes when there is active peripheral polyarthritis and in association with presumably early phases of the disease,[182] especially in association with early Reiter's syndrome or dysentery with polyarthritis.

CLINICAL FEATURES OF CARDIAC LESIONS. In many patients there is evidence of active carditis before aortic regurgitation appears. Precordial pain, pericardial friction rubs, marked tachycardia, cardiac enlargement not explained by hypertension, or other recognizable forms of heart disease and varying P-R intervals greater than 0.24 sec are frequently described, usually when patients have active peripheral arthritis and/or spondylitis with fever and increased erythrocyte sedimentation rates.[182] Remarkably few critical studies have been made of myocardial function in patients with AS before evidence of aortic insufficiency draws attention to cardiac involvement, but it is clear that cardiomyopathy may precede valvular involvement.[188] The usual cardiac features of AS are the gradual evolution of aortic regurgitation and varying degrees of atrioventricular block. The prevalence of the valve lesion is related to the duration of spondylitis and peripheral joint involvement, reaching an incidence in one series of 10 per cent in those with spondylitis for 30 years or more and of 18 per cent if peripheral joint involvement was also present. The prevalence of AV block in each of the above groups was 8.5 and 15.5 per cent, respectively.[182]

When aortic regurgitation is first recognized, the aortic second sound is characteristically accentuated as in syphilitic aortitis, and at this time systolic murmurs are trivial or absent. The aortic lesions tend to progress slowly, and free aortic regurgitation may not occur until as many as 7 years later, at which time the aortic second sound frequently disappears and loud harsh systolic murmurs are transmitted to the neck as the valve cusps become sclerosed. Austin Flint murmurs may also develop. Clinical and postmortem findings indicate that the cardiovascular lesions of some patients with AS may antedate articular disease and may regress spontaneously.[183,187] In one long follow-up of 97 patients with AS, of whom 14 had cardiovascular lesions, aortic regurgitation occurred in 10 patients. Mitral regurgitation and atrioventricular block

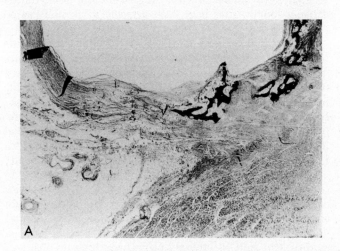

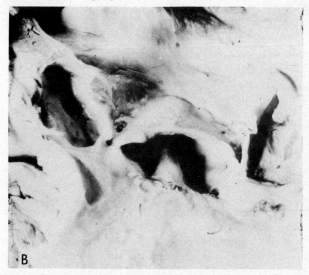

FIGURE 48–9   A, Base of left aortic cusp. Calcification, fibrosis, and vascularization at base of valve, with medial hypertrophy of arterioles (H and E, ×12). B, Aortic valve. Separation of cusps at commissure, with fenestration of free margins of cusps. Small, firm band of tissue connects lower portions of cusps. (From Davidson, P., et al.: Cardiac and aortic lesions in rheumatoid spondylitis. Mayo Clin. Proc. *38*:427, 1963.)

appeared as isolated findings in 1 and 3 patients, respectively. Nine of the 14 patients had peripheral arthritis, and 3 had iritis.[183] Anterior uveitis and extraspinal disease may also precede the articular lesions of AS by months or years. Hence the discovery of isolated aortic regurgitation in young or middle-aged men requires that AS be considered in the differential diagnosis. In addition, the aortic regurgitation of AS is now well documented to occur in so-called "secondary" forms of the disease such as spondylitis associated with psoriasis, regional enteritis,[183] ulcerative colitis,[189] and Reiter's disease.[190]

Aortic valve replacement (p. 1114) has been performed successfully in several centers, and patients with AS may be suitable candidates when such a procedure is indicated.[191] Cardiac pacemakers have been implanted for atrioventricular block.[183]

Reiter's Disease

Cardiac involvement in the acute stages of Reiter's disease has been described frequently and consists most commonly of acute pericarditis, apical systolic murmurs and gallops, prolongation of the P-R interval, and flattening of T waves. These changes disappear rapidly, and long-term follow-up of large series reveals only an occasional case of cardiac failure or third-degree atrioventricular block.[192] This acute form of Reiter's disease usually features nonspecific urethritis, nonsuppurative migratory polyarthritis, conjunctivitis, circinate balanitis, and keratoderma blenorrhagica. Initial attacks usually subside spontaneously, but second attacks occur in about 15 per cent of cases and chronic manifestations (almost always in B27-positive individuals[193]) may then ensue, with recurrent anterior uveitis, painful mutilating deformities of the feet, sacroiliitis, spondylitis, atrioventricular block, and an aortic valve lesion leading to aortic and occasionally to mitral regurgitation.[194–197]

Postmortem studies of the aortic valves have shown the cusps to be thickened, with rolled edges, and the aorta to incur changes similar if not identical to the lesions described in AS.[197,198]

The development of Reiter's disease in patients with *Yersinia* arthritis has prompted careful studies of the role of the B27 antigen in the frequency of expression of various clinical features of the syndrome.[199–203] In 5 of 49 patients who were B27-positive, carditis developed, two cases with "significant murmurs," one with friction rub, and two with transient cardiac enlargement, as evident on chest roentgenography.[180]

RHEUMATOID ARTHRITIS

PATHOLOGY. The heart is frequently involved in the inflammatory process of rheumatoid arthritis (RA), yet its function is seldom compromised by the lesions produced. The exudative type of rheumatoid inflammation affects the pericardial surfaces, producing a fibrinous pericarditis that is usually low-grade and subclinical. Pericardial inflammation becomes symptomatic and clinically significant in its more florid form, usually as part of a severe vasculitis (Chap. 43).

The most characteristic pathological lesion of RA, the nodular granuloma, involves the myocardium, endocardium, and valves of the heart.[204,205] The extent of this kind of involvement is generally proportionate to the severity of the disease and is almost always associated with diffusely distributed rheumatoid nodules, subcutaneously and elsewhere. These granulomas rarely compromise the function of the myocardium, however, nor do they often affect the function of the heart valves unless they become large and numerous enough to distort them (Fig. 48–10).

Diffuse arteritis, when present, affects small vessels, causing round cell infiltration, edema, fibrosis, and proliferation of the intima. Such involvement of the pericardial vessels may be extensive when it reflects an intense systemic form of RA, and the disease may begin in the pericardium before the joints become involved. Coronary arteritis is often observed at necropsy in severe RA, but it very rarely results in clinically apparent myocardial ischemia.

Although usually asymptomatic, the clinical syndromes of rheumatoid heart disease are well known and have been well described.[206–209] The more one keeps in mind the frequent participation of the connective tissues of the heart in the rheumatoid process, the more frequently will the alert clinician detect evidence of such involvement.

Clinical Features

PERICARDITIS (see also p. 1512). The frequency of rheumatoid pericarditis in necropsy studies ranges from 11 to 50 per cent, with an overall estimate of about 30 per cent.[209] Clinically, the diagnosis of pericarditis is made in about 2 per cent of cases in the adult form and in about 6 per cent in the juvenile form of RA. In careful studies of the more severe forms of the disease which require hospital admission, approximately 10 per cent of patients with RA have clinical evidence of rheumatoid pericarditis during the lifetime course of their disease. Part of the disparity between clinical and autopsy findings is due to the fact that the chest pain may be overshadowed by arthritic pains and may be masked by antirheumatic agents or mistaken for arthritic pain in neighboring joints. In addition, when symptoms of chest pain are lacking, careful and frequent auscultation for pericardial friction rubs is usually omitted. In controlled studies when signs of pericarditis have been actively sought, rubs have been detected in as many as 30 per cent of patients.[209]

The pathophysiology of the acute fibrinous pericarditis of RA is not clear, but in severe cases the pericardial fluid, like synovial fluid, shows decreased hemolytic complement (CH_{50}) and C3 levels. Immunofluorescence staining of the pericardium shows plasma cell infiltration and deposits of IgG, IgM, IgA, or C3 in the pericardial vessels.[210] Moreover, the polymorphonuclear leukocytes in the pericardial fluid may show cytoplasmic inclusions which stain for IgM, indicative of ingested immune complexes such as are also seen in the polymorphonuclear cells of synovial fluid in the same patients.[211] These findings are associated with extremely low levels of glucose, indicative of active phagocytosis, as observed in pleural and synovial rheumatoid fluids. About half the patients with overt rheumatoid pericarditis also have rheumatoid pleural and lung lesions.

With the availability of noninvasive cardiac procedures such as echocardiography, the diagnosis of pericardial involvement is being made earlier and more often.[212,213] In a

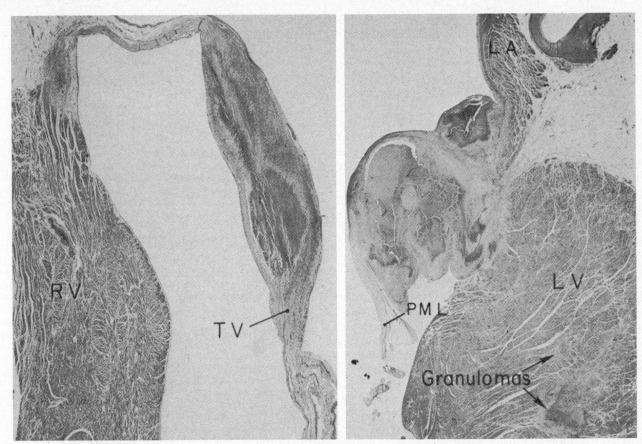

FIGURE 48–10 *Left*, Tricuspid value (TV) leaflet. Typical rheumatoid granuloma is located within substance of leaflet. RV indicates right ventricle (H and E, ×12). *Right*, Mitral valve. Section includes posterior mitral leaflet (PML) and adjacent portions of left atrial (LA) and left ventricular (LV) walls. Large rheumatoid granuloma is located within proximal three-fourths of posterior leaflet. Smaller nodule involves endocardium of left atrium as well. Two rheumatoid granulomas are located within the left ventricular wall (H and E, ×6.5). (From Roberts, W. C., et al.: Cardiac valvular lesions in rheumatoid arthritis. Arch. Intern. Med. *122*:141, 1968. Copyright 1968, American Medical Association.)

recent series of patients with RA studied by echocardiography, pericardial effusion was demonstrated in 30 per cent of all patients studied and in 50 per cent of those with subcutaneous nodules.[212] This incidence is as high as the reported frequency of postmortem findings of rheumatoid pericarditis.

Pericarditis may appear without relation to the duration of RA and sometimes may even be the harbinger of the onset of a severe form of the disease. It occurs most often in middle-aged men in whom arthritis was of acute onset. Most often, the clinical course is benign, and symptoms and signs will respond to moderate amounts of prednisone. Occasionally, however, the disease may be more protracted and severe, leading to cardiac tamponade and constrictive pericarditis.

In its florid form the disease has the usual symptoms and signs of pericarditis, and when persistent, it imitates closely tuberculous pericarditis, from which it must be carefully differentiated. Although some fatal cases have been described in which a true pancarditis was present,[214] such cases are exceptional, and even severe rheumatoid pericarditis usually spares myocardial and endocardial function.

Pericardial fluid is of considerable diagnostic value in cases in which the etiology of the pericarditis may be in doubt. The features of the pericardial fluid in RF have been noted above. In some cases, a high level of cholesterol has been found.[215] Such instances of so-called "cholesterol pericarditis" are probably due to poor absorption of lipid from pericardial effusions by the thickened pericardium in RA and in other forms of chronic pericarditis, which leads to the concentration and precipitation of cholesterol.

Treatment of rheumatoid pericarditis is the same as that for the arthritic disease. Although corticosteroids tend to be used more liberally in pericarditis to suppress inflammation, there is no evidence that such suppression will prevent adhesive or constrictive pericarditis. When tamponade occurs, surgical intervention is necessary, and pericardiectomy may be required. Needle pericardiocentesis is usually inadequate or difficult because of the thick, loculated nature of the effusion, and usually more vigorous procedures aimed at pericardial drainage by indwelling catheter or partial pericardiectomy are necessary.

RHEUMATOID MYOCARDITIS. Except for rare cases of myocarditis with diffuse granulomas or amyloid infiltration of the myocardium associated with very severe RA, myocarditis is mostly nonspecific and subclinical in the great majority of patients. The histological lesions may be focal or generalized infiltrations of lymphocytes, plasma cells, palisading histiocytes, and fibroblasts.[205] The incidence of myocarditis in autopsies of rheumatoid arthritis patients is reported as 19 per cent. Most of such cases are associated with severe arthritis, vasculitis, and endocarditis or pericarditis.

Whether drug toxicity, superimposed viral infection, or corticosteroid therapy may have caused some reported cases of severe myocarditis rather than primary rheumatoid disease cannot be determined with certainty. Although left ventricular function may be compromised by a variety of pathological processes in severe rheumatoid arthritis, the typical case is remarkable for its characteristic sparing of the myocardial musculature despite extensive involvement of the fibrous structures of the heart. Nevertheless, when there are unusually severe systemic manifestations of rheumatoid arthritis, rheumatoid pancarditis with congestive heart failure has been well described and confirmed by necropsy. Such patients exhibit the whole spectrum of rheumatoid inflammation of the heart.[214]

CORONARY ARTERY DISEASE. The incidence of coronary artery disease is higher in rheumatoid arthritis patients than in matched controls.[206,208] Clinicopathological correlation suggests that the nature of the coronary artery disease analyzed in some studies is probably rheumatoid rather than arteriosclerotic. Coronary arteritis is observed in about 20 per cent of rheumatoid arthritis patients at autopsy. This arteritis is probably a manifestation of generalized vasculitis often seen in RA. Inflammation with edema of the intima of the artery may lead to severe narrowing or occlusion of its lumen, to necrosis, and to angina or infarction. Nevertheless, myocardial necrosis secondary to this form of arteritis is rare.

VALVULAR AND ENDOCARDIAL LESIONS. As in myocarditis, the histological picture of the valves and adjacent endocardial areas of patients with RA shows nonspecific inflammation with fibrotic and sclerotic changes and infiltrations of histiocytes, plasma cells, lymphocytes, and occasional eosinophils.[204,205] The most characteristic lesions, however, are granulomas resembling rheumatoid nodules. Usually these do not interfere with valvular function unless they reach large enough proportions to produce frank valvular regurgitation by destroying the base of the valve and its cusps. Such regurgitation may be of sufficient magnitude and rapidity of onset to cause severe cardiac decompensation and death[216] (Chap. 32).

All valves may be involved, but the descending order of frequency is mitral, aortic, tricuspid, and pulmonary. Chronic endocarditis and valvular fibrosis was observed in 6 per cent of one series of hospitalized cases of severe RA.[208] Echocardiographic studies have shown a significant slowing of mitral valve movement in RA patients correlating with the duration of the disease and the extent of the formation of subcutaneous nodules.[213] It is not clear whether left ventricular disease can be excluded as a cause contributing to this finding or whether it is due entirely to intrinsic involvement of the mitral valve alone. At least in a few well-described cases, however, mitral and aortic valvular deformity with marked regurgitation due to rheumatoid nodules was the characteristic pathological picture.[214]

ELECTROCARDIOGRAPHIC ABNORMALITIES. Studies of the electrocardiogram in patients with RA and in matched controls show that first-degree atrioventricular block is the most significant finding in RA.[206] Complete heart block causing Adams-Stokes syndrome has been de-

scribed, and other abnormalities include left bundle branch block, atrial fibrillation, and atrial and ventricular ectopic beats. Abnormal T waves, however, do not occur more frequently than in controls and are of little value in the diagnosis of rheumatoid heart disease despite the frequency of rheumatoid pericarditis.[209]

The Vasculitis Syndromes

Etiology. Most of the clinical manifestations of periarteritis nodosa, systemic lupus erythematosus (SLE), and several other forms of diffuse vasculitis may be produced by infections such as hepatitis B, in which massive and persistent antigenemia gives rise to circulating immune complexes, the qualitative and quantitative features of which determine the localization and character of the vascular lesions. It has also become clear that bacterial endocarditis, like hepatitis B, produces many of the varied glomerular lesions of SLE, produces large and small lesions of polyarteritis, and produces serological findings similar to those of SLE.[217-220]

In addition to infectious agents as a cause of immune complex disease, the prolonged administration of certain drugs can produce most, if not all, of the features of SLE (drug-induced lupus). Procainamide is the most notorious offender, but hydralazine, phenytoin (Dilantin), and several other anticonvulsants, isoniazide, sulfonamides, and several other drugs administered for prolonged periods may produce features of SLE.[221,222] Whereas true SLE nephritis is rare in drug-induced lupus, cases are now reported in which the entire syndrome has evolved when the drug has been given long enough and in sufficient doses. In one fatal case, a patient was reported to have ingested enormous amounts of procainamide during 9 years of continuous therapy; the full-blown syndrome was proved at autopsy, including lupus nephritis and Libman-Sacks endocarditis, and the serological features were characteristic.[223]

As in the case of the seronegative spondyloarthropathies (see above), only a small portion of the syndromes recognized can be shown to be due to specific infectious agents or drugs. Most cases of large-vessel polyarteritis, or the small-vessel and capillary diffuse vasculitis of SLE, must be considered idiopathic, but a careful search for known infectious agents capable of producing persistent antigenemia and for a history of drug therapy should be undertaken before one resorts to an idiopathic, descriptive diagnosis.

Systemic Lupus Erythematosus

Pathological Features. The hallmark of this disease is the presence of a number of antibodies to nuclear components, the antinuclear antibodies (ANA), which participate in the pathogenesis of SLE by forming antigen-antibody-complement complexes that are found in many of the lesions. These complexes tend to be trapped by vascular and glomerular basement membranes and to produce, through complement activation, lesions affecting small vessels and capillaries. In experimental immune complex disease in animals and in serum sickness in humans, inflammation of joints, skin, pleura, pericardium, brain, kidneys, and other systems occurs because of the persistent excess antigenemia and subsequent circulating immune complexes. These and probably other hyperimmune phenomena explain many of the protean clinical manifestations of SLE. Although anti-heart antibodies have been described in the sera of patients with SLE, they bear no clear relationship to the frequency and severity of cardiac lesions and may be a result rather than a cause of cardiac inflammation, presumably owing to release of myocardial antigens into the circulation.[224]

CARDIAC ABNORMALITIES. Because the basic anatomical lesion of SLE is a diffuse microvasculitis,[225,225a] the heart is almost always found to be involved at autopsy.[226] The clinical manifestations, however, are usually overshadowed by the symptoms and signs related to involvement of other organs, and attention is drawn to the heart only when the lesions of pericarditis, myocarditis, or endocarditis are florid. Clinical evidence of cardiac abnormalities has been observed, however, in as many as 50 to 60 per cent of cases in two large series.[227,228] As methodology becomes more sophisticated, detection of cardiac involvement begins to approach that found at necropsy (see below).

Pericarditis. This is found in approximately two-thirds to three-fourths of autopsies and is perhaps the commonest cardiac lesion of SLE (p. 1511).[226–231] The acute pericardial inflammation may extend into the sinoatrial and atrioventricular nodes, with destruction of conducting fibers.[232–235] Pericardial fluid may be clear or sanguineous and has a high protein content. Effusions may be voluminous and occasionally cause tamponade. Histologically, the pericardium shows fibrinoid degeneration, edema, and necrosis of connective tissue when the process is acute, and various stages of fibrosis with the formation of adhesions are found during the healing or chronic phase. Constrictive pericarditis occurs only rarely; however, pericardial tamponade and constrictive pericarditis both have been reported in cases of procainamide-induced lupus erythematosus.[236,237] Pericarditis, like arthritis, tends to be episodic and to heal well in remissions rather than to become chronic and sclerosing.[238]

Myocarditis. Subclinical myocarditis is common. Its severity is proportionate to the severity of the systemic disease process. The lesions observed at autopsy consist of fibrinoid necrosis involving interstitial tissues and blood vessels, and only rarely are the cardiac myofibrils destroyed. Small vessel changes include an arteriopathy of vessels 0.1 to 1.0 mm in diameter. The abnormal vessels are located in the conduction system of patients selected for study because of the presence of arrhythmias. Segmental arteritis and periarteritis with some occlusions of the arterial lumen and small areas of fibrosis distal to the obstruction are found. Involvement of the atrioventricular as well as the sinoatrial node in the inflammatory process of SLE has been shown at autopsy in a death due to arrhythmia in a 24-year-old man.[233] Rare cases of myocardial infarction, presumably due to arteritis of larger coronary vessels, have been reported.[239,240] Atherosclerotic coronary disease is being reported somewhat more frequently than might be expected in patients with SLE treated with corticosteroids, possibly related to worsening of hypertension in such patients.[241] Cardiac enlargement is frequent.[242]

Endocarditis. This is the most characteristic cardiac lesion of SLE.[225,226] The Libman-Sacks[243] verrucous valvular lesions are wartlike, varying from pinhead size to 3 to 4 mm. The lesions may be discrete or in clumps and are composed of degenerating valve tissue apparently extruded beyond the endothelium and accompanied by some fibrosis of the underlying leaflet. The lesions usually contain granular, basophilic masses of cellular debris, the characteristic so-called "hematoxylin bodies" composed of basophilic fragments in the cytoplasm of cells. They may be found anywhere on the endocardial surface of the heart but are most common in the angles of the atrioventricular valves and on the underside of the base of the mitral valve. They may also extend onto the chordae tendineae or papillary muscles. Generalized involvement of the entire thickness of the heart valves with inflammatory and fibrous changes may also occur. Aortic valve involvement is rare but has been well described.[244] Despite the frequency and extent of the endocardial lesions of SLE, they do not often profoundly affect the function of the valves and, unlike rheu-

matic fever, do not produce serious regurgitation during the acute phase of the disease. Only rarely do they lead to marked scarring and deformity during healing, requiring valve replacement.[245]

CLINICAL FEATURES. Although autopsy shows that at least two-thirds of patients have pericarditis at some time during the course of SLE, only one-third have recognizable symptoms and signs during life.[227–231] Typical pericardial pain may occur, but often the friction rubs, characteristic electrocardiographic changes, or enlargement of the cardiac silhouette on chest x-ray due to pericardial effusion may be found in the absence of symptoms, and therefore evidence of pericarditis should always be suspected and sought in *all* patients with SLE, even in those without clinical manifestations. Cardiac tamponade is rare but can occur, requiring repeated aspirations of fluid.[231] Systolic and diastolic murmurs at the mitral area, and less often at the aortic area, seem to come and go during the course of acute exacerbations of the disease and are presumably due to Libman-Sacks endocarditis. However, at autopsy the presence of these lesions is not always confirmed, and other factors such as anemia, tachycardia, fever, myocarditis, transient papillary muscle dysfunction, and the adventitious sounds of pleuropericarditis must be considered. Hemodynamically significant and permanent valvular regurgitation from lupus carditis is rare, but such cases have been reported and have even required valve replacement.[245]

Congestive heart failure due to SLE is also uncommon except when associated with hypertension secondary to renal disease. Heart failure may be mistakenly diagnosed in the presence of edema due to renal disease or pericardial effusion or both. Clinically apparent myocarditis, like that of rheumatic fever, producing tachycardia, gallop rhythm, and cardiac dilatation, is a feature of very toxic cases of SLE when high fever and other multisystem manifestations of acute vasculitis are present. Arrhythmias are also relatively uncommon and consist of atrial flutter and fibrillation with varying degrees of atrioventricular block.[232] Attention has been called to the development of congenital complete heart block, a "lupus-like syndrome," and pericarditis in infants born to mothers with active SLE.[246,247] The observation suggests that transplacental transfer of abnormal antibodies (or small immune complexes) may be of pathogenetic importance in these cases. During examination of a pregnant woman with SLE, fetal bradycardia should be recognized as a possible complication of lupus rather than fetal distress from other causes.

Echocardiography may be useful in SLE for demonstrating pericardial involvement and for evaluating valve function in the presence of various murmurs.[238,245,248] Extensive hemodynamic studies carried out on a group of five patients who had had SLE for 2½ to 7 years prior to heart catheterization and who had no obvious clinical findings of cardiac involvement showed considerable evidence of impairment of myocardial function.[249]

TREATMENT. To the extent that their antiinflammatory effect can control active myocarditis, corticosteroids may be necessary to manage severe cardiac involvement in SLE. Control of hypertension is also very helpful in the treatment and prevention of congestive heart failure. There is no evidence that corticosteroid treatment can prevent the rare cases of constrictive pericarditis or valvular deformity.[241] Although the inflammatory reaction may be dramatically suppressed, the basic disease process and tissue injury are not altered by corticosteroid therapy, which is at most supportive and sometimes causes problems (hypertension and fluid retention). Immunosuppressive therapy is usually reserved for the most severe, corticosteroid-resistant forms of the disease and especially for renal involvement. Death from the cardiac disease of SLE compared with other causes of fatality in this disease is rare, so that cardiac manifestations usually do not determine the choice of antiinflammatory therapy.

PERIARTERITIS NODOSA

As noted above, necrotizing inflammation of blood vessels is a common finding in immune complex diseases of known and unknown etiologies; however, because the origin and nature of the offending agent is unknown in most instances, the vasculitides continue to be classified on the basis of their histological and clinical features. These depend largely upon the size of the involved blood vessels, their anatomical sites, the stage of the inflammation, and the characteristics of the lesions.

The clinical features of most cases fit into one of the following five major categories: periarteritis nodosa, allergic granulomatosis, Wegener's granulomatosis, hypersensitivity vasculitis, and giant cell arteritis.[250]

Pathological Features. The muscular arteries, adjacent veins, and occasionally arterioles and venules (but not the capillaries) are involved in a necrotizing inflammation. Segments of vessels, at times only part of the circumference being affected, are involved in the lesions, especially at the bifurcation of arteries. Small aneurysms may form and rupture. In the acute stage of inflammation the lesions contain predominantly polymorphonuclear leukocytes, whereas in chronic lesions mononuclear cell infiltration and partial healing are apparent. However, both phases may be present at once, suggesting repeated or continuous insults.

The lesions are commonly found in the coronary arteries as well as kidneys, muscles, and vasa nervorum, but the lungs are usually spared. *Myocardial infarction* is therefore relatively common, and this leads to patchy myocardial fibrosis and left ventricular enlargement. The latter is also secondary to hypertension, frequently present owing to renal involvement. Hemorrhage into the pericardial sac with tamponade and death, inflammatory pericarditis, or uremic pericarditis are causes of pericardial involvement. Endocardial or valvular lesions do not occur unless the papillary muscle is injured by ischemia.

CLINICAL FEATURES. Periarteritis nodosa may occur at any age, produces fever and multisystem involvement, and may persist for months or years. Pericarditis may be clinically evident, frequently associated with pleuritis, but is not a prominent feature of the disease. Chest pain due to true angina pectoris is also relatively rare[251,252] despite the occurrence of myocardial infarction. In one series of 41 cases of periarteritis nodosa and myocardial infarction, only 3 were diagnosed clinically.[251] The most common form of heart involvement is congestive failure and hypertension due to renal disease, which causes most deaths.[251,252] Cardiac arrhythmias, most often atrial flutter and fibrillation, can occur. Death from ruptured aneurysms, particularly gastrointestinal bleeding, is not uncommon.

Kawasaki Disease (see also p. 1053). In recent years, Kawasaki and others have delineated a periarteritis-like vasculitis in Japanese infants. It is a complication of an acute febrile disease that they have called "mucocutaneous lymph node syndrome";[253,254] more recently this has become known as Kawasaki disease.[255] A polyarteritic syndrome occurs in approximately 2 per cent of infants following an acute mucocutaneous exanthematous febrile illness. Severe arteritis of the larger coronary arteries and of arteries of other organs results in rapid or sudden death from cardiac arrhythmias or massive myocardial infarction. Aneurysms of the coronary, brachial, iliac, and other vessels can be observed in the acute stage of the disease but may cause late-stage arterial aneurysms in children. The disease has been reported from Hawaii, continental United States, Canada, Greece, and Korea. Previously reported cases of "infantile periarteritis nodosa with coronary artery involvement" from the United States may be identical with Kawasaki disease.[255]

Laboratory Findings. Most helpful diagnostically is angiography when it reveals the characteristic multiple small aneurysms at branch points of mesenteric, renal, and other arteries (Fig. 48–11). The diagnosis may be quite difficult to establish in the absence of this finding, and biopsies of clinically involved tissues are usually necessary to establish the diagnosis. "Blind" muscle biopsy is positive in fewer than one-third of cases later confirmed. Hepatitis B soluble antigen is found in the blood of increasing numbers of patients with periarteritis nodosa in recently reported series, and this antigen has been identified in vascular lesions along with immunoglobulin and complement.[256,257] Other infectious diseases associated with prolonged antigenemia have been also identified as causes of polyarteritis, such as cytomegalovirus infections and trichinosis.[258,259]

COURSE AND TREATMENT. The prognosis of periarteritis nodosa is grave; one-half to two-thirds of patients die within a year when series comprised hospitalized cases. Treatment with corticosteroids is frequently followed by temporary improvement on doses of 40 to 60 mg of prednisone or prednisolone per day. Five-year survival of untreated patients is estimated at 13 per cent. Studies with immunosuppressive drugs have been encouraging in appar-

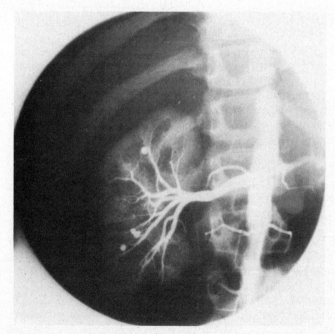

FIGURE 48–11 Renal artery angiogram in a 13-year-old boy with periarteritis nodosa. (From Stollerman, G. H.: Rheumatic Fever and Streptococcal Infection. New York, by permission of Grune and Stratton, 1975.)

ently prolonging the course in some cases, but adequate controlled studies have not been made.[260]

OTHER FORMS OF DIFFUSE VASCULITIS

Allergic Granulomatosis. This disease involves the vessels of the heart in the same way as periarteritis nodosa but eosinophils tend to be more abundant in the lesions, and granulomatous collections of epithelioid and giant cells are formed, accounting for the name of the condition.[260] Pulmonary involvement dominates the clinical picture, and patients tend to have a history of respiratory infection, asthma, and fever, often with a striking peripheral eosinophilia.

Wegener's Granulomatosis. This syndrome is distinguished by necrotizing granulomas of the upper respiratory tract, especially the destructive lesions of the nasopharynx and paranasal sinuses, middle ear, and bronchial tree. Necrotizing inflammation extends into the smaller pulmonary vessels of the lungs and other organs, particularly the kidneys. Pericardial and myocardial involvement is not uncommon, but the clinical picture is dominated by respiratory and renal involvement, without which the diagnosis cannot be made. The special feature of treatment is the encouraging response of this particular syndrome to cyclophosphamide therapy, resulting in dramatic remissions, often complete, and in prolonged survival.[260-262]

Hypersensitivity Vasculitis.[263] Hypersensitivity vasculitis is also called small-vessel vasculitis or angiitis and is characterized by involvement of arterioles, venules, and capillaries only. The presence of antigen-antibody complexes in the lesions all tend to be of the same age. It is difficult to tell at the inception of the disease whether it is part of a larger syndrome, such as SLE, subacute infective endocarditis, mixed cryoglobulinemia, Henoch-Schönlein purpura, or a drug reaction except by the course and distinguishing features of the other syndromes. Hypersensitivity vasculitis is the most common form of immune complex disease. Muscular and large arteries are spared, so that the tissue lesions are due to microinfarcts and hemorrhagic and exudative reactions at the capillary level rather than to thrombosis of large vessels with resulting ischemia and necrosis. The most common cardiac finding is pericarditis, but such involvement occurs along with that of many other organs, skin, mucous membranes, joints, and so on.

Giant Cell Arteritis.[260,264,265] Giant cell arteritis, also called cranial or temporal arteritis, affects predominantly older individuals. Large or medium-sized arteries, including the superficial temporal artery, are involved without small-vessel or capillary lesions. The lesions are usually cellular and granulomatous and contain multinucleated giant cells. Involvement of the arteries is spotty and segmented and tends to produce thrombosis at the site of involvement. The aorta is often involved, and aneurysms and dissection can result (p. 1560). External and internal carotids and vertebral arteries can be affected, and thrombosis of the ophthalmic or central retinal artery leads to blindness. Thrombosis of the coronary, iliac, femoral, or mesenteric arteries produces ischemia and infarctions.

Often the polymyalgia rheumatica syndrome is an associated finding. It is characterized by pain and stiffness in the neck and shoulders, upper arms, hips, and thighs. Joint and muscle pain and tenderness may be severe. Headache is characteristically associated with tender and thickened temporal arteries. The erythrocyte sedimentation rate is strikingly elevated owing primarily to a marked increase in the serum alpha-2 globulins. Myocarditis due to giant cell arteritis has been reported only rarely despite the frequently described association of this form of vasculitis with polymyalgia rheumatica.[264] Myocarditis may be present, however, even though clinically unsuspected, as was shown recently in an autopsy on a patient with giant cell arteritis involving primarily the aorta and lower extremities who died of a cerebral hemorrhage.[264] The lesions were difficult to distinguish from viral myocarditis, and, indeed, it is noteworthy that the polymyalgia rheumatica syndrome has been described in association with hepatitis B virus infection.[266] The dramatic response of all symptoms to relatively small doses of corticosteroids (15 to 20 mg per day of prednisone) is a good therapeutic test for the syndrome, and treatment with corticosteroids usually completely suppresses the symptoms and signs within a few days. After a few weeks the dose may be tapered to a maintenance dose of approximately 10 mg per day which will usually suffice to control the disease, and eventually treatment may be discontinued altogether in most patients.

PROGRESSIVE SYSTEMIC SCLEROSIS (DIFFUSE SCLERODERMA)

Progressive systemic sclerosis (PSS) is an insidious, chronic, fibrosing condition that presents as progressive tightening and thickening of the skin (scleroderma), developing over a period of many years. Raynaud's phenomena occur at some time in almost all patients. Visceral involvement may occur at any time during the course of the disease, affecting the gastrointestinal tract, lungs, heart or kidney. Much attention has been given to the classification of various subgroups of this syndrome that include patients with diffuse scleroderma, those without diffuse skin changes but with other shared features, such as calcinosis, Raynaud's phenomena, esophageal dyskinesia, sclerodactyly, and telangiectasia (the CREST syndrome), and those with features overlapping polymyositis or systemic lupus erythematosus or both. The implications of these classifications are dealt with elsewhere.[267-269]

Pathological Features and Pathogenesis. In contrast to the acute exudative forms of vasculitis associated with the necrotizing lesions described above, PSS seems to be a disease at the opposite end of the inflammatory scale, where very slow scarring and fibrosis results from gradual obliteration of small vessels. It is difficult to classify PSS pathophysiologically because the cause of the extensive fibrosis is not known. Hereditary factors have not been identified. Qualitative abnormalities of collagen are not documented. The disease apparently results from injury at the level of very small arteries, 150 to 500 μm in diameter, and capillaries are gradually obliterated.[270,271] Early in the course of the lesions, mononuclear cell infiltrates occur around small arteries and in the interstitium. The basement membrane of the capillaries appears thickened. Fibroblastic proliferation and overproduction of collagen result from the low-grade inflammatory process. Narrowing and obliteration of small arteries result in decreased vascularization of the skin, skeletal muscles, lung, and heart, followed by fibrosis. The interlobular arteries of the kidney are involved by intensive intimal proliferation, which causes the most serious complication of the disease, namely, rapid renal failure often with severe hypertension.

Biopsies of apparently unaffected muscles show basement membrane changes in capillaries with marked reduction in their numbers per unit area of muscle, suggesting that an early stage of involvement is at the level of the endothelial cell–fibroblast membrane.[271] Autopsy studies have shown pericarditis or pericardial effusions in about one-half of patients; the most common pathological lesions are fibrous adhesions resulting in obliteration of the pericardial sac.

CARDIAC LESIONS. The importance of primary cardiac involvement in the natural history of the disease has been repeatedly emphasized.[269,272,273] Heart involvement is a frequent cause of death and second only to involvement of the kidneys as a factor shortening the survival of patients with this disease.[274] Confusion concerning the question of primary involvement of the heart by the sclerosing process has been caused by the frequency of cor pulmonale resulting from pulmonary involvement of PSS and severe hypertension and hypertensive heart disease resulting from the renal involvement. Cardiac involvement without kidney involvement occurs in approximately 12 per cent of patients and shortens survival.

"Scleroderma heart" is primarily a myocardial disease, and the heart's small vessels are all vulnerable to the sclerosing process. Atherosclerosis of the major coronary arteries occurs to the same degree in patients with PSS as in age and sex-matched controls. PSS patients, however, have much more intimal sclerosis of the small coronary arteries than do controls,[275,276] and such involvement may lead to ischemia, small infarctions, and fibrosis. The combination of vascular insufficiency and fibrosis produces a cardiomyopathy with congestive heart failure and conduction system abnormalities.[277,278] Acute and chronic pericarditis, even in the absence of uremia, is common but usually asymptomatic. At times the resulting effusion can be large enough to cause tamponade,[279] although this degree of effusion is rare. Pericardial fluid, when obtainable, has the features of an exudate but lacks evidence of autoantibodies, immune complexes, or complement depletion, such as that seen in rheumatoid arthritis or SLE.[280] Endocardial involvement is rare, and the deformities of mitral and aortic valves that have been reported probably have little hemodynamic significance.

CLINICAL FEATURES. The primary clinical manifestations of scleroderma heart disease are those of pericarditis and congestive heart failure. In one series, pericarditis patients had a 7-year cumulative survival rate of 33 per cent, whereas none of the PSS patients with heart failure survived for 7 years.[281] Men have significantly worse survival rates than women, as do blacks and older patients. Although cardiac symptoms may appear months or even years before the skin is involved, as a rule overt heart disease is not a prominent part of the clinical picture of PSS until late in its course, when myocardial involvement and resultant heart failure indicate a grim prognosis. Pericarditis, however, may be intermittently symptomatic for long periods of time.

When dyspnea with exertion or at rest occurs in the patient with PSS, primary myocardial failure must be distinguished from myocardial failure secondary to hypertension from renal disease and pulmonary insufficiency from pulmonary fibrosis due to PSS. Cardiac murmurs are not usually due to valvular deformity but to cardiac dilatation and to anemia or to papillary weakness. Chest pain simulating ischemic heart disease as well as typical pericardial pain may occur. Right ventricular failure is a feature of pulmonary hypertension with or without myocardial involvement. Angina pectoris has been described in a patient who showed normal large coronary arteries on angiographic studies, and in another patient with anginal pain and scleroderma, the large coronary arteries were patent, but a slow flow velocity of the dye was observed in the vessels.[282] Such hemodynamic findings associated with biventricular dysfunction and with left ventricular hypokinesia are consistent with the small vessel involvement of PSS.

The *roentgenogram of the chest* may reveal cardiac enlargement from pericardial effusion, cardiomyopathy, or hypertension. The electrocardiographic findings are also nonspecific and may, indeed, be normal when the heart is seriously involved. All degrees of atrioventricular conduction blocks, right and left ventricular hypertrophy, and all varieties of arrhythmias have been described,[283,284] but conduction defects are found most often in patients with the primary cardiomyopathy of PSS.[278]

Echocardiographic studies revealed patterns consistent with a congestive cardiomyopathy or a restrictive cardiomyopathy (p. 128).[285] Echocardiographic abnormalities were reported in 37 (69 per cent) of a series of 54 patients with PSS, and in 22 of these, pericardial effusion was noted, although it was suspected clinically in only 7.[286]

TREATMENT. Many drugs have been used for the treatment of PSS but without significant or prolonged effect. The value of corticosteroids is limited to improvement of the early edematous phase of the disease, but this effect on the heart has not been systematically evaluated and probably will not influence the eventual course of the disease. Captopril has been observed to control the severe accelerated hypertension associated with the renovascular disease of scleroderma and to relieve the digital vasospasm of Raynaud's phenomena.[287]

POLYMYOSITIS AND DERMATOMYOSITIS
(See also p. 1715)

Polymyositis is a diffuse inflammatory disease of unknown cause affecting primarily proximal striated muscles and various connective tissues of the body, especially skin and joints.[288-292] When the disease involves the skin, it is called *dermatomyositis*. Polymyositis may be due to a pathological process common to several etiologies because it is seen in association with a variety of syndromes. It is grouped with the connective tissue or rheumatic diseases because of its overlapping clinical and laboratory features, especially when it is associated with rheumatoid arthritis and progressive systemic sclerosis but also with systemic lupus erythematosus or polyarteritis. Involvement of the heart in polymyositis has just begun to be fully appreciated in the past decade and was mentioned in earlier publications only as a rare finding, if at all.

Pathological Features. Polymyositis is either increasing in incidence or is being more frequently diagnosed, and it is now recognized as one of the most common myopathies.[293] The principal changes in muscle tissue consist of widespread destruction of muscle fibers with phagocytosis of destroyed cells. There may be focal infiltrates of inflammatory cells, such as lymphocytes, mononuclear leukocytes, plasma cells, and, only rarely, neutrophilic leukocytes. Regeneration of destroyed muscle in the form of proliferating sarcolemmal nuclei, basophilic sarcoplasm, and new myofibrils is a prominent feature. Residual muscle fibers may be small. In any given biopsy specimen, either degeneration of muscle fibers or infiltrations of inflammatory cells may predominate. In electron microscopic studies, the most significant changes, in addition to those in muscle fibers, are found in the endothelium and basement membrane of capillaries and small arterioles, much like those described in scleroderma and SLE. Inclusions in the cytoplasm of endothelial cells that are identical to those found in SLE and scleroderma have been described.[294]

PATHOLOGY OF THE HEART.[295-304] The cardiac lesions involve the conducting system predominantly but also can produce an extensive cardiomyopathy and pericarditis. The latter may appear far more often than would be suspected on clinical grounds. The cardiac valves and coronary arteries are spared except in overlap syndromes. The sinoatrial node shows conspicuous fibrosis, swelling and degeneration of collagen, and focal or complete replacement. The fibrosis extends into the adjacent myocardium of the right atrium. The atrioventricular node, bundle of His, and both bundle branches all may be involved in the degenerative and fibrotic process (Fig. 48–12). Cardiac muscle fibers in the atria and ventricles are replaced in scattered areas by fibrosis, and, in some cases, the pattern of focal myocardial necrosis and inflammation is the same as that seen in skeletal muscle.[296] Pericarditis is described more often clinically than pathologically.

CLINICAL FEATURES. Almost all authors comment on the rarity of cardiovascular manifestations in polymyositis, and, indeed, the best reported studies of survivorship do not relate death to cardiac causes but

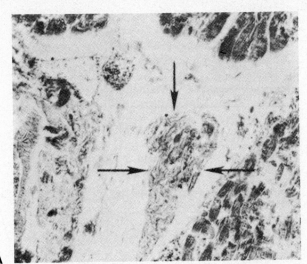

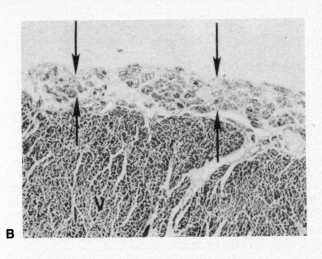

FIGURE 48–12   *A*, First part of right bundle branch (arrows). Note presence of only a few remaining cells in right bundle branch (Gomori's trichrome stain, original magnification ×150). *B*, Periphery of posterior fibers of left bundle branch (arrows), showing considerable fibrosis and loss of cells. V = ventricular myocardium (Gomori's trichrome stain, original magnification ×45). (From Lightfoot, P. R., et al.: Chronic dermatomyositis with intermittent trifascicular block. An electrophysiologic conduction system correlation. Chest *71*:413, 1977.)

rather to pneumonitis, which is relatively common from aspiration secondary to respiratory muscle weakness and dysphagia.[293] However, there have been informal reports indicating a much higher frequency of cardiac involvement in polymyositis than was previously appreciated. When standard 12-lead electrocardiograms are analyzed systematically, arrhythmias may be quite frequent;[304,305] these usually consist of supraventricular tachycardia, but ventricular tachycardia and advanced heart block associated with syncope or cardiac arrest have also been observed. Deaths have been attributed directly to cardiac failure or arrhythmias or both in some cases, and cardiac muscle histology has been found to be abnormal on autopsy.

TREATMENT. Corticosteroids and immunosuppressive drugs may be of benefit in the treatment of polymyositis-dermatomyositis,[290] but only a controlled prospective study can settle this issue. The course of the disease may not be truly modified by corticosteroids, but the complications of muscle weakness, especially of the respiratory and deglutitional muscles, which lead to pulmonary disease and death, might be diminished by the frequent improvement of muscle strength observed after this treatment.

In the absence of malignancy, survival statistics are favorable for all groups (87 to 91 per cent) in several studies. The leading causes of death, which in one series[290] were metastatic malignancy (24 per cent), sepsis (19 per cent), profound muscular weakness (9.5 per cent), and cardiovascular and cerebrovascular disorders (unspecified percentage), suggest that at least some of these may be modified by therapy and management to improve the prognosis.

HERITABLE DISORDERS OF CONNECTIVE TISSUE

The heritable disorders of connective tissue are characterized by a definable mode of inheritance and by the clinical expression of a generalized defect of some connective tissue element. This group of disorders includes Marfan syndrome, osteogenesis imperfecta, Ehlers-Danlos syndrome, and pseudoxanthoma elasticum, as well as Hurler syndrome and the other mucopolysaccharidoses.[305]

Involvement of the connective tissues of the large arteries, cardiac valves, and other cardiac connective tissue elements determines the cardiovascular manifestations of these disorders. The spectrum of cardiovascular involvement is broad and includes characteristic pathological changes of minimal clinical import as well as of major catastrophic valvular incompetence, aortic dissection, and death. In a number of these disorders, recent investigations of the metabolism and biochemistry of connective tissue have clarified the defects; in others, the basic abnormality remains obscure.[306]

In addition, there are some patients who manifest no or only subtle extracardiac changes of the generalized connective tissue disorders but who display pathological and clinical cardiovascular disease indistinguishable from the generalized disorders. Whether these patients represent a forme fruste of the generalized disease process or they express the limited response of the cardiovascular connective tissue to varied insults is not clear. Patients with myxomatous degeneration of connective tissue of the mitral and aortic valves and those with cystic medial necrosis with involvement of the aortic annulus are included in this group (Chap. 45).[307,308]

THE MARFAN SYNDROME[305]

The Marfan syndrome (also see p. 1620) is a generalized abnormality of connective tissue with major clinical features involving the skeletal, ocular, and cardiovascular systems. The typical skeletal manifestations include excessive limb length, arachnodactyly, loose-jointedness, kyphoscoliosis, and anterior chest deformity. Affected individuals are characteristically tall with long, thin extremities and show weakness of joint capsules, ligaments, tendons, and fascia that results in joint dislocation, hernia, and kyphoscoliosis. A sparsity of subcutaneous fat is a striking feature. The ocular manifestations include defective suspensory ligaments of the lens and subsequent ectopia lentis. The excessive length of the eyeball and involvement of the connective tissue of the retina contribute to the severe myopia and retinal detachment that is often found.

Involvement of the cardiovascular system includes aortic aneurysm with dissection, aortic insufficiency from dilation of both the aortic root and the annulus or from myxomatous involvement of the leaflets themselves and myxomatous degeneration of the mitral valve and its apparatus with secondary mitral incompetence (Fig. 48–13).

The Marfan syndrome exhibits simple mendelian autoso-

THE MARFAN SYNDROME

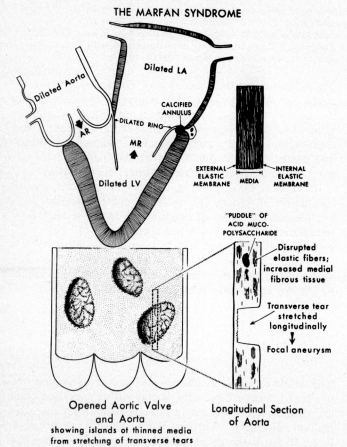

Opened Aortic Valve and Aorta
showing islands ot thinned media from stretching of transverse tears

Longitudinal Section of Aorta

FIGURE 48–13 The various cardiovascular abnormalities found in Marfan's syndrome. The aortic regurgitation appears to be related primarily to dilatation of the aorta. The mitral regurgitation probably results from a combination of factors: dilatation of the left ventricular cavity, altering the papillary muscle–mitral leaflet angle; dilatation of the mitral annulus; calcification of the mitral annulus; and elongation of the mitral leaflets and chordae, allowing prolapse of the leaflets into the left atrium during ventricular systole. *Top right,* Longitudinal section of normal aorta. *Bottom right,* Longitudinal section in a patient with Marfan's syndrome. There is severe loss of elastic fibers, deposition of abnormal amounts of acid mucopolysaccharide material, and tears in the wall. The tears expand to cause the islands of thinning seen in the view of the opened aortic valve and aorta. (From Roberts, W. C., et al.: Nonrheumatic valvular cardiac disease. A clinicopathologic survey of 27 different conditions causing valvular dysfunction. *In* Likoff, W. (ed.): Valvular Heart Disease. Philadelphia, F. A. Davis Co., 1973, p. 368.)

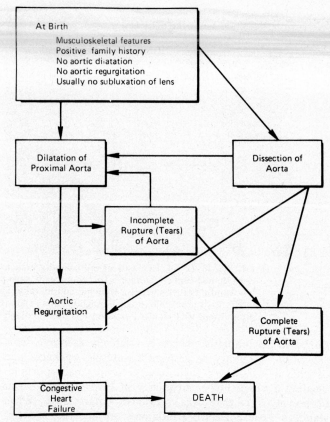

FIGURE 48–14 Schema of development of cardiovascular complications in the Marfan syndrome. (Reproduced with permission from Roberts, W. C.: Am. Heart J. *104*:115, 1982.)

mal dominant inheritance with variable phenotypic expression (Chap. 47). According to McKusick, 15 per cent of all cases are de novo mutations, and this likelihood increases with increasing paternal age.[305] The diagnosis of the Marfan syndrome is most secure when a positive family history of the disease is present or ectopia lentis is found in conjunction with the classic musculoskeletal or cardiovascular changes.[305,309,309a]

PATHOLOGICAL FEATURES. The pathological changes seen in patients with the Marfan syndrome[305,307,309–323] are most striking in the ascending aorta and annulus (p. 1556, Fig. 48–14). In patients with long-term aortic regurgitation, the proximal aorta is diffusely dilated along with the aortic annulus and sinuses of Valsalva. Dilatation of the pulmonary artery also occurs. Chronic aortic dissection and transverse tears without dissection are also found. Histologically, advanced changes include fragmented and sparse elastic tissue in the tunica media, with irregular whorls of smooth muscle and increased amounts of collagen. The vasa vasorum are dilated. The tunica media is interspersed with cystic vacuoles of metachromatically staining material, probably mucopolysaccharide. Inflammation is conspicuously absent. In patients succumbing to acute dissection, earlier changes in the aorta have been studied and reveal cystic medial necrosis and moderate degeneration of elastic elements with disorganization of the smooth muscle bundles. Faults in the media are seen that contain a mucopolysaccharide-rich ground substance. The left ventricle is often enlarged and hypertrophied, reflecting the

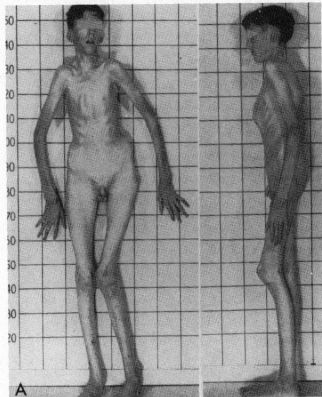
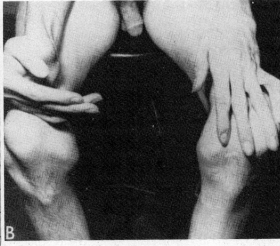

FIGURE 48–15 A, Eleven-year-old boy with Marfan's syndrome. Note excessive length of lower compared with upper segment; the extremities are very long. B, Arachnodactyly. (From McKusick, V.A.: Heritable Disorders of Connective Tissue, 4th ed. St. Louis, The C.V. Mosby Co., 1972.)

degree and duration of the hemodynamic burden imposed by aortic or mitral incompetence.

More recently, the pathological changes and clinical significance of primary valvular abnormalities of the Marfan syndrome have been recognized. Changes in the mitral valve have included ballooning and redundant cusps, fenestrations in the leaflets, elongated and thinned chordae tendineae, and occasionally ruptured and thickened valve cusps with rolled edges. Thin, shiny, diaphanous leaflets are also described. Similar changes in the aortic valve cusps have also been reported. The histological changes include disruption and loss of normal valvular architecture, increase in mucopolysaccharide ground substance, cystic degeneration, and loss of cellularity. These changes are similar to those found in cystic medial necrosis of the aorta. These valvular changes have been termed myxomatous degeneration.

James and coworkers studied the atrioventricular conduction system in two patients with the Marfan syndrome and clinical cardiac conduction abnormalities.[310] Medial degeneration, hyperplasia, and intimal proliferation with luminal narrowing were present in the nutrient arteries of the sinoatrial and atrioventricular nodes as well as in the intramyocardial arteries.

CLINICAL FEATURES. In this generalized disorder of connective tissue, there are ocular and skeletal as well as cardiovascular abnormalities. Weakness of the supporting tissues causes bilateral subluxation of the lens, minor degrees of which can be appreciated by slit-lamp examination. Increased length of the extremities, with an abnormally low ratio of the upper segment (crown to pubic symphysis) to the lower segment (lower than 0.84 in whites and 0.79 in blacks), very long "spider" fingers

(arachnodactyly), long metacarpols, pectus carinatum, and pectus excavatum are other important features (Fig. 48–15).

Cardiovascular complications of the Marfan syndrome occur in 30 to 60 per cent of patients in different series. The poor prognosis in patients with the Marfan syndrome reflects the cardiovascular complications and the progressive nature of the lesions. Of 257 patients with the Marfan syndrome followed between 1939 and 1970, the average age at death of the 72 deceased patients was 32 years. Of 56 patients who died, the cause of death in 52 was cardiovascular complications, with aortic dilatation, rupture, and/or dissection accounting for 80 per cent of these.[311] In a study of the Marfan syndrome in infancy and childhood, 61 per cent of patients had cardiac abnormalities.[312,313] Mitral valve disease with mitral regurgitation was the most common lesion found (47 per cent). Mitral systolic clicks with late systolic murmurs were the most common signs. Generally the prognosis is good when isolated mitral valve involvement occurs. Severe mitral and aortic regurgitation may develop, however, requiring valve replacement.[313,314,314a]

During the course of the disease, the ascending aorta becomes dilated with worsening regurgitation, and the likelihood of rupture or dissection increases. In addition to signs and symptoms of left heart failure, chest pain with anginal features is often observed in the Marfan syndrome. This symptom may be secondary to aortic regurgitation, dilatation of the aorta, or coronary ostial involvement.

Systolic honks and musical murmurs may be heard. If chordae or leaflets rupture, loud thrills and longer murmurs may be heard. An echocardiographic study of 26 patients with clinical evidence of the Marfan syndrome showed 12 patients with isolated dysfunction of the mitral valve apparatus. Four patients demonstrated widening of the aortic root as well as abnormality of the mitral valve, and four patients showed abnormality of the aortic root alone.[315]

Infective endocarditis involving the mitral valve in patients with the Marfan syndrome is well documented, and this process has accounted for a significant number of deaths.[305,311,316,317]

PATHOGENESIS AND MANAGEMENT. The biochemical lesion of the Marfan syndrome remains undefined, but as emphasized by McKusick[305,305a] and Bowers[309] the cardiovascular manifestations most likely reflect the response of defective connective tissue to prolonged hemodynamic stresses. Theoretical considerations have prompted the use of the beta-adrenergic blocking agent propranolol in patients with the Marfan syndrome who manifest early signs of aortic dilatation. The murmur of aortic regurgitation, dilatation of the aorta on radiographic examination, and echocardiographic evidence of an enlarged aorta may serve as guides to the initiation and effectiveness of therapy.[315,319] Conclusive evidence of the efficacy of this therapy remains to be established.

The underlying connective tissue defect presents a considerable obstacle to surgical therapy. Although prosthetic valves are favored, not uncommonly they become dislodged. Aortic valve replacement and graft reconstruction of the ascending aorta have proved successful in the management of aortic regurgitation and congestive heart failure with and without aortic dissection.[320] Recurrent dissection, valvular incompetence, and progressive dilatation of any remaining native aorta have been late complications.[307] Elective prophylactic surgery of a greatly enlarged or enlarging aorta found on serial echocardiography in asymptomatic persons can be carried out at a relatively low risk and may prolong survival.[323]

The increasing recognition of mitral valve involvement in the Marfan syndrome that is morphologically indistinguishable from the mitral valve prolapse syndrome makes antibiotic prophylaxis of infective endocarditis appear to be warranted in these patients (p. 1094).

OSTEOGENESIS IMPERFECTA[324]

Osteogenesis imperfecta is a generalized disorder of connective tissue with major involvement of the bones, teeth, saliva, and inner ear. The disease involves other connective tissue elements as well, including fascia and tendons. The ascending aorta, the aortic valve and its annulus, and the mitral valve apparatus are the cardiovascular structures most commonly affected. The incidence of cardiovascular involvement is unknown but is probably low.

Osteogenesis imperfecta is inherited as an autosomal dominant trait with a wide range of phenotypic expression (Chap. 47). This variability has led to the clinical classifications of osteogenesis imperfecta congenita and tarda. In addition, there is most likely a second disorder presenting as osteogenesis imperfecta congenita inherited as an autosomal recessive.

Osteogenesis imperfecta congenita is characterized by extremely brittle bones and subsequent intrauterine fractures. The soft, membranous skull offers little protection at birth, and intracranial hemorrhage is common. The extremities are short and often bowed. Respiratory difficulty often occurs secondary to rib fractures and flail chest. All bones are poorly calcified, and the sclera is blue. Prolonged survival is rare.

In osteogenesis imperfecta tarda, a wide range of symptoms and signs is seen. In childhood, repeated fractures from trivial trauma are the hallmarks of the disease. Severe osteoporosis, lax ligaments and

tendons, and repeated fractures lead to skeletal deformities, including small stature; bowed, misshapen long bones; and scolioses.

Involvement of the middle ear and petrous bone leads to early deafness. Blue sclera is the ocular hallmark of the disease, although it is not invariably present. The skin is thin and appears atrophic. A qualitative platelet abnormality and abnormal vessels may result in a bleeding diathesis. Although the basic defect in osteogenesis imperfecta is not clearly defined, recent investigations suggest that an abnormal ratio of molecular types of collagen is present. Fibroblasts from some patients synthesize decreased amounts of type I collagen, an important component of the osteoid matrix of bone.[322,323]

PATHOLOGICAL FEATURES. The connective tissues of the aorta, valve leaflets, and mitral apparatus are selectively involved in osteogenesis imperfecta as in Marfan's syndrome and probably for the same reasons.[305,323-326] Changes of cystic medial necrosis are seen in the aorta. The valve leaflets appear acellular, and cystic faults are present, containing metachromatically staining material — changes indistinguishable from myxomatous degeneration. Fenestrated aortic and mitral valve leaflets; ruptured chordae tendineae; and ballooning, torn, and redundant valve leaflets are described. The aorta and its annulus may be dilated, and aneurysms of the sinuses of Valsalva may be present.[325,326]

CLINICAL FEATURES. In adults the clinical features of cardiovascular involvement include aortic regurgitation, most often from dilatation of the aortic root and the annulus. The hemodynamic burden may be progressive, requiring valve replacement. Although cystic medial necrosis of the aorta is seen, aortic dissection has not been reported. Patients may present with sudden congestive heart failure secondary to chordal rupture and mitral regurgitation, or mitral regurgitation of less catastrophic onset may occur. The age at onset is variable and probably reflects the severity of the connective tissue disorder. Two cases of infective endocarditis in osteogenesis imperfecta have been reported.[305,324] Aortic dilatation may be conspicuous by chest roentgenogram without obvious valvular insufficiency.

MANAGEMENT. Management includes routine therapy of congestive heart failure. Successful prosthetic valve replacement is hampered by postoperative bleeding and by poor native connective tissue at the suture sites.[327,328] Prophylaxis for endocarditis appears warranted in clinically recognizable valvular disease.

EHLERS-DANLOS SYNDROME

The Ehlers-Danlos syndrome is a heterogeneous group of disorders of connective tissue that is characterized by hyperelasticity and fragility of the skin; hyperextensibility of the joints; easy bruisability; ocular abnormalities including blue sclera, microcornea, and ectopia lentis; and variable involvement of the respiratory, alimentary, and cardiovascular systems.

Recent biochemical studies have identified distinct abnormalities of collagen synthesis in Ehlers-Danlos syndrome. These findings have included abnormal ratios of collagen types and enzyme deficiencies that affect both normal collagen cross-linking and the conversion of collagen precursor to mature collagen fibers.[322] These studies have supported the clinical impression of distinct phenotypic patterns; seven types are recognized at present. The mode of inheritance is variable.

Histological studies of the cardiovascular lesions of the Ehlers-Danlos syndrome are scarce. Lesions similar to cystic medial necrosis have been described in the aorta in one case.[329] Although many congenital abnormalities of the cardiovascular system have been reported in this syndrome, including tetralogy of Fallot, atrial septal defect, and pulmonary artery and aortic arch anomalies, most authorities believe that these are coincidental and not reflections of the underlying disorder.[305]

CARDIOVASCULAR MANIFESTATIONS. Aortic dissection and spontaneous rupture and dissection of other large arteries with exsanguination are reported in the Ehlers-Danlos syndrome.[330] These episodes may be spontaneous or precipitated by minimal trauma, and significant morbidity secondary to arterial catheterization is reported. Dilatation of the aortic root and sinuses of Valsalva with aortic regurgitation occur.[331] Extensive reviews of patients with Ehlers-Danlos syndrome report various cardiovascular abnormalities, including atrioventricular conduction defects, mitral valve murmurs, nonspecific systolic murmurs, and aortic regurgitation.[332] Some of these findings have been attributed to the deformities of the chest wall found in this disorder.[333] More recently, however, reports of mitral valve murmurs and echocardiographic evidence of prolapse of the mitral valve have suggested widespread involvement of the cardiac connective tissue, and the occurrence of conduction abnormalities in Ehlers-Danlos syndrome has been emphasized. These include right bundle branch block, incomplete right bundle branch block, and left anterior hemiblock alone and with right bundle branch block.[334,335] The histological nature of the valvular and conduction tissue abnormalities remains unknown. Endocarditis prophylaxis in cases of mitral valve involvement is recommended.

PSEUDOXANTHOMA ELASTICUM[305]

Pseudoxanthoma elasticum is an inherited disorder of connective tissue with major involvement of the skin, eyes, and gastrointestinal and cardiovascular systems. The basic defect is thought to be a dysplasia or abiotrophy of elastic tissue. Although originally described as a disorder of the skin and the mesenchymal elements of the eye, involvement of the heart and the peripheral and visceral vasculature is responsible for the more serious manifestations of the disorder, including gastrointestinal hemorrhage, hypertension, congestive heart failure, premature myocardial infarction, peripheral vascular disease, and sudden death.

Pseudoxanthoma elasticum appears to be a heterogeneous group of disorders that Pope has divided into four types according to clinical patterns and modes of inheritance.[336,337] The basic biochemical lesion remains undefined, but in some types autosomal recessive inheritance suggests an enzymatic defect and in others with dominant inheritance, a structural defect.

PATHOLOGICAL FEATURES. Pathological studies of the cardiovascular system are not numerous, but distinctive lesions of the heart, arteries, and arterioles have been described. In the vessels the elastic membrane is often disrupted, and elastic fibers are increased, often shortened, wrinkled, and degenerated, and show an unusual propensity to calcify. Fibrous proliferation of media and intima may severely narrow the lumen.[338] Pathological studies of the heart reveal changes similar to those in the vessels.[339,340] The valve leaflets are also involved, and the cusps may be rolled or thickened; mitral valve prolapse is a common finding.[341] Endocardium of both the ventricle and the atrium is involved. Microscopically, the endocardium ex-

hibits nodular plaques of altered and increased elastic tissue and collagen fibers. Involvement of conducting tissue is also described. Biopsy of the coronary artery has revealed changes indistinguishable from those of peripheral vessels.[342]

CLINICAL FEATURES. Clinically, pseudoxanthoma elasticum is characterized by thickened, coarse, and grooved skin having a leathery and "crepelike" appearance. The skin is lax and redundant with prominent folds. The face, neck, axillae, and inguinal folds are most commonly involved. Mucous membranes of the mouth and stomach may also show changes. The hallmarks of ocular involvement are angioid streaking and chorioretinitis with subsequent visual impairment. Skin changes may be obvious or evident only microscopically, and they usually appear in the second decade. Prominent visceral involvement, however, may occur despite trivial skin changes.

The clinical cardiovascular manifestations of pseudoxanthoma elasticum parallel the pathological changes described. The spectrum includes peripheral vascular disease, hypertension, coronary artery disease, restriction to filling due to subendocardial fibrosis with congestive heart failure, and the clinical manifestations of prolapse of the mitral valve.[341] Symptoms and physical findings appear in the second and third decades.

Intermittent claudication was present in 18 per cent of patients in one large study.[343] A distinctive feature of pseudoxanthoma elasticum is involvement of the arteries of the upper extremities, which distinguishes it from typical atherosclerosis. Physical examination reveals decreased pulses and atrophic changes. The pulse wave is often reduced in amplitude with a slow rise and plateau. Roentgenograms often show calcification of limb arteries.

Both the extraparenchymal and the intraparenchymal renal arteries may be involved in the vasculopathy of pseudoxanthoma elasticum, and the compromised renal blood flow is the most likely cause of the hypertension, often seen in adolescents and young adults.

The incidence of angina is quite variable in large studies of pseudoxanthoma elasticum. In a study of 200 cases, angina was reported in 29 per cent.[343] Acute myocardial infarction and sudden death are not common but are well-documented complications in the second and third decades.[344,345]

Congestive heart failure is an uncommon but recognized manifestation. Murmurs of mitral regurgitation, aortic stenosis, and aortic regurgitation are described.[346] Dilatation of the aorta or its annulus is not a feature of pseudoxanthoma elasticum. The congestive heart failure is probably multifactorial. The hemodynamic burdens imposed by the vascular lesions, combined with the endocardial fibroelastic changes,[345] may be the mechanism of congestive heart failure. However, the role of hypertension and coronary artery disease in cardiac pump function may also be significant. Recently, prolapse of the mitral valve has been described in one type of pseudoxanthoma elasticum.[336]

MANAGEMENT. There is no specific management for the cardiovascular complications of this disorder. Angina, hypertension, and congestive heart failure are managed conventionally. Intractable angina and the Leriche syndrome have been treated with vascular bypass surgery.[342]

HURLER SYNDROME AND OTHER MUCOPOLYSACCHARIDOSES

Hurler syndrome is the prototype of a group of disorders characterized by the abnormal metabolism of mucopolysaccharides. The accumulation of these moieties in mesenchymal cells and their excess urinary excretion serve to identify and classify the disorders. In several forms the enzymatic defect has been identified and the pathogenesis more clearly defined.

Pathological Features. The pathological hallmark of the disease is the presence of Hurler cells, connective tissue cells laden with the mucopolysaccharide moieties heparin sulfate and dermatan sulfate. These cells are found in the connective tissue stroma of many organs. Recently, cells containing intralysosomal collagen fibers have been described in the cardiac valves of patients with Hurler syndrome.[347]

The morphological changes in the heart are striking.[347-350] Grossly, the valves are thickened with fibrous nodules at the closure lines. Aneurysmal dilatations of the leaflets are also seen. The chordae tendineae are also thickened, resembling endocardial fibroelastosis. The cardiac chambers are enlarged. Microscopically, valve thickening is due to the presence of classic Hurler cells, cells with granular inclusions, and an increase in the extracellular collagenous matrix. Increased amounts of collagen and occasional clear cells are responsible for chordal and endocardial thickening. The myocardial cells are relatively spared, but the interstitium may contain Hurler cells. Narrowing of the coronary arteries is seen.

Clinical Features. Patients with classic Hurler syndrome are characterized by dwarfism, corneal clouding, mental retardation, skeletal malformations, hepatosplenomegaly, and cardiovascular lesions. Dermatan sulfate and heparin sulfate are excreted in the urine, and the activity of α-L-iduronidase, a lysosomal hydrolase, is decreased in the fibroblasts of these patients. The condition demonstrates autosomal recessive inheritance and results in early death, most often from respiratory and cardiovascular complications.

Cardiovascular Manifestations.[350-353] Clinically, symptoms of congestive heart failure and ischemic heart disease are most common and are important factors in the poor survival of individuals with Hurler syndrome. In one report 26 of 75 deaths were secondary to congestive heart failure, and 7 additional deaths were sudden. The morphological studies illustrating involvement of conduction tissue suggest arrhythmia as a possible cause of sudden death. Hypertension is also commonly seen, but the cause is unknown. The heart is enlarged on physical examination and chest roentgenogram. Murmurs of mitral regurgitation, aortic stenosis, and aortic regurgitation are often heard. The distorted and thickened mitral valve may produce hemodynamic stenosis. In 15 patients studied by cardiac catheterization,[351] only 1 of whom had clinical congestive heart failure, both systemic and pulmonary hypertension were common. Elevated left ventricular end-diastolic pressures were present in 5 of 9 patients. Angina pectoris occurs in children with Hurler syndrome.

Valvular lesions, thickened, noncompliant endocardium, hypertension, and severely compromised coronary circulation are the features that collectively produce congestive heart failure in Hurler syndrome and its variants. The four mucopolysaccharidoses that involve the cardiovascular system are Hurler syndrome, Hurler-Scheie syndrome, Hunter syndrome, and Morquio syndrome.[351]

Management. Treatment of these disorders with plasma in an effort to replace the deficient or defective enzyme has been reported. There is no specific treatment for the cardiovascular complications of the mucopolysaccharidoses, and early death has underscored the poor response to conventional therapy.

References

RHEUMATIC DISEASES

1. Stollerman, G. H.: Rheumatic Fever and Streptococcal Infection. New York, Grune and Stratton, 1975.
2. Halsey, R. H.: Heart disease in children of school age. J.A.M.A. *77*:672, 1921.
3. Rammelkamp. C. H., Denny, F. W., and Wannamaker, L. W.: Studies on the epidemiology of rheumatic fever in the armed services. *In* Thomas, L. (ed.): Rheumatic Fever. Minneapolis, University of Minnesota Press, 1952, pp. 72–89.
4. Frank, P. F., Stollerman, G. H., and Miller, L. F.: Protection of a military population from rheumatic fever. J.A.M.A. *193*:775, 1965.
5. Gordis, L.: Effectiveness of comprehensive-care programs in preventing rheumatic fever. N. Engl. J. Med. *289*:331, 1973.
6. Miller, R. A., Stamler, J., Smith, J. M., Milne, W. S., Paul, M. H., Abrams, I., Hastreiter, A. R., Restivo, R. M., and DeBoer, L.: The detection of heart disease in children. Results of mass field trials with use of tape-recorded heart sounds. II. The Michigan City study. Circulation *32*:956, 1965.
7. Stamler, J.: Cardiovascular diseases in the United States. Am. J. Cardiol. *10*: 319, 1962.
8. Argarwal, B. L.: Rheumatic heart disease unabated in developing countries. Lancet *2*:910, 1981.
9. Stetson, C. A.: The relation of antibody response to rheumatic fever. *In* McCarty, M. (ed.): Streptococcal Infections. New York, Columbia University Press, 1954, pp. 208–218.
10. Rammelkamp, C. H., Jr.: The Lewis A. Conner Memorial Lecture. Rheumatic heart disease—A challenge. Circulation *17*:842, 1958.
11. Siegel, A. C., Johnson, E. E., and Stollerman, G. H.: Controlled studies of streptococcal pharyngitis in a pediatric population. I. Factors related to the attack rate of rheumatic fever. N. Engl. J. Med. *265*:559, 1961.
12. Stollerman, G. H.: Factors determining the attack rate of rheumatic fever. J.A.M.A. *177*:823, 1961.
13. Stollerman, G. H., Siegel, A. C., and Johnson, E. E.: Variable epidemiology of streptococcal disease and the changing pattern of rheumatic fever. Mod. Concepts Cardiovasc. Dis. *34*:45, 1965.
14. Kaplan, E. L., Top, F. H., Dudding, B. A., and Wannamaker, L. W.: Diagnosis of streptococcal pharyngitis: Differentiation of active infection from the carrier state in the symptomatic child. J. Infect. Dis. *123*:490, 1971.
15. Top, F. H., Wannamaker, L. W., Maxted, W. R., and Anthony, G. V.: M antigens among group A streptococci isolated from skin lesions. J. Exp. Med. *126*:667, 1967.
16. Stollerman, G. H.: Nephritogenic and rheumatogenic group A streptococci. J. Infect. Dis. *120*:258, 1969.
17. Wannamaker, L. W.: Medical progress. Differences between streptococcal infections of the throat and of the skin. N. Engl. J. Med. *282*:23 and 78, 1970.
18. Wannamaker, L. W.: The chain that links the heart to the throat. Circulation *48*:9, 1973.
19. Bisno, A. L., Pearce, I. A., Wall, H. P., Moody, M. D. and Stollerman, G. H.: Contrasting epidemiology of acute rheumatic fever and acute glomerulonephritis. Nature of the antecedent streptococcal infection. N. Engl. J. Med. *283*:561, 1970.
20. Poon-King, T., Mohammed, I., Cox, R., Potter, E. V., Simon, N. M., Siegel, A. C., and Earle, D. P.: Recurrent epidemic nephritis in South Trinidad, N. Engl. J. Med. *277*:728, 1967.
21. Potter, E. V., Svartman, M., Poon-King, T., and Earle, D. P.: The families of patients with acute rheumatic fever or glomerulonephritis in Trinidad. Am. J. Epidemiol. *106*:130, 1977.
22. Widdowson, J.P., Maxted, W. R., Notley, C. M., and Pinney, A. M.: The antibody responses in man to infection with different serotypes of group A streptococci. J. Med. Microbiol. *7*:483, 1974.
23. Bisno, A. L.: The concept of rheumatogenic and nonrheumatogenic group A streptococci. *In* McCarty, M., and Zabriskie, J. B. (eds.): Streptococcal Diseases and the Immune reponse. New York, Academic Press, 1980, p. 789.
24. Stollerman, G. H.: Global changes in group A streptococcal diseases and strategies for their prevension. Adv. Intern. Med. *27*:373, 1982.
25. Stollerman, G. H.: The streptococcus, rheumatic fever and rheumatic heart disease. *In* Shaper, A. G., Hutt, M. S. R., and Fejfar, Z. (eds.): Cardiovascular Disease in the Tropics. London, British Medical Associates, 1974.
26. Sanyal, S. K., Thapar, M. K., Ahmed, S. H., Hooja, V., and Tewari, P.: The initial attack of acute rheumatic fever during childhood in North India. A prospective study of the clinical profile. Circulation *49*:7, 1974.
27. Taranta, A.: Rheumatic fever in children and adolescents. A long-term epidemiologic study of subsequent prophylaxis, streptococcal infections, and clinical sequelae. IV. Relation of the rheumatic fever recurrence rate per streptococcal infection to the titers of streptococcal antibodies. Ann. Intern. Med. *60*(Suppl. 5):47, 1964.
28. Taranta, A., Kleinberg, E., Feinstein, A. R., Wood, H. F., Tursky, E., and Simpson, R.: Rheumatic fever in children and adolescents. A long-term epidemiologic study of subsequent prophylaxis, streptococcal infections, and clinical sequelae. V. Relation of the rheumatic fever recurrence rate per streptococcal infection to pre-existing clinical features of the patients. Ann. Intern. Med. *60* (Suppl. 5):58, 1964.
29. Johnson, E. E., Stollerman, G. H., and Grossman, B. J.: Rheumatic recurrences in patients not receiving continuous prophylaxis. J.A.M.A. *190*:407, 1964.

30. Taranta, A.: Rheumatic fever made difficult. A critical review of pathogenetic theories. Paediatrician 5:74, 1976.

31. Markowitz, M.: Cultures of the respiratory tract in pediatric practice. Am. J. Dis. Child. 105:12, 1963.

32. Rantz, L. A., Boisvert, P. J., and Spink, W. W.: Etiology and pathogenesis of rheumatic fever. Arch. Intern. Med. 76:131, 1945.

33. Zagala, J. G., and Feinstein, A. R.: The preceding illness of acute rheumatic fever. J.A.M.A. 179:863, 1962.

34. Grossman, B. J., and Stamler, J.: Potential preventability of first attacks of acute rheumatic fever in children. J.A.M.A. 183:985, 1963.

35. Rammelkamp, C. H., Jr.: Epidemiology of streptococcal infections. Harvey Lecture Series 51:113, 1955–1956.

36. Stollerman, G. H.: The epidemiology of primary and secondary rheumatic fever. In Uhr, J. W. (ed.): The Streptococcus, Rheumatic Fever and Glomerulonephritis. Baltimore, Williams and Wilkins, 1964, pp. 311–337.

37. Green, C. A.: Researches into aetiology of acute rheumatism; rheumatic carditis. Postmortem investigation of nine consecutive cases. Ann. Rheum. Dis. 1:86, 1939.

38. Collis, W. R. F.: Bacteriology of rheumatic fever. Lancet 2:817, 1939.

39. Watson, R. F., Hirst, G. K., and Lancefield, R. C.: Bacteriological studies of cardiac tissues obtained at autopsy from eleven patients dying with rheumatic fever. Arthr. Rheum. 4:74, 1961.

40. Yoshimoya, S., and Pope, R. M.: Detection of immune complexes in acute rheumatic fever and their relationship to HLA-B5. J. Clin. Invest. 65:136, 1980.

41. Gray, E. D., Wannamaker, L. W., Ayoub, E. M., Kholy, A. E., and Abdin, Z. H.: Cellular immune responses to extracellular streptococcal products in rheumatic heart disease. J. Clin. Invest. 68:665, 1982.

42. Kaplan, M. H., Meyeserian, M., and Kushner, I.: Immunologic studies of heart tissue. IV. Serologic reactions with human heart tissue as revealed by immunofluorescent methods: Isoimmune, Wassermann, and auto-immune reactions. J. Exp. Med. 113:17, 1961.

43. Burgio, G. R., Severi, F., Vaccaro, R., and Rossoni, R.: Antibodies reacting with heart tissue in the course of rheumatic fever in children. Schweiz. Med. Wschr. 96:431, 1966.

44. Hess, E. V., Fink, C. W., Taranta, A., and Ziff, M.: Heart muscle antibodies in rheumatic fever and other diseases. J. Clin. Invest. 43:886, 1964.

45. Ehrenfeld, E. N., Gery, I., and Davies, A. M.: Specific antibodies in heart disease. Lancet 1:1138, 1961.

46. Kaplan, M. H.: Immunologic relation of streptococcal and tissue antigens. I. Properties of an antigen in certain strains of group A streptococci exhibiting an immunologic cross-reaction with human heart tissue. J. Immunol. 90:595, 1963.

47. Kaplan, M. H., and Suchy, M. L.: Immunologic relation of streptococcal and tissue antigens. II. Cross reactions of antisera to mammalian heart tissue with a cell wall constituent of certain strains of group A streptococci. J. Exp. Med. 119:643, 1964.

48. Zabriskie, J. B., and Freimer, E. H.: An immunological relationship between the group A streptococcus and mammalian muscle. J. Exp. Med. 124:661, 1966.

49. Lyampert, I. M., Danilova, T. A., Borodyuk, N. A., and Beletskaya, L. V.: Mechanism of formation of antibodies to heart tissue in immunization with group A streptococci. Folia Biol. 12:108, 1966.

50. Lyampert, I. M., Vvedenskaya, O. I., and Danilova, T. A.: Study on streptococcus group A antigens common with heart tissue elements. Immunology 11:313, 1966.

51. Goldstein, I., Halpern, B., and Robert, L.: Immunological relationship between streptococcus A polysaccharide and the structual glycoproteins of heart valves. Nature 213:44, 1967.

52. Sandson, J., Hammerman, D., Janis, R., and Rojkind, M.: Immunologic and chemical similarities between the streptococcus and human connective tissue. Trans. Assoc. Am. Phys. 81:249, 1968.

53. Bisno, A. L., Wood, J. W., Lawson, J., Roy, S., Beachey, E. H., and Stollerman, G. H.: Antigens in urine of patients with glomerulonephritis and in normal human serum which cross-react with group A streptococci: Identification and partial characterization. J. Lab. Clin. Med. 91:500, 1978.

54. van de Rijn, I., Zabriskie, J. B., and McCarty, M.: Group A streptococcal antigens cross-reactive with myocardium. Purification of heart-reactive antibody and isolation and characterization of the streptococcal antigen. J. Exp. Med. 146:579, 1977.

55. Beachey, E. H., Stollerman, G. H., Chiang, E. Y., Chiang, T. M., Seyer, J. M., and Kang, A. H.: Purification and properties of M protein extracted from group A streptococci with pepsin: Covalent structure of the amino terminal region of type 24 M antigen. J. Exp. Med. 145:1469, 1977.

56. Stollerman, G. H.: Streptococcal vaccines revisited. J. Lab. Clin. Med. 91:872, 1978.

57. Husby, G., van de Rijn, I., Zabriskie, J. B., Abdin, Z. H., and Williams, R. C.: Antibodies reacting with cytoplasm of subthalamic and caudate nuclei neurons in chorea and acute rheumatic fever. J. Exp. Med. 144:1094, 1976.

58. Zabriskie, J. B., Hsu, K. C., and Seegal, B.C.: Heart-reactive antibody associated with rheumatic fever: Characterization and diagnostic significance. Clin. Exp. Immunol. 7:147, 1970.

59. Yang, L. C., Soprey, P. R., Wittner, M. K., and Fox, E. N.: Streptococcal-induced cell-mediated immune destruction of cardiac myofibers in vitro. J. Exp. Med. 146:344, 1977.

60. Beachey, E. H., and Stollerman, G. H.: Mediation of cytotoxic effects of streptococcal M protein by non-type-specific antibody in human sera. J. Clin. Invest. 52:2563, 1973.

61. Zimmerman, R. A., Auernheimer, A. H., and Taranta, A.: Precipitating antibody to group A streptococcal polysaccharide in humans. J. Immunol. 107:832, 1971.

62. Ayoub, E. M., Taranta, A., and Bartley, T. D.: Effect of valvular surgery on antibody to the group A streptococcal carbohydrate. Circulation 50:144, 1974.

63. Taranta, A., Torosdag, S., Metrakos, J., Jegier, W., and Uchida, I.: Rheumatic fever in monozygotic and dizygotic twins. In Proceedings of the Tenth International Congress of Rheumatology. Torino, Minerva Medica, 1961, pp. 96–98.

64. Stollerman, G. H.: Hypersensitivity and antibody responses in streptococcal disease. In Wannamaker, L. W., and Masten, J. M. (eds.): Streptococci and Streptococcal Diseases. Recognition, Understanding, and Management. New York, Academic Press, 1972, pp. 501–513.

65. Kuhns, W. J., and McCarty, M.: Studies of diphtheria antitoxin in rheumatic fever subjects. Analysis of reactions to the Schick test and of antitoxin responses following hyperimmunization with diphtheria toxoid. J. Clin. Invest. 33:759, 1954.

66. Neumann, E.: Die Picrocarminfarbung und ihre Anwendung auf die Entzündungslehre. Arch. Mikr. Anat. (Bonn) 25:130, 1880.

67. Neumann, E.: Zur Kenntnis der fibrinoiden Degeneration des Bindegewebes bei Entzündungen. Virchow Arch. Pathol. Anat. 144:201, 1896.

68. Talalaev, V. T. (Talalajew, W. T.): Der akute Rheumatismus. Klin. Wochenschr. 8:124, 1929.

69. Klinge, F.: Der Rheumatismus. Munich, J. Bergmann, 1933.

70. Aschoff, L.: Zur Myocarditisfrage. Verhandl. Dtsch. Pathol. Ges. 8:46, 1904–1905.

71. Gross, L., and Ehrlich, J. C.: Studies on the myocardial Aschoff body. II. Life cycle, sites of predilection and relation to clinical course of rheumatic fever. Am. J. Pathol. 10:489, 1934.

72. Murphy, G. E.: Nature of rheumatic heart disease with special reference to myocardial disease and heart failure. Medicine 39:289, 1960.

73. Gitlin, D., Craig, J. M., and Janeway, J. A.: Studies on the nature of fibrinoid in the collagen diseases. Am. J. Pathol. 33:55, 1957.

74. Vazquez, J. J., and Dixon, F. J.: Immunohistochemical analysis of lesions associated with "fibrinoid change." Arch. Pathol. 66:504, 1958.

75. Wagner, B. M.: Studies in rheumatic fever. III. Histochemical reactivity of the Aschoff body. Ann. N.Y. Acad. Sci. 86:992, 1960.

76. Aschoff, L.: The rheumatic nodules in the heart. Ann. Rheum. Dis. 1:161, 1939.

77. Sokoloff, L.: The pathogenesis of rheumatic fever. In Mills, L. C., and Mayer, J. H. (eds.): Inflammation and Diseases of Connective Tissue. Philadelphia, W. B. Saunders Co., 1961, p. 135.

78. Pienaar, J. G., and Price, H. M.: Ultrastructure and origin of the Anitschkow cell. Am. J. Pathol. 51:1063, 1967.

79. Kuschner, M., Ferrer, M. I., Harvey, R. M., and Wylie, R. H.: Rheumatic carditis in surgically removed appendages. Am. Heart J. 43:286, 1952.

80. Virmani, R., and Roberts, W. C.: Aschoff bodies in operatively excised atrial appendages and in papillary muscles. Frequency and clinical significance. Circulation 55:559, 1977.

81. Roberts, W. C., and Virmani, R.: Aschoff bodies at necropsy in valvular heart disease. Evidence from an analysis of 543 patients over 14 years of age that rheumatic heart disease, at least anatomically, is a disease of the mitral valve. Circulation 57:803, 1978.

82. Stollerman, G. H., Lynch, W. F., Dolman, M. A., Young, D., and Schwedel, J. B.: Immunologic evidence of streptococcal infection in patients undergoing mitral commissurotomy. Circulation 15:267, 1957.

83. Lanningan, R.: Cardiac Pathology. London, Butterworth and Co., 1966.

84. Coombs, C. F.: The myocardial lesions of the rheumatic infection. Br. Med. J. 2:1513, 1907.

85. Reubner, B.: The relationship between muscle damage and the Aschoff cell in rheumatic carditis. J. Pathol. Bacteriol. 68:101, 1954.

86. Gross, L., and Friedberg, C. K.: Lesions of the cardiac valve rings in rheumatic fever. Am. J. Pathol. 12:469, 1936.

87. Pappenheimer, A. M., and Von Glahn, W. C.: Studies on the pathology of rheumatic fever. Two cases presenting unusual cardiovascular lesions. Am. J. Pathol. 3:583, 1927.

88. Gross, L., Kugel, M. A., and Epstein, E. Z.: Lesions of the coronary arteries and their branches in rheumatic fever. Am. J. Pathol. 11:253, 1935.

89. Bayred, E. D.: Hematologic complications of cardiac surgery. Adv. Intern. Med. 19:57, 1974.

90. Steele, P. P., Weily, H. S., Davies, H., and Genton, E.: Platelet survival in patients with rheumatic heart disease. N. Engl. J. Med. 290:537, 1974.

91. Coombs, C. F.: The microscopic or "submiliary" nodules of active rheumatic carditis. J. Pathol. Bacteriol. 15:489, 1910–1911.

92. Winkelman, N. W., and Eckel, J. L.: The brain in acute rheumatic fever. Nonsuppurative meningoencephalitis rheumatica. Arch. Neurol. Psychiatr. 28:844, 1932.

93. Neubuerger, K. T.: The brain in rheumatic fever. Dis. Nerv. Syst. 8:259, 1947.

94. Costero, I.: Cerebral lesions responsible for death of patients with active rheumatic fever. Arch. Neurol. Psychiatr. 62:48, 1949.

95. Buchanan, D. N.: Pathologic changes in chorea. Am. J. Dis. Child. 62:443, 1941.

96. Kernohan, J. W., Woltman, H. W., and Barnes, A. R.: Involvement of the

nervous system associated with endocarditis. Neuropsychiatric and neuropathologic observations in 42 cases of fatal outcome. Arch. Neurol. Psychiatr. 42:789, 1939.

97. Rammelkamp, C. H., Jr., and Stolzer, B. L.: The latent period before the onset of acute rheumatic fever. Yale J. Biol. Med. 34:386, 1961.

98. Deliee, E. M., Dodge, K. G., and McEwen, C.: The prognostic significance of age at onset in initial attacks of rheumatic fever. Am. Heart J. 26:681, 1943.

99. Feinstein, A. R., and Spagnuolo, M.: The clinical patterns of acute rheumatic fever: A reappraisal. Medicine 41:279, 1962.

100. Pader, E., and Elster, S. K.: Studies of acute rheumatic fever in the adult. I. Clinical and laboratory manifestations in thirty patients. Am. J. Med. 26:424, 1959.

101. Ben-Dov, I., and Berry, E.: Acute rheumatic fever in adults over the age of 45 years: An analysis of 23 patients together with a review of the literature. Semin. Arthritis Rheum. 10:100, 1980.

102. United Kingdom and United States Joint Report on Rheumatic Fever: The treatment of acute rheumatic fever in children. A cooperative clinical trial of ACTH, cortisone and aspirin. Circulation 11:343, 1955.

103. United Kingdom and United States Joint Report on Rheumatic Heart Disease: The evolution of rheumatic heart disease in children. Five-year report of a cooperative clinical trial of ACTH, cortisone and aspirin. Circulation 22:503, 1960.

103a.Bittl, J. A., and Perloff, J. K.: Chronic post-rheumatic fever arthropathy of Jaccoud. Am. Heart J. 105:515, 1983.

104. United Kingdom and United States Joint Report on Rheumatic Heart Disease: The natural history of rheumatic fever and rheumatic heart disease. Ten-year report of a cooperative clinical trial of ACTH, cortisone and aspirin. Circulation 32:457, 1965.

105. Massell, B. V., Fyler, D. C., and Roy, S. B.: The clinical picture of rheumatic fever. Diagnosis, immediate prognosis, course and therapeutic implications. Am. J. Cardiol. 1:436, 1958.

106. Feinstein, A. R., and DiMassa, R.: The unheard diastolic murmur in acute rheumatic fever. N. Engl. J. Med. 260:1331, 1959.

107. Combined Rheumatic Fever Study Group, 1960: A comparison of the effect of prednisone and acetylsalicylic acid on the incidence of residual rheumatic heart disease. N. Engl. J. Med. 262:895, 1960.

108. Combined Rheumatic Fever Study Group, 1965: A comparison of the short-term, intensive prednisone and acetylsalicylic acid therapy in the treatment of acute rheumatic fever. N. Engl. J. Med. 272:63, 1965.

109. Robinson, R. W.: Effect of atropine upon the prolongation of the P-R interval found in acute rheumatic fever and certain vagotonic persons. Am. Heart J. 29:378, 1945.

110. Lenox, C. C., Zuberbuhler, J. R., Park, S. C., Neches, W. H., Mathews, R. A., and Zoltun, R.: Arrhythmias and Stokes-Adams attacks in acute rheumatic fever. Pediatrics 61:599, 1979.

111. Meynet, P.: Rheumatisme articulaire subaigu avec production de tumeurs multiples dans les tissus fibreux periarticulaires et sur le perioste d'un grand numbre d'os. Lyons Med. 19:495, 1875.

112. Cheadle, W. B.: Various Manifestations of the Rheumatic State as Exemplified in Childhood and Early Life. London, Smith, Elder, 1889.

113. Baldwin, J. S., Kerr, J. M., Kuttner, A. G., and Doyle, E. F.: Observations on rheumatic nodules over a 30-year period. J. Pediatr. 56:465, 1960.

114. Burke, J. B.: Erythema marginatum. Arch. Dis. Child. 30:359, 1955.

115. Diamond, E. F., and Tentler, R.: The electroencephalogram in rheumatic fever. J.A.M.A. 182:685, 1962.

116. Lessof, M. H., and Bywaters, E. G. L.: The duration of chorea. Br. Med. J. 1: 1520, 1956.

117. Taranta, A., and Stollerman, G. H.: The relationship of Sydenham's chorea to infection with group A streptococci Am. J. Med. 20:170, 1956.

118. Bland, E. F.: Chorea as a manifestation of rheumatic fever. A long-term perspective. Trans Am. Clin. Climatol. Assoc. 73:209, 1961.

119. Doliopoulos, T.: Abdominal pain in rheumatic fever. Rheumatism 7:42, 1951.

120. Coburn, A. F.: The Factor of Infection in the Rheumatic State. Baltimore, Williams and Wilkins, 1931.

121. Goldring, D., Behrer, M. R., Brown, G., and Elliott, G.: Rheumatic pneumonitis. Part II. Report on the clinical and laboratory findings in twenty-three patients. J. Pediatr. 53:547, 1958.

122. Bisno, A. L., and Stollerman, G. H.: Streptococcal antibodies in the diagnosis of rheumatic fever. In Cohen, A. S. (ed.): Laboratory Diagnostic Procedures in the Rheumatic Diseases. 2nd ed. Boston, Little, Brown and Co., 1974.

123. Rantz, L. A., Randall, E., and Rantz, H. H.: Antistreptolysin "O." A study of this antibody in health and in hemolytic streptococcus respiratory disease in man. Am. J. Med. 5:3, 1948.

124. Wannamaker, L. W.: Streptococcal deoxyribonucleases. In Uhr, J. W. (ed.): The Streptococcus, Rheumatic Fever and Glomerulonephritis. Baltimore, Williams and Wilkins, 1964, pp. 140–165.

125. Bergner-Rabinowitz, S., Ofek, I., Fleiderman, S., Zohar, M., Rabinowitz, K., and Ginsburg, I.: Evaluation of streptozyme and antistreptolysin O tests in streptococcal pyoderma nephritis. Appl. Microbiol. 26:56, 1973.

126. Bisno, A. L., and Ofek, I.: Serologic diagnosis of streptococcal infection. Comparison of a rapid hemagglutination technique with conventional antibody tests. Am. J. Dis. Child. 127:676, 1974.

127. Gewurz, H., Mold, C., Siegel, J., and Fiedel, B.: C-reactive protein and the acute phase response. Adv. Intern. Med. 27:345, 1982.

128. Mauer, A. M.: The early anemia of acute rheumatic fever. Pediatrics 27:707, 1961.

129. Mirowski, M., Rosenstein, B. J., and Markowitz, M.: A comparison of atrioventricular conduction in normal children and in patients with rheumatic fever, glomerulonephritis, and acute febrile illnesses. A quantitative study with determination of the P-R index. Pediatrics 33:334, 1964.

130. Feinstein, A. R., and DiMassa, R.: Prognostic significance of valvular involvement in acute rheumatic fever. N. Engl. J. Med. 260:1001, 1959.

131. Feinstein, A. R., Wood, H. F., Spagnuolo, M., Taranta, A., Jonas, S., Kleinberg, E., and Tursky, E.: Rheumatic fever in children and adolescents. VII. Cardiac changes and sequelae. Ann. Intern. Med. 60(Suppl. 5):87, 1964.

132. Jones, T. D.: The diagnosis of rheumatic fever. J.A.M.A. 126:481, 1944.

133. Jones Criteria (revised) for guidance in the diagnosis of rheumatic fever. Circulation 32:664, 1965.

134. Trentham, D. E., McCravey, J. W., and Masi, A. T.: Low-dose penicillin for gonococcal arthritis. A comparative therapy trial. J.A.M.A. 236:2410, 1976.

135. Stollerman, G. H.: Penicillin-sensitive gonococci and polyarthritis (editorial). J.A.M.A. 236:2433, 1976.

136. Williams, R. C., Jr., and Kunkel, H. C.: Rheumatoid factor, complement and conglutinin aberrations in patients with subacute bacterial endocarditis. J. Clin. Invest. 41:666, 1962.

137. Greenberg, M. S.: Ear lobe histiocytosis as a clue to the diagnosis of subacute bacterial endocarditis. Ann. Intern. Med. 61:124, 1964.

138. Kantor, T. G., and Tanner, M.: Rubella arthritis and rheumatoid arthritis. Arthritis Rheum. 5:378, 1962.

139. Dull, H. B.: Vaccinology and selected virus diseases. Adv. Intern. Med. 17: 143, 1971.

140. Uzsoy, N. K.: The coexistence of rheumatic heart disease and sickle cell anemia. Am. J. Med. Sci. 246:462, 1963.

141. Wiernik, P. H.: Rheumatic heart disease occurring in sickle cell disease and trait. South. Med. J. 61:404, 1968.

142. Mazzara, J. T., Burns, G. C., Mueller, H. S., and Ayres, S. M.: Coexistence of sickle cell anemia and rheumatic heart disease. N.Y. State J. Med. 71:2426, 1971.

143. Calabro, J. J., and Marchesane, J. M.: Juvenile rheumatoid arthritis. N. Engl. J. Med. 277:696, 1967.

144. Silverstein, M. N., and Kelly, P. J.: Bone and joint involvement in acute leukemia. Rheumatism 21:67, 1965.

145. Brodie, H. R., and Marchessault, V.: Acute benign pericarditis caused by Coxsackie virus Group B. N. Engl. J. Med. 262:1278, 1960.

146. Wolff, L., and Wolff, R.: Diseases of the pericardium. Ann. Rev. Med. 16:21, 1965.

147. Keith, J. D.: Congenital mitral insufficiency. Progr. Cardiovasc. Dis. 5:264, 1962.

148. Taranta, A., Spagnuolo, M., and Feinstein, A. R.: "Chronic" rheumatic fever. Ann. Intern. Med. 56:367, 1962.

149. McIntosch, R., and Wood, C. L.: Rheumatic infections occurring in the first three years of life. Am. J. Dis. Child. 49:835, 1935.

150. Rosenthal, A., Czoniczer, G., and Massell, B. F.: Rheumatic fever under three years of age. A report of ten cases. Pediatrics 41:612, 1968.

151. Feinstein, A. R., and Spagnuolo, M.: The duration of activity in acute rheumatic fever. J.A.M.A. 175:1117, 1961.

152. Ellis, L. B.: Recurrent mitral stenosis. Mod. Concepts Cardiovasc. Dis. 33: 851, 1964.

153. Wood, H. F., Simpson, R., Feinstein, A. R., Taranta, A., Tursky, E., and Stollerman, G. H.: Rheumatic fever in children and adolescents. I. Description of the investigative techniques and of the population studied. Ann. Intern. Med. 60(Suppl. 5):6, 1964.

154. Stollerman, G. H.: Prognosis and treatment of acute rheumatic fever: The possible effect of treatment on subsequent cardiac disease. Progr. Cardiovasc. Dis. 3:193, 1960.

155. Chen, S. C., Donahoe, J. R., and Fagan, L. F.: Rheumatic fever in children. A follow-up study with emphasis on cardiac sequelae. Jpn. Heart J. 22:167, 1981.

156. Vaisman, S., Guasch, J., Vignau, A. Correa, E., Schuster, A., Mortimer, E. A., Jr., and Rammelkamp, C. H., Jr.: The failure of penicillin to alter acute rheumatic valvulitis. J.A.M.A. 194:1284, 1965.

157. Stolzer, B. L., Houser, H. B., and Clark, E. J.: Therapeutic agents in rheumatic carditis. Comparative effects of acetylsalicylic acid, corticotropin, and cortisone. Arch. Intern. Med. 95:677, 1955.

158. Czoniczer, G., Amezcua, F., Pelargonio, S., and Massell, B. F.: Therapy of severe rheumatic carditis. Comparison of adrenocortical steroids and aspirin. Circulation 29:813, 1964.

159. Tierney, R. C., and Kaplan, S.: Treatment of Sydenham's chorea. Am. J. Dis. Child. 109:408, 1965.

160. Lockman, L. A.: Movement disorders. In Swaiman, K., and Wright, F. (eds.): Practice of Pediatric Neurology. St. Louis, The C. V. Mosby Co., 1975.

161. Shields, W. D., and Bray, P. F.: A danger of haloperidol therapy in children. J. Pediatr. 88:301, 1976.

162. Massell, B. F., Sturgis, G. P., Knobloch, J. D., Steeper, R. B., Hall, T. N., and Norcross, P.: Prevention of rheumatic fever by prompt penicillin therapy of hemolytic streptococci respiratory infections. J.A.M.A. 146:1469, 1951.

163. Stollerman, G. H., Rusoff, J. H., and Hirschfeld, I.: Prophylaxis against group A streptococci in rheumatic fever. The use of single monthly injections of benzathine penicillin G. N. Engl. J. Med. 252:787, 1955.

164. Albam, B., Epstein, J. A., Feinstein, A. R., Gavrin, J. B., Jonas, S., Kleinberg, E., Simpson, R., Spagnuolo, M., Stollerman, G. H., Taranta, A. Tursky, E., and Wood, H. F.: Rheumatic fever in children and adolescents. A long-term

epidemiologic study of subsequent prophylaxis, streptococcal infections, and clinical sequelae. Ann. Intern. Med. 60(Suppl. 5): No. 2, Part II, 1964.

165. American Heart Association, Committee on Rheumatic Fever and Bacterial Endocarditis: Prevention of rheumatic fever. Circulation 55:1, 1977.

166. Guthe, T., Idsoe, O., and Willcox, R. R.: Untoward penicillin reactions. Bull. WHO 19:427, 1958.

167. Feinstein, A. R., Wood, H. F., Spagnuolo, M., Taranta, A., Tursky, E., and Kleinberg, E.: Oral prophylaxis of recurrent rheumatic fever: Sulfadiazine vs. a double daily dose of penicillin. J.A.M.A. 188:489, 1964.

168. Stahlman, M. T., and Denny, F. W., Jr.: The prophylaxis of streptococcal infection in patients with rheumatic fever: A comparison between sulfadiazine and erythromycin. Am. J. Dis. Child. 98:66, 1959.

169. Wannamaker, L. W., Rammelkamp, C. H., Jr., Denny, F. W., Brink, W. R., Houser, H. B., Hahn, E. O., and Dingle, J. H.: Prophylaxis of acute rheumatic fever by treatment of the preceding streptococcal infection with various amounts of depot penicillin. Am. J. Med. 10:673, 1951.

170. Wannamaker, L. W., Denny, F. W., Perry, W. D., Rammelkamp, C. H., Jr., Eckhardt, G. C., Houser, H. B., and Hahn, E. O.: The effect of penicillin prophylaxis on streptococcal disease rates and the carrier state. N. Engl. J. Med. 249:1, 1953.

171. Bernstein, S. H., Feldman, H. A., Harper, O. F., and Klingensmith, W. H.: Mass oral penicillin prophylaxis in control of streptococcal disease. Arch. Intern. Med. 93:894, 1954.

172. Morris, A. J., and Rammelkamp, C. H., Jr.: Benzathine penicillin G in the prevention of streptococci infections. J.A.M.A. 165:664, 1957.

173. Davis, J., and Schmidt, W. C.: Benzathine penicillin G. Its effectiveness in the prevention of streptococcal infections in a heavily exposed population. N. Engl. J. Med. 256:339, 1957.

174. Beachey, E. H., Stollerman, G. H., Johnson, R. H., et al.: Human immune response to immunization with a structurally defined polypeptide fragment of streptococcal M protein. J. Exp. Med. 150:862, 179.

175. Hasty, D. L., Beachey, E. H., Simpson, W. A., et al.: Hybridoma antibodies against protective and nonprotective antigenic determinants of a structurally defined polypeptide fragment of streptococcal M protein. J. Exp. Med. 155:1010, 1982.

176. Land, M. A., and Bisno, A. L. Acute rheumatic fever. A vanishing disease in suburbia. J.A.M.A. 249:895, 1983.

177. Moll, J. M. H., Haslock, I., Macrae, I. F., and Wright, V.: Associations between ankylosing spondylitis, psoriatic arthritis, Reiter's disease, the intestinal arthropathies, and Behçet's syndrome. Medicine 53:343, 1974.

178. Bluestone, R., and Pearson, C. M.: Ankylosing spondylitis and Reiter's syndrome: Their interrelationships and association with HLA B27. Adv. Intern. Med. 22:1, 1977.

179. Khan, A., and Khan, M. K.: Diagnostic value of HLA-B27 testing in ankylosing spondylitis and Reiter's syndrome. Ann. Intern. Med. 96:70, 1982.

180. Laitinen, O., Leirisalo, M., and Skylv, G.: Relation between HLA-B27 and clinical features in patients with Yersinia arthritis. Arthr. Rheum. 20:1121, 1977.

181. Schachter, J.: Can chlamydial infections cause rheumatic disease? In Dumonde, D. C. (ed.): Infection and Immunology in Rheumatic Diseases. Oxford, Blackwell Scientific Publications, 1976, pp. 151–157.

182. Graham, D. C., and Smythe, H. A.: The carditis and aortitis of ankylosing spondylitis. Bull. Rheum. Dis. 9:171, 1958.

183. Thomas, D., Hill, W., Geddes, R., Sheppard, M., Arnold, J., Fritzsche, J., and Brooks, P. M.: Early detection of aortic dilatation in ankylosing spondylitis using echocardiography. Aut. N.Z.J. Med. 12:10, 1982.

184. Stewart, S. R., Robbins, D. L., and Castles, J. J.: Acute fulminant aortic and mitral insufficiency in ankylosing spondylitis. N. Engl. J. Med. 42:901, 1978.

185. Roberts, W. C., Hollingsworth, J. F., Bulkley, B. H., Jaffe, R. B., Epstein, S. E., and Stinson, E. B.: Combined mitral and aortic regurgitation in ankylosing spondylitis. Angiographic and anatomic features. Am. J. Med. 56:237, 1974.

186. Nitter-Hauge, S., and Otterstad, J. E.: Characteristics of atrioventricular conduction disturbances in ankylosing spondylitis (Mo. Bechterew). Acta Med. Scand. 210:197, 200, 1981.

187. Bulkley, B. H., and Roberts, W. C.: Ankylosing spondylitis and aortic regurgitation. Description of the characteristic cardiovascular lesion from study of eight necropsy patients. Circulation 48:1014, 1973.

188. Takkunen, J., Vuopala, U., and Isomaki, H.: Cardiomyopathy in ankylosing spondylitis. I. Medical history and results of clinical examination in a series of 55 patients. Ann. Clin. Res. 2:106, 1970.

189. Cowan, G. O.: Aortic incompetence associated with ulcerative colitis and ankylosing spondylitis. Proc. Roy. Soc. Med. 63:4, 1970.

190. Good, A. E.: Reiter's disease: A review with special attention to cardiovascular and neurologic sequelae. Semin. Arthr. Rheum. 3:253, 1974.

191. Malette, W. G., Eiseman, B., Danielson, G. K., Mozzoleni, A., and Rams, J. J.: Rheumatoid spondylitis and aortic insufficiency. An operable combination. J. Thorac. Cardiovasc. Surg. 57:471, 1969.

192. Sairanen, E., Paronen, I., and Mahonen, H.: Reiter's syndrome: A follow-up study. Acta Med. Scand. 185:57, 1969.

193. Calin, A., and Fries, I. F.: An experimental epidemic of Reiter's syndrome revisited. Follow-up evidence on genetic and environmental factors. Ann. Intern. Med. 84:564, 1976.

194. Cliff, J. M.: Spinal bony bridging and carditis in Reiter's disease. Ann. Rheum. Dis. 30:171, 1971.

195. Rodnan, G. P., Benedek, T. G., Shaver, J. A., and Fennell, R. H., Jr.: Reiter's syndrome and aortic insufficiency. J.A.M.A. 189:889, 1964.

196. Paulus, H. E., Pearson, C. M., and Pitts, W., Jr.: Aortic insufficiency in five patients with Reiter's syndrome: A detailed clinical and pathological study. Am. J. Med. 53:464, 1972.

197. Collins, P.: Aortic incompetence and active myocarditis in Reiter's disease. Br. J. Vener. Dis. 48:300, 1972.

198. Neu, L. T., Jr., Reider, R. A., and Mack, R. E.: Cardiac involvement in Reiter's disease: Report of a case with review of the literature. Ann. Intern. Med. 53:215, 1960.

199. Arvastson, B., Damgaard, K., and Winblad, S.: Clinical symptoms of infection with Yersinia enterocolitica. Scand. J. Infect. Dis. 3:37, 1971.

200. Ahvonen, P., Sievers, K., and Aho, K.: Arthritis associated with Yersinia enterocolitica infection. Acta Rheum. Scand. 15:232, 1969.

201. Ahvonen, P., Hiisi-Brummer, L., and Aho, K.: Electrocardiographic abnormalities and arthritis in patients with Yersinia enterocolitica infection. Ann. Clin. Res. 3:69, 1971.

202. Aho, K., Ahvonen, P., and Lassus, A.: HLA B27 in reactive arthritis. A study of Yersinia arthritis and Reiter's disease. Arthritis Rheum. 17:521, 1974.

203. Hakansson, U., Eitrem, R., Löw, B., and Winblad, S. W.: HLA-antigen B27 in cases with joint affections in an outbreak in salmonellosis. Scand. J. Infect. Dis. 8:245, 1976.

204. Cruickshank, B.: Heart lesions in rheumatoid disease. J. Pathol. Bacteriol. 76:223, 1958.

205. Lannigan, R.: Cardiac Pathology. London, Butterworth and Co., 1966.

206. Cathcart, E. S., and Spodick, D. H.: Rheumatoid heart disease. A study of the incidence and nature of cardiac lesions in rheumatoid arthritis. N. Engl. J. Med. 266:959, 1962.

207. Bonfiglio, T., and Ativater, E. C.: Heart disease in patients with seropositive rheumatoid arthritis. A controlled autopsy study and review. Arch. Intern. Med. 124:714, 1969.

208. Lebowitz, W. B.: The heart in rheumatoid arthritis (rheumatoid disease). A clinical and pathological study of sixty-two cases. Ann. Intern. Med. 58:102, 1963.

209. Khan, A. H., Spodick, D. H.: Rheumatoid heart disease. Semin. Arthritis Rheum. 1:327, 1972.

210. Butman, S., Espinoza, L. R., Del Carpio, J., and Osterland, C. K.: Rheumatoid pericarditis. Rapid deterioration with evidence of local vasculitis. J.A.M.A. 238:2394, 1977.

211. Liss, J. P., and Bachmann, W. T.: Rheumatoid constrictive pericarditis, treated by pericardiectomy. Report of a case and review of the literature. Arthritis Rheum. 13:869, 1970.

212. Bacon, P. A., and Gibson, D. G.: Cardiac involvement in rheumatoid arthritis. An echocardiographic study. Ann. Rheum. Dis. 33:20, 1974.

213. MacDonald, W. J., Jr., Crawford, M. H., Klippel, J. H., Zvaifler, N. J., and O'Rourke, R. A.: Echocardiographic assessment of cardiac structure and function in patients with rheumatoid arthritis. Am. J. Med. 63:890, 1977.

214. Roberts, W. C., Kehoe, J. A., and Carpenter, D. F.: Cardiac valvular lesions in rheumatoid arthritis. Arch. Intern. Med. 122:141, 1968.

215. Kindred, L. H., Heilbrun, A., and Dunn, M.: Cholesterol pericarditis associated with rheumatoid arthritis. Treatment by pericardiectomy. Am. J. Cardiol. 23:464, 1969.

216. Linch, D. C., Gillmer, D. J., Whimster, W. F., and Keates, J. R. W.: Rheumatoid aortic valve prolapse requiring emergency valve replacement. Br. Heart J. 43:237, 1980.

217. Reed, W. P., and Williams, R. C.: Immune complexes in infectious diseases. Adv. Intern. Med. 22:49, 1977.

218. Oldstone, M. B. A., and Dixon, F. J.: Immune complex disease in chronic viral infections. J. Exp. Med. 134(Suppl.):32S, 1971.

219. Christian, C. L.: Systemic lupus erythematosus and type C RNA viruses (editorial). N. Engl. J. Med. 295:501, 1976.

220. Agnello, V.: Complement deficiency states. Medicine 57:1, 1978.

221. Lee, S. L., and Chase, P. H.: Drug-induced systemic lupus erythematosus: A critical review. Semin. Arthritis Rheum. 5:83, 1975.

222. Stevens, M. B.: Procainamide-induced lupus. Johns Hopkins Med. J. 138:289, 1976.

223. Levo, Y., Pick, A. I., Avidor, I., and Ben-Bassat, M.: Clinicopathological study of a patient with procainamide-induced systemic lupus erythematosus. Ann. Rheum. Dis. 35:181, 1976.

224. Das, S. K., and Cassidy, J. T.: Antiheart antibodies in patients with systemic lupus erythematosus. Am. J. Med. Sci. 265:275, 1973.

225. Klemperer, P., Pollack, A., and Baehr, G.: Pathology of disseminated lupus erythematosus. Arch. Pathol. 32:569, 1941.

225a. Liberthson, R. R., Homcy, C., Fallon, J. T., Gross, S., Leppo, J., and Miller, L.: Systemic lupus erythematosus and heart disease. Primary Cardiol. 9:77, 1983.

226. Gross, L.: Cardiac lesions in Libman-Sacks disease with consideration of its relationship to acute diffuse lupus erythematosus. Am. J. Pathol. 16:375, 1940.

227. Harvey, A. M., Shulman, L. E., Tumulty, P. A., Conley, C. L., and Schoenrich, E. H.: Systemic lupus erythematosus: A review of the literature and clinical analyses of 138 cases. Medicine 33:291, 1954.

228. Hejtmancik, M. R., Wright, J. C., Quint, R., and Jennings, F.: The cardiovascular manifestations of systemic lupus erythematosus. Am. Heart J. 68:119, 1964.

229. Dubois, E. L.: Lupus Erythematosus; A Review of the Current Status of Discoid and Systemic Lupus Erythematosus and Their Variants. 2nd ed. Los Angeles, University of Southern California Press, 1974.

230. Brigden, W., Bywaters, E. G., Lessof, M. H., and Ross, I. P.: The heart in systemic lupus erythematosus. Br. Heart J. 22:1, 1960.

231. Kong, T. Q., Kellum, R. E., and Haserick, J. R.: Clinical diagnosis of cardiac involvement in systemic lupus erythematosus. A correlation of clinical and autopsy findings in thirty patients. Circulation 26:7, 1962.

232. James, T. N., Rupe, C. E., and Monto, R. W.: Pathology of the cardiac conduction system in systemic lupus erythematosus. Ann. Intern. Med. 63: 402, 1965.

233. Ito, K., Yokoyama, N., Hashida, J., Kajiwara, N., and Okada, R.: A case of lupus erythematosus with arrhythmias. A complete morphological study of the conduction system. Jpn. Heart J. 15:92, 1974.

234. Bharati, S., de la Fuente, D. J., Kallen, R. J., Freij, Y., and Lev, M.: Conduction system in systemic lupus erythematosus with atrioventricular block. Am. J. Cardiol. 35:299, 1975.

235. Wray, R., and Iveson, M.: Complete heart block and systemic lupus erythematosus. Br. Heart J. 37:982, 1975.

236. Sunder, S. K., and Shah, A.: Constrictive pericarditis in procainamide-induced lupus erythematosus syndrome. Am. J. Cardiol. 36:960, 1975.

237. Ghose, M. K.: Pericardial tamponade. A presenting manifestation of procainamide-induced lupus erythematosus. Am. J. Med. 58:581, 1975.

238. Elkayam, U., Weiss, S., and Laniado, S.: Pericardial effusion and mitral valve involvement in systemic lupus erythematosus: Echocardiographic study. Ann. Rheum. Dis. 36:349, 1977.

239. Bonfiglio, T. A., Botti, R. E., and Hagstrom, J. W.: Coronary arteritis, occlusion and myocardial infarction due to lupus erythematosus. Am. Heart J. 83: 153, 1972.

240. Benisch, B. M., and Pervez, N.: Coronary artery vasculitis and myocardial infarction with systemic lupus erythematosus. N.Y. State J. Med. 74:873, 1974.

241. Bulkley, B. H., and Roberts, W. C.: The heart in systemic lupus erythematosus and the changes induced in it by corticosteroid therapy: A study of 36 necropsy patients. Am. J. Med. 58:243, 1975.

242. del Rio, A., Vázquez, J. J., Sobrino, J. A., Gil, A., Barbado, J., Maté, I., and Ortiz-Vázquez, J.: Myocardial involvement in systemic lupus erythematosus: A noninvasive study of left ventricular function. Chest 74:414, 1978.

243. Libman, E., and Sacks, B.: A hitherto undescribed form of valvular and mitral endocarditis. Arch. Intern. Med. 33:701, 1924.

244. Rawsthorne, L., Ptacin, M. J., Choi, H., Olinger, G. N., and Bamrah, V. S.: Lupus valvulitis necessitating double valve replacement. Arthritis Rheum. 24: 561, 1981.

245. Paget, S. A., Bulkley, B. H., Grauer, L. E., and Seningen, R.: Mitral valve disease os sytemic lupus erythematosus. A cause of severe congestive heart failure reversed by valve replacement. Am. J. Med. 59:134, 1975.

246. McCue, C. M., Mantakus, M. E., Tingelstad, J. B., and Ruddy, S.: Congenital heart block in newborns of mothers with connective tissue disease. Circulation 56:82, 1977.

247. Doshi, N., Smith, B., and Klionsky, B.: Congenital pericarditis due to maternal lupus erythematosus. J. Pediatr. 96:699, 1980.

248. Maniscalco, B. S., Felner, J. M., McCans, J. L., and Chiapella, J. A.: Echocadiographic abnormalities in systemic lupus erythematosus. Circulation 52(Suppl. 2):211, 1975.

249. Strauer, B. E., Brune, I., Schenk, H., Knoll, D., and Perings, E.: Lupus cardiomyopathy: Cardiac mechanics, hemodynamics, and coronary blood flow in uncomplicated systemic lupus erythematosus. Am. Heart J. 92:715, 1976.

250. Zeek, P. M.: Periarteritis nodosa and other forms of necrotizing angiitis. N. Engl. J. Med. 148:764, 1953.

251. Holsinger, D. R., Osmundsen, P. J., and Edwards, J. E.: The heart in periarteritis nodosa. Circulation 25:610, 1962.

252. Griffith, G. C., and Vural, I. L.: Polyarteritis nodosa: Correlation of clinical and postmortem findings in 17 cases. Circulation 3:481, 1951.

253. Kawasaki, T., Kosaki, F., Okawa, S., Shigematsu, I., and Yanagawa, H.: A new infantile acute febrile mucocutaneous lymph node syndrome (MLNS) prevailing in Japan. Pediatrics 54:271, 1974.

254. Onouchi, Z., Tomizawa, N., Goto, M., Nakata, K., Fukuda, M., and Goto, M.: Cardiac involvement and prognosis in acute mucocutaneous lymph node syndrome. Chest 68:297, 1975.

255. Landing, B. H., and Larson, E. J.: Are infantile periarteritis nodosa with coronary artery involvement and fatal mucocutaneous lymph node syndrome the same? Comparison of 20 patients from North America with patients from Hawaii and Japan. Pediatrics 59:651, 1977.

256. Duffy, J., Lidsky, M. D., Sharp, J. T., Davis, J. S., Person, D. A., Hollinger, F. B., and Kyung-Whan, M.: Polyarthritis, polyarteritis and hepatitis B. Medicine 55:19, 1976.

257. Michalak, T.: Immune complexes of hepatitis B surface antigen in the pathogenesis of periarteritis nodosa. A study of seven necropsy cases. Am. J. Pathol. 90:619, 1978.

258. Doherty, M., and Bradfield, J. W.: Polyarteritis nodosa associated with acute cytomegalovirus infection. Ann. Rheum. Dis. 40:419, 1981.

259. Frayha, R. A.: Trichinosis-related polyarteritis nodosa. Am. J. Med. 71:307, 1981.

260. Cupps, T. R., and Fauci, A. S.: The vasculitis syndromes. Adv. Intern. Med. 27:315, 1982.

261. Novack, S. N., and Pearson, C. M.: Cyclophosphamide therapy in Wegener's granulomatosis. N. Engl. J. Med. 284:938, 1971.

262. Forstot, J. Z., Overlie, P. A., Neufeld, G. K., Harmon, C. E., and Forstot, S. L.: Cardiac complications of Wegener Granulomatosis: A case report of complete heart block and review of the literature. Semin. Arthritis Rheum. 10: 148, 1980.

263. Sams, W. M., Jr., Claman, H. N., and Kohler, P. F.: Human necrotizing vasculitis: Immunoglobulins and complement in vessel walls of cutaneous lesions and normal skin. J. Invest. Derm. 64:441, 1975.

264. Huston, K. A., and Hunder, G. G.: Giant cell (cranial) arteritis: A clinical review. Am. Heart J. 100:99, 1980.

265. Klein, R. G., Hunder, G. G., Stanson, A. W., and Sheps, S. G.: Large artery involvement in giant cell (temporal) arteritis. Ann. Intern. Med. 83:806, 1975.

266. Bacon, P. A., Doherty, S. M., and Zuckerman, A. J.: Hepatitis-B antibody in polymyalgia rheumatica. Lancet 2:476, 1975.

267. Campbell, P. M., and LeRoy, E. C.: Pathogenesis of systemic sclerosis: A vascular hypothesis. Semin. Arthritis Rheum. 4:351, 1975.

268. Masi, A. T., and Rodnan, G. P.: Preliminary criteria for the classification of systemic sclerosis (scleroderma). Bull. Rheum. Dis. 31:1, 1981.

269. Botstein, G. R., and LeRoy, E. C.: Primary heart disease in systemic sclerosis (scleroderma): Advances in clinical and pathologic features, pathogenesis, and new therapeutic approaches. Am. Heart J. 102:913, 1981.

270. Norton, W. L., and Nardo, J. M.: Vascular disease in progressive systemic sclerosis (scleroderma). Ann. Intern. Med. 73:317, 1970.

271. Norton, W. L., Hurd, E. R., Lewis, D. C., and Ziff, M.: Evidence of microvascular injury in scleroderma and systemic lupus erythematosus: Quantitative study of the microvascular bed. J. Lab. Clin. Med. 71:919, 1968.

272. Weiss, S., Stead, E., Warren, J., and Bailey, O.: Scleroderma heart disease. Arch. Intern. Med. 71:749, 1943.

273. Oram, S., and Stokes, W.: The heart in scleroderma. Br. Heart J. 23:243, 1961.

274. Medsger, T. A., Jr., Masi, A. T., Rodnan, G. P., Benedek, T. G., and Robinson, H.: Survival with systemic sclerosis (scleroderma). A life-table analysis of clinical and demographic factors in 309 patients. Ann. Intern. Med. 75:369, 1971.

275. Bulkley, B. H., Ridolfi, R. L., Salyer, W. R., and Hutchins, G.: Myocardial lesions of progressive systemic sclerosis. A cause of cardiac dysfunction. Circulation 53:483, 1976.

276. D'Angelo, W. A., Fries, J. F., Masi, A. T., and Shulman, L. E.: Pathologic observations in systemic sclerosis (scleroderma). A study of 58 autopsy cases and 58 matched controls. Am. J. Med. 46:428, 1969.

277. James T. N.: De subitaneis mortibus. VIII. Coronary arteries and conduction system in scleroderma heart disease. Circulation 50:844, 1974.

278. Roberts, N. K., Cabeen, W. R., Jr., Moss, J., Clements, P. J., and Furst, D. E.: The prevalence of conduction defects and cardiac arrhythmias in progressive systemic sclerosis. Ann. Intern. Med. 94:38, 1981.

279. McWhorter, J. E., and LeRoy, E. C.: Pericardial disease in scleroderma (systemic sclerosis). Am. J. Med. 57:566, 1974.

280. Gladman, D. D., Gordon, D. A., Urowitz, M. B., and Levy, H. L.: Pericardial fluid analysis in scleroderma (systemic sclerosis). Am. J. Med. 60:1064, 1976.

281. Medsger, T. A., Jr., and Masi, A. T.: Survival with scleroderma. II. A life-table analysis of clinical and demographic factors in 358 male U.S. veteran patients. J. Chron. Dis. 26:647, 1973.

282. Gupta, M. P., Zoneraich, S., Zeitlin, W., Zoneraich, O., and D'Angelo, W. A.: Scleroderma heart disease with slow flow velocity in coronary arteries. Chest 67:116, 1975.

283. Ridolfi, R. L., Bulkley, B. H., and Hutchins, G. M.: The cardiac conduction system in progressive systemic sclerosis. Clinical and pathologic features of 35 patients. Am. J. Med. 61:361, 1976.

284. Escudero, A., and McDevitt, E.: The electrocardiogram in scleroderma: Analysis of 60 cases and reviews of the literature. Am. Heart J. 56:846, 1958.

285. Eggebrecht, R. F., and Kleiger, R. E.: Echocardiographic patterns in scleroderma. Chest 71:47, 1977.

286. Smith, J. W., Clements, P. J., Levisman, J., Furst, D., and Ross, M.: Echocardiographic features of progressive systemic sclerosis (PSS). Correlation with hemodynamic and postmortem studies. Am. J. Med. 66:28, 1979.

287. Whitman, H. H., Case, D. B., Laragh, J. H., Christian, C. C., Botstein, G., Marica, H., and Leroy, E. C.: Variable response to oral angiotensin-converting enzyme blocade in hypertensive scleroderma patients. Arthritis Rheum. 25: 241, 1982.

288. Adams, R. D.: The pathological substratum of polymyositis. In Pearson, C. M., and Mostofi, F. K. (eds.): The Striated Muscle. Baltimore, Williams and Wilkins, 1973, p. 292.

289. Bohan, A., and Peter, J. B.: Polymyositis and dermatomyositis. N. Engl. J. Med. 292:344 and 403, 1975.

290. Bohan, A., Peter, J. B., and Bowman, R. L., and Pearson, C. M.: A computer assisted analysis of 153 patients with polymyositis and dermatomyositis. Medicine 56:255, 1977.

291. Bunch, T. W., Tancredi, R. G., and Lie, J. T.: Pulmonary hypertension in polymyositis. Chest 79:105, 1981.

292. Singsen, B., Goldreyer, B., Stanton, R., and Hanson, V.: Childhood polymyositis with cardiac conduction defects. Am. J. Dis. Child. 130:72, 1976.

293. Medsger, T. A., Jr., Robinson, H., and Masi, A. T.: Factors affecting survivorship in polymyositis. A life-table study of 124 patients. Arthritis Rheum. 14: 249, 1971.

294. Norton, W. L., Velayos, E., and Robison, L.: Endothelial inclusions in dermatomyositis. Ann. Rheum. Dis. 29:67, 1970.

295. Barnard, B. G., Rankin, A. M., and Robertson, J. H.: Polymyositis: Report on 3 cases from West Africa. Br. Med. J. 1:1473, 1960.

296. Hill, D. L., and Barrows, H. S.: Identical skeletal and cardiac muscle involvement in a case of fatal polymyositis. Arch. Neurol. 19:545, 1968.

297. Schaumburg, H. H., Melsen, S. L., and Yurchak, P. M.: Heart block in polymyositis. N. Engl. J. Med. 284:480, 1971.

298. Lynch, P. G.: Cardiac involvement in chronic polymyositis. Br. Heart J. 33: 416, 1971.

299. Lightfoot, P. R., Bharati, S., and Lev, M.: Chronic dermatomyositis with intermittent trifascicular block. An electrophysiologic conduction system correlation. Chest 71:413, 1977.

300. Oppenheim, H.: Zur Dermatomyositis. Berlin. Klin. Wochenschr. 36:805, 1899.

301. Sheard, C., Jr.: Dermatomyositis. Arch. Inter. Med. 88:640, 1951.

302. Garcin, R., Lapresle, J., Gruner, J., and Scherrer, J.: Les polymyosites. Rev. Neurol. 92:465, 1955.

303. Oka, M., and Raasakka, T.: Cardiac involvement in polymyositis. Scand J. Rheumatol. 7:203, 1978.

304. Reid, J. M., and Murdoch, R.: Polymyositis and complete heart block. Br. Heart J. 41:628, 1979.

305. McKusick, V. A.: Heritable Disorders of Connective Tissue. 4th ed. St. Louis, The C. V. Mosby Co., 1972.

305a. Pyeritz, R. E., and McKusick, V. A.: Basic defects in the Marfan syndrome. N. Engl. J. Med. 305:1101, 1981.

306. Uitto, J., and Lichtenstein, J. R.: Defects in the biochemistry of collagen in diseases of connective tissue. J. Invest. Dermatol. 66:59, 1976.

307. Roberts, W. C., and Honig, H. S.: The spectrum of cardiovascular disease in the Marfan syndrome: A clinico-morphologic study of 18 necropsy patients and comparison to 151 previously reported necropsy patients. Am. Heart J. 104:115, 1982.

308. Chapman, D. W., Beazley, H. L., Petersen, P. K., et al.: Annulo-aortic ectasia with cystic medial necrosis. Diagnosis and surgical treatment. Am. J. Cardiol. 16:679, 1965.

309. Bowers, D.: Pathogenesis of primary abnormalities of the mitral valve in the Marfan's syndrome. Br. Heart J. 31:679, 1969.

309a. Missri, J. C., and Swett, D. D., Jr.: Marfan syndrome: A review Cardiovasc. Rev. Rep. 3:1645, 1982.

310. James, T. N., Frame, B., and Schatz, I. J.: Pathology of cardiac conduction system in Marfan's syndrome. Arch. Intern. Med. 114:339, 1964.

311. Murdoch, J. L., Walker, B. A., and Halpern, B. I., Kuzma, J. W., and McKusick, V. A.: Life expectancy and causes of death in the Marfan syndrome. N. Engl. J. Med. 286:804, 1972.

312. Phornphutkul, C., Rosenthal, A., and Nadas, A.: Cardiac manifestation of Marfan syndrome in infancy and childhood. Circulation 47:587, 1973.

313. Simpson, J. W., Nora, J. J., and McNamara, D. G.: Marfan syndrome and mitral valve disease: Acute surgical emergencies. Am. Heart J. 77:96, 1969.

314. Nelson, R. M., and Vaughn, C. C.: Double valve replacement in Marfan's syndrome. J. Thorac. Cardiovasc. Surg. 57:732, 1969.

314a. Pyeritz, R. E., and Wappel, M. A.: Mitral valve dysfunction in the Marfan syndrome. Clinical and echocardiographic study of prevalence and natural history. Am. J. Med. 74:797, 1983.

315. Spangler, R. D., Nora, J. J., Lortscher, R. H., Wolfe, R. W., and Okin, J. T.: Echocardiography in Marfan's syndrome. Chest 69:72, 1976.

316. Wunsch, C. M., Steinmetz, E. F., and Fisch, C.: Marfan's syndrome and subacute bacterial endocarditis. Am. J. Cardiol. 15:102, 1965.

317. Dowling, J. N., Lee, W. S., Sacco, R. J., and Ho, H.: Endocarditis caused by Neisseria mucosa in Marfan syndrome. Ann. Intern. Med. 18:641, 1974.

318. Prokop, E. K., Palmer, R. F., and Wheat, M. W., Jr.: Hydrodynamic forces in dissecting aneurysms. In-vitro studies in a Tygon model and in dog aortas. Circ. Res. 27:121, 1970.

319. Halpern, B. L., Char, F., and Murdoch, J. L.: A prospectus on the prevention of aortic rupture in the Marfan syndrome with data on the survivorship without treatment. Johns Hopkins Med. J. 129:123, 1971.

320. Symbas, P. N., Baldwin, B. J., and Silvermin, M. E.: Marfan's syndrome with aneurysms of ascending aorta and aortic regurgitation: Surgical treatment and new histochemical observations. Am. J. Cardiol. 25:483, 1970.

321. Symbas, P. N., Raizner, A. E., and Tyras, D. A.: Aneurysms of all sinuses of Valsalva in patients with Marfan's syndrome: An unusual late complication following replacement of aortic valve and ascending aorta for aortic regurgitation and fusiform aneurysm of ascending aorta. Ann. Surg. 174:902, 1971.

322. Hirst, A. E., and Gore, I.: Marfan's syndrome: A review. Prog. Cardiovasc. Dis. 16:187, 1973.

323. Donaldson, R. M., Olsen, E. G. J., Emanuel, R. W., and Ross, D. N.: Management of cardiovascular complications in Marfan syndrome. Lancet 2:1178, 1980.

324. Remigio, P. A., and Grinvalsky, H. J.: Osteogenesis imperfecta congenita. Association with conspicuous extraskeletal connective tissue dysplasia. Am. J. Dis. Child. 119:524, 1970.

325. Criscitello, M. G., Ronan, J. A., Jr., Besterman, E. M., and Schoenwetter, W.: Cardiovascular abnormalities in osteogenesis imperfecta. Circulation 31:255, 1965.

326. Heppner, R., Babitt, H., Bianchine, J., and Warbasse, R.: Aortic regurgitation and aneurysm of sinus of Valsalva associated with osteogenesis imperfecta. Am. J. Cardiol. 31:654, 1973.

327. Weisinger, B., Glassman, E., Spencer, F., and Bergner, A.: Successful aortic valve replacement for aortic regurgitation associated with osteogenesis imperfecta. Br. Heart J. 37:475, 1975.

328. Wood, S. J., Thomas, J., and Braimbridge, M. V.: Mitral valve disease and open heart surgery in osteogenesis imperfecta tarda. Br. Heart J. 35:103, 1973.

329. Madison, W. M., Bradley, E., and Castillo, A.: Ehlers-Danlos syndrome with cardiac involvement. Am. J. Cardiol. 11:689, 1963.

330. McFarland, W., and Fuller, D.: Mortality in Ehlers-Danlos syndrome due to spontaneous rupture of large arteries. N. Engl. J. Med. 271:1309, 1964.

331. Edmondson, P., Nellen, M., and Ross, D. N.: Aortic valve replacement in a case of Ehlers-Danlos syndrome. Br. Heart J. 42:103, 1979.

332. Cupo, L. N., Pyeritz, R. E., Olson, J. L., McPhee, S. J., Hutchins, G. M., and McKusick, V. A.: Ehlers-Danlos syndrome with abnormal collagen fibrils, sinus of Valsalva aneurysms, myocardial infarction, panacinar emphysema and cerebral heterotopias. Am. J. Med. 72:1051, 1981.

333. Antani, J., and Srinivas, H. V.: Ehlers-Danlos syndrome and cardiovascular abnormalities. Chest 63:214, 1973.

334. Jaffe, A. S., Geltman, E. M., Rodey, G. E., and Vitto, J.: A consistent manifestation of type IV Ehlers-Danlos syndrome. The pathogenetic role of the abnormal production of type III collagen. Circulation 64:121, 1981.

335. Come, P. C., Fortuin, N. J., White, R. K. Jr., and McKusick, V.A.: Echocardiographic assessment of cardiovascular abnormalities in the Marfan syndrome. Comparison with clinical findings and with roentgenographic estimation of aortic root size. Am. J. Med. 74:465, 1983.

336. Pope, F. M.: Two types of autosomal recessive pseudoxanthoma elasticum. Arch. Dermatol. 110:209, 1974.

337. Pope, F. M.: Two types of autosomal dominant pseudoxanthoma elasticum. J. Med. Genet. 11:152, 1974.

338. Mendelsohn, G., Bulkley, B. H., and Hutchins, G. M.: Cardiovascular manifestations of pseudoxanthoma elasticum. Arch. Pathol. Lab. Med. 102:298, 1978.

339. Akhtar, M., and Brody, H.: Elastic tissue in pseudoxanthoma elasticum: Ultrastructural study of endocardial lesions. Arch. Pathol. 99:667, 1975.

340. Huang, S. N., Steel, H. D., and Kumar, G.: Ultrastructural changes of elastic fibers in pseudoxanthoma elasticum: A study of histogenesis. Arch. Pathol. 83:108, 1967.

341. Lebwohl, M. G., Distefano, D., Prioleau, P. G., Uram, M., Yannuzi, L. A., and Fleischmajer, R.: Pseudoxanthoma elasticum and mitral valve prolapse. N. Engl. J. Med. 307:228, 1982.

342. Bete, J., Banas, J., Jr., Moran, J., Pinn, V., and Levine, H. J.: Coronary artery disease in an 18-year-old girl with pseudoxanthoma elasticum: Successful surgical therapy. Am. J. Cardiol. 36:515, 1975.

343. Eddy, D. D., and Farber, E. M.: Pseudoxanthoma elasticum: Internal manifestations. A report of cases and a statistical review of the literature. Arch. Dermatol. 86:729, 1962.

344. Schachner, L., and Young, D.: Pseudoxanthoma elasticum with severe cardiovascular disease in a child. Am. J. Dis. Child. 127:571, 1974.

345. Navarro-Lopez, F., Llorian, A., Ferrer-Roca, O., Betriu, A., and Sanz, G.: Restrictive cardiomyopathy in pseudoxanthoma elasticum. Chest 78:113, 1980.

346. Coffman, J. D., and Sommers, S.: Familial pseudoxanthoma elasticum and valvular heart disease. Circulation 19:242, 1959.

347. Renteria, V. G., and Ferrans, V. J.: Intracellular collagen fibrils in cardiac valves of patients with the Hurler syndrome. Lab. Invest. 34:263, 1976.

348. Renteria, V. G., Ferrans, V. J., and Roberts, W. C.: The heart in the Hurler syndrome: Gross, histologic and ultrastructural observations in five necropsy cases. Am. J. Cardiol. 38:487, 1976.

349. Okada, R., Rosenthal, I. M., Scaravelli, G., and Lev, M.: A histopathologic study of the heart in gargoylism. Arch. Pathol. 84:20, 1967.

350. Krovetz, L. J., Lorincz, A. E., and Schiebler, G. L.: Cardiovascular manifestations of the Hurler syndrome: Hemodynamic and angiocardiographic observations in 15 patients. Circulation 31:132, 1965.

351. Factor, S. M., Biempica, L., and Goldfischer, S.: Coronary intimal sclerosis in Morquio's syndrome. Virchows Arch. 379:1, 1978.

352. Brosius, F. C., III, and Roberts, W. C.: Coronary artery disease in the Hurler syndrome. Qualitative and quantitative analysis of the extent of coronary narrowing at necropsy in six children. Am. J. Cardiol. 47:649, 1981.

353. Johnson, G. L., Vine, D. L., Cottrill, C. M., and Noonan, J. A.: Echocardiographic mitral valve deformity in mucopolysaccharidosis. Pediatrics 67:401, 1981.

49 HEMATOLOGIC-ONCOLOGIC DISORDERS AND HEART DISEASE

by David S. Rosenthal, M.D., Robert I. Handin, M.D., and Eugene Braunwald, M.D.

During the past two decades, the increased frequency of cardiovascular abnormalities in patients with hematologic and neoplastic disorders, as well as of hematologic disorders in patients treated for a variety of cardiovascular diseases, has led to more frequent interaction between these two specialties. Hematologist-oncologists frequently require the consultation of cardiologists for clinical problems ranging from the interpretation of abnormal physical, electrocardiographic, and echocardiographic changes in patients with neoplastic hematologic disorders to advise about the treatment of heart failure, pericardial effusion, or other cardiac complications that are frequent in patients with anemia and hematologic malignancies. Conversely, hematologic complications occur quite frequently in cardiac patients. Blood dyscrasias are rather common complications of cardiac medications, prosthetic heart valves, and cardiovascular surgery. The convergence of interests between these fields inspired an innovative monograph devoted to the hematologic complications of cardiac disorders.[1]

ANEMIA AND CARDIOVASCULAR DISORDERS

Anemia is one of the most common causes of increased cardiac output, sometimes resulting in high output failure. As discussed in Chapter 24, the combination of tissue hypoxia and reduced blood viscosity leads to decreased systemic vascular resistance, which is associated with an increase in cardiac output.[1-3] Acutely induced anemia reduces coronary vascular resistance (Fig. 24–2, p. 810), while chronic anemia enhances the growth of intercoronary collaterals.[4] All signs and symptoms of cardiovascular disease usually disappear when the hemoglobin concentration is restored to normal. The gradual development of anemia may lead to cardiac hypertrophy[3] and in experimental animals has been associated with high catecholamine levels in plasma and urine but decreased levels in myocardial tissue.[5]

CARDIAC SYMPTOMS OF ANEMIA. The symptoms of reduced cardiac reserve, fatigue, exertional dyspnea, and edema depend on the severity of the anemia and the presence of an underlying cardiovascular disorder such as myocardial or valvular heart disease. Castle and Minot[6] showed that severely anemic patients without heart disease have few if any symptoms. When hemoglobin values decline below 7 gm/dl, resting cardiac output increases.[2,7-9] There is general agreement that symptoms depend not only on the severity of the anemia but also on (1) the rapidity with which it develops, (2) the physical activity of the patient, and (3) the coexistence of underlying cardiac or coronary artery pathology. For example, in the presence of coronary artery disease, anemia lowers the threshold for development of angina pectoris, so that patients with mild anemia may have an increased frequency of anginal episodes. The following queries are usually posed by the clinician: (1) At what level does an individual become symptomatic with anemia? (2) Has the anemia developed acutely or chronically? (3) Are the cardiac symptoms due to the anemia alone or secondary to underlying heart disease? (4) Can the murmur and the electrocardiographic changes detected in the anemic patient be distinguished from those due to intrinsic cardiac disease?

If the anemia has developed gradually, patients with less than 7 gm Hb/dl may be able to compensate sufficiently to carry out all but the most strenuous activity. Although uncommon, severe congestive heart failure with pulmonary edema can occur solely on the basis of severe anemia (Hb less than 4 gm/dl in the absence of antecedent heart disease). It may be difficult to distinguish congestive heart failure secondary to chronic anemia from that related to myocardial infiltration with iron, i.e., to hemosiderosis resulting from multiple transfusions (p. 1682). However, the symptoms of reduced cardiac reserve secondary to anemia alone are usually relieved when the anemia is corrected and a normal red cell mass has been restored.

OXYGEN DISSOCIATION AND LEVELS OF 2,3-DIPHOSPHOGLYCERATE IN RED CELLS

To account for the circulatory adaptation that occurs in chronic anemia, it is important to realize that factors other than the hemoglobin concentration and blood flow play a role in the quantity of oxygen delivered to tissues. These include tissue oxygen tension and the position of the hemoglobin-oxygen dissociation curve (Fig. 49–1). Normally, 1 gm of hemoglobin binds 1.34 ml of O_2. With a hemoglobin concentration of 15 gm/dl, 100 ml of arterial blood contains 20 ml of O_2. As can be calculated from the hemoglobin-oxygen dissociation curve (Fig. 49–2), 100 ml of mixed venous blood having a pO_2 of 40 mm Hg will contain 15.5 ml of O_2. The difference, i.e., 4.5 ml of O_2 per 100 ml of arterial blood, would be available for delivery to tissues. If the body depended only upon the cardiac output to sustain oxygen delivery in the anemic state, blood flow would have to double in order to preserve tissue oxygenation when the hemoglobin declined from 15 to 7.5 gm/dl.

However, in most patients with anemia, the hemoglobin-oxygen dissociation curve is shifted to the right and more oxygen is released from hemoglobin as the pO_2 declines. The intracellular concentration of 2,3-diphosphoglycerate (2,3-DPG), which is known to vary in the red cells in a number of disease states,[10,11] profoundly affects the binding and release of oxygen by hemoglobin. Deoxygenated hemoglobin, which is more alkaline than oxyhemoglobin, stimulates increased production of 2,3-DPG, a by-product of glycolysis. As a consequence, the intraerythrocytic ratio of deoxy- to oxyhemoglobin serves as a critical regulator of 2,3-DPG concentration. For example, the decreased oxygen affinity seen in chronic anemia can be accounted for by this increase in red cell 2,3-DPG. As shown in Figure 49–1, at a normal arterial pO_2, arterial oxygen saturation remains high despite the reduction in oxygen affinity. However, at the lower

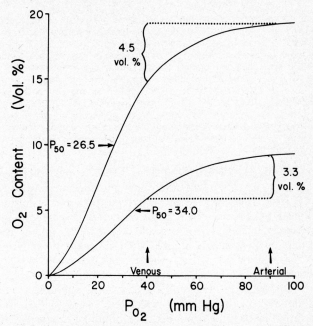

FIGURE 49–2 Enhancement of oxygen unloading by decreased red cell oxygen affinity in anemia with an increase in P_{50} from 26.5 to 34.0 (From Klocke, R. A.: Oxygen transport and 2,3-diphosphoglycerate. Chest 62:795, 1972.)

pO_2 in the venous blood, elevated 2,3-DPG displaces the hemoglobin-oxygen dissociation curve to the right, enabling greater release of oxygen from the cells at any level of pO_2. Oski has calculated that decreased oxygen affinity mediated by increased red cell 2,3-DPG may compensate for up to half the oxygen deficit in anemia.[12] High levels of 2,3-DPG have also been found in subjects exposed to altitude[13] and in patients with pulmonary disease.[14]

The position of the oxygen-hemoglobin dissociation curve can be expressed by the P_{50}, i.e., the partial pressure of O_2 at which hemoglobin is 50 per cent saturated. A reduction of the oxygen affinity of hemoglobin, i.e., a shift to the right of the dissociation curve, is reflected in an elevation of the P_{50}. With a P_{50} of 34 mm Hg (instead of the normal P_{50} of 26.5 mm Hg), 3.3 ml of O_2 is unloaded per 100 ml of blood. As a consequence, an anemic individual with a 50 per cent reduction in red cell mass would suffer only a 27 per cent reduction in oxygen unloading (Fig. 49–2).

Figure 49–3 summarizes the factors responsible for oxygenation and response to hypoxia. Oxygen delivery to the metabolizing tissues depends directly on three principal factors: (1) blood flow, (2) hemo-

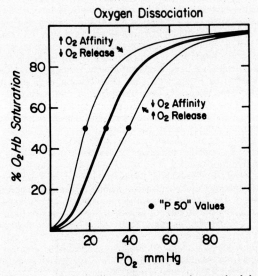

FIGURE 49–1 Oxygen dissociation curve of normal adult blood. P_{50} is the oxygen tension at 50 per cent oxygen saturation (normal = 27 mm Hg). With a shift to the right, oxygen affinity of hemoglobin decreases, releasing additional oxygen at a given tension. With a shift to the left, the opposite occurs. (From Oski, F.: The role of 2,3-DPG and oxygen delivery to tissues. In Jepson, J. H., and Frankl, W. (eds.): Haematological Complications in Cardiac Practice, Philadelphia, W. B. Saunders Co., 1975, p. 79.)

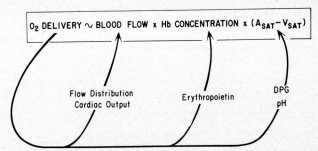

FIGURE 49–3 Oxygen delivery to an organ is directly proportional to (1) blood flow, (2) hemoglobin (Hb) concentration, and (3) the difference in oxygen saturation of the arterial and venous blood ($A_{sat} - V_{sat}$). Patients with various types of hypoxia may compensate in the following ways: (1) the distribution of blood flow may be altered to maintain oxygenation of vital organs; total cardiac output increases when hypoxia is severe; (2) increased erythropoietin production stimulates erythropoiesis; (3) oxygen unloading is enhanced by a shift to the right in the oxygen dissociation curve, mediated by red blood cell pH and 2,3-DPG. (From Bunn, H. F. in Petersdorf, R. L., et al. (eds.): In Harrison's Principles of Internal Medicine. 10th ed., McGraw-Hill Book Co., New York, 1983, p. 285.)

globin concentration (i.e., the oxygen-carrying capacity of the blood, and (3) the oxygen unloading per unit of blood, as represented by the difference between arterial and venous oxygen saturations. Each of these three independent factors is influenced in various ways. Blood flow to any tissue is a function of total cardiac output and its fractional distribution. The red cell mass is regulated by erythropoietin in response to tissue oxygenation. The position of the oxyhemoglobin dissociation curve is determined primarily by red cell 2,3-DPG levels and blood pH. Chronic anemia is usually well tolerated when these compensatory mechanisms operate effectively, i.e., with an increased cardiac output and redistribution of blood flow, as well as decreased oxygen affinity.

CARDIAC EXAMINATION. The cardiac enlargement that develops with severe, chronic anemia usually results from dilatation, eccentric hypertrophy, and a normal ratio of wall thickness to cavity diameter. The precordium is usually hyperactive. Third and fourth heart sounds are frequently present and a midsystolic murmur, maximal at the left sternal border, is usually audible.[15,16] The systolic murmur is probably secondary to the combined effects of increased velocity of blood flow across the pulmonary and aortic valve orifices and reduced blood viscosity. Less frequently, an early and mid-diastolic rumbling murmur may be heard at the apex or along the left sternal border. These diastolic murmurs are probably related to the increased blood flow across the mitral or tricuspid valves and may be difficult to distinguish from the murmurs of mitral or tricuspid stenosis. Accurate diagnosis may require echocardiography or auscultation after correction of the anemia.

Cardiac Disorders Associated with Hemolytic Anemias

The classification of common hemolytic anemias is presented in Table 49–1. This discussion will focus on (1) two of the common hemoglobinopathies, sickle cell anemia and the thalassemic syndromes, which frequently affect the heart; (2) the traumatic hemolytic anemias secondary to valvular heart disease, intracardiac prostheses, and cardiopulmonary bypass; and (3) the immunohemolytic anemias.

TABLE 49–1 CLASSIFICATION OF HEMOLYTIC ANEMIAS

I. **Extrinsic Causes of Hemolysis**
Immunohemolytic Anemias
Idiopathic (primary)
Secondary
Systemic lupus erythematosus
Other immune disorders
Infections: Infectious mononucleosis
Mycoplasma pneumonia
Leukemia
Other tumors
Drugs (see Table 49–10)
Traumatic (Microangiopathic) Hemolytic Anemia
Burns
Disseminated intravascular coagulation
Thrombotic thrombocytopenia purpura
Malignant hypertension
Metastatic carcinoma
Valvular heart disease
II. **Intrinsic Red Cell Abnormalities**
Membrane Disorders
Hereditary spherocytosis
Paroxysmal nocturnal hemoglobinuria
Hemoglobinopathies
Sickle cell anemia and other hemoglobinopathies
Thalassemias
Enzyme Deficiencies
G-6-PD deficiency
Pyruvate kinase deficiency

Hemolytic anemias are usually characterized by marked reticulocytosis and erythroid hyperplasia of the bone marrow. Indirect bilirubinemia, increased serum lactic acid dehydrogenase, and reduced haptoglobin are common findings in all hemolytic anemias. If lysis of red cells occurs within the circulation (intravascular hemolytic anemia), hemoglobinemia and hemoglobinuria may occur and will reflect the severity of hemolysis. Specific laboratory investigations will identify the type of hemolytic anemia, e.g., positive antiglobulin (or Coombs') test in immunohemolytic anemia, increased red cell osmotic fragility in hereditary spherocytosis, and abnormal hemoglobin electrophoresis in sickle cell anemia and the thalassemic syndromes. Acquired hemolytic anemias may occur rather precipitously. The symptoms of acute hemolytic anemia may closely resemble acute blood loss with peripheral vasoconstriction, hypotension, tachycardia, fatigue, lightheadedness, and dyspnea on exertion.

HEMOGLOBINOPATHIES

Sickle Cell Disease. Sickle hemoglobin results from a change in the sixth amino acid of the beta chain from glutamic acid to valine ($\alpha_2\beta_2^{6\ glu\ \rightarrow\ val}$); 8 to 10 per cent of black Americans are heterozygous for this trait. In certain regions of central Africa, the gene frequency is as high as 20 per cent. It is likely that the high frequency of hemoglobin S in these areas of Africa is associated with resistance to or protecti on against falciparum malaria. With decreased oxygen tension, red cells containing hemoglobin S acquire an elongated crescent (sickle) shape. Electron microscopy demonstrates bundles of fibers running parallel to the long axis of the cells.[17] If sickle cells are reoxygenated within a short period of time, they can reform their normal red cell shape. As red cells remain sickled in vivo, however, the membranes become damaged and rigid, resulting eventually in irreversibly sickled cells that may block small blood vessels and have a shortened survival. The continuous formation and destruction of irreversibly sickled cells may contribute to the symptoms of sickle cell disease. Factors that decrease oxygen affinity, such as acidosis and increased red cell 2,3-DPG (Fig. 49–1), lead to deoxygenation of hemoglobin and promote the formation of sickled cells.

The heterozygote is not anemic and rarely has symptoms, except at high altitudes or as a result of marked hypoxia. In contrast, the signs and symptoms of the homozygous state of sickle cell anemia (SS) begin at about six months of age, when the switch from fetal to adult hemoglobin production is completed. Clinical syndromes of sickle cell anemia are related to (1) constitutional manifestations, (2) hemolytic anemia with the occurrence of aplastic crises, and (3) vessel occlusion caused by the sickled cells. The constitutional symptoms include impairment of growth and development and increased tendencies toward infection; the latter is partially attributed to inability of the spleen to clear blood-borne bacteria. The spleen may be massively enlarged in infancy, but with repeated infarction it gradually becomes a small nubbin of fibrous tissue.[18] The anemia may be aggravated if the patient becomes folate-deficient or if infection suppresses erythropoiesis.

The vasoocclusive phenomena, the primary cause of morbidity and mortality, fall into two major classes—painful crises and chronic organ damage.[17,19] The painful crises may occur in any part of the body and can mimic the chest pain of ischemic heart disease, the acute abdomen of appendicitis, or renal colic. Chronic organ damage occurs when there is marked stasis of red cells, particularly in organs in which oxygen uptake is high. Repeated vasoocclusive events may lead to fibrosis and eventually organ failure. The tissues most commonly affected include the retina, renal medulla, cerebral cortex, and bone.

The cardiopulmonary system is frequently involved in sickle cell anemia.[19a] As in other chronic anemias, both cardiac output and oxygen extraction by tissues are increased, and reduced oxygen content of the red cells leads to further sickling. In addition, for any given level of the hematocrit, the auscultatory findings associated with anemia and the elevation of cardiac output are greater for sickle cell anemia[9,20] than for other anemias (Fig. 49–4). The normal left ventricle is able to tolerate the volume overload of chronic, moderately severe anemia for indefinite periods without any deterioration of functional capacity (Chap. 24). When cardiac decompensation occurs in patients with sickle cell anemia or other forms of chronic anemia, it is usually the result of other coexisting complications or the presence of underlying cardiovascular abnormalities. For example, deaths secondary to congestive heart failure occurring in children and young adults with sickle cell anemia are usually precipitated by chronic renal failure, pulmonary thrombosis, or infections.[21,22]

Pulmonary infarction, commonly encountered, is probably due to thrombosis in situ rather than to embolization. Although infrequent, fat and marrow emboli to the lungs have been reported, the latter resulting from necrosis in the marrow caused by sickling in the marrow sinusoids. Patients with sickle cell anemia are unusually susceptible to infection. In addition, damage to the lung caused by repeated vascular insults creates a suitable medium for bacterial growth; as a consequence, pneumonia is a frequent and serious complication. Mortality and morbidity are high in the setting of pneumonia and hypoxia; treatment of these complications must be immediate and vigorous. However, it may be difficult to differentiate pulmonary infection from infarction in patients with sickle cell anemia. Although impairment of pulmonary function in sickle cell anemia is quite common, pulmonary hypertension and cor pulmonale are rarely encountered.[20,23]

Echocardiographic measurements performed in sickle cell patients with cardiac symptoms can document depressed left ventricular performance.[24,25] More oxygen is extracted by the myocardium than by any other tissue, and transmural myocardial infarction due to in situ thrombosis by sickled cells occurs rarely. However, infarction of the papillary muscles of the heart may occur.[26] The papillary muscles are at the terminal portion of the coronary

circulation, where collaterals are very poor and hypoxia is marked.

Almost all patients with sickle cell anemia ultimately develop cardiac enlargement,[27] and at autopsy striking increases in heart weights are found in a majority of patients, despite the absence of other causes such as hypertension or atherosclerosis. Histologic study has suggested that the increased heart weight is secondary to fibrosis, presumably caused by the combination of anemia and papillary muscle infarction. Despite the poor oxygen delivery, the presence of sickle hemoglobin does not increase the incidence of coronary artery disease.[28] In occasional patients who have received multiple blood transfusions, myocardial iron deposition (hemosiderosis) may also contribute to the impairment of cardiac function. However, this complication occurs much less frequently in sickle cell anemia than in homozygous thalassemia.

Biventricular enlargement, systolic and diastolic murmurs, and electrocardiographic changes such as nonspecific ST and T changes, decreased QRS amplitude, and AV conduction disturbance are common and may suggest the presence of congenital or rheumatic valvular heart disease.[1]

A number of other syndromes involve sickle cell hemoglobin(s), including SF, S thalassemia (SThal), SC, and SD. The clinical severity of these other syndromes is variable but may sometimes approach that of SS disease. The order of clinical severity of these syndromes is SS > SD > SThal > SC > SA.[29] This order correlates roughly with in vitro tests of sickling.

Thalassemic Syndromes. The thalassemias are a group of inherited disorders caused by an imbalance in the synthesis of hemoglobin chains, rather than a single amino acid substitution as in sickle cell disease. The two principal types are referred to as α-thalassemia, in which alpha chain synthesis is absent or reduced, and β-thalassemia, in which beta chain synthesis is absent or reduced. The homozygous form of β-thalassemia is also referred to as Cooley's or Mediterranean anemia and is common in individuals of Greek and Italian descent. The α-thalassemias are most common in Oriental individuals. Heterozygous α- and β-thalassemias are also common in American blacks, particularly in association with sickle cell trait. The clinical heterogeneity in the thalassemias is due in part to a variety of molecular lesions that impair synthesis of globin subunits.[17] The net result in both types of thalassemia is decreased production of hemoglobin A and therefore hemoglobin-deficient red cells that are both microcytic and hypochromic. In addition, the red cells are target-shaped and demonstrate basophilic stippling.

The diagnosis of β-thalassemia is confirmed by quantitative hemoglobin electrophoresis in which Hb A is decreased or absent and Hb A_2 and HB F are increased. The anemia in homozygous β-thalassemia results from a combination of hemolysis and ineffective erythropoiesis. Children have a characteristic "chipmunk" appearance due to marked hyperplasia of the marrow in the facial bones and massive hepatosplenomegaly owing to extramedullary hematopoiesis. Occasionally, the expanding marrow extrudes from the ribs, sternum, and vertebrae, forming a mass resembling a lymphoma as seen on chest roentgenogram.

CARDIAC ABNORMALITIES IN THALASSEMIA.
Iron overload leads to cutaneous siderosis and damage to many organs, including the heart.[30-35] Cardiac siderosis is a frequent problem in thalassemia but not in sickle cell anemia. It results from the combination of extravascular hemolysis, frequent transfusion therapy and an inappropriate increase in intestinal iron absorption.[32] As a consequence, cardiac failure and arrhythmias are the most common causes of death in children with Cooley's anemia.[31,33] Although the anemia per se undoubtedly contributes to

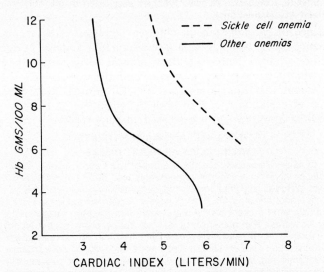

FIGURE 49–4 Relation between hemoglobin concentration and cardiac index at rest in several types of anemia. At any given level of hemoglobin the cardiac index is more elevated in sickle cell anemia (broken line) than in other anemias. (From Varat, M. A., et al.: Cardiovascular effects of anemia. Am. Heart J. *83*:415, 1972.)

the cardiomegaly, iron overload of the heart is the most likely cause of myocardial damage.

Prior to the era of hypertransfusion and chelation therapy, patients with transfusion-dependent, chronic severe refractory thalassemia regularly manifested cardiac involvement, which was the most common cause of death, usually in the second decade of life. Congestive heart failure developed at an average age of 16 years. Death from heart failure occurred often within months. Occasional patients died suddenly, presumably of an arrhythmia. Intensive treatment of heart failure and antiarrhythmic therapy does not appear to have changed the natural history. At postmortem examination widespread iron deposition characteristic of hemochromatosis was found in all viscera, including the heart, which was hypertrophied and sometimes double the normal weight; it was stained a deep brown, with large amounts of iron in myocardial cells, demonstrated by staining with Prussian blue. The sinoatrial node is spared, but the A-V node is frequently involved. Cardiac dysfunction appeared to depend on the quantity of iron deposited in the ventricles. It has been suggested that myocardial damage results from iron-induced release of acid hydrolases from lysosomes.[14]

Pericarditis occurs in about half of all patients with thalassemia and is often recurrent and associated with fever, precordial pain and electrocardiographic changes characteristic of acute pericarditis[30] (p. 1474). Pericardial effusion is common; occasionally creation of a pericardial window is necessary for tamponade or recurrent pericardial effusion.

The electrocardiogram often shows left ventricular hypertrophy, nonspecific ST-T wave abnormalities, supraventricular or ventricular premature contractions, and first- or second-degree A-V block. The His bundle electrogram may show prolongation of the P-H interval, signifying an abnormality of conduction through the A-V node. The chest roentgenogram may show slight to moderate cardiac enlargement. The echocardiogram may disclose enlargement of left ventricular end-diastolic dimensions, left atrial and aortic root dimensions, and increased thickness of the left ventricular wall. A normal or elevated cardiac index with moderate elevations of the left ventricular end-diastolic pressure are the usual findings at cardiac catheterization. The ejection fraction may be reduced and the end-systolic volume increased.

There has been substantial interest in defining abnormalities of cardiac performance non-invasively in asymptomatic patients. Valdes-Cruz et al. have reported that in asymptomatic children with thalassemia major[36] the left ventricular posterior wall thinned more slowly than normal during diastole. Borow et al., utilizing a noninvasively determined index of left ventricular function that relates ventricular fractional shortening to end-systolic pressure (Fig. 14–15, p. 481, and Fig. 14–18, p. 482), identified preclinical left ventricular dysfunction (Fig. 49–5); this approach may be useful in the serial assessment of left ventricular contractility in response to chelation therapy (p. 1684).[37]

Supportive therapy, consisting primarily of an adequate transfusion program and even hypertransfusions, splenectomy, and early treatment of infections, has prolonged the life of patients with thalassemia. Roentgenographic evi-

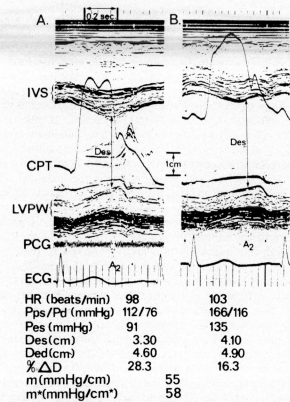

	A	B
HR (beats/min)	98	103
Pps/Pd (mmHg)	112/76	166/116
Pes (mmHg)	91	135
Des(cm)	3.30	4.10
Ded(cm)	4.60	4.90
%ΔD	28.3	16.3
m(mmHg/cm)	55	
m*(mmHg/cm*)	58	

FIGURE 49–5 Recordings from a 16-year old patient with thalassemia major during baseline conditions (A) and at peak methoxamine effect (B). Both the actual and corrected slope values (m and m*) were abnormal despite normal resting fractional shortening (%ΔD). The 44 mm Hg increase in end-systolic pressure (Pes) resulted in a 0.80-cm increase in end-systolic dimension (Des). For the control population, a comparable change in Pes resulted in a 0.40 ± 0.05-cm increase in Des. IVS = interventricular septum; LVPW = left ventricular posterior wall; A_2 = aortic component of the second heart sound; HR = heart rate; Pps = peak systolic pressure; Pd = aortic diastolic pressure; %ΔD = per cent fractional shortening; m = slope; m* = corrected slope. (Reproduced with permission from Borow, K. M., Propper, R., Bierman, F. Z., et al.: The left ventricular end-systolic pressure-dimensions relation in patients with thalassemia major. A new noninvasive method for assessing contractile state. Circulation *66*:980, 1982, by permission of the American Heart Association, Inc.)

dence of cardiomegaly in children regresses with maintenance of the hemoglobin above 10 gm/dl.[35] Indeed, in one study, 4 of 7 patients with significant cardiomegaly had normal heart size one week after multiple transfusions had brought the hemoglobin level to near-normal levels. The use of chelating agents in both the treatment and prevention of iron overload is discussed on page 1684.

HEMOLYTIC ANEMIA IN PATIENTS WITH VALVULAR HEART DISEASE

In 1964, Dameshek described a patient with aortic, mitral, and tricuspid stenosis and mitral regurgitation who had hemolytic anemia with distorted and fragmented red cells, including helmet cells, burr cells, and schistocytes.[38] At autopsy, numerous calcified excrescences were present on the mitral valve and the free margins of the aortic valve. The presence of excess iron deposits in the kidney suggested intravascular hemolysis, but it could not be established whether the cardiac abnormalities were the cause. Subsequently, shortened red cell survival was demonstrated in other patients with aortic valve disease, some of whom had anemia.[39] In patients with rheumatic aortic valve disease, red cell survival may be significantly reduced during periods of exercise.[40] Although this form of hemolytic anemia is probably uncommon, it should be considered in patients with unexplained anemia and valvular heart disease.

Hemolytic Anemia During Cardiac Surgery. In the past, hemolysis frequently occurred as a consequence of extracorporeal circulation. When the blood of many donors must be transfused or is mixed in a pump-oxygenator, as may be the case in patients undergoing cardiac surgery, the question arises whether the samples should be cross-matched with each other as well as with the patient. The plasma of one donor may contain a potent antibody that might interact with cells from a donor who has the antigen specific for that antibody. Although infrequent, this phenomenon may explain some mild-to-moderate hemolysis and hemoglobinemia seen following cardiopulmonary bypass.

With the use of earlier heart-lung machines, red cells became damaged as they passed through the pump oxygenator, presumably as a result of shear forces leading to slight hemolysis and resulting in hemoglobinemia and hemoglobinuria. This problem has been largely obviated with newer machines, which also require little if any blood for priming. As a consequence, hemolytic complications have become far less frequent.[41] In addition, the use of autologous blood and blood aspirated and filtered for re-use during and following operation has been helpful in this regard.[42]

Hemolytic Anemia Following Cardiac Surgery. In 1954, following the surgical implantation of Hufnagel valves in the descending aorta for the treatment of aortic regurgitation, a significant number of patients developed anemia,[43] presumably on a hemolytic basis. When, in dogs, the Hufnagel valve was placed between the left ventricle and the aorta, red cell survival measured by chromium-51 was greatly reduced, and intravascular hemolysis commonly occurred. It was postulated that either red cells were traumatized by being forced between the rigid ball and valve casing or the red cell membrane was damaged, causing antigenic changes that could lead to antierythrocyte antibodies.[44]

The exact nature of the hemolytic anemia associated with intracardiac prostheses was not really appreciated until Sayed et al. noted the development of a chronic and severe hemolytic anemia characterized by microangiopathic red cell changes (consisting of fragmented cells, burr cells, and schistocytes) in a patient following a Teflon patch repair of an ostium primum atrial septal defect (Fig. 49–6).[45] Chromium-51 red cell survival studies confirmed that not only autologous red cells but also donor cells had a short-

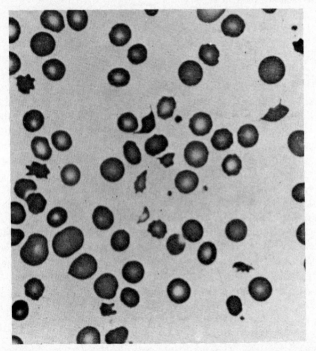

FIGURE 49–6 Peripheral blood smear of patient with microangiopathic hemolytic anemia secondary to abnormal prosthetic valve (× **1000**).

TABLE 49–2 CARDIAC CAUSES OF MICROANGIOPATHIC HEMOLYTIC ANEMIA

Intracardiac and intravascular prostheses
Unsuccessful mitral valvuloplasty
Patch repairs for ostium primum defects
Repair of tetralogy of Fallot
Severe aortic valve disease
Ruptured aneurysms of sinus of Valsalva
Coarctation of aorta
Idiopathic hypertrophic subaortic stenosis

ened half-life, indicating a defect *extrinsic* to the red cell. In keeping with intravascular hemolysis, high concentrations of hemoglobin in the plasma and urine were noted along with hemosiderinuria. At reoperation, the surgeons noted a jet of blood that regurgitated through a cleft in the mitral valve that had been impinging on the prosthetic interatrial Teflon patch. Part of the septum had become denuded of endothelium and had formed a small cul-de-sac in contact with a jet of blood. Repair of the cul-de-sac and re-endothelialization of the area were followed by cessation of the hemolysis. Microangiopathic hemolytic anemia has now been reported with many cardiac defects (Table 49–2).

The incidence of microangiopathic hemolytic anemia following valvular surgery depends on many variables, including the specific operation, the surgical technique, and the tests used to determine hemolysis. The reported incidences vary from 4 per cent to 73 per cent.[46,47] In the latter study, red cell life span was determined in patients with aortic valve disease or valve replacement and the results compared with those in normal subjects. In many instances, diurnal variations occur with greater intravascular hemolysis during physical activity.[48]

The *clinical presentation* may be sudden or gradual. There is usually no associated splenomegaly. Rarely a vicious circle develops in a patient with a paravalvular leak: the resultant shear stress produces hemolytic anemia, which increases stroke volume and stress, which, in turn, intensifies the anemia. While it is agreed that direct mechanical trauma to the red cells is the cause of the hemolysis, the relative contributions of valve closure, denuded endothelium, turbulence, and the development of antierythrocyte autoantibodies is uncertain. Pirofsky et al. described seven patients with hemolytic anemia that developed within two weeks of aortic valve replacement.[49] Six had positive antiglobulin (Coombs') tests; the material that coated the erythrocyte was identified as an erythrocyte autoantibody; therapy with corticosteroids helped to correct the hemolysis in four patients. Although these and other studies raised the possibility of an immune reaction created by the artificial valve, the vast majority of patients have a negative antiglobulin test. It is likely that in some instances the hemolytic anemia observed in the early postoperative period is due simply to multiple transfusions during the operative procedure or to the lymphocyte-splenomegaly syndrome (post–pump-oxygenator syndrome) associated with cytomegaloviral infection.

Turbulence is the most common feature of all hemolytic anemias due to valvular disease and cardiac surgery. For example, following insertion of a prosthetic valve, paravalvular regurgitation will increase the stroke volume and therefore the turbulence through the narrowed orifice. Experiments in vitro have demonstrated that shearing stresses in excess of 3000 dynes/cm² can easily cause hemolysis and that such degrees of stress may readily develop in the presence of defects causing regurgitation from the aorta to the left ventricle.[50] This degree of shearing stress can also be seen in situations in which the lumen of the aortic valve prosthesis is small relative to the stroke volume or where the ball is relatively large for the diameter of the aorta. Although much less common, similar phenomena can occur with prosthetic mitral valves.

The definitive treatment of this hemolytic syndrome consists of surgical repair of the cardiac abnormality, i.e., either replacement or correction of the prosthesis or correction of the paravalvular leak. If a patient is not readily operable, rest will alleviate the condition; iron and folate replacement may be helpful. Treatment with corticosteroids is usually of no benefit.

Hemosiderosis and Hemochromatosis
(see also p. 1425)

A number of disease states are characterized by excessive iron stores in the body. The deposition of significant amounts of iron in the myocardium, liver, and pancreas may lead to varying degrees of dysfunction of these organs.[51] Insofar as the heart is concerned, myocardial deposits of iron may lead to congestive heart failure, conduction disturbances, and arrhythmias. Significant siderosis is most often encountered in patients with idiopathic hemochromatosis or in anemic patients with large and long-standing transfusion requirements.

Patients with *idiopathic hemochromatosis* absorb inappropriately large quantities of iron from the gastrointestinal tract. This inherited disorder with variable clinical expression develops slowly and depends, in part, upon environmental factors, such as the magnitude of dietary intake of iron, the quantity of alcohol intake, and the severity of any underlying liver disease. An association between hemochromatosis and HLA-A3 and HLA-B14 antigens has been described.[52] Prior to the histocompatibility studies, idiopathic hemochromatosis was thought to be autosomal-dominant. HLA subtyping has now suggested a recessive mode of transmission, has linked the disease with chromosome 6, and has helped to distinguish idiopathic hemochromatosis from iron overload secondary to liver disease.[53]

Clinical manifestations of hemochromatosis occur more frequently in men than in women. The disease rarely manifests itself before the age of 20 years and reaches its peak incidence in the fifth decade. Diabetes is the most common initial manifestation, occurring in half the patients. The classic clinical presentation includes increased pigmentation of the skin, hepatomegaly, and cardiac dysfunction. Loss of libido and other endocrinopathies, such as hypopituitarism, may also become apparent. Cellular damage results from iron-induced release of lysosomal acid hydrolases.[54]

The incidence of cardiac symptoms increases with time.[54,55] Dyspnea, edema, and ascites are noted early in the course in 15 to 20 per cent of the patients, but eventually about one third develop symptoms referable to the heart and approximately the same fraction eventually die of cardiac

failure.[55] Arrhythmias are common and include paroxysmal atrial tachycardia and flutter, chronic atrial fibrillation, and frequent premature ventricular contractions; varying degrees of AV block have also been noted. Heart block and arrhythmias are often associated with iron deposits in the AV node[56] and supraventricular arrhythmias with iron deposition in the atria. Low voltage and nonspecific T wave changes are also frequently present.

Radiographic studies in symptomatic patients usually reveal a globular heart with biventricular enlargement and poor pulsations. Some patients may have elevated right ventricular and right atrial pressures[57] consequent to the restrictive cardiomyopathy secondary to iron deposition in the myocardium, as well as involvement of the pericardium itself.

TRANSFUSIONAL HEMOSIDEROSIS. This may become a clinical problem in patients with severe chronic anemia who survive long enough to accumulate toxic quantities of iron from transfused blood. For example, patients with thalassemia major, chronic refractory anemias, myeloid metaplasia, pure red cell aplasia, and aplastic anemia may accumulate 50 gm of iron from transfusions, resulting in a variety of clinical problems similar to those encountered in idiopathic hemochromatosis. Indeed, children with β-thalassemia major maintained on hypertransfusion programs, while spared the cardiac consequences of severe anemia, generally die of heart failure as a consequence of myocardial siderosis in their second decade of life.[31,33] In adults with chronic anemias, cardiac iron deposition secondary to transfusional hemosiderosis, may contribute to cardiovascular disability, which is often inappropriately attributed solely to high-output heart failure. Undoubtedly, the combination of impaired cardiac function secondary to iron deposition and the increased burden on the heart imposed by the persistent, partly treated anemia is responsible.

In a review of 135 hearts studied at autopsy, composed of 4 patients with hemochromatosis and 131 with chronic anemia requiring repeated transfusions, 19 were found to have cardiac iron deposits.[58] Among the patients with leukemia in this series, only 7 per cent lived long enough to develop cardiac iron deposits, whereas 30 per cent of those with refractory anemias who required repeated transfusions did so. Grossly visible iron deposits in the heart were always associated with a prior history of cardiac dysfunction and usually of chronic cardiac failure. The iron deposits were usually most extensive in idiopathic hemochromatosis and in patients who received more than 100 units of blood, without evidence of blood loss. In patients with cardiac hemosiderosis, histological examination revealed that the ventricular free walls and septum contained heavier deposits than did the atrial walls (Fig. 49–7). The quantity of iron in the various layers of the ventricular myocardium is quite variable. The epicardium and the papillary muscles contain the most iron, the subendocardium intermediate, and the midmyocardium and conduction tissue the least.

It is often difficult to determine whether myocardial dysfunction results from the chronic anemia or the presence of myocardial hemosiderosis. With the use of atomic absorption spectrophotometry, the exact concentrations of iron can be determined in various body organs or tissues.

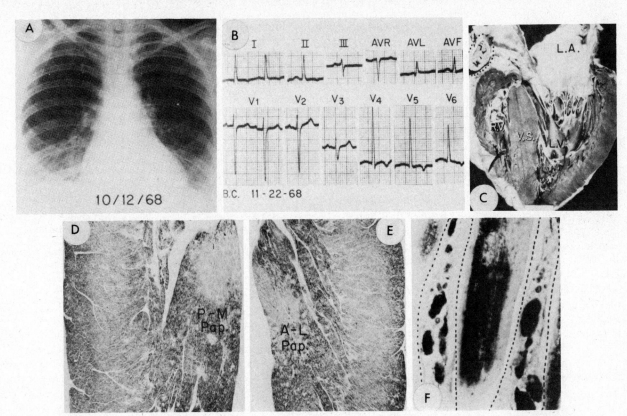

FIGURE 49–7 Observations in a 42-year-old woman with sickle cell anemia who developed congestive heart failure after cumulative transfusions of 260 units of blood. At the time of her death, she had received a total of 359 units of blood (90 gm iron). *A*, Chest roentgenogram two weeks prior to death, showing cardiomegaly. *B*, Ischemic ST and T wave changes can be seen on the electrocardiogram. *C*, At autopsy the walls of the right (R.V.) and left (L.V.) ventricles, left atrium (L.A.), and atrial and ventricular (V.S.) septa were rusty brown owing to extensive iron deposits. The right atrial wall (partially enclosed by dotted line), in contrast, was tan; only minute particles of iron were present on microscopic examination. *D* and *E*, Large areas of replacement fibrosis (pale areas) were present in both left ventricular papillary muscles. *F*, Severely degenerated myocardial fibers (enclosed by dotted lines) that also contained iron deposits were often found adjacent to viable myocardial fibers. (Prussian blue stains.) (From Buja, L. M., and Roberts, W. C.: Iron in the heart. Am. J. Med. *51*:209, 1971.)

Rarely is iron deposition found solely in the heart. Since the liver is easily accessible by biopsy and its iron concentration is closely related to that in the myocardium, liver biopsy appears to be a convenient way of confirming a diagnosis of myocardial siderosis. In some patients, it may be possible by echocardiography to detect early left ventricular dysfunction prior to the development of symptoms.[34,59] In a group of patients with severe β-thalassemia or transfusion-dependent anemias without clinical cardiac symptoms, left ventricular dysfunction measured by radionuclide cineangiography was demonstrated during exercise but not at rest.[59] Noninvasive assessment of the left ventricular end-systolic pressure-dimension relation (using a methoxamine challenge) can identify preclinical left ventricular dysfunction not evident from resting or dynamic exercise studies and not due to chronic anemia per se. This technique may be a very sensitive way of following therapies of iron overload diseases to prevent cardiac complications.

Since the "iron heart is not a strong heart, but a weak one,"[58] and the majority of patients with myocardial siderosis ultimately die of irreversible cardiac failure and arrhythmias, reversal of the iron overload should be attempted. In patients with idiopathic hemochromatosis, it is possible to mobilize iron stores by repeated phlebotomies, and this is the preferred mode of therapy.[60,61] Decrease in hepatic iron stores and fibrosis, improvement of liver function, amelioration of diabetes, and reversal of cardiomyopathy have all occurred. Since the average patient with idiopathic hemochromatosis has 20 to 40 gm of stored iron, a weekly to bimonthly phlebotomy schedule usually has to be continued for two to three years. Initially the hematocrit will drop but will then return toward normal despite repeated phlebotomies. Removal of excess body iron by phlebotomy has been possible even in patients with hematocrits as low as 30 per cent.

The distribution of tissue iron differs somewhat between individuals with idiopathic hematochromatosis and those with transfusion siderosis, who have relatively more iron stored in the reticuloendothelial cells. However, in the latter with repeated transfusions, organ dysfunction does occur in a pattern similar to that in idiopathic hemochromatosis.[62] Phlebotomy is, of course, not a therapeutic alternative in the management of iron overload due to the chronic administration of blood transfusions for the treatment of anemia. Chelation therapy, on the other hand, is the only available approach for the removal of iron in these anemic patients.[63,64]

Desferrioxamine B is the most widely studied iron chelator; this hydroxamic acid compound initially isolated from

Streptomyces has a very high affinity for trivalent iron, with a binding capacity of 9.3 mg of iron per 100 mg. It must be administered parenterally, and most of the chelated iron is excreted in the urine within four hours following injection. Initial studies with intramuscular desferrioxamine were unsuccessful in achieving sustained negative iron balance. However, the addition of oral ascorbic acid doubles iron excretion,[64] and when ascorbic acid loading is combined with the continuous, subcutaneous administration of desferrioxamine, negative iron balance can be achieved in children with thalassemia.[65] However, ascorbate supplementation in patients with iron overload may be hazardous. Clinical cardiotoxicity manifested by fatal congestive heart failure and arrhythmias has been reported in patients treated simultaneously with ascorbic acid and desferrioxamine. Not only does ascorbate make more cellular iron available for chelation, but it also liberates free intracellular iron, which can generate membrane-damaging free oxygen radicals.[66] Although effective chelation can also be achieved in adults with various types of severe transfusional hemosiderosis, it is not clear whether this therapy will reverse the endocrine, hepatic, and myocardial dysfunction.

DISORDERS ASSOCIATED WITH ABNORMAL FLOW DISTRIBUTION OR INCREASED VISCOSITY

As discussed above, oxygen delivery to an organ or tissue is directly proportional to blood flow, hemoglobin concentration, and the difference in oxygen saturation of arterial and venous blood (Fig. 49–3). Anemic patients compensate by increased blood flow, in part due to reduced blood viscosity, and enhance oxygen delivery through elevated levels of red cell 2,3-DPG. In contrast, conditions associated with increased viscosity cause an increase in resistance to flow and a reduction in blood flow. Disorders with increased viscosity and abnormal blood rheology include the erythrocytoses, such as polycythemia vera, and disease states associated with hypergammaglobulinemia, such as multiple myeloma and cryoglobulinema.

Polycythemia

Polycythemia is characterized by an increase in red blood cells as measured by hematocrit, hemoglobin, or red blood cell count.[67] However, the terms *polycythemia* and its synonym, *erythrocytosis*, do not refer to a specific disease entity but to a variety of conditions. As presented in Table 49–3, a distinction is made between absolute and relative polycythemias. The former refers to the conditions in which there is an absolute increase in red cell mass (as measured by ^{51}Cr labeling or other dilution techniques). Absolute polycythemias, in turn, are subclassified as primary or secondary, depending upon whether the elevation in red cell mass is autonomous (primary) or under hormonal (erythropoietin) control. Primary polycythemia, i.e., polycythemia vera, is part of the spectrum of the myeloproliferative disorders. Secondary polycythemia is further classified into those disorders that cause an approp riate increase in erythropoietin secretion (e.g., disorders associ-

TABLE 49–3   CLASSIFICATION OF POLYCYTHEMIAS

I. Absolute Polycythemia
  Primary: Polycythemia vera
  Secondary
    Decreased oxygen transport—appropriate erythropoietin stimulation
    Cyanotic congenital heart disease (R → L shunts)
    Pulmonary arteriovenous fistula
    High altitude
    Impaired ventilation (e.g., chronic obstructive pulmonary disease, pickwickian syndrome)
    Impaired hemoglobin function (e.g., congenital methemoglobinemia, congenital hemoglobinopathy with high oxygen affinity, excessive cigarette smoking [CO-Hb]

    Inappropriate erythropoietin production (unrelated to oxygen transport)
    Malignant tumors: kidney, liver, adrenal, lung
    Benign tumors: uterine fibroids, cerebellar, hemangioma, pheochromocytoma, Cushing's syndrome
    Renal: cysts, hydronephrosis, Bartter's syndrome, transplantation

II. Relative Polycythemia
  Stress (Gaisböck's syndrome), dehydration, diuretic therapy, burns, adrenocortical insufficiency

ated with hypoxia, such as cyanotic forms of congenital heart disease and pulmonary disease) and those in which there is an inappropriate increase in erythropoietin production, as occurs with tumors and a variety of renal diseases. In the relative polycythemias, the red cell mass is normal but plasma volume is decreased, producing elevations of hematocrit, hemoglobin, and red cell count (Fig. 49–8).

Although the symptoms of secondary polycythemia depend on the underlying disease state, they are also usually a consequence of increased blood volume and viscosity; the latter increases exponentially with increases in hematocrit.[68] When flow rate through a capillary tube is determined at various levels of hematocrit, flow decreases as an essentially linear function of hematocrit (Fig. 49–8). The

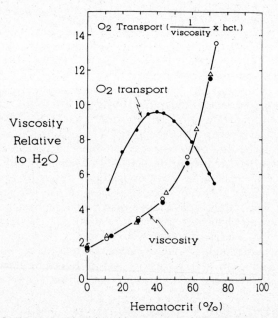

FIGURE 49–8   Viscosity of heparinized normal blood related to hematocrit. Viscosity was measured with an Ostwald viscosimeter at 37° C and expressed in relation to viscosity of water. Oxygen transport was calculated from the product of hematocrit and 1/viscosity and is recorded in arbitrary units. (From Williams, W. J. (ed.): Hematology. 2nd ed. New York, McGraw-Hill Book Co., 1977, p. 256.)

product of flow rate and arterial oxygen content provides a relative measure of the rate of oxygen transport through a single blood vessel; the hematocrit level is optimal just below 40 per cent. Oxygen delivery to the body depends on the product of total blood flow and the oxygen content of arterial blood, which tends to be high in polycythemia vera, in which blood volume, cardiac output, and oxygen content of arterial blood are all elevated, despite the increase in viscosity.

While the increased oxygen content, increased blood volume, and increased cardiac output in polycythemia vera are not required for adequate tissue oxygenation, in the polycythemias secondary to hypoxemia the increased blood oxygen content and increased cardiac output improve oxygen delivery.

Polycythemia Vera.[69] In 1892, Vaquez described a patient with persistent erythrocytosis whom he considered to have had a congenital cardiac lesion, which was subsequently not revealed at autopsy.[70] Osler further delineated the clinical picture as a specific disease,[71] and later Turk associated the findings not with erythrocytosis alone but with a panmyelosis with increased granulocytes and platelets.[72] Although the pathogenesis of polycythemia vera is not understood, it has been classified as a myeloproliferative disorder. All hematopoietic cells are monoclonal by assays of glucose-6-phosphate dehydrogenase (G-6-PD) isozymes,[73] an enzymatic marker that has been used as evidence for the clonal origin of a tumor. In patients who are heterozygous for G-6-PD, normal tissues will possess both isoenzymes A (phenotype: Gd-A) and B (phenotype: Gd-B). The presence of only one isoenzyme in the neoplastic cells of such a patient strongly supports the clonal origin of the neoplasm or, in this case, the disease polycythemia vera. Thus, erythropoietin is not the stimulus for increased red cell production; indeed, erythropoietin concentrations are frequently abnormally low in this condition.

Polycythemia vera is distinguishable from the secondary polycythemias by the various laboratory tests described in Table 49–4. Berlin has suggested a "decision tree" (Fig. 49–9) for the evaluation of patients with an elevated hematocrit, and the Polycythemia Vera Study Group has established the following major and minor criteria for diagnosis:[74]

If the erythrocytosis is accompanied by an increased red cell mass, arterial oxygen saturation less than 92 per cent, and splenomegaly, the diagnosis of polycythemia vera is confirmed. In the absence of splenomegaly, any two of the following laboratory findings satisfy the diagnostic criteria: thrombocytosis, leukocytosis (in the absence of infection), elevated neutrophil alkaline phosphatase activity, or a combination of elevated serum B_{12} concentration and unsaturated B_{12} binding capacity.

Clinical symptoms may be divided into those secondary to the in-

TABLE 49–4 DIFFERENTIATION OF POLYCYTHEMIA VERA AND SECONDARY ERYTHROCYTOSIS

FINDING	POLYCYTHEMIA VERA	SECONDARY POLYCYTHEMIA
Pruritus	Present	Absent
WBC	Increased in 80%	Normal
Platelets	Increased in 50%	Normal
Basophils	Increased	Normal
Splenomegaly	Present in 75%	Absent
Hepatomegaly	Present in 35%	Absent
Serum uric acid	Increased	Increased
Leukocyte alkaline phosphatase activity	Increased in 80%	Normal
Serum B_{12} binding capacity	Increased in 75%	Normal
Serum histamine	Increased	Normal
Bone marrow	Hyperplasia of all elements	Erythroid hyperplasia
Erythropoietin	Normal to decreased	Normal to increased

creased red cell mass and increased blood volume, including headache, plethora, pruritus, dyspnea, and bleeding; those due to increased blood viscosity, including paresthesias and thrombosis; and those due to hypermetabolism, including weight loss despite a good appetite and night sweats. *Angina pectoris, intermittent claudication, and arterial hypertension occur frequently.*

It seems paradoxical that bleeding and thrombosis are both complications of the disease; each occurs in 33 to 50 per cent of patients and they are the major causes of morbidity and mortality. Bleeding is caused by the distention of veins and capillaries by the increased blood volume, by defective platelet function, or both. Thrombosis has been thought to be related to increased blood viscosity, thrombocytosis, and abnormally increased aggregation of platelets. Thrombotic sites include coronary and cerebral arteries as well as those in the extremities. Thrombosis of mesenteric and portal veins also occurs but is less frequent. The operative morbidity in patients with polycythemia vera who are inadequately treated is high. Anesthesia and the stress of operation further increase the likelihood of hemorrhagic and thrombotic events in the immediate postoperative period.

Treatment is aimed primarily at decreasing the potential for both hemorrhage and thrombosis by decreasing viscosity through phlebotomy and by the administration of radioactive phosphorus or chemotherapy to control the proliferation of red cells, white cells, and platelets.

Mechanisms of Symptoms. The clinical severity of polycythemia is usually related to the degree of hypervolemia and increased viscosity.[68,69,75] In older patients with underlying atherosclerotic vascular disease, the cardiac output tends not to be elevated, and, as a consequence of the increased viscosity without increased flow, there

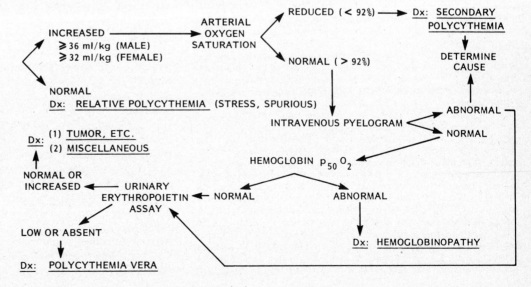

FIGURE 49–9 Decision tree for the evaluation of an elevated hematocrit. (From Berlin, N.: Diagnosis and classification of the polycythemias. Semin. Hematol. *12:*339, 1976.)

may be a higher incidence of ischemic episodes. In vitro studies suggest that white cells can contribute significantly to blood viscosity,[76] and, since leukocytosis is characteristic of polycythemia vera, white cells undoubtedly play a role in the elevated blood viscosity characteristic of this disease.

Cerebral blood flow is significantly reduced and is associated with cerebral symptoms in about half of patients with hematocrits averaging 53.6 per cent, confirming the relationship between cerebral vascular insufficiency and blood viscosity.[77,78] By lowering the hematocrit to 45.5 per cent, viscosity declines by 30 per cent and cerebral blood increases by 73 per cent. With hematocrit values ranging from 46 to 52 per cent, cerebral blood flow is still lower than normal, suggesting that even slight increases in red cell mass may interfere with cerebral perfusion. These studies suggest that patients with polycythemia vera should undergo phlebotomy until hematocrit levels reach the low 40s rather than the previously recommended level of approximately 45 per cent.

Secondary Polycythemias. The secondary polycythemias are logically divided into two subgroups: those in which the increased red cell mass compensates for a reduction in oxygen transport with appropriate stimulation by erythropoietin, and those in which erythrocytosis is associated with an inappropriate increase in erythropoietin production (Table 49–3). It has been suggested that with any hypoxic stimulus the production of an enzyme in the kidney, erythrogenin, becomes stimulated and generates erythropoietin by acting enzymatically on a proposed plasma protein substrate, which may be of hepatic origin.

If an individual living at sea level is transported to a high altitude, a rise in hemoglobin concentration occurs,[79] accompanied by an increase in urinary erythropoietin. Similarly, with severe degrees of chronic hypoxemia in chronic obstructive pulmonary disease, an arterial pO_2 less than 60 mm Hg usually leads to an increase in red cell mass. Although in some instances the hemoglobin has been reported to be as high as 24 gm/dl and the hematocrit as high as 75 per cent, in most patients with polycythemia secondary to chronic obstructive lung disease, the hematocrit does not exceed 57 per cent and the hemoglobin 17 gm/dl.[80] In cyanotic congenital heart disease, red cell mass increases as resting arterial oxygen saturation falls (p. 949). Hematocrits as high as 86 per cent may be seen with red blood cell masses almost three times normal.[81] Plasma volume may be diminished, but total blood volume remains significantly elevated because of the striking elevations of red cell mass. The most common congenital malformations producing these elevations include tetralogy of Fallot, transposition of the great arteries, and persistent truncus arteriosus.

Signs and symptoms of hyperviscosity will generally occur as the hematocrit increases above 60 per cent; cardiac function may be compromised because of both the constant volume load and the augmented vascular resistance secondary to the increased viscosity of the blood. Ruddy cyanosis, headache, dizziness, roaring in the ears, thrombotic episodes, and bleeding are major clinical findings and may be treated with phlebotomy.[82] Careful monitoring during phlebotomy is necessary, and acute reduction of blood volume may have to be overcome by replacement of volume with plasma expanders.[83] Following isovolemic phlebotomy, reducing the hematocrit from the 70s to the 60s, cardiac output rises, and, despite the fall in arterial oxygen content, systemic oxygen transport will usually increase. These favorable changes are attributed to the reduced blood viscosity and vascular resistance. Although the erythrocytosis is a homeostatic mechanism compensating for the chronic arterial hypoxemia, greatly increased hematocrits (with values exceeding 70 per cent) are generally undesirable.

The optimal level of hematocrit for patients with cyanotic congenital heart disease and other chronically hypoxemic states is poorly defined and presents an interesting and perplexing dilemma. The clinical presentation of the patient must be carefully considered. Reduction of cerebral blood flow occurs in secondary erythrocytosis as well as polycythemia vera and improves with phlebotomy.[84,85] If phlebotomy is deemed necessary, close monitoring of the patient's blood pressure, heart rate, arterial oxygen saturation, and general condition is necessary. As might be expected from the decreased oxygen transport associated with right-to-left shunts, the P_{50} and red cell 2,3-DPG are increased, but there is great variability in the relationship between decreased arterial oxygen tension and the rise in P_{50} and red cell 2,3-DPG.[86] Successful surgical correction of the cardiac defect will result in a normalization of the saturation and remove the neces-

sity for the adaptive mechanism; hematocrit and blood volume will return to normal.

In 1966, it first became recognized that a hemoglobin variant with *increased* oxygen affinity could be associated with erythrocytosis.[87] These variants, which generally have amino acid substitutions at structural sites crucial to hemoglobin function, now number over 40. They are transmitted in an autosomal dominant fashion and cause a shift in the oxygen dissociation curve to the left with reduced level of P_{50}. The shift to the left of the oxygen-hemoglobin dissociation curve results in a marked reduction in the oxygen extraction by the tissues. Increased hemoglobin concentration and blood flow are available compensatory mechanisms to maintain oxygen delivery (Fig. 49–3). However, the primary response appears to be erythrocytosis mediated by increases in erythropoietin.[88] Cardiac output is usually normal.[89] Polycythemia constitutes the primary adjustment for oxygen delivery in patients with these hemoglobin variants. They do not have any increased incidence of myocardial ischemia or other forms of organ hypoxia.[90]

True erythrocytosis without demonstrable cause, other than excessive cigar and cigarette smoking, has also been noted in a significant number of individuals.[91] All had elevated levels of carboxyhemoglobin with shifts of the hemoglobin-oxygen dissociation curve to the left, resulting in the stimulation of erythropoiesis. In most cases of polycythemia secondary to inappropriate erythropoietin production, such as tumors, renal cysts, and hydronephrosis, and red cell mass, although increased, does not generally cause symptoms of hyperviscosity.

Relative Polycythemia. Relative polycythemia is a distinct and commonly encountered entity that is also referred to as spurious polycythemia, Gaisböck's syndrome, polycythemia hypertonica, pseudopolycythemia, and stress erythrocytosis. It is not a primary disease process and may be merely a physiological state in which the plasma volume is slightly reduced and the red cell mass slightly increased. The hematocrit rarely exceeds 60 per cent, and other blood constituents are normal. This disorder can be distinguished from polycythemia vera by measurement of red cell mass which, by definition, is normal in relative polycythemia and elevated in polycythemia vera. Patients are often hypertensive, prone to thromboembolic complications,[92] and obese. These complications appear to be unrelated to the hematological changes, and reduction of red cell mass by phlebotomy or chemotherapy is not appropriate. When present, the hypertension and thromboembolic complications should be treated in the usual manner.

NEOPLASTIC DISEASES

Primary tumors of the heart (Chap. 42) are quite rare, occurring at a frequency of 0.0017 to 0.1 per cent of autopsies. Metastatic tumors to the pericardium or heart are far more common, ranging from 1.5 to 20.6 per cent (average 6 per cent) in autopsies on patients with malignant diseases. Metastases usually occur to the pericardium (p. 1507) and myocardium and rarely involve the valves or endocardium; the right side of the heart appears to be affected more frequently than the left.[93,94] Solitary metastases to the heart are rare; co-existence with metastases to other organs is usual. Metastatic nodules in the heart are generally multiple (Figs. 49–10 and 49–11), but they may become diffuse and lead to the manifestations of a restrictive cardiomyopathy (p. 1422). The mode of spread may be by direct extension, as occurs in lung cancer; via the hematogenous route, as in malignant melanoma; or through lymphatic channels, as in lymphoma.

The most common primary tumor producing cardiac metastases is bronchogenic carcinoma (Fig. 49–10), with carcinoma of the breast, malignant melanoma, lymphomas, and leukemias next in order of frequency (Table 49–5).[93–97] At autopsy, 15 to 35 per cent of patients dying with primary lung cancer show cardiac involvement, while over 60 per cent of patients with melanoma will have cardiac metastases.[95] Hematological malignancies, especially lympho-

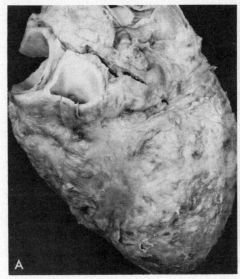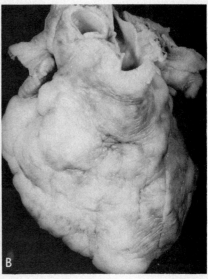

FIGURE 49–10 Metastatic carcinoma of the pericardium in two patients with bronchogenic carcinoma. *A,* The tumor nodules are obscured by fibrinous exudate. *B,* Extensive metastatic nodules. (From Edwards, J. E.: Effects of malignant noncardiac tumors upon the cardiovascular system. *In* Brest, A. N. (ed.): Cardiovascular Clinics. Vol. 4. Philadelphia, F. A. Davis, 1972, p. 282.)

mas, have been reported to account for 15 per cent of all metastases to the heart and pericardium.[96] Of patients dying of malignant lymphomas, approximately 15 per cent have cardiac involvement with tumor.

CLINICAL MANIFESTATIONS. Many metastatic cardiac lesions are clinically silent and are found only at necropsy.[97] For example, despite massive heart involvement with melanoma ("charcoal heart"), there may be little evidence of cardiac dysfunction.[98] The most common clinical manifestations result from pericardial effusion, tachyarrhythmias, AV block,[99] or congestive heart failure. Metastatic cardiac disease is rarely the presenting symptom of the primary tumor. The mode of spread may be by direct extension via the hematogenous route or through lymphatic channels. Routine chest radiographs, nuclide imaging with gallium or thallium, and/or echocardiography are sometimes helpful in diagnosis.[100–103] Osteogenic sarcoma, which may metastasize to the heart, is unique because the metastases contain bone and may be radiographically visible.[104]

In recent years, aggressive chemotherapy and mega-voltage therapy have led to more favorable response rates in patients with various malignancies, such as Hodgkin's disease, non-Hodgkin's lymphoma, testicular tumors, and the leukemias. With the development of high remission rates and apparent cure, i.e., permanent remission in some instances, cardiac toxicity related to both forms of therapy has received significant attention. Anthracyclines and other therapeutic agents may cause a fatal cardiomyopathy (p. 1690), while irradiation of mediastinal structures may lead to pericarditis (p. 1689) and coronary artery obstruction. Cardiac metastases are usually a late phenomenon in most malignancies, but, in view of the prolonged remissions frequently obtained, it has become increasingly important to prevent, detect, and treat these cardiac complications.

Pericardial Involvement (see also p. 1507). The clinical syndromes of cardiovascular involvement in malignancies are listed in Table 49–6. Signs and symptoms of pericarditis with pericardial effusion and cardiac tamponade occur particularly in patients with carcinoma of the lung and breast, as well as in Hodgkin's disease, non-Hodgkin's lymphoma,[105] and the leukemias, particularly acute myelogenous, lymphoblastic leukemia and the blast crisis of chronic myelogenous leukemia.[106] Pericardial involvement is usually diagnosed premortem because of the resultant symptomatology and the radiographic picture. Clinically, the involvement takes the form of either cardiac tamponade or adhesive pericarditis, associated with extensive nodular tumor infiltration of the pericardium.[107] The finding of chylous pericardial effusion is usually characteristic of lymphomatous involvement.[108] Echocardiography is a key tool in the diagnosis of neoplastic involvement of the pericardium. With increased use of serial M-mode echocardiography in patients with advanced malignant disease, the incidence of pericardial effusions appears to be much

FIGURE 49–11 Sections of left ventricle showing metastatic nodules in the myocardium. Tumor was primary in a bronchus. (From Edwards, J. E.: Effects of malignant noncardiac tumors upon the cardiovascular system. *In* Brest, A. N. (ed.): Cardiovascular Clinics. Vol. 4. Philadelphia, F. A. Davis, 1972, p. 282.)

TABLE 49–5 METASTATIC CARDIAC DISEASE

TUMOR TYPE	TOTAL No.	HEART METASTASES	PERICARDIAL METASTASES	HEART AND PERICARDIAL METASTASES
Bronchogenic carcinoma	402	43 (10.2)	66 (15.7)	23 (5.4)
Breast carcinoma	289	24 (8.3)	34 (11.8)	3 (1.4)
Malignant melanoma	59	20 (34.0)	14 (23.7)	12 (20.4)
Colonic carcinoma	214	2 (0.9)	6 (2.8)	0
Esophageal carcinoma	65	5 (7.7)	5 (7.7)	2 (3.6)
Hypernephroma	95	5 (5.3)	0	0
Ovarian carcinoma	115	6 (5.7)	8 (7.0)	3 (2.6)
Prostatic carcinoma	186	5 (2.7)	2 (1.0)	0
Gastric carcinoma	308	11 (3.6)	10 (3.2)	3 (0.9)
Sarcoma*	207	19 (9.2)	19 (9.2)	8 (3.9)
Hodgkin's disease	75	—	11 (14.6)	—
Acute leukemia	420	227 (53.9)	95 (22.4)	—
Total	2,435	367 (15.1)	270 (11.1)	54 (2.2)

*Reticulum cell and lymphosarcoma
Note: Numbers in parentheses represent percentages.
Reproduced with permission from Applefeld, M. M., and Pollock, S. H.: Cardiac disease in patients who have malignancies. Current Problems in Cardiology, Vol. 4. Chicago, Year Book Medical Publishers, 1980, p. 5.

higher than was previously thought.[102] Pericardiocentesis may be necessary to differentiate tumor from radiation effect.[109]

Pericardial tumor or fibrosis secondary to radiation therapy may mimic chronic constrictive pericarditis or chronic effusive pericardial disease and cause problems in differential diagnosis (p. 1509). In patients with carcinoma of the lung, Hodgkin's disease, and non-Hodgkin's lymphoma, radiation-induced pericarditis is common, and it was believed that it could be differentiated from tumor involvement because it occurred usually within a year after irradiation of the chest. It has become clear, however, that radiation-induced pericarditis may occur as late as eight years following therapy.[110] In patients with leukemia, massive involvement of the pericardium and epicardium is a common finding at autopsy;[111,112] the extent of infiltration is usually related to the degree of elevation of circulating white cells. Leukemic infiltration is more common in the acute leukemias and in the blast-crisis phase of chronic myelogenous leukemia.

Vena Caval Obstruction. The superior vena cava syndrome, resulting from tumor obstruction of the superior vena cava, is also a recognized complication of patients with carcinoma of the lung and malignant lymphoma.[113] Enlarged mediastinal nodes or the primary tumor itself may impinge on or even occlude the superior vena cava, causing dyspnea, distention of neck veins, edema of the face and arm, proptosis, headache, and syncope. Because

TABLE 49–6 CLINICAL MANIFESTATIONS OF CARDIAC INVOLVEMENT IN MALIGNANT DISEASE

Pericardial Involvement
  Pericarditis
  Cardiac tamponade
Superior Vena Cava Syndrome
Arrhythmias
  Supraventricular tachycardia
  Carotid sinus syncope
  Atrioventricular block
Cardiomegaly and Congestive Heart Failure
Unexplained Heart Murmur
Unexplained Hypotension
Bacterial and Nonbacterial Endocarditis

of the potential severity and life-threatening nature of this problem, local irradiation therapy may have to be initiated prior to any diagnostic procedure. Similar enlargement of nodes or tumor may cause obstruction of the inferior vena cava with massive leg edema, congestive hepatomegaly, and hypotension.

Electrocardiographic and Roentgenographic Findings. *Arrhythmias* and a wide variety of electrocardiographic changes are common in patients with metastatic disease. While they may certainly be caused by tumor involvement of the heart, they are more commonly due to concomitant factors, such as altered electrolyte concentrations, anemia, and hypoxia. Nonspecific ST-T wave changes, low voltage, and sinus tachycardia are frequent electrocardiographic abnormalities, and they are not diagnostic.[113a] It may be clinically difficult to determine whether any electrocardiographic abnormality is attributable to cardiac metastases or is due to an associated cardiac problem, irradiation, or the cardiotoxic effect of drugs. Indeed, in comparing 137 patients with lymphoma with or without cardiac involvement, an equal incidence of abnormal electrocardiographic findings was noted.[103] Atrial arrhythmias, such as fibrillation and flutter, may occur secondary to neoplastic involvement of autonomic fibers supplying the atria or invasion by tumor of the coronary vessels perfusing the atria with resulting atrial infarction, as well as to neoplastic infiltration of the atrial myocardium or of the sinus node. Similarly, electrocardiographic changes of acute myocardial infarction can be produced by tumor infiltration or hemorrhage into the ventricle or occlusion of one of the coronary arteries. Occasionally, the exact area of tumor involvement may be pinpointed by the acute electrocardiographic changes. Involvement of the AV node is a rare cause of complete heart block but may be the presenting symptom of the tumor.[114] In addition, tumor involvement of cervical lymph nodes without mediastinal involvement has been associated with carotid sinus syncope.[115]

Roentgenographic evidence of cardiac enlargement and the development of congestive heart failure may be the only clinical signs of cardiac involvement in some patients with malignant involvement of the heart. Unexplained pan-

or late-systolic murmurs may occur with intraluminal invasion or external compression of the carotid or pulmonary arteries by the tumor.[116] In addition to coincidental atherosclerosis, coronary artery disease in cancer patients can be caused by tumor emboli, by extrinsic compression of the coronary arteries or ostia, or by thromboemboli brought about by tumor-associated coagulation disorders.

In a study of 816 patients with solid tumors, 33 (4 per cent) died of *myocardial infarction*.[117] Patients with carcinoma of the lung, malignant lymphoma, and leukemia were most commonly afflicted; less affected were patients with cancer of the breast and gastrointestinal tract and malignant melanoma.[118] The most common cause of tumor-related myocardial infarction is extrinsic compression of a coronary artery, occurring in 60 per cent, whereas tumor emboli are responsible for about 35 per cent. Widespread thromboses, including coronary artery thromboses as a result of disseminated intravascular coagulation, occasionally occur in patients with metastatic tumors, most commonly mucin-secreting adenocarcinomas. Half of all patients with acute myocardial infarction secondary to malignant disease had a history of typical chest pain prior to death. The occurrence of acute myocardial infarction in a patient with advanced malignant disease is a particularly poor prognostic sign, with more than two thirds of the patients dying within three weeks of the event. In general, however, the etiology of coronary artery disease in patients with cancer is most likely coincidental spontaneous atherosclerosis.[119]

Nonbacterial Thrombotic Endocarditis. *Nonbacterial endocarditis* occurs with various forms of malignant disease, especially adenocarcinoma, leukemia, and lymphoma, and may be diagnosed only at autopsy.[120] The incidence in adult deaths is at least 1.6 per cent and the pathogenesis unclear. Nonbacterial thrombotic endocarditis is most frequently associated with Hodgkin's disease, carcinoma of the pancreas, stomach, colon, and lung, and the rare condition of acute eosinophilic leukemia. There is evidence that immune complexes, elicited by the underlying malignant process, play an important role in the pathogenesis of thrombus formation in nonbacterial thrombotic endocarditis.[121] The exact relationship between the latter and endomyocardial fibrosis is unclear, but there is a high level of association between eosinophilia in the bone marrow and peripheral blood and the occurrence of endomyocardial fibrosis,[122] which may cause restrictive cardiomyopathy (p. 1422). Ever since Loffler described the entity "endocarditis perietalis fibroplastica" with eosinophilia, this association has been interesting but unclear. In some patients, the cardiac manifestations predominate, most commonly cardiomegaly, congestive heart failure, arrhythmias, and heart murmurs, whereas in others all the symptoms are secondary to the leukemia. Pathologically, these syndromes are characterized by local or widespread eosinophilic infiltrates with fibrous scarring and thickening of the endocardium, including the atrioventricular valves. The pathogenesis of this disorder is poorly understood, but similar clinical pathological features are seen with tropical infestations such as filariasis, status asthmaticus, polyarteritis nodosa, and antituberculosis chemotherapy, all conditions associated with eosinophilia. Many cases may have a chronic and insidious course, but death is usually the direct result of cardiac involvement.[123]

CARDIAC EFFECTS OF RADIATION THERAPY AND CHEMOTHERAPY

With the advent of intensive radiation therapy and aggressive chemotherapy, cardiac toxicity of antitumor treatment has increased greatly. The heart had been considered to be one of the most radioresistant organs in the thorax, as well as being spared from most of the side effects of chemotherapy. However, the incidence of cardiovascular complications has risen sharply with curative forms of radiation therapy for Hodgkin's disease and non-Hodgkin's lymphoma and the addition of one of the most potent families of chemotherapeutic agents, the anthracyclines.

RADIATION THERAPY

Acute and chronic forms of pericarditis are the most common cardiovascular complications of radiation therapy[123a] (Table 49–7). The incidence following radiotherapy depends upon how carefully it is searched for. Acute pericarditis occurs in 10 to 15 per cent of patients with Hodgkin's disease receiving over 4000 rads to the mediastinum.[124] These episodes are characterized by fever, pleuritic pain, pericardial friction rub, and electrocardiographic and echocardiographic changes typical of pericardial disease (p. 1474). The time from completion of radiotherapy to the clinical onset of pericarditis ranges from 0 to 85 months, with the peak incidence occurring between 5 and 9 months. However, with longer follow-up of cured patients, symptoms may not develop for 8 to 10 years.[110,125] The incidence of pericarditis appears to be a function of the fractional and total dose of radiation to the pericardium and the amount of the heart irradiated. When the entire dose of radiation is delivered through an anterior port, the incidence of pericarditis is increased. However, when chest irradiation is given in divided doses to an anterior and a posterior port and with a subcarinal shield, the incidence of pericarditis has decreased to 2.5 per cent, without increasing the risk of relapse of Hodgkin's disease. If the entire heart receives therapeutic doses of radiation, up to 50 per cent of patients may develop pericardial complications.[126] With large mediastinal masses, to ensure adequate therapy, whole heart irradiation has been replaced with cu-

TABLE 49–7 CLASSIFICATION OF RADIATION-RELATED CARDIAC DISEASE

I. Acute pericarditis (caused by necrosis of tumor adjacent to the heart)
II. Delayed pericarditis
   A. Acute radiation-induced pericarditis, without effusion
   B. Acute radiation-induced pericarditis, with effusion, with/without cardiac tamponade
   C. Chronic effusive pericarditis
   D. Effusive-constrictive pericarditis
   E. Chronic pericardial constriction
   F. Occult constrictive pericarditis
III. Myocardial fibrosis
IV. Occlusive coronary artery disease
V. Conduction abnormalities
VI. Valvular regurgitation or stenosis

Reproduced with permission from Applefeld, M. M., and Pollock, S. H.: Cardiac disease in patients who have malignancies. Current Problems in Cardiology, Vol. 4. Chicago, Year Book Medical Publishers, 1980. p. 5.

rative forms of chemotherapy. It has been suggested that routine follow-up during the first year after irradiation should consist of frequent chest roentgenograms. If any evidence of increased cardiac diameter is noted, or if a patient develops clinical manifestations suggestive of pericarditis or pericardial effusion and there is no reason to suspect another cause of pericarditis, patients may be treated symptomatically but occasionally may require pericardiocentesis and/or pericardiectomy.[109,110,127] It is anticipated that, with current changes in radiotherapeutic techniques and available curative chemotherapy, the incidence of pericarditis will continue to decline.

Documented instances of clinical disease resulting from radiation damage to the myocardium and endocardium are quite rare.[124,128] Radiation-induced endocardial fibrosis may cause manifestations of a restrictive cardiomyopathy (p. 1422) and a variety of nonspecific electrocardiographic changes, as well as varying degrees of AV block,[129,] mitral regurgitation secondary to papillary muscle dysfunction, and aortic regurgitation as a consequence of endocardial valvular thickening. The onset of new murmurs occurring after radiation therapy should alert the physician to these possibilities. In an autopsy study of the cardiac effects of radiation exposure, three fourths of the patients exposed to more than 3500 rads, with a field resulting in more exposure of the anterior thorax, develop interstitial myocardial fibrosis, with more extensive involvement of the right than the left ventricle. Functional abnormalities demonstrated by echocardiography and radionuclide angiocardiography may occur 5 to 15 years after radiation but as with pericarditis should become less frequent with new techniques of radiotherapy.[129a]

Since the report by Cohn et al.[128] in 1967 of a 15-year-old boy suffering a fatal myocardial infarction 16 months after receiving 4000 rads to the heart for Hodgkin's disease, a number of similar occurrences have been reported.[110,129-131,131a] Although coronary artery disease is common, supportive evidence for radiation-induced coronary artery disease includes (1) its occurrence in subjects who are very young and without predisposing factors with disease limited to coronary vessels in the beam of radiation, (2) lack of atherosclerosis in arteries not exposed to irradiation, (3) reports of occlusive lesions in other arteries such as the carotid artery following irradiation,[132] (4) presence of distinctive pathological changes, and (5) production of similar lesions in experimental models.

Occlusive coronary and carotid artery disease following irradiation generally occurs from 6 to 12 years after exposure. In rabbits, 2500 rads has produced coronary atherosclerosis that is quite similar to human coronary artery disease.[133] Rabbits do not develop radiation-induced atherosclerosis unless they also receive a diet high in lipids and cholesterol, which by itself is insufficient to produce the atherosclerotic lesion. However, the coronary artery lesions presumably induced by radiotherapy appear to be distinct pathologically and contain severe medial and adventitial fibrosis in continuity with overlying epicardial fibrous tissue and a marked paucity of lipid in the intimal lesions.[130,134] In affected young patients examined at autopsy, the proximal portion of the arteries is significantly more narrowed than the distal. In addition, there is significant loss of smooth muscle cells from the media.[134]

Radiation-induced coronary artery or carotid artery occlusion may require surgical treatment. Because of the relatively low incidence of this complication and the concern that reduced radiation might impair chances of effective treatment of the neoplastic process requiring irradiation, no systematic attempts have been made to try to prevent this complication other than considering chemotherapeutic alternatives if whole-heart irradiation is deemed necessary to "cure" the disease.

CARDIOTOXICITY OF CHEMOTHERAPY FOR NEOPLASTIC DISEASE

For many years, the only notable cardiovascular complications of chemotherapy for neoplastic disease were the orthostatic hypotension[135] and the rare myocardial infarction[136] that occurred in the course of therapy with vincristine, a periwinkle alkaloid, and the interstitial disease and mild pulmonary hypertension secondary to the pulmonary fibrosis created by bleomycin or busulfan.[137] However, with the advent of the anthracycline group of drugs (doxorubicin, daunorubicin), the incidence of cardiac toxicity as a consequence of chemotherapy for neoplastic disease has increased greatly. Doxorubicin (Fig. 49-12) is a glycoside antibiotic, the potent antitumor effect of which is thought to be due to its ability to inhibit nucleic acid synthesis by binding to both strands of the DNA helix, intercalating between base pairs and thereby inhibiting the normal function of DNA and RNA polymerases. Doxorubicin has received more attention than the related compound daunorubicin because of its wider spectrum of antitumor activity in solid tumors and hematologic malignancies.[138] Complete remissions in 30 to 40 per cent of patients with Hodgkin's disease and non-Hodgkin's lymphoma and all types of acute leukemia have been reported with the single agent doxorubicin. Its effectiveness is enhanced by combination with other chemotherapeutic agents. Remission rates of 60 to 80 per cent are obtained in adults with leukemias when it is combined with cytosine arabinoside, and with lymphomas when used together with bleomycin, cyclophosphamide, vincristine, and corticosteroids.[139]

The majority of the toxic manifestations—alopecia, gastrointestinal distress, myelosuppression, and mucositis—produced by these drugs were predicted by animal studies.

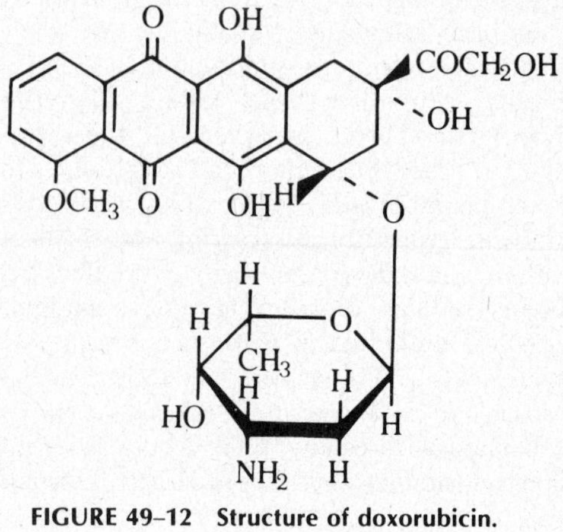

FIGURE 49-12   Structure of doxorubicin.

Not predicted, however, was the occurrence of cardiac toxicity and the interactions with radiation therapy. Arrhythmias, including supraventricular tachyarrhythmias, premature atrial and ventricular contractions, abnormalities of conduction such as left axis deviation, decreased QRS voltage, and a variety of nonspecific ST-segment and T-wave abnormalities, occur in approximately 11 per cent of patients, with a range from 0 to 41.2 per cent.[139,140] These electrocardiographic changes are usually transient, may occur even at low doses of doxorubicin, and usually are seen within several days after administration of the drug. Sudden death has been reported.[141]

Cardiomyopathy and congestive heart failure occurring during anthracycline therapy usually develop suddenly; the clinical manifestations consist of sinus tachycardia, tachypnea, cardiomegaly, peripheral and pulmonary edema, hepatomegaly, venous congestion, and pleural effusion. The cardiomyopathy is usually secondary to a cumulative effect of the drug, occurring with increasing frequency at higher doses of doxorubicin. Congestive heart failure occurs from 9 to 192 days, with a median of 34 days after the administration of the last dose. The congestive heart failure is refractory to therapy; when it is severe, survival is short, usually less than two weeks.[142] Pathological examination discloses enlarged, pale, flabby hearts with ventricular dilatation. Mural thrombi are occasionally found, but the coronary arteries and cardiac valves appear normal. Light microscopy reveals a severe cardiomyopathy with a reduction of the number of myocardial cells and the remaining cells showing degenerative changes. Electron microscopy shows extensive reduction in the number of myofibrillar bundles, myofibrillar lysis, and distortion and disruption of the Z-lines; the mitochondria are swollen with disrupted cristae and contain inclusion bodies[140,142] (Fig. 49–13).

The incidence of cardiomyopathy with doxorubicin administration is 1.7 per cent and with daunorubicin 4.4 per cent. It is fatal in over half the cases.[139] There is a clear

TABLE 49–8 CORRELATION OF CARDIOMYOPATHY AND THE TOTAL DOSE OF ADRIAMYCIN IN ADULTS

TOTAL DOSE (mg/M²)	PATIENTS AT RISK	PATIENTS WITH CMY	FREQUENCY (PER CENT)
< 450	738	0	0
451–500	26	0	0
501–550	32	3	9
551–600	15	3	20
> 600	37	15	41
Total > 550	52	18	35
Total < 550	796	3	0.4

CMY = cardiomyopathy.

dose-related incidence of anthracycline cardiomyopathy. There were no cases of cardiomyopathy in 764 patients who received less than a cumulative dose of 500 mg/M², but a progressively increased frequency with higher doses was noted[142] (Table 49–8). It is therefore recommended that cumulative doses of doxorubicin be held to less than 450 to 500 mg/M² and 500 to 600 mg/M² of daunorubicin. However, with increasing frequency, cardiomyopathies are being reported with dosages less than 450 mg/M² of doxorubicin.[140,142,143] It has been suggested that the use of these agents in combination with other modalities of therapy, such as radiation or cyclophosphamide, may have been synergistic in the pathogenesis of the cardiomyopathy in some patients.[134,143–146] Both radiation and cyclophosphamide alone have been described as potentially cardiotoxic.

There is no established mechanism for doxorubicin cardiotoxicity, although numerous proposals have been put forward.[147] For example, lipid peroxidation may be caused by the binding of DNA by the drug, specifically bound to spectrin, actin, or cardiolipin.[148] Doxorubicin inhibits ATP production, interferes with the sarcolemmal sodium-potassium pump, inhibits oxidative phosphorylation, may provoke an autoimmune response, binds to DNA precursors, interferes with mitochondrial respiration by inhibiting coenzyme Q, and causes myocardial necrosis by allowing the build-up of high concentrations of calcium in myocardial cells.[149]

Because of the high incidence of toxicity, numerous approaches have been suggested for early detection of this complication and for predicting susceptible patients.[150,151] Noninvasive studies include serial follow-up of systolic time intervals, particularly the PEP/LVET ratio (p. 54) and radionuclide cineangiography (p. 360). The *PEP/LVET* was thought to be a sensitive parameter for monitoring toxicity. However, this has not held up in further study and, in fact, is criticized because false-positive changes may be responsible for the improper withholding of further doxorubicin therapy that is potentially life saving.[152,153] *Radionuclide angiography* appears to provide a sensitive and reproducible measurement of left ventricular dysfunction due to doxorubicin cardiotoxicity.[150] Sequential studies demonstrate the frequent presence of subclinical left ventricular abnormalities.[154] There may be, however, an increased incidence of abnormal results that may not be clinically significant if the studies are performed after exercise.[155] *Endomyocardial biopsy* (p. 297) appears at present to be more diagnostic of toxicity than any of the noninvasive evaluations. In the hands of trained personnel, it has become a safe procedure.[156] Administration of doxoru-

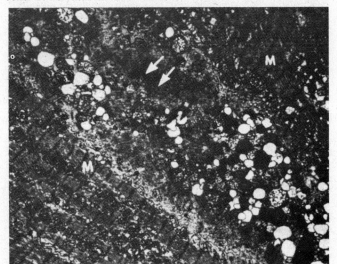

FIGURE 49–13 Myofibrillar loss (white arrows) and sarcotubular swelling (black arrows) are characteristic findings in patients who develop congestive heart failure during doxorubicin therapy. Juxtaposition of normal myocytes (M) and destroyed cells demonstrates microscopic focality of lesion. Histopathologic assessment may also be used to titrate dosage. (Reproduced with permission from Greene, H. L., Reich, S. D., and Dalen, J. E.: How to minimize doxorubicin toxicity. J. Cardiovasc. Med. 7:306, 1982.)

TABLE 49–9   RISK FACTORS FOR DOXORUBICIN CARDIOTOXICITY

Cumulative dose (> 550/M^2)
Age extremes
Preexistent coronary artery disease
Hypertension
Metastatic pericardial or myocardial disease
Prior mediastinal irradiation
Coexistent chemotherapy with alkylating agents

bicin was associated with a dose-related increase in the degree of myocyte damage; drug-associated degenerative changes were identified in 27 of 129 patients at doses greater than or equal to 240 mg/M.^{2} Simultaneous studies of endomyocardial biopsy and radionuclide cineangiography demonstrate good correlation. While the noninvasive studies reveal an accelerating decrease in myocardial function with levels exceeding 400 mg/M^2, biopsy studies show a fairly constant progression of myocardial damage as a function of cumulative dose.[155,157] These findings suggest that compensatory mechanisms are available to maintain myocardial function despite pathological damage. Prospective studies in young patients indicate that up to one half of patients who have received the drug, although asymptomatic cardiac-wise, may have impairment of left ventricular function, which may or may not be permanent. Additional information needed is the long-term follow-up of treated patients.

Certain risk factors for developing drug cardiotoxicity have been suggested (Table 49–9) and include advanced age, coincident coronary artery disease, uncontrolled hypertension, mediastinal irradiation, metastatic involvement of the pericardium or heart, and coexistent chemotherapy with cyclophosphamide or other alkylating agents.[153,158]

PREVENTION OF DOXORUBICIN TOXICITY.[105] Several possibilities for preventing doxorubicin-induced cardiotoxicity have been suggested. The use of free radical scavengers (vitamin E),[149] sulfhydryl compounds,[159] coenzyme Q10 (a mitochondrial quinone),[160] and cardiac glycosides[161] have all been reported to lessen cardiac toxicity; prospective studies to determine the efficacy of these interventions are underway. Reducing peak blood levels of the drug appears to offer the best reduction of cardiac toxicity. In a controlled study monitoring cardiac toxicity by noninvasive techniques as well as by endomyocardial biopsy, drug-related damage was significantly reduced but not eliminated when the drug was administered by prolonged continuous intravenous infusion rather than by bolus injection; the reduced toxicity clearly appears to be related to reduced peak plasma levels. Antitumor activity does not appear to be compromised by this technique of administration.[162]

Other Antineoplastic Agents.   Fatal cardiomyopathies have been reported secondary to high doses of intravenous cyclophosphamide.[146] In contrast to doxorubicin cardiotoxicity, the effect of cyclophosphamide is fairly acute and not due to a cumulative dose. It causes a reduction of ECG voltage and reduction of systolic function on echocardiography. Although mortality is appreciable, survivors exhibit no residual cardiac abnormalities.[163] AMSA, an acridine derivative, is an experimental chemotherapeutic agent recently found to have significant cardiac abnormal-

ities, including congestive heart failure and arrhythmias, reversible with discontinuation of the drug.[164]

HEMATOLOGIC ABNORMALITIES RELATED TO CARDIAC MEDICATION

Blood dyscrasias are frequent complications of drugs used in the treatment of cardiac disorders. The development of an unexplained anemia, granulocytopenia, or thrombocytopenia in a patient receiving a diuretic, antihypertensive, or antiarrhythmic agent should immediately arouse the suspicion that a drug used in the treatment of cardiac disease might be responsible.

Many different types of blood dyscrasias occur secondary to drug ingestion. The anemias include the aplastic, hemolytic, megaloblastic, and sideroblastic types; there may be granulocytopenia and agranulocytosis, thrombocytopenia, thrombocytosis, defects of platelet function, and a variety of miscellaneous disorders (Table 49–10). The mechanisms include suppression of one or more of the three cellular elements in the bone marrow, as well as a variety of immune phenomena with increased peripheral destruction of the formed elements. The drug effect may be dose-related or idiosyncratic.

Aplastic Anemia. Many chemical agents are capable of suppressing marrow function and producing hypoplasia or even aplasia. Chloramphenicol, benzene, cytostatic agents used in malignancies, and phenylbutazone are the most common drugs implicated. Less frequently, and perhaps less well documented, are antibiotics such as sulfonamides, hypoglycemic agents, and insecticides. The antiarrhythmic agent phenytoin (p. 661), the diuretic agent acetazolamide, and the newer angiotensin-converting enzyme inhibitor captopril[165] (p. 539) are among the medications leading to such reactions in cardiac patients. The onset of aplastic anemia is usually insidious, and the symptoms are directly related to the degree of pancytopenia. If the causative agent is immediately discontinued upon the appearance of the blood dyscrasia, it will usually be reversed.

Megaloblastic Anemia. A pancytopenia characterized by macrocytic red cells owing to impairment of DNA synthesis may be caused by vitamin B_{12} or folate deficiency, or by purine and pyrimidine inhibitors. Most commonly, drugs cause megaloblastic anemia by impairing the absorption of folic acid or acting as folate antagonists. Phenytoin (p. 661), oral contraceptives, and a variety of other drugs can impair folate absorption by interfering with liver conjugases necessary for the breakdown of the polyglutamate structure of naturally occurring folates to the monoglutamate form appropriate for absorption through the gastrointestinal tract. Triamterene, a potassium-sparing diuretic (p. 533), is a pteridine analogue and has antifolate activity, similar to aminopterin, in vitro. Its propensity to produce a megaloblastic anemia is probably dose-related.

Immunohemolytic Anemias. Drug-induced immunohemolytic anemias have been known for over 30 years, but their mechanism has only recently become clear. There are four different causes for the development of a positive direct Coombs' or antiglobulin test, two of which involve cardiac medication: The first mechanism, which is uncommon, involves some drugs, including quinidine and the sulfonamides, which bind to plasma proteins and thereby become antigenic. The resultant antigen-antibody complex may deposit on the red cell surface and cause agglutinability by anticomplement sera. Hemolysis may be severe, but rapid improvement follows withdrawal of the drug. The second type of positive Coombs' test involves the antihypertensive drug alpha-methyldopa (p. 915).[166] The analog L-dopa, administered to patients with Parkinson's disease, also causes a positive Coombs' test. The mechanism of antibody formation is unknown, but presumably antibody induced by alpha-methyldopa has affinity for the Rh locus of the red cell, in a manner similar to that of IgG antibodies in idiopathic immunohemolytic anemia. The frequency of positive Coombs' test varies from 11 per cent for patients who are receiving 0.75 gm per day for over three months to 40 per cent for those on 2 gm for the same period of time. Fortunately, the affinity of

TABLE 49–10 BLOOD DYSCRASIAS ASSOCIATED WITH CARDIAC MEDICATION

	ANEMIA			NEUTROPENIA	THROMBOCYTOPENIA	OTHER
	Aplastic	*Megaloblastic*	*Hemolytic*			
Antiarrhythmic						
Ajmaline	−	−	−	+	−	−
Digitoxin	−	−	−	−	+	L
Phenytoin	+	+	−	+	+	L,P
Procainamide	−	−	−	+(A)	−	−
Propranolol	−	−	−	+	−	−
Quinidine	−	−	+	+	+	−
Anticoagulants						
Heparin	+*	−	−	−	+	−
Phenindione	−	−	−	+	−	−
Antihypertensives						
Captopril	+	−	−	+	+	−
Glutethimide	+*	−	−	−	−	P
Hydralazine	−	−	−	−	+	L
Methyldopa	−	−	+	+	+	P
Reserpine	−	−	−	−	+	−
Diuretics						
Acetazolamide	+	−	−	+	+	−
Chlorothiazide	−	−	−	−	+	−
Chlorthalidone	−	−	−	+	+	−
Diazoxide	−	−	−	−	+	−
Ethacrynic acid	−	−	−	+	−	−
Hydrochlorothiazide	−	−	−	+	−	−
Mercurials	−	−	−	+	+	−
Spironolactone	−	−	−	−	+	−
Triamterene	−	+	−	−	−	−
Coronary Dilators						
Amyl nitrite	−	−	−	−	−	M
Nitroglycerin	−	−	−	−	−	M
Other						
Amrinone	−	−	−	−	+	−

*Pure red cell aplasia. L = Lupus-like syndrome; P = porphyria; A = agranulocytosis; M = methemoglobinemia.

the alpha-methyldopa antibody for red cells is low, and fewer than 1 per cent of patients developing a positive antiglobulin test develop significant hemolytic anemia. Nonetheless, alpha-methyldopa leads all other drugs in causing immunohemolytic anemias. On withdrawal of the drug, the hemolysis will improve within 1 or 2 weeks, with full recovery in 1 month, but the positive Coombs' test may persist for 6 to 24 months. A positive Coombs' test without hemolysis is not an indication for discontinuing alpha-methyldopa if its administration is otherwise indicated in the treatment of hypertension. The third mechanism of drug-related positive antiglobulin reactions is represented by penicillin, in which the drug binds to the red cell membranes, creating a cell-drug complex and antigenic stimulation of an IgG antibody. The fourth mechanism involves cephalothin, which is bound to the red cell membrane; normal serum proteins adhere nonspecifically to red cell membranes.

Granulocytopenia and Agranulocytosis. Reduction in circulating neutrophils is the most common toxic hematologic effect of drugs. It may be secondary to depression of the marrow or it may be an immune mechanism with peripheral destruction. When there is immune suppression, examination of the marrow reveals active myeloid precursors, while absence of myeloid elements suggests suppression of synthesis. Pisciotta has demonstrated that the marrow-depressive effect is dose-related.[167] Anticoagulants such as pheninone, antiarrhythmias such as procainamide, antihypertensives such as captopril, and diuretics such as the thiazides have all been reported to produce granulocytopenia. *Procainamide* is the most frequent and dangerous cardiac drug implicated in granulocytopenia.[168] Presenting symptoms may include a sore throat, ulcerations of mucous membranes, fever, malaise, fatigue, and weakness; there may be a rebound with a leukemoid picture after discontinuation of the drug. Because laboratory tests are not conclusive for white cell antibodies, accurate definition of the immune mechanism responsible for white cell destruction remains unclear.

Drug-Induced Thrombocytopenia. Many of the drugs used to treat cardiovascular disorders may cause thrombocytopenia, either by a direct effect on the bone marrow or by inducing the formation of drug-specific antibody. For example, the thiazide diuretics (p. 533) directly suppress megakaryocyte production. Thiazide-induced throm-

bocytopenia is usually mild, with the platelet count rarely falling below 50,000/μl. It is unique, since it persists for six to eight weeks after drug withdrawal. Amrinone thrombocytopenia is less well studied but is clearly related to the dose of drug administered and is related to peripheral destruction of platelets.[169] Other common agents like alcohol and some estrogen preparations may cause thrombocytopenia by a direct marrow effect.

Shortened platelet survival secondary to antibody or complement binding to platelets can cause severe thrombocytopenia and life-threatening hemorrhage. The onset is abrupt and is not related to the dose of medication or the duration of its use. In most cases of immunologic thrombocytopenia, the offending agent induces a specific antibody. The resulting drug-antibody complex then binds to the platelet and thereby shortens its survival. Quinidine was one of the first cardiac drugs producing this response and is one of the most well-studied causes of thrombocytopenia. The defect can be transferred to a normal individual by the administration of serum from a patient with quinidine-induced thrombocytopenia, followed by challenge of the normal subjects with quinidine.[170] A similar defect can be caused by antibodies to quinine, including the small quantities present in tonic drinks.[171] Acetaminophen, a common analgesic given to cardiac patients, acetazolamide, digitoxin, phenytoin, ethacrynic acid, alpha-methyldopa, and spironolactone have all been implicated in various cases of drug-induced thrombocytopenia, although the mechanism has not always been well-defined.

Although in vitro laboratory tests for drug-dependent platelet antibody are available, the results do not always correlate with clinical events. The best proof of drug-induced thrombocytopenia is prompt recovery of the platelet count after drug withdrawal, followed by a second episode of thrombocytopenia after readministration of the suspected drug. (Because of the potential hazard, the drug challenge is not always undertaken.) If serious hemorrhage persists following drug withdrawal, additional treatment with 1 mg/kg prednisone or its equivalent may be necessary. Corticosteroids may hasten the return of a normal platelet count and may also protect capillaries and small vessels even without altering the platelet count. Platelet transfusions are not usually helpful but can be tried in desperate situations with life-threatening hemorrhage. They are most useful if thrombocytopenia persists well after the drug-antibody complex has been cleared. In this situation, some patients have had a gratifying elevation in platelet count.

The commonly used anticoagulant *heparin* is one of the most important causes of thrombocytopenia in cardiac patients. The incidence varies from 5 to 25 per cent of patients receiving heparin, is more common in patients receiving heparin derived from beef lung, and has been associated with all modes and doses of heparin administration.[172] Heparin has a direct platelet-aggregating effect that may contribute to thrombocytopenia. This property is most marked in those fractions with highest molecular weight and lowest affinity for antithrombin.[173] There is an increase in platelet-associated immunoglobulin in many of the cases, suggesting an immune etiology. However, the nature of the offending antigen in heparin and its relationship to the biologically active heparin fractions remain unclear. In addition, some patients with heparin-induced thrombocytopenia develop paradoxical thrombosis and disseminated intravascular coagulation. The development of thromboembolism in association with thrombocytopenia is unique to heparin.

Other Cardiac Drug Hematologic Abnormalities. Amyl nitrite, sodium nitrite, and nitroglycerin can oxidize hemoglobin to methemoglobin, which cannot effectively carry oxygen. The patient with methemoglobinemia has a cyanotic appearance but has a normal pO_2 and will not improve his color with oxygen therapy. Although normal adults can get symptomatic methemoglobinemia, most cases occur when children accidentally ingest medications prescribed for adults. Occasionally, adults with mild congenital methemoglobinemia will become markedly symptomatic when exposed to small doses of these same medications. With the current availability of intravenous nitroglycerin, this complication may become more frequent.[174] If venous blood is chocolate brown and the color remains after the blood is shaken in air, the diagnosis of methemoglobinemia is almost certain. The diagnosis is confirmed by the addition of a few drops of 10 per cent potassium cyanide, which results in the rapid production of the bright red cyanmethemoglobin. Symptoms are nonspecific and consist of dyspnea, headache, fatigue, and dizziness. They are usually self-limited if the responsible drugs are discontinued, since normal red cells can enzymatically reduce the methemoglobin. In severe cases or in patients with enzyme defects, methylene blue may be administered to stimulate reduction of the methemoglobin.

Other medications may interfere with oxygen delivery to tissues. For example, nitroprusside used in the treatment of hypertensive emergencies (Chap. 27) or for reduction of afterload in the management of heart failure (p. 537) may cause symptoms such as fatigue, nausea, abnormal behavior, and muscle spasm due to the reaction of the agent with oxyhemoglobin and the resultant production of cyanmethemoglobin and free cyanide ions.[175]

Hydralazine, procainamide, and rarely phenytoin can cause a lupus erythematosus–like syndrome, with urticaria, erythema multiforme, photosensitivity, delirium, and immune-mediated blood cell destruction. Although patients with drug-induced lupus have positive antinuclear antibody tests and many of the clinical manifestations of SLE, they do not usually have renal impairment, and all the symptoms remit within several months if the drugs are discontinued. The syndrome is of particular importance in cardiac patients, since the onset of chest pain, pleurisy, or pericardial effusion in the patient with heart disease could lead to an erroneous diagnosis unless drug-induced lupus is suspected.

THROMBOSIS, ANTICOAGULATION, AND BLEEDING IN HEART DISEASE

PATHOGENESIS OF THROMBOSIS

More than a century ago, Virchow proposed that thrombosis resulted from a combination of three factors: local vessel or tissue injury, circulatory stasis, and alterations in blood coagulability.[176] Since that time, both clinical observations on patients with thromboembolism and research on thrombosis have upheld these basic principles. The composition of thrombi varies with their anatomical site and depends upon the velocity of blood flow. In arteries, they consist of aggregated platelets with few fibrin strands, giving them a white appearance. Venous thrombi, which form in areas where the velocity of blood flow is slower, are made up of fibrin strands and entrapped red cells, giving them a red appearance. The role of platelets in venous thrombi is not clear, although platelets may provide the initial nidus for thrombus formation and can be seen at the head of thrombi, where they attach to damaged endothelium on venous valves.

To understand the development of thrombi, it is important to understand the normal hemostatic mechanism, its limiting reactions, and its inhibitors. Thrombosis has, in fact, been defined as blood coagulation occurring in the wrong place or at the wrong time. The sequence of events in clotting can be divided into: (1) formation of the platelet plug—platelet adhesion and aggregation; (2) the platelet release reaction; (3) the generation of thrombin; (4) the formation of the fibrin clot; and (5) dissolution of the fibrin clot through the fibrinolytic system.

Platelet Aggregation, Platelet Release, and Thrombin Generation. Following vascular injury, platelets adhere to exposed subendothelial collagen or to noncollagenous microfibrils (Fig. 49–14). Activated platelets release ADP and other mediators, which cause circulating platelets to be attracted to the traumatic site, beginning the formation of a "platelet plug."[175,178,179] As a result of endothelial cell

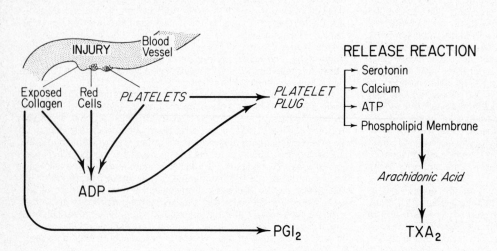

FIGURE 49-14 Diagram of the hemostatic reaction at the site of injury, showing the role of platelets. TXA_2 thromboxane; PGI_2 prostacyclin.

injury and platelet activation, metabolites of arachidonic acid—prostaglandins and thromboxanes—are formed that regulate platelet release and aggregation. Prostacyclin (PGI_2), produced by endothelial cells, is a potent inhibitor of platelet aggregation, while thromboxane (TXA_2), a product of arachidonic acid metabolism in the platelet, causes platelet release and aggregation.[179] In addition, platelets may serve as a site for the rapid activation of clotting factors.[177] There is evidence that prothrombin conversion to thrombin occurs several thousand times faster on platelets than in plasma.

As the platelet plug is being formed, exposed collagen and tissue thromboplastin from the damaged vessel activate the plasma coagulation system, leading to thrombin generation and fibrin formation (Fig. 49–15). There are two closely intertwined pathways for thrombin formation. They both involve the limited proteolysis of inactive precursors or proenzymes to produce active enzymes, which, in turn, proteolyze additional molecules in an enzymatic cascade. The reactions are carefully regulated by lipid and protein cofactors and plasma inhibitors so that sufficient thrombin is generated for local fibrin deposition without systemic coagulation. The intrinsic pathway is initiated by Hageman factor (Factor XII) contact with collagen. The activation of Factor XII is facilitated by two cofactors, high molecular weight kininogen and prekallikrein. Activated Hageman factor fragments then activate Factor XI, which, in concert with Factors IX and VIII, activates Factor X. In the extrinsic or tissue factor–dependent pathway, Factor VII forms a complex with tissue factor which can directly activate Factor X. Activated Factor X (X_a), in conjunction with Factor V, converts prothrombin to thrombin (Fig. 49–14). Formation of small amounts of thrombin accelerates further platelet aggregation and release and, eventually, more thrombin production.

Formation of Fibrin Clot. Once thrombin is formed, it attacks the fibrinogen molecule, converting it to fibrin with release of two fragments, fibrinopeptides A and B. As fibrin is laid down, the hemostatic plug is strengthened and stabilized by Factor XIII, which catalyzes covalent cross-links between polymerized fibrin molecules. The resultant clot becomes mechanically strong and able to withstand the trauma of collisional events within the vascular system.

Dissolution of the Fibrin Clot via the Fibrinolytic System. Plasminogen is normally incorporated into the fibrin clot and is ready to be activated to plasmin, an enzyme capable of fibrinolysis. Endothelial cells secrete a plasminogen activator that diffuses into the clot to initiate fibrinolysis. Fibrinolysis remains localized to the clot because of the high local concentration of plasminogen within the clot and the presence in plasma of the alpha$_2$ plasmin inhibitor,[180] which

rapidly neutralizes any free plasmin. There has been a great deal of recent interest in the fibrinolytic system and its role in thrombosis, since patients have been described with recurrent thromboembolism who have either a deficiency of venous plasminogen activator or abnormal plasminogen molecules that resist activation and have reduced fibrinolytic potential.[181,182] In addition, pharmacologic agents that can activate the fibrinolytic system, such as urokinase or streptokinase, are under study for the treatment of venous and arterial thrombosis and embolism (see below).

Laboratory Tests—Hemostasis and Thrombosis. The integrity of the clotting mechanism can be evaluated by various laboratory studies. Platelet function can be screened by a simple bleeding time. In addition, studies of platelet aggregation and measurement of platelet release reactions after exposure to aggregating agents can serve as useful indicators of abnormal platelet physiology. Abnormalities of the intrinsic coagulation pathway can be detected by the partial thromboplastin time (PTT), while the extrinsic pathway is screened with the prothrombin time (PT). These tests are most useful for evaluating hemostatic failure and bleeding disorders and are of little help in the diagnosis of thromboembolism. Newer tests that can detect platelet secretion and activation of plasma coagulation and may be useful in patients with thromboembolism are discussed below.

THE HYPERCOAGULABLE STATE

In addition to tissue injury and changes in the vessel wall, a number of changes in the blood itself may predispose patients to thrombosis. These are collectively referred to as "the hypercoagulable state"[183] and include (1) abnormalities in blood flow, (2) decreased concentration of clotting inhibitors, (3) abnormal platelet release and aggregation, (4) delayed or impaired clearance of activated factors, and (5) defects in the fibrinolytic system (Table 49–11).

Abnormal Blood Flow. Although stasis alone does not ordinarily produce venous thrombosis, it is definitely a contributing factor. Many of the clinical disorders associated with abnormal blood flow and thrombosis have been previously discussed in this chapter and include sickle cell disease, the polycythemias, and hyperviscosity syndromes. In addition, the occurrence of thromboembolism in pregnancy or following the use of oral contraceptives may be related, in part, to changes in blood flow. There is increasing clinical evidence suggesting that exogenous estrogens used in contraception, in the therapy of prostatic carcinoma, in the treatment of endometriosis, or as prophylaxis for atherosclerosis may increase the incidence of thromboembolic disease.[184,185] In addition, during pregnancy, the frequency of thromboembolism increases slightly with each trimester but is highest during the early postpartum period, a time of maximal estrogen secretion.[186] Estrogen and progesterone have major effects on

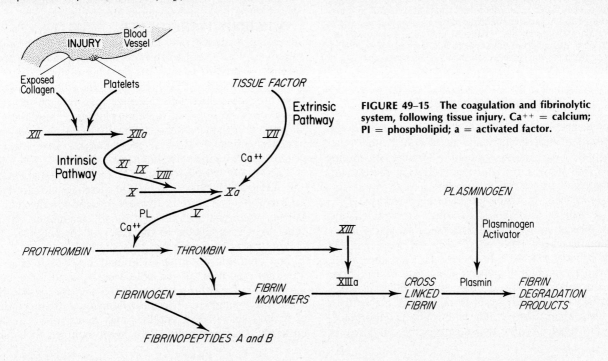

FIGURE 49–15 The coagulation and fibrinolytic system, following tissue injury. Ca^{++} = calcium; PI = phospholipid; a = activated factor.

TABLE 49–11   HEMATOLOGIC ABNORMALITIES THAT INCREASE
THE RISK OF THROMBOEMBOLISM

Abnormal blood flow
Decreased levels of inhibitors
  Antithrombin deficiency or dysfunction
  Protein C deficiency
Impaired platelet release and aggregation
Thrombocytosis in myeloproliferative disorders
Impaired clearance of activated factors
Impaired fibrinolytic activity
  Abnormal fibrinogen
  Decreased vascular plasminogen activator
    content/release
  Abnormal plasminogen

blood flow and rheology. For example, they reduce both venous flow velocity and distensibility in the lower limbs and red cell deformability, the latter leading to increased blood viscosity and increased pulmonary capillary blood volume as well as a minor increase in pulmonary artery pressure. As discussed below, oral contraceptives have multiple effects on the coagulation system that could account for their association with thromboembolism.

Decreased Level of Inhibitors.   As previously pointed out, many coagulation proteins exist in the circulation as proenzymes, which are then cleaved to form the active clotting factors. There are several inhibitors in blood that can inactivate active clotting proteins by forming a stable but inactive complex (Table 49–13). The most well described is *antithrombin*, which binds to coagulation proteins such as thrombin, X_a, IX_a, XI_a, and XII_a. Its activity is markedly enhanced by the mucopolysaccharide heparin. In fact, the heparin cofactor activity of antithrombin is thought to account for the majority of heparin's anticoagulant activity. Deficient or biochemically abnormal antithrombin molecules have been reported in families with increased thrombosis.[186] The inheritance pattern is thought to be autosomal dominant with variable penetrance. Almost 70 per cent of patients with the deficiency have a thrombotic tendency. Levels of antithrombin III may fall slightly during active thrombosis, and it has been suggested that this reduction could perpetuate a thrombotic tendency. Heparin normally activates antithrombin activity, and markedly reduced levels of antithrombin III could explain rare cases of heparin resistance. It is still unclear, however, what activates antithrombin in vivo, although heparin-like molecules have been isolated from cell surfaces and vessel walls.

Recently, another clinically important inhibitor, *protein C*, has been discovered. Protein C is a vitamin K–dependent protease that is activated by thrombin after it is bound to an endothelial cell protein, thrombomodulin. Activated protein C can then inactivate Factors V and VIII and slow down coagulation reactions. Absence of this protein could lead to unchecked coagulation, by allowing excess thrombin generation and thrombosis.[187] At least one large family with this defect has been described to date.[188] Protein C also has some poorly understood profibrinolytic activity, which may help limit the size of thrombi.[189]

Platelets and Thrombosis

As noted, platelets adhere to microfibrils exposed in vessels denuded of endothelium and to ulcerated atherosclerotic plaques.[190] As previously noted, a number of complex biochemical pathways are activated following platelet adhesion that lead to platelet aggregation and release.[177] Imbalance or defects in these biochemical pathways could lead to bleeding or thrombosis. Although most platelet aggregation defects are associated with bleeding, spontaneous aggregation has been reported to occur in some patients with thrombotic states.[191] In disorders associated with thrombocytosis, including polycythemia vera, essential or primary thrombocytosis, and other myeloproliferative disorders in which the incidence of thrombosis is higher than normal, such abnormalities may be of clinical importance. Wu demonstrated platelet hyperaggregability in vitro in

thrombocytosis due to myeloproliferative disorders but not in patients with reactive thrombocytosis.[192]

Assays for measuring components that are part of the "platelet release reaction" are now available.[193] Increased levels of two of these proteins, Platelet Factor four (PF-4) and beta-thromboglobulin (B-TG), have been reported in patients with disseminated intravascular coagulation and with venous or arterial thrombosis, pulmonary emboli, prosthetic cardiac valves, and severe cardiorespiratory failure. In addition, marked elevations are found in a significant number of patients with acute myocardial infarction, as well as in patients with angina pectoris or with exercise-induced ischemia.[194] In some studies, B-TG levels have been shown to correlate with the vascular complications that occur in diabetes.[195] While these studies of PF-4 and B-TG are of considerable interest and represent an important area for further investigation, at the present time it is unclear whether they represent the cause or the effect of thrombotic and vascular disease.

Platelets also serve as a potential link in supporting the concept that stress causes ischemic heart disease. Friedman and Rosenman observed that most of their myocardial infarction–prone patients were of the "type A" behavioral pattern (p. 1826) and exhibited accelerated clotting times and increased circulating catecholamines.[196] Epinephrine and norepinephrine are potent platelet-aggregating agents, making them more responsive to ADP and thrombin. Activation of the sympathoadrenal system might be implicated in the pathogenesis of coronary artery thrombosis by increasing arterial pressure, platelet aggregation, coronary vascular tone, and circulating free fatty acids, which all may act in concert to increase the severity of myocardial ischemia.

IMPAIRED CLEARANCE OF ACTIVATED FACTORS.   The liver and reticuloendothelial systems normally remove activated clotting factors and plasminogen activators as well as soluble fibrin complexes from the circulation. Liver disease (cirrhosis, viral hepatitis, and so on) can impair the clearance mechanism and lead to widespread thrombosis and systemic fibrinolysis.

IMPAIRED FIBRINOLYTIC ACTIVITY.   There is increasing evidence that abnormalities in the fibrinolytic system may also lead to thrombosis. As mentioned above, absence of protein C may reduce fibrinolytic activity and lead to thrombosis (Table 49–12). In addition, patients have been described with defective plasminogen molecules that cannot be fully activated to plasmin,[181] and there are patients with reduced venous content[180] and release of plasminogen activator. Most of these patients have recurrent venous thrombosis and pulmonary embolism.

TESTS OF POSSIBLE USE IN THE DIAGNOSIS OF THROMBOSIS.   Although there are no firmly established diagnostic tests that are specific for thromboembolism, there are a number of blood coagulation changes that may be applicable to the study of thrombosis. These include fibrin monomer complexes, fibrinopeptides A and B, and the fibrin-fibrinogen degradation products (Fig. 49–15). More recently, assays have been reported for circulating thrombin-antithrombin complexes and for prothrombin activation fragments. The measurement of these products of various coagulation reactions may be useful in the diagnosis of thromboembolism and, when coupled with radio-

TABLE 49–12   CHARACTERISTICS OF THE COAGULATION PROTEIN INHIBITORS

NAME	MECHANISM OF ACTION	ACTIVATOR	DIAGNOSTIC TEST	CLINICAL DISORDER
Antithrombin III	Complexes with thrombin, X_a, and other serine proteases	Heparin	Immunoassay: Rate of thrombin neutralization $\pm$ heparin	Reduction or dysfunction causes recurrent venous arterial thrombosis
Protein C	Proteolyzes Factors V and VIII	Thrombin and thrombomodulin on the endothelial cell surface	Immunoassay	Decrease causes venous thromboembolism
α_2 plasmin inhibitor	Complexes with plasmin	None	Immunoassay	Absence causes rapid fibrinolysis, bleeding

isotope labeling studies utilizing coagulation proteins like fibrinogen or plasminogen, may localize the site of a thrombus. The fibrinopeptide A radioimmunoassay has been most widely employed and is elevated in patients with venous thrombosis and pulmonary embolism and promptly returns to normal following administration of heparin. Unfortunately, many nonspecific stimuli also raise the plasma fibrinopeptide A level, and the test is not yet clinically useful.[183]

EFFECTS OF ORAL CONTRACEPTIVES ON COAGULATION.

Ingestion of oral contraceptives raises the risk of thromboembolism in young women and provides an interesting model for a drug-induced hypercoagulable state. Many of the blood changes discussed previously are induced by the use of oral contraceptives. In addition, the clinical and epidemiologic studies have firmly linked pill use to certain thrombotic and vascular complications. Venous thrombosis and embolism, myocardial infarction, and cerebrovascular disease, as well as other thromboembolic phenomena in young women, have all been attributed to oral contraceptives.[184,185] The presumed mechanisms include effects of the drug on the coagulation profile, i.e., high platelet counts, short partial thromboplastin times, elevation of the concentrations of various clotting factors, increased platelet adhesiveness, lowered levels of antithrombin III[183–186] (Table 49–12) and decreased clearance of activated clotting factors. In addition, since exogenous estrogens alter the endothelium of the cervix and endometrium, it is possible that similar changes may occur in vascular endothelium, causing an injury site—the first step in the formation of a thrombus. Thus, there is a definite hazard of vascular complications and thrombosis associated with the use of oral contraceptive agents. However, some of the risks, like venous thromboembolism, may be no greater than the risks associated with pregnancy itself.[186] Since the risks are not uniformly distributed among oral contraceptive users, attention must also be directed toward identifying the subpopulations that are especially prone to these thromboembolic complications. These include all women exceeding 35 years of age and women of any age with one of the other risk factors for atherosclerosis (i.e., cigarette smoking, hypertension, or hypercholesterolemia), or a history of a clotting disorder. In addition to their effect on the clotting system, oral contraceptives may enhance the risk of the development or exacerbation of hypertension (p. 873).

In conclusion, the following alterations in the blood have been shown to be associated with either an increased risk of thromboembolism or active thrombosis: (1) reduced antithrombin III, (2) reduced fibrinolytic activity, (3) increased platelet aggregation, (4) increased PF-4, (5) increased B-TG, (6) fibrin-monomer complexes, (7) fibrinopeptides, and (8) fibrin-fibrinogen degradation products.

Anticoagulants and Platelet Suppression

Anticoagulant therapy with heparin or warfarin is clearly of benefit in the treatment and prevention of venous thrombosis but is of limited value in patients at risk of arterial thrombosis. Parenteral heparin is effective in the treatment of thrombophlebitis and pulmonary embolism (p. 1588) and in prevention of thromboembolic events in bedridden or inactive patients, including those with heart failure (Chap. 16) and acute myocardial infarction (p. 1304). Warfarin and related coumarin drugs have the same spectrum of effects; however, their action is delayed and they are less potent than heparin. Advantages are their effectiveness following oral administration and their usefulness when long-term prophylaxis is needed, as in patients with artificial heart valves and vascular prostheses. Platelet-suppressive agents, aspirin, dipyridamole, and sulfinpyrazone, because of their ability to inhibit the platelet release reaction and aggregation, are useful to postoperative patients with prosthetic heart valves and in patients with coronary and cerebral artery disease.

HEPARIN. Heparin, a naturally occurring sulfated mucopolysaccharide, is a powerful anticoagulant acting at several sites in the clotting schema. Most important is the inhibition of activated Factor X and thrombin, accomplished by increasing the neutralizing effect of antithrombin III–heparin cofactors.[198] It is the most useful drug available for the prophylaxis and treatment of venous thromboembolism.[199] Mortality and morbidity rates have been markedly reduced in patients with acute pulmonary embolism (Chap. 46).

Studies in large numbers of postoperative patients have confirmed that low-dose prophylaxis reduces the incidence of deep-vein thrombosis and the mortality from subsequent pulmonary embolism.[200] The dosage required for the treatment of established thromboembolism is higher than that needed for prophylaxis because of the need to reduce the rate of thrombin generation. In addition, inhibitors like PF-4 released from activated platelets may partially neutralize heparin. The current recommended dose for treatment of patients with thromboembolism is 20,000 to 30,000 U/24 hr by continuous intravenous infusion or enough to keep the partial thromboplastin time at 1.5 to 2 times the control level.[201] Hemorrhagic complications are reduced with the use of continuous intravenous infusion of heparin.

Although prophylaxis of venous thrombosis with heparin has been widely employed in postoperative patients for over 40 years, not until 1970 was there any firm evidence to support its use.[198-201] Many clinical trials support the use of subcutaneous low-dose heparin in preventing postoperative deaths due to pulmonary embolism. In other clinical situations, such as following hip surgery or myocardial infarction, the regimen has been less successful. The dosage recommended in prophylaxis is approximately half that of the therapeutic dose—that is, 10,000 to 15,000 U/24 hr, given subcutaneously in two or three divided doses.

ORAL ANTICOAGULANTS. Warfarin and its derivatives prevent vitamin K–dependent carboxylation of glutamic acid residues on the prothrombin complex proteins in the liver. As a result, the activity of clotting Factors II, VII, IX, and X is markedly reduced, which impairs fibrin formation and the growth of thrombi. The primary indications for long-term therapy with these agents are venous thrombosis in the leg and pulmonary embolism after the patient has initially received intravenous heparin.[202] In patients with hemodynamically significant mitral stenosis, particularly those with transient or permanent atrial fibrillation and in those with prosthetic heart valves, embolic episodes are minimized by permanent treatment with oral anticoagulants (Chap. 32). In addition, oral anticoagulants are useful after an acute arterial embolic episode and after hip surgery. Their long-term use in cerebrovascular disease and after myocardial infarction is still controversial, and they may actually be dangerous in patients with completed strokes.

The starting dose of the commonly used agent warfarin is 10 mg/24 hr for three to four days, with a maintenance dose between 3 and 8 mg/24 hr, depending upon the individual patient. Prothrombin times are usually kept at 2 to 2.5 times those of control. Complications include significant bleeding, as with heparin, as well as failure of anticoagulation with rethrombosis. Both of these complications may occur because of the addition or omission of other medications that may potentiate or antagonize the effect of warfarin (Table 49–13). Prolonged prothrombin times and bleeding may also occur with infection, liver disease, cardiac failure, alcoholic excess, or radical alteration in the diet with resultant change in the microbial intestinal flora. Despite careful control of the prothrombin time, the incidence of serious hemorrhage is 5 to 10 per cent per patient-year at risk and the incidence of fatal complications 0.5 to 1 per cent per patient-year. Newer immunoas-

TABLE 49–13   INTERACTION OF COMMONLY USED DRUGS WITH COUMARIN DERIVATIVES

POTENTIATE	ANTAGONIZE
Phenylbutazone	Barbiturates
Salicylates	*Other*:
Thyroid	chronic alcohol
Other:	allopurinol
acute alcohol	cholestyramine
anabolic steroids	diuretics
antibiotics	glutethimide
antiplatelet drugs	nortriptyline
clofibrate	rifampin
phenytoin	
oral hypoglycemic agents	
quinidine sulfate	
sulfonamides	

says that can monitor the concentration of normal and abnormal prothrombin and the assays that detect prothrombin activation fragments or thrombin-antithrombin complexes may provide better ways to monitor warfarin dose and both improve its efficacy as an antithrombotic agent and reduce the incidence of bleeding.

THROMBOLYTIC THERAPY. Drugs that activate the fibrinolytic system can be administered to patients to hasten the resoultion of established thrombi. The mechanism of action of these drugs is outlined in Figure 49–16. Streptokinase (SK), a bacterial product, forms a complex with plasminogen which then activates additional plasminogen molecules. Urokinase (UK), derived from cultured kidney cells, directly activates plasminogen. Both of these agents have been used to treat patients with acute arterial thrombosis and massive pulmonary embolism. Since these drugs cause severe hypofibrinogenemia, bleeding is a potential complication. Intracoronary infusion of SK or UK is less hazardous and has been used to restore the patency of arteriovenous shunts or to reverse acute coronary occlusion (pp. 336 and 1324).

One potentially important new development is the successful commercial production of tissue plasminogen activator (TPA) using recombinant DNA technology. Since TPA must bind to fibrin to initiate fibrinolysis, it may selectively lyse thrombi without causing systemic fibrinogen depletion and bleeding. It is likely that systemic fibrinolytic therapy with TPA will become available for clinical studies.

PLATELET INHIBITORS. Because of the role of platelets in normal hemostasis and thrombosis, a number of drugs that interfere with platelet function in vitro have undergone clinical trials. Three agents have been shown to have some benefit: (1) aspirin, (2) sulfinpyrazone, and (3) dipyridamole (Table 49–14). Although the latter's precise

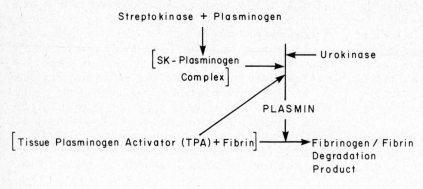

FIGURE 49–16 Mechanism of action of three fibrinolytic agents. Urokinase, which directly activates plasminogen; streptokinase (SK), which complexes to plasminogen; and tissue plasminogen activator (TPA), which requires fibrin to effectively activate plasminogen.

TABLE 49–14 ACTION OF ANTIPLATELET DRUGS

	ASPIRIN	DIPYRIDAMOLE	SULFINPYRAZONE
Mode of action	Irreversible acetylation of cyclooxygenase	Inhibition of platelet cAMP phosphodiesterase	Transient inhibition of cyclooxygenase (in vitro)
			? effect on platelet-vessel wall interaction
Laboratory effects on platelets*			
Aggregation	↓	0 (at clinical levels)	0
Adhesion	0	↓	?
Survival	0	↑	↑
Bleeding time	↑	0	0
Effects on clinical thromboembolism†			
Ischemia heart disease	−	−	+
Cerebrovascular disease	+	−	+ / −
Venous thrombosis	+ / −	−	+ / −
Prosthetic surfaces			
Heart valves	−	+ with warfarin	+ with warfarin
	+ with warfarin		
	+ with heparin		
Shunts	+		+
Arterial prostheses			−
Coronary artery bypass‡ graft patency	+	+	

*(↓) diminished; (↑) prolonged; (0) no effect
†(+) improved; (−) not improved; (+ / −) conflicting data or positive trends without statistical significance
‡Combined therapy with aspirin and dipyridamole.
Modified from Schafer, A. I., and Handin, R. I.: The role of platelets in thrombotic and vascular disease. Prog. Cardiovasc. Dis. 22:31–52, 1979.

site of action is still unclear, the first two agents interfere with normal platelet synthesis of prostaglandins and thromboxane[179] (Fig. 49–17). Platelet survival in patients with valvular heart disease and with prosthetic valves is significantly shortened, presumably because of platelet aggregation on, or consumption by, the abnormal surface. Antiplatelet medication may prevent these interactions that shorten platelet survival, and they are often given in addition to oral anticoagulants. Platelet survival is also shortened in cerebrovascular disease, and a recent study demonstrated aspirin's effectiveness in reducing complications of threatened strokes in men.[204]

Because of the postulated relationship between platelet aggregation and myocardial infarction, many studies are in progress to determine the benefit of platelet inhibition in coronary artery disease. One study using sulfinpyrazone claimed a reduction in mortality from sudden death in the first year after myocardial infarction, but the interpretation of the results has been disputed. The mechanism for this supposedly beneficial effect and the reproducibility of this finding are still unknown.[205] Dipyridamole appears to suppress experimentally induced arteriosclerosis in an animal model. Although there is no evidence for a similar effect in humans, the drug has been successful in reducing embolization from prosthetic valves, and the combination of aspirin and dipyridamole may improve coronary bypass graft patency.[206]

Bleeding Due to Platelet Dysfunction. Qualitative defects of platelet function, associated with normal platelet counts but prolonged bleeding time and decreased aggregation, are being noted with increasing frequency. The most common causes include abnormalities in platelet production or response to thromboxane A_2, or defects in the platelet packaging and storage of adenine nucleotides or other granule contents—storage pool disease. The most common cause of a decrease in TXA_2 production is the ingestion of nonsteroidal anti-inflammatory agents like aspirin, indomethacin, or ibuprofen. In fact, as discussed above, the antiplatelet effect of these drugs is being exploited as a means to prevent thromboembolism. One unavoidable side effect is the development of mild to moderate bleeding and the exacerbation of bleeding from organic lesions or at the

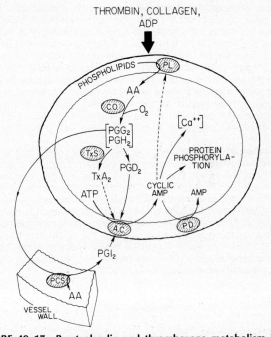

FIGURE 49–17 Prostaglandin and thromboxane metabolism in the platelet and vessel wall. The major platelet product is thromboxane A_2, a vasoconstrictor and platelet activator that inhibits adenylate cyclase, and the major vessel wall product PGI_2, a vasodilator and platelet inhibitor that stimulates adenylate cyclase and increases cyclic AMP. Hatched circles represent major control and synthetic enzymes. *PL* (phospholipase) releases the precursor arachidonic acid (AA) from membrane phospholipid. *CO* (cyclo-oxygenase) oxygenates AA to produce the prostaglandin intermediate PGG_2. *TxS* (thromboxane synthetase) converts PGG_2 to thromboxane A_2. *PCS* (prostacyclin synthetase) converts PGG_2 to PGI_2 in the endothelial cell. *AC* (adenylate cyclase) converts ATP to cyclic AMP, which inhibits platelet activation. *PD* (phosphodiesterase) breaks down cyclic AMP. Antiplatelet drugs exert their effects via these enzymes. Aspirin irreversibly inhibits CO and abolishes thromboxane production. Sulfinpyrazone also inhibits CO, although its effect is more short-lived. Dipyridamole (Persantine) blocks PD and prevents breakdown of cyclic AMP. Newer drugs which inhibit TxS or inhibit PL have not yet undergone extensive clinical testing.

time of major surgery. The most effective screening test is the bleeding time and the most effective therapy withdrawal of the drug. Aspirin is unique as it is an irreversible inhibitor of the platelet cyclooxygenase enzyme, and its effect persists for the life of the platelet, i.e., for up to seven days after drug withdrawal. The effects of the other drugs are more moderate and disappear within several hours to a day following drug withdrawal.

Bleeding Associated with Cardiac Surgery. Abnormal bleeding may occur in patients with cyanotic congenital heart disease; it can be severe and even fatal. A wide variety of coagulation defects has been demonstrated, including hypofibrinogenemia, thrombocytopenia, prolonged prothrombin time, shortened euglobulin clot lysis, poor clot retraction, elevated levels of fibrinogen degradation products, disseminated intravascular coagulation, impaired platelet adhesiveness, decreased platelet factor 3, and shortened platelet survival.[207-211] Thrombocytopenia and hypofibrinogenemia correlate with the degree of reduced arterial oxygen saturation and directly with the severity of the secondary polycythemia and the resultant increased blood viscosity.[209] Thus, the bleeding may be due to one or more of the coagulation defects just noted or to polycythemia, as discussed earlier (p. 1686). In patients with cyanotic congenital heart disease and coagulation defects, phlebotomy should be carried out cautiously and in small amounts, with saline replacement prior to operation to reduce viscosity and postoperative bleeding.

Uncontrolled bleeding occurring in patients with heart disease immediately following extracorporeal circulation has been thought to be due to thrombocytopenia and disseminated intravascular coagulation.[210] In addition, platelets may undergo reversible aggregation and release after contact with the extracorporeal device, yet continue to circulate, although their hemostatic potential is diminished.[210] Fibrin degradation products are found in high concentrations in chest tube drainage but not in the systemic circulation, suggesting that fibrinolysis may be localized to the thorax.[210] Thrombocytopenia, however, may be quite severe, beginning as early as the commencement of cardiac bypass or as late as the third postoperative day.[211] Platelets can aggregate on the surface of the extracorporeal apparatus which is exposed to the blood, and they may be consumed without causing generalized disseminated intravascular coagulation. The resultant bleeding disorder, which can be life-threatening in the early postoperative period, can usually be treated effectively with platelet concentrates.

In addition, bleeding following cardiopulmonary bypass may be due to unneutralized heparin.[210,211] Usually 200 U/kg of heparin is administered during the course of open heart surgery, and this is neutralized by an equal dose of protamine sulfate. It is possible that with this regimen, significant amounts of unneutralized heparin will persist and may be responsible for continued bleeding. Therefore, it is advisable to obtain an activated partial thromboplastin time if bleeding persists and continue to administer protamine until the partial thromboplastin time returns to normal.[212] Prosthetic valves themselves can cause thrombocytopenia and a shortened platelet survival following interaction of platelets with the valve surface.

References

1. Jepson, J. H., and Frankl, W. S.: Hematological Complications in Cardiac Practice. Philadelphia, W. B. Saunders Co., 1975.
2. Graettinger, J. S., Parsons, R. L., and Campbell, J. A.: A correlation of clinical and hemodynamic studies in patients with mild and severe anemia with and without congestive failure. Ann. Intern. Med. 58:617, 1963.
3. Levine, S. A.: Clinical Heart Disease. Philadelphia, W. B. Saunders Co., 1937, p. 50.
4. Eckstein, R. W.: Development of interarterial coronary anastomoses by chronic anemia. Disappearance following correction of anemia. Circ. Res. 3:306, 1955.
5. Rossi, M. A., Carillo, S. V., and Oliveria, J. S. M.: The effect of iron deficiency anemia in the rat on catecholamine levels and heart morphology. Cardiovasc. Res. 15:313, 1981.
6. Castle, W. B., and Minot, G. R.: Pathological Physiology and Clinical Description of the Anemias. New York, Oxford University Press, 1936, p. 2.
7. Blumgart, H. D., and Altschule, M. D.: Clinical significance of cardiac and respiratory adjustments in chronic anemia. Blood 3:329, 1948.
8. Duke, M., and Abelmann, W. H.: The hemodynamic response to chronic anemia. Circulation 39:503, 1969.
9. Varat, M. A., Adolph, R. J., and Fowler, N. O.: Cardiovascular effects of anemia. Am. Heart J. 83:415, 1972.
10. Torrance, J. D., Jacobs, P., Restrepo, A., Eschbach, J., Lenfant, C., and

11. Finch, C. A.: Intraerythrocyte adaptation to anemia. N. Engl. J. Med. 283:165, 1970.
11. Koch, H. H., and Schrofer, W.: Kompensatorische Veranderungen der erythrocytaren 2,3-DPG Konzentration bei Anamien und Polyglobulien. Monatsschr. Kinderheilkd. 121:392, 1973.
12. Oski, F. A., Marshall, B. D., Cohen, P. J., Sugerman, H. J., and Miller, L. D.: Exercise with anemia. The role of the left or right shifted oxygen-hemoglobin equilibrium curve. Ann. Intern. Med. 74:44, 1971.
13. Lenfant, C., Torrance, J., English, E., Finch, C. A., Reyafarje, C., Ramos, J., and Faura, J.: Effect of altitude on the oxygen binding by hemoglobin and on organic phosphate levels. J. Clin. Invest. 47:2652, 1968.
14. Oski, F. A., Gottlieb, A. J., Delivoria-Papadopoulos, M., and Miller, W. W.: Red-cell 2,3-diphosphoglycerate levels in subjects with chronic hypoxemia. N. Engl. J. Med. 280:1165, 1969.
15. Hunter, A.: The heart in anemia. Q. J. Med. 15:107, 1946.
16. Harris, T. N., Friedman, S., Tuncali, M. T., and Hallidie-Smith, K. A.: Comparison of innocent murmurs of childhood with cardiac murmurs in high output states. Pediatrics 33:341, 1964.
17. Braunwald, E.: Cyanosis, hypoxia, and polycythemia. In Petersdorf, R. F., et al.: Harrison's Principles of Internal Medicine. 10th ed. New York, McGraw-Hill, 1983, pp. 162.
18. Pearson, H. A., Spencer, R. P., and Cornelius, E. A.: Functional asplenia in sickle cell anemia. N. Engl. J. Med. 281:923, 1969.
19. Serjeant, G. R.: The Clinical Features of Sickle Cell Disease. Clinical Studies, Vol. 4. Amsterdam, North-Holland Publishing Co., 1974.
19a. Denenberg, B. S., Criner, G., Jones, R., and Spann, J. F.: Cardiac function in sickle cell anemia. Am. J. Cardiol. 51:1674, 1983.
20. Shubin, H., Kaufmann, R., Shapiro, M., and Levinson, D. C.: Cardiovascular findings in children with sickle cell anemia. Am. J. Cardiol. 6:875, 1960.
21. Perrine, R. P., Pembrey, M. E., John, P., Perrine, J. S., and Shoup, F.: Natural history of sickle cell anemia in Saudi Arabs; A study of 270 subjects. Ann. Intern. Med. 88:1, 1978.
22. Gerry, J. L., Bulkley, B. H., and Huktchins, G. M.: Clinicopathologic analysis of cardiac dysfunction in 52 patients with sickle cell anemia. Am. J. Cardiol. 42:211, 1978.
23. Donald, K. W., Bishop, J. M., Cumming, G., and Wade, O. L.: The effect of exercise on the cardiac output and circulatory dynamics of normal subjects. Clin. Sci. 14:37, 1955.
24. Rees, A. H., Stefadouras, M. A., Strong, W. B., Miller, M. D., Gilman, P., Rigby, J. A., and McFarlane, J.: Left ventricular performance in children with homozygous sickle cell anemias. Br. Heart J. 40:690, 1978.
25. Val-Mejias, J., Lee, W. K., Weisse, A. B., and Regan, T. J.: Left ventricular performance during and after sickle cell crisis. Am. Heart J. 97:589, 1979.
26. Rubler, S., and Fleischer, R. A.: Sickle cell states and cardiomyopathy. Sudden death due to pulmonary thrombosis and infarction. Am. J. Cardiol. 19:867, 1967.
27. Higgins, W. H., Jr.: The heart in sickle cell anemia. South. Med. J. 42:39, 1949.
28. Burnheimer, J., and Haywood, L. J.: Prevalence of hemoglobinopathies in patients with ischemic heart disease. J. Natl. Med. Assoc. 68:312, 1976.
29. Bookchin, R. M., and Nagel, R. L.: Ligand induced conformational dependence of hemoglobin in sickling interactions. J. Molec. Biol. 60:262, 1971.
30. Master, J., Engle, M. A., Stern, G., and Smith, C. H.: Cardiac complications of chronic severe refractory anemia with hemochromatosis. I. Acute pericarditis of unknown etiology. J. Pediatr. 58:455, 1961.
31. Ohene-Frempong, K., and Schwartz, E.: Clinical features of thalassemia. Pediatr. Clin. North Am. 27:403–420, 1980.
32. Henrich, H. C., and Gabbe, E. E.: Absorption of inorganic and food iron in children with heterozygous and homozygous beta-thalassemia. Z. Kinderheilk. 115:1, 1973.
33. Engel, M. A., Erlandson, M., and Smith, C. H.: Late cardiac complications of chronic severe refractory anemia with hemochromatosis. Circulation 30:698, 1964.
34. Ehlers, K. H., Levin, A. R., Klein, A. A., Markenson, A. L., O'Loughlin, J. E., and Engle, M. A.: The cardiac manifestations of thalassemia major: Natual history, noninvasive cardiac diagnostic studies and results of cardiac catheterization. In Engle, M. A. (ed.): Pediatric Cardiovascular Disease. Cardiovascular Clinics II (No. 2). Philadelphia, F. A. Davis Co., 1981, pp. 171–186.
35. Tahernia, A. C., and Vazirian, S.: Cardiac aspects of Cooley's anemia. South. Med J. 70:396, 1977.
36. Valdes-Cruz, L. M., Reinecke, C., Rutkowski, M., Dudell, G. G., Goldberg, S. J., Allen, H. D., Schu, D. J., and Piomelli, S.: Preclinical abnormal segmental cardiac manifestations of thalassemia major in children on transfusion-chelation therapy: Echographic alterations of left ventricular posterior wall contraction and relaxation patterns. Am. Heart J. 103:505, 1982.
37. Borow, K. M., Propper, R., Bierman, F. Z., et al.: The left ventricular end-systolic pressure-dimensions relation in patients with thalassemia major. A new noninvasive method for assessing contractile state. Circulation 66:980, 1982.
38. Dameshek, W., and Roth, S. I.: Case Records of the Massachusetts General Hospital — Weekly Clinicopathological Exercises. Case 52. N. Engl. J. Med. 271:898, 1964.
39. Westring, D. W.: Aortic valve disease and hemolytic anemia. Ann. Intern. Med. 65:203, 1966.

40. Miller, D. S., Mengel, C. E., Kremer, W. B., Gutterman, J., and Senningen, R.: Intravascular hemolysis in a patients with valvular heart disease. Ann. Intern. Med. 65:210, 1966.

41. Cooley, D. A., Bloodwell, R. D., and Beall, A. C.: Cardiac valve replacement without blood transfusions. J.A.M.A. 213:1032, 1970.

42. Hallowell, P., Bland, J. H., Buckley, M. J., and Lowenstein, E.: Transfusion of fresh autologous blood in open heart surgery: Method for reducing blood bank requirements. J. Thorac. Cardiovasc. Surg. 64:941, 1972.

43. Ruse, J. C., Hufnagel, C. A., Freis, C. D., Harvey, W. P., and Partonope, E. A.: The hemodynamic alterations produced by a plastic valvular prosthesis for severe aortic insufficiency in man. J. Lab. Clin. Med. 33:891, 1954.

44. Stohlman, F., Sarnoff, S. J., Case, R. B., and Ness, A. T.: Hemolytic syndrome following the insertion of a lucite ball valve prosthesis into the cardiovascular system. Circulation 13:586, 1956.

45. Sayed, H. M., Dacie, J. V., Handley, D. A., Lewis, S. M., and Cleland, W. P.: Hemolytic anemia of mechanical origin after open-heart surgery. Thorax 16: 356, 1961.

46. Dacie, J. V.: The Hemolytic Anemias. Part III. 2nd ed. New York, Grune and Stratton, 1967, p. 957.

47. Brodeur, M. T. H., Sutherland, D. W., Koler, R. D., Starr, A., Kimsey, J. A., and Griswold, H. E.: Red blood cell survival in patients with aortic valvular disease and ball valve prostheses. Circulation 32:570, 1965.

48. Sears, A. D., and Crosby, W. H.: Intravascular hemolysis due to intracardiac prosthetic devices. Diurnal variations related to activity. Am. J. Med. 39:341, 1965.

49. Pirofsky, B., Sutherland, D. W., Starr, A., and Griswold, H. E.: Hemolytic anemia complicating aortic-valve surgery. N. Engl. J. Med. 272:235, 1965.

50. Nevaril, C. G., Lynch, E. C., Alfrey, C. P., Jr., and Hellums, J.: Erythrocyte damage and destruction induced by shearing stress. J. Lab. Clin. Med. 71:784, 1968.

51. Schafer, A. I.: Iron overload. In Fairbanks, V. F. (ed.): Current Hematology. New York, John Wiley and Sons, 1981, pp. 191–218.

52. Simon, M., Bourel, M., Fauchet, R., et al.: Association of HLA-A3 and HLA-B14 antigens with idiopathic hemochromatosis. Gut 17:332, 1976.

53. Edwards, C. Q., Dadone, M. M., Skolnick, M. H., and Kushner, J. P.: Hereditary Hemochromatosis. Clin. Hematol. 11:411–435, 1982.

54. Swan, W. G. A., and Dewar, H. A.: The heart in hemochromatosis. Br. Heart J. 14:117, 1952.

55. Finch, S. C., and Finch, C. A.: Idiopathic hemochromatosis, an iron storage disease. Medicine 34:381, 1955.

56. James, T. N.: Pathology of the cardiac conduction system in hemochromatosis. N. Engl. J. Med. 271:92, 1964.

57. Wasserman, A. J., Richardson, D. W., Baird, C. L., and Wyso, E. M.: Cardiac hemochromatosis simulating constrictive pericarditis. Am. J. Med. 32:316, 1962.

58. Buja, L. M., and Roberts, W. C.: Iron in the heart. Etiology and clinical significance. Am. J. Med. 51:209, 1971.

59. Leon, M. B., Borer, J. S., Bacharach, S. L., Green, M. V., Benz, E. J., Griffith, P., and Neinhuis, A. W.: Detection of early cardiac dysfunction in patients with severe beta thalassemia and chronic iron overload. N. Engl. J. Med. 301: 1143–1148, 1979.

60. Easley, R. M., Schreiner, B. F., and Yu, P. N.: Reversible cardiomyopathy associated with hemochromatosis. N. Engl. J. Med. 287:866, 1972.

61. Skinner, C., and Kenmore, C. F.: Haemochromatosis presenting as congestive cardiomyopathy and responding to venesection. Br. Heart J. 35:466, 1973.

62. Schafer, A. I., Cheron, R. G., Dluhy, R., Cooper, B., Gleason, R. E., Soeldner, J. S., and Bunn, H. F.: Clinical consequences of acquired transfusional iron overload in adults. N. Engl. J. Med. 304:319–324, 1981.

63. Ley, T. J., Griffith, D., and Nienhuis, A. W.: Transfusion haemosiderosis and chelation therapy. Clin. Haematol. 11:437–464, 1982.

64. Schafer, A. I.: Treatment of iron overload with parenteral deferoxamines. In Update III to Isselbacher, K. J. (ed.): Harrison's Principles of Internal Medicine. New York, McGraw-Hill, 1982, pp. 157–166.

65. Cohen, A., and Schwartz, E.: Iron chelation therapy with deferoxamine in Cooley anemia. J. Pediatr. 92:643–647, 1978.

66. Nienhuis, A. W.: Vitamin C and iron. N. Engl. J. Med. 304:170–171, 1981.

67. Bunn, H. F.: Disorders of hemoglobin structure, function and synthesis. In Petersdorf, R. G., et al.: Harrison's Principles of Internal Medicine. 10th ed. New York, McGraw-Hill, 1983, pp. 1875.

68. Castle, W. B., and Jandl, J. H.: Blood viscosity and blood volume: Opposing influences upon oxygen transport in polycythemia. Semin. Hematol. 3:193, 1966.

69. Adamson, J. W.: Polycythemia vera. In Petersdorf, R. G., et al.: Harrison's Principles of Internal Medicine. 10th ed. New York, McGraw-Hill, 1983, pp. 1917.

70. Vaquez, H.: Sur une forme speciale de cyanose s'accompagnant d'hyperglobulie excessive et persistente. Compt. Rend. Soc. Biol. 4:384, 1892.

71. Osler, W.: Chronic cyanosis with polycythemia and enlarged spleen; A new clinical entity. Am. J. Med. Sci. 126:187, 1903.

72. Turk, W.: Beitrage zur Kenntnis des Symptomabbildes PKolyzythamie mit Mitztumor und Zyanose. Wien. Klin. Wochenschr. 17:153, 1904.

73. Adamson, J. W., and Fialkow, P. J.: Polycythemia vera: Stem-cell and probable clinical origin of the disease. N. Engl. J. Med. 245:913, 1976.

74. Berlin, N.: Diagnosis and classification of the polycythemias. Semin. Hematol. 12:339, 1976.

75. Dintenfass, L.: Viscosity and clotting of blood in venous thrombosis and coronary occlusion. Circ. Res. 14:1, 1964.

76. Dintenfass, L.: Viscosity of the packed red and white blood cells. Exp. Molec. Pathol. 4:597, 1965.

77. Thomas, D. J., Marshall, J., Russell, R. W., Wetherley-Mein, G., duBoulay, G. H., Pearson, T. C., Symon, L., and Zilkha, E.: Cerebral blood flow in polycythemia. Lancet 2:161, 1977.

78. Thomas, D. J., Marshall, J., Russell, R. W., Wetherley-Mein, G., duBoulay, G. H., Pearson, T. C., Symon, L., and Zilkha, E.: Effect of hematocrit on cerebral blood flow in man. Lancet 2:941, 1977.

79. Torrance, J. D., L'enfant, C., and Cruz, J.: Oxygen transport mechanisms in residents at high altitude. Respir. Physiol. 11:1, 1970.

80. Balcerzak, S. P., and Bromberg, P. A.: Secondary polycythemia. Semin. Hematol. 12:353, 1976.

81. Rosenthal, A., Button, L. N., and Nathan, D. G.: Blood volume changes in cyanotic congenital heart disease. Am. J. Cardiol. 29:162, 1971.

82. Golde, D. W., Hocking, W. G., Koeffler, H. P., and Adamson, J. W.: Polycythemia: Mechanism and management. Ann. Intern. Med. 95:71–871, 1981.

83. Rosenthal, A., Nathan, D. G., Marty, A. T., Button, L. N., Miettinen, O. S., and Nadas, A. S.: Acute hemodynamic effects of red cell production in polycythemia of cyanotic congenital heart disease. Circulation 42:297, 1970.

84. Willison, J. R., Thomas, D. J., duBoulay, G. H., et al.: Effect of high hematocrit on alertness. Lancet 1:846–848, 1980.

85. York, E. L., Junes, R. L., Menon, D., and Sproule, B. J.: Effects of secondary polycythemia on cerebral blood flow in chronic obstructive pulmonary disease. Am. Rev. Respir. Dis. 121:813–818, 1980.

86. Rosenthal, A., Mentzer, W. C., and Eisenstein, E. B.: The role of red blood cell organic phosphates in adaptation to congenital heart disease. Pediatrics 47: 537, 1971.

87. Clarache, S., Weatherall, D. J., and Clegg, J. B.: Polycythemia associated with a hemoglobinopathy. J. Clin. Invest. 45:813, 1966.

88. Adamson, J. W., and Finch, C. A.: Erythropoietin and the polycythemias. Ann. N.Y. Acad. Sci. 149:560, 1968.

89. Bromberg, P. A., Padilla, F., Boy, J. T., and Balcerzak, S. P.: Effect of a new hemoglobin (Hb Little Rock) on the physiology of oxygen delivery. J. Lab. Clin. Med. 78:837, 1971.

90. Chrache, S., Achuff, S., Winslow, R., Adamson, J., and Chevernick, P.: Variability of the homeostatic response to P50. Blood 52:1156, 1978.

91. Smith, J., and Landow, S. A.: Smoker's polycythemia. N. Engl. J. Med. 298:6, 1978.

92. Weinreb, N. J., and Shih, C. F.: Spurious polycythemia. Semin. Hematol. 12: 397–407, 1975.

93. Cohen, G. U., Perry, T. M., and Evans, J. M.: Neoplastic invasion of the heart and pericardium. Ann. Intern. Med. 42:12381, 1955.

94. Heath, D.: Pathology of cardiac tumors. Am. J. Cardiol. 21:315, 1968.

95. Roberts, W. C., Glancy, D. L., and DeVita, V. T.: Heart in malignant lymphoma. A study of 196 autopsy cases. Am. J. Cardiol. 22:85, 1968.

96. Petersen, C. D., Robinson, Q. A., and Kurnich, J. E.: Involvement of the heart and pericardium in the malignant lymphomas. Am. J. Med. Sci. 272:161, 1976.

97. Strauss, B. L., Matthews, M. J., and Cohen, M. H.: Cardiac metastases in lung cancer. Chest 71:607, 1977.

98. Waller, B. F., Gottdiener, J. S., Virmni, R., and Roberts, W. C.: Structure-function correlations in cardiovascular and pulmonary diseases—The charcoal heart. Chest 77:671, 1980.

99. Almange, C., Lebrestec, T., Louvet, M., Courgeon, P., Guerin, D., and Leborgne, P.: Bloc auriculo-ventriculaire complet par metastase cardiaque: A propos d'une observation. Sem. Hop. Paris 54:1419, 1978.

100. Lubell, D. L., and Goldfarb, C. R.: Metastatic cardiac tumor demonstrated by 201 thallium scan. Chest 78:98, 1980.

101. McDonnell, P. J., Becker, L. C., and Bulkley, B. H.: Thallium imaging in cardiac lymphoma. Am. Heart J. 101:809, 1981.

102. Markiewics, Q., Glatstein, E., London, E. J., and Popp, R. L.: Echocardiographic detection of pericardial effusion and pericardial thickening in malignant lymphoma. Radiology 123:161, 1977.

103. Lindsay, J., Goldberg, S. D., and Roberts, W. C.: Electrocardiogram in neoplastic and hematologic disorders. In Rios, J. C. (ed.): Controversies in Cardiology. Philadelphia, F. A. Davis Co., 1977, p. 225.

104. Seibert, K. A., Rettenmier, C. W., Waller, B. F., Battle, W. E., Levine, A. S., and Roberts, W. C.: Osteogenic sarcoma metastatic to the heart. Am. J. Med. 73:136, 1982.

105. Lloyd, E. A., and Curcio, C. A.: Lymphoma of the heart as an unusual cause of pericardial effusion. S. Afr. Med. J. 58:937, 1980.

106. Gunz, F. W., and Baikie, A. G. (eds.): Leukemia. New York, Grune and Stratton, 1974, pp. 255, 287–288.

107. Katz, R. J., Simms, E. B., DiBianco, R., et al.: Pericardial tamponade in lung cancer: Diagnosis, management and response to treatment. Am. J. Med. (in press).

108. Barton, J. C., and Durant, J. R.: Isolated chylopericardium associated with lymphoma. South. Med. J. 73:1551, 1980.

109. Posner, M. R., Cohen, G. I., and Skarin, A. T.: Pericardial disease in patients with cancer. The differentiation of malignant from idiopathic and radiation-induced pericarditis. Am. J. Med. 71:407, 1981.

110. Applefeld, M. M., and Spicer, K. M., Slawson, R. G., Singleton, R. T.,

Wesely, M., and Wiernick, P. H.: The long-term cardiac effects of radiotherapy in patients treated for Hodgkin's disease. Cancer Treat. Rep. 66: 1003, 1982.

111. Roberts, W. C., Bodey, G. P., and Wertlake, P. T.: The heart in acute leukemia. A study of 420 autopsy cases. Am. J. Cardiol. 21:388, 1968.

112. Wiernik, P. H., Sutherland, J. C., and Steelmiller, B. K.: Clinically significant cardiac infiltration in acute leukemia, lymphocytic lymphoma and plasma cell myeloma. Med. Pediatr. Oncol. 2:75, 1976.

113. Perez, C. A., Presant, C. A., and Amburg, A. L.: Management of superior vena cava syndrome. Semin. Oncol. 5:123, 1978.

113a. Koiwaya, Y., Nakamura, M., and Yamamoto, K.: Progressive ECG alterations in metastatic cardiac mural tumor. Am. Heart J. 105:339, 1983.

114. Cole, T. O., Attah, E. B., and Onyemelukwe, G. C.: Burkitt's lymphoma presenting with heart block. Br. Heart J. 37:94, 1975.

115. Ballentyne, F., VanderArk, C. R., and Holick, M.: Carotid sinus syncope and cervical lymphoma. Wis. Med. J. 74:91, 1975.

116. O'Neill, M. O., Marshall, A. J., and Watt, I.: Occult cardiac metastasis and mitral reflux. Br. J. Radiol. 52:669, 1979.

117. Inagaki, J., Rodriguez, V., and Body, G. P.: Causes of death in cancer patients. Cancer 33:568, 1974.

118. Kopelson, G., and Herwig, K. J.: The etiologies of coronary artery disease in cancer patients. Int. J. Radiol. Oncol. Biol. Phys. 4:895, 1978.

119. Stewart, J. R., and Fajardo, L. F.: Cancer and coronary artery disease. Int. J. Rad. Oncol. Biol. Phys. 11:915–916, 1978.

120. Deppisch, L. M., and Fayemi, A. O.: Non-bacteria thrombotic endocarditis. Am. Heart J. 92:723, 1976.

121. Lehto, V. P., Stenman, S., and Somer, T.: Immunohistological studies on valvular vegetations in nonbacterial thrombotic endocarditis. Arch. Pathol. Microbiol. Scand. 90:207, 1982.

122. Yam, L. T., Li, C. Y., Necheles, T. F., and Katayama, I.: Pseudo eosinophilic, eosinophilic endocarditis and eosinophilic leukemia. Am. J. Med. 53:193, 1972.

123. Oakley, C. M., and Olsen, E. G. J.: Eosinophilia and heart disease. Br. Heart J. 39:233, 1977.

123a. Applefeld, M. M., and Wiernik, P. H.: Cardiac disease after radiation therapy for Hodgkin's disease: Analysis of 48 patients. Am. J. Cardiol. 51:1679, 1983.

124. Taymor-Luria, H., Kohn, K., and Pasternak, R. C.: Radiation heart disease. J. Cardiovasc. Med. 8:113, 1983.

125. Applefeld, M. M., Cole, J. F., Pollock, S. H., Sutton, F. J., Slawson, R. G., Singleton, R. T., and Wiernik, P. H.: The late appearance of chronic pericardial disease in patients treated by radiotherapy for Hodgkin's disease. Ann. Intern. Med. 94:338, 1981.

126. Carmel, R. J., and Kaplan, H. S.: Mantle irradiation in Hodgkin's disease. Cancer 37:2813, 1976.

127. Morton, D. L., Glancy, D. L., Joseph, W. L., and Adkins, P. C.: Management of patients with radiation-induced pericarditis with effusion: A note on the development of aortic regurgitation in two of them. Chest 64:291, 1973.

128. Cohn, K. E., Stewart, J. R., Fajardo, L. F., and Hancock, E. W.: Heart disease following radiation. Medicine 46:281, 1967.

129. Cohen, S. I., Bharati, S., Glass, J., and Lev, M.: Radiotherapy as a cause of complete atrioventricular block in Hodgkin's Disease. Arch. Int. Med. 141: 676, 1981.

129a. Gottdiener, J. S., Katin, M. J. Borer, J. S., Bacharach, S. L., and Green, M. V.: Late cardiac effects of therapeutic mediastinal irradiation: Assessment by echocardiography and radionuclide angiography. N. Engl. J. Med. 308:569, 1983.

130. McReynolds, R. A., Gold, G. L., and Roberts, W. C.: Coronary heart disease after mediastinal irradiation for Hodgkin's disease. Am. J. Med. 60:39, 1976.

131. Iqbal, S. M., Hanson, E. L., and Gensini, G. D.: Bypass graft for coronary arterial stenosis following radiation therapy. Chest 71:664, 1977.

131a. Miller, D. D., Waters, D. D., Dangoisse, V., and David, P. R.: Symptomatic coronary artery spasm following radiotherapy for Hodgkin's disease. Chest 83: 284, 1983.

132. Silverberg, G. O., Britt, R. H., and Goffinet, D. R.: Radiation-induced carotid artery disease. Cancer 41:130, 1978.

133. Amromin, G. D., Gildenhorn, H. C., and Solomon, R. D.: The synergism of x-irradiation ad cholesterol-fat feeding on the development of coronary artery lesions. J. Atheroscler. Res. 4:325, 1975.

134. Brosius, F. C., Waller, B. F., and Roberts, W. C.: Radiation heart disease: Analysis of 16 young (aged 15 to 33 years) necropsy patients who received over 3500 rads to the heart. Am. J. Med. 70:519–530, 1981.

135. Carmichael, S. M., Eagleton, L., Ayers, C. R., and Mohler, D.: Orthostatic hypotension during vincristine therapy. Arch. Intern. Med. 126:290, 1970.

136. Mandel, E. M., Lewinski, U., and Djaldetti, M.: Vincristine-induced myocardial infarction. Cancer 36:1979, 1975.

137. Schoenberger, C. I., and Crystal, R.: Update IV to Isselbacker, K. J. (ed.): Harrison's Principles of Internal Medicine. New York, McGraw-Hill, 1982, pp. 49–74.

138. Young, R. C., Oxuls, R. F., and Myers, C. E.: The anthracycline antineoplastic drugs. N. Engl. J. Med. 305:139, 1981.

139. Lenaz, L., and Page, J. A.: Cardiotoxicity of adriamycin and related anthracyclines. Cancer Treat. Rev. 3:111, 1976.

140. Ali, M. K., Soto, P. A., Maroongroge, D., Bekheit-Saad, S., Buzdar, A. U., Blumenschein, G. R., Hortobagyi, G. N., Tashima, C. K., Wiseman, C. L., and Shullenberger, C. C.: Electrocardiographic changes after adriamycin chemotherapy. Cancer 43:465, 1979.

141. Wortman, J. E., Lucas, V. S., Jr., Schuster, E., Thiele, D., and Logue, G. L.: Sudden death during doxorubicin administration. Cancer 44:1588, 1979.

142. Greene, H. L., Reich, S. D., and Dalen, J. E.: How to minimize doxorubicin toxicity. J. Cardiovasc. Med. 7:306, 1982.

143. Merrill, J., Greco, F. A., Zimbler, H., Brereton, H. D., Lambert, J. D., and Pomeroy, T. C.: Adriamycin and radiation: Synergistic cardiotoxicity. Ann. Intern. Med. 82:122, 1975.

144. Fajardo, L. F., and Stewart, J. R.: Pathogenesis of radiation-induced myocardial fibrosis. Lab. Invest. 29:244, 1973.

145. O'Connell, T. X., and Berenbaum, M. D.: Cardiac and pulmonary effects of high doses of cyclophosphamide and isophosphamide. Cancer Res. 34:1586, 1974.

146. Mills, B. A., and Roberts, R. W.: Cyclophosphamide-induced cardiomyopathy. A report of two cases and a review of the English literature. Cancer 43:2223–2226, 1979.

147. Tritton, T. R., Murphree, S. A., and Sartorelli, A. C.: Adriamycin: A proposal on the specificity of drug action. Biochem. Biophys. Res. Commun. 84:802, 1978.

148. Lewis, W., Kleinerman, J. and Poszkin, S.: Interaction of adriamycin in vitro with cardiac myofibrillar proteins. Circ. Res. 50:547, 1982.

149. Myers, C. E., McGuire, W. P., Liss, R. H., Ifrim, I., Grotzmyer, K., and Young, R. C.: The role of lipid peroxidation in cardiac toxicity and tumor response. Science 197:165, 1977.

150. Alexander, J., Dainiak, T., Berger, H. J., Goldman, L., Johnstone, D., Reduto, L., Duffy, T., Schwartz, P., Gottschalk, A., and Zaret, B. L.: Serial assessment of doxorubicin cardiotoxicity with quantitative radionuclide angiocardiography. N. Engl. J. Med. 300:278, 1979.

151. Biancaniello, T., Meyer, R. A., Wong, K. Y., Sager, C., and Kaplan, S.: Doxorubicin cardiotoxicity in children. J. Pediatr. 97:45, 1980.

152. Henderson, I. C., Sloss, L. J., Jaffe, N., Blum, R. H., and Frei, E.: Serial studies of cardiac function in patients receiving adriamycin. Cancer Treat. Rep. 62:923, 1978.

153. Applefeld, M. M., and Pollock, S. H.: Cardiac disease in patients who have malignancies. Current Problems in Cardiology, Vol. 4. Chicago, Year Book Medical Publishers, 1980.

154. Gottdiener, J. S., Mathisen, D. J., Borer, J. S., Bonow, R. O., Myers, C. E., Barr, L. H., Schwartz, D. E., Bacharach, S. L., Green, M. V., and Rosenberg, S. A.: Doxorubicin cardiotoxicity: Assessment of late left ventricular dysfunction by radionuclide cineangiography. Ann. Intern. Med. 94:430, 1981.

155. Mason, J. W., Bristow, M. R., Billingham, M. E., and Daniels, J. R.: Invasive and non-invasive methods of assessing cardiotoxic effects in man: Superiority of histopathologic assessment using endomyocardial biopsy. Cancer Treat. Rep. 62:857, 1978.

156. Bristow, M. R., Mason, J. W., Billingham, M. E., and Daniels, J. R.: Doxorubicin cardiomyopathy. Evaluation by phonocardiography, endomyocardial biopsy and cardiac catheterization. Ann. Intern. Med. 88:168, 1978.

157. Bristow, M. R., Mason, J. W., Billingham, M. E., and Daniels, J. R.: Dose effect and structure-function relationships in doxorubicin cardiomyopathy. Am. Heart J. 102:709, 1981.

158. Von Hoff, D. D., Layard, M. W., Basa, P., Davis, H. L., Von Hoff, A. L., Rozencweig, M., and Muggia, F. M.: Risk factors for doxorubicin-induced congestive heart failure. Ann. Intern. Med. 91:710, 1979.

159. Doroshow, H. J., Locker, G. Y., Ifrim, I., and Myers, C. E.: Prevention of doxorubicin cardiac toxicity in the mouse by N-acetylcysteine. J. Clin. Invest. 68:1053, 1981.

160. Cortes, E. P., Gupta, M., Chew, C., Amin, V. C., and Folker, K.: Adriamycin cardiotoxicity: Early detection by systolic time interval and possible prevention by Coenzyme Q. Cancer Treat. Rep. 62:887, 1978.

161. Somberg, J., Cagin, N., Levitt, L. B., et al.: Blockade of tissue uptake of the antineoplastic agent, doxorubicin. J. Pharmacol. Exp. Ther. 204:226, 1978.

162. Legla, S. S., Benjamin, R. S., MacKay, B., Ewer, M., Wallace, S., Valdirieso, M., Rasmussen, S. L., Blumenschein, G. R., and Freireich, E. J.: Reduction of doxorubicin cardiotoxicity by prolonged continuous intravenous infusion. Ann. Intern. Med. 96:133, 1982.

163. Gottdiener, J. S., Appelbaum, F. R., Ferrans, V. J., Deiseroth, A., and Ziegler, J.: Cardiotoxicity associated with high dose cyclophosphamide therapy. Arch. Intern. Med. 141:758, 1981.

164. Steinherz, L. J., Steinherz, P. G., Mangiacasale, D., Tan, C., and Miller, D. R.: Cardiac abnormalities after AMSA administration. Cancer Treat. Rep. 66: 483, 1982.

165. Gavras, I., Graff, L. G., Rose, B. D., McKenna, J. M., Brunner, H. R., and Gavras, H.: Fatal pancytopenia associated with the use of captopril. Ann. Intern. Med. 94:58–59, 1981.

166. Lundh, B., and Hasselgren, K. H.: Hematological side effects from antihypertensive drugs. Acta Med. Scand. (Suppl. 628):73, 1979.

167. Pisciotta, A. V.: Drug-induced leukopenia and aplastic anemia. Clin. Pharmacol. Ther. 12:13, 1971.

168. deGruchy, G. C.: Agranulocytosis. In deGruchy, G. C. (ed.): Drug-induced Blood Disorders. London, Blackwell, 1975, pp. 76–117.

169. Ansell, J., McCue, J., Tiarks, C., Prilla, N., Rybak, M. E., and Benotti, J.: Amrinone-induced thrombocytopenia. Blood 58(Suppl. 1):187a, 1981.

170. Shulman, N. R.: Immunologic reactions to drugs. N. Engl. J. Med. 247:409,1972.

171. Belkin, G. A.: Cocktail purpura: An unusual cause of quinine sensitivity. Ann. Intern. Med. 66:583, 1967.

172. Bell, W. R., Tomasulo, P. A., Alvirx, B. N., and Duffy, J. P.: Thrombocytope-

nia occurring during the administration of heparin. A prospective study in 52 patients. Ann. Intern. Med. 85:155, 1976.

173. Salzman, E. W., Rosenberg, R. D., Smith, M. H., Lindon, J. N., and Favreau, L.: Effect of heparin and heparin fractions on platelet aggregation. J. Clin. Invest. 65:64, 1980.

174. Gibson, G. R., Hunter, J. B., Raabe, D. S., Manjoney, D. L., and Ittlema, F. P.: Methemoalbuminemia produced by high dose intravenous nitroglycerin. Ann. Intern. Med. 96:615–616, 1982.

175. Palmer, R. F., and Lasseter, R. C.: Drug therapy: Sodium nitroprusside. N. Engl. J. Med. 292:294, 1975.

176. Virchow, R.: Gesammelte Abhandlungen zur wissenschaftlichen Medizin. Frankfurt, Meidenger Sohn, 1856.

177. Weiss, H. J.: Platelet physiology and abnormalities of platelet function. N. Engl. J. Med. 293:531, 1975.

178. Weiss, H. J.: Antiplatelet agents: Current status in treating cardiovascular disease. J. Cardiovasc. Med., 5:921, 1980.

179. Mehta, J., and Mehta, P.: Platelets and prostaglandins in cardiovascular disease. Mt. Kisko, N.Y., Futura Publishing, 1981.

180. Aoki, N., Saito, H., Kamiya, T., Koie, K., Sakata, Y., and Ksbakukra, M.: Congenital deficiency of α 2 plasmin inhibitor associated with a severe hemorrhagic tendency. J. Clin. Invest. 63:877, 1979.

181. Aoki, N., Muroi, M., Sakata, Y., Yoshida, N., and Matsuda, M.: Abnormal plasminogen. A hereditary molecular abnormality found in a patient with recurrent thrombosis. J. Clin. Invest. 61:1186, 1978.

182. Stead, N., Kinney, T., Bauer, K., Lewis, J., Shipman, M., Campbell, E., Rosenberg, R., and Pizzo, S.: Familial thrombosis secondary to diminished vascular plasminogen activator. Blood 58(Suppl. 1):540a, 1981.

183. Hirsh, J.: Hypercoagulability. Semin. Hematol. 14:409, 1977.

184. Dear, H. D., and Jones, W. B.: Myocardial infarction associated with the use of oral contraceptives. Ann. Intern. Med. 74:236, 1971.

185. Masi, A. T., and Dugdale, M.: Cerebrovascular disease associated with the use of oral contraceptives. Ann. Intern. Med. 72:111, 1970.

186. Handin, R. I.: Thromboembolic complications of pregnancy and oral contraceptives. Prog. Cardiovasc. Dis. 16:395, 1974.

187. Sas, G., Pepper, D. S., and Cash, J. D.: Plasma and serum antithrombin III: Differentiation by crossed immunoelectrophoresis. Thromb. Res. 6:87, 1975.

188. Esmon, C. T., and Owen, W. G.: Identification of an endothelial cell co-factor for thrombin-catalyzed activation of protein C. Proc. Natl. Acad. Sci. USA 78: 2249, 1981.

189. Griffin, J. H., Evat, B., Zimmerman, T. S., Kleiss, A. J., and Wideman, C.: Deficiency of protein C in congenital thrombotic disease. J. Clin. Invest. 68: 1370, 1981.

190. Comp, P. C., Esmon, C. T.: Generation of fibrinolytic activity by infusion of activated protein C into dogs. J. Clin. Invest. 68:1221, 1981.

191. Stemerman, M. B., Baumgartner, H. J. R., and Spaet, T. H.: The subendothelial microfibril and platelet adhesion. Lab. Invest. 24:179, 1971.

192. Wu, K. K., Barnes, R. W., and Hoak, J. C.: Platelet hyperaggregability in idiopathic recurrent deep vein thrombosis. Circulation 53:687, 1976.

193. Wu, K. K.: Platelet hyperaggregability and thrombosis in patients with thrombocythemia. Ann. Intern. Med. 88:7, 1978.

194. Bolton, A. E., Ludlam, C. A., Pepper, D. S., Moore, S., and Cahs, J. D.: A radioimmunoassay for platelet factor 4. Thromb. Res. 8:51, 1976.

195. Handin, R. I., McDonough, M., and Lesch, M.: Elevation of platelet factor found in acute myocardial infarction: Measurement by radioimmunoassay. J. Lab. Clin. Med. 91:340, 1978.

196. Mustard, J. F., and Packham, M. A.: Platelets and diabetes mellitus. N. Engl. J. Med. 297:1345, 1978.

197. Friedman, M., and Rosenman, R. H.: Type A Behaviour and Your Heart. London, Wildwood House, 1974.

198. Rosenberg, R. D.: The function of heparin. In Kakkar, V. V., and Thomas, D. P. (eds.): Heparin: Chemistry and Clinical Usage. London, Academic Press, 1976. p. 101.

199. Thomas, D. P.: Heparin and venous thromboembolism. Semin. Hematol. 15:1, 1978.

200. Lahnborg, G., Bergstrom, K., and Furman, L.: Effect of low dose haparin on incidence of postoperative pulmonary embolism detected by photoscanning. Lancet 1:329, 1974.

201. An International Multicentre Trial: Prevention of fatal postoperative pulmonary embolism by low doses of heparin. Lancet 2:45, 1975.

202. Brozuric, M.: Oral anticoagulants in clinical practice. Semin. Hematol. 15:27, 1978.

203. Berger, S., and Solomon, E. W.: Thromboembolic complications of prosthetic devices. Prog. Hemost. Thromb. 2:273, 1974.

204. The Canadian Cooperative Study Group: A randomized trial of aspirin and sulfinpyrazone in threatened stroke. N. Engl. J. Med. 299:53, 1978.

205. The Anturane Reinfarction Trial Research Group: Sulfinpyrazone in the prevention of sudden death after myocardial infarction. N. Engl. J. Med. 302: 250, 1980.

206. Cheseboro, J. H., Clements, I. P., Fuster, V., Elverback, L. R., Smith, H. C., Bardsley, W. T., Frye, R. L., Holmes, D. R., Jr., Vlietstra, R. E., Pluth, J. R., Wallace, R. B., Puga, F. J., Orszulak, T. A., Piehler, J. M., Schaff, H. V., and Danielson, G. K.: A platelet-inhibitor-drug trial in coronary-artery bypass operations: Benefit of perioperative dipyridamole and aspirin therapy on early postoperative vein-graft patency. N. Engl. J. Med. 307:73, 1982.

207. Goldschmidt, B., Sarkadi, B., Gardos, G., and Matlary, A.: Platelet production and survival in cyanotic congenital heart disease. Scand. J. Haematol. 13 :10, 1974.

208. Bhargava, M., Sangal, S. K., Thapar, M. K., Kumar, S., and Hooja, V.: Impairment of platelet adhesiveness and platelet factor 3 activity in cyanotic congenital heart disease. Acta Haematol. 55:216, 1976.

209. Gupta, B., Jindal, S. K., Mohanty, D., Das, K. C., Bidwal, P. S., and Wahi, P. L.: Abnormalities of haemostasis associated with congenital heart disease. Indian Heart J. 29:27, 1977.

210. Bick, R. L., Arbegast, N., Crawford, L., Holerman, M., Adams, T., and Schmalhorst, W.: Hemostatic defects induced by cardiopulmonary bypass. Vasc. Surg. 9:228, 1975.

211. Umlas, J.: Fibrinolysis and disseminated intravascular coagulation in open heart surgery. Transfusion 16:460, 1976.

212. Moriau, M., Masure, R., Horlet, A., Debeys, C., Chalant, C., Panlot, R., Jaumain, P., Servage-Kestens, Y., Ravaux, A., Louis, A., and Goenen, M.: Haemostasis disorders in open heart surgery with extracorporeal circulation. Vox Sang. 32:41, 1977.

50 NEUROLOGICAL DISORDERS AND HEART DISEASE

by Joseph K. Perloff, M.D.

Cardiovascular disorders occur as consequences of diseases of the nervous system, and, conversely, disorders of the nervous system can be secondary to heart disease. This chapter concentrates on the interplay between cardiology and neurology and focuses on seven general topics: (1) major heredofamilial neuromyopathic disorders in which cardiac disease is an inherent part, (2) less common neuromyopathic diseases that are sometimes associated with disorders of the heart, (3) neuromuscular disorders presenting as cardiomyopathy, (4) electrocardiographic and vasomotor abnormalities accompanying cerebrovascular accidents, (5) cardiac complications of drugs used in treating neuromuscular diseases, and (6) neurological complications of therapy for cardiovascular disease. Cardiac causes of syncope are discussed in Chapter 28. Neurological complications associated with congenital and acquired heart disease are discussed in the chapters dealing with the specific disorders.

MAJOR HEREDOFAMILIAL NEUROMYOPATHIC DISORDERS

Involvement of the heart is an inherent part of three major heredofamilial neuromyopathic disorders—the progressive muscular dystrophies, myotonic dystrophy, and Friedreich's ataxia.[1] The majority of nonmyotonic progressive muscular dystrophies fall into the following categories:

1. X-linked progressive muscular dystrophy

A. Early onset, rapidly progressive (classic Duchenne's dystrophy)
B. Late onset, slowly progressive (Becker's muscular dystrophy)
2. Early onset, slowly progressive dystrophy (autosomal recessive)
3. Limb-girdle dystrophy of Erb
4. Facioscapulohumeral dystrophy of Landouzy-Déjérine

Evidence of cardiovascular disease—subtle or overt—has been found in each of these major categories, although with varying frequency and severity.[1]

Progressive Muscular Dystrophies

X-LINKED PROGRESSIVE MUSCULAR DYSTROPHY

Classic Duchenne's muscular dystrophy is sex-linked recessive, transmitted by the mother to one half of her sons as overt disease, and to half of her daughters as a carrier state.[1,2] (For a discussion of this mode of inheritance, see pp. 1608 and 1624.) Because of its recessive inheritance and an apparently very high new mutation rate, sporadic cases are as frequent as 30 per cent. Pseudohypertrophy of the ca especially marked early in the course of the disease, and weakness and contractures result in talipes equinovarus (Fig. 50–1). Dystrophy of chest muscles and diaphragm (Fig. 50–2) interferes with coughing and breathing. Patients are likely to succumb to pulmonary infection in the second decade, although cardiac disease is an

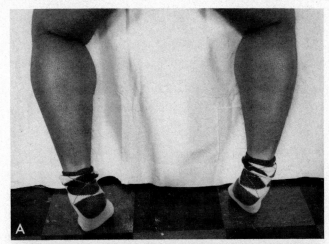

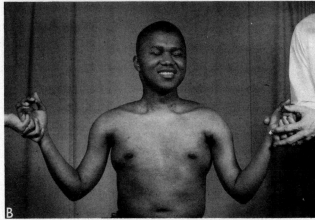

FIGURE 50–1 *A*, Classic Duchenne's progressive muscular dystrophy in a 14-year-old boy with typical calf pseudohypertrophy. The feet show talipes equinovarus. *B*, The deltoid and pectoral muscles exhibit striking pseudohypertrophy. (From Perloff, J. K.: The myocardial disease of heredofamilial neuromyopathies. *In* Fowler, N. O. (ed.): Myocardial Disease. New York, 1973, by permission of Grune and Stratton.)

important and, at times, dramatic cause of death.[1] Rapidly progressive preterminal heart failure may follow years of circulatory stability during which the only suspicion of cardiac involvement is the abnormal electrocardiogram.

Physical and radiographic examinations of the heart are often altered by thoracic deformities and diaphragmatic dystrophy (Fig. 50–2). A decrease in anteroposterior chest dimensions may be responsible for a systolic impulse at the left sternal edge, a grade 1 to 3/6, short, impure, midsystolic murmur in the second left intercostal space, and a loud pulmonic component of the second heart sound (palpable and audible).[1,3] These signs should not be taken as evidence of pulmonary hypertension. There is an increased prevalence of both third and fourth heart sounds (quadruple rhythms), and occasionally a patient has mitral regurgitation not because of heart failure but because of dystrophic scarring of a papillary muscle and adjacent left ventricular wall.[4,5] An increase in transverse heart size may be caused by high diaphragm (Fig. 50–2) or narrow anteroposterior chest dimensions rather than by ventricular dilatation.

Heart rates tend to be rapid, with patients exhibiting persistent or labile sinus tachycardia.[1,4] The combination of excessive rate acceleration after atropine followed by effec-

tive slowing with propranolol seems to discount the role of the parasympathetic nervous system and implicate augmented sympathetic activity as the cause of the resting tachycardia in Duchenne's dystrophy.[6] In addition, a variety of tachyarrhythmias occur, including ectopic atrial and ventricular beats, atrial flutter, paroxysmal ventricular tachycardia, and exaggerated irritability during cardiac catheterization.[1] Degeneration of nerve fibers to the cardiac nodes has not been consistently found at necropsy,[4] and occlusive disease of small coronary arteries to the sinoatrial and atrioventricular nodes appears to be rare[4,7] (Fig. 50–3).

By far the most reliable tool in suspecting cardiac involvement is the electrocardiogram.[1,4,8–11] Although a variety of neuromyopathic disorders are associated with abnormal scalar electrocardiograms, only one, the classic X-linked pseudohypertrophic dystrophy of Duchenne, results in a distinctive, recurrent, uniform electrocardiographic pattern (Fig. 50–4); the vectorcardiogram is a useful supplement to the scalar electrocardiogram.[12,13]

Tall R waves over the right precordium with increased R/S amplitude ratios, and deep Q waves in limb leads and over the left lateral precordium form a distinctive pattern (Fig. 50–4),[4,8] which is also occasionally found in female carriers.[10,14,15] At times, the deep Q waves coexist with al-

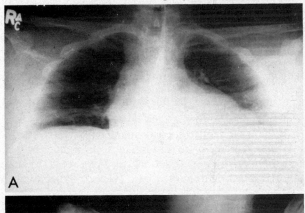

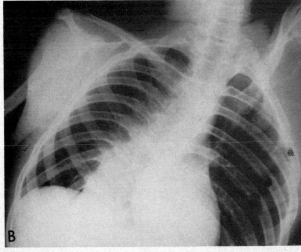

FIGURE 50–2 Roentgenograms of two patients with classic X-linked Duchenne's muscular dystrophy. *A*, Nine-year-old boy with striking symmetrical elevation of the diaphragm (diaphragmatic dystrophy). The transverse dimensions of the heart are accordingly increased. *B*, Eleven-year-old boy with distortion of the heart because of marked scoliosis to the right. (From Perloff, J. K.: The myocardial disease of heredofamilial neuromyopathies. *In* Fowler, N. O. (ed.): Myocardial Disease. New York, 1973, by permission of Grune and Stratton.)

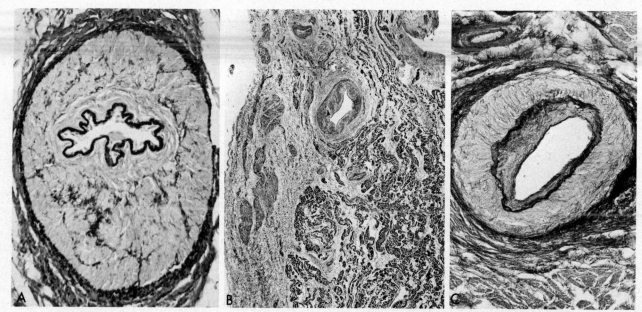

FIGURE 50–3 Small intramural coronary arteries in X-linked Duchenne's dystrophy. *A,* Small coronary artery from the left atrium of an 18-year-old boy. There is severe hypertrophy of the media with marked luminal narrowing (Verhoeff–van Gieson elastic tissue stains). *B,* Section from the right atrium in the region of the sinus node in the same patient. The neurogenic fibers of the sinus node are seen as well as an intramural coronary artery that has a thick wall and slightly narrowed lumen. Staining disclosed increased quantities of mucopolysaccharides in the vessel wall. *C,* Right atrial intramural coronary artery from a 12-year-old boy. The vessel exhibits a thick media and intima and a narrowed lumen (elastic tissue stain). (From Perloff, J. K., et al.: The distinctive electrocardiogram of Duchenne's muscular dystrophy. Am. J. Med. *42:*179, 1967.)

tered shapes of right precordial R waves (RSr'or polyphasic R waves). The electrocardiographic changes in Duchenne's dystrophy are *not* related to thoracic deformity, thoracic muscle atrophy, or pulmonary hypertension; to hypertrophy of the right ventricle, crista supraventricularis, or interventricular septum; or to abnormalities in right ventricular conduction.[1,4] Striking abnormalities have been found in small intramural coronary arteries (severe hypertrophy of

the media with luminal narrowing) (Fig. 50–3), but the arteriopathy was not related to the electrocardiographic pattern or to the distribution of myocardial dystrophy[4,16] (see below). The occurrence of identical electrocardiograms in siblings with Duchenne's dystrophy implies a genetic determinant of the distinctive patterns.

The prominent anterior forces (anterior shift of the QRS vector loop) appear to represent a relative loss of

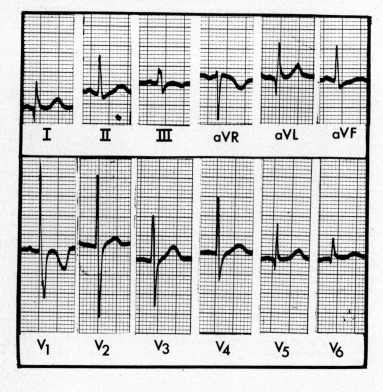

FIGURE 50–4 Electrocardiogram from a 12-year-old boy with classic Duchenne's progressive dystrophy. There is a tall R wave in lead V₁ in addition to deep Q waves in leads I and aVL. At necropsy myocardial dystrophy was found to be confined to the posterolateral left ventricular wall. (From Perloff, J. K.: The distinctive electrocardiogram of Duchenne's muscular dystrophy. Am. J. Med. *42:*179, 1967.)

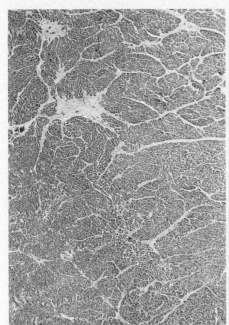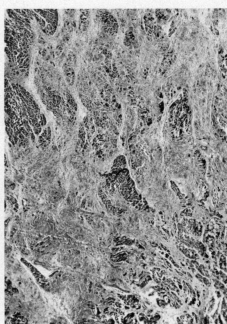

FIGURE 50–5 Photomicrographs from an 18-year-old boy who died of classic Duchenne's progressive muscular dystrophy. The ventricular septum (left) shows only a few microscopic scars, whereas the posterobasal left ventricular wall (right) is extensively scarred (hematoxylin and eosin stains). (From Perloff, J. K., et al.: The distinctive electrocardiogram of Duchenne's muscular dystrophy. Am. J. Med. *42*:179, 1967.)

posterobasal electrical activity, as in strictly posterior myocardial infarction,[1,4,13,17] and the Q waves may reflect lateral or diaphragmatic extension.[4,13] Necropsy studies have disclosed selective transmural scarring of the posterobasal left ventricle with or without lateral or inferior wall extension (Figs. 50–5 and 50–6), providing acceptable electrocardiographic/vectorcardiographic/necropsy correlations.[4,5,16] Positron computed tomography using F-18 deoxyglucose and

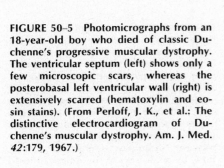

FIGURE 50–6 Diagram of the left side of the heart illustrating the location of myocardial dystrophy at necropsy. Scarring was limited to the posterolateral wall of the left ventricle. No significant scarring was observed in the inferior wall or in the ventricular septum. A papillary muscle was scarred in one patient who had clinical mitral regurgitation. (Courtesy of William C. Roberts, M.D., Pathology Branch, National Heart, Lung and Blood Institute, Bethesda, Maryland.)

N-13 ammonia has identified a regional metabolic abnormality in the posterior and posterolateral left ventricular wall.[18] Thus, the cardiomyopathy of Duchenne's dystrophy appears to be a unique form of heart disease in which a specific segment of ventricular myocardium is genetically labeled as the target site. Dystrophic involvement of the posterobasal left ventricle and contiguous posterior papillary muscle may cause mitral regurgitation (papillary muscle dysfunction),[4] sometimes with mitral prolapse seen on echocardiography.[5,19] Evaluation of left ventricular function by echocardiography provides additional information, especially on wall motion.[20]

Enzymes of skeletal muscle are copiously released into the plasma in Duchenne's dystrophy. This release, especially of creatine kinase, has been used to identify active systemic myopathy. However, the use of enzyme or isoenzyme quantification has not proved useful in detecting myocardial dystrophy.[1] It was hoped that distinctive isozyme profiles—both lactic dehydrogenase (LDH) and MB creatine phosphokinase (CPK)—might be used to identify active myocardial dystrophy, but these enzymes originate in dystrophic skeletal muscle and merely resemble those of cardiac muscle, compromising the specificity of the determinations.[2,21] Further, coronary sinus catheterization has not convincingly documented myocardial release of enzymes.[1] Measurement of creatine kinase has been established as a means of identifying "preclinical" systemic dystrophy in male siblings of propositi[22] and in female carriers in families with Duchenne's progressive muscular dystrophy.[14,15,23] The majority (about two-thirds) of female carriers of X-linked muscular dystrophy have elevated serum creatine kinase.[21] These female carriers sometimes manifest occult or overt muscle weakness and calf pseudohypertrophy[15,24] in addition to electrocardiographic evidence of cardiac involvement.[10,14,15]

SLOWLY PROGRESSIVE MUSCULAR DYSTROPHY OF EARLY ONSET.[25,26] Dystrophy with the phenotype of Duchenne may be slowly progressive and either early-onset, autosomal recessive, or late-onset, X-linked recessive (Becker's dystrophy) (Fig. 50–7). When family ped-

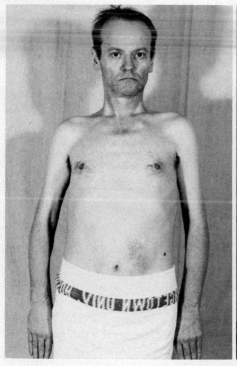
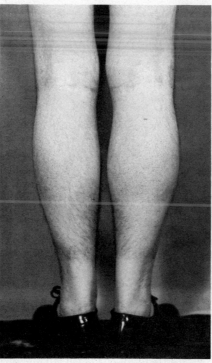

FIGURE 50–7 A 40-year-old man believed to have late-onset, slowly progressive Duchenne's muscular dystrophy (Becker's dystrophy). He died because of cardiomyopathy and complete heart block (see Fig. 49–12). Dystrophy of shoulder girdle, arms, pelvic girdle, and proximal leg muscle is seen, with mild asymmetrical pseudohypertrophy of the calves. (From Perloff, J. K., et al.: The cardiomyopathy of progressive muscular dystrophy. Circulation *33*:625, 1966, by permission of the American Heart Association, Inc.)

igrees are deficient, it is difficult to distinguish these two subvarieties from each other or from limb-girdle dystrophy of Erb with calf pseudohypertrophy.[1] Such patients may not only have cardiomyopathy[27] but stand a good chance of dying from it[1] (Fig. 50–8). The type of cardiac involvement differs from classic Duchenne's dystrophy.[1] The ventricles dilate and fail (biventricular dystrophy) with abnormalities of infranodal conduction (left bundle branch block and complete heart block) (Fig. 50–8).[1] In families with Becker's X-linked muscular dystrophy, congestive cardiomyopathy may appear in one member while other members are clinically spared.[27]

LIMB-GIRDLE DYSTROPHY OF ERB. Transmission is typically autosomal recessive, with insidious onset usually in the second decade.[28] Dystrophy of the hip girdle usually precedes involvement of the shoulders (Fig. 50–9A). Calf pseudohypertrophy occurs, but this is relatively late in onset and mild to moderate in degree[28] (Fig. 50–10). Progression is slow, but the majority of affected individuals are incapacitated within two decades. Although cardiac involvement is infrequent and seldom severe, it is expressed as (1) disturbances in rhythm and conduction, namely, sinus bradycardia (sick sinoatrial node), (2) atrial flutter (tachycardia), (3) first-degree heart block (abnormal atrioventricular node), and (4) complete right bundle branch block, QRS prolongation, and complete heart block (infranodal disease) (Table 50–1). Sporadic patients with limb-girdle dystrophy of Erb have both cardiomyopathy *and* extensive disease of the cardiac conducting system (sinus node, atrioventricular node, and infranodal tissue).[29,30]

TABLE 50–1 NEUROMUSCULAR
DISEASES WITH COMPLETE HEART BLOCK

Myotonic muscular dystrophy
Kearns-Sayre syndrome
X-linked humeroperoneal dystrophy
Peroneal muscular atrophy
Limb-girdle dystrophy

FACIOSCAPULOHUMERAL DYSTROPHY (LANDOUZY-DÉJÉRINE). Transmission is autosomal dominant (equal incidence in males and females) with onset from the first to fourth decades. Dystrophy begins in the shoulder girdle (scapulohumeral) (Fig. 50–9B) with inevitable progression to the muscles of facial expression (thus "*facio*scapulohumeral"). There is subsequent spread to the pelvic girdle. Myocardial involvement in facioscapulohumeral dystrophy seldom occurs and as a rule is clinically unimportant,[1] but sporadic examples have been cited.[31,32]

The most dramatic and intriguing cardiac disorder associated with facioscapulohumeral dystrophy is permanent paralysis of the atria (atrial standstill).[33] It is of interest that the first documentation of atrial paralysis was in a patient with facioscapulohumeral muscular dystrophy.[34] Criteria for the diagnosis include absence of P waves on scalar, esophageal, and intracardiac electrocardiograms, lack of atrial response to direct (intracardiac) electrical stimulation, absence of *a* waves in the jugular venous and right atrial pressure pulses, a supraventricular QRS, and immobility of the atria on fluoroscopy.[33,35]

Myotonic Muscular Dystrophy

Myotonic dystrophy (dystrophia myotonica, myotonia atrophica, or Steinert's disease) is a slowly progressive, multisystem, autosomal dominant disorder.[36,37] Clinical manifestations characteristically appear in the third or fourth decade,[38] although occasional cases are seen in childhood and infancy. Myotonia (delayed relaxation after contraction) can be provoked by voluntary, mechanical, or electrical stimulation of muscles of the hands, forearms, tongue, and jaw. The myotonic response is typically elicited by tapping the thenar eminence (percussion myotonia), especially after the patient rapidly opens and closes the fist. Dystrophy (atrophy or wasting) is initially found

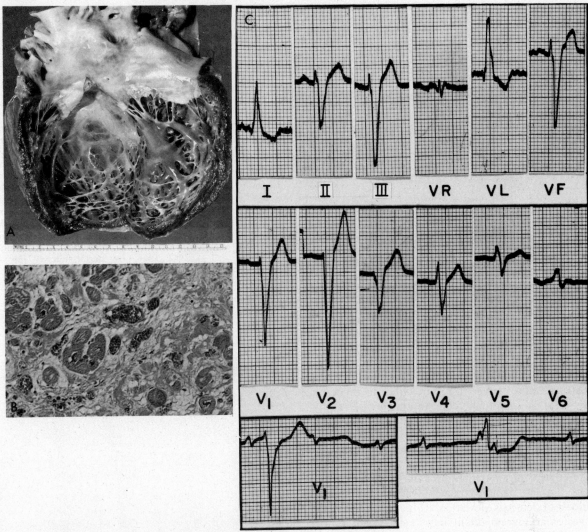

FIGURE 50–8 Gross and microscopic cardiac pathological specimens and the electrocardiogram from a 45-year-old man with late-onset, slowly progressive Becker's muscular dystrophy. *A,* Dilated, flabby left ventricle with focal endocardial thickening. The left atrium is also dilated. *B,* Microscopic section from the left ventricle shows marked confluent scarring with variations in fiber size; there was no significant coronary artery disease. *C,* Electrocardiogram recorded at age 40 years. The 12-lead tracing shows left-axis deviation, a QRS of 0.14 sec, small q waves in leads I and aVL and loss of R-wave amplitude in leads V_2 and V_3. The lower tracings, taken 4 years later (a year before death), show complete heart block with a variable QRS configuration. (From Perloff, J. K., et al.: The cardiomyopathy of progressive muscular dystrophy. Circulation *33*:625, 1966, by permission of the American Heart Association, Inc.)

in forearms, neck (especially sternocleidomastoid), and face (expressionless myopathic facies) (Fig. 50–11).[36,38] There is subsequent disturbance of the extensors of the knees and hips and dorsiflexors of the feet.[38] Myotonic dystrophy is a systemic disease that includes important nonmyotonic/nonmyopathic features: cataracts, gonadal atrophy, frontal baldness or thinning of hair (Fig. 50–11), and disease of muscles of the upper gastrointestinal tract.[36,38] Appropriate to this discussion is the cardiac involvement which has been known since the descriptions of Griffith in 1911.[39] Myotonia congenita (Thomsen's disease) with rare exception[40] does not involve the heart and is otherwise distinct from myotonic dystrophy.[41]

Apart from electrocardiographic abnormalities (see below), there is usually little overt clinical evidence of heart disease.[38,41–44] Even so, myotonic dystrophy may *present* as cardiac disease before the neuromuscular diagnosis has

been established.[37,38,42,45–47] Cardiac involvement selectively disturbs impulse formation and conduction (Table 50–2).[37–39,41–44,46,48–57] Despite light microscopic[43,47,49,58] and ultrastructural abnormalities,[59,60] clinically detectable myocardi-

TABLE 50–2 ELECTROCARDIOGRAPHIC ABNORMALITIES IN MYOTONIC MUSCULAR DYSTROPHY

Disorders of impulse formation
  Sinus bradycardia
  Atrial flutter
  Atrial fibrillation
  Ventricular tachycardia
Disturbances in conduction
  AV nodal (P-R prolongation)
  Intra-His
  Infra-His (LAD, LBBB, RBBB,
    complete heart block)

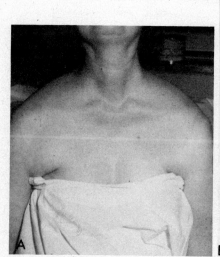
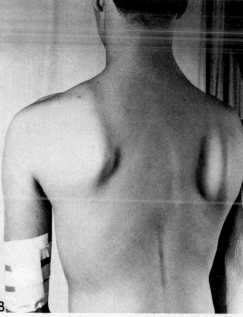

FIGURE 50–9 *A*, Woman with typical limb-girdle dystrophy (Erb's) showing involvement of the shoulder girdle. The proximal leg muscles and pelvic girdle were also involved, but her face was completely spared. *B*, Young man with facio-scapulohumeral dystrophy (Landouzy-Déjérine) involving the shoulder girdle, proximal arm muscle (bandage at biopsy site), and face (not shown). (From Perloff, J. K., et al.: The cardiomyopathy of progressive muscular dystrophy. Circulation *33*:625, 1966, by permission of the American Heart Association, Inc.)

al disease is not a feature of myotonic dystrophy.[51] Nor is myocardial myotonia known to occur, either in myotonic dystrophy[49,61] or in myotonia congenita (Thomsen's disease). The earliest and most common electrocardiographic abnormalities are sinus bradycardia and prolongation of the P-R interval. Bradycardia[54] may be punctuated by episodes of tachycardia (atrial flutter or fibrillation).[37,38,41,47,62] The most frequent infranodal abnormality is defective conduction in the left bundle branch system (left bundle branch block or left-axis deviation) (Fig. 50–12),[37,41,42,44,51] and the vectorcardiogram often shows evidence of abnormal intraventricular conduction.[41,43,51,62] Left bundle branch block may initially be intermittent.[62] Both procainamide and phenytoin are used as antimyotonic agents.[46] However, it is preferable to use phenytoin, which shortens the atrioventricular nodal refractory period and has little or no effect on infranodal conduction; procainamide prolongs both AV nodal and infranodal conduction.[46] In addition to the disorders in rhythm and conduction listed in Table 50–2, low-voltage P waves, ST-segment abnormalities, and flattening or inversion of T waves occur.[37,42] Occasionally the electrocardiogram exhibits a pattern resembling myocardial infarction.[42]

Patients may manifest cardiomegaly without symptoms;[38,62] bradycardia may contribute to or be responsible for the enlargement.[49] There is a tendency for the systemic arterial pressure to be relatively low.[41,47] Recurrent syncope occurs because of complete heart block (Stokes-Adams attacks) or sinus bradycardia (Table 50–2),[38,45] and sudden death is a hazard.[36,42,47,50,58,62] Insertion of a transvenous right ventricular pacemaker is desirable in patients with serious bradyarrhythmias associated with this disease.[43,48,53]

In addition to intrinsic heart disease, patients with myotonic muscular dystrophy are at risk because of abnormalities of the neuromuscular apparatus of respiration.[36,38] Alveolar hypoventilation may result in hypercapnia and hypoxemia. There are several reports of prolapse of the mi-

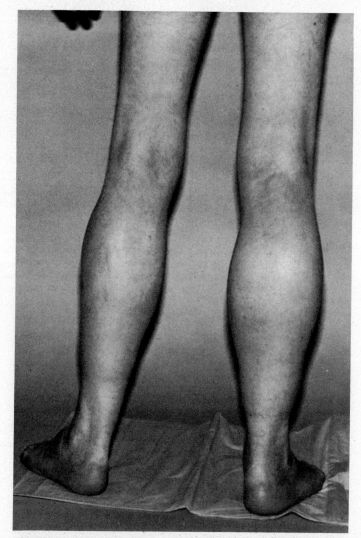

FIGURE 50–10   Asymmetrical calf pseudohypertrophy in a 52-year-old man with Erb's dystrophy.

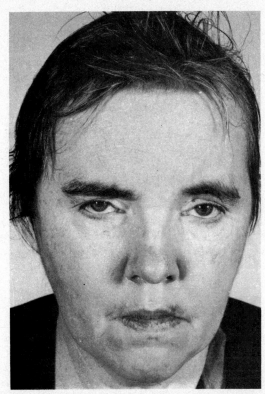

FIGURE 50–11 Fifty-year-old woman with myotonic muscular dystrophy, typical expressionless myopathic facies, and thinning of the frontal hair. (From Perloff, J. K., et al.: Uncommon or commonly unrecognized causes of heart failure. Prog. Cardiovasc. Dis. *12*:409, 1970, by permission of Grune and Stratton.)

tral valve in myotonic dystrophy, but it is unclear whether or not the relationship is coincidental.[18,63–65]

The combination of sinus bradycardia, tachycardia (atrial flutter/fibrillation), P-R interval prolongation, left/right bundle branch block, left-axis deviation, and complete heart block[65a] is an aggregate of related disorders of the sinus node, atrioventricular node, and infranodal conduction tissues analogous to the "sick sinus syndrome" in much older subjects. The heart disease of myotonic dystrophy may therefore take the form of premature aging of impulse

regulation and conduction. Other features of premature aging occur in myotonic dystrophy, namely, a decrease in gonadal function, thinning of the hair, frontal baldness, and cataracts.

Friedreich's Ataxia

Friedreich's ataxia is a progressive heredofamilial disorder characterized by neurological disease and a cardiomyopathy.[66–70] Nicolaus Friedreich, in a series of five papers between 1863 and 1877, described a specific form of spinal degeneration with distinctive clinical and pathological features encountered in nine members of three sibships.[71] Despite a century of lively interest, Friedreich's ataxia has resisted precise clinical and biochemical definition,[70,72] and there is still disagreement on where this spinocerebellar degenerative disease fits within the complex framework of hereditary ataxias.[67] Phenotypically similar disorders (Charcot-Marie-Tooth disease,[73] cerebellar ataxia, Roussy-Levy syndrome,[74] and familial spastic paralysis) are sometimes found within the same family pedigree.[75] Charcot-Marie-Tooth disease, i.e., peroneal muscular atrophy, progresses more slowly than Friedreich's disease, has a better prognosis, is usually devoid of heart disease,[73] but occasionally is accompanied by high-degree heart block (p. 730). The ataxia of Marie is cerebellar rather than spinal and has no known association with heart disease.[75] Refsum's disease, an inborn error of lipid metabolism (phytanic acid), involves the heart and is occasionally mistaken for Friedreich's ataxia.[76]

The typical neuropathological findings identify Friedreich's disease principally as a spinal disorder with degeneration of posterior columns, spinocerebellar tracts, and pyramidal tracts.[67] The disease is inherited as an autosomal recessive trait. The onset is usually before the end of puberty and virtually never after age 20 years. Once the disorder begins, there are no remissions but, instead, relentlessly progressive ataxia of gait and muscle weakness, first of the lower limbs and then of all four extremities. Dysarthria is present very early. Pes cavus (Friedreich's foot) (Fig. 50–13) and kyphoscoliosis develop within 2 years of onset. In addition, somewhat fewer than half the

FIGURE 50–12 Electrocardiogram from a 41-year-old woman with myotonic muscular dystrophy. The P-R interval is 0.28 sec. The QRS complex exhibits left-axis deviation (left anterior hemiblock).

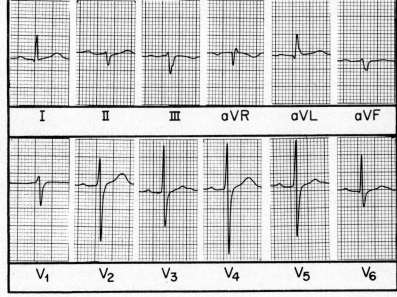

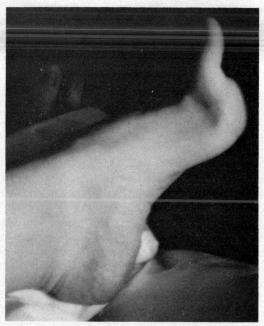

FIGURE 50–13   Typical "Friedreich's foot" showing pes cavus and hammer toe. (From Perloff, J. K., et al.: Uncommon or commonly unrecognized causes of heart failure. Prog. Cardiovasc. Dis. *12*:409, 1970, by permission of Grune and Stratton.)

patients have nystagmus.[77] Abnormal amounts of skeletal muscle enzymes are not consistently released into the circulation because the disorder is essentially neurological rather than myopathic.[78]

It is now estimated that 10 to 50 per cent of patients have cardiac symptoms,[79,80] nearly 100 per cent have abnormalities of electrocardiogram, vectorcardiogram, or echocardiogram (Fig. 50–14), one-half to two-thirds die of cardiac disorders,[80] and virtually all cases studied at necropsy have involvement of the heart.[80,82] In the usual clinical pattern, progressively severe ataxia occurs long before symptomatic heart disease.[83] Rarely, however, evidence of cardiac disease precedes the neurological manifestations.[75,84,85] There is no necessary relationship between the severity of cardiac involvement and the degree of neurological impairment.[84] Severe scoliosis, together with neuromuscular impairment of respiratory muscles, leads to impairment of lung function that varies from mild to severe.[86] It is of further interest that cardiac abnormalities are sometimes found in neurologically normal siblings.[75]

Inappropriate tachycardia is relatively common at rest, with changes in position, and with slight stress.[75,87] Occasional patients experience chest pain that resembles angina pectoris or myocardial infarction,[75,81,82,88] but there is no relationship among chest pain, electrocardiographic patterns, and the coronary arteriopathy of Friedreich's ataxia (see later). One child 6 years of age died following severe chest pain and at necropsy was found to have normal coronary arteries and no infarction. Symptomatic congestive heart failure is rare before puberty.[80] Midsystolic murmurs, usually grade 2 or 3 of 6, may relate either to the kyphoscoliosis or hypertrophic obstructive cardiomyopathy (see later). In this regard, the systemic arterial pulse may exhibit a typical rapid upstroke.[87]

The electrocardiogram is likely to be abnormal soon after if not at the onset of the neurological disease even in young children. Electrocardiographic alterations fall into two categories: (1) disturbances in rhythm, and (2) abnormalities in QRS-T patterns. Inappropriate sinus tachycardia[75,81,83,89,90] has been attributed to increased stimulation by the sympathetic nervous system.[75] Other rhythm disturbances include supraventricular and ventricular ectopic beats, paroxysmal atrial tachycardia, atrial fibrillation, and atrial flutter.[75,81,83,89,90] The commonest abnormality of the QRS-T in the standard scalar electrocardiogram is left ventricular hypertrophy (both voltage and repolarization criteria) or nonspecific ST–T-wave changes.[75,81,83,88–90] Occasionally there are electrocardiographic signs of right ventricular or biventricular hypertrophy, despite little or no necropsy evidence of right ventricular involvement.[90] Vectorcardiographic studies support these conclusions and in addition display QRS vector loops that are often irregular and altered by continuous abnormalities during the course of inscription.[88]

It is no mere coincidence that left ventricular hypertrophy is a common feature of the electrocardiogram. There is now substantial evidence that the cardiomyopathy of Friedreich's ataxia *is* hypertrophic, usually symmetrical (concentric) (Fig. 50–14*B*) and less commonly asymmetrical (disproportionate septal thickness) (Figs. 50–15, 50–16).[66,67,69,84,91–98] Obstruction to left ventricular outflow can be present, absent, or provocable.[66,67,84] The echocardiogram in Friedreich's ataxia identifies cardiac abnormalities in a high percentage of patients (upwards of 90 per

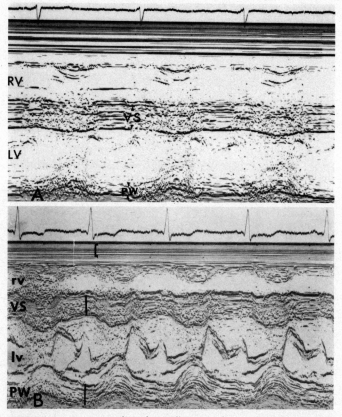

FIGURE 50–14   M-mode echocardiograms from two patients with Friedreich's ataxia. *A*, Thirty-nine-year-old man. The ventricular septum (VS) is disproportionately thick compared with the left ventricular posterior wall (PW). *B*, Twelve-year-old girl. There is symmetrical increase in the thickness of the ventricular septum (VS) and left ventricular posterior wall (PW).

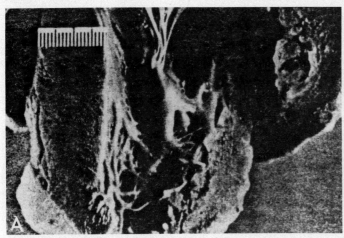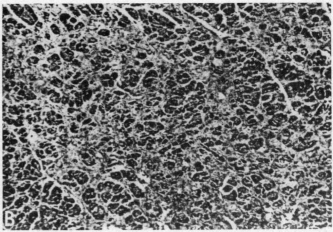

FIGURE 50–15 A. Heart of patient with Friedreich's ataxia showing the hypertrophy of the septum (ruler), which measures 2 cm in thickness. The left ventricular free wall, to the right side of the septum, is 1.4 cm thick. B, Left ventricle showing marked interstitial fibrosis and the hypertrophy of the myocardial fibers. (Mason's trichrome ×33.) (Reproduced with permission from Lamarche, J. B., Cote, M., and Lemieux, B.: The cardiomyopathy of Friedreich's ataxia. Neurology 7:389, 1980.)

cent)[66,67,95,97–99] (Fig. 50–14). The tracings are characterized by ventricular septal hypertrophy, hypertrophy of the left ventricular free wall, and occasionally an abnormal ratio of septal to posterior wall thickness.[67,91,95] The echocardiograms may exhibit all of the typical features of hypertrophic obstructive cardiomyopathy (p. 1415), that is, asymmetrical septal hypertrophy, hypokinetic septum, and systolic anterior motion of the anterior mitral leaflet.[66,91,95,97,98] However, the extensive septal cellular disarray that is a hallmark of typical genetic hypertrophic cardiomyopathy has not been described in necropsy reports.[75,80,81,100–102]

If the cardiac involvement in Friedreich's ataxia is hypertrophic, what is the connection between this form of cardiomyopathy and the neurological disease? The sympathetic nervous system may be the link. Increased sympathetic activity (catecholamines)[103] or an abnormal response by developing myocardium (receptor sites) has been proposed as a pathogenetic mechanism in genetic hypertrophic cardiomyopathy with asymmetrical septal hypertrophy and septal cellular disarray.[104] In Friedreich's ataxia, the sympathetic nervous system has been implicated in the pathogenesis of the cardiac involvement since 1938,[100] and more recently increased sympathetic stimulation has been held responsible for the inappropriate sinus tachycardia.[75]

In addition to disease of the myocardium, attention has been called to abnormalities of coronary arteries that may show all stages of luminal narrowing, from trivial intimal proliferation to complete obliteration.[75,80–83,105] Particular attention has been paid to involvement of small intramural coronary arteries,[105] but large and medium-sized branches can also be affected.[75,80] The vessels exhibit neither thrombi nor atheroma,[75,80,81] and a relationship between coronary arteriopathy and the diabetes mellitus that sometimes occurs with Friedreich's ataxia is unsubstantiated.[75,81,106] Although no theory can ignore the striking coronary arteriopathy, the coronary disorder does not appear to be the cause of the myocardial disease.

SPORADIC NEUROMUSCULAR DISEASES SOMETIMES ASSOCIATED WITH CARDIAC DISORDERS

PERONEAL MUSCULAR ATROPHY (CHARCOT-MARIE-TOOTH DISEASE)

Peroneal muscular atrophy, which is believed to be related to Friedreich's ataxia, is a slowly progressive neurogenic disorder principally affecting distal muscles of the legs and, occasionally, intrinsic muscles of the hands.[107–109] Although cardiac disease is commonly associated with Friedreich's ataxia, as noted, peroneal muscular atrophy seldom involves the heart.[74] In 1961 a single case was identified, with atrial flutter and heart failure.[108] A decade then passed before additional reports appeared of a family with peroneal muscular atrophy and disturbances of cardiac impulse formation and conduction.[110,111] The propositus in these latter reports, a man of 41 years, had experienced dizziness for 2 years and was found to have sinus

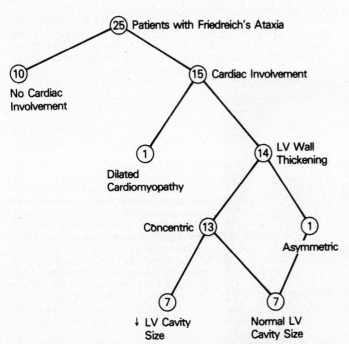

FIGURE 50–16 Flow diagram summarizing echocardiographic data in 25 patients with Friedreich's ataxia. LV, left ventricular; ↓, decreased. (Reproduced with permission from Gottdiener, J. S., Hawley, R. J., Maron, B. J., et al.: Characteristics of the cardiac hypertrophy in Friedreich's ataxia. Am. Heart J. 103:525, 1982.)

bradycardia, complete right bundle branch block, and left-axis deviation. Admission to hospital was preceded by a Stokes-Adams attack caused by complete heart block (Table 50–1). The patient had a sick sinus node (sinus bradycardia) with infranodal disease (right bundle branch block and left-axis deviation), culminating in complete (infranodal) heart block. It is of interest that 10 members of three generations were affected; in some, heart block and peroneal muscular atrophy coexisted; in others, right bundle branch block occurred alone; and in one, peroneal muscular atrophy occurred without a conduction defect.[110] If this family represents an example of heredofamilial neuromuscular disease with involvement of the heart, the cardiac disorder seems to have been confined to the sinus node and conduction system, leaving the myocardium clinically uninvolved.

X-LINKED HUMEROPERONEAL DYSTROPHY

This disorder is characterized by slowly progressive muscle weakness most marked in the humeral muscles (less in peroneals), with heel cord and elbow contractures developing in the first decade of life and stabilizing near the end of the second decade.[112,113] The X-linked scapuloperoneal syndrome is believed to be nosologically similar if not identical,[113–115] but an autosomal dominant scapuloperoneal syndrome has also been described with a high incidence of cardiomyopathy.[114] Characteristic cardiac involvement takes the form of atrial arrhythmias, atrial paralysis (standstill), and profound bradycardia and high-degree heart block (Table 49–1).[112,113,115–117] Electrocardiograms show abnormally small P waves, P-R interval prolongation (atrioventricular node), atrial fibrillation, atrial flutter, permanent atrial paralysis with slow junctional pacemaker, and complete atrioventricular block (infranodal).[112] H-V intervals are prolonged. Exploration of the right atrium with an electrode catheter revealed no atrial electrical activity, and stimulation of the right atrium induced no electrical response.[112] It is of interest that ventricular function appears to be normal. Accordingly, cardiac involvement in this X-linked form of muscular dystrophy seems to represent primarily disease of atrial muscle (atrial standstill) with sinus bradycardia, atrial fibrillation, and atrial flutter, together with evidence of fibroskeletal disease (AV node disease represented by P-R interval prolongation and infranodal disease represented by H-V prolongation or heart block).

CENTRONUCLEAR MYOPATHY

In 1966 the first description was published of a congenital myopathy histologically characterized by central nuclei in 85 per cent of skeletal muscle fibers.[118] A number of identical cases have subsequently been reported.[119–121] Centronuclear myopathy typically exhibits a slow but progressive wasting and weakness of skeletal muscle, be-

ginning at birth. Ptosis of the eyelids is the rule, and patients are hyporeflexic or areflexic. Serum creatine kinase is released from diseased skeletal muscle. The electroencephalogram is usually abnormal, and seizures have been described. The central or internal location of nuclei in a high percentage of skeletal muscle fibers is the dominant histological abnormality, giving the disease its name. In addition, pronounced variation of diameter of muscle fibers is often found. Familial occurrence is known, but the mode of inheritance is unclear because pedigree data are insufficient. Two brothers with centronuclear myopathy were reported; both had cardiomyopathy, which caused death in one.[119] At necropsy there was diffuse cardiac dilatation and extensive fibrosis. Even though the total number of cases is small, there is presumptive evidence that centronuclear myopathy may be associated with a cardiomyopathy that can cause death at an early age. It is a point of interest that in one study on skeletal muscle in patients with idiopathic cardiomyopathy, numerous internal nuclei were visible in an illustrated figure;[121] apparently, centronuclear myopathy had occurred as cardiomyopathy before the neuromuscular disease was diagnosed.

KEARNS-SAYRE SYNDROME (PROGRESSIVE EXTERNAL OPHTHALMOPLEGIA WITH PIGMENTARY RETINOPATHY; OCULOCRANIOSOMATIC SYNDROME)

In 1958, Kearns and Sayre identified the triad of progressive external ophthalmoplegia, atypical pigmentary retinopathy, and heart block.[122] Subsequent observations established the Kearns-Sayre syndrome as nosologically distinct among the many neuromuscular disorders characterized by progressive external ophthalmoplegia (Fig. 50–17).[123] In the original description of Kearns and Sayre, both reported patients had complete heart block, and one of them died of it.[122] Kearns predicted that prognosis would be determined by the heart block and was proved correct (Table 50–1),[29,124,125] but with notable exceptions.[126] In many cases, there is evidence of a widespread neurological disorder. Although multisystem neurological diseases are frequently hereditary, the Kearns-Sayre syndrome is believed to be acquired, beginning before age 20 years and involving the sexes equally.[123]

Morphological alterations in skeletal muscle are characterized by ragged-red fibers in the trichrome stain.[123] Whether the progressive external ophthalmoplegia is neurogenic or myopathic in origin has long been debated, and doubt has been cast upon the criteria for making this distinction in ocular muscles. Similarly, it is necessary to ask whether involvement of the heart represents a neural or muscle disorder.[127] Even though the term "cardiomyopathy" has been loosely applied,[123] there is reason to believe that the cardiac disease primari-

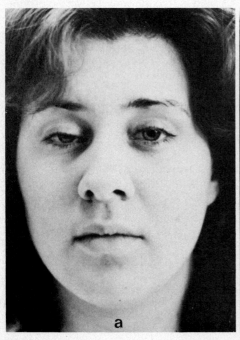 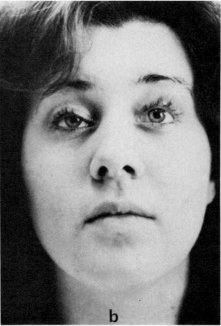

FIGURE 50–17 An eighteen-year-old girl with Kearns-Sayre syndrome and bilateral asymmetric ptosis. Within 24 months, her electrocardiogram changed from normal to bifascicular showing block (complete right bundle branch block and left anterior fascicular block). *A,* The asymmetric ptosis when the patient looks straight ahead. *B,* The ptosis of the right lid persists when the patient looks up. She also had atypical pigmentary retinopathy.

ly, if not exclusively, afflicts the specialized conduction pathways rather than the myocardium.[127] Despite ultrastructural changes, clinically detectable myocardial disease is not a feature of the Kearns-Sayre syndrome.[125] All signs thus far support the view that cardiac involvement in this disorder is "neurogenic" rather than myopathic and that two alterations in cardiac conduction coexist: a gradual progressive impairment of infranodal conduction (left anterior hemiblock, right bundle branch block, complete heart block) and a concomitant enhancement of AV nodal conduction.[127,128]

A convincing morphological basis for impaired infranodal conduction in Kearns-Sayre syndrome was demonstrated in a patient whose electrophysiological study had shown trifascicular block (right bundle branch block, left anterior hemiblock, and a very prolonged H-V interval).[128] At necropsy, there were extensive changes in the distal portion of the bundle of His, extending to the origins of the bundle branches.[128] Recently, evidence of enhanced AV nodal conduction was identified with bundle of His electrocardiography.[127] A short or relatively short P-R interval should therefore not be taken as evidence against the risk inherent in trifascicular disease in patients with Kearns-Sayre syndrome with right bundle branch block and left anterior hemiblock.[127]

Myasthenia Gravis. The association of myocardial disease with thymoma, especially malignant thymoma, is generally accepted. The association of myasthenia gravis with heart disease is less clear, despite a considerable body of suggestive information.[129] A specific cardiac pathological condition for this neuromuscular disorder is unproven in spite of clinical, electrocardiographic, vectorcardiographic, and necropsy data implicating the myocardium.[129]

McArdle's Syndrome. This condition is a metabolic myopathy (muscle phosphorylase deficiency) resulting in inadequate skeletal muscle glycolysis.[130] The disease is clinically manifested by exercise intolerance due to muscle cramps. The electrocardiogram may reveal sinus bradycardia, increased QRS voltage, and P-R interval prolongation.[130] The disorder differs from another metabolic myopathy characterized by mitochondrial myopathy of skeletal and cardiac muscle with storage of glycogen and lipid and exercise-induced lactic acidemia.[131]

GUILLAIN-BARRÉ SYNDROME

The Guillain-Barré syndrome, or Landry's ascending paralysis, is characterized by an elevated cerebrospinal fluid protein concentration without increase in the number of white blood cells at a normal pressure. The protein-cell dissociation in the spinal fluid is necessary for the diagnosis. The motor paralysis is flaccid and has a considerable tendency to ascend, hence the eponym of Landry. Involvement of thoracic muscle makes assisted ventilation necessary. Despite the use of mechanical ventilation, the Guillain-Barré syndrome is fatal in approximately 20 per cent of children who manifest significant involvement of trunk muscles and who develop respiratory insufficiency.[132]

When sudden death occurs, postmortem studies have shed no light on the cause. There is evidence, however, that deaths are often related to arrhythmias.[132-135] Bradyarrhythmias (sinus arrest, complete heart block), tachyarrhythmias (supraventricular and ventricular), as well as premature atrial and ventricular beats, are relatively frequent and are enhanced by use of a respirator.[134,135] Pacemaker support has been required because of recurrent asystole.[135] In one patient, tracheal aspiration (tracheostomy) produced an idioventricular rhythm of 40 beats/min, which reverted to sinus rhythm when aspiration was stopped.[132] Cardiac monitoring is wise, especially when the Guillain-Barré syndrome is sufficiently severe to warrant assisted ventilation.[132,134]

NEUROMUSCULAR DISORDERS PRESENTING AS CARDIOMYOPATHY

Heart block (selective involvement of the specialized conduction system) is occasionally the presenting problem in patients subsequently found to have neuromuscular disorders, such as Kearns-Sayre syndrome, myotonic muscular dystrophy, or the X-linked humeroperoneal syndrome (previously discussed) (Table 50–1).[29,116,122] Other patients

are seen with disease of the cardiac conduction system *plus* cardiomyopathy and are found to have neuromuscular disorders such as limb-girdle dystrophy of Erb.[30] Still others show cardiomyopathy alone and are found to have skeletal muscle disease either on careful study or with subsequent development of clinical disease.[85] Thus, occasional patients with little or no clinical evidence of a systemic neuromuscular disorder come to attention initially because of overt cardiac disease.[136]

Evans commented on skeletal muscle involvement in idiopathic cardiomyopathy more than 30 years ago.[137] Patients with idiopathic congestive cardiomyopathy have been found to exhibit histological evidence of centronuclear myopathy.[120,121] In addition, occasionally mothers of patients with classic X-linked Duchenne's muscular dystrophy have cardiomyopathy with mild or occult clinical evidence of systemic muscle involvement.[2,10,14,15] Hypertrophic cardiomyopathy is a primary disease of cardiac muscle. Nevertheless, abnormalities of skeletal muscle have been found on electromyography and on both light and electron microscopic studies of biopsy material.[138,139] The conclusion should not be overstated, but occasionally it might prove useful to consider coexisting neuromuscular disease as the underlying cause in relatively young patients with sinoatrial or atrioventricular conduction disease or with idiopathic congestive cardiomyopathy.

Polymyositis (also see p. 1664)

Polymyositis occurs in both adults and children and, when accompanied by the characteristic skin rash, is designated *dermatomyositis* because the muscle disease appears to be the same in either case.[140,141] Patients develop symmetrical muscle weakness, especially in the limb-girdle and anterior neck flexors.[140] When the disorder occurs without rash, a mistaken diagnosis of muscular dystrophy may be made, especially in children. On muscle biopsy and at necropsy, diffuse interstitial and perivascular mononuclear cell infiltration and fiber necrosis, usually with multivacuolated fibers showing regeneration, degeneration, and fibrosis, are seen.[140] Electromyography discloses fractionation of the motor unit (small amplitude, excessive motor action potentials on slight voluntary effort, and fibrillations).[140] Cardiac involvement is believed to occur only rarely in childhood polymyositis but may merely be clinically occult.[141] In adults, the infrequency of symptomatic involvement of the heart contrasts with a relatively high incidence of electrocardiographic abnormalities, especially rhythm and conduction disturbances,[140] that take the form of atrial fibrillation or flutter, premature beats (atrial and ventricular), multifocal atrial tachycardia, impaired AV conduction (first-, second-, and third-degree heart block), and abnormalities of infranodal conduction (left-axis deviation and bundle branch block).[140,141]

At necropsy, infiltration, degeneration, and fibrous replacement of sinoatrial node, distal bundle of His, and left and right bundle branches wholly or in part underlie the conduction defects.[140,141] In addition to the occasional occurrence of fibrinous pericarditis, pathological changes in the myocardium are usually similar to those in skeletal muscle, including diffuse mononuclear cell infiltration and myofiber degeneration, regeneration, and fibrosis.[140] It would seem that these abnormalities should manifest themselves clinically as congestive heart failure—and this may be so—but recent echocardiographic studies have identified a high incidence of *enhanced* left ventricular function.[140] If these puzzling observations are correct, the mechanism is not known. Prolapse of the mitral valve has also been recorded,[140] but it is unclear whether polymyositis is causal or coincidental.

Periodic Paralysis

This disorder, characterized by recurrent attacks of flaccid weakness, is accompanied by either abnormally high or abnormally low levels of serum potassium.[142] In the hypokalemic type,[143] attacks typically begin in late childhood or adolescence, usually occur at night, tend to be severe, and last a day or longer. In the hyperkalemic type, onset is at a younger age, and attacks occur more frequently but tend to be milder and shorter (minutes or hours). Many features are common to both varieties of periodic paralysis: familial occurrence (autosomal dominant inheritance), heightened susceptibility immediately after ceasing strenuous exercise, termination of incipient attacks by *mild* exercise, onset of weakness in the lower extremities with progression to arms (but not to respiratory muscles), intensification by cold, and persistent weakness between attacks when potassium levels may be normal.[142,144]

It is hardly a surprise that the electrocardiogram exhibits peaked T waves during hyperkalemia and low-voltage T waves (and digitalis sensitivity) during hypokalemia. More to the point are the cardiac arrhythmias, potentially lethal, especially in hyperkalemic (but sometimes during normokalemic) periodic paralysis. Noteworthy are ventricular ectopic beats (unifocal or multiform), ventricular bigeminy, bidirectional ventricular tachycardia, and fusion between sinus beats and one or both of the two forms of bidirectional ventricular beats, producing multiform complexes.[142,144,145] Hypokalemic attacks are best treated with oral potassium chloride (KCl) and hyperkalemic episodes with glucose and insulin. It must be noted that administration of potassium and antiarrhythmics does not always suppress the ventricular electrical instability.[145]

Alcoholic Cardiomyopathy (also see p. 1406)

The dilated (congestive) cardiomyopathy associated with chronic ingestion of large amounts of ethyl alcohol rarely exists with liver cirrhosis but may be accompanied by skeletal myopathy and disorders of the central nervous system.[146-149] The low incidence of peripheral neuritis supports the view that the cardiac abnormality does not depend upon malnutrition.[146] Chronic alcoholics in the withdrawal state are susceptible to convulsions ("rum fits").[147] The teratogenic potential of alcohol, exemplified by the fetal alcohol syndrome, afflicts the central nervous system but not the fetal myocardium.[150]

ELECTROCARDIOGRAPHIC AND VASOMOTOR ABNORMALITIES ACCOMPANYING CEREBROVASCULAR ACCIDENTS

A connection between certain acute cerebral disorders—subdural hematoma, spontaneous subarachnoid hemorrhage, intracranial hemorrhage, and cerebral thrombosis or embolus—and overt cardiovascular abnormalities has been recognized for nearly 100 years.[151] Bradycardia and a rise in systemic arterial blood pressures were known to Harvey Cushing at the turn of the century.[152] Interestingly, intense cerebral compression in rats evoked within minutes marked systemic arteriolar constriction, systemic arterial hypertension, pulmonary venous hypertension, and hemorrhagic pulmonary edema.[153] In human subjects, brain stem hemorrhage appears to be associated with noncardiogenic pulmonary edema.[154] The question of a relationship between head trauma and cardiac arrhythmias was posed 50 years ago.[155] The principal cardiac abnormalities in these settings are essentially electrocardiographic and fall into two groups: disturbances in rhythm and conduction and abnormalities of repolarization.

Electrocardiographic Abnormalities. An appreciation of these abnormal electrocardiograms is essential if diagnostic errors are to be avoided. Approximately 90 per cent of patients with acute cerebrovascular accidents, especially cerebral or subarachnoid hemorrhage, exhibit electrocardiographic abnormalities during the first 3 days of observation.[154,156-163] *Acute subdural hematoma* may be accompanied by both brady- and tachyarrhythmias, including sinus bradycardia (sometimes profound), sinus tachycardia,

atrial arrhythmias (ectopic beats, fibrillation, flutter, or supraventricular tachycardia), ventricular arrhythmias (ectopic beats or ventricular tachycardia or fibrillation), and abnormalities in atrioventricular conduction.[151]

Spontaneous *subarachnoid or intracranial hemorrhage* may also be accompanied by bradycardia (occasionally tachycardia), but the most marked electrocardiographic features are abnormalities of repolarization closely simulating ischemic heart disease.[154,158-160,164] Similar electrographic changes occasionally occur with space-occupying lesions (brain tumors)[160] or cervical laminectomy.[165] ST-segment displacement (principally elevation) and T-wave inversions suggest recent myocardial infarction. Although the T waves may merely be flat or with shallow negativity (chiefly in leads I and aVL and in the left precordium), they may instead be deeply and symmetrically inverted, indistinguishable from the pattern sometimes seen in acute myocardial infarction (Fig. 50–18).[154,159] At necropsy, the coronary arteries and ventricular myocardium can be normal despite these electrocardiographic signs. Less commonly, tall, upright T waves occur as a manifestation of intracranial disease (subdural hematoma, tumor, or head trauma).[160] In addition to abnormalities of ST segments and T waves, prominent U waves and Q-T interval prolongation are commonly seen in patients with spontaneous intracranial or subarachnoid hemorrhage, and occasionally the amplitude of the P waves increases.[154] The mechanisms for these varied electrocardiographic abnormalities are unclear,[166] but they are related, at least in part, to the location of the intracranial hemorrhage.[154] Ventricular ectopic beats are common after an acute cerebrovascular accident, predisposing to ventricular tachycardia.[157] The tendency for the QT interval to prolong reinforces this predisposition.[156,167]

Coexistence of Cerebrovascular and Coronary Disease. It is true that acute cerebrovascular accidents are sometimes responsible for disturbances in cardiac rhythm and conduction and for repolarization abnormalities that resemble myocardial ischemia or infarction in patients without other evidence of heart disease. However, it is not surprising that cerebrovascular and cardiovascular disease often coexist. This coexistence takes a variety of forms,

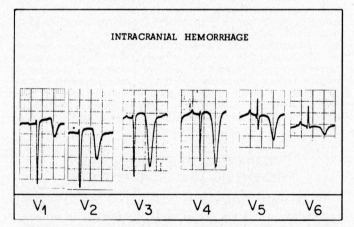

FIGURE 50–18 Deep, symmetrical T-wave inversions in precordial leads of a patient with a cerebral hemorrhage. (Courtesy of Dr. John H. Phillips, Tulane Medical Center, New Orleans, Louisiana.)

some subtle and overlooked and some quite apparent. Prospective studies have disclosed a 12 to 30 per cent incidence of recent myocardial infarction in patients with acute cerebrovascular accidents. In the majority, the only clinical evidence of an acute cardiac infarct was the electrocardiogram and serum enzymes, without which the diagnoses might not have come to light.[162,168] Moreover, many, if not most, of these patients had enzymatic but not convincing electrocardiographic evidence of recent myocardial infarction. Rarely, inverted T waves of a prior infarction become upright after a cerebrovascular accident, "normalizing" the electrocardiogram.[169] Release of MB (cardiac-specific) creatine kinase is more likely to be helpful than the electrocardiogram, which can be abnormal without infarction and nondiagnostic despite enzymatic evidence of myocardial damage. Nevertheless, patients with elevated serum creatine kinase levels are twice as likely to have ST-segment depressions, T-wave inversions, conduction defects, and atrial fibrillation than those with normal CPK, and the mortality in these subjects is relatively high, 53 to 66 per cent.[162-164,166,168] The association of atherosclerotic cerebrovascular and coronary artery disease is no surprise, since the two groups of disorders are prevalent in the same patient population and have common risk factors, such as diabetes, hyperlipidemia, and cigarette smoking, and especially systemic hypertension.

Cerebral Emboli. The combination of stroke and heart disease is also seen in young adults and even in children, though much less frequently. Cerebral emboli caused by mitral stenosis with atrial fibrillation (intermittent or chronic) are constant threats regardless of the patient's age. The focal neurological signs in occasional patients with prolapse of the mitral valve are believed to be embolic.[168,170] *Myxoma of the left atrium*, aside from producing syncope due to mitral orifice obstruction, results in peripheral emboli in about 45 per cent of cases (p. 1460); the brain is affected in half of these. Moreover, cardiac myxomas occasionally are seen initially by neurologists because of predominantly or exclusively neurological manifestations.[171] Left ventricular mural thrombi with systemic (and therefore cerebral) emboli are most frequent in the setting of healed adult myocardial infarction, especially when accompanied by segmental akinesis, dyskinesis, or frank ventricular aneurysm (Chap. 37). However, mural thrombi are common in cardiomyopathy during either the active subacute phase or the healed chronic phase, regardless of the patient's age (Chap. 41). Infants with endocardial fibroelastosis of the dilated type may suffer strokes caused by cerebral emboli from left ventricular endocardial thrombi (p. 1049).[172]

Neurological complications of diagnostic cardiac catheterization are infrequent but are usually due to emboli and relatively rarely to reactions to contrast media.[173]

Not so rare are transient cerebral ischemic events (focal cerebrovascular insufficiency or diffuse cerebral ischemia, manifested by dizziness, giddiness, or syncope) provoked by bradyarrhythmias or high-degree heart block in older subjects.[174] Twenty-four hour ambulatory electrocardiographic monitoring has revealed hemodynamically significant arrhythmias in approximately one-third of adults with transient neurological symptoms.[175]

In addition to cardiac chambers as sources, cerebral emboli originate from heart valves or systemic veins (paradoxical embolus). Valve emboli related to cardiac surgery can occur either during the actual repair (thrombotic or calcific fragments) or after insertion of a rigid prosthesis, especially in the mitral location. Open operation has made the former rare, and anticoagulants coupled with improved prostheses have minimized the latter (p. 1086). When unrelated to cardiac surgery, cerebral emboli of valvular origin are typified by the septic embolus of infective endocarditis (p. 1154), which is relatively common, and by the bland embolus of noninfective thrombotic deposits (socalled marantic endocarditis, especially on the aortic valve), which is commoner than clinically recognized.[176] *Drug abuse* not only causes infective endocarditis, but, depending upon the drug and vehicle (embolization of foreign matter), is also associated with intracranial or subarachnoid hemorrhage, cerebral emboli, ischemic stroke, and systemic hypertension.[177] The stage is set for *paradoxical emboli* when systemic venous blood freely enters the systemic arterial circulation (the right-to-left shunts of cyanotic congenital heart disease). The infrequency of such emboli is explained by the low incidence of a source, since the relevant age group rarely has systemic phlebothrombosis or thrombophlebitis. An exception is the multigravida with an ostium secundum atrial septal defect in whom there may be inferior vena caval to left atrial streaming despite low pulmonary vascular resistance and a large left-to-right shunt.

Focal discrete neurological deficits (sudden weakness of a hand or foot, isolated homonymous visual field defects, and so on) are well-known sequelae of cerebral emboli. Less well known are diffuse cerebral symptoms believed to result from recurrences of multiple small (cortical) emboli, causing agitated confusion, dulled sensorium, and seizures.[178] In addition, septic emboli may give rise to intracranial bleeding—after a misleading interval of quiescence—or cerebral abscess.

Apart from systemic emboli, cerebral disease and cardiac disease interrelate in several other settings, each of which can occur in the young. Cerebral trauma, by causing intracranial hemorrhage, cerebral edema, and/or subdural hematoma, can result in disturbances of cardiac rhythm and conduction and in abnormalities of repolarization, as cited earlier. In addition, subarachnoid hemorrhage in coarctation of the aorta results from spontaneous rupture of an aneurysm of the circle of Willis, a disaster that surgical repair of the coarctation does not necessarily preclude.[172]

Cyanotic congenital heart disease can be associated with neurological manifestations—most dramatically, hemiplegia—owing either to an excessive red cell mass or to a red cell mass that is inadequate for tissue needs (erythrocytosis with relative anemia).[179] The cyanotic, hyperpneic spells in Fallot's tetralogy cause not only transient syncope and seizures (see below) but also, rarely, hemiplegia.[172] Brain damage and mental retardation (recurrent cerebral hypoxia), venous sinus thromboses (especially after prolonged hypoxic spells), cerebral (paradoxical) embolism, and brain abscess add to the list of serious central nervous system complications in cyanotic congenital heart disease.[172]

CARDIAC COMPLICATIONS OF DRUGS USED IN TREATING NEUROMUSCULAR DISEASE

Another interplay between neuromuscular and cardiovascular disease results from the cardiac complications of certain drugs used by the neurologist. Inflammatory retroperitoneal fibrosis occurs in patients taking methysergide for migraine headache,[180,181] and there is evidence of similar fibrotic disease of the pleura, great arteries, cardiac valves, and endocardium. The lesions chiefly involve the left side of the heart.[180] Fibrotic thickening has been described in the aortic and mitral valves, chordae tendineae, tips of papillary muscles, and, to a lesser extent, left ventricular endocardium; the aortic root and the left coronary ostium were densely scarred. Constrictive pericarditis has also been reported in a patient taking methysergide.[182] It is of interest that methysergide-induced lesions do not appear to damage the valve structure; instead, the fibrotic and thickened appearance of the leaflets is caused by a layer of fresh collagen deposited on the surface of otherwise unharmed cusps.[180] Both grossly and microscopically these findings are similar to those occurring in carcinoid.[183] The mechanism by which methysergide exerts its effect on cardiac tissue is unknown, but it has been theorized that the chemical similarity of methysergide and serotonin may in part provide the answer.

The aortic valve lesion induced by methysergide is both stenotic and incompetent; the clinically overt mitral lesion is generally regurgitation, although the gross appearance of the valve suggests stenosis as well. If methysergide is continued, the valvular abnormalities progress, but, in at least some patients, regression or complete disappearance—at least of the cardiac murmurs—has followed discontinuance of the drug.[180]

Parkinsonism is another disease in which drugs employed for neurological treatment may cause cardiac complications.[184,185] In Parkinson's disease, neurons are selectively destroyed (by unknown causes) and therefore cannot release the neurotransmitter dopamine. Accordingly, levodopa (L-dopa), the precursor of dopamine, is used in treatment. Since no less than 1 per cent of oral levodopa penetrates the blood-brain barrier, relatively large doses are required for a therapeutic response, and such doses are seldom tolerated without side effects. L-Dopa tends to provoke hypotension (both supine and postural) as well as ventricular ectopic beats. Accordingly, the drug must be used cautiously in patients with cerebral ischemia, angina, recent myocardial infarction, or cardiac arrhythmias, even though after weeks (sometimes months) tolerance improves and side effects diminish. The cardiovascular effects are mediated by the actions of L-dopa on both the central and the peripheral nervous systems.

Bromocriptine, an ergot derivative, stimulates dopamine-sensitive receptors and is also useful in parkinsonism.[186] Bromocriptine can cause a significant postural fall in blood pressure in parkinsonian patients treated with large amounts of the drug, and a hypotensive effect can persist for as long as 6 weeks. Rarely, severe hypotension, both supine and erect, occurs even after initial doses of bromocriptine. The site of action of the hypotensive effect of bromocriptine is speculative.[186]

NEUROLOGICAL COMPLICATIONS OF THERAPY FOR CARDIOVASCULAR DISEASE

Certain forms of treatment for cardiovascular disease can leave serious neurological sequelae in their wake. Cardiopulmonary arrest with resuscitation is a dramatic example.[187,188] The depth and duration of postarrest coma correlate significantly with poor neurological prognosis. Ninety per cent of patients with good central nervous system recovery are alert within 18 hours after resuscitation. Prolonged coma, motor unresponsiveness, absent pupillary light reflexes, and absent oculocephalic responses are closely associated with poor prospects for neurological recovery. The comatose "survivors" of cardiopulmonary resuscitation pose the important ethical problem of when to withdraw life support measures.

Electrical or pharmacological cardioversion for chronic atrial fibrillation with normal mitral valve rarely gives rise to systemic emboli (probably less than 1 per cent),[189] but if emboli occur, they do so either at the moment of reversion to sinus rhythm or subsequently at the time of return to atrial fibrillation. Thus, if prophylactic anticoagulants are used in this setting, they must not only precede cardioversion but must also be maintained until stable sinus rhythm seems assured. Cerebral air embolism during the course of cardiopulmonary bypass is now rare, indeed. When this complication occurs, even profound degrees of cerebral depression are sometimes followed by gratifying recovery.

Several commonly used cardiac drugs have important although relatively rare untoward central nervous system effects. Lidocaine neurotoxicity includes drowsiness, dizziness, dysarthria, blurred vision, muscular fasciculations, and, occasionally, convulsive seizures.[190] Propranolol, in addition to causing drowsiness and lightheadedness, occasionally provokes mental depression.[191] Quinidine and procainamide may interfere with neuromuscular transmission (anticholinergic properties), can produce myasthenia-like weakness in patients with peripheral neuropathy,[192] can unmask previously unsuspected myasthenia gravis, or can exacerbate previously well-controlled symptoms.[193] Even digitalis glycosides are not immune from neurotoxic effects (p. 525), producing—although rarely—colored vision, toxic psychosis, and delirium. In the words of William Withering, "The Foxglove when given in very large and quickly repeated doses occasions . . . giddiness, confused vision, objects appearing green or yellow; . . . cold sweats, convulsions, syncope, death."[194] Ischemic stroke is associated with prolonged half-life of digitalis glycosides, resulting in reduced tolerance.[195]

CARDIAC SYNCOPE (See pp. 935 to 938)

References

1. Perloff, J. K., deLeon, A. C., and O'Doherty, D.: The cardiomyopathy of progressive muscular dystrophy. Circulation 33:625, 1966.
2. Pearson, C. M.: Muscular dystrophy. Am. J. Med. 35:632, 1963.
3. deLeon, A. C., Perloff, J. K., Twigg, H., and Hajd, M.: The straight back syndrome—Clinical cardiovascular manifestations. Circulation 32:193, 1965.
4. Perloff, J. K., Roberts, W. C., deLeon, A. C., and O'Doherty, D.: The

distinctive electrocardiogram of Duchenne's progressive muscular dystrophy. Am. J. Med. 42:179, 1967.

5. Sanyal, S. K., Johnson, W. W., Dische, M. R., Pitner, S. E., and Beard, C.: Dystrophic degeneration of papillary muscle and ventricular myocardium. A basis for mitral value prolapse in Duchenne's muscular dystrophy. Circulation 62:430, 1980.

6. Perloff, J. K.: The myocardial disease of heredofamilial neuromyopathies. In Fowler, N. (ed.): Myocardial Disease. New York, Grune and Stratton, 1973.

7. James, T. N.: Observations on the cardiovascular involvement, including the cardiac conduction system, in progressive muscular dystrophy. Am. Heart J. 63:48, 1962.

8. Slucka, C.: The electrocardiogram in Duchenne's progressive muscular dystrophy. Circulation 38:933, 1968.

9. Skyring, A., and McKusick, V. A.: Clinical, genetic and electrocardiographic studies in childhood muscular dystrophy. Am. J. Med. Sci. 242:54, 1961.

10. Mann, O., deLeon, A. C., Perloff, J. K., Simanis, J., and Horrigan, F. D.: Duchenne's muscular dystrophy: The electrocardiogram in female relatives. Am. J. Med. Sci. 255:376, 1968.

11. Leth, A., and Wulff, K.: Myocardiopathy in Duchenne's progressive muscular dystrophy. Acta Paediatr. Scand. 65:28, 1976.

12. Ronan, J. A., Perloff, J. K., Bowen, P. J., and Mann, O.: The vectorcardiogram in Duchenne's progressive muscular dystrophy. Am. Heart J. 84:588, 1972.

13. Fitch, C. W., and Ainger, L. E.: The Frank vectorcardiogram and the electrocardiogram in Duchenne muscular dystrophy. Circulation 35:1124, 1967.

14. Lane, R. J. M., Gardner-Medwin, D., and Roses, A. D.: Electrocardiographic abnormalities in carriers of Duchenne muscular dystrophy. Neurology 30:497, 1980.

15. Yoshioka, M.: Clinically manifesting carriers in Duchenne muscular dystrophy. Clin. Genet. 20:6, 1981.

16. Rubler, S., Perloff, J. K., and Roberts, W. C.: Clinical Pathological Conference—Duchenne's muscular dystrophy. Am. Heart J. 94:776, 1977.

17. Perloff, J. K.: Recognition of strictly posterior myocardial infarction by conventional scalar electrocardiography. Circulation 30:706, 1964.

18. Henze, E., Perloff, J. K., and Schelbert, H. R.: Alterations of regional myocardial perfusion and metabolism in Duchenne's muscular dystrophy detected by positron computed tomography. Circulation 64:279, 1981.

19. Reeves, W. C., Griggs, R., Nanda, N. C., Thomson, K., and Gramiak, R.: Echocardiographic evaluation of cardiac abnormalities in Duchenne's dystrophy and myotonic muscular dystrophy. Arch. Neurol. 37:273, 1980.

20. Farah, M. G., Evans, E. B., and Visnos, P. J.: Echocardiographic evaluation of left ventricular function in Duchenne's muscular dystrophy. Am. J. Med. 69:248, 1980.

21. Pennington, R. J. T.: Serum enzymes. In Rowland, L. P. (ed.): Pathogenesis of Human Muscular Dystrophies. Amsterdam-Oxford, Excerpta Medica, 1977.

22. Fowler, W. M., and Pearson, C. M.: Diagnostic and prognostic signficance of serum enzyme: I. Muscular dystrophy. Arch. Phys. Med. 45:125, 1964.

23. Wilson, K. M., Evans, K. A., and Carter, C. O.: Creatine kinase levels in women who carry genes for three types of muscular dystrophy. Br. Med. J. 1:750, 1965.

24. Fowler, W. M., Gardner, G. W., Taylor, R. G., Scavarda, A., and Busheikin, J. B.: Quantitative measurements in female siblings and mothers of boys with Duchenne dystrophy. Arch. Phys. Med. Rehab. 50:301, 1969.

25. Mabry, C. C., Roeckel, L. E., Munich, R. L., and Robertson, D.: X-linked pseudo-hypertrophic muscular dystrophy with a late onset and slow progression. N. Engl. J. Med. 273:1062, 1965.

26. Zellweger, H., and Hanson, J. W.: Slowly progressive X-linked recessive muscular dystrophy. Arch. Intern. Med. 120:525, 1967.

27. Katiyar, B. C., Misia, S., Somani, P. N., and Chaterji, A. M.: Congestive cardiomyopathy in a family of Becker's X-linked muscular dystrophy. Postgrad. Med. J. 53:12, 1977.

28. Jackson, C. E., and Strehler, D. A.: Limb-girdle muscular dystrophy: Clinical manifestations and detection of pre-clinical disease. Pediatrics 41:495, 1968.

29. Lambert, C. D., and Fairfax, A. J.: Neurological associations of chronic heart block. J. Neurol. Neurosurg. Psychiatr. 39:571, 1976.

30. Fairfax, A. J., and Lambert, C. D.: Neurological aspects of sinoatrial heart block. J. Neurol. Neurosurg. Psychiatr. 39:576, 1976.

31. Lisan, P., Anbriglia, J., and Likoff, W.: Myocardial disease associated with progressive muscular dystrophy. Am. Heart J. 57:913, 1959.

32. Gailani, S., Danowski, T. S., and Fisher, D. S.: Muscular dystrophy. Circulation 17:583, 1958.

33. Baldwin, A. J., Talley, R. C., Johnson, C., and Nutter, D. O.: Permanent paralysis of the atrium in a patient with facioscapulohumeral muscular dystrophy. Am. J. Cardiol. 31:649, 1973.

34. Bloomfield, D. A., and Sinclair-Smith, B. C.: Persistent atrial standstill. Am. J. Med. 39:335, 1965.

35. Ruff, P., Leier, C. V., and Schaal, S. F.: Temporary atrial standstill. Am. Heart J. 98:412, 1979.

36. Kohn, N. N., Faires, J. S., and Rodman, T.: Unusual manifestations due to involvement of involuntary muscle in dystrophia myotonica. N. Engl. J. Med. 271:1179, 1964.

37. Payne, C. A., and Greenfield, J. C.: Electrocardiographic abnormalities associated with myotonic dystrophy. Am. Heart J. 65:536, 1963.

38. Church, S. C.: The heart in myotonia atrophica. Arch. Intern. Med. 119:176, 1967.

39. Griffith, T. W.: On myotonia. Q. J. Med. 5:229, 1911.

40. Anderson, M.: Probable Thomsen's disease with cardiac involvement. J. Neurol. 214:301, 1977.

41. Orndahl, G., Thulesius, O., Enestrom, S., and Dehlin, O.: The heart in myotonic disease. Acta Med. Scand. 176:479, 1964.

42. Fearington, E. L., Gibson, T. C., and Churchill, R. E.: Vectorcardiographic and electrocardiographic findings in myotonia atrophica; A study employing the Frank lead system. Am. Heart J. 67:599, 1964.

43. Uemura, N., Tanaka, H., Niimura, T., Hashiguchi, N., Yoshimura, M., Terashi, S., and Kanehisa, T.: Electrophysiological and histological abnormalities of the heart in myotonic dystrophy. Am. Heart J. 86:616, 1973.

44. Josephson, M. E., Caracta, A. R., Gallagher, J. J., and Damato, A. N.: Site of conduction disturbances in a family with myotonic dystrophy. Am. J. Cardiol. 32:114, 1973.

45. Petkovich, N. J., Dunn, M., and Reed, W.: Myotonia dystrophica with A-V dissociation and Stokes-Adams attacks. Am. Heart J. 68:391, 1964.

46. Griggs, R. C., Davis, R. J., Anderson, D. C., and Dove, J. T.: Cardiac conduction in myotonic dystrophy. Am. J. Med. 59:37, 1975.

47. Holt, J. M., and Lambert, E. H. N.: Heart disease as presenting features of myotonia atrophica. Br. Heart J. 26:433, 1964.

48. Clements, S. D., Colmers, R. A., and Hurst, J. W.: Myotonia dystrophica: Ventricular arrhythmias, intraventricular conduction abnormalities, atrioventricular block and Stokes-Adams attacks successfully treated with permanent transvenous pacemaker. Am. J. Cardiol. 37:933, 1976.

49. Kennel, A. J., Titus, J. L., and Merideth, J.: Pathologic findings in the atrioventricular conduction system in myotonic dystrophy. Mayo Clin. Proc. 49:838, 1974.

50. Litchfield, J. A.: A-V dissociation in dystrophia myotonica. Br. Heart J. 15:357, 1953.

51. Roberts, N. K., Cabeen, W. R., and Perloff, J. K.: The cardiac disease of myotonic muscular dystrophy. Am. J. Cardiol. 47:421, 1981.

52. Prystowsky, E. N., Pritchett, E. L. C., Roses, A. D., and Gallagher, J.: The natural history of conduction system disease in myotonic muscular dystrophy as determined by serial electrophysiologic studies. Circulation 60:1360, 1979.

53. Komajda, M., Frank, R., Vedel, J., Fontaine, C., Petitot, J. C., and Grosgogeat, Y.: Intracardiac conduction defects in dystrophia myotonica. Br. Heart J. 43:315, 1980.

54. Atarashi, H., Saito, H., Hoki, H., and Hayakawa, H.: Myotonic dystrophy associated with sick sinus syndrome. Jpn. Circ. J. 45:763, 1981.

55. Gottdiener, J. S., Hawley, R. V., DiBianco, R., Fletcher, R. D., and Engel, W. K.: Left ventricular relaxation, mitral valve prolapse and intracardiac conduction in myotonia atrophica. Am. Heart J. 104:77, 1982.

56. Thomson, A. M. P.: Dystrophia cordis myotonica studied by serial histology of the pacemaker and conducting system. J. Pathol. Bacteriol. 96:285, 1968.

57. Cannon, P. J.: The heart and lungs in myotonic muscular dystrophy. Am. J. Med. 32:765, 1962.

58. Fisch, C., and Evans, P. V.: The heart in dystrophia myotonica: Report of an autopsied case. N. Engl. J. Med. 251:527, 1954.

59. Bulloch, R. T., Davis, J. L., and Hara, M.: Dystrophia myotonica with heart block. A light and electron microscopic study. Arch. Pathol. 84:130, 1967.

60. Motta, J., Guilleminault, C., Billingham, M., Barry, W., and Mason, J.: Cardiac abnormalities in myotonic dystrophy. Am. J. Med. 67:467, 1979.

61. Saloman, J., and Easley, R. M.: Cardiovascular abnormalities in myotonic dystrophy. Chest 64:135, 1973.

62. Miller, P. B.: Myotonic muscular dystrophy with electrocardiographic abnormalities. Am. Heart J. 63:704, 1962.

63. Winters, S. J., Schreiner, B., Griggs, R. C., Rowley, P., and Nanda, N. C.: Familial mitral valve prolapse and myotonic dystrophy. Ann. Intern. Med. 85:19, 1976.

64. Strasberg, B., Kanakis, C., Dhingra, R. C., and Rosen, K. M.: Myotonia dystrophica and mitral valve prolapse. Chest 78:845, 1980.

65. Morris, L. K., Cuetter, A. C., and Gunderson, C. H.: Myotonic dystrophy, mitral valve prolapse and cerebral embolism. Stroke 13:93, 1980.

65a. Lev, M., Bump, T., Bauernfeind, R. A., and Bharati, S.: Dystrophica myotonia: Correlative electrocardiographic, electrophysiologic and conduction system study. J. Am. Coll. Cardiol. 1:682, 1983.

66. Gottdiener, J. S., Hawley, R. U., Maron, B. J., Bertorini, T. F., and Engle, W. K.: Characteristics of the cardiac hypertrophy in Friedreich's ataxia. Am. Heart J. 103:525, 1982.

67. Pasternac, A., Krol, R., Petitclerc, R., Harvey, C., Andermann, E., and Barbeau, A.: Hypertrophic cardiomyopathy in Friedreich's ataxia: Symmetric or asymmetric? Can. J. Neurol. Sci. 7:379, 1980.

68. Harding, A. E.: Friedreich's ataxia: A clinical and genetic study of 90 families with an analysis of early diagnostic criteria and intrafamilial clustering of clinical features. Brain 104:589, 1981.

69. Barbeau, H.: Friedreich's ataxia 1980. An overview of the pathophysiology. Can. J. Neurol. Sci. 7:455, 1980.

70. Azari, J., Reisine, T., Barbeau, A., Yamamura, H. I., and Huxtable, R.: The Syrian golden hamster: A model for the cardiomyopathy of Friedreich's ataxia. Can. J. Neurol. Sci. 6:223, 1979.

71. Friedreich, N.: Über degenerative Atrophie der spinalen Hinterstrange. Virchows Arch. Pathol. Anat. 26:391, 433, 1863.

72. Walker, J. L., Chamberlain, S., and Robinson, N.: Lipids and lipoproteins in Friedreich's ataxia. J. Neurol. Neurosurg. Psychiatry 43:111, 1980.

73. Isner, J. M., Hawley, R. J., Weintraub, A. M., and Engel, W. K.: Cardiac

findings in Charcot-Marie-Tooth disease. Arch. Intern. Med. *139*:1161, 1979.

74. Kriel, R. L., Cliffer, K. D., Berry, J., Sung, J. H., and Bland, C. S.: Investigation of a family with hypertrophic neuropathy resembling Roussy-Levy syndrome. Clinical, electrophysiologic, histologic and biochemical studies. Neurology *24*:801, 1974.

75. Thoren, C.: Cardiomyopathy in Friedreich's ataxia. Acta Paediatr. (Suppl.) *153*: 1, 1964.

76. Richterich, R., Van Mechelen, P., and Rossi, E.: Refsum's disease. Am. J. Med. *29*:230, 1965.

77. Geoffroy, G., Barbeau, A., Breton, G., Lemieux, B., Aube, M., Leger, C., and Bouchard, J. T.: Clinical description and roentgenologic evaluation of patients with Friedreich's ataxia. Can. Sci. Neurol. *3*:279, 1976.

78. Butterworth, R. F., Shapcott, D., Melancon, S., Breton, G., Geoffroy, G., Lemieux, B., and Barbeau, A.: Clinical laboratory findings in Friedreich's ataxia. J. Can. Sci. Neurol. *3*:335, 1976.

79. Cote, M., Davignon, A., Elias, G., Solignac, A., Geoffroy, G., Lemieux, B., and Barbeau, A.: Hemodynamic findings in Friedreich's ataxia. J. Can. Sci. Neurol. *3*:333, 1976.

80. Hewer, R. L.: The heart in Friedreich's ataxia. Br. Heart J. *31*:5, 1969.

81. Ivemark, B., and Thoren, C.: Pathology of the heart in Friedreich's ataxia. Acta Med. Scand. *175*:227, 1964.

82. Gauthier, E. J.: Cardiac disease in Friedreich's ataxia. Ann. Intern. Med. *60*: 892, 1964.

83. Thilenius, O. G., and Gross, B. J.: Friedreich's ataxia with heart disease in children. Pediatrics *27*:246, 1961.

84. Ruschhaupt, D. G., Thilenius, O. G., and Cassels, D. E.: Friedreich's ataxia associated with idiopathic hypertrophic subaortic stenosis. Am. Heart J. *84*:95, 1972.

85. Berg, R. A., Kaplan, H. M., Jarrett, P. B., and Molthan, M. E.: Friedreich's ataxia with acute cardiomyopathy. Am. J. Dis. Child. *134*:390, 1980.

86. Cote, M., Bureau, M., Leger, C., Martin, J., Gattiker, H., Cimon, M., Larose, A., and Lemieux, B.: Evolution of cardio-pulmonary involvement in Friedreich's ataxia. J. Can. Sci. Neurol. *6*:151, 1979.

87. Cote, M., Davignon, A., Pecko-Drouin, K., Solignac, A., Geoffroy, G., Lemieux, B., and Barbeau, A.: Cardiological signs and symptoms in Friedreich's ataxia. J. Can. Sci. Neurol. *3*:319, 1976.

88. Gregorini, L., Valentini, R., and Libretti, A.: The vectorcardiogram in Friedreich's ataxia. Am. Heart J. *87*:158, 1974.

89. Boyer, S. H., Chisholm, A. W., and McKusick, V. A.: Cardiac aspects of Friedreich's ataxia. Circulation *25*:493, 1962.

90. Malo, S., Latour, Y., Cote, M., Geoffroy, G., Lemieux, B., and Barbeau, A.: Electrocardiographic and vectorcardiographic findings in Friedreich's ataxia. J. Can. Sci. Neurol. *3*:323, 1976.

91. Smith, E. R., Sangalang, V. E., Heffernan, L. P., Welch, J. P., and Flemington, C. S.: Hypertrophic cardiomyopathy: The heart disease of Friedreich's ataxia. Am. Heart J. *94*:428, 1977.

92. Soulié, P., Vernant, P., and Gaudeau, S.: Le coeur dans la maladie de Friedreich: Étude hémodynamique droite et gauche. Mal. Cardiov. *7*:369, 1966.

93. Gach, J. V., Andriange, M., and Franck, G.: Hypertrophic obstructive cardiomyopathy and Friedreich's ataxia: Report of a case and review of literature. Am. J. Cardiol. *27*:436, 1971.

94. Boehm, T. M., Dickerson, R. B., and Glasser, S. P.: Hypertrophic subaortic stenosis occurring in a patient with Friedreich's ataxia. Am. J. Med. Sci. *260*: 279, 1970.

95. Gattiker, H. F., Davignon, A., Bozio, A., Batlle-Diaz, J., Geoffroy, G., Lemieux, B., and Barbeau, A.: Echocardiographic findings in Friedreich's ataxia. Can. J. Neurol. Sci. *3*:329, 1976.

96. Griggs, R. C.: Hypertrophy and cardiomyopathy in the neuromuscular diseases. Cir. Res. *35*(Suppl. 2):145, 1974.

97. Weiss, E., Kronzon, I., Winer, H. E., and Berger, A. R.: Echocardiographic observations in patients with Friedreich's ataxia. Am. J. Med. Sci. *282*:136, 1981.

98. Sutton, M. A., Olukotun, A. Y., Tajik, A. J., Lovett, J. L., and Giuliani, E. R.: Left ventricular function in Friedreich's ataxia. Br. Heart J. *44*:309, 1980.

99. Pernot, C.: La myocardiopathie de la maladie de Friedreich. Arch. Fr. Pediatr. *36*:11, 1979.

100. Hartman, J. M., and Booth, R. W.: Friedreich's ataxia: A neurocardiac disease. Am. Heart J. *60*:716, 1960.

101. Sanchez-Casis, G., Cote, M., and Barbeau, A.: Pathology of the heart in Friedreich's ataxia: Review of the literature and report of one case. J. Can. Sci. Neurol. *3*:349, 1976.

102. Lamarche, J. B., Cote, M., and Lemieux, B.: The cardiomyopathy of Friedreich's ataxia: Morphologic observations in three cases. Can. J. Neurol. Sci. *7*: 389, 1980.

103. Goodwin, J. F.: Prospects and predictions for the cardiomyopathies. Circulation *50*:210, 1974.

104. Perloff, J. K.: Pathogenesis of hypertrophic cardiomyopathy. Am. Heart J. *101*: 219, 1981.

105. James, T. N., and Fisch, C.: Observations on the cardiovascular involvement in Friedreich's ataxia. Am. Heart. J. *66*:164, 1963.

106. Barbeau, A.: Friedreich's ataxia 1976—An overview. Can. J. Neurol. Sci. *3*: 389, 1976.

107. Spillane, J. D.: Familial pes cavus and absent ankle jerks. Its relationship with Friedreich's disease and peroneal muscular atrophy. Brain *63*:275, 1940.

108. Leak, D.: Paroxysmal atrial flutter in peroneal muscular atrophy. Br. Heart J. *23*:326, 1961.

109. Roth, M.: Relationship between hereditary ataxia and peroneal muscular atrophy. Brain *71*:416, 1948.

110. Littler, W. A.: Heart block and peroneal muscular atrophy. Q. J. Med. *39*:431, 1970.

111. Kay, J. M., Littler, W. A., and Meade, J. B.: Ultrastructure of myocardium in familial heart block and peroneal muscular atrophy. Br. Heart J. *34*:1081, 1972.

112. Waters, D. D., Nutter, D. O., Hopkins, L. C., and Dorney, E. R.: Cardiac features of an unusual X-linked humeroperoneal muscular disease. N. Engl. J. Med. *293*:1017, 1975.

113. Hassan, Z., Fastabend, C. P., Mohanty, P. K., and Isaacs, E. R.: Atrioventricular block and supraventricular arrhythmias with X-linked muscular dystrophy. Circulation *60*:1365, 1979.

114. Chakrabarti, A., and Pearce, J. M.: Scapuloperoneal syndrome with cardiomyopathy. J. Neurol. Neurosurg. Psychiatry *44*:1146, 1981.

115. Thomas, P. K., Schott, G. D., and Morgan-Hughes, J. A.: Adult-onset scapuloperoneal myopathy. J. Neurol. Neurosurg. Psychiatry *38*:1008, 1975.

116. Thomas, P. K., Calne, D. P., and Elliott, C. F.: X-linked scapuloperoneal syndrome. J. Neurol. Neurosurg. Psychiatry *35*:208, 1972.

117. Hopkins, L. C., Jackson, J. H., and Elsas, L. J.: Emery-Dreifuss humeroperoneal muscular dystrophy: An X-linked myopathy with unusual contractures and bradycardia. Ann. Neurol. *10*:230, 1981.

118. Spiro, A. J., Shy, G. M., and Gonatas, N. K.: Myotubular myopathy. Arch. Neurol. *14*:1, 1966.

119. Verhiest, W., Brucher, J. M., Goddeeris, P., Lauweryns, J., and DeGeest, H.: Familial centronuclear myopathy associated with cardiomyopathy. Br. Heart J. *38*:504, 1976.

120. Bethlem, J., VanWijngaarden, G. K., Meijerae, F. H., and Hulfmann, W. C.: Neuromuscular disease with type I fiberatrophy centronuclei and myotube-like structures. Neurology *19*:705, 1969.

121. Shafiq, S. A., Sande, M. A., Carruthers. R. R., Killip, T., and Milhorat, A. T.: Skeletal muscle in idiopathic cardiomyopathy. J. Neurol. Sci. *15*:303, 1972.

122. Kearns, T. P., and Sayre, G. P.: Retinitis pigmentosa, external ophthalmoplegia, and complete heart block. Arch. Ophthalmol. *60*:280, 1958.

123. Berenberg, R. A., Pellock, J. M., DiMauro, S., Schotland, D. L., Bonilla, E., Eastwood, A., Hays, A., Vicale, C. T., Behrens, M., Chutorian, A., and Rowland, L. P.: Lumping or splitting? "Ophthalmoplegia-plus" or Kearns-Sayre syndrome? Ann. Neurol. *1*:37, 1977.

124. Lowes, M: Chronic progressive external ophthalmoplegia, pigmentary retinopathy and heart block. (Kearns-Sayre syndrome). Acta Ophthalmol. *53*: 610, 1975.

125. Charles, R., Holt, S., Kay, J. M., Epstein, E. J., and Rees, J. R.: Myocardial ultrastructure and the development of atrioventricular block in Kearns-Sayre syndrome. Circulation *63*:214, 1981.

126. Coulter, D. L., and Allen, R. J.: Abrupt neurological deterioration in children with Kearns-Sayre syndrome. Arch. Neurol. *38*:247, 1981.

127. Roberts, N. K., Perloff, J. K., and Kark, P.: Cardiac conduction in Kearns-Sayre syndrome. Am. J. Cardiol. *44*:1396, 1979.

128. Clark, D. S., Meyerburg, R. J., Morales, R. R., Befeler, B., Hernandez, F. A., and Gelband, H.: Heart block and Kearns-Sayre: Electrophysiologic-pathologic correlation. Chest *68*:727, 1975.

129. Gibson, T. C.: The heart in myasthenia gravis. Am. Heart J. *90*:389, 1975.

130. Ratinov, G., Baker, W. P., and Swaiman, K. F.: McArdle's syndrome with previously unreported electrocardiographic and serum enzyme abnormalities. Ann. Intern. Med. *62*:328, 1965.

131. Sengers, R. C. A., ter Haar, B. G. A., Trijbels, J. M. F., Willems, J. L., and Daniels, O. Congenital cataract and mitochondrial myopathy of skeletal and heart muscle associated with lactic acidosis after exercise. J. Pediatr. *86*:873, 1975.

132. Emmons, P. R., Blume, W. T., and DuShane, J. W.: Cardiac monitoring and demand pacemaker in Guillain-Barré syndrome. Arch. Neurol. *32*:59, 1975.

133. Fave, H., Foex, P., and Guggisberg, M.: Use of demand pacemaker in a case of Guillain-Barré syndrome. Lancet *1*:1062, 1970.

134. Stewart, I. M.: Arrhythmias in the Guillain-Barré syndrome. Br. Med. J. *2*: 665, 1973.

135. Greenland, P., and Griggs, R. C.: Arrhythmic complications in the Guillain-Barré syndrome. Arch. Intern. Med. *140*:1053, 1980.

136. Isaacs, H., and Muncke, G.: Idiopathic cardiomyopathy and skeletal muscle abnormality. Am. Heart J. *90*:767, 1975.

137. Evans, W.: Familial cardiomegaly. Br. Heart J. *11*:68, 1949.

138. Smith, E. R., Heffernan, L. P., Sangalang, V. E., Vaughan, L. M., and Flemington, C. S.: Voluntary muscle involvement in hypertrophic cardiomyopathy. Ann. Intern. Med. *85*:566, 1976.

139. Darsee, J. E., Nutter, D. O., Hopkins, L. C., and Heymsfield, S. B.: Neurogenic skeletal myopathy in patients with primary cardiomyopathy. Circulation *59*: 492, 1979.

140. Gottdiener, J. S., Sherber, H. S., Hawley, R. J., and Engel, W. K.: Cardiac manifestations in polymyositis. Am. J. Cardiol. *41*:1141, 1978.

141. Singsen, B., Goldreyer, B., Stanton, R., and Hanson, V.: Childhood polymyositis with cardiac conduction defects. Am. J. Dis. Child. *130*:72, 1976.

142. Lisak, R. P., Lebeau, J., Tucker, S. H., and Rowland, L. P.: Hyperkalemic periodic paralysis and cardiac arrhythmias. Neurology *22*:810, 1972.

143. Buruma, O. J., Schipperheyn, J. J., and Bots, G. T.: Heart muscle disease in familial hypokalaemic periodic paralysis. Circulation *64*:12, 1981.

144. Klein, R., Ganelin, R., Marks, J. F., Usher, P., and Richards, C.: Periodic paralysis with cardiac arrhythmia. J. Pediatr. 62:371, 1963:

145. Kastor, J. A., and Goldreyer, B. N.: Ventricular origin of bidirectional tachycardia. Circulation 48:897, 1973.

146. Regan, T. J.: Alcoholic cardiomyopathy. In Fowler, N. O. (ed): Myocardial Disease. New York, Grune and Stratton, 1973.

147. Meyer, J. G., and Urban, K.: Electrolyte changes and acid-base balance after alcohol withdrawal. With special reference to rum fits and magnesium depletion. J. Neurol. 215:135, 1977.

148. Rubin, E.: Alcoholic myopathy in heart and skeletal muscle. N. Engl. J. Med. 301:28, 1979.

149. Regan, T. J., Haider, B., Ahmed, S. S., Lyons, M. M., Oldewurtel, H. A., and Ettinger, P. O.: Whiskey and the Heart. Cardiovasc. Med. 2:165, 1977.

150. Clarren, S. K., and Smith D. W.: The fetal alcohol syndrome. N. Engl. J. Med. 298:1063, 1978.

151. VanderArk, G. D.: Cardiovascular changes with acute subdural hematoma. Surg. Neurol. 3:305, 1975.

152. Cushing, H.: Concerning a definite regulatory mechanism of the vasomotor center which controls blood pressure during cerebral compression. Bull. Johns Hopkins Hosp. 12:390, 1901.

153. Chen, H. I., Liao, J. F., Kuo, L., and Ho, S. T.: Centrogenic pulmonary hemorrhagic edema induced by cerebral compression in rats. Circ. Res. 47:366, 1980.

154. Yamour, B. J., Sridharan, M. R., Rice, J. F., and Flowers, N. C.: Electrocardiographic changes in cerebrovascular hemorrhage. Am. Heart J. 99:294, 1980.

155. Bramwell, C.: Can head injury cause auricular fibrillation? Lancet 1:8, 1934.

156. Carruth, J. E., and Silverman, M. E.: Torsade de pointe atypical ventricular tachycardia complicating subarachnoid hemorrhage. Chest 78:886, 1980.

157. Mikolich, J. R., Jacobs, W. C., and Fletcher, G. F.: Cardiac arrhythmi as in patients with acute cerebrovascular accidents. J.A.M.A. 246:1314, 1981.

158. Harries, A. D.: Subarachnoid haemorrhage and the electrocardiogram. Postgrad. Med. J. 57:294, 1981.

159. Goldberger, A. L.: Recognition of ECG pseudoinfarct patterns. Mod. Concepts Cardiovasc. Dis. 49:13, 1980.

160. Burch, G. E., and Phillips, J. H.: The large upright T wave as an electrocardiographic manifestation of intracranial disease. South. Med. J. 61:331, 1968.

161. Taylor, A. L., and Fozzard, H. A.: Ventricular arrhythmias associated with CNS disease. Arch. Intern. Med. 142:232, 1982.

162. Dimant, J., and Grob, D.: Electrocardiographic changes and myocardial damage in patients with acute cerebrovascular accidents. Stroke 8:448, 1977.

163. Britton, M., de Faire, U., Helmers, C., Miah, K., Ryding, C., and Wester, P. O.: Arrhythmias in patients with acute cerebrovascular disease. Acta Med. Scand. 205:425, 1979.

164. Gascon, P., Ley, T. J., Toltzis, R. J., and Bonow, R. O.: Spontaneous subarachnoid hemorrhage simulating acute transmural myocardial infarction. Am. Heart J. 105:511, 1983.

165. Baur, H. R., Gobel, F. L., and Pierach, C. A.: Electrocardiographic changes after cervical laminectomy. Int. J. Cardiol. 1:37, 1981.

166. Goldman, M. R., Rogers, E. L., and Rogers, M. C.: Subarachnoid hemmorrhage: Association with unusual electrocardiographic changes. J.A.M.A. 234:957, 1975.

167. Frank, E., Tew, J. M., and Pagani, L.: The prolonged Q-T syndrome presenting as a focal neurological lesion. Surg. Neurol. 16:333, 1981.

168. Chin, P. L., Kaminski, J., and Rout, N.: Myocardial infarction coincident with cerebrovascular accidents in the elderly. Age Ageing 6:29, 1977.

169. Gould, L., Reddy, R. C., Kollali, M., Singh, B. K., and Zen, B.: Electrocardiographic normalization after cerebral vascular accident. J. Electrocardiol. 14:191, 1981.

170. Barnett, H. J. M., Boughner, D. R., Taylor, D. W., Cooper, P. E., Kostuk, W. J., and Nichol, P. M.: Further evidence relating mitral valve prolapse to cerebral ischemic events. N. Engl. J. Med. 302:139, 1980.

171. Yufe, R., Karpati, G., and Carpenter, S.: Cardiac myxoma: A diagnostic challenge for the neurologist. Neurology 26:1060, 1976.

172. Perloff, J. K.: The Clinical Recognition of Congenital Heart Disease. 2nd Ed. Philadelphia, W. B. Saunders Co., 1978.

173. Dawson, D. M., and Fischer, E. G.: Neurologic complications of cardiac catheterization. Neurology 27:496, 1977.

174. Walter, P. W., Reid, S. D., and Wenger, N. K.: Transient cerebral ischemia due to arrhythmia. Ann. Intern. Med. 72:471, 1970.

175. Luxon, L. M., Crowther, A., Harrison, M. J., and Coltart, D. J.: Controlled study of 24-hour ambulatory electrocardiographic monitoring in patients with transient neurological symptoms. J. Neurol. Neurosurg. Psychiatry 43:37, 1980.

176. Baron, K. D., Siqueira, E., and Hirano, A.: Cerebral embolism caused by nonbacterial thrombotic endocarditis. Neurology 10:391, 1960.

177. Caplan, L. R., Hier, D. B., and Banks, G.: Stroke and drug abuse. Current Conc. Cerebrovasc. Dis. 17:9, 1982.

178. Dodge, R. P., Richardson, E. P., and Victor, M.: Recurrent convulsive seizures as a sequel to cerebral infarction. Brain 77:610, 1959.

179. Rosenthal, A., Nathan, D. G., Marty, A. T., Button, L. N., Miettinen, O. S., and Nadas, A. S.: Acute hemodynamic effects of red cell volume reduction in polycythemia of cyanotic congenital heart disease. Circulation 42:297, 1970.

180. Bana, D. S., MacNeal, P. S., LeCompte, P. M., Shah, Y., and Graham, J. R.: Cardiac murmurs and endocardial fibrosis associated with methysergide therapy. Am. Heart J. 88:640, 1974.

181. Graham, J. R., Suby, H. I., LeCompte, P. M., and Sadowsky, N. L.: Fibrotic disorders associated with methysergide therapy for headaches. N. Engl. J. Med. 274:359, 1966.

182. Orlando, R. C., Moyer, P., and Barnett, T. B.: Methysergide therapy and constrictive pericarditis. Ann. Intern. Med. 88:213, 1978.

183. Roberts, W. C., and Sjoerdsma, A.: The cardiac disease associated with the carcinoid syndrome (carcinoid heart disease). Am. J. Med. 36:5, 1964.

184. Thorner, M. O.: Dopamine—An important neurotransmitter in the autonomic nervous system. Lancet 1:662, 1975.

185. Calne, D. B., Brennan, J., Spiers, A. S. D., and Stern, G. M.: Hypotension caused by L-dopa. Br. Med. J. 1:474, 1970.

186. Greenacre, J. K., Teychenne, T. F., Petrie, A., Calne, D. B., Leigh, P. N., and Reid, J. L.: The cardiovascular effects of bromocriptine in Parkinsonism. Br. J. Clin. Pharmacol. 3:571, 1976.

187. Snyder, B. D., Ramierz-Lassepas, M., and Lippert, D. M.: Neurologic status and prognosis after cardiopulmonary arrest. Neurology 27:807, 1977.

188. Caronna, J. J., and Finklestein, S.: Neurological syndromes after cardiac arrest. Curr. Concepts Cerebrovasc. Dis. (Stroke) 13:9, 1978.

189. Lown, B.: Electrical reversion of cardiac arrhythmias. Br. Heart J. 29:469, 1967.

190. Benorvitz, N. L.: Clinical applications of the pharmocokinetics of lidocaine. Cardiovasc. Clin. 6:77, 1974.

191. Greenblatt, D. J., and Koch-Weser, J.: Adverse reactions to propranolol in hospital medical patients. Am. Heart J. 86:478, 1973.

192. Niakan, E., Bertorini, T. E., Acchiardo, S. R., and Werner, M. F.: Procainamide-induced myasthenia-like weakness in a patient with peripheral neuropathy. Arch. Neurol. 38:378, 1981.

193. Kornfeld, P., Horowitz, S. H., Genkins, G., and Paptestas, A. E.: Myasthenia gravis unmasked by antiarrhythmic agents. Mt. Sinai J. Med. 43:10, 1976.

194. Withering W.: An account of the Foxglove. In Willius, F. A., and Keys, T. E.: Classics of Cardiology. Vol. 1. New York, Dover Publications, 1941, p. 232.

195. Weidler, D. J., Jallad, N. S., Keener, D. B., Das, S. K., and Wagner, J. G.: The effects of acute focal cerebral ischemia on digoxin toxicity and pharmacokinetics. Pharmacology 20:188, 1980.

51

ENDOCRINE AND NUTRITIONAL DISORDERS AND HEART DISEASE

by Gordon H. Williams, M.D., and Eugene Braunwald, M.D.

In 1835, Robert Graves described "three cases of violent and long-continued palpitation in females" with thyrotoxicosis.[1] Twenty years later, Thomas Addison reported that patients with disease of the "suprarenal capsules" had a "pulse, small and feeble . . . excessively soft and compressible." As the disease progressed "the body wastes . . . the pulse becomes smaller and weaker, and . . . the patient at length gradually sinks and expires."[2] Thus, since the mid-19th century, it has been known that deranged hormonal secretion can significantly alter cardiovascular function. However, only in the last few decades with the advent of techniques to measure the concentration of circulating hormones has the magnitude of the endocrine system's influence on cardiovascular function been generally appreciated. The purpose of this chapter is to summarize the more important cardiovascular manifestations of endocrine and nutritional diseases.

ACROMEGALY

The anterior pituitary gland secretes at least seven polypeptide hormones. Four (ACTH, FSH, LH, and TSH) primarily produce their biological effect indirectly by altering hormonal secretion from a specific target gland (adrenal cortex, gonad, and thyroid). Thus, the pathophysiological manifestations of a derangement in their secretion are the same as those of their target organs and will be discussed later. There are no cardiovascular manifestations of altered prolactin secretion or growth hormone deficiency; however, acromegaly (growth hormone excess) is associated with a number of clinical signs and symptoms related to the cardiovascular system.

Action of Growth Hormone. Growth hormone influences many metabolic processes, but its net effect is anabolic. Thus, when growth hormone is administered to a growth hormone–deficient individual, positive nitrogen balance, accompanied by retention of calcium, sodium, potassium, magnesium, and chloride, is manifest within days.[3,4] While many facets of nitrogen metabolism following administration of growth hormone have been studied, its primary effect has not been assessed definitively. Growth hormone increases the synthesis of both transfer and messenger RNA.[5] It reduces the breakdown of amino acids to urea and increases the transport of amino acids into skeletal and cardiac muscle, thus augmenting the substrate available for protein synthesis.[6] However, direct measurement of intracellular amino acid content has not documented the increase expected if these actions were the only ones responsible for the increased protein synthesis.

Growth hormone also induces changes in both fat and carbohydrate metabolism.[7,8] When administered acutely, it increases the uptake and utilization of glucose by fat cells, thus increasing lipogenesis. However, when administered chronically, it promotes lipolysis, thus increasing plasma free fatty acid levels and their oxidation and promoting ketogenesis, particularly in diabetic patients or animals. Growth hormone reduces glucose uptake by fat and muscle cells, increases gluconeogenesis, and increases peripheral resistance to insulin; as a consequence, plasma glucose levels rise. Because of this reduced tissue uptake of glucose and the increased blood levels of free fatty acids and ketones, those tissues, like the myocardium, that are able to use these latter compounds as energy substrates, do so.[9] Growth hormone can also increase the synthesis and/or accumulation of sulfated mucopolysaccharides in connective tissue.

Clinical and Biochemical Manifestations. Acromegaly is almost invariably the result of a growth hormone–producing chromophobic or eosinophilic pituitary adenoma. Characteristically, the disease is a slowly progressive one with signs and symptoms often predating diagnosis by more than 10 years. The striking physical findings (broad, spadelike hands and feet) are the result of growth hormone's effect on bone, muscle, and connective tissue. Osteoarthritis is common, as is organomegaly, hypertrichosis, hyperhidrosis, and modest weight gain.[4]

A derangement in carbohydrate metabolism is the most common metabolic consequence of chronic overproduction of growth hormone. Impaired glucose tolerance is found in half the patients, and hyperinsulinism is present in nearly all; thus, a state of insulin resistance exists. However, clinical diabetes mellitus is present in only 10 per cent of patients, which suggests that only those who are predisposed and have limited insulin reserve actually develop overt disease.[10] While it might be anticipated that hyperlipidemia would be common in acromegaly, it is in fact infrequently observed except in patients with clinical diabetes mellitus.[10,11] Even in these patients, it is probably secondary to the decreased secretion of insulin rather than to the increased secretion of growth hormone.

Cardiovascular Manifestations

The cardiac manifestations of acromegaly include cardiac enlargement which is greater than would be anticipated for the generalized organomegaly. In addition, the frequency of a number of other cardiovascular disorders is increased in acromegaly: hypertension, premature coronary artery disease, congestive heart failure, and cardiac arrhythmias, particularly frequent ventricular premature beats and intraventricular conduction defects.[12-14] Indeed, because of the frequent occurrence of congestive heart failure and cardiac arrhythmias in patients who otherwise have no predisposing factors (e.g., no hypertension or arteriosclerosis), it has been suggested that a specific acromegalic cardiomyopathy exists[15] (see below).

CARDIOMEGALY. Nearly all patients with acromegaly have cardiomegaly (Fig. 51–1), particularly after the fifth decade.[16] Echocardiographic assessment suggests that frequently there is an increase in cardiac mass with little other evidence of cardiac disease.[17,17a] Although the cardiomegaly may be related to the generalized effect of growth hormone on protein synthesis, some data suggest that other factors may also be important. For example, enlargement of the heart is often greater than that of other organs. Furthermore, there is no direct relationship between the degree of cardiomegaly and the level of circulating growth hormone.[14] While there is a correlation between the duration of acromegaly and cardiac hypertrophy,[15] other factors which may be important in the genesis of cardiomegaly include hypertension and atherosclerosis, both of which occur with increased frequency in acromegaly. Focal cardiac interstitial fibrosis and a myocarditis with lymphocytic infiltrate also have been reported in the majority of cases.[15,18] The former is probably due to the effect of growth hormone on collagen synthesis. Recently, it has

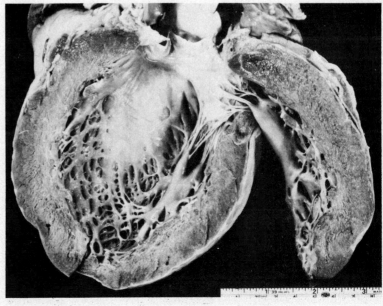

FIGURE 51–1 Opened left ventricle of the heart, showing the marked dilatation and hypertrophy, with fibrosis in the left septal endocardium. (From Rossi, L., et al.: Dysrhythmias and sudden death in acromegalic heart disease. A clinicopathologic study. Chest 72:496, 1977.)

been reported that small vessel disease of the myocardium occasionally may be present.[15] The resultant dysfunction in cardiac contraction secondary to any of these pathological changes could also contribute to the cardiac hypertrophy. Finally, cardiomyopathy characteristic of acromegaly may also contribute to the cardiomegaly.

HYPERTENSION. Hypertension is the most common cardiovascular manifestation of acromegaly, occurring in 15 to 50 per cent of patients if individuals with hypopituitarism are excluded. Hypertensive acromegalic patients tend to be older and to have had their acromegaly longer than nonhypertensive acromegalic patients. The underlying pathophysiology is uncertain. Most investigators either have searched for factors other than growth hormone that could cause hypertension or have attempted to determine how growth hormone itself may produce hypertension. Early studies suggested that the urine of patients with hypertension and acromegaly contains a specific pressor substance that was not derived from the pituitary gland and that was not a catecholamine;[19] however, these findings have not been confirmed. In many respects patients with acromegaly appear to be volume-expanded; the presence of an increase in glomerular filtration rate, renal plasma flow, extracellular fluid volume and sodium space, and reduction in plasma renin activity all support this hypothesis.[20–22] Thus, several studies have assessed the secretion of aldosterone in acromegaly; while increased secretion has been reported, this is an uncommon finding.[21–23] What does appear to occur frequently in acromegalics, however, is a change in tissue responsiveness to angiotensin II. Thus, on a sodium-restricted intake the response of aldosterone production to angiotensin II is decreased, but the vasoconstrictor response is increased when compared to normal subjects. This abnormality is present in both hypertensive and normotensive acromegalics.[24] Whether this is related to the pathogenesis of the elevated arterial pressure or simply a reflection of an expanded extracellular fluid volume is unclear.

A number of studies have suggested that growth hormone itself may be responsible for the hypertension. Thus, pituitary irradiation or hypophysectomy significantly reduces arterial pressure in hypertensive acromegalic patients, even when full glucocorticoid replacement is carried out.[24] Indeed, the apparent volume expansion may be directly related to the elevated growth hormone levels, since administration of growth hormone can produce retention of sodium and expansion of extracellular fluid volume.[25] It has been proposed that the pathophysiology of the hypertension in acromegaly may be similar to that in essential hypertension. In both conditions, initially there may be an elevation of cardiac output secondary to an expansion of extracellular fluid volume (Chap. 26). This could lead to a rise in arterial pressure and, finally, to changes in the peripheral vasculature producing fixed hypertension.

Early studies suggested that the presence of hypertension was a poor prognostic sign in acromegalic patients. Recent observations, however, are that the hypertension usually is mild, uncomplicated, and readily responsive to drugs.[14] This discrepancy may reflect the greater severity of the acromegalic process in earlier studies and the recognition now of the disorder at an earlier stage, rather than a change in the course of the disease.

ATHEROSCLEROSIS. Since growth hormone produces significant alterations in carbohydrate and lipid metabolism as well as hypertension, it is not surprising that premature atherosclerosis occurs in patients with acromegaly. What is uncertain is its frequency. One recent report suggests that major coronary disease may be present in only 10 per cent of acromegalics.[15] Coronary atherosclerosis could also contribute to the cardiomegaly observed in these patients.

ACROMEGALIC CARDIOMYOPATHY. Some patients with acromegaly without evidence of hypertension or atherosclerosis have significant cardiac dysfunction.[15] They primarily have either cardiomegaly, congestive heart failure, and/or cardiac dysrhythmias;[18] the congestive heart

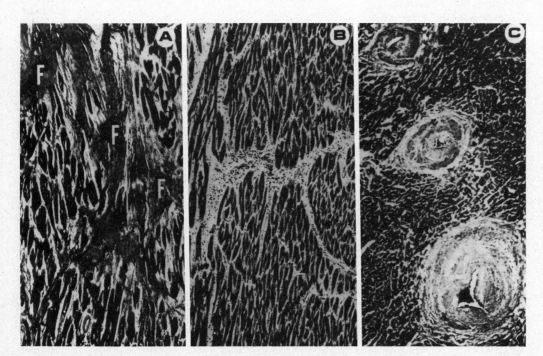

FIGURE 51–2 Histopathological features of acromegalic heart disease. *A,* Nonspecific myocardial hypertrophy and interstitial fibrosis (F). *B,* Myocarditis with predominantly lymphomononuclear cell infiltrate. *C,* Small vessel disease (proliferative fibrous wall thickening) of intramural coronary artery branches. (Reproduced with permission from Lie, J.T.: Acromegaly and heart disease. Primary Cardiol. 7:53, 1981. Copyright PW Communications, Inc.)

failure is particularly resistant to conventional therapy. It has been suggested that these are manifestations of an acromegalic cardiomyopathy which is related to the higher collagen content per gram of heart than in normal myocardium.[27] Histological observations show cellular hypertrophy, patchy fibrosis, and myofibrillar degeneration (Fig. 51–2). Sudden death has been associated with inflammatory and degenerative damage to the sinoatrial perinodal nerve plexus and degeneration of the AV node.[18]

It is not clear whether acromegalic cardiomyopathy is a specific entity. The evidence in favor of this position is indirect and comes from four types of observations: (1) Nearly 50 per cent of acromegalic patients have electrocardiographic abnormalities.[12,13,28] The most common findings are ST-segment depression with or without T-wave abnormalities, patterns consistent with left ventricular hypertrophy, intraventricular conduction disturbances—specifically, bundle branch block—and, infrequently, supraventricular or ventricular ectopic rhythms. While hypertension or other signs of atherosclerosis are present in many, 10 to 20 per cent of patients with acromegaly and electrocardiographic changes have no evidence of these conditions. (2) Ten to 20 per cent of acromegalics have overt congestive heart failure. In perhaps a fourth of these there is no known predisposing cause. (3) The majority of patients with acromegaly but without hypertension or atherosclerosis have subclinical evidence for cardiac dysfunction, as manifested by a shortening of the left ventricular ejection time (LVET), prolongation of the preejection period (PEP), and an elevation of the PEP/LVET ratio[29] (p. 54).[4] Approximately half of all patients with acromegaly, including patients without hypertension, have echocardiographic evidence of left ventricular hypertrophy.[30] These patients have growth hormone levels that are significantly higher than those of patients without left ventricular hypertrophy. Half of the patients with left ventricular hypertrophy exhibit asymmetrical septal hypertrophy, and these patients have a significantly greater percentage of internal dimensional shortening during systole than either the patients with concentric hypertrophy or those without left ventricular hypertrophy.

Diagnosis and Treatment

The *diagnosis* of acromegaly is established by documenting the nonsuppressibility of serum growth hormone levels following glucose loading.[4] In most laboratories, growth hormone concentrations in normal subjects are less than 2 ng/ml 120 minutes after the oral administration of 100 gm of glucose. It is also important to evaluate the integrity of the other pituitary hormones and, in hypertensive patients, to rule out an associated pheochromocytoma or aldosteronoma. The presence of sinus tachycardia or atrial fibrillation in a patient with acromegaly warrants a careful search for co-existing hyperthyroidism.

Surgery and irradiation remain the mainstays of treatment. The surgical approach is more often transsphenoidal[31] rather than transfrontal; heavy particle (proton beam) instead of conventional irradiation is being used with increasing frequency.[32] Preliminary studies suggest that growth hormone can be suppressed in some acromegalics with the dopamine agonist, bromocriptine. Whether this agent has any effect on tumor growth, however, is unclear.

Acromegalic patients with cardiovascular abnormalities usually respond to conventional therapeutic measures for hypertension, heart failure, or arrhythmias. Two caveats: (1) those with hypertension appear to be particularly responsive to volume-depleting maneuvers, i.e., diuretics and sodium restriction, perhaps even more so than patients with essential hypertension; and (2) some patients with congestive heart failure, primarily those *without* underlying hypertensive heart disease (i.e., those who are considered to have acromegalic cardiomyopathy), appear to be particularly resistant to therapy.

THYROID DISEASE

Thyroid hormone has a profound effect on a number of metabolic processes in virtually all tissues, with the heart being particularly sensitive to its effects. Therefore, it is not surprising that thyroid dysfunction can produce dramatic cardiovascular effects, often mimicking primary cardiac disease.

Action of Thyroid Hormone. Two biologically active hormones are secreted by the thyroid: thyroxine (T4) and triiodothyronine (T3). The relative importance of T4 and T3 in mediating the effects of thyroid hormone is being actively investigated. The question is not completely resolved, though most studies support the hypothesis that T3 is the final mediator and that T4 is a prohormone.[33] Major support for this position comes from the universal presence of T3 but not T4 nuclear receptors in tissues responsive to thyroid hormones.[34]

Even though the mechanism of action of thyroid hormone has been intensively investigated over the past three decades, uncertainty still exists about its principal effects. Most studies have provided data to support one of two general hypotheses. The older hypothesis suggests that thyroid hormone alters cellular metabolism by a direct action on mitochondria and is supported by studies showing (1) uncoupling of oxidative phosphorylation in isolated mitochondria by thyroxine; (2) increased total body oxygen consumption by thyroid hormone; and (3) increased substrate utilization with little generation of high-energy phosphate by thyroid hormone.[35] However, the following findings oppose this hypothesis: (1) the dose of thyroxine necessary to produce uncoupling of oxidative phosphorylation is more than 100 times the physiological dose; (2) the administration of dinitrophenol, a compound that also uncouples oxidative phosphorylation, does not induce a euthyroid state in hypothyroid animals[36]; and (3) it is possible that the uncoupling of oxidative phosphorylation may actually be an artifact of the in vitro systems.[37]

The second hypothesis, which has gained increasing support and is more likely to be correct, proposes that the major site of initiation of action of thyroid hormone is on the cell nucleus.[38] It has been observed that thyroid hormone is specifically bound to a chromatin-bound nonhistone nucleoprotein in the nucleus. As a result of that binding, alterations occur in protein synthesis, leading to many of the biochemical and metabolic effects observed with thyroxine administration. According to this hypothesis, the increased oxygen consumption results not from a direct interaction between thyroid hormone and mitochondria but rather indirectly via an increase in mitochondrial protein synthesis secondary to the effect of the thyroid hormone on the nucleus. Support for this hypothesis comes from several sources: (1) specific binding of T3 and, much less strongly, of T4 to nuclear receptor sites has been documented; (2) those tissues sensitive to thyroid hormone have nuclear binding sites; (3) the addition of thyroid hormone in vitro produces an increase in O_2 consumption only after a significant time lag; (4) an early metabolic effect of thyroxine is an increased rate of incorporation of a labeled precursor into nuclear RNA; (5) inhibitors of protein synthesis prevent many, if not most, of thyroid hormone's effects; and (6) treatment of hypothyroid animals with T3 causes increases in in vivo synthesis of specific messenger RNA's in several tissues including the heart.[39]

Edelman and Ismail-Beigi have extended this hypothesis one step further.[40] They postulated that not only does thyroid hormone enhance protein synthesis, but it specifically increases the activity of Na+-K+-ATPase. Thus, the augmented hydrolysis of ATP at the site of the sodium pump in the sarcolemma stimulates cellular (mitochondrial) oxygen consumption. Support for this hypothesis includes the observations that (1) hypothyroid rats treated with T3 exhibit a reduction in active sodium transport in crude homogenates and membrane-rich fractions and a decrease in intracellular Na+/K+ ratio in liver, diaphragm, and kidney,[41-42] and (2) the number of renal Na+ pump sites and the incorporation of radiolabeled methionine into renal cortical Na+-K+-ATPase are both increased, suggesting an increase in protein synthesis as the primary event.[41,42] Some reports, however, have suggested that the effect of thyroid hormone on cellular respiration cannot be entirely secondary to a change in the activity of this enzyme[44,45]

RELATION BETWEEN THE THYROID AND THE SYMPATHETIC NERVOUS SYSTEM

While the effects of thyroid hormone on the heart are varied and complex, it has been proposed that some of them are indirect, being secondary to changes in the activity of the sympathetic nervous system (Table 51-1). For example, many of the cardiovascular effects of hyperthyroidism, i.e., tachycardia, systolic hypertension, increased cardiac output, and myocardial contractility, can be abolished or reduced by blocking the activity of the sympathetic nervous system.[46] It has been proposed that thyroid hormone may alter the relationship between the sympathetic nervous and cardiovascular systems, either by increasing the activity of the sympathoadrenal system, or enhancing the response of cardiac tissue to normal sympathetic stimulation. Also, it has been suggested that sympathetic stimuli merely exert a direct additive effect on cardiovascular function above that produced by thyroid hormone. On the other hand, there is also evidence that hyperthyroidism reduces the sensitivity of cardiac tissue to sympathetic stimuli.[47]

Thus, the results of experiments on the relationship between the sympathoadrenal system and hyperthyroidism have evoked considerable controversy. On one hand, the plasma and urine levels of norepinephrine, epinephrine, and dopamine-β-hydroxylase are either low or normal in hyperthyroidism and either normal or elevated in hypothyroidism,[48-50] which suggests that the sympathomimetic features of hyperthyroidism cannot be explained by a simple change in adrenergic activity. On the other hand, we observed in a study on conscious, instrumented dogs rendered hyperthyroid that the reductions of heart rate and myocardial contractility induced by propranolol were greater than they were in the euthyroid state, a finding which indicates that the contribution of adrenergic stimulation to heart rate and myocardial contractility is greater in the hyperthyroid than the euthyroid state. However, the levels of heart rate and contractility following beta blockade were still greater when the dogs were hyperthyroid than when they were euthyroid, providing support for the concept that thyroid hormone exerts a direct effect on cardiac function, independent of any effect on the sympatho-adrenal system.[51]

After 50 years of investigation, disagreement still exists regarding a possible role for thyroid hormone in enhancing cardiac responses to catecholamines. Early studies reported an augmented sensitivity,[52] but later investigations suggested no significant displacement of the dose-response relationship.[53] In a study using fetal mouse hearts in tissue culture to avoid the problems of the delayed effect of thyroid hormone and the difficulty of interpreting the results using tissue obtained from animals with experimental hyperthyroidism, it was shown that T3 shifts the catecholamine dose-response curve to the left and that this increase in sensitivity is specific for those agents which stimulate beta receptors.[54,55] In support of this finding are the observations that there is an increase in either the number or the affinity of cardiac beta receptors after administration of thyroid hormone.[56-59] Further support comes from the study by Guarnieri et al., who showed that hyperthyroid rats have an enhanced activation of protein kinase and contractile response following administration of threshold doses of the beta-adrenergic agonist, isoproterenol.[60] In the aforementioned study on conscious hyperthyroid dogs,[51] however, we found no alteration in the sensitivity of the inotropic response to isoproterenol and norepinephrine.

The reasons for the conflicting results in this area may be related to the specificity of the technique used to assess beta-receptor activity, since it has been postulated that thyroid hormone influences the interconversion of alpha and beta receptors. Thus, rat atria obtained from hypothyroid animals have increased alpha and decreased beta receptor activity,[61] and there is evidence that hyperthyroidism produces the opposite effect.[56] Thus, if the agent used to determine adrenergic receptor activity were not highly specific for beta receptors, incorrect conclusions could be drawn.

TABLE 51-1   CLINICAL FEATURES OF HYPERTHYROIDISM*

DIRECT THYROID HORMONE EFFECT†	BETA-ADRENERGIC-LIKE EFFECT†
Resting heart rate > 90/min (90%)	Resting heart rate > 90/min (90%)
Palpitations (85%)	**Palpitations (85%)**
Atrial fibrillation (10%)	**Exertional dyspnea (80%)**
Pedal edema (30%)	**Increased pulse pressure (systolic hypertension)**
Increased oxygen consumption (basal metabolism)	**Active apical impulse**
Weight loss	**Loud first heart sound and pulmonic component of second heart sound**
Skeletal muscle myopathy	
Increased bone turnover (occasional osteoporosis or hypercalcemia)	**Midsystolic murmur, usually basal**
	Third heart sound (occasional)
Fine skin	**Means-Lerman scratch (rare)‡**
Fine brittle hair	Tremor
Brittle nails	Brisk reflexes
Oligo- or amenorrhea	Increased perspiration
Increased bowel frequency	Heat intolerance
	Insomnia
	Anxiety
	Stare, lid lag§

*Cardiac response to hyperthyroidism and symptoms of hyperthyroidism that mimic those of heart disease are shown in boldface type. The numbers in parentheses are approximate prevalences of the findings, compiled from several large series. Goiter is almost always present, though in elderly patients the thyroid enlargement may be minimal or absent.

†Both types of effects contribute to the tachycardia and palpitations.

‡A systolic scratch or click in the second left intercostal space that is probably generated by the pleura and pericardium rubbing together.

§These reflect upper-lid retraction. Infiltrative ophthalmyopathy with exophthalmos is found only when Graves' disease is the cause of the hyperthyroidism and is not related to the hyperthyroid state per se.

Reproduced with permission from Kaplan, M. M.: The thyroid and the heart: How do they interact? J. Cardiovasc. Med. 7:893, 1982.

EFFECT OF THYROID HORMONE ON THE HEART

There is evidence that thyroid hormone may alter cardiac function directly. Thus, the addition of thyroid to fragments of chick embryonic heart increases the rate of beating of the cells.[62] Additionally, the increased heart rate and myocardial contractility observed in experimental hyperthyroidism are not completely reversed by either sympathetic or parasympathetic blockade.[47,51] Finally, thyroxine enhances the rate of contraction of cardiac muscle even in the presence of adrenergic blockade.[63] Right ventricular papillary muscles isolated from cats rendered hyperthyroid exhibited augmented myocardial contractility, as reflected in an upward shift of the myocardial force-velocity curve,[47] with a greatly increased velocity of myocardial fiber shortening, a reduced time to peak tension during isometric contraction, and an augmented peak tension development (Fig. 51-3). Prior catecholamine depletion by pretreatment of the hyperthyroid cats with reserpine did not alter this inotropic effect of hyperthyroidism, providing further evidence for a direct cardiac effect.[47] Assessment of this hypothesis in the intact conscious calf recently has been performed. The results suggest that the major actions of thyroxine on the left ventricle are (1) a direct positive inotropic effect and (2) an increase in the size of the ventricular cavity without a change in the end-diastolic pressure or length of the sarcomere in diastole.[64]

The available data suggest that the direct effect of thyroid hormone on the heart is mediated via a change in protein synthesis.[64a,64b] Thyroid hormone increases the activity of the sodium pump in myocardial cells as it does in other tissues. Philipson and Edelman have documented that the activity of both the Na^+-K^+-ATPase and the K^+-dependent p-nitrophenyl phosphatase in the heart is increased by more than 50 per cent when T3 is administered

to hypothyroid rats.[65] The hearts of euthyroid rabbits rendered hyperthyroid exhibited a doubling of myofibrillar ATPase activity.[66] Reverse T3 (a biologically inactive analog) has no effect. Curfman et al. have suggested that this increased activity is the result of an increase in the number of functional enzyme complexes.[67] There is evidence that thyroid hormone both increases the synthesis of myosin and alters its structure, increasing its contractile properties,[68] particularly by increasing the more mobile myosin isoenzyme as determined by polyacrylamide gel electrophoresis.[68-70] The heart appears to respond to thyrotoxicosis by enhancing synthesis of a myosin isoenzyme with a fast ATPase activity.[66,69] The augmented myosin ATPase activity appears to contribute to the enhanced contractile response of the hyperthyroid heart, since the activity level of this enzyme is thought to regulate the rate of turnover of actin-myosin cross-bridge links in cardiac muscle. However, this is probably not the principal cause, since administration of exogenous thyroid can stimulate contractility before any change in the myosin ATPase activity occurs.[71] The sarcoplasmic reticulum isolated from hyperthyroid dogs and rabbits accumulates and exchanges calcium at an increased rate,[72] resulting in increased availability of calcium to the myofibrils during activation, as well as an enhanced rate of myofibrillar relaxation.

The tachycardia observed in hyperthyroidism appears to be due to a combination of an increased rate of diastolic depolarization and a decreased duration of the action potential in the sinoatrial node cells.[73] The propensity for the development of atrial fibrillation may be due to the shortened refractory period of atrial cells.[74]

Hyperthyroidism

Hyperthyroidism is the clinical state resulting from the excess production of triiodothyronine, thyroxine, or both. The most common cause is a diffuse toxic goiter (Graves' disease). Although the etiology of this condition is still unkown, the hyperproduction of T4 and T3 are thought to result from circulating IgG autoantibodies that bind to the thyrotropin receptor on the thyroid gland. The second most common form of hyperthyroidism is nodular toxic goiter, a condition in which localized areas of the gland function excessively and autonomously. Less common causes include a single toxic adenoma, ingestion of excessive amounts of thyroid hormone, and subacute thyroiditis, in which there may be a self-limited phase of hyperthyroidism. Rarely, hyperthyroidism may also occur as a result of the production of thyroid hormone by a thyroid carcinoma or production of a thyrotropic substance (probably HCG) by a hydatidiform mole or choriocarcinoma.

Hyperthyroidism is a relatively common disease, occurring four to eight times more commonly in women than in men, with a peak incidence in the third and fourth decades. The commonly associated signs and symptoms include fatigue, hyperactivity, insomnia, heat intolerance, palpitations, dyspnea, increased appetite with weight loss, nocturia, diarrhea, oligomenorrhea, muscle weakness, tremor, emotional lability, increased heart rate, systolic hypertension, hyperthermia, warm moist skin, lid lag, stare, and brisk reflexes. In the vast majority of cases a goiter can be palpated. Hyperthyroidism in childhood occurs most frequently just before or during adolescence. It is usually associated with a diffuse goiter. The most common early manifestations of juvenile hyperthyroid patients are excessive movements and emotional lability.

T3 levels are invariably elevated and serum T4 levels are usually increased as well. In addition to the signs and symptoms directly related to increased production of thyroid hormone, patients with Graves' disease often have exophthalmos and occasionally circumscribed areas of thickening of the skin, particularly of the lower extremities; presumably these are related to the immunological aspects of the disease.

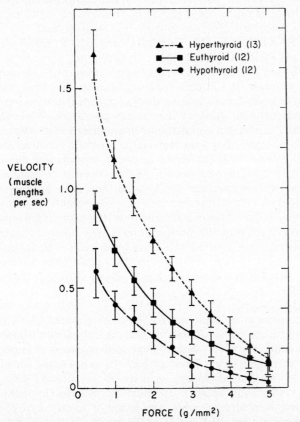

FIGURE 51-3 The average force-velocity relationship for papillary muscles from hyperthyroid, euthyroid, and hypothyroid cats. Initial velocity of shortening is normalized in terms of muscle lengths per second; load, corrected for cross-sectional area of individual muscles is expressed in gm/mm². Brackets represent ± SEM. (From Buccino, R. A., Spann, J. F., Poole, P. E., and Braunwald, E.: Influence of the thyroid state on the intrinsic contractile properties and the energy stores of the myocardium. J. Clin. Invest. *46*:1669, 1967.)

Particularly in older patients, the typical clinical picture is occasionally absent.[75] In these individuals with so-called *apathetic hyperthyroidism*, few clinical manifestations are apparent except in cardiovascular function. Thus, cardiac arrhythmias and heart failure resistant to conventional forms of therapy are common.

CARDIOVASCULAR MANIFESTATIONS. The heart is among the most responsive organs in thyroid disease, and cardiovascular signs and symptoms are therefore important clinical features of hyperthyroidism. Palpitations, dyspnea, tachycardia, and systolic hypertension are common findings. Diastolic hypertension can also occur. Typically, there is a hyperactive precordium with a loud first heart sound, an accentuated pulmonic component of the second heart sound, and a third heart sound; occasionally, a systolic ejection click is heard. Midsystolic murmurs along the left sternal border are common and a systolic scratch, the so-called Means-Lerman scratch, is occasionally heard in the second left intercostal space during expiration. It is presumed to be secondary to the rubbing together of normal pleural and pericardial surfaces by the hyperdynamic heart.

As would be anticipated, and as described in greater detail on page 812, cardiac and stroke volume index, mean systolic ejection rate, and coronary blood flow[75a] are all increased, the systolic ejection period and preejection period are abbreviated, the pulse pressure is widened, and systemic vascular resistance is reduced in hyperthyroidism.[76,77] It has been suggested that many of the changes in cardiac function are secondary to the increased metabolic demands of peripheral tissue. However, the increase in cardiac output is greater than would be predicted on the basis of the increased total body oxygen consumption, supporting the view that thyroid hormone exerts a direct cardiac stimulant action independent of its effect on general tissue metabolism.

Roentgenographic and electrocardiographic changes are common but are nonspecific in hyperthyroidism.[78] Thus, the left ventricle, aorta, and the pulmonary artery are prominent, and, in some cases, there is generalized cardiac enlargement, which may be accompanied by signs and symptoms of heart failure. In patients with sinus rhythm, the magnitude of the tachycardia, in general, parallels the severity of the disease. Sinus tachycardia, i.e., a rate exceeding 100/min, is present in 40 per cent of patients with hyperthyroidism, occurring most frequently in the younger age groups. About 15 per cent of patients with hyperthyroidism have persistent atrial fibrillation, which is often heralded by one or more transient episodes of this arrhythmia.[28] There is shortening of the AV conduction time and functional refractory period, resulting in an increased frequency at which the AV conduction system transmits rapid atrial impulses.[79] Intra-atrial conduction disturbances, manifested by prolongation or notching of the P wave and prolongation of the P-R interval in the absence of treatment with digitalis, occur in 15 per cent and 5 per cent of patients with hyperthyroidism, respectively. Occasionally, second or third degree heart block may result.[80] The cause of the AV conduction disturbance is not clear, since animal experiments have shown that the functional refractory period of the AV conduction system and the conduction time were shortened in dogs with hyperthyroidism and prolonged in dogs with hypothyroidism.[79] Intraventricular conduction disturbances, most commonly right bundle

branch block, occur in about 15 per cent of patients with hyperthyroidism without associated heart disease of other etiology.[81] Paroxysmal supraventricular tachycardia and flutter are rare in hyperthyroidism.

Both angina pectoris and congestive heart failure occur in patients with hyperthyroidism, and for many years it was assumed that these were seen only in the presence of underlying cardiovascular disease. Support for this position came primarily from the absence of these symptoms in young persons with significant hyperthyroidism. Recently, however, three lines of evidence have suggested otherwise. First, congestive heart failure has been produced in experimental animals by simply administering thyroxine. Secondly, infants with neonatal thyrotoxicosis without underlying cardiac disease may develop congestive heart failure[82]; and finally, abnormal left ventricular function observed during exercise in hyperthyroid subjects is not reversed by beta blockade but is reversed by treating the hyperthyroidism.[83] Thus, when it is severe enough, thyrotoxicosis can overtax even the normal heart, although, in most instances, the development of clinical manifestations of heart failure and myocardial ischemia in patients with hyperthyroidism signifies the presence of underlying cardiac or coronary vascular disease.

Finally, mitral valve prolapse has been associated with hyperthyroidism. In a recent report, 19 of 40 patients with hyperthyroidism had auscultatory and echocardiographic evidence of mitral valve prolapse. This is a frequency more than twice that observed in euthyroid individuals.[84]

TREATMENT OF CARDIOVASCULAR DISEASE IN HYPERTHYROIDISM. Hyperthyroid patients with cardiovascular disease are particularly resistant to therapy. For example, it has been well documented that both congestive heart failure and cardiac arrhythmias are resistant to conventional doses of the cardiac glycosides. While the specific mechanisms underlying these altered responses remain obscure, they may be related to both systemic and local effects.[85,86] First, serum levels of digitalis are diminished in hyperthyroidism, not because there is an augmentation of its metabolism but because there is an increase in its volume of distribution. Second, experimental hyperthyroidism reduces the enhancement of the myocardial contractile force and the prolongation of the atrioventricular nodal refractory period produced by digitalis.[86] Because of this decreased sensitivity to cardiac glycosides, toxicity may develop at a dose that has relatively little therapeutic effect.

DIAGNOSIS AND THERAPY. The diagnosis of hyperthyroidism is made on the basis of elevated levels of thyroid hormone in the blood. Because only serum triiodothyronine, T3, is elevated in some individuals, it is important to obtain serum levels of *both* T3 and T4 and an index of the thyroid-binding capacity of the patient's serum (resin thyroxine uptake). In most laboratories hyperthyroidism is confirmed when the levels of serum thyroxine are greater than 10.5 μg/dl or T3 levels are greater than 180 ng/dl with normal resin thyroxine uptakes. Occasionally, patients will have hyperthyroidism with both T3 and T4 within the normal range. If suspected, confirmation may be obtained by measuring the TSH (thyroid stimulating hormone) response to TRH (thyrotropin releasing hormone), which should be blunted in hyperthyroidism. Such has recently been reported in four patients with unexplained atrial fibrillation.[87] However, caution needs to be exercised in using this test, since false-positive results are common.

Prompt treatment of the hyperthyroid state can significantly reduce, if not eliminate, the associated cardiovascular symptoms. About half of patients with concurrent onset of hyperthyroidism and angina pectoris experience complete remission of symptoms after treatment of hyperthyroidism.[88] Furthermore, 62 per cent of 163 thyrotoxic patients with atrial fibrillation sustained for one week or longer were found to revert spontaneously to sinus rhythm when they became euthyroid.[89] Arterial embolization is not common in patients with thyrotoxicosis and atrial fibrillation, but it does occur. In one series, 8 per cent of 262 patients with both conditions had embolization.[90] Thus, it is important to determine quickly whether hyperthyroidism is present in patients with cardiovascular disease, since treatment often results in dramatic improvement. In elderly patients with apathetic hyperthyroidism, cardiovascular manifestations, specifically atrial fibrillation and/or congestive heart failure, predominate and therefore evaluation of thyroid function in such patients is particularly important. However, it should be noted that these individuals are particularly resistant to cardiac glycosides.

The definitive treatment of hyperthyroidism is surgical removal of the gland or irradiation using [131]I. In severely ill patients, particularly those with thyroid storm or significant cardiovascular symptoms or both, neither of these therapies is appropriate. Thus, medical therapy is directed at reducing both the production and biological effect of thyroid hormone. Since many of the cardiovascular symptoms of thyrotoxicosis are related to increased beta-adrenergic activity, treatment with beta-adrenergic blocking agents has been useful.[91] Tachycardia, palpitations, tremor, restlessness, muscle weakness, and heat intolerance are reversed by these agents, which offer the additional benefit of inhibiting the conversion of thyroxine to the biologically active T3 in peripheral tissues.

Beta-blockers can be administered orally or intravenously, but since this drug interferes with the effects of sympathetic stimulation on the heart, it must be used with caution in patients with congestive heart failure. However, if the heart failure is in part related to the tachycardia, beta-blockade may be beneficial. These agents can be administered in small doses while the patient is under close observation and being treated with digitalis and diuretics and reduction in physical activity. Beta-blocking drugs and cardiac glycosides act synergistically to slow ventricular rate in atrial fibrillation by increasing the refractoriness of the atrioventricular conduction system. Thus, the combination may allow a beneficial effect that would require toxic doses of either agent used alone. Beta-adrenergic blockade also improves many of the peripheral manifestations of thyrotoxicosis and in a double-blind controlled study has been shown to reduce tremor, stare, hyperreflexia, lid lag, and globe lag.[92]

While beta-adrenergic blockade can produce significant improvement of the cardiovascular status in patients with hyperthyroidism, correction of the basic metabolic defect requires specific therapy directed at reducing the production of thyroid hormone.[77] The most useful agents are among the thionamides, such as propylthiouracil. These drugs should be administered concurrently with a beta-

blocking agent so as to reduce the total production of thyroid hormone. The usual starting dose of propylthiouracil is 300 to 800 mg in divided doses daily; it not only reduces thyroid hormone production but also has the advantage of reducing the peripheral conversion of thyroxine into T3. Usual maintenance doses range from 50 to 300 mg. The thionamides are not without risk, since between 1 and 5 per cent of patients have significant side effects — usually gastrointestinal disturbances or a suppression of the bone marrow; infrequently, a generalized vasculitis has been reported.

Iodine, most commonly administered in the form of two drops of saturated solution of potassium iodide three times daily, inhibits the release of thyroid hormones from the thyrotoxic gland, and its beneficial effects occur rapidly, indeed, more rapidly than those of agents that inhibit the synthesis of the hormone. It is therefore useful in the rapid amelioration of the hyperthyroid state in patients with thyroid heart disease. It may also be utilized along with antithyroid agents to control thyrotoxicosis following ^{131}I treatment until the radioiodine has had time to take effect. Most hyperthyroid patients, however, escape from the effects of iodide after 10 to 14 days.

Hypothyroidism

Hypothyroidism results from reduced secretion of both thyroxine and T3, occurring in most cases as a consequence of destruction of the thyroid gland itself, usually by an inflammatory process. In some cases, it is secondary to decreased secretion of thyrotropin, due to either pituitary or hypothalamic disease. In secondary hypothyroidism, the signs and symptoms associated with deficiency of other pituitary hormones are also usually present. The incidence of hypothyroidism peaks between the ages of 30 and 60 years and is twice as common in women as in men. The following signs and symptoms are common: cold intolerance, dryness of the skin, weakness, impairment of memory, personality changes, shortness of breath, constipation, hoarseness, menorrhagia and other forms of menstrual dysfunction, and, occasionally, heart failure. In addition, in the more severe forms of the disease, there is facial puffiness, particularly around the eyes, a characteristic nonpitting form of edema (myxedema) of the lower extremities, slow speech, decreased hearing, and a yellow hue to the skin due to decreased conversion of carotene into vitamin A. These signs and symptoms may be present for years before treatment is initiated, particularly in patients in whom the disease has developed gradually.

Infants with severe congenital hypothyroidism may have a cardiac murmur, pallor, hepatomegaly, and edema. These manifestations appear before the signs of congenital hypothyroidism, which may not be apparent until one to three months of age, and which include retarded growth and development, with persistence of infantile features, a protuberant tongue, sluggish movements with poor muscle tone, coarse hair, cool skin, hypothermia, and constipation.[93]

CARDIOVASCULAR MANIFESTATIONS. The heart in overt myxedema is often pale, flabby, and grossly dilated. Histological examination discloses myofibrillar swelling, loss of striations, and interstitial fibrosis.[94] With the development of methods that reliably and easily measure the circulating levels of thyroid hormone, the diagnosis of hypothyroidism is being made with increasing frequency at an earlier stage of the disease. Treatment is therefore also initiated earlier, resulting in a reduction in the incidence of cardiovascular signs and symptoms. Thus, the classic findings of cardiac enlargement, cardiac dilatation, significant bradycardia, weak arterial pulses, hypotension, distant heart sounds, low electrocardiographic voltages, nonpitting facial and peripheral edema, and evidence of congestive heart failure, such as ascites, orthopnea, and paroxysmal dyspnea, are now seen only infrequently. However, exertional dyspnea and easy fatigability continue to be common complaints.

Myxedema is associated with increased capillary permeability and subsequent leakage of protein into the interstitial space, resulting in pericardial effusion, a common clinical finding in overt myxedema, occurring in about one third of all patients[95] (p. 1515). Rarely, it is complicated by cardiac tamponade.[96] Cardiomegaly on chest radiograph and low voltage in the electrocardiogram are not reliable indicators of pericardial effusion; echocardiography is the most useful method of establishing the diagnosis[95] (p. 1478). The effusions disappear with thyroid replacement therapy.[97]

The electrocardiographic changes observed in patients with hypothyroidism other than sinus bradycardia include prolongation of the Q-T interval, but since the T-wave amplitude is low, precise measurement of this interval is often impossible.[28] The P-wave amplitude is usually very low, and in some cases this wave is not even discernible. Sinus tachycardia is very rare, whereas bradycardia is common. It is possible that hypothermia may contribute to reentrant ventricular arrhythmias by slowing the heart rate and increasing the duration of the QRS and the Q-T intervals.[28] The incidence of atrioventricular and intraventricular conduction disturbances is about three times greater in patients with myxedema than in the general population.[98] Other electrocardiographic changes are those associated with pericardial effusion.[28,97] Thus, flattening or inversion of the T waves and low P-, QRS-, and T-wave amplitudes are commonly observed in patients with pericardial effusion. In most cases these revert to normal with the removal of the fluid. In some cases, however, the electrocardiographic changes persist even though the pericardial fluid is removed, which suggests that the lack of thyroid hormone may produce a primary myocardial abnormality.[99] Incomplete or complete right bundle branch block has been observed, but other forms of arrhythmias are uncommon.

Cardiovascular manifestations of congenital hypothyroidism are similar except for the rarity of pericardial effusion. Thus, the size of the left ventricle, its capacity and the posterior wall thickness are all lower in the hypothyroid infant. Since heart rate is also lower, cardiac output is reduced. There is also a prolongation of the preejection period of the left ventricle.[100]

MYOCARDIAL EFFECTS. Hypothyroid patients have reduced cardiac output, stroke volume, and blood and plasma volumes.[101] Circulation time is prolonged, but right and left heart filling pressures are usually within normal limits unless they are elevated by the pericardial effusion. There is a redistribution of blood flow with mild reductions in cerebral and renal flow and significant reductions in cutaneous flow.[102] A delay in the relaxation of skeletal muscle is a well-known finding in hypothyroidism; measurements of isovolumetric relaxation time, by a combination of apex cardiography and phonocardiography, have revealed a prolongation of this interval with an abbreviation to normal during thyroxine replacement.[103] In addition, there is lengthening of the preejection period and an increased ratio of the preejection period to the left ventricular ejection time (PEP/LVET); these changes are the opposite of those observed in hyperthyroidism.[104]

Cardiac muscle isolated from cats with experimentally produced hypothyroidism exhibited reduced contractility, characterized by a depression of the myocardial force-velocity curve, a reduction of the rate of tension development, and a prolongation of the contractile response (see Fig. 51–3).

There is little evidence from either experimental or clinical studies that congestive heart failure is common in myxedema or that it occurs in the absence of other cardiac disease.[105] Presumably, the depressed myocardial contractility is sufficient to sustain the reduced workload placed on the heart in hypothyroidism. However, it may be difficult to distinguish between the heart in myxedema and heart failure.[94] Dyspnea, edema, effusions, cardiomegaly, and T wave changes occur in both conditions. In left heart failure, pulmonary artery pressure is usually elevated during exercise, cardiac output fails to rise normally, and the Valsalva response is normal, while the opposite occurs in myxedema.[106] The hemodynamic changes in myxedema respond to thyroid hormone administration.

Cardiac catecholamine levels are not reduced in hypothyroidism. Whether a change in the binding of catecholamine receptors or the total number of myocardial receptors is altered has yet to be established. However, it is unlikely that a significant alteration in adrenergic nervous system is responsible for the change in myocardial contractility. Indeed, neither the sensitivity of the mechanical performance of the heart to exogenous catecholamines or sympathetic nerve stimulation[107] nor the response of adenylate cyclase to graded doses of norepinephrine is altered in hypothyroidism.[108] A more likely explanation is related to the direct effect of thyroid hormone on the contractile process itself. In experimental hypothyroidism, calcium in isolated myocardial sarcoplasmic reticulum particles is reduced, which may explain the altered contractile state.[72] As noted above, thyroid hormone can affect the quantity and function of myosin ATPase activity through a change in protein synthesis. The activity of cardiac myosin ATPase[109] and the rate of calcium uptake and the calcium-dependent ATP hydrolysis by isolated myocardial sarcoplasmic reticulum in the excitation-contraction-relaxation process[72] are reduced in hypothyroidism.

ATHEROSCLEROSIS. It has been suggested that patients with hypothyroidism are at increased risk of developing atherosclerosis, since this disease is accompanied by significant changes in lipid metabolism. Thus, hypercholesterolemia, hypertriglyceridemia, and impairment in free fatty acid mobilization, all associated with development of premature coronary artery disease, are found in patients with hypothyroidism. Support for this hypothesis has come from several sources, including the documentation that coronary atherosclerosis occurs with twice the frequency in patients with myxedema than in age- and sex-matched controls and that the development of atherosclerosis in cholesterol-fed animals is enhanced by the presence of hypothyroidism and reduced when thyroid hormone is administered.[110–112] Additionally, it has recently been reported that hypothyroidism has a deleterious effect in dogs in whom a myocardial infarction has been induced. Infarct size was increased, dysrhythmias were more severe, and abnormalities in the microvasculature were present.[113] Yet myocardial infarction and angina pectoris are relatively uncommon occurrences in patients with hypothyroidism.[114]

The latter was present in only 7 per cent of a group of patients with hypothyroidism.[115] This low frequency of cardiac complications from atherosclerosis may simply reflect the decreased metabolic demands on the myocardium in hypothyroidism. A definitive study which examines the frequency of atherosclerosis in euthyroid individuals and persons who are now euthyroid but had once been myxedematous has not been reported. However, in one series of treated hypothyroid patients, angina pectoris improved more frequently than it became worse,[111] suggesting that the development of lipid abnormalities may not have the same implications in hypothyroid as in euthyroid individuals.

OTHER METABOLIC CHANGES

The evaluation of patients with myxedema and chest pain is complicated by the known effects of hypothyroidism on serum enzyme concentrations commonly used to assess myocardial damage. Thus, creatine kinase (CK), lactic dehydrogenase (LDH), and serum glutamic oxaloacetic transaminase (SGOT) may be moderately or significantly elevated in hypothyroidism.[116] The mechanism for the elevated enzymes is uncertain, but it may be related to mild cardiac or skeletal muscle damage with release of enzymes, decreased clearance of normal enzyme concentrations, or hepatic damage and congestion. The third possibility is unlikely, since the LDH isoenzyme pattern is similar to that seen in acute myocardial infarction, and serum glutamic pyruvic transaminase (SGPT) is not elevated. Treatment with thyroid hormone reverses the enzyme abnormalities usually within days to weeks.

DIAGNOSIS AND TREATMENT OF HYPOTHYROIDISM

Caution must be exercised in treating hypothyroid patients who are elderly and who may have underlying organic heart disease, to avoid precipitating myocardial infarction or severe congestive heart failure; a slow replacement program is indicated in these individuals.

Some have suggested using T3 rather than thyroxine to treat patients with myxedema; since it has a shorter half-life, if toxic effects develop, they will be dissipated more quickly. However, because it has a quicker onset of action, T3 also induces complications more rapidly. Thus, it appears to us more desirable to treat myxedema with thyroxine, usually beginning with a dose as small as 0.0125 mg daily and doubling this dose every 14 days until a dose of 0.1 to 0.125 mg is reached. During this process the patient's cardiovascular status is monitored frequently, and, if untoward events occur, the dose is reduced or maintained constant. Recently, the measurement of serum TSH levels has become readily available as a biochemical marker of adequacy of the replacement therapy.

The treatment of congestive heart failure is particularly difficult in patients with myxedema, both because of the effect of thyroid hormone on the heart and because the heart's response to cardiac glycosides is altered.[85,117] Patients with severe angina pectoris and untreated myxedema pose a difficult clinical dilemma because angina may be exacerbated by thyroid hormone replacement, and the usual medical management of angina with propranolol may induce severe bradycardia. Coronary arteriography often shows severe coronary artery disease in these patients, and an excellent surgical team can perform successful coronary revascularization with minimal thyroid replacement. Full thyroid replacement can then be safely achieved during the postoperative period, without the recurrence of angina.[118,119]

An increasingly common problem in ill patients is the so-called euthyroid sick syndrome. This occurs in acutely or chronically ill patients who have low serum T4 and T3 levels yet do not have hypothyroidism. The low T3 levels are secondary to decreased extrathyroidal conversion of T4 to T3. The low T4's are often due to a decrease in the concentration of thyroxine binding globulin, resulting in a decrease in total but only minimal changes in the free hormone levels. In very severe illness, there can be central (CNS) suppression of TSH release and an induced secondary hypothyroid state. Prolonged dopamine infusions can produce this situation also, by direct suppression of TSH secretion. In the euthyroid sick syndrome the serum TSH will be normal, whereas in hypothyroidism TSH will be increased, thus providing a biochemical mechanism for distinguishing them.[120]

DISEASES OF THE ADRENAL CORTEX

Since Addison's description in 1849 of adrenal insufficiency,[2] it has been appreciated that steroids secreted by the adrenal cortex exert a significant effect on the cardiovascular system, primarily by altering blood pressure. Adrenal insufficiency is characterized by significant hypotension, while excessive production of adrenal steroids is often accompanied by hypertension.

Three classes of steroids are secreted by the adrenal cortex: glucocorticoids, e.g., cortisol; mineralocorticoids, e.g., aldosterone; and androgens, e.g., dehydroepiandrosterone. In this section, the physiology and pathophysiology of glucocorticoid and mineralocorticoid secretion will be addressed.

HORMONE ACTIONS

Cortisol. Cortisol, the primary glucocorticoid, is synthesized from cholesterol in the inner layers of the adrenal cortex by a series of enzymatic transformations. After release into the circulation, it is bound to a high-affinity, low-capacity globulin, transcortin. Thus, most of the circulating cortisol is biologically inactive. The daily secretion rate of cortisol ranges from 15 to 30 mg with a pronounced diurnal cycle. Its average plasma concentration is 15 μg/dl in the morning, falling to 5 μg/dl by early evening.[121] The fundamental mechanism of action of the glucocorticoids is similar to that of other steroid hormones. They enter a target tissue by diffusion and combine with a specific high-affinity cytoplasmic receptor protein. The receptor-cortisol complex is then transferred to specific acceptor sites on nuclear chromatin tissue, where it produces an increase in RNA and later protein synthesis.

The division of adrenal steroids into glucocorticoids and mineralocorticoids is somewhat arbitrary in that most glucocorticoids have some mineralocorticoid-like properties and vice versa. The major action of glucocorticoids is to promote gluconeogenesis, and, in that respect, they are both catabolic and anti-insulin. They mobilize amino acid precursors from peripheral supporting structures, such as bone, skin, muscle, and connective tissue, and inhibit protein synthesis and amino acid uptake in these same tissues. Gluconeogenesis is also indirectly enhanced by an increase in glucagon secretion secondary to the glucocorticoid-induced hyperaminoacidemia.

Glucocorticoids also have anti-inflammatory properties related both to their effects on the microvasculature and the lymphatic system. They maintain normal vascular responsiveness to circulating vasoconstrictors, such as norepinephrine, and have a major effect on both the distribution and excretion of body water. For example, patients with Addison's disease cannot effectively excrete a water load. Finally, they can alter calcium absorption from the gastrointestinal tract by interfering with the activation of vitamin D in the liver and/or blocking its effect on the gastrointestinal tract.[121]

Cortisol secretion by the adrenal cortex is primarily under the control of a negative feedback loop involving the adrenal cortex and the pituitary gland. Thus, as cortisol concentrations fall, ACTH secretion from the pituitary increases, stimulating the adrenal cortex to produce more cortisol and vice versa. The hypothalamus also interacts with this system by releasing corticotropin-releasing hormone, thus modifying ACTH release and the response of the pituitary to the inhibitory effect of cortisol. In addition to this primary negative feedback loop, there is an intrinsic diurnal rhythm in the release of both ACTH and cortisol, probably mediated by changes in the release of corticotropin-releasing hormone from the hypothalamus.

Aldosterone. The major mineralocorticoid produced by the human adrenal gland is aldosterone. It is also synthesized from cholesterol but almost exclusively in the outer layer (glomerulosa) of the adrenal cortex. Aldosterone has two important functions: (1) it is a major regulator of extracellular fluid volume by its effect on sodium retention, and (2) it is a major determinant of potassium metabolism. Aldosterone acts predominantly on the distal convoluted tubule and/or collecting duct of the kidney where it promotes the reabsorption of sodium. Potassium then diffuses into the lumen of the tubules because of the change in electrochemical gradient produced by the active reabsorption of the positively charged sodium ion. Hydrogen ion may also be more freely excreted due to this change in the electrochemical gradient. While aldosterone also acts on salivary and sweat glands and on the endothelial cells of the gastrointestinal tract, these have little impact on total body sodium and potassium homeostasis.

There are three well-defined control mechanisms for aldosterone release.[121]

1. The renin-angiotensin system is the major system for the control of extracellular fluid volume by regulating aldosterone secretion. Aldosterone is linked in a negative feedback loop with the renin-angiotensin system. Thus, during periods registered as volume deficiency there is an increased release of the enzyme renin from the juxtaglomerular cells of the kidney. Renin then increases the production of angiotensin I from its substrate. Angiotensin I is rapidly converted into the biologically active angiotensin II, which increases aldosterone secretion. Angiotensin II also produces vasoconstriction, thereby raising blood pressure and reducing blood flow to a variety of tissues, especially the kidney.

2. Potassium ion also regulates aldosterone secretion independent of the renin-angiotensin system; elevation of potassium concentration increases aldosterone secretion and vice versa. The adrenal cortex is very sensitive to changes in potassium concentration with as little as a 0.1 mEq/l increment producing significant changes in the plasma aldosterone levels.

3. ACTH also has been documented to affect aldosterone secretion profoundly. However, because the control of aldosterone release is not appreciably altered in patients who have been on long-term steroid therapy, ACTH probably has a smaller role than the other two factors in maintaining normal aldosterone secretion. Finally, the prior dietary intake of both sodium and potassium alters the magnitude of the aldosterone response to acute stimulation, sodium restriction, and potassium loading, both enhancing the response of the adrenal.

Diseases of the adrenal cortex, therefore, primarily affect the cardiovascular system via changes in blood pressure or volume homeostasis. Three specific conditions will be discussed next: glucocorticoid excess (Cushing's syndrome), mineralocorticoid excess (primary aldosteronism), and adrenal insufficiency (Addison's disease).

Cushing's Syndrome (See also p. 885)

In 1932 Harvey Cushing reported a syndrome characterized by truncal obesity, hypertension, fatigue, weakness, amenorrhea, hirsutism, purple abdominal striae, glucosuria, edema, and osteoporosis.[122] Since his original description, a number of specific causes for this syndrome have been described. However, the majority are secondary to bilateral adrenal hyperplasia, with the predominant feature being excess production of glucocorticoids and androgens.[123] Some cases are due to ACTH-producing tumors, of either the pituitary gland (Cushing's disease) or nonendocrine tissue (ectopic ACTH production). Fifteen to 20 per cent of the cases are due to primary adrenal neoplasia, either adenoma or carcinoma. Three times as many women as men are afflicted and the onset is usually in the third or fourth decade of life. Most patients have the typical body habitus: central obesity and slender extremities with proximal muscle weakness. Hypertension is present in 80 to 90 per cent of patients and diabetes occurs in 20 per cent, probably in those individuals with a predisposition.[121,123] Evidence of androgen excess may also be present including hirsutism, amenorrhea, clitoromegaly, and, in some cases, deepening of the voice. The majority of patients also have significant emotional changes ranging from lability of mood to severe depression, confusion, or even frank psychosis.

Laboratory tests disclose evidence of excess production of both glucocorticoids and androgens in the majority of cases. Thus, urinary metabolites of these steroids, 17-ketosteroids and 17-hydroxy-steroids, are characteristically elevated. Most patients show some evidence of glycosuria or hyperglycemia. There is usually generalized osteoporosis, most marked in the spine and pelvis; polycythemia is frequently encountered. In severe cases, hypokalemia, a mineralocorticoid manifestation, may also occur.

CARDIOVASCULAR MANIFESTATIONS. Prior to the development of effective treatment for Cushing's syndrome, accelerated atherosclerosis was a common finding. Early death from either myocardial infarction, congestive heart failure, or stroke usually occurred. While the pathophysiology of the accelerated atherosclerosis is not clear, the hypertensive process probably contributes. However, it is unlikely to be the sole reason, since the hypertension of patients with primary aldosteronism may be as significant and yet atherosclerosis is unusual. Part of the atherosclerotic changes may be mediated by the lipid-mobilizing effect of cortisol. Chronic excess production of cortisol leads to hyperlipidemia and hypercholesterolemia, both of which may promote the development of atherosclerosis.[124]

The pathophysiology of the hypertension in Cushing's syndrome has been much debated. Early studies suggested that it was secondary to volume expansion due to cortisol's mineralocorticoid properties. However, recent studies have not supported this hypothesis. Alternative hypotheses include glucocorticoid potentiation of response of vascular smooth muscle to vasoconstrictive agents[125] and ACTH- or cortisol-induced increases in renin substrate.[126] The latter thesis suggests that the increased blood pressure is secondary to increased generation of angiotensin II. Thus, the pathophysiology of the hypertension may be multifactoral, being related to volume expansion, increased production of vasoactive agents, e.g., angiotensin II, and increased sensitivity of vascular smooth muscle to vasoactive agents.

Hemodynamic, electrocardiographic, and roentgenographic studies of patients with Cushing's syndrome have revealed no specific abnormalities except those that are, in general, associated with either hypertension or hypokalemia. The P-R interval tends to be shorter than normal.

DIAGNOSIS AND TREATMENT. The diagnosis of Cushing's syndrome is established by the lack of appropriate suppression of cortisol secretion by dexamethasone. The best screening test is the administration of 1 mg of dexamethasone at bedtime with measurement of plasma cortisol between 7 and 10 A.M. the next morning. In normal subjects cortisol levels will be less than 5 μg/dl. Some patients, particularly the obese, may have false-positive responses, but false-negative responses occur only rarely. The definitive diagnosis of Cushing's syndrome is made by administration of 0.5 mg of dexamethasone every 6 hours for two days with measurement either of plasma cortisol levels at the end of the second day (normal < 5μg/dl) or of the 24 hour 17-OH excretory rate on the second day of dexamethasone supression (normal < 3 mg/24 hr).[127]

Therapy of Cushing's syndrome is usually directed at the specific cause. Thus, patients with adrenal carcinoma or adenoma are treated surgically. In some cases, patients with adrenal carcinoma have nonresectable lesions and therefore surgery is combined with chemotherapy. The treatment of patients with bilateral hyperplasia is controversial, since the etiology is often unknown. In some centers, bilateral adrenalectomy is the treatment of choice, while in others, therapy directed at the pituitary (either surgery or irradiation) is used.[128]

The treatment of cardiovascular abnormalities associated with Cushing's syndrome is directed at lowering blood pressure and correcting the hypokalemia if present. Caution should be exercised in treating the hypertension with potassium-losing diuretics because of the tendency for these patients to develop hypokalemia. Thus, potassium-sparing diuretics or potassium supplements should be administered. In many cases, the hypertension may be more specifically treated with agents that block the action or production of renin, such as beta blockers (e.g., propranolol) or converting enzyme inhibitors (e.g., captopril). As in all clinical conditions in which hypokalemia may be present, cardiac glycosides should be used with caution in patients with Cushing's syndrome.

Hyperaldosteronism
(See also p. 883)

Clinical and Biochemical Manifestations. Aldosteronism is a syndrome associated with hypersecretion of aldosterone. Primary aldosteronism signifies that the stimulus for the excess aldosterone production resides within the adrenal. In secondary aldosteronism, the stimulus is of extra-adrenal origin. These two conditions have similar effects on potassium metabolism.

In patients with primary aldosteronism, which most commonly is due to an aldosterone-producing adrenal adenoma, hypertension, hypokalemia, and metabolic alkalosis are common.[129,130] Polyuria may exist because of the hypokalemia, and glucose intolerance is increased in frequency. Muscle cramps due to the hypokalemia may be present, but little else distinguishes this from other forms of hypertension. Laboratory studies confirm the presence of hypokalemic alkalosis with a low specific gravity of urine and normal levels of adrenal glucocorticoids. The incidence of primary aldosteronism is between 0.5 and 2 per cent of the hypertensive population and occurs twice as frequently in females as in males, with an initial presentation usually between the ages of 30 and 50 years.[121]

CARDIOVASCULAR MANIFESTATIONS. Many of the cardiovascular effects of aldosteronism are nonspecific, being related to aldosterone's effect on atrial pressure and potassium balance. Thus, T wave flattening or U wave prominence on the electrocardiogram (p. 236) and the presence of premature ventricular contractions and other arrhythmias due to hypokalemia are observed.[28] Evidence of left ventricular hypertrophy, either on the electrocardiogram or on the chest roentgenogram, may also be present in patients with long-standing hypertension and hyperaldosteronism. Malignant hypertension and changes in renal function secondary to severe hypertensive angiopathy are infrequent.

DIAGNOSIS AND TREATMENT. The diagnosis of primary aldosteronism is made by the presence of diastolic hypertension without edema, hypersecretion of aldosterone that fails to suppress appropriately during volume expansion, hyposecretion of renin, and hypokalemia with inappropriate urinary potassium loss during salt loading. The state of the renin-angiotensin system is often used to distinguish primary aldosteronism from other conditions that produce hypertension and hypokalemia. For example, hypertension and hypokalemia may be part of the clinical picture of secondary aldosteronism that accompanies malignant or accelerated hypertension or is associated with renal artery stenosis. Secondary aldosteronism can be readily distinguished from primary aldosteronism by the plasma renin activity, which is elevated in the former and reduced in the latter. However, the combination of hypertension and a low plasma renin activity does not necessarily mean primary aldosteronism. Between 15 and 30 per cent of patients with essential hypertension have low renin levels, so-called "low renin" essential hypertension.[131] These patients have been extensively evaluated for excess mineralocorticoid secretion; however, no definitive evidence for such exists (Chap. 26).

The principal treatment for primary aldosteronism is surgical removal of the aldosterone-producing adenoma. In some cases, this is not possible because of the excessive risk imposed by the general physical status of the patient; then, spironolactone, which pharmacologically blocks the effects of aldosterone, is used long-term. This form of therapy may be of limited benefit in males, since compliance is reduced by the undesirable side effects of gynecomastia and impotency, particularly when doses greater than 200 mg per day are required.[132]

Although congestive heart failure occurs infrequently in patients with primary aldosteronism, treatment of patients with this condition with cardiac glycosides must be cautious because of the hypokalemia.

In some patients, primary aldosteronism is not due to a solitary adenoma but to bilateral hyperplasia.[121] While the clinical characteristics of these two conditions are similar, their responses to surgery are different. In both cases hypokalemia is corrected, but patients with bilateral hyperplasia often do not exhibit reduction in arterial pressure. Patients with bilateral hyperplasia are best treated with spironolactone and other antihypertensive agents. Thus, preoperative distinction between bilateral hyperplasia and an adrenal adenoma using adrenal venography or adrenal scanning is important.

Adrenal Insufficiency

Hypofunction of the adrenal cortex includes all conditions in which the level of secretion of adrenal steroids is less than the needs of the body. There are two major categories: those associated with primary damage to the adrenal cortex, and those associated with secondary failure due to the lack of a stimulator such as ACTH. Clinically, patients with adrenal insufficiency can be divided into four types:[121] (1) the most common, primary insufficiency (Addison's disease); (2) secondary insufficiency due to a lack of ACTH; (3) selective hypoaldosteronism; and (4) enzyme deficiency (congenital adrenal hyperplasia).

Clinical and Biochemical Manifestations. Addison's disease may occur at any age and affects both sexes equally. It is commonly due to a destructive process involving both adrenal glands, sometimes infectious, but most often idiopathic atrophy, probably autoimmune in nature. Nearly all patients with primary adrenal insufficiency have weakness, increased skin pigmentation, significant weight loss, anorexia, nausea, vomiting, and hypotension, particularly postural. A significant minority also complain of abdominal pain, salt craving, and diarrhea or constipation. In mild forms, baseline laboratory studies are usually within normal limits. However, as the disease progresses, there is a gradual reduction in serum levels of sodium, chloride, and bicarbonate and an increase in potassium. The hyponatremia is due to extravascular loss of sodium, both into the urine (because of aldosterone deficiency) and into the intracellular compartment. The hyperkalemia is due both to the deficiency of aldosterone and to the impaired glomerular filtration rate and acidosis present in these patients. Other nonspecific findings include a reduction in basal metabolic rate with normal thyroid function and a normocytic anemia with relative lymphocytosis. While Addison's disease is often thought of as a common cause of significant eosinophilia, this is observed only occasionally.

Cardiovascular Manifestations. The most common cardiovascular finding in adrenal insufficiency is arterial hypotension. In severe cases, the pressure may be in the range of 80/50 mm Hg, with postural accentuation. Indeed, syncope occurs in a significant percentage of patients. In severe cases, heart size and peripheral pulses decrease. The electrocardiogram is abnormal in the majority of patients with Addison's disease.[28] The most common abnormalities are low or inverted T waves, sinus bradycardia, prolonged $Q-T_c$ interval, and low voltage. Conduction defects also occur, with first-degree block present in 20 per cent of patients. Changes secondary to the hyperkalemia are not common even though the serum potassium levels may be elevated. It is of interest that the electrocardiographic abnormalities, other than those secondary to hyperkalemia, do not respond to mineralocorticoids but require glucocorticoid replacement. Cardiac failure in prolonged adrenocortical insufficiency has also been reported.[28a]

Diagnosis and Treatment. Decreased response of the adrenal cortex to ACTH establishes the diagnosis of Addison's disease. The best screening test is the administration of synthetic ACTH (cosyntropin), 0.25 mg IM or IV, with measurement of plasma cortisol levels 30 and 60 minutes later. Cortisol levels double or increase by 10 μg/dl in normal subjects. Definitive evaluation is by prolonged (usually 24-hour) infusion of ACTH with assessment of either plasma cortisol or excretion of 17-hydroxysteroids or both.[121]

It is possible to differentiate primary adrenal insufficiency from secondary adrenal insufficiency, isolated hypoaldosteronism, or congenital adrenal hyperplasia because one of the adrenal hormonal functions is normal in each of the latter three conditions. Thus, in secondary adrenal insufficiency due to ACTH deficiency, aldosterone secretion is normal and the biochemical effects of mineralocorticoid deficiency, i.e., hyperkalemia, are not present. In isolated hypoaldosteronism, glucocorticoid function is normal. Female patients with congenital adrenal hyperplasia have evidence of androgen excess, such as virilization and hirsutism, and hypertension may also be present with a deficiency of 11-hydroxylase[133] (p. 887).

An increasingly common form of hypoaldosteronism is that associated with hyporeninism. Most commonly, this syndrome is observed in older diabetic patients with a mild degree of renal impairment and hypertension; acidosis is also common. Usually, these patients present with unexplained hyperkalemia. The cause is unknown but may be secondary to damage to the juxtaglomerular apparatus and/or reduced conversion of a renin precursor into the active enzyme.[134]

The treatment of adrenal insufficiency is accomplished by replacement of the deficient steroid. In adults with primary or secondary insufficiency, hydrocortisone, 20 to 30 mg daily, is administered in divided doses, usually two thirds in the morning and one third in midafternoon. In those patients with associated aldosterone deficiency, 9-α-fluorohydrocortisone, 0.05 to 0.10 mg daily, is given. During periods of significant stress (surgery, infection, or trauma), the dose of glucocorticoids should be increased. Occasionally, acute adrenal insufficiency in patients who previously had apparently normal adrenal function, is precipitated by the stress of cardiac surgery.[135]

PHEOCHROMOCYTOMA
(Also see p. 885)

In 1859, Oliver and Shafer demonstrated that adrenal extract raised blood pressure when injected into experimental animals. In 1901, one active ingredient, epinephrine, was isolated and characterized and in 1922 a syndrome of paroxysmal hypertension associated with an adrenal medullary tumor, pheochromocytoma, was reported.

EFFECTS OF CATECHOLAMINES ON
THE CARDIOVASCULAR SYSTEM

The adrenal medulla and sympathetic nervous system are linked morphologically, biochemically, and physiologically and are often referred to as the sympathoadrenal system.[136] The sympathoadrenal system differs from other endocrine systems in several respects, including the fact that plasma levels of the secretory product, catecholamines, are not regulated by a direct feedback mechanism. Instead, catecholamine secretion is the efferent branch of a reflex arc involv-

ing centers in the brain stem, the hypothalamus, and perhaps the cerebral cortex as well. The human adrenal medulla contains about 1 mg of catecholamine per gram of tissue, approximately 85 per cent of which is epinephrine. The strategic location of the adrenal medullary cells within the cortex is associated with their capacity to form epinephrine, since high-dose glucocorticoids induce the formation of phenylethanolamine-N-methyl-transferase, the enzyme needed to convert norepinephrine into epinephrine.[137]

In addition to their important effects on the cardiovascular system, catecholamines also have significant metabolic effects, stimulating glycogenolysis and gluconeogenesis, that is, increasing the production of glucose from glycogen and amino acid precursors and stimulating lipolysis, thereby mobilizing free fatty acids and inhibiting secretion of insulin. The absence of the adrenal medulla does not produce definable disease in humans. However, the presence of a hormonally active adrenal medullary tumor produces a number of significant findings.

Clinical and Biochemical Manifestations. A pheochromocytoma is a catecholamine-producing tumor derived from chromaffin cells. Those arising from extra-adrenal chromaffin cells are called nonadrenal pheochromocytomas or paraganglionomas. Probably less than 0.1 per cent of patients with hypertension have a pheochromocytoma. Despite the fact that it is an uncommon disease, pheochromocytomas generate a great deal of interest, largely because the morbidity and mortality associated with these tumors are significant, with detection often resulting in cure. Pheochromocytomas are highly vascular tumors; less than 10 per cent are malignant as indicated by local invasion or metastasis, but, as with other endocrine tumors, malignancy cannot always be determined by microscopic appearance alone.

While the vast majority of tumors occur sporadically, approximately 5 per cent are inherited as an autosomal trait, of which they are often part of a pluriglandular neoplastic syndrome[138] which, in addition to pheochromocytoma, may consist of medullary carcinoma of the thyroid, parathyroidadenoma, and retinal or cerebellar hemangioblastomas. Most pheochromocytomas are solitary adrenal tumors, with 10 per cent being bilateral and 10 per cent nonadrenal. However, in the familial form of pheochromocytoma nearly half the patients have bilateral adrenal tumors.

The features that suggest pheochromocytoma in hypertensive patients are (1) paroxysmal attacks of any kind, (2) headaches, (3) excessive sweating, (4) signs of hypermetabolism, (5) orthostatic hypotension, and (6) unusual blood pressure elevations to trauma or operation.[136,139] Many of the features are similar to those of hyperthyroidism. While paroxysmal attacks are the hallmark of pheochromocytoma, more than half the patients have fixed hypertension and nearly 10 per cent are normotensive.

CARDIOVASCULAR MANIFESTATIONS. Hypertension is the major cardiovascular manifestation of pheochromocytoma. Its lability sometimes distinguishes it from other forms of hypertension; however, only clinical awareness of the entity and specific laboratory testing permit establishment of the proper diagnosis. The lability of blood pressure in patients with pheochromocytoma has been suggested to be due not only to episodic discharge of catecholamines but also to a reduction in plasma volume, as well as to impaired sympathetic reflexes. Recent studies have indicated that an absolute reduction of plasma volume exists in only a minority of cases,[140,141] but a number of observations suggest that chronic volume depletion is present. For example, alpha-adrenergic blockade or removal of the tumor produces severe hypotension, which is correctable by volume expansion.[136,142] Cardiac output has been reported to be normal, whereas heart rate is increased and orthostatic hypotension is accompanied by decreased stroke volume and inadequate adjustments in peripheral resistance indicative of impaired peripheral vascular reflexes.[141]

The electrocardiogram is abnormal in as many as 75 per cent of the patients with pheochromocytoma.[28] The changes consist of T-wave inversion, left ventricular hypertro-

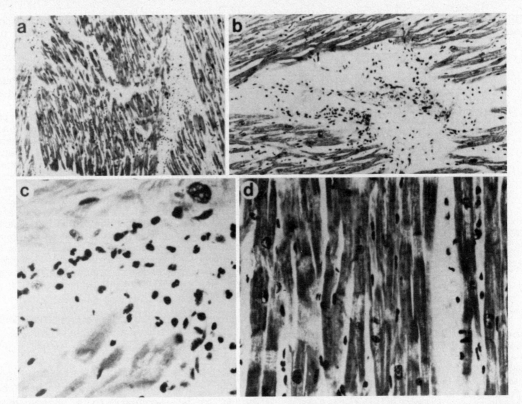

FIGURE 51–4 Left ventricular myocardium with acute myocarditis and contraction band necrosis in a patient with pheochromocytoma dying of catecholamine crisis. *a*, Diffuse infiltration by inflammatory cells through myocardium. *b*, Perivascular inflammation. *c*, Close-up of the inflammatory infiltrate. *d*, Contraction-band necrosis of myocytes. (Hematoxylin and eosin stains; original magnification × 20 (a), × 45 (b), × 540 (c), × 330 (d)). (Reproduced with permission from McManus, B. M., Fleury, T. A., and Roberts, W. C.: Fatal catecholamine crisis in pheochromocytoma: Curable cause of cardiac arrest. Am. Heart J. *102*:930, 1981.)

phy, sinus tachycardia, and, in some cases, other alterations in rhythm, such as frequent supraventricular ectopic beats or paroxysmal supraventricular tachycardia. When arterial pressure increases markedly, changes suggestive of myocardial damage, including transient ST-segment elevations, marked diffuse T-wave inversions, and depression of ST-segments are present. These changes are usually transient, and the electrocardiographic pattern reverts to normal after removal of the tumor or pharmacological blockade.[143] Some of the electrocardiographic abnormalities are presumably due to hypertensive heart disease or myocardial ischemia. However, a specific catecholamine-induced myocarditis has also been suggested.[144]

The echocardiogram during a hypertensive crisis may show systolic anterior involvement of the anterior mitral leaflet, paradoxical septal motion and proximal exclusion of the posterior wall.[145]

Myocarditis. Pathologically, the myocarditis consists of focal necrosis with infiltration of inflammatory cells, perivascular inflammation, and contraction band necrosis[146] (Fig. 51–4), finally resulting in fibrosis. In one study, 50 per cent of patients who died from pheochromocytoma had myocarditis,[140] usually accompanied by left ventricular failure and pulmonary edema. Although coronary atherosclerosis is usually present, medial thickening is the most characteristic lesion of the coronary arteries. The high catecholamine levels may have been the cause, since similar lesions were found in rats exposed to high levels of norepinephrine.

DIAGNOSIS AND TREATMENT. The diagnosis of pheochromocytoma is established by documenting increased urinary, blood, or platelet levels of catecholamines or one of their metabolites.[142,147–149] Three tests are commonly employed: (1) total catecholamines, (2) vanillylmandelic acid (VMA); and (3) metanephrine. The latter two are metabolites of catecholamine and were first used to screen for pheochromocytoma because they are present in greater quantities. When reliably performed, these tests are probably equivalent in accuracy. The probability of a pheochromocytoma being present in a hypertensive patient with a single normal urine level is less than 5 per cent. It is most desirable to measure both the catecholamines and one of the two metabolites, preferably metanephrine, in screening for pheochromocytoma. If the blood pressure fluctuates it is particularly important to collect the urine at a time the pressure is elevated. Specific pharmacological tests to screen for pheochromocytoma are of limited benefit, usually hazardous, and therefore warranted only in unusual circumstances. Recently, clonidine has been proposed as a useful definitive test for pheochromocytoma. Normal subjects suppress catecholamine levels following clonidine administration via stimulation of central alpha-adrenergic receptors; patients with pheochromocytoma do not[150] (Fig. 51–5). Unfortunately, profound and prolonged hypotension has been reported in some patients during the course of this test.

Once the diagnosis of pheochromocytoma is established, specific pharmacological blockade should be initiated.[151] Phenoxybenzamine hydrochloride should be begun, with the initial dose 10 mg q 12 hr; the dose is then gradually increased every two to three days until the arterial pressure is restored to normal. However, it should be noted that alpha-adrenergic blockade may induce a decline in ar-

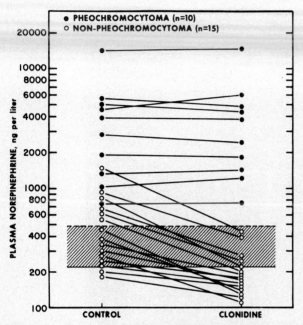

FIGURE 51–5 Plasma norepinephrine values in individual patients before and three hours after a single oral dose of clonidine (0.3 mg). The hatched area represents the mean of values obtained from 60 adult healthy subjects (+3 S.D.). To convert norepinephrine values to nanomoles per liter, multiply by 0.006. (Reproduced with permission from Bravo, E. L., Tarazi, R. C., Fouad, F. M.,et al: Clonidine-suppression test: A useful aid in the diagnosis of pheochromocytoma. N. Engl. J. Med. *305*:623, 1981.)

terial pressure accompanied by serious postural hypotension, presumably because of the vasodilatation occurring in the presence of hypovolemia. This hypotensive response can be prevented by adequate sodium intake; if it is very striking, the infusion of saline may be required. Adequate control of arterial pressure is essential prior to any arteriographic procedure, before initiating beta-receptor blockade, and before operation.

Beta-adrenergic blockade is useful in patients with pheochromocytoma who have significant tachycardia, palpitations, and catecholamine-induced arrhythmias. However, beta blockade with a drug affecting beta-2 receptors must *not* be initiated prior to adequate alpha blockade, since severe *hypertension* may occur as a result of the unopposed alpha-stimulating activity of the circulating catecholamines.

Definitive treatment is surgical removal of the tumor, usually after localization with CAT scan, arteriography, or scanning using an ^{131}I-derivative of guanethidine as the scanning agent.[152] In those patients with inoperable lesions, long-term use of the combination of alpha- and beta-adrenergic blockers has been helpful. Drugs that inhibit the biosynthesis of catecholamines, such as alpha-methyltyrosine, have also been used in patients with malignant pheochromocytoma.[142,153]

PARATHYROID DISEASE

Disordered parathyroid secretion is associated with two cardiovascular disturbances, cardiac arrythmias and hypertension. Changes in calcium metabolism as well as a direct effect of parathyroid hormone on the heart appear to be responsible.

Clinical and Biochemical Manifestations. Parathyroid hormone (PTH) is a single-chain polypeptide of 84 amino acids. Its major biological effect is to increase mobilization of calcium into the extracellular fluid from a variety of tissues; this action is linked in a negative feedback loop with serum unbound calcium concentration. Thus, an increase in serum calcium concentration reduces parathyroid hormone release and vice versa.[154] PTH also increases urinary excretion of phosphate, augments bone resorption and reduces the urinary excretion of calcium. It also indirectly increases the absorption of calcium from the gastrointestinal tract by increasing the rate of conversion of 25-hydroxy vitamin D into the biologically active 1,25-dihydroxy vitamin D.[155]

Hyperparathyroidism, the excess production of parathyroid hormone, is usually secondary to a solitary parathyroid adenoma. Occasionally, generalized parathyroid hyperplasia exists, and, infrequently, carcinoma of the parathyroid gland is found. In many cases, hyperparathyroidism is asymptomatic; 10 to 20 per cent of patients are first diagnosed as the result of a routine chemical screening test.[156]

The signs and symptoms of hyperparathyroidism are related to direct effects of PTH on kidney or bone or those associated with the hypercalcemia. Nearly half the patients have signs and symptoms of renal dysfunction, such as polyuria, nocturia, renal stones, and, in severe cases, nephrocalcinosis and renal failure. In many patients, there are also nonspecific joint and back symptoms, and in unusual circumstances spontaneous fractures occur. Hypercalcemia reduces the excitability of the neuromuscular system, which can lead to such diverse effects as significant myocardial dysfunction and decreased auditory acuity.

CARDIOVASCULAR MANIFESTATIONS
OF HYPERPARATHYROIDISM
(See also page 887)

CARDIAC EFFECTS. Until recently, most of the effects of parathyroid hormone on the heart have been assumed to be secondary to a change in extracellular calcium. It has now been documented that PTH also has a direct effect on the heart resulting in an increased beating rate of isolated heart cells and a positive inotropic action.[157,158] These effects are probably mediated by PTH binding to specific receptors, leading to an increased entry of calcium into the heart cell and by PTH increasing the release of endogenous myocardial norepinephrine. The direct effect of PTH may be deleterious, since it causes early death in rat heart cells and may be directly responsible for the increased accumulation of calcium in dystrophic muscles and for the heart damage found in uremia.[157,159] On the other hand, hypoparathyroidism may cause a dilated cardiomyopathy, caused presumably by hypocalcemia, but perhaps also by hypomagnesemia and reduced circulating PTH.[160]

In addition to any direct action of PTH on the heart, hypercalcemia also has an adverse effect. Chronic hypercalcemia from a variety of causes is associated with increased deposition of calcium in the fibrous skeleton of the heart and valvular cusps as well as in coronary arteries and in myocardial fibers[161] (Figs. 51–6 and 51–7).

The plateau of the action potential of cardiac fibers is prolonged by low and shortened by high extracellular calcium concentrations (Chap. 19). Lengthening of the plateau prolongs the duration of the action potential, whereas shortening of the plateau has the opposite effect. These changes in duration of action potential are accompanied by corresponding changes in the duration of the refractory period, of the ST segment, and of the Q-T interval.[28,162] Thus, the major electrocardiographic change in hypercalcemia is shortening of the Q-T interval. Less frequently, disorders of intraventricular conduction have been reported with shortening of the P-R interval.[28] Complete heart block occurs only rarely.

HYPERTENSION. Hypercalcemic patients detected by routine serum calcium screening techniques have higher

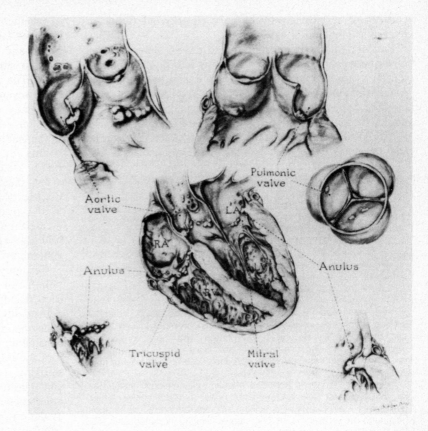

FIGURE 51–6 Drawing of heart showing distribution of calcific deposits in the tricuspid and mitral valve anuli and at the bases of both pulmonic and aortic valve cusps in a 43-year-old woman with hypercalcemia secondary to primary hyperparathyroidism. (Reproduced with permission from Roberts, W. C., and Waller, B. F.: Effect of chronic hypercalcemia on the heart: An analysis of 18 necropsy patients. Am. J. Med. *71*:371, 1981.)

arterial pressure than do matched normocalcemic subjects;[163,164] the pathophysiology of the hypertension may be related to one or more factors. For example, hypercalcemia produces nephrocalcinosis, which may lead to renal failure and hypertension. Thus, reversal of hypertension after successful parathyroid surgery is more likely to occur when renal function is normal. Elevated serum calcium also increases myocardial contractility, peripheral resistance, and release of or vascular sensitivity to vasoconstrictor agents, such as angiotensin II and norepinephrine.[165] While hypercalcemia can increase cardiac contractility and arterial pressure acutely,[166] it is unlikely that this action produces a significant alteration in cardiac output or performance in the absence of PTH on a chronic basis. Thus, an elevation of peripheral resistance is the most likely cause of the hypertension associated with hyperparathyroidism. Resnick has concluded that primary hyperparathyroidism is frequently associated with hypertension. While the mechanism of hypertension in these patients remains to be elucidated, it (1) may be renin-dependent, (2) is associated with and apparently caused by increased circulating PTH rather than hypercalciuria, and (3) is curable surgically in a significant number of patients.[167]

DIAGNOSIS AND TREATMENT

If hypercalcemia is *not* due to primary hyperparathyroidism, circulating concentration of parathyroid hormone should be suppressed. Thus, an elevated or even a normal concentration of parathyroid hormone in the presence of hypercalcemia establishes the diagnosis of hyperparathyroidism; many patients with this condition manifest hypercalcemia for the first time after starting thiazide therapy for treatment of the associated hypertension. Treatment

FIGURE 51–7 Longitudinal section of wall of left atrium (LA) and left ventricle (LV) showing heavy calcific deposits in the mitral anular region and also some deposits in the adjacent coronary artery. *a*, radiography; *b*, gross photograph of same area. (Reproduced with permission from Roberts, W. C., and Waller, B. F.: Effect of chronic hypercalcemia on the heart: An analysis of 18 necropsy patients. Am. J. Med. *71*:371, 1981.)

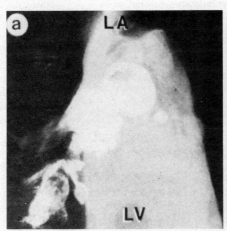
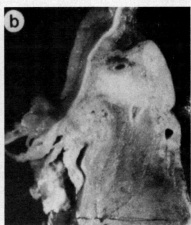

consists of surgical removal of the parathyroid tumor or hyperplastic glands.

Patients with hypertension should have a determination of serum calcium levels before therapy is begun. If thiazide diuretics are used in treatment, determination of serum calcium should be repeated every six months. If thiazide-induced hypercalcemia occurs, the serum calcium should be determined for two to three months after discontinuing the thiazides. Persistence of the hypercalcemia suggests that the patient has primary hyperparathyroidism.[163]

DIABETES MELLITUS

Diabetes mellitus is one of the leading public health problems in the industrialized world, and it has a profound effect on the cardiovascular system. Nearly 10 million people are afflicted with this disease in the United States; it is the eighth health-related cause of death. Nearly all the morbidity from diabetes is related to cardiovascular dysfunction, either coronary artery disease or renal failure secondary to vascular disease.

Actions of Insulin. Insulin is a double-chain polypeptide derived from proinsulin, which is synthesized in the islet cells of the pancreas. Many stimuli, such as glucose, glucagon, amino acids, catecholamines, and gastrointestinal hormones, can promote insulin secretion, which usually occurs in two phases. The rapid early phase releases preformed insulin stored in granules in the beta cells, while the prolonged late phase results from increased biosynthesis of insulin.[168,169]

Insulin is an anabolic hormone affecting all metabolic substrates, i.e., carbohydrates, fats, and proteins, as well as nucleic acids. All target tissues for insulin have specific membrane-bound receptors; thus, binding to the receptor is the first step in initiating its metabolic effect. Cahill and his colleagues have popularized the concept that insulin is the "fed" hormone.[170] Thus, the ingestion of fuel substances provokes a rapid rise in the concentration of circulating insulin, which then facilitates the transfer of these substances into their respective depots. According to this theory, in the fasted state insulin levels are low; as a result, there is increased gluconeogenesis by the liver, decreased lipogenesis with lipolysis and fatty acid release from fat tissue, and decreased glucose uptake in cardiac and skeletal muscle. On the other hand, in the fed state insulin levels are high; gluconeogenesis by the liver is reduced; and in cardiac and skeletal muscle, there is increased glucose and amino acid uptake and increased protein synthesis. In adipose tissue, there is increased glucose and triglyceride uptake, lipogenesis, and absence of release of fatty acids.

In the patient with diabetes, because there is decreased insulin release in response to the ingested fuel, there is a delay in the uptake and the disposal of these fuels into their respective depots, which leads to abnormal circulating levels of the substrates. The increased concentrations of lipids in the circulation may be the underlying pathophysiological effect producing a number of the clinical complications of diabetes mellitus.

Clinical and Biochemical Manifestations. In the past several years, our understanding of the pathogenesis of diabetes mellitus has been significantly altered. Several lines of evidence suggest that in many instances the juvenile form may be infectious in origin, while in most cases the adult onset is probably the result of a genetic predisposition.[171]

Most of the signs and symptoms of this disease either are related to the increased levels of blood glucose or are secondary to changes in the cardiovascular system. Thus, the classic presenting symptoms (observed in about 25 per cent of patients) are polyuria, polydipsia, and polyphagia, all due to the glucosuria. The major pathophysiological consequence of diabetes mellitus is related to changes in the vascular system. The specific target organs include the heart, the eye, the kidney, and the peripheral vasculature.

Cardiovascular Changes in Diabetes

PATHOLOGY. The vascular disease associated with diabetes mellitus can be nonspecific (atherosclerosis and arteriosclerosis) or specific (microangiopathic or endotheli-

al proliferative changes of arterioles). The former primarily involves large vessels (especially in the lower extremities), heart, and brain of older patients, while the latter is localized to small vessels and may be seen in patients of all ages. The atherosclerosis tends to be more extensive and more severe than in nondiabetics, resulting in an increased frequency of myocardial infarction and cerebral and peripheral vascular disease.[172] Indeed, coronary heart disease is the leading cause of death among adult diabetics and accounts for about three times as many deaths among diabetics as among nondiabetics. The incidence of coronary artery disease correlates more closely with the duration of diabetes than with the severity of the diabetes. Of interest is the recent documentation that diabetics have an increased mortality for noncardiovascular diseases (e.g., cancer) as well.[173] The mechanism(s) responsible for this generalized increased mortality is unclear.

Certainly, diabetes should be considered to be a separate risk factor for coronary heart disease[174] (p. 1217). Since each risk factor for vascular disease is thought to add independently (though not equally) to the likelihood for the development of ischemic disease, the diabetic should be considered a high-risk patient in whom all correctable factors should be managed. It is logical to approach cigarette smoking and even moderate elevation of blood pressure and plasma lipids more intensively in diabetic than in nondiabetic patients. Contraceptive drugs that suppress ovulation probably should be avoided, since they may contribute to the metabolic abnormalities that underlie their increased risk for vascular disease. The obese diabetic patient should lose weight; this is often accompanied by gratifying improvement of hypertension, hyperglycemia, hyperinsulinemia, and hypertriglyceridemia.[174]

The microangiopathy produces a characteristic thickening of the basement membrane of the capillaries in the retina, conjunctiva, glomerulus, brain, pancreas, and myocardium.[175] In some cases, there is also proliferation of the epithelial cells leading to occlusion of small arterioles, similar to that observed in immune arteritis.

CARDIAC INVOLVEMENT. Not only is the frequency of acute myocardial infarction increased in diabetic patients,[176] but also the treatment of the infarct is more complicated than in the nondiabetic patient. Patients with acute myocardial infarction and with poor control of the diabetes before hospital admission exhibit a significantly higher mortality than those with good control, but there appears to be no significant difference in mortality between well-controlled diabetics and nondiabetics. Thus, these patients' precarious metabolic status and the difficulty of adjusting insulin therapy to prevent ketoacidosis while not precipitating hypoglycemia probably contribute to the increased mortality from acute myocardial infarction.[177]

The occurrence of a myocardial infarction has a distinctly adverse effect on carbohydrate and fat metabolism[178] and often leads to stimulation of the sympathetic nervous system and increased catecholamine concentration (p. 1276). Subsequent increases in circulating free fatty acid levels and reductions in glucose tolerance appear to be related to a number of physiological functions—adipose tissue lipolysis, hepatic and muscle glycogenolysis, catecholamine-induced suppression of insulin release, and increased circulating concentrations of growth hormone and cortisol. The net result is that carbohydrate intolerance is common following a myocardial infarction, even in nondiabetics. Also, the high concentrations of free fatty acid in the acute phases of a myocardial infarction may lead to ventricular arrhythmias.[179] The suppression of insulin release as a consequence of increased catecholamine activity may decrease glucose utilization by a myocardium that may require this fuel for glycolytic activity.[180]

Diabetic patients with acute myocardial infarction differ from nondiabetics in that their pain patterns are more variable, and infarction may actually occur without pain. Also, survival after infarction is more limited than in the nondiabetics.[181]

Peripheral somatic neuropathy is a common complication of diabetes mellitus; also, diabetic autonomic neuropathy leading to diarrhea, vomiting, and other gastrointestinal disturbances is well known in this disease. Cardiac autonomic dysfunction also exists in many diabetic patients.[182] Occasionally, it may be present before clinical symptoms of generalized autonomic neuropathy are demonstrable.[183] Furthermore, the neuropathy may involve the sympathetic nervous system and/or the parasympathetic nervous system. Indeed, it may become so severe as to lead to total cardiac denervation.[184] These changes in adrenergic nervous system function result in tachycardia and a fixed, rapid heart rate that barely responds to physiological stimuli, such as the Valsalva maneuver, carotid sinus pressure, or tilting, or to drugs, such as phenylephrine, atropine, or propranolol. Rarely, these denervated hearts develop arrhythmias.

Congestive Heart Failure. Insulin-dependent diabetes mellitus appears to increase the likelihood of the development of congestive heart failure from all causes. The role of diabetes in congestive heart failure in the Framingham study was analyzed,[185] and the risk of developing heart failure was found to be increased substantially. Even when patients with prior coronary or rheumatic heart disease were excluded, diabetic subjects had a four- to five-fold increased risk of congestive heart failure. Furthermore, this increased risk persisted after age, blood pressure, weight, and cholesterol values, as well as coronary heart disease, were taken into account. On the basis of these findings it appeared that the excessive risk of heart failure in diabetic patients is caused by factors other than accelerated atherogenesis and coronary heart disease. One suggested possibility is a diabetes-induced cardiomyopathy.[184a]

A statistically significant increase in the frequency of diabetes in patients with idiopathic cardiomyopathy has been reported.[174,186] These patients had serious congestive heart failure, which was difficult to control and invariably at autopsy showed patent large coronary arteries but abnormalities in the small intramural coronary vessels, including intimal fibroblastic thickening and hyaline deposits, as well as inflammatory changes. In contrast, small vessel disease was rare in patients with cardiomyopathy without diabetes. In addition, significant extravascular deposition was noted of collagen, triglyceride, and cholesterol, which may have contributed to the cardiomyopathy. These findings further supported the idea that diabetic patients can develop myocardial disease without large coronary artery involvement, possibly owing to pathological changes in small coronary vessels, but there is considerable

dispute concerning the role, if any, of involvement of the latter.

Further clinical evidence for a diabetic cardiomyopathy came from the observations of Regan et al.[187] They studied a group of diabetic patients without evident heart failure who exhibited an elevation of left ventricular end-diastolic pressure and of the left ventricular end-diastolic pressure/volume ratio. Increments of afterload effected an abnormal increase of filling pressure without an increase in stroke volume, compared to normal subjects, consistent with a preclinical cardiomyopathy. Left ventricular biopsy in two patients without ventricular decompensation showed interstitial deposition of collagen with relatively normal muscle cells. These findings suggest a nonischemic myopathic process.

An abnormality of left ventricular function in diabetes is also reflected in the shortening of the left ventricular ejection time, the prolongation of the preejection period, and the elevation of the ratio of the preejection period to the left ventricular ejection time (PEP/LVET).[188] Left ventricular function has also been assessed by echocardiography in diabetic patients with microangiopathy, defined as proteinuria exceeding 3 gm/24 hr, or proliferative retinopathy, but without angina, previous myocardial infarction, hypertension, or alcoholism and with normal electrocardiograms and chest radiographs.[189] Diabetics with microangiopathy had impaired left ventricular function, whereas those with uncomplicated diabetes exhibited normal function. This finding supports the existence of a specific diabetic cardiomyopathy associated with microangiopathy rather than secondary to a metabolic defect.[190] This association between microangiopathy and impaired left ventricular function may help to explain the high incidence of cardiogenic shock, congestive heart failure, and mortality which has been reported in some series of myocardial infarction in diabetics. There is also now accumulated a large body of evidence that impaired left ventricular diastolic function, reflected in a reduced rate of left ventricular wall thinning and dimension increase, may be present in many asymptomatic diabetic patients,[191] particularly those with severe microvascular complications.[192]

In postmortem studies of 11 diabetic patients, of whom 9 were without significant obstructive disease of the proximal coronary arteries and who had died of cardiac failure, all exhibited positive periodic acid–Schiff staining material in the interstitium, but none had luminal narrowing of the intramural vessels. Collagen accumulation was present in perivascular loci, between the myofibers, or as replacement fibrosis. Multiple samples of left ventricle and septum revealed abnormally increased deposits of triglyceride and cholesterol.[187] Thus these observations, taken in toto, suggest that a diffuse abnormality, either extravascular or involving the microvasculature, may be the basis for the cardiomyopathic features of diabetes. Hypertension appears to accelerate this process, as severe interstitial fibrosis, focal scars, and myocytolytic activity were significantly more frequent in hypertensive diabetics with chronic heart failure examined at postmortem than in normotensive diabetics[193] (Fig. 51–8).

In order to gain a better understanding of diabetic cardiomyopathy, a mild, noninsulin-requiring, alloxan diabetes was produced in dogs.[194] Despite similar end-diastolic

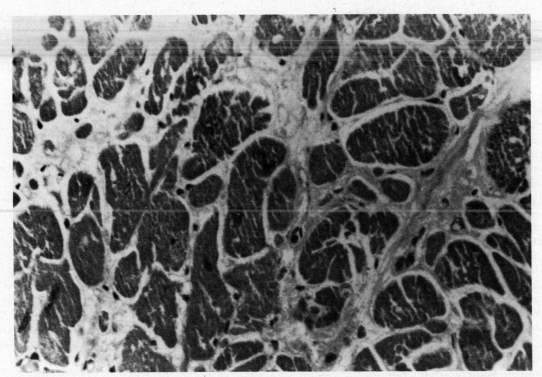

FIGURE 51–8 This section of left ventricular myocardium from a 46-year-old white male (at death) who had insulin-dependent diabetes for 20 years. It demonstrates diffuse interstitial fibrosis. There is marked variability of myocardial cell size, with virtually every cell surrounded by dense collagen. This abnormality is a characteristic feature of the hypertensive-diabetic heart (hematoxylin-eosin; original magnification × 250). (Reproduced with permission from Factor, S. M., Minase, T., and Sonnenblick, E. H.: Clinical and morphological features of human hypertensive-diabetic cardiomyopathy. Am. Heart J. *99*:446, 1980.)

pressures, the end-diastolic volume and stroke volume were significantly less than in control dogs. During acute volume expansion of the ventricle with saline, the end-diastolic pressure increment in diabetic dogs was twice that observed in control dogs. These responses were attributed to an increased stiffness of the left ventricle that was apparently due to accumulation of glycoproteins in the interstitium, measured by periodic acid–Schiff staining. Similar abnormalities were observed in dogs with diabetes that occurred spontaneously. During infusion of ^{14}C-l-oleic acid, fatty acid incorporation, which was predominantly into phospholipid in the control dogs, was diverted to triglyceride in the diabetic dogs; analysis of lipids in the left ventricle revealed elevated concentrations of triglyceride and cholesterol despite normal plasma levels. Thus, these experimental observations support the hypothesis that chronic diabetes mellitus can alter myocardial composition and function independent of its vascular and acute metabolic effects. In this model, therapy with insulin for one year did not reverse all of the myocardial abnormalities.[195] Additional experimental studies suggest, however, that adequate control of the hyperglycemia may reverse the process. In the streptozotocin-induced diabetic rat, there is a significant decrease in contractile protein ATPase activity, resulting in a slowing of relaxation and a depression of shortening velocity.[196] Treatment with insulin acutely—less than one week—did not modify these abnormalities. However, treatment for one month completely reversed them.[197] Whether the different effect of insulin therapy in these studies is related to species differences or differing methods to induce the diabetic state is uncertain.

Other (nondiabetic) cardiomyopathies may exhibit similar hemodynamic abnormalities; an abnormal rise of ventricular filling pressure without a stroke volume increase in response to afterload increments has also been observed in the preclinical phase of alcoholic cardiomyopathy,[198] in which the interstitium is also altered.[199] More severely altered interstitial changes may be the predominant lesion in the incipient stages of amyloid heart disease.[199]

Diabetes mellitus is associated with another form of cardiomyopathy. Approximately half the infants of diabetic mothers have either radiographic cardiomegaly or clinical features suggesting congestive heart failure.[200] The cardiomyopathy in these infants may be transient and secondary to hematological, respiratory, and metabolic problems or a more protracted form of nonobstructive or obstructive hypertrophic cardiomyopathy, which appears to be secondary to maternal hormonal influences and to be reversible.

Electrocardiographic changes are commonly observed in patients with diabetes.[28] While many of the changes are predictable on the basis of the associated hypertension or coronary artery disease, in some there is an unexplained diffuse T-wave abnormality that may be related to the cardiomyopathy.

VASCULAR DISEASE. Peripheral vascular disease is a frequent and significant manifestation of diabetes mellitus, often leading to gangrene and amputation of the lower extremity. The smaller arteries below the knee are more likely to be involved in patients with diabetes in contrast to iliac or femoral artery disease in nondiabetic patients. Cerebral vascular disease is also more frequent, with a greater incidence of cerebral infarction though not cerebral hemorrhage. The increased atherosclerosis of the cerebral vessels and the proliferative changes in the cerebral arterioles both contribute to this increased rate of infarction.

The renal vasculature is affected in a number of ways: atherosclerosis is common in the larger vessels, with proliferative endothelial changes occurring in small vessels. Third, capillary basement membrane thickening is common, particularly in the glomerular tuft where a pathognomonic change—nodular glomerulosclerosis—is often found. These vascular changes, in concert with parenchymal changes secondary to pyelonephritis, lead to a variety of renal disorders, including the nephrotic syndrome, hypertension, and renal failure.

Most studies have reported an increased incidence of hypertension in diabetes, in part related to renal disease. Volume overload may be an additional factor contributing to the hypertension, since many diabetic patients have low renin levels; often the hypertension is best managed by diuretics and sodium restriction. Indeed, more than one third of diabetic patients have hypertension, an incidence that is higher than that of the general population. It is possible to explain the increased susceptibility of diabetics to arteriosclerotic cardiovascular disease in large measure by the increased incidence of hypertension.

DIAGNOSIS AND TREATMENT OF DIABETES MELLITUS

It is generally agreed that therapy directed at the control of excessive fatty acid mobilization and oxidation and protein catabolism is essential in the treatment of diabetes mellitus. On the other hand, disagreement still exists regarding the usefulness of treating asymptomatic hyperglycemia. Recently, it has been documented that the synthesis of polyols and basement membrane glycoproteins is increased by hyperglycemia.[175,201] Thus, "tight control" of blood glucose may be important if the long-term complications of diabetes mellitus are to be reduced.

Diet, insulin, and oral hypoglycemic agents have been the mainstays of treatment. However, a controversy has arisen concerning the efficacy of oral hypoglycemic agents, such as the sulfonylureas.[202,203] While hyperglycemia is better controlled with these agents than it is with diet alone, an increased frequency of myocardial infarction has been reported. Although the interpretation and implications of these findings are still controversial, there is some experimental evidence suggesting that sulfonylureas may have an adverse effect on the myocardium. Wu and colleagues have reported increased "stiffness" of the myocardium secondary to interstitial accumulation of periodic acid–Schiff staining material which reduced left ventricular function in dogs treated with tolbutamide.[204]

On the basis of available information, in our judgment the only patients with diabetes who should use oral hypoglycemic agents are those who are not ketosis-prone, whose hyperglycemia cannot be controlled with diet alone, and who are unwilling or unable to receive insulin injections. It should also be recognized that beta-adrenergic blockers reduce the hyperglycemic reaction to stress, and it is possible that beta-adrenergic blocker therapy may require a downward adjustment of insulin dosage, since patients receiving beta blockers may be more susceptible to hypoglycemia. Since many of the symptoms of which the hypoglycemic patient is aware are due to the effects of the epinephrine which is released, both physician and patient must be alert to the possibility that hypoglycemia occurring in the beta blocker–treated diabetic may be relatively asymptomatic. Since certain diuretics, such as the thiazides and furosemide, may result in hypokalemia, and because hypokalemia can inhibit insulin release, these drugs may intensify the glucose intolerance of diabetic patients.

In patients with diabetes mellitus and impairment of left ventricular function, a sudden increase in the glucose concentration of extracellular fluid, as occurs with the development of insulin deficiency, may result in the movement of fluid from the intracellular to the extracellular space and an intensification of heart failure. This responds to the lowering of blood glucose concentration by insulin.[205]

OBESITY

There are two types of obesity: adult-onset and lifelong. Adult-onset obesity is extremely common, probably occurring to a varying extent in nearly all individuals in developed countries. Its clinical course consists of normal weight patterns during childhood and adolescence, with a gradual increase in weight beginning between 20 and 40 years of age; it reflects an imbalance between caloric intake and utilization.[206] Much less frequent is lifelong obesity, characterized by the development of obesity early in childhood, with significant increase in weight during adolescence and, in the female, during and after pregnancy. These individuals are usually grossly obese, weighing more than 150 per cent of their ideal weight as adults.

Hirsch and coworkers have documented an increase both in the size and the number of adipose cells in individuals with lifelong obesity, while in adult-onset obesity, only an increase in cell size occurs.[207] With weight reduction the size of the adipose cells decreases in both conditions; however, the number does not change in either. Whether in lifelong obesity the increased number of adipose cells is determined by genetic or environmental factors is uncertain. However, it has been documented that there is no significant change in the number of adipose cells when obesity develops after late childhood in both experimental animals and humans. On the other hand, some evidence suggests that early infant feeding habits may significantly alter their number.[208] The metabolic consequences of obesity include decreased sensitivity to insulin, with resultant hyperinsulinemia, glucose intolerance, hypercholesterolemia, hypertriglyceridemia, and hyperaminoacidemia.

CARDIOVASCULAR CONSEQUENCES OF SEVERE OBESITY

It is well known from a variety of statistical data that marked obesity is accompanied by an increased morbidity and excessive mortality, a large portion of which is related to cardiovascular abnormalities. *Hypertension* is common in the grossly obese,[208a] although it must be recognized that indirect measurement of blood pressure frequently leads to overestimation of the arterial pressure by the standard cuff method (p. 22). Nonetheless, direct measurement of arterial pressure frequently shows moderate elevations that can usually be promptly restored to normal by means of weight reduction and salt restriction.

Evidence of circulatory dysfunction in the massively obese, associated with cardiac enlargement during life and at autopsy, was first described by Smith and Willius in 1933.[209] It is now widely appreciated that massive obesity is accompanied by a marked increase in blood volume and cardiac output, which are proportional to the excess of body weight;[210–212] the hematocrit is often slightly elevated as well. The elevated cardiac output is secondary to an increased stroke volume, since heart rate is normal; the cardiac output rises normally during exercise. Left ventricular filling pressures are at or close to the upper limits of normal in the supine position in the basal state, but increase with passive leg raising, and reach strikingly elevated levels during exercise. These increases in ventricular filling pressure are associated with a high resting central blood volume, which also increases significantly with exertion. The maximum velocity of myocardial fiber shortening and the ratio of stroke work index to left ventricular end-diastolic pressure were reduced, even in relatively young obese persons, without any other evidence of heart disease[211] (Fig. 51–9). Massive edema may occur as a consequence of the elevated ventricular filling pressure, despite elevation of the cardiac output.

Examination of the gross and microscopic anatomy of the heart in patients with marked chronic obesity showed heart weight to be considerably greater than predicted for

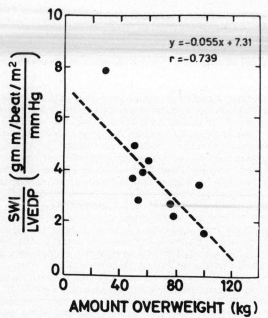

$$y = -0.055x + 7.31$$
$$r = -0.739$$

FIGURE 51–9 The significant negative correlation between the ratio of the stroke work index (SWI) to the left ventricular end-diastolic pressure (LVEDP) and the amounts of overweight shows that the higher the degree of obesity, the greater the impairment of left ventricular function. (Reproduced with permission from Divitiis, O., Fazio, S., Petitto, M., et al: Obesity and cardiac function. Circulation **64**:477, 1981, by permission of the American Heart Association, Inc.)

ideal body weight, with marked left ventricular hypertrophy and, in a few instances, right ventricular hypertrophy as well.[212a] This increase in cardiac weight is not due to excess epicardial fat and fatty infiltration of the myocardium, which were previously considered to be the principal features of the obese heart.[213] Thus, when these clinical, hemodynamic, and pathological observations are taken together, it appears that manifestations of myocardial dysfunction occur in very obese subjects without evidence of other heart disease and that in the absence of the obesity hypoventilation syndrome (p. 1596), cor pulmonale is not a presenting feature.

Heart failure in the markedly obese is usually chronic. The pulmonary and systemic congestion with symptoms of dyspnea and edema are, at first, simply related to the reductions in ventricular compliance and elevations of filling pressures. Later, these symptoms are related also to increases in ventricular end-diastolic volume and the reduction of myocardial contractility. Thus, the marked chronic elevation of cardiac work, i.e., of cardiac output and arterial pressure, ultimately leads to heart failure.

Fortunately, weight reduction is beneficial in the majority of patients, even those with heart failure. It usually improves the exercise capacity of patients with chronic exogenous obesity and decreases total body oxygen uptake, the cardiothoracic ratio on chest roentgenogram, systemic arterial pressure, blood volume, cardiac output, arteriovenous oxygen difference, and left ventricular filling pressure at rest.[210] However, evidence of left ventricular dysfunction persists, as reflected in the elevation of left ventricular filling pressure with exercise.[214,215]

Treatment of heart failure in these patients consists of maintenance of the reduced body weight, dietary sodium restriction, cardiac glycosides, and diuretics. Often, patients with massive obesity have associated arteriosclerotic coronary artery disease and the salutary results of weight reduction may be particularly striking in them.

TREATMENT

Most cases of adult-onset obesity are the result of imbalance between intake and output. Thus, reduction of intake is the most significant factor in treating this disease. While abnormalities in endocrine function, particularly of the thyroid or adrenal, have often been implicated in the pathophysiology of obesity, this thesis is rarely substantiated by detailed evaluation. The amount and rate of weight loss with a given level of caloric restrictions depends on the degree of energy expenditure. Energy expenditure depends on both the physical activity and mass of the individual. Thus, with a fixed level of intake and activity, the rate of weight loss decreases as the total weight decreases. There is no evidence that a specific type of diet has any intrinsic benefit except as it is related to its caloric content. Thus, the claim that high protein diets are more efficacious is related not to their caloric content but rather to the accompanying ketosis that suppresses appetite.

MALNUTRITION

Malnutrition, particularly protein-calorie deficiency, is prevalent in many underdeveloped areas of the world. However, in recent years, it has also become a concern in developed countries in those individuals who have chronic diseases, in whom it exists as a result of both anorexia and hypermetabolism. The clinical picture is similar to adult kwashiorkor reported from underdeveloped countries, described below.

Protein-calorie malnutrition of childhood refers to syndromes of nutritional deficiency, which range from marasmus to kwashiorkor and which result from a stress like a serious infection superimposed upon an inadequate diet.[93] *Marasmus* is a state of malnutrition in an infant who has been weaned early and fed a diet grossly deficient in calories, protein, and other essential nutrients. *Kwashiorkor* usually occurs in children 1 to 4 years of age and is due to deficiency of protein relative to calories.

The circulatory status of patients with severe nutritional depletion and electrolyte imbalance is precarious; the cardiac output, systolic pressure, and pulse pressure are abnormally low and there may be massive, generalized edema; the P-R interval may be shortened. There is loss of subcutaneous fat and general wasting and atrophy of most organs, including the heart, which is thin-walled, pale, and flabby on gross examination. Histological study reveals atrophy of the muscle fibers, sometimes with interstitial edema. In experimental chronic protein-calorie undernutrition, not only is the heart atrophic, but also left ventricular function may be abnormal. In the dog, there are reductions in left ventricular compliance and contractility,[216] whereas in the rat this apparently does not occur, although there is striking atrophy of the heart.[217] The treatment of the dehydrated or severely anemic patient with protein-calorie malnutrition involves correction of hematological, fluid, and electrolyte imbalance and the treatment of infection. Congestive failure can be avoided if care is taken to avoid overloading with sodium, water, or blood. Digitalis must be given cautiously when these patients are in heart failure because of their sensitivity to glycosides.

In parts of the world where pediatric kwashiorkor is common, there are also cases of adults with similar clinical features.[218] These features include loss of subcutaneous fat and muscle with edema, weakness, depression, anorexia, diarrhea, abdominal distention, hair loss, and thinning of the skin. Classically, plasma albumin and amino acid levels are low, as are serum concentrations of sodium, magnesium, and phosphorus. Urinary excretion of nitrogen is reduced, as is total body potassium. On the other hand, total body and extracellular water and plasma volume are usually increased. The primary pathophysiological event is protein malnutrition. All the clinical signs and symptoms are related to this basic defect.

MALNUTRITION IN CARDIAC DISEASE

Assessment of protein-calorie nutritional status in cardiac patients has not been extensively evaluated. However, during the last two decades there has been an increasing awareness that some patients with cardiovascular disease have clinical features similar to those described above. In these cases, instead of involuntary protein deprivation, anorexia plays a significant role. For example, chronic congestive heart failure leads to cellular hypoxia as well as hypermetabolism. Gastrointestinal hypoxia produces anorexia, which then initiates a vicious circle. Decreased protein intake produces cardiac atrophy and increasing congestive heart failure, which produces more cellular hypoxia, greater anorexia, and finally death.[219]

A similar condition has been described in some patients undergoing open heart surgery for correction of rheumatic valvular disease. In some malnourished patients, the mortality reaches 20 per cent, significantly greater than the 1 to 2 per cent in normally nourished patients undergoing the same procedure. The underlying pathophysiology is uncertain but probably includes (1) decreased cardiac mass, (2) reduction of biosynthetic activity of liver, (3) poor healing due to reduced levels of substrate, and (4) impairment of cell-mediated immunity.[219,220] As a result, wound healing is retarded, skin ulcers occur, and requirements for artificial ventilation are prolonged. Abel and colleagues have suggested that hyperalimentation in the immediate postoperative period does not significantly alter the increased morbidity.[219] This has led Blackburn et al. to suggest that both preoperative and concurrent nutritional support is necessary[220] (Fig. 51–10). However, definitive studies to distinguish between nutritional status and severity of the cardiovascular disease as the cause for the increased morbidity have not been reported.

CARDIOVASCULAR MANIFESTATIONS OF VITAMIN DEFICIENCY

Thiamine Deficiency (see p. 814)
Other Vitamin Deficiencies. Deficiencies of other vitamins have not led to specifically definable cardiovascular abnormalities, except for the hypocalcemia-accompanied vitamin D deficiency. However, vitamin deficiencies, particularly of the B group and folic acid, have been diagnosed with increasing frequency in patients with cardiovascular disease. For example, nearly a third of infants and children with congenital heart disease have been reported to be deficient in a number of the B vitamins.[221] Folic acid deficiency has been documented in a significant number of patients with congestive heart failure. While the deficient state may simply be related to decreased intake, abnormal intestinal absorption or increased rates of excretion may also contribute.

ALTERATIONS IN GONADAL HORMONE SECRETION

There are no specific cardiovascular abnormalities associated with altered gonadal function even though the heart does contain androgen receptors, whose function has not been defined.[222] However, the effect of sex steroids on the development of atherosclerosis has been the subject of intensive investigation over the past decade.

GONADAL FUNCTION AND CARDIOVASCULAR DISEASE

Middle-aged men are at a higher risk for developing cardiovascular disease than age-matched women. Because the discrepancy between male and female mortality disappears in older, postmenopausal women, some investigators have suggested that estrogen reduces the rate of development of coronary atherosclerosis. Support for this thesis includes the observation that total cholesterol is lower and HDL cholesterol is higher in postmenopausal women who are taking estrogens than in those who are not.[223,224] Additionally, the risk ratio for coronary artery disease death is only 0.43 in postmenopausal estrogen users compared to nonusers[225] (p. 1218). Several studies, however, have provided evidence against this thesis. First, it has been documented that the development of coronary artery disease in women who underwent hysterectomies and were also castrated is no different than in age-matched noncastrated women.[226] Second, widespread use of oral contraceptives, most of which contain estrogen, has proved that estrogen administration is not without cardiovascular risk, since it can increase total cholesterol and beta-lipoprotein (LDL) cholesterol and decrease alpha-lipoprotein (HDL) cholesterol in premenopausal females.[227,228] Additionally, it has been

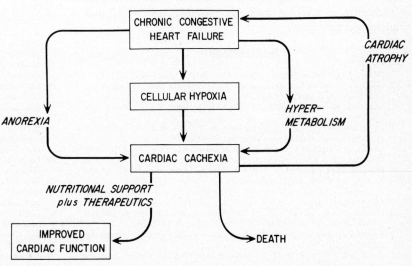

FIGURE 51–10 Pathogenesis of cardiac cachexia. A positive feedback loop forms a vicious circle that leads to irreversible protein malnutrition. Heart failure therapy must begin and forced feeding must be initiated to reduce morbidity and mortality. (From Blackburn, G. L., et al.: Nutritional support in cardiac cachexia. J. Thorac. Cardiovasc. Surg. 73:494, 1977.)

shown to increase the degree of abnormality in post-exercise electrocardiograms in those individuals who had abnormal tests prior to estrogen therapy.[229]

This has led some investigators to suggest that it is not the increased estrogen but the decreased testosterone that is protective to women. They base this theory on the documented reduction in serum cholesterol levels and incidence of atherosclerosis in castrated men and the positive correlation between plasma testosterone and high density lipoprotein cholesterol levels.[230] However, the similar frequency of coronary artery disease in postmenopausal women and men of similar age with significantly different testosterone levels is unexplained.

CARDIOVASCULAR EFFECTS OF ORAL CONTRACEPTIVES

Within the last decade, several studies have documented that in some patients the use of oral contraceptives is accompanied by an increased risk of cardiovascular morbidity and mortality in premenopausal females.[227-229,231] Specifically, there is an increased frequency of diabetes mellitus, hypertension, and thromboembolic disease. While the increased risk is small, nevertheless caution in the use of oral contraceptive agents by individuals who may be predisposed to the development of these diseases is warranted.

HYPERTENSION (see also p. 873). The hypertension associated with estrogen administration is probably related to its effect in modifying the production of renin substrate by the liver.[232] It has been clearly documented that oral contraceptives increase the concentration of renin substrate and blood angiotensin II.[233] However, most individuals do not develop clinical hypertension, which suggests that a counter-regulatory mechanism(s) is activated, reducing the vascular effect of angiotensin II. Alternatively, blood pressure may increase in all patients, but only the predisposed will develop hypertension. Thus, individuals who have a personal or family history of renal disease are more likely to develop hypertension with estrogen administration.

THROMBOEMBOLIC DISEASE. At least two clearly defined alterations in the clotting system are produced by oral contraceptive agents; either or both could be responsible for the increased frequency of thromboembolic disease.[231] First, estrogen enhances the biosynthesis of a number of the clotting factors by the liver. Second, oral contraceptives increase both the viscosity of blood and platelet adhesiveness.

References

1. Graves, R. J.: Clinical lectures. London Med. Surg. J. (Part II):7, 516, 1835.
2. Addison, T.: On the Constitutional and Local Effects of Disease of the Suprarenal Capsules. London, Highley, 1855.
3. Sonenberg, M., and Cohen, H.: Growth hormone. Ann. N.Y. Acad. Sci. 148:291, 1968.
4. Daughaday, W. H.: The adenohypophysis. In Williams, R. H. (ed.): Textbook of Endocrinology, Philadelphia, W. B. Saunders Co., 1974, p. 31.
5. Korner, A.: Anabolic action of growth hormone. Ann. N.Y. Acad. Sci. 148:408, 1968.
6. Frelin, C.: The regulation of protein turnover in newborn rat heart cell cultures. J. Biol. Chem. 255:11149, 1980.
7. Goodman, H. M.: Growth hormone and the metabolism of carbohydrate and lipid in adipose tissue. Ann. N.Y. Acad. Sci. 148:419, 1968.
8. Mautalen, C. A., Mellinger, R. C., and Smith, R. W., Jr.: Lipolytic effect of growth hormone in acromegaly. J. Clin. Endocrinol. 28:1031, 1968.
9. Randle, P. J., and Morgan, H. E.: Regulation of glucose uptake by muscle. Vitam. Horm. 20:199, 249, 1962.
10. Coggeshall, C., and Root, H. F.: Acromegaly and diabetes mellitus. Endocrinology 26:1, 1940.

11. Aloia, J. F., Roginsky, M. D., and Field, R. A.: Absence of hyperlipidemia in acromegaly. J. Clin. Endocrinol. 35:921, 1972.
12. Courville, C., and Mason, V. R.: The heart in acromegaly. Arch. Intern. Med. 61:704, 1938.
13. Hejtmancik, M. R., Bradfield, J. Y., and Hermann, G. R.: Acromegaly and the heart: A clinical and pathologic study. Ann. Intern. Med. 34:1445, 1951.
14. McGuffin, W. L., Sherman, B. M., Roth, J., Gorden, P., Kahn, C. R., Roberts, W. C., and Frommer, P. L.: Acromegaly and cardiovascular disorders. Ann. Intern. Med. 81:11, 1974.
15. Lie, J. T., and Grossman, S. J.: Pathology of the heart in acromegaly: Anatomic findings in 27 autopsied patients. Am. Heart J. 100:41, 1980.
16. Mather, H. M., Boyd, M. J., and Jenkins, J. S.: Heart size and function in acromegaly. Br. Heart J. 41:697, 1979.
17. Savage, D. D., Henry, W. L., Eastman, R. C., Borer, J. S., and Gorden, P.: Echocardiographic assessment of cardiac anatomy and function in acromegalic patients. Am. J. Med. 67:823, 1979.
17a. Csanady, M., Gaspar, L., Hogye, M., Hogye, M., and Gruber, N.: The heart in acromegaly: An echocardiographic study. Intern. J. Cardiol. 2:349, 1983.
18. Rossi, L., Thiene, G., Caregaro, L., Giordano, R., and Lauro, S.: Dysrhythmias and sudden death in acromegalic heart disease. A clinicopathologic study. Chest 72:495, 1977.
19. Hamwi, G. J., Skillman, T. G., and Tufts, K. C., Jr.: Acromegaly. Am. J. Med. 29:690, 1960.
20. Falkheden, T., and Sjögren, B.: Extracellular fluid volume and renal function in pituitary insufficiency and acromegaly. Acta Endocrinol. 46:80, 1964.
21. Cain, J. P., Williams, G. H., and Dluhy, R. G.: Plasma renin activity and aldosterone secretion in patients with acromegaly, J. Clin. Endocrinol. 34:73, 1972.
22. Strauch, G., Vallotton, M. B., and Touitou, Y.: The renin-angiotensin-aldosterone system in normotensive and hypertensive patients with acromegaly. N. Engl. J. Med. 287:795, 1972.
23. Dluhy, R. G., and Williams, G. H.: Primary aldosteronism in a hypertensive acromegalic patient. J. Clin. Endocrinol. 29:1319, 1969.
24. Moore, T. J., Thein-Wai, W., Dluhy, R. G., Dawson-Hughes, B. F., Hollenberg, N. K., and Williams, G. H.: Abnormal adrenal and vascular responses to angiotensin II and an angiotensin antagonist in acromegaly. J. Clin. Endocrinol. Metab. 51:215, 1980.
25. Souadjian, J. V., and Schirger, A.: Hypertension in acromegaly. Am. J. Med. Sci. 254:629, 1967.
26. Biglieri, E. G., Watlington, C. O., and Forsham, P. H.: Sodium retention with human growth hormone and its subfractions. J. Clin. Endocrinol. 21:361, 1961.
27. Kellgron, J. A., Ball, J., and Tutton, G. K.: The articular and other limb changes in acromegaly. Q. J. Med. 21:405, 1952.
28. Surawicz, B., and Mangiardi, M. L.: Electrocardiogram in endocrine and metabolic disorders. In Rios, J. C. (ed.): Clinical Electrocardiographic Correlations. Philadelphia, F. A. Davis, 1977, p. 243.
28a. Knowlton, A. I., and Baer, L.: Cardiac failure in Addison's disease. Am. J. Med. 74:829, 1983.
29. Jonas, E. A., Aloia, J. F., and Lane, F. J.: Evidence of subclinical heart muscle dysfunction in acromegaly. Chest 67:190, 1975.
30. Smallridge, R. C., Rajfer, S., Davis, J., and Schaaf, M.: Acromegaly and the heart. Am. J. Med. 66:22, 1979.
31. Hardy, J.: Trans-sphenoidal microsurgical removal of pituitary microadenoma. Progr. Neurol. Surg. 6:200, 1975.
32. Kjellberg, R. M. Proton-beam therapy in acromegaly. N. Engl. J. Med. 278:689, 1968.
33. Schimmel, M., and Utiger, R. D.: Thyroidal and peripheral production of thyroid hormones. Review of recent findings and their clinical implications. Ann. Intern. Med. 87:760, 1977.
34. Kaplan, M. M.: The thyroid and the heart; how do they interact? J. Cardiovasc. Med., 7:893, 1982.
35. Lardy, H. A., and Feldott, H. G.: Metabolic effects of thyroxine in vitro. Ann. N.Y. Acad. Sci. 54:636, 1951.
36. Tata, J., Ernster, L., and Lindberg, O.: The action of thyroid hormones at the cell level. Biochem. J. 86:408, 1963.
37. Stocker, W. W., Samaha, F. J., and Degroot, L. J.: Coupled oxidative phosphorylation in muscle of thyrotoxic patients. Am. J. Med. 44:900, 1968.
38. Oppenheimer, J. H., Schwartz, H. L., Surks, M. I., Koerner, D., and Dillmann, W. H.: Nuclear receptors and the initiation of thyroid hormone action. In Greep, R. O. (ed.): Recent Progress in Hormone Research. New York, Academic Press, 1976, p. 529.
39. Seelig, S., Liaw, C., Towle, H. C., and Oppenheimer, J. H.: Thyroid hormone attenuates and augments hepatic gene expression at a pretranslational level. Proc. Natl. Acad. Sci. USA 78:4733–4737, 1981.
40. Edelman, I. S., and Ismail-Beigi, F.: Thyroid thermogenesis and active sodium transport. Recent Progr. Horm. Res. 30:235, 1974.
41. Asano, Y., Liberman, U. A., and Edelman, I. S.: Thyroid thermogenesis: Relationships between Na^+-dependent respiration and $Na^+ + K^+$-adenosine triphosphatase activity in rat skeletal muscle. J. Clin. Invest. 57:368, 1976.
42. Lo, C. S., August, T. R., Liberman, U. A., and Edelman, I. S.: Dependence of renal ($Na^+ + K^+$) adenosine triphosphatase activity on thyroid status. J. Biol. Chem. 251:7826, 1976.
43. Lo, C. S., and Edelman, I. S.: Effect of triiodothyronine on the synthesis and degradation of renal cortical ($Na^+ + K^+$) adenosine triphosphatase. J. Biol. Chem. 251:7834, 1976.

44. Fain, J. N., and Rosenthal, J. W.: Calorigenic action of triiodothyronine on white cells: Effects of ouabain, oligomycin, and cathecholamines. Endocrinology 89:1205, 1971.
45. Primack, M. P., and Buchanan, J. L.: Control of oxygen consumption in liver slices from normal and T4-treated rats. Endocrinology 95:619, 1974.
46. Knight, R. A.: The use of spinal anesthesia to control sympathetic overactivity in hyperthyroidism. Anesthesiology 6:225, 1945.
47. Buccino, R. A., Spann, J. F., Pool, P. E., and Braunwald, E.: Influence of the thyroid state on the intrinsic contractile properties and the energy stores of the myocardium. J. Clin. Invest. 46:1669, 1967.
48. Bayliss, R. I. S., and Edwards, O. M.: Urinary excretion of free catecholamines in Graves' disease. Endocrinology 49:167, 1971.
49. Christensen, H. J.: Plasma noradrenaline and adrenaline in patients with thyrotoxicosis and myxoedema. Clin. Sci. Molec. Med. 45:163, 1973.
50. Nishizawa, Y., Hamada, N., Fujii, S., Morii, H., Okuda, K., and Wada, M.: Serum dopamine-beta-hydroxylase activity in thyroid disorders. J. Clin. Endocrinol. Metab. 39:599, 1974.
51. Rutherford, J. P., Vatner, S. F., and Braunwald, E.: Adrenergic control of myocardial contractility in conscious hypertrophied dogs. Am. J. Physiol. 237:590, 1980.
52. Brester, W. R., Isaacs, J. R., and Osgood, P. F.: The hemodynamic and metabolic interrelationships in the activity of epinephrine, norepinephrine, and the thyroid hormones. Circulation 13:1, 1956.
53. Van Der Schoot, J. B., and Moran, N. C.: An experimental evaluation of the reported influence of thyroxine on the cardiovascular effects of catecholamines. J. Pharmacol. Exp. Ther. 149:336, 1965.
54. Wildenthal, K.: Studies of isolated fetal mouse hearts in organ culture: Evidence for a direct effect of triiodothyronine in enhancing cardiac responsiveness to norepinephrine. J. Clin. Invest. 51:2702, 1972.
55. Wildenthal, K.: Studies on fetal mouse hearts in organ culture: Influence of prolonged exposure to triiodothyronine on cardiac responsiveness to isoproterenol, glucagon, theophylline, acetylcholine, and dibutyryl cyclic 3', 5'-adenosine monophosphate. J. Pharmacol. Exp. Ther. 109:272, 1974.
56. Williams, L. T., Lefkowitz, R. J., Watanbe, A. M., Hathaway, D. R., and Besch, H. R.: Thyroid hormone regulation of beta-adrenergic receptor number. J. Biol. Chem. 252:2787, 1977.
57. Scarpace, P. J., and Abrass, I. B.: Thyroid hormone regulation of rat heart, lymphocyte, and lung beta-adrenergic receptors. Endocrinology 108:1007, 1981.
58. Whitsett, J. A., Pollinger, J., and Matz, S.: β-adrenergic receptors and catecholamine sensitive adenylate cyclase in developing rat ventricular myocardium: Effect of thyroid status. Pediatr. Res. 16:463, 1982.
59. Tse, J., Wrenn, R. W., and Kuo, J. F.: Thyroxine-induced changes in characteristics and activities of beta-adrenergic receptors and adenosine 3', 5'-monophosphate and guanosine 3', 5'-monophosphate systems in the heart may be related to reputed catecholamine supersensitivity in hyperthyroidism. Endocrinology 107:6, 1980.
60. Guarnieri, T., Filburn, C. R., Beard, E. S., and Lakatta, E. G.: Enhanced contractile response and protein kinase activation to threshold levels of β-adrenergic stimulation in hyperthyroid rat heart. J. Clin. Invest. 65:861, 1980.
61. Kunos, G., Vermes-Kunos, I., and Nickerson, M.: Effects of thyroid state on adrenoreceptor properties. Nature 250:779, 1974.
62. Markowitz, C., and Yater, W. M.: Response of explanted cardiac muscle to thyroxine. Am. J. Physiol. 100:162, 1932.
63. Murayama, M., and Goodkind, M. J.: Effect of thyroid hormone on the frequency-force relationship of atrial myocardium from the guinea pig. Circ. Res. 23:743, 1968.
64. Goldman, S., Olajos, M., Friedman, H., Roeske, W. R., and Morkin, E.: Left ventricular performance in conscious thyrotoxic calves. Am. J. Physiol. 242:H113, 1982.
64a. Morkin, E., Flink, I. L., and Goldman, S.: Biochemical and physiologic effects of thyroid hormone on cardiac performance. Prog. Cardiovasc. Dis. 25:435, 1983.
64b. Banerjee, S. K.: Comparative studies of atrial and ventricular myosin from normal, thyrotoxic, and thyroidectomized rabbits. Circ. Res. 52:131, 1983.
65. Philipson, K. D., and Edelman, I. S.: Thyroid hormone control of Na+-K+-ATPase and K+-dependent phosphatase in rat heart. Am. J. Physiol. 232:C196, 1977.
66. Litten, R. Z., Martin, B. J., Howe, E. R., Alpert, N. R., and Solaro, R. J.: Phosphorylation and adenosine triphosphate activity of myofibrils from thyrotoxic rabbit hearts. Circ. Res. 48:498, 1981.
67. Curfman, G. D., Crowley, T. J., and Smith, T. W.: Thyroid-induced alterations in myocardial sodium- and potassium-activated adenosine triphosphatase, monovalent cation active transport and cardiac glycoside binding. J. Clin. Invest. 59:586, 1977.
68. Banerjee, S. K., Flink, I. L., and Morkin, E.: Enzymatic properties of native and N-ethylmaleimide-modified cardiac myosin from normal and thyrotoxic rabbits. Circ. Res. 39:319, 1976.
69. Litten, R. Z., III, Martin, B. J., Low, R. B., and Alpert, N. R.: Altered myosin isozyme patterns from pressure-overloaded and thyrotoxic hypertrophied rabbit hearts. Circ. Res. 50:856, 1982.
70. Chizzonite, R. A., Everett, A. W., Clark, W. A., Jakovcic, S., Rabinowitz, M., and Zak, R.: Isolation and characterization of two molecular variants of myosin heavy chain from rabbit ventricle. Change in their content during normal growth and after treatment with thyroid hormone. J. Biol. Chem. 257:2056, 1982.
71. Goodkind, M. J., Dambach, G. E., Thyrum, P. T., and Luchi, R. J.: Effect of thyroxine on ventricular myocardial contractility of ATPase activity in guinea pigs. Am. J. Physiol. 226:66, 1974.
72. Suko, J.: The calcium pump of cardiac sarcoplasmic reticulum. Functional alterations at different levels of thyroid state in rabbits. J. Physiol. (Lond.) 228:563, 1973.
73. Johnson, P. N., Freedberg, A. S., and Marshall, J. M.: Action of thyroid hormone on the transmembrane potentials from sinoatrial cells and atrial muscle cells in isolated atria of rabbits. Cardiology 58:273, 1973.
74. Arnsdorf, M. D., and Childers, R. W.: Atrial electrophysiology in experimental hyperthyroidism in rabbits. Circ. Res. 26:575, 1970.
75. Davis, P. J., and Davis, F. B.: Hyperthyroidism in patients over the age of 60 years. Medicine 53:161, 1974.
75a. Talafih, K., Briden, K. L., and Weiss, H. R.: Thyroxine-induced hypertrophy of the rabbit heart. Effect on regional oxygen extraction, flow, and oxygen consumption. Circ. Res. 52:272, 1983.
76. Hillis, W. S., Bremmer, W. F., Lawrie, T. D. V., and Thomson, J. A.: Systolic time intervals in thyroid disease. Clin. Endocrinol. 4:617, 1975.
77. Cohen, M. V., Schulman, I. C., Spenillo, A., and Surks, M. I.: Effects of thyroid hormone on left ventricular function in patients treated for thyrotoxicosis. Am. J. Cardiol. 48:33, 1981.
78. Hoffman, I., and Lowrey, R. D.: The electrocardiogram in thyrotoxicosis. Am. J. Cardiol. 6:893, 1960.
79. Goel, B. G., Hanson, C. S., and Han, J.: A-V conduction in hyper- and hypothyroid dogs. Am. Heart J. 83:504, 1972.
80. Miller, R. H., Corcoran, F. H., and Baker, W. P.: Second and third degree atrioventricular block with Graves' disease: A case report and review of the literature. PACE 3:702, 1980.
81. Benker, V. G., Preiss, H., and Kreuser, H.: EKG—Veranderungen Hyperthyreose. Untersuchungen as 542 Patienten. Z. Kardiol. 63:799, 1974.
82. Shapiro, S., Steier, M., and Dimich, I.: Congestive heart failure in neonatal thyrotoxicosis. A curable cause of heart failure in the newborn. Clin. Pediatr. 14:1155, 1975.
83. Forfar, J. C., Muir, A. L., Sawers, S. A., and Toft, A. D.: Abnormal left ventricular function in hyperthyroidism: Evidence for a possible reversible cardiomyopathy. N. Engl. J. Med. 307:1165, 1982.
84. Channick, B. J., Adlin, E. V., Marks, A. D., Denenberg, B. S., McDonough, M. T., Chakko, C. S., and Spann, J. F.: Hyperthyroidism and mitral-valve prolapse. N. Engl. J. Med. 305:497, 1981.
85. Doherty, J. E., and Perkins, W. H.: Digoxin metabolism in hypo- and hyperthyroidism. Studies with tritiated digoxin in thyroid disease. Ann. Intern. Med. 64:489, 1966.
86. Morrow, D. H., Gaffney, T. E., and Braunwald, E.: Studies on digitalis. VIII. Effect of autonomic innervation and of myocardial catecholamine stores upon the cardiac action of ouabain. J. Pharmacol. Exp. Ther. 140:236, 1963.
87. Forfar, J. C., Feek, C. M., Miller, H. C., and Toft, A. D.: Atrial fibrillation and isolated suppression of the pituitary-thyroid axis: Response to specific antithyroid therapy. Int. J. Cardiol. 1:43, 1981.
88. Sandler, G., and Wilson, G. M.: The nature and prognosis of heart disease in thyrotoxicosis. A review of 150 patients treated with 131I. Q. J. Med. 28:347, 1959.
89. Nakazawa, H. K., Sakurai, K., Hamada, N., Momotani, N., and Ito, K.: Management of atrial fibrillation in the post-thyrotoxic state. Am. J. Med. 72:903–906, 1982.
90. Staffurth, J. S., Gibberd, M. C., and Fui, S. T.: Arterial embolism in thyrotoxicosis with atrial fibrillation. Br. Med. J. 2:688, 1977.
91. Ingbar, S. H.: The role of antiadrenergic agents in the management of thyrotoxicosis. Cardiovasc. Rev. Rep. 2:683, 1981.
92. Grossman, W., Robin, N. I., Johnson, L. W., Brooks, H., Selenkow, H. A., and Dexter, L.: Effects of beta blockade on the peripheral manifestations of thyrotoxicosis. Ann. Intern. Med. 74:875, 1971.
93. Whittemore, R., and Caddell, J. L.: Metabolic and nutritional diseases. In Moss, A., et al. (eds.): Heart Disease in Infants, Children and Adolescents. Baltimore, Williams and Wilkins, 1977, p. 887.
94. Skelton, C. L., and Sonnenblick, E. H.: Cardiovascular system in hypothyroidism. In Werner, S. C., and Ingbar, S. H. (eds.): The Thyroid. 2nd Ed. New York, Harper and Row, 1962, p. 873.
95. Kerber, R. E., and Sherman, B.: Echocardiographic evaluation of pericardial effusion in myxedema. Incidence and biochemical and clinical correlations. Circulation 52:823, 1975.
96. Smolar, E. N., Rubin, J. E., Avramides, A., and Carter, A. C.: Cardiac tamponade in primary myxedema and review of the literature. Am. J. Med. Sci. 272:345, 1976.
97. Khaleeli, A. A., and Memon, N.: Factors affecting resolution of pericardial effusions in primary hypothyroidism: A clinical, biochemical and echocardiographic study. Postgrad. Med. J. 58:1073, 1982.
98. Vanhaelst, I., and Neve, P.: Coronary artery disease in hypothyroidism. Lancet 2:800, 1967.
99. Aber, C. P., and Thompson, G. S.: Factors associated with cardiac enlargement in myxedema. Br. Heart J. 25:421, 1963.
100. Fouron, J. C., Bourgin, J. H., Letarte, J., Dussault, J. H., Ducharme, G., and Davignon, A.: Cardiac dimensions and myocardial function of infants with congential hypothyroidism: An echocardiographic study. Br. Heart J. 47:584, 1982.
101. Graettinger, J. S., Muenster, J. J., and Checchia, C.: A correlation of clinical and hemodynamic studies in patients with hypothyroidism. J. Clin. Invest. 37:502, 1958.

102. Stewart, J. H., and Evans, W. F.: Peripheral blood flow in myxedema. Arch. Intern. Med. *69*:808, 1942.

103. Manns, J. J., Shepherd, A. M. M., Crooks, J., and Adamson, D. B.: Measurement of cardiac muscle relaxation in hypothyroidism. Br. Med. J. *1*:1366, 1976.

104. Hillis, W. S., Bremner, W. F., Lawrie, T. D. V., and Thomson, J. A.: Systolic time intervals in thyroid disease. Clin. Endocrinol. *4*:617, 1975.

105. Aber, C. P., and Thompson, G. S.: The heart in hypothyroidism. Am. Heart J. *68*:429, 1964.

106. McBrion, D. J., and Hindle, W.: Myxoedema and heart failure. Lancet *1*:1065, 1963.

107. Margolius, H. S., and Gaffney, T. E.: Effects of injected norepinephrine and sympathetic nerve stimulation in hypothyroid and hyperthyroid dogs. J. Pharmacol. Exp. Ther. *149*:329, 1965.

108. Levey, G. S., Skelton, C. L., and Epstein, S. E.: Decreased myocardial adenyl cyclase activity in hypothyroidism. J. Clin. Invest. *48*:2244, 1969.

109. Rovetto, M. J., Hjarmarson, A. C., and Morgan, H. E.: Hormonal control of cardiac myosin adenosine triphosphate in the rat. Circ. Res. *31*:397, 1972.

110. Steinberg, A. D.: Myxedema and coronary artery disease—a comparative autopsy study. Ann. Intern. Med. *68*:338, 1968.

111. Myasnikov, A. L., and Zaitzev, V. F.: The influence of thyroid hormones on cholesterol metabolism in experimental atherosclerosis in rabbits. J. Atheroscler. Res. *3*:295, 1963.

112. Vanhaelst, L., Neve, P., Chailly, P., and Bastenie, P. A.: Coronary-artery disease in hypothyroidism. Lancet *2*:800, 1967.

113. Karlsberg, R. P., Friscia, D. A., Aronow, W. S., and Sekhon, S. S.: Deleterious influence of hypothyroidism on evolving myocardial infarction in conscious dogs. J. Clin. Invest. *67*:1024, 1981.

114. Littman, D. S., Jeffers, W. A., and Rose, E.: The infrequency of myocardial infarction in patients with thyrotoxicosis. Am. J. Med. Sci. *233*:10, 1957.

115. Keating, F. R., Parkin, T. W., Selby, J. B., and Dickinson, L. S.: Treatment of heart disease associated with myxedema. Progr. Cardiovasc. Dis. *3*:364, 1960.

116. Griffiths, P. D.: Serum enzymes in diseases of the thyroid gland. J. Clin. Pathol. *18*:660, 1965.

117. Morrow, D. H., Gaffney, T. E., and Braunwald, E.: Studies on digitalis. VII. Influence of hyper- and hypothyroidism in the myocardial response to ouabain. J. Pharmacol. Exp. Ther. *140*:324, 1963.

118. Paino, T. D., Rogers, W. J., Baxley, W. A., and Russell, R. O.: Coronary arterial surgery in patients with incapacitating angina pectoris and myxedema. Am. J. Cardiol. *40*:226, 1977.

119. Hay, I. D., Duick, D. S., Vlietstra, R. E., Maloney, J. D., and Pluth, J. R.: Thyroxine therapy in hypothyroid patients undergoing coronary revascularization: A retrospective analysis. Ann. Intern. Med. *95*:456, 1981.

120. Kaplan, M. M., Larsen, P. R., Crantz, F. R., Dzau, V. J., and Rossing, T. H.: Prevalence of abnormal thyroid function test results in patients with acute medical illnesses. Am. J. Med. *72*:9, 1982.

121. Williams, G. H., and Dluhy, R. G.: Diseases of the adrenal cortex. *In* Thorn, G. W., Adams, R. D., Braunwald, E., Isselbacher, K. J., and Petersdorf, R. G. (eds.): Harrison's Principles of Internal Medicine, 10th ed. New York, McGraw-Hill Book Co., 1983 (in press).

122. Cushing, H.: The basophil adenomas of the pituitary body and their clinical manifestations (pituitary basophilism). Bull. Johns Hopkins Hosp. *50*:137, 1932.

123. Liddle, G. W.: Pathogenesis of glucocorticoid disorders. Am. J. Med. *53*:638, 1972.

124. Soffer, L. J., Iannaecone, A., and Gabrilove, J. L.: Cushing's syndrome (study of 50 patients). Am. J. Med. *45*:116, 1961.

125. Kalsner, S.: Mechanism of hydrocortisone potentiation of response to epinephrine and norepinephrine in rabbit aorta. Circ. Res. *24*:383, 1969.

126. Krakoff, L., Nicolis, G., and Amsel, B.: Pathogenesis of hypertension in Cushing's syndrome. Am. J. Med. *58*:216, 1975.

127. Liddle, C. W.: Tests of pituitary-adrenal suppressibility in the diagnosis of Cushing's syndrome. J. Clin. Endocrinol. *20*:1539, 1960.

128. Tyrrel, J. B., Brooks, R. M., Fitzgerald, P. A., Cofoid, P. B., Forsham, P. H., and Wilson, C. B.: Cushing's disease: Selective transsphenoidal resection of pituitary microadenomas. N. Engl. J. Med. *298*:753, 1978.

129. Conn, J. W.: Primary aldosteronism, a new clinical syndrome. J. Lab. Clin. Med. *45*:3, 1955.

130. Cain, J. P., Tuck, M. L., Williams, G. H., Dluhy, R. G., and Rosenoff, S. H.: The regulation of aldosterone secretion in primary aldosteronism. Am. J. Med. *53*:637, 1972.

131. Tuck, M. L., Williams, G. H., Cain, J. P., Sullivan, J. M., and Dluhy, R. G.: The relationship of age, diastolic blood pressure, and known duration of hypertension to the presence of low-renin essential hypertension. Am. J. Cardiol. *22*:637, 1973.

132. Rose, L. I., Underwood, R. H., Newmark, S. R., Kisch, E. S., and Williams, G. H.: Pathophysiology of spironolactone-induced gynecomastia. Ann. Intern. Med. *87*:398, 1977.

133. Bongiovanni, A. M., and Eberlein, W. R.: Disorders of adrenal steroid biogenesis. Recent Prog. Horm. Res. *23*:375, 1967.

134. Schambelan, M., Sebastian, A., and Biglieri, E. G.: Prevalence, pathogenesis and functional significance of aldosterone deficiency in hyperkalemic patients with chronic renal insufficiency. Kidney Int. *17*:89, 1980.

135. Alford, W. C., Meador, C. K., Mihalevich, J., Burrus, G. R., Glassford, D. M., Stoney, W. S., and Thomas, C. S.: Acute adrenal insufficiency following cardiac surgical procedures. J. Thorac. Cardiovasc. Surg. *78*:489, 1979.

136. Levine, R. J., and Landsberg, L.: Catecholamine and the adrenal medulla. *In*

137. Bondy, P. K. (ed.): Duncan's Diseases of Metabolism. Philadelphia, W. B. Saunders Co., 1974, p. 1181.

138. Wurtman, R. J., and Axelrod, J.: Control of enzymatic synthesis of adrenaline in the adrenal medulla by adrenal cortical steroids. J. Biol. Chem. *241*:2301, 1966.

139. Goldsmith, R. E.: Polyendocrine syndromes and the heart. Primary Cardiol. *7*: 153, 1981.

140. DeLarue, N. C., Morrow, J. D., Kerr, J. H., and Colapinto, R. F.: Pheochromocytoma in the modern context. Can. J. Surg. *21*:387, 1978.

141. Sjoerdsma, A., Engelman, K., and Waldmann, T. A.: Pheochromocytoma: Current concepts of diagnosis and treatment. Ann. Intern. Med. *65*:1302,1966.

142. Levenson, J. A., Safar, M. E., London, G. M., and Simon, A. C.: Haemodynamics in patients with phaeochromocytoma. Clin. Sci. *58*:349, 1980.

143. Melmon, K. L.: The adrenals: Catecholamines and adrenal medulla. *In* Williams, R. H. (ed.): Textbook of Endocrinology. Philadelphia, W. B. Saunders Co., 1974, p. 283.

144. Cheng, T. O., and Bashour, T. T.: Striking electrocardiographic changes associated with pheochromocytoma. N. Engl. J. Med. *274*:1102, 1966.

145. Van Vliet, P. D., Burchell, H. B., and Titus, J. L.: Myocarditis associated with pheochromocytoma. N. Engl. J. Med. *274*:1102, 1966.

146. Cueto, L., Arriaga, J., and Zinser, J.: Echocardiographic changes in pheochromocytoma. Chest *76*:600, 1979.

147. McManus, B. M., Fleury, T. A., and Roberts, W. C.: Fatal catecholamine crisis in pheochromocytoma: Curable form of cardiac arrest. Am. Heart J. *102*:930, 1981.

148. Jones, D. H., Allison, D. J., Hamilton, C. A., and Reid, J. L.: Selective venous sampling in the diagnosis and localization of phaeochromocytoma. Clin. Endocrinol. *10*:179, 1979.

149. Bravo, E. L., Tarazi, R. C., Gifford, R. W., and Stewart, B. H.: Circulating and urinary catecholamines in pheochromocytoma: Diagnostic and pathophysiologic implications. N. Engl. J. Med. *301*:682, 1979.

150. Zweifler, A. J., and Julius, S.: Increased platelet catecholamine content in pheochromocytoma: A diagnostic test in patients with elevated plasma catecholamines. N. Engl. J. Med. *306*:890, 1982.

151. Bravo, E. L., Tarazi, R. C., Fouad, F. M., Vidt, D. G., and Gifford, Jr., R. W.: Clonidine-suppression test: A useful aid in the diagnosis of pheochromocytoma. N. Engl. J. Med. *305*:623, 1981.

152. Crago, R. M., Eckholdt, J. W., and Wiswell, J. G.: Pheochromocytoma: Treatment with alpha and beta adrenergic blocking drugs. J.A.M.A. *202*:870, 1967.

153. Sisson, J. C., Frager, M. S., Valk, T. W., Gross, M. D., Swanson, D. P., Wieland, D. M., Tobes, M. C., Beierwaltes, W. H., and Thompson, N. W.: Scintigraphic localization of pheochromocytoma. N. Engl. J. Med. *305*:12,1981.

154. Hengstmann, J. H., Gugler, R., and Dengler, H. J.: Malignant pheochromocytoma. Effect of oral α-methyl-p-tyrosine upon catecholamine metabolism. Klin. Wochenschr. *57*:351, 1979.

155. Keutmann, H. T., Dawson, B. F., and Aurbach, G. D.: Structure, synthesis, and mechanism of action of parathyroid hormone. Recent Prog. Horm. Res. *28*:353, 1972.

156. Rasmussen, H., and Wong, M.: Hormonal control of the renal conversion of 25-hydroxycholecalciferol to 1,25-dihydroxycholecalciferol. J. Clin. Invest. *51*: 2502, 1972.

157. Habener, J. F., and Potts, J. T.: Parathyroid physiology and primary hyperparathyroidism . *In* Avioli, L. V., and Krane, S. M. (eds.): Metabolic Bone Disease. Vol. 2. New York, Academic Press, 1978.

158. Bogin, E., Massry, S. G., and Harary, I.: Effect of parathyroid hormone on rat heart cells. J. Clin. Invest. *67*:1215, 1981.

159. Katoh, Y., Klein, K. L., Kaplan, R. A., Sanborn, W. G., and Kurokawa, K.: Parathyroid hormone has a positive inotropic action in the rat. Endocrinology *109*:2252, 1981.

160. Palmieri, G. M., Nutting, D. F., Bhattacharya, S. K., Bertorini, T. E., and Williams, J. C.: Parathyroid ablation in dystrophic hamsters: Effects of Ca content and histology of heart, diaphragm, and rectus femoris. J. Clin. Invest. *68*:646, 1981.

161. Giles, T. D., Iteld, B. J., and Rires, K. L.: The cardiomyopathy of hypoparathyroidism. Chest *79*:225, 1981.

162. Roberts, W. C., and Waller, B. F.: Effect of chronic hypercalcemia on the heart: An analysis of 18 necropsy patients. Am. J. Med. *71*:371, 1981.

163. Surawicz, B.: Relationship between electrocardiogram and electrolytes. Am. Heart J. *73*:814, 1967.

164. Kleerekoper, M., Rao, D. S., and Frame, B.: Hypercalcemia, hyperparathyroidism and hypertension. Cardiovasc. Med. *3*:1283, 1978.

165. Christensson, T., Hellstrom, K., and Wengle, B.: Blood pressure in subjects with hypercalcemia and primary hyperparathyroidism detected in a health screening program. Eur. J. Clin. Invest. *7*:109, 1977.

166. Weidmann, P., Massry, S. G., and Coburn, J. W.: Blood pressure effects of acute hypercalcemia. Ann. Intern. Med. *76*:741, 1972.

167. Sialer, S., McKenna, D. H., Corliss, R. J., et al.: Systemic and coronary hemodynamic effects of intravenous administration of calcium chloride. Arch. Int. Pharmacodyn. *169*:177, 1967.

168. Resnick, L. M.: Calcium, parathyroid disease, and hypertension. Cardiovasc. Rev. Rep. *3*:1341, 1982.

169. Grodsky, G. M., Curry, D. L., Landahl, H., and Bennett, L.: Further studies on the dynamic aspects of insulin release in vitro with evidence for a two-compartmental storage system. Acta Diabetol. Lat. *1* (Suppl.):554, 1969.

170. Cerasi, E.: An analogue computer model for the insulin response to glucose infusion. Acta Endocrinol. (Kbh.)*55*:163, 1967.

171. Cahill, G. F., Jr.: Physiology of insulin in man. Diabetes *20*:785, 1971.

171. Rimoin, D. L.: Inheritance in diabetes mellitus. Med. Clin. North Am. 55:807, 1971.
172. Waller, B. F., Palumbo, P. J., Lie, J. T., and Roberts, W. C.: Status of the coronary arteries at necropsy in diabetes mellitus with onset after age 30 years: Analysis of 229 diabetic patients with and without clinical evidence of coronary heart disease and comparison to 183 control subjects. Am. J. Med. 69: 498, 1980.
173. Yano, K., Kagan, A., McGee, D., and Rhoads, G. G.: Glucose intolerance and nine-year mortality in Japanese men in Hawaii. Am. J. Med. 72:71, 1982.
174. Zoneraich, S.: Diabetes and the Heart. Springfield, Ill., Charles C. Thomas, 1978, p. 303.
175. Factor, S. M., Okun, E. M., and Minase, T.: Capillary microaneurysms in the human heart. N. Engl. J. Med. 302:384, 1980.
176. Bryfogle, J. W., and Bradley, R. F.: The vascular complications of diabetes mellitus. A clinical study. Diabetes 6:159, 1957.
177. Harrower, A. D. B., and Clarke, B. F.: Experience of coronary care in diabetes. Br. Med. J. 1:126, 1976.
178. Oliver, M. F.: Metabolic response during impending myocardial infarction. II. Clinical implications. Circulation 42:981, 1970.
179. Oliver, M. F., Rowe, M. J., Luxton, M. R., Miller, N. E., and Neilson, J. M.: Effect of reducing circulating free fatty acids on ventricular arrhythmias during myocardial infarction and on ST-segment depression during exercise-induced ischemia. In Braunwald, E. (ed.): Protection of the Ischemic Myocardium. American Heart Association Monograph No. 48, 1976, p. 210.
180. Opie, L. H., Tansey, M. J., and Kennelly, B. M.: The heart in diabetes melli-tus. Acute myocardial infarction and diabetes. II. S. Afr. Med. J. 56:256, 1979.
181. Beard, O. W., Hipp, H. R., Robins, M., and Verzolini, V. R.: Survival in myocardial infarction. Am. Heart J. 73:317, 1967.
182. Smith, S. E., Smith, S. A., and Brown, P. M.: Cardiac autonomic dysfunction in patients with diabetic retinopathy. Diabetologia 21:525, 1981.
183. Pfeifer, M. A., Cook, D., Brodsky, J., Tice, D., Reenan, A., Swedine, S., Halter, J. B., and Porte, J. R.: Quantitative evaluation of cardiac parasympathetic activity in normal and diabetic man. Diabetes 31:339, 1982.
184. Lloyd-Mostyn, R. H., and Watkins, P. J.: Total cardiac denervation in diabetic autonomic neuropathy. Diabetes 25:748, 1976.
184a. Vered, Z., Battler, A., Segal, P., Liberman, D., Yerushalmi, Y., Berezin, M., and Neufeld, H. N.: Exercise induced left ventricular dysfunction in young asymptomatic male diabetic patients. A diabetic cardiomyopathy. J. Am. Coll. Cardiol. 1:723, 1983.
185. Kannel, W. B., Hjortland, M., and Castelli, W. P.: The role of diabetes in congestive heart failure: the Framingham study. Am. J. Cardiol. 34:29, 1974.
186. Hamby, R. I., Zoneraich, S., and Sherman, L.: Diabetic cardiomyopathy. J.A.M.A. 229:1749, 1974.
187. Regan, T. J., Lyons, M. M., Ahmed, S. S., Levinson, G. E., Oldewurtel, H. A., Ahman, M. R., and Haider, B.: Evidence for cardiomyopathy in familial diabetes mellitus. J. Clin. Invest. 60:885, 1977.
188. Ahmed, S. S., Jaferi, G. A., Narang, R. M., and Regan, T. J.: Preclinical abnormality of left ventricular function in diabetes mellitus. Am. Heart J. 89: 153, 1975.
189. Seneviratne, B. I. B.: Diabetic cardiomyopathy: The preclinical phase. Br. Med. J. 1:1444, 1977.
190. A. D'Elia, J. A., Weinrauch, L. A., Healy, R. W., Libertino, T. A., Bradley, R. F., and Leland, O. S.: Myocardial dysfunction without coronary artery disease in diabetic renal failure. Am. J. Cardiol. 43:193, 1979.
191. Shapiro, L. M., Howat, A. P., and Calter, M. M.: Left ventricular function in diabetes mellitus. I: Methodology, and prevalence and spectrum of abnormalities. Br. Heart J. 45:122, 1981.
192. Shapiro, L. M.: Echocardiographic features of impaired ventricular function in diabetes mellitus. Br. Heart J. 47:439, 1982.
193. Factor, S. M., Minase, T., and Sonnenblick, E. H.: Clinical and morphological features of human hypertensive-diabetic cardiomyopathy. Am. Heart J. 99:446, 1980.
194. Regan, T. J., Ettinger, P. O., Khan, M. I., Jesrani, M. U., Lyons, M. M., Oldewurtel, H. A., and Weber, M.: Altered myocardial function and metabolism in chronic diabetes mellitus without ischemia in dogs. Circ. Res. 35:222, 1974.
195. Regan, T. J., Wu, C. F., Yeh, C. K., Oldewurtel, H. A., and Haider, B.: Myocardial composition and function in diabetes: The effects of chronic insulin use. Circ. Res. 49:1268, 1981.
196. Malhotra, A., Penpargkul, S., Fein, F. S., Sonnenblick, E. H., and Scheuer, J.: The effect of streptozotocin-induced diabetes in rats on cardiac contractile proteins. Circ. Res. 49:1243, 1981.
197. Fein, F. S., Strobeck, J. E., Malhotra, A., Scheuer, J., and Sonnenblick, E. H.: Reversibility of diabetic cardiomyopathy with insulin in rats. Circ. Res. 49:1251, 1981.
198. Regan, T. J., Levinson, G. E., Oldewurtel, H. A., Frank, M. J., Weisse, A. B., and Moschos, C. B.: Ventricular function in noncardiacs with alcohol fatty liver. The role of ethanol in the production of cardiomyopathy. J. Clin. Invest. 48:397, 1969.
199. Regan, T. J., Wu, C. F., Weisse, A. B., Moschos, C. B., Haider, B., Ahmed, S., and Lyons, M. M.: Acute myocardial infarction in toxic cardiomyopathy without coronary obstruction. Circulation 51:453, 1975.
200. Wolfe, R. R., and Way, G. L.: Cardiomyopathies in infants of diabetic mothers. Johns Hopkins Med. J. 140:177, 1977.
201. Gabbay, K. H., and O'Sullivan, J. B.: The sorbitol pathway. Enzyme localization and content in normal and diabetic nerve and cord. Diabetes 17:239,1968.
202. University Group Diabetes Program: A study of the effect of hypoglycemic

agents on vascular complications in patients with adult-onset diabetes. Diabetes 19 (Suppl. II):474, 1970.
203. University Group Diabetes Program: A study of the effects of hypoglycemic agents on vascular complications in patients with adult-onset diabetes. V. Evaluation of phenformin therapy. Diabetes 24(Suppl. I):65, 1975.
204. Wu, C. F., Haider, B., Ahmed, S. S., Oldewurtel, H. A., Lyons, M. M., and Regan, T. J.: The effects of tolbutamide on the myocardium in experimental diabetes. Circulation 55:200, 1977.
205. Axelrod, L.: Response of congestive heart failure to correction of hyperglycemia in the presence of diabetic nephropathy. N. Engl. J. Med. 293:1243, 1975.
206. Salans, L. B.: Obesity and the adipose cell. In Bondy, P. K., and Rosenberg, L. E. (eds.): Metabolic Control and Disease. 9th ed. Philadelphia, W. B. Saunders Co., 1980, p. 510.
207. Hirsch, J., and Knittle, J.: Cell lipid content and cell number in obese and nonobese human adipose tissue. J. Clin. Invest. 45:1023, 1966.
208. Hirsch, J., and Knittle, J. L.: Cellularity of obese and nonobese human adipose tissue. Fed. Proc. 29:1516, 1970.
208a. Messerli, F. H., Sundgaard-Riise, K., Reisin, E., Dreslinski, G., Dunn, F. G., and Frohlich, E.: Disparate cardiovascular effects of obesity and arterial hypertension. Am. J. Med. 74:808, 1983.
209. Smith, H. L., and Willius, R. A.: Adiposity of the heart. A clinical and pathologic study of one hundred and thirty-six obese patients. Arch. Intern. Med. 52:911, 1933.
210. Kaltman, A. J., and Goldring, R. M.: Role of circulatory congestion in the cardiorespiratory failure of obesity. Am. J. Med. 60:645, 1976.
211. De Divitiis, O., Fazio, S., Petitto, M., Maddalena, G., Contaldo, F., and Mancini, M.: Obesity and cardiac function. Circulation 64:477, 1981.
212. Messerli, F. H., Ventura, H. O., Reisin, E., Dreslinski, G. R., Dunn, F. G., MacPhee, A. A., and Frohlich, E. D.: Borderline hypertension and obesity: Two prehypertensive states with elevated cardiac output. Circulation 66:55,1982.
212a. Ventura, H. O., Messerli, F. H., Dunn, F. G., and Frohlich, E. D.: Left ventricular hypertrophy in obesity: Discrepancy between echo and electrocardiogram. J. Am. Coll. Cardiol. 1:682, 1983.
213. Amad, K. H., Brennan, J. C., and Alexander, J. K.: The cardiac pathology of chronic exogenous obesity. Circulation 32:740, 1965.
214. Alexander, J. K., and Peterson, K. L.: Cardiovascular effects of weight reduction. Circulation 40:310, 1972.
215. Backman, L., Freyschuss, U., Hallberg, D., and Melcher, A.: Reversibility of cardiovascular changes in extreme obesity: Effects of weight reduction through jejunoileostomy. Acta Med. Scand. 205:367, 1979.
216. Abel, R. M., Grimes, J. B., Alonso, D., Alonso, M., and Gay, W. A., Jr.: Adverse hemodynamic and ultrastructural changes in dog hearts subjected to protein-calorie malnutrition. Am. Heart J. 97:733, 1979.
217. Nutter, D. O., Murray, T. G., Heymsfield, S. T., and Fuller, E. O.: The effect of chronic protein-calorie undernutrition in the rat on myocardial function and cardiac function. Cir. Res. 45:144, 1979.
218. Gillanders, A. D.: Nutritional heart disease. Br. Heart J. 13:177, 1951.
219. Abel, R. M., Fischer, J. E., Buckley, M. J., Barnett, G. O., and Austen, W. G.: Malnutrition in cardiac surgical patients. Arch. Surg. 111:45, 1976.
220. Blackburn, G. L., Gibbons, G. W., Bothe, A., Benotti, P. N., Harken, D. E., and McEnany, T. M.: Nutritional support in cardiac cachexia. J. Thorac. Cardiovasc. Surg. 73:489, 1977.
221. Steier, M., Lopez, R., and Cooperman, J. M.: Riboflavin deficiency in infants and children with heart disease. Am. Heart J. 92:139, 1976.
222. McGill, Jr., H. C., Anselmo, V. C., Buchanan, J. M., and Sheridan, P. J.: The heart is a target organ for androgen. Science 207:775, 1980.
223. Barrett-Connor, E., Brown, W. V., Turner, J., Austin, M., and Criqui, M. H.: Heart disease risk factors and hormone use in postmenopausal women. J.A.M.A. 241:2167, 1979.
224. Wallace, R. B., Hoover, J., Barrett-Connor, E., Rifkind, B. M., Hunninghake, D. B., MacKenthun, A., and Heiss, G.: Altered plasma lipid and lipo-protein levels associated with oral contraceptive and estrogen use. Lancet 2:112, 1979.
225. Ross, R. K., Paganini-Hill, A., Mack, T. M., and Arthur, M., and Henderson, B. E.: Menopausal oestrogen therapy and protection from death from ischaemic heart disease. Lancet 1:858, 1981.
226. Ritterband, A. B., Jaffee, I. A., and Densen, P. M.: Gonadal function and the development of coronary heart disease. Circulation 27:237, 1963.
227. The Coronary Drug Project: Initial findings leading to modifications of its research protocol. J.A.M.A. 214:1303, 1970.
228. Webber, L. S., Hunter, S. M., Baugh, J. G., Srinivasan, S. R., Sklov, M. C., and Berenson, G. S.: The interaction of cigarette smoking, oral contraceptive use, and cardiovascular risk factor variables in children: The Bogalusa Heart Study. Am. J. Publ. Health 72:266, 1982.
229. Jaffe, M. D.: Effect of oestrogens on postexercise electrocardiogram. Br. Heart J. 38:1299, 1976.
230. Gutai, J., LaPorte, R., Kuller, L., Dai, W., Falvo-Gerard, L., and Caggiula, A.: Plasma testosterone, high density lipoprotein cholesterol and other lipoprotein fractions. Am. J. Cardiol. 48:897, 1981.
231. Wood, J. E.: The cardiovascular effects of oral contraceptives. Mod. Concepts Cardiovasc. Dis. 41:37, 1972.
232. Boyd, W. N., Burden, R. P., and Aber, G. M.: Intrarenal vascular changes in patients receiving estrogen-containing compounds—A clinical, histological and angiographic study. Q. J. Med. 44:415, 1975.
233. Hollenberg, N. K., Williams, G. H., Burger, B., Chenitz, W., Hooshmand, I., and Adams, D. F.: Renal blood flow and its response to A II: An interaction between oral contraceptive agents, sodium intake and the renin-angiotensin system in healthy young women. Circ. Res. 38:35, 1976.

52 RENAL DISORDERS AND HEART DISEASE

by Eugene Braunwald, M.D., and Michael N. Gottlieb, M.D.

There is an intimate relation between disorders of the heart and of the kidneys. Some of the principal clinical manifestations of impairment of the heart's performance as a pump result from the renal retention of sodium and water; a number of diseases of the heart, such as infective endocarditis and cardiogenic shock, may result in serious renal disease. Conversely, chronic renal failure frequently results in hypertension and lipid abnormalities, which often lead to accelerated atherosclerosis so that coronary artery disease is a common cause of death in patients being treated for chronic renal insufficiency. Also, uremia may result in pericarditis and thereby lead to cardiac tamponade or constrictive pericarditis; renal failure may also cause secondary hyperparathyroidism, which can produce cardiac calcification with a variety of disturbances of cardiac function.

EFFECTS OF CARDIAC DISEASE ON RENAL FUNCTION

Changes in Renal Function and Electrolyte Balance in Heart Failure

The pathophysiology of congestive heart failure is described in Chapters 13 and 15; and the use of diuretics in treating heart failure is discussed in Chapter 16; the alterations in renal function are reviewed here. J. P. Peters at Yale is credited with the concept that the kidney in heart failure is physiologically similar to the kidney in hypovolemia, both states a consequence of inadequate cardiac output. Retention of salt and water occurs in an attempt to restore the effective arterial blood volume, an as yet poorly defined parameter of the filling of the arterial tree, related in some manner to the ratio of the arterial blood volume to the capacity of the vascular bed.

Modulation of the tubular transport of sodium provides the most important mechanism for regulation of sodium excretion. The proximal tubule is the primary site for sodium reabsorption in the nephron, with approximately 60 per cent of filtered sodium being reabsorbed isotonically at this site. As shown in Figure 52–1, blood enters the nephron at the afferent arteriole, passes through the glomerulus to the efferent arteriole, and moves on to a network of peritubular capillaries. The current concepts of the forces governing the proximal tubular reabsorption of sodium in the normal state and in heart failure are shown in Figure 52–2. As cardiac output falls, several stimuli—including augmented alpha-adrenergic neural activity, circulating catecholamines, and increased circulating and locally produced angiotensin II—cause renal vasoconstriction, particularly of the efferent arterioles (Fig. 52–3). As a consequence, the glomerular filtration rate declines, but there is a proportionately greater fall in renal blood flow, and, therefore, filtration fraction—i.e., the ratio of glomerular filtration rate to renal blood flow—rises. This results in an elevation of the protein concentration in the peritubular capillaries and a decline in the postglomerular capillary hydrostatic pressure; thus, the transcapillary hydraulic pressure gradient falls.

The combination of these two events, i.e., the reduction of peritubular capillary hydrostatic pressure and an elevation of peritubular oncotic pressure, enhances the peritubular capillary uptake of proximal tubular fluid and thereby increases the absolute quantity of sodium reabsorbed by the proximal tubule.[1,2] An additional proposed mechanism for sodium retention in heart failure is the redistribution of blood flow from cortical to juxtamedullary nephrons that have longer loops of Henle and that, therefore, are capable of greater sodium reabsorption.

In addition to the more avid sodium reabsorption in the proximal convoluted tubule, increased sodium reabsorption also occurs in distal nephron sites, including the collecting duct segments. This results from the operation of Starling forces, i.e., a lowering of capillary hydrostatic pressure and an elevation of oncotic pressure, such as those described for the proximal tubule; in addition, the action of aldosterone, whose sodium reabsorption action is limited to the

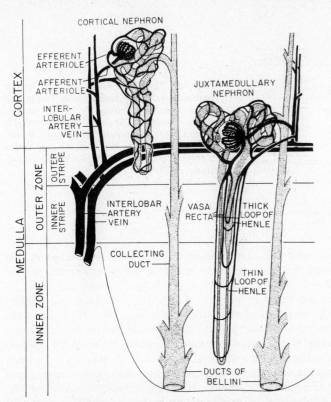

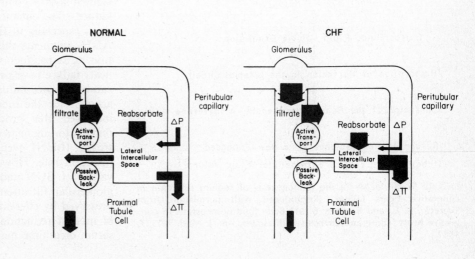

FIGURE 52–1 Anatomy of the kidney, emphasizing comparison of the blood supplies of cortical and juxtamedullary nephrons. (Reproduced with permission from Pitts, R. F.: Physiology of the Kidney and Body Fluids. 3rd ed. Copyright 1974 by Year Book Medical Publishers, Inc., Chicago.)

terminal segment of the nephron, the distal tubule, and the collecting duct system, has been recognized as an important factor in the sodium retention associated with congestive heart failure. The absolute concentration of circulating aldosterone is increased in some patients with congestive heart failure because of a combination of the stimulation of production by the renin-angiotensin axis and the diminished metabolism of aldosterone. In acute heart failure, decreased renal perfusion (whether caused by a reduction in total cardiac output or by a decrease in the renal fraction of the cardiac output) activates the juxtaglomerular appa-

ratus to enhance renin release, which in turn augments the generation of angiotensin II, the stimulus for aldosterone secretion and thus for retention of sodium[3] (Figure 26–21, p. 868). Angiotensin II, both circulating and locally produced, also plays a role in the constriction of efferent arterioles and the resultant elevation in the filtration fraction, discussed above. Indeed, the administration of angiotensin II–converting enzyme inhibitor in heart failure markedly increases renal blood flow and glomerular filtration with return of filtration fraction toward normal and usually induces a natriuresis. The impairment in aldosterone biodegradation that sometimes occurs in heart failure is consequent to hepatic congestion, as well as reduced splanchnic blood flow secondary to reduced cardiac output and splanchic vasoconstriction.[4]

The renal retention of sodium expands extracellular fluid volume and tends to return the renin-angiotensin-aldosterone system toward normal. For that reason, circulating angiotensin II and aldosterone concentrations are frequently normal in chronic stable heart failure, although they tend to be high relative to the expanded extracellular fluid volume (Figs. 52–4 and 52–5). In terminal heart failure, however, with further impairment of renal perfusion, the production of renin is again enhanced, despite the expansion of extracellular fluid volume.

The role of other vasoactive substances, such as prostaglandins, kallikreins, and kinins, has yet to be determined, but they have also been implicated as factors in sodium balance.[5,6] Intrarenal prostaglandins act to oppose the actions of angiotensin II on the renal vascular bed.[7] In heart failure, infusion of prostaglandin A_2 may enhance sodium excretion,[8] whereas inhibition of prostaglandin synthesis by means of prostaglandin synthesis inhibitors such as indomethacin may enhance arteriolar resistance, depress glomerular filtration rate, and increase sodium retention.[9]

The mechanisms for *water retention* in congestive heart failure are outlined in Figure 52–6. Enhanced proximal reabsorption, together with a decline in glomerular filtration rate, results in a fall in the delivery of tubular fluid to the diluting segments of the nephron;[10] in addition, with a reduction in renal blood flow, renal medullary blood flow is diminished, which also results in a decreased capacity of the nephron to excrete water.[1] The lowered effective arteri-

FIGURE 52–2 Peritubular control of proximal tubule fluid reabsorption. Current concept of the role of peritubular capillary physical forces in the regulation of proximal tubule fluid reabsorption in the normal state (*left*) and in the patient with congestive heart failure (*right*). ΔP and $\Delta \pi$ are, respectively, the transcapillary hydraulic and oncotic pressure differences operating across the peritubular capillary. The increase in filtration fraction causes $\Delta \pi$ to rise in heart failure. The increase in renal vascular resistance in CHF is thought to reduce ΔP. Both the increase in $\Delta \pi$ and the fall in ΔP serve to enhance peritubular capillary uptake of proximal reabsorbate and thus increase absolute sodium reabsorption by the proximal tubule. (From Humes, H. D., et al.: The kidney in congestive heart failure. *In* Brenner, B. M., and Stein, J. H. [eds.]: Sodium and Water Homeostasis. New York, Churchill Livingstone, 1978, p. 51.)

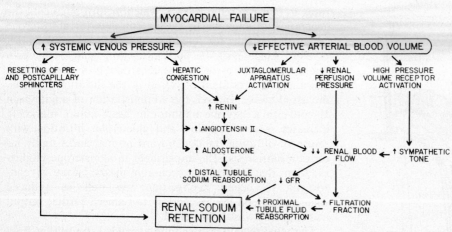

FIGURE 52–3 Summary of the major pathophysiological mechanisms leading to renal sodium retention in heart failure. (From Humes, H. D., et al.: The kidney in congestive heart failure. *In* Brenner, B. M., and Stein, J. H. [eds.]: Sodium and Water Homeostasis. New York, Churchill Livingstone, 1978, p. 51.)

al blood volume serves as a nonosmotic stimulus to enhanced release of antidiuretic hormone, which favors water retention. Furthermore, heart failure stimulates the sensation of thirst;[11] angiotensin II, acting centrally, may also be responsible for stimulating the thirst mechanism.[12] A number of nonosmotic stimuli for release of antidiuretic hormone (ADH), such as discomfort, anxiety, beta-adrenergic agonists, and central nervous system depressants, including barbiturates and narcotics, are commonly present in congestive heart failure. There is a high incidence of inappropriately elevated ADH secretion, which plays an important role in the dilutional hypoosmolality present in many patients with heart failure.[13,14]

The elevated peripheral venous pressure characteristic of heart failure also causes a reflex resetting of pre- and postcapillary resistance in the systemic vascular bed, so that the transudation of fluid into the interstitial space is favored,[15] which tends to lower blood volume and thereby enhances sodium retention. Elevated systemic venous pressure transmitted to the ostium of the thoracic duct impedes lymphatic drainage, enhancing the formation of edema and decreasing intravascular volume. In short-term

experiments, distention of the atria activates receptors that may be considered to monitor atrial and intrathoracic blood volume. Activation of these receptors and vagal afferent fibers reduces renal vascular resistance and inhibits the secretion of antidiuretic hormone, thus augmenting the excretion of sodium and water (p. 462).[16] However, a resetting of the atrial pressure receptors occurs with chronic cardiac failure and atrial distention. In animals with heart failure secondary to experimental pulmonic stenosis and tricuspid regurgitation, the spontaneous activity of the atrial receptors was found to be depressed,[17,18] and in dogs with heart failure caused by an aortocaval fistula, the water diuretic response to left atrial distention is blunted.[19] This attenuated sensitivity of venous and atrial pressure receptors may be responsible for reduced renal vasodilatation (i.e., a higher renal vascular resistance), which, in turn, contributes to salt and water retention in heart failure by mitigating the diuresis and natriuresis that would otherwise accompany the volume expansion and atrial distention characteristic of heart failure.

Total body *sodium* is uniformly elevated in edematous patients with congestive heart failure[20] and total body water is usually increased to an even greater extent. The serum concentration is thus usually slightly reduced in heart failure; in some patients with severe heart failure, it is greatly reduced. Furthermore, sodium may become osmotically inactivated in edema,[21] perhaps by binding to chondroitin sulfate[22] as well as to other polyelectrolytes.

PRERENAL AZOTEMIA IN HEART FAILURE. Azotemia is a common finding in severe congestive heart failure.[23] The enhanced water reabsorption in the collecting duct, especially in the presence of inappropriately elevated ADH, augments the passive reabsorption of urea. In addition, urea production may be enhanced in some forms of heart failure[24]—especially in acute myocardial infarction; a catabolic state induced by the stress of heart failure may account for the increased urea load. The combination of increased urea production and decreased excretion (secondary to augmented reabsorption) elevates blood urea nitrogen (BUN) even prior to a reduction of glomerular filtration rate. However, the principal mechanism for elevation of BUN and serum creatinine is reduction of the glomerular filtration rate. As already noted, the latter is preserved by efferent arteriolar constriction in the presence of modest reductions in renal plasma flow, and therefore serum creatinine may remain normal until, in severe heart

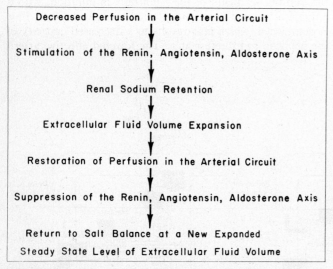

FIGURE 52–4 Stages in the pathogenesis of sodium retention in congestive heart failure. (Reproduced with permission from Skorecki, K. L., and Brenner, B. M.: Body fluid homeostasis in congestive heart failure and cirrhosis with ascites. Am. J. Med. *72*:323, 1982.)

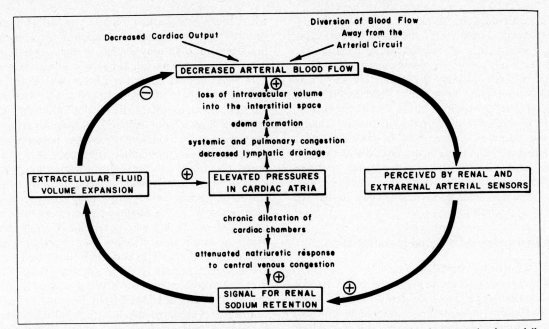

FIGURE 52–5 Sensing mechanisms that initiate and maintain renal sodium retention in congestive heart failure. (Reproduced with permission from Skorecki, K. L., and Brenner, B. M.: Body fluid homeostasis in congestive heart failure and cirrhosis with ascites. Am. J. Med. 72:323, 1982.)

failure, there are marked reductions in renal plasma flow, constriction of afferent arterioles, and reduction of glomerular filtration rate. Thus, an elevation of serum creatinine is usually a sign of advanced heart failure. It is not uncommon in heart failure for the BUN/creatinine ratio to exceed 10 to 1. In severe heart failure, when glomerular filtration rate declines, the BUN may exceed 100 mg/dl and the serum creatinine, 4 mg/dl.

Prerenal azotemia of this degree is a poor prognostic sign in heart failure. Treatment should be directed at improvement of cardiac function, as outlined in Chapter 16.

HEART FAILURE IN PATIENTS WITH RENAL DISEASE. The improved therapy of heart failure (Chap. 16) has prolonged the life of many patients with the combination of cardiac failure and chronic renal disease. In many such patients, the intrinsic renal disease is not severe enough to cause salt, water, or nitrogen retention in the presence of a normal cardiac output. However, when heart failure and the attendant alterations in renal hemodynam-

ics described above are superimposed on intrinsic renal disease, serious problems in salt, water, and nitrogen retention readily occur. Hemodialysis with ultrafiltration or peritoneal dialysis can be effective in the management of this combination of disorders.

POTASSIUM BALANCE IN HEART FAILURE. Mild hypokalemia is a relatively common finding in patients with congestive heart failure, as a consequence of the distal tubular exchange of sodium for potassium and hydrogen under the influence of excess aldosterone. In addition, since all of the major diuretics (other than spironolactone, triamterene, and amiloride) inhibit sodium chloride reabsorption proximal to the site of action of aldosterone in the distal tubule, they increase the delivery of sodium to the distal tubule, enhancing the likelihood of the exchange of sodium for hydrogen and potassium (p. 531). Therefore, serum potassium should be monitored in patients with congestive heart failure to ascertain the need for potassium replacement therapy. Since potassium excretion is aug-

FIGURE 52–6 Summary of the major pathophysiological mechanisms leading to water retention in congestive heart failure. (From Humes, H. D., et al.: The kidney in congestive heart failure. *In* Brenner, B. M., and Stein, J. H. [eds.]: Sodium and Water Homeostasis. New York, Churchill Livingstone, 1978, p. 51.)

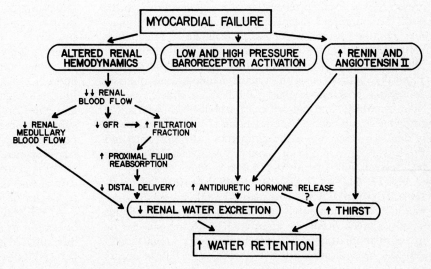

mented and accompanied by alkalosis, any necessary potassium replacement should be in the form of potassium chloride rather than potassium bicarbonate or gluconate.

In the end stage of chronic congestive heart failure, prerenal azotemia and oliguria may become severe enough to limit the ability to excrete potassium. Fundamentally, at this stage the delivery of sodium to the distal tubule is so low, even in the presence of diuretics, that its exchange with potassium becomes reduced and hyperkalemia may develop. In patients with severe heart failure and progressive azotemia and oliguria, potassium-sparing diuretics (spironolactone, amiloride, and triamterene) must be used with caution, if at all, since these agents may hasten the development of hyperkalemia.

Cardiac Disorders with Renal Manifestations

INFECTIVE ENDOCARDITIS   (see also Chap. 33.) The association between glomerulonephritis and bacterial endocarditis has been appreciated for many years. In 1920, prior to the availability of antibiotics and when infective endocarditis was uniformly fatal, 11 per cent of patients with this infection ultimately died of renal failure.[25] It was initially thought that the glomerular lesion was secondary to septic embolization to the kidneys from infected valvular vegetations, but little firm evidence supports this theory. Instead, the pathogenesis of the renal lesions appears to be more in keeping with the generally accepted pathogenesis of most types of glomerulonephritis.[26] Soluble antigenic components of the infecting organism and antibody directed against these antigens have been demonstrated in the glomeruli.[27] As indicated in Chapter 33, many organisms have been responsible for the infective endocarditis that may be associated with glomerulonephritis. By immunofluorescence, the presence of immune complexes and the third component of complement (C3) can be demonstrated in the glomeruli of patients with endocarditis and glomerulonephritis;[27] early in the course, there is a decline in the serum level of C3 and of another component of the complement system, C1q. It now appears that the glomerular lesion of endocarditis results from the deposition of immune complexes along the glomerular basement membrane and in the mesangium.

The most commonly observed abnormality by light microscopy is a focal, proliferative glomerulonephritis, often with focal fibrinoid necrosis. Less commonly, the lesions may be more diffuse, and in some instances extracapillary epithelial proliferation (crescents), such as that seen in rapidly progressive glomerulonephritis, has been observed.[27] Clinically, patients have the typical manifestations of acute or rapidly progressive renal failure, often with hypertension, hematuria, and red cell casts, usually without marked proteinuria and edema. The retention of sodium and water is due to reductions in the glomerular filtration rate and the fractional excretion of sodium.[28] Azotemia is generally progressive, unless rapid bacteriological cure occurs.

ACUTE RENAL FAILURE SECONDARY TO CARDIOGENIC SHOCK   (see also p. 587). Prerenal azotemia and, less commonly, acute renal failure (acute tubular necrosis) may occur in association with massive acute myocardial infarction. The mechanism of prerenal azotemia has been discussed above. Acute renal failure occurs

when there is a marked, sudden reduction of renal perfusion.[29] The myoglobinuria accompanying excessive myocardial necrosis may play a contributory role. It is critically important to distinguish between prerenal azotemia and acute renal failure, since the former will generally respond to measures that improve cardiac output, whereas acute renal failure, once established, is a more serious problem that will usually not respond to extrarenal manipulation. Brief periods of modest hypotension (generally lasting less than an hour) often elicit reversible derangements, but more prolonged or profound hypotension lasting for 1 hour or more usually leads to acute tubular necrosis.

The distinction between prerenal azotemia and acute tubular necrosis in the oliguric patient (i.e., urine output less than 400 ml/24 hr) can generally be made by measurements of serum urea nitrogen and creatinine and the sodium, urea, and creatinine concentrations and osmolality of a concurrent sample of urine. In the absence of recent diuretic therapy, patients with prerenal azotemia retain their ability to conserve sodium; therefore, urinary sodium concentration is low, usually less than 20 mEq/liter. Tubular function is well preserved, as reflected in urine osmolality exceeding 500 mOsm, and the urinary/plasma ratios for urea and creatinine exceed 8 and 40, respectively. The BUN is more than 10 times the serum creatinine concentration.

In acute tubular necrosis, tubular function is impaired and the urinary sodium concentration generally exceeds 40 mEq/liter; the impairment of tubular function is also reflected in a urine osmolality less than 350 mOsm; the urinary/plasma values for urea and creatinine are below 2 and 20, respectively; and the BUN exceeds the serum creatinine by a ratio of less than 10 to 1. The urinary sediment may also be helpful in the differential diagnosis; patients with prerenal azotemia usually have a relatively clear sediment with a few granular or hyaline casts, whereas those with acute tubular necrosis have many tubular cells and casts in the urine.

As in patients with other causes of acute renal failure, the treatment of acute renal failure secondary to myocardial infarction and pump failure consists of controlling fluid intake to levels in accord with urinary output and insensible losses, as well as modifying the dosages of medications that are excreted by the kidneys, observing the patient closely for hyperkalemia, and intervening with dialysis for severe hyperkalemia or azotemia. In general, dialytic therapy, either hemodialysis or peritoneal dialysis, is initiated when serum creatinine levels reach 8 to 10 mg/dl and no reversible component for the renal failure is apparent. In addition, efforts must be made to maintain left ventricular filling pressure at levels that will optimize cardiac output and therefore renal perfusion (18 to 22 mm Hg). Given sufficient time and with no other associated problems, the prognosis for acute renal failure, when appropriately treated, is excellent.[29] However, when failure of the cardiac pump is severe enough to lead to acute renal failure, myocardial insufficiency rather than the renal failure is the determinant of the patient's poor prognosis.

ATHEROEMBOLIC DISEASE. Atheromatous embolization to the kidneys, which results in chronic, fibrotic, interstitial disease, is relatively uncommon.[30,31] It may occur spontaneously but more commonly follows operation on the aorta and renal arteries and catheter manipulation and aortography in patients with severe atheromatous disease of the aorta (p. 1566). Patchy areas of necrosis develop, followed by fibrosis with cholesterol clefts, as well as the response of a foreign body containing multinucleated giant cells. The disorder may be suspected if there has been some manipulation of the atheromatous aorta preceding the onset of progressive renal insufficiency. Examination of the urine is sometimes helpful in confirming the diagnosis; when it is allowed to sediment, fat will be found floating at the top. Treatment consists of avoiding further arterial and aortic manipulation, but progressive destruction of renal tissue occurs with subsequent renal insufficiency; the prognosis for improvement of renal function is guarded.

EFFECTS OF RENAL DISEASE ON THE CARDIOVASCULAR SYSTEM

The successful treatment of end-stage renal disease by dialysis and transplantation is widely considered to be one of the major advances of modern medicine. However, the mortality rate for patients treated by chronic hemodialysis still remains approximately 10 per cent per year.[32] Cardiovascular disease is the principal cause of mortality in these patients, accounting for 50 to 60 per cent of deaths,[33] compared with less than 15 per cent of deaths in age-corrected control populations. Myocardial infarction accounts for 25 to 30 per cent of deaths,[34] and cerebrovascular disease, for 10 to 15 per cent.

As shown in Figure 52–7 and Table 52–1, numerous risk factors for atherosclerosis have been identified in patients with end-stage renal disease.[35] These patients have a high incidence of complex premature ventricular contractions,[36] and in those with angina pectoris that is refractory to medical therapy, coronary bypass surgery has been carried out successfully.[37,38] In addition, angina unassociated with coronary atherosclerosis, presumably related to the combination of severe hypertension, left ventricular hypertrophy, and anemia, has been reported in chronic renal failure.[39]

TABLE 52–1   POSSIBLE CAUSES OF HEART FAILURE IN RENAL INSUFFICIENCY

Hypertension	Increased ventricular afterload
Hypervolemia	Increased ventricular preload
Anemia	Increased cardiac work (high output state)
Lipid abnormalities	Increased atherogenesis
Pericarditis	Restriction of ventricular filling
Ionic alterations	Negative inotropic effect
Hyperkalemia	
Hypocalcemia	
Hypermagnesemia	
Metabolic acidosis	
Disordered calcium and vitamin D metabolism	(A) Metastatic calcification (cardiac and vascular)
	(B) ? Vitamin D deficiency cardiomyopathy
Arteriovenous shunt for hemodialysis	Increased cardiac work (high output state)
Thiamine depletion by dialysis	Increased cardiac work (high output state)
Beriberi (?)	
Uremic toxins (?)	Depressed contractility; ? cardiomyopathy

Hypertension (See also Chap. 26)

Few patients develop chronic renal failure requiring dialysis without experiencing hypertension, which is probably the most important risk factor in the development of atherosclerotic cardiovascular disease. Hemodynamic studies in patients with end-stage renal disease have shown an elevated cardiac index and mean arterial pressure but a normal systemic vascular resistance.[40] The elevated cardiac index and normal systemic vascular resistance are related to the anemia; when the anemia is corrected, the cardiac index falls, and both arterial pressure and systemic vascular resistance rise.[41] The majority of patients with end-stage renal failure who develop hypertension have so-called *volume-dependent hypertension* (Chap. 26). Many studies in patients with end-stage renal failure have shown that arterial pressure is exquisitely dependent on blood volume[42–45] and that blood pressure control may be achieved by ultrafiltration during dialysis and control of salt and water intake in the interdialytic interval[42] (Fig. 52–8). However, a minority of patients with chronic renal failure have hyper-

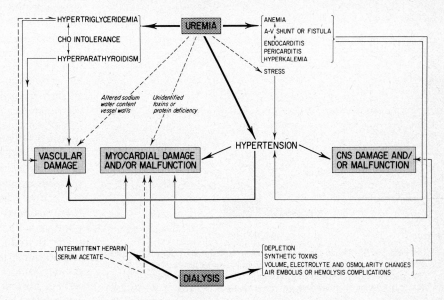

FIGURE 52–7 Risk factors for cardiovascular disease associated with chronic renal failure. CHO = carbohydrate; CNS = central nervous system. (From Lazarus, J. M., and Kjellstrand, C. M.: Dialysis: Medical aspects. *In* Brenner, B. M., and Rector, F. C. (eds.): The Kidney. Philadelphia, W. B. Saunders Co., 1980.)

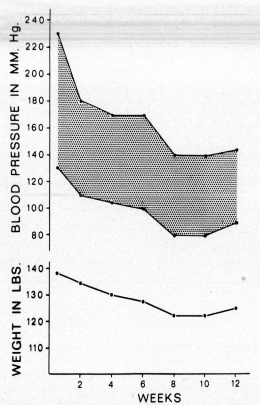

FIGURE 52–8 Blood pressure response to achievement of dry weight in a typical patient with volume-mediated hypertension. (From Vertes, V., et al.: Hypertension in end-stage renal disease. N. Engl. J. Med. *280*:978, 1969.)

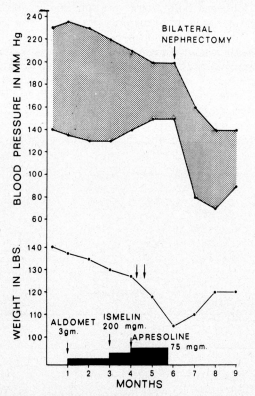

FIGURE 52–9 Blood pressure response to intensive dialysis, antihypertensive drug therapy, and, finally, bilateral nephrectomy in a typical patient with renin-mediated hypertension. (From Vertes, V., et al.: Hypertension in end-stage renal disease. N. Engl. J. Med. *280*: 978, 1969.)

tension that is not volume-related but instead is secondary to elevation of plasma renin activity; the hypertension is uncontrollable by lowering blood volume but does respond to bilateral nephrectomy with consequent reduction in plasma renin activity (Fig. 52–9). Dustan and Page demonstrated the volume-dependent nature of hypertension but also showed that arterial pressure was higher for any given volume when the kidneys were present than after they had been removed.[42] Subsequently, a significant correlation between *plasma renin* levels and arterial pressure was demonstrated.[46] The importance of plasma renin is reflected also in observations on patients with renal failure, hypertension, and expanded blood volume who exhibited renin values which, although normal, were higher than expected for the expanded state of their extracellular volume and which therefore may have contributed to the maintenance of hypertension.[47]

A third mechanism, which operates in patients whose blood pressure cannot be controlled either by volume reduction or bilateral nephrectomy or explained by elevations in plasma renin activity, may be related to *sympathetically mediated vasoconstriction*. Reduced baroreceptor activity has been demonstrated in patients with chronic renal failure by their response to the inhalation of amyl nitrite and the Valsalva maneuver.[48,49] Inhalation of amyl nitrite results in peripheral vasodilation and therefore a fall in blood pressure, which normally results in reflex vasoconstriction and tachycardia. A blunted response in heart rate elevation is taken as evidence of reduced baroreceptor function. Autonomic insufficiency, as evidenced by an inadequate response to the Valsalva maneuver, is said to be present if both bradycardia and arterial pressure overshoot are absent after release of forced expiration against a standard pressure (40 mm Hg) for a set time (12 sec). Many patients with renal insufficiency whose hypertension is caused by sympathetically mediated vasoconstriction exhibit an exaggerated response to the cold pressor test and elevated plasma levels of dopamine beta-hydroxylase as indices of increased adrenergic function but become hypotensive during dialysis.

A fourth possible mechanism of hypertension in patients with renal failure is the *secretion of pressor substances not related to the renin-angiotensin system*. A pressor substance that differs from and is a more potent constrictor than angiotensin II has been isolated from the blood of dogs with bilateral, surgically induced renal artery stenosis.[50] The identity of this substance and its role in hypertension associated with human renal disease remains to be elucidated. A fifth mechanism that has been proposed is the *absence of vasodepressor substances* of renal origin, such as the prostaglandins, which may play a role in the genesis of renoprival hypertension.[51,52]

TREATMENT. Since volume-dependent hypertension is the most common mechanism in patients with chronic renal disease, the reduction of plasma volume should be the central theme in the management of hypertension in these patients. Before renal function has deteriorated to the point at which dialysis is required, an attempt should be made to reduce plasma volume, but not to the point at which glomerular filtration will decline further; dietary sodium should be restricted to the lowest level consistent with a normal sodium balance. However, since many patients may have difficulty with this degree of sodium restriction on a long-term basis, and since they may have an inability to excrete even this low quantity of sodium, it is often necessary to add diuretics. Generally, for patients with creatinine clearances exceeding 40 ml/min, thiazide diuretics are effective. However, when the glomerular filtration rate falls below this level, furosemide is required, sometimes in very high doses.

If the arterial pressure remains elevated despite sodium restriction and diuretic agents, antihypertensive agents are generally effective. These include clonidine, alpha-methyldopa, propranolol, hydralazine, prazosin (and, for the patient refractory to these agents, minoxidil). Sympatholytic agents such as guanethidine are not advisable, since they may be associated with particularly profound postural changes in blood pressure in patients with renal failure.

The problem of the control of hypertension is simpler in patients with chronic renal failure who are maintained on intermittent hemodialysis. In addition to dietary restriction of sodium intake, lowering of blood volume by ultrafiltration during hemodialysis may be employed (Fig. 52–8). In patients in whom volume reduction does not control blood pressure, pharmacological treatment is indicated. Agents such as alpha-methyldopa and propranolol lower plasma renin activity, but vasodilators (hydralazine and minoxidil) may have to be added;[53,54] it is unusual to encounter patients with renal insufficiency who do not respond to a combination of minoxidil and propranolol. However, minoxidil may induce a pericardial effusion, and patients receiving this medication should be monitored by echocardiography to determine the presence of free pericardial fluid that may develop during therapy; it generally resolves within 1 month after withdrawal of the drug.[55]

Angiotensin-converting enzyme inhibitors appear to be particularly useful antihypertensive agents in patients with renal insufficiency (p. 921). Bilateral nephrectomy[56] is employed only in those patients who do not respond to antihypertensive drugs, cannot comply with antihypertensive regimens, or have intolerable side effects of antihypertensive medication. Although aggressive therapy of hypertension for the patient with renin-mediated malignant hypertension may transiently compromise renal function to the point at which dialysis is required, the increased survival associated with control of the hypertension[57] outweighs the risks attending maintenance hemodialysis.

HYPERTENSION FOLLOWING RENAL TRANSPLANTATION. Hypertension occurs in 30 to 80 per cent of patients in the post-transplant period.[58] Multiple factors have been implicated in its etiology, including acute and chronic rejection,[59] recurrent disease in the transplanted kidney,[60] stenosis of the transplanted renal artery,[61] and large doses of steroids.[59] During acute rejection episodes, the levels of renin and angiotensin are markedly elevated. In addition, the renin-angiotensin-aldosterone system appears to be of pathogenic importance in the hypertension associated with stenosis of the artery to the transplanted kidney, a complication that occurs in 10 per cent of the transplant population,[61] as well as in some patients in whom the diseased native kidneys release renin.

The treatment of hypertension in the post-transplant period depends on elucidating the underlying mechanisms of the disorder. In patients with severe refractory hypertension that cannot be ascribed to rejection, angiography and determination of renin activity in venous blood both from the native and the transplanted kidneys are indicated. Surgical revision of a stenosed renal artery or nephrectomy of the native kidney may be in order.

Whereas hypertriglyceridemia is the predominant lipid abnormality in patients with chronic renal failure (see below), hypercholesterolemia Types IIA and B tend to predominate following renal allotransplantation, although in some transplanted patients hypertriglyceridemia persists.[62] The etiology of these lipid abnormalities in the post-transplant period is unclear, but they may be related to the large doses of glucocorticoids administered to these patients.[62] In view of the combination of hypertension and lipid abnormalities in a substantial fraction of patients following transplantation, it is not surprising that coronary atherosclerosis accounts for more deaths than any disease process other than infection.[63]

Lipid Abnormalities

Hypertriglyceridemia with elevations of very low density lipoproteins (VLDL), i.e., Type IV hyperlipoproteinemia (p. 1215), is common in patients with chronic renal failure. Bagdade et al. studied both undialyzed and dialyzed patients with uremia not associated with the nephrotic syndrome and found the plasma triglyceride concentrations to be elevated in both groups.[64] There appears to be no relation between the duration of dialysis or the etiology of the renal disease and the severity of the hyperlipidemia. A second abnormality in lipid metabolism, *reduced concentration of high density lipoprotein (HDL) cholesterol*, has also been documented in chronic renal failure,[64,65] a finding of potential importance in view of the strong negative correlation between HDL concentration and the risk of the development of ischemic heart disease (p. 1211). An inverse correlation has been noted between plasma triglyceride and HDL cholesterol levels in both uremic and nonuremic subjects.[65]

Several suggestions have been proposed to explain the elevation of plasma triglycerides in chronic renal failure. The first is that the increased hepatic synthesis of triglycerides, presumably secondary to insulin resistance and the resultant elevated levels of plasma insulin, and/or of abnormally high levels of growth hormone—both of which occur in renal failure—causes increased release of fatty acids from adipose tissue. A second possibility, for which there is increasing evidence,[66,67] centers on deficiencies in lipoprotein lipase and hepatic triglyceride lipase, known to be necessary for the removal of triglycerides from plasma and their ultimate catabolism; this deficiency may also result from elevated insulin levels, from direct inhibition of these lipases by a nondialyzable factor in uremic serum,[67] or from a deficiency of apoprotein CII in both HDL and VLDL.[68] The reduction of hepatic triglyceride lipase[69] and lipoprotein lipase[70] causes a defect in the catabolism of triglyceride-rich lipoproteins, which in turn leads to the accumulation of VLDL[71] and of enrichment of intermediate-density lipoprotein and low-density lipoproteins with triglyceride; it is also associated with the appearance of apoprotein B48, an increased concentration of apoprotein AIV, and the presence in LDL of apoproteins C and E (proteins not normally found in LDL). It has been suggested that these abnormal substances may be atherogenic.[67]

In one study, HDL cholesterol was significantly reduced in patients with renal failure on chronic hemodialysis (average, 26 mg/dl) compared with normal persons (average, 52 mg/dl).[66] This reduction of HDL was due to a reduced protein content of all its subfractions. Apoprotein electrophoresis showed an increase in "arginine-rich" peptide in the VLDL and the HDL fraction and, as noted, a reduction of apoprotein CII, which is transferred to VLDL from HDL[72] and which functions as an activator of the enzyme lipoprotein lipase.[73]

Treatment. The standard dietary therapy of patients with Type IV hyperlipoproteinemia in the absence of renal failure consists of weight reduction, limitation of alcohol intake, a reduction in carbohydrate consumption, and, if these measures are inadequate, the administration of clofibrate (p. 1226).[74] In patients with chronic renal failure, the lipid abnormality is not usually associated with excessive body weight or alcohol consumption, and reduction in carbohydrate intake is somewhat difficult to achieve owing to the limitations imposed on the patient's diet by virtue of the reduced protein intake. A reasonable therapeutic approach is to provide caloric replacement through increases in polyunsaturated fat in the diet.[75] With this diet, a significant reduction in plasma triglyceride levels has been observed, both in conservatively treated patients with chronic renal failure and in patients on dialysis.[76]

Clofibrate is normally metabolized by the kidney, and active metabolites can accumulate in patients with severely compromised renal function; patients with renal failure may develop severe myositis in association with the ingestion of the usual doses of this drug.[77] A reduction in total dosage of clofibrate to 1.5 gm per week may lead to a lowering of plasma triglyceride concentration without producing myositis. However, even with this reduced dosage, an increase in serum creatine kinase levels has been reported, presumably as a consequence of damage to skeletal muscle.[77]

Hemodialysis

Technical Considerations. Hemodialysis may accomplish three objectives. It may (1) remove solutes, (2) alter the electrolyte concentration of the patient's extracellular fluid, and (3) remove as much as 1 liter of extracellular fluid per hour. These three processes should be viewed as being essentially independent of one another, and it is often desirable, in the course of a single dialysis, to carry out only one or two of these three functions.

Patients with heart failure, circulatory congestion, or hypertension often derive benefit from removal of fluid by ultrafiltration during the course of hemodialysis. This must be carefully done, since normotensive patients may become hypotensive with removal of excess fluid.[78] Echocardiography is a useful noninvasive method for evaluating left ventricular function serially during hemodialysis; it can distinguish between left ventricular failure, decreased left ventricular compliance, and fluid overload.[79-81]

Electrolyte Shifts. In manipulating electrolyte concentrations, it is important to appreciate that most dialysates contain 1.5 to 3.0 mEq/liter of potassium and 3 to 3.5 mEq/liter of calcium (6 to 7 mg/dl of ionized Ca^{++}). Since most patients commence dialysis with some elevation of serum potassium, the serum potassium may fall precipitously when dialysis begins, whereas the concentration of ionized calcium rises, setting the stage for digitalis intoxication in digitalized patients (p. 523). The likelihood of this complication is enhanced by any digoxin excess, which might come about if the dosage has not been adjusted downward to take into consideration the markedly prolonged half-life of this drug in patients with renal failure (p. 514). In patients on hemodialysis who are not hypoxemic, myocardial performance, as reflected in the echocardiogram, often improves; this may be related to a reduction in serum potassium and an elevation of calcium.[80]

Arteriovenous Fistulas. To achieve vascular access to dialysis, an arteriovenous fistula must be created. These shunts have a flow rate of 250 to 750 ml/minute and thereby add to the cardiac workload. As discussed on page 814, in association with the anemia characteristic of chronic renal failure, this may contribute to the development of high-output heart failure.[82] In our experience, this form of heart failure can be readily controlled if any excess fluid accumulation is prevented by ultrafiltration during dialysis and if the anemia is partially treated by transfusion. Obviously, it is desirable to have only a single vascular access site present in a patient at any one time and to limit the size of the anastomosis to the smallest required for successful dialysis. The contribution of the fistula to the heart failure state can be determined by studying the effect of occlusion of the fistula on left ventricular function, as assessed by echocardiography or radionuclide ventriculography.[78]

Infection is a major complication of arteriovenous shunts and may become metastatic. Septic pulmonary emboli and infective endocarditis, most often staphylococcal, have been reported.[83] Since patients on hemodialysis often have functional systolic and occasionally even diastolic murmurs, which may change with the patient's altered hemodynamic status, the diagnosis of endocarditis may be missed. Therefore, the *early* diagnosis of endocarditis in patients with infected vascular access sites depends on a high index of clinical suspicion and the immediate obtaining of blood cultures. However, the diagnosis of infective endocarditis may be difficult, since an infected vascular access site without infection of the endocardium can also give rise to positive blood cultures.

Hypoxemia. A fall in arterial oxygen tension of 10 to 15 mm Hg occurs frequently within the first 30 minutes of hemodialysis and persists throughout the procedure.[84] This event is obviously undesirable in patients with heart or lung disease and may lead to serious hypoxemia in patients with even mild arterial desaturation at the commencement of the hemodialysis. Together with the electrolyte changes which occur during hemodialysis referred to above, it may lower the threshold for the development of arrhythmias. Also, the PEP/LVET ratio (p. 54) may increase significantly during dialysis,[85,86] an increase which correlates significantly with the fall in arterial oxygen tension, suggesting that the latter actually impairs left ventricular function.

The mechanism responsible for the decline in arterial pO_2 is in some dispute. It has been reported that activation of complement leads to aggregation of neutrophils in the lungs that interfere with normal oxygenation.[87] An alternative explanation is that it is due to physiological hypoventilation secondary to the diffusion of carbon dioxide across the dialyzer.[85] Whatever the mechanism, patients with impaired pulmonary function and severe heart disease should be monitored for arterial hypoxemia during the early phase of dialysis and may require inhalation of oxygen-enriched mixtures during the procedure.

Potassium Balance

Life-threatening hyperkalemia may occur in acute oliguric renal failure, in end-stage chronic renal failure, and, rarely, in terminal heart failure (p. 500). The principal detrimental effect of hyperkalemia is in its electrical effect on the heart. The progressive electrocardiographic abnormalities associated with hyperkalemia are illustrated in Figures 7–43 (p. 236). Generally, the earliest electrocardiographic sign of hyperkalemia is peaking of the T waves, followed progressively by an increase in T-wave amplitude, a widening of the QRS complex, and loss of atrial activity. Finally, with extreme hyperkalemia, a sine wave pattern is noted on the electrocardiogram, followed by cardiac arrest.[88] Unfortunately, however, only a rough correlation exists between the level of serum potassium and the electrocardiographic changes, although in any given patient, directional changes in the serum potassium can be estimated from the electrocardiogram. Even severe hyperkalemia per se produces few if any symptoms; occasionally, weakness of skeletal muscles or dyspnea presumably secondary to paralysis of respiratory muscles may be noted.

TREATMENT. Severe hyperkalemia is a medical emergency, and its treatment can generally be divided into acute and chronic phases. The most rapid means of counteracting the toxic cardiac effects of potassium is with the administration of intravenous calcium, given in the form of 10 to 20 ml of 10 per cent *calcium chloride* with electrocardiographic monitoring to assure that the electrocardiographic signs of hyperkalemia have been reversed. While administration of calcium chloride is an effective emergency measure, it does not lower the elevated serum potassium concentration.

The second aspect of therapy relies upon lowering the serum potassium. In patients with hyperkalemia and acidosis, *sodium bicarbonate* causes a fall in serum potassium; the usual dose is 1 to 2 ampoules (44 to 88 mEq) administered intravenously. The combination of *glucose and insulin* will also result in a redistribution of potassium from the extracellular to the intracellular space; the usual dose is 50 ml of 50 per cent glucose with 10 units of regular insulin, intravenously. The effects of alkalinization or glucose and insulin administration can be observed within 15 to 30 minutes and may last for several hours. Although these forms of therapy are useful for rapidly lowering the serum potassium concentration, they do *not* lower total body potassium stores.

Further treatment of hyperkalemia involves removal of potassium from the body, which can be accomplished by the administration of *cation exchange resins* by mouth or enema. The resin most commonly employed is sodium polystyrene sulfonate (Kayexalate), 1 gm of which exchanges approximately 1 mEq of sodium for potassium. The usual dose is 50 gm two or three times daily. When

administered by mouth, it is desirable to accompany it with an osmotic cathartic to prevent intestinal obstruction as a consequence of inspissation of the resin in the gut.

The most effective means of reducing the body's potassium stores is by means of *dialysis*, either hemodialysis or peritoneal dialysis. However, when using these modalities care must be exercised not to lower the serum potassium too precipitously, especially in those patients who are receiving cardiac glycosides. This can be accomplished by beginning with a dialysis solution having a potassium concentration of approximately 4 mEq/liter and then progressively lowering it as the serum potassium declines.

Secondary Hyperparathyroidism

Ectopic calcification in a variety of tissues, including the heart and arterial bed, is a common manifestation of secondary hyperparathyroidism, which is a frequent complication of chronic renal failure. Involvement of the sinoatrial and atrioventricular nodes, the valvular annuli and cusps (particularly the mitral annulus,[88a,88b]), the intima and media of epicardial coronary arteries, the interventricular septum, and the ventricular myocardium similar to that illustrated in Figures 51–6 and 51–7 (p. 1737)[89–91] has been described; clinical and electrocardiographic changes include left ventricular failure and varying degrees of atrioventricular block.[92,93] As many as half the patients on maintenance hemodialysis have been reported to have radiological evidence of arterial calcification;[94,95] calcium deposition is generally in the media, leading to Mönckeberg sclerosis.[96] Calcium deposition may be associated with almost complete obliteration of the vascular lumen and may result in ischemia and, ultimately, gangrene of tissue distal to the involved vessels.[94–97]

The most effective *treatment* of secondary hyperparathyroidism consists of renal transplantation or subtotal parathyroidectomy. The latter procedure has been shown to improve cardiac contractility.[97] For patients maintained on dialysis, dietary phosphate restriction, the use of non-absorbable aluminum-containing antacids and the use of dihydrotachysterol (DHT), a synthetic analog of vitamin D, given in doses of 0.125 to 0.5 mg/24 hr, are also useful measures.[98] Recently, the active form of vitamin D, 1,25-dihydroxycholecalciferol, has become available commercially.

Uremic Pericarditis (See also p. 1505)

Pericarditis is a common complication of both acute and chronic renal failure. Prior to the era of dialysis, the appearance of pericarditis in the uremic patient was generally taken as a sign of limited life expectancy.[99] Its incidence varies among different series, but it has been reported to occur in up to 50 per cent of patients at the initiation of dialysis;[100] its incidence appears to be declining with the increasing use of early dialysis prior to the development of advanced uremia. The mechanism of development of pericarditis is not clear, but it is probably related to the accumulation of uremic toxin(s), which is responsible for an inflammatory serositis. The serositis most commonly involves the pericardium but can also involve the pleura.[101] Fibrinous pleuritis, pleural friction rubs,[102] hemorrhagic pleural effusion,[103] and pneumonitis[101] have also been reported to occur in uremia.

Three and a half per cent of the patients accepted for dialysis at the Brigham and Women's Hospital during a 5-year period developed clinical evidence of pericarditis and pericardial effusion while on dialytic therapy.[104] Pericarditis occurring in patients with stable chronic dialysis may be related to inadequate dialysis or to an intercurrent illness, such as a viral infection. In patients with renal failure, pericarditis is frequently preceded by an otherwise benign respiratory tract infection; infection with cytomegalovirus and other conditions such as systemic lupus erythematosus and acute myocardial infarction have also been implicated as causes.[105]

The clinical features of uremic pericarditis are summarized in Table 52–2. The diagnosis is made by the same clinical criteria used for other forms of pericarditis, i.e., chest pain generally ameliorated by sitting up and leaning forward, typical electrocardiographic and echocardiographic changes, increases in heart size on chest roentgenogram, and evidence of circulatory embarrassment with severe pericarditis. With echocardiography, a surprisingly high incidence (32 per cent) of small, asymptomatic, pericardial effusions was found in our institution in patients on chronic maintenance hemodialysis,[110] a finding in concert with those of other observers.[111] The development of hypotension during dialysis, which cannot be readily attributed to changes in intravascular volume, is a useful clue to the presence of significant pericardial effusion. However, the diagnosis of pericarditis may sometimes be made in error. Uremic patients frequently develop a systolic ejection murmur, most probably related to the high-output state secondary to chronic anemia. Occasionally, patients with chronic renal failure and hypertension develop diastolic blowing murmurs of aortic regurgitation, and the combination of these two murmurs may be mistaken for a to-and-fro pericardial friction rub.

Cardiac tamponade is the major and a potentially lethal complication of pericarditis. Pericardial fluid is generally exudative and bloody,[100,101] and the heparinization required for hemodialysis may cause serious bleeding into the pericardial cavity in patients with pericarditis. Therefore, it is important to avoid systemic heparinization during hemodialysis in the presence of active pericarditis and large effusions. However, systemic heparinization can be used safely in patients with small pericardial effusions without associated physical signs and symptoms of active pericarditis. The development of *chronic constrictive pericarditis* is an

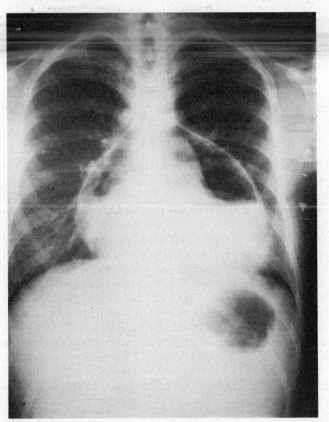

FIGURE 52–10   Chest roentgenogram showing air-fluid level in the pericardial space of a patient with a uremic pericardial effusion, following instillation of air and removal of pericardial fluid.

unusual complication of uremic pericarditis. It developed in 2 of 25 patients at the Brigham and Women's Hospital with prior severe effusions;[104] other centers report a similarly low incidence.

Treatment.   Management of the patient with asymptomatic pericardial effusion should consist of vigorous hemodialysis and the use of regional heparinization (see below). Uremic pericarditis complicated by tamponade or persistent large effusion should be treated with immediate pericardiocentesis, coupled with vigorous hemodialysis; this results in a very high rate of resolution.[100,104] The placement of air into the pericardial space has the advantage of limiting the apposition of visceral and parietal pericardial surfaces and providing an air-fluid level, thereby allowing the rate of reaccumulation of fluid to be followed readily on a routine chest roentgenogram (Fig. 52–10). The instillation of corticosteroids into the pericardial cavity,[112] the use of oral indomethacin, catheter drainage of the pericardial effusion,[113] and the construction of a pericardial window have all been advocated. The early use of pericardial stripping for the treatment of uremic pericardial effusion has been suggested.[114] However, because of the rarity of the development of constrictive pericarditis, we believe that *prophylactic* pericardiectomy is not justified.

It is our practice to treat uremic pericarditis by vigorous dialysis and catheter drainage of the pericardial space with the instillation of air. However, placement of the catheter into the pericardial cavity should be attempted only by persons experienced in this technique, and in our institution it is performed by cardiothoracic surgeons. The use of the local instillation of nonabsorbable steroids or the sys-

TABLE 52–2   CLINICAL FEATURES OF UREMIC PERICARDITIS*

FEATURE	FREQUENCY (%)
Pain	66
Pericardial friction rub	93
Fever	84
Leukocytosis	56
Arrhythmias	23
Hypotension	56
Hepatomegaly	60
Elevated venous pressure	71
Abnormal electrocardiogram	90
Enlarged cardiac silhouette	96

*Adapted from Lowenthal,[106] Comty et al.,[107] Ribot,[108] and Silverberg et al.[109]

temic use of indomethacin or both may be of additional benefit, but more experience with these modalities is required. Pericardial stripping is the treatment of choice in patients with subacute or chronic constrictive pericarditis secondary to uremia.[104,106,115]

Cardiac Infections in Renal Failure. Patients with chronic renal failure on hemodialysis are compromised hosts with impairment of most immunological defense mechanisms. Infections are responsible for about one-fifth of all deaths in these patients. Arteriovenous shunts and fistulas are particularly susceptible to bacterial infections and, as already pointed out, may result in septicemia and infective endocarditis. Viral or purulent pericarditis is another common infection in patients with chronic renal failure and may be confused with uremic pericarditis. Patients with transplanted kidneys on immunosuppressive therapy have a particularly high risk of infection.

MANAGEMENT OF PATIENTS WITH CARDIAC DISEASE IN RENAL FAILURE

The generally greater availability of dialysis facilities and the broadened criteria for acceptance of patients into treatment programs for end-stage renal disease have resulted in a patient population in whom other diseases, including cardiac disease which may require surgical treatment, may be present. The high frequency of coronary artery disease that develops among patients with renal failure and the occasional presence of coexisting valvular heart disease often lead to a consideration of cardiopulmonary bypass among these patients. Patients on maintenance hemodialysis can undergo major operations without a great excess of mortality or morbidity,[116] and several series have been published documenting the ability of patients with renal failure to tolerate open heart surgery, both coronary renovascularization and valve replacement.[117,118] It has been our experience that among patients with end-stage renal disease, cardiac operations may be performed with equal success regardless of whether the renal failure has been treated by dialysis or transplantation.[119,120]

The major problems associated with operation in patients with chronic renal failure include the development of hyperkalemia, fluid overload, and arrhythmias. However, with the appropriate use of hemodialysis both before and after operation and careful monitoring of the patient's hemodynamic status and electrolytes, the excess risks of operation have been contained. Although many observers feel that patients who have severely impaired renal failure but who do not yet require hemodialysis may undergo cardiac surgery without hemodialysis, it is our policy to dialyze patients with less than 20 per cent of normal glomerular filtration rate on several occasions on the days preceding and following such operations.

The management of patients with hypertrophic obstructive cardiomyopathy (p. 1409) and chronic renal failure presents a unique problem. It is well established that these patients are particularly sensitive to acute changes in blood volume and to tachyarrhythmias. During hemodialysis, blood volume is ordinarily reduced. Although most patients tolerate this volume depletion without difficulty, those with hypertrophic cardiomyopathy often develop an acute increase in obstruction to left ventricular outflow. In our experience, this complication can be avoided by using

dialysis apparatus requiring a low extracorporeal volume and having precise control of ultrafiltration. In addition, these patients are treated with propranolol and transfused to maintain the hematocrit in the range of 30 per cent.

Modification of Common Cardiac Medications in Patients with Renal Failure

Since many drugs (and/or their active metabolites) used in the treatment of heart disease are excreted by the kidney, renal failure affects the pharmacokinetics of many agents, including those commonly used to treat heart disease.

CARDIAC GLYCOSIDES (also see p. 514). *Digoxin* is filtered in the glomeruli, and the excretion of digoxin by the kidneys is directly proportional to the glomerular filtration rate. It is not altered by the rate of urine flow and therefore by the administration of diuretics;[121] only very small quantities of digoxin may be secreted by the distal convoluted tubule.[122] The ratio of the clearance of digoxin to endogenous creatine is 0.8 and the percentage of the body's total stores of digoxin lost per day can be calculated as $14 + 0.2 \times$ creatinine clearance in milliliters per minute. Thus, 85 per cent of administered digoxin is normally excreted in the urine, most in unchanged form, and only 10 to 15 per cent is eliminated in the stool through biliary excretion. Normally, 38 per cent of the body's stores of digoxin are either metabolized or excreted per day,[123] whereas in anephric patients, 14 per cent of total body digoxin stores are eliminated per day via the biliary tree. Therefore, in the patient without significant renal function, digoxin elimination is reduced to approximately 37 per cent of normal, and digoxin dosage should be modified accordingly.

In patients with end-stage renal disease requiring treatment with digoxin, it is our policy to use a loading dose of 0.25 mg and maintenance doses of 0.125 mg every other day. Digoxin levels are determined 1 week later, and, depending on the clinical response, the dose is modified, often upward, to 0.125 mg orally daily. In contrast to digoxin, the half-life of *digitoxin* is not greatly affected by impaired renal function,[124] and therefore the dosage does not need to be altered in patients with renal failure. Because of high tissue and protein binding of both digoxin and digitoxin, little removal occurs with either hemo- or peritoneal dialysis.[125] Therefore, these methods are ineffective in the treatment of digitalis intoxication.

ANTIARRHYTHMIC DRUGS (see also Chap. 21). The dose of *procainamide* must be modified in patients with end-stage renal disease because this drug is normally eliminated by both renal excretion and hepatic metabolism. Procainamide is readily dialyzable.[126]

Quinidine is metabolized by a variety of tissues, including the liver, mostly to hydroxy derivatives; no specific modification of the dose is necessary in patients with impaired renal function. Since quinidine is 80 per cent protein-bound[127] and is widely distributed in tissue, clearance by dialysis would be expected to be quite poor; indeed, clearances by peritoneal dialysis have been measured and found to be less than 10 ml/min.[128]

The half-life of *lidocaine* is about 1 hour, and its deactivation depends largely on hepatic metabolism; no dosage modification is necessary in patients with renal failure.[129]

No data are available on its dialyzability, but, because of a high degree of protein-binding (approximately 60 per cent),[130] it is probably poor.

The liver is also the principal site of inactivation of *phenytoin*.[131] Because of the diminished protein-binding of the drug in patients with renal failure, therapeutic and toxic levels may be achieved at lower doses than those used in patients with renal function.[132] Therefore, the usual dosage should be reduced by one third in patients with creatinine clearance below 30 ml/min. As is the case for most of the antiarrhythmic agents, phenytoin is poorly dialyzed.[133]

Propranolol is used extensively in patients with renal failure for its effects on arterial pressure, angina pectoris, and, less commonly, cardiac arrhythmias. Since it is metabolized primarily by the liver, its half-life is not altered by renal failure.[134,135] It is largely (90 per cent) protein-bound and has a large volume of distribution;[136] therefore, it is not surprising that it is poorly dialyzed.

Heart Failure Secondary to Renal Failure

Chronic renal failure can impair cardiac performance by a variety of mechanisms, many of which result from an augmentation of cardiac work (Table 52–1). It has been found that there is an increased left ventricular stroke work index and left ventricular end-diastolic pressure and size in many patients with end-stage renal disease.[79,137,138] In addition, an increase in pulmonary capillary permeability tending to lead to pulmonary edema, even in the absence of elevation of pulmonary capillary wedge pressure, has been reported in renal insufficiency as well.[139] Impairment of cardiac performance also occurs secondary to ischemic heart disease as a consequence of the accelerated atherogenesis referred to earlier (p. 1753). The possibility must be considered that dialysis results in the depletion of essential substances; thus, the water-soluble vitamins are dialyzable, and it has been suggested that their loss can lead to beriberi heart disease.[140] Therefore, it seems desirable to provide supplements of these vitamins for patients who are on maintenance hemodialysis. It is possible that long-term dialysis leads to depletion of other, as yet unidentified substances necessary for normal cardiac performance, but this has not been established.

The possibility that the uremic state depresses myocardial function is intriguing. As early as 1944, Raab suggested that specific myocardial toxins might be present in uremia.[141] Recently, depression of cardiac function in isolated rat heart preparations perfused with urea, creatinine, guanidinosuccinic acid, and methyl-guanidine, singly and in combination, has been reported.[142] Similarly, a depression of myocardial contractility has been demonstrated in a guinea pig model of uremia secondary to acute obstructive renal failure.[143]

Uremia produces serious disturbances in monovalent cation transport. Red blood cells, leukocytes, lung, and bone from patients with renal insufficiency have an elevated sodium content and a reduction in ouabain-sensitive Na-K–activated ATPase activity.[144,145] It is possible that this same fundamental abnormality is responsible for the observed reduction in human skeletal muscle transmembrane potential, which returns toward normal with vigorous hemodialysis.

The presence of a *cardiomyopathy* in uremic patients has been suggested, but its existence as a specific entity has been difficult to document in view of the many other possible causes of abnormal cardiac function in such patients.[146,147] Although reversibility of myocardial dysfunction with treatment of uremia is not clear,[148] there is suggestive evidence that it can occur. In one study, patients with severe cardiomyopathy and uremia were reported to have developed their cardiac disease while on low-protein diets prior to initiation of hemodialysis, and all had striking clinical improvement with dialysis.[149] In another, hemodialysis raised the left ventricular ejection fraction, both acutely and chronically,[150] whereas in a third, left ventricular function improved following renal transplantation.[137]

References

1. Skorecki, K. L., and Brenner, B. M.: Body fluid homeostasis in congestive heart failure and cirrhosis with ascites. Am. J. Med. *72*:323, 1982.
2. Hostetter, T. H., Pfeffer, J. M., Pfeffer, M. A., Braunwald, E., and Brenner, B. M.: Cardiorenal hemodynamics and sodium excretion in rats with myocardial infarction. Am. J. Physiol. 1983, in press.
3. Watkins, L., Burton, J. A., Cant, J. R., Smith, F. W., and Barger, A. C.: The renin-angiotensin-aldosterone system in congestive heart failure in conscious dogs. J. Clin. Invest. *57*:1606, 1976.
4. Higgins, C. B., Vatner, S. F., Franklin, D., and Braunwald, E.: Effects of experimentally produced heart failure on the peripheral vascular response to severe exercise in conscious dogs. Circ. Res. *31*:186, 1972.
5. McGiff, J., and Itskovitz, H. D.: Prostaglandin and the kidney. Circ. Res. *33*:479, 1973.
6. Mills, I. H., MacFarlane, N. A. A., Ward, P. E., and Obika, L. F. O.: The renal kallikrein-kinin system and the regulation of salt and water excretion. Fed. Proc. *35*:181, 1976.
7. Ichikawa, I., Pfeffer, J. M., Pfeffer, M. A., Hostetter, T. H., Braunwald, E., and Brenner, B. M.: Glomerular response to severe congestive heart failure in the rat. Proceedings, 15th Annual Meeting of the American Society of Nephrology, 152a, 1982.
8. DiPerri, T., Forconi, S., Puccetti, F., Vittoria, A., and Guerrini, M.: Effects of prostaglandin A$_1$ on renal handling of salt and water in congestive heart failure. J. Cardiovasc. Pharm. *2*:215, 1980.
9. Boudreau, R. J., and Mandin, H.: The role of prostaglandins in the regulation of renal function during chronic pericardial tamponade. Effect of indomethacin and arachidonic acid on renal function in cardiac edema. Circ. Res. *26*:867A, 1978.
10. Berliner, R. W., and Davidson, P. G.: Production of hypertonic urine in the absence of pituitary antidiuretic hormone. J. Clin. Invest. *36*:1416, 1957.
11. Fitzsimmons, J. T.: Thirst. Physiol. Rev. *52*:468, 1972.
12. Fitzsimmons, J. T., and Simons, B. J.: The effect on drinking in the rat of intravenous infusion of angiotensin given alone or in combination with other stimuli of thirst. J. Physiol. (Lond.) *203*:45, 1969.
13. Riegger, G. A. J., Liebau, G., and Kochsiek, K.: Antidiuretic hormone in congestive heart failure. Am. J. Med. *72*:49, 1982.
14. Szatalowicz, V. L., Arnold, P. E., Chaimovitz, C., Bichet, D., Bert, T., and Schrier, R. W.: Radioimmunoassay of plasma arginine vasopressin in hyponatremic patients with congestive heart failure. N. Engl. J. Med. *305*:263, 1981.
15. Oberg, B.: Effects of cardiovascular reflexes on net capillary fluid transfer. Acta Physiol. Scand. (Suppl.) *62*:229, 1964.
16. Braunwald, E., Ross, J., Jr., and Sonnenblick, E. H.: Mechanisms of Contraction in the Normal and Failing Heart. 2nd ed. Boston, Little, Brown, 1976, pp. 250–254.
17. Greenberg, T. T., Richmond, W. H., Stocking, R. A., Gupta, P. D., Meehan, J. P., and Henry, J. P.: Impaired arterial stretch receptor responses in dogs with heart failure due to tricuspid insufficiency and pulmonary artery stenosis. Circ. Res. *32*:424, 1973.
18. Zucker, I. H., Earle, A. M., and Gilmore, J. P.: The mechanism of adaptation of left atrial stretch receptors in dogs with chronic congestive heart failure. J. Clin. Invest. *60*:323, 1977.
19. Zucker, I. H., Share, L., and Gilmore, J. P.: Renal effects of left atrial distention in dogs with chronic congestive heart failure. Am. J. Physiol. *236*:H554, 1979.
20. Birkenfeld, L. W., Liebman, J., O'Meara, M. P., and Edelman, I. S.: Total exchangeable sodium, total exchangeable potassium, and total body water in edematous patients with cirrhosis of the liver and congestive heart failure. J. Clin. Invest. *37*:687, 1958.
21. Carroll, H. J., Gotterer, R., and Altshuler, B.: Exchangeable sodium, body potassium, and body water in previously edematous cardiac patients. Evidence for osmotic inactivation of cation. Circulation *32*:185, 1965.
22. Farber, S. J., and Schubert, M.: The binding of cations by chondroitin sulfate. J. Clin. Invest. *36*:1715, 1957.

23. Hricik, D. E., and Kassirer, J. P.: Azotemia in cardiac failure. J. Cardiovasc. Med. 8:397, 1983.

24. Domenet, J. G., and Evans, D. W.: Uremia in congestive heart failure. Q. J. Med. 38:117, 1969.

25. Baehr, G., and Laude, H.: Glomerulonephritis as a complication of subacute streptococcus endocarditis. J.A.M.A. 75:789, 1920.

26. Glassock, R. J.: Pathophysiology of glomerular diseases. In Brenner, B. M., and Rector, F. C. (eds.): The Kidney. 2nd ed. Philadelphia, W. B. Saunders Co., 1980.

27. Gutman, R. A., Striker, G. E., Gilliland, B. C., and Cutler, R. E.: The immune complex glomerulonephritis of bacterial endocarditis. Medicine 51:1, 1972.

28. Coggins, C. H.: Nephrotic and nephritic edema. In Brenner, B. M., and Stein, J. H. (eds.): Sodium and Water Homeostasis. New York, Churchill Livingstone, 1978, p. 117.

29. Levinsky, N. G., Alexander, E. A., and Venkatachalam, M. A.: Acute renal failure. In Brenner, B. M., and Rector, F. C. (eds.): The Kidney. 2nd ed. Philadelphia, W. B. Saunders Co., 1980.

30. Harrington, J. T., Sommers, S. C., and Kassirer, J. P.: Atheromatous emboli with progressive renal failure. Renal arteriography as the probable inciting factor. Ann. Intern. Med. 68:152, 1968.

31. Kassirer, J. P.: Atheroembolic renal disease. N. Engl. J. Med. 280:812, 1969.

32. Strange, P. V., and Sumner, A. T.: Predicting treatment costs and life expectancy for end-stage renal disease. N. Engl. J. Med. 298:372, 1978.

33. Lindner, A., Charra, B., Sherrard, D. J., and Scribner, B. H.: Accelerated atherosclerosis in prolonged maintenance hemodialysis. N. Engl. J. Med. 290:697, 1974.

34. Lazarus, J. M., Lowrie, E. G., Hampers, C. L., and Merrill, J. P.: Cardiovascular disease in uremic patients on hemodialysis. Kidney Int. 7 (Suppl. 2):S167, 1975.

35. Friedman, H. S., Shah, B. N., Kim, H. J. G., Bove, L. A., Del Monte, M. M., and Smith, A. J.: Clinical study of the cardiac findings in patients with chronic maintenance hemodialysis: The relationship to coronary risk factors. Clin. Nephrol. 16:75, 1981.

36. deMello, V. R., Malone, D., Thanovaro, S., Kleiger, R. E., Kessler, G., and Oliver, G. C.: Cardiac arrhythmias in end-stage renal disease. South. Med. J. 74:178, 1981.

37. Zawada, E. T., Jr., Stinson, J. B., and Done, G.: New perspectives on coronary artery disease in hemodialysis patients. South. Med. J. 75:694, 1982.

38. Francis, G. S., Conty, C. M., Sharma, B., and Helseth, H. K.: Myocardial revascularization in chronic renal disease patients. In Love, J. (ed.): Cardiac Surgery in Patients with Chronic Renal Disease. Mt. Kisco, N.Y., Futura Publishing Co., 1982, pp. 115–134.

39. Roig, E., Betriu, A., Castaner, A., Magrina, J., Sanz, G., and Navarrlo-Lopez, F.: Disabling angina pectoris with normal coronary arteries in patients undergoing long-term hemodialysis. Am. J. Med. 71:431, 1981.

40. Kim, K. E., Onesti, G., and Schwartz, A. B.: Hemodynamics of hypertension in chronic end-stage renal disease. Circulation 467:456, 1972.

41. Kim, K. E., Onesti, G., and Schwartz, A. B.: Hemodynamic alterations in hypertension of chronic end-stage renal disease. In Onesti, G., Kim, K. E., and Moyer, J. H. (eds.): Hypertension: Mechanisms and Management. New York, Grune and Stratton, 1973, p. 609.

42. Dustan, H. P., and Page, I. H.: Some factors in renal and renoprival hypertension. J. Lab. Clin. Med. 64:948, 1964.

43. Vertes, V., Cangiano, J. L., Berman, L. B., and Gould, A.: Hypertension in end-stage renal disease. N. Engl. J. Med. 280:978, 1969.

44. DePlanque, B. A., Mulder, E., and Mees, E. J. D.: The behavior of blood and extracellular volume in hypertensive patients with renal insufficiency. Acta Med. Scand. 186:75, 1969.

45. Lazarus, J. M., Hampers, C. L., and Merrill, J. P.: Hypertension and chronic renal failure. Treatment with hemodialysis and nephrectomy. Arch. Intern. Med. 133:1059, 1974.

46. Wilkinson, R., Scott, D. F., Uldall, P. R., Kerr, D. N. S., and Swinney, J.: Plasma renin and exchangeable sodium in the hypertension of chronic renal failure. The effect of bilateral nephrectomy. Q. J. Med. 39:377, 1970.

47. Cangiano, J. L., Ramirez-Muxo, O., Ramirez-Gonzalez, R., Trevino, A., and Campos, J. A.: Normal renin uremic hypertension. Arch. Intern. med. 136:17, 1976.

48. Lazarus, J. M., Hampers, C. L., Lowrie, E. G., and Merrill, J. P.: Baroreceptor activity in normotensive and hypertensive uremic patients. Circulation 47:1015, 1973.

49. Lilley, J. J., Golden, J., and Stone, R. A.: Adrenergic regulation of blood pressure in chronic renal failure. J. Clin. Invest. 57:1190, 1976.

50. Grollman, A., and Krishnamurty, V. S. R.: A new pressor agent of renal origin: Its differentiation from renin and angiotensin. Am. J. Physiol. 221:1499, 1971.

51. Muirhead, E. E., Brown, G. B., Germain, G. S., and Leach, B. E.: The renal medulla as an antihypertensive organ. J. Lab. Clin. med. 76:641, 1970.

52. Lee, J. B., and Mookerjee, B. K.: The renal prostaglandins as etiologic factors in human essential hypertension. Fact or fantasy? Cardiovasc. Med. 1:302, 1976.

53. Hull, A. R., Long, D. L., Prati, R. C., Pettinger, W. A., and Parker, T. F., III: The control of hypertension in patients undergoing regular maintenance dialysis. Kidney Int. 7 (Suppl. 2):S184, 1975.

54. Briggs, W. A., Lowenthal, D. T., Cirksina, W. J., Price, W. E., Gibson, T. P., and Flamenbaum, W.: Propranolol in hypertensive dialysis patients: Efficacy and compliance. Clin. Pharmacol. Ther. 18:606, 1975.

55. Gelfand, M. C., Horton, J., Gottlieb, M., Winchester, J. F., Lowrie, E. G., Farate, A., Miller, D., Lazarus, J. M., and Schreiner, G. E.: Asymptomatic pericardial effusion—A possible complication of minoxidil therapy in patients with chronic renal failure. Abstracts, Sixth International Congress of Nephrology, Montreal, 1978, p. B23.

56. Lazarus, J. M., Hampers, C. L., Bennett, A. H., VanDam, L. D., and Merrill, J. P.: Urgent bilateral nephrectomy for severe hypertension. Ann. Intern. Med. 76:733, 1972.

57. Woods, T. W., Blythe, W. B., and Huffines, W. D.: Malignant hypertension and renal insufficiency. N. Engl. J. Med. 291:10, 1974.

58. Bachy, C., Alexandre, G. P. J., and van Ypersele de Strihou, C.: Hypertension after renal transplantation. Br. Med. J. 2:1287, 1976.

59. Popovtzer, M. M., Pinnggera, W., Katz, F. H., Corman, J. L., Robinette, J., Lanois, B., Halgrimson, C. G., and Starzl, T. E.: Variations in arterial blood pressure after kidney transplantation: Relation to renal function, plasma renin activity and the dose of prednisone. Circulation 47:1297, 1973.

60. McPhaul, J. J., Jr., Thompson, A. L., Jr., Lordon, R. E., Klebanoff, G., Cosimi, A. B., de Lemos, R., and Smith, R. B.: Evidence suggesting persistence of nephritogenic immunopathologic mechanisms in patients receiving renal allografts. J. Clin. Invest. 52:1059, 1973.

61. Lacombe, M.: Arterial stenosis complicating allotransplantation in man. Ann. Surg. 181:283, 1975.

62. Ibels, L. S., Alfrey, A. C., and Weil, R., III: Hyperlipidemia in adult, pediatric and diabetic transplant recipients. Am. J. Med. 64:634, 1978.

63. Matas, A. J., Simmons, R. L., Buselmeier, T. J., Kjellstrand, C. M., and Najarian, J. S.: The fate of patients surviving three years after renal transplantation. Surgery 80:390, 1976.

64. Bagdade, J., Casaretto, A., and Albers, J.: Effects of chronic uremia, hemodialysis and renal transplantation on plasma lipids and lipoproteins in man. J. Lab. Clin. Med. 87:37, 1976.

65. Brunzell, J. D., Albers, J. J., Haas, L. B., Goldberg, A. P., Agode, L., and Sherrard, D. J.: Prevalence of serum lipid abnormalities in chronic hemodialysis. Metabolism 26:903, 1977.

66. Rapoport, J., Aviram, M., Chaimovitz, C., and Brook, J. G.: Defective high density lipoprotein composition in patients on chronic hemodialysis. N. Engl. J. Med. 299:1326, 1978.

67. Nestel, P. J., Fidge, N. H., and Tan, M. H.: Increased lipoprotein-remnant formation in chronic renal failure. N. Engl. J. Med. 307:329, 1982.

68. Murase, T., Cattran, D. C., Pakenstein, B., and Steiner, G.: Inhibition of lipoprotein lipase by uremic serum. A possible cause of hypertriglyceridemia. Metabolism 24:1279, 1975.

69. Mordasini, R., Frey, F., Flury, W., Klose, G., and Greten, H.: Selective deficiency of hepatic triglyceride lipase in uremia patients. N. Engl. J. Med. 297:1362, 1977.

70. Goldberg, A. P., Sherrard, D. J., and Brunzell, J.: Hypertriglyceridemia in hemodialysis patients; dual defect of adipose tissue lipoprotein lipase. Clin. Res. 24:361A, 1976.

71. Cattran, D. C., Fenton, S. S. A., Wilson, D. R., and Steiner, G.: Defective triglyceride removal in lipemia associated with peritoneal dialysis and haemodialysis. Ann. Intern. Med. 85:29, 1976.

72. Havel, R. J., Kane, J. P., and Kashyap, M. L.: Interchange of apolipoproteins between chylomicrons and high density lipoproteins during alimentary lipemia in man. J. Clin. Invest. 52:32, 1973.

73. LaRosa, J. C., Levy, R. I., Herbert, P., Lux, S. E., and Fredrickson, D. S.: A specific apoprotein activator for lipoprotein lipase. Biochem. Biophys. Res. Commun. 41:57, 1970.

74. Fisher, W. R., and Truitt, D. H.: The common hyperlipoproteinemias. Ann. Intern. Med. 85:497, 1976.

75. Uraemia, lipoproteins and atherosclerosis. Lancet 2:1151, 1981.

76. Sanfelippo, M. L., Swensen, R. S., and Reaven, G. M.: Reduction of plasma triglycerides by diet in subjects with chronic renal failure. Kidney Int. 11:54, 1977.

77. Goldberg, A. P., Sherrard, D. J., Haas, L. B., and Brunzell, J. D.: Control of clofibrate toxicity in uremic hypertriglyceridemia. Clin. Pharmacol. Ther. 21:317, 1977.

78. Eiser, A. R., and Swartz, C. E.: Hemodialysis and peritoneal dialysis in patients with cardiac disease. In Lowenthal, D. T. (ed.): Management of the Cardiac Patient with Renal Failure. Philadelphia, F. A., Davis Co., 1981, pp. 78–80.

79. Kleiger, R. E., deMello, V. R., Malone, D., Fernandes, J., Thanavaro, S., Connors, J. P., and Oliver G. C.: Left ventricular function in end-stage renal disease. Echocardiographic classification. South. Med. J. 74:819, 1981.

80. Chaignon, M., Chen, W.-T., Tarazi, R. C., Nakamoto, S., and Salcedo, E.: Acute effects of hemodialysis on echographic-determined cardiac performance: Improved contractility resulting with serum increased calcium with reduced potassium despite hypovolemic-reduced cardiac output. Am. Heart J. 103:374, 1982.

81. Cini, G., Camici, M., Pentimone, F., and Palla, R.: Echocardiographic hemodynamic study during ultrafiltration sequential dialysis. Nephron 30:124, 1982.

82. Arduson, C. B., Codd, J. R., Graff, R. A., Grace, M. A., Harter, H. R., and Newton, W. T.: Cardiac failure in upper extremity arteriovenous dialysis fistulae. Arch. Intern. Med. 136:292, 1976.

83. Nsouli, K. A., Lazarus, J. M., Schoenbaum, S. C., Gottlieb, M. N., Lowrie, E. G., and Shocair, M.: Bacteremic infection in hemodialysis. Arch. Intern. Med. 139:1255, 1979.

84. Aurigemma, N. M., Feldman, N. T., Gottlieb, M. N., Ingram, R. H., Lazarus, J. M., and Lowrie, E. G.: Arterial oxygenation during hemodialysis. N. Engl. J. Med. 297:871, 1977.

85. Mahajan, S., Kinhal, V., Gardiner, H., Briggs, W., and McDonald, F.: Cardiac functional changes during hemodialysis. Proc. Clin. Dial. Transplant Forum 7:99, 1977.

86. Thayssen, P., Anderson, K. H., and Pindborg, T.: Non-invasive monitoring of cardiac function during haemodialysis. Scand. J. Urol. Nephrol. 15:313, 1981.

87. Craddock, P. R., Fehr, J., Brigham, K. L., Dronenberg, R. S., and Jacob, H. S.: Complement and leukocyte mediated pulmonary dysfunction in hemodialysis. N. Engl. J. Med. 296:769, 1977.

88. Fisch, C.: Relation of electrolyte disturbances to cardiac arrhythmias. Circulation 47:408, 1973.

88a. D'Cruz, I. A., Jain, M., Fishman, S., Abrahams, C., and Kathpalia, S.: Calcification of the mitral region in patients with chronic renal failure: 2-D echocardiographic, hormonal and autopsy correlation. J. Am. Coll. Cardiol. 1:625, 1983.

88b. Nestico, P. F., DePace, N. L., Kotler, M. N., Rose, L. I., Brezin, J. H., Swartz, C., Mintz, G., and Schwartz, A. B.: Calcium and phosphorus metabolism in dialysis patients with and without mitral anular calcium. Analysis of 30 patients. Am. J. Cardiol. 51:497, 1983.

89. Roberts, W. C., and Waller, B. F.: Effect of chronic hypercalcemia on the heart. An analysis of 18 necropsy patients. Am. J. Med. 71:371, 1981.

90. Depace, N. L., Rohrer, A. H., Kotler, M. N., Brezin, J. H., and Parry, W. R.: Rapidly progressing, massive mitral annular calcification. Arch. Intern. Med. 141:1663, 1981.

91. Jain, M. C., D'Cruz, I., and Kathpalia, S.: Chronic renal failure: Intracardiac calcification. Primary Cardiol. Clin. 4:27, 1981.

92. Terman, D. S., Alfrey, A. C., Hammond, W. S., Donndelinger, T., Ogden, D. A., and Holmes, J. H.: Cardiac calcification in uremia. A clinical, biochemical and pathologic study. Am. J. Med. 50:744, 1971.

93. Arora, K., Lacy, J. P., Schacht, R. A., Martin, D. G., and Gutch, C. F.: Calcific cardiomyopathy in advanced renal failure. Arch. Intern. Med. 135:603, 1975.

94. Friedman, S. A., Novak, S., and Thompson, G. E.: Arterial calcification and gangrene in uremia. N. Engl. J. Med. 280:1392, 1969.

95. Rosen, H., Friedman, S. A., Raizner, A. E., and Gerstmann, K.: Azotemic arteriopathy. Am. Heart J. 84:250, 1972.

96. Ejerblad, S., Ericsson, J. L. E., and Eriksson, I.: Arterial lesions of the radial artery in uraemic patients. Acta. Chir. Scand. 145:415, 1979.

97. Drueke, T., Fleury, J., Toure, Y., deVernejoul, P., Fauchet, M., Lesourd, P., LePailleur, C., and Crosnier, J.: Effect of parathyroidectomy on left ventricular function in haemodialysis patients. Lancet 1:112, 1980.

98. Verberckmoes, R., Bouillon, R., and Krempien, B.: Disappearance of vascular calcifications during treatment of renal osteodystrophy. Ann. Intern. Med. 82:529, 1975.

99. Wacker, W., and Merrill, J. P.: Uremic pericarditis in acute and chronic renal failure. J.A.M.A. 156:764, 1954.

100. Bailey, G. L., Hampers, C. L., Hager, E. B., and Merrill, J. P.: Uremic pericarditis: Clinical features and management. Circulation 38:582, 1968.

101. Hoops, H. C., and Wissler, R. W.: Uremic pneumonitis. Am. J. Pathol. 31:361, 1955.

102. Nidus, B. D., Matalon, R., Cantazino, D., and Eisinger, R. P.: Uremic pleuritis—A clinicopathological entity. N. Engl. J. Med. 281:255, 1969.

103. Galen, M. A., Steinberg, S. M., Lowrie, E. G., Lazarus, J. M., Hampers, C. L., and Merrill, J. P.: Hemorrhagic pleural effusions in patients undergoing chronic hemodialysis. Ann. Intern. Med. 82:359, 1975.

104. Goldberg, M., Lazarus, J. M., Gottlieb, M. N., Lowrie, E. G., and Merrill, J. P.: Treatment of uremic pericardial effusion. Proc. Clin. Dial. Transplant Forum 5:20, 1975.

105. Hampers, C. L., Schupak, E., Lowrie, E. G., and Lazarus, J. M.: Long Term Hemodialysis. 2nd ed. New York, Grune and Stratton, 1973, p. 80.

106. Kotler, M. N., and Parry, W. R.: Pericardial disease in chronic renal failure. In Lowenthal, D. T. (ed.): Management of the Cardiac Patient in Renal Failure. Philadelphia, F. A. Davis Co., 1981, pp. 78–80.

107. Comty, C. M., Cohen, S. L., and Shapiro, F. L.: Pericarditis in chronic uremia and its sequels. Ann. Intern. Med. 75:173, 1971.

108. Ribot, S., Frankel, H. J., and Gielchinsky, I.: Treatment of uremic pericarditis. Clin. Nephrol. 2:127, 1974.

109. Silverberg, S., Oreopoulos, D. G., and Wise, D. J.: Pericarditis in patients undergoing long-term hemodialysis and peritoneal dialysis. Incidence, complications and management. Am. J. Med. 63:874, 1977.

110. Lazarus, J. M., Gottlieb, M. N., Lowrie, E. G., Teicholtz, L., and Merrill, J. P.: Echocardiographic findings in stable hemodialysis patients. Proc. Clin. Dial. Transplant Forum 6:53, 1976.

111. Kleiman, J. H., Motta, J., London, E., Pennell, J. P., and Popp, R. L.: Pericardial effusions in patients with end-stage renal disease. Br. Heart J. 40:190, 1978.

112. Fuller, T. J., Knochel, J. P., Brennan, J. P., Tetnu, C. D., and White, M. G.: Reversal of intractable uremic pericarditis by triamcinolone hexacetonide. Arch. Intern. Med. 136:979, 1976.

113. Buselmeier, T. J., Simmons, R. L., Najarian, J. S., Mauer, S. M., Matas, A. J., and Kjellstrand, C. M.: Uremic pericardial effusion: Treatment by catheter drainage and local nonabsorbable steroid administration. Nephron 16:371, 1976.

114. Connors, J. P., Kleiger, R. E., Shaw, R. C., Voiles, J. D., Clark, R. E., Harter, H., and Roper, C. L.: The indications for pericardiectomy in the uremic pericardial effusion. Surgery 80:689, 1976.

115. Pillay, V. K. G., Sarpel, S. C., and Kurtzman, N. A.: Subacute constrictive uremic pericarditis: Survival after pericardiectomy. J.A.M.A. 235:1351, 1976.

116. Hampers, C. L., Bailey, G. L., Hager, E. B., VanDam, L. D., and Merrill, J. P.: Major surgery in patients on maintenance hemodialysis. Am. J. Surg. 115:747, 1968.

117. Crawford, F. A., Jr., Selby, J. H., Jr., Bower, J. D., and Lehan, D. H.: Coronary revascularization in patients maintained on chronic hemodialysis. Circulation 56:684, 1977.

118. Connors, J. P., and Shaw, R. C.: Considerations in the management of open-heart surgery in uremic patients. J. Thorac. Cardiovasc. Surg. 75:400, 1978.

119. Lamberti, J. J., Jr., Cohn, L. H., and Collins, J. J., Jr.: Cardiac surgery in patients undergoing renal dialysis or transplantation. Ann. Thorac. Surg. 19:135, 1975.

120. Chawla, R., Gailiunas, P., Jr., Lazarus, J. M., Gottlieb, M. N., Lowrie, E. G., Collins, J. J., and Merrill, J. P.: Cardiopulmonary bypass surgery in chronic hemodialysis and transplant patients. Trans. Am. Soc. Artif. Intern. Organs 23:694, 1977.

121. Falch, D.: The influence of kidney function, body size and age on plasma concentration and urinary excretion of digoxin. Acta Med. Scand. 194:251, 1973.

122. Steiness, E.: Renal tubular secretion of digoxin. Circulation 50:103, 1974.

123. Jelliffe, R. W.: An improved method of digoxin therapy. Ann. Intern. Med. 69:703, 1968.

124. Rasmussen, K., Jervell, J., Storstein, L., and Gjerdrum, K.: Digitoxin kinetics in patients with impaired renal function. Clin. Pharmacol. Ther. 13:6, 1972.

125. Ackerman, G. L., Doherty, J. F., and Flanigan, W. J.: Peritoneal dialysis and hemodialysis of tritiated digoxin. Ann. Intern. Med. 67:718, 1967.

126. Gibson, T. P., Lowenthal, D. T., Nelson, H. A., and Briggs, W. A.: Elimination of procainamide in end-stage renal failure. Clin. Pharmacol. Ther. 17:321, 1975.

127. Conn, H. L., and Luchi, R. J.: Some quantitative aspects of the binding of quinidine and related quinolone compounds by human serum albumin. J. Clin. Invest. 40:509, 1961.

128. Donadu, J. V., Whelton, A., and Kazyak, I.: Quinidine therapy and peritoneal dialysis in acute renal failure. Lancet 1:375, 1968.

129. Thompson, P. D., Melmon, K. L., Richardson, J. A., Cohn, K., Steinbrunn, W., Cudikee, R., and Rowland, M.: Lidocaine pharmacokinetics in advanced heart failure, liver disease and renal failure in humans. Ann. Intern. Med. 78:499, 1973.

130. Eriksson, E., Granberg, P., and Ortengren, B.: Study of renal excretion of prilocaine and lidocaine. Acta Chir. Scand. 358(Suppl):55, 1966.

131. Letteri, J. M., Mellk, H., Louis, S., Kutti, H., Durante, P., and Glazko, A.: Diphenylhydantoin metabolism in uremia. N. Engl. J. Med. 285:648, 1971.

132. Reidenberg, M. M., Odar-Cederlof, I., VonBahr, C., Borga, M. L., and Sjoqvist, F.: Protein binding of diphenylhydantoin and dimethylimipramine in plasma from patients with poor renal function. N. Engl. J. Med. 285:264, 1971.

133. Anderson, R. J., Gambertoglio, J. G., and Schrier, R. W.: Clinical Use of Drugs in Renal Failure. Springfield, Ill., Charles C Thomas, 1976, p. 251.

134. Evans, G. H., Nies, A. S., and Shand, D. G.: The disposition of propranolol. J. Pharmacol. Exp. Ther. 186:114, 1973.

135. Thompson, P. D., Joekes A. M., and Foulkes, D. M.: Pharmacodynamics of propranolol in renal failure. Br. Med. J. 2:434, 1972.

136. Shand, D. G., Wed, A. J. J., Vestal, R. E., Wilkinson, G. R., and Branch, R. A.: Pharmacokinetic and pharmacodynamic factors determining variations in propranolol responsiveness. In Braunwald, E. (ed.): Beta-Adrenergic Blockade. New York, Elsevier, 1978, pp. 74–80.

137. Lai, K. N., Barnden, L., and Mathew, T. H.: Effect of renal transplantation on left ventricular function in hemodialysis patients. Clin. Nephrol. 18:74, 1982.

138. Capelli, J. P., and Kasparian, H.: Cardiac work demands and left ventricular function in end-stage renal disease. Ann. Intern. Med. 86:261, 1977.

139. Crosbie, W. A., Snowden, S., and Parsons, V.: Changes in lung capillary permeability in renal failure. Br. Med. J. 4:388, 1972.

140. Gotloib, L., and Servadio, C.: A possible case of beriberi heart failure in a chronic hemodialysis patient. Nephron 14:293, 1975.

141. Raab, W.: Cardiotoxic substances in the blood and heart muscle in uremia. J. Lab. Clin. Med. 29:715, 1944.

142. Scheuer, J., and Stezoski, S. W.: The effects of uremic components on cardiac function and metabolism. J. Mol. Cell. Cardiol. 5:287, 1973.

143. Reicker, G., Velker, W., and Strauer, B. E.: Cardiac and circulatory disorders in renal insufficiency. In Uraemia: An International Conference on Pathogenesis, Diagnosis and Therapy. London, Churchill Livingstone, 1971, pp. 72–78.

144. Welt, L. G., Smith, E. K. M., Dunn, M. J., Czerwinski, A., Proctor, H., Cole, C., Balfo, J. W., and Gitelman, H. J.: Membrane transport defect: The sick cell. Tr. Assoc. Am. Physicians 80:217, 1967.

145. Patrick, J., and Jones, N. F.: Cell sodium, potassium and water in uremia and the effects of regular dialysis as studied in the leukocyte. Clin. Sci. Mol. Med. 46:583, 1974.

146. Prosser, D., and Parsons, V.: The case for a specific uremic myocardiopathy. Nephron 15:4, 1975.

147. Gueron, M., Berlyne, C. M., Nord, E., and BenAri, J.: The case against the existence of a specific uraemic myocardiopathy. Nephron 15:2, 1975.

148. Drüeke, T., Le Pailleur, C., Meilhac, B., Kontoudis, C., Zingraff, J., DiMatteo, J., and Crosnier, J.: Congestive cardiomyopathy in uremic patients on long-term haemodialysis. Br. Med. J. 1:350, 1977.

149. Bailey, G. L., Hampers, C. L., and Merrill, J. P.: Reversible cardiomyopathy in uremia. Tr. Am. Soc. Artif. Intern. Organs 13:263, 1967.

150. Hung, J., Harris, P. J., Uren, R. F., Tiller, D. J., and Kelly, D. T.: Uremic cardiomyopathy—Effect of hemodialysis on left ventricular function in end-stage renal failure. N. Engl. J. Med. 302:547, 1980.

53 PREGNANCY AND CARDIOVASCULAR DISEASE

by Joseph K. Perloff, M.D.

IMPORTANCE OF THE PROBLEM

For statistical information to be meaningful it must take into consideration the population under study, since figures vary widely, especially in comparisons between populations of developed and underdeveloped countries. In India, for example, acute and chronic rheumatic heart disease still constitute a major health problem in the pregnant woman. In Venezuela and Argentina, the relatively high prevalence of Chagas' disease materially increases the probability of Chagasic cardiomyopathy among pregnant women.[1] In Western Europe and North America, maternal mortality from all causes has been steadily decreasing for decades. This favorable trend has resulted mainly from control of noncardiac causes of maternal death, especially preeclampsia, hemorrhage, and infection. During the first half of this century, approximately 1 to 4 per cent of pregnancies in the United States and Western Europe were complicated by cardiac disease, 90 per cent of which was rheumatic.[2] As a consequence of the decline in incidence of chronic rheumatic heart disease among pregnant patients, this condition now represents no more than 75 per cent of the cardiac disorders complicating pregnancy.[2]

Congenital heart disease previously constituted most of the 10 per cent of nonrheumatic heart disease complicating pregnancy. In recent years, the relative frequency of rheumatic and congenital heart disease in childbearing women has undergone a change. Although the number of pregnant women with rheumatic heart disease has declined, as pointed out above, the number of pregnant women with congenital heart disease has increased, because the natural rate of occurrence of congenital heart disease remains relatively constant at 0.8 per cent of live births and because, in addition, successful cardiac surgery has produced a new population of patients—the postoperative cardiac patient.[3, 3a] Operative intervention in childhood has permitted increasing numbers of women with congenital heart disease to reach childbearing age, including those with anomalies that heretofore would not have permitted survival beyond childhood.[3] Systemic hypertension, apart from coarctation of the aorta, may antedate pregnancy or appear for the first time during gestation. Preeclampsia is more frequent in pregnant patients with preexisting hypertension than in initially normotensive pregnant women.[4] Cardiomyopathy complicating pregnancy chiefly takes the form of postpartum or peripartum inflammatory disease of the myocardium.[5-7]

CARDIOPULMONARY CHANGES IN NORMAL PREGNANCY

Rational management of heart disease in pregnancy presupposes an understanding of the circulatory adaptations to the normal gravid state (Table 53–1).[8–11a] To describe these adaptive responses, four variables must be characterized: the time of onset of the adaptive change, the magnitude of the change, the time when the change reaches its peak, and the behavior of the adaptive response after it has reached its maximum deviation from the nonpregnant state. These data should be based upon serial studies in the same patients in order to circumvent the problem of variation among individuals.[12–14]

Cardiac Output

It is generally agreed that a rise in cardiac output is well under way by the end of the first trimester.[2,12–17] The peak increment—on the order of 30 to 50 per cent—is reached by the twentieth to twenty-fourth week of gestation.[2,12–14,16] Up to the twentieth week, an increase in heart rate is responsible for the augmented cardiac output, but thereafter an increase in stroke volume contributes.[14] Once the maximum cardiac output is achieved, the level is maintained

TABLE 53–1   CIRCULATORY CHANGES IN NORMAL PREGNANCY

Cardiac output	↑ 30 to 50%
Stroke volume	↑
Heart rate	↑ Average 10 beats/min
Blood volume	↑ 40 to 50%
Systemic blood pressure	↓ Slightly until term
Systemic vascular resistance	↓
Pulmonary vascular resistance	↓

throughout the course of pregnancy[2,12,16] when output is measured with the patient in the lateral recumbent but not in the supine position. The older belief that the elevated cardiac output declined toward the end of gestation[18] has been resolved by taking into account the position of the patient (supine or lateral) and the mechanical effects of the gravid uterus.[2,13,14,17,19-25] Early studies showing a late fall in cardiac output were performed with patients in the supine position.

It has long been known that the gravid uterus can exert profound mechanical effects simply by virtue of its weight and size and the position of the patient. When the uterus is manually lifted away from the inferior cava during cesarean section, the caval pressure falls dramatically, as it does when the patient turns on her side (Fig. 53–1).[19] When the cava is manually compressed under direct vision, complete occlusion produces a pressure equal to but not greater than that found in the supine position before delivery. These observations imply that complete caval occlusion occurs in supine patients late in pregnancy. Predelivery caval angiograms confirm complete occlusion in the majority of patients studied while supine and caval patency when patients were restudied in the lateral position. Venous return during caval occlusion is channeled via the azygous, lumbar, and paraspinal veins. The fall in caval pressure that occurs when the position is changed from supine to lateral is consistently accompanied by a reciprocal rise in cardiac output. Echocardiographic determinations of cardiac output at term have confirmed that when patients turn from supine to lateral recumbence, the output rises appreciably.[13,14,17] Interestingly, these postural hemodynamic changes appear to be attenuated when the fetal head is engaged in the pelvis, thus rendering the uterus less mobile.[19] In addition to its effect on the cava, the gravid uterus partially compresses the abdominal aorta and displaces it laterally.[24]

As a rule, the normal fall in cardiac output in the supine position is not associated with a decline in systemic blood pressure, implying that peripheral vascular resistance rises appropriately.[2,19] In fact, brachial arterial pressure in the

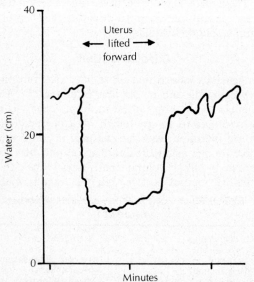

FIGURE 53–1 Effect on the inferior cava pressure of lifting the gravid uterus forward before opening the uterus at cesarean section. (From Kerr, M. G.: The mechanical effects of the gravid uterus in late pregnancy. J. Obstet. Gynecol. Br. Comm. *72*:513, 1965.)

left lateral position may be lower than in the supine position, even after the twenty-eighth week.[20,21] However, there is a tendency for a supine related fall in femoral arterial pressure.[22] An occasional patient experiences lightheadedness or frank syncope when supine; arterial pressure becomes depressed, and the heart rate slows, i.e., bradycardiac syncope occurs.[2,19,26] This is the most dramatic form of the so-called supine hypotensive syndrome of pregnancy, which can be promptly relieved simply by turning the patient on her side. Postural shock is a special problem when it manifests itself under anesthesia, which sometimes abolishes the compensatory peripheral vasoconstriction required to maintain systemic blood pressure in the supine position.[19]

The 30 to 50 per cent rise in resting cardiac output which occurs during pregnancy is accompanied by increments in stroke volume[2,13,14,16,17] but not necessarily in ejection fraction and mean velocity of circumferential fiber shortening.[13,17] An adaptive increase in left ventricular mass accompanies an increase in end-diastolic volume.[13] The magnitude and time course of these variables generally approximate the changes in cardiac output.[13,14,17] In addition, there is a rise in resting heart rate (average 10 beats per minute), which remains relatively constant in both supine and lateral recumbency, even at term.[2,13,19] Despite supine caval compression and a fall in cardiac output, the heart rate does not usually accelerate in this position. Failure to accelerate appears to be a feature of caval occlusion and has been demonstrated in nonpregnant patients undergoing laparotomy.[19]

Blood Volume and Intravascular Pressures

Blood volume is consistently elevated in normal pregnancy; plasma volume begins to rise as early as 6 weeks of gestation and increases rapidly until about midpregnancy and then more slowly until term. Total red cell volume, in contrast, increases steadily throughout pregnancy.[27] The relative difference between the increment in plasma volume (50 per cent) and that of red cell mass (20 to 40 per cent) accounts for the "physiologic anemia" of pregnancy. The increase in total blood volume is on the order of 40 to 50 per cent. The increment is higher in twin pregnancy than in single pregnancy and greater in multigravidas than in primigravidas.[2,28] Importantly, the time course of the changes in blood volume does not parallel the variations in cardiac output.[16] The average increase in exchangeable sodium is about 500 to 600 mEq, and in the average pregnant woman total body water increases by about 8.5 liters.[2]

Systemic arterial blood pressure declines slightly in early pregnancy. Systolic pressure falls from the nonpregnant level, and there is a somewhat greater reduction in diastolic pressure, resulting in a slight increase in pulse pressure that reflects the augmentation of stroke volume.[13,14] Both systolic and diastolic pressures tend to return toward nonpregnant levels before term.[2,29] Peripheral vascular resistance and mean arterial pressure appear to be lowest when cardiac output is maximal. Both maternal age and parity affect blood pressure during pregnancy. Systolic and diastolic pressures within a given age group decrease as parity increases, with the greatest difference observed between primiparas and multiparas; within each parity level, arterial pressures increase in older gravidas.[29] The effect of cigarette smoking on blood pressure is noteworthy. Smoking one to two cigarettes causes a prompt, short-term elevation in blood pressure and, in late pregnancy, a significant increase in fetal heart rate and a reduction in fetal breathing movements (see below).[30,31]

Pulmonary arterial systolic, diastolic, and mean pressures remain unchanged during the course of normal pregnancy despite the increased cardiac output, implying a reciprocal decline in pulmonary vascular resistance.[2,18] Thus, the right ventricle, like the left, handles an augmented volume but ejects this load at a normal systolic pressure. The increased work performed by both ventricles thus represents pure volume overload.[18]

Peripheral edema is a normal occurrence in uncomplicated pregnancy and can occur in the absence of either cardiac or renal disease.[2] Increased tissue hydration is considered universal in normal pregnancy, and clinical edema is found in 50 to 80 per cent of healthy gravid women.[32] The frequency of peripheral edema increases with maternal age, especially over 30 years. The presence and degree of edema are chiefly attributable to the increase in body water and total exchangeable sodium. In the third trimester there is the additive effect of increased venous pressure in the lower extremities in the supine and especially in the standing posture;[2] this is produced by compression of the inferior vena cava by the gravid uterus, particularly in the face of increased uterine blood flow draining into the inferior cava (see below). Varicosities are not normal features of pregnancy, but the above factors predispose to them.

Light to moderate exercise during uncomplicated pregnancy provokes an appropriate rise in cardiac output. The increments in cardiac output relative to oxygen consumption are normal and constant in all stages of pregnancy.[33] However, since the resting cardiac output is increased, the circulatory demands of exercise for any given workload are additive, implying that maximum cardiac output is reached at a correspondingly lower work level in pregnancy than in the nonpregnant state.[34]

Effects of Labor and Delivery

Labor and delivery initiate circulatory responses that are best understood when consideration is given to the method of delivery, the maternal posture, and the type and amount of sedation and anesthesia. In lightly sedated but unanesthetized women who deliver vaginally, maternal hemodynamics vary at different stages of labor according to the intensity and frequency of uterine contractions. The contracting uterus finds its support in the retrouterine fulcrum formed by the most protruding segment of lumbar lordosis (L_4-L_5).[24] During major uterine contractions, mean systemic arterial pressure rises approximately 10 per cent, and a significant amount of blood (estimated at 300 to 500 ml) is expressed into the maternal circulation.[23] The increment in venous return and the transient increase in heart rate result in augmentation of cardiac output (15 to 20 per cent) followed by reflex bradycardia.[2,23]

Contraction of the uterus also results in extrinsic compression of the aorta, particularly in the supine position.[23] This, combined with compression of the uterine vasculature within the contracting wall, transiently diverts cardiac output from the uterus and lower extremities with each contraction.[18] The rises in cardiac output and systemic arterial pressure indicate an increase in cardiac work. Caudal anesthesia does not affect the hemodynamic changes caused by uterine contraction per se, but the elevation of cardiac output during periods of uterine quiescence is abolished, since that rise is largely a response to pain and apprehension.[2]

The circulatory changes immediately following delivery are necessarily influenced by the amount of blood loss, which averages 500 ml or more with vaginal delivery and approximates 1000 ml with cesarean section. The pregnant woman tolerates such losses without ill effect, which is understandable, since the loss is in large part a desirable corrective for the increased blood volume accumulated during pregnancy. Accordingly, gestational hypervolemia can be looked upon as a safeguard against maternal blood loss at delivery, and normal maternal blood loss can be looked on as a corrective against the no longer needed gestational hypervolemia.[18] Nevertheless, the early puerperium is generally characterized by bradycardia, regardless of anesthetic technique, and a rise in cardiac output of about 10 to 20 per cent above predelivery levels.[2,35] Cardiac output begins to increase immediately after delivery as a consequence of the relief of inferior vena cava compression by the gravid uterus, and, along with puerperal bradycardia, this increase may persist for 2 weeks. A transient postpartal increase in blood volume has been attributed to both the autotransfusion from the contracting uterus and the absorption into the circulation of extracellular fluid accumulated during gestation. Puerperal diuresis then reduces total body water, and nongravid blood volume is restored 4 to 6 weeks after delivery.[2] However, this transient rise in blood volume is not a necessary feature of the early puerperium. Apart from blood loss during delivery, good renal function appears to be capable of rapid clearance of excess extracellular fluid without a detectable rise in blood volume.[28]

MECHANISM OF CIRCULATORY CHANGES

The circulatory changes of normal pregnancy described above can be looked upon from two points of view: either as responses that precede and therefore anticipate the needs of the growing fetus or as adaptive responses to the metabolic and nutritional needs of the fetus.[16] The increases in body water, blood volume, cardiac output, heart rate, and stroke volume and the fall in peripheral vascular resistance begin by the end of the first trimester, i.e., before fetal metabolic demands are fully evident.[2,12–17,36] Further, the time courses of changes in cardiac output and in blood volume are not parallel, so the former does not depend entirely upon the latter.[16] The timing and magnitude of the hemodynamic changes of normal pregnancy therefore precede and for a time exceed the demands of the fetus, whose needs are nicely anticipated. Similarly, the hypothesis that the placenta acts as a large arteriovenous fistula provoking most if not all of the above circulatory responses is not borne out, because hemodynamic changes begin before the placenta is well enough developed to function as a fistula.[16] If neither the metabolic and nutritional needs of the fetus nor the effect of the placenta as a fistula initiates the cardiocirculatory changes of pregnancy, what are the alternatives? Ovarian and/or placental sex steroids may play pivotal roles. Estrogen administration to pregnant ewes causes an increase in heart rate, cardiac output, and blood flow to the breast, uterus, and skin, whereas peripheral vascular resistance declines.[37,38] Moreover, estrogens have been found to increase myocardial contractility by what may be a direct effect on the contractile proteins.[39] Estrogen and progesterone concentrations rise progressively during gestation, and, by stimulating an increase in circulating levels of aldosterone, serve to promote retention of sodium and an increase of total body water.[40] Progesterone also causes venous relaxation, thereby increasing vascular capacity and promoting fluid retention.[41]

The importance of hormonal effects on circulatory physiology early in the course of normal pregnancy should not obscure the roles of a host of other factors that contribute in varying degrees as pregnancy proceeds into the second and third trimesters. Growth of the uterus, placenta, and breasts is associated with an increase in vascular capacity and in total circulating blood volume.[16] There is a general correlation between total blood volume and the weight of the products of conception.[28] Moreover, in the supine position in late pregnancy, the ability to excrete large water loads is limited.[19]

THE AORTA IN PREGNANCY

The morphology of the aorta in normal pregnancy has been the subject of several studies but with conflicting results. Significant and specific changes were found in the aortic media of pregnant rabbits, and similar alterations have been described in the aorta of gravid women. Histochemical changes varied according to the duration of pregnancy and included fragmentation of reticular fibers, decrease in acid mucopolysaccharides, loss of the normal corrugation (wavy pattern) of elastic fibers, and both hypertrophy and hyperplasia of smooth muscle cells. These biochemical and morphological alterations in the aortic wall have been attributed to hormonal effects,[42] but the findings have not been confirmed.[43]

RESPIRATORY CHANGES IN NORMAL PREGNANCY

Changes in the control of respiration, in lung volumes and mechanics, and in acid-base balance normally occur during pregnancy (Table 53–2). In addition, the placenta provides the means for the critical interplay between maternal and fetal gas exchange. Thus, respiratory physiology of the normal pregnant state may be appropriately considered from two points of view, namely, changes in maternal respiration and maternal/fetal respiratory interactions.[34,44]

Resting oxygen consumption rises progressively during the course of normal pregnancy, reaching a maximum of about 30 per cent near term.[44] Hyperventilation, which is consistently present, is manifested by an increase in minute ventilation that both precedes the rise in oxygen consumption and is approximately twice its magnitude. The increase in resting minute ventilation begins early in pregnancy and reaches a maximum of approximately 40 to 50 per cent in the last 4 weeks of gestation. Hyperventilation is believed to be mediated primarily by progesterone. The hormonally mediated hyperventilation and hypocapnia of pregnancy are associated with renal excretion of HCO_3, so that pH is maintained within the normal range. Thus, compensated respiratory alkalosis is the principal acid-base pattern of normal pregnancy.[44]

During mild to moderate exercise in the first two trimesters, the ventilatory response is similar to that occurring in the nonpregnant state.[34,44] In the last trimester, however, exercise-induced increments in minute ventilation and oxygen consumption are greater in magnitude.[45]

The functional residual capacity (lung volume at the end of quiet expiration) falls as the gravid uterus elevates the diaphragm. However, this fall is accompanied by an increase in inspiratory capacity, so that total lung capacity is reduced little, if at all.[44,46,47] Pulmonary capillary blood volume is not increased in normal pregnant women,[46] and pulmonary compliance remains normal.[44]

There is a decrease in *total* pulmonary respiratory resistance to approximately one-half that in the nongravid state.[44] This reduction is almost entirely the result of diminished airway resistance per se, suggesting a hormonally mediated effect on tracheobronchial smooth muscle tone and an increase in airway cross-sectional area.[44]

Although pulmonary compliance remains normal during pregnancy, the work of breathing increases,[48] owing partly to hyperventilation and partly to the extra work required to displace the diaphragm as the uterus enlarges. Because of the reduction in airway resistance, only a small increase in the work of quiet breathing occurs during normal gestation.[44]

Placental production of progesterone contributes to maternal hyperventilation, favoring the transfer of carbon dioxide from fetal to maternal blood. The placenta has sometimes been considered functionally analogous to the lung,[49] but there are significant differences. Placental oxygen transfer is facilitated by the relatively higher affinity of fetal hemoglobin for oxygen. However, hemoglobin concentration and the rates of uterine and umbilical blood flow are more important determinants of the rate of placental oxygen transfer.

Cardiorespiratory Symptoms and Signs in Normal Pregnancy

Normal uncomplicated pregnancy is accompanied by symptoms, physical signs, and electrocardiographic, roent-

TABLE 53–2   RESPIRATORY CHANGES IN NORMAL PREGNANCY

O₂ consumption	↑
Minute ventilation	↑
Functional residual capacity	↓
Inspiratory capacity	↑
Vital capacity	Unchanged
Total lung capacity	Unchanged
Pulmonary compliance	Unchanged
Airway resistance	↓
Compensated respiratory alkalosis	

TABLE 53–3   CARDIORESPIRATORY SYMPTOMS AND SIGNS IN NORMAL PREGNANCY

Dyspnea
Hyperventilation
Easy fatigability
Decreased exercise tolerance
Lightheadedness
Syncope
Peripheral edema
Basilar rales
Small waterhammer pulse
Prominent jugular venous *a-v* crests and *x-y* troughs
Brisk, displaced left ventricular impulse
Right ventricular impulse
Increased first heart sound
Persistently split second heart sound
Third heart sound
Pulmonic midsystolic murmur
Supraclavicular systolic murmur
Continuous murmurs
ECG changes in rhythm, axis, and repolarization
X-ray—lateral displacement of apex, increased lung markings

genographic, and echocardiographic changes that simulate heart disease and can be erroneously attributed to it (Table 53–3). The circulatory and respiratory changes occurring during normal pregnancy described above provide an explanation for these findings.

Dyspnea, easy fatigability, and a reduction in exercise tolerance are relatively common.[12] In late pregnancy, the supine hypotensive syndrome (see above) occasionally causes lightheadedness or even syncope.[19] On physical examination, the combination of basilar rales (that disappear after coughing or deep breathing) and peripheral edema may be misleading. The systemic arterial pulse often exhibits a brisk rise and collapse (small waterhammer) beginning as early as the end of the first trimester,[50] findings in accord with augmented stroke volume, and echocardiographic registration of increased systolic motion of the aortic root.[17] Arterial pulsations can sometimes be palpated in the fingertips.

On *precordial palpation* (p. 26) there is generally a brisk, nonsustained left ventricular impulse that may be displaced to the left and often also an impulse over the right ventricle (mid to lower left sternal edge) and pulmonary trunk (second left intercostal space).[50] However, as pregnancy progresses, enlargement of the breasts and abdomen makes these signs difficult to elicit.

The *jugular venous pulse* (p. 20) is more easily seen during pregnancy, with clearly defined and relatively prominent *a* and *v* peaks and brisk *x* and *y* descents. The mean jugular venous pressure, as estimated from the superficial jugular vein, remains normal.

AUSCULTATORY FINDINGS. During normal gestation these start at the end of the first trimester, disappear (with few exceptions) a week after delivery, and include variations in heart sounds and the presence of systolic and continuous murmurs.[50,51] The *first heart sound* is increased in intensity (tachycardia and increased left ventricular contractility) and is often prominently split. The *second heart sound*, at least toward the end of pregnancy, tends to exhibit persistent expiratory splitting, especially when patients are examined in the lateral position. However, the supine position may restore the splitting to normal, owing to decreased venous return caused by uterine compression of the inferior vena cava. Since *third heart sounds* are common in normal young nonpregnant women, it is not surprising that the increased rate of atrioventricular flow during pregnancy would augment the intensity of these sounds.[50] Occasionally, a prominent third heart sound is followed by brief, soft, low-frequency after-vibrations that can be mistaken for a short mid-diastolic murmur. With this exception, diastolic murmurs are not features of uncomplicated pregnancy. Fourth heart sounds seldom occur in healthy young persons, male or female, and should not occur during normal pregnancy. Low-frequency oscillations with the timing of fourth heart sounds are occasionally recorded with appropriate phonocardiographic filters, but these vibrations are seldom audible.[50]

Murmurs. Two types of functional (innocent) *systolic murmurs* occur in healthy nonpregnant women, and these murmurs increase in intensity and prevalence during pregnancy.[52] The innocent or normal pulmonic midsystolic murmur (maximal in the second left intercostal space) represents audible vibrations caused by right ventricular ejection into the pulmonary trunk; innocent or normal supraclavicular systolic murmurs originate in brachiocephalic arteries at their points of branching from the aortic arch.[53] Both these murmurs are midsystolic, beginning after the first heart sound and terminating before the second, and both are understandably augmented by the increased cardiac output and stroke volume during pregnancy. The pulmonic midsystolic murmur seldom exceeds grade 3 (of six), but the supraclavicular systolic murmur may exceed grade 4 and occasionally radiates, with attenuation, below the clavicles. A third innocent murmur, this one peculiar to pregnancy—the *mammary souffle*—can be either systolic or continuous. The mammary souffle, like all arterial murmurs, is louder in systole whether or not it is continuous, and at times it is confined to systole.[53,54] This murmur is heard over the breasts late in pregnancy, but especially in the postpartum period in lactating women. There is a tendency for the murmur to be loudest in the second or third right or left intercostal spaces bilaterally. The souffle is best heard with the patient supine and may vanish altogether in the upright position, with firm pressure of the stethoscope or with digital compression adjacent to the site of auscultation. In addition, the day-to-day or cycle-to-cycle variation of the murmur and its permanent disappearance following termination of lactation are reassuring features of normality. A second and far more common continuous murmur is the *venous hum* (p. 30). The hum is relatively frequent in nonpregnant young women and, if properly sought, is almost universal during gestation. Rarely, the hum is loud enough to radiate beneath the clavicle, but wherever heard, it promptly vanishes with compression of the ipsilateral deep jugular vein.

Some murmurs caused by organic heart disease increase in intensity during pregnancy owing to the increase in cardiac output and stroke volume associated with the gravid state. The murmurs of pulmonic stenosis and aortic stenosis fall into this category; the murmur of mitral stenosis is especially accentuated because the increased blood flow and the shortening of diastolic filling time as the heart rate increases combine to augment the rate of flow across the mitral valve.

The diminution or disappearance of organic murmurs during pregnancy is less well-known but equally important.[51] The decrease in peripheral vascular resistance that accompanies pregnancy may cause the murmurs of aortic regurgitation or mitral regurgitation to soften or even disappear.[55] Prolapse of the mitral valve is relatively common in healthy young women (p. 1089), and the auscultatory hallmarks—the systolic click(s) and late systolic murmur—vary with alterations in left ventricular volume and shape.[56] The increase in left ventricular internal dimensions and volume at end diastole during pregnancy[17] may be enough to attenuate or abolish both the click(s) and late systolic murmur.[57] Similarly, the systolic murmur of hypertrophic obstructive cardiomyopathy may decrease or vanish as the left ventricle handles a larger volume during gestation (p. 1409).[58]

ELECTROCARDIOGRAPHIC CHANGES. The electrocardiogram in normal pregnant women may exhibit changes in rate, rhythm, P-R interval, QRS axis, ST segment, T wave, and Q-T interval.[59] Heart rate increases (see above), accounting for a slight decrease in PR interval and QT interval.[60] Premature atrial and ventricular beats are relatively frequent, and apparently innocent ventricular bigeminy sometimes occurs. Reentrant supraventricular tachycardia is most common in normal young women, and pregnancy lowers the threshold for recurrences in susceptible patients.[2] The P wave exhibits no change in amplitude, duration, or axis. The QRS amplitude and duration remain unaltered but not the axis, which may undergo a leftward shift averaging 40 degress in the third trimester.[60] The axis sometimes becomes more vertical somewhat near term as the fetus descends into the pelvis. A small Q wave may accompany T-wave inversions in lead III; deep inspiration tends to decrease or abolish both these changes.[2] Apart from this slight leftward shift of the T axis in the third trimester, there are no significant changes in amplitude, duration, or axis of the T wave,[60] with the following exception. Occasionally, slight, transient ST-segment depressions and T-wave inversions occur in limb and precordial leads and may recur during subsequent pregnancies in the same patient.[61] The mechanism is unknown. Atrioventricular conduction is seldom altered in normal pregnancy except for the slight decrease in P-R interval. In a study of 26,000 electrocardiograms in pregnant women with no other demonstrable heart disease, there were six examples of second-degree atrioventricular block of the Wenckebach type[62] (p. 731). An early report of paroxysmal ventricular tachycardia in a normal young pregnant woman probably represented a misdiagnosis of the Wolff-Parkinson-White syndrome.[63,64]

CHEST X-RAY. Radiation exposure is avoided in pregnant women, so there is relatively little information on plain film radiography. As pregnancy advances, elevation of the diaphragm results in a relatively horizontal cardiac position (upward and lateral displacement of the apex), with an increase in the cardiothoracic ratio.[2] The left cardiac silhouette straightens, and the vascular soft-tissue densities increase slightly.[2] Straightening of the left heart border as well as radiographic prominence of the main pulmonary artery is usually attributable to the hyperlordosis of pregnancy.[65]

ECHOCARDIOGRAM. Since echocardiography can be used with impunity during pregnancy, it is important to recognize that increases in stroke volume, cardiac output, ventricular volumes, and internal dimensions at end diastole are normal and expected (see above).

HEART DISEASE IN WOMEN OF CHILDBEARING AGE

The cardiocirculatory and respiratory changes and the symptoms and signs that accompany normal pregnancy set the stage for discussing the clinical manifestations of heart disease in the gravid woman. Cardiac disease can preexist the pregnancy or be induced by the gravid state (pre-eclampsia/eclampsia, thromboembolic disease, possibly peripartum cardiomyopathy, and rarely, dissecting aneurysm). The types of cardiac disorders—acquired, congenital, or developmental—that are of the greatest clinical importance during pregnancy are obviously those most likely to occur in young women.[66] In addition, as has already been pointed out, cardiac surgery has produced a new and increasing patient population—the postoperative cardiac patient of childbearing age.[3] The prevailing patterns of heart disease vary geographically and socioeconomically and have changed during the course of time, especially in the last two decades.[2,67,68] It was long considered a truism that rheumatic mitral stenosis constituted the principle cardiac threat in pregnancy, since the most common form of heart disease in young women was the result of rheumatic fever, and its most common morphological expression, mitral stenosis, is a condition in which the female:male ratio of incidence is 4:1. However, although mitral stenosis is still the most frequent valvular abnormality in pregnancy, there has been a progressive decline since the early 1960's in both the incidence and the severity of rheumatic heart disease in prenatal clinics.[69]

Acute Rheumatic Fever (see p. 1641)

Acute rheumatic fever, especially the first episode, has its peak incidence before puberty, but because of recurrence, an occasional young woman conceives during the active phase of the rheumatic disease. Although there is no acceptable evidence that pregnancy per se predisposes to active rheumatic fever, evidence of recurrence is sometimes found during gestation.[70]

Chorea as a manifestation of active rheumatic fever has been reported during pregnancy,[70] and about two-thirds of women with chorea gravidarum have histories of prior chorea or rheumatic fever.[72] However, there are reports of women who manifest chorea during consecutive pregnancies but are otherwise free of it and, rarely, free of clinical evidence of rheumatic heart disease.[71] Chorea is more likely to occur in primigravidas, and in about half the instances it begins in the first trimester. Chorea remits prior to delivery in approximately one-third of the patients and shortly thereafter in the remainder.[72] Severe chorea has been accompanied by spontaneous abortion, premature labor, intrauterine fetal death, maternal heart failure, hyperpyrexia, and profound exhaustion. Termination of pregnancy is indicated when severe chorea is accompanied by violent, uncontrollable movements, agitation, and psychiatric disturbances.[72]

Active rheumatic carditis is a serious complication of pregnancy. Patients may die suddenly during labor or shortly after delivery, and a number of fatal cases have been reported without preexisting rheumatic valvular heart disease.[2] Conversely, active rheumatic carditis may initiate or aggravate heart failure in patients with established rheumatic valvular disease.

Chronic Rheumatic Valvular Disease
(See also Chap. 32)

MITRAL STENOSIS. Chronic rheumatic valvular heart disease in pregnancy is represented by pure or predominant mitral stenosis in 90 per cent of cases, by mitral regurgitation in about 6 to 7 per cent, and by aortic regurgitation/stenosis in the remainder.[2] In most cases women with rheumatic valvular disease—mild, moderate, and even severe—can be managed through relatively uneventful pregnancy and delivery. Nevertheless, these patients run the risk of complications, the majority relating to mitral stenosis and taking the form of pulmonary venous congestion (cough, breathlessness, orthopnea, paroxysmal nocturnal dyspnea, or pulmonary edema); sudden brisk hemoptysis (hemorrhage from varicosed bronchial veins); and, less commonly, atrial fibrillation, systemic or pulmonary emboli, and infective endocarditis.[2,73] One or more of these complications occur in about one-fourth of pregnant women with chronic rheumatic heart disease, but the incidence has declined in the past decade.[67,68]

The basic hemodynamic defect in mitral stenosis is the impediment to effective emptying of the left atrium. This defect is aggravated by at least two of the normal cardiocirculatory responses to pregnancy, namely, the increased cardiac output and the increase in heart rate, both of which augment the left atrioventricular pressure gradient and increase left atrial, pulmonary venous, and capillary pressures. Should atrial fibrillation supervene, the hemodynamic burden is compounded by the loss of left atrial contraction and often by a further acceleration of heart rate (and consequent reduction in the duration of diastole). Generally, the smaller the stenotic mitral orifice, the more likely symptomatic pulmonary venous congestion and its sequelae.

The woman with mitral stenosis faces hazards during pregnancy in addition to those of pulmonary congestion. These include right ventricular failure, thromboembolism, and pulmonary arterial hypertension. Right ventricular failure is, of course, undesirable in its own right, but especially during gestation because of the tendency of the pregnant woman to develop peripheral edema and varicose veins. Moreover, chronic peripheral venous stasis increases the risk of pulmonary embolism. Severe pulmonary hypertension—or, more precisely, high pulmonary vascular resistance—exposes the gravid female to special risks.[53,74] Physiological adaptations to fluctuations in cardiac output are limited; an increase in venous return is accompanied by a rise in pulmonary arterial pressure and/or further right ventricular failure; physical effort, stress, or excitement may provoke syncope due to acute right ventricular failure and little or no increase in cardiac output in the face of a fall in systemic vascular resistance. Pulmonary emboli are more likely to occur and more apt to be serious, if not lethal.

OTHER VALVULAR LESIONS. Patients with pure or predominant *rheumatic mitral regurgitation*, especially those with sinus rhythm, usually accommodate to the increased cardiac output and tachycardia of normal pregnancy. The left ventricle copes comparatively well with the increment in volume; the increase in heart rate is little or no handicap, and pulmonary hypertension is uncommon, but infective endocarditis is a real risk. Acute augmentation of mitral regurgitation due to rupture of chordae tendineae in the setting of rheumatic mitral valve disease is almost always a sequel of infective endocarditis.[75,76] As described below, spontaneous chordal rupture occurs in a different setting.[77,78]

Rheumatic aortic valve disease is usually accompanied by mitral valve disease, and the hemodynamic consequences of pregnancy must be considered in this light. The responses to isolated pure aortic regurgitation or aortic stenosis are discussed later.

Rheumatic tricuspid stenosis seldom occurs without associated mitral stenosis.[79] In this setting the aortic valve can be purely incompetent, can be purely stenotic, or can have varying combinations of each, but it is seldom normal. Obstruction of the tricuspid orifice serves to increase systemic venous pressure, promote peripheral edema, aggravate varices, and limit cardiac output, both at rest and with effort or stress.

The *time course of symptoms* complicating chronic rheumatic valvular disease, especially mitral stenosis, is noteworthy. Heart failure can occur at any stage, but the incidence rises as pregnancy progresses;[80] this trend continues to term because, as already discussed, cardiac output does not fall prior to delivery. The frequency of pulmonary venous congestion in patients with mitral stenosis increases with maternal age and parity, doubling when women over 30 years of age are compared with those younger than 20 years of age, especially during or after the third pregnancy.[2] It is important to emphasize, however, that previously asymptomatic women with rheumatic mitral stenosis and less than 30 years of age may also develop unanticipated acute pulmonary edema during pregnancy. This is usually provoked by undue effort or emotional stress, paroxysms of sinus or atrial tachycardia, or upper respiratory infections, but sometimes no apparent precipitating cause can be identified.[2]

Labor can also aggravate preexisting heart failure, but heart failure seldom has its onset during labor, especially if the pregnancy has been well managed. Therefore, the patient whose rheumatic valvular heart disease is well compensated at term can anticipate labor with little fear. However, the rapidly changing physiological adjustments during the puerperium (see above) are not without risk.

Congenital Heart Disease (See also Chap. 30)

Survival to adulthood of patients with congenital heart disease occurs as a result of natural selection or because of surgical intervention. Operation not only increases the life span of patients with anomalies in which there is an inherent tendency toward survival to adulthood but also permits increasing numbers of patients with disorders that were previously fatal in childhood to reach adult life.[3,81,82] **COMMON CONGENITAL DEFECTS.** Common congenital cardiac defects in which adult survival can be anticipated, in order of female prevalence, are ostium secundum atrial septal defect, patent ductus arteriosus, valvular pulmonic stenosis, ventricular septal defect with pulmonic stenosis, functionally normal bicuspid aortic valve, valvular aortic stenosis, aortic regurgitation, and coarctation of the aorta.

Ostium secundum atrial septal defect (p. 1027) remains one of the most common forms of congenital heart disease found in adults. Since the natural history spans the childbearing age, and since the majority of patients are female,[53] the anomaly is of special importance in any consideration of congenital heart disease and pregnancy.[53,81,83] The great majority of women with uncomplicated ostium secundum atrial septal defects endure the hemodynamic burden of pregnancy—even multiple pregnancies—with relatively little difficulty.[2,53] Infective endocarditis poses little or no threat unless there is associated prolapse of the mitral valve with incompetence.[56]

The most important practical concerns in pregnant women with atrial septal defect are pulmonary hypertension, right ventricular failure, and atrial arrhythmias. After the fourth decade, atrial arrhythmias—fibrillation, flutter, or paroxysmal supraventricular tachycardia—increase in frequency and represent serious complications leading to disability and cardiac failure.[53,83] Peripheral edema predisposes to thromboembolism, which may enter the systemic circulation as a paradoxical embolus; death has occurred in this setting, even during the puerperium.[2] Pulmonary hypertension is a relatively late occurrence in ostium secundum atrial septal defect and is seldom a complicating issue in pregnant women below age 30 years. A much higher incidence and earlier onset occur among patients with atrial septal defect who are born at high altitudes.[84] Although an occasional woman with pulmonary hypertension complicating ostium secundum atrial septal defect tolerates pregnancy with surprisingly little difficulty, this is the exception and not the rule.[85]

Patent ductus arteriosus (p. 1038) also predominates in females.[41,53] Beginning with the third decade, an increasing number of patients with large shunts develop cardiac failure, whereas those with small communications remain asymptomatic.[53] The incidence of large patent ductus arteriosus with suprasystemic pulmonary vascular resistance and right-to-left shunt is relatively infrequent. Happily, the combination of patent ductus arteriosus and pregnancy is becoming of less and less practical importance, since the clinical diagnosis of patent ductus is simple, and surgical division is safe, routine, and curative in childhood.

The response to pregnancy in patients with patent ductus arteriosus depends in large part upon where in the spectrum of the lesion gestation occurs. The asymptomatic young woman with a small or moderate-sized patent ductus arteriosus and normal pulmonary arterial pressure experiences uncomplicated pregnancy,[2] although such patients are at risk to develop infective endocarditis (see below). Left ventricular failure may occur or be aggravated during pregnancy in the presence of a large ductus and left-to-right shunt. In patients with large patent ductus arteriosus, pulmonary hypertension, and reversed shunts, right ventricular failure and maternal mortality are distinct threats. Rarely, such patients experience uneventful pregnancies.[2]

Isolated *valvular pulmonic stenosis* (p. 1037) is a relatively common congenital cardiac defect occurring with equal frequency in males and females. Survival into adulthood is comparatively frequent, even though signs of the anomaly are usually present from infancy. In one review of 69 anatomically proven unoperated cases, the average age of death was 26 years.[53] The tendency for the pulmonary valve to grow in proportion to the increase in body size may in part account for this. The majority of patients with pulmonic stenosis proceed through infancy and childhood with little handicap. The increased cardiac output of pregnancy augments the burden on an already pressure-loaded right ventricle, but in young asymptomatic women with mild to moderate and occasionally even severe pulmonic stenosis, pregnancy is, as a rule, satisfactorily tolerated.[2] In view of the relatively conspicuous murmur, the safety and simplicity of diagnostic confirmation, and the low risk of surgical correction, patients with moderate to severe pulmonic stenosis should, and now usually do, undergo operation long before pregnancy, preferably in childhood.

Isolated *ventricular septal defect* (p. 1033) is one of the most common congenital cardiac malformations, occurring with equal prevalence in males and females, although in one series, the majority of patients over age 20 years were women.[53] However, this anomaly is of relatively little importance as a potential complication of pregnancy because of its infrequency in adults. As many as 45 per cent of ventricular septal defects close spontaneously; in patients with large nonrestrictive defects not surgically corrected, either congestive heart failure causes death in infancy or the left-to-right shunts become reduced because of a decrease in ventricular septal defect size, a rise in pulmonary vascular resistance, or the development of obstruction to right ventricular outflow (see below). The occasional acyanotic adult survivor with little or no pulmonary hypertension will tolerate pregnancy in accordance with the magnitude of the left-to-right shunt and the functional state of the left ventricle. In women with relatively large shunts, the added volume load of pregnancy can cause heart failure, and sporadic deaths have been reported as a result of antepartum cardiac failure and postpartum paradoxical embolism.[2] There is a risk of infective endocarditis in patients with this anomaly.

Although isolated ventricular septal defects, irrespective of size, are seldom seen in adults, when large ventricular septal defects are associated with appropriate degrees of pulmonic stenosis, prolonged survival is relatively frequent. Thus, a number of patients with ventricular septal defect and pulmonic stenosis reach childbearing age.

A large ventricular septal defect with obstruction to right ventricular outflow that offers resistance at or above systemic levels, i.e., *tetralogy of Fallot* is the most common congenital anomaly associated with cyanosis in adults with congenital heart disease[53] (p. 1034). Adult survival with this combination of lesions implies a degree of obstruction to right ventricular outflow that permits pulmonary blood flow that is adequate for oxygenation but is not enough to overload the left ventricle. Despite an increased tendency for adult survival, women with cyanotic tetralogy of Fallot seldom have normal full-term pregnancies; their offspring have low birth weights, an observation in accord with the generalization (discussed below) that infants born of cyanotic mothers are typically small for gestational age (see later).[53,86-88] The magnitude of the right-to-left shunt varies inversely with the systemic vascular resistance in patients with tetralogy of Fallot. In pregnancy, the decrease in pe-

ripheral vascular resistance coupled with the increase in cardiac output (and venous return to the obstructed right ventricle) results in a larger right-to-left shunt, a fall in systemic arterial oxygen saturation, deeper cyanosis, and a rising hematocrit. Although full-term pregnancies occur occasionally, the risk to both mother and child is considerable, as discussed below. The labile hemodynamic adjustments during the immediate postpartum period place the patient at further risk. A sudden reduction in systemic vascular resistance may provoke intense, and occasionally fatal, cyanosis and syncope.[2] In addition, there is the risk of infective endocarditis.

In women with pulmonary vascular obstructive disease associated with *Eisenmenger's complex*, i.e., large, nonrestrictive ventricular septal defects with pulmonary vascular resistance at or above systemic levels,[53] (p. 832) hemoptysis may recur or first appear during gestation.[89] The level of the pulmonary vascular resistance is the chief determinant of the risk of pregnancy.[90,91] Maternal mortality has been estimated at 30 to 70 per cent, and death may occur during either the gestational period or the puerperium.[91,92] A number of physiological changes in pregnancy conspire as potential threats. A fall in systemic vascular resistance augments the right-to-left shunt, reduces the arterial oxygen saturation, and increases the hematocrit, just as in the case of tetralogy of Fallot. Conversely, bearing down during labor, by increasing systemic vascular resistance, can suddenly depress cardiac output and provoke syncope with dangerous sequelae. Thus, fluctuations in systemic vascular resistance, cardiac output, and blood volume are tolerated poorly, since the fixed pulmonary resistance permits little or no circulatory reserve. It has further been proposed that widespread thromboses in already compromised small pulmonary arteries and arterioles sometimes result in a rapid postpartum increase in pulmonary vascular obstruction.[91]

Congenital aortic valve disease—Functionally normal bicuspid aortic valve, aortic stenosis, or aortic regurgitation—predominates in males, but this does not reduce the importance of these lesions when they occur in individual pregnant females. A *functionally normal bicuspid aortic valve* is perhaps the most common congenital anomaly of the heart or great arteries.[93] The high susceptibility to infective endocarditis poses a constant threat. Since it is unlikely that an isolated, functionally normal, congenital bicuspid aortic valve would be identified in a young woman before or during pregnancy, the presence of the anomaly may rarely announce itself after delivery because of infective endocarditis which may be accompanied by the sudden appearance of aortic regurgitation.[94]

Congenital valvular aortic stenosis (p. 1026) results from progressive fibrosis and calcification of an initially functionally normal bicuspid valve or from a valve that is inherently obstructed from birth.[53] The fixed obstruction to left ventricular outflow resulting from aortic stenosis imposes a pressure load upon the left ventricle. Pregnancy, by adding the stress of increased cardiac output to an already pressure-loaded left ventricle, increases the transaortic gradient and the left ventricular systolic pressure and work. Patients with mild to moderate aortic stenosis tolerate pregnancy relatively well, but infective endocarditis following delivery remains a risk irrespective of severity. An occasional patient who has asymptomatic severe aortic stenosis prior to conception remains symptom-free throughout pregnancy,[2] but the risk is ever-present, reserve is limited, and syncope, especially after effort or excitement, may first appear during gestation. Should cerebral symptoms, dyspnea, or angina precede conception or develop during early pregnancy, serious sequelae can be anticipated. In any event, abrupt, strenuous, or isometric exercise should be scrupulously avoided.

Like aortic valve lesions, *coarctation of the aortic isthmus* (p. 1038), with or without a coexisting bicuspid aortic valve, occurs predominantly in males.[53] The majority of patients without surgical correction live to adulthood, but only a minority reach 40 years of age. Major symptoms in uncorrected coarctation derive from four complications: congestive heart failure, rupture of the aorta or dissecting aneurysm, infective endocarditis (usually at the site of a bicuspid valve), and cerebral hemorrhage. Beyond infancy, the incidence of cardiac failure peaks after the second decade. Rupture of the aorta or dissecting aneurysm is a dramatic complication that occurs most frequently in the third and fourth decades, whereas cerebral hemorrhage is most common in the second and third decades. Intracranial hemorrhage is usually due to rupture of an aneurysm of the circle of Willis. The behavior of the arterial pressure in pregnancy complicating coarctation of the aorta is analogous to that occurring in normal pregnancy, i.e., the directional changes are similar but from an initially higher level.[53] The risk of complications increases in pregnant women with uncorrected coarctation, and, not surprisingly, death has been reported from rupture of the aorta, cerebrovascular accidents, congestive heart failure, pulmonary edema, and infective endocarditis of a bicuspid aortic valve.[2,95] Overall maternal mortality is estimated at 3.5 per cent[2,96] and morbidity, i.e., cardiovascular complications without death, at 90 per cent.[97,98]

Surgical correction of coarctation of the aorta is now generally performed in children around the age of 4 years, so that more and more patients born with this anomaly are reaching childbearing age *after* having undergone operative repair. Even so, there is the persistent risk of the coexisting bicuspid aortic valve and of late recurrence of systemic hypertension. Also, it is not likely that the threat of rupture of an aneurysm of the circle of Willis is abolished by surgical repair of coarctation.[3]

UNCOMMON CONGENITAL DEFECTS

Some uncommon congenital cardiac defects with expected survival to adulthood are listed in Table 53-4. Pure *congenital aortic regurgitation* (p. 1105), generally due to a bicuspid aortic valve, varies from the trivial to the severe, with all gradations in between. Although the risk of infective endocarditis is present irrespective of severity, pregnancy is otherwise tolerated well, especially in women with mild to moderate regurgitation but also in those with severe incompetence, in whom symptoms are absent prior to pregnancy and in whom left ventricular end-diastolic pressure is normal. The increase in cardiac output during gestation is generally handled well, and its effects are in part corrected by both the fall in systemic vascular resistance and the acceleration in heart rate accompanied by an abbreviation of diastole, which serve to decrease the volume of regurgitant flow. However, in patients with free aortic regurgitation who are symptomatic before conception, especially if the left ventricular end-diastolic pressure is elevated, progressive left ventricular failure can be anticipated during the course of gestation. Similar considerations apply to rheumatic aortic regurgitation.

Uncomplicated *situs inversus* carries no risk, since the heart and circulation are otherwise anatomically and physiologically normal.

TABLE 53-4 UNCOMMON CONGENITAL CARDIAC DEFECTS IN WHICH ADULT SURVIVAL IS EXPECTED

Aortic regurgitation
Situs inversus (mirror-image dextrocardia)
Situs solitus with right thoracic heart
Congenital complete heart block
Congenitally corrected transposition of the great arteries
Idiopathic dilatation of the pulmonary trunk
Congenital pulmonary valve regurgitation
Ebstein's anomaly of the tricuspid valve
Primary pulmonary hypertension
Congenital pulmonary arteriovenous fistula
Lutembacher's syndrome
Coronary arteriovenous fistula

Situs solitus with a right cardiac apex is almost invariably complicated by additional congenital cardiac malformations, the presence and degree of which determine the response to pregnancy. The commonest coexisting anomalies are congenitally corrected transposition of the great arteries, pulmonic stenosis, and ventricular septal defect.[53] The isolated association of corrected transposition, mild pulmonic stenosis, small ventricular septal defect, or a left-to-right interatrial shunt poses little or no problem, but severe pulmonic stenosis with reversed ventricular or atrial shunts involves the risks of anomalies producing cyanosis cited above.

Congenital complete heart block (p. 1043) has no sex predilection, and the natural history generally justifies cautious optimism;[53,99] pregnancy is usually uneventful in otherwise normal women with congenital complete heart block, although there are a few reports of women in whom Stokes-Adams attacks first appeared during gestation.[2,53] It is noteworthy that the functional state of the heart can apparently remain unimpaired when a pregnant woman has an artificial fixed-rate pacemaker.[100]

In *congenitally corrected transposition of the great arteries* (p. 1003), the response to pregnancy is determined by the type and degree of coexisting anomalies that are usually present and most commonly consist of prolonged atrioventricular conduction, incompetence of the systemic atrioventricular valve, ventricular septal defect, and pulmonic stenosis.[53]

Ebstein's anomaly of the tricuspid valve (p. 1040) involves males and females equally and is sometimes compatible with a relatively long and active life;[53] successful pregnancies have been reported in women with Ebstein's anomaly,[101] but gestation poses a number of potential hazards. The functionally inadequate right ventricle, already burdened by tricuspid regurgitation, copes poorly with the increased cardiac output of pregnancy. Recurrent episodes of supraventricular tachycardia, atrial fibrillation, or atrial flutter occur in about one-third of nongravid patients with Ebstein's anomaly and are not likely to be well tolerated during pregnancy, especially when preexcitation (Wolff-Parkinson-White bypass tracts) permits very rapid ventricular rates.[53,64] Cyanosis due to reversed interatrial shunting may first appear in pregnancy during an episode of rapid heart action, especially when acute right ventricular failure is provoked.[53] Chronic cyanosis diminishes the probability of successful gestation and introduces the risk of paradoxical embolism.

The risks of pregnancy in *primary pulmonary hypertension* are formidable,[74] and the disorder is most frequent in young women, with a female:male ratio of 5:1 (p. 836).[53] Sudden death can be precipitated by a variety of stresses that would ordinarily be considered innocuous, and maternal mortality is about 50 per cent.[2,53,74] Effort syncope, chest pain, dyspnea, weakness, and fatigue may first appear during pregnancy, and, as expected, mortality is highest in symptomatic women.[53] The increase in cardiac output and fall in systemic vascular resistance are badly tolerated in the face of the high fixed pulmonary vascular resistance. Labor and the puerperium are even more critical times.

Developmental Defects

Two cardiac disorders that might be called "developmental"—prolapse of the mitral valve and Marfan's syndrome—may complicate pregnancy. About 6 per cent of echocardiograms in presumably normal young females reveal *prolapse of the mitral valve* (p. 1089).[56] These estimates place prolapse of the mitral valve among the commonest clinical cardiac abnormalities (if, in fact, all gradations of echocardiographic prolapse can be called abnormal). The increased cardiac output and reduced systemic vascular resistance characteristic of normal pregnancy serve to diminish leaflet/chordal redundancy and attenuate prolapse; the late systolic murmur may soften or disappear, and the clicks may soften or disappear altogether. Under these circumstances, a diagnosis of mitral prolapse may be clinically impossible (or at least impractical). Yet prolapse is susceptible to infective endocarditis, certainly when accompanied by mitral regurgitation, and bacteremia may occur during labor and delivery. Spontaneous, i.e., noninfectious, rupture of chordae tendineae occasionally complicates mitral prolapse,[56] but it is not yet clear whether the presumed connective tissue changes in pregnancy or the stress of labor and delivery or both increase susceptibility to this complication.[78] A more practical issue is the frequency of disturbances in cardiac rhythm. The commonest sustained tachyarrhythmia is supraventricular tachycardia,[56] an undesirable occurrence during pregnancy, especially toward term, labor, or delivery.

Classic *Marfan syndrome* (p. 1665) has been reported in approximately 4 per cent of patients with prolapse of the mitral valve;[56] conversely, nearly all patients with Marfan syndrome have prolapse of the mitral valve. Myxomatous degeneration of both the aortic and the mitral valves is associated with diaphanous thinning of elongated chordae tendineae. The mitral annulus may be remarkably dilated as a part of the connective tissue defect, and the aortic sinuses and aortic root share in this disorder. Dissection of the aorta is uncommon in nonhypertensive women of childbearing age, but when it does occur it is associated with pregnancy at least half the time;[102,103] structural alterations in the aortic wall during gestation are believed to be responsible,[2,102] and Marfan syndrome, with its inherent abnormality of the aortic media, predisposes to aortic dissection.

Accordingly, the pregnant female with Marfan syndrome is at increased risk,[104] apart from and in addition to the complications associated with the abnormality of the mitral and aortic valves (regurgitation and infective endocarditis). Importantly, the strain of labor and delivery is not necessarily a precipitating factor in aortic dissection, since rupture occurs most commonly in the third trimester or in the first stage of labor.[102]

Cardiomyopathies

The cardiomyopathies are important in pregnancy chiefly with respect to *postpartum* or *peripartum cardiomyopathy*, the term applied to a form of idiopathic congestive cardiomyopathy (p. 1400) beginning in the last month of gestation or the first few months after delivery.[1,5–7,104a] The incidence is low, but the maternal consequences can be dire. At necropsy, cardiac enlargement and mural thrombi have been found with histologic evidence of degeneration and fibrosis of myocardial fibers.[5,6] The etiology of the disorder is unknown, but the probability of its occurrence is increased if a gravid woman of age 30 years or more is experiencing her third or subsequent pregnancy, is pregnant with twins, or has toxemia.[2,5,6] Malnutrition can aggravate the disease but is not a necessary ingredient in its cause or progression. The current consensus is that patients presenting with idiopathic heart failure in the last trimester or in the puerperium are probably examples of dilated preexisting cardiomyopathy that was unrecognized before pregnancy. Even so, the precipitating causes of overt heart failure are unknown. However, in Nigeria, a uniquely high incidence of peripartum heart failure has been related to the custom of ingesting an excessive amount of local lake salt for 40 days postpartum under conditions which diminish evaporative water loss.[105] The long-term prognosis in peripartum cardiomyopathy relates to the rapidity and degree with which heart size returns to normal in response to conventional treatment (Fig. 53–2).[5,6] Patients who maintain cardiomegaly for 6 months or more have an extremely poor prognosis.[5,6] There is a tendency for recurrence of the syndrome in subsequent pregnancies, especially in patients with persistent cardiomegaly.[5,6]

Hypertrophic obstructive cardiomyopathy (p. 1409) is affected by a number of hemodynamic variables that exist during the course of normal pregnancy, labor, and delivery.[2,106] As a rule, gestation is tolerated well.[107] As discussed in Chapter 40, the degree of obstruction to left ventricular outflow is determined chiefly by the interplay among three variables—the left ventricular end-diastolic dimensions (volume), the systemic vascular resistance, and the inotropic state of the left ventricle. During pregnancy, the increase in cardiac output (and left ventricular diastolic volume) should reduce the obstruction, but the fall in systemic vascular resistance counteracts this effect.[106] When mitral regurgitation complicates the syndrome, the hemodynamic effects of pregnancy may dramatically increase its severity, so that pulmonary congestion supervenes.[106] In

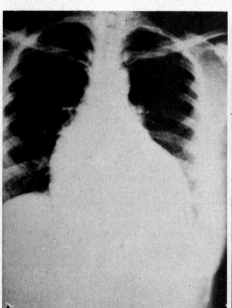
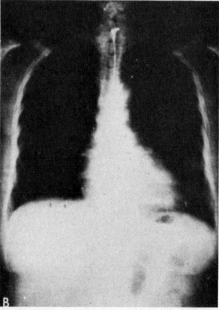

FIGURE 53–2 *A*, Admission chest roentgenogram showing cardiomegaly in a patient with peripartum cardiomyopathy, *B*, Normal heart size in same patient 6 months later. (From Demakis, J. G., et al.: Natural course of peripartum cardiomyopathy. *Circulation 44*:1053, 1971, by permission of the American Heart Association, Inc.)

later pregnancy, compression of the inferior vena cava in the supine position by the gravid uterus decreases venous return and left ventricular volume and accordingly augments the obstruction of left ventricular outflow; patients are therefore well advised to avoid the supine position. A number of opposing variables came into play during labor. The adrenergic stimulation associated with pain and emotional stress, together with the Valsalva maneuver (bearing down), serves to increase outflow obstruction, but the rise in central blood volume during active uterine contraction has the opposite effect.[106] Moreover, the rapid decline in blood volume in the puerperium[29] can reduce left ventricular internal dimensions and intensify the obstruction. In addition, the frequency of coexisting mitral regurgitation exposes patients to the risk of infective endocarditis.

Hypertension (See also p. 888)

Central to the issue of hypertension during gestation are the problems of the previously hypertensive woman who becomes pregnant, the problem of the hypertension of preeclampsia in women who were previously normotensive, and the occurrence of preeclampsia in previously hypertensive women.[108] The incidence of hypertension during pregnancy from all causes has been estimated at 6 per cent, and in about one-fourth of these, elevated blood pressure preceded pregnancy.[2,109] Untoward events related to hypertension in pregnancy are greater in black than in white women.[110,111] The changes in systemic blood pressure that characterize normotensive pregnancy also occur in a significant number of pregnant women with essential hypertension.[2] Thus, the systolic pressure may fall 20 to 30 mm Hg, and the diastolic may decline 10 to 15 mm Hg in the first trimester. There are important variations, however. In some patients, the blood pressure remains unchanged, in others it increases, and in still others blood pressure normalizes during gestation but returns to the preexisting hypertensive levels in the third trimester or after delivery.[112] Gravid women with labile blood pressure generally experience uncomplicated pregnancies, but some develop sustained hypertension late in gestation.[2] Although this labile elevation of pressure is likely to normalize following delivery, a substantial portion of such patients manifest persistent hypertension years later. Criteria for the diagnosis of hypertension usually include a consistent rise in blood pressure of 30/15 mm Hg or an absolute level of greater than 140/90 mm Hg or both (Chap. 26).

As a general rule, maternal prognosis is excellent in women whose arterial pressure is below 160/100 mm Hg during the first 20 weeks of pregnancy,[2] provided renal and cardiac functions are good and preeclampsia does not develop. Conversely, more severe hypertension early in gestation exposes both mother and fetus to increasing risk and requires special medical and obstetrical care.

Treatment. Physical activity should be restricted; anxiety should be controlled with sedatives; long periods of bed rest should be imposed; and sodium restriction, diuretics, and antihypertensive agents (hydralazine, beta blockade, or methyl dopa) should be employed.[2,112] Successful pregnancy is possible even in women who have experienced malignant hypertension, provided that blood pressure is controlled during gestation.[114] However, even mild

hypertension is a risk to the fetus (see below).[115] In selecting appropriate pharmacological treatment, it should be borne in mind that there is evidence of a significant deficit in intravascular volume in many hypertensive pregnant women, especially those with severe preeclampsia or with preeclampsia superimposed upon chronic hypertension.[116] Accordingly, diuretics must be used judiciously because of the risk of decreased plasma volume and uterine (placental) blood flow.[112,113] Unless the hypertension is severe, it is advisable to decrease or discontinue treatment 2 to 3 days before delivery. One major objective of early vigorous treatment of hypertension is the prevention of preeclampsia, which puts the fetus at serious risk, even if the high blood pressure is subsequently reduced.

Preeclampsia

This condition is characterized by normal blood pressure before pregnancy and during the first half of gestation but a rise in blood pressure in the second half, especially during the third trimester. The earlier preeclampsia occurs in the pregnancy, the greater the risk to both mother and fetus.[109] Preeclampsia is more frequent in primiparas, in twin pregnancies, and in women with a history of toxemia or hypertension. Indeed, preexisting moderate essential hypertension is complicated by preeclampsia in 10 to 20 per cent of cases; in this situation, blood pressure is elevated early in pregnancy with a substantial increase in the third trimester. Progression to eclampsia is ominous, with a 5 to 10 per cent maternal mortality and a 20 to 25 per cent fetal mortality. If preeclampsia does not subside within a few days of hospitalization (during which bed rest, sedation, sodium restriction, and pharmacological control of blood pressure are prescribed), the pregnancy should be interrupted as soon as possible by cesarean section unless term is sufficiently near for induction of labor. It has been emphasized that the premature infant of a preeclamptic mother has a better chance in a neonatal intensive care unit than in utero.

It is important to distinguish between edema of the lower extremities of normal pregnancy and the periorbital and hand edema of toxemia (preeclampsia and eclampsia).[112] Similarly, *proteinuria* must be properly interpreted; it usually appears in toxemia *after* the rise in systemic arterial pressure and the development of edema.[112] In a normotensive pregnant woman without edema, proteinuria is more likely due to genitourinary tract infection.[112] Thus, the proteinuria of toxemia must be distinguished from pyelonephritis, and the edema of pregnancy must be separated from the edema of toxemia.

Considerable attention has been focused on the important questions of whether pregnancy permanently aggravates systemic hypertension and whether preeclampsia in previously normotensive women predisposes to the late postpartum development of sustained hypertension. It is current consensus that essential hypertension, at least in white women, is not generally aggravated by pregnancy unless there is superimposed toxemia.[2] The long-term effects of toxemia are more controversial. White women with a history of documented preeclampsia in their first pregnancy have the same prognosis for sustained hypertension or for survival as white women of the same age with no history of preeclampsia. On the other hand, there is a significant increase in the prevalence of sustained hypertension among black women who had preeclampsia as primiparas and among both black and white women who had preeclampsia as multiparas. These observations suggest that toxemia of pregnancy, when it occurs in black women in any pregnancy or in white women after their first pregnancy, marks a tendency for the development of chronic sustained hypertension in later life.[117] Toxemia *per se*, i.e., independent of the presence and degree of systemic hypertension, can result in acute pulmonary edema and T-wave inversions in the electrocardiogram.[2] Cardiac size is not significantly increased in these patients, and the pulmonary edema has been ascribed to retention of fluid and perhaps to effects on pulmonary capillary permeability.[2]

Vascular spasm is an important component of the toxemic state. Approximately one-third of patients with fatal eclampsia (hypertension, edema, proteinuria, and convulsions) were found at autopsy to have contraction band necrosis, a lesion secondary to coronary reflow after periods of no flow.[118] This finding suggests that coronary spasm may be common in patients who die of eclampsia.[118]

Arrhythmias

During pregnancy arrhythmias fall into two general categories: (1) those occurring in the course of an otherwise normal, uncomplicated gestation and (2) those associated with certain cardiac diseases that are likely to be found in women of childbearing age. The type and prevalence of rhythm disturbances are yet to be firmly identified by continuous monitoring of gravid females at different stages of gestation, labor, and the puerperium. Nevertheless, routine electrocardiographic and clinical examination has disclosed a number of arrhythmias in healthy pregnant women. Palpitations caused by premature beats are relatively common during gestation and the puerperium.[59] The premature beats may arise in the atria, the atrioventricular junction, or infranodal sites (ventricular) and occasionally produce bigeminy or trigeminy.

The sporadic occurrence of premature beats is of no clinical importance, especially if they are not subjectively disturbing and if the patient is reassured of their innocence. The most likely sustained arrhythmia in pregnancy is reentrant paroxysmal supraventricular tachycardia, since this rhythm disturbance is relatively common and has its peak incidence in young women. During the obstetrical history, the physician should inquire about prior paroxysmal rapid heart action, since reentrant supraventricular tachycardia often begins in the teens or earlier, forewarning of potential recurrences to which pregnancy predisposes, especially in the third trimester.[59,119] As a rule, the clinical manifestations, pharmacological management, and response to therapy are similar to conventional experience in nonpregnant women, but occurrences close to term, during labor, or in the puerperium are potentially hazardous. Rarely, supraventricular tachycardia is refractory to standard drug therapy. In one such instance, the patient underwent cardioversion seven times during three successive pregnancies with no apparent ill effect on the fetus.[119]

Occasional premature ventricular beats, even with bigeminy or trigeminy, are generally unimportant in the pregnant woman without evident organic heart disease, but multiform beats or repetitive firing—especially toward term or in the puerperium—should arouse suspicion of peripartum cardiomyopathy. Atrial flutter or atrial fibrillation is for all practical purposes evidence of coexisting organic heart disease, either acquired (most commonly rheumatic mitral stenosis) or congenital (especially ostium secundum atrial septal defect, or Ebstein's anomaly of the tricuspid valve). The Wolff-Parkinson-White syndrome with attacks of paroxysmal supraventricular tachycardia or atrial fibrillation at a very rapid ventricular rate (p. 712) may occur during pregnancy.[120]

Venous Disease

The gravid state, and especially repeated pregnancies, predisposes to peripheral venous disease and thromboembolism. If short-term anticoagulants are required, heparin is the drug of choice. The problems of long-term anticoagulant therapy are dealt with below. Increased venous pressure in the lower extremities is an important factor in the development of varicosities. In addition, a prolonged and difficult labor has been implicated as a cause of pelvic vein thrombosis.[2] In either case, overt or occult pulmonary emboli are potential threats. Multiple recurrent pulmonary emboli—insidious or overt—can result in a clinical picture closely resembling if not indistinguishable from primary pulmonary hypertension (pp. 836 and 1597).[121] Symptoms of venous disease or of pulmonary embolism or of both may begin within a few months after delivery or may be delayed for years.[2] In fact, there is a significant increase in the incidence of superficial and deep phlebitis of leg veins during the first four postpartum weeks. Oral contraceptives in the postpartum period should be avoided, not only because of the added risk of venous thrombosis and pulmonary embolism, but because of evidence that an already elevated pulmonary vascular resistance may rapidly increase in women on anovulatory pills even in the absence of identifiable thromboembolism.[122]

Pregnancy After Cardiac Surgery

One of the most important relationships between pregnancy and heart disease involves a new and increasing population—the postoperative cardiac patient.[3] Those who previously would not have reached childbearing age or who might have done so physiologically ill equipped for pregnancy are now presenting postoperatively for obstetrical and cardiological care.

Although cardiac surgery can be performed *during* gestation (see below), the objective of operative intervention should be anticipatory, i.e., to increase the safety and success of pregnancy and the subsequent health of both mother and child.[96] However, it is important to bear in mind that with few exceptions cardiac surgery is not curative, and both the patient and the physician must recognize the need for continuing medical care. The form of management is determined by the presence, type, and degree of postoperative cardiac and vascular residua and sequelae. On the other hand, serious cardiovascular disease can appreciably reduce sexual and ovarian function, and successful cardiac surgery may increase fertility.[96] Relief of cyanosis may not only permit a woman to conceive but substantially improves stability of the pregnancy and the probability of delivery at or near term.[96] Thus, there is general agreement that cardiac surgery *prior* to pregnancy may be enormously beneficial. For example, the complication rate during pregnancy in surgically treated women with previously symptomatic mitral stenosis is reduced significantly.[2,96,124] Uncomplicated gestation has followed intracardiac repair of tetralogy of Fallot, one woman sustaining five pregnancies without incident.[125]

There are special problems in the management of pregnant women with *prosthetic cardiac valves*, namely the risk of infective endocarditis from potential bacteremia during labor and delivery, the risk to the mother of thromboembolism, and the risk to the fetus of anticoagulants, both coumarin-related vitamin K antagonists and heparin.[124-137] The methods of prophylaxis for infective endocarditis are conventional (see below), but anticoagulants pose serious problems that require refined judgment and meticulous care (p. 1778). In pregnant women with rigid prosthetic valves, omission of anticoagulants substantially increases the probability of systemic embolism.[126-128,131] Although anticoagulants do not eliminate thromboembolic complications, the risk is higher in pregnant women with prosthetic valves in whom anticoagulants are discontinued than in those who continue to take the drugs or who have never received them.[131,136] The responses may in part be affected by the relative state of hypercoagulability believed to exist during pregnancy.[126,128] Although the use of oral anticoagulants benefits the mother, the drugs readily cross the placental barrier and expose the fetus to appreciable risks.[126,128,131,134,135,137-139]

Of nearly 450 reported pregnancies in which coumarin derivatives were used, at most two-thirds resulted in apparently normal infants.[139] When coumadin was given in the first trimester, the commonest disorder was what has been called "warfarin embryopathy" or chondrodysplasia punctata[137-139]. Features include saddle nose, hypoplasia of nares and air passages resulting in upper airway obstruction and neonatal respiratory distress, hypertelorism, frontal bossing, short neck, short stature, and stippled epiphyses (punctata).[137-139] Even in the second and the third trimesters, coumadin administration is hardly devoid of fetal risks, which consist of spontaneous abortion, stillbirth, or live offspring with significant abnormalities in one-third of cases.[139] In addition to the ongoing risk of hemorrhagic complications, malformations include optic atrophy, microphthalmia, deafness, malformed ears, low weight for gestational age, dwarfism, dystrophic nails with short fingers, and central nervous system defects, especially mental retardation, microcephaly, hydrocephalus, mengingocele, and cerebral atrophy.[139]

With the hope of circumventing these risks, heparin, which does not cross the placenta, has been proposed during the first or first and second trimesters.[126,135] However, the drug is relatively cumbersome to administer and control, the incidence of maternal hemorrhagic complications is not greater than with coumadin,[139a] but isolated use in the first trimester still results in an overall neonatal morbidity and mortality of 36 per cent—prematurity, death with prematurity, or stillbirth.[139] Apart from the risks of placental or fetal hemorrhage, the chelating effects of heparin (calcium and other cations) with intrauterine deficiencies have been proposed as causes of fetal injury.[139]

Despite the Scylla of maternal thromboembolism and the Charybdis of fetal death or malformation, anticoagulants are routinely employed in the pregnant woman with rigid prosthetic cardiac valves. Heparin in the first trimester does not appear to be superior to coumadin throughout.[139] When coumadin is used, meticulous regulation should maintain the prothrombin time at one and one half times and certainly less than twice the control time.

Management of anticoagulants at the end of pregnancy is much clearer than at the beginning. The hazard of fetal hemorrhage is increased by the obligatory trauma of labor and delivery. During the last 2 weeks of pregnancy, coumadin should be replaced by heparin.[132,133] At the earliest onset of labor or in anticipation of it, and through delivery, protamine is administered and heparin is discontinued. The timing of these events is more readily controlled if labor is induced electively. Should spontaneous labor begin in a patient receiving oral anticoagulants, administration of fresh frozen plasma is desirable.[132] Under these circumstances, birth by cesarean section is said to be associated with a lower risk of fetal death than that by vaginal delivery.[126] If elective cesarean section is planned for any reason, anticoagulants are discontinued 2 to 3 days before delivery.[128] Twenty-four hours after delivery, anticoagulants should be resumed, some clinicians recommending resumption with heparin and gradual replacement by oral anticoagulants.[130,133] In any event, breast feeding should be avoided because oral anticoagulants are secreted in the milk.[2] Antiplatelet agents have been suggested instead of oral anticoagulants in pregnant women with prosthetic heart valves, but the safety and effectiveness of these agents are unproved.[126,127] The availability and value of porcine and human cadaver tissue valves which are nonthrombogenic and which do not require anticoagulant treatment should largely obviate this problem. Although many surgeons continue to prefer rigid prostheses, these devices should, if at all possible, be avoided in women of childbearing age (p. 1086).

The interaction between pregnancy and maternal heart disease—preoperative or postoperative—has thus far focused on gestation, delivery, and the puerperium (see above), and there is general agreement that each of these periods entails an added risk in patients with certain types of organic heart disease. It is also important to ask whether pregnancy, once successfully concluded, alters the subsequent course of maternal heart disease. It has been stated without apparent irony that " . . . most physicians have believed that a woman's impaired cardiac reserve is like a bank account that is irreversibly depleted by the cost of pregnancy."[140] Current opinion does not support this view, at least for rheumatic heart disease.[141] Women with significant impairment of cardiac reserve are at higher risk *during* their pregnancies, but if they survive, no long-term harmful effects have been identified except those attendant on the postpartum exertion necessary for the care of another child.[140] Studies have not provided convincing evidence of a remote adverse effect of pregnancy on the course of chronic rheumatic valvular disease[2,141-143], except in certain underdeveloped countries.[144]

Other Forms of Heart Disease

Atherosclerosis of the large extramural coronary arteries is rare in young menstruating women who have no major risk factors. However, there are a number of reports of postpartum myocardial infarction secondary to coronary thrombosis, but with otherwise normal coronary arteries.[145,146] Occasional examples have been reported of pregnancy complicated by still other forms of heart disease, e.g., luetic heart disease, acute or chronic pericarditis,[2] and Takayasu's disease.[147] These and other sporadic disorders, while individually important, have little collective impact and will not be dealt with further here.

MANAGEMENT OF THE MOTHER WITH HEART DISEASE

Care of the expectant mother with heart disease is based upon a number of simple principles. Maternal mortality varies directly with functional class (Table 53–5). The mother's cardiac reserve is inherently limited by her heart disease and is called upon to meet the additional circulatory demands of pregnancy. This challenge can almost always be met by minimizing unnecessary demands upon the circulation and by meticulous medical management of the cardiovascular disease per se. In so doing, a place can be made for pregnancy within the framework of a limited cardiovascular reserve. Conversely, interruption of pregnancy as a means of preserving or restoring cardiac compensation is seldom warranted. If the decision is made to terminate pregnancy on other grounds, the interruption should be done when safest, i.e., during the first trimester. However, in the presence of a few cardiovascular lesions, child-bearing imposes such a significant threat to maternal survival that interruption of pregnancy is recommended. These include women whose pulmonary vascular resistance is at or above systemic resistance, women with Marfan's syndrome, and women with persistent cardiomegaly following peripartum cardiomyopathy.

Factors that serve to aggravate the heart disease and needlessly encroach on cardiac reserve should be identified, removed, or at least minimized (Table 53–6). Anxiety is a tangible source of stress, especially in the primipara who anticipates the new experience of pregnancy in the face of her heart disease. Reassurance begins with a frank, clear, but euphemistic appraisal designed to remove fear of the unknown. The expectant mother should be told what to expect during each stage of pregnancy through labor, delivery, and the puerperium. Coordination between obstetrician and cardiologist is obligatory to provide intelligent care and to assure that the patient does not receive conflicting and therefore disturbing information. Acute and often unnecessary anxiety can provoke pulmonary edema in young women with mitral stenosis whether or not they are pregnant. The reassurance that the pain of labor and

TABLE 53–6   FACTORS THAT AGGRAVATE MATERNAL HEART DISEASE

Anxiety
Retention of sodium and water
Sudden, strenuous, or isometric exercise
Heat and humidity
Anemia
Pyelonephritis
Lower respiratory infection
Hyperthyroidism
Arrhythmias
Thromboembolism

delivery will be relieved is especially important. Thus, "natural childbirth" should be discouraged.

The tendency for body water and total exchangeable sodium to increase in the normal gravid woman must be reckoned with in the pregnant cardiac patient; initial restriction of sodium followed by judicious use of diuretics prevents these increases from reaching undesirable proportions. Body weight should be carefully recorded each morning before breakfast. Not only is weight an important means to detect excess sodium and water retention, but excess dry body weight (obesity) is also a cardiocirculatory burden that is best minimized. Since exercise augments an already increased basal cardiac output, the pregnant cardiac patient should avoid abrupt, strenuous, or isometric effort; should rest an hour or two during the day, preferably in the early afternoon; and should be assured of a restful night even if sedatives are required. Gradations clearly exist. The asymptomatic patient with physiologically mild cardiac disease, e.g., mild isolated mitral regurgitation, needs little or no restriction, whereas the symptomatic pregnant patient with serious cardiac compromise may require prolonged hospitalization with complete bed rest.[78] The psychological impact of hospitalization for this purpose must, of course, be balanced against the anticipated benefits.

Certain environmental conditions exert important effects on the heart and circulation and may initiate or intensify heart failure in susceptible individuals. The combination of heat and humidity increases the hemodynamic burden,[148] and may serve as an important aggravating cause of heart failure in an otherwise stable pregnant cardiac patient.[1] Since gestation is normally accompanied by a high–cardiac output state (p. 1763) and greater heat production owing to the metabolic activity of the products of conception, increased skin blood flow and a cool, dry environment are required for dissipation of heat and proper regulation of body temperature. Pregnancy, heat, and humidity independently increase resting cardiac output;[148] the additive effects decrease cardiac reserve, so an air-conditioned environment can be therapeutic.

Alcohol decreases cardiac output in patients with heart disease.[149] When used in moderation, it may be helpful in the relief of anxiety, but excessive use must be avoided. Alcohol solutions are sometimes used intravenously to stop premature labor. In addition to the deleterious effect on cardiac performance which may result (p. 1406), large volumes of hypertonic solution are occasionally administered for this purpose, a practice hazardous to the patient with heart disease. Coexisting noncardiac diseases may also exert undesirable circulatory effects, especially in the

TABLE 53–5

MATERNAL MORTALITY ACCORDING TO FUNCTIONAL CLASS[2,52]

Classes I and II	Classes III and IV
0.4%	6.8%

FETAL MORTALITY ACCORDING TO FUNCTIONAL CLASS[2]

Class I	Class IV
NIL	30%

pregnant cardiac patient. *Anemia* is a case in point and with rare exception can be corrected by oral iron. Pathological anemia must be distinguished from the "physiologic" anemia of pregnancy (see above), but even the latter can be deleterious in patients with marginal ventricular function. *Infection*, especially pyelonephritis, is relatively common during pregnancy and the postpartum period, so the index of suspicion should be appropriately high.[112] *Lower respiratory infection*, though coincidental, poses special problems in the pregnant cardiac patient with marginally elevated or increased pulmonary venous pressure. Epidemic *influenza* is associated with greater morbidity and mortality during pregnancy and is especially dangerous to women with mitral stenosis.[150] Vaccination with a killed vaccine is recommended for these patients.

Hyperthyroidism may not be as readily suspected because of the hyperkinetic circulation of pregnancy, but the effect is no less harmful, since the two hypermetabolic states (Chap. 24) conspire to reduce cardiac reserve. *Arrhythmias* should be anticipated and appropriate drugs used prophylactically. A history of recurrent supraventricular tachycardia in a previously healthy woman or reports of recurrent atrial fibrillation in a pregnant patient with mitral stenosis dictate the use of digoxin. Quinidine has been incriminated as a cause of premature labor,[59] but the drug has only minimal oxytocic effect and then not until spontaneous uterine contractions have begun.[2] The inherent tendency for stasis in leg veins and the attendant risk of thromboembolism can be minimized in a number of relatively simple ways. Aside from judicious use of sodium restriction and diuretics, the patient should be given detailed instructions on leg care, i.e., passive standing should be avoided, the supine position should be minimized (supine vena caval compression), the knees should be straightened when sitting (the legs need not be uncomfortably elevated), and ambulation should begin as soon as practical after delivery. In high-risk cases in which there is a history of thromboembolism, administration of prophylactic heparin within 24 hours after delivery has been advised.[151] The risks of oral anticoagulants, especially to the fetus, were discussed above.

Medical Management

With this background, let us now turn to the medical (i.e., nonsurgical) management of heart disease per se during pregnancy, labor, delivery, and the puerperium. Because of the hazards of radiation, chest roentgenography, cardiac catheterization, and angiography are usually deferred until after the completion of pregnancy. Treatment of occult congestive heart failure is important, but the management of acute pulmonary edema is pivotal, since this complication ranks as the greatest single cause of maternal cardiac mortality, accounting for 50 per cent of deaths in pregnant women with rheumatic heart disease.[2,144] The detection of incipient pulmonary congestion in the pregnant cardiac patient is essential. At each visit evidence must be sought by means of history and physical examination for developing pulmonary and peripheral venous congestion. A change in exercise tolerance or a sudden gain in weight requires explanation. Since the basal circulatory burden is elevated beginning in the first trimes-

ter, symptoms of reduced cardiac reserve can become manifest early in women with severe heart disease. Cardiac failure is best treated promptly and vigorously with marked restriction of physical activity, even bed rest, in addition to digitalis, diuretics, and salt restriction. Aggravating or precipitating causes should be diligently sought and corrected,[80] as emphasized earlier.

Comment was made (see above) on elective induction of labor near term in preeclampsia and in order to provide controlled timing when anticoagulants are administered to pregnant women with prosthetic valves. However, induction of labor well before term is not an appropriate method of delivery for the pregnant cardiac patient and, in fact, may increase the risk of heart failure. It is still the consensus that a spontaneous term vaginal delivery with adequate relief of pain and apprehension, performed with the aid of an experienced obstetrical anesthesiologist, is the method of choice in the pregnant woman with heart disease. The importance of the relief of pain and anxiety should be underscored. Cesarean section using epidural anesthesia[92] or thiopental, nitrous oxide, and succinylcholine anesthesia has been proposed for selected seriously ill pregnant cardiac patients.[152]

Infective endocarditis following uncomplicated vaginal delivery is rare.[153] Blood cultures taken at intervals during labor and delivery have not confirmed that bacteremia is a natural or necessary occurrence,[2] and some authorities have indicated that antibiotic prophylaxis is not necessary at the time of delivery in cardiac patients.[153] However, in pregnant women with cardiac lesions susceptible to infective endocarditis, it is not prudent to assume that delivery will be uncomplicated. Accordingly, prophylactic antibiotics (p. 1175) are recommended from the onset of labor through the fourth to sixth postpartum day.[2]

Cardiac Surgery

Fortunately, the issue of whether or not cardiac surgery is required in the pregnant cardiac patient seldom arises. When the problem is posed, it is almost always in women with rheumatic mitral stenosis[2,68,154,155] and only rarely in those with congenital heart disease.[83,96] Mitral valvotomy (without use of extracorporeal circulation) probably has a role, albeit a limited one. The most defensible indications are intractable (medically refractory) pulmonary edema and persistent massive hemoptysis in a patient with proven severe mitral stenosis.[2,68] Many cardiologists and obstetricians agree that, whenever possible, premature termination of pregnancy is preferable to cardiac surgery in patients with life-threatening heart failure that is unresponsive to medical management. Although valvotomy has been carried out at various stages in pregnancy, it is desirable to proceed as early as possible. The use of a pump oxygenator and extracorporeal circulation introduces a major variable of a completely different order of magnitude—the high risk of fetal mortality, which is greater than 30 per cent.[68,83,155] Moreover, even if the fetus survives, it may be born deformed.[93] Sporadic reports exist, however, of patients with mitral stenosis and intractable pulmonary edema responding to emergency open mitral valvotomy during the third trimester and subsequently delivering a normal infant at term.[155] On one occasion, cesarean section was successfully performed while the mother was on cardiopulmonary bypass.[156] When confronted with the rare catastrophe of sudden maternal death, consideration must be given to immediate postmortem cesarean section. About 150 postmortem cesarean sections have been reported, with an infant survival of approximately 15 per cent.[157]

EFFECTS OF MATERNAL HEART DISEASE ON THE FETUS

In the pregnant woman with heart disease, the lives of both the mother and the fetus are at stake, and it is now appropriate to summarize the effects of maternal cardiac disease on the fetus,[11a] even though a number of points have already been made. The fetus is exposed both to immediate risks that threaten its viability and to remote risks that express themselves as congenital malformations. Normal uterine blood flow and normal placental function are fundamental determinants of the intrauterine milieu upon which fetal integrity largely depends. Maternal heart disease, by reducing uterine blood flow and by altering the physiology of the placenta, threatens the growth, development, and viability of the fetus. Moreover, the fetus is at independent risk of congenital malformations which can result from genetic transmission of certain types of maternal heart disease or from transplacental transfer of teratogens, often in the form of drugs used in treating the pregnant cardiac patient.

In addition, certain factors unrelated to heart disease per se threaten the fetus and should not be disregarded. The fetal alcohol syndrome is a major risk in pregnant women who consume the equivalent of 90 ml or more of absolute alcohol per day, but lower levels of consumption may impose some risk.[158] Cigarette smoking throughout pregnancy can damage the umbilical artery and vein and the vessels of placental villi.[159] The placentas are relatively small and poorly vascularized, birth weights are low for gestational age, and there is increased risk of first trimester abortion, stillbirth, prematurity, and perinatal mortality.[29,159,160] Occasionally, supine vena caval obstruction results in a reduction in cardiac output sufficient to cause fetal hypoxia, but this effect is transient and readily reversed merely by having the mother turn on her side.[19]

The effects of maternal heart disease itself and the effects of the medical and surgical interventions employed to treat the cardiac disorder are of the greatest importance for fetal survival. The functional class of the mother materially influences fetal mortality; the risk varies from virtually nil in the asymptomatic pregnant woman with heart disease (Class I) to nearly 30 per cent in gravid women who are symptomatic at rest (Class IV) (Table 53–5).[2,52] There is no evidence, however, that live offspring of such women have a higher incidence of congenital malformations.

Certain types of heart disease pose greater threats than others to the fetus. *Systemic hypertension*, independent of the high risk of preeclampsia,[2,161] is associated with intrauterine growth retardation and an increased incidence of stillbirths and perinatal mortality.[2,108,110,162] The absolute level of blood pressure need not be great to increase fetal mortality. If the diastolic level exceeds 84 mm Hg at any time during gestation, the risk to the fetus increases, even more so when proteinuria is present.[163] In the United States, annual fetal attrition due to maternal hypertension is about 10,000.[164] *Maternal congenital heart disease* threatens the fetus in a number of respects. Aside from its effect on the functional class of the mother (see above), there is a material risk of genetic transmission (Chap. 47). Congenital cardiac defects have been found in 13.8 per cent of infants born of mothers with congenital heart disease, regardless of whether or not they had been operated upon.[165] Surgical correction, by permitting more patients to reach maturity, necessarily increases the number of women who will produce children at increased risk of congenital cardiac anomalies.[3]

Maternal cyanosis substantially increases fetal risk, even though in cyanotic forms of congenital heart disease, certain responses serve to facilitate delivery of oxygen to the fetus.[165,166] Systemic arterial hypoxemia increases red cell mass and oxygen-carrying capacity of the blood and displaces the whole blood–oxyhemoglobin dissociation curve to the right.[166] The placenta is proportionately larger in infants of hypoxic mothers, and it has been shown that the fetus responds to severe maternal hypoxemia by increasing 2, 3-DPG, and decreasing red cell oxygen affinity, thus facilitating the release of oxygen to the tissues.[165]

Despite these compensatory mechanisms, the vast majority of infants born to mothers with cyanosis are dysmature (small for gestational age)[96] or premature (gestation less than 37 weeks). In addition, there is a high rate of spontaneous abortion, the incidence of which increases in parallel with the mother's hematocrit; however, even in the presence of relatively mild cyanosis, the spontaneous abortion rate exceeds 50 per cent.[96]

Cardiovascular Drugs in Pregnancy

The response of the pregnant patient to cardiovascular drugs is important in a number of respects, especially the effect on uteroplacental blood flow, the effect on the tone of uterine muscle (and therefore on labor), and the effect on the fetus.[167] Transplacental transfer of drugs such as oral anticoagulants, together with the ill effects on the fetus of heparin, even though it does not cross the placental barrier, have already been discussed (p. 1775). The breast-fed neonate is also vulnerable to the drugs that the mother is taking, since a number of potentially harmful drugs are excreted in the milk.[2] As a matter of principle, it is desirable to minimize or avoid drug administration in the first trimester of pregnancy during fetal organogenesis.

Alpha-adrenergic stimulants, beta-adrenergic agonists, and drugs with combined alpha and beta effects influence both uterine blood flow and contraction. A vasoconstrictor given to a hypotensive pregnant patient is likely to increase uteroplacental blood flow by raising perfusion pressure, whereas the converse is the case when vasoconstriction is induced by administering such a drug to a normotensive subject. Beta-adrenergic agonists such as isoproterenol inhibit contraction of smooth muscle and accordingly depress both spontaneous and oxytocin-stimulated uterine contraction.[167] The unstressed heart rate of the fetus and neonate are under minimal beta-adrenergic control,[168] and offspring of propranolol-treated mothers have not manifested cardiac effects attributable to beta blockade.[167] Nevertheless, blockade of the humoral stimulation of beta-adrenergic receptor sites removes a potentially important reserve response to acute fetal stress and therefore seems undesirable under certain circumstances of fetal adaptation.[167] Propranolol increases uterine activity, an effect more pronounced in nonpregnant than in pregnant women.[169] The drug also crosses the placenta and is secreted in breast milk, thus potentially affecting fetal and neonatal heart rate and respiration.

Blood concentrations of *digitalis* are significantly lower in pregnant women than in nonpregnant patients receiving the same dose.[167] The glycosides freely cross the placental barrier, but there is no evidence of a harmful effect on the fetus.[170,171] Interestingly, digitalis not only increases the force of myocardial contraction but also may have a similar effect on the myomentrium.[172] It is not yet clear whether this effect accounts for the clinical impression that digitalized patients have shorter labors.

Inhibitors of prostaglandin synthesis—aspirin, indomethacin, and naproxen—are sometimes recommended for delaying premature labor.[173] These drugs interfere with uterine contractility and with maternal, fetal, and neonatal platelet function and are capable of constricting the fetal ductus with significant elevation of pulmonary arterial pressure.[173]

Diuretics administered in late pregnancy produce no apparent ill effects. However, in early gestation, care should be taken not to give diuretics injudiciously merely because of the presence of the mild ankle edema so common in normal pregnancy. An inappropriate reduction in maternal plasma volume is undesirable and potentially harmful to the fetus.[113] Antiarrhythmic agents such as quinidine, procainamide, lidocaine, and phenytoin have not been found to have adverse effects on the fetus but are best avoided during the first trimester as a matter of principle.[2] Disopyramide has been reported to initiate uterine contractions in the thirty-second week of pregnancy.[174] Antibiotics cross the placenta but are apparently not teratogenic, although tetracyclines given in late pregnancy can cause discoloration of the infant's teeth, and prolonged administration of streptomycin increases the risk of damage to the eighth cranial nerve of the fetus.[2] Morphine significantly reduces fetal heart rate and causes respiratory depression in the newborn. Prednisone has been held responsible for depressing placental function.[2] The high risk to the fetus of oral anticoagulants and heparin has been discussed and includes both the risk to fetal viability (fatal hemorrhage) and the teratogenic hazard.[130,131,137-139] Oral anticoagulants are secreted in the milk, but heparin is not. Open heart surgery carried out on the mother imposes a substantial risk to the life and normal development of the fetus.

References

1. Perloff, J. K., Lindgren, K. M., and Groves, B. M.: Uncommon or commonly unrecognized causes of heart failure. Prog. Cardiovasc. Dis. 12:409, 1970.
2. Szekely, P., and Snaith, L.: Heart Disease and Pregnancy. Edinburgh and London, Churchill-Livingstone, 1974.
3. Perloff, J. K.: Late postoperative concerns in adults with congenital heart disease. In Pediatric Cardiovascular Disease. Philadelphia, F.A. Davis Co., 1981.
3a. Engle, M. A., and Perloff, J. K. (eds.): Symposium on postoperative congenital heart disease in adults. Am. J. Cardiol. 50:541, 1982.
4. Chesley, L. C., Cosgrove, R. A., and Annito, J. E.: A follow-up study of eclamptic women. Am. J. Obstet. Gynecol. 83:1360, 1962.
5. Demakis, J. G., and Rahimtoola, S. H.: Peripartum cardiomyopathy. Circulation 44:964, 1971.
6. Demakis, J. G., Rahimtoola, S. H., Sutton, G. C., Meadows, W. R., Szanto, P. B., Tobin, J. R., and Gunnar, R. M.: Natural course of peripartum cardiomyopathy. Circulation 44:1053, 1971.
7. Burch, G. E.: Heart disease and pregnancy. Am. Heart J. 93:104, 1977.
8. Metcalf, J., and Ueland, K.: Maternal cardiovascular adjustments to pregnancy. Prog. Cardiovasc. Dis. 16:363, 1974.
9. Lees, M. M.: Central circulatory responses in normotensive and hypertensive pregnancy. Postgrad. Med. J. 55:311, 1979.
10. Spielman, F. J., and Popio, K. A.: Pregnancy and heart disease (key references). Circulation 65:831, 1982.
11. Leman, R. B., and Assey, M. E.: Heart disease and pregnancy. South. Med. J. 74:944, 1981.
11a. Elkayam, U., and Gleicher, N.: Cardiac Problems in Pregnancy. New York, Alan R. Liss, Inc., 1982.
12. Ueland, K., Novy, M. J., Peterson, E. N., and Metcalfe, J.: Maternal cardiovascular dynamics. IV. The influence of gestational age on the maternal cardiovascular response to posture and exercise. Am. J. Obstet. Gynecol. 104:856, 1969.
13. Katz, R., Karliner, J. S., and Resnik, R.: Effects of a natural volume overload state (pregnancy) on left ventricular performance in normal human subjects. Circulation 58:434, 1978.
14. Lavid-Meeter, K., van de Ley, G., Bom T. H., Wladimiroff, J. W., and Roelandt, J.: Cardiocirculatory adjustments during pregnancy—An echocardiographic study. Clin. Cardiol. 2:328, 1979.
15. Atkins, H. J., Watt, J. M., Milan, P., Davies, P., and Crawford, J. S.: A longitudinal study of cardiovascular dynamic changes throughout pregnancy. Eur. J. Obstet. Gynaecol. Reprod. Biol. 12:215, 1981.
16. Lees, M. M., Taylor, S. H., Scott, D. B., and Kerr, M. G.: A study of cardiac output at rest throughout pregnancy. J. Obstet. Gynec. Br. Comm. 74:319, 1967.
17. Rubler, S., Damani, P. M., and Pinto, E. R.: Cardiac size and performance during pregnancy estimated with echocardiography. Am. J. Cardiol. 40:534, 1977.
18. Rose, D. J., Bader, M. E., Bader, R. A., and Braunwald, E.: Catheterization

19. Kerr, M. G.: The mechanical effects of the gravid uterus in late pregnancy. J. Obstet. Gynecol. Br. Comm. 72:513, 1965.
20. Van Donsen, P. W., Eskes, T. K., Martin, D. B., and Van Hof, M. A.: Postural blood pressure differences in pregnancy. Am. J. Obstet. Gynecol. 138:1, 1980.
21. Atkins, H. J., Watt, J. M., Milan, P., Davies, P., and Crawford, J. S.: The influence of posture upon cardiovascular dynamics throughout pregnancy. Eur. J. Obstet. Gynaecol. Reprod. Biol. 12:357, 1981.
22. Marx, G. F., Husain, F. J., and Shian, H. F.: Brachial and femoral blood pressures during the prenatal period. Am. J. Obstet. Gynecol. 136:11, 1980.
23. Ueland, K., and Hansen, J. M.: Maternal cardiovascular dynamics. II. Posture and uterine contractions. Am. J. Obstet. Gynecol. 103:1, 1969.
24. Bieniarz, J., Crottogini, J. K., Curuchet, E., Romero-Salinas, G., Yoshida, T., Poseiro, J. J., and Caldeyro-Barcia, R.: Aortocaval compression by the uterus in late human pregnancy. II. An arteriographic study. Am. J. Obstet. Gynecol. 100:203, 1968.
25. Blake, S., O'Neill, H., and MacDonald, D.: Haemodynamic effects of pregnancy in patients with heart failure. Br. Heart J. 47:495, 1982.
26. Kim, Y. I., Chandra, P., and Marx, G. F.: Successful management of severe aortocaval compression in twin pregnancy. Obstet. Gynecol. 46:362, 1975.
27. Lund, C. J., and Donovan, J. C.: Blood volume during pregnancy. Significance of plasma and red cell volume. Am. J. Obstet. Gynecol. 98:393, 1967.
28. Ueland, K.: Maternal cardiovascular dynamics. VII. Intrapartum blood volume changes. Am. J. Obstet. Gynecol. 126:671, 1976.
29. Christianson, R. E.: Studies on blood pressure during pregnancy. I. Influence of parity and age. Am. J. Obstet. Gynecol. 125:509, 1976.
30. Biggs, J. S. G.: Blood pressure changes following smoking in pregnancy. Aust. N. Z. J. Obstet. Gynaecol. 15:204, 1975.
31. Ritchie, K.: The fetal response to changes in the composition of maternal inspired air in human pregnancy. Semin. Perinatol. 4:295, 1980.
32. Robertson, E. G.: The natural history of oedema during pregnancy. J. Obstet Gynecol. Br. Comm. 78:520, 1971.
33. Artal, R., Platt, L. D., Sperling, M., Kammula, R. K., Jilek, J., and Nakamura, R.: Maternal cardiovascular and metabolic responses in normal pregnancy. Am. J. Obstet. Gynecol. 140:123, 1981.
34. Guzman, C. A., and Caplan, R.: Cardiorespiratory response to exercise during pregnancy. Am. J. Obstet. Gynecol. 108:600, 1970.
35. Ueland, K., and Hansen, J. M.: Maternal cardiovascular dynamics. III. Labor and delivery under local and caudal analgesia. Am. J. Obstet. Gynecol. 103:8, 1969.
36. Liebson, P. R., Mann, L. I., Evans, M. I., Duchin, S., and Arditi, L.: Cardiac performance during pregnancy. Serial evaluation using external systolic time intervals. Am. J. Obstet. Gynecol. 122:1, 1975.
37. King, T. M., Whitehorn, W. V., and Reeves, B.: Effects of estrogen on composition and function of cardiac muscle. Am. J. Physiol. 196:1282, 1959.
38. Ueland K., and Parer, J. T.: Effects of estrogens on the cardiovascular system of the ewe. Am. J. Obstet. Gynecol. 96:400, 1966.
39. Csapo, A.: Actomyosin formation by estrogen action. Am. J. Physiol. 162:406, 1950.
40. Hytten, F. E., and Thompson, A. M.: Water and electrolytes in pregnancy. Br. Med. Bull. 24:15, 1958.
41. Wood, J. E.: The cardiovascular effects of oral contraceptives. Mod. Concepts Cardiovasc. Dis. 41:37, 1972.
42. Manalo-Estrella, P., and Barker, A. E.: Histopathologic findings in human aortic media associated with pregnancy. A study of 16 cases. Arch. Pathol. 83:336, 1967.
43. Cavanzo, F. J., and Taylor, H. B.: Effect of pregnancy on the human aorta and its relationship to dissecting aneurysms. Am. J. Obstet. Gynecol. 105:567, 1969.
44. Novy, M. J., and Edwards, M. J.: Respiratory problems in pregnancy. Am. J. Obstet. Gynecol. 99:1024, 1967.
45. Pernoll, M. L., Metcalfe, J., Schlenker, T. L., Welch, J. E., and Matsumoto, J. A.: Oxygen consumption at rest and during exercise in pregnancy. Respir. Physiol. 25:285, 1975.
46. Gazioglu, K., Kaltreider, N. L., Rosen, M., and Yu, P. N.: Pulmonary function during pregnancy in normal women and in patients with cardiopulmonary disease. Thorax 25:445, 1970.
47. Pernoll, M. L., Metcalfe, J., Kovach, P. A., Wachtel, R., and Dunham, M. J.: Ventilation during rest and exercise in pregnancy and postpartum. Respir. Physiol. 25:295, 1975.
48. Bader, R. A., Bader, M. E., and Rose, D. J.: The oxygen cost of breathing in dyspnoeic subjects as studied in normal pregnant women. Clin. Sci. 18:223, 1959.
49. Burwell, C. S., and Metcalfe, J.: Heart Disease and Pregnancy. Physiology and Management. Boston, Little, Brown & Co., 1958.
50. Cutforth, R., and MacDonald, C. B.: Heart sounds and murmurs in pregnancy. Am. Heart J. 71:741, 1966.
51. Goldberg, L. M., and Uhland, H.: Heart murmurs in pregnancy: A phonocardiographic study of their development, progression, and regression. Dis. Chest 52:381, 1967.
52. Selzer, A.: Risks of pregnancy in women with cardiac disease. J.A.M.A. 238:892, 1977.
53. Perloff, J. K.: The Clinical Recognition of Congenital Heart Disease. 2nd ed. Philadelphia, W. B. Saunders Co., 1978.

54. Tabatznik, B., Randall, T. W., and Hersch, C.: The mammary souffle of pregnancy and lactation. Circulation 22:1069, 1960.
55. Marcus, F. I., Ewy, F. A., O'Rourke, R. A., Walsh, B., and Bleich, A. C.: The effect of pregnancy on murmurs of mitral and aortic regurgitation. Circulation 41:795, 1970.
56. Devereux, R. B., Perloff, J. K., Reichek, N., and Josephson, M. E.: Mitral valve prolapse. Circulation 54:3, 1976.
57. Haas, J. M.: The effect of pregnancy on the midsystolic click and murmur of the prolapsing posterior leaflet of the mitral valve. Am. Heart J. 92:407, 1976.
58. Kolibash, A. J., Ruiz, D. E., and Lewis, R. P.: Idiopathic hypertrophic subaortic stenosis in pregnancy. Ann. Intern. Med. 82:791, 1975.
59. Bellet, S.: Essentials of Cardiac Arrhythmias. Diagnosis and Management. Philadelphia, W. B. Saunders Co., 1972.
60. Carruth, J. E., Mirvis, S. B., Brogan, D. R., and Wenger, N. K.: The electrocardiogram in normal pregnancy. Am. Heart J. 102:1075, 1981.
61. Boyle, D. M., and Lloyd-Jones, L. L.: The electrocardiographic ST segment in pregnancy. J. Obstet. Gynecol. Br. Comm. 73:986, 1966.
62. Copeland, G. D., and Stern, T. N.: Wenckebach periods in pregnancy and puerperium. Am. Heart J. 56:291, 1958.
63. McMillan, T. M., and Bellet, S.: Ventricular paroxysmal tachycardia: Report of a case in a pregnant girl of 16 years with apparently normal heart. Am. Heart J. 7:70, 1931.
64. Gallagher, J. J., Gilbert M., and Sverson, R. H.: Wolff-Parkinson-White syndrome. The problems, evaluation and surgical correction. Circulation 51:767, 1975.
65. Turner, A. F.: The chest radiograph in pregnancy. Clin. Obstet. Gynecol. 18:65, 1975.
66. Petch, M. C.: Cardiac disease in pregnancy. Postgrad. Med. J. 55:315, 1979.
67. Besterman, E.: The changing face of acute rheumatic fever. Br. Heart J. 32:579, 1970.
68. Szekely, P., Turner, R., and Snaith, L.: Pregnancy and the changing pattern of rheumatic heart disease. Brit. Heart J. 35:1293, 1973.
69. Chesley, L. C.: Severe rheumatic cardiac disease and pregnancy: The ultimate prognosis. Am. J. Obstet. Gynecol. 136:552, 1980.
70. Ueland, K., and Metcalfe, J.: Acute rheumatic fever in pregnancy. Am. J. Obstet. Gynecol. 95:586, 1966.
71. Lewis, B. V., and Parsons, M.: Chorea gravidarum. Lancet 1:284, 1966.
72. Barnes, C. C.: Medical Disorders in Obstetric Practice. 3rd ed. Oxford, Blackwell Scientific Publishers, 1970.
73. Wood, P.: An appreciation of mitral stenosis. Br. Med. J. 1:1051, 1113, 1954.
74. Nielsen, N. C., and Fabricius, J.: Primary pulmonary hypertension with special reference to prognosis. Acta Med. Scand. 170:731, 1961.
75. Ronan, J. A., Steelman, R. B., DeLeon, A. C., Waters, T. J., Perloff, J. K., and Harvey, W. P.: The clinical diagnosis of acute severe mitral insufficiency. Am. J. Cardiol. 27:284, 1971.
76. Reichek, N., Shelburne, J. C., and Perloff, J. K.: Clinical aspects of rheumatic valvular disease. Prog. Cardiovasc. Dis. 15:491, 1973.
77. Roberts, W. C., and Perloff, J. K.: Mitral valvular disease. A clinicopathologic survey of the conditions causing the mitral valve to function abnormally. Ann. Intern. Med. 77:939, 1972.
78. Caves, P. K., and Paneth, M.: Acute mitral regurgitation in pregnancy due to ruptured chordae tendineae. Br. Heart J. 34:541, 1972.
79. Perloff, J. K., and Harvey, W. P.: Clinical recognition of tricuspid stenosis. Circulation 22:346, 1960.
80. Selzer, A.: When is cardiac surgery necessary during pregnancy? J. Cardiovasc. Med. 7:1332, 1982.
81. Perloff, J. K.: Congenital heart disease. In Beeson, P. B., and McDermott, W.: Textbook of Medicine. 16th ed. Philadelphia, W. B. Saunders Co., 1982.
82. Perloff, J. K., and Lindgren, K. M.: Adult survival in congenital heart disease. Geriatrics 29:93, 94, 99, 1974.
83. Cannell, D. E., and Vernon, C. P.: Congenital heart disease and pregnancy. Am. J. Obstet. Gynecol. 85:744, 1963.
84. Khoury, G. H., and Hawes, C. R.: Atrial septal defect associated with pulmonary hypertension in children living at high altitudes. J. Pediat. 70:432, 1967.
85. Arias, F.: Maternal death in a patient with Eisenmenger's syndrome. Obstet. Gynecol. 50:76, 1977.
86. Meyer, E. C., Tulsky, A. S., Sigmann, P., and Siber, E. N.: Pregnancy in the presence of tetralogy of Fallot. Am. J. Cardiol. 14:874, 1964.
87. Jacoby, W. J.: Pregnancy with tetralogy and pentalogy of Fallot. Am. J. Cardiol. 14:866, 1964.
88. Leibbrandt, G., Münch, U., and Gander, M.: Two successful pregnancies in a patient with single ventricle and transposition of the great arteries. Intl. J. Cardiol. 1:257, 1982.
89. Haroutunian, L. M., and Neill, C. A.: Pulmonary complications of congenital heart disease: Hemoptysis. Am. Heart J. 84:540, 1972.
90. Naeye, R. L., Hagstrom, J. W. C., and Talmadge, B. R.: Postpartum death with maternal congenital heart disease. Circulation 36:304, 1967.
91. Pitts, J. A., Crosby, W. M., and Basta, L. L.: Eisenmenger's syndrome in pregnancy: Does heparin prophylaxis improve the maternal mortality rate? Am. Heart J. 93:321, 1977.
92. Spinnato, J. A., Kraynak, B. J., and Cooper, M. W.: Eisenmenger's syndrome in pregnancy. New Engl. J. Med. 304:1215, 1981.
93. Roberts, W. C.: The congenitally bicuspid aortic valve. Am. J. Cardiol. 26:72, 1970.
94. Morganroth, J., Perloff, J. K., Zeldis, S. M., and Dunkman, W. V.: Acute severe aortic regurgitation. Ann. Intern. Med. 87:223, 1977.
95. Deal, K., and Wooley, C. F.: Coarctation of aorta and pregnancy. Ann. Intern. Med. 78:706, 1973.
96. Ueland, K.: Cardiac surgery and pregnancy. Am. J. Obstet. Gynecol. 92:148, 1965.
97. Barash, P. G., Hobbins, J. C., Hook, R., Stansel, H. C., Whittmore, R., and Hehre, F. W.: Management of coarctation of the aorta during pregnancy. J. Thorac. Cardiovasc. Surg. 69:781, 1975.
98. Mortensen, J. D., and Joelsson, I.: Coarctation of the aorta in pregnancy. J.A.M.A. 191:596, 1965.
99. Kenmure, A. C. F., and Cameron, A. J. V.: Congenital complete heart block in pregnancy. Br. Heart J. 29:910, 1967.
100. Shouse, E. E., and Acker, G. E.: Pregnancy and delivery in a patient with external-internal cardiac pacemaker. Obstet. Gynecol. 24:817, 1964.
101. Littler, W. A.: Successful pregnancy in a patient with Ebstein's anomaly. Br. Heart J. 32:711, 1970.
102. Anagnostopoulos, C. E., Prabhakar, M., and Kittle, C. F.: Aortic dissections and dissecting aneurysms. Am. J. Cardiol. 30:263, 1972.
103. Wilson, S. K., and Hutchins, G. M.: Aortic dissecting aneurysms: Causative factors in 204 subjects. Arch. Pathol. Lab. Med. 106:175, 1982.
104. Huseybe, K. O., Wolff, H. J., and Friedman, L.: Aortic dissection in pregnancy: A case of Marfan's syndrome. Am. Heart J. 55:662, 1958.
104a.Cepin, D., James, F., and Carabello, B. A.: Left ventricular function in peripartum cardiomyopathy. Chest 83:701, 1983.
105. Fillmore, S. J., and Parry, E. H. O.: The evolution of peripartal heart failure in Zaria, Nigeria. Circulation 56:1058, 1977.
106. Kolibash, A. J., Ruiz, D. E., and Lewis, R. P.: Idiopathic hypertrophic subaortic stenosis in pregnancy. Ann. Intern. Med. 82:791, 1975.
107. Oakley, G. D. G., McGarry, K., Limb, D. G., and Oakley, C. M.: Management of pregnancy in patients with hypertrophic cardiomyopathy. Br. Med. J. 1:1749, 1979.
108. Gant, N. F., and Worley, R. J.: Hypertension in Pregnancy: Concepts and Management. New York, Appleton-Century-Crofts, 1980.
109. Lin, C. C., Lindheimer, M. D., River, P., and Moawad, A. H.: Fetal outcome in hypertensive disorders of pregnancy. Am. J. Obstet. Gynecol. 142:255, 1982.
110. Page, E. W., and Christianson, R.: Influence of blood pressure changes with and without proteinuria upon outcome of pregnancy. Am. J. Obstet. Gynecol. 126:821, 1976.
111. Finnerty, F. A.: Hypertension is different in blacks. J.A.M.A. 216:1634, 1971.
112. Finnerty, F. A.: Hypertension and pregnancy. J. Cardiovasc. Med. 5:559, 1980.
113. Lindheimer, M. D., and Katz, A. I.: Sodium and diuretics in pregnancy. N. Engl. J. Med. 288:891, 1973.
114. Weir, R. J., and Willocks, J.: A successful pregnancy following malignant phase hypertension. Brit. J. Obstet. Gynecol. 83:584, 1976.
115. Silverstone, A., Trudinger, B. J., Lewis, P. J., and Bulpitt, C. J.: Maternal hypertension and intrauterine fetal death in midpregnancy. Br. J. Obstet. Gynaecol. 87:457, 1980.
116. Soffronoff, E. C., Kaufmann, B. M., and Connaughton, J. F.: Intravascular volume determinations and fetal outcome in hypertensive diseases of pregnancy. Am. J. Obstet. Gynecol. 127:4, 1977.
117. Chesley, L. C., Annitto, J. E., and Cosgrove, R. A.: The remote prognosis of eclamptic women: Sixth periodic report. Am. J. Obstet. Gynecol. 124:446, 1976.
118. Bauer, T. W., Moore, G. W., and Hutchins, G. M.: Morphologic evidence for coronary artery spasm in eclampsia. Circulation 65:255, 1982.
119. Schroeder, J. S., and Harrison, D. C.: Repeated cardioversion during pregnancy. Am. J. Cardiol. 27:445, 1971.
120. Gleicher, N., Meller, J., Sandler, R. Z., and Sullum, S.: Wolf-Parkinson-White syndrome in pregnancy. Obstet. Gynecol. 58:748, 1981.
121. Perloff, J. K.: Auscultatory and phonocardiographic manifestations of pulmonary hypertension. Prog. Cardiovasc. Dis. 9:303, 1967.
122. Oakley, C., and Somerville, J.: Oral contraceptives and progressive pulmonary vascular disease. Lancet 1:890, 1968.
123. Mendelson, C. L.: Medical care, cardiovascular surgery and obstetric management as related to maternal and fetal welfare. In Mendelson, C. L.: Cardiac Disease in Pregnancy. Philadelphia, F. A. Davis Co., 1960, pp. 218–255.
124. Wallace, W. A., Harken, D. E., and Ellis, L. B.: Pregnancy following closed mitral valvuloplasty. J.A.M.A. 217:297, 1971.
125. Ralstin, J. H., and Dunn, M.: Pregnancies after surgical correction of tetralogy of Fallot. J.A.M.A. 235:2627, 1976.
126. Limet R., and Grondin, C. M.: Cardiac valve prostheses, anticoagulation, and pregnancy. Ann. Thorac. Surg. 23:337, 1977.
127. Taguchi, K.: Pregnancy in patients with a prosthetic heart valve. Surg. Gynecol. Obstet. 145:206, 1977.
128. Ibarra-Perez, C., Arevalo-Toledo, N., Cadena, O. A., and Noriega-Guerra, L.: The course of pregnancy in patients with artificial heart valves. Am. J. Med. 61:504, 1976.
129. Ibarra-Perez, C., and Bosque-Ruiz, M.: Pregnancy in six patients with Starr-Edwards heart valve prostheses. Am. J. Cardiol. 30:565, 1972.
130. Chew, P. C. T., and Ratnam, S. S.: Pregnancies in patients with prosthetic heart valves: A review and report of two further cases. Aust. N. Z. J. Obstet. Gynaecol. 15:150, 1975.
131. Buxbaum, A., Aygen, M. M., Sajhin, W., Levy, M. J., and Ekerling, B.: Pregnancy in patients with prosthetic heart valves. Chest 59:639, 1971.
132. McCans, J. L., and Wenger, N. K.: Problems in management of the pregnant

patient with rheumatic heart disease and valve prosthesis. South. Med. J. 69: 1007, 1976.

133. Saka, D. M., and Marx, G. F.: Management of a patient with cardiac valve prosthesis. Anesth. Analg. Curr. Res. 55:214, 1976.

134. Palacios-Macedo, X., Diaz-Devis, C., and Escudero, J.: Fetal risk with the use of coumarin anticoagulant agent in pregnant patients with intracardiac ball valve prosthesis. Am. J. Cardiol. 24:853, 1969.

135. Hirsh, J., Cade, J. K., and Gallus, A. S.: Anticoagulants in pregnancy: A review of indications and complications. Am. Heart J. 83:301, 1972.

136. Casanegra, P., Aviles, G., Maturana, G., and Dubernet, J.: Cardiovascular management of pregnant women with a heart valve prosthesis. Am. J. Cardiol. 36:802, 1975.

137. Pettifor, J. M., and Benson, R.: Congenital malformations associated with the administration of oral anticoagulants during pregnancy. J. Pediatr. 86:459, 1975.

138. Shaul, W. L., Emery, H., and Hall, J. G.: Chondrodysplasia punctata and maternal warfarin use during pregnancy. Am. J. Dis. Child. 129:360, 1975.

139. Hall, J. G., Pauli, R. M., and Wilson, K. M.: Maternal and fetal sequelae of anticoagulation during pregnancy. Am. J. Med. 68:122, 1980.

139a.Hull, R., Delmore, T., Carter, C., Hirsh, J., Genton, E., Gent, M., Turpie, G., and McLaughlin, D.: Adjusted subcutaneous heparin versus warfarin sodium in the long-term treatment of venous thrombosis. N. Engl. J. Med. 306:189, 1982.

140. Chesley, L. C.: Rheumatic cardiac disease in pregnancy. Obstet. Gynecol. 46:699, 1975.

141. Chesley, L. C.: Severe rheumatic cardiac disease and pregnancy. Am. J. Obstet. Gynecol. 136:552, 1979.

142. Boyer, N. H., and Nadas, A. S.: The ultimate effect of pregnancy on rheumatic heart disease. Ann. Intern. Med. 20:99, 1944.

143. Maynard, E. P., and Grover, Z.: The effect of childbearing on the course of rheumatic heart disease: A 25-year study. Ann. Intern. Med. 52:163, 1960.

144. Cole, T. O., and Adaleye, J. A.: Rheumatic heart disease and pregnancy in Nigerian women. Clin. Cardiol. 5:280, 1982.

145. Henion, W. A., Hilal, A., Matthew, P. K., Lazarus, A., and Cohen, J.: Postpartum myocardial infarction. N. Y. State J. Med. 82:57, 1982.

146. Ciraulo, D. A., and Markovitz, A.: Myocardial infarction in pregnancy associated with a coronary artery thrombus. Arch. Intern. Med. 139:1046, 1979.

147. Hauth, J. C., Cunningham, F. G., and Young, P. K.: Takayasu's syndrome in pregnancy. Obstet. Gynecol. 50:373, 1977.

148. Burch, G. E., and Giles, T. D.: The burden of a hot humid environment on the heart. Mod. Concepts Cardiovasc. Dis. 39:115, 1970.

149. Gould, L., Zahir, M., DeMartino, A., and Gomprecht, R. F.: Cardiac effects of a cocktail. J.A.M.A. 218:1799, 1971.

150. Stevens, K. M.: Cardiac stroke volume as a determinant of influenzal fatality. N. Engl. J. Med. 295:1363, 1976.

151. Jackson, P.: Puerperal thromboembolic disease in high risk cases. Br. Med. J. 1:263, 1973.

152. Ueland, K., Hansen, J., Eng, M., Kaloppa, R., and Parer, J. T.: Maternal cardiovascular dynamics. V. Cesarean section under thiopental, nitrous oxide and succinylcholine anesthesia. Am. J. Obstet. Gynecol. 108:615, 1970.

153. Kaplan, E. L., Anthony, B. F., Bisno, A., Durack, D., Hauser, H., Millard, H. D., Sanford, J., Shulman, S. T., Stillerman, M., Taranta, A., and Wenger, N.: Prevention of bacterial endocarditis. Circulation 56:139A, 1977.

154. Kay, C. F., and Smith, K.: Surgery in the pregnant cardiac patient. Am. J. Cardiol. 12:293, 1963.

155. Salomon, J., Yortner, R., and Levy, M. J.: Open heart surgery during pregnancy—Case report. Vasc. Surg. 9:257, 1975.

156. Martin, M. C., Pernoll, M. L., Boruszak, A. N., Jones, J. W., and Lo Cicero, J.: Cesarian section while on cardiac bypass. Obstet. Gynecol. 57:41-S, 1981.

157. Wever, C. E.: Postmortem cesarean section: Review of the literature and case reports. Am. J. Obstet. Gynecol. 110:158, 1971.

158. Clarren, S. K., and Smith, D. W.: The fetal alcohol syndrome. N. Engl. J. Med. 298:1063, 1978.

159. Amussen, I.: Fetal cardiovascular system as influenced by maternal smoking. Clin. Cardiol. 2:246, 1979.

160. Meyer, M. B., and Tonascia, J. A.: Maternal smoking, pregnancy complications and perinatal mortality. Am. J. Obstet. Gynecol. 128:494, 1977.

161. Valentine, B. H., and Baker, J. L.: Treatment of recurrent pregnancy hypertension by prophylactic anticoagulation. Br. J. Obstet. Gynecol. 84:309, 1977.

162. Redman, C. W. G., Beilin, L. J., Bonnar, J., and Ounsted, M. K.: Fetal outcome in trial of antihypertensive treatment in pregnancy. Lancet 2:753, 1976.

163. Friedman, E. A., and Neff, R. K.: Hypertension-hypotension in pregnancy. Correlation with fetal outcome. J.A.M.A. 239:2249, 1978.

164. Chesley, L. C.: Hypertensive Disorders in Pregnancy. New York, Appleton-Century-Crofts. 1978.

165. Whittemore, R., Hobbins, J. C. and Engle, M. A.: Pregnancy and its outcome in women with and without surgical treatment of congenital heart disease. Am. J. Cardiol. 50:641, 1982.

166. Novy, M. J., Peterson, E. N., and Metcalfe, J.: Respiratory characteristics of maternal and fetal blood in cyanotic congenital heart disease. Am. J. Obstet. Gynecol. 100:821, 1968.

167. Brinkman, C. R., and Woods, J. R.: Effects of cardiovascular drugs during pregnancy. Cardiovasc. Med. 1:231, 1976.

168. Nuwayhid, B., Brinkman, C. R., Su, C., Bevan, J. A., and Assali, N. S.: Development of autonomic control of fetal circulation. Am J. Physiol. 228:337, 1975.

169. Pruyn, C. S., Phelan, J. P., and Buchanan, G. C.: Long-term propranalol therapy in pregnancy: Maternal and fetal outcome. Am. J. Obstet. Gynecol. 135:485, 1979.

170. Okita, G. T., Plotz, E. J., and Davis, M. E.: Placental transfer of radioactive digitoxin in pregnant women and its fetal distribution. Circ. Res. 4:376, 1956.

171. Rogers, M. C., Willerson, J. T., Goldblatt, A., and Smith, T. W.: Serum digoxin concentrations in the human fetus, neonate and infant. N. Engl. J. Med. 287:1010, 1972.

172. Norris, P. R.: The action of cardiac glycosides on the human uterus. J. Obstet. Gynecol. Br. Comm. 68:916, 1961.

173. Rudolph, A. M.: Effects of aspirin and acetaminophen in pregnancy and in the newborn. Arch. Intern. Med. 141:358, 1981.

174. Leonard, R. F., Braun, T. E., and Levy, A. M.: Initiation of uterine contractions by disopyramide during pregnancy. N. Engl. J. Med. 299:84, 1978.

54 RELATIONSHIP BETWEEN DISEASES OF THE HEART AND LUNGS

by E. Regis McFadden, Jr., M.D., and Roland H. Ingram, Jr., M.D.

Because of the integrated nature of the function of the heart and lungs, it is difficult for one component to be compromised without altering the physiology of the other. In fact, with chronic disease originating in either the heart or the lungs, there is both subjective and objective evidence of dysfunction in both systems. While a great deal is known about right ventricular hypertrophy or dilatation secondary to lung disease (e.g., cor pulmonale, Chapter 46) and pulmonary malfunction in acute left ventricular failure (e.g., pulmonary edema, Chapter 17), many other pathophysiological interfaces between the cardiovascular and pulmonary systems exist clinically. The purposes of this chapter are to explore these interactions and to detail their mechanisms as far as they are known.

MECHANISMS BY WHICH HEART DISEASE LEADS TO LUNG DYSFUNCTION

Cardiac disease can alter lung function or induce pulmonary disease through the effects of (1) pulmonary venous hypertension from elevated left ventricular end-diastolic and/or left atrial pressures[1-15]; (2) compression of mediastinal structures, airways, or lung by global cardiomegaly, pericardial and pleural effusions, and specific chamber enlargement[16-20]; (3) pharmacological agents used to treat cardiac disease, such as beta antagonists, diuretics, nitrates, and others[21-26]; and (4) miscellaneous phenomena such as hemoptysis due to cardiac disease giving rise to

blood pneumonias. Of these, the most important factor is pulmonary venous hypertension.

Increased Pulmonary Venous Pressure

Physiologically significant increases in left ventricular end-diastolic or left atrial pressures are invariably transmitted retrogradely to the pulmonary vasculature and, in addition to producing pulmonary arterial hypertension, evoke one or more of the stages of pulmonary edema formation, i.e., increased lymph flow, interstitial edema, or alveolar edema (Chapter 17). The magnitude and duration of the pulmonary venous hypertension then determines the extent to which the lung is affected. If the changes in pressure are acute and modest in degree, then vascular engorgement and perivascular and interstitial edema predominate. In these circumstances the effects on the lung tend to be subtle. If the venous pressure changes are chronic, then the changes in lung function are more easily measured because, in addition to the above, anatomical changes such as fibrosis, medial hypertrophy, and intimal thickening may develop in the arteries and veins, airways narrow from peribronchiolar and mucosal edema, and the interstitial edema within the parenchyma may eventually be replaced by fibrosis.[27,28] In rare instances, the last can be so severe that dense calcification and actual bone formation can develop.[29] Thus, it is not possible to elevate pulmonary venous pressures without altering lung function. The *lung* is the organ that undergoes the anatomical and physiological disturbances responsible for dyspnea, chest tightness, and cough.

ALTERATIONS IN PULMONARY MECHANICS.
From a mechanical standpoint, patients with chronically elevated pulmonary venous pressure can be characterized as having "restrictive ventilatory defects," i.e., loss of lung volume. Typically, vital capacity is reduced, residual volume and functional residual capacity are normal or nearly so, and total lung capacity is less than predicted.[6–10,30,31] The reduction in total lung capacity results from replacement of the air in the lung with either blood or interstitial fluid, with resulting changes in the elastic properties of the pulmonary parenchyma. As pulmonary venous hypertension (hence, interstitial and alveolar wall edema) advances, the lung becomes stiffer or less compliant. As this process worsens, air trapping can occur because of earlier than normal closure of dependent airways, and residual volume may actually increase as total lung capacity decreases.[5]

The progressive changes in lung size and recoil tend to increase the pleural pressures required to efffect respiration, thus elevating the work of breathing[8] and thereby leading to tachypnea with a low tidal volume and high respiratory frequency (Fig. 15–2. p. 493).[32]

In addition to volume loss, there is evidence that pulmonary vascular congestion and edema can interfere with peripheral airway function.[5,33–39] Studies in animals have shown that the resistance in distal airways increases to a greater degree in response to elevations of left atrial pressure than does total airway resistance and that with sustained increases of pressure pulmonary changes are slow to resolve. These findings suggest that engorgement of the blood vessels within the confines of the bronchovascular sheath can encroach upon the lumina of the airways and promote edema formation, which can persist for considerable periods. Such observations provide the basis for understanding disturbances in ventilation-perfusion relationships that can often be profound in pulmonary congestion or edema.

ALTERATIONS IN THE DISTRIBUTION OF VENTILATION AND PERFUSION.
The mechanical factor that determines the distribution of ventilation within the lung is the product of the resistance of the bronchi and the compliance of the alveolar units subtended to them. This product is called a time constant ($R \times C = \tau$), and in the normal lung the regional values for τ are nearly equal so that all the alveoli fill and empty synchronously when respiration is initiated at functional residual capacity.[40] However, because of the above derangements in compliance and resistance, in heart disease inter- and intraregional nonhomogeneities develop and result in maldistribution of inspired air. Regional alveolar hypoxia then ensues with its attendant sequelae.[41] The maldistribution becomes more severe with increases in respiratory frequency,[41,42] thus the exercise performance of affected patients is also altered.

The disease in the pulmonary vessels gives rise to abnormal distribution of perfusion, with a reversal of the normal apex-to-base gradient (Fig. 46–5, p. 1576), i.e., the apical lung zones are perfused more than the basilar lung zones.[11–15] The extent of reversal correlates well with increases in pulmonary capillary wedge pressure.[11,12,14] Although there is evidence that the arterioles in the basilar zones of the lung are more responsive to hypoxia than are their apical counterparts in normal subjects,[43] breathing 100 per cent oxygen in mitral stenosis does not completely correct the abnormal distribution of blood flow,[44] suggesting that hypoxic vasoconstriction is not the sole cause for the reversed flow pattern. Acute perivascular edema probably accounts for some of the changes in the flow pattern, but, in chronic pulmonary venous hypertension, structural vascular alterations develop (p. 829) and play a prominent role. These pathological changes tend to be more severe in the basilar zones.[44,45] The overall physiological consequences of all these abnormalities are mismatched ventilation-perfusion relationships that result in widened alveolar-arterial differences for oxygen, arterial hypoxemia, and enlarged dead space-tidal volume ratios.[30]

An additional factor often considered to *cause* the reductions in arterial oxygen content and partial pressure seen in heart disease is a depressed partial pressure of oxygen in the mixed venous blood.[46,47] However, for several reasons, consideration of this factor as a cause of arterial hypoxemia leads to circular and nonproductive reasoning. In normal subjects engaging in heavy exercise at sea level while breathing air, the mixed venous oxygen content diminishes to extremely low values, yet the arterial content remains normal. Hence low values for mixed venous oxygen do not a priori cause a lower than normal arterial value. However, when there is abnormal gas exchange in the lung, whether due to ventilation-perfusion abnormalities or shunt, low arterial oxygen contents result in lower mixed venous values at any given oxygen consumption and cardiac output. Basically, then, the values for mixed venous oxygen are the most dependent of the variables affecting heart-lung interrelations and are the result of oxygen transfer in the lung, cardiac output, and peripheral tissue metabolic consumption of oxygen. Therefore, this factor should always be considered as a *consequence* of hypoxemia rather than as a principal cause.

ALTERATIONS IN ARTERIAL BLOOD GASES.
The extent to which arterial blood gases are disturbed depends upon the severity and suddenness of the rise in left-side pressures. In acute pulmonary edema secondary to left ventricular decompensation, gas exchange can be so severely compromised that frank respiratory failure can result. Aberman and Fulop, in a prospective study of 50 consecutive cases of pulmonary edema, demonstrated that, prior to treatment, affected patients as a group had severe hypoxemia and either metabolic or combined metabolic and respiratory acidosis.[48] In this study, 58 per cent of the patients had values for arterial pO_2 that were less than 50 mm Hg, and 83 per cent had acidemia with a pH less than 7.36. Hypoxemia was most severe in the patients with the greatest acidosis. Twenty-three patients had hypocapnia, 12 were eucapnic, and 11 had arterial CO_2 tensions in excess of 45 mm Hg. The hypercapnic patients did not have a greater incidence of underlying chronic airway obstruction than those without CO_2 retention. The arterial CO_2 tensions and pH rapidly returned to normal, with resolution of alveolar hypoventilation resulting from alveolar flooding and interstitial edema, and with the disappearance of the lactic acidosis secondary to the low cardiac output state.

RESPIRATORY RESPONSE TO EXERCISE.
The abnormalities in mechanics and gas-exchanging function of the lung described thus far are related to the degree and chronicity of the elevated pulmonary capillary pressures.

Since there are further increases in pulmonary venous hypertension with exercise in congestive heart failure, one would anticipate that the degree of pulmonary dysfunction would increase in direct proportion to the degree of acute change.[49]

With physical exertion in patients with pulmonary venous hypertension, left atrial and pulmonary artery pressures rise, causing transudation of fluid from the intravascular space so that pulmonary extravascular fluid volume increases.[4] Concomitantly, the lung becomes stiffer, and the work of breathing and resistance to air flow greatly increase.[50,51] Presumably as a result of these factors, these patients ventilate at higher frequencies for any given level of oxygen consumption, so the ventilation equivalent $\dot{V}_E/VO_2$ is abnormal,[52] and maximal oxygen uptakes reduced.[53] Some studies have demonstrated that dead space ventilation in patients with mitral stenosis is greater both at rest and with exercise than in normal subjects.[30,54]

The effects of exercise on arterial O_2 tensions in patients with pulmonary venous hypertension are inconsistent. Some investigators have noted decreases,[55] while others have reported no change.[52] These discrepancies result in part from the fact that a change in pulmonary blood flow distribution occurs that could possibly offset the effect of an increase in wasted ventilation with exercise. The previously described resting reversal of the normal pulmonary blood flow distribution pattern can return toward normal during physical exertion in some patients, resulting in relative increases in basilar perfusion.[56] Under these circumstances one would expect to find an improvement in gas exchange to the extent that basilar lung units are ventilated. Despite the above derangements, exercise limitations per se in patients with congestive heart failure or mitral stenosis do not appear to be related simply to the level of the pulmonary venous pressure that is reached. Rather, it seems that a complex interaction of respiratory, cardiac, and peripheral mechanisms is involved.

INTRATHORACIC SPACE-OCCUPYING EFFECTS

Heart disease can alter lung function or produce pulmonary symptoms directly, by compression of mediastinal structures such as the trachea, major bronchi, and esophagus, and indirectly, through the effects of pleural effusions. Partial obstruction of the esophagus can occasionally interfere with deglutition and give rise to aspiration pneumonias. The consequences of compressive effects of major airways are much more severe in infants, compared with older children and adults.

In infants, vascular abnormalities such as vascular ring (p. 1013) can produce tracheal obstruction with dyspnea, wheezing, use of accessory muscles of respiration, and a crowing stridor on both inspiration and expiration.[16] There is commonly a history of recurrent pulmonary infections and the condition is frequently misdiagnosed as croup, bronchitis, or asthma. Bronchial obstruction may occur as a result of any cardiac condition in which there is a large left-to-right shunt, but it is most commonly due to a ventricular septal defect or to a large patent ductus arteriosus.[17,18] Also, any condition associated with massive cardiomegaly, particularly a greatly enlarged left atrium, as occurs in some patients with severe mitral regurgitation (p. 1083), may compress the bronchi. With large left-to-right shunts, the dilated pulmonary artery and the distended left atrium can cause atelectasis or hyperinflation, depending upon the degree of obstruction.[17] Sites of predilection are the left main, left upper, and right middle lobe bronchi.[17] With massive cardiomegaly, the left main bronchus may be completely obstructed, with resulting atelectasis of the left lung.[17]

Because the magnitude of the left-to-right shunt is limited by the high pulmonary vascular resistance in the neonatal period, bronchial obstruction from this mechanism is rare in this age period. The peak

incidence of bronchial obstruction occurs between two and nine months of age when pulmonary artery pressure tends to rise. Other cardiac abnormalities that cause compression of major airways via large pulmonary arteries and distended left atria, with or without left ventricular decompensation, are anomalous pulmonary venous drainage, cor triatriatum, and left atrial obstruction due to a supravalvular mitral ring or congenital mitral stenosis.[19] In adults it has long been recognized that massive cardiomegaly or pericardial effusions can compress the left lower lobe and so give rise to Ewart's sign (dullness, bronchial breathing, and increased tactile fremitus near the angle of the scapula). Hypoventilation of the entire left lung has also been reported.

Lung function in patients with pleural effusion has not been extensively studied, but the available data suggest that effusions, if large enough, can act as space-occupying lesions that limit lung volume and gas exchange.[57,58] In pleuritis regional lung function deteriorates as the result of resolved pleural effusions. Both blood flow and ventilation are shifted away from the lung base on the involved side.[59]

EFFECTS ON LUNG FUNCTION OF DRUGS USED TO TREAT HEART DISEASE

Of all the agents in use for the treatment of cardiac disease, the ones that have received the most attention for their potentially harmful pulmonary effects are the beta-antagonists. While there is no doubt that beta-adrenergic receptor blockade in asthmatic subjects may cause precipitous and prolonged airway narrowing and an increased sensitivity of the tracheobronchial tree to other constrictor stimuli,[21,60,61] responses in normal subjects and in patients with other forms of obstructive airway disease have been conflicting. Recent evidence based upon an extensive evaluation of the pressure-flow-volume interrelationships of the lung demonstrates that the intravenous administration of 20 mg of propranolol is entirely innocuous in normal subjects.[62] This is not true in patients with hay fever or chronic obstructive lung disease.

For reasons not completely understood, some patients with chronic bronchitis are hyperresponsive to constrictor stimuli and, when given beta blockers, develop severe bronchoconstriction.[61,63,64] Similarly, asymptomatic nonasthmatic first-degree relatives of asthmatics and individuals with atopic histories but without asthma may behave similarly.[61] These effects are also seen with agents purported to be more selective beta blockers. Unfortunately, in the doses required for treatment of angina in the majority of patients, the so-called cardioselective beta blockers (beta$_1$) produce sufficient beta$_2$ blockade that bronchoconstriction may still be a troublesome side effect in susceptible patients. Thus, the advantages of the "cardioselective" beta blockers exist only when very small doses of these agents are employed.

Beta-adrenergic blockers, in addition to producing acute bronchospasm in asthmatics, have also been found to worsen airway function in individuals with nonspecific chronic obstructive lung disease.[63-65] In fact, even small quantities of these drugs absorbed from remote sites can have adverse effects; for example, the conjunctival instillation of timolol has been reported to worsen lung function in susceptible individuals.[65] Therefore, these drugs should be used with care, and careful pulmonary and allergic histories should be routinely sought before one prescribes these agents. The *calcium-channel blocking agents* have not been shown to have any adverse pulmonary effects.[66] Hence, these drugs may be the treatment of choice for myocardial ischemia in patients with coexisting primary airway disease who otherwise would receive beta blockers.

Sodium nitroprusside, nitroglycerin, dopamine, and *hydralazine* can all have adverse effects on gas exchange in patients with left-sided heart disease.[23,25,67-69] These agents have been shown to cause a fall in arterial oxygen tension despite improving cardiac hemodynamics. Usually, the depression in O_2 is modest ($\leq$ 10 mm Hg) and is believed to be secondary to alterations in ventilation-perfusion relationships, i.e., it is caused by improved perfusion of poorly ventilated alveoli.

Compensatory alveolar hypoventilation with CO_2 retention has been reported to occur rarely in patients with cardiac disease who have developed severe metabolic alkalosis secondary to diuretics that increase potassium excretion.[70] Severe H^+ and Cl^- depletion, together with dehydration, appears to be responsible.

The effects of therapeutic doses of morphine on lung function are controversial. Some authors have warned against the use of this drug in patients with myocardial infarction or acute pulmonary edema because of its tendency to interfere with gas exchange by ventilatory depression.[71] While there is little doubt that this does occur in some individuals, it has been shown that 15 mg of morphine administered by intramuscular injection are well tolerated in both groups of patients.[24,72] Arterial pO_2 falls 2 to 3 mm Hg and CO_2 increases 4 to 5 mm Hg within an hour of receiving an intramuscular injection.[24,72] However, it should be noted that the respiratory depression produced by morphine may be potentiated by lidocaine, and the adverse effects of morphine on gas exchange in patients with preexisting chronic obstructive lung disease who develop an acute myocardial infarction can be dramatic.

PULMONARY EFFECTS SECONDARY TO SPECIFIC CARDIAC DISORDERS

MITRAL STENOSIS AND CONGESTIVE HEART FAILURE

In view of the similarity of the effects of mitral stenosis and left ventricular failure on pulmonary vascular pressures, they are discussed together. Because much of the general information regarding the pulmonary alterations in these conditions is presented elsewhere (pp. 492 and 1066), this section will focus primarily on the degree and kinds of lung dysfunction that occur in relation to the functional cardiac classification.[30,31]

When the underlying condition is mild with no limitation on ordinary activity (Class I), then, generally speaking, lung function tends to be relatively normal at rest (Figs. 54–1 and 54–2). Vital capacity may be slightly reduced and the alveolar-arterial gradient for O_2 may be increased. As the disease process worsens, and the patient's symptomatic disability increases, virtually all aspects of lung function deteriorate. Vital capacity, forced expiratory flow rates and volumes, maximum breathing capacity, dynamic compliance, resting diffusing capacities, and arterial oxygen tensions all fall progressively, while airway resistance and alveolar-arterial gradients for O_2 rise.[30,31] These measurements correlate well with the increase in pulmonary artery pressure and pulmonary vascular resistance.

Patients with Class IV disability generally have severely compromised lung function.[72a] Mean values for vital capacity are 60 to 70 per cent of predicted values, while flow rates in the midvital capacity tend to be around 30 per cent of expected normal. Diffusing capacity tends to be abnormally low and about one-half that observed in Class I, while dynamic compliance is severely reduced, being only one-third of its previous value. Arterial oxygen tensions range between 58 and 75 mm Hg (normal = 95 ± 5 mm Hg), and the alveolar-arterial gradients for O_2 lie between 30 and 41 mm Hg (normal ≤ 20 mm Hg).

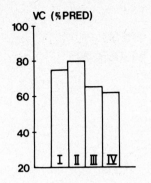

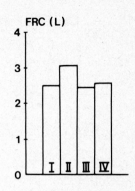

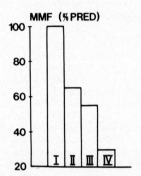

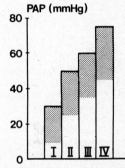

FIGURE 54–1 Alterations in pulmonary mechanics and pulmonary artery pressures observed in the various clinical stages of mitral stenosis. The heights of the bars represent mean values. VC = vital capacity; FRC = functional residual capacity; MMF = maximum midexpiratory flow rate; PAP = pulmonary artery pressure. In the PAP graph the top of the shaded area represents the systolic pressure and the bottom, the diastolic pressure. Roman numerals represent stages of increasing clinical disability. (Data redrawn from Palmer, W. H., et al.: Disturbances of pulmonary function in mitral valve disease. Canad. Med. Assoc. J. *89*:744, 1963.)

The changes in dynamic compliance (i.e., compliance measured during tidal respiration) vary inversely with pulmonary capillary wedge pressures.[9,10] When compliance is normal at rest, as it tends to be in patients with Class I and II disability, pulmonary wedge pressure tends to be normal; as wedge pressure rises with progression of the disease, or with exercise, dynamic compliance falls (Fig. 54–3).

Measurements of the static pressure-volume (recoil) properties have shown that the lungs of patients with mitral stenosis are altered in a distinct manner.[7,73] As can be seen in Figure 54–4*A*, elastic recoil is increased at high lung volumes, is normal at functional residual capacity, and then becomes abnormally low as residual volume is

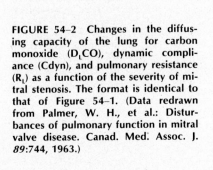

FIGURE 54–2 Changes in the diffusing capacity of the lung for carbon monoxide (D_LCO), dynamic compliance (Cdyn), and pulmonary resistance (R_L) as a function of the severity of mitral stenosis. The format is identical to that of Figure 54–1. (Data redrawn from Palmer, W. H., et al.: Disturbances of pulmonary function in mitral valve disease. Canad. Med. Assoc. J. *89*:744, 1963.)

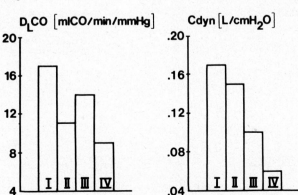

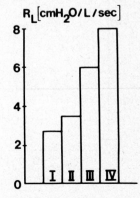

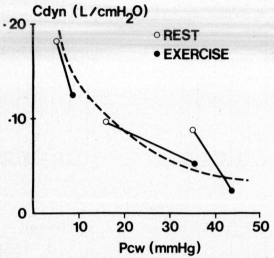

FIGURE 54-3 Relationships between pulmonary capillary wedge pressure (Pcw) and dynamic compliance (Cdyn) in patients with pulmonary venous hypertension. The dashed line is a schematic representation of the overall relationship. (Data from Saxton, G. A., Jr., et al.: The relationship of pulmonary compliance to pulmonary vascular pressures in patients with heart disease. J. Clin. Invest. *35*:611, 1965, and White, H. C., et al.: Lung compliance in patients with mitral stenosis. Clin. Sci. *17*:667, 1958.) The three sets of data points demonstrate the effects on dynamic compliance of acutely increasing pulmonary capillary wedge pressure with exercise. (Data from Saxton, G. A., Jr., et al., as cited.)

approached. This is unlike the situation seen in either atrial septal defect or pulmonary fibrosis (Fig. 54-4*B*). It has been suggested that vascular plethora accounts for the loss of recoil at small lung volumes and that pulmonary fibrosis produces the increased retractive forces at the larger volumes. Regardless of the mechanism involved, this type of change in elastic properties helps to explain why functional residual capacity and residual volume can remain normal in the presence of a reduced total lung capacity. In the case of functional residual capacity, the resting mechanical balance of the respiratory system, set by the tendency of the lung to recoil and the chest wall to spring outward, appears intact. With respect to residual volume, it can be seen that two forces (airway compression from

engorgement or edema of the vascular sheath and loss of recoil with resultant loss of radial traction of the airways) combine to promote early airway closure with air trapping.[5] In addition to these functional abnormalities it has been suggested that there is a disturbance of respiratory muscle function in patients with mitral valve disease.[73]

Collins and colleagues evaluated airway function in 72 patients with left-sided valvular and ischemic heart disease who were free of symptoms and demonstrated that, as a group, these individuals had lower values for standard spirometric indices (forced vital capacity [FVC] and one-second forced expiratory volumes [FEV$_1$]) than did healthy subjects. These findings were taken as evidence of airway obstruction, but the FEV$_1$/FVC ratio averaged 0.75. This value is within normal limits for a population of this age and implies that the lungs were emptying normally but from a lower volume. The significance of these findings is that they are consistent with the observations of the Framingham study[74] that reductions in vital capacity can predict the development of congestive heart failure. In 5209 persons evaluated over an 18-year period, the risk of congestive heart failure varied in inverse proportion to vital capacity. Both a persistently low and a recent fall in vital capacity were associated with increased risk. Among persons with ischemic heart disease, hypertension, or rheumatic heart disease, chances of developing congestive failure were doubled in men and tripled in women with low vital capacities. It is possible that a reduction of vital capacity is not a "risk factor" for heart failure in the classic sense that cigarette smoking is a risk factor for ischemic heart disease, but actually represents a manifestation of heart failure that is not otherwise evident clinically.

MYOCARDIAL INFARCTION (See also page 1276)

Arterial hypoxemia and abnormalities in regional ventilation-perfusion relations and pulmonary mechanics regularly occur in patients with acute myocardial infarction and unstable angina as well as in experimentally provoked coronary insufficiency.[34–39,75–77] The sequence of events is believed to be left ventricular dysfunction from either left ventricular failure and/or a reduction in ventricular com-

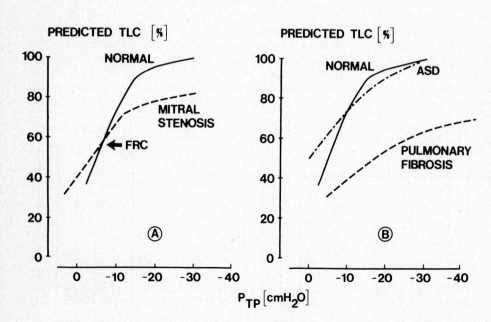

FIGURE 54-4 Comparison of the static pressure-volume relationships of the lung in normal subjects and in patients with (*A*) mitral stenosis and (*B*) atrial septal defects (ASD) and pulmonary fibrosis. TLC = total lung capacity; P$_{TP}$ = transpulmonary pressure; FRC = functional residual capacity. (Data redrawn from Wood, T. E., et al.: Mechanics of breathing in mitral stenosis. Am. Rev. Resp. Dis. *104*:52, 1971.)

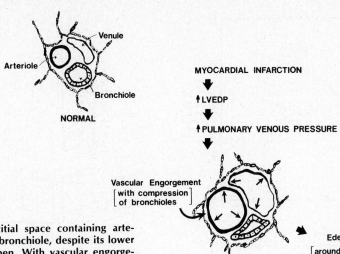

FIGURE 54–5 Normally the loose interstitial space containing arterioles, venules, and bronchioles allows the bronchiole, despite its lower intraluminal pressure, to remain widely open. With vascular engorgement, the dilated venules and arterioles compress the bronchiole, causing an increase in the resistance of these airways. With interstitial edema, the lumina of all structures are compromised.

pliance, leading to acute elevations in end-diastolic pressure with subsequent development of pulmonary vascular congestion and edema that lasts for hours or up to two days in uncomplicated cases. With the onset of edema, the arterioles and bronchioles become compressed, causing the pathogenetic sequence discussed earlier. As this occurs, there is widespread closure of dependent airways with resultant arterial hypoxemia[39,75] (Fig. 54–5). Several studies have demonstrated that after a myocardial infarction or during an episode of prolonged myocardial ischemia, the lung volume at which airway closure begins can encroach upon, or even exceed, functional residual capacity.[39,75] Therefore, during normal respiration, some alveoli are not ventilated and act as anatomical shunts. More severe elevation of pulmonary capillary pressure results in alveolar flooding (Chap. 17).

In addition to alterations in gas exchange, myocardial ischemia and/or infarction may cause acute elevations in airway resistance and reductions in pulmonary compliance[36,37] (Figs. 54–6 and 54–7). A schematic representation of the pulmonary consequences of vascular engorgement, interstitial edema, and alveolar flooding is contained in Figure 54–8. Many patients with coronary artery disease are cigarette smokers and frequently show the changes in pulmonary function resulting therefrom, including elevated residual volume, reduced air flow rates, and increasingly abnormal dynamic compliance with increasing respiratory frequency. In most patients with acute myocardial ischemia it is difficult to distinguish between the various causes of impaired lung function, but the contribution of acute myocardial ischemia can be assessed by repeating the measurements after the cessation of the acute episode and return of the hemodynamics to the baseline state. It is also difficult to determine whether the changes in mechanics and gas exchange are secondary to left ventricular dysfunction or to other factors, such as smoking. One method is to observe whether acute improvement follows the administration of diuretics.[75]

CONGENITAL HEART DISEASE

It is convenient to discuss congenital heart disease in terms of the effects of left-to-right and right-to-left intracardiac shunts on pulmo-

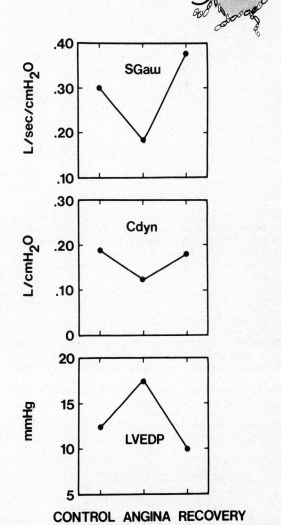

CONTROL ANGINA RECOVERY

FIGURE 54–6 Interrelationships between heart and lung function during induced myocardial ischemia. SGaw = specific conductance (the reciprocal of airway resistance corrected for the volume at which it was measured); Cdyn = dynamic compliance; LVEDP = left ventricular end-diastolic pressure. The data points are mean values during a control period (left), during the induction of angina (center), and during recovery (right). (Data redrawn from Pepine, C. J., and Wiener, L.: Relationship of anginal symptoms to lung mechanisms during myocardial ischemia. Circulation 46:863, 1972, by permission of the American Heart Association, Inc.)

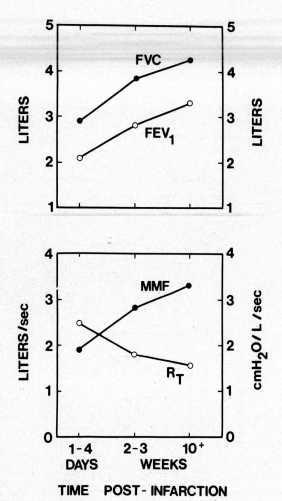

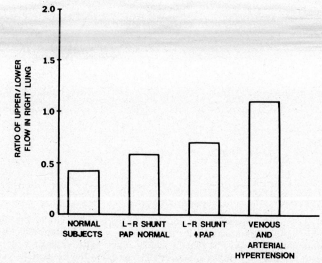

FIGURE 54–9 Alterations in regional pulmonary blood flow in patients with congenital heart disease. PAP = pulmonary artery pressure. (Redrawn from Friedman, W. F., Braunwald, E., and Morrow, A. G.: Alterations in regional pulmonary blood flow in patients with congenital heart disease studied by radioisotope scanning. Circulation *37*:747, 1968, by permission of the American Heart Association, Inc.)

TIME POST- INFARCTION

FIGURE 54–7 Changes in pulmonary mechanics observed at various times following an acute myocardial infarction. FVC = forced vital capacity; FEV_1 = one-second forced expiratory volume; MMF = maximum midexpiratory flow rates; R_T = total respiratory resistance. (Data redrawn from Interiano, B., et al.: Interrelation between alterations in pulmonary mechanics and hemodynamics in acute myocardial infarction. J. Clin. Invest. *52*:1994, 1973.)

nary blood flow from atrial septal defects are more extensive and can be related to the level of pulmonary hypertension.[81] In those patients in whom the mean pulmonary artery pressure is normal, the only change observed is an increase in diffusing capacity. Thus when pulmonary blood flow is abnormally high but vascular pressures are normal, pulmonary mechanics are normal. However, when both blood flow and pressures are increased, lung function deteriorates. Consequently, in those patients with modest pulmonary hypertension, there is an overt decrease in maximum expiratory flows at all lung volumes and some reduction in static compliance, in addition to the increased diffusing capacity (Fig. 54–4*B*). However, when pulmonary hypertension becomes severe, air flow rates are markedly depressed, elastic recoil and lung volumes are sharply reduced, airway resistance is elevated, and diffusing capacity becomes normal.

Alterations in regional pulmonary blood flow have been recorded in patients with both atrial and ventricular septal defects.[82,83] Typically, abnormalities characterized by increased pulmonary blood flow or elevated pulmonary arterial pressures, or both, increase the ratio of pulmonary blood flow in the lung apices relative to that in the dependent lung zones (Fig. 54–9). Studies of regional lung function in patients with ventricular septal defect have demonstrated mildly abnormal ventilation-perfusion relationships. Ventilation to the left lung tends to be depressed slightly while perfusion is slightly increased.[83] These changes improve with closure of the defect.

Patients with right-to-left intracardiac shunts tend to have normal pulmonary mechanics.[84] However, there are abnormalities in regional lung function and ventilatory control mechanisms.[85,86] Individuals with tetralogy of Fallot have been reported to have a high incidence of hyperperfusion of one lung relative to the other.[85] The significance of this observation with respect to regional gas exchange has not been evaluated, but it is known that children with this condition lack carotid body sensitivity to arterial hypoxemia.[86] As a result, the superimposition of alveolar hypoxia from lung disease or anesthesia may threaten life by aggravating systemic hypoxia to intolerable levels. The mechanism responsible for the blunting of the ventilatory responses to hypoxia in patients with congenital cyanotic heart disease is not clear, but recent evidence suggests it may represent an acquired adaptation to prolonged hypoxemia, because the defect disappears with surgical correction of the cardiac abnormalities.[86]

nary function. Frequently, signs of obstructive lung disease such as wheezing, use of accessory muscles of respiration, hyperinflation, and lobar emphysema will dominate the clinical course of infants with ventricular septal defects and large left-to-right shunts (p. 963).[78,79] The airway obstruction in these patients can be due to compression of airways by enlarged pulmonary arteries or cardiac chambers, and to an increase in small airway resistance as the result of accumulation of peribronchiolar fluid. Pulmonary compliance is also decreased.[80]

Infants with atrial septal defects have also been reported to have low values for dynamic compliance.[80] However, in older children and adults the respiratory consequences of a chronic increase in pulmo-

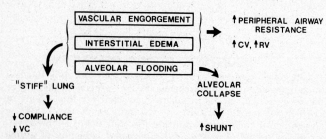

FIGURE 54–8 The functional alterations resulting from vascular engorgement, interstitial edema, and alveolar flooding are shown schematically.

CARDIOGENIC SHOCK (See page 583)

As noted previously, respiratory insufficiency with abnormal gas exchange frequently develops in conjunction with acute myocardial infarction or pulmonary edema. Usually the mechanisms are related to

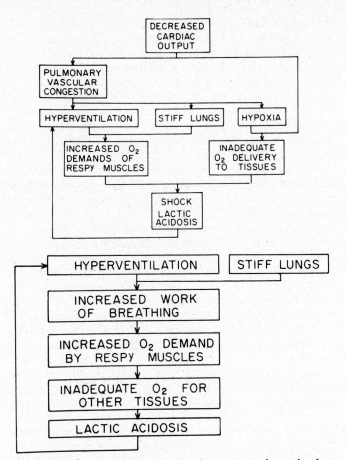

FIGURE 54–10 *Top,* Schema showing how oxygen demands of respiratory muscles can contribute to cardiogenic shock in the face of decreased cardiac output. *Bottom,* Vicious circle whereby hyperventilation and increased work of breathing contribute to O_2 lack and lactic acidosis, which in turn further increases ventilation and respiratory work. (From Macklem, P. T.: Respiratory muscles: The vital pump. Chest *78*:753, 1980.)

alterations in ventilation-perfusion relationships from interstitial edema and alveolar flooding, but new evidence suggests that other factors may also play a role.[87] In situations in which the cardiac output is low, the work of breathing increases substantially because of the hyperventilation induced by hypoxemia and acidemia and because of the mechanical alterations secondary to pulmonary vascular congestion. However, despite the increase in energy demands and expenditure, the blood supply to the respiratory muscles may be reduced because of the very low cardiac output, thus limiting their perfusion. Respiratory muscle fatigue may then occur, leading to respiratory failure. This train of events is shown schematically in Figure 54–10.

CARDINAL MANIFESTATIONS OF HEART VERSUS LUNG DISEASE

Because of the functional interrelations of the heart and lungs, it is not surprising that the cardinal symptoms of heart and lung disease are similar: dyspnea, cough, chest pain, and hemoptysis. It is likely that cough and dyspnea appear only with lung dysfunction, whether it is primary or solely secondary to cardiac dysfunction. Hence, their etiology cannot be clearly distinguished in many instances. In contrast, chest pain and hemoptysis have features characteristic enough to provide a better idea of the primary process.

DYSPNEA (See also pp. 4 and 493)

It is frequently difficult to differentiate cardiac from pulmonary causes of dyspnea.[72a,87a] In actual practice the major functional classifications of patients with either heart or lung disease are based largely upon the degree of exertion necessary to produce breathlessness (p. 12). Such classifications provide no differentiation between primary heart and lung disease. Furthermore, they cannot be rigidly applied as quantitators of disease in either system. For example, a conditioned athlete who begins to develop dyspnea during previously tolerated activity may have a more serious disturbance than a sedentary person who complains of greater breathlessness with much less exertion. On the other hand, other diseases, such as musculoskeletal disorders, may prevent a level of activity that would be necessary to produce dyspnea.

Lest all appear hopeless, in most patients the cause of dyspnea can usually be clearly identified. Thus, a patient with systemic hypertension, an enlarged left ventricle, an S_3 gallop, and bilateral inspiratory rales should not present a problem in identification of left ventricular failure as the cause of dyspnea. In like manner, a long-term smoker with chronic bronchitis, a normal cardiac silhouette, severe hyperinflation, and airway obstruction undoubtedly has sufficient lung disease to account for the shortness of breath. Any number of such clear-cut examples could be cited by a physician with only limited clinical experience.

However, an overweight, middle-aged, male cigarette smoker, with mild chronic bronchitis and mild systemic hypertension, who begins to complain of dyspnea during previously tolerated activity presents a challenging problem. Neither history nor physical examination may reveal sufficient abnormalities to account for symptoms, and laboratory results may be within normal limits. In such an instance complete pulmonary function testing, including arterial blood gas determinations before, during, and after exercise, electrocardiographic stress testing, and cardiac catheterization at rest and during exercise, may be needed in order to identify the process accounting for his exertional dyspnea. Usually, however, such an extensive workup is not necessary and utilization of simple tests and therapeutic trials will suffice.

For example, mild airway obstruction that responds briskly to bronchodilators would justify a trial of sympathomimetic bronchodilators. If this treatment, along with smoking cessation, controlled symptoms, it would seem likely that lung disease predominated. If pulmonary function testing showed no response to the short-term administration of bronchodilators, it would seem reasonable to administer diuretics with or without cardiac glycosides in a therapeutic trial. Regression of symptoms with this treatment would point toward congestive failure as the cause for his complaints. Given the age and risk factors for the patient in question, an electrocardiographic stress test would be reasonable to perform, either before or after the therapeutic trials. If positive, the question would be whether painless myocardial ischemia were leading to transient elevation of left ventricular diastolic pressure during exertion. In the latter instance, pretreatment with nitroglycerin and repeat of the exercise challenge might help to indicate whether myocardial ischemia were accounting for his exertional dyspnea.

Another type of difficulty is presented by the patient with both left ventricular failure and chronic obstructive airway disease who has worsening dyspnea. The question is whether the lung or the heart process or both have worsened. If an endobronchial infection caused worsening of the lung disease with increasing hypoxemia and hypercapnia, cardiac arrhythmias would ensue directly and secondary to lowering of the therapeutic index for digitalis. Attention might then be directed toward the heart disease as the initiating event, when, in fact, respiratory failure secondary to the endobronchial infection was the primary culprit. A history of increased cough and purulent sputum production at the onset of worsening should allow identification of the initiating event. Absence of such a history and minimal increases in arterial pCO_2 would suggest that the heart was the primary offender.

A patient with acute respiratory failure may suffer myocardial infarction with associated electrocardiographic and enzyme changes. This would not necessarily indicate that a primary cardiac process initiated the sequence of events, since an acute myocardial infarction can occur during an episode of respiratory failure. Our experience indicates that acute myocardial infarction is far more common in patients with acute-on-chronic respiratory failure than was previously thought. While both the cardiac and respiratory problems require treatment, the therapeutic situation is fraught with competing rationales. Morphine would be clearly contraindicated from the standpoint of the respiratory failure, but some means of pain and anxiety control is needed for the myocardial infarction. There is no clear answer for this dilemma, unless the patient is already being supported by a mechanical ventilator. Sympathomimetics are clearly indicated for bronchodilation and increased mucociliary clearance, yet may precipitate or worsen dangerous cardiac arrhythmias and increase the area of ischemic injury. Electrocardiographic monitoring is helpful in anticipating and adjusting treatment to correct arrhythmias. Diuretics present a different problem: If left ventricular failure is present, diuretics are indicated; if not, dehydration resulting from diuresis increases sputum viscosity and interferes with bronchopulmonary drainage. Accurate monitoring of pulmonary capillary wedge pressure can aid in making the appropriate therapeutic decision.

Several patterns of *dyspnea* are thought to be more indicative of heart than lung disease; paroxysmal nocturnal dyspnea occurring after a person falls asleep has been considered indicative of left ventricular failure. However, if such paroxysms of dyspnea occur shortly after assumption of the supine posture and are relieved by cough with expectoration of substantial quantities of sputum, it is likely that bronchitis with accumulated secretions rather than heart failure is responsible.

An additional form of paroxysmal nocturnal dyspnea with wheezing occurs in asthmatics and is thought to be related to the lowering of the firing threshold of subepithelial irritant receptors in the tracheobronchial tree.[88] The brisk response of this symptom to inhaled bronchodilators is distinctive.

Orthopnea is another symptom mainly indicating congestive heart failure, yet patients with this symptom frequently have severe chronic airway obstruction rather than primary heart disease. This usually occurs in patients with severe hyperinflation who must use their accessory muscles of respiration. In order for these muscles to assist in breathing, the patient's arms must be braced at his sides. This is apparent on simple inspection and makes it likely that the discomfort experienced in the supine posture is due to the loss of the contribution of the accessory muscles of inspiration. The confusion between a pulmonary and cardiac cause of orthopnea is occasionally compounded by the fact that these patients sit up most of the night and develop dependent edema in the absence of elevations of central venous pressure. A clue to the presence of normal central venous pressure in such patients, indicative of a pulmonary origin, is the brisk collapse of the neck veins during inspiration.

An additional yet rare form of orthopnea is that associated with bilateral diaphragmatic paralysis. In this condition, in the supine posture, there is a paradoxical inward abdominal motion with inspiration, indicating that the weight of the abdominal contents pressing upon the paralyzed diaphragm results in ascent of this structure further into the chest when intrathoracic pressures become negative. The characteristic inward abdominal motion with inspiration and the onset of dyspnea immediately upon assuming the supine posture, along with absence of signs of left ventricular failure or lung disease, usually suffice to suggest this diagnosis.

Cheyne-Stokes respiration (p. 499), a breathing pattern characteristic of left ventricular failure, results in orthopnea and may even awaken the patient from sleep during the hyperpneic phase. This breathing pattern almost never occurs as a consequence of lung disease alone, hence its presence is practically diagnostic of left ventricular failure if there is no central nervous system process to account for it. Occasionally, patients with heart failure who have Cheyne-Stokes respiration may awaken at night during the hyperventilatory phase of their periodic respiration and complain of dyspnea. This phenomenon should be distinguished from paroxysmal nocturnal dyspnea.[89]

Another form of dyspnea that awakens patients from sleep is sleep apnea with arousal. This disorder is caused by cessation of respiratory efforts due to central nervous system causes (central apnea), ineffective respiration because of upper airway obstruction (obstructive apnea), or a combination of both. These disorders can lead to cor pulmonale and are discussed in Chapter 46.

Two uncommon patterns of breathlessness are sufficiently distinct to have received separate designations: trepopnea and platypnea. *Trepopnea* refers to breathlessness that is limited to one lateral decubitus position. Although originally described for heart disease and attributed to distortion of great vessels in one posture versus the other, the symptom also occurs in patients with lung disease; its cause is not clear, but it may be related to the observation that patients with predominantly unilateral lung disease have lower arterial oxygen tensions when they lie in the lateral decubitus position with the more severely affected lung down.[90] *Platypnea* refers to breathlessness that is present only in the upright position and that promptly abates upon assumption of the supine posture.[91,92] It was originally described in severe chronic obstructive lung disease and was attributed to decreased perfusion of Zone 2 (see Fig. 17–4, p. 564) with consequent enlargement of Zone 1 due to increased alveolar pressures. This results in an increase of wasted (dead space) ventilation in the upright posture but no change in arterial pO_2. Platypnea in association with increasing hypoxia has also been described in several cyanotic forms of congenital heart disease[93,94] and has been attributed to a reduction in systemic arterial pressure and venous return, with blood taking the course of least resistance from the right side to the aorta. In the past several years two patients with both heart and lung disease have been shown to exhibit orthostatic hypoxemia and platypnea.[95,96] These patients had the rare combination of pneumonectomy and atrial septal defect. It has been proposed that pressure from the right hydrothorax pressing upon the right atrium increased right atrial pressures, resulting in a larger right-to-left shunt.

CHEST PAIN (See also page 5)

The differentiation between cardiac and pulmonary causes of chest pain is usually easily made. Key diagnostic features are the location, character, and behavior of the pain. Although pleural pain can occur anywhere between the lower neck and lower abdomen because of the many spinal cord segments that innervate the parietal pleura, it is usually easy to distinguish because of its sharp superficial lancinating characteristics and its aggravation by deep inspiration and cough. The pulmonary parenchyma and bronchi are devoid of pain fibers; however, there is often a scratchy and nagging substernal discomfort in association with both acute and chronic bronchitis. This is not of the same character as myocardial pain and should never serve as a source of confusion.

Acute spontaneous pneumomediastinum is a relatively rare condition that produces severe and sudden substernal chest pain that may mimic myocardial infarction or even dissection of the aorta.[91] In addition, like spontaneous pneumothorax, which may coexist, pneumomediastinum is occasionally associated with electrocardiographic abnormalities consisting of vertical axis, poor R-wave progression in the precordial leads, precordial ST-segment elevation, and T-wave inversion.[97-99] Like the pain of pericarditis, it is aggravated by deep breathing, swallowing, and lying down and is relieved by sitting up and leaning forward. Points of differentiation are that acute spontaneous pneumomediastinum occurs almost exclusively in young adults and is commonly accompanied by sore throat and dysphagia.

Recognition of pneumomediastinum depends upon the detection of subcutaneous emphysema, especially in the neck, on physical examination and demonstration of free air within the borders of the mediastinum by chest radiographs. Often the victims of this condition experience a peculiar crunching or crackling sound synchronous with the heart beat (Hamman sign). When this condition is suspected and the diagnostic signs are absent, lateral radiographs of the chest and neck should be obtained. Air between the mediastinal and cervical fascial layers is often seen on lateral films when none of the classic signs are positive.[100]

HEMOPTYSIS

Clinically, the expectoration of blood occurs in one of five ways; the form taken may provide a clue as to wheth-

er the underlying process is primarily from cardiac or pulmonary pathology. For example, pink frothy sputum is pathognomonic of *pulmonary edema.* Deep rust-colored sputum typifies *bacterial pneumonia.* Blood streaked on the surface of mucus is usually associated with *bronchitis,* or bleeding from endobronchial tumors. Dark blood intermixed with sputum to give a "currant jelly" appearance is seen with *pulmonary infarction* and necrotizing pneumonias. Finally, quantities of bright red blood indicate bleeding from enlarged bronchial vessels; this is the form often associated with long-standing *cardiac dysfunction.* Here the differential diagnosis includes bronchiectasis and granulomatous endobronchial and parenchymal disease, such as tuberculosis. Again, as above, the combination of the clinical history, physical examination, and chest radiography should establish the correct diagnosis.

The incidence of a cardiovascular cause has varied from 1.4 to 7 per cent among patients with hemoptysis in several series[101-104]; thus, although a relatively uncommon complication, it is one that is potentially lethal. Well-recognized cardiovascular causes include mitral stenosis and congenital heart disease.[105] In the second category, hemoptysis has been most frequently described in pulmonary vascular obstructive disease, including Eisenmenger syndrome, but it also occurs in patients with pulmonary venous congestion. Generally, the hemoptysis is secondary to bleeding from enlarged tortuous bronchial vessels and thrombotic lesions in the small pulmonary arteries.

An uncommon complication of heart disease is occult pulmonary hemorrhage in patients on anticoagulant therapy.[106] This syndrome is characterized by dyspnea, unexplained acute anemia, and alveolar infiltrates on chest roentgenogram.

COUGH

Cough is perhaps the most common clinical manifestation of primary respiratory disease, and the most frequent initiating stimulus is the presence of secretions in the tracheobronchial tree. When cough is a prominent symptom associated with primary heart disease, it is most often due to some secondary intrabronchial process, such as congestion of mucosal vessels or the presence of secretions or edema. However, as already suggested, bronchial deformation due to cardiac enlargement can stimulate subepithelial irritant receptors and initiate cough that is usually nonproductive. An enlarged left atrium caused by mitral valve disease is a common cause of nonproductive cough, and cough may also be a manifestation of progression of left heart failure. Thus, in the final analysis, there is no reasonable way to assess whether a nonproductive cough is predominantly due to heart versus lung disease when both conditions are present.

ARRHYTHMIAS IN PATIENTS WITH LUNG DISEASE

Arrhythmias occur as frequently in patients with acute respiratory failure complicating the obstructive pulmonary syndromes as in those with acute myocardial infarction.[107-113] A variety of supraventricular arrhythmias, such as paroxysmal supraventricular tachycardia, atrial flutter, multifocal atrial tachycardia, and atrioventricular junctional tachycardia, have been reported. In addition, ventricular arrhythmias such as bigeminy, atrioventricular dissociation, idioventricular rhythm, ventricular tachycardia, and fibrillation have been observed as well. These arrhythmias usually develop in association with episodes of increasing hypoxemia with or without hypercapnia, particularly during sleep. The nocturnal hypoxia that develops in patients with chronic airway obstruction predisposes them to atrial and ventricular arrhythmias.[114] Similar problems occur in patients with sleep apnea; arrhythmias can be prevented or diminished by nocturnal oxygen therapy. Cardiac arrhythmias may also be provoked by reducing arterial CO_2 tension during ventilatory support, particularly in patients with renal compensation for chronic hypercapnia.[109]

The precise cause of the arrhythmias is not known. It has been suggested that the severe hypoxemia, hypercapnia, and changes in pH common in respiratory failure alter the automaticity of the cardiac conducting tissue or permit the development of reentry circuits. Other factors, such as the catecholamines, theophylline, glucocorticoids, and diuretics used to treat the respiratory symptoms and right heart failure, alone or in combination with the blood gas abnormalities, can also reduce electrical stability either directly or secondarily through their effects on cellular ion transport. In addition some evidence indicates that the sinus node may be damaged in patients with cor pulmonale.[115]

Although the use of cardiac glycosides to control atrial arrhythmias is well established, their role in the treatment of cor pulmonale is ambiguous and controversial. A review of the literature suggests that patients with pulmonary disease may be more susceptible to the toxic effects of cardiac glycosides than patients without primary airway or parenchymal disease (p. 521).[116] However, few studies correlating the effects of digitalis with pulmonary status have characterized the type of respiratory illness present or controlled for concurrent unrelated left ventricular disease. Thus, our current state of knowledge suggests that digitalis be used with caution in patients with respiratory failure; to minimize the risk of toxicity, the specific therapeutic goal should be defined as clearly as possible. Frequent observation and regulation of dosage must be undertaken.

CARDIAC EFFECTS OF DRUGS AND OTHER MODALITIES USED TO TREAT LUNG DISORDERS

Of the various agents currently in use in the treatment of obstructive lung disease, only two classes (adrenergic stimulants and methylxanthines) have significant cardiovascular effects.

ADRENERGIC STIMULANTS

This class of compounds consists of catecholamines (norepinephrine, epinephrine, isoproterenol, and isoetharine), resorcinols (metaproterenol and terbutaline), saligenins (albuterol), and ephedrine which act through stimulation of adrenergic receptors.[117] In 1948, Ahlquist demonstrated that the response to adrenergic drugs appears to be mediated through at least two receptor systems (α and β).[118] Stimulation of α receptors is associated with vasoconstriction, increased uterine activity, and relaxation of

intestinal muscle, while stimulation of the β receptors results in inhibition of smooth muscle contraction in the respiratory tract, uterus, and blood vessels and positive inotropic and chronotropic cardiac stimulation. Later, Lands and colleagues demonstrated that beta-adrenergic effects could be differentiated further into β_1 and β_2: β_1 agonists cause cardiac stimulation and β_2 agonists produce bronchodilatation and vasodilation.[119]

Given this information, one can easily appreciate that the perfect agent in this class would be one with pure β_2 activity. Unfortunately, no such compound exists. However, isoetharine, terbutaline, metaproterenol, and albuterol have more β_2 selectivity than the others.[117]

In isolated cardiac tissues, albuterol and terbutaline are much less active than isoproterenol and metaproterenol. The available data indicate that albuterol has minimal cardiac effects, irrespective of the route of administration, whereas terbutaline by intravenous injection may produce a reflex increase in heart rate secondary to its vasodilator activity. Metaproterenol has little cardiac-sparing effect when given orally, but it is usually well tolerated by inhalation. It is of interest that albuterol has been shown to be useful in the treatment of chronic heart failure presumably by reducing afterload by vasodilatation.[120]

In patients with symptomatic obstructive lung disease coexistent with an ischemic or hypertensive cardiomyopathy, aerosols of selective β_2 agonists such as albuterol can be used with safety, and this is the preferred mode of therapy. We have yet to observe the precipitation of an arrhythmia or worsening of hypertension or angina with albuterol aerosols, although this has occurred with the oral use of such agents. Since only micrograms of these drugs are nebulized and milligrams are ingested, presumably this behavior reflects the substantial differences in the quantity of medication absorbed systemically between the two routes.

A particularly difficult clinical problem is posed by the patient with the combination of reactive airways and severely symptomatic angina with or without arrhythmias. One solution is to employ a β_1 antagonist to control the cardiac symptoms and a β_2 agonist to treat the airways in an effort to avoid the undesirable β_1-induced cardiac stimulation and β_2-blockade–induced bronchoconstriction. A word of caution should be interjected, however; this course of action is not without the potential hazards of excessive cardiac stimulation and bronchoconstriction initially, so that the patient's cardiac and pulmonary status should be carefully monitored until the safety and efficacy of the final dosage of both drugs have been determined. Any change in dose of either agent should also be followed objectively.

Another potential solution is to treat the angina pectoris with a calcium-channel blocker. Although these drugs can attenuate the airway obstruction that follows certain constrictor stimuli in asthmatics,[66] they have no effect on resting airway tone and are not bronchodilators. Hence, should there be an acute exacerbation of airway obstruction, a bronchodilator would be required. It has not yet been determined whether the calcium-channel blocker would protect against any cardiac stimulation that might occur as a consequence of the administration of beta-adrenergic agonists. Further, it is not known how this class of compounds interacts with the effects of sympathomimetics and/or methylxanthines on airway smooth muscle.

The toxicity of *halogenated hydrocarbon propellants* has been extensively studied and it has become clear that these agents are not "inert" as was once believed, but neither do they appear to be potentially fatal in patients with lung disease.[120–124] In experimental animals these compounds can sensitize the myocardium to the arrhythmogenic effects of sympathomimetics, but data from many studies in humans indicate that extremely high levels of these compounds are required.[120–122,125] Hence, it appears that only the most flagrant abuse of pressurized aerosols will result in blood concentrations high enough to have this effect.

METHYLXANTHINES

In general, theophylline is safer than the catecholamines and has been shown to improve the performance of both ventricles in patients with obstructive lung disease.[126] However, it also has potentially serious side effects. Like the catecholamines, methylxanthines increase left ventricular work, and relative myocardial ischemia may be produced even though mild coronary artery dilation may also occur. Because theophylline is typically well tolerated, its potential for abuse is high. Until measurements of serum levels became widely available, aminophylline was usually administered in a fixed amount, and if the desired effect was not forthcoming, the dose was increased until toxic side effects were observed. The hazard of this approach can be readily appreciated, and it is not surprising that aminophylline administration has been implicated as a predisposing factor in 60 per cent of the cases of cardiac arrest in one study involving patients in intensive care units.[127]

The therapeutic range for theophylline lies between 10 and 20 μg/ml, and this can be readily achieved in most patients with an intravenous infusion of aminophylline, 5 to 6 mg/kg. However, there is great variability among patients in the metabolism of this drug and the half-life is markedly prolonged in patients with congestive heart failure, acute pulmonary edema, chronic obstructive lung disease, or liver disease. Thus, therapy must be individualized and frequent assessment of serum concentration is required.

POSITIVE END-EXPIRATORY PRESSURE

It has long been noted that high inflation pressures during mechanical ventilation with or without positive end-expiratory pressure (PEEP) are associated with a fall in blood pressure. Changes in each of the two determinants of blood pressure (cardiac output and peripheral vascular resistance) have been considered to be responsible.

Of the two possible causes, much more attention has appropriately been focused upon the diminution in cardiac output. Several reasons have been proposed for a fall in cardiac output during mechanical ventilation with PEEP, one of which is that the positive airway pressure, with secondary increases in pleural pressure, simply increases the impedance to venous return (p. 435). While this is undoubtedly a contributory factor, a surprising experimental finding was an increase in left-sided filling pressures (mean left atrial and left ventricular end-diastolic).[128] Higher filling pressures and decreased cardiac output indicated an alteration in left ventricular function. With positive intrapleural pressures it was important that cardiac chamber pressures be analyzed in terms of true, transmural (i.e., inside minus outside) distending forces. Earlier experimental studies assumed that intrapleural pressure was a reasonable estimate of the pressure surrounding the heart. Based on this assumption, the following sequence evolved: (1) increases in lung volume with PEEP increase pulmonary vascular resistance; (2) this results in an increase in right ventricular pressures which, in turn, displaces the interventricular septum to encroach upon the left ventricular cavity; (3) left ventricular diastolic filling thus becomes impaired, leading to a smaller end-diastolic volume at higher pressures[129]; (4) the subsequent stroke volume is smaller and contributes to the decrease in cardiac output. Previous considerations of humoral factors that might impair cardiac contractility were eliminated by the appropriate experiments. These experimental results in animals have now been supported by clinical studies.[130] Thus the idea of "ventricular interdependence" as a contributor to diminution in cardiac output and the hypotension seen with PEEP appears to be supported in a clinical setting.

As attractive as these ideas may be, further experimental evidence has been obtained that indicates that pericardial pressures are much greater than pleural pressures, leading to the view that the heart is directly compressed[131,132] by the hyperinflated lung to impair filling without alteration of the left ventricular volume versus transmural pressure relationship. This controversy is not yet settled and may revolve around the validity of any technique to assess pericardial pressure with accuracy. Nonetheless, despite lack of unanimity concerning transmural pressure, it is agreed that diastolic filling of the left ventricle is impaired; thus, stroke volume is diminished with PEEP.

Experimental studies of the decrease in peripheral vascular resistance with lung hyperinflation have suggested that humoral agents are released to account for this finding, but vascularly isolated and perfused limbs and muscles also decrease their resistance. Hence, humoral factors alone cannot account for the hypotension. When the vagus nerves from the lung are interrupted, hyperinflation of the lung no longer results in a diminution in peripheral vascular tone.[133] Thus, a reflex mechanism is also a likely contributor. With regard to the clinical relevance of these experiments, however, the very large alveolar pressures required to produce this change are greater than those likely to be seen during mechanical ventilation.

PREOPERATIVE PULMONARY EVALUATION FOR CARDIAC SURGERY

Although pulmonary complications in the postoperative period are more common in patients with preexisting lung disease,[134] it is not possible to predict the risk precisely based upon preoperative pulmonary function testing. An additional concern arises when pulmonary resection is contemplated. Here the issue is whether sufficient pulmonary reserve will be left following surgery; rather elaborate preoperative assessments have been proposed.[135,136] Despite these recommendations, most surgeons simply observe the patient's tolerance to climb two flights of stairs.

This empirical assessment of integrated heart-lung function clearly has no place in the evaluation of most candidates for cardiac surgery, since such patients usually have sufficient cardiac embarrassment that angina or dyspnea during exercise is a problem that will likely be alleviated by the surgical procedure. Even extensive pulmonary function testing may be of little help, since, as already discussed, the effects of heart disease on pulmonary function can be prominent enough to mimic primary lung disease. This is particularly true in patients with longstanding pulmonary venous hypertension.

The major issues, then, are whether there is coexisting primary lung disease that will not be improved by surgery and whether the lung dysfunction will contribute to the likelihood of postoperative mortality and morbidity. There are no prospective studies to provide guidelines in the resolution of this issue. Usually, however, complete clinical assessment, including pulmonary function testing and blood gas determinations at rest and during exercise, suffices in discovering whether there is coexisting lung disease. For example, marked air trapping, severe hypoxemia, and hypercapnia in a patient at rest point toward primary lung dysfunction. Alternatively, the development, or worsening, of pulmonary mechanical and gas-exchange abnormalities during exercise in a patient with a surgically correctable heart disease, who shows only subtle changes in lung function at rest, implicates heart disease as the primary problem. In the latter circumstance, cardiac surgery would be expected to improve lung function to the extent that cardiac function improved; in the former case, surgery is particularly hazardous.

In general, if there is primary lung disease, pulmonary function testing gives a good quantitative assessment of its severity, and this information has some value in predicting whether a patient is likely to tolerate cardiac surgery. When the vital capacity and flow rates are 80 per cent or more of their predicted values, there is little cause for concern from the point of view of pulmonary function.[137] On the other hand, if the values for these indices fall below 50 per cent of predicted values, the possibility of postoperative respiratory insufficiency and death increases.[137] However, since the approach to postoperative intensive care for the pulmonary complications of cardiac surgery is improving dramatically, it is likely that the risk of cardiac surgery in patients with impaired pulmonary function will diminish in the future.

RESPIRATORY CARE
AFTER CARDIAC SURGERY

The major respiratory problems that arise in the period immediately after cardiac surgery are related to (1) the thoracotomy itself; (2) the use of drugs in the postoperative period; (3) the effects of cardiopulmonary bypass on the lungs; (4) the effects of coexisting morbid processes, such as chronic airway obstruction; and (5) the transitory effects on the heart of the surgical intervention.

Certainly the disruption of the chest wall by either a lateral thoracotomy or a median sternotomy interferes with its movement; a clouded sensorium caused by medications and self-imposed restriction of movement to avoid pain further contribute to impairment of chest wall motion and may lead to atelectasis. Perhaps even more important, the pain, sedatives, and mechanical restriction lead to an impaired coughing mechanism and the patient's reluctance even to try coughing, and as a consequence, secretions accumulate. These problems are often managed by leaving the endotracheal tube in place and providing mechanical ventilatory assistance in the first few postoperative hours. During this time the tracheobronchial tree is periodically suctioned to remove secretions, and sufficient tidal volumes are provided to prevent atelectasis.

Some patients develop the adult respiratory distress syndrome (Chapters 17 and 18), characterized by increasing intrapulmonary shunting, decreasing lung compliance, and diffuse alveolar infiltrates. This syndrome, which may not develop fully until 24 hours after operation, has been attributed to the use of the extracorporeal membrane oxygenator and perfusion pump and has therefore been referred to as "pump lung." Many theories have been proposed regarding the pathogenesis, yet no single factor has been firmly identified. It is our impression that the incidence of this syndrome has diminished in recent years, perhaps related to shorter bypass times. The pathophysiology and management are detailed in Chapter 18.

Extra attention and effort should be directed toward the postoperative management of the patient with chronic obstruction of the airways by using bronchodilators, by encouraging cough, and, when possible, by the application of physical therapy techniques for mobilization of secretions.

References

1. Glauser, F. L., Hoshiko, M., Watanabe, M., and Wilson, A. F.: Physiologic changes associated with increasing pulmonary wedge pressures in the dog. Respiratory 31:459, 1974.
2. Gump, F. E., Zikria, B. A., and Mashima, Y.: The effect of interstitial edema on pulmonary function in the dog. J. Trauma 12:764, 1972.
3. Hauge, A., Bφ, G., and Waaler, B. A.: Interrelations between pulmonary liquid volumes and lung compliance. J. Appl. Physiol. 38:608, 1975.
4. Luepker, R., Liander, B., Korsgren, M., and Varnauskas, E.: Pulmonary intravascular and extravascular fluid volumes in exercising cardiac patients. Circulation 44:626, 1971.
5. Collins, J. V., Clark, T. J. H., and Brown, D. J.: Airway function in healthy subjects and in patients with left heart disease. Clin. Sci. Molec. Med. 49:217, 1975.
6. Frank, N. R., Lyons, H. A., Siebens, A. A., and Nealon, T. F.: Pulmonary compliance in patients with cardiac disease. Am. J. Med. 22:516, 1957.
7. Wood, T. E., McLeod, P., Anthonisen, N. R., and Macklem, P. T.: Mechanics of breathing in mitral stenosis. Am. Rev. Resp. Dis. 104:52, 1971.
8. Marshall, R., McIlroy, M. B., and Christie, R. V.: The work of breathing in mitral stenosis. Clin. Sci. 13:137, 1954.
9. White, H. C., Butler, J., and Donald, K. W.: Lung compliance in patients with mitral stenosis. Clin. Sci. 17:667, 1958.
10. Saxton, G. A., Jr., Rabinowitz, M., Dexter, L., and Haynes, F.: The relationship of pulmonary compliance to pulmonary vascular pressures in patients with heart disease. J. Clin. Invest. 35:611, 1965.
11. James, A. E., Jr., Cooper, M., White, R. I., and Wagner, H. N., Jr.: Perfusion changes on lungs in patients with congestive heart failure. Radiology 100:99, 1971.
12. Giuntini, C., Mariani, M., Barsotti, A., Fazio, F., and Santolicandro, A.: Factors affecting regional pulmonary blood flow in left heart valvular disease. Am. J. Med. 57:421, 1974.
13. Dawson, A., Rocamora, J. M., and Morgan, J. R.: Regional lung function in chronic pulmonary congestion with and without mitral stenosis. Am. Rev. Resp. Dis. 113:51, 1976.
14. Pain, M. C. F., Bucens, D., Cade, J. F., and Sloman, J. G.: Regional lung function in patients with mitral stenosis. Aust. N.Z. J. Med. 3:228, 1972.
15. Hughes, J. M. B., Glazier, J. B., Rosenzweig, D. Y., and West, J. B.: Factors determining the distribution of pulmonary blood flow in patients with raised pulmonary venous pressure. Clin. Sci. 37:847, 1969.
16. Blumenthal, S., and Ravitch, M. M.: Seminar on aortic vascular rings and other anomalies of the aortic arch. Pediatrics 20:896, 1957.
17. Stranger, P., Lucas, R. V., Jr., and Edwards, J. E.: Anatomic factors causing respiratory distress in acyanotic congenital cardiac disease: Special reference to bronchial obstruction. Pediatrics 43:760, 1969.
18. Bryk, D.: Atelectasis, emphysema, and heart disease. Am. J. Dis. Child. 110:100, 1965.
19. Moss, A. J., and McDonald, L. V.: Cardiac disease in the wheezing child. Chest 71:187, 1977.
20. Spellberg, R. D., Surprenant, E. L., and O'Reilly, R. J.: Hypoventilation of left lung in acquired heart disease. Am. J. Roentgenol. Radium Ther. Nucl. Med. 118:785, 1973.
21. Ryo, U. Y., and Townley, R. G.: Comparison of respiratory and cardiovascular effects of isoproterenol, propranolol, and practolol in asthmatic and normal subjects. J. Allergy Clin. Immunol. 57:12, 1976.
22. Nordstrom, L. A., MacDonald, F., and Gobel, F. L.: Effect of propranolol on respiratory function and exercise tolerance in patients with chronic obstructive lung disease. Chest 67:287, 1975.
23. Mookherjee, S., Fuleihan, D., Warner, R. A., Vardan, S., and Obeid, A. I.: Effects of sublingual nitroglycerine on resting pulmonary gas exchange and hemodynamics in man. Circulation 57:106, 1978.
24. Hoel, B. L., Bay, G., and Refsum, H. E.: The effects of morphine on the arterial and mixed venous blood gas state and on the hemodynamics in patients with clinical pulmonary congestion. Acta Med. Scand. 190:549, 1971.
25. Huckauf, H., Ramdohr, B., and Schroder, R.: Dopamine induced hypoxemia in patients with left heart failure. Int. J. Clin. Pharmacol. 14:217, 1976.
26. Goldring, R. M., Cannon, P. J., Heinemann, H. O., and Fishman, A. P.: Respiratory adjustment to chronic metabolic alkalosis in man. J. Clin. Invest. 47:118, 1968.
27. Turino, G. M., and Fishman, A. P.: The congested lung. J. Chron. Dis. 9:510, 1959.
28. Heard, B. E., Steiner, R. E., Herdon, A., and Gleason, D.: Oedema and fibrosis of the lungs in left ventricular failure. Br. J. Radiol. 41:161, 1968.
29. Galloway, R. W., Epstein, E. J., and Coulshed, N.: Pulmonary ossific nodules in mitral valve disease. Br. Heart J. 23:297, 1961.
30. Friedman, B. L., Macias, D. J., and Yu, P. N.: Pulmonary function studies in patients with mitral stenosis. Am. Rev. Tuberc. 79:265, 1959.
31. Palmer, W. H., Gee, J. B. L., and Bates, D. V.: Disturbances of pulmonary function in mitral valve disease. Canad. Med. Assoc. J. 89:744, 1963.
32. Milic-Emili, J., and Petit, J. M.: Mechanical efficiency of breathing. J. Appl. Physiol. 15:359, 1960.
33. Hogg, J. C., Agarawal, J. B., Gardiner, A. J. S., Palmer, W. H., and Macklem, P. T.: Distribution of airway resistance with developing pulmonary edema in dogs. J. Appl. Physiol. 32:20, 1972.
34. Sutherland, P. W., Cade, J. F., and Pain, M. C. F.: Pulmonary extravascular fluid volume and hypoxaemia in myocardial infarction. Aust. N.Z. J. Med. 1:141, 1971.
35. Tattersfield, A. E., McNicol, M. W., and Sillett, R. W.: Relationship between haemodynamic and respiratory function in patients with myocardial infarction and left ventricular failure. Clin. Sci. 42:751, 1972.
36. Pepine, C. J., and Wiener, L.: Relationship of anginal symptoms to lung mechanics during myocardial ischemia. Circulation 46:863, 1972.
37. Interiano, B., Hyde, R., Hodges, M., and Yu, P. N.: Interrelation between alterations in pulmonary mechanics and hemodynamics in acute myocardial infarction. J. Clin. Invest. 52:1994, 1973.
38. Al Bazzar, F. J., and Kazemi, H.: Arterial hypoxemia and distribution of perfusion after uncomplicated myocardial infarction. Am. Rev. Resp. Dis. 106:721, 1972.
39. Demedts, M., Sniderman, A., Utz, G., Palmer, W. H., and Becklake, M. R.: Lung volumes including closing volume and arterial blood gas measurements in acute ischaemic left heart failure. Bull. Physiopathol. Resp. 10:11, 1974.
40. Otis, A. B., McKerrow, C. B., Bartlett, R. A., Mead, J., McIlroy, M. B., Silverstone, N. J., and Radford, E. P., Jr.: Mechanical factors in distribution of pulmonary ventilation. J. Appl. Physiol. 8:427, 1956.
41. Raine, J., and Bishop, J. M.: The distribution of alveolar ventilation in mitral stenosis at rest and after exercise. Clin. Sci. 24:63, 1963.
42. Ingram, R. H., Jr., and Schilder, D. P.: Association of a decrease in dynamic compliance with a change in gas distribution. J. Appl. Physiol. 23:911, 1967.
43. Dawson, A.: Regional pulmonary blood flow in sitting and supine man during and after acute hypoxia. J. Clin. Invest. 48:301, 1969.

44. Dawson, A., Kaneko, K., and McGregor, M.: Regional lung function in patients with mitral stenosis studied with xenon[133] during air and oxygen breathing. J. Clin. Invest. 44:999, 1965.

45. Wagenvoort, C. A., Heath, D., and Edwards, J. E.: The Pathology of the Pulmonary Vasculature, Springfield, Ill., Charles C Thomas, 1964, p. 186.

46. Kelman, G. R., Nunn, J. F., Prys-Roberts, C., and Greenbaum, R.: The influence of cardiac output on arterial oxygenation: A theoretical study. Br. J. Anaesthesiol. 39:450, 1967.

47. Tenny, S. M.: A theoretical analysis of the relationship between venous blood and mean tissue oxygen pressures. Resp. Physiol. 20:283, 1974.

48. Aberman, A., and Fulop, M.: The metabolic and respiratory acidosis of acute pulmonary edema. Ann. Intern. Med. 76:173, 1972.

49. Ingram, R. H., Jr., and McFadden, E. R., Jr.: Respiratory changes during exercise in patients with pulmonary venous hypertension. Progr. Cardiovasc. Dis. 19:109, 1976.

50. Hayward, G. W., and Knotts, J. M. S.: The effect of exercise on lung distensibility and respiratory work in mitral stenosis. Br. Heart J. 17:303, 1955.

51. Gilbert, R., and Auchincloss, J. H., Jr.: Cardiac and pulmonary function at the exercise breaking point in cardiac patients. Am. J. Med. Sci. 257:370, 1969.

52. Jebavy, P., Widimsky, J., and Stanek, V.: Distribution of inspired gas and pulmonary diffusing capacity at rest and during graded exercise in patients with mitral stenosis. Respiration 28:216, 1971.

53. Auchincloss, J. H., Jr., Gilbert, R., and Baule, G. H.: Unsteady state measurement of oxygen transfer in patients with rheumatic heart disease. Clin. Sci. 39:21, 1970.

54. Goodenday, L. S., Simon, G., Craig, H., and Dalby, L.: Abnormal distribution of pulmonary blood flow in aortic valve disease. Relation between pulmonary function and chest radiograph. Br. Heart J. 32:406, 1970.

55. Hurych, J., Widimsky, J., and Kasalicky, J.: Pulmonary gas exchange at rest and during exercise in patients with mitral stenosis. Bull. Physiopathol. Resp. 2:472, 1966.

56. Bjure, J., Liander, B., and Widimsky, J.: Effect of exercise on distribution of pulmonary blood flow in patients with mitral stenosis. Br. Heart J. 33:438, 1971.

57. Yoo, O. H., and Ting, E. Y.: The effect of pleural effusions on lung function. Am. Rev. Resp. Dis. 89:55, 1964.

58. Anthonisen, N. R., and Martin, R. R.: Regional lung function in pleural effusion. Am. Rev. Resp. Dis. 116:201, 1977.

59. Davidson, F. F., and Glazier, J. B.: Unilateral pleuritis and regional lung function. Ann. Intern. Med. 77:37, 1972.

60. MacDonald, A. J., Ingram, C. G., and McNeil, R. S.: The effect of propranolol on airway resistance. Br. J. Anaesthesiol. 39:919, 1967.

61. Zaid, G., and Beall, G. N.: Bronchial response to beta-adrenergic blockade. N. Engl. J. Med. 275:580, 1966.

62. Tattersfield, R. E., Leaver, D. G., and Pride, N. B.: Effects of β-adrenergic blockade and stimulation on normal human airways. J. Appl. Physiol. 35:613, 1973.

63. Wunderlich, J., Macha, H. N., Wudicke, H., and Huckauf, H.: Beta adrenergic blockers and terbutaline in patients with chronic obstructive lung disease. Chest 78:714, 1980.

64. Tivenius, L.: Effects of multiple doses of metoprolol and propranolol on ventilatory function in patients with chronic obstructive lung disease. Scand. J. Resp. Dis. 57:190, 1976.

65. McMahon, C. D., Shaffer, R. N., Hoskins, H. D., and Hetherington, J.: Adverse effects experienced by patients taking timolol. Am. J. Ophthalmol. 88:736, 1979.

66. McFadden, E. R.: Calcium-channel blocking agents and asthma. Ann. Intern. Med. 95:232, 1981.

67. Mookherjee, S., Warner, R., Keighley, J., and Obeid, A.: Worsening of ventilation perfusion relationship in the lungs in the face of hemodynamic improvement during nitroprusside infusion. Am. J. Cardiol. 39:282, 1977.

68. Pierpont, G., Hale, K. A., Franciosa, J. A., and Cohn, J. N.: Effects of vasodilators on pulmonary hemodynamics and gas exchange in left ventricular failure. Am. Heart J. 49:208, 1980.

69. Chick, J. W., Kochukoshy, K. N., Matsumoto, S., and Leach, J. K.: The effect of nitroglycerine on gas exchange, hemodynamics, and oxygen transport in patients with chronic obstructive pulmonary disease. Am. J. Med. Sci. 276:105, 1978.

70. Tuller, M. A., and Mehdi, F.: Compensatory hypoventilation and hypercapnia in primary metabolic alkalosis. Am. J. Med. 501:281, 1971.

71. Nagle, R. E., and Pilcher, J.: Respiratory and circulatory effects of pentazocine. Review of analgesics used after myocardial infarction. Br. Heart J. 34:244, 1972.

72. Hoel, B. L., and Refsum, H. E.: The effect of morphine on arterial blood gases in patients with acute myocardial infarction. Acta Med. Scand. 186:511, 1969.

72a. Nery, L. E., Wasserman, K., French, W., Oren, A., and Davis, J. A.: Contrasting cardiovascular and respiratory responses to exercise in mitral valve and chronic obstructive pulmonary diseases. Chest 83:446, 1983.

73. DeTroyer, A., Estenne, M., and Yernault, J. C.: Disturbance of respiratory muscle function in patients with mitral valve disease. Am. J. Med. 69:867, 1980.

74. Kannel, W. B., Seidman, J. M., Fercho, W., and Castelli, W. P.: Vital capacity and congestive heart failure. The Framingham study. Circulation 49:1160, 1974.

75. Hales, C. A., and Kazemi, H.: Small-airways function in myocardial infarction. N. Engl. Med. 290:761, 1974.

76. Rotsztain, A., Shugoll, G. I., and Lloyd, R. A.: Hypoxemia in acute myocardial infarction and in coronary insufficiency. Am. J. Med. Sci. 266:255, 1973.

77. Biddle, T. L., Khanna, P., Yu, P. N., Hodges, M., and Shah, P. M.: Lung water in patients with acute myocardial infarction. Circulation 49:115, 1974.

78. Hordof, A. J., Mellins, R. B., Gersony, W. M., and Steeg, C. N.: Reversibility of chronic obstructive lung disease in infants following repair of ventricular septal defect. J. Pediatr. 90:187, 1977.

79. Howlett, G.: Lung mechanics in normal infants and infants with congenital heart disease. Arch. Dis. Child. 471:707, 1972.

80. Bancalari, E., Jesse, M. J., Gelband, H., and Garcia, O.: Lung mechanics in congenital heart disease with increased and decreased pulmonary blood flow. J. Pediatr. 90:192, 1977.

81. De Troyer, A., Yernault, J. C., and Englert, M.: Mechanics of breathing in patients with atrial septal defect. Am. Rev. Resp. Dis. 115:413, 1977.

82. Friedman, W. F., Braunwald, E., and Morrow, A. G.: Alterations in regional pulmonary blood flow in patients with congenital heart disease studied by radioisotope scanning. Circulation 37:747, 1968.

83. Sade, R. M., Williams, R. G., Castaneda, A. R., and Treves, S.: Abnormalities of regional lung function associated with ventricular septal defect and pulmonary artery band. J. Thorac. Cardiovasc. Surg. 71:572, 1976.

84. Bates, D. V., Macklem, P. T., and Christie, R. V.: Respiratory function in disease. 2nd ed. Philadelphia, W. B. Saunders Co., 1971, p. 351.

85. Gates, G. F., Orme, H. W., and Dore, E. K.: The hyperperfused lung. Detection in congenital heart disease. J.A.M.A. 233:782, 1975.

86. Edelman, N. H., Lahiri, S., Braudo, L., Cherniack, N. S., and Fishman, A. P.: The blunted ventilatory response to hypoxia in cyanotic congenital heart disease. N. Engl. J. Med. 282:405, 1970.

87. Aubier, M., Trippenbach, T., and Roussos, C.: Respiratory muscle fatigue during cardiogenic shock. J. Appl. Physiol. Resp. Environ. Exercise Physiol. 51:499, 1981.

87a. Loke, J.: Distinguishing cardiac versus pulmonary limitation in exercise performance. Chest 83:441, 1983.

88. De Vries, K., Goei, J. T., Booy-Noord, H., and Orie, N. G. M.: Changes during 24 hours in the lung function and histamine hyperreactivity of the bronchial tree in asthmatic and bronchitic patients. Int. Arch. Allergy 20:93, 1962.

89. Rees, P. J., and Clark, T. J. H.: Paroxysmal nocturnal dyspnea and periodic respiration. Lancet 2:1315, 1979.

90. Zorck, M. B., Pontoppidan, H., and Kazemi, H.: The effect of lateral positions on gas exchange in pulmonary disease. Am. Rev. Resp. Dis. 110:49, 1974.

91. Altman, M., and Robin, E. D.: Platypnea: Diffuse zone I phenomenon? N. Engl. J. Med. 281:1347, 1969.

92. Robin, E. D., and Altman, M.: By a waterfall: "Zone I and Zone II phenomena" in obstructive lung disease. Am. J. Med. Sci. 258:219, 1969.

93. Montgomery, G. E., Geraci, J. E., Parker, R. L., and Wood, E. H.: The arterial oxygen saturation in cyanotic types of congenital heart disease. Proc. Staff Meet. Mayo Clin. 23:169, 1948.

94. Lurie, P. R.: Postural effects in tetralogy of Fallot. Am. J. Med. 10:297, 1953.

95. Schnabel, T. G., Jr., Ratto, O., Kirby, C. K., Johnson, J., and Comroe, J. H., Jr.: Postural cyanosis and angina pectoris following pneumonectomy: Relief by closure of an interatrial septal defect. J. Thorac. Surg. 32:246, 1956.

96. Begin, R.: Platypnea after pneumonectomy. N. Engl. J. Med. 293:342, 1975.

97. Munsell, W. P.: Pneumomediastinum. J.A.M.A. 202:689, 1967.

98. Copeland, R. B., and Omenn, G. S.: Electrocardiograms suggestive of coronary artery disease in pneumothorax. Arch. Intern. Med. 25:151, 1970.

99. Littmann, D.: Electrocardiographic phenomena associated with spontaneous pneumothorax and mediastinal emphysema. J. Med. Sci. 212:682, 1946.

100. Millard, C. E.: Pneumomediastinum. Dis. Chest 56:297, 1969.

101. Heller, R.: The significance of hemoptysis. Tubercle 27:70, 1946.

102. Abbott, D. A.: The clinical significance of pulmonary hemorrhage: A study of 1,316 patients with chest disease. Dis. Chest 14:824, 1948.

103. Levitt, N.: Clinical significance of hemoptysis. J. Mich. State Med. Soc. 50:606, 1951.

104. Souders, C. R., and Smith, A. T.: The clinical significance of hemoptysis. J.A.M.A. 150:746, 1952.

105. Haroutunian, L. M., and Neill, C. A.: Pulmonary complications of congenital heart disease: Hemoptysis. Am. Heart J. 84:540, 1972.

106. Finley, T. N., Aronow, A., Cosentino, A. M., and Golde, D. W.: Occult pulmonary hemorrhage in anticoagulated patients. Am. Rev. Resp. Dis. 112:23, 1975.

107. Corazza, L. J., and Pastor, B. H.: Cardiac arrhythmias in chronic cor pulmonale. N. Engl. J. Med. 259:862, 1958.

108. Shine, K. I., Kastor, J. A., and Yurchak, P. M.: Multifocal atrial tachycardia. Clinical and electrocardiographic features in 32 patients. N. Engl. J. Med. 279:344, 1968.

109. Ayres, S. M., and Grace, W. J.: Inappropriate ventilation and hypoxemia as causes of cardiac arrhythmias. The control of arrhythmias without antiarrhythmic drugs. Am. J. Med. 46:495, 1969.

110. Kleiger, R. E., and Senior, R. M.: Long-term electrocardiographic monitoring of ambulatory patients with chronic airway obstruction. Chest 65:483, 1974.

111. Hudson, L. D., Kurt, T. L., Petty, T. L., and Genton, E.: Arrhythmias associated with acute respiratory failure in patients with chronic airway obstruction. Chest 63:661, 1973.

112. Holford, F. D., and Mithoefer, J. C.: Cardiac arrhythmias in hospitalized pa-

tients with chronic obstructive pulmonary disease. Am. Rev. Resp. Dis. *108*: 979, 1973.

113. Sideris, D. A., Katsadoros, D. P., Valianos, G., and Assioura, A.: Type of cardiac dysrhythmias in respiratory failure. Am. Heart J. *89*:32, 1975.

114. Tirlapur, V. G., and Mir, M. A.: Nocturnal hypoxemia and associated electrocardiographic changes in patients with chronic obstructive airway disease. N. Engl. J. Med. *306*:125, 1982.

115. Thomas, M. A., and Wee, A. S. T.: The sinus node in cor pulmonale. Isr. J. Med. Sci. *5*:831, 1969.

116. Green, L. H., and Smith, T. W.: The use of digitalis in patients with pulmonary disease. Ann. Intern. Med. *87*:459, 1977.

117. McFadden, E. R., Jr.: Beta 2 receptor agonists: Metabolism and pharmacology. J. Allergy Clin. Immunol. *68*:91, 1981.

118. Ahlquist, R. P.: A study of the adrenotropic receptors. Am. J. Physiol. *153*: 586, 1948.

119. Lands, A. M., Arnold, A., McAuliff, J. P., Luduena, F. P., and Brown, T. G.: Differentiation of receptor systems activated by sympathomimetic amines. Nature *214*:597, 1967.

120. Bourdillon, P. D. V., Dawson, J. R., Foale, R. A., Timmis, A. D., Poole-Wilson, P. A., and Sutton, J. C.: Salbutamol in treatment of heart failure. Br. Heart J. *43*:206, 1980.

121. Brooks, S. M., Mintz, S., and Weiss, E.: Changes occurring after freon inhalation. Am. Rev. Resp. Dis. *105*:640, 1972.

122. Clark, D. G., and Tinston, D. J.: Cardiac effects of isoproterenol, hypoxia, hypercapnia, and fluorocarbon propellents and their use in asthma inhalers. Ann. Allergy *30*:536, 1972.

123. Fabel, H., Wettengel, R., and Hartmann, W.: Myokardischamie und Arrhythmien durch den Gebrauch von Dosieraerosolen beim Menschen? Dtsch. Med. Wschr. *97*:428, 1972.

124. Silverglade, A.: Cardiac toxicity of aerosol propellents. J.A.M.A. *222*:827, 1972.

125. Speizer, F. E., Wegman, D. H., and Ramirez, A.: Palpitation rates associated with fluorocarbon exposure in a hospital setting. New Engl. J. Med. *292*:624, 1975.

126. Matthay, R. A., Berger, H. J., Loke, J., Gottschalk, A., and Zaret, B. L.: Ef-

fect of aminophylline upon right and left ventricular performance in chronic obstructive pulmonary disease. Am. J. Med. *65*:903, 1978.

127. Camarata, S. J., Weil, M. H., and Hanashiro, D. K.: Cardiac arrest in the critically ill. A study of predisposing causes in 132 patients. Circulation *44*: 688, 1971.

128. Scharf, S. M., Caldini, P., and Ingram, R. H., Jr.: Cardiovascular effects of increasing airway pressure in the dog. Am. J. Physiol. *232*:435, 1977.

129. Haynes, J. B., Carson, S. D., Whitney, W. P., Zerbe, G. O., Hyers, T. M., and Steele, P.: Positive end-expiratory pressure shifts and left ventricular diastolic pressure-area curves. J. Appl. Physiol. Resp. Environ. Exercise Physiol. *48*: 670, 1980.

130. Jardin, F., Farcot, J. C., Boisante, L., Curien, N., Margairaz, A., and Bourdarias, J. P.: Influence of positive end-expiratory pressures on left ventricular performance. N. Engl. J. Med. *304*:387, 1981.

131. Wise, R. A., Robotham, J. L., Bromberger-Barnea, B., and Permutt, S.: Effect of PEEP on left ventricular function in right-heart–bypassed dogs. J. Appl. Physiol. Resp. Environ. Exercise Physiol. *51*:541, 1981.

132. Fewell, J. E., Abendschein, D. R., Carlson, C. J., Rapaport, E., and Murray, J.: Mechanism of decreased right and left ventricular end-diastolic volumes during continuous positive-pressure ventilation in dogs. Circ. Res. *47*:467, 1980.

133. Cassidy, S. S., Eschenbacher, W. L., and Johnson, R. L., Jr.: Reflex cardiovascular depression during unilateral lung hyperinflation in the dog. J. Clin. Invest. *64*:620, 1979.

134. Gaensler, E. A., and Weisel, R. D.: The risks of abdominal and thoracic surgery in COPD. Postgrad. Med. *54*:183, 1973.

135. Olsen, G. N., Block, A. J., and Tobias, J. A.: Prediction of postpneumonectomy pulmonary function using quantitative macroaggregate lung scanning. Chest *66*:13, 1974.

136. Tisi, G. M.: Preoperative evaluation of pulmonary function. *In* Isselbacher, K. J., et al. (eds.): Principles of Internal Medicine, Update III. New York, McGraw-Hill Book Co., 1982, p. 101.

137. Mittman, C.: Assessment of operative risk in thoracic surgery. Am. Rev. Resp. Dis. *84*:197, 1961.

55

GENERAL PRINCIPLES OF CARDIAC SURGERY

by John W. Kirklin, M.D., Eugene H. Blackstone, M.D., and James K. Kirklin, M.D.

Cardiac surgery, like other forms of surgery, is advised for any given patient when the surgical risks to survival and useful life are fewer than those of nonsurgical treatment. Ideally, cardiac surgery should have a *hospital mortality* rate *approaching zero** and should prevent *premature late death.*** When these criteria are associated with full functional capacity, the operation is considered *curative.* In some patients, cure may be unattainable, and for them a life expectancy and a functional capacity better than that imposed by the disease itself are sought (*palliative* operation).

The purpose of this chapter is to describe the general aspects of cardiac surgery that affect early and late results and to provide insight into some of the mechanisms underlying its current problems.

PREOPERATIVE CONDITIONS AFFECTING EARLY AND LATE RESULTS OF CARDIAC SURGERY

The Lesion

The early and late results of cardiac surgery depend significantly upon the specific cardiac lesion being treated.

---

*By this is meant a hospital mortality rate whose lower 70 per cent confidence limit (CL) is less than 1 per cent and whose upper one is less than 5 per cent.

**By this is meant an actuarial survival rate whose upper 70 per cent CL or 1 standard deviation overlaps the survival rate of an age-sex-race-matched general population.

For example, hospital mortality approaches zero for the repair of uncomplicated atrial septal defects (hospital mortality, 0.9 per cent; 70 per cent CL, 0.4 to 1.8 per cent*) and for coronary artery bypass grafting (0.7 per cent; 70 per cent CL, 0.6 to 0.9 per cent), whereas that for primary combined aortic and mitral valve replacement is 4 per cent (70 per cent CL, 3 to 7 per cent) and that for an operation such as the modified Fontan procedure for single ventricle and other types of complex congenital heart disease other than tricuspid atresia is 29 per cent (70 per cent CL, 17 to 49 per cent).

The early and late risks of cardiac surgery may, in the case of some lesions, result from the noncorrectable (by current techniques) aspects of their morphology or from morphology that is manageable only by methods that themselves have important risks. For example, extensive three-vessel coronary artery disease with a left ventricular ejection fraction of 0.2 or less results in a significant risk for premature late death in the postoperative period because of surgically untreatable left ventricular scarring. Similarly, survival and salvage of left ventricular function after acute revascularization following acute myocardial infarction with cardiogenic shock may be limited by the amount of irreversible myocardial injury. Atrioventricular (AV) septal (canal) defects with severe left AV valve regur-

---

*70 per cent CL = 70 per cent confidence limit, analogous to 1 standard deviation. The representative hospital mortalities presented are from the Department of Surgery, University of Alabama in Birmingham (UAB), unless otherwise stated.

gitation may continue to have severe left AV valve regurgitation after repair because of leaflet deficiency. Tetralogy of Fallot with a very small pulmonary annulus requires either a transannular patch with its resultant pulmonary valvular regurgitation and consequent damaging effect on the right ventricle or an orthotopic or bypassing pulmonary valve replacement with its long-term uncertainties.

However, it is not only the complexity of the cardiac condition itself that increases the risks. It also may be that patients with a particular lesion have come to operation unusually ill, especially young, or with other major associated cardiac conditions. In the case of some lesions (for example, mitral and aortic regurgitation), the apparently unfavorable effect of the lesion on late mortality may be related in large part to the lesion's damaging influence on ventricular structure and function. The increased risks of operation for some lesions may be related to the complexity of the operation required or to lack of knowledge about some particular aspect of postoperative care, rather than to risk factors within the patient. All of these considerations make multivariate analysis necessary to the development of an understanding of the lesion's effect on the results of operation.

Ventricular Structure and Function

THE SECONDARY CARDIOMYOPATHIES. One of the most important limitations of the surgical treatment of heart disease may be the damage already sustained by the ventricles by the time the operation is undertaken. This *secondary cardiomyopathy* is produced by a chronic pressure or volume overload (p. 449) or by acute or chronic myocardial ischemia. It is sometimes forgotten that the *right*, as well as the left ventricle is subject to these damaging effects; the time required for the development of secondary right ventricular cardiomyopathy, however, seems to be somewhat longer than in the case of the left ventricle.

An early response to volume or pressure overload or to myocardial scarring is increased ventricular mass. This results initially from myocardial cell hypertrophy. In the case of volume overload, the increased ventricular mass is primarily associated with greater ventricular volume at any given diastolic pressure. In the case of pressure overload, it is mainly linked with increased ventricular wall thickness. When the volume or pressure overload or ischemic damage is inordinate or prolonged, mitochondrial changes occur as well as disruption of sarcomeres and fiber disarray.

Modest increase in ventricular mass may not impair ventricular systolic or diastolic function. In fact, it may be compensatory and preserve function, such as occurs in aortic stenosis when the increased left ventricular wall thickness maintains nearly normal systolic wall stress (and thus afterload) despite elevated left ventricular systolic pressure (p. 453).[1] When the hypertrophy no longer keeps pace with the ventricular overload, such as in the afterload mismatch of long-standing aortic stenosis, ventricular systolic and diastolic functions are adversely affected even though degenerative myocardial changes are not present. When myocardial degenerative changes are present, contractility is usually impaired in proportion to the extent and severity of the degenerative changes.

All of these factors are of great surgical importance because of the tendency of the secondary cardiomyopathy to become irreversible. If only hypertrophy is present, the ventricular mass regresses toward but not *to* a normal state, and systolic and diastolic functions are improved and may become normal. Degenerative changes are irreversible, and in their presence the regression of ventricular mass toward a normal state is more limited. When degenerative changes are extensive, little regression of mass occurs, contractility remains impaired postoperatively, and symptomatic improvement is limited. Several months or years after operation, extreme secondary cardiomyopathy may worsen in spite of mechanical relief of the defect, resulting in further impairment of systolic and diastolic function, increasing symptoms, increasing ventricular electrical instability, and premature late death.

These phenomena must be taken into consideration in choosing the time of operation for many forms of congenital and acquired heart disease. In delaying operation, the disadvantages of the progression of the secondary cardiomyopathy must be weighed against the advantages of continued medical therapy or of awaiting improved surgical methods.

VOLUME OVERLOAD (see also p. 453). Ventricular volume overload, in surgically treatable states, exists when the ventricular stroke volume is greater than net forward systemic blood flow. The return toward but not to normal ventricular mass when volume overload has been of brief duration ($\pm$ 30 days) was demonstrated experimentally by Papadimitriou and colleagues[2] (Table 55–1). When this kind of regression occurs in humans after an operation, premature late death is infrequent and the functional results are good. When regression of the secondary cardiomyopathy does not take place, or particularly when the cardiomyopathy increases postoperatively, premature late death is common.

Since myocardial biopsies are rarely performed in surgical patients, and death followed by autopsies is rather infrequent, much of the evidence for a cardiomyopathy secondary to chronic volume overload is circumstantial and is based upon the observation of depressed ventricular systolic function and advanced functional disability in patients with volume-overloaded ventricles. In this regard, it is noteworthy that patients with depressed left ventricular systolic function in whom aortic valve replacement has been carried out for aortic regurgitation have a lower 5-year survival rate after hospital dismissal than do patients whose systolic function is normal preoperatively (Fig. 55–1A).[3] In such patients, depressed preoperative exercise capacity (or increased NYHA Functional Class) still further depresses the late survival rate (Figs. 55–1B, 55–2, and 55–3).[3,4,5] Poor functional capacity or depressed systolic function in the preoperative period also predisposes to lack of improvement of ventricular diastolic function late in the postoperative period (Fig. 55–4)[5,6] (see also p. 454).

Patients with *atrial septal defect* (ASD) have a *volume overload* of the *right ventricle*, and the same type of *secondary* cardiomyopathy slowly develops in time. Thus, older patients with ASD have more severe symptoms preoperatively than younger ones (Table 55–2), symptomatic patients undergoing repair of their ASD are older than asymptomatic ones, and the right ventricular systolic func-

TABLE 55–1 MEASUREMENTS IN NORMAL DOGS; IN DOGS WITH SURGICALLY CREATED LARGE AORTOCAVAL FISTULA OF ±30 DAYS' DURATION; AND IN DOGS 3 MONTHS AND 6 MONTHS AFTER FISTULA CLOSURE

	BODY WEIGHT (KG)	HEART RATE (BEATS/MIN)	LEFT VENTRICULAR END-DIASTOLIC PRESSURE (MM HG)	CARDIAC INDEX (ML/MIN/KG)	LEFT VENTRICLE WEIGHT (GM/KG)
Normal (8)	21.3 ± 3.3	88 ± 27	5 ± 3	134 ± 41	4.19 ± 0.47
Patent fistula (7)	21.1 ± 2.9	124 ± 18	31 ± 7	459 ± 135	5.34 ± 0.34
p value compared with normal dogs	NS	<0.01	<0.001	<0.001	<0.001
Fistula closed at 3 mos (5)	20.6 ± 1.3	67 ± 10	6 ± 2	130 ± 26	5.25 ± 0.16
p value compared with normal dogs	NS	NS	NS	NS	<0.001
p value compared with dogs with patent fistulas	NS	<0.001	<0.001	<0.001	NS
Fistula closed at 6 mos (6)	22.5 ± 2.4	82 ± 29	7 ± 1.4	186 ± 64	4.82 ± 0.54
p value compared with normal dogs	NS	NS	NS	NS	<0.05
p value compared with dogs with patent fistulas	NS	<0.01	<0.001	<0.001	NS

All values are means ± SD. The number of dogs studied is given in parentheses. NS = nonsignificant; SD = standard deviation; mos = months. (Modified from Papadimitriou, J. M., et al.: Regression of left ventricular dilation and hypertrophy after removal of volume overload. Circ. Res. *35*:127, 1974.)

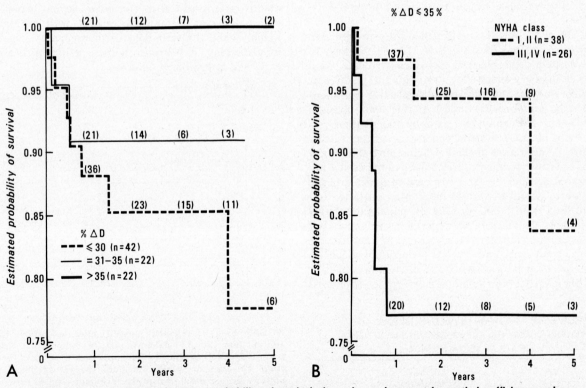

FIGURE 55–1 *A,* Relation between probability of survival after valve replacement for aortic insufficiency and preoperative per cent change of left ventricular dimension (% Δ D), an index of systolic function. Patients with low values, and thus diminished systolic function, have significantly decreased probability of survival (p < 0.05). (Numbers in parentheses are numbers of patients at risk at each interval.) *B,* Relation between preoperative NYHA functional classification and probability of survival after valve replacement for aortic insufficiency in patients with preoperatively depressed left ventricular systolic function. Patients in Functional Class I or II had longer survival than those in Class III or IV (p = 0.05). (From Cunha, C. L. P., Giuliani, E. R., Fuster, V., Seward, J. B., Brandenburg, R. O., and McGoon, D. C.: Preoperative M-mode echocardiography as a predictor of surgical results in chronic aortic insufficiency. J. Thorac. Cardiovasc. Surg. *79*:256, 1980.)

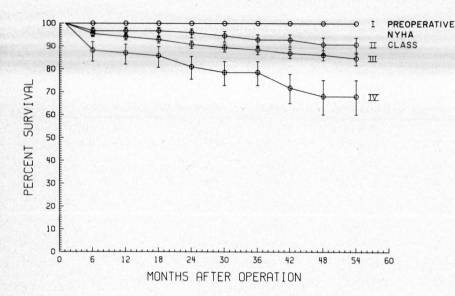

FIGURE 55–2 Actuarial survival of hospital survivors after aortic, mitral, or aortic and mitral valve replacement, according to the preoperative NYHA Functional Class. These relations hold for any of these subgroups. The vertical bars enclose the 70 per cent confidence limits (1 standard deviation). (From Karp, R. B., Cyrus, R. J., Blackstone, E. H., Kirklin, J. W., Kouchoukos, N. T., and Pacifico, A. D.: The Bjork-Shiley valve. J. Thorac. Cardiovasc. Surg. *81*:602, 1981.)

tion is less efficient in the older patient (Table 55–3).[7] When this secondary right ventricular cardiomyopathy is long-standing, it is apt to be irreversible, as it is in other types of secondary cardiomyopathy. Thus, only about 20 per cent of older patients have nearly normal right ventricular end-diastolic volume late after repair of their ASD, and only about 60 per cent of patients aged 10 years at operation experienced a return to a nearly normal state (Table 55–4).[8]

Sometimes overlooked is the fact that patients with *congenital tricuspid atresia* (p. 984) have volume overload of the left ventricle. This chamber provides systemic blood flow plus pulmonary blood flow (through the ventricular septal defect and the diminutive and ineffective right ventricle into the pulmonary arteries) in this malformation. The overload is frequently increased by the surgical creation in early life of a systemic–pulmonary artery shunt. The gradual deterioration of these patients after the second decade of life, their frequent development of increasing mitral regurgitation, and the poor response of patients in the third or fourth decades of life to the Fontan operation (diversion of vena caval blood into the left pulmonary artery) are all probably the result of the progressing secondary left ventricular cardiomyopathy that develops. In contrast, the surprisingly good long-term survival of such individuals after the Fontan repair[9] (closure of the shunts and direct or indirect right atrial to pulmonary artery anastomosis)

when it is done in the first decade of life is probably due as much to the relief of the left ventricular volume overload as to the ablation of cyanosis.

Other lesions resulting in chronic left or right ventricular volume overload, with all its implications for the development of a secondary cardiomyopathy, include ventricular septal defect, aortopulmonary window, large patent ductus arteriosus, atrioventricular septal (canal) defect, and post-repair tetralogy of Fallot with a transannular patch. When the secondary cardiomyopathy is severe and long-standing, it becomes in these lesions also a cause of early and late surgical failures.

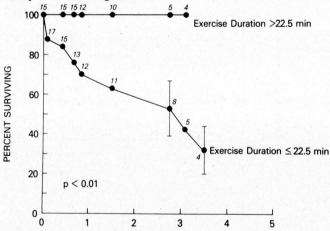

FIGURE 55–3 Actuarial survival after operation for aortic regurgitation in 32 patients, all of whom had subnormal preoperative left ventricular fractional shortening (less than 29 per cent), an index of systolic function. The vertical lines with bars indicate the standard error of the technique. The 15 patients whose exercise duration was greater than 22.5 minutes had significantly preoperative better survival than the 17 patients whose exercise duration was 22.5 minutes or less. The number of patients at risk is indicated at each interval. (From Bonow, R. O., Borer, J. S., Rosing, D. R., Henry, W. L., Pearlman, A. S., McIntosh, C. L., Morrow, A. G., and Epstein, S. E.: Preoperative exercise capacity in symptomatic patients with aortic regurgitation as a predictor of postoperative left ventricular function and long-term prognosis. Circulation *62*:1280, 1980, by permission of the American Heart Association, Inc.)

TABLE 55–2   RELATION BETWEEN SYMPTOMS (NYHA FUNCTIONAL CLASS) AND AGE AT OPERATION FOR REPAIR OF ATRIAL SEPTAL DEFECT

NYHA FUNCTIONAL CLASS AT TIME OF OPERATION	AGE (YRS) AT OPERATION		
	Mean	*Median*	*Range*
I	16	12	3.3–63
II	32	30	4.2–72
III	50	54	0.9–68
IV	51	57	2.2–66

From Kirklin, J. W.: Unpublished data, 1967–1979, n = 340.

A special situation exists when the ventricular volume overload is from mitral or tricuspid valve regurgitation, because of the favorable effect on afterload of the abnormally rapid decrease in ventricular volume and increase in wall thickness during each systole (Fig. 55–5).[10] This masks the developing left ventricular secondary cardiomyopathy until very late in the natural history of the disease by improving apparent left ventricular systolic function. Surgical correction of the AV valve regurgitation may unmask the secondary cardiomyopathy and show it to be more advanced than suspected preoperatively (Fig. 55–6.)[11] As in other situations, the cardiomyopathy may then progress and may result in worsening left ventricular systolic

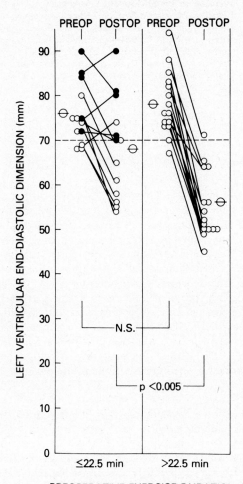

PREOP POSTOP PREOP POSTOP

≤22.5 min   >22.5 min

PREOPERATIVE EXERCISE DURATION

FIGURE 55–4 Changes in echocardiographic left ventricular end-diastolic dimension (an index of diastolic function) as a result of operation in symptomatic patients undergoing valve replacement for aortic regurgitation, according to preoperative exercise duration. Patients who completed Stage I before operation (more than 22.5 minutes) had a greater decrease in diastolic size late in the postoperative period than patients who could not complete Stage I (22.5 minutes or less). The dashed line at 70 mm indicates the value of postoperative diastolic dimension above which patients have been shown to be at high risk of subsequent death from congestive heart failure. ◯-alive; ●-late death from congestive heart failure: N.S.-not significant. (From Bonow, R. O., Borer, J. S., Rosing, D. R., Henry, W. L., Pearlman, A. S., McIntosh, C. L., Morrow, A. G., and Epstein, S. E.: Preoperative exercise capacity in symptomatic patients with aortic regurgitation as a predictor of postoperative left ventricular function and long-term prognosis. Circulation *62*:1280, 1980, by permission of the American Heart Association, Inc.)

TABLE 55–3 OLDER AGE AND DECREASED RIGHT VENTRICULAR SYSTOLIC FUNCTION IN SYMPTOMATIC PATIENTS WITH ATRIAL SEPTAL DEFECTS

GROUP	AGE, YEARS (MEAN VALUE)	RIGHT VENTRICULAR EJECTION FRACTION (MEAN VALUE)
Asymptomatic	25	64%
Symptomatic	52	36%

From Liberthson, R. R., Boucher, C. A., Strauss, H. W., Dinsmore, R. E., McKusick, K. A., and Pohost, G. M.: Right ventricular function in adult atrial septal defect. Am. J. Cardiol. *47*:56, 1981.

and diastolic function late in the postoperative period and in premature late death.

PRESSURE OVERLOAD. The chronic pressure overload of abnormally high intraventricular systolic pressure initially produces hypertrophy of myocardial cells and increased ventricular mass and wall thickness. Initially, the increase in wall thickness results in continued normal left ventricular afterload, a process called *afterload matching* (p. 452).[1] In this situation, the systolic function returns toward normal after surgical relief of the pressure overload.

Late in the course of a chronic pressure overload (Fig. 13–9, p. 453), or at birth in the case of the pressure overload produced by some kinds of congenital heart disease (Table 55–5), the increase in wall thickness may be insufficient to normalize ventricular afterload, a condition of *afterload* mismatch.[12,13] Ventricular systolic function is thereby reduced. When the afterload mismatch is a long-standing phenomenon, secondary cardiomyopathy develops. In such situations, the advanced cardiomyopathy is associated with degenerative myocardial structural changes[14] and reduced *myocardial contractility*. These may *not* regress after surgical relief of the pressure overload.

Chronic left ventricular pressure overload is present in all forms of left ventricular outflow tract obstruction (subaortic, valvular, and supravalvular aortic stenosis), in aortic coarctation, and in systemic arterial hypertension. Chronic right ventricular pressure overload occurs in all forms of right ventricular outflow obstruction, including tetralogy of Fallot and pulmonary stenosis with intact septum. It is also present in pulmonary hypertension from any cause.

ISCHEMIC CARDIOMYOPATHY (see also p. 1364). Myocardial infarction in patients with ischemic heart dis-

TABLE 55–4 LATE POSTOPERATIVE RIGHT VENTRICULAR FUNCTION AFTER REPAIR OF ATRIAL SEPTAL DEFECT

AGE AT OPERATION (YEARS)	n	PROPORTION WITH NEAR NORMAL RV END-DIASTOLIC VOLUME
< 10	11	64% (CL, 44%–81%)
> 25	14	21% (CL, 10%–38%)

p = 0.04;
CL = 70% confidence limits;
RV = right ventricular.
(From Pearlman, A. S., Borer, J. S., Clark, C. E., Henry, W. L., Redwood, D. R., Morrow, A. G., Epstein, S. E., Burn, C., Cohen, E., and McKay, F. J.: Abnormal right ventricular size and ventricular septal motion after atrial septal defect closure. Am. J. Cardiol. *41*:295, 1978.)

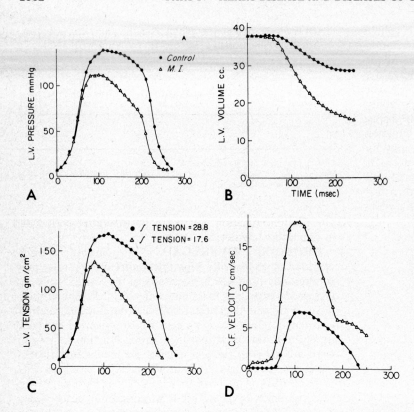

FIGURE 55–5   *A*, Experimental demonstration of the effect of mitral regurgitation on left ventricular (LV) afterload by the rapid reduction of volume during systole, *B*, and by decrease in wall tension, *C*. The result is an increase in systolic function as expressed by the mean velocity of circumferential fiber shortening (CF), *D*. (From Urschel, C. W., Covell, J. W., Sonnenblick, E. H., Ross, J., Jr., and Braunwald, E.: Myocardial mechanics in aortic and mitral valvular regurgitation: The concept of instantaneous impedance as a determinant of the performance of the intact heart. J. Clin. Invest. *47*:867, 1968.)

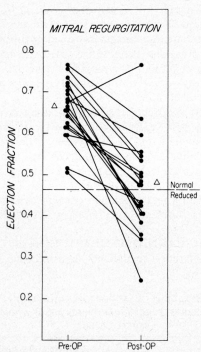

FIGURE 55–6   Ventricular systolic function (expressed as ejection fraction) before and early after mitral valve replacement for mitral regurgitation. Individual values are shown, and mean values are expressed by (Δ). Although all patients had an ejection fraction that was at least normal preoperatively, half had a postoperative ejection fraction below normal. (The lower limit of normal [0.50] is represented by a broken line.) All but one had a decrease in ejection fraction after operation. (From Boucher, C. A., Bingham, J. B., Osbakken, M. D., Okada, R. D., Strauss, H. W., Black, P. C., Levine, F. H., Phillips, H. R., and Pohost, G. M.: Early changes in left ventricular size and function after correction of left ventricular volume overload. Am. J. Cardiol. *47*:991, 1981.)

ease results in ventricular scars of variable size and homogeneity. Nonhomogeneous scars (viable myocardial cells scattered through the area of myocardial scarring) may be small, or they may be extensive and involve a large segment of the ventricle. It is not yet clear to what extent myocardial revascularization can improve the function in such areas of ischemic scarring, by its effect on the viable muscle cells in the areas. The myocardial scar may be essentially homogeneous and transmural and devoid of viable myocardial cells. When such a scar is large, it is usually dyskinetic and is properly called a *left ventricular aneurysm*. Not only is recovery of function after revascularization theoretically impossible, but also the coronary artery to the area has usually been destroyed in the necrotic process.

These regional ischemic changes in left ventricular structure and function have a secondary effect on the nonscarred (but sometimes ischemic during stress) portions of the left ventricle. A pressure overload of the remainder of the ventricle probably results from the regional abnormalities in the scarred areas and their effect on the geometry of the ventricle (an increase in ventricular volume and a resulting augmentation of wall tension, according to the Law of Laplace, p. 431), with the same opportunities for development and progression of the secondary cardiomyopathy as exists in general for pressure-overloaded ventricles.

Secondary Subsystem Abnormalities of Structure and Function

The Lungs.   Abnormalities in structure and function of the lungs are commonly involved in early and late deaths after cardiac surgery. This involvement results in part from the vulnerability of the lungs to the damaging effects of cardiopulmonary bypass (see below) and in part from the

TABLE 55–5 LEFT VENTRICULAR SYSTOLIC FUNCTION (EJECTION FRACTION) IN COARCTATION OF THE AORTA

AGE (WEEKS)	LV MASS	LV EJECTION FRACTION	COMMENT
< 2	Normal	Severely depressed	Afterload mismatch
4 < 24	Increased	Mildly depressed	Afterload match

LV = left ventricular. (From Graham, T. P., Jr., Atwood, G. F., Boerth, R. C., Boucek, R. J., Jr., and Smith, C. W.: Right and left heart size and function in infants with symptomatic coarctation. Circulation 56:641, 1977, by permission of the American Heart Association, Inc.)

frequency with which they have preoperative abnormalities of structure and function.

Hypertensive pulmonary vascular disease complicates many kinds of congenital heart disease (pp. 832 and 950). It is reversible in infants after correction of the underlying congenital cardiac malformation under many circumstances[15,16] (p. 950) (Fig. 55–7), but in older patients, when advanced, it persists after operation and may progress to cause premature late death. The classic description of the various stages of this kind of pulmonary vascular disease by Heath and Edwards,[17] supplemented by the more recent morphometric studies by Reid and colleagues,[18] has provided an excellent morphological understanding of the condition. Although there is a correlation between this morphology and the calculated pulmonary vascular resistance, it is not sufficiently strong to allow exact prediction of one from the other.[19]

When hypertensive pulmonary vascular disease becomes severe, the reactivity of the pulmonary vascular bed to physiological stimuli such as exercise disappears. In this situation, characterized by moderate or severe elevation of pulmonary vascular resistance, an increase in pulmonary blood flow in response to exercise cannot occur. As long as there is a defect or communication between the pulmonary and systemic circulations, systemic blood flow can be augmented during exercise by right-to-left shunting, although arterial desaturation results. If the defect is closed, the opportunity for augmentation of systemic blood flow by right-to-left shunting is lost, and there is a risk of sudden death during exercise or stress resulting from an in-

ability to increase systemic and thus coronary blood flow because of the high, nonyielding ("fixed") pulmonary vascular resistance. Therefore, pulmonary vascular disease of such severity is a contraindication to repair of the defect.

A similar but usually less severe type of pulmonary vascular disease develops gradually in patients with *chronically elevated left atrial pressure*, generally from mitral stenosis (p. 830). Although in unusual cases advanced morphological changes are present, more commonly a large element of arteriolar spasm is present. This is evident from the fact that pulmonary arteriolar resistance usually falls immediately after left atrial pressure is reduced by mitral valvotomy or replacement.[5,20]

Pulmonary vascular disease of a different type may be present in patients with *cyanotic congenital heart disease.* Although it has some of the features of hypertensive pulmonary vascular disease, thrombotic occlusive lesions are a major component of this abnormality and tend to be more extensive the more advanced the cyanotic congenital heart disease and its accompanying polycythemia.[21] In some patients, particularly those in whom congenital pulmonary atresia is a part of the malformation, congenital stenoses in the small and large branches of the pulmonary arterial tree, as well as hypertrophy of the distal pulmonary arteriolar walls, add to the hypertensive effect of the pulmonary vasculature.[22] These changes, *in toto*, must be evaluated and considered preoperatively in deciding upon the probable early and late results of cardiac surgery in an individual patient with cyanotic congenital heart disease.

Pulmonary disease unrelated to the cardiac disease may

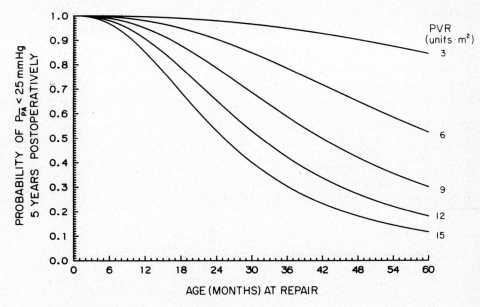

FIGURE 55–7 Probability of mean pulmonary artery pressure less than 25 mm Hg, 5 or more years after repair of ventricular septal defect. Age at operation is along the horizontal axis. The family of curves represents levels of preoperative pulmonary vascular resistance (units · meter²). Note the high probability in infants, even when PVR is high, and the low probability when PVR is high in older patients. (Nomogram from Blackstone, E. H., Kirklin, J. W., Bradley, E. L., DuShane, J. W., and Appelbaum, A.: Optimal age and results in repair of large ventricular septal defects. J. Thorac. Cardiovasc. Surg. 72:661, 1976.)

also be present and may complicate the early and late postoperative period. The most common of these is *chronic obstructive pulmonary disease.* Its presence affects not only the risk of cardiac surgery, and thus the indications for it, but also the postoperative management of the patient.

The Kidneys (see also Chap. 52). Preexisting *chronic renal disease* increases the risk of developing acute renal dysfunction and renal failure early in the postoperative period and thus affects patient management in this period and the risk of the operation.[23,24] *Cyanotic congenital heart disease* predisposes the patient to acute renal failure early postoperatively, probably because such a patient gradually develops morphological renal abnormalities.[25] *Preoperative chronic congestive heart failure* likewise predisposes to acute renal failure soon after operation, most likely because of the abnormalities of renal function and structure that result from this state.

The Blood. The *polycythemia* secondary to cyanotic congenital heart disease (pp. 949 and 1686) is overcome immediately at the start of cardiopulmonary bypass by the hemodilution that is used. However, most patients who were polycythemic preoperatively have a greater than usual tendency to bleed in the perioperative period. Special preventive measures are required.

Long-standing *congestive heart failure* with hepatic congestion may reduce hepatic synthesis of normal clotting factors and thereby increase the tendency for bleeding after cardiopulmonary bypass. Because of the current prevalence of *aspirin ingestion* and the use of other drugs that affect platelet function, preoperative laboratory determination of bleeding time is advisable in most patients.

The Liver. Even mild preexisting liver disease increases the risk of acute hepatic failure early after cardiac surgery. Thus, its presence must be taken into account in planning the conduct of the operation and management in the early postoperative period.

The Brain. Patients who have recovered virtually completely from a hemiplegic episode prior to their cardiac surgery may have a temporary reappearance of the hemi-plegic signs and symptoms immediately after cardiac surgery using cardiopulmonary bypass. This does not necessarily indicate that a new neurological injury has occurred, and recovery from this temporary relapse is usually rapid.

Because of the largely nonpulsatile nature of perfusion during cardiopulmonary bypass, patients with significant carotid artery stenosis may be at increased risk for ischemic neurological injury during and after operation. Thus, signs and symptoms of cerebrovascular insufficiency should be sought in adult patients with generalized atherosclerosis so that proper preoperative evaluation and intraoperative management may be employed to minimize the risk of neurological injury.

Other Factors Affecting The Outcome of Surgery

Preoperative Symptomatic State. Advanced preoperative symptoms affect the early results of cardiac surgery because they are usually associated with impaired ventricular systolic and diastolic performance, as well as other organ dysfunction. They affect late results because of their implications with regard to the secondary cardiomyopathy.

As an example of the effect on early results, in infants less than 3 months old, at least between 1967 and 1978, the hospital mortality was directly related to the preoperative symptomatic state[26] (Table 55–6). As another instance, the preoperative symptomatic state of the patient undergoing aortic valve replacement (isolated or combined with mitral valve replacement) affects the probability of early postoperative death from cardiac causes (Fig. 55–8). Aortic valve replacement, isolated or combined with mitral valve replacement, exemplifies the effect of preoperative symptoms on late results as well (Fig. 55–2).

Age of the Patient. Very young age and very old age are incremental risks for hospital death under many circumstances. This does not mean that hospital mortality is necessarily higher in the very young and the very old. It

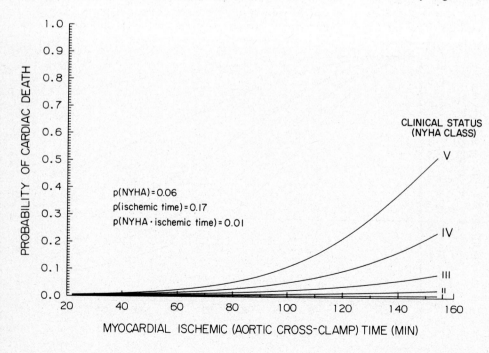

p(NYHA) = 0.06
p(ischemic time) = 0.17
p(NYHA · ischemic time) = 0.01

CLINICAL STATUS
(NYHA CLASS)

V

IV

III

II

PROBABILITY OF CARDIAC DEATH

MYOCARDIAL ISCHEMIC (AORTIC CROSS-CLAMP) TIME (MIN)

FIGURE 55–8 Relation of preoperative clinical status and myocardial ischemic (aortic cross-clamp) time to probability of cardiac death after primary or secondary, isolated or combined, aortic valve replacement, UAB[19] (n = 1,042, 1975 to July 1979).

TABLE 55–6 THE RELATION OF PREOPERATIVE SYMPTOMATIC CLASS TO HOSPITAL DEATH AFTER INTRACARDIAC OPERATION IN THE FIRST 3 MONTHS OF LIFE

PREOPERATIVE CLASS	n	HOSPITAL DEATHS		
		n	%	70% CL (%)
II	15	3	20	9–36
III	68	15	22	17–28
IV	68	37	54	47–94
V	23	20	87	75–94
Total	174	75	43	39–47

p(chi-square) for table < 0.0001.
CL = confidence limits.
UAB, 1967 to July 1981. Classes II, III, IV correspond to the NYHA Class, and Class V indicates preoperative shock or metabolic acidosis.
(From Kirklin, J. K., Blackstone, E. H., Kirklin, J. W., McKay, R., Pacifico, A. D., and Bargeron, L. M., Jr.: Intracardiac surgery in infants under age 3 months: Incremental risk factors for hospital mortality. Am. J. Cardiol. *48*:500, 1981.)

means only that it is *more difficult* to obtain very low hospital mortality rates in these two groups.

The incremental risk of very young age (less than about 6 months) is probably related to the very young patient's increased sensitivity to the damaging effects of cardiopulmonary bypass (see below). For many lesions, however, appropriate knowledge and experience can neutralize this incremental risk (Fig. 55–9).[27]

Date of Operation. The knowledge and techniques of cardiac surgery continue to improve. As a result, both the early and the late results of cardiac surgery improve with time (Fig. 55–9).[28] This makes comparisons between nonconcurrent clinical studies hazardous, unless a specific effort is made to take into account these changes with time.

Institution of Operation. There are true institutional (and surgeon-to-surgeon) differences in the early and late results of cardiac surgery. These are related to variations in knowledge, technique, and experience. Since these differences are generally identified by comparisons between two or more prospective but not necessarily concurrent clinical studies involving a more or less heterogeneous population, the comparisons must be done with great care and full knowledge of the multivariate nature of the determinants of these results. For example, a preliminary comparison of the results of coronary artery bypass grafting in hospital A and in hospital B may indicate that the hospital mortality rate is the same in the two institutions. The conclusion might be drawn that the quality of work in the two hospitals is similar. However, analysis of the two patient populations may show a much higher proportion of patients with moderately or severely depressed left ventricular function in hospital B, which is an incremental risk factor for hospital death even when the patient is in highly knowledgeable and experienced hands. The conclusion would be that the quality of the work in hospital B was in fact superior.

Comments. It is evident that a very large number of preoperative variables affect the results of cardiac surgery. This must be taken into account in estimating the risks, and thus the advisability of, surgical treatment for an individual patient. In addition, the complexities of *comparative* analysis of results are apparent from this and from the large number of intraoperative variables that also affect results (see below). Such comparative studies must therefore be based upon precise and extensive data gathering, sophisticated and multivariate statistical methods, and a contemplative analysis of the results.

INTRAOPERATIVE CONDITIONS AFFECTING EARLY AND LATE RESULTS

Cardiopulmonary Bypass (CPB)

CPB could be considered a safe support system for clinical cardiac surgery, judging from the fact that the hospital mortality for coronary artery bypass grafting (CABG) in recent years approaches zero. However, there are important damaging effects of CPB that contribute to in-hospital morbidity and mortality and must be considered in early postoperative management.

The manifestations of the damaging effects of CPB include an abnormal tendency to bleed externally and into tissues; a diffuse or whole-body "inflammatory reaction," characterized by increased capillary permeability with con-

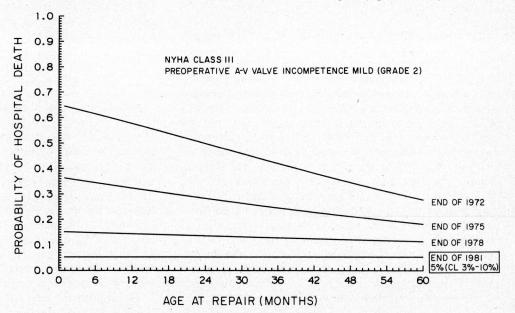

FIGURE 55–9 Probability of hospital death after repair of uncomplicated AV septal defects *with* interventricular communication ("complete AV canal defect"). Note that by 1981, hospital mortality was 5 per cent, and the incremental risk of young age was neutralized (70 per cent confidence limits are available but not shown). (From Studer, M., Blackstone, E. H., Kirklin, J. W., Pacifico, A. D., Soto, B., Chung, G. K. T., Kirklin J. K., and Bargeron, L. M., Jr.: Determinants of early and late results of repair of atrioventricular septal (canal) defects. J. Thorac. Cardiovasc. Surg. *84*: 523, 1982.)

sequent transcapillary plasma loss, increased interstitial fluid, leukocytosis, and fever; renal dysfunction; peripheral and perhaps central vasoconstriction, which persists a variable time after CPB and results in both hemodynamic and metabolic problems; breakdown of red blood cells, resulting in hemoglobinemia, hemoglobinuria, and anemia; and perhaps increased susceptibility to infection. These all contribute to organ and subsystem dysfunction early postoperatively, a state that some call "postperfusion syndrome," or "postpump syndrome." The fact that most patients convalesce normally after CPB attests only to patients' ability to compensate for these damaging effects and not to their absence. The uncommon occurrence of severe pulmonary edema without elevated left atrial pressure (p. 566), severe bleeding diatheses, and transient subtle neurological changes occasionally brings these abnormalities of CPB forcefully to attention. Much of the current residual morbidity and mortality from open heart operations is secondary to these poorly understood changes produced by CPB.

The possible *mechanisms for the damaging effect* are the exposure of blood to an abnormal environment and altered arterial blood flow patterns. The first of these, the exposure of blood, has a particularly powerful and generalized influence on the organism. During CPB, blood is *exposed to nonendothelial surfaces*. This exposure has direct and indirect effects on *platelets*, which result in platelet clumping and embolization, a reduction in the number of platelets,[29] and a reduction in their important adhesive and aggregating properties.[30] These phenomena have a number of important secondary effects. *Proteins* are damaged by blood exposure to nonphysiologic surfaces. Some degree of protein denaturation occurs, the lipoproteins liberating free fat in the process.[31] Fat microemboli result. Damage to *proteins* that are *part of the humoral amplification system* has particularly complex and widespread effects. Probably an initiating event in this process is the activating of *Hageman factor (Factor XII)*.[32,33] This initiates the cascade of the coagulation humoral amplification system, which consumes the coagulation factors to a varying degree.[29,34] Also activated to a varying degree are the *fibrinolytic system*,[35] the *complement system*,[36,37,38,39] and the *kallikrein-bradykinin system*.[40,41,42]

The adverse effects of activation of the complement system may be particularly important. The complement cascade, once activated, results in a complex of glycoproteins (called C5 to C9) that aid in membrane lysis and phagocytosis. It results also in the production of powerful anaphylatoxins (called C3a and C3b), which increase vascular permeability, cause smooth muscle contraction, mediate leukocyte chemotaxis, and facilitate leukocyte aggregation and enzyme release.[43,44,45] The usefulness of these reactions as a response to localized injury is obvious, but the production of a *whole-body inflammatory reaction* (as reflected by complement activation) may be severely detrimental. As a part of this, the anaphylatoxins stimulate polymorphonuclear aggregation, which with shear stress damage (also occurring during CPB) results in the *pulmonary sequestration of leukocytes*.[46,47] This sequestration and the pulmonary endothelial injury from activated platelets[48] probably in large measure account for the variable degree of pulmonary dysfunction seen in most patients after CPB.

Shear stresses are generated during CPB by blood pumps, suction systems, abrupt acceleration and deceleration of blood, and cavitation around the end of the arterial cannula. These are part of the abnormal environment encountered by the blood. Shear stresses damage leukocytes,[46] already subjected to other injurious effects, and erythrocytes.[49] Damage to erythrocytes results in hemolysis and elevation of serum hemoglobin levels.[50]

Part of the abnormal environment of blood is its encounter with *abnormal substances* (air bubbles, bits of fibrin and tissue debris, platelet aggregates, and defoaming agents), which are incorporated into blood and may form microemboli. Thus, some degree of microembolization occurs during each operation with CPB, and this is generally greatest during the first 10 or 15 minutes of the perfusion.[51]

Arterial blood flow patterns during CPB are variable. Most CPB for cardiac surgery is conducted with roller pumps; the arterial blood flow is nearly linear (nonpulsatile), and the arterial pressure pulse is very small. This is an alteration from the normal state, in which the arterial pulse pressure is about one-third the systolic blood pressure. However, it remains controversial whether pulsatile flow, which can be used during CPB, results in fewer functional derangements than does nonpulsatile flow.[52,53]

There are some incremental risk factors that increase the probability of important clinical manifestations resulting from CPB. One is the *duration of CPB*. In adults the probability of demonstrable structural or functional damage increases as the perfusion extends beyond about 150 minutes. Another is the *age of the patient*. The probability of damage appears to increase in patients under 6 months of age and even more so in those under 3 months.[26] The probability of damage may also be greater in the very elderly. These two risk factors, duration of CPB and age, probably interact, so that in small infants the probability of demonstrable damage from more than 90 to 120 minutes of CPB seems to be as great as from over 150 minutes of CPB in adults. Possibly, the *cardiac defect* being treated is influential. Preoperatively cyanotic patients seem more susceptible to the damaging effects of CPB. Other factors that may affect the probability of a demonstrable damaging effect include the *perfusion flow rate*, the *composition of the perfusate*, the *oxygenating surface*, and the *temperature of the patient* during the perfusion. These variables also interact with one another.

Profound Hypothermia and Total Circulatory Arrest

An alternative method to continuous CPB for cardiac surgery is the use of profound hypothermia and a continuous period of total circulatory arrest during the repair. The method is used routinely for infant cardiac surgery by some surgeons and by most surgeons for a few special situations at any age. This technique provides optimal surgical exposure in a field uncluttered by cannulae, which accounts for its use by many in infant cardiac surgery. In this method, the patient's body temperature is reduced to about 20°C by a sequential combination of surface cooling and then further "core cooling" by a cold perfusate during CPB[54] or by "core cooling" only.[55] Total circulatory arrest times of 30 to 75 minutes have been used.

The hypothesis underlying the use of this method is that there is a "safe" duration of total circulatory arrest (this is, one characterized by absence of functional or structural derangements in the early or late postoperative period) and that the "safe" duration is inversely related to body temperature during the arrest period. It is further hypothesized that hypothermia, without itself producing damage, reduces metabolic activity to the extent that the available small energy stores in the various organs maintain cell viability throughout the ischemic period of total circulatory arrest and thus allow normal structure and function to return during reperfusion. The brain is the organ most rapidly damaged by total circulatory arrest, and its "safe total circulatory arrest time" is considered the factor limiting the time of the arrest period.

The accumulated experimental data[56-61] indicate that 30 minutes of total circulatory arrest at 20°C are in fact "safe" (using the criterion given earlier). Clinical experiences[61-63] support this idea. However, there is uncertainty regarding the safety of longer periods of circulatory arrest. Seizures or choreoathetoid movements or both, usually but not always transient, develop in up to 10 per cent of such patients.[62-65] Probably the more important evidences of brain damage, including impaired intellectual development, develop in an increasingly larger proportion of the patients as the length of total circulatory arrest is extended beyond 30 minutes and particularly when it is extended beyond 45 minutes.[66]

For these reasons, we use total circulatory arrest very infrequently in cardiac surgery, even in infants. In part this is because of concerns about the damaging effects of total circulatory arrest; in part because of the greatly improved exposure during CPB obtained by current methods of cannulation;[19] and in part because of an apparent reduction in the damaging effects of CPB in infants because of present techniques.[26]

Myocardial Ischemia

In the early years of cardiac surgery, little was made of the *possibility that low cardiac output in the early postoperative period was related to the perioperative development of myocardial necrosis* (or infarction). Then in 1967, Taber and colleagues described scattered areas of myocardial necrosis estimated to involve about 30 per cent of the left ventricular myocardium in patients dying early after cardiac operations, and implicated this as the etiology of the patients' low cardiac output and death.[67] Najafi and colleagues showed in 1967 that acute diffuse subendocardial myocardial infarction was a frequent finding in patients dying early after valve replacement and suggested that this was related to methods of intraoperative management of the myocardium.[68,69] When coronary artery bypass grafting began in the early 1970's, cardiologists and cardiac surgeons noted that a disturbingly high proportion of patients developed perioperatively (during or within 48 hours of operation) a transmural myocardial infarct.[70,71] Soon it was shown that the development of transmural myocardial infarction was not limited to patients undergoing coronary artery bypass grafting but was a complication of cardiac surgery in general.[72,73] The rarely occurring extreme form of ischemic damage, "stone heart,"[74] was recognized at about that time as occurring during reperfusion and has been confirmed to be essentially massive ischemic contracture.[75,76]

Unfortunately, almost all kinds of cardiac operations done with the help of CPB require that the aorta be cross-

clamped during at least part of the repair. The aortic cross-clamping stops coronary blood flow, since the arterial input from the pump-oxygenator comes into the aorta distal to the cross-clamping. Aortic cross-clamping has the favorable effect of improving exposure for the cardiac operation by stopping the coronary flow and by preventing any leakage back into the heart through the aortic valve. Another result is that cardiac action lessens and eventually stops, which facilitates the technical aspects of the operation. Aortic cross-clamping has the disadvantage of producing immediate and global myocardial ischemia. The phenomena that follow this include (1) myocardial edema, (2) functional depression without permanent structural damage, and (3) myocardial cell death.

Myocardial edema results in part from the same factors that increase interstitial fluid throughout the body during CPB (see earlier section). It is increased by episodes of global myocardial ischemia and thus is present to some degree in nearly all hearts after aortic cross-clamping. This results not only from the tendency to interstitial edema upon reperfusion but also from cellular edema and swelling. The latter is from depletion of energy stores and impairment of active membrane transport of ions[77] and from intracellular production of new osmotically active molecules by ischemic metabolic conversion of osmotically less active larger molecules.[78] Myocardial edema, when sufficiently severe, reduces ventricular diastolic function by lessening compliance (distensibility). This tends to reduce preload and thus stroke volume and cardiac output.

Temporary functional depression (reduced myocardial contractility) without permanent structural or biochemical damage probably occurs after even short periods of aortic cross-clamping with any method of myocardial protection.[79] This depression has been difficult to define and quantitate. However, it is probably related to the inevitable, but reversible, consequences of an ischemic period. Lactate accumulates in the tissue, and intracellular pH falls[80] as tissue pO_2 falls with ischemia and energy depletion. Adenosine triphosphate (ATP) levels decline, and the reduction is greater the longer the duration of ischemia.[81,82] The calcium content of isolated mitochondria rises.[83]

Myocardial cell death is the most important result of global myocardial ischemia and occurs commonly as a complication of cardiac surgery before cold cardioplegia.[84] Its importance is underscored by the facts that cardiac output in the early postoperative period is inversely proportional to the extent of the myocardial necrosis, no matter what the method of myocardial protection, and thus that the amount of myocardial necrosis is a determinant of the patient's early postoperative condition and probability of survival (Fig. 55-10). Myocardial cell death is often difficult to identify by routine light microscopy after global ischemia *without* reperfusion.[85] Special techniques, however, do demonstrate discrete loss of glycogen[85,86] and vague changes in the density of affected fibers. Electron microscopy shows uniform and readily recognizable changes, including relaxation of myofibrils, prominent I bands, virtual absence of glycogen, and margination of nuclear chromatin (p. 1264).

With reperfusion, irreversibly damaged myocardial cells undergo further changes, easily seen even by light microscopy, including a disruption of the regular myofibrillar pattern and the presence of prominent *contraction bands*[87]

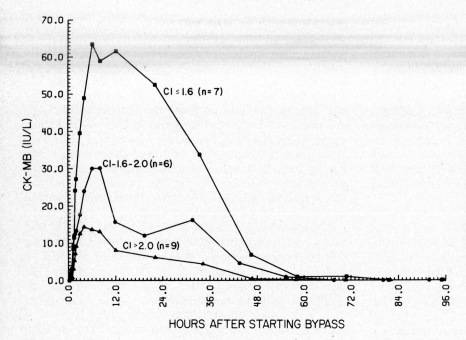

FIGURE 55–10 The relation of extent of perioperative myocardial necrosis (reflected in the blood CK-MB isoenzyme values along the vertical axis) and the early postoperative cardiac index (CI in liters· min^{-1}· meter^{-2}) in 22 consecutive patients undergoing mitral valve replacement at UAB in 1975, using simple cold ischemic arrest. Geometric mean values are portrayed. Note the very high levels of CK-MB in patients with low cardiac output (1.6 or less) and the low levels in patients with large cardiac output (more than 2.0). The overall correlation of CK-MB (duration, peak, and integrated area) and cardiac index is r = −0.4 and p = 0.04. (From Kirklin, J. W., and Barratt-Boyes, B. G.: Textbook of Cardiac Surgery. New York, John Wiley and Sons [in preparation].)

(the prerequisite of which is cell death). During cardiac surgery, reperfusion of a heart that has been severely damaged by ischemia may produce a sudden massive palpable *contracture*[74,75,76] (localized or global "stone heart"), which may seem to the surgeon to be simply ventricular fibrillation but which is not. This is *not* the true contracture (or rigor) of ischemia[84] but is a phenomenon of reperfusion of a ventricle that has experienced severe ischemic damage. This may be the gross analogue of the contraction bands observed microscopically. With reperfusion, calcium accumulations become abnormally high in the mitochondria,[88,89] secondary to an accelerated entry of calcium ions into the cells. This accelerated entry results from loss of membrane selective permeability properties in the presence of a reduced capacity for the control of cytoplasmic calcium concentration by the sodium-calcium pump, believed to be the result of low levels of ATP[90] (p. 1253).

The incidence and extent of perioperative ischemic myocardial necrosis are significantly related to the *duration of the global myocardial ischemia*, no matter what method of myocardial protection is used.[91] When the myocardium is hypothermic during the ischemic period, the proportion of cells dying in any given ischemic time is less, such that the degree of damage is directly related to myocardial temperature during the period of global ischemia.[92] When the heart's electromechanical activity is stopped shortly after the start of global ischemia ("cardioplegia"), myocardial necrosis is still further reduced.

Myocardial Protection. A number of methods for *myocardial protection* during cardiac surgery have been used, but in recent years most surgeons have turned to the technique of myocardial preservation with cold and cardioplegia. This method takes advantage of the protective effect of cold and of sudden cessation of electromechanical activity. It greatly extends the "safe" time of global myocardial ischemia (ischemia without myocardial necrosis). The data on humans indicate that with this method no significant myocardial necrosis or permanent functional damage results from total myocardial ischemia for up to 120 minutes, if the preoperative myocardial reserves are good

(i.e., NYHA Functional Class I or II). However, decreased preoperative myocardial reserves (presumably present in patients in NYHA Functional Classes III and IV) appear to lower the safe time limits of cold cardioplegia, and the data suggest that only about 80 minutes are allowed in patients with advanced heart failure (Fig. 55–8).

The most commonly used cardioplegic agent at present is potassium, in concentrations of 15 to 35 mEq. Potassium in this concentration blocks the initial "fast" (inward sodium current) phase of myocardial cellular depolarization. Even with this concentration of potassium, electromechanical activity can persist or return in the presence of agents such as catecholamines, which "open" the latter "slow" (inward calcium and sodium current) phase of myocardial cellular depolarization on which potassium has no effect, and when noncoronary collateral flow is large. Proper methodology overcomes these potential problems. The cardioplegic vehicle is either asanguineous (some type of buffered electrolyte solution usually containing mannitol) or sanguineous (made up of blood from the pump-oxygenator). It is delivered into the aortic root, or directly into the coronary ostia, at a temperature of about 4°C. Infusions are repeated about every 30 minutes during the ischemic period.

Completeness of Repair

It is sometimes forgotten that a poor hemodynamic state early in the postoperative period may be related, in part at least, to an incomplete surgical procedure (such as replacement of only one valve when two are significantly abnormal in function, very incomplete myocardial revascularization, incomplete repair of a large ventricular septal defect, the leaving of important right ventricular outflow tract obstruction in the repair of tetralogy of Fallot, and so forth). This emphasizes the need for complete knowledge of the preoperative cardiac conditions, a wise assessment of the surgical procedures needed to correct them, and a skillful and determined surgical effort to carry out a completely corrective procedure.

CONVALESCENCE AND CARE AFTER CARDIAC SURGERY

The primary determinants of the success of a cardiac operation are events in the operating room. However, every cardiac surgical patient requires postoperative care. Unfortunately, all invasive monitoring and some that is noninvasive (for example, the recording of an electrocardiogram without proper grounding), as well as all interventions, involve risks of varying magnitude to the patient. They should, therefore, be used only when the probability of postoperative problems is greater than their inherent risks.

After cardiac operations, the combination of the basic cardiac disease, the cardiac trauma of the operation, and the whole-body response to cardiopulmonary bypass (CPB) creates special problems. The problems related to CPB are particularly complex (see earlier section). Many conceptual, scientific, and management errors are made by failing to realize that humans during and for a time after CPB are in a special biological situation to which the knowledge and rules derived for "intact" humans may or *may not* apply. Fortunately, in spite of these problems, many cardiac operations are now almost without risk (risk approaches zero). Postoperative care can be quite simple for patients undergoing these operations. Yet certain situations still have an appreciable probability of hospital death or morbidity, and in them more extensive monitoring and interventions are needed.

The patient may be considered as a complex integrated system composed of a number of separate but interrelated subsystems (i.e., cardiovascular, pulmonary, renal, nervous, and alimentary). The care of such a patient can be accomplished effectively utilizing a "subsystems analysis" approach.[93] This commences in the operating room as CPB is discontinued and continues into the early and late postoperative period.

An *uncomplicated or normal convalescence* is one devoid of any findings or events that increase the probability of hospital death or of important complications or of a suboptimal late result. As long as this pattern of normal convalescence continues, monitoring, testing, and interventions can safely be minimized. Alertness to deviations from the pattern of an uncomplicated convalescence is required, as these are an indication for greater intensity of observation and treatment.

Cardiovascular Subsystem

Most perioperative complications, hospital deaths, and late failures after cardiac surgery are in some way a failure of the cardiovascular subsystem. An understanding of its function and postoperative management is therefore necessary.

Convalescence can be considered normal with regard to the cardiovascular subsystem when the cardiac output is adequate for the metabolic needs of the organism. The output can be evaluated either by measuring the cardiac output or by assessing its adequacy, or by both methods. Cardiac output may be measured by indocyanine green indicator dilution techniques or by thermodilution. The former has the advantage that residual intracardiac shunts can be detected by the contour of the indicator dilution curve or by double sampling techniques. The adequacy of cardiac output is assessed by evaluation of the pedal pulses and skin temperature, urine flow, and mixed venous oxygen levels, and these methods are generally highly reliable. Arterial blood pressure is ordinarily an insensitive guide to cardiac performance early in the postoperative period, chiefly because the systemic vascular resistance is unusually high. However, arterial hypotension is always an indication for intense evaluation, and the patient cannot be considered to be convalescing normally when mean arterial blood pressure is less than 10 per cent below normal for age.

The treatment of *inadequate cardiac output* is directed at increasing the output by manipulation of preload, afterload, the contractile state, and heart rate and at improving tissue oxygen levels by other means as well. When cardiac output is low, preload is made appropriate by increasing blood volume until the higher of the two atrial pressures is approximately 15 mm Hg. If the wall thickness of the left ventricle is unusually great, or its contractility or compliance or both are decreased, it may be helpful to take mean left atrial pressure to 20 mm Hg. When the right ventricle is the limiting one, right atrial pressure usually can advantageously be taken only to approximately 18 mm Hg. Above these levels, a fall in cardiac output may occur.

Afterload reduction (p. 534) can often be used to improve cardiac performance early after cardiac surgery. When the left ventricular performance is the limiting one, and systemic arterial blood pressure is more than approximately 10 per cent above normal, its afterload should be reduced by lowering arterial blood pressure to between normal and 10 per cent above normal, generally with nitroprusside. However, vasodilator therapy, which results in a mean arterial blood pressure lower than normal, often is associated with a reduction in cardiac output and is dangerous.[94] Rarely, in patients with severe long-standing mitral valve disease or congenital heart disease with pulmonary vascular obstructive changes, right ventricular dysfunction associated with elevated pulmonary artery pressure may limit cardiac performance, and reduction of right ventricular afterload with vasodilator agents is indicated.

Heart rate is optimized as necessary. For patients in sinus or junctional rhythm, atrial pacing is used; if atrial fibrillation is present, ventricular pacing is used; and if AV dissociation is the rhythm, AV sequential pacing is used. If tachyarrhythmias are present, control is usually obtained by pharmacological means or by specialized pacing methods.[95]

If these relatively simple measures do not bring cardiac output to an adequate level, administration of catecholamines or intraaortic balloon pumping (IABP) is used. The former is chosen in infants and children, in adults without major myocardial necrosis and with only mild or moderate impairments, and in those with a contraindication to IABP. If catecholamines are indicated, dopamine (p. 542) is begun at low doses, which can be increased up to 15 μg $\cdot$ kg^{-1} $\cdot$ min^{-1} if needed. When dopamine is not effective, dobutamine (p. 543) is added, and the dosages are similar. Dobutamine is a potent inotropic agent that usually does not increase systemic or pulmonary vascular resistance and has less tendency to produce tachycardia.

Epinephrine, isoproterenol, and norepinephrine are now rarely used. However, in the presence of predominantly right ventricular dysfunction and decreased or normal heart rate, isoproterenol may be the preferred drug because of its favorable effect on pulmonary vascular resistance. When catecholamines are administered, and a satisfactory response obtained, 8 to 12 hours later an aggressive and persistent effort is begun *gradually* to reduce and finally discontinue them.

In adults, if adjustment of preload, afterload, and heart rate and modest doses (2.5 to 5 $\mu g \cdot kg^{-1} \cdot min^{-1}$) of dopamine do not result in adequate cardiac performance, intraaortic balloon pumping (IABP) (p. 593) is considered. If a strong suspicion of myocardial necrosis exists or if ventricular electrical instability is present, IABP is preferable to catecholamines as *initial* treatment.

While efforts are being made to increase cardiac output, the tissue and mixed venous oxygen levels should also be raised by attention to the other variables represented in the Fick equation. The blood hemoglobin is kept above 10 to 12 gm $\cdot dl^{-1}$ by administration of packed red blood cells or whole blood, and the PaO_2 is maintained at 100 to 200 mm Hg by increasing the fractional concentration of oxygen in the inspired air. Unduly high oxygen consumption ($\dot{V}O_2$) is prevented while the patient is on a ventilator, by use of sedation or paralyzing drugs, to prevent restlessness or agitation. Hyperthermia (rectal or central temperature $\geq 39.7°C$, or 103.5°F) is treated vigorously.

Postoperative morbidity and mortality can result from *cardiac arrhythmias*. These may occur when the cardiac subsystem has been otherwise functioning normally or as a complication of low cardiac output. They may be the manifestation of a severe secondary cardiomyopathy. Atrial and ventricular pacing wires, routinely placed at operation and left for 5 to 10 postoperative days, are of utmost importance in the diagnosis[96] and treatment[97,98] of postoperative arrhythmias.[95]

Ventricular electrical instability, which includes *premature ventricular contractions* (PVC's) and *ventricular tachycardia*, is an extremely important arrhythmia. Although controversy exists concerning the proportion of patients with PVC's who develop ventricular fibrillation, it may be that this potential exists in any patient who has significant intermittent or continuous ventricular electrical instability. Therefore, the electrocardiogram is monitored continuously for at least 48 hours in all patients, and ventricular electrical instability is treated vigorously by the methods generally used in other settings (p. 720).

Various *atrial arrhythmias* may complicate the postoperative period. *Atrial fibrillation* (p. 699) is treated initially with digitalis. If it persists until the seventh postoperative day in patients who have not been in atrial fibrillation preoperatively, electroversion should usually be carried out. *Atrial flutter* (p. 697), formerly a difficult arrhythmia to manage postoperatively, is now usually converted to sinus rhythm by rapid atrial pacing (via the two implanted atrial wires) at the so-called critical pacing rate with sudden cessation of pacing after about 20 seconds.[95] Digoxin is begun and continued for 6 weeks. Procainamide is begun and continued for 8 weeks, with a switch to quinidine if long-term drug therapy is indicated. *Paroxysmal atrial contractions* (PAC's) (p. 694) may trigger or lead to atrial fibrillation, and, therefore, an attempt is made to suppress them

with atrial pacing, digoxin, procainamide (Pronestyl), or quinidine. *Paroxysmal atrial tachycardia* (PAT) (p. 702) is usually first treated by rapid atrial pacing and then sudden cessation.[95] If this is unsuccessful, intravenous propranolol, verapamil, or digoxin is usually successful. If PAT is recurrent or refractory to treatment, continuous rapid atrial pacing at approximately 100 beats faster than the intrinsic atrial rate is employed to produce and sustain a 2:1 block. Patients who have had PAT generally should receive digoxin for about 6 weeks.

When the onset of a supraventricular tachyarrhythmia is accompanied by significant hemodynamic deterioration, prompt cardioversion (p. 669) is indicated if atrial wires are not in place.

Renal Subsystem

Convalescence after cardiac surgery can be considered uncomplicated when urine volume is "adequate". Useful but somewhat arbitrary criteria are that it be greater than 500 ml $\cdot$ 24 hours$^{-1}\cdot$ meter^{-2} or 167 ml $\cdot$ 8 hours$^{-1}\cdot$ meter^{-2} or 20 ml $\cdot$ hr$^{-1}\cdot$ meter^{-2}. Solute excretion must also be "adequate," and the convalescence is abnormal when solute excretion is insufficient to keep serum potassium levels below 5 mEq $\cdot$ liter^{-1}, blood urea nitrogen (BUN) levels below 40 mg $\cdot$ dl^{-1}, and creatinine levels below 1.5 mg $\cdot$ dl^{-1}. Others use different criteria. Convalescence cannot be considered normal when the urine is pink but without red blood cells early in the postoperative period, for this indicates an inordinate and potentially dangerous amount of hemolysis (free plasma hemoglobin levels >40 mg $\cdot$ dl^{-1}).

As a guide to the continuing evaluation of the renal subsystem, a urinary catheter is inserted in the operating room preoperatively and left for 24 to 48 hours to monitor urine flow. Serum potassium is measured every 4 hours during the first 24 postoperative hours, and if convalescence is not normal, every 8 hours for at least the next 48 hours. Serum creatinine and BUN are measured each morning for at least the first 48 hours.

Acute renal failure after cardiac surgery is rare in adults, occurring in fewer than 0.1 per cent of patients undergoing operations such as coronary artery bypass grafting, but may occur in 8 to 10 per cent of infants undergoing open intracardiac operations.[99,100] It is usually associated with low cardiac output initially, but rarely may happen when the other criteria of cardiac subsystem performance are satisfactory.[24,100,101]

The probability of acute renal failure after surgery with CPB is also influenced by certain incremental risk factors other than low cardiac output:

1. *Young age*: One reason for the apparently increased incidence in infants (noted above) is the higher proportion in this age group of seriously ill patients with low cardiac output early in the postoperative period. The immaturity of the kidney in infants and young children, resulting in less ability to concentrate the urine, may also predispose them to acute renal failure. Infants may develop more tissue hypoxia during and early after CPB than do older patients, with a resultant increased production of potassium, urea nitrogen, and other substances, some of which may be nephrotoxic.

2. *Cyanotic heart disease*: Acute renal failure is more likely to occur after operations for cyanotic heart disease.[25] A renal lesion is known to exist in many such patients preoperatively.

3. *Preoperative impairment of renal function* considerably increases the risk of acute renal failure early in the postoperative period.[23,101] Therefore, a part of the preoperative evaluation should be the determination of renal function.

4. A *long period* of *CPB* (> 180 minutes in adults, less than this in infants and small children) probably increases the risk of acute renal failure.

5. The additional risk from *profound hypothermia and total circulatory arrest* is not known, nor is that of long periods of *reduced flow* during *hypothermic CPB*. However, flows 1.6 liter $\cdot$ min^{-1} $\cdot$ m^{-2} or more at 28°C and mean arterial blood pressure 30 mm Hg or more during CPB at moderate hypothermia seem adequate to minimize acute renal failure.[24]

6. A *high plasma hemoglobin level* (> 40 mg $\cdot$ dl^{-1}) during and early after CPB probably increases the risk of acute renal failure.

7. The suggestion that a *whole blood prime* is an incremental risk is supported by several studies.[102,103]

8. *Aminoglycosides* (gentamicin) and some other antibiotics may increase the risk of acute renal failure after CPB.

Acute renal failure may develop within 12 to 48 hours after operation. Its first effect is resistant oliguria of increasing severity, resulting in very rapidly rising serum potassium levels (probably because of the acute loss of potassium from hemolyzing red blood cells and from the whole-body loss of intracellular potassium that characterizes the perioperative period in patients who have been on CPB) and more slowly rising BUN and creatinine levels. Although this form of acute renal failure is rarely the primary mode of death, it complicates recovery in a major way unless effective interventions are promptly made. It is the type usually seen in infants. A less lethal form becomes apparent on the third or fourth postoperative day. This manifests itself by a progressive rise in BUN and creatinine levels, which peak at 80 to 120 and 5 to 8 mg $\cdot$ dl^{-1}, respectively, about 7 to 10 days postoperatively. There is often little or no oliguria, and hyperkalemia greater than 5 mEq $\cdot$ liter^{-1} does not usually develop. Spontaneous resolution usually follows, and as long as the patient's clinical condition is satisfactory, urine flow is adequate, and BUN and creatinine levels eventually begin to fall, dialysis is not indicated.

When *oliguria* occurs early postoperatively, *cardiac preload performance* should be optimized (see above). Intravenous *furosemide* (1 mg $\cdot$ kg^{-1}) is sometimes administered. If a good response is obtained, this is repeated every 6 hours for 3 days. If a response to furosemide is not obtained, the dose is doubled, and then quadrupled, and then 8 mg $\cdot$ kg^{-1} is given. When the *serum potassium* level rises above *5.5 mEq $\cdot$ l^{-1}*, *glucose-insulin solution* is given *intravenously* and *sodium polystyrene sulfonate (Kayexalate) enemas* are used.

Unless oliguria and hyperkalemia respond to treatment within a few hours, and especially in infants, the nephrologist should proceed immediately with dialysis. Usually, peritoneal dialysis is used early postoperatively, particularly in infants.[104] In older patients hemodialysis may be substituted for peritoneal dialysis after a few days if acute renal failure persists. With these measures many patients can be maintained in good condition until cardiac and renal functions improve and ultimately recover fully.[100]

Pulmonary Subsystem

Patients are extubated early after cardiac surgery, as soon as the effects of the anesthetic agents have disappeared, when normal convalescence is likely. In patients undergoing *closed* operations, including infants, this usually means extubation in the operating room. After *open* operations of an uncomplicated nature, such as repair of simple congenital lesions, coronary artery bypass grafting, or isolated valve replacement or valvotomy, patients, including infants, are usually extubated within 4 to 8 hours postoperatively. Following complex open operations, ventilation is continued at least overnight, and the patient is not extubated until the appropriate criteria are met.

While intubated, the patient is ventilated with a volume-controlled respirator that provides *intermittent positive pressure breathing* (IPPB). It should be equipped with valves that allow the patient to breathe himself, when he will, in between the *intermittent mandatory ventilation* (IMV) from the ventilator. The IMV is reduced gradually as soon as spontaneous breathing is sufficient, to accustom the patient to breathing again and to gain the hemodynamic advantages of the negative intrapleural pressures that develop during spontaneous inspiration. *Positive end-expiratory pressure* (PEEP) should be used in most patients. PEEP is preferred because of the studies that suggest larger lung volumes and fewer perfused but nonventilated alveoli during ventilation and smaller alveolar-arterial oxygen differences (A-a) pO$_2$ after extubation when it is used.[105] PEEP is not used in patients with chronic obstructive lung disease (for fear of air-trapping and rupturing a bulla with consequent pneumothorax), in infants who have undergone interatrial transposition of venous return, Fontan's operation, or a superior vena caval–right atrial anastomosis (to avoid still further elevation of jugular venous pressure). While the patient is intubated and ventilated, the inspired gases are warmed and humidified. Appropriate aspiration of the trachea, turning of the patient, and chest physiotherapy are carried out. After extubation, which should be done as soon as possible, *reintubation* is usually not necessary when the patient truly meets the criteria for extubation. However, when the work of breathing is excessive, when CO$_2$ retention is enough to produce significant respiratory acidosis, or when the patient is becoming exhausted by ventilatory efforts, reintubation is indicated. When the situation is borderline, careful observation by senior members of the team is required for proper decision-making.

Other Subsystems

Abnormalities of the other subsystems are infrequent during convalescence from cardiac surgery using a pump-oxygenator. Therefore, management of them is relatively straightforward.

Because of the increase in extracellular fluid and total exchangeable sodium and the decrease in exchangeable potassium that develop during CPB, early postoperative *fluid administration* must be precise. For approximately 48 hours after operation, no sodium is administered, and 500 ml · 24 hours^{-1}· meter^{-2} of water (as 5 per cent glucose in water) are given intravenously.[106]

Some *metabolic acidosis* (base deficit > 2 mEq · 1^{-1})[107] may be present during the early hours after intracardiac surgery, even when the patient is convalescing normally. It is left untreated if the arterial pH is 7.4 or greater and P$_a$CO$_2$ is 30 mm Hg or more. If in this circumstance PaCO$_2$ is less than 30 mm Hg, the base deficit is treated *before* adjusting the PaCO$_2$ appropriately upward. When pH is less than about 7.35, the base deficit is treated. However, if convalescence is otherwise normal, treatment is delayed for 4 to 8 hours in adults and 2 to 4 hours in infants, by which time the acidosis may have cleared spontaneously. In infants particularly, it is best to avoid this additional sodium load whenever possible.

A mild *metabolic alkalosis* may be present 24 hours after operation in normally convalescing patients, probably related, in part at least, to the sodium load contained in the anticoagulant solution of the banked blood. It is self-correcting under these circumstances and is not treated.

Body temperature may become severely elevated in the first 48 postoperative hours, particularly in infants, as discussed earlier. It is usually a manifestation of a profound reaction to cardiopulmonary bypass, although infection, reaction to homologous blood, or brain stem damage are other possible etiological factors. Its identification and vigorous treatment are important, because the prognosis for patients with it is otherwise poor. Whenever the usually monitored rectal temperature becomes abnormally high during the first 48 postoperative hours ($\geq$ 39.5°C, or 103°F), an esophageal thermistor should be introduced because the central ("core") temperature may be even higher than rectal temperature under these circumstances. When the central temperature exceeds 39.5°C, or 103°F, vigorous antipyretic measures are initiated.

Patients after cardiopulmonary bypass who are convalescing normally frequently have persistent temperature elevations ($\geq$ 38.8°C, or 102°F) for 7 to 10 days after operation in the absence of infection. This febrile response appears to be a direct response to the effects of bypass and is a self-limiting process that does not require special therapy.[108] Such patients should be examined for signs of infection, but in the absence of clinical evidence of infection, extensive laboratory investigation is usually not warranted.

Bleeding tendency of some degree develops in all patients who have been on CPB, as most of the clotting factors are abnormal for a time. In spite of this, good hemostasis can be obtained in the operating room in almost all patients, although great patience and care are often required. Special hematologic investigation and treatment are seldom needed, and minimal blood administration should be possible in the operating room and intensive care unit in most uncomplicated cases.

Drainage from the chest tubes is monitored postoperatively. Uncommonly, the drainage is excessive, and then prompt reoperation is indicated. Under proper circumstances, this should be necessary in only 1 or 2 per cent of patients. When rather rigorous criteria for reoperation are used, reentries are usually done within 3 to 4 hours of the patient's leaving the operating room, while the patients are

in good condition, and without the disadvantages of the infusion of large volumes of homologous blood.

References

1. Ross, J., Jr.: Afterload mismatch and preload reserve: A conceptual framework for the analysis of ventricular function. Prog. Cardiovasc. Dis. *18*:255, 1976.
2. Papadimitriou, J. M., Hopkins, B. E., and Taylor, R. R.: Regression of left ventricular dilation and hypertrophy after removal of volume overload. Circ. Res. *35*:127, 1974.
3. Cunha, C. L. P., Giuliani, E. R., Fuster, V., Seward, J. B., Brandenburg, R. O., and McGoon, D. C.: Preoperative M-mode echocardiography as a predictor of surgical results in chronic aortic insufficiency. J. Thorac. Cardiovasc. Surg. *79*:256, 1980.
4. Karp, R. B., Cyrus, R. J., Blackstone, E. H., Kirklin, J. W., Kouchoukos, N. T., and Pacifico, A. D.: The Bjork-Shiley valve. J. Thorac. Cardiovasc. Surg. *81*:602, 1981.
5. Bonow, R. O., Borer, J. S., Rosing, D. R., Henry, W. L., Pearlman, A. S., McIntosh, C. L., Morrow, A. G., and Epstein, S. E.: Preoperative exercise capacity in symptomatic patients with aortic regurgitation as a predictor of postoperative left ventricular function and long-term prognosis. Circulation *62*:1280, 1980.
6. Gault, J. H., Covell, J. W., Braunwald, E., and Ross, J., Jr.: Left ventricular performance following correction of free aortic regurgitation. Circulation *47*:773, 1970.
7. Liberthson, R. R., Boucher, C. A., Strauss, H. W., Dinsmore, R. E., McKusick, K. A., and Pohost, G. M.: Right ventricular function in adult atrial septal defect. Am. J. Cardiol. *47*:56, 1981.
8. Pearlman, A. S., Borer, J. S., Clark, C. E., Henry, W. L., Redwood, D. R., Morrow, A. G., Epstein, S. E., Burn, C., Cohen, E., and McKay, F. J.: Abnormal right ventricular size and ventricular septal motion after atrial septal defect closure. Am. J. Cardiol. *41*:295, 1978.
9. Fontan, F. M., DeVille, C., Quaegebeur, J., Ottenkamp, J., Choussat, A., and Brom, G. A.: Repair of tricuspid atresia in 100 patients. J. Thorac. Cardiovasc. Surg. (in press).
10. Urschel, C. W., Covell, J. W., Sonnenblick, E. H., Ross, J., Jr., and Braunwald, E.: Myocardial mechanics in aortic and mitral valvular regurgitation: The concept of instantaneous impedance as a determinant of the performance of the intact heart. J. Clin. Invest. *47*:867, 1968.
11. Boucher, C. A., Bingham, J. B., Osbakken, M. D., Okada, R. D., Strauss, H. W., Block, P. C., Levine, F. H., Phillips, H. R., and Pohost, G. M.: Early changes in left ventricular size and function after correction of left ventricular volume overload. Am. J. Cardiol. *47*:991, 1981.
12. Carabello, B. A., Green, L. H., Grossman, W., Cohn, L. H., Koster, J. K., and Collins, J. J., Jr.: Hemodynamic determinants of prognosis of aortic valve replacement in critical aortic stenosis and advanced congestive heart failure. Circulation *62*:42, 1980.
13. Graham, T. P., Jr., Atwood, G. F., Boerth, R. C., Boucek, R. J., Jr., and Smith, C. W.: Right and left heart size and function in infants with symptomatic coarctation. Circulation *56*:641, 1977.
14. Schwarz, F., Schaper, J., Flameng, W., and Herhlein, F. W.: Correlation between left ventricular function and myocardial ultrastructure in patients with aortic valve disease. Circulation *53* and *54* (Suppl. II):II-67, 1976 (abstract).
15. DuShane, J. W., and Kirklin, J. W.: Late results of the repair of ventricular septal defect on pulmonary vascular disease. *In* Kirklin, J. W. (ed.): Advances in Cardiovascular Surgery. New York, Grune and Stratton, 1973, p. 9.
16. Blackstone, E. H., Kirklin, J. W., Bradley, E. L., DuShane, J. W., and Appelbaum, A.: Optimal age and results in repair of large ventricular septal defects. J. Thorac. Cardiovasc. Surg. *72*:661, 1976.
17. Heath, D., and Edwards, J. E.: The pathology of hypertensive pulmonary vascular disease. A description of six grades of structural changes in the pulmonary arteries with special reference to congenital cardiac septal defects. Circulation *18*:533, 1958.
18. Hislop, A., Haworth, S. G., Shinebourne, E. A., and Reid, L.: Quantitative structural analysis of pulmonary vessels in isolated ventricular septal defects in infancy. Br. Heart J. *37*:1014, 1975.
19. Kirklin, J. W., and Barratt-Boyes, B. G.: Textbook of Cardiac Surgery. New York, John Wiley and Sons (in preparation).
20. Ellis, F. H., Jr., Kirklin, J. W., Parker, R. L., Burchell, H. B., and Wood, E. H.: Mitral commissurotomy. Arch. Intern. Med. *94*:774, 1954.
21. Best, P. V., and Heath, D.: Pulmonary thrombosis in cyanotic congenital heart disease without pulmonary hypertension. J. Pathol. Bacteriol. *75*:281, 1958.
22. Haworth, S. G., Rees, P. G., Taylor, J. F. N., Macartney, F. J., de Leval, M., and Stark, J.: Pulmonary atresia with ventricular septal defect and major aortopulmonary collateral arteries. Br. Heart J. *45*:133, 1981.
23. Abel, R. M., Buckley, M. J., Austen, W. G., Barratt, G. O., Beck, C. H., Jr., and Fisher, J. E.: Etiology, incidence, and prognosis of renal failure following cardiac operations. J. Thorac. Cardiovasc. Surg. *71*:323, 1976.
24. Hilberman, M., Myers, B. D., Carrier, B. J., Derby, G., Jamison, R. L., and Stinson, E. B.: Acute renal failure following cardiac surgery. J. Thorac. Cardiovasc. Surg. *77*:880, 1979.
25. Tanaka, J., Yasui, H., Nakano, E., Sese, A., Matsui, K., Takeda, Y., and

Tokunaga, K.: Predisposing factors of renal dysfunction following total correction of tetralogy of Fallot in the adult. J. Thorac. Cardiovasc. Surg. *80*:135, 1980.

26. Kirklin, J. K., Blackstone, E. H., Kirklin, J. W., McKay, R., Pacifico, A. D., and Bargeron, L. M., Jr.: Intracardiac surgery in infants under age 3 months: Incremental risk factors for hospital mortality. Am. J. Cardiol. *48*:500, 1981.

27. Rizzoli, G., Blackstone, E. H., Kirklin, J. W., Pacifico, A. D., and Bargeron, L. M., Jr.: Incremental risk factors in hospital mortality rate after repair of ventricular septal defect. J. Thorac. Cardiovasc. Surg. *80*:494, 1980.

28. Studer, M., Blackstone, E. H., Kirklin, J. W., Pacifico, A. D., Soto, B., Chung, G. K. T., Kirklin, J. K., and Bargeron, L. M., Jr.: Determinants of early and late results of repair of atrioventricular septal (canal) defects. J. Thorac. Cardiovasc. Surg. *84*:523, 1982.

29. Kalter, R. D., Saul, C. M., Wetstein, L., Soriano, C., and Reiss, R. F.: Cardiopulmonary bypass. Associated hemostatic abnormalities. J. Thorac. Cardiovasc. Surg. *77*:428, 1979.

30. Eisenhart, C.: Expression of the uncertainties of final results. Science *160*:1201, 1968.

31. Lee, W. H., Jr., Krumbhoar, D., Fonkalsrud, E. W., Schjeide, O. A., and Maloney, J. V., Jr.: Denaturation of plasma proteins as a cause of morbidity and death after intracardiac operations. Surgery *50*:29, 1961.

32. Feijen, J.: Thrombogenesis caused by blood-foreign surface interaction. *In* Kenedi, R. M., Courtney, J. M., Gaylor, J. D. S., and Gilchrist, T. (eds.): Artificial Organs. Baltimore, University Park Press, 1977, pp. 235–247.

33. Verska, J. J.: Control of heparinization by activated clotting time during bypass with improved postoperative hemostasis. Ann. Thorac. Surg. *24*:170, 1977.

34. Davies, G. C., Sobel, M., and Salzman, E. W.: Elevated plasma fibrinopeptide A and thromboxane B₂ levels during cardiopulmonary bypass. Circulation *61*:808, 1980.

35. Lambert, C. J., Marengo-Rowe, A. J., Leveson, J. E., Green, R. H., Theile, J. P., Geisler, G. F., Adam, M., and Mitchel, B. F.: The treatment of postperfusion bleeding using epsilon-aminocaproic acid, cryoprecipitate, fresh-frozen plasma, and protamine sulfate. Ann. Thorac. Surg. *28*:440, 1979.

36. Chenoweth, D. E., Cooper, S. W., Hugli, T. E., Stewart, R. W., Blackstone, E. H., and Kirklin, J. W.: Complement activation during cardiopulmonary bypass: Evidence for generation of C3a and C5a anaphylatoxins. N. Engl. J. Med. *304*:497, 1981.

37. Hairston, P., Manos, J. P., Graber, C. D., and Lee, W. H., Jr.: Depression of immunologic surveillance by pump-oxygenator perfusion. J. Surg. Res. *9*:587, 1969.

38. Hammerschmidt, D. E., Stroncek, D. F., Bowers, T. K., Lammi-Keefe, C. J., Kurth, D. M., Ozalins, A., Nicoloff, D. M., Lillehei, R. C., Craddock, P. R., and Jacob, H. S.: Complement activation and neutropenia occurring during cardiopulmonary bypass. J. Thorac. Cardiovasc. Surg. *81*:370, 1981.

39. Parker, D. J., Cantrell, J. W., Karp, R. B., Stroud, R. M., and Digerness, S. B.: Changes in serum complement and immunoglobulins following cardiopulmonary bypass. Surgery *71*:824, 1972.

40. Ellison, N., Behar, M., MacVaugh, H., III, and Marshall, B. E.: Bradykinin, plasma protein fraction and hypotension. Ann. Thorac. Surg. *29*:15, 1980.

41. Friedli, B., Kent, G., and Olley, P. M.: Inactivation of bradykinin in the pulmonary vascular bed of newborn and fetal lambs. Circ. Res. *33*:421, 1973.

42. Pang, L. M., Stalcup, S. A., Lipset, J. S., Hayes, C. J., Bowman, F. O., Jr., and Mellins, R. B.: Increased circulating bradykinin during hypothermia and cardiopulmonary bypass in children. Circulation *60*:1503, 1979.

43. Grant, J. A., Dupree, E., Goldman, A. S., Schultz, D. R., and Jackson, A. L.: Complement-mediated release of histamine from human leukocytes. J. Immunol. *114*:1101, 1975.

44. Goldstein, I. M., Brai, M., Osler, A. G., and Weissman, G.: Lysosomal enzyme release from human leukocytes: Mediation by the alternate pathway of complement activation. J. Immunol. *111*:33, 1973.

45. Hugli, T.: Chemical aspects of the serum anaphylatoxins. Contemp. Top. Mol. Immunol. *7*:181, 1978.

46. Martin, R. R.: Alterations in leukocyte structure and function due to mechanical trauma. *In* Hwang, N. H. C., Gross, D. R., and Patel, D. J. (eds.): Quantitative Cardiovascular Studies: Clinical and Research Applications of Engineering Principles. Baltimore, University Park Press, 1979, pp. 419–454.

47. Wilson, J. W.: Pulmonary morphologic changes due to extracorporeal circulation: A model for the "the shock lung" at cellular level in humans. *In* Forscher, B. K., Lillehei, R. C., and Stubbs, S. S. (eds.): Shock in Low- and High-Flow States. Proceedings of a Symposium at Brook Lodge, Augusta, Michigan. Amsterdam, Excerpta Medica, 1972, pp. 160–171.

48. Jorgensen, L., Hovig, T., Towsell, H. C., and Mustard, J. F.: Adenosine diphosphate–induced platelet aggregation and vascular injury in swine and rabbit. Am. J. Pathol. *61*:161, 1970.

49. Solen, K. A., Whiffen, J. D., and Lightfoot, E. N.: The effect of shear, specific surface, and air interface on the development of blood emboli and hemolysis. J. Biomed. Materials Res. *12*:381, 1978.

50. DeVenuto, F., Friedman, H. I., Neville, J. R., and Peck, C. C.: Appraisal of hemoglobin solution as a blood substitute. Surg. Gynecol. Obstet. *149*:417, 1979.

51. Clark, R. E., Beauchamp, R. A., Magrath, R. A., Brooks, J. D., Ferguson, T. B., and Weldon, C. S.: Comparison of bubble and membrane oxygenators in short and long perfusions. J. Thorac. Cardiovasc. Surg. *78*:655, 1979.

52. Mavroudis, C.: To pulse or not to pulse. Ann. Thorac. Surg. *25*:259, 1978.

53. Singh, R. K. K., Barratt-Boyes, B. G., and Harris, E. A.: Does pulsatile flow improve perfusion during hypothermic cardiopulmonary bypass? J. Thorac. Cardiovasc. Surg. *79*:827, 1980.

54. Barratt-Boyes, B. G., Simpson, M. M., and Neutze, J. M.: Intracardiac surgery in neonates and infants using deep hypothermia. Circulation *61* and *62* (Suppl. III):III-73, 1970.

55. Hamilton, D. I., Shackleton, J., Rees, G. J., and Abbott, T.: Experience with deep hypothermia in infancy using core cooling. *In* Barratt-Boyes, B. G., Neutze, J. M., and Harris, E. A. (eds.): Heart Disease in Infancy. Baltimore, Williams and Wilkins Co., 1973, pp. 52–64.

56. Folkerth, T. L., Angell, W. W., Fosburg, R. G., and Oury, J. H.: Effect of deep hypothermia, limited cardiopulmonary bypass, and total arrest on growing puppies. *In* Recent Advances in Studies on Cardiac Structure and Metabolism. Vol. 10. Baltimore, University Park Press, 1975, pp. 411–421.

57. Fisk, G. C., Wright, J. S., Turner, B. B., Baker, DeC., Hicks, R. G., Lethlean, A. K., Stacey, R. B., Lawrence, J. C., Lawrie, G. M., Kalnins, I., and Rose, M.: Cerebral effects of circulatory arrest at 20°C in the infant pig. Anaesth. Intensive Care *2*:33, 1974.

58. Fisk, G. C., Wright, J. S., Hicks, R. G., Anderson, R. M., Turner, B. B., Baker, W., Lawrence, J. C., Stacey, R. B., Lawrie, G. M., Kalvins, I., and Rose, M.: The influence of duration of circulatory arrest at 20°C on cerebral changes. Anaesth. Intensive Care *4*:126, 1976.

59. Kramer, R. S., Sanders, A. P., Lesage, A. M., Woodhall, B., and Sealy, W. C.: The effect of profound hypothermia on preservation of cerebral ATP content during circulatory arrest. J. Thorac. Cardiovasc. Surg. *56*:699, 1968.

60. Wolin, L. R., Massopust, L. C., Jr., and White, R. J.: Behavioral effects of autocerebral perfusion, hypothermia and arrest of cerebral blood flow in the rhesus monkey. Exp. Neurol. *39*:336, 1973.

61. Messmer, B. J., Schallberger, U., Gattiker, R., and Senning, A.: Psychomotor and intellectual development after deep hypothermia and circulatory arrest in early infancy. J. Thorac. Cardiovasc. Surg. *72*:495, 1976.

62. Clarkson, P. M., MacArthur, B. A., Barratt-Boyes, B. G., Whitlock, R. M., and Neutze, J. M.: Developmental progress following cardiac surgery in infancy using profound hypothermia and circulatory arrest. Circulation *62*:855, 1980.

63. Stewart, R. W., Blackstone, E. H., Kirklin, J. W., and Pacifico, A. D.: Clinical experiences in profound hypothermia and total circulatory arrest (unpublished data).

64. Brunberg, J. A., Reilly, E. L., and Doty, D. B.: Central nervous system consequences in infants of cardiac surgery using deep hypothermia and circulatory arrest. Circulation *49* and *50* (Suppl. II):II-60, 1973.

65. Bergouignan, M., Fontan, F., Trarieux, M., and Julien, J.: Syndromes choreiformes de l'enfant au decours d'interventions cardiochirurgicales sous hypothermie profonde. Rev. Neurol. (Paris) *105*:48, 1961.

66. Treasure, T., Garcia, J. H., Conger, K. A., Blackstone, E. H., and Kirklin, J. W.: Effect of hypothermic circulatory arrest time on cerebral function, morphology and biochemistry: An experimental study. Circulation (abstract) *66* (Suppl. II):II-152, 1982.

67. Taber, R. E., Morales, A. R., and Fine, G.: Myocardial necrosis and the postoperative low-cardiac-output syndrome. Ann. Thorac. Surg. *4*:12, 1967.

68. Henson, D. E., Najafi, H., Callaghan, R., Coogan, P., Julian, O. C., and Eisenstein, R.: Myocardial lesions following open heart surgery. Arch. Pathol. *88*:423, 1969.

69. Najafi, H., Henson, D., Dye, W. S., Javid, H., Hunter, J. A., Callaghan, R., Eisenstein, R., and Julian, O. C.: Left ventricular hemorrhagic necrosis. Ann. Thorac. Surg. *7*:550, 1969.

70. Assad-Morell, J. L., Wallace, R. B., Elveback, L. R., Gau, G. T., Connolly, D. C., Barnhorst, D. A., Pluth, J. R., and Danielson, G. K.: Serum enzyme data in diagnosis of myocardial infarction during or early after aorta-coronary saphenous vein bypass graft operations. J. Thorac. Cardiovasc. Surg. *69*:851, 1975.

71. Brewer, D. L., Bilbro, R. H., and Bartel, A. G.: Myocardial infarction as a complication of coronary bypass surgery. Circulation *47*:58, 1973.

72. Hultgren, H. N., Miyagawa, M., Buch, W., and Angell, W. W.: Ischemic myocardial injury during cardiopulmonary bypass surgery. Am. Heart J. *85*:167, 1973.

73. Roberts, W. C., Bulkley, B. H., and Morrow, A. G.: Pathologic anatomy of cardiac valve replacement: A study of 224 necrosy patients. Prog. Cardiovasc. Dis. *15*:539, 1973.

74. Cooley, D. A., Reul, G. J., and Wukasch, D. C.: Ischemic contracture of the heart: "Stone heart." Am. J. Cardiol. *29*:575, 1972.

75. Katz, A. M., and Tada, M.: The "stone heart" and other challenges to the biochemist. Am. J. Cardiol. *39*:1073, 1977.

76. Lie, J. T., and Sun, S. C.: Ultrastructure of ischemic contracture of the left ventricle ("stone heart"). Mayo Clin. Proc. *51*:785, 1976.

77. Leaf, A.: Maintenance of concentration gradients and regulation of cell volume. Ann. N.Y. Acad. Sci. *72*:396, 1959.

78. Tranum-Jensen, J., Janse, M. J., Fiolet, J. W. T., Krieger, W. J. G., D'Alnoncourt, C. H., and Durrer, D.: Tissue osmolality, cell swelling, and reperfusion in acute regional myocardial ischemia in the isolated porcine heart. Circ. Res. *49*:364, 1981.

79. Lucas, S. K., Elmer, E. B., Flaherty, J. T., Prodromos, C. C., Bulkley, B. H., Gott, V. L., and Gardner, T. J.: Effects of multiple-dose potassium cardioplegia on myocardial ischemia, return of ventricular function, and ultrastructural preservation. J. Thorac. Cardiovasc. Surg. *80*:102, 1980.

80. Neely, J. R., Liedtke, A. J., Whitman, J. T., and Rovelto, M. J.: Relationship between coronary flow and adenosine triphosphate production from glycolysis and oxidative metabolism. *In* Roy, D. C., and Harris, P. (eds.): The Cardiac Sarcoplasm. Vol 8. Baltimore, University Park Press, 1975, p. 301.

81. Hearse, D. J., Garlick, P. B., and Humphrey, S. M.: Ischemic contracture of the myocardium: Mechanisms and prevention. Am. J. Cardiol. *39*:986, 1977.

82. Schaper, J., Mulch, J., Winkler, B., and Shaper, W.: Ultrastructural, functional, and biochemical criteria for estimation of reversibility of ischemic injury: A study on the effects of global ischemia on the isolated dog heart. J. Mol. Cell. Cardiol. *11*:521, 1979.

83. Chance, B.: The energy-linked reactions of calcium with mitochrondria. J. Biol. Chem. *240*:2729, 1965.

84. Sapsford, R. N., Blackstone, E. H., Kirklin, J. W., Karp, R. B., Kouchoukos, N. T., Pacifico, A. D., Roe, C. R., and Bradley, E. L.: Coronary perfusion versus cold ischemic arrest during aortic valve surgery; a randomized study. Circulation *49*:1190, 1974.

85. Jennings, R. B., Sommer, H. M., Herdson, P. B., and Kaltenback, J. P.: Ischemic injury of myocardium. Ann. N. Y. Acad. Sci. *156*:61, 1969.

86. Moulder, P. V., Blackstone, E. H., Eckner, F. A. O., and Lev, M.: Pressure derivative loop for left ventricular resuscitation. Arch. Surg. *96*:323, 1968.

87. Martin, A. M., Jr., and Hackel, D. B.: An electron microscopic study of the progression of myocardial lesions in the dog after hemorrhage shock. Lab. Invest. *15*:243, 1966.

88. Isom, O. W., Kutin, W. D., Falk, E. A., and Spencer, F. C.: Patterns of myocardial metabolism during cardiopulmonary bypass and coronary perfusion. J. Thorac. Cardiovasc. Surg. *66*:705, 1973.

89. Shen, A. C., and Jennings, R. B.: Myocardial calcium and magnesium in acute ischemic injury. Am. J. Pathol. *67*:417, 1972.

90. Nayler, W. G., Poole-Wilson, P. A., and Williams, A.: Hypoxia and calcium J. Mol. Cell. Cardiol. *11*:683, 1979.

91. Jennings, R. B., Sommers, H. M., Smyth, G. A., Flack, H. A., and Linn, H.: Myocardial necrosis induced by temporary occlusion of a coronary artery in the dog. Arch. Pathol. *70*:82, 1960.

92. Hearse, D. J., Stewart, D. A., and Braimbridge, M. V.: Cellular protection during myocardial ischemia. The development and characterization of a procedure for the induction of reversible ischemic arrest. Circulation *54*:193, 1976.

93. Kirklin, J. W.: Systems Analysis in Surgical Patients with Particular Attention to the Cardiac and Pulmonary Subsystems (Macewen Memorial Lecture). Glasgow, University of Glasgow Press, 1970.

94. Stinson, E. B., Holloway, E. L., and Derby, G. C.: Control of myocardial performance early after open-heart operations by vasodilator treatment. J. Thorac. Cardiovasc. Surg. *73*:523, 1977.

95. Waldo, A. L., and MacLean, W. A. H.: Diagnosis and Treatment of Cardiac Arrhythmias following Open Heart Surgery. Emphasis on the Use of Atrial and Ventricular Epicardial Wire Electrodes. New York, Futura Publishing Company, 1980.

96. Waldo, A. L., Ross, S. M., and Kaiser, G. A.: The epicardial electrogram in the diagnosis of cardiac arrhythmias following cardiac surgery. Geriatrics *26*:108, 1971.

97. Friesen, W. G., Woodson, R. D., Ames, A. W., Herr, R. H., Starr, A., and Kassebaum, D. G.: A hemodynamic comparison of atrial and ventricular pacing in postoperative cardiac surgical patients. J. Thorac. Cardiovasc. Surg. *55*:271, 1968.

98. Waldo, A. L., MacLean, W. A. H., Karp, R. B., Kouchoukos, N. T., and James, T. N.: Sustained rapid atrial pacing to control supraventricular tachycardias following open heart surgery. Circulation *51* and *52* (Suppl. II):II–13, 1975.

99. Chesney, R. W., Kaplan, B. S., Freedom, R. M., Haller, J. A., and Drummond, K. N.: Acute renal failure: An important complication of cardiac surgery in infants. J. Pediatr. *87*:381, 1975.

100. Srinivasan, V., Levinsky, L., Choh, J. H., Baliah, T., and Subramanian, S.: Renal failure following intracardiac surgery in infants—Improved survival with early dialysis: Indications and results. J. Pediatr. (in press).

101. Bourgeois, B. F. D., Donath, A., Paunier, L., and Rouge, J.-C.: Effects of cardiac surgery on renal functions in children. J. Thorac. Cardiovasc. Surg. *77*:283, 1979.

102. German, J. C., Chalmers, G. S., Hirai, J., Nrisingha, M. D., Wakabayashi, A., and Connolly, J. E.: Comparison of nonpulsatile and pulsatile extracorporeal circulation on renal tissue perfusion. Chest *61*:65, 1972.

103. Williams, G. D., Seifen, A. B., Lawson, N. W., Norton, J. B., Readinger, R. I., Dungan, T. W., and Callaway, J. K.: Pulsatile perfusion versus conventional high-flow nonpulsatile perfusion for rapid core cooling and rewarming of infants for circulatory arrest in cardiac operation. J. Thorac. Cardiovasc. Surg. *78*:667, 1979.

104. Norman, J. C., McDonald, H. P., and Sloan, H.: The early and aggressive treatment of acute renal failure following cardiopulmonary bypass with continuous peritoneal dialysis. Surgery *56*:240, 1964.

105. Ashbaugh, D. G., and Petty, T. L.: Positive end-expiratory pressure. J. Thorac. Cardiovasc. Surg. *65*:165, 1979.

106. Sturtz, G. S., Kirklin, J. W., Burke, E. C., and Power, M. H.: Water metabolism after cardiac operations involving a Gibbon-type pump-oxygenator. I. Daily water metabolism, obligatory water losses, and requirements. Circulation. *16*:988, 1957.

107. Astrup, P., Andersen, O. S., Jorgenson, K., and Engel, K.: The acid-base metabolism. A new approach. Lancet *1*:1035, 1960.

108. Livelli, F. D., Jr., Johnson, R. A., McEnany, M. T., Sherman, E., Newell, J., Block, P. C., and DeSanctis, R. W.: Unexplained in-hospital fever following cardiac surgery. Circulation *57*:968, 1978.

56 GENERAL ANESTHESIA AND NONCARDIAC SURGERY IN PATIENTS WITH HEART DISEASE

by Marshall A. Wolf, M.D., and Eugene Braunwald, M.D.

The cardiovascular system of patients undergoing general anesthesia and noncardiac surgical procedures is subject to multiple stresses due to depression of myocardial contractility and respiration as well as fluctuations in temperature, arterial pressure, ventricular filling pressure, blood volume and activity of the autonomic nervous system. Complications of anesthesia and operation, such as hemorrhage, infection, fever, pulmonary embolism, and myocardial infarction, impose additional burdens on the cardiovascular system. The patient with cardiac disease who is compensated preoperatively may be unable to meet these increased demands during the perioperative period, in which case heart failure, myocardial ischemia, and/or arrhythmias may develop.[1,1a] As a consequence, one-fourth to one-half of all deaths in most series of noncardiac operations result from cardiovascular complications.

Since both the frequency and seriousness of cardiovascular complications of anesthesia and operation are considerably increased in the patient with known cardiovascular disease, one must appreciate the magnitude of these risks in order to reduce cardiovascular morbidity and mortality. In addition, both the life expectancy and quality of life of the patient must be taken into account. For instance, a high surgical risk may be difficult to justify if the cardiac condition precludes a survival period sufficient to allow the patient to reap the benefits of the surgical procedure, should the outcome be successful. In addition, the dangers and disability of the disease for which an operation is being proposed must also be balanced against the risk of the operation itself. In assessing the latter, the skills of the surgical and anesthesia teams must be taken into account.

ANESTHESIA

Changes in cardiovascular function during general anesthesia are due to many factors, including direct effects of the anesthetic agent(s) on the heart and indirect effects mediated primarily through the autonomic nervous system. In addition, if respiration is inadequately maintained, the resulting hypoxia, hypercarbia, and acidosis may further depress myocardial contractility and increase cardiac irritability. The interplay of all these variables may produce changes in arterial and central venous pressures, cardiac output, and rate and rhythm. To minimize the risk of operation in the patient with a compromised cardiovascular system, it is essential to minimize these fluctuations.[2]

CARDIOVASCULAR EFFECTS OF ANESTHESIA. Most general anesthetic agents depress myocardial contractility (Table 56–1). Studies on isolated cardiac muscle demonstrate a range of depressant effects, with agents such as halothane and methoxyflurane being the most depressant[3] and diethyl ether, nitrous oxide, and cyclopropane having the least effect on cardiac contractility. Superimposed on this direct myocardial depression, however, are alterations of the sympathetic nervous system, which may change the degree of depression observed in vivo. Thus, halothane, which produces minimal stimulation of sympathetic activity, may cause hypotension when administered

1815

TABLE 56–1   CARDIOVASCULAR EFFECTS OF VARIOUS ANESTHETIC AGENTS

	MORPHINE	HALOTHANE	NITROUS OXIDE	ENFLURANE	ETHER
Blood pressure	— ↓	↓	—	— ↓	—
Heart rate	↓	— ↑	↓	↑	↑
Myocardial contractility	—	↓↓	↓	↓	↓
Systemic vascular resistance	↓	↓↓	↑	↓	↓
Cardiac output	— ↑	↓	↓	↑	—

From Sanfelippo, J. F.: Noncardiac surgery and anesthesia in patients with heart disease. Pract. Ther. 26:204, 1982.

in sufficient concentrations, whereas cycloproprane and ether, which induce considerable sympathetic discharge, are less likely to do so. Halothane depresses myocardial contractility apparently by inhibiting actinomyosin ATPase and interfering with calcium release from the sarcoplasmic reticulum.[4] The myocardial depressant actions of halothane, enflurane, isoflurane, and methoxyflurane are similar and are dose-dependent. Therefore, light halothane anesthesia, in a dose range of 0.3 to 0.5 per cent, is effective in producing minimal myocardial depression and vasodilatation. Enflurane anesthesia is also well tolerated by cardiac patients,[5] particularly when its concentration can be minimized by combining it with 40 per cent nitrous oxide and when good muscle relaxation is produced by a muscle relaxant, such as pancuronium.

Some of the newer anesthetic combinations, such as droperidol and fentanyl (Innovar) or nitrous oxide and pancuronium, cause minimal depression of cardiac contractility and may be excellent for the patient with impaired myocardial function.[6] A disadvantage associated with the use of such anesthetic combinations is the inability to lighten the level of anesthesia quickly, as can be done with inhalation anesthesia.

Anesthesia with narcotics is an excellent option in poor-risk cardiac patients. With this approach, anesthesia is induced with nitrous oxide, relatively large sequential doses of a narcotic (generally 1 to 2 mg/kg morphine or fentanyl [up to 60 μg/kg]), and a muscle relaxant. Hypotension is rare, and the respiratory depression caused by the narcotic can be avoided with controlled respiration. Upon termination of the operation, any residual narcotic depression can be reversed with a narcotic antagonist.

Intravenous thiopental is a satisfactory agent for induction, especially in the apprehensive patient with a history of arrhythmias. However, the myocardial depression and vasodilatation associated with thiopental may be poorly tolerated by patients with fixed cardiac outputs and secondary vasoconstriction. In such patients, induction with ketamine, up to 2 mg/kg intravenously, may be more desirable.[7] Ketamine does not stimulate catecholamine secretion but exerts a cocaine-like effect, preventing the uptake of catecholamines at postganglionic sympathetic nerve terminals and thereby causing mild sympathetic stimulation. Ketamine is relatively contraindicated in patients with hypertension as well as in those with mitral stenosis who may tolerate poorly the tachycardia which this agent produces. Because it is important to avoid hypotension and increased right-to-left shunting in patients with cyanotic congenital heart disease, induction with an agent such as

ketamine, which allows a high concentration of oxygen and does not cause hypotension in anesthetic dose ranges, is particularly desirable.[7,8]

Regardless of the anesthetic or anesthetic combination used, it is desirable to induce a light state of anesthesia in the cardiac patient. However, it is possible to err on this side as well; when anesthesia is too light, endotracheal intubation or skin incision can elicit sympathomimetic discharge, with tachycardia, hypertension, and increased systemic vascular resistance depressing cardiac output in patients with impaired cardiac reserve; the hypertension may require treatment with nitroprusside or nitroglycerin.

SELECTION OF ANESTHETIC AGENT(S). The anesthesiologist, especially one who is experienced in cardiac surgery, is more qualified than the internist-cardiologist to select the appropriate anesthetic agent(s) for the cardiac patient undergoing noncardiac surgery. The physician's role is to advise the anesthesiologist as to the nature and severity of the patient's cardiac disease and to detect and, during the preoperative period, to correct factors such as hypovolemia, arrhythmias, hypoxemia, or acid-base and electrolyte imbalance that can complicate and increase the risk of anesthesia.

Since anesthetic agents vary considerably in their tendency to depress cardiac function and to enhance the potency of various arrhythmogenic stimuli,[9] it might be predicted that the choice of anesthetic agent would markedly affect morbidity and mortality from anesthesia in patients with underlying cardiovascular disease. However, several series have failed to demonstrate a significant effect of the choice of anesthetic on the outcome of operation in such patients.[10–15] It is clear that careful monitoring of arterial pressure and respiratory status and their maintenance within narrow and normal limits are more critical than the agent or agents employed.

Muscle relaxants are frequently used during moderate anesthesia and require controlled ventilation. Succinylcholine may stimulate the parasympathetic nervous system and produce bradycardia, especially when repeated doses are used, while d-tubocurarine frequently causes hypotension. Pancuronium bromide produces mild stimulation of heart rate and blood pressure and is often used for cardiac patients. Another excellent agent for the patient with heart disease is metocurine, which has minimal effects on cardiovascular dynamics. Quinidine may markedly prolong the physiologic half-life of muscle relaxants, and prolonged postoperative support may be required in patients receiving this antiarrhythmic agent.

Alternatives to general anesthesia are spinal, epidural, or

regional anesthesia, since these modes cause little myocardial depression, although the attendant sympathetic blockade may produce significant hypotension, especially in the hypovolemic patient. There is less post-operative heart failure with spinal or epidural anesthesia than with general anesthesia. However, the lower mortality often attributed to spinal and epidural anesthesia is probably a function of the type of operation in which they are employed; they are often used for less extensive surgical procedures but rarely used for high abdominal or thoracic surgery, which present the greatest risk to patients with cardiovascular disease. For operations on the extremities, nerve block anesthesia is satisfactory, while for operations involving the prostate, spine, and lower limbs, spinal or epidural anesthesia may be ideal, if care is taken to avoid hypotension. Epidural anesthesia takes effect more slowly than spinal anesthesia and thus allows more time to prevent or correct hypotension by means of volume expansion or a vasopressor. Local anesthesia, without epinephrine, can be used for minor operations. Major ophthalmic surgery can be performed with local anesthesia with very low risk.[16]

ANESTHETIC TECHNIQUES. Excitement, hypoxia, and catecholamine release during induction of anesthesia may elevate arterial pressure. Although arterial pO_2 and pCO_2 may be adequately maintained during anesthesia, they may become temporarily abnormal during intubation. In addition, in lightly anesthetized patients, intubation may produce arrhythmias by sympathetic stimulation and/or elevation of arterial pressure. Endotracheal suction during anesthesia may also induce arrhythmias; a period of hyperventilation with a high concentration of oxygen and limiting the duration of aspiration and the associated anoxia to 5 to 10 seconds may reduce such rhythm disturbances. Adequate ventilation and oxygenation must be assured throughout the anesthetic period and states of hypoxia, acidosis, and alkalosis prevented.

In patients with severe underlying heart disease, it is mandatory to monitor cardiac function during anesthesia,[17] including cardiac rate and rhythm and directly recorded arterial blood pressure. A radial artery line permits not only intraarterial monitoring of pressure but also frequent sampling for determination of blood gases. Indirect (cuff) blood pressure measurements in the presence of peripheral vasoconstriction may grossly underestimate true arterial pressure. Monitoring of the pulmonary artery (or, preferably, pulmonary artery wedge) pressure and cardiac output is often desirable in patients who are critically ill, who have marginal cardiovascular reserve, who are to undergo prolonged operative procedures in which blood losses might occur, and in whom hypotensive anesthesia is to be employed. Both pulmonary artery wedge pressure and cardiac output can be measured with the aid of a multiple-lumen balloon flotation catheter (Swan-Ganz) and the thermodilution method (Chap. 9). In seriously ill patients, urine output should be monitored with a Foley catheter.

ARRHYTHMIAS AND ANESTHESIA. Alterations in cardiac rhythm are extremely common in the perioperative period.[18,19] Arrhythmias are most likely to occur in patients with severe coronary atherosclerosis or calcific aortic stenosis. They are most common in patients with preoperative arrhythmias and are observed most frequently during induction and intubation.[20] Fortunately, most arrhythmias observed intraoperatively are of little clinical significance and rarely require more specific treatment than alterations in anesthetic management during the surgical procedure. Common arrhythmias are sinus bradycardia and nodal rhythm, related presumably to excessive vagal tone.[2] Often these arrhythmias will respond to lightening the depth of anesthesia, the administration of atropine, or both. Many other arrhythmias observed during anesthesia are the consequence of an augmentation of sympathetic activity; the latter is usually a response to hypoxia, hypercarbia, or light anesthesia. Certain surgical manipulations, such as tracheal intubation, eye manipulation, or traction on cerebral or visceral structures, may also induce transient arrhythmias.

Anesthetic agents may sensitize the heart to the increased sympathetic stimuli experienced during operation. In animals, general anesthesia lowers the arrhythmia threshold. This effect is most marked with chloroform, cyclopropane, and trichloroethylene; moderate with halothane; and minimal with methoxyflurane, fluroxene, diethyl ether, enflurane, and isoflurane.[7,21] In most cases, these arrhythmias respond to alterations in the depth of anesthesia; correction of hypoxia, hypoventilation, or hypovolemia; and termination of the precipitating surgical manipulation. Only when arrhythmias cannot be corrected by these measures or by adjusting the depth of anesthesia should they be treated with the usual antiarrhythmic agents (Chap. 20).

Patients with heart disease tolerate tachycardia less well than do normal individuals.[20,22] Coronary blood flow occurs during diastole and patients with coronary artery disease may develop severe ischemia during tachycardia owing to the attendant reduction in the duration of diastole. Patients with mitral stenosis, in whom the transvalvular pressure gradient and therefore the pulmonary capillary pressure is a function of diastolic filling time, are also intolerant of tachyarrhythmias (p. 1065). In such cases preoperative digitalization may be justified, especially in those with a history of atrial fibrillation or other supraventricular tachyarrhythmias.

THE OPERATION

A number of studies, most of them uncontrolled retrospective reviews, have examined the association between surgical risk and underlying cardiovascular status.[11–15,23] Results have been similar to those reported in Goldman's prospective series.[10,24] The magnitude of operative risk, especially in patients with cardiovascular disease, may be surprisingly great—often exceeding 35 per cent in patients with recent myocardial infarction. It is sometimes argued that such statistics are no longer valid, since more recent improvements in surgical and anesthetic techniques have markedly reduced perioperative mortality. However, except for two uncontrolled studies that employed intensive hemodynamic monitoring,[25,26] the incidence of perioperative myocardial infarction and cardiac death among patients with underlying heart disease has not changed significantly during the last 25 years nor has a significant reduction in mortality as a result of changes in anesthetic technique been documented.[10–15]

THE NATURE OF THE OPERATION. The extent to which cardiovascular disease contributes to a patient's risk varies greatly depending on the nature of the surgical procedure.[11,15,27] For example, Skinner and Pearce demonstrated minimal and equal mortality in patients with and without cardiac disease subjected to herniorrhaphy or transurethral prostatic resection (Fig. 56–1).[27] In contrast, mortality among cardiac patients subjected to cholecystectomy, subtotal gastrectomy, or bowel resection was twice that of patients without heart disease. Among patients who have had previous myocardial infarctions,[11,14] major vascular surgery is associated with a two- to threefold increase in risk, while results of surgery involving the extremities do not appear to be affected.

Emergency operation is associated with a greatly increased mortality in patients with cardiovascular disease. Skinner and Pearce[27] noted that mortality from cholecystectomy among cardiac patients was 10 per cent for an elective procedure versus 29 per cent when it was carried out on an emergency basis. Similar differences were noted for bowel resections (18 vs. 50 per cent) and other intraperitoneal operations (21 vs. 47 per cent). In Goldman's series[10] patients over 40 years of age who underwent emergency major surgery experienced a fourfold greater incidence of postoperative infarction or cardiac death—an increased risk that remains highly significant after multivariate analysis.[24] Obviously, while it is always desirable to avoid emergency operation, this is especially important in the patient with cardiac disease.

THE DURATION OF OPERATION. The relationship between the duration of anesthesia and the risk of cardiovascular mortality and morbidity is uncertain. Although it is generally assumed that the longer the operation, the greater the hazard to the patient with cardiovascular disease, this relation is, in part, confounded by the fact that more serious operations frequently take longer. It is of interest that in Skinner and Pearce's study, when the influence of the duration of operation was examined for the same surgical procedure, there was actually an inverse relationship between mortality and duration.[27] Tarhan et al. also noted no greater incidence of reinfarction as duration of anesthesia increased.[14] On the other hand, Steen and associates, who limited their analysis to patients with previous myocardial infarction, found that in

procedures involving the aorta, thorax, and upper abdomen, mortality was a function of the duration of anesthesia.[11] Goldman et al. noted an increased risk of heart failure but not infarction or cardiac death when surgery lasted more than 5 hours.[10]

UNDERLYING CARDIOVASCULAR DISEASE

ISCHEMIC HEART DISEASE

Ischemic heart disease is a major determinant of perioperative morbidity and mortality. The incidence of perioperative myocardial infarction is increased 10- to 50-fold in patients who have previously suffered infarcts.[15] Patients undergoing general anesthesia soon after myocardial infarction are at particularly high risk of reinfarction. Tarhan et al. noted a 37 per cent reinfarction rate in patients operated on within 3 months of a previous myocardial infarction; this rate fell to 16 per cent when the operation was performed 3 to 6 months after the prior attack, and to 5 per cent when surgery was performed more than 6 months after the initial infarct.[14] Several other studies have confirmed a similar high risk when operation is performed within the first 6 months after myocardial infarction.[10–13,15] Obviously, whenever possible, elective surgery should be avoided during this period.

Innovations in anesthetic techniques during the last two decades may have reduced the risk of intraoperative infarction, but they have had little effect on postoperative infarction and the overall incidence of perioperative events. In 1978, Steen et al. documented new, perioperative infarctions in 36 of 587 patients (6.1 per cent) who had previous infarctions[11;] a similar study from the same institution carried out seven years earlier noted perioperative reinfarctions in 28 of 422 patients (6.6 per cent)[14] (Table 56–2).

Myocardial infarction occurring in the perioperative period is often painless[14,28;] indeed, half of Goldman's patients described no chest discomfort in association with their infarctions,[10] and only 11 of the 28 patients in Steen's series who experienced postoperative reinfarction gave a history of chest pain.[11] Obviously, then, the incidence of perioperative infarction will be underestimated if electrocardiograms are not obtained routinely during the postoperative period. Furthermore, the electrocardiogram detects only a fraction of infarcts, and it is likely that if the incidence of infarction were determined by more sensitive methods, such as serial estimations of serum creatine kinase (MB fraction), it would be even higher. Seventy per cent of perioperative infarcts occur within the first six days, with the peak incidence on the third day.[29]

While the mortality for patients experiencing an initial infarction during the perioperative period is similar to that for the general population with a first infarction, the risk of a second infarction occurring in the perioperative period is substantially greater.[14,30] Mortality among patients suffering a postoperative myocardial infarction *without* a prior infarction was 26.6 per cent, whereas mortality among those *with* a prior infarction was 2.5 times higher (64.1 per cent). It is discouraging that the management of patients experiencing a second infarct in an intensive care setting, who are presumably receiving excellent care, does not appear to have reduced this high mortality significantly.[11]

Two recent studies utilizing intensive intraoperative and

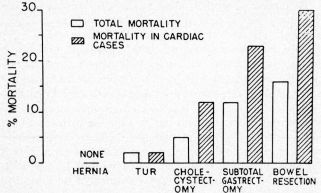

FIGURE 56–1 A comparison of surgical mortality in cardiac cases with total surgical mortality in five selected operations. TUR = transurethral prostatic resection. (From Skinner, J. F., and Pearce, M. L.: Surgical risk in the cardiac patient. J. Chron. Dis. *17*:57, 1964. Copyright 1964, Pergamon Press, Ltd.)

TABLE 56–2 EFFECT OF A PREVIOUS MYOCARDIAL INFARCTION ON INCIDENCE OF PERIOPERATIVE MYOCARDIAL INFARCTION AND ON MORTALITY

| AUTHOR | YEAR OF STUDY | NO. OF PATIENTS | | PATIENTS WITH NEW POSTOPERATIVE INFARCTION | | MORTALITY (%) |
		Previous Infarction	No Previous Infarction	History of Previous Infarction(%)	No History of Previous Infarction(%)	
Knapp[23]	1962	427	8,557	6.0	0.7	58
Topkins[13]	1964	658	12,054	6.5	0.7	70
Tarhan[14]	1972	422	32,455	6.6	0.1	54
Steen[11]	1978	587	—	6.1	—	69
AVERAGES				6.4	0.4	63

Reproduced with permission from Salem, D. N., et al.: Management of cardiac disease in the general surgical patient. *In* Harvey, W. P. (ed.): Current Problems in Cardiology. Vol. 5. Copyright © 1980 by Year Book Medical Publishers, Inc., Chicago.

postoperative hemodynamic monitoring have reported a much lower incidence of perioperative myocardial infarction. Wells and Kaplan reported a series of 48 patients who underwent noncardiac surgery 3 months after infarction; there were no reinfarctions, although 15 per cent of the patients experienced significant arrhythmias.[25] In Rao and El-Etr's series, only 7.8 per cent of 38 patients operated within 3 months of a previous infarct experienced reinfarction; the 59 patients who underwent surgery 3 to 6 months after their previous infarction experienced an infarction rate of 3.4 per cent.[26]

Patients with ischemic heart disease tolerate unplanned, sustained intraoperative hypotension poorly, presumably because it intensifies ischemia in marginally perfused tissue. Conversely, patients suffering an intraoperative infarction may experience unexplained hypotension. Mauney et al. described a fourfold greater incidence of intraoperative hypotension in those patients who suffered a perioperative infarction.[30] Steen et al. noted a 15.2 per cent infarction rate in patients in whom systolic pressure decreased by at least 30 per cent for at least 10 minutes or more during anesthesia vs. a 3.2 per cent infarction rate in patients who did not experience such a pressure drop.[11] While it has been presumed that hypotension was the inciting event for the infarction in these patients, the possibility that it was the *consequence* of the infarct has not been excluded.

The role of coronary artery bypass grafting in altering the mortality and morbidity from general anesthesia and surgery in the patient with manifest coronary artery disease is still unclear. Several studies have suggested that patients who had coronary artery bypass surgery may be at reduced risk from subsequent major noncardiac surgery[31–36]; however, controlled studies are needed to establish the validity of these observations.

HYPERTENSION

Patients with mild to moderate essential hypertension, uncomplicated by congestive heart failure, renal failure, or coronary artery disease, can be expected to tolerate the stresses of general anesthesia and operation as well as normotensive patients.[37–39] However, hypertensive patients are subject to more frequent and wider swings of pressure during anesthesia and operation.[40] Hypertensive episodes are more likely to occur during induction and intubation but can be minimized with careful technique,[41] while hypotensive episodes may result from the hypovolemia that is common among hypertensive patients treated with diuretics.[42] Halothane anesthesia, which causes vasodilation as well as myocardial depression, is particularly likely to elicit intraoperative hypotension in these patients.

Controversy continues concerning management with antihypertensive medications during the perioperative period. Early studies, emphasizing the hazards of hypotension that occur during general anesthesia,[43,44] suggested that this tendency was increased by treatment with *reserpine* and led to the recommendation that reserpine be discontinued about 10 days prior to planned general anesthesia. However, several investigators have shown that the fluctuations of arterial pressure are *not* greater in hypertensive patients who received reserpine than in those who did not.[45–47] Indeed, Prys-Roberts et al. have demonstrated that patients with well-controlled hypertension whose drug therapy was maintained up to and including the day of operation were more stable during anesthesia than were patients with untreated hypertension.[47,48]

More recently, a controversy reminiscent of that engendered by reserpine has developed concerning the maintenance of *propranolol* therapy in the immediate preoperative period. On the basis of several case reports, Viljoen et al. suggested that propranolol might significantly increase the myocardial depression produced by most anesthetic agents and recommended that the drug be withdrawn at least 2 weeks before operation.[49] However, subsequent studies have documented no adverse reactions in patients undergoing cardiopulmonary bypass while receiving propranolol.[50–52] Actually, it has been suggested that beta-adrenergic blocking agents reduce the incidence of intraoperative arrhythmias and myocardial ischemia.[41] Patients taking propranolol had no adverse reactions during anesthesia and vascular surgery, and Prys-Roberts concluded that "for patients with hypertension or ischemic heart disease, maintenance of beta receptor blocking therapy through the period of anesthesia and surgery, far from causing adverse reactions, may be beneficial."[48] Indeed, sudden withdrawal of beta-adrenergic blockers in patients with ischemic heart disease who have been receiving these drugs on a chronic basis may cause a rebound effect, with intensification of the severity of ischemia; for this reason it now seems most unwise to withdraw these agents during the preoperative period,[50–54] and it is our policy not to do so.

VALVULAR HEART DISEASE

Patients with valvular heart disease undergoing anesthesia and operation are subject to many potential hazards:

heart failure, infection, tachycardia, and embolization. As might be expected, patients with no or only mild limitation of activity (i.e., those in New York Heart Association [NYHA] Class I or II) tolerate operation well and probably require little more than prophylaxis for infective endocarditis. Those with more serious impairment of cardiac reserve (i.e., those in NYHA Class III or IV) tolerate major noncardiac surgery poorly, and their prognosis for surviving the operation is distinctly worse.[27] As is the case for patients with rheumatic heart disease who face the stress of pregnancy (Chap. 53), the risk of operation depends on the functional state of the heart. Patients with symptomatic critical aortic or mitral stenosis are especially prone to sudden death or acute pulmonary edema during the perioperative period; this may occur if demands on cardiac output are suddenly increased or if atrial fibrillation is precipitated by anesthesia or operation. Every effort should be made to treat heart failure preoperatively. Patients with severe failure and valvular regurgitation may benefit from intraoperative hemodynamic monitoring, afterload reduction, and preload augmentation,[55] while those with severe stenotic or regurgitant valve disease should undergo corrective valvular surgery prior to an elective operation.

Patients with *hypertrophic cardiomyopathy* are intolerant of hypovolemia, which may lead to both a reduction in the elevated preload necessary to maintain cardiac output and an increase in the obstruction to left ventricular outflow. Agents such as halothane and spinal anesthesia, which cause peripheral vasodilatation, may be particularly poorly tolerated by such patients. Intraoperative monitoring of right and left ventricular filling pressures will minimize the chance of hemodynamic compromise in patients with outflow tract obstruction.

Most patients with prosthetic heart valves receive *anticoagulants* on a chronic basis to prevent thromboembolic complications (p. 1086). If these medications are continued through the operative period, hemostasis, hematoma formation, and persistent postoperative bleeding may ensue. Anticoagulants can be temporarily discontinued during the perioperative period with minimal risk of thrombosis. In a study by Tinker and Tarhan, no thromboembolic complications occurred in 159 patients with prosthetic valves undergoing 180 noncardiac operations when anticoagulants were discontinued an average of 2.9 days preoperatively and resumed 2.7 days postoperatively.[56] Using a similar approach, Katholi et al. did not observe thromboembolic complications in 25 operations on patients with prosthetic aortic valves[57]; however, two such complications occurred in the 10 patients with mitral valve prostheses when anticoagulants were discontinued for noncardiac surgery, although these patients had Kay-Shiley caged-disk valves, which are associated with a somewhat higher risk of thromboembolic complications. Because there is a distinct risk of hemorrhagic complications in patients whose anticoagulants have been discontinued for only 2 or 3 days,[56] prothrombin time should be restored to within 20 per cent of normal before one proceeds with noncardiac surgery.[16]

Patients with valvular disease and prosthetic heart valves should receive *prophylactic antibiotics* for surgical procedures likely to be complicated by bacteremias.[58] These include incision and drainage of an infected site; oral, low-

er gastrointestinal, and gallbladder surgery; and genitourinary procedures. Penicillin can be used prior to surgery involving the upper respiratory tract, with erythromycin or vancomycin an acceptable alternative for patients with a penicillin allergy. For gastrointestinal and genitourinary surgery, which can be complicated by either enterococci or gram-negative bacteremia, gentamicin or streptomycin are required in addition to penicillin. (Suggested doses are given on page 1176.) The value of antibiotic prophylaxis in patients with mitral valve prolapse remains controversial. Although small series of patients with endocarditis involving such valves have been reported, the absolute incidence is quite low given the prevalence of this abnormality in the adult population. Nonetheless, on the basis of available information, we recommend prophylaxis for these patients (p. 1094).

CONGENITAL HEART DISEASE

Depending on the nature of the malformation, the patient with congenital heart disease may be subject to one or more potentially serious complications such as infection, bleeding, hypoxemia, and paradoxical embolization during general anesthesia and operation. As is the case for patients with valvular heart disease, patients with congenital heart disease who are to undergo a surgical procedure require prophylaxis to prevent bacterial endocarditis. Patients with cyanotic congenital heart disease and secondary polycythemia are at increased risk of intraoperative and postoperative hemorrhage as a consequence of coagulation defects and thrombocytopenia (p. 1700); this risk can be reduced with careful preoperative phlebotomy, usually to a hematocrit of 50 to 55 per cent.[59]

Patients with cyanotic congenital heart disease tolerate systemic hypotension poorly, since this increases the right-to-left shunt and the severity of hypoxemia. Anesthetic agents such as halothane or spinal anesthesia that cause peripheral vasodilatation are especially hazardous, while ketamine, which has a sympathomimetic effect, is often desirable in these patients.[8] Occasionally, infusion of a vasoconstrictor such as phenylephrine may be required to raise systemic vascular resistance and thereby decrease the magnitude of the right-to-left shunt. Because patients with right-to-left shunts are subject to the risk of paradoxical emboli, including air emboli, meticulous techniques with regard to intravenous solutions and injections are mandatory to prevent such complications.

CONGESTIVE HEART FAILURE

Congestive heart failure is a major determinant of risk, irrespective of the nature of the underlying heart disorder. Skinner and Pearce found a highly significant correlation between NYHA classification and mortality for major noncardiac surgery: 4 per cent in NYHA Class I patients, 11 per cent in Class II, 24 per cent in Class III, and 67 per cent in Class IV patients.[27] Goldman et al. noted a similar association in that the presence of a third heart sound or pulmonary congestion had a marked adverse effect on perioperative mortality.[24] Since the perioperative mortality rate appears to depend more on the patient's condition at the time of operation than on the most severe depression of cardiovascular status the patient has ever experienced, treatment of congestive heart failure prior to contemplated major elective noncardiac surgery is clearly advisable. However, since such a therapeutic regimen almost always includes a diuretic, hypovolemia and hypokalemia are frequent problems for patients treated just prior to operation. It is therefore desirable, if possible, to stabilize the patient's condition by treating heart failure for approximately one week rather than for only one or two days prior to the contemplated operation. In addition, the anesthetic agent for the patient who is in or has just recovered from congestive heart failure should be selected with these risks in mind. Thus, halothane, because of its associated myocardial depression and vasodilatation, might be tolerated less well in such patients than would ketamine, which maintains systemic vascular resistance and arterial pressure.

HEART BLOCK AND PACEMAKERS

The patient with heart block must respond to the demands for an increased cardiac output by augmenting stroke volume, but this compensatory response is prevented in many patients by a concurrent impairment of cardiac contractility. In addition, most anesthetic agents depress myocardial contractility and/or produce peripheral vasodilatation. Furthermore, anesthesia may depress further the automaticity and therefore the ventricular rate of the patient with heart block. Thus, patients with untreated complete heart block may be unable to meet the increased demands placed on the cardiovascular system by anesthesia and operation, and a permanent or temporary pacemaker should be inserted prior to general anesthesia, even in asymptomatic patients (Chap. 22).

A more difficult problem is presented by the patient with chronic bifascicular block.[60–67] A significant fraction of patients developing this abnormality in the course of an acute myocardial infarction progress to complete heart block often accompanied by sudden severe hemodynamic compromise (p. 1287). In several series, a progression from bifascicular to complete heart block has not been documented during the perioperative period in patients without a previous history of third-degree heart block.[10] Therefore, we do not recommend prophylactic pacemaker placement for such patients nor for patients with first-degree atrioventricular (AV) block or Type I second-degree AV block (Wenckebach), although a pacemaker should always be available in the operating room for emergency placement. However, in patients with bifascicular block, with Type II second-degree AV block, or with a history of unexplained syncope or transient third-degree AV block, the risk is much higher, and a temporary pacemaker should be inserted preoperatively. Also, the appearance of new bifascicular block in the immediate postoperative period justifies insertion of a temporary demand pacemaker, since the incidence of subsequent complete AV block is high in this group.[64,67]

When a patient with a permanent pacemaker in situ is about to undergo operation, the device should be carefully evaluated (Chap. 22) to insure that it is functioning properly preoperatively. Demand pacemakers are sensitive to electromagnetic interference, such as that produced by the electrocautery, which may result in failure to pace. The danger of this potentially hazardous interaction can be reduced by placing the indifferent plate of the cautery unit as far as possible from the lead and pulse generator, and the electrocautery should be used in brief bursts rather than continuously.[63] Also, a magnet should be available in the operating room to convert the pacemaker from the demand to the fixed-rate mode. Since the cautery may also interfere with the electrocardiographic monitor and render it temporarily uninterpretable, arterial pressure should be monitored directly during the interval when the cautery is being used.

Preoperative Digitalization

As noted, heart failure greatly increases the risk of anesthesia and operation[24,27] and digitalis glycosides are indicated in the preoperative management of most of these patients. Similarly, patients with atrial fibrillation or a history of recurrent atrial fibrillation or other supraventricular tachyarrhythmia should be digitalized before operation to reduce the ventricular rate or the likelihood of the recurrence of the arrhythmia. Additional indications for preoperative digitalization are unclear and highly controversial.

Proponents of prophylactic digitalization argue that all patients who are at risk of developing heart failure or arrhythmias intra- or postoperatively should receive this drug.[65,66,68] Their recommendations are based on a number of considerations: (1) anesthetic agents are myocardial depressants, and digitalis drugs can reduce this negative inotropic effect[69;–71] (2) digitalis may prevent or at least control the excessive ventricular rate that may develop in patients with supraventricular arrhythmias complicating the postoperative course, especially after cardiac or thoracic surgery, even in patients with no history of previous arrhythmias; (3) the metabolic rate is increased in the postoperative patient, and the patient with borderline cardiac compensation may be better able to tolerate this stress after digitalization.[72] Thus, Deutsch and Dalen have suggested that digitalis therapy be initiated prior to operation for all patients with ischemic heart disease or cardiac enlargement or hypertrophy.[65]

On the other hand, Selzer and Cohn[73] have emphasized the potential hazards of prophylactic digitalization: (1) it is difficult to select optimal digitalizing and maintenance doses in patients with sinus rhythm without cardiac failure; (2) hypoxia and hypokalemia, both common in the postoperative patient, increase the likelihood of digitalis toxicity; (3) despite the theoretical considerations expressed above, it has not been clearly established whether preoperative digitalization actually decreases the incidence of or increases the control of heart rate in postoperative supraventricular tachycardias.

The information currently available does not permit an unequivocal resolution of this controversy. At present, we recommend preoperative digitalization in (1) patients with overt congestive heart failure or a history of heart failure who have not had corrective cardiac surgery; (2) patients with a history of recurrent supraventricular tachyarrhythmias; (3) patients with moderate or severe valvular heart disease; and (4) elderly patients who are to undergo pneumonectomy even in the absence of overt heart disease. We do *not* believe that digitalis is necessary for patients with previous myocardial infarction without apparent left ventricular dysfunction, nor should it be given only for the purpose of counteracting the cardiac depression caused by anesthetics.[74] Careful postoperative monitoring and prompt digitalization when failure or arrhythmias develop is recommended for patients with less severe cardiac disease.

Postoperative Arrhythmias

Arrhythmias are very common after operation and are often a manifestation of a noncardiac complication such as bleeding, infection, or an acid-base or electrolyte imbalance occurring in a patient with heart disease. Management of these arrhythmias often requires recognition and correction of these extracardiac factors.

To assess the clinical correlates and therapeutic outcome of new postoperative supraventricular tachyarrhythmias, Goldman prospectively followed 916 patients who were in sinus rhythm throughout the course of major noncardiac surgery.[75] The 35 patients who developed new postoperative supraventricular tachyarrhythmias (4 per cent of the 916) frequently had concurrent medical problems: 46 per cent had acute cardiac conditions, 31 per cent had major infections, 29 per cent had preexisting hypotension, 26 per cent had anemia, 23 per cent had metabolic derangements, 23 per cent had received parenteral drug therapy, and 20 per cent were hypoxic. Forty per cent of the patients required no new therapy with cardiac medications, and only two required electrical cardioverson; the arrhythmias of all treated patients reverted to sinus rhythm. No deaths were related to the supraventricular tachyarrhythmias per se, but half the patients in whom these arrhythmias occurred died as a result of the concurrent medical problems. Goldman concluded that the onset of a new postoperative supraventricular tachyarrhythmia should prompt a search for remediable medical problems. Direct antiarrhythmic therapy is often unnecessary and is usually secondary in importance to correction of the underlying cause of the arrhythmia.

Sinus tachycardia is the most common rhythm disturbance in the postoperative patient. Multiple noncardiac etiologies have been identified, including hypo- or hypervolemia, fever, anemia, hypoxemia, pulmonary emboli, pain, anxiety, infection, hypotension, and electrolyte abnormalities (especially hypokalemia). These noncardiac etiologies are much more common causes of sinus tachycardia in the postoperative cardiac patient than is either myocardial infarction or heart failure. Sinus tachycardia not due to congestive heart failure will not slow with cardiac glycosides. The therapeutic/toxic ratio of these drugs is actually reduced by most of the above-mentioned noncardiac causes of sinus tachycardia and therefore, digitalis drugs are not considered appropriate therapeutic agents for postoperative patients unless the sinus tachycardia is likely to be caused by impaired cardiac function.

Atrial fibrillation is also a common postoperative arrhythmia. Atrial dilatation, which lowers the threshold for development of this arrhythmia, may result from heart failure, mitral valve disease, and/or hypervolemia. Noncardiac precipitant causes include pneumonia, atelectasis, and pulmonary emboli. Mowry and Reynolds observed atrial fibrillation in 19 per cent of all patients after pneumonectomy; it occurred in 23 per cent of patients after left pneumonectomy, in 14 per cent after right pneumonectomy, and in 28 per cent of patients 50 years of age or over.[76] Initially, treatment of the postoperative patient with atrial fibrillation should be a digitalis glycoside; in addition, a beta-adrenergic blocker or verapamil can be used to help gain rapid control of the ventricular rate. Cardioversion is usually delayed until the precipitating factors have been eliminated, since the patient who is cardioverted prior to clearing the atelectasis or pneumonia frequently reverts to atrial fibrillation, while the patient whose pulmonary problem or congestive heart failure is adequately treated often reverts spontaneously to sinus rhythm.

Atrial flutter, which may be the initial manifestation of pulmonary embolism,[77] is often poorly tolerated because of the rapid ventricular rate and the difficult pharmacological management. Cardioversion is usually the treatment of choice, along with quinidine or procainamide administered to prevent recurrences (p. 698).

THE ROLE OF THE MEDICAL CONSULTANT

The physician called upon to evaluate a patient with suspected or overt cardiac disease prior to elective or emergency noncardiac surgery must first determine whether cardiovascular disease is present and, if it is, must identify those factors that may increase the risk of operation. It may be necessary to invest considerable time and effort to prepare the patient for operation. In addition, the patient must be followed carefully after operation to detect and manage the cardiac problems that frequently complicate the postoperative period.

ESTIMATION OF RISK. A few patients have such compelling reasons for operation, e.g., rupturing aortic aneurysm, perforated or necrotic bowel, life-threatening hemorrhage, or some forms of intestinal obstruction, that estimation of operative risk is an academic exercise, since failure to operate almost certainly dooms the patient. Often, however, the timing or even the performance of an operation is elective, and under these circumstances estimation of risk is an important aspect of the medical consultant's role. Certain cardiovascular problems such as recent myocardial infarction (less than 3 months), overt congestive heart failure, and severe mitral or aortic stenosis are absolute contraindications to truly *elective* surgery. Relative contraindications include more remote myocardial infarction (3 to 6 months earlier), angina pectoris, mild heart failure, cyanotic congenital heart disease with severe polycythemia and a coagulation abnormality. Several other problems should be recognized and treated prior to operation: anemia, hypovolemia, polycythemia, pulmonary disease causing hypoxemia, adrenal hyporesponsiveness secondary to chronic administration of adrenal steroids, hypertension, electrolyte abnormalities, as well as the entire gamut of cardiac arrhythmias. Considerable judgment must be exercised when one or more of the above-mentioned contraindications are present and when a patient requires prompt surgical treatment but the situation is not a true emergency, as for neoplastic disease.

To identify those preoperative factors associated with the development of cardiac complications after major noncardiac operation, Goldman et al. prospectively studied

TABLE 56–3 CARDIAC RISK FACTORS AND CARDIAC RISK CLASSES
DERIVED BY SUMMATING TOTAL POINTS FOR CARDIAC RISK FACTORS*

MEANS OF EVALUATION	FINDING	NO. OF POINTS
History	Myocardial infarction < 6 months prior to surgery	10
	Age > 70	5
Physical examination	S_3 gallop or jugular venous distention	11
	Signs of aortic stenosis	3
ECG	*Any* rhythm other than sinus rhythm or	7
	Premature atrial contractions on last preoperative ECG	
	More then 5 premature contractions per minute on	
	any previous ECG	7
Laboratory data	Po_2 < 60; Pco_2 > 50;	
	K^+ < 3.0; HCO_3 > 20;	
	BUN > 50; creatinine >; 3.0.	
	Abnormal SGOT or signs of chronic liver disease	3
Operation	Emergency	4
	Intraperitoneal, thoracic, or major vascular procedure	3
	TOTAL	53

CLASS	NO. OF POINTS	NO OR MINOR COMPLICATIONS (%)	LIFE-THREATENING COMPLICATIONS†(%)	CARDIAC DEATH (%)
I	0–5	99	0.7	0.2
II	6–12	93	5	2
III	13–25	86	11	2
IV	26	22	22	56

*Data from Goldman, L., et al.: N. Engl. J. Med. *297*:845, 1977, and Goldman, L., et al.: Medicine *57*:357, 1978.
†Myocardial infarction, ventricular tachycardia, pulmonary edema.

1001 patients over 40 years of age.[24] Using multivariate discriminant analysis, they identified nine independent significant correlates of life-threatening and fatal cardiac complications, weighed these factors based on their relative significance as predictors of cardiac outcome, and devised a scale for predicting perioperative risk (Table 56–3). They then separated patients into four classes of varying risk and found that 10 of the 19 postoperative cardiac fatalities occurred in the 118 patients at highest risk. Notably, *unimportant* factors included smoking, glucose intolerance, hyperlipidemia, hypertension, peripheral atherosclerotic vascular disease, angina, and remote myocardial infarction. The predictive value of the Goldman index was confirmed by Weathers and Paine; 20 of the 23 perioperative cardiovascular deaths occurred in patients in Goldman Classes III and IV.[78]

Several of the factors involved in determining the cardiac risk index are potentially controllable, such as the third heart sound, jugular venous distention, recent myocardial infarction, and poor general medical condition. Thus, elective surgery should be delayed until congestive heart failure has been treated, the patient's general medical condition has improved, and (if possible) 6 months have elapsed since a previous myocardial infarction. Several studies have suggested that preoperative cardiac catheterization in high-risk patients allows the adjustment of preload, afterload, and inotropic state to optimize cardiac performance.[79,80] Coronary arteriography might be advisable to distinguish patients with ischemic heart disease from those without clinical evidence of heart disease but with positive exercise tests and/or evidence of other vascular disease who are to undergo major elective noncardiac surgery. Such an approach would allow identification of high-risk patients, and performing coronary revascularization first and/or careful hemodynamic monitoring dur-ing the noncardiac surgery in these patients might reduce operative mortality[36,79;–82] however, the value of this more aggressive approach has not yet been established.[83]

PREPARATION OF THE PATIENT FOR ANESTHESIA AND OPERATION

Careful preparation of the cardiac patient for operation may diminish the frequency and seriousness of intraoperative and postoperative complications.[84] Since many of these complications are the result of hypotension, hypoxemia, or both, every effort should be made to diminish the incidence, duration, and severity of these stresses. Adequate preparation for an elective operation may require days to weeks. The medical consultant should not hesitate to urge postponement or cancellation of an elective operation in order to have sufficient time to institute measures necessary to minimize the risk. In addition to providing a detailed general medical assessment, the consultant physician should take the following steps during this preoperative period:

1. Obtain a careful medication history. This should include current medications in order to identify those drugs which might interact with anesthetic agents. In particular, the patient's experiences during prior surgery, especially adverse reactions to previously employed anesthetic techniques and agents should be identified as should allergies and drug reactions.

2. Treat congestive heart failure without inducing hypovolemia or electrolyte imbalance.

3. Correct anemia or polycythemia. When anemia is severe in the patient with heart failure or cardiomegaly, packed red cells should be given in place of whole blood. Phlebotomy may be helpful in minimizing the hemorrhagic and thrombotic complications of polycythemia. Particular

care must be taken to avoid dehydration in polycythemic patients.

4. Control arrhythmias.

5. Check or insert pacemaker.

6. Adjust antihypertensive medications to achieve good control.

7. Correct acid-base and electrolyte disturbances. Hypokalemia predisposes to arrhythmias and sensitizes the myocardium to the toxic effects of digitalis, while hyponatremia may predispose to hypotension.

8. Adjust anticoagulant therapy for patients with prosthetic valves.

9. Estimate and, if necessary, improve pulmonary function.

10. Provide appropriate antibiotic coverage for the patient with valvular or congenital heart disease.

11. In consultation with the anesthetist and the surgeon, determine the variables to be monitored intraoperatively and discuss the choice of anesthetic agents.

POSTOPERATIVE MEDICAL COMPLICATIONS

Cardiac complications occur much more frequently during the postoperative period than during the intraoperative period. Peak incidence of myocardial infarction is on the third postoperative day, and electrocardiograms should be obtained daily for the first 4 to 5 days after operation in patients with previous myocardial infarction or who have experienced intraoperative hypotension. Because anemia, hypo- and hypervolemia, hypoxemia, fever, and electrolyte abnormalities may be poorly tolerated by patients with a compromised cardiovascular system, these abnormalities should be watched for and corrected if present. Arrhythmias require prompt recognition and management. Agitation and psychosis are common in patients with life-threatening illnesses who undergo general anesthesia and major surgery (particularly the elderly) and may impose an additional cardiovascular stress. Postoperative thromboembolic disease is more frequent and often of greater clinical severity in patients with heart disease. Measures to minimize thromboembolic complications include early ambulation, exercise of the lower extremities while the patient is in bed, use of elastic stockings, and small (mini) doses of heparin (Chap. 46).

Pulmonary parenchymal complications also occur more frequently in cardiac than in noncardiac patients, perhaps because of the chronic pulmonary congestion characterizing the former. Thoracic operations add to the risk of ventilatory disturbances because they interfere with movements of the chest wall and impair the patient's ability to cough and eliminate secretions. Postoperative pulmonary complications may be diminished by postural drainage, by the inspiration of humidified air, and by the use of bronchodilators in patients with postoperative bronchospasm; the value of the routine use of antibiotics is controversial. In patients with suspected respiratory failure, measurements of ventilation and arterial blood gases are mandatory as a guide to therapy.

Prompt recognition and management of the multiple problems that may complicate the postoperative period are possible only if the physician closely follows the patient throughout convalescence. All too often the patient with heart disease is appropriately prepared for a noncardiac operation and survives the procedure but is not followed adequately during the early postoperative period, when the risk of serious complications still exists.

References

1. Glasser, S. P. (ed.): Noncardiac Surgery in the Cardiac Patient. Mt. Kisco, N.Y., Futura Publishing Co., 1983.

1a. Hillis, L. D., and Cohn, P. F.: Noncardiac surgery in patients with coronary artery disease: Risks, precautions and perioperative management. Arch. Intern. Med. 138:972, 1978.

2. Kaplan, J. A. (ed.): Cardiac Anesthesia. New York, Grune and Stratton, 1979.

3. Sorensen, B., Rasmussen, J. P., Dauchot, P. J., and Regula, G.: Cardiac function during induction and early anesthesia with methoxyflurane. An evaluation using systolic time intervals and pressure time indices. Acta Anaesth. Scand. 22:615, 1978.

4. Ngai, S. H.: Current concepts in anesthesiology. Effects of anesthetics on various organs. N. Engl. J. Med. 302:564, 1980.

5. Christensen, V., Sorensen, M. B., Klauber, P. V., and Skovsted, P.: Haemodynamic effects of enflurane in patients with valvular heart disease. Acta Anaesth. Scand. 67:34, 1978.

6. Bille-Brahe, N. E., Sorensen, M. B., Mondorf, T., and Engell, H. C.: Central haemodynamics during induction of neurolept anaesthesia in patients with arteriosclerotic heart disease. Acta Anaesth. Scand. Suppl. 67:47, 1978.

7. Friedberg, C. K.: Surgical procedures in the cardiac patient (Chap. 49). In Diseases of the Heart. 3rd ed. Philadelphia, W. B. Saunders Co., 1966.

8. Radney, P. A., Arai, T., and Nagashima, H.: Ketamine-gallamine anesthesia for great-vessel operations in infants. Anesth. Analg. 53:365, 1974.

9. Hug, C. C., Jr.: Pharmacology—anesthetic drugs. In Kaplan, J. A. (ed.): Cardiac Anesthesia. New York, Grune and Stratton, 1979, p. 3.

10. Goldman, L., Caldera, D. L., Southwick, F. S., Nussbaum, S. R., Murray, B., O'Malley, T. A., Goroll, A. H., Caplan, C. H., Nolan, J., Burke, D. S., Krogstad, D., Carabello, B., and Slater, E. E.: Cardiac risk factors and complications in non-cardiac surgery. Medicine 57:357, 1978.

11. Steen, P. A., Tinker, J. H., and Tarhan, S.: Myocardial reinfarction after anesthesia and surgery. J.A.M.A. 239:2566, 1978.

12. Arkins, R., Smessaert, A. A., and Hicks, R. G.: Mortality and morbidity in surgical patients with coronary heart disease. J.A.M.A. 190:485, 1964.

13. Topkins, M. J., and Artusio, J. F., Jr.: Myocardial infarction and surgery: A five year study. Anesth. Analg. 43:716, 1964.

14. Tarhan, S., Moffitt, E. A., Taylor, W. F., and Giulioni, E. R.: Myocardial infarction after general anesthesia. J.A.M.A. 220:1451, 1972.

15. Knorring, J.: Postoperative myocardial infarction: A prospective study in a high-risk group of surgical patients. Surgery 90:55, 1981.

16. Tinker, J. H., Noback, C. R., Vlietstra, R. E., and Frye, R. L.: Management of patients with heart disease for noncardiac surgery. J.A.M.A. 246:1348, 1981.

17. Kaplan, J. A., and Dunbar, R. W.: Anesthesia for noncardiac surgery in patients with cardiac disease. In Kaplan, J. A. (ed.): Cardiac Anesthesia. New York, Grune and Stratton, 1979, p. 377.

18. Katz, R. L., and Bigger, J. T., Jr.: Cardiac arrhythmias during anesthesia and operation. Anesthesiology 33:193, 1970.

19. Vanik, P. E., and Davis, H. S.: Cardiac arrhythmias during halothane anesthesia. Anesth. Analg. 47:299, 1968.

20. Walton, H. J., Cross, P., and Pollack, E. W.: Ventricular cardiac arrhythmias during anesthesia: Feasibility of preoperative recognition. South Med. J. 75:27, 1982.

21. Joas, T. A., and Stevens, W. C.: Comparison of the arrhythmic doses of epinephrine during forane, halothane and fluroxene anesthesia in dogs. Anesthesiology 35:48, 1971.

22. Narahara, K. A., and Blettel, M. L.: Effect of rate on left ventricular volumes and ejection fraction during chronic ventricular pacing. Circulation 67:323, 1983.

23. Knapp, R. B., Topkins, M. J., and Artusio, J. F., Jr.: The cerebrovascular accident and coronary occlusion in anesthesia. J.A.M.A. 182:332, 1962.

24. Goldman, L., Caldera, D. L., Nussbaum, S. R., Southwick, F. S., Krogstad, D., Murray, B., Burke, D. S., O'Malley, T. A., Goroll, A. H., Caplan, C. H., Nolan, J., Carabello, B., and Slater, E. E.: Multifactorial index of cardiac risk in noncardiac surgical procedures. N. Engl. J. Med. 297:845, 1977.

25. Wells, P. H., and Kaplan, J. A.: Optimal management of patients with ischemic heart disease for noncardiac surgery by complementary anesthesiologist and cardiologist interaction. Am. Heart J. 102:1029, 1981.

26. Rao, T. L. K., and El-Etr, A. A.: Myocardial reinfarction following anesthesia in patients with recent infarction. Anesth. Analg. 60:271, 1981.

27. Skinner, J. F., and Pearce, M. L.: Surgical risk in the cardiac patient. J. Chron. Dis. 17:57, 1964.

28. Driscoll, A. C., Hobika, J. H., Etsten, B. E., and Proger, S.: Clinically unrecognized myocardial infarction following surgery. N. Engl. J. Med. 264:633, 1961.

29. Salem, D. N., Homans, D. C., and Isner, J. M.: Management of cardiac disease in the general surgical patient. In Harvey, W. P. (ed.): Current Problems in Cardiology Vol. 5. Chicago, Year Book Medical Publishers, Inc., 1980.

30. Mauney, F. M., Jr., Ebert, P. A., and Sabiston, D. C., Jr.: Postoperative myocardial infarction: A study of predisposing factors, diagnosis and mortality in a high risk group of surgical patients. Ann. Surg. *172*:497, 1970.

31. McCollum, C. H., Garcia-Rinaldi, R., Graham, J. M., and DeBakey, M. E.: Myocardial revascularization prior to subsequent major surgery in patients with coronary artery disease. Surgery *81*:302, 1977.

32. Mahar, L. J., Steen, P. A., Tinker, H. H., Vlietstra, R. E., Smith, H. C., and Pluth, J. R.: Perioperative myocardial infarction in patients with coronary artery disease with and without aorta-coronary artery bypass grafts. J. Thorac. Cardiovasc. Surg. *76*:533, 1978.

33. Scher, K., and Tice, D. A.: Operative risk in patients with previous coronary bypass. Arch. Surg. *111*:807, 1976.

34. Edwards, W. H., Mulhern, J. L., and Wolher, W. E.: Vascular reconstructive surgery following myocardial revascularization. Ann. Surg. *187*:653, 1978.

35. Crawford, E. S., Morris, G. C., Howell J. F., et al.: Operative risk in patients with previous coronary artery bypass. Ann. Thorac. Surg. *26*:215, 1978.

36. Fudge, T. L., McKinnon, W. M. P., Schoettle, P., Ochsner, J. L., and Mills, N. L.: Improve operative risk after myocardial revascularization. South. Med. J. *74*:799, 1981.

37. Goldman, L., and Caldera, D. L.: Risks of general anesthesia and elective surgery in the hypertensive patient. Anesthesiology *50*:285, 1979.

38. Chamberlain, D. A., and Edmunds-Seal, J.: Effects of surgery under general anesthesia on the electrocardiogram in ischemic heart disease and hypertension. Br. Med. J. *2*:784, 1964.

39. Rosen, M., Mushin, W. W., Kilpatrick, G. S., Campbell, H., Davies, L. G. G., and Harrison, E.: Study of myocardial ischemia in surgical patients. Br. Med. J. *2*:1415, 1966.

40. Seltzer, J. L., Gerson, J. I., and Grogono, A. W.: Hypertension in the perioperative period. N. Y. State J. Med. *80*:29, 1980.

41. Prys-Roberts, C., Greene, L. T., Meloche, R., and Foex, P.: Studies of anesthesia in relation to hypertension. II: Hemodynamic consequences of induction and endotracheal intubation. Br. J. Anesth. *43*:531, 1971.

42. Tarazi, R. C., Frohlich, E. D., and Dustan, H. P.: Plasma volume in man with essential hypertension. N. Engl. J. Med. *278*:762, 1968.

43. Foster, M. W., Jr., and Gayle, R. F., Jr.: Dangers in combining reserpine with electroconvulsive therapy. J.A.M.A. *159*:1520, 1955.

44. Ziegler, C. H., and Lovette, J. B.: Operative complications after therapy with reserpine and reserpine compounds. J.A.M.A. *176*:916, 1961.

45. Katz, R. L., Weintraub, H. D., and Papper, E. M.: Anesthesia, surgery and rauwolfia. Anesthesiology *25*:142, 1964.

46. Munson, W. M., and Jenicek, J. A.: Effect of anesthetic agents on patients receiving reserpine therapy. Anesthesiology *23*:741, 1962.

47. Prys-Roberts, C., Meloche, R., and Foex, P.: Studies of anesthesia in relation to hypertension. 1. Cardiovascular responses of treated and untreated patients. Br. J. Anesth. *43*:122, 1971.

48. Prys-Roberts, C.: Medical problems of surgical patients. Hypertension and ischaemic heart disease. Ann. R. Coll. Surg. Engl. *58*:465, 1976.

49. Viljoen, J. F., Estafanous, G., and Kellner, G. A.: Propranolol and cardiac surgery. J. Thorac. Cardiovasc. Surg. *64*:826, 1972.

50. Caralps, J. M., Mulet, J., Wienke, H. R., Moran, J. M., and Pifarre, R.: Results of coronary artery surgery in patients receiving propranolol. J. Thorac. Cardiovasc. Surg. *67*:526, 1974.

51. Kaplan, J. A., Dunbar, R. W., Bland, J. W., Sumpter, R., and Jones, E. L.: Propranolol and cardiac surgery: A problem for the anesthesiologist. Anesth. Analg. *54*:571, 1975.

52. Should propranolol be stopped before surgery? Med. Lett. *18*:41, 1976.

53. Goldman, L.: Noncardiac surgery in patients receiving propranolol. Case reports and a recommended approach. Arch. Intern. Med. *141*:193, 1981.

54. Goldman, L.: Noncardiac surgery in patients receiving propranol. Arch. Intern. Med. *141*:193, 1981.

55. Stone, J. G., Hoar, P. F., Calabro, J. R., DePetrillo, M. A., and Bendixen, H. H.: Afterload reduction and preload augmentation improve the anesthetic management of patients with cardiac failure and valvular regurgitation. Anesth. Analg. *59*:737, 1980.

56. Tinker, J. H., and Tarhan, S.: Discontinuing anticoagulant therapy in surgical patients with cardiac valve prostheses. J.A.M.A. *239*:738, 1978.

57. Katholi, R. E., Nolan, S. P., and McGuire, L. B.: Living with prosthetic heart valves. Subsequent noncardiac operations and the risk of thromboembolism or hemorrhage. Am. Heart J. *92*:162, 1976.

58. Kaplan, E. L., Anthony, B. F., and Bishop, A.: Prevention of bacterial endocarditis. Circulation *56*:139A, 1977.

59. Sommerville, J., McDonald, L., and Edgill, M.: Postoperative haemorrhage and related abnormalities of blood coagulation in cyanotic congenital heart disease. Br. Heart J. *27*:440, 1965.

60. Berg, G. R., and Kotler, M. N.: The significance of bilateral bundle branch block in the preoperative patient. Chest *59*:62, 1971.

61. Kunstadt, D., Punja, M., Cagin, N., Fernandez, P., Levitt, B., and Yuceoglu, Y. Z.: Bifascicular block: A clinical and electrophysiologic study. Am. Heart J. *86*:173, 1973.

62. Rooney, S. M., Goldiner, P. L., and Muss, E.: Relationship of right bundle branch block and marked left axis deviation to complete heart block during general anesthesia. Anesthesiology *44*:64, 1976.

63. Simon, A. B.: Perioperative management of the pacemaker patient. Anesthesiology *46*:127, 1977.

64. Logue, R. B., and Kaplan, J. A.: The cardiac patient and noncardiac surgery. *In* Harvey, W. P. (ed.): Current Problems in Cardiology. Vol. 7. Chicago, Year Book Medical Publishers, Inc., 1982.

65. Deutsch, S., and Dalen, J. E.: Indications for prophylactic digitalization. Anesthesiology *30*:648, 1969.

66. Dalen, J. E., and Dexter, L.: Operation in the patient with heart disease. *In* Conn, H. L. (ed.): Cardiovascular Diseases. Philadelphia, Lea & Febiger Co., 1971.

67. Perlroth, M. G., and Hultgren, H. N.: The cardiac patient and general surgery. J.A.M.A. *233*:1279, 1979.

68. Wheat, M. W., Jr., and Burford, T. H.: Digitalis in surgery: Extension of classical indications. J. Thorac. Cardiovasc. Surg. *41*:162, 1961.

69. Goldberg, A. H., Maling, H. M., and Gaffney, T. E.: The effect of digoxin pretreatment in heart contractile force during thiopental infusion in dogs. Anesthesiology *22*:974, 1961.

70. Goldberg, A. H., Maling, H. M., and Gaffney, T. E.: The value of prophylactic digitalization in halothane anesthesia. Anesthesiology *23*:207, 1962.

71. Shimosato, S. A., and Etsten, B.: Performance of digitalized heart during halothane anesthesia. Anesthesiology *24*:41, 1963.

72. Bille-Brahe, N. E.: Digitalization of surgical patients with impaired left ventricular function. Danish Med. Bull. *29*:45, 1982.

73. Selzer, A., and Cohn, K. E.: Some thoughts concerning the prophylactic use of digitalis. Am. J. Cardiol. *26*sf,1 :214, 1970.

74. Foex, P.: Preoperative assessment of the patient with cardiovascular disease. Br. J. Anaesth. *53*:731, 1981.

75. Goldman, L.: Supraventricular tachyarrhythmias in hospitalized adults after surgery. Chest *73*:450, 1978.

76. Mowry, F. M., and Reynolds, E. W.: Cardiac rhythm disturbances complicating resectional surgery of the lung. Ann. Intern. Med. *61*:688, 1964.

77. Johnson, J. C., Flowers, N. C., and Horan, L. G.: Unexplained atrial flutter: A frequent herald of pulmonary embolism. Chest *60*:29, 1971.

78. Weathers, L. W., and Paine, R.: The risk of surgery in cardiac patients. Ann. Intern. Med. *2*:57, 1981.

79. DelGuercio, L. R. M., and Cohn, J. D.: Monitoring operative risk in the elderly. J.A.M.A. *243*:1350, 1980.

80. Babu, S. C., Sharma, P. V. P., and Raciti, A.: Operability with safety is increased in patients with peripheral vascular disease. Arch. Surg. *115*:1384, 1980.

81. Gage, A. A., Bhayana, J. N., Balu, V., and Hook, N.: Assessment of cardiac risk in surgical patients. Arch. Surg. *112*:1488, 1977.

82. Hertzer, N. R., Young, J. R., Kramer, J. R., Phillips, D. F., deWolfe, V. G., Ruschhaupt, W. F., and Beven, E. G.: Routine coronary angiography prior to elective aortic reconstruction. Arch. Surg. *114*:1336, 1979.

83. Bille-Brahe, N. E., and Eickhoff, J. H.: Measurement of central haemodynamic parameters during preoperative exercise testing in patients suspected of arteriosclerotic heart disease. Acta Chir. Scand. *502*:38, 1980.

84. Abrams, L. M., and Chambers, D. A.: Preoperative management. *In* Kaplan, J. A. (ed.): Cardiac Anesthesia, New York, Grune and Stratton, 1979, p. 169.

57

EMOTION, PSYCHIATRIC DISORDERS, AND THE HEART

by Thomas P. Hackett, M.D., and Jerrold F. Rosenbaum, M.D.

"Every affection of the mind that is attended with either pain or pleasure, hope or fear, is the cause of an agitation whose influence extends to the heart."

WILLIAM HARVEY, EXERCITATIO DE MOTU CORDIS ET SANGUINIS, 1628[1]

Although few would disclaim Harvey's sentiment, the precise nature of the link between the mind and heart disease remains to be defined. Substantial evidence exists to indicate associations between psychosocial stresses and coronary artery disease, hypertension, arrhythmia, and sudden death, but the intervening variables that mediate pathological changes have yet to be subjected to rigorous, prospective study. In this chapter these and other issues relevant to the interface between cardiology and psychiatry are discussed.

PSYCHIATRIC ASPECTS OF CORONARY ARTERY DISEASE

Psychosocial Factors

Clinicians have long suspected that the accumulation of small stresses from longstanding conflicts can augment the development of cardiovascular disease, most especially of essential hypertension and coronary atherosclerosis. In the 1910 Lumleian lecture, Sir William Osler, commenting on physicians with angina pectoris, said, ". . . the outstanding feature was the incessant treadmill of practice; and yet if hard work—that 'badge of our tribe'—was alone responsible, would there not be a great many more cases? Every one of these men had an additional factor—worry; in not a single case under fifty years of age was this feature ab-

sent. . . ."[2] Three decades later, Flanders Dunbar gave the following capsule description of patients with coronary artery disease: "They are compulsive, have a tendency to work long hours and not take vacations, a tendency to seize authority; dislike of sharing responsibility, . . . articulate, . . . few neurotic traits, . . . a tendency to depression which is rarely admitted to, . . . a tendency to minimize symptoms, . . . self-neglect. . . ."[3] This sketch of the coronary patient, consumed in work and beset by worry, has been recognized and redrawn by many clinicians.

Although researchers have examined the roles of life dissatisfaction, acute stress, personal loss, sociological factors, and personality traits in coronary artery disease, much time and effort have also been devoted to describing a personality behavior pattern characteristic of the overworked and anxious coronary patient. Friedman and Rosenman developed the concept of a "coronary-prone behavior pattern," which they termed *Type A behavior*.[4] Over the last two decades they have relentlessly investigated the association between Type A behavior and coronary artery disease and have concluded that Type A behavior is as significant as any of the major risk factors of coronary artery disease, such as cigarette smoking, hypercholesterolemia, and hypertension; Friedman defines Type A behavior as "a characteristic action-emotion complex" found in people who are constantly struggling to reach poorly defined goals in the shortest time possible.[4] In his opinion, the most critical aspects of Type A behavior patterns are excesses of competitiveness, pace, and aggression. Diagnostic indicators of Type A behavior are listed in Table 57–1. Type B individuals exhibit the opposite type of behavior; they are relaxed, unhurried, and less aggressive. Although they may be interested in success, and may indeed be successful, in most instances they do not struggle so vigorously as Type A individuals in pursuit of this goal.

In the Western Collaborative Group Study (WCGS)[5] male subjects were sorted into groups on the basis of the prominence of Type A behavior patterns, measured in an interview designed to test the behavior of each subject. The study was conducted in double-blind fashion; neither the rating team nor the medical examiner had knowledge of all risk factors. Follow-up at 4½, 6½, and 8½ years revealed that men with coronary-prone Type A behavior at entry experienced 1.7 to 4.5 times the rate of new coronary diseases as did Type B men (Fig. 57–1).

Research data from various other demographical and geographical settings consistently relate Type A behavior to coronary artery disease.[6] Investigations in Europe, Australia, and Israel point to the cross-cultural relevance of some aspects of such behavior.[7] Other studies have shown that the Type A pattern appears to be specifically related to atherosclerosis. Individuals with other diseases, such as lung disease and cancer, tend to include an equal distribution of Types A and B.[7,8] Jenkins feels that there is a strong link between Type A behavior and the clinical emergence of myocardial infarction and coronary artery disease and that Type A behavior has "about the same strength of associations with coronary artery disease prevalence and incidence as do other standard risk factors."[7] This point of view is now shared by a number of experienced cardiologists.[9] Some studies have attempted to correlate anxiety and neuroticism with coronary artery disease.[6] These studies are all retrospective and tend to indicate that these variables are more predictive of angina pectoris than of myocardial infarction. Friedman and his associates provided advice and instructions designed to diminish Type A behavior to 600 patients who had suffered a myocardial infarction. After 1 year the rate of nonfatal infarction was significantly lower among subjects who received behavioral and cardiological counseling than among those who received cardiological counseling on the usually accepted risk factors alone.[10]

Stress and life change have largely been investigated by means of the Holmes and Rahe Schedule of Recent Experience.[11-13] A number of studies[7,12-14] have shown that the Holmes-Rahe scores for myocardial infarction victims in a 6-month period prior to infarction were two to three times greater than those for a control group. This association of life change with the presence of coronary artery disease supports the findings reported in the admirable studies in England by Rees and Lutkins[15] and by Parkes and colleagues,[16] which indicate increased mortality during the first year of bereavement among widowers, widows, and other relatives close to the deceased, and of Engel[17,18] and Greene et al.[19] of loss preceding sudden death from coronary artery disease. However, many of these studies may be challenged because of their retrospective nature. One prospective study by Theorell et al.[20] showed no connec-

TABLE 57–1 DIAGNOSTIC INDICATORS OF TYPE A BEHAVIOR

Time Urgency

A. Psychomotor manifestations
1. Characteristic facial tautness expressing tension
2. Rapid horizontal eyeball movements during ordinary conversation
3. Rapid eye blinking (over 40 blinks/min)
4. Knee jiggling or rapid vigorous tapping of fingers
5. Rapid, frequently dysrhythmic speech involving elimination of terminal words of sentences
6. Lip clicking during ordinary speaking
7. Rapid ticlike eyebrow lifting
8. Head nodding when speaking
9. Sucking in of air during speech
10. Humming (tuneless)
11. Speech hurrying
12. Tense posture
13. Motorization accompanying responses
14. Expiratory sighing
15. Rapid body movements
B. Direct behavioral tests
1. The interviewer, in posing a question whose answer is already clear from its contents, hesitates, becomes laboriously tedious or repetitive, and then stammers. The subject interrupts the stammering with his answer.
C. Physiological indicators
1. Periorbital pigmentation
2. Excessive forehead and upper lip perspiration
D. Significant biographical content
1. Self-awareness of presence of Type A behavior
2. Polyphasic activities (e.g., reads while driving, reads while using electric shaver, and thinks of other matters during conversation with others)
3. Walks fast, eats fast, and does not dawdle at table
4. Subject makes fetish of always being on time under all circumstances
5. Has been told by spouse to slow down in working and living habits
6. Difficulty in sitting and doing nothing
7. Subject habitually substitutes numerals for metaphors in his speech

Excessive Competitiveness and Hostility

A. Psychomotor manifestations
1. Characteristic facial set exhibiting aggression and hostility (eye and jaw muscles)
2. Characteristic ticlike drawing back of corner of lips, almost exposing teeth
3. Hostile, jarring laugh
4. Use of clenched fist and table pounding or excessively forceful use of hands and fingers
5. Explosive, staccato, frequently unpleasant-sounding voice
6. Frequent use of obscenity
7. Subject exhibits irritation and rage when asked about some past events in which he became angered
B. Direct behavioral tests
1. The interviewer directly challenges the validity of some comment or behavior that the subject has reported. The subject reacts in a hostile or unpleasant manner.
2. The interviewer questions the subject about his views on politics, races, women, or competitors. The subject responds with absolute, almost angry generalizations.
C. Significant biographical content
1. The subject reports that he is irritated if kept waiting for any reason or if driving behind a car moving too slowly in his view
2. The subject expresses general distrust of other people's motives (e.g., distrust of altruism)
3. The subject reports that he almost always plays any type of game to win (even with young children)

Modified from Friedman, M., et al.: Circulation *66*:83, 1982, by permission of the American Heart Association, Inc.

tion between a high life change score and the incidence of acute myocardial infarction.

Attempts have also been made to correlate coronary artery disease with *life or work dissatisfaction*. Wolf described a Sisyphean pattern, in which the individual "strives without joy."[21] Rarely is this individual rewarded by the satisfaction of accomplishment. Instead he doggedly toils on to

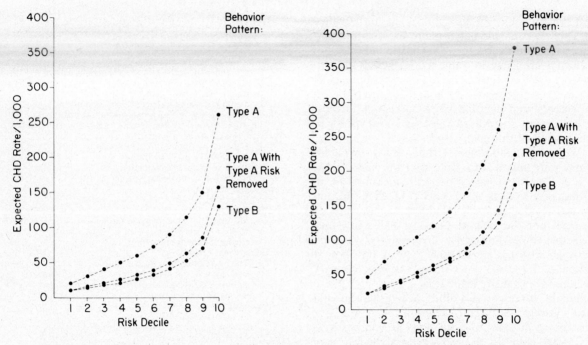

FIGURE 57–1   Expected rates of coronary heart disease in 8.5 years by decile of estimated risk for WCGS men ages 39 to 49 (*A*) and 50 to 59 (*B*). (From Brand, R. J., Rosenman, R. H., Sholtz, R. I., and Friedman, M.: Multivariate prediction of coronary heart disease in the Western Collaborative Group Study compared to the findings of the Framingham study. Circulation, *53*:348, 1976, by permission of the American Heart Association, Inc.)

a state of "psychic exhaustion" or "emotional drain" described by both Wolf[21] and Bruhn[22] as a precursor to myocardial infarction and sudden death. Their evidence, although retrospectively collected and therefore only suggestive, is at the same time compelling.

Response to Symptoms

The most important psychological danger to the patient with acute myocardial infarction is *delay*—the time interval from symptom onset to arrival at a medical facility (Chaps. 23 and 38). Median delay times in recent studies range from 2.9 to 5.1 hours (Fig. 57–2).[23–25] The enormity of this problem becomes apparent when one realizes that 55 to 80 per cent of deaths from myocardial infarction occur within 4 hours of the onset of symptoms;[26] thus the lives of many of these victims might have been saved had they responded in time.

What accounts for this delay? Can it be explained on the basis of an educative or cognitive deficit?[27] In three independent studies, delay time did not correlate significantly with educational level, occupation, socioeconomic class, or past history of heart disease.[23–25] In our study at the Massachusetts General Hospital, delay tended to diminish as the severity of symptoms mounted; however, according to the Peale score,[23] there was no relationship between delay time and the severity of the disease. Individuals who recognized the true source of their pain came sooner than did those who displaced the cause of pain to the gastrointestinal system. Patients who interpreted the symptoms as totally unrelated to their hearts delayed the longest. Considerable time was usually wasted in trying to decide what action to take. The victim's friends and associates appear to be more effective at reducing delay than are husbands or wives. Individuals who experience myocardial infarction

at their place of employment reach the hospital most swiftly because they may be ordered to do so by a plant supervisor or nurse. Although spouses are less effective catalysts than are foremen or supervisors, some take the initiative

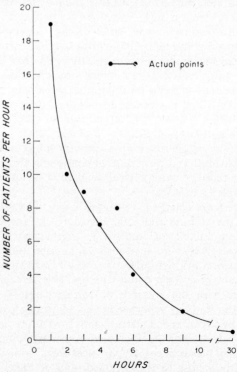

FIGURE 57–2   Rate at which patients seek medical care as a function of time from onset of coronary symptoms. (From Hackett, T. P., and Cassem, N. H.: Factors contributing to delay in responding to the signs and symptoms of acute myocardial infarction. Am. J. Cardiol., *24*:651, 1969.)

by calling an ambulance or a doctor, despite patient protest.

Why does the stricken patient fail to take energetic corrective action in his own behalf? With the abundance of information available to the lay public, replete with examples of public figures who have recovered from myocardial infarction, a more appropriate and salubrious response might be expected. Although there is no specific answer to this question, the defense of denial has been used as a partial explanation.[23] *Denial* has been cited as the most common human reaction to situations of life stress[28] and is defined as the conscious or unconscious repudiation of part or all of the total available meaning of an event in order to allay fear, anxiety, or other unpleasant effects.[29] At its simplest, it is the negation of personal danger (i.e., "This can't be happening to me"). *Displacement* is another form of denial (i.e., "This pain must be indigestion"). *Rationalization* is still another (i.e., "This pain can't be a heart attack; I'm too young"). The list of variations continues, but the goal is the same—to reduce or eliminate the threat. Myocardial infarction presents a profound threat to life. Even survival, in the minds of many, carries the toll of permanent cardiac impairment. For some people, to acknowledge that chest pain may herald myocardial infarction is tantamount to accepting a grim future. It is necessary to correct such misconceptions in order to prevent what is clearly inordinate delay.

In an effort to reduce delay, physicians should attempt to dispel the myth of automatic invalidism after myocardial infarction by stressing to both patient and family that many patients are able to return to their previous occupations and to resume essentially unaltered life styles. The public must also be introduced to a simple set of specific guidelines outlining the type, duration, and variation in symptoms of myocardial infarction and the urgent need for immediate medical consultation if and when such symptoms appear. The possibility of both delay and denial by the patient must be anticipated, and friends and family must be encouraged to respond to these symptoms by seeking assistance despite possible protest.

Hospitalization

EMERGENCY WARD. Most hospitals provide immediate care for people entering with chest pain, enabling patients to be seen by a physician before nonessential information is obtained. The emergency ward experience is generally brief and reassuring. Despite the patient's rapid transit through this area, three aspects deserve attention:

1. The patient should be given a clear account of what is happening to him, and any questions he or she may ask should be answered. A direct relationship seems to exist between uncertainty and anxiety, so that as long as presentation of the medical facts is buttressed by as much reassurance as one can reasonably provide, the patient will benefit from the truth.

2. Administering the sacrament of the sick to Catholic patients is not as stressful an experience as it may appear.[30] The critical variable here is the attitude of the priest; if he is friendly and emphasizes the routine nature of the procedure, the patient's response is apt to be positive.

3. The coronary care unit should be carefully described to the patient ahead of time, especially if it is windowless or unusual in any other way.

PROBLEMS IN THE CORONARY CARE UNIT (CCU). The cardiac monitor is central to the experience of a patient in the CCU. When continuous monitoring was first introduced, many conjectured that the restraint of the leads, audible "beeps," and visible electrocardiograms would induce considerable anxiety in the patient. However, our findings[31] and those of others[32,33] demonstrate that the monitor may be more reassuring than frightening to the cardiac patient, in large part because of the way in which the monitor is introduced. In our unit the nurses have referred to it as a "mechanical guardian angel" and have told the patient, "As long as you're hooked up with this machine, you can't die if you try"—a remarkably effective stratagem.

Witnessing a cardiac arrest is judged by the staff to be the most distressing event in the CCU. In a study of patients who watched a resuscitation effort, only 20 per cent of the spectators *admitted* to being frightened by the scene.[31] Although all patients were impressed by the speedy response of the drill team to the alarm and many were equally impressed by the brevity of resuscitation, the most common general response was *anger* directed toward the patient in cardiac arrest. The usefulness of anger is not difficult to discover. If an anxious person can be made angry—a more controllable and more acceptable emotion than anxiety—his apprehension declines. Lack of identification with the arrest victim further reduces anxiety. Although empathy for the patient in cardiac arrest was expressed by all, only rarely did a patient identify with him, even when the victim and observer were of the same sex and of similar age and social background. The typical response of the patient witnessing cardiac arrest is an attempt to grasp the most comforting meaning from the event while denying its more threatening aspects. That this is not always effective is demonstrated by Bruhn's report of anxiety and elevated systolic pressure in patients who had viewed a fatal arrest.[34] Requests for tranquilizers and pain medication increase in the wake of an arrest. In one study in which CCU patients were asked whether they would prefer to be in a single room or in a two- or four-bed ward should they require subsequent hospitalization, all chose the latter except those who had seen an arrest—these patients chose single rooms.[31]

The experience of cardiac arrest itself is almost always clouded by amnesia. Nine of 10 patients remember nothing specific about the event.[31] We have found nothing to support the observations of Kübler-Ross, who has described several "afterlife experiences" in a dream state during the period of arrest.[35]

An early report on the psychological state of survivors of cardiac arrest provided a grim picture of life after resuscitation.[36] These survivors appeared to be suffering from traumatic neurosis. Chronically anxious and depressed, they complained of feeling different from others, as though, like Lazarus, they had returned from the dead. Subsequent reports have not supported this early observation.[37,38] Indeed, there appears to be a remarkable absence of emotional debility in some patients who survive cardiac arrest. Dobson and his coworkers, who have followed a series of survivors for some years after cardiac arrest, report a uniformly good long-term response and emphasize the importance of informing the patient about what has happened.[38] It is helpful to stress the routine nature of resuscitation and that it does not necessarily alter the patient's prognosis.

Although most patients in the CCU are anxious, particularly in the first 2 days, few openly complain of anxiety or appear unduly apprehensive to their attending physician. If questioned closely, patients may admit to feelings of anxiety, but the tendency is to minimize this affect, as though its presence were cowardly. Although depression is usually not a cause for concern in the CCU, patients begin to experience a sense of sadness toward the end of their stay, when the critical period has passed, and they begin to assess their future. This is essentially a reactive depression, a quite normal response under the circumstances and one that typically occurs in individuals who have sustained loss. In this case it is the loss of the sense of health and intactness; rarely is the depression pathological (Fig. 57–3). Delirium, so common in the surgical intensive care unit, is seldom a problem in the CCU. It occurs in fewer than 1 per cent of the patients.[39]

The defense of denial (defined earlier) is a common adaptive process in patients who face danger. In situations of stress, denial can lower the sense of tension, both psychologically and physiologically. An unexpected finding in one study was the inverse relationship between denial and mortality in the CCU.[31] Individuals who denied being frightened, minimized the seriousness of their illness, displayed a fatalistic attitude, and gave the appearance of being unruffled tended to survive the CCU experience in larger numbers than did those who worried constantly and seemed unable to deny their distress. Although denial can play the role of enemy to the myocardial infarction victim in delaying his arrival in the emergency ward, it can also serve as an ally in the CCU.

PSYCHOLOGICAL MANAGEMENT IN THE CCU
(See also Chap. 38)

Patient Education and Clarification of the Patient's Condition.   Informing the patient about the facts of his illness and about the function of equipment and purpose

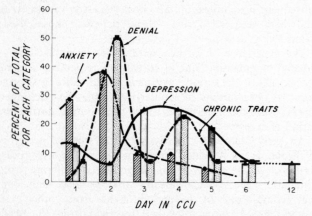

FIGURE 57–3   Hypothetical schedule of onset of emotional and behavioral reactions of a coronary care unit (CCU) patient. (From Cassem, N. H., and Hackett, T. P.: Psychiatric consultation in a coronary care unit. Ann. Intern. Med., *75*:9, 1971.)

of procedures is becoming common practice. Lack of information, partial disclosures, and conspiracies of silence detract from the doctor-patient relationship.[40] The side effects of medication should be explained, as should the reason for performing certain procedures, such as hourly determination of vital signs. While clarifying medical issues and misconceptions, it is also possible to impart a sense of enlightened optimism by mentioning, for example, that the Boston Marathon has been successfully completed by individuals who have suffered myocardial infarction.

Predicting that an event will produce anxiety is as good as saying that such anxiety is normal. Thus, the anxiety loses its sting. A good example of this is to anticipate that the sound of the alarm buzzer in the CCU will provoke anxiety and to point out that the alarm is usually activated by a loose electrode. Similarly, if the patient is warned that he will feel anxious upon being transferred out of the CCU, even when he is fully aware that the move is a sign of improvement, he will view his anxiety as legitimate, and its impact will be reduced.

Medication.   Assuming that all patients in the CCU are anxious, no matter how calm they appear, we routinely order an antianxiety agent on a regular, not on an as-needed (p.r.n.), basis. "As-needed" ordering should be avoided, because patients will seldom ask for a tranquilizer. If pain medication is on order, patients will choose it over an anxiolytic, even though their primary complaint is anxiety. To many patients, to request a tranquilizer is somehow to admit a weakness. Diazepam, 2 to 10 mg orally four times a day, or chlordiazepoxide, 5 to 25 mg orally four times a day, is the optimal range of doses of choice. We prefer the benzodiazepines to the more traditional phenobarbital, because they produce less mental confusion (less sedation) and interfere less with sodium warfarin (Coumadin). A hypnotic dose of the medication can be obtained by doubling the sedative dose at bedtime.

Although acute anxiety or panic spells are seldom seen in the CCU, they can easily be dealt with by increasing the dose of benzodiazepine (diazepam, 20 mg orally stat or 5 to 10 mg intravenously). As the patient regains his calm, a careful examination should be carried out to determine the source of fear, if possible. Proper reassurance cannot be given until the nature of this fear is learned. Should the panic attack herald an acute psychosis (agitation, delusions, hallucinations), haloperidol, 1 to 5 mg orally four times a day, is the treatment of choice. It is, of course, imperative to enlist psychiatric consultation whenever panic or psychosis occurs.

Treatment of *depression* in the CCU should be negotiated without medication. As discussed below, tricyclic antidepressants, monoamine oxidase inhibitors, and phenothiazines present risks when used in patients with cardiovascular disorders. It should be noted that the depression one encounters in the CCU is reactive in nature and is normal under the circumstances; however, if the physician feels that the depression is more serious than this, he should immediately request an examination by a psychiatric consultant.

TRANSFER FROM THE CORONARY CARE UNIT. The transition from CCU to the "stepdown unit" should be presented to the patient as a graduation exercise—tangible reassurance that progress has been made. Departing from the CCU, however, is not an unmixed blessing. The patient leaves the security provided by close nursing care, a doctor within calling distance, and in some instances, the "guardian angel" presence of the monitor. All these factors may contribute to the sense of vulnerability and the apprehension which occur at the time of transition from the CCU. The elevated levels of urinary catecholamines at this time[41] may reflect this increase in anxiety.

The increasing use of submaximal exercise electrocardiograms and [201]thallium perfusion scans prior to hospital discharge (p. 1293) provides reassurance to patients, since it demonstrates to them their capacity to perform physical activity. Frequently, it allows the physician to inform the patient that objective measurements (response of heart rate, blood pressure, electrocardiogram, and myocardial perfusion) indicate that physical activity is *not* harmful.

Convalescence

PROBLEMS OF CONVALESCENCE. Of the many thousands of patients who survive acute myocardial infarctions each year, many do not return to work because of psychological invalidism. More important than the income lost unnecessarily is the emotional suffering these patients experience. The extent of this suffering can be exemplified by a study of 24 patients interviewed between 3 and 9 months after their discharge from the hospital.[42] At this early point in their convalescence, 21 rated themselves as anxious or depressed; 18 were judged by the examiner to require either a tranquilizer or an antidepressant. Sleep disturbances occurred in 15 patients, and disruptive family quarrels over aspects of convalescence took place in 18 cases. These patients consistently tended to minimize symptoms during follow-up examinations, to retain harmful habits, and to avoid taking sedatives. Eleven patients did not return to work—nine for psychological reasons. Those who did resume part- or full-time employment experienced anxiety, augmentation of angina, or dyspnea.

Although there are many and diverse causes for distress in cardiac convalescence, a common denominator to all is *depression*. The post–myocardial infarction depression, as mentioned earlier, is a normal reaction to loss. Even in uncomplicated cases, the sense of loss is present, although in a symbolic rather than a real way. The individual who has sustained a myocardial infarction feels vulnerable. His immortality and sense of physical intactness have been challenged, and some refer to this vulnerability as "ego infarction."[43] When the myocardial infarction is complicated, and the individual is left with sequelae such as angina, congestive heart failure, or arrhythmias, depression and the feeling of hopelessness may be compounded. In general the depression tends to be self-limited and improves during the first month at home, beginning with the individual's realization that he is able to negotiate walks around the house and short flights of stairs and, sometimes even more importantly, to experience human contact without suffering undue strain. By the time sexual intercourse can be resumed, the patient is generally sound enough to commence work, at which point the road to normal functioning is more easily traversed.

The term "homecoming depression" has been used to describe the initial stages of the post–myocardial infarction depression,[42] typically manifest during the first week after the patient has returned home. It is heralded by the complaint of exertional weakness—a symptom which the patient considers to be a harbinger of cardiac decline. Even minimal activity such as a walk to the front door or a stroll in the garden may produce a disproportionate sense of weakness. Since the feeling of weakness does not relent with the passage of days, the patient may think that his heart is more damaged than he was led to believe, and this symptom becomes the nucleus around which other depressive symptoms collect. A pervasive sense of gloom and hopelessness is accompanied by an inability to control tearfulness. A change in sleeping pattern—one of the most sensitive indicators of depression—is present, as well as anorexia or hyperphagia, irritability, withdrawal, anhedonia (loss of pleasure in acts that normally give pleasure), and loss of a sense of humor. A basic sense of anxiety accompanies the depression, and although the individual may not be oppressed by a sense of impending death, the thought of his own demise hovers in the back of his mind. Once the full-blown picture sets in, the depression is often recognized by the spouse, through whom it may be relayed to the physician.

Myths about myocardial infarction abound, reinforcing the victim's fears. Many patients are embarrassed to ask about them. Some common myths include the following: (1) The victim of myocardial infarction is "over the hill"; he not only has reached maturity but also has entered physical and psychological senium. (2) Excitement must be avoided; it is risky to watch exciting sporting events. (3) Arms must be kept below the head (said to apply to any activity from plastering a ceiling to raising one's hand to take an oath). (4) All isometric effort is contraindicated. (5) Driving a car is apt to produce angina or a recurrent myocardial infarct. (6) Sex is a thing of the past; death is apt to take place at the moment of orgasm. (7) Deep sleep is dangerous; hypnotics should be avoided; sudden death is more apt to occur in sound than in light sleep. (8) Beware of anniversaries; there is a strong possibility of recurrence around the time of one's first infarction or around the anniversary of the death of a loved one from myocardial infarction. Some of these myths are based on fact; others are entirely fallacious. In either case, every effort should be made to anticipate these concerns and to counteract them.

MANAGEMENT ISSUES IN CONVALESCENCE

Patient Education. Education is a principal factor in the treatment of post–myocardial infarction depression. At the time of discharge the physician should confer with the patient and his or her spouse to outline the main problems of convalescence. The patient should be informed that weakness can be expected because of the time spent in bed. Bed rest can produce a weekly loss of strength of about 10 to 15 per cent secondary to muscle atrophy and a reduction in maximal oxygen uptake. The physician should also point out that depression following myocardial infarction is a normal response which usually disappears spontaneously within 2 or 3 months.

We have found that although coronary patients often know something about the cause of infarction (a "plugged vessel"), many have no conception of how it heals; some individuals even believe there is no healing, picturing the heart with a perpetual leak in the pumping system. During the discharge discussion the patient might be asked to draw a heart, illustrating his or her concept of infarction and of healing. This can serve as an embarkation point for a more detailed discussion of the mechanics of a heart attack and the nature of recovery.

Since there is a great deal of misunderstanding about the safety of sexual activity during convalescence, it should be pointed out to the patient that coital death is unusual. In the study by Ueno which is most often cited, coition accounted for 0.6 per cent of endogenous sudden deaths,[44] most of which occurred in the setting of extramarital intercourse. Males were an average of 13 years older than their companions, and one-third were inebriated at the time of intercourse. Hellerstein and Friedman have reported that the equivalent cost in oxygen of maximal activity during intercourse approximates 6 calories per minute.[45] During foreplay and afterplay about 4.5 calories per minute are consumed. According to these calculations the demand placed upon the heart by sexual intercourse is equal to that of a brisk walk around the block or of climbing one flight of stairs. Although Hellerstein and Friedman have been criticized for generalizing from too small and too unique a sample, their findings do offer an estimation of the energy levels involved in sexual activity.

Activity and Physical Conditioning (see also Chap. 40). Convalescents from a myocardial infarction usually state that inactivity is their greatest source of frustration. No sedentary pastime can diminish the boredom of idle days. Since physical activities require different levels of exertion, most questions posed by patients in the first 2 months of convalscence pertain to the cost of an activity in terms of cardiovascular strain. One of the best available systems for quantifying the energy spent in various activities and for translating it into understandable units for the patient is the metabolic equivalents system (METS).[46] The physician or a cardiac nurse should instruct the patient and spouse about the MET system and set up a program of graduated activity so that a goal can be set for each day. Activity, no matter how trivial it may seem, provides an excellent prophylaxis against depression. A physical conditioning program gives the patient a sense of participating in his recovery rather than of being the passive recipient of care. Confidence in his performance is restored as the patient watches his potential to perform various activities expand.[47]

Group Activities. It has been reported that group meetings of post–myocardial infarction patients may be helpful during convalescence.[48] The purpose here is educational rather than psychotherapeutic; the meetings take place regularly every week for 12 weeks and are conducted by a professional (a physician or nurse clinician) with the goal of exchanging information and sharing experiences. Although their value remains to be rigorously demonstrated, these groups are enthusiastically endorsed by the individuals who participate in them.

Medication. The use of antianxiety agents such as the benzodiazepines can be helpful during convalescence of cardiac patients. It should be emphasized to the patient that his state of mind as well as his physical health contributes to his rehabilitation and that tranquilizers are an cumstances, such as driving in traffic, anxious feelings are bound to emerge. Until the patient has developed his own method of coping with nervousness, anxiolytics are a helpful adjunct. The dosage is the same as that used in the CCU (p. 1830). (Antidepressants will be discussed later in this chapter.)

Telephone Follow-up. A nurse clinician can be available for a specific period of time during the day to receive telephone calls from patients or she can make weekly follow-up calls to the patient and spouse to provide information about diet, sexual problems, permissible activity, and the like.

Relaxation Techniques and Autohypnosis. Relaxation techniques are increasingly advocated and are probably helpful. Publications describing the relaxation response are available, and the technique can easily be learned by the patient.[49] Autohypnosis is a potent tool for the promotion of relaxation in receptive subjects. However, both relaxation and hypnosis tend to be more attractive to those self-reliant individuals who are also most apt to participate in physical conditioning therapy programs.

Psychotherapy. Since the post–myocardial infarction depression is essentially self-limited, psychotherapy is necessary only for those who fail to improve after 2 to 3 months. Patients who complain of a persistent loss of libido, impotence, anorexia, and disturbed sleep or those who develop hypochondriacal complaints can frequently benefit from psychotherapy.

CARDIAC SURGERY AND POSTOPERATIVE DELIRIUM

Along with its many benefits, open-heart surgery also presents the problem of postoperative delirium. For this reason recent psychiatric studies have focused more attention on the postcardiotomy patient than on all other surgical patients combined.

THE COURSE AND NATURE OF POSTCARDIOTOMY DELIRIUM. Delirium is defined as a clouding of consciousness accompanied by hyperalertness or agitation. Its hallmark is disorientation in time, place, or person. Perceptual distortions in the form of illusions, delusions, or hallucinations may also be present, accounting for the use of the term postoperative "psychosis." The true incidence of postoperative delirium is difficult to determine because the criteria for recognition vary so widely. It has been reported to range from 13 to 100 per cent, depending upon how the investigator defines the condition.[50,51]

The typical post-cardiotomy delirium begins after a clear period of 1 to 2 days following surgery. When this "civil interval" ends, the patient becomes confused and then delirious. In this state he may remove intravenous catheters, attempt to leave the unit, and behave in a generally disruptive and potentially dangerous way. The delirium usually subsides within 3 days and is seldom seen after transfer from the recovery room.[52]

PSYCHOSOCIAL INFLUENCES ON POSTOPERATIVE DELIRIUM. In an effort to devise strategies to prevent postoperative delirium, predisposing factors have been examined. Age was found to be one such factor—the older the patient, the more apt he is to become delirious. A past history of postoperative delirium also increases the likelihood of recurrence. A history of schizophrenia or major affective disease does not predispose a patient to delirium following surgery, but a current psychiatric problem or a past history of addiction to alcohol or drugs does increase the risk. Evidence of cortical impairment, as disclosed by a neurological examination or psychological testing can also predispose an individual to delirium.[53]

POSSIBLE CAUSES OF POSTOPERATIVE DELIRIUM. Various types of cardiac surgery present different risks. For example, in one study, the incidence of delirium was 36 per cent following multiple valve replacement, 35 per cent following aortic valve replacement, 22 per cent following mitral valve replacement, 9 per cent following mitral commissurotomy, and 8 per cent following repair of a congenital defect.[52] For those diseases classified by the New York Heart Association Functional and Therapeutic Indices, there is a significant relationship between the extent of illness and the development of delirium.[52] Abram states that the high incidence of delirium is attributed to a number of factors about which few investigators agree.[54] Some cite the length of time on cardiopulmonary bypass as a principal risk factor; others claim that the monotony of the surgical intensive care unit results in sensory deprivation which may produce delirium; sleep deprivation and abnormal sensory input have been implicated by others. As the data accumulate, the etiological significance of organic factors increases. Delirium is evidently only one manifestation of a more general neurological impairment, such as an acute but transient organic brain syndrome.

According to Heller and his colleagues, both the incidence and the severity of delirium following cardiac procedures appear to be declining.[52] Of a number of possible reasons, the most important is a reduction in the time the patient must spend undergoing cardiopulmonary bypass. Also, the attention most surgical services now give to preoperative educational programs is of considerable importance. Usually staffed by nurses, their teaching efforts inform the patient about what can be expected from surgery.

Preoperative depression does not bode well for the postoperative course. Individuals who view their future without hope or who actively wish to die may indirectly contribute to their own mortality.[29] The highest incidence of postoperative mortality and morbidity occurs in patients who are depressed *before* the operation or who deny anxiety even though they are obviously apprehensive.[55,56]

MEASURES TO REDUCE THE INCIDENCE AND/OR SEVERITY OF POSTOPERATIVE DELIRIUM. Several prophylactic measures can reduce the incidence and/or severity of postoperative delirium:

1. Get to know the patient and instill a sense of trust in the doctor-patient relationship.

2. Educate the patient with regard to short-term discomforts in the surgical intensive care unit and clarify misconceptions about the ultimate course of the illness.

3. Arrange a preoperative visit to the surgical intensive care unit to familiarize the patient with the environment and the staff.

4. Forewarn the patient that he will feel strange at some point in the unit and that delirium might develop—a delirium which would be both normal and transient, not insanity.

5. Arrange a prompt postoperative visit by the individual responsible for preoperative educational programs to discuss possible problems.

6. Instruct the family about the value of frequent visits in providing round-the-clock orientation.

7. Provide sedation if necessary; haloperidol (1 to 3 mg two or three times a day) is the preferred agent, with a low incidence of cardiovascular effects, few interactions with cardiovascular drugs, and little or no autonomic receptor blockade.

EMOTIONS AND CARDIAC DYSFUNCTION

Emotions are experienced both psychologically and physiologically. Although the variety of cognitive representations of feelings is extensive (anger, fear, anxiety, joy), the body's repertory of autonomic responses is more limited. Emotional arousal, through centrally triggered sympathetic discharge, is manifest in the cardiovascular system in much the same way as physical stress or exercise: tachycardia, elevated blood pressure, increased oxygen consumption, changes in cardiac output and peripheral resistance, increased muscle blood flow, and decreased renal and splanchnic blood flow.[57] The cardiovascular consequences of emotion, as distinct from those of exercise, may be more deleterious because of the absence of associated muscular activity.

The sympathetically mediated release of epinephrine and norepinephrine has predictable effects on the myocardium, increasing oxygen demand as well as myocardial irritability. Just as physical exertion can represent a significant threat to the patient with diminished myocardial or coronary vascular reserve, emotional stress can intensify heart failure or ischemia by augmenting cardiac demands.[58–60] As Chambers and Reiser and others have described, emotional stress and traumatic life events very often precede cardiac decompensation and congestive heart failure.[58,60]

Emotional stress and anxiety have been associated with a variety of *arrhythmias*,[61] most importantly premature ventricular contractions, ventricular tachycardia, and ventricular fibrillation.[57,62] Although the risk of serious arrhythmia is greatest for the diseased or ischemic myocardium, psychophysiological arrhythmias have been observed in individuals with no apparent heart disease but with manifest emotional stress. Reich and coworkers reported that 25 of 117 patients with life-threatening ventricular arrhythmias lacked evidence of an acute myocardial infarction but had experienced acute emotional distress as an apparent precipitant.[63] This subject is discussed in detail in Chapter 23.

Using ambulatory electrocardiographic monitoring, Taggart and colleagues recorded the electrocardiograms of 32 normal individuals and 24 patients with coronary artery disease while they drove in busy city traffic.[64] Both groups showed increased heart rates, sometimes exceeding 140 beats per minute. ST-segment changes not related to tachycardia developed in 3 of 32 drivers. In 13 of those with coronary artery disease, the ST-segment and T-wave abnormalities increased. Five developed multiple ventricular ectopic beats. In another study, 23 normal subjects, most of whom were physicians speaking at medical meetings, and a second group of 7 speakers with coronary artery disease were monitored.[65] Heart rates of up to 180 beats/min, as well as elevations of plasma catecholamine and free fatty acid concentration were observed in both groups. Ischemic ST-segment depression occurred in six of the seven coronary subjects. More than six ectopic beats per minute were recorded in six of the normal subjects while they were speaking. Five of the seven coronary subjects had multiple or multifocal ventricular ectopic beats. A beta-blocking agent suppressed the tachycardia and electrocardiographic changes in both groups. Lown and colleagues studied a man with normal coronary arteries and cardiac function in whom ventricular fibrillation and cardiac arrest and, following recovery, ventricular premature beats were provoked by psychophysiological stress.[62] Beta blockade and other measures to reduce sympathetic activity attenuated the arrhythmia.

Despite the apparent importance of peripheral sympathetic activity in emotionally induced arrhythmia, Lown and coworkers have reported data implicating central neural mechanisms as primary in triggering, via sympathetic efferents, the aberrant electrical activity.[66] In animals, hypothalamic and stellate ganglion stimulation has produced ventricular fibrillation that was abolished with beta-adrenergic blockade.[67] In the presence of an electrically unstable heart, a diseased myocardium, or coronary artery disease, psychological distress is a potentially lethal stimulus.

In addition to the sympathetically mediated ventricular irritability and increased oxygen demand, life-threatening "vagal reaction" leading to bradycardia and circulatory collapse has been reported.[68] The parasympathetic or vagal response to emotional stimuli producing decreased heart rate, fall in arterial pressure, and syncope in some individuals is a familiar syndrome, although not in itself as a cause of sudden death.

Although a major stressful life event, such as hearing of a loved one's demise, could be the proximal "cause" of death, more often the terminal stress is not in itself extraordinary; rather, as reported by Greene and coworkers, the scenario in the weeks preceding the final stressful event is one of increased emotionally vulnerability, often following a series of losses, with chronic depression, fatigue, frustration, or disappointment.[19] This observation is reminiscent of other theories of the emotional vulnerability to serious illness resulting from feelings of hopelessness and the "giving-up–given-up" response.[69] For example, a patient with a perceived loss in professional or job status, possibly having had a prior myocardial infarction, feeling sad and discouraged, becomes angry or anxious while performing an ordinary stressful task, such as income tax preparation, triggering a fatal arrhythmia. The notion that preceding stressful life events, whether losses or positive life changes, lays the physiological foundation for sudden death is supported by Rahe's data measuring accumulated life change units (Table 57–2).[70]

One implication of the foregoing for the clinical management of the cardiac patient is the necessity to be alert for signs of depression and fatigue, for reports of recent major life events, and for indications of anxiety-provoking circumstances in the patient's life. In addition, the physician can counsel the patient to avoid stressful settings when possible and encourage conscious control over emotional arousal ("Is this worth dying for?") when necessary. Other

TABLE 57–2   LIFE CHANGE EVENTS IN MEN AND THEIR WEIGHTS IN LIFE CHANGE UNITS (LCU) SCALED FOR FINLAND

EVENT	FINNISH LCU WEIGHT
Health	
Recent illness (in bed for a week or hospitalization)	62
Change in heavy physical work or exercise	19
Change in sleeping habits	15
Change in eating habits	11
Work	
Recently out of work	50
Recently fired from work	50
Retirement from farming, forestry, or industry	40
Change to new type of work	36
Change in work responsibilities	29
Troubles with boss	22
Work or life going well (awards, achievements, etc.)	20
Correspondence courses (home study)	17
Change in hours of work a day	13
Home and Family	
Concern over health of family member	54
Recently married	50
Separation from wife due to marital problems	48
Gaining a new family member (in the home)	39
Separation from wife due to work	34
Engaged to be married	32
New home improvements	26
Son or daughter leaving home	23
Wife began or ended work	23
Troubles with in-laws	22
Change in get-togethers with friends	21
Change to a new residence	15
Change in get-togethers with relatives	13
Vacation	11
Personal and Social	
Death of wife	105
Divorce	80
Held in jail	64
Sexual difficulties	41
Change in number of arguments with wife	40
Death of a close relative	39
Financial difficulties	38
Major decisions regarding the future	38
Death of a close friend	34
Unpaid bills leading to threatened legal action	26
Recent purchases worth more than 8000 Fmk ($2000)	22
Change in religious or political convictions	20
Change in personal habits	12
Recent purchases worth less than 8000 Fmk	11
Minor violations of the law	7

Rahe, R. H., et al.: Subjects' recent life changes and coronary heart disease in Finland. Am. J. Psychiatry *130*:1223, 1973.

strategies to diminish the impact of emotional stress include relaxation training, anxiolytics (e.g., the benzodiazepines) in small doses as needed, and in the absence of contraindications, administration of beta-adrenergic blocking drugs. The cardiac patient who manifests sustained depression should be referred for psychiatric consultation as a prophylactic and therapeutic measure.

PSYCHIATRIC ISSUES IN HYPERTENSION

EMOTIONAL FACTORS IN ESSENTIAL HYPERTENSION.   Though definitive study of the causes of hypertension remains to be done, reports so far indicate associations between elevated arterial pressure and a variety of environmental and psychological conditions. Environmental factors, including diet (salt), social conditions, life changes, psychological conflicts, and psychophysiological mechanisms, have been estimated as contributing substantially to the etiology of essential hypertension.[71] These factors are also discussed in Chapter 26.

SOCIOCULTURAL FACTORS. Henry and Cassel observed that blood pressure levels were lower in groups or societies based on firm traditions and stable social structures.[72] In societies in which traditions were disintegrating or in those in transition, arterial pressures for the populations rose (e.g., southern Black society in the late 1950's). Blood pressure has been reported as higher in city than in rural dwellers.[73] Harburg et al. described one city in which citizens in the higher crime and lower socioeconomic district had significantly elevated levels of blood pressure,[74] apparently confirming earlier cross-cultural observations that hypertension was more prevalent in societies dominated by social stress and conflict.[75]

In the most intriguing animal study of social factors involved in elevated arterial pressure, Henry et al. manipulated social interactions of mice by crowding them into small boxes, building a system of tunnel-connected cages that forced frequent confrontations, exposing the mice to a cat for 6 to 12 months, and introducing isolation-reared mice into the regular population. The resultant territorial conflict and concomitant constant defensive vigilance resulted in relatively sustained increases in blood pressure.[76]

PSYCHOLOGICAL FACTORS. Life changes and traumatic life events have been associated with the onset of sustained hypertension[77] and with the shift from the benign to the malignant form of the disease.[78] In addition, specific personality traits have been implicated as contributory to essential hypertension. Despite the subjective and anecdotal nature of descriptions of hypertensive individuals, the following characteristics are consistently noted: The hypertensive person manifests a desire to please, a wish to be liked; however, while outwardly calm, the internal stance is that of suppressed anger, tension, and suspicion.[79–81] Presumably these traits derive from early experience with individuals (parents) on whom the person depended and toward whom anger and hostility could not be expressed, because of the real or imagined threat of loss of love. The desire to please and be approved of by authority figures, combined with a rebellious "ready-to-fight" unconscious posture, was felt to be characteristic of many individuals with essential hypertension.

Wolf and Wolff found that in subjects with restrained hostility or anxiety, peripheral vascular resistance rises without change in cardiac output.[82] These individuals were thought to be blood pressure "responders," especially in situations that triggered repressed hostile feelings. Hypertension, therefore, had an adaptive quality, in that a rise in blood pressure could be seen as a preparation to deal with a threat. Alexander, describing the conflict between aggressive feelings and dependence on the object of the aggression, viewed sustained hypertension as a permanent "emergency state," emotionally triggered and physically expressed.[79] Several studies have demonstrated increases in diastolic pressure with inhibited anger[83,84] or with deferential behavior.[85]

Most data indicate that certain traits may be associated with hypertension, but their role in etiology is unclear; certainly many individuals with similar characteristics never become hypertensive. Ostfeld and Lebovitz[86] failed to show personality differences between renovascular and essential hypertensives and have criticized the "specific conflict" notion of a hypertensive personality.[87] Another difficulty with studies of psychological aspects of hypertension is their failure to differentiate labile from sustained hypertensives. The labile group may experience transient rises in stressful situations (e.g., blood pressure–taking by a physician) but are normotensive in other settings. As a result, repeated readings of blood pressure are necessary for the diagnosis of essential hypertension.

PSYCHOPHYSIOLOGICAL FACTORS. Many environmental and psychological factors can cause acute elevations of baseline blood pressure in both normotensive and hypertensive individuals. It is normal for arterial pressure to fluctuate during the course of a day[88]; however, elevated blood pressure is more prevalent, for example, in generally stressful occupations such as air traffic controllers.[89] The common denominator in cases of hypertension may be "stress" in a nonspecific sense, since stressful events (often idiosyncratic in impact, such as life trauma, social and interpersonal conflicts, and unacknowledged and unexpressed emotion) generate sympathetically mediated vasoconstriction and other autonomic responses that may well have a greater and more sustained impact on blood pressure in individuals predisposed to hypertension. Brod and colleagues have found that the vasoconstrictive response to stress is more prolonged in hypertensive than in normotensive subjects.[90,91] Lacy's notion of an "autonomic response specificity" suggests that constitutionally predisposed individuals respond to specific and general stress with acute and sustained elevations of arterial pressure.[92] The finding that normotensive sons of essential hypertensives react more readily to stress with elevations of blood pressure is of interest in this regard.[93]

Cardiovascular reaction patterns to stress vary in animals and humans, but operant conditioning studies have demonstrated that animals can be conditioned to experience blood pressure elevations in response to specific and general stimuli.[94] For humans as well, Shapiro et al. have reported that subjects in the laboratory could learn to elevate their blood pressure without changes in heart rate.[95]

BEHAVIORAL THERAPY. Since psychophysiological data implicate stress, autonomic arousal, and conditioned learning as causes of blood pressure elevation, various types of behavioral therapy—relaxation, meditation, and biofeedback—have been applied to hypertensives.[96–98] Although it would be of great benefit if these nonpharmacological treatments were effective, especially for the borderline hypertensive, clinical studies suggest only a minor role for behavioral regimens at this time. However, the fact that these treatments are without risk and are associated with an increased sense of well-being renders them appropriate adjunctive modalities despite the modest claims of the data so far reported.

Benson has hypothesized that a variety of techniques, including relaxation exercises, meditation, yoga, and hypnosis, have the ability to evoke an integrated hypothalamic "relaxation response" that results in reduced heart rate, blood pressure, and respiratory rate as well as the subjective feeling of relaxation.[49] Shapiro et al. have noted that relaxation-induced blood pressure changes are small but statistically significant, ranging from 7/4 to 37/22 mm Hg; the higher the pretreatment pressure, the greater the decrease with relaxation. If subjects discontinued the regimen, values returned to baseline levels.[98] A fall in adrenergic activity, as reflected in lower dopamine beta-hydroxylase levels, in patients performing an Eastern meditation exercise has been reported.[99] One well-constructed series of studies, including some 12-month follow-ups, control groups, and cross-over treatment of controls, and based on a program of relaxation and galvanic skin response biofeedback, demonstrated an average decrease in blood pressure of 27/15 mm Hg and decreased requirements for medication.[100,101] Using an ambulatory monitoring device, one group has demonstrated sustained blood pressure decreases during the work day for essential hypertensives trained in relaxation.[102]

When an individual is made aware of changes in blood pressure by means of visual or auditory biofeedback, he becomes able, through unknown mechanisms, to use this sensory input to alter his own blood pressure. The results of blood pressure biofeedback also vary, ranging from virtually no change to sustained decreases of 18/8 mm Hg.[103]

PSYCHOTHERAPY. Before the era of antihypertensive medication, Reiser et al. reported decreased arterial pressure and symptomatic improvement in a group of 98 hypertensive patients receiving varying degrees of supportive psychotherapy.[77] This salutary effect of a constant, supportive relationship with the physician should not be discounted.

PATIENT COMPLIANCE WITH ANTIHYPERTENSIVE TREATMENT. Reviews of the issue of noncompliance underscore the significance, magnitude, and complexity of this problem.[104–107] Sackett has noted over 200 reported determinants of noncompliance, including educational, demographic, personality, and prescribing factors.[108] Patients with relatively high levels of physical complaints and those with attitudes of suspiciousness have a high incidence of poor compliance.[109] Surveys consistently estimate that 30 to 50 per cent of hypertensive patients neglect their treatment, even as public awareness of the dangers of "high blood pressure" increases.[106,109a] Physicians are generally unable to predict and recognize those who do not follow instructions[110] and too often attribute the cause of the problem to the patient's lack of responsibility.

Attempts to understand adherence to medical regimens using the sociobehavioral "health belief model" emphasize the patient's (1) estimate of personal vulnerability to and seriousness of the disease; (2) perception of the efficacy and feasibility of the treatment; and (3) internal and external motivations to treatment, such as the desire to relieve symptoms or to avoid the sick role (internal), or as a response to public health campaigns (external).[104] Although all these factors were deemed relevant when studied retrospectively, recent prospective work has confirmed only the "attitude toward the sick role" as predictive of compliance —those who perceive social and interpersonal consequences of illness as negative are likely to comply with treatment.[108]

Efforts to indict any one factor as the "cause" of noncompliance will be inadequate given the individual variability of patients' personalities and manners of coping with adversity. Some patients do not follow directions because of lack of concern or low anxiety levels, whereas others manifest a denial and rationalization response because of high levels of anxiety. Engendering increased concern is to no avail in the latter type of patient. A sufficiently independent patient will appreciate the opportunity to monitor his own blood pressure and be "responsible" for his treatment, whereas dependent patients will require more nurturing and didactic care and frequent follow-up visits.

The following factors are generally acknowledged as useful in maintaining patient compliance with treatment programs:

1. Creating a doctor-patient relationship characterized by mutual trust and a sense of alliance or working together to solve the problem.[109a,111]

2. Providing sufficient time with a care-giver (whether physician, physician's assistant, or nurse clinician).[112,113]

3. Prescribing an effective yet simple treatment regimen and making sure the patient understands the regimen before he leaves the office or clinic.[106]

4. Adapting dosage schedules to the patient's daily routine or habits.[114]

5. Educating and enlisting the help of family members, especially spouses (who may also deny the importance of treatment).

6. Anticipating with the patient possible side effects of medications and how these will be handled.

7. Offering assistance on follow-up visits to the patient who has had difficulty adhering to the treatment program.

8. Monitoring compliance (e.g., pill counts) and attempting to adapt the interpersonal approach to the noncompliant patient's needs and fears.

PSYCHIATRIC COMPLICATIONS OF ANTIHYPERTENSIVE MEDICATIONS (see also Chap. 27). Medications used to treat hypertension have neuropsychiatric effects, primarily depression. Rauwolfia alkaloids such as reserpine, which deplete central intraneuronal stores of catecholamines, can result in severe depressive illness that may endure well beyond withdrawal from the medication.[115] These agents are rarely used at present, but when the physician does wish to prescribe one of them, patients having suffered prior depressions should be screened, because of their increased vulnerability to this drug-induced affective illness. Alpha-methyldopa has also been associated with depression and other psychiatric symptoms (lethargy, insomnia, decreased mental acuity)[116–118] as well as confusional states in conjunction with haloperidol[119] and lithium.[120] Patients on alpha-methyldopa are at greater risk for lithium toxicity. Those taking propranolol may experience increased lethargy, mental slowing, and occasionally clinical depression. Hydralazine also induces lethargy and drowsiness. Drugs that cause impotence such as guanethidine or alpha-methyldopa may secondarily precipitate depression in the emotionally vulnerable patient. Diuretics are associated with mental changes, primarily as the result of electrolyte disturbances.

A variety of interactions with psychotropic medication may occur with antihypertensive agents.[121] The antipsychotics potentiate the hypotensive effects of reserpine, alpha-methyldopa, hydralazine, and propranolol, and, except for molindone, antagonize guanethidine.

The tricyclic antidepressants generally interfere with drugs that require uptake into adrenergic nerve terminals, blocking the action, for example, of guanethidine with the possibility of causing severe withdrawal hypotension and impeding the efficacy of clonidine.[123] These antidepressants may also interact centrally with alpha-methyldopa, reserpine, and propranolol, resulting in diminished blood pressure control.[124] The newer agent, mianserin, is reported at this early date to be free of the above interactions.[125] Initially, the tricyclics may cause hypertension when reserpine is administered. The monoamine oxidase inhibitors increase the hypotensive effects of diuretics and hydralazine but can lead to acute hypertension when administered with guanethidine, alpha-methyldopa, or reserpine.

For patients taking lithium and such diuretics as the thiazides, which act on the distal tubule, sodium loss in the distal tubule results in the reabsorption of lithium proximally and hence in elevated lithium levels.[126] Higher blood lithium levels increase the risk of side effects and toxicity. When such a combination is necessary, lithium dosages must be lowered and levels must be monitored. In addition, increased vigilance must be kept concerning other potential causes of additional sodium loss, such as sweating or diarrhea.

PSYCHOPATHOLOGY AND CARDIAC SYMPTOMS

Patients with any of a number of psychiatric disorders may attribute their distress to alterations of body function and may seek treatment from the nonpsychiatric physician; furthermore, objective physical symptoms may derive from specific functional conditions, as in the case of bursts of tachycardia from attacks of panic or anxiety. Estimates of the prevalence in cardiological practices of patients with anxiety-derived complaints range from 10 to 14 per cent.[127] The heart is a frequent focus of emotionally based complaints, not only because of its actual response to psychological stress but also because of its psychological and symbolic importance. Recognition of the psychiatric component of patients' complaints is a crucial task for the physician. The anxious and depressed patient suffers no less than the patient with a primary physical illness, and many of the psychiatric conditions underlying the distress can respond dramatically to prompt treatment; for others, proper management can greatly improve the quality of life. Finally, diagnosis of relevant psychological factors may obviate medical or surgical interventions and their attendant morbidity.

Anxiety Disorders

Anxiety may be defined as a psychological and physiological response similar to fear but in response to internal stimuli or inappropriate to the reality of external stimuli; it may be a life-long constant *trait* or a transient *state* relative to specific life events. The psychological component of the anxiety experience includes such descriptors as dread, edginess, nervousness, tension, or worry. Among the physical signs and symptoms, generally consequent to sympathetic arousal, are chest pain or tightness, diaphoresis, dyspnea, faintness, fatigue, flushing, muscle tension, palpitations, queasy stomach, tachycardia, tachypnea, and tremulousness.

Although the experience of anxiety is universal, pathological anxiety—an anxiety disorder capable of significantly impairing or restricting the life of a patient—is estimated to afflict between 2 and 4 per cent of the general population.[128] Anxiety symptoms are a particularly prominent component of phobic disorders such as agoraphobia (fear of being alone or in public), social phobia (fear of scrutiny by others), and simple phobias (e.g., insects, elevators), as well as post-traumat-

ic stress disorder (e.g., following military combat) and obsessive-compulsive disorder. For patients seeking treatment from the nonpsychiatric physician, the more common syndromes encountered, however, are generalized anxiety disorder and panic disorder.

Generalized Anxiety Disorder.   The patient with generalized anxiety manifests such persistent anxiety symptoms as ubiquitous uneasiness, moist palms, a worried look, and difficulty in falling asleep. Although often chronic or life-long, the signs of motor tension, autonomic hyperactivity, and apprehension may emerge only during discrete periods or be of clinical significance only during times of relative exacerbation. The variety of bodily symptoms, particularly in the cardiovascular system, lead many sufferers to seek a primary medical cause.

Panic Disorder.   Patients with panic disorder experience recurrent panic (anxiety) attacks—the sudden, often spontaneous onset of massive autonomic, particularly sympathetic, arousal accompanied by a feeling of terror or impending doom. Although the predominant symptom may vary, the usual bodily response to panic includes symptoms suggestive of heart disease, such as dyspnea, hyperventilation, chest pain, tachycardia, palpitations, tremulousness, dizziness, faintness, hot and cold flashes, and diaphoresis. The typical behavioral response is to flee home or to a safe or familiar place.

Patients having panic attacks have little if any conscious control over the experience. Those unfamiliar with the syndrome believe they are stricken with a myocardial infarction, stroke, or other life-threatening condition. For patients with ischemic heart disease or myocardial electrical instability, the sympathetic arousal is indeed life-threatening. In addition to the exceptional distress of the condition, untreated panic disorder often leads to agoraphobia. After a period of avoiding places with restricted escape (in the event of an attack), such as public transportation, tunnels, traffic congestion, and crowded stores, sufferers may become homebound. A secondary generalized or anticipatory anxiety may follow the onset of panic attacks, and depressive signs and symptoms also can occur.

Panic disorder occurs twice as frequently in women as men,[129] often has its onset in early adulthood, is more common in family members of patients with the disorder,[129] and is associated with an excess mortality,[130] particularly in men. As with affective illness, the disorder may be recurrent or chronic, mild or severe.

Early attempts to elucidate the physiology of panic attacks have drawn on the work of Pitts and McClure,[131,132] who, by infusing intravenous sodium lactate, provoked attacks in those with the disorder, and on the report by Frohlich[133] of patients with hyperdynamic beta-adrenergic circulatory state who experienced dramatic emotional responses to isoproterenol. A more recent hypothesis based on neurophysiological studies and effects of psychotropic drugs implicates a central site, possibly the locus ceruleus,[134] as the "trigger" mechanism generating sympathetic arousal peripherally and a cortical response of terror or need to flee.

Differential Diagnosis of Anxiety Disorders.   Patients with anxiety disorders account for a significant percentage of general medical and cardiological practices.[127] The list of possible medical illnesses producing symptoms mimicking anxiety or panic is extensive. Any condition that leads to sympathetic discharge or causes such symptoms as tremors, dizziness, respiratory distress, tachycardia, or restlessness may resemble an anxiety state.

A thorough yet efficient medical evaluation includes the following considerations.[135] In a patient with a known medical illness, that ailment (including its possible symptoms, complications, and treatment) should be suspect. For the apparently well patient, beyond a general review of symptoms and physical examination, particular scrutiny should be directed at conditions commonly associated with anxiety: arrhythmias, excessive ingestion of caffeine or other stimulants, drug or alcohol withdrawal, thyroid abnormalities (especially hyperthyroidism), and hypoglycemia. Additional evaluation directed toward the patient's "somatic locus"[136] of anxiety—the system most prominently affected (e.g., cardiovascular, respiratory, gastrointestinal)—affords the greatest yield from investigations.

The mitral valve prolapse syndrome (p. 1089) appears to be approximately twice as prevalent in patients with panic disorder compared with the normal population.[129,137] Whether this association represents a cause and effect relationship is unclear, since patients with prolapse of the mitral valve and panic disorder cannot be distinguished from those with panic disorder alone by family history studies,[129] response to lactate infusion,[138] or efficacy of psychotropic drug treatment.[138] On the other hand, patients with prolapse of the mitral valve alone are significantly affected, with increased arrhythmias, by psychological stress and anxiety.[139]

TREATMENT. For patients with emergence of anxiety symptoms during or following a life crisis, explanation and reassurance of their physical well-being and a sympathetic attitude are important, with referral for supportive or brief psychotherapeutic intervention when necessary. Generalized anxiety symptoms abate and become more tolerable with the use of anxiolytics, preferably the benzodiazepines, since others such as barbiturates are more sedative, more lethal in overdose, and more physically addicting. The dose should be titrated to help the patient to manage, not eliminate, his symptoms and should be administered on an as-needed basis with daily limits. Some evidence indicates that patients with more prominent "somatic" or bodily symptoms from anxiety do well with varying doses of a beta-adrenergic blocker.[140] Relaxation training is helpful for many anxious patients. Psychodynamic and behavioral therapy offers relief for patients with specific conflicts associated with their symptoms.

Panic attacks are only partially attenuated by anxiolytics, but these agents often will not prevent attacks. Certain antidepressants, however, especially the tricyclic imipramine and the monoamine oxidase inhibitor phenelzine, usually at full antidepressant dosages, are frequently successful in abolishing anxiety attacks after 2 to 4 weeks of treatment.[141] A beta-adrenergic blocker may serve some patients as a second-line treatment of panic disorder.[140]

Depression

Sadness and grief, the normal human emotional responses to loss, are distinct from clinical depressive illness. Depression may be associated with an antecedent loss but constitutes a unique constellation of psychological and vegetative features. The cardiologist should be familiar with the presentation of depression, not only because it frequently coexists with chronic or serious illness but also because depressed patients, particularly older ones, experience an increase in physical symptoms which they attribute to bodily illness. A depressed patient, feeling fatigue or chest pain, not infrequently presents with cardiac complaints.

The following signs and symptoms are the most sensitive indicators of the presence of a clinical depressive illness: early morning awakening and disturbance of sleep continuity (or hypersomnia); tearfulness, sadness, or crying spells; loss of appetite and weight; loss of energy, ability to concentrate, and sexual interest; and loss of interest in usually pleasurable activities. Psychomotor retardation with prolonged response latency to questions and immobile or sad facies, may be observed in some, whereas a hand-wringing motor restlessness or agitation is prominent in others. The psychological state is one of despair, hopelessness, and helplessness, with marked loss of self-esteem and feelings of guilt and worthlessness.

TREATMENT. For patients suffering sadness or grief, the sense of personal injury and loss following the death of a loved one, job loss, or convalescence from myocardial infarction often will resolve with support, understanding, and time. Depressive illness, unlike grief, generally requires biological therapy. In most cases (80 to 90 per cent), depression will respond to antidepressant medication or, in severe or refractory cases, electroconvulsive therapy.[121]

Hypochondriasis

The cardiologist will most certainly be faced with the patient whose anxious overconcern extends to a morbid preoccupation with bodily functions and fear of illness. The hypochondriac often firmly believes that he is sick and that the physician has overlooked the urgency of his complaints, which may be monosymptomatic or may include multiple organ systems with minimal physical findings. Kenyon estimates that 85 per cent of cases of hypochondriasis are secondary to anxiety states, depressive illness, and other emotional disorders.[142] Reports of pain, the most frequent hypochondriacal symptom, may resolve if any underlying affective illness is treated. Cardiac symptoms often reflect an unrecognized anxiety disorder with tachycardia, palpitations, pain, and increased cardiac awareness.

Cardiac neurosis refers to hypochondriacal concern, usually in the setting of recovery from myocardial infarction or other cardiac illness, with obsessive focus on heart symptoms and exaggerated restriction of daily functioning. The syndrome may be iatrogenic, deriving from

incomplete explanation to the patient of his condition. Signs and symptoms of depressive illness should be reviewed, since cardiac neurosis may be a "depressive equivalent," that is, the somatic expression of an underlying change of mood. A treatable anxiety disorder, causing cardiac symptoms, may have been overlooked in the patient with a cardiac neurotic behavior pattern. When the patient's symptoms and disability are not secondary to misunderstanding, depression, or anxiety, the physician should seek to enhance the patient's ability to cope by *prescribing* graduated tasks or stepwise goals to achieve the appropriate level of activity.

Cardiac neurosis should not be taken lightly at its onset, since it may herald a chronic pattern of hypochondriacal behavior and unwarranted invalidism. The likelihood that the syndrome reflects a massive defensive effort to deal with underlying inadequacies emphasizes the value of early psychiatric referral.

A *conversion (hysterical) symptom* is an unexplained medical symptom involving motor function or sensation. This condition arises for a variety of psychological and interpersonal reasons which must be discovered on psychiatric examination. Prominent in medical and psychiatric lore is the concept of an anniversary reaction, the development of a conversion symptom (e.g., chest pain) at the same time of year as a prior traumatic event, such as death of a loved one from myocardial infarction.

CARDIOVASCULAR EFFECTS OF PSYCHOTROPIC AGENTS

Psychotropic medications, frequently administered to the elderly and those with or at risk for heart disease, have a significant impact on the cardiovascular system. Since untreated psychiatric illness carries its own morbidity and mortality and can also exacerbate cardiac illness (e.g., exhaustion from mania), the risks and benefits of medication must be carefully weighed. The following section describes the important cardiovascular effects of psychotropic drugs.

Antidepressants

In the late 1950's, the development of effective antidepressant pharmacotherapy heralded a significantly improved quality of life for those suffering from clinical depressive syndromes. The monoamine oxidase inhibitors (MAOI) and a few years later the tricyclic antidepressants (TCA) were the first consistently effective pharmacological interventions in the treatment of mood disorders. More recently, a number of agents with chemical structures distinct from TCA are being explored and introduced in hopes of achieving therapeutic benefits without such adverse effects as cardiotoxicity. Current hypotheses suggest that TCA and the newer antidepressants combat depression by increasing the activity of such central neurotransmitters as norepinephrine and serotonin either by blocking re-uptake from synaptic clefts or by binding to presynaptic (α_2) receptors.

TRICYCLIC ANTIDEPRESSANTS. Of significant benefit in 60 to 80 per cent of severe depressions,[121] TCA remain in wide use as acute and maintenance treatment for mood disorders. Their pharmacological effects are wide-ranging, acting on many systems in addition to the central nervous system. Their impact on the cardiovascular system has been viewed as a major limitation on the use of these medications, especially in patients with cardiac illness and depression.[143-145] For example, a higher than expected incidence of sudden death had been noted in patients with acute cardiovascular disorders who received these drugs, especially amitriptyline.[146-148] In clinical and laboratory studies, TCA have a variety of pharmacological actions beside their effect on catecholamine reabsorption by the adrenergic neuron. These include anticholinergic activity, quinidine-like effects (depressing conduction velocity and myocardial contractility) and alpha-adrenergic blocking properties, and it is clinically relevant that these actions vary among the TCA.

Electrocardiographic Changes. Electrocardiographic abnormalities with TCA include widened QRS complexes, increased P-R and Q-T intervals, ST-segment and T-wave changes, atrioventricular (Fig. 57–4) and intraventricular conduction defects, and tachycardia and bradycardia.[149–151] The most common changes at therapeutic doses (75 to 250 mg/day for imipramine) in healthy individuals are reversible T-wave changes and tachycardia. The latter occurred in 30 per cent of individuals on amitriptyline in one study.[152] Some increase in heart rate probably occurs and remains for the duration of treatment in every patient receiving these medications. At toxic levels, which can last for 3 to 4 days after overdose,[153] any and all types of arrhythmias may occur.[154] Although the reported frequency of serious TCA-induced electrocardiographic change varies with the population and the specific drug, for older patients with cardiac disease, in one report, the risk involved is up to 10 times greater than in young, healthy individuals.[147]

The pharmacological properties responsible for the electrocardiographic changes are principally anticholinergic effects and Type I antiarrhythmic activity (quinidine-like effects, p. 652). The former is probably the main direct factor in the drug-induced tachycardia. TCA have atropine-like effects that cause partial vagal blockade and tachycardia, of particular concern in patients with ischemic heart disease and congestive heart failure. Amitriptyline is the most anticholinergic TCA, followed in order by

doxepin, nortriptyline, imipramine, and desipramine,[155] the last being the TCA of choice in patients requiring a minimum of anticholinergic effects. In cases of TCA toxicity, temporary inprovement in tachycardia is attained with physostigmine,[156] the drug of choice to reverse the central nervous system "atropine psychosis."[157] Propranolol has also been suggested as useful in modifying TCA-induced tachycardia.[152]

TCA resemble quinidine in the capacity to delay cardiac conduction.[149,158,159] His bundle electrocardiography has demonstrated prolonged distal (H-V) conduction time for imipramine, nortriptyline, and amitriptyline.[160]

For the majority of patients at therapeutic, not toxic, doses and plasma levels of TCA, the quinidine-like side effects are of little clinical consequence. Bigger and colleagues have suggested that imipramine could actually be effective as an antiarrhythmic, like quinidine or procainamide, since it is a potent antiarrhythmic drug with a long duration of action and relatively few major adverse effects.[158,159,161,161a] Certainly, for patients on TCA, dosage levels of these antiarrhythmics should be lowered. For patients with preexisting conduction delay, institution of TCA treatment should be approached with caution, given the risk of increased or complete heart block and subsequent ventricular arrhythmia. Therefore, in patients over 40, a pretreatment electrocardiogram should be obtained with particular attention to the presence of intraventricular or atrioventricular block; on repeat study after treatment is initiated, one should be alert for a prolonged Q-T interval corrected for rate $(Q-T_c)$.[162] In the event of TCA overdose, cardiac arrhythmias should be managed in a manner similar to quinidine toxicity.

Doxepin has been touted as the TCA of choice for treatment of depression in patients with intraventricular or

FIGURE 57–4 *Top,* Concentration of imipramine and its psychoactive metabolite desmethylimipramine plotted against days after beginning drug administration during two separate treatment courses. Solid bars indicate the occurrence of 2:1 atrioventricular block. *Bottom,* Concentration of imipramine and desmethylimipramine plotted against hours after discontinuation of drug treatment. Solid bars indicate the period of continuous 2:1 atrioventricular block. Stippled bars indicate intermittent periods of 2:1 atrioventricular block. (From Kantor, S. J., et al.: Imipramine-induced heart block. J.A.M.A., *231*:1364, 1975. Copyright 1975, American Medical Association.)

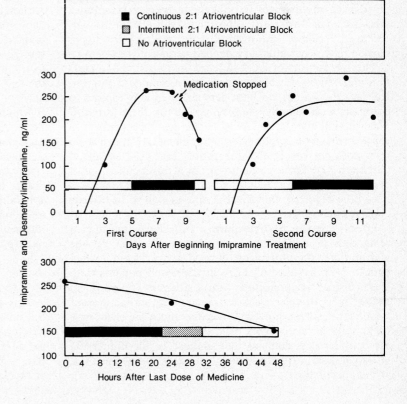

atrioventricular conduction disturbances. This claim is controversial, resting in part on poorly controlled data that may primarily reflect the propensity of doxepin to achieve lower plasma levels than other TCA at similar oral doses. Despite this and other evidence that doxepin does indeed have some impact on cardiac conduction,[163] a number of reports of a relative advantage lend support to the practice of selecting doxepin as the TCA of choice for these patients. The argument may become moot with the introduction of newer agents without these effects.

Despite the general safety of TCA for most patients, idiosyncratic vulnerability to serious (ventricular) arrhythmia may be encountered.[164] In patients receiving TCA (or other psychotropic drugs) who experience a life-threatening arrhythmia, administration of the suspected drug in the course of electrophysiological study may identify those in whom administration of the agent may be fatal or in whom it may be unrelated to the arrhythmia that was experienced.[165]

Effects on Blood Pressure. Postural hypotension is a common complication of TCA treatment.[152,166] Although the postural decrease in pressure does not differ significantly according to age, the experience of symptoms and such untoward consequences as fractures and lacerations from falling is greater among the elderly.[167,168] Although up to 20 per cent of patients on TCA may suffer postural hypotension, there is a markedly increased prevalence among those with left ventricular impairment or those on cardiovascular medication.[167]

For most patients who experience a postural change upon initiation of TCA treatment, the *symptoms* of orthostatic hypotension usually improve or disappear over days to weeks, despite persistence of a measurable postural drop in pressure.[168] The dosages at which orthostatic changes occur are usually well below therapeutic levels, and increasing doses to the therapeutic range (e.g., 100 to 200 mg/day of imipramine) is unlikely to worsen symptoms, whereas small downward adjustments will afford little advantage.[168] Some improvement in measurable hypotension may occur after an extended period of treatment.

The mechanism of TCA-induced hypotension is uncertain, but affinity for alpha-adrenergic receptors in the central nervous system has been demonstrated and appears to correlate with the hypotensive effects of these drugs.[169] Nortriptyline is the TCA with the least propensity to cause orthostatic hypotension, particularly if the plasma level does not exceed the therapeutic limit (150 ng/ml).[168] Although *hypertension* resulting from a therapeutic dose of TCA alone is a theoretical possibility, and a few cases have been reported, this effect is rare enough to be of little clinical significance.[152]

Effects on the Myocardium. TCA have long had a reputation of exerting a direct depressant effect on the myocardium, an impression derived largely from animal data.[144,152] In a study of TCA in depressed patients with heart disease, radionuclide ventriculograms revealed no change in ventricular ejection fraction with antidepressant treatment,[170] suggesting that a negative inotropic effect may occur only at toxic doses. The conclusions of this study are considered preliminary but underscore the impression of exaggerated early concerns about cardiotoxicity of TCA at therapeutic doses.

MONOAMINE OXIDASE INHIBITORS (MAOI). The renewed popularity of these medications, which block the oxidative deamination of norepinephrine, epinephrine, serotonin, and other amines by the enzyme monoamine oxidase, derives from their efficacy in treating panic disorder, atypical depressions, and some TCA-refractory depressed patients. A cardiovascular limitation to their use is their ability to cause severe orthostatic hypotension. Presumably, this is related to a "false neurotransmitter" effect, either from the drug itself or from the buildup of other nonvasoactive amines. Because of this property, pargyline has found a place in the treatment of hypertension.

The greatest risk of MAOI (e.g., phenelzine, tranylcypromine, and isocarboxazid), especially for cardiac patients, is the acute hypertensive crisis and the complications concomitant with ingestion of tyramine-containing foods and beverages or the administration of sympathomimetic medications. The failure of liver and intestinal MAO to deaminate tyramine in such foods as cheeses, red wine, yogurt, and chicken liver leads to a tyramine-induced release of adrenergic neurotransmitters. Arrhythmias may occur in addition to hypertension. These reactions, although rare, justify caution in prescribing MAOI to patients with serious cardiac disease. This is unfortunate, because they lack the anticholinergic and other cardiotoxic properties of TCA.[121]

Antihypertensive agents such as reserpine and guanethidine, which acutely release vasoactive amines, and alphamethyldopa, which is converted to sympathomimetic amines, should also be avoided by patients receiving MAOI. In the event of hypertensive crisis with MAOI, an alpha-adrenergic blocking drug, such as phentolamine, should be administered.

NEWER ANTIDEPRESSANTS. A number of new antidepressant compounds with a variety of chemical structures are available for clinical and experimental use. Although none are more effective than TCA in treating depression, their main attraction is the possibility of diminished side effects, particularly cardiotoxic ones. Although the claims of relative cardiac safety appear justified for many of these agents, they have not been subjected to the extensive clinical and laboratory scrutiny that the TCA have.

Maprotiline and amoxapine, for example, although heralded as producing low cardiotoxicity, have anticholinergic and other effects similar to those of TCA. Trazodone, however, is virtually devoid of anticholinergic properties but does pose some risk of postural hypotension. Other compounds without anticholinergic effects are zimelidine, fluvoxamine, and bupropion; those with minimal anticholinergic effects include nomifensine and mianserin. These agents appear to present a very low risk of cardiotoxicity.[171]

The Antipsychotics

This group of psychotropic agents includes the phenothiazines, thioxanthenes, butyrophenones, dibenzepins, and indolones. They are often dramatically effective in abating the severity of symptoms in psychotic episodes. Their action is presumed to be related to their common property of blocking central dopamine receptors.

With the widespread use of the phenothiazines have come reports of sudden death. Since some of the fatalities occurred in young and apparently healthy individuals, cardiovascular effects, especially arrhythmias, have been implicated.[150,172,173] Nearly all such reports were of patients taking either thioridazine or chlorpromazine. Other cardiovascular complications of the antipsychotics derive from central and peripheral alpha-blocking and anticholinergic effects, producing orthostatic hypotension and tachycardia.

Electrocardiographic Changes. The phenothiazines have been associated with a variety of electrocardiographic changes,[150,174] including prolongation of P-R and Q-T intervals, widened QRS complex, ST-segment depression, T-wave changes (usually blunting and widening), variable degrees of heart block, and serious ventricular arrhythmias.[150] The T-wave alterations, benign and reversible, are the most common ECG changes. Accentuated U waves occur with thioridazine. Electrocardiographic changes in general are associated with the phenothiazines of the aliphatic (chlorpromazine) and piperidine (thioridazine) types.

Alpha-adrenergic Blocking Effects. The antipsychotics, especially the aliphatic and piperidine phenothiazines, have both central and peripheral alpha-adrenergic blocking properties[175] in addition to their ability to block dopamine. This property correlates with the degree of hypotension and sedation associated with the specific agent and is of a greater degree than the mild alpha-blocking properties of the TCA but is minimal in the butyrophenone haloperidol. Severe hypotension, which occurs with an overdose, should not be treated with epinephrine or with agents having both alpha and beta effects, since increased hypotension can result; instead, alpha-adrenergic pressors such as norepinephrine should be employed.

Anticholinergic Activity. With the exception of thioridazine, the antipsychotics have less anticholinergic activity than TCA.[176] Nonetheless, they produce sufficient vagal blockade, especially in overdose, to be of clinical significance. This effect is often compounded by the administration of antiparkinsonian agents, such as benztropine or trihexyphenidyl, which also inhibit cholinergic activity.

Other Cardiovascular Effects. Quinidine-like activity has been reported for some of the phenothiazines.[150,174] A toxic cardiomyopathy has been associated with phenothiazine administration,[172,173] and congestive heart failure may be exacerbated by a negative inotropic effect. Changes in intracellular potassium ion concentration have been proposed to explain some phenothiazine-induced electrocardiographic changes.[174] Depression of autonomic midbrain centers and alterations in adrenal medulla secretion have also been implicated in phenothiazine-induced hypotension.[172]

Choice of Antipsychotic. The incidence of adverse cardiac effects of antipsychotics is increased in patients with cardiovascular disease, in the elderly, in higher doses, in synergy with other drugs (especially TCA), and with intramuscular administration. The nonphenothiazines such as haloperidol, molindone, loxapine, and thiothixene have not been shown to have cardiotoxic effects. The high-potency phenothiazines of the piperazine type (e.g., fluphenazine) induce minimal adverse cardiac reactions. Haloperidol, a very high-potency antipsychotic with low anticholinergic[176] and alpha-blocking properties,[169] is often the drug of choice for treating the psychotic or severely agitated cardiac patient; recent reports describe successful intravenous administration in life-threatening states of delirium.[177] Thioridazine, on the other hand, should be avoided in the treatment of cardiac patients.

Lithium

Lithium carbonate is valuable in the management of patients with mood disorders, especially manic-depressive illness. The major toxic effects are neurological and require frequent monitoring of plasma levels. Although prescribing information has generally implied that lithium is cardiotoxic, a variety of reports have indicated its relative cardiac safety.[178,179] The negative response to this drug derives in part from its unrestricted use as a salt substitute in the 1940's, with subsequent morbidity and mortality from lithium poisoning. Reported cardiovascular complications—hypotension, circulatory collapse, and arrhythmia—were agonal events in patients in prolonged coma.[180] In the majority of patients receiving lithium, the drug appears to cause minimal cardiotoxicity and is not associated with blood pressure changes. Congestive heart failure and myocarditis are rare. Instances of syncope secondary to sinus node dysfunction have been reported consequent to lithium treatment.[181]

Electrocardiographic Changes. T-wave changes, similar to those in hypokalemia and possibly related to displacement of intracellular potassium by lithium ions, occurs in virtually all patients treated with this drug.[182] Decreased amplitude, flattening, and even inversion of T waves are considered to be benign and reversible effects that generally do not constitute a reason to discontinue treatment. Individual case reports of arrhythmias, including conduction defects and increased frequency of extrasystoles, suggest that some patients may show idiosyncratic sensitivity to lithium.[178,183] Cases of disordered sinus node function in patients receiving lithium have also been registered.[178,184]

Toxic Effects. The primary concern for cardiac patients is the development of lithium toxicity—nausea, vomiting, diarrhea, ataxia, slurred speech, convulsions, coma, and death—resulting from failure to maintain adequate renal clearance. The patient with congestive heart failure is particularly vulnerable, because of decreased glomerular filtration rate, dietary restriction of sodium chloride, and use of diuretics. The thiazide diuretics elevate plasma lithium significantly and necessitate downward adjustment of daily doses and close monitoring of drug levels.[126] It is good practice to evaluate cardiac parameters carefully before and after initiating lithium treatment for patients with cardiac disease.[184]

Electroconvulsive Therapy (ECT)

Because it is the most consistently effective treatment for severe depression and does not have the cardiotoxic effects of TCA, electroconvulsive therapy has been advocated as the antidepressant therapy of choice for cardiac patients. It should be remembered, however, that ECT is not an entirely benign treatment. Enhanced sympathetic activity following induction of the seizure leads to brief periods of occasionally serious hypertension and arrhythmias.[185-187] Myocardial infarctions following ECT have been reported.[188] The type of barbiturate anesthesia used is also a factor in cardiac morbidity.[189] Careful monitoring and the use of a rapid-acting antihypertensive, such as nitroprusside, can help avert the complications of hypertension. Since the general mortality from ECT is quite low (0.2 to 0.3 per cent)[190] and since depression carries its own mortality, ECT should be considered in treating the severely depressed cardiac patient.

References

1. Harvey, W.: Exercitatio de motu cordis et sanguinis. Cited in Jenkins, C. D.: Behavioral risk factors in coronary artery disease. Ann. Rev. Med. 29:543, 1978.
2. Osler, W.: The Lumleian lectures on angina pectoris. Delivered before the Royal College of Physicians of London. Lancet 1:939, 1910.
3. Dunbar, F.: Psychosomatic Diagnosis. New York, Paul B. Hoeber, Inc., 1943, p. 309.
4. Friedman, M.: Pathogenesis of Coronary Artery Disease. New York, McGraw-Hill Book Co., 1969.
5. Rosenman, R. H., Brand, R. J., Jenkins, C. D., Friedman, M., Straus, R., and Wurm, M.: Coronary heart disease in the Western Collaborative Group Study: Final follow-up experience of 8½ years. J.A.M.A. 233:872, 1975.
6. Jenkins, C. D.: Recent evidence supporting psychologic and social risk factors for coronary disease. N. Engl. J. Med. 294:987, 1976.
7. Jenkins, C. D.: Behavioral risk factors in coronary artery disease. Ann. Rev. Med. 29:543, 1978.
8. Kenigsberg, D., Zyzanski, S. J., Jenkins, C. D., Wardwell, W. I., and Licciardello, A. T.: The coronary prone behavior pattern in hospitalized patients with and without coronary heart disease. Psychosom. Med. 36:344, 1974.
9. Review Panel on Coronary-Prone Behavior and Coronary Heart Disease: Coronary-prone behavior and coronary heart disease: A critical study. Circulation 63:1199, 1981.
10. Friedman, M., Thoresen, C. E., Gill, J. J., Ulmer, D., Thompson, L., Powell, L., Price, V., Elek, S. R., Rabin, D. D., Breall, W. S., Piaget, G., Dixon, T., Bourg, E., Levy, R. A., and Tasto, D. L.: Feasibility of altering Type A behavior pattern after myocardial infarction. Recurrent coronary prevention project study: Methods, baseline results and preliminary findings. Circulation 66:83, 1982.
11. Holmes, T. H., and Rahe, R. H.: The social readjustment rating scale. J. Psychosom. Res. 11:213, 1967.
12. Rahe, R. H., and Lind, E.: Psychosocial factors and sudden cardiac death: A pilot study. J. Psychosom. Res. 15:19, 1971.
13. Rahe, R. H., and Paasikivi, J.: Psychosocial factors and myocardial infarction: An outpatient study in Sweden. J. Psychosom. Res. 15:33, 1971.
14. Rahe, R. H., Bennett, L., Romo, M., Siltanen, P., and Arthur, R. J.: Subjects' recent life changes and coronary heart disease in Finland. Am. J. Psychiatr. 130:1222, 1973.
15. Rees, W. D., and Lutkins, S. G.: Mortality of bereavement. Br. Med. J. 4:13, 1967.
16. Parkes, C. M., Benjamin, B., and Fitzgerald, R. G.: Broken heart: A statistical study of increased mortality among widowers. Br. Med. J. 1:740, 1969.
17. Engel, G. L.: Sudden death and the medical model in psychiatry. Can. Psychiatr. Assoc. J. 15:527, 1970.
18. Engel, G. L.: Sudden and rapid death during psychological stress—folklore or folk wisdom? Ann. Intern. Med. 74:771, 1971.
19. Greene, W. A., Goldstein, S., and Moss, A. J.: Psychosocial aspects of sudden death—a preliminary report. Arch. Int. Med. 129:725, 1972.
20. Theorell, T., Lind, E., and Floderus, B.: The relationship of disturbing life changes and emotions to the early development of myocardial infarction and other serious illnesses. Int. J. Epidemiol. 4:281, 1975.
21. Wolf, S.: The end of the rope: The role of the brain in cardiac death. Can. Med. Assoc. J. 97:1022, 1967.
22. Bruhn, J. G., Paredes, A., Adsett, C. A., and Wolf, S.: Psychological predictors of sudden death in myocardial infarction. J. Psychosom. Res. 18:187, 1974.
23. Hackett, T. P., and Cassem, N. H.: Factors contributing to delay in responding to the signs and symptoms of acute myocardial infarction. Am. J. Cardiol. 24:651, 1969.
24. Moss, A. J., and Goldstein, S.: The pre-hospital phase of acute myocardial infarction. Circulation 41:737, 1970.
25. Simon, A. B., Feinleib, M., and Thompson, H. K.: Components of delay in the pre-hospital phase of acute myocardial infarction. Am. J. Cardiol. 30:476, 1972.
26. Wallace, W. A., and Yu, P. N.: Sudden death and the pre-hospital phase of acute myocardial infarction. Ann. Rev. Med. 26:1, 1975.
27. Sjögren, A., Erhardt, L. R., and Theorell, T.: Circumstances around the onset of a myocardial infarction. Acta Med. Scand. 205:287, 1979.

28. Hamburg, D. A., Coelho, G. V., and Adams, J. E.: Coping and Adaptation. New York, Basic Books, Inc., 1974.
29. Weisman, A. D., and Hackett, T. P.: The predilection to death. Psychosom. Med. 23:232, 1961.
30. Cassem, N. H., Wishnie, H. A., and Hackett, T. P.: How coronary patients respond to last rites. Postgrad. Med. 45:147, 1969.
31. Hackett, T. P., Cassem, N. H., and Wishnie, H. A.: The coronary care unit: An appraisal of its psychological hazards. New Engl. J. Med. 279:1365, 1968.
32. Cay, E. L., Vetter, N., Philip, A. E., and Dugard, P.: Psychological reactions to a coronary care unit. J. Psychosom. Res. 16:425, 1972.
33. Dominian, J., and Dobson, M.: Study of patients' psychological attitudes to a coronary care unit. Br. Med. J. 4:795, 1969.
34. Bruhn, J. G., Thurman, A. E., Jr., Chandler, B. C., and Bruce, T. A.: Patients' reactions to death in a coronary care unit. J. Psychosom. Res. 14:65, 1970.
35. Kübler-Ross, E.: Death does not exist. J. Holistic Health 2:60, 1977.
36. Druss, R. G., and Kornfeld, D. S.: Survivors of cardiac arrest: Psychiatric study. J.A.M.A. 201:291, 1967.
37. Hackett, T. P.: The Lazarus complex revisited. Ann. Intern. Med. 76:135, 1972.
38. Dobson, M., Tattersfield, A. E., Adler, M. M., and McNicol, M. W.: Attitudes and long-term adjustment of patients surviving cardiac arrest. Br. Med. J. 3:207, 1971.
39. Parker, D. L., and Hodge, J. R.: Delirium in the coronary care unit. J.A.M.A. 201:702, 1967.
40. Farber, I. J.: Hospitalized cardiac patient: Some psychological aspects. N.Y. State J. Med. 78:2045, 1978.
41. Klein, R. F., Kliner, V. A., Zipes, D. P., Troyer, W. G., Jr., and Wallace, A. G.: Transfer from a coronary care unit. Arch. Intern. Med. 122:104, 1968.
42. Wishnie, H. A., Hackett, T. P., and Cassem, N. H.: Psychological hazards of convalescence following myocardial infarction. J.A.M.A. 215:1292, 1971.
43. Cassem, N. H., and Hackett, T. P.: Psychological rehabilitation of myocardial infarction patients in the acute phase. Heart Lung 2:383, 1973.
44. Ueno, M.: The so-called coition death. Jap. J. Leg. Med. 17:330, 1963.
45. Hellerstein, H. K., and Friedman, E. H.: Sexual activity and the post-coronary patient. Arch. Intern. Med. 125:987, 1970.
46. Naughton, J.: The effects of acute and chronic exercise on cardiac patients. In Naughton, J. P., and Hellerstein, H. K. (eds.): Exercise Testing and Exercise Training in Coronary Heart Disease. New York, Academic Press, 1973.
47. Hackett, T. P., and Cassem, N. H.: Psychological adaptation to convalescence in myocardial infarction patients. In Naughton, J. P., and Hellerstein, H. K. (eds.): Exercise Testing and Exercise Training in Coronary Heart Disease. New York, Academic Press, 1973.
48. Bilodeau, C. J., and Hackett, T. P.: Issues raised in a group setting by patients recovering from initial myocardial infarction. Am. J. Psychiatry 128:73, 1971.
49. Benson, H.: The Relaxation Response. New York, William Morrow and Co., 1975.
50. Gilberstadt, H., and Sako, Y.: Intellectual and personality changes following open-heart surgery. Arch. Gen. Psychiatry 16:210, 1967.
51. Kimball, C. P.: Psychological responses to the experience of open-heart surgery. Am. J. Psychiatry 126:348, 1969.
52. Heller, S. S., Frank, K. S., Malm, J. R., Bowman, F. O., Harris, P. D., Charlton, M. H., and Kornfeld, D. S.: Psychiatric complications of open-heart surgery: A re-examination. N. Engl. J. Med. 283:1015, 1970.
53. Surman, O. S.: The surgical patient. In Hackett, T. P., and Cassem, E. H. (eds.): MGH Handbook of General Hospital Psychiatry. St. Louis, C. V. Mosby Co., 1978.
54. Abram, H. S.: Psychological reaction to cardiac operation: A historical perspective. Int. J. Psychiat. Med. 1:277, 1970.
55. Kimball, C. P.: Psychological responses to the experience of open-heart surgery. Am. J. Psychiatry 126:348, 1969.
56. Kimball, C. P.: The experience of cardiac surgery: Psychological patterns and predictions of outcome. Presented at the 9th European Conference on Psychosomatic Research. Vienna, April 30, 1972.
57. Bove, A. A.: The cardiovascular response to stress. Psychosomatics 18:13, 1977.
58. Chambers, W. N., and Reiser, M. F.: Emotional stress and the precipitation of congestive heart failure. Psychosom. Med. 15:38, 1953.
59. Klein, R. F., Garrity, T. F., and Gelein, J.: Emotional adjustment and catecholamine excretion during early recovery from myocardial infarction. J. Psychosom. Res. 18:425, 1974.
60. Bishop, L. F., and Reichert, P.: Emotion and heart failure. Psychosomatics 12:412, 1971.
61. Regestein, Q. R.: Relationships between psychological factors and cardiac rhythm and electrical disturbances. Compr. Psychiatry 16:137, 1975.
62. Lown, B., Temte, J. V., Reich, P., Gaughan, C., Regestein, Q. R., and Hai, H.: Basis for recurring ventricular fibrillation in the absence of coronary heart disease and its management. N. Engl. J. Med. 294:623, 1976.
63. Reich, P., DeSilva, R. A., Lown, B., and Murawski, B. J.: Acute psychological disturbance preceding life-threatening arrhythmias. J.A.M.A. 246:233, 1981.
64. Taggart, P., Gibbons, D., and Somerville, W.: Some effects of motor-car driving on the normal and abnormal heart. Br. Med. J. 4:130, 1969.
65. Taggart, P., Carruthers, M., and Somerville, W.: Electrocardiogram, plasma catecholamines, and lipids, and their modification by oxyprenolol when speaking before an audience. Lancet 2:341, 1973.
66. Lown, B., and DeSilva, R. A.: Roles of psychologic stress and autonomic ner-

vous system changes in provocation of ventricular premature complexes. Am. J. Cardiol. *41*:979, 1978.

67. Verrier, R. L., Calvert, A., and Lown, B.: The effect of posterior hypothalamic stimulation on ventricular fibrillation threshold. Am. J. Physiol. *228*:923, 1975.

68. Schlesinger, Z., Barzilay, J., Stryjer, D., and Almog, C. H.: Life-threatening "vagal reaction" to emotional stimuli. Isr. J. Med. Sci. *13*:59, 1977.

69. Engel, G.: A life setting conducive to illness: The giving-up—given-up complex. Ann. Intern. Med. *69*:293, 1968.

70. Rahe, R., and Romo, M.: Recent life changes and the onset of myocardial infarction and sudden death in Helsinki. *In* Gunderson, E. K., and Rahe, R. (eds.): Life Stress and Illness. Springfield, Ill., Charles C Thomas, 1974, p. 105.

71. Weiner, H.: Essential hypertension. *In* Weiner, H.: Psychobiology and Human Disease. New York, Elsevier-North Holland, Inc., 1977, p. 116.

72. Henry, J. P., and Cassel, J. C.: Psychological factors in essential hypertension. Recent epidemiologic and animal experimental evidence. Am. J. Epidemiol. *90*: 171, 1969.

73. Stamler, J., Stamler, R., and Pullman, T.: The Epidemiology of Essential Hypertension. New York, Grune and Stratton, 1967.

74. Harburg, E., Erfurt, J. C., Hauenstein, L. S., Chape, C., Schull, W. J., and Schork, M. A.: Socio-ecological stress, suppressed hostility, skin color, and black-white male blood pressure: Detroit. Psychosom. Med. *35*:276, 1973.

75. Donnison, C. P.: Blood pressure in the African native, its bearing on the etiology of hyperpiesia and arteriosclerosis. Lancet *1*:6, 1929.

76. Henry, J. P., Meehan, J. P., and Stephens, P. M.: The use of psychosocial stimuli to induce prolonged hypertension in mice. Psychosom. Med. *29*:408, 1967.

77. Reiser, M. F., Brust, A. A., and Ferris, E. B., Jr.: Life situations, emotions and the course of patients with arterial hypertension. Psychosom. Med. *13*:133, 1951.

78. Reiser, M. F., Rosenbaum, M., and Ferris, E. B., Jr.: Psychological mechanisms in malignant hypertension. Psychosom. Med. *13*:147, 1951.

79. Alexander, F.: Psychosomatic Medicine. New York, W. W. Norton, 1950.

80. Binger, C. A., Ackerman, N. W., Cohn, A. E., Chroeder, H. A., and Steele, J. M.: Personality in Arterial Hypertension. New York, Brunner, 1945.

81. Weiss, E.: Psychosomatic aspects of hypertension. J.A.M.A. *120*:1081, 1942.

82. Wolf, S., and Wolff, H. G.: A summary of experimental evidence relating life stress to the pathogenesis of essential hypertension in man. *In* Bell, E. T. (ed.): Hypertension. Minneapolis, University of Minnesota Press, 1951.

83. Oken, D.: An experimental study of suppressed anger and blood pressure. Arch. Gen. Psychiatry *2*:441, 1960.

84. Wolff, H. G.: Stress and Disease. Springfield, Ill., Charles C Thomas, 1953.

85. Pilowsky, I., Spalding, D., Shaw, J., and Korner, P. I.: Hypertension and personality. Psychosom. Med. *35*:15, 1973.

86. Ostfeld, A. M., and Lebovitz, B. Z.: Personality factors and pressor mechanisms in renal and essential hypertension. Arch. Intern. Med. *104*:497, 1959.

87. Ostfeld, A. M.: Editorial: What's the payoff in hypertension research? Psychosom. Med. *35*:1, 1973.

88. Sokolow, M., Werdegar, D., Perloff, D. B., Cowan, R. M., and Brenenstuhl, H.: Preliminary studies relating portably recorded blood pressures to daily life events in patients with essential hypertension. Bibl. Psychiatr. *144*:164, 1970.

89. Cobb, S., and Rose, R. M.: Hypertension, peptic ulcer and diabetes in air traffic controllers. J.A.M.A. *224*:489, 1973.

90. Brod, J., Fencl, V., Hejl, Z., and Jirka, J.: Circulatory changes underlying blood pressure elevation during acute emotional stress (mental arithmetic) in normotensive and hypertensive subjects. Clin. Sci. *18*:269, 1959.

91. Brod, J.: Hemodynamics and emotional stress. Bibl. Psychiatr. *144*:13, 1970.

92. Lacey, J. I., Bateman, D. E., and Van Lehn, R.: Autonomic response specificity: An experimental study. Psychosom. Med. *15*:8, 1953.

93. Doyle, A. E., and Fraser, J. R. E.: Essential hypertension and inheritance of vascular reactivity. Lancet *2*:509, 1961.

94. Gantt, W. H.: Cardiovascular component of the conditioned reflex to pain, food and other stimuli. Physiol. Rev. *40*(Suppl. 4):266, 1960.

95. Shapiro, D., Tursky, B., and Schwartz, G. E.: Differentiation of heart rate and blood pressure in man by operant conditioning. Psychosom. Med. *32*:417, 1970.

96. Blanchard, E. B., and Miller, S. T.: Psychological treatment of cardiovascular disease. Arch. Gen. Psychiatry *34*:1402, 1977.

97. Jacob, R. G., Kraemer, H. C., and Agras, S.: Relaxation therapy in the treatment of hypertension: A review. Arch. Gen. Psychiatry *34*:1417, 1977.

98. Shapiro, A. P., Schwartz, G. E., Ferguson, D. C. E., Redmond, D. P., and Weiss, S. M.: Behavioral methods in the treatment of hypertension: A review of their clinical status. Ann. Intern. Med. *86*:626, 1977.

99. Stone, R. A., and DeLeo, J.: Psychotherapeutic control of hypertension. N. Engl. J. Med. *294*:80, 1976.

100. Patel, C. H.: 12 month follow-up of yoga and bio-feedback in the management of hypertension. Lancet *1*:62, 1975.

101. Patel, C. H., and North, W. R. S.: Randomized controlled trial of yoga and bio-feedback in management of hypertension. Lancet *2*:93, 1975.

102. Southam, M. A., Agras, W. S., Taylor, C. B., and Kraemer, H. C.: Relaxation training, blood pressure lowering during the working day. Arch. Gen. Psychiatry *39*:715, 1982.

103. Kristt, D. A., and Engel, B. T.: Learned control of blood pressure in patients with high blood pressure. Circulation *51*:370, 1975.

104. Becker, M. H., and Maiman, L. A.: Sociobehavioral determinants of compliance with health and medical care recommendations. Med. Care *13*:10, 1975.

105. Blackwell, B.: Drug therapy: Patient compliance. New Engl. J. Med. *289*:249, 1973.

106. Gillum, R. F., and Barsky, A. J.: Diagnosis and management of patient noncompliance. J.A.M.A. *228*:1563, 1974.

107. Haynes, R. B.: A critical review of the "determinants" of patient compliance with therapeutic regimens. *In* Sackett, D. L., and Haynes, R. B. (eds.): Compliance with Therapeutic Regimens. Baltimore, Johns Hopkins University Press, 1976, p. 26.

108. Sackett, D. L.: Patients and therapies: Getting the two together. N. Engl. J. Med. *298*:278, 1978.

109. Zacest, R., Barrow, C. G., O'Halloran, M. W., and Wilson, L. L: Relationship of psychological factors to failure of antihypertensive drug treatment. Aust. N. Z. J. Med. *11*:501, 1981.

109a. National Heart and Lung Institute: National Heart and Lung Institute's hypertension detection and follow-up study. Cited in Hypertension: Getting—and keeping—it under control. Med. World News *17*:52, 1976.

110. Mushlin, A. I., and Appel, F. A.: Diagnosing potential noncompliance: Physicians' ability in a behavioral dimension of medical care. Arch. Intern. Med. *137*:318, 1977.

111. Schmidt, D. D.: Patient compliance: The effect of the doctor as a therapeutic agent. J. Fam. Pract. *4*:853, 1977.

112. Finnerty, F. A., Jr., Mattie, E. C., and Finnerty, F. A., III: Hypertension in the inner city. I. Analysis of clinic dropouts. Circulation *47*:73, 1973.

113. Finnerty, F. A., Jr., Shaw, L. W., and Himmelsbach, C. K.: Hypertension in the inner city, II. Detection and follow-up. Circulation *47*:76, 1973.

114. Haynes, R. B., Sackett, D. L., Gibson, E. S., Taylor, D. W., Hackett, B. C., Roberts, R. S., and Johnson, A. L.: Improvement of medication compliance in uncontrolled hypertension. Lancet *1*:1265, 1976.

115. Goodwin, F. K., and Bunney, W. E.: Depressions following reserpine: A reevaluation. Semin. Psychiatry *3*:435, 1971.

116. Hamilton, M., and Kopelman, H.: Treatment of severe hypertension with methyldopa. Br. Med. J. *1*:151, 1963.

117. Smirk, H.: Hypotensive action of methyldopa. Br. Med. J. *1*:146, 1963.

118. Alder, S.: Methyldopa-induced decrease in mental activity. J.A.M.A. *230*:1428, 1974.

119. Thornton, W. E.: Dementia induced by methyldopa with haloperidol. N. Engl. J. Med. *294*:1222, 1976.

120. O'Regan, J. B.: Adverse interaction of lithium carbonate and methyldopa. Can. Med. Assoc. J. *115*:385, 1976.

121. Baldessarini, R. J.: Chemotherapy in Psychiatry. Cambridge, Harvard University Press, 1977.

122. Simpson, L. L.: Combined use of molindone and guanethidine in patients with schizophrenia and hypertension. Am. J. Psychiatry *136*:1410, 1979.

123. Von Zwieten, P. A.: Interaction between centrally acting hypotensive drugs and tricyclic antidepressants. Arch. Int. Pharmacodyn. Ther. *214*:12, 1975.

124. Risch, C. S., Groom, G. P., and Janowsky, D. S.: The effects of psychotropic drugs on the cardiovascular system. J. Clin. Psychiatry *43*:16, 1982.

125. Burgess, C. D., Turner, P., Wadsworth, J.: Cardiovascular responses to mianserin hydrochloride: A comparison with tricyclic antidepressant drugs. Br. J. Clin. Pharmacol. *5*(Suppl. 1):215, 1978.

126. Himmelhoch, J. M., Poust, R. I., Mallinger, A. G., Hanin, I., and Neil, J. F.: Adjustment of lithium dose during lithium-chlorothiazide therapy. Clin. Pharmacol. Ther. *22*:225, 1977.

127. Marks, I., and Lader, M.: Anxiety states (anxiety neurosis): A review. J. Nerv. Ment. Dis. *156*:3, 1973.

128. Diagnostic and Statistical Manual of Mental Disorders. (3rd ed.) Washington, D.C., American Psychiatric Association, 1980.

129. Crowe, R. R., Pauls, D. L., Slymen, D. J., and Noyes, R.: A family study of anxiety neurosis: Morbidity in families with and without mitral valve prolapse. Arch. Gen. Psychiatry *37*:701, 1982.

130. Coryell, W., Noyes, R., and Clancy, J.: Excess mortality in panic disorder. Arch. Gen. Psychiatry *39*:701, 1982.

131. Pitts, F. N., and McClure, J. N.: Lactate metabolism in anxiety neurosis. N. Engl. J. Med. *277*:1329, 1967.

132. Pitts, F. N.: Biochemical factors in anxiety neurosis. Behav. Sci. *16*:82, 1971.

133. Frohlich, E. D., Tarazi, R. C., and Dustan, H. P.: Hyperdynamic β-adrenergic circulatory state: Increased beta receptor responsiveness. Arch. Intern. Med. *123*:1, 1969.

134. Hoehn-Saric, R.: Neurotransmitters in anxiety. Arch. Gen. Psychiatry *39*:735, 1982.

135. Rosenbaum, J. F.: The drug treatment of anxiety. N. Engl. J. Med. *306*:401, 1982.

136. Rosenbaum, J. F.: Anxiety. *In* Lazare, A. (ed.): Outpatient Psychiatry: Diagnosis and Treatment. Baltimore, Williams and Wilkins Co., 1979, pp. 252–256.

137. Weinstein, G., Allen, G., and Ford, C. V.: Anxiety and mitral valve prolapse syndrome. J. Clin. Psychiatry *43*:33, 1982.

138. Gorman, J. M., Fyer, A. F., Gliklich, J., King, D., and Klein, D. F.: Effect of sodium lactate on patients with panic disorder and mitral valve prolapse. Am. J. Psychiatry *138*:247, 1981.

139. Combs, R. L., Shah, P. M., Klorman, R. S., and Klorman, R.: Effects of psychological stress on click and rhythm in mitral valve prolapse. Am. Heart J. *99*:714, 1980.

140. Schuckit, M. A.: Current therapeutic options in the management of typical anxiety. J. Clin. Psychiatry *42*:15, 1981.

141. Sheehan, D. V., Ballenger, J., and Jacobsen, G.: Treatment of endogenous anx-

iety with phobic, hysterical, and hypochondriacal symptoms. Arch. Gen. Psychiatry *37*:51, 1980.

142. Kenyon, F. E.: Hypochondriacal states. Br. J. Psychiatry *129*:1, 1976.

143. Muller, O. F., Goodman, N., and Bellet, S.: The hypotensive effect of imipramine hydrochloride in patients with cardiovascular disease. Clin. Pharmacol. Ther. *2*:300, 1961.

144. Robinson, D. S., and Barker, E: Tricyclic antidepressant cardiotoxicity. J.A.M.A. *236*:2089, 1976.

145. Carlsson, A.: Pharmacological depletion of catecholamine stores. Pharmacol. Rev. *18*:541, 1966.

146. Coull, D. C., Crooks, J., Dingwall-Fordyce, I., Scott, A. M., and Weir, R. D.: Amitriptyline and cardiac disease, risk of sudden death identified by monitoring system. Lancet *2*:590, 1970.

147. Swett, C. P., Jr., and Shader, R. I.: Cardiac side effects and sudden death in hospitalized psychiatric patients. Dis. Nerv. Syst. *38*:69, 1977.

148. Moir, D. C., Crooks, J., Cornwell, W. B., O'Malley, K., Dingwall-Fordyce, I., Turnbull, M. J., and Weir, R. D.: Cardiotoxicity of amitriptyline. Lancet *2*: 561, 1972.

149. Ziegler, V. E., Co, B. T., and Biggs, J. T.: Electrocardiographic findings in patients undergoing amitriptyline treatment. Dis. Nerv. Syst. *38*:697, 1977.

150. Fowler, N. O., McCall, D., Chou, T., Holmes, J. C., and Hanenson, I. B.: Electrocardiographic changes and cardiac arrhythmias in patients receiving psychotropic drugs. Am. J. Cardiol. *37*:223, 1976.

151. Marshall, J. B., and Forker, A. D.: Cardiovascular effects of tricyclic antidepressant drugs: Therapeutic usage, overdose, and management of complications. Am. Heart J. *103*:401, 1982.

152. Jefferson, J. W.: A review of the cardiovascular effects and toxicity of tricyclic antidepressants. Psychosom. Med. *37*:160, 1975.

153. Spiker, D. G., and Biggs, J. T.: Tricyclic antidepressants: Prolonged plasma levels after overdose. J.A.M.A. *236*:1711, 1976.

154. Siddiqui, J. H., Vakassi, M. M., and Ghani, M. F.: Cardiac effects of amitriptyline overdosage. Curr. Ther. Res. *22*:321, 1977.

155. Snyder, S., and Yamamura, H.: Antidepressants and the muscarinic acetylcholine receptor. Arch. Gen. Psychiatry *34*:236, 1977.

156. Tobis, J., and Das, B.: Cardiac complications in amitriptyline poisoning: Successful treatment with physostigmine. J.A.M.A. *235*:1474, 1976.

157. Granacher, R. P., and Baldessarini, R. J.: Physostigmine: Its use in acute anticholinergic syndrome with antidepressant and antiparkinson drugs. Arch. Gen. Psychiatry *32*:375, 1975.

158. Bigger, J. T., Jr., Giardina, E. G. V., Perel, J. M., Kantor, S. J., and Glassman, A. H.: Cardiac antiarrhythmic effect of imipramine hydrochloride. N. Engl. J. Med. *296*:206, 1977.

159. Giardina, E.-G. V., Bigger, J. T., Jr., Glassman, A. H., Perel, J. M., and Kantor, S. J.: The electrocardiographic and antiarrhythmic effects of imipramine hydrochloride at therapeutic plasma concentrations. Circulation *60*:1045, 1979.

160. Burrows, G. D., Vohra, J., Hunt, D., Sloman, J. G., Scoggins, B. A., and Davies, B.: Cardiac effects of different tricyclic antidepressant drugs. Br. J. Psychiatry *129*:335, 1976.

161. Giardina, E.-G. V., and Bigger, J. T.: Antiarrhythmic effect of imipramine hydrochloride in patients with ventricular premature complexes without psychological depression. Am. J. Cardiol. *50*:172, 1982.

161a. Veith, R. C., Raskind, M. A., Caldwell, J. H., Barns, R. F., Gumbrecht, G., and Ritchie, J. L.: Cardiovascular effects of tricyclic antidepressants in depressed patients with chronic heart failure. N. Engl. J. Med. *306*:954, 1982.

162. Rainey, J. M., Pohl, R. B., and Bilolikar, S. G.: The QT interval in drug-free depressed patients. J. Clin. Psychiatry *43*:39, 1982.

163. Brennan, F. J.: Electrophysiologic effects of imipramine and doxepin on normal and depressed cardiac Purkinje fibers. Am. J. Cardiol. *46*:599, 1980.

164. Marshall, J. B., and Forker, A. D.: Cardiovascular effects of tricyclic antidepressant drugs: Therapeutic usage, overdose, and management of complications. Am. Heart J. *103*:401, 1982.

165. Magorien, R. D., Jewell, G. M., Schaal, S. F., and Leier, C. V.: Electrophysiologic studies of perphenazine and protriptyline in a patient with psychotropic drug-induced ventricular fibrillation. Am. J. Med. *67*:353, 1979.

166. Burckhardt, D., Raeder, E., Müller, V., Imhof, P., and Neubauer, H.: Cardiovascular effects of tricyclic and tetracyclic antidepressants. J.A.M.A. *239*:213, 1978.

167. Glassman, A. H., Walsh, T. W., Roose, S. P., Rosenfeld, M. A., Bruno, R. L., Bigger, J. T., Jr., and Giardina, E. V.: Factors related to orthostatic hypotension associated with tricyclic antidepressants. J. Clin. Psychiatry *43*:35, 1982.

168. Glassman, A. H., and Bigger, T.: Cardiovascular effects of therapeutic doses of tricyclic antidepressants. Arch. Gen. Psychiatry *38*:815, 1981.

169. U'Prichard, D. C., Greenberg, D. A., Sheehan, P. P., and Snyder, S. H.: Tricyclic antidepressants: Therapeutic properties and affinity for alpha-noradrenergic receptor binding sites in the brain. Science *199*:197, 1978.

170. Veith, R. C., Raskind, M. A., Caldwell, J. H., Barnes, R. F., Gumbrecht, G., and Ritchie, J. L.: Cardiovascular effects of tricyclic antidepressants in depressed patients with chronic heart disease. N. Engl. J. Med. *306*:954, 1982.

171. Feighner, J. P.: Clinical efficacy of the newer antidepressants. J. Clin. Psychopharm. *1*:23, 1981.

172. Leestma, J. E., and Koenig, K. L.: Sudden death and phenothiazines: A current controversy. Arch. Gen. Pyschiatry *18*:137, 1968.

173. Alexander, C. S., and Niño, A.: Cardiovascular complications in young patients taking psychotropic drugs: A preliminary report. Am. Heart J. *78*:757, 1969.

174. Chouinard, G., and Annable, L.: Phenothiazine-induced ECG abnormalities: Effect of a glucose load. Arch. Gen. Psychiatry *34*:951, 1977.

175. Peroutka, S. J., U'Prichard, D. C., Greenberg, D. A., and Snyder, S. H.: Neuroleptic drug interactions with norepinephrine alpha receptor binding-sites in rat brain. Neuropharmacology *16*:549, 1977.

176. Snyder, S., Greenberg, D., and Yamamura, H. I.: Anti-schizophrenic drugs and brain cholinergic receptors. Arch. Gen. Psychiatry *31*:58, 1974.

177. Sos, J., and Cassem, N. H.: The intravenous use of haloperidol for acute delirium in intensive care settings. *In* Speidel, H., and Rodewald, G. (eds.): Psychic and Neurologic Dysfunctions after Open Heart Surgery. Stuttgart, Georg Thieme Verlag, 1980.

178. Tilkian, A. G., Schroeder, J. S., Kao, J. J., and Hultgren, H. N.: The cardiovascular effects of lithium in man: Review of the literature. Am. J. Med. *61*: 665, 1976.

179. Jefferson, J. W., and Greist, J. H.: Primer of Lithium Therapy. Baltimore, Williams and Wilkins Co., 1977.

180. Gershon, S., and Shopsin, B.: Lithium: Its Role in Psychiatric Research and Treatment. New York, Plenum Press, 1973, P. 108.

181. Hagman, A., Arnman, K., and Rydén, L.: Syncope caused by lithium treatment: Report on two cases and a prospective investigation of the prevalence of lithium-induced sinus node dysfunction. Acta Med. Scand. *205*:467, 1979.

182. Demers, R. G., and Heninger, G. R.: Electrocardiographic T-wave changes during lithium carbonate treatment. J.A.M.A. *218*:381, 1971.

183. Tilkian, A. G., Schroeder, J. S., Kao, J., and Hultgren, H.: Effect of lithium on cardiovascular performance: Report on extended ambulatory monitoring and exercise testing before and during lithium therapy. Am. J. Cardiol. *38*:701, 1976.

184. Mitchell, J. E., and MacKenzie, T.: Cardiac effects of lithium in man: a review. J. Clin. Psychiatry *43*:47, 1982.

185. Anton, A. H., Uy, D. S., and Redderson, C. L.: Autonomic blockade and the cardiovascular and catecholamine response to electroshock. Anesth. Analg. *56*: 46, 1977.

186. Arneson, G. A., and Butler, T.: Cardiac arrest and electroshock therapy. Am. J. Psychiatry *117*:1020, 1961.

187. McKenna, G., Engle, R. P., Jr., Brooks, H. N., and Dolen, J.: Cardiac arrhythmias during electroshock therapy: Significance, prevention, and treatment. Am. J. Psychiatry *127*:530, 1970.

188. Hussar, A. E., and Pachter, M.: Myocardial infarction and fatal coronary insufficiency during electroconvulsive therapy. J.A.M.A. *204*:1004, 1968.

189. Pitts, F. N., Jr., Desmarais, G. M., Stewart, W., and Schaberg, W.: Induction of anesthesia with methohexital and thiopental in electroconvulsive therapy. N. Engl. J. Med. *273*:353, 1965.

190. Kalinowsky, L. B.: The convulsive therapies. *In* Freedman, A. M., Kaplan, H. I., and Saddock, B. J. (eds.): Comprehensive Textbook of Psychiatry/II. Baltimore, Williams and Wilkins Co., 1975.

INDEX

Pages in *italics* indicate illustrations. Page numbers followed by t indicate tables.